A CATALOGUE OF

Seventeenth Century
Printed Books

IN THE NATIONAL LIBRARY OF MEDICINE

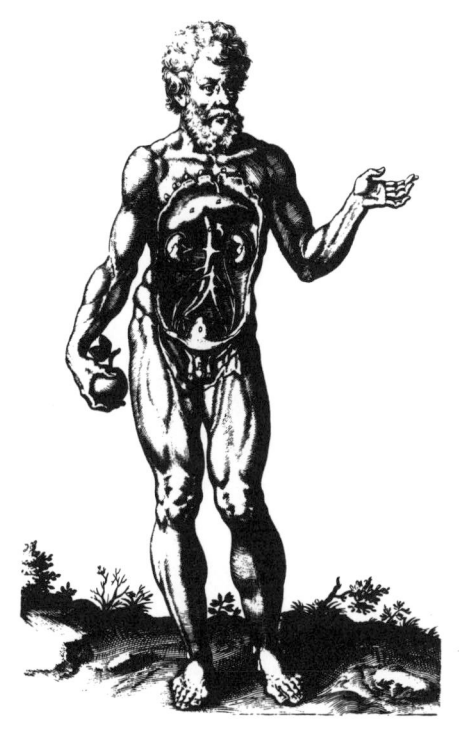 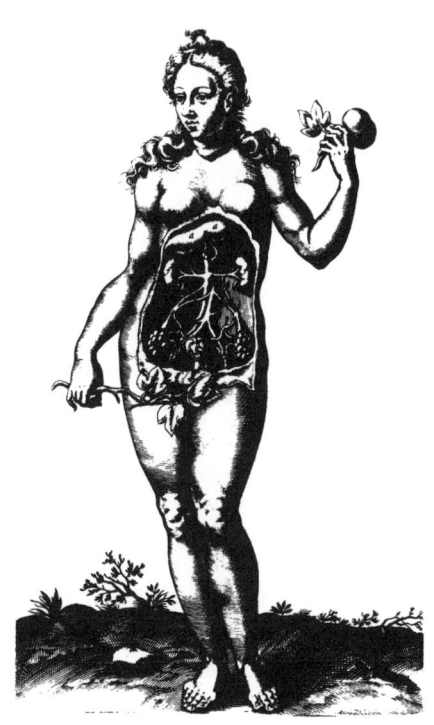

Compiled by Peter Krivatsy

U.S. DEPARTMENT OF HEALTH AND HUMAN SERVICES

Public Health Service
National Institutes of Health

National Library of Medicine
Bethesda, Maryland

1989

NIH Publication No. 89-2619

National Library of Medicine Cataloging in Publication

National Library of Medicine (U.S.)
    A catalogue of seventeenth century printed books in
the National Library of Medicine/compiled by Peter
Krivatsy. —
    Bethesda, Md.: U.S. Dept. of Health and Human
Services, Public Health Service, National Institutes
of Health, National Library of Medicine, 1989.
    (NIH publication; no. 89-2619) Bibliography: p. 1.
Bibliography of Medicine 2. Libraries, Medical-
Maryland-catalogs. I. Krivatsy, Peter, 1922-II. Title. III.
Series.

Z 675.M4 N278cf

Source of title-page figure: Jourdain Guibelet, *Trois discours philosophiques* (1603; entry 5081), facing
p. 133^v and p. 134^r.

Contents

Preface

This is the fifth in a series of book catalogues of pre-19th century holdings in the National Library of Medicine. Its predecessors are:

Dorothy Schullian and Francis E. Sommer, *A Catalogue of Incunabula and Manuscripts in the Army Medical Library* (1950)

Richard J. Durling, *A Catalogue of 16th Century Printed Books in the National Library of Medicine* (1967)

Peter Krivatsy, *A Catalogue of Incunabula and 16th Century Printed Books in the National Library of Medicine,* First Supplement (1971)

John B. Blake, *A Short Title Catalogue of 18th Century Printed Books in the National Library of Medicine* (1979)

These catalogues record nearly 45,000 works that were published between the invention of printing and 1801 and that are now held by NLM. The book catalogues were prepared in order to make these holdings known and accessible to scholars around the world.

The holdings of NLM, including the records here, are also available in the CATLINE (CATalog on LINE) database and in a microfiche catalogue derived from CATLINE.

There are advantages to each of the formats. The book catalogues and microfiche are inexpensive and individual scholars can add them to their personal libraries. Their convenience also comes at a price, namely, the book catalogues do eventually go out of print and cannot be readily updated by the inclusion of subsequent additions to the Library.

The CATLINE database is updated frequently and, most importantly, permits searching that could not be undertaken in a book catalogue at all or only with great labor. For example, one can easily retrieve all of the citations to works published in a given language in a particular decade. Searching CATLINE on NLM's MEDLARS system is made easier by using the software package GRATEFUL MED, a personal computer based searching interface. For information on access to CATLINE and on GRATEFUL MED, contact the MEDLARS Management Section, Bibliographic Services Division, National Library of Medicine, 8600 Rockville Pike, Bethesda, MD 20894.

The present catalogue has been prepared by Peter Krivatsy. His work is a major contribution to the dissemination of information about the holdings of the National Library of Medicine. In addition, we hope and expect that it will serve as a contribution to the History of Medicine in particular and to 17th-century scholarship in general.

Donald A. B. Lindberg, M.D.
DIRECTOR

Introduction

This catalogue lists about 13,300 books printed between 1601 and 1700. Included are monographs, dissertations and corresponding program disputations, broadsides, pamphlets, and serials.

Entries are chiefly by author, editor, or compiler but occasionally by corporate body responsible for the work, and in some cases by a title created for a format, such as pharmacopoeia. Title entries are used also but only as a last resort. Aside from this infrequent practice, titles do not have separate entries.

Entries were established following the rules of the American Library Association's *Rules for Author and Title Entries* (2nd ed., 1949). Exceptions to these guidelines are that names of corporate bodies are used in the form current at the time the work was published and that entries under place names have been changed to those of the institutions themselves. The Library of Congress, *Rules for Descriptive Cataloging* (1949) were used with one exception: accents of Greek words were used as they appeared in each book. Most authors' names are listed in the vernacular form with *see* references for more complicated (usually Latin) names.

Entries are arranged in alphabetical order according to the American Library Association, *Rules for Filing Catalog Cards* (1942). These rules are closely followed, for example, unlauts are filed as *ae*, *oe*, or *ue*.

Collation is by printed pages or printed leaves. In unpaged and unfoliated books the total number of printed pages or leaves is given within square brackets. Intermediate blank pages are counted but blank leaves are not.

Manual indexes of printers and publishers and vernacular imprints are maintained in the History of Medicine Division. Scholars who wish to use them may visit the Division or write: Chief, History of Medicine Division, National Library of Medicine, Bethesda, MD 20894. Interested persons may also write to this address for further information on searching NLM's online catalog, CATLINE, by place and language of publication and by printer's name.

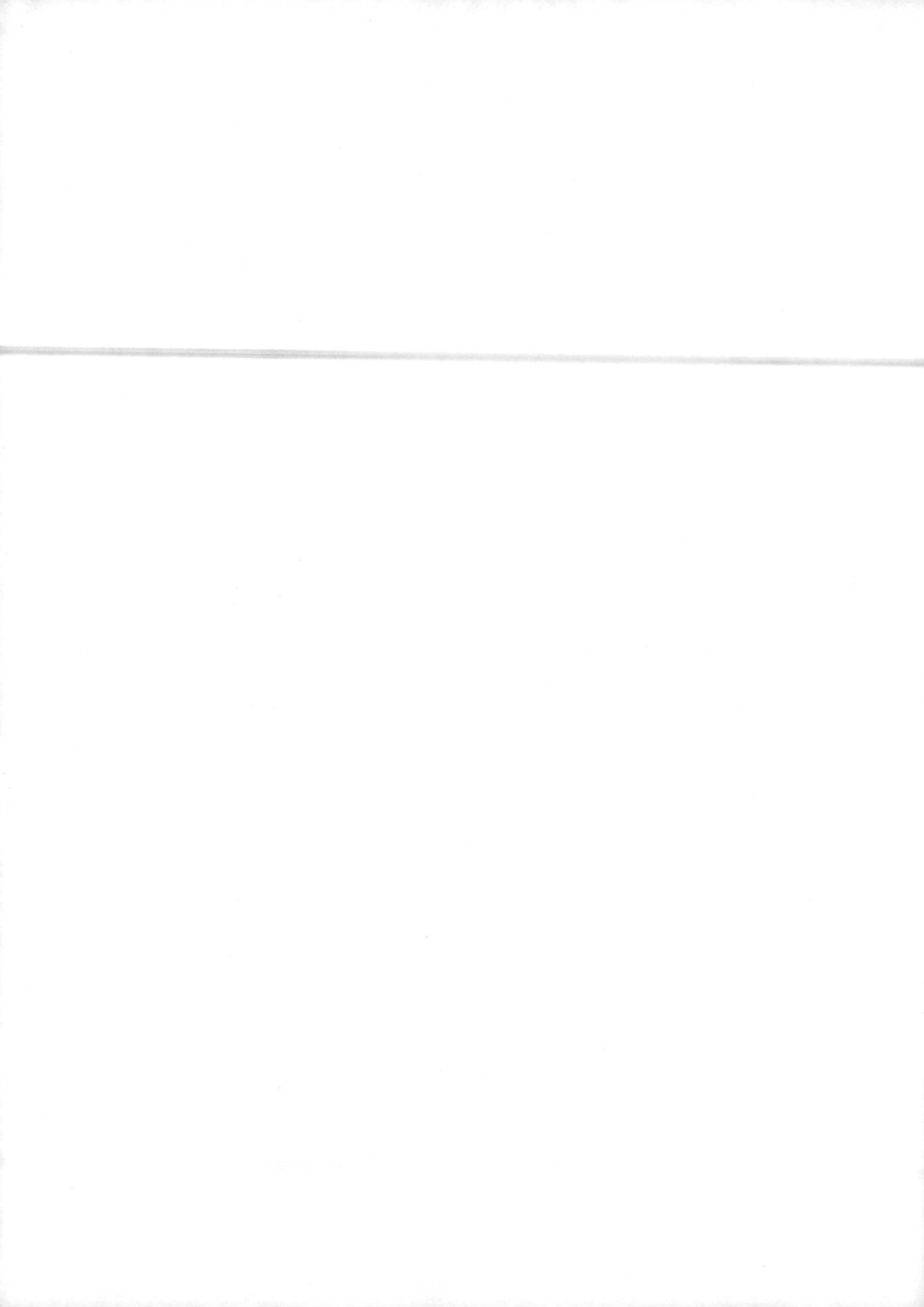

References

Adam
Adam, Melchior. *Vitae Germanorum medicorum; qui seculo superiori, et quod excurrit, claruerunt, congestae, et ad annum usque MDCXX, deductae . . .* 3d ed., rev. Frankfurt am Main, 1706.

Arents
Arents, George. *Tobacco; Its History Illustrated by the Books, Manuscripts and Engravings in the Library of George Arents, Jr.* 5 vols. New York, 1937-52.

Astruc
Astruc, Jean. *Mémoires pour servir a l'histoire de le Faculté de medecine de Montpellier.* Paris, 1767.

Aveling
Aveling, James Hobson. *The Chamberlens and the Midwifery Forceps.* London, 1882.

Baumgartner-Fulton
Baumgartner, Leona, and John F. Fulton. *A Bibliography of the Poem, "Syphilis", sive Morbus Gallicus by Girolamo Fracastoro, of Verona.* New Haven, 1935.

Barbier
Barbier, Antoine Alexandre. *Dictionnaire des ouvrages anonymes.* 4 vols. Paris, 1872-79.

Benzing (A)
Benzing, Josef. *Die Buchdrucker des 16. und 17. Jahrhunderts im deutschen Sprachgebiet.* Beiträge zum Buch- und Bibliothekswesen, vol. 12. Wiesbaden, 1963.

Benzing (B)
——— "Die deutschen Verleger des 16. und 17. Jahrhunderts." *Archiv für Geschichte des Buchwesens,* 2 (1959-60): 445-509.

Bibl.Belg.
Bibliotheca Belgica. Bibliographie générale des Pays-Bas. Ghent, 1880-1979.

Bibl.Med Neerland.
Nederlandsche Maatschapij tot Bevordering der Geneeskunst. *Catalogus; van de Bibliotheek der Nederlandsche Maatschappij tot Bevordering der Geneeskunst in briukleen vereenigd met de Bibliotheek der Universiteit van Amsterdam.* 2 vols. Amsterdam, 1930-49.

Bibl.Osler.
Osler, Sir William, bart. *Bibliotheca Osleriana; A Catalogue of Books Illustrating the History of Medicine and Science.* Oxford, 1929.

Bibl.Portug.
Academia das Ciencias de Lisboa. *Bibliografia geral portuguesa.* 2 vols. Lisbon, 1941-42.

Biog.méd.
Dictionnaire des sciences médicales. Biographie médicale. 7 vols. Paris, 1820-25.

Biologie médicale
Biologie médicale. Revue bimestrielle des sciences biologigues. 60 vols. Paris, 1903-71.

Blanck
Blanck, Georg Friedrich August. *Die mecklenburgischen Aerzte von den ältesten Zeiten bis zur Gegenwart.* Schwerin, 1901.

Bouvet
Bouvet, Maurice. *Les Rouvière.* Paris, 1959.

Bowes
Bowes, Robert. *A Catalogue of Books Printed at or Relating to the University, Town & County of Cambridge from 1521 to 1893.* Cambridge, 1894.

BNC
Bibliothèque nationale. Département des imprimés. *Catalogue général des livres imprimés de la Bibiothèque nationale.* Paris, 1897-.

BMC
British Museum. Dept. of Printed Books. *General Catalogue of Printed Books . . . to 1955.* 263 vols. London, 1959-66.

Brown
Brown, Horatio Robert Forbes. *The Venetian Printing Press.* London, 1891.

Brunet
Brunet, Jacques Charles. *Mauel du libraire et de l'amateur de livres.* 5th ed. augm. 6 vols. Paris, 1860-65.

Burckhardt — Burckhardt, Albrecht. *Geschichte der Medizinischen Fakultät zu Basel, 1460-1900.* Basel, 1917.

Caillet — Caillet, Albert Louis. *Manuel bibliographique des sciences psychiques ou occultes.* 3 vols. Paris, 1912.

Carrère — Carrère, Joseph Berthélemy François. *Bibliothèque littéraire historique et critique de la médecine ancienne et moderne.* 2 vols. Paris, 1776.

Choulant-Frank — Choulant, Johann Ludwig. *History and Bibliography of Anatomic Illustration.* Translated and annotated by Mortimer Frank. New York, 1962.

Cinelli Calvoil — Cinelli Calvoli, Giovanni. *Biblioteca volante de Gio. Cinelli Calvoli.* 2d ed. 4 vols. Venice, 1734-47.

Comrie — Comrie, John Dixon. *History of Scottish Medicine.* 2 vols. London, 1932.

Copinger — Copinger, Harold Bernard. *The Elzevier Press; A Handlist of the Productions of the Elzevier Presses at Leyden, Amsterdam, the Hague and Utrecht.* London, 1927.

Cosenza — Cosenza, Mario Emilio. *Biographical and Bibliographical Dictionary of the Italian Humanists and of the World of Classical Scholarship in Italy, 1300-1800.* 2d ed., rev. and enl. 6 vols. Boston, 1962-67.

Cushing — Cushing, Harvey Williams. *A Bio-bibliography of Andreas Vesalius.* 2d ed. Hamden, Conn., 1962.

DAL — Holzmann, Michael. *Deutsches Anonymenlexikon.* 7 vols. Weimar, 1902-28.

DBF — *Dictionnaire de biographie francaise* Paris, 1933-.

DG — *Deutscher Gesamtkatalog.* Edited by Preussischen Staatsbibliothek. Berlin, 1931.

Diels — Diels, Hermann. *Die Handschriften der antiken Ärzte.* 2 vols. Berlin, 1905-06.

Dobell — Dobell, Clifford. *Antony van Leeuwenhoek and His "Little Animals".* London, 1932.

Doe — Doe, Janet. *A Bibliography of the Works of Ambroise Paré.* New York Academy of Medicine Library. History of Medicine Series, no. 4. Chicago, 1937.

Durling — Durling, Richard J., comp. *A Catalogue of Sixteenth Century Printed Books in the National Library of Medicine.* Bethesda, Md., 1967.

Duveen — Duveen, Denis I. *Bibliotheca alchemica et chemica.* London, 1949.

Eloy — Eloy, Nicolas François Joseph. *Dictionnaire historique de la médecine ancienne et moderne.* 4 vols. Mons, 1778.

Facciolatie — Facciolatie, Jacopo. *Fasti Gymnasii Patavini.* 3 vols. Padua, 1757.

Feindel — Willis, Thomas. *The Anatomy of the Brain and Nerves.* Edited by William Feindel. 2 vols. Montreal, 1965 [i.e. 1966].

Ferguson (A) — Young, James, and John Ferguson. *Bibliotheca chemica.* 2 vols. Glasgow, 1906.

Ferguson (B) — Ferguson, John. "The Secrets of Alexis . . ." *Proc. Roy. Soc. Med., Sect. Hist. Med.* 24 (1931):225-246.

Finlayson — Finlayson, James. *Account of the Life and Works of Maister Peter Lowe.* Glasgow, 1889.

Foerster — Foerster, Richard, ed. *Scriptores physiognomici Graeci et Latini.* 2 vols. Leipzig, 1893.

Forbes — Forbes, Robert James. *Short History of the Art of Distillation, from the Beginnings up to the Death of Cellier Blumenthal.* Leiden, 1948.

Frati — Frati, Carlo. *Bibliografia Malpighiana; catalogo descrittivo delle opere a stampa di Mercello Malpighi e degli scritti che lo riguardano.* London, [1960]

Friedenwald — Friedenwald, Harry. *Jewish Luminaries in Medical History . . . and a Catalogue of Works Bearing on the Subject of the Jews and Medicine from the Private Library of Harry Friedenwald.* Baltimore, 1946.

Fulton (A) — Fulton, John Farquhar. *A Bibliography of the Honourable Robert Boyle.* 2d ed. Oxford, 1961.

Fulton (B)	——— *A Bibliography of Two Oxford Physiologists; Richard Lower and John Mayow.* Oxford, 1935.	**Husner**	Husner, Fritz. *Verzeichnis der Basler Medizinischen Universitätsschriften von 1575-1829.* Basel, 1942.
Gibson	Gibson, R.W. *Francis Bacon; a Bibliography of His Works and of Baconiana to the Year 1750.* Oxford, 1950.	**Index-Catalogue**	*Index-Catalogue of the Library of the Surgeon-General's Office, United States Army.* 1st-4th series. 58 vols. Washington, 1880-1955.
Goldsmith	Goldsmith, V.F. *A Short Title Catalogue of French Books, 1601-1700, in the Library of the British Museum.* Folkestone, 1969-73.	**Jöcher**	Jöcher, Christian Gottlieb. *Allgemeines Gelehrten-Lexicon.* 4 vols. Leipzig, 1750-51. *Fortsetzung und Ergänzungen.* 7 vols. Leipzig, 1784-1897.
Gurlt	Gurlt, Ernst Julius. *Geschichte der Chirurgie und ihrer Ausübung; Volkschirurgie, Alterthum, Mittelalter, Renaissance.* 3 vols. Berlin, 1898.	**Kestner**	Kestner, Christian Wilhelm. *Medicinisches Gelehrten-Lexicon.* Jena, 1740.
Haller	Haller, Albrecht von. *Bibliotheca medicinae practicae qua scripta ad partem medicinae practicam facientia . . . recensentur.* 4 vols. Basel, 1776-88.	**Keynes (A)**	Keynes, Geoffrey Langdon. *A Bibliography of Dr. Robert Hooke.* Oxford, 1960.
Halkett-Laing	Halkett, Samuel and John Laing. *Dictionary of Anonymous and Pseudonymous English Literature.* New and enl. ed. 9 vols. Edinburgh and London, 1926-62.	**Keynes (B)**	——— *A Bibliography of Sir Thomas Browne.* 2d ed., rev. and augm. Oxford, 1968.
Heffter	Heffter, Johann Karl. *Museum disputatorium physico-medicum tripartitum.* New ed. 2 vols. Zittau, 1763-64.	**Keynes (C)**	——— *A Bibliography of Sir William Petty.* Oxford, 1971.
Henrey	Henrey, Blanche. *British Botanical and Horticultural Literature before 1800.* 3 vols. London and New York, 1975.	**Keynes (D)**	——— *A Bibliography of the Writings of Dr. William Harvey, 1573 [sic]-1657.* 2d ed., rev. Cambridge, 1953.
Hernández Morejón	Hernández Morejón, Antonio. *Historia bibliográfica de la medicina española.* 7 vols. Madrid, 1842-52.	**Keynes (E)**	——— *Dr. Timothie Bright, 1550-1615; A Survey of His Life with a Bibliography of His Writings.* Wellcome Historical Medical Library. Publications, n.s. 1. London, 1962.
Hirsch	Hirsch, August. *Biographisches Lexikon der hervorragenden Ärzte aller Zeiten und Völker.* 2d ed. 6 vols. Berlin, 1929-35.	**Keynes (F)**	——— *John Ray; A Bibliography.* London, [1951].
Hoffmann	Hoffmann, Samuel Friedrich Wilhelm. *Bibliographisches Lexicon der gesammten Literatur der Griechen.* 2d ed. 3 vols. Amsterdam, 1961.	**Kośmiński**	Kośmiński, Stanisaw Lubicz. *Sownik lekarzów polskich.* Warsaw, 1883-[88].
Hull	Hull, Charles Henry, ed. *The Economic Writings of Sir William Petty.* 2 vols. Cambridge, 1899.	**Krieg**	Krieg, Michael o. *Mehr nicht erschienen; ein Verzeichnis unvollendet gebliebener Druckwerke.* 2 vols. Bibliotheca bibliographica, vol. 2. Bad Bocklet, 1954-58.
Hunt	Hunt, Rachel McMasters Miller. *Catalogue of Botanical Books in the Collection of Rachel McMasters Miller Hunt.* 3 vols. Pittsburgh, 1958-61.	**Kühn**	Galenus. *Opera omnia.* Edited by Karl Gottlog Kühn. 20 vols. Medicorum Graecorum opera quae exstant, vol. 1-20. Leipzig, 1821-33.
		Lawn	Lawn, Brian. *The Salernitan Questions; An Introduction to the History of*

	Medieval and Renaissance Problem Literature. Oxford, 1963.
Lepreux	Lepreux, Georges. *Gallia typographica; ou, Répertoire biographique et chronologique de tous les imprimeurs de France depuis les origines de l'imprimerie jusqu' à la révolution.* 5 vols. Paris, 1900-12.
Linde	Linde, Antonius van der. *Balthasar Bekker; bibliografie.* 's-Gravenhage, 1869.
Linden	Linden, Joannes Antonides van der. *Lindenius renovatus; sive . . . De Scriptis Medicis Libri Duo.* Nuremberg, 1686.
Littré	Hippocrates. *Oeuvres complètes d'Hippocrate.* Translated by E. Littré. 10 vols. Paris, 1839-61.
Lowndes	Lowndes, William Thomas. *The Bibliographer's Manual of English Literature.* New ed., rev., cor. and enl. 4 vols. London, 1857-64.
Madan	Madan, Falconer. *The Early Oxford Press; A Bibliography of Printing and Publishing at Oxford, 1468-1640.* Oxford, 1895.
Mazzuchelli	Mazzuchelli, Giammaria, conte. *Gli scrittori d'Italia.* 2 vols. Brescia, 1753-63.
Medina	Medina, José Toribio. *La imprenta en México, 1539-1821.* 8 vols. Santiago, 1908-12.
Melzi	Melzi, Gaetano, conte. *Dizionario di opere anonime e pseudonime di scrittori italiani, o come che sia aventi relazione all'Italia.* 3 vols. Milano, 1848-59.
Mennessier de la Lance	Mennesier de la Lance, Gabriel René. *Essai de bibliographie hippique donnant la description détaillée des ouvrages publiés ou traduits en latin et en français sur le cheval et la cavalerie.* 2 vols. Paris, 1915-17.
Mueller	Mueller, Wolf. *Bibliographie des Kaffee, des Kakao, der Schokolade, des Tee und deren Surrogate bis zum Jahre 1900.* Bad Bocklet, 1960.
Munk	Munk, William. *The Roll of the Royal College of Physicians of London.* 2d ed., rev. and enl. 6 vols. London, 1878-82.
NDB	*Neue deutsche Biographie, hrsg. von der Historischen Kommission bei der Bayerischen Akademie der Wissenschaften.* Berlin, [1953-].
Nicaise	Guy de Chauliac. *La grande chirurgie, composée en l'an 1363.* Edited by E. Nicaise. Paris, 1890.
Nissen	Nissen, Claus. *Die botanische Buchillustration; ihre Geschichte und Bibliographie.* 2 vols. Stuttgart, 1951.
NUC	*The National Union Catalog. Pre-1956 Imprints; A Cumulative Author List Representing Library of Congress Printed Cards and Titles Reported by Other American Libraries.* 754 vols. London, 1968-81.
Palau	Palau y Dulcet, Antonio. *Manual del librero hispano-americano.* 2d ed., corr. and aug. 28 vols. Barcelona, 1948-77.
Papadopoli	Papadopoli, Niccolò Comneno. *Historia Gymnasii Patavini . . . Cum auctario de claris cum professoribus tum alumnis ejusdem.* 2 vols. Venetiis, 1726.
Passano	Passano, Giovanni Battista. *Dizionario di opere anonime e pseudonime in supplemento a quello di Gaetano Melzi.* Ancoma, 1887.
Pauly	Pauly, Alphonse. *Bibliographie des sciences médicales.* Paris, 1874.
Pauly-Wissowa	Pauly, August Friedrich von. *Real-Encyclopädie der classischen Altertumswiseensachaft.* Edited by Georg Wissowa. 24 vols. Stuttgart, 1894-1963.
Peréz	Peréz Pastor, Critóbal. *Bibliografia madrileña; ó, Descripción de las obras imprésas en Madrid.* 3 vols. Madrid, 1891-1907.
Pescetto	Pescetto, G.B. *Biografia medica Ligure.* Genova, 1846.
Plessner	Plessner, Martin. *Vorsokratische Philosophie und griechische Alchemie in arabisch-lateinischer Überlieferung.* Wiesbaden, 1975.
Power	Power, Sir D'Arcy. *Selected Writings, 1877-1930.* Oxford, 1931.
Poynter	Poynter, Frederick Noël Lawrence. *A Bibliography of Gervase Markham.* Oxford, 1962.

Pritzel — Pritzel, Georg August. *Thesaurus literaturae botanicae omnium gentium.* Leipzig 1872-[77]

Proksch — Proksch, Johann Karl. *Die Litteratur über die venerischen Krankheiten.* 3 vols. Bonn, 1889-91.

Rahir — Rahir, Edouard. *Catalogue d'une collection unique de volumes imprimés par les Elzevier.* Paris, 1896.

Renouard — Renouard, Philippe. *Imprimeurs parisiens . . . depuis l'introduction de l'imprimerie à Paris (1470) jusqua' à la fin du xvi siècle.* Paris, 1898.

Rogent and Duràn — Rogent, Elíes, and Duràn, Estanislau. *Bibliografía de les impressions Lul-lianes.* Barcelona, 1927.

Sabattini — Sabattini, Gino. *Bibliografia di opere antiche e moderne di chiromanzia e sulla chiromanzia.* [Bologna] 1946.

Sabin — Sabin, Joseph. *Bibliotheca Americana. A Dictionary of Books Relating to America, from its Discovery to the Present Time.* 29 vols. New York, 1868-1936.

Sargent — Sargent, Charles Sprague, and Ethelyn Maria Tucker. *Catalogue of the Library of the Arnold Arboretum of Harvard University.* 2 vols. Cambridge, 1914-17.

Schmieder — Schmieder, Karl Christoph. *Geschichte der Alchemie.* Halle, 1832.

Sherrington — Sherrington, Sir Charles Scott. *The Endeavour of Jean Fernel, with a List of the Editions of His Writings.* Cambridge, 1946.

Sivette — Silvette, Herbert. *Catalogue of the Works of Philemon Holland . . . 1600-1940.* Charlottesville, Va., 1940.

Smith — Smith, Sir Frederick. *The Early History of Veterinary Literature and Its British Development.* 4 vols. London, 1919-33.

Sorbelli — Sorbelli, Albano. *Storia della stampa in Bologna.* Bologna, [1929].

Spencer — Spencer, Herbert Ritchie. *The History of British Midwifery from 1650 to 1800.* London, 1927.

STC (A) — Pollard, Alfred William, and Redgrave, G.R., comp. *A Short-title Catalogue of Books Printed in England, Scotland, & Ireland and of English Books Printed Abroad, 1475-1640.* London, 1926. 2d ed. rev. and enl. by W.A. Jackson, F.S. Ferguson, and Katherine F. Pantzer. London, 1976-1986.

STC (B) — Wing, Donald Goodard, comp. *Short-title Catalogue of Books Printed in England, Scotland, Ireland, Wales, and British America and of English Books Printed in Other Countries, 1641-1700.* New York, 1945-51 [and] 2d ed. 1972- .

Steinschneider — Steinschneider, Moritz. *Die hebraeischen Uebersetzungen des Mittelalters und die Juden als Dolmetscher.* 2 vols. Berlin, 1893.

Stübler — Stübler, Eberhard. *Leonhart Fuchs, Leben und Werk.* Munich, 1928. Münchener Beiträge zur Geschichte und Literatur der Naturwissenschaften und Medizin, Heft 13/14. Munich, 1928.

Sudhoff (A) — Sudhoff, Karl. *Bibliographia Paracelsica.* Graz, 1958.

Sudhoff (B) — ——— *Versuch einer Kritik der Echtheit der Paracelsischen Schriften.* 2 vols. Berlin, 1894-99.

Szinnyei — Szinnyei, József. *Bibliotheca Hungarica historiae naturalis et matheseos. Magyarország természettudományi és mathematikai könyvészete, 1472-1875.* Budapest, 1878.

Thieme-Becker — Thieme, Ulrich, and Becker, Felix, ed. *Allgemeines Lexikon der bildenden Künstler von der Antike bis zur Gegenwart.* 37 vols. Leipzig, 1907-50.

Thorndike — Thorndike, Lynn. *A History of Magic and Experimental Science.* 8 vols. New York, [1923-58].

Toppi — Toppi, Nicolò. *Biblioteca Napoletana . . . Dalle loro origini, per tutto l'anno 1678.* Naples, 1678.

Waller — Uppsala. Universitet. Bibliotek. *Bibliotheca Walleriana. The Books Illustrating the History of Medicine and Science Collected by Dr. Erik Waller and Bequeathed to the Library of the Royal University of Uppsala.* Acta Bibliotecae R. Universitatis Upsaliensis, vols. 8-9. Stockholm, 1955.

Watt Watt, Robert. *Bibliotheca Britannica; or, A General Index to British and Foreign Literature.* 4 vols. Edinburgh, 1824.

Weller Weller, Emil Ottokar. *Die falschen und fingierten Druckorte.* 2d ed., enl. and imp. 2 vols. Leipzig, 1864.

Wellcome Wellcome Historical Medical Library, London. *A Catalogue of Printed Books . . .* I. Books Printed before 1641 . . . [II, III. Books Printed from 1641 to 1850. A-E, F-L.] London, 1962- .

Wilkin Wilkin, Simon, ed. *The Works of Sir Thomas Browne.* 3 vols. London, 1894-1900.

Willems Willems, Alphonse. *Les Elzevier; histoire et annales typographiques.* Brussels, 1880.

Wood Wood, Anthony à. Athenae Oxonienses. *An Exact History of All the Writers and Bishops Who Have Had Their Education in the University of Oxford. To Which Are Added the Fasti, or Annals of the Said University.* 5 vols. London, 1813-20.

Zedler Zedler, Johann Heinrich. *Grosses vollständiges Universal-Lexikon.* 64 vols. Graz, 1961-64.

A

A., D. [*fl. ca.* 1685] *tr. See* Boyle, *Hon.* R. Apparatus ad historiam naturalem sanguinis humani. 1684, 1685, 1686 [and] De specificorum remediorum cum corpusculari philosophia concordia. 1686, 1687 [and] Tentamen prologicum. 1686 [and] Tractatus de ipsa natura. 1688.

A., F., *M. D. See* Le Parnasse assiegé. 1697.

A., I., *M. D., tr. See* Dariot, C. Die gulden Arch, 1614.

A., I. S., *D. M. See* Valles, F. de. Methodus medendi. 1651.

A., J. D. Thom. *See* Thom, J. D.

A., T. *See* Read, A. Most excellent and approved medicines. 1652.

A.D.A.S. *See* Leti, Gregorio [1630-1701]

A.E.B.D.C.I. *See* I., A.E.B.D.C.

A. M. *See* M., A.

A. P. *See* Porchon, Ant.

A. T. *See* T., A., practitioner in physicke and chirurgerie.

A. V. V. V. *See* V., A. V. V.

AALBORG, Niels Michelsen [1562-1645] Medicin eller laege-boog. Deelt udi fem smaa bøger. De indeholdis i den I. bog. Om menniskens sundhed ... II. Om atskillige siuger at curere ... III. Om nogle synderlige urters kraffter ... IV. Om den laegedom som huert menniske altid haffuer hos sig selff. V. Om spaede børns siuger [Ex Joh. Witichio] ... Nu anden gang forbedret ... [Kiøbenhaffn] Tyge Nielssøn, 1640.

[24], 323, [13] p. 16 cm. [1]

Each book has special title page. Book 2 is dated 1638.

With this is bound Flemlose, P. J. En elementisch oc jordisch astrologia [1644]

AALSTIUS, Joannes [*fl.* 1693] *See* Bekker, B. Brief ... aan ... Joannes Aalstius. 1693.

AANMERKINGEN op de staatkundige bedenking, rakende het verschil tusschen den ... Bonaventura Dortmont ... en ... Fredericus Ruysch ... mitsgaders Mr. Andries Boekelman ... Amsterdam, Anthony Lescailje, 1677.

23 p. 16 cm. [2]

AARDIGE duyvelary, voorvallende in dese dagen. Begrepen in een brief van een heer te Amsterdam, geschreven aan een van sijn vrienden te Leeuwaerden, in Vriesland. [Rotterdam? 1691?]

45 p. 19 cm. [3]

Not in Linde.

Concerns controversy with Balthasar Bekker.

With this is bound Vervolg van de Aardige duyvelary. 1691.

ABANO, Pietro d' [1250-1315?] Conciliator enucleatus; seu, Differentiarum philosophicarum et medicarum Petri Apponensis compendium opera Gregorii Horstii ... editum. Giessae Hassorum, Casparus Chemlinus, 1615.

[4], 156 p. 20 cm. [4]

Imperfect: p. 9-16, 53-54, 59-60 wanting; p. 55-56 mutilated.

Colophon at end of the first section dated 1614.

In two sections, each with special half title (Conciliatoris enucleati, seu differentiarum ... in compendium redactarum pars prior medicinam theoreticam illustrans [-posterior medicinam practicam illustrans] in incluta Academia Giessena publice disputandi gratia ... anno MDCXIV [-MDCXV] proposita. Directore & praeside Gregorio Horstio ...) and consisting of three "exercitationes." Each exercitatio has a different respondent.

—[The same.] Ed. nova. Giessae, Casparus Chemlinus, 1621.

[16], 279 p. 16 cm. [5]

—De diebus decretoriis. *See* Imbrasius, *of Ephesus.* Prognostica de decubitu.

—*tr. See* Bovio, Z. T. Melampigo. 1617, 1626.

—*See* Mesuë [924 *or* 5-1015] Opera. 1602, 1623.

—*as subject. See* Gockel, E. Enchiridion medico-practicum de peste. 1669.

ABATI, Baldo Angelo [16th cent.] De admirabili viperae natura, & de mirificis ejusdem facultatibus liber ... Noribergae, Recusus, sumptibus & typis Sebastiani Heusleri, 1603.

[16], 125 (i.e. 133), [10] p. illus. 20 cm. **[6]**

—[The same.] Hagae Comitis, Sam. Broun, 1660.

[26], 186, [26] p. illus. 14 cm. **[7]**

ABBAMA, Fredericus [*fl.* 1631] *respondent. See* Burgersdijck, F. P., *praeses*. Collegium physicum. 1642.

ABBATIA, Antonius de. Send-Brieff von Verwandelung der Metallen. *In* Drey vortreffliche und noch nie im Druck gewesene chymische Bücher. 1670.

ABBATIUS, Baldus Angelus. *See* Abati, Baldo Angelo [16th cent]

ABBAZIO, Baldo Angelo. *See* Abati, Baldo Angelo [16th cent]

ABBÉ, P. L'. *See* Labbé, Pierre [1596-1678]

'ABD al-MALIK IBN ZUHR IBN 'ABD al-MALIK, Abū Marwān. *See* Avenzoar [*d. ca.* 1162]

'ABD al-RAHMĀN IBN ABĪ BAKR, Jalāl al-Dīn, al-Suyūtī. *See* al-Suyūtī [1445-1505]

'ABD al-RAHMĀN IBN MUHAMMAD, *called* Ibn Wāfid [999-1068] *See* Mesuë [924 *or* 5-1015] Opera. 1602, 1623.

ABEILLE, Scipion [*d.* 1697] L'anatomie de la teste, et de ses parties ... Paris, Laurent d'Houry, 1689.

[12], 84 p.; 130 (i.e. 128), [4] p. 15 cm. **[8]**

Part [2] has special title page: Chapitre singulier tiré de Guidon ... en deux parties, & enrichi de vers.

—Le parfait chirurgien d'armée, le traité des playes d'arquebusade, le chapitre singulier tiré de Guidon, l'anatomie de la teste et de ses parties. Pour l'instruction des étudians en chirurgie ... Paris, Jean Guignard, 1696.

[14], 224 p. 16 cm. **[9]**

Contains 4 treatises; [2-4] have special title pages and [2-3] are dated 1695.

ABEL, Jakob [*fl.* 1655] *respondent.* Jacobus Abel ... De phtisi dissertationem ... discutiendam offero ... Basilae, Typis Georgii Deckeri [1655]

[20] p. 20 cm. **[10]**

Diss.—Basel.

ABEN EZRA, Abraham ben Meïr. *See* Ibn Ezra, Abraham ben Meïr [1092-1167]

ABENGUEFIT. *See* 'Abd al-Rahmān ibn Muhammad, *called* Ibn Wāfid [999-1068]

ABERCROMBY, David [*d.* 1701 *or* 2?] Opuscula medica hactenus edita. I. De luis venereae absque salivatione mercuriali, curatione, II. De modo curandi bubonis venerei & tutiore salivationis methodo. (Nunc primum editum) III. De varietate, ac variatione pulsus. IV. De dignoscendis medicis plantarum, ac corporum quorumcumque virtutibus ex solo capore ... Londini, Impensis Samuelis Smith, 1687.

1 v. 16 cm. **[11]**

Various pagings.

Parts [3-4] have special title pages with date altered by hand from MDCLXXXV to MDCLXXXVII.

Part [3] has title: De variatione, ac varietate pulsus observationes ... Part [4] has title: Nova medicinae tum practicae, tum speculativae clavis.

—De variatione, ac varietate pulsus observationes. Accessit ejusdem authoris Nova medicinae tum speculativae, tum practicae clavis. Sive ars explorandi medicas plantarum ac corporum quorumcumque facultates ex solo sapore. Londini, Impensis Samuelis Smith, 1685.

[12], 54 p.; [12], 36, [4] p. 16 cm. **[12]**

In 2 parts. Part [2] has special title page.

Published also as parts 3-4 of his Opuscula medica, 1687.

—Fur academicus. Amstelodami, Apud Abrahamum Wolfgang, 1689.

[20], 319, [21] p. 14 cm. **[13]**

—Tuta, ac efficax luis venereae, saepe absque mercurio, ac semper absque salivatione mercuriali, curandae methodus ... Londini, Impensis Samuelis Smith, 1684.

[14], 79, [17] p. 16 cm. **[14]**

"A catalogue of late physick books sold by Samuel Smith": [8] p. at end.

—[Dutch tr.] De Spaanse pok-meester, beschryvende den oorsprong, oorsaak en regte genesing der pokken, als mede der zaaddruppers, chankers, klapooren, invallen der neuse, pynen en kalk der beenderen. In't Engels beschreven door David Abercromby ... en ... vertaalt en vermeerdert door Jan Babtista Lusart ... Amsterdam, Jan ten Hoorn, 1691.

[16], 400 p. 16 cm. **[15]**

Added engraved title page.

—[FRENCH TR.] Methode asseurée & efficace pour guerir la maladie venerienne sans salivation mercurielle. Composée en latin par un celebre medecin d'Angleterre, & nouvellement mise en françois. Par le Sr. G. B. De S. Romain ... Paris, Laurent d'Houry, 1690.

[24], 128 p.   16 cm.   [16]

"Dissertation sur la cure du bubon venerien, & sur la plus sûre methode de la salivation": p. 108-128. The second treatise is a translation of Abercromby's De modo curandi bubonis venerei & tutiore salivationis methodo.

ABERGLAUBE und Zauberey. *See* ANHORN VON HARTWISS, B. Magiologia. 1674.

ABGETROCKNETE Thränen. 1698. *See* PASSAU, Diocese.

ABHANDLUNG dreyer . . . Instrumenten. 1688. *See* ALENCE, J. d'.

ABHENGUEFIT. *See* ʿABD AL-RAḤMĀN IBN MUḤAMMAD, *called* IBN WĀFID [999-1068]

ABHOMERON. *See* AVENZOAR [*d. ca.* 1162]

ABRAAM TORTUOSIENSIS. *See* ABRAHAM BEN SHEM-TOB [13th cent]

ABRAHAM A SANCTA CLARA, *Father* [1644-1709] Danck und Denckzahl dess Achten gegen dem Drey; das ist, Ein kleine Schluss-Predig, so in der Octav dess solennem Danck-Fests zu der Allerheiligisten Dreyfaltigkeit, mitten in der Statt Wienn auff offentlichem Platz bey einer unglaubigen Menge Volcks gehalten worden . . . Saltzburg, Melchior Haan, 1687.

[2], 13, [1] p.   19 cm.   [17]

—Oesterreichisches Deo Gratias; das ist, Ein aussführliche Beschreibung eines Hochfeyerlichen Danck-Fests, welches zu Ehren der Allerheiligsten Dreyfaltigkeit wegen gnädiger Abwendung der über uns verhängten schwären Straff der Pest in der . . . Statt Wienn, den 17. Junii Anno 1680, durch die Löbl. N. O. Herrn Land- Ständ höchst-aufferbäulich angestellt worden; sambt einer kurtzen Predig . . . in Mitte der Statt . . . vorgetragen durch Pr. Fr. Abraham à S. Clara . . . Saltzburg, Melchior Haan, 1688.

[2], 16 [1] p.   19 cm.   [18]

ABRAHAM AVENARE. *See* IBN EZRA, Abraham ben Meïr [1092-1167]

ABRAHAM BEN EZRA. *See* IBN EZRA, Abraham ben Meïr [1092-1167]

ABRAHAM BEN MEÏR ABEN EZRA. *See* IBN EZRA, Abraham ben Meïr [1092-1167]

ABRAHAM BEN SHEM-TOB [13th cent.] *See* MESUË [924 *or* 5-1015] Opera. 1602, 1623.

ABRAHAM DA TORTOSA. *See* ABRAHAM BEN SHEM-TOB [13th cent.]

ABRAHAM ECCHELLENSIS [*d.* 1664] *tr. See* AL-SUYŪTĪ. De proprietatibus ac virtutibus medicis animalium. 1647.

ABRAHAM IBN EZRA. *See* IBN EZRA, Abraham ben Meïr [1092-1167]

ABRAHAM JUDAEUS [1092-1167] *See* IBN EZRA, Abraham ben Meïr [1092-1167]

ABRAHAM JUDAEUS TORTUOSENSIS. *See* ABRAHAM BEN SHEM-TOB [13th cent.]

ABREGÉ d'anatomie. 1667. *See* PILES, R. de.

ABREU, ALEXO DE [1568-1630] Tratado de las siete enfermedades, de la inflammacion universal del higado, zirbo, pyloron, y riñones, y de la obstrucion, de la satiriasi, de la terciana y febre maligna, y passion hipocondriaca. Lleva otros tres tratados, del mal de loanda, del guzano, y de las fuentes y sedales . . . Lisboa, Pedro Craesbeeck, 1623.

[24], 228 ll.   20 cm.   [19]

Leaves 25-28 misbound after l. 32.

ABŪ al-KĀSIM KHALAF IBN AL-ʿABBĀS, AL-ZAHRĀWĪ. *See* ABULCASIS [936?-1013?]

ABŪ al-MUTARRIF ʿABD al-RAHMĀN IBN MUHAMMAD IBN ʿABD al-KARĪM IBN YAHYA IBN al-WĀFID al-LAKHMĪ. *See* ʿABD al-RAḤMĀN IBN MUHAMMAD, *called* IBN WĀFID [999-1068]

ABŪ al-QĀSIM KHALAF IBN ʿABBĀS, al-ZAHRĀWĪ. *See* ABULCASIS [936?-1013?]

ABŪ al-WĀLID MUHAMMAD IBN AHMAD, *called* Ibn Rushd. *See* AVERROËS [1126-1198].

ABŪ ʿALĪ AL-ḤUSAIN IBN ʿABD ALLĀH. *See* AVICENNA [980?-1037]

ABŪ BAKR MUḤAMMAD IBN ZAKARĪYĀ, al-Rāzī. *See* MUḤAMMAD IBN ZAKARĪYĀ, Abū Bakr, al-Rāzī [865-925]

ABŪ MARWĀN ‘ABD AL-MALIK IBN ABĪ BAKR IBN MUḤAMMAD IBN MARWĀN IBN ZUHR. *See* AVENZOAR [*d. ca.* 1162]

ABŪ MŪSĀ JĀBIR IBN ḤAYYĀN. *See* JĀBIR IBN ḤAIYĀN, al-Ṭarasūsī.

ABŪ YA‘KUB ISHAK IBN SULAIMĀN, al-Isra‘īlī. *See* ISRAELI, Isaac [*ca.* 832–*ca.* 932]

ABU YŪSUF YA‘KŪB IBN ISḤĀK IBN ṢUB-BĀH, al-Kindī. *See* YA‘KUB IBN ISḤĀK IBN ṢUB-BĀH, Abū Yūsuf, al-Kindi [*d. ca.* 873]

ABŪ ZAKARĪYĀ YAḤYA YŪḤANNĀ IBN MASAWAIH. *See* MESUË [*d.* 857]

ABULCASIS [936?-1013?] Liber servitoris. *In* MESUË [924 *or* 5-1015] Opera. 1602, 1623.

—*See* DALECHAMPS, J. Chirurgie françoise. 1610.

ABYNZOAR. *See* AVENZOAR [*d. ca.* 1162]

ACACIA, MARTINUS [1539-1588] *See* AKAKIA, Martin [1539-1588]

ACADEMIA ALBERTINA. *See* ALBERTUS-UNIVERSITÄT.

ACADEMIA ALDORFIANA. *See* PICCART, M. Oratio academica qua Altorfinam Norimbergensium Academiam metu luis per contagium invectae dilabentem. 1612.

ACADEMIA ALTFORIANA. *See* ACADEMIA ALDORFIANA.

ACADEMIA CAESAREA-LEOPOLDINO NATURAE CURIOSORUM. *See* ACADEMIA NATURAE CURIOSORUM.

ACADEMIA FRANEKERANA. Acclamationes, ad ... D. Nicolaum Blancardum L. A. magistrum, medicinae doct ... cum illi ex auctoritate ... Frisiae ordinum solenniter linguae & historiae Graecae professio demandaretur ... Franekerae, Johannes Wellens, 1670.

[8] p.   20 cm.   [**20**]

ACADEMIA FRISIAE. *See* ACADEMIA FRANEKERANA.

ACADEMIA HAVNIENSIS. *See* UNIVERSITAS REGIA HAFNIENSIS. Facultas medica.

ACADEMIA IMPERIALIS LEOPOLDINA NATURAE CURIOSORUM. *See* ACADEMIA NATURAE CURIOSORUM.

ACADEMIA JULIA. *See* JULIUS UNIVERSITÄT, Helmstedt.

ACADEMIA JULIA CAROLINA. *See* JULIUS UNIVERSITÄT, Helmstedt.

ACADEMIA LIPSIENSIS. *See* UNIVERSITÄT LEIPZIG.

ACADEMIA LUGDUNO-BATAVA. *See* RIJKSUNIVERSITEIT TE LEIDEN.

ACADEMIA NATURAE CURIOSORUM. Academiae Naturae Curiosorum ortus, leges, catalogus. Noribergae, 1683.

[56] p.   20 cm.   [**21**]
Signatures: A-C⁴, D²; A-B⁴; C:C⁶.
Part [2] and [3] have special title pages.

—*See* MISCELLANEA CURIOSA; Miscellanea medicophysica Academiae Naturae curiosorum Germaniae [Annus primus] 1672.

—*as subject. See* WEDEL, G.W. Opiologia ad mentem Academiae Naturae Curiosorum. 1674, 1682.

ACADEMIA PHILOEXOTICORUM NATURAE ET ARTIS, BRESCIA. *See* ACCADEMIA DEI FILOSOTICI, Brescia.

ACADEMIA REGIA HAFNIENSIS. *See* UNIVERSITAS REGIA HAFNIENSIS. Facultas medica.

ACADEMIA REGIOMONTANA. *See* ALBERTUS-UNIVERSITÄT.

ACADEMIA TÜBINGENSIS. *See* EBERHARD-KARLS-UNIVERSITÄT Tübingen.

ACADÉMIE CHIMIQUE, CHAMBÉRY. *See* COPPONAY DE GRIMALDY, D. de. Etablissement du laboratoire de S.A.R. 1684.

ACADEMIE CHYMIQUE DE SAVOYE. *See* ACADÉMIE CHIMIQUE, Chambéry.

ACADÉMIE DE FRANCE À ROME. *See* GENGA, B. Anatomia per uso et intelligenza del disegno. 1691.

ACADÉMIE DE PEINTURE, SCULPTURE, ARCHITECTURE ÉTABLIE À ROME. *See* ACADÉMIE DE FRANCE À ROME.

ACADÉMIE ROYALE DES SCIENCES, Paris. Memoires for a natural history of animals. Being the anatomical descriptions of several animals dissected by the Royal Academy at Paris. Englished by A.P. SRS ... [n.p.] 1687.

> [14], 3-267, [13] p.; 40 p.   plates.   30 cm.
>   **[22]**

Engraved title page.
Translation by Alexander Pitfield from the Mémoires of Claude Perrault.
"The measure of the earth" (2d group of paging) has caption title and was translated by Richard Waller.

—[The same.] Memoir's [sic] for a natural history of animals. Containing the anatomical descriptions of several creatures dissected by the Royal Academy of Sciences at Paris. Englished by Alexander Pitfield ... To which is added an account of The measure of a degree of a great circle of the earth ... Englished by Richard Waller, S. R. S. London, Printed by Joseph Streater, and sold by T. Basset, J. Robinson, B. Aylmer, Joh. Southby and W. Canning, 1688.

> [17], 3-267, [13] p.; [2], 40 p.   plates.   31 cm.
>   **[23]**

Added engraved title page.
The text is of the same setting as the 1687 ed.
"The measure of the earth" (2d group of paging) has special title page.

—*See* [PERRAULT, C.] Description anatomique de divers animaux dissequez dans l'Academie royale des sciences. 1682.

ACAKIA, MARTIN [1539-1588] *See* AKAKIA, Martin [1539-1588]

ACAMPO, SIMONE [1532-*ca.* 1592] Commentaria in libros Galeni De differentiis febrium, in textus 13, nempe a tex. 46, usque ad tex. 58, tertii libri Artis medicinalis. In librum De tumoribus praeter naturam ... A Simone Acampo juniore ... recognito, & in lucem edito. Neapoli, Ex typographia Secundini Roncalioli, 1642.

> [8], 454; 320, [16] p.   22 cm.   **[24]**

ACAMPO, SIMONE [*fl.* 1642] *ed. See* ACAMPO, S. [1532-*ca.* 1592] Commentaria in libros Galeni De differentiis febrium. 1642.

ACCADEMIA DEI FILESOTICI, BRESCIA. *See* ACTA NOVAE ACADEMIAE PHILEXOTICORUM NATURAE ET ARTIS. 1687.

ACCADEMIA DEI LINCEI, ROME. *See* HERNÁNDEZ, F. Rerum medicarum Novae Hispaniae thesaurus. 1628.

ACCADEMIA DEL CIMENTO, FLORENCE. Saggi di naturali esperienze fatte nell'Accademia del Cimento ... Firenze, Giuseppe Cocchini, 1667.

> [15], cclxix, [16] p.   illus.   36 cm.   **[25]**

Written by Lorenzo Magalotti, the secretary of the academy.

—[English tr.] Essayes of natural experiments made in the Academia del Cimento ... Written in Italian by the secretary of that academy [i.e. Lorenzo Magalotti]. Englished by Richard Waller ... London, Benjamin Alsop, 1684.

> [24], 160 (i.e. 164), [10] p.   plates.   23 cm.
>   **[26]**

Added engraved title page.

ACCADEMIA DI FRANCIA IN ROMA. *See* ACADÉMIE DE FRANCE À ROME ...

ACCLAMATIONES, ad ... D. Nicolaum Blancardum. *See* ACADEMIA FRANEKERANA.

ACCOLTI, PIETRO [*fl.* 1625] Lo inganno degl'occhi, prospettiva practica ... Firenze, Pietro Cecconcelli, 1625.

> [12], 152 p.   diagrs., plate.   29 cm.   **[27]**

The ACCOMPLISH'D lady's delight in preserving, physick, beautifying and cookery. Containing, I. The art of preserving and candying fruits ... II. The physical cabinet, or excellent receipts in physick ... together with ... New and excellent secrets and experiments in the art of angling. III. The compleat cooks guide ... London, B. Harris, 1675.

> [7], 382, [10] p.   front., plates.   15 cm.   **[28]**

Added engraved title page.
Imperfect: p. [203] mutilated.
Items 2 and 3, and the "New ... art of angling" have special title pages.
The epistle dedicatory, signed by T.P., i.e. Hannah Woolley?

The ACCOMPLISHED ladies rich closet of rarities. 1696. *See* [SHIRLEY, J.]

The ACCOMPLISHT physician. 1670. *See* [MERRET, C.]

An ACCOMPT of some books. I. Marc. Malpigii . . . Dissertatio epistolica de bombyce . . . [London, 1669]

987-990 p.   23 cm.   [29]

Caption title.

A review of Malpighi's De bombyce detached from Philosophical Transactions, 1669, vol. 4.

Bound with Malpighi, M. Praeclarissimo . . . viro D. Jacobo Sponio. [1684]

ACEVEDO, MANUEL D'. *See* AZEVEDO, Manoel de, *Father* [d. 1672].

ACHEMONE. *See* BOVIO, Z. T. Melampigo. 1617, 1626.

ACHMET f. SIERIM. *See* AHMAD IBN SIRIN [fl. 813-833]

ACHOLZIUS, JOHANNES. *See* AICHHOLTZ, JOHANN [1520-1588]

ACHT, JOHANN. *See* ECHT, JOHANN [1515?-ca. 1568]

ACKER, JOHANN [fl. 1681] respondent. *See* MATTHAEUS, P., *praeses.* Disputatio medica de chylo. 1681.

ACKER, NIKOLAUS. *See* AGER, Nikolaus [1568-1634]

ACOLUTH, ANDREAS [1654-1704] De אורד'ם ה מ'ד ר ם sive, Aquis amaris maledictionem inferentibus, vulgo dictis zelotypiae, et Num. V. v. ii. usque ad finem cap. descriptis, ex anatolica antiquitate, hoc est: fontibus sacris, eorundemque variis tum orientalibus, tum occidentalibus versionibus, Thalmude utroque, & omnium aetatum Hebraeis exegetis, homiletis, philosophis, kabbalistis, atque Masora, erutum, adeoque Judaeorum in textus sacros commentandi rationem multiplicem ostendens philologema. Lipsiae, Typis Justini Brandii, 1682.

[48], 480 p.   21 cm.   [30]

Added engraved title page.

ACOLUTH, JOHANNES [fl. 1679] respondent. *See* ETTMÜLLER, M., *praeses.* Virtutem opii diaphoreticam. 1679.

ACOSTA, CRISTÓBAL. *See* COSTA, Christovam da [ca. 1540-1599]

ACOSTA, JOSÉ DE [ca. 1539-1600] The naturall and morall historie of the Est and West Indies. Intreating of the remarkeable things of heaven, of the elements, mettalls, plants and beasts which are proper to that country . . . Written in Spanish . . . and translated into English by E. G. London, Printed by Val. Sims for Edward Blount and William Aspley, 1604.

[6], 590, [14] p.   19 cm.   [31]

Translation sometimes attributed to Edward Grimstone.

STC 94.

ACOSTA, JUAN DUARTE NÚÑEZ. *See* NÚÑEZ DE ACOSTA, Duarte [fl. 1653-1681]

A COSTA, ROMANUS. *See* COSTA, Romanus a [fl. ca. 1620]

ACQUAPENDENTE, GIROLAMO FABRICI D'. *See* FABRICIUS, Hieronymus, ab Aquapendente [ca. 1533-1619]

ACTA eruditorum anno 1682-1700. Lipsiae, Prostant apud J. Grassium & J. F. Gletitschium, typis Christophori Güntheri [Christiani Goezii, Joh. Grossii haeredes & Joh. Thom. Fritschium, Johannis Georgii] 1682-1700.

21 v.   illus., plates.   22 cm.   [32]

Imperfect: Anno 1695 wanting.

ACTA medica & philosophica Hafniensia ann. 1671 [-1679] 1673-1680. *See* BARTHOLIN, T., ed.

ACTA novae Academiae Philexoticorum Naturae et Artis. 1686 . . . Brixiae, Apud Jo. Mariam Ricciardum, 1687.

[8], 3-241, [5] p.   illus., plates.   17 cm.   [33]

Dedicatory epistle by Ermete Francesco Lantana.

ACTEN gemässe relatio facti. *See* SCHMIDTS, M., *defendant.*

ACTON, GEORGE [fl. ca. 1669] A letter in answer to certain quaeries and objections made by a learned Galenist against the theorie and practice of chymical physick. Wherein the right method of curing of diseases is demonstrated; the possibility of an universal medicine evinced; and chymical physick vindicated . . . London, Printed by William Godbid for Walter Kettleby, 1670.

[2], 14 p.   20 cm.   [34]

—Physical reflections upon a letter written by J. Denis . . . to Monsieur de Montmor . . . concerning a new way of curing sundry diseases by transfusion of blood . . . London, Printed by T.R. for J. Martyn, 1668.

[6], 10 p.   21 cm.   [35]

ACTUARIUS, JOANNES. *See* JOANNES ACTUARIUS [13th cent.]

ACUENZA Y MOSA, PEDRO. *See* AQUENZA Y MOSSA, Pedro [*fl.* 1696-1726]

AD Theriacae Andromachi singularia schediasma. Lesznae, Typis Vetterianis, 1642.

    80p. 16 cm   [36]
    Sometimes attributed to Joannes Jonstonus.

ADAM, MELCHIOR [1551-1622] Vitae Germanorum medicorum: qui seculo superiori, et quod excurrit, claruerunt . . . Haidelbergae, Impensis heredum Jonae Rosae, excudit Johannes Georgius Geyder, 1620.

    [32], 451, [27] p. 19 cm.   [37]

ADAMANTIUS. La physionomie; ou, Des indices que la nature a mis au corps humain par où l'on peut descouvrir les moeurs, & les inclinations d'un chacun. Avec un traitté de la divination par les palpitations, & un autre par les marques naturelles. Le tout traduit du grec d'Adamantius & de Melampe, par Henry de Boyvin du Vauroüy . . . Paris, Toussainct du Bray, 1635.

    [16], 282 p. 18 cm.   [38]
    Translations of Adamantius' Physiognomica (an epitome of the Physiognomica of Antonius Polemo); and of Melampus' De divinatione per palpitationes and De naevis corporis. Cf. Foerster; Pauly-Wissowa, v. 21, col. 1345-1348.

ADAMI, JACOB CHRISTIAN [*fl.*1690] *respondent. See* PETRI VON HARTENFELS, G.C., *praeses.* Disputatio inauguralis medica, de phlegmone. 1690.

ADAMI, JOHANN SAMUEL [1638-1713] Misanders [*pseud.*] Theatrum tragicum; oder. Eröffnete Schau-Bühne, allerhand . . . Trauer- und Todes-Fälle, die sich . . . nahe und ferne, begeben haben, und auff 369 Titul sich erstrecken . . . Dresden, Verlegt von Johann Christoph Miethen, und Joh. Christoph Zimmermannen, 1695.

    [37], 1040, [71] p. front. 17 cm.   [39]

ADAMI, JOHANN STEPHAN [*fl.*1684] *respondent.* Dissertationem inauguralem de osse cordis cervi . . . publicae censurae submittit Johannes Stephanus Adami . . . Giessae Hassorum, Literis Academicis Kargerianis, 1684.

    16 p. 20 cm.   [40]
    Diss.—Giessen.

ADAMI, TOBIAS [1581-1643] *ed. See* CAMPENELLA, T. De sensu rerum et magia. 1620.

ADAMS, THOMAS [*fl.*1612-1653] Mystical bedlam; or, The world of mad-men . . . London, By George Purslowe, for Clement Knight, 1615.

    [6], 82 p. 18 cm.   [41]
    Imperfect: upper margins trimmed.
    STC 124.

ADAMUS, JOHANNES STEPHANUS. *See* ADAMI, Johann Stephan [*fl.*1684]

ADELGEHR, LAURENTIUS [*fl.* 1626] *respondent.* De pleuritide dissertationem . . . proponit . . . Laurentius Adelgehr . . . Argentorati, 1626.

    [20] p. 19 cm.   [42]
    Diss.—Strasbourg.

ADELUNG, JOHANN CHRISTOPH. *See* ADLUNG, Johann Christoph [1648-1681]

ADER, GUILLAUME [*b.* 1578] De la methode de consulter les maladies chirurgicales. *In* Chaumette, A. Le parfaict chirurgien. 1628.

—De pestis cognitione, praevisione, & remediis. Praelectiones in libellulum redactae . . . Tolosae, Typis Raim. Colomerii, 1628.

    [12], 96 p. 15 cm.   [43]

—Enarrationes, de aegrotis, et morbis in Evangelio. Opus in miraculorum Christi Domini amplitudinem Ecclesiae Christianae elimatum . . . Tolosae, Apud Dominicum & PETRUM BOSC, 1620.

    [24], 458, [6] p. 18 cm.   [44]

—[The same.] . . . 1621.   [45]

—[The same.] . . . Tolosae, Typis Raymundi Colomerii, 1623.   [46]

ADLUNG, JOHANN CHRISTOPH [1648-1681], *praeses.* Miraculosa eaque catholica in piscina Bethesdea morborum cura exercitatione philologica descripta . . . [Erfurti] Typis Kirschianis [1676]

    [16] p. 19 cm.   [47]
    Diss.—Erfurt (N. C. Nicolai, *respondent*)

—*respondent.* Febris infantum purpurata dissertatione inaugurali descripta . . . Erfurti, Typis Kirschianis [1676]

    24 p. 18 cm.   [48]
    Diss. — Erfurt.

—*respondent. See* PURPIUS, A., *praeses.* Exercitatio academica prior. 1669 [AND] Exercitatio academica posterior. 1669.

Les ADMIRABLES qualitez du kinkina, confirmées par plusieurs experiences, et la maniere de s'en servir dans toutes les fiévres pour toute sorte d'âge, de sexe, & de complexions. Paris, Martin Jouvenel, 1689.

    [24], 164, [2], 4 p.   16 cm.   **[49]**
A treatise on quinine, as used by Robert Talbor.

    —[The same.] . . . 1694.   **[50]**
Sig. 04 (blank) wanting.

    —[Italian tr.] La kinakina, e le di lei stupende qualità, con la maniera di servirsene, in tutte le febbri, per ogni sorte d'età, sesso, e complessione, aggiuntovi il nuovo metodo scuoperto dal . . . Elvetio, per servirsi di quell 'efficacissimo rimedio, senza nulla prendere per bocca. Il tutto portato dal francese in italiano . . . Parma, Guiseppe dall'Oglio, e Francesco Maria Rosati, 1694.

    [14], xvii, [1], 154, [1] p.   16 cm.   **[51]**
Translation by Carlo Ricani of Les admirables qualitez du kinkina, and J.A. Helvétius' Methode pour guerir toute sorte de fievres.

ADMIRANDA rerum admirabilium encomia. Sive diserta & amoena Pallas disserens seria sub ludicra specie. Hoc est, dissertationum ludicararum, nec non amoenitatum scriptores varii . . . Noviomagi Batavorum, Typis Reineri Smetii, 1666.

    [12], 660 p.   14 cm.   **[52]**
Added engraved title page.
Includes: Hieronymi Cardani Podagrae encomium, Bilibaldi Pirckheimeri Apologia podagrae, Guillelmi Menapi Encomium febris quartanae, Jacobi Gutherii Tiresias seu caecitatis encomium.

    —[The same.] . . . 1676.   **[53]**
Added engraved title page, with new illustration, dated 1677. A page for page reprint of the 1666 edition.

ADMONITIO . . . De via ad aurum potabile . . . [Argentorati, Sumptib. haeredum Eberhardi Zetzneri, 1661]

    382–393 p., vol. 6.   20 cm. (*In* Zetzner, Lazarus, *ed.* Theatrum chemicum. Argentorati, 1659–61)   **[54]**
Caption and running title.

ADOLPHI, CHRISTIAN MICHAEL [1676–1753] *respondent.* Specimen physicum de siderum influxu

. . . publicae censurae . . . expositum, a M. Christiano Michaele Adolphi . . . respondente Justino Wachtelio . . . Lipsiae, Literis Christoph. Fleischeri [1700]

    [16] p.   19 cm.   **[55]**
Diss.—Leipzig (J. Wachtel, *respondent*)

    —*See* ORTLOB, J.F., *praeses.* Dissertatio medica de tono & atonia. 1700.

ADRIAANSZ, PIETER, *tr. See* PORTAL, P. De practyk der vroed' meesters, en vroed' vrouwen. 1690.

ADVICE to a physician. 1695. *See* [WALDSCHMIDT, J.J.]

ADVIS sur la peste. 1606. *See* ELLAIN, N.

AEGIDUS DE VADIS [*fl.* 1521?] Dialogus inter naturam et filium philosophiae . . .

    85–109 p., vol. 2, table. 20 cm. (*In* Zetzner, Lazarus, *ed.* Theatrum chemicum. Argentorati, 1659–61)   **[56]**
Caption title.
Edited by Bernard Georges Penot.

AEGIDIUS ROMANUS. *See* COLONNA, Egidio [1247?–1316]

AEGINETA I. *See* SCHULTZ, Gottfried [1643–1698]

AEGINETA, PAULUS. *See* PAULUS AEGINETA.

AEGYDIUS DE VADIS. *See* AEGIDIUS DE VADIS [*fl.* 1521?]

AELIANUS, CLAUDIUS. Περὶ ζώων ἰδιότητος βιβλία ιξ' . . . De animalium natura libri XVII. Petro Gillio . . . & Conrado Gesnero . . . interpretibus . . . Genevae, Apud Joann. Tornaesium, 1611.

    [8], 1018, [94] p.   13 cm.   **[57]**
In Greek and Latin.
Previously published under title: De historia animalium libri XVII.

AEN den eedelen Cocceaanschen docter. [n. p., 1677]

    [4] p.   16 cm.   **[58]**
Caption title.
A poem against Andreas Boekelman.

AENGELEN, PIETER VAN [*fl.* 1662] Herbarius kruyt en bloem-hof. Of de natuerlijcke secreten en verborgentheden . . . Het eerste [-derde] deel. Amsterdam, Broer en Ian Ioosten Appelaer, 1663.

    3 pts. in 1 v.   16 cm.   **[59]**

Part 2 has special title page: Instructie van het herbariseren, of hoveniers oeffeninge; om thuynen en boomgaerden te bereyden . . . Part 3 has special title page: De mede-lydige Samaritaen, of de heydensche wonde-meester.

AENHANGHSEL van verscheyden sonderlinge secreten. *See* BATEN, C. Secreet-boeck. 1650, 1656, 1661.

AEOLUS. *See* FÜRST, Johann Zacharias [*fl.* 1674–1692]

AEPLINIUS, GEORG FRIEDRICH [1657–1721] *respondent. See* WEDEL, G. W., *praeses.* Disputatio inauguralis medica, de catarrho suffocativo. 1680.

—Dissertatio medica, aegrum incubo laborantem sistens. 1678.

—*See* FASCH, A. H. Augustinus Henricus Faschius . . . decanus salutem . . . precatur lectori benevolo! 1681.

AESOPUS. [Fabularum selectarum partes duae Graecolatinae. Ingolstadii, Sartorius, 1606?]
[3], 148, [5] p.   13 cm.   [60]
Imperfect: title page wanting.
Title supplied from Hoffmann, vol. 1, p. 69.
Also published in 1618. Cf. DG, vol. 2, col. 115.
Text in Greek and Latin.
Original binding bears date 1621.
Bound with Goclenius, R. Uranoscopiae. 1608.

AETIUS, *of Amida. See* DALECHAMPS, J. Chirurgie françoise. 1610.

AETIUS ANTIOCHENUS. *See* AETIUS, *of Amida.*

AEZIO, CLETO. *See* CLETI, Ezio [*fl.* 1621]

AFFORTY, FRANÇOIS [*fl.* 1673–*ca.* 1733] *respondent. See* BIENDISANT, C., *praeses.* Quaestio medica. 1674.

AGER, JOHANN HEINRICH [*fl.* 1671] *respondent.* Disputatio medica inauguralis de varicibus . . . Argentorati, Literis Johannis Wilhelmi Tidemanni, 1671.
29 (i.e. 20) p.   19 cm.   [61]
Diss. — Strasbourg.

AGER, NIKOLAUS [1568–1634]

Dissertations — Strasbourg

—*praeses.* Decas quaestionum physicarum de somno . . . Argentorati, Typis Johannis Andreae, 1623.
[16] p.   20 cm.   [62]
J. K. Böringer, *respondent.*

—Disputatio physica de auditu . . . Argentorati, Excudebat Marcus ab Heyden [1621]
[11] p.   20 cm.   [63]
H. Itzstein, *respondent.*

—Disputatio physica de luna . . . Argentorati, Paulus Ledertz, 1626.
[12] p.   20 cm.   [64]
D. Kober, *respondent.*

—Disputatio physica . . . de mente humana . . . Argentorati, Typis Johannis Reppii, 1626.
[8] p.   20 cm.   [65]
J. Fritsch, *respondent.*

—Disputatio physica de monstris et prodigiis . . . Argentorati, Typis Johannis Reppii, 1625.
[8] p.   19 cm.   [66]
K. Tilger, *respondent.*

Disputatio physica de nutritione . . . Argentorati, Typis Hollandi Findleri, 1624.
[18] p.   20 cm.   [67]
J. G. Halbmayer, *respondent.*

—Disputatio physica de somno . . . Argentorati, Conradus Scher, 1621.
[7] p.   19 cm.   [68]
M. Listemann, *respondent.*

—Disputatio physica de somno, insomniis et vigilia . . . Argentorati, Typis Hollandi Findleri, 1623.
[28] p.   20 cm.   [69]
D. Killman, *respondent.*

—Disputatio physica de visu et visione . . . Argentorati, Typis Hollandi Findleri, 1623.
[11] p.   20 cm.   [70]
J. P. Bartsch, *respondent.*

—ed. *See* RYFF, W. H. Newe aussgerüste deütsche Apoteck. 1602.

AGER, NIKOLAUS [*fl.* 1623–1624] *respondent. See* SEBISCH, M. [1578–1674?] *praeses.* Disputatio de diebus criticis prior. 1626 [and] Exercitationes medicae. 1639.

AGERIUS, NICOLAUS. *See* AGER, Nikolaus [1568–1634]

AGESILAUS. *See* GERBEZIUS, MARCUS [*ca.* 1658–1718]

AGGRAVI, GIOVANNI FRANCESCO [*fl.* 1664] Antilucerna fisica oroscopante. La conservatione della sanità, con amplificatione formalizzata nella pluralità dell'universali . . . Padova, Mattio Cadorin, 1664.

[16], 280 p.   22 cm.   [71]

Engraved title page. Added general title.

—Protolume chimico e cheggiante di condupplicati paraphrasi . . . Venetia, Abbondio Menafoglio, 1682.

[12], 365, [7] p.   17 cm.   [72]

—Trattato della sovrana medicina curativa universale, d'ogn'infermità illetale, reativo magistero, chimicamente edutto, dall'arcanizzato spirito aureo detto, Rosa solis . . . Venetia, Iseppo Prodocimo, 1682.

[24], 473, [7] p.   13 cm.   [73]

AGNEAU, DAVID L'. *See* LAGNEAU, David [*ca.* 1590-1659]

AGOSTI, LEONARDO [*d.* 1660] L'antimedicina, cioè che a gl'infermi non si de' trarr'il sangue, prohibir'il vino, nè dar medicine . . . Bergamo, Marc' Antonio Rossi, 1654.

[8], 36 p.   21 cm.   [74]

—Il medico de grandi . . . Bergamo. Heredi di Marc'Antonio Rossi, 1659.

[15], 39 p.   21 cm.   [75]

AGRAVI, GIOVAN FRANCESCO. *See* AGGRAVI, Giovanni Francesco [*fl.* 1664]

AGRICOLA, GEORG [1494-1555] De re metallica libri XII . . . Quibus accesserunt hac ult. ed., tractatus ejusdem argumenti, ab eodem conscripti, sequentes. De animantibus subterraneis. Lib. I. De ortu & causis subterraneorum. Lib. V. De natura eorum quae effluunt ex terra. Lib. IV. De natura fossilium. Lib. X. De veteribus & novis metallis. Lib. II. Bermannus; sive, De re metallica, dialogus. Lib. I. . . . Basileae, Sumptibus & typis Emmanuelis König, 1657.

[14], 708, [90] p.   illus., plates.   34 cm.   [76]

AGRICOLA, GEORG ANDREAS [1672-1738] *respondent. See* BERGER, J. G. von, *praeses.* De succi nutricii per nervos transitu. 1695; HOFFMANN, F. [1660-1742] *praeses.* Disputatio medica inauguralis, de salubritate fluxus haemorrhoidalis. 1697.

AGRICOLA, JOHANN [1589-1643] Chirurgia parva, das ist: Wundartzney, darinnen alle Wunden, sie kommen wie sie wollen, mit Fleiss beschrieben worden, wie sich ein Wundartzt darbey verhalten,

und solche curirn solle . . . Nürnberg, In Verlegung Wolffgang Endters, 1643.

[23], 914, [14] p.   front. (port.)   15 cm.   [77]

Added engraved title page, illustrated.
Errata: p. [14]

—[The same.] . . . Nürnberg, In Verlegung Christoph Endters, 1674.

[21], 799, [13 +] p.   front. (port.)   17 cm.   [78]

Imperfect: added engraved title page and all leaves following sig. 3E6 wanting.

—Deutlich- und wolgegründeter Anmerckungen über die chymische Artzneyen, Johannis Popii, erst- und anderer Theil . . . Nunmehr zum andernmal von vielen Fehlern gereiniget, und mit neuen . . . Anmerckungen Joh. Helfrici Jungkens . . . vermehrt, und auf vielfältiges Begehren, an den Tag gelegt. Nürnberg, In Verlegung Johann Ziegers, Gedruckt by Johann Michael Spörlin, 1686.

[7], 1096, [24] p.   front. (port.)   22 cm.   [79]

Added engraved title page.

—Institutiones chirurgicae; oder, Newe Feldscherer Kunst. Darin ein Feldscherer, Wundartzt oder Balbierer gründlich unterrichtet wird, wie er sich in allen Wunden . . . im verbinden und heilen verhalten soll . . . Franckfurt, Bey Clemens Schleichen, und Peter de Zetter, 1634.

200 p.   14 cm.   [80]

—Kurtzer aber doch gründtlicher Bericht, von dieser jetzt herumschleichenden unnd flechtenden Kranckheit der rothen Ruhr. Auch mit kurtzer Andeutung eines Febris malignae epidemialis, welches sich zugleich mit Sehen und Spüren lest, welcher Gestalt man sich beydes praeserviren unnd curiren könne . . . Erffurdt, Gedruckt bey Johan. Röhbock, in Verlegung Johannis Bürckners, 1616.

[102] p.   16 cm.   [81]

AGRICOLA, JOHANN CHRISTIAN [*fl.* 1652] *respondent. See* DEUSING, A., *praeses.* Disputationum anatomicarum nona. 1652.

AGRICOLA, JOHANN GEORG [1558-1633] Cervi excoriati et dissecti in medicina usus. Das ist: Kurtze Beschreibung welcher Gestalt dess zu gewisser Zeit gefangenen Hirschens fürnembste Glieder in der Artzney zugebrauchen; und erstlich: was Massen dass abgenommene und zubereite Geweyhe in mancherley dess Leibs Beschwerungen beyzubringen . . . Amberg, Michael Forster, 1603.

[24], 120, [3] p.   20 cm.   [82]

—Cervi cum integri et vivi natura et proprietas: tum excoriati, et dissecti, in medicina usus. Das ist: Aussführliche Beschreibung dess gantzen lebendigen Hirschens, seiner Natur, und Eygenschafften: dann ferrner welcher Gestalt dess zu gewisser Zeit gefangenen Hirschens fürnembste Glieder in der Artzney zugebrauchen. Erstlich zwar: was Massen das abgenommene, unnd zu bereitte Geweyhe in mancherley dess menschlichen Leibs Beschwerungen beyzubringen . . . [Amberg, Gertruckt und verlegt durch Michael Forstern, 1617]

[56], 244, [11], p.   20 cm.   [83]

AGRICOLA, JOHANN WILHELM [*fl.* 1645] *respondent. See* SEBISCH, M. [1578-1674?] *praeses.* Disputatio de naturalibus facultatibus prima [-octava & ultima] 1644 [i.e. 1645]

AGRIPPA, LIVIO [*fl.* 1599] Discorso . . . sopra la natura, & complessione humana . . . [Roma, Per gli heredi di Nicolò Mutii, 1601]

16 p.   illus.   20 cm.   [84]
Imperfect: p. 7-[9] mutilated.

—[The same.] *In* PORTA, G. B. della. Della fisionomia dell'huomo. 1644, 1668.

AGRIPPA, LIVIO LUIGI. *See* AGRIPPA, Livio [*fl.* 1599]

AGRIPPA, LUIGI. *See* AGRIPPA, Livio [*fl.* 1599]

AGRIPPA VON NETTESHEIM, HEINRICH CORNELIUS [1486-1535] De incertitudine & vanitate omnium scientiarum & artium liber . . . Accedunt duo ejusdem auctoris libelli; quorum unus est De nobilitate & praecellentia foeminei sexus, ejusdemque supra virilem eminentia; alter De martrimonio seu conjugio . . . Lugduni Batavorum, Excudebat Severinus Matthaei, pro officinis Abrahami Commelini & Davidis Lopes de Haro, 1643.

[16], 359 (i.e. 356) p.   14 cm.   [85]
Added engraved title page dated 1644.

—[The same.] . . . Ed. ult. . . . Hagae-Comitum, Ex typographia Adriani Vlacq, 1653.

[24], 501 (i.e. 503) p.;   48 p.   14 cm.   [86]

Imperfect: p. 123-4 wanting; supplied in photocopy from College of Physicians of Philadelphia library.
De nobilitate & praecellentia foeminei sexus . . . has special title page.

—[English tr.] The vanity of arts and sciences . . . London, Printed by J. C. for Samuel Speed, 1676.

[19], 368 p.   front. (port.)   20 cm.   [87]
A different translation from the 1575 edition.

—[The same.] . . . London, Printed by R.E. for R.B. and are to be sold by C. Blount, 1684.

[19], 368 p.   front. (port.)   19 cm.   [88]
Imprint date altered by hand from 1684 to 1686.
Imperfect: signatures F3, L4-5 wanting.
A page for page reprint of the 1676 edition.

—[French tr.] Paradoxe sur l'incertitude, vanité & abus des sciences. Traduitte en françois . . . [par Louis Turquet de Mayerne]. [Paris] 1603.

[20], 737 (i.e. 747) p.   15 cm.   [89]

—In Artem brevem R. Lullii commentaria. *In* LULL, R. Opera. 1617, 1651.

—Three books of occult philosophy . . . Translated out of the Latin . . . by J[ohn] F[rench] London, Printed by R. W. for Gregory Moule, 1651.

[27], 583, [12] p.   front. (port.), illus., plates. 19 cm.   [90]

—*See* POTIER, P. Insignes curationes. 1625.

AGÜERO, BARTOLOMÉ HIDALGO DE [1530 or 1-1597]. Tesoro de la verdadera cirugia y via particular contra la comun . . . Corr . . . in esta ult. imp. . . . Valencia, Claudio Macè, 1654.

[12], 400 + p.   31 cm.   [91]
Imperfect: p. 37-52, p. 107-134 and all after p. 400 wanting.

AGUILON, FRANÇOIS D' [1566-1617] Opticorum libri sex philosophis juxta ac mathematicis utiles. Antverpiae, Ex Officina Plantiniana, apud viduam et filios Jo. Moreti, 1613.

[48], 684, [43] p.   illus., diagrs.   36 cm.[92]
Engraved title page.

AGUIRRE, JUAN. *See* MARTÍNEZ DE ZALDUENDO Y AGUIRRE, Juan [*fl.* 1696]

AHMAD IBN SEIRIM. *See* AḤMAD IBN SĪRĪN [*fl.* 813-833]

AḤMAD IBN SĪRĪN [*fl.* 813-833]. Oneirocritica. *See* ARTEMIDORUS DALDIANUS. Artemidori Daldiani & Achmetis Sereimi f. Oneirocritica. 1603.

—Traumbuch. *See* COLER, J. Oeconomia ruralis. 1645.

AHRNDS, EBERHARD [*fl.* 1695] *respondent. See* MEIER, G., *praeses*. Rationale de virginis partu cogitationes. 1695.

AHUMADA, PEDRO DE, [*fl.* 1653] Question en la qual se intenta averiguar como, y de que venas, y de que partes se deba sangrar en las enfermedades que curamos, segun la idea, y naturaleza de la enfermedad . . . Sevilla, Juan Gomez de Blas [1653]
    [2], 13 (i.e. 16) ll.   20 cm.   **[93]**

AICARDO, PAOLO [*d.* 1607] *ed. See* MERCURIALE, G. De morbis cutaneis. 1601.

AICHHOLTZ, JOHANN [1520-1588] *See* SCHOLTZ, L. Consiliorum medicinalium . . . liber singularis. 1610.

AICHOLZ, JOHANN EMERICH. *See* AICHHOLTZ, Johann [1520-1588]

AIGENTLICHER Abriss der neuen im Spital aufgehengten Tafeln. *See* PFANN, J. Biblische Emblemata und Figuren. 1626.

AIGNAN, FRANÇOIS, 1644-1709. L'ancienne medecine a la mode; ou, Le sentiment uniforme d'Hippocrate & de Galien sur les acides & les alkalis . . . Paris, Laurent d'Houry, 1693.
    [8], 219, [3] p.   17 cm.   **[94]**

— Le prestre medecin; ou, Discours physique sur l'établissement de la medecine. Avec un traité du caffé & du thé de France, selon le systeme d'Hippocrate . . . Paris, Laurent d'Houry, 1696.
    [36], 263, [1] p.   17 cm.   **[95]**
    Errata: p. [264]

AIGNEAU, JUSRUA L'. *See* LAGNEAU, Justus [*fl.* 17th cent.]

AILIANOS. *See* AELIANUS, Claudius.

AILLEBOUST, JEAN D'. Portentosum lithopaedion. *In* Augenio, O. Epistolarum et consultationum medicinalium prioris tomi libri XII. 1602; Collectanea de diuturna graviditate. 1662; Rousset, F. Exsectio foetus vivi ex matre viva sine alterutrius vitae periculo. 1601.

AILLY, PIERRE D' [*ca.* 1620-1684] *tr. See* [PLAZZONI, F.] Traité des blesseures et playes faites par armes a feu. 1668.

AIROLDI, GIOVANNI PIETRO. *ed. See* GALENUS. [Selected works. Latin.] Francisci Vallesii . . . Commentaria illustria, in Cl. Galeni Pergameni libros. 1645.

AKAKIA, MARTIN [1539-1588] *See* SCHOLTZ, L. Consiliorum medicinalium . . . liber singularis. 1610.

ALAIMO, MARCO ANTONIO, 1590-1662. Consigli politico-medici . . . Composti d'ordine dell'illustriss. senato palerminato, per l'occorrenti necessità di peste . . . Ne'quali si donano le vere regole, e profittevoli ordinationi, cavati dall'infelici eventi delle passate pestilenze . . . Palermo, Nicolò Bua, 1652.
    [3], 12, 460, [32] p.   20 cm.   **[96]**

—Consultatio. Pro ulceris syriaci nunc vagantis curatione . . . Panhormi, Sumptibus Petri Orlandi, typis Alphonsi de Insula, 1632.
    [7], 196 p.   21 cm.   **[97]**
    With this is bound: Macherone, P. Responsa medica. 1630.

—Discorso. . . intorno alla preservatione del morbo contagioso, e mortale, che regna al presente in Palermo, & in altre città, e terre del regno di Sicilia . . . Palermo, Angelo Orlandi, 1625.
    144 p.   20 cm.   **[98]**

ALAIN DE LILLIE. *See* ALANUS, *Bp. of Auxerre* [*d.* 1212]

ALANUS, *Bp. of Auxerre* [*d.* 1212] Dicta . . . de lapide philosophico, e Germanico idiomate Latine reddita, per Justum a Balbian . . .
    722-734 p., vol. 3.   20 cm. (*In* Zetzner, Lazarus, *ed.* Theatrum chemicum. Argentorati, 1659-61)   **[99]**
    Caption title.

ALANUS DE INSULIS. *See* ALANUS, *Bp. of Auxerre* [*d.* 1212]

ALARD, WILHELM [1572-1645] Panacea sacra, das ist: Heylsame, wolbewehrte Seelenartzney, gegen die Pestilentz, und alle ihre Zufälle: auss der vollen und reichen Apoteken dess heiligen Geistes, von den krefftigsten Wurtzeln, Kräutern und Blumen dess Paradeises göttliches Worts, mit Fleiss zusammen gezogen, und zu diesen gebrechlichen Zeiten, frommen Christen zur wolgemeinten Erinnerung, in Druck gegeben . . . Hamburg, Philip von Ohr, 1605.
    [84] p.   20 cm.   **[100]**

ALARY, BARTHÉLEMY [*fl.* 1685] La guerison assurée des fievres tierces, doubles tierces, en deux jours, quartes & doubles quartes, en quatre. Par le remede provençal en tablettes, que le sieur B. Alary . . . fait & distribue . . . Paris, Chez l'auteur, 1685.

[16], 98, [4] p. port. 15 cm. **[101]**

Half-title: Le remede provencal en tablettes pour la guerison de toutes les fiévres intermittentes.

ALBAMA, FREDERICUS. *See* ABBAMA, Fredericus [*fl.* 1631]]

ALBANESE, GUIDO ANTONIO [*d.* 1657] Aphorismorum Hippocratis expositio peripatetica . . . Patavii, Typis Pauli Frambotti, 1649.

163 p. 22 cm. **[102]**

Includes Latin text of books 1 and 2 of the Aphorismi, in the version of Niccolò Leoniceno.

ALBECKH, ERNEST JOSEPH [*fl.* 1688-1689] *respondent. See* CAMERARIUS, E. R., *praeses.* Dissertatio medica inauguralis, de glandulis. 1689; Expositio medica casus de aegritudine animi. 1688.

ALBENGNEFIT. *See* 'ABD AL-RAḤMĀN IBN MUḤAMMAD, *called* IBN WĀFID [999-1068]

ALBENGUEFIT. *See* 'ABD AL-RAḤMĀN IBN MUḤAMMAD, *called* IBN WĀFID [999-1068]

ALBERDING, ADRIAAN VAN [*fl.* 1678[*respondent.* Disputatio medica inauguralis de arthritide . . . Trajecti ad Rhenum, Ex officina Guilielmi a Walchren, 1678.

[15] p. 21 cm. **[103]**

Diss.—Utrecht.

ALBERT THE GREAT. *See* ALBERTUS MAGNUS, *Saint, Bp. of Ratisbon* [1193?-1280]

ALBERT VON BOLLSTAEDT. *See* ALBERTUS MAGNUS, *Saint, Bb. of Ratisbon* [1193?-1280]

ALBERT, GEORG. *See* STÜBNER, Albert Georg [*fl.* 1699-1700]

ALBERTI, HEINRICH CHRISTOPH [*fl.* 1682-1693] *praeses.* Disquisitio inauguralis medica, de bilis natura et usu medico . . . Erfordiae, Stannô Groschiano [1691]

32 p. 18 cm. **[104]**

Diss.—Erfurt (W. Cordes, *respondent*)

—*respondent. See* WIDMARCKTER, K., *praeses.* Dissertatio inauguralis medica de inflammatione. 1682.

ALBERTI, JULIUS GOTTFRIED [*fl.* 1674] *respondent. See* MEIBOM, H., *praeses.* Disputatio medica inauguralis de ulcerum natura et curatione in genere. 1674.

ALBERTI, SALOMON [1540-1600] *See* SENNERT, D. De scorbuto tractatus. 1624.

ALBERTI, VALENTINO [1635-1697] Disquisitio physiologica de intellectione altera, quae est de verbo mentis . . . Lipsiae, Typis Johannis Baueri [1659]

[12] p. 18 cm. **[105]**

Diss. pro loco—Leipzig.

Dissertations—Leipzig

—*praeses.* De sternutatione, disputationem physicam . . . P. P. Gottfredus Sigismundus Birnbaum . . . Lipsiae, Literis Johann-Erici Hahnii [1671]

[16] p. 19 cm. **[106]**

G. S. Birnbaum, *respondent.*

—Disputatio physica de qualitatibus occultis in genere . . . Lipsiae, Literis Johann-Erici Hahnii [1661]

[16] p. 20 cm. **[107]**

M. Heer, *respondent.*

—Dissertatio physica de oscitatione . . . Lipsiae, Literis Christophori Fleischeri [1685]

[16] p. 20 cm. **[108]**

J. B. Beutler, *respondent.*

—Dissertationem historico-physicam de pluvia prodigiosa . . . publico . . . examini submittit Fridrich-Augustus Janus . . . Lipsiae, Literis Johannis Erici Hahnii [1667]

[32] p. 20 cm. **[109]**

F. A. Jahn, *respondent.*

—[The same.] . . . Lipsiae, Recusa literis Johannis Erici Hahnii, 1674.

[32] p. 20 cm. **[110]**

Diss. 1667. F. A. Jahn, *respondent.*

ALBERTINA. *See* ALBERTUS-UNIVERSITÄT.

ALBERTINI, ANNIBALE, 16th-17th cent. De affectionibus cordis. Libri tres. Quorum primus agit de naturalibus. Secundus & tertius de pręternaturalibus, de palpitione nempe, & syncope, atque earum curatione . . . Venetiis, Apud Joannem Guerilium, 1618.

[40], 405, [1] p. 21 cm. **[111]**

—[The same.] . . . Caesenae, Apud Nerium, 1648.

[32], 335 p.   21 cm.   [112]

Imperfect: p. 321-322 wanting.

ALBERTUS MAGNUS, *Saint, Bp. of Ratisbon* [1193?-1280] De secretis mulierum libellus, scholiis auctus, & a mendis repurgatus. Ejusdem De virtutibus herbarum, lapidum, animalium quorundam libellus. Item, De mirabilibus mundi, ac de quibusdam effectibus causatis a quibusdam animalibus, &c. Adjecimus & ob materiae similitudinem Michaëlis Scoti . . . De secretis naturae opusculum . . . Argentorati, per Lazarum Zetznerum, 1601.

391, [9] p.   12 cm.   [113]

Includes his De horis dierum & nocticum.

—[The same.] . . . Argentorati, Per Lazarum Zetznerum, 1607.

390, [9] p.   12 cm.   [114]

A reprint of the 1601 edition.

—[The same.] . . . Argentorati, Per Lazarum Zetznerum, 1615.

390, [9] p.   12 cm.   [115]

A reissue of the 1607 edition with new title page.

—Tractatus Henrici de Saxonia, Alberti Magni discipuli, de secretis mulierum, in Germania nunquam editus. Accessit insuper ejusdem De virtutibus herbarum, lapidum, quorundam animalium, aliorumque libellus. Francofurti, Excudebat Johannes Bringerus, opera & impensa Petri Musculi, 1615.

411 p.   14 cm.   [116]

"Alberti Magni De virtutibus herbarum, lapidum, & animalium": p. 291-343; "Alberti Magni De horis dierum & noctium": p. 344-347; "Alberti Magni De mirabilibus mundi": p. 347-411.

With this is bound (as issued?): Scott, M. Tractatus . . . de secretis naturae. 1615.

—De secretis mulierum libellus, scholiis auctus, & a mendis repurgatus. Ejusdem De virtutibus herbarum, lapidum, & animalium quorundam libellus. Item De mirabilibus mundi, ac de quibusdam effectibus causatis a quibusdam animalibus, &c. Adjecimus & ob materiae similitudinem Michaelis Scoti philosophi, De secretis naturae opusculum . . . Argentorati, Sumptibus haeredum Lazari Zetzneri, 1637.

340, [9] p.   13 cm.   [117]

Text as in the 1615 Strasbourg edition.
"Alberti Magni Libellus de horis dierum & nocticum": p. 164-166.

—[The same.] De secretis mulierum. Item De virtutibus herbarum lapidum et animalium. Amstelodami, Apud Jodocum Janssonium, 1643.

366, [9] p.   13 cm.   [118]

Engraved title page.
"Alberti Magni Libellus de mirabilibus mundi": p. 175-223; "Michaëlis Scoti Libellus de secretis naturae": p. 224-366.

—[The same.] . . . 1648.

358, [13] p.   14 cm.   [119]

Engraved title page.
"Alberti Magni Libellus de mirabilibus mundi": p. 170-218; "Michaëlis Scoti Libellus de secretis naturae": p. 219-358.

—[The same.] . . . 1665.

358, [14] p.   14 cm.   [120]

Engraved title page.
A reprint of the 1648 edition.

—[The same.] . . . Amstelodami, Apud Joannem Ravesteinium, 1665.

329, [4] p.   14 cm.   [121]

Engraved title page.
"Alberti Magni Libellus de mirabilibus mundi": p. 158-203; "Michaëlis Scoti Libellus de secretis naturae": p. 204-329.

—[The same.] . . . Amstelodami, Apud Henricum et Theod. Boom, 1669.

329, [6] p.   14 cm.   [122]

Engraved title page.
A reprint of the 1665 edition.

—[German tr.] Von den Geheimnissen derer Weiber: wie auch von den Tugenden derer Kräuter, Steine und Thiere: und den Wunderwercken der Welt. Samt Michaël Scoti Büchlein von den Geheimnissen der Natur. Wie solche Anfangs zu Amsterdam in Latein heraus gegeben, anietzo aber . . . in die hochteutsche Sprache übersetzet. Nürnberg, In Verlegung Johann Hofmanns, 1678.

[1], 550, [24] p.   15 cm.   [123]

Added engraved title page.
Imperfect: p. 355-6 mutilated.
Translation of the author's three works: De secretis mulierum, Liber aggregationis and De mirabilibus mundi, and Michael Scott's De secretis naturae.

—Von Weibern und Geburten der Kinder, samt denen darzu gehörigen Arzneyen, und Unterricht, wie sich sowohl die Gebährenden verhalten, als auch die Hebammen . . . ihren Dienst recht verrichten sollen. Nebst einer Erklärung von den Tugenden der vornehmsten Kräuter, und Von Kraft und Würkung der Edelgesteine; item, Von Art und Natur etlicher

Thiere, aus Apollinaris [pseud. i.e. Walther Hermenius Ryff] Grossen Kräuter-Buch gezogen; und demenoch ein bewährtes Mittel für die Pestilenz, und wie man sich wegen des Aderlassens verhalten solle, noch beygefügt. Nebst denen Landleuten zum Nutzen wieder aufs neue eingerichtet, und mit darzu dienlichen Figuren ausgezieret. [n.p., 16--?]

106, [4] p. illus. 17 cm. [124]

A collection of works originally edited by W.H. Ryff under title: Ein newer Albertus Magnus.

Translation of the author's De secretis mulierum and his Liber aggregationis, to which are added two anonymous works: Das fünfte Buch . . . von viel köstlichen Arzneystücken, besonders Aqua Vitae, und Das sechste Buch . . . Eine Ordnung wie man sich in der Zeit der Pestilentz, mit Essen und Trinken verhalten soll.

—[The same.] Ein newer Albertus Magnus, von Weybern und Geburten der Kinder, sampt ihren Artzneyen. Auch von Tugenden etlicher fürnemer Kreüter und von Krafft der edlen Gestein. Von Art und Natur etlicher Thier. Mit sampt einem bewerten Regiment für die Pestilentz. Alles auffs new gebessert durch Q. Apollinarem [pseud. i.e. Walther Hermenius Ryff] [Augspurg, Bey David Francken] 1608.

48, [2] ll. illus. 21 cm. [125]

Imperfect: leaves 2-3 wanting.
A reprint of the 1567 edition.
Bound with Sechs Bücher auserlesener Artzney und Kunst-Stück. 1613.

—[The same.] Albertus Magnus. Daruth der Fruwens ere Heimlicheit, thofellige Schwackheit, unde Arstedye; dartho mennigerley Krüder, Eddelstene unde deerte Ardt unde Natur: ock Rath yegen de Pestilentz, und vam Aderlatende kan gelehret werden. Uppet nye mit Flythe dörchgesehen, unde mit einer Vörrede van Alberti Magni herkumpft und letiende vormehrt, unde also in de sassische Sprake gebrocht. Hamborch, 1613.

[8], 145, [6] p. illus. 16 cm. [126]

A low-German version of the collection of works originally edited in German by W.H. Ryff under title: Ein newer Albertus Magnus. The German version also appeared, with added material, under title: Albertus Magnus. Daraus man alle Heimligkeit dess weiblichen Geschlechts erkennen kan.
Bound with Aristoteles. Problemata. 1604.

—[The same.] . . . Von Weiberen und Geburten der Kinder, sampt ihren Artzneyen. Auch Von Tugenden etlicher fürnehmer Kräutter, und Von Krafft der edlen Gestein. Item, Von Art und Natur etlicher Thier, mit sampt einem bewärten Regiment für die Pestilentz. Alles auffs new gebessert durch Q. Apollinarem [pseud. i.e. Walther Hermenius Ryff] Strassburg, Marx von der Heyden, 1629.

ciiii, [6] p. illus. 16 cm. [127]

—[The same.] . . . Von Weiberen und Geburten der Kinder, sampt ihren Artzneyen. Auch Von Tugenden etlicher fürnemmen Kräuter, und von Krafft der edlen Gestein, von Art und Natur etlicher Thier. Mit sampt einem bewerten Regiment für die Pestilentz. Alles auffs new wider gebessert und vermehrt. [n.p.] 1659.

110 (i.e. 106), [5] p. illus. 17 cm. [128]

Bound with Arnaldus de Villanova. Practica medica. 1619.

—Speculum astronomiae: nunc primum e ms. codice in lucem editum. Praemittuntur autem ejusdem authoris libelli, De virtutibus herbarum, lapidum, &c. Lugduni, 1615.

166 (i.e. 168) p. 12 cm. [129]

Contents.—Liber aggregationis; seu, Liber secretorum de virtutibus herbarum, lapidum & animalium quorumdam.—De mirabilibus mundi.—Speculum astronomiae.

—[English tr.] The secrets . . . Of the vertues of hearbs, stones, and certain beasts. Whereunto is newly added a short discourse of the seven planets governing the nativities of children. Also a book of the same authour, Of the marvailous things of the world, and of certaine things caused of certaine beasts. London, Printed by R. Cotes, to be sold by Fulke Clifton, 1650.

[125] p. 15 cm. [130]

Reprint of the edition published by W. Jaggard in 1599 and 1617. Wing A875I.

—[Italian tr.] Alberto Magno. Diviso in libri tre, nel primo si tratta della virtù delle herbe. Nel secondo della virtù delle pietre. Et nel terzo la virtù di alcuni animali. Di nuovo con somma diligentia stampato, & ricorretto. Venetia, Domenico Imberti, 1610.

[61] p. 15 cm. [131]

"Delle virtu delli ogli": p. 55-61.
Imperfect: sig. D1 wanting.

—Compendium . . . de ortu & metallorum materia, supra quam spagyricus radicalia principia fundet.

123-126 p., vol. 2. 20 cm. (In Zetzner, Lazarus, ed. Theatrum chemicum. Argentorati, 1659-61) [132]

Caption title.

—De alchemia praefatio.

423-458 p., vol. 2. 20 cm. (*In* Zetzner, Lazarus, *ed.* Theatrum chemicum. Argentorati, 1659-61)   [133]

Caption title.

—De concordantia philosophorum de lapide [&] ... Compositum de compositis [&] ... Liber octo capitulorum, de lapide philosophorum.

809-862 p., vol. 4. 20 cm. (*In* Zetzner, Lazarus, *ed.* Theatrum chemicum. Argentorati, 1659-61)   [134]

Caption titles.

—De virtutibus herbarum. *In* Longinus, C., *ed.* Trinum magicum; sive, Secretorum magicorum opus. 1616, 1673.

—Secretorum tractatus ...

121-130 p., vol. 3. 17 cm. (*In* Artis auriferae, Basileae, 1610)   [135]

Caption title.

—*See* CAMPANELLA, T. Astrologicorum libri VII. 1630.

ALBERTUS, KONRAD [*fl.* 1622] *respondent. See* WENCK, G., *praeses.* Disputatio philosophica de praecipua passione mobilis. 1622.

ALBERTUS, MARTINUS. *See* Hildebrand, W. Neu vermehrt ... Kunst und Wunderbuch. 1690.

ALBERTUS UNIVERSITÄT. Medizinische Fakultät. Decanus senior ... & professores Facultatis Medicae in Academia Regiomontana ad disputationem inauguralem ... Petri Thofals ... officiose invitant. [Regiomonti] Praelo Eusneriano [*ca.* 1672]

[8] p. 20 cm.   [136]

Friedrich Reusner was active between 1666 and 1678. Benzing (A) p. 246.

Program—Königsberg (with vita of P. Thofall)

—*See* BECKHER, D. Historia morbi Academici Regiomontani. 1649.

ALBINEUS, NATHAN. *See* AUBIGNÉ DE LA FOSSE, Nathan [1601-1669?]

ALBINUS, BERNHARD [1653-1721] Demonstrationibus anatomicis in corpore masculino ... invitat Bernh. Albinus ... Francofurti ad Oderam, Literis Christophori Zeitleri, 1683.

[8] p. 19 cm.   [137]

—Disputatio medica, de fonticulis ... Francofurti ad Viadrum, Literis Christophori Zeitleri [1681]

16 p. 18 cm.   [138]

Diss. pro loco—Frankfurt an der Oder (J.F. Ortlob, *respondent*)

Dissertations—Frankfurt an der Oder

— *praes.* De tabaco ... Francofurti ad Viadrum, Literis Christophori Zeitleri [1695]

32 p. 20 cm.   [139]

J.G. Letsch, *respondent.*

—Delineatio medica inauguralis de apoplexia ... Francofurti cis Viadrum, Typis Christophori Zeitleri [1695]

[20] p. 20 cm.   [140]

P. Liege, *respondent.*

—Disputatio inauguralis medico-chirurgica de paracentesi thoracis et abdominis ... Francofurti ad Oderam, Typis Christophori Zeitleri [1687]

22 p. 19 cm.   [141]

E. Heinsius, *respondent.*

—Disputatio medica inauguralis de atrophia ... Francofurti ad Viadrum, Typis Christophori Zeitleri [1684]

32 p. 20 cm.   [142]

G. G. Knobeloch, *respondent.*

—Disputatio medica inauguralis, de elephantiasi ... Francofurti ad Oderam, Typis Johannis Coepselii [1694]

[4], 28 p. 20 cm.   [143]

N. Gerlach, *respondent.*

—Disputatio medica inauguralis de sterilitate ... Francofurti, Typis Christoph. Andreae Zeitleri junioris, 1693.

31, [1] p. 20 cm.   [144]

Diss. 1683. S. Reuter, *respondent.*

—Disputatio solennis medica de vomica pulmonum ... Francofurti ad Viadrum, Literis Christophori Zeitleri [1693]

16 p. 20 cm.   [145]

J. F. Praetorius, *respondent.*

—Disputatione medica inauguralis de melancholia ... Francofurti ad Oderam, Typis Christophori Zeitleri [1687]

[39] p. 19 cm.   [146]

G. C. Wolff, *respondent.*

—Dissertatio de cervo corde glande plumbea trajecto ... Francofurti ad Viadrum, Typis Christophori Zeitleri, 1689.
    [26] p. plate. 19 cm.   [147]
    Diss. 1686. G. C. Wolff, *respondent.*

—Dissertatio de fonte sacro Freienwaldensi ... Francofurti ad Oderam, Literis Christophori Zeitleri [1685]
    [2], 34 p. 20 cm.   [148]
    P. E. Friederich, *respondent.*

—Dissertatio de phosphoro liquido & solido ... Francofurti ad Oderam, Typis Zeitlerianis [1688]
    [56] p. 20 cm.   [149]
    J. C. Kletwich, *respondent.*

—Dissertatio de thee ... publico examini exhibebit ... Johannes Melchior Genge ... Francofurti ad Oderam, Typis Christophori Zeitleri [1684]
    31 p. 20 cm.   [150]
    J. M. Genge, *respondent.*

—[The same.]   [151]
    The respondent's name is spelled Benge.

—Dissertatio de venenis ... Francofurti ad Viadrum, Literis Christophori Zeitleri [1682]
    24 p. 19 cm.   [152]
    J. C. Mentzel, *respondent.*

—Dissertatio inauguralis de fame canina ... Francofurti ad Viadrum, Literis Christophori Zeitleri [1691]
    24 p. 20 cm.   [153]
    K. L. Neccer, *respondent.*

—Dissertatio inauguralis de pravitate sanguinis ... Francofurti ad Viadrum, Literis Christoph. Zeitleri [1689]
    63 p. 20 cm.   [154]
    J. G. Slötel, *respondent.*

—Dissertatio inauguralis de tarantismo ... Francofurti, Typis Christoph. Andr. Zeitleri [1691]
    [39] p. 19 cm.   [155]
    N. B. N. de Pivier, *respondent.*

—Dissertatio inauguralis medica, de abortu ... Francofurti ad Viadrum, Literis Christophori Zeitleri [1697]
    [4], 26, [2] p. 21 cm.   [156]
    J. G. von Bergen.

—Dissertatio inauguralis medica de incubo ... Francofurti ad Viadrum, Literis Christophori Zeitleri [1691]
    [24] p. 19 cm.   [157]
    C. G. Wenzlovius, *respondent.*

—Dissertatio inauguralis medica, de mania ... Francofurti ad Viadrum, Praelo Johann. Coepselii [1692]
    [1], 25 p. 20 cm.   [158]
    D. Nicolaus, *respondent.*

—Dissertatio inauguralis medica, de pleuritide vera ... Francofurti ad Viadrum, Typis Johannis Coepselii [1696]
    24 p. 20 cm.   [159]
    W. H. Baurmeister, *respondent.*

—Dissertatio inauguralis medico chirurgica de catarrhacta ... Francofurti ad Viadrum, Literis Christophori Zeitleri [1695]
    [3], 27, [1] p. plate. 20 cm.   [160]
    L. D. Gosky, *respondent.*

—Dissertatio inauguralis medico-chirurgica, de polypis ... Francofurti ad Viadrum, Literis Christophori Zeitleri [1695]
    [1], 26 p. 20 cm.   [161]
    J. M. Welsch, *respondent.*

—Dissertatio medica de pica ... Francofurti ad Viadrum, Literis Christophori Zeitleri [1691]
    38 p. 20 cm.   [162]
    D. Christiani, *respondent.*

—Dissertatio medica inauguralis, de missione sanguinis ... Francofurti ad Oderam, Typis Christophori Zeitleri [1686]
    46, [2] p. 20 cm.   [163]
    P. E. Friederich, *respondent.*

—Dissertatio medica inauguralis, de partu difficili ... Francofurti ad Viadrum, Literis Christophori Zeitleri [1696]
    30 p. 21 cm.   [164]
    J. G. Letsch, *respondent.*

—Dissertatio medica inauguralis, de partu naturali ... Francofurti ad Viadrum, Literis Joh. Coepselii [1697]
    24 p. 21 cm.   [165]
    J. W. Koch, *respondent.*

—Dissertatio medica inauguralis de salivatione mercuriali ... Francofurti ad Oderam, Imprimebat Christophorus Zeitlerus [1689]

[1], 55 p.   19 cm.   [166]

G. K. de Horn, *respondent.*

—Dissertatio solennis medica de cardialgia ... Francofurti ad Viadrum, Typis Johannis Coepselii [1691]

22 p.   20 cm.   [167]

J. F. Hamel, *respondent.*

—Dissertatio solennis medica, de febre quartana intermittente ... Francofurti ad Viadrum, Literis Christophori Zeitleri [1694]

30 p.   20 cm.   [168]

J. J. Chüden, *respondent.*

—Dissertatio solennis medica, de hydrophobia ... submittit Johannes Melchior Benge [sic] Francofurti ad Viadrum, Typis Johannis Coepselii [1687]

[32] p.   19 cm.   [169]

J. M. Genge, *respondent.*

—Dissertationem anatomico-medicam de poris humani corporis ... publicae ... disquisitioni sistet ... Gustavus Daniel Lipstörp ... Francofurti ad Oderam, Literis Christophori Zeitleri [1685]

[8], 72 p.   19 cm.   [170]

G. D. Lipstorp, *respondent.*

—Dissertationem chirurgico-medicam de paronychia ... praeside Dn. Bernhardo Albino ... publicae ... indagationi permittet Nicolaus Privigyei ... Francofurti ad Viadrum, Typis Christophori Zeitleri [1694]

24 p.   20 cm.   [171]

M. Privigyei, *respondent.*

—Dissertationem diaeteticam de affectibus animi ... publicae eruditorum censurae submittet ... Joh. Fridericus Ortlob ... Francofurti, Typis Christoph. Andr. Zeitleri, 1690.

21, [2] p.   19 cm.   [172]

Diss. 1681. J. F. Ortlob, *respondent.*

—Dissertationem medicam de cantharidibus ... publicae ... censurae submittet ... Ernestus Heinsius ... Francofurti ad Oderam, Typis Zeitlerianis [1687]

35 p.   20 cm.   [173]

E. Heinsius, *respondent.*

—Exercitationem medicam de dysenteria ... publicis ventilationibus submittet ... Daniel Luge ... Francofurti ad Viadrinum, Typis Johannis Coepselii [1693]

[21] p.   19 cm.   [174]

D. Luge, *respondent.*

—Inauguralis dissertatio medica de somnambulatione ... Francofurti ad Viadrum, Literis Christoph. Zeitleri [1689]

38 p.   20 cm.   [175]

T. Latimer, *respondent.*

—*respondent.* Disputatio medica inauguralis de catalepsi ... Lugduni Batavorum, Apud viduam & haeredes Johannis Elsevirii, 1676.

[16] p.   22 cm.   [176]

Diss. — Leyden.

—[The same.] Francofurti ad Viadrum, Literis Christophori Zeitleri, de novo impressa anno 1690.

[12] p.   20 cm.   [177]

Diss. — Leyden, 1676.

—*See* CRAANEN, T. Disputatio medica de epilepsia. 1690.

ALBINUS, BERNHARD FRIEDRICH. *See* ALBINUS, Bernhard [1653–1721]

ALBINUS, JAKOB [*fl.* 1611–1620] *respondent.* Praecidanea ... de scorbuto ... Basileae, Typis Joan. Jacobi Genathii [1614]

[16] p.   22 cm.   [178]

Diss. — Basel.

—*See* ARNISAEUS, H. Disputatio medica therapeutica. [1611]

ALBINUS, JOHANN SAMUEL [*fl.* 1638] *respondent. See* ROLFINCK, W., *praeses.* Disputatio inauguralis de pleuritide. 1638.

ALBINUS, SEBASTIAN [17th cent.] Kurtzer Bericht und Handgrieff, wie man mit denen Personen ... so etwan in eusserste Wassers-Gefahr ... gerathen, nicht zu lange im Wasser gelegen: doch gleichsam für Tod heraus gezogen werden, gebähren und umbgehen solle ... Jetzo abermahl aufs neue gedruckt. [n.p.] 1675.

[23] p.   16 cm.   [179]

"Joan. Schenk à Graffenberg lib. 2. Observation medicinalium observatione 18. aqua suffoc: & liberat.": p. [13-16]

ALBIUS, THOMAS. *See* WHITE, Thomas [1593-1676]

ALBOSIUS, JOANNES. *See* AILLEBOUST, Jean d'.

ALBRECHT, JOHANN GÜNTHER [*fl.* 1696] *respondent. See* PETERMANN, A., *praes.* Scrutinium icteri ex calculis vesiculae fellis occasione casus cujusdam singularis. 1696.

ALBRECHT, JOHANN PETER [1647-1724] *tr. See* BLANKAART, S. Newe Kunst-Kammer de Chirurgie. 1688; BONTEKOE, C. Neues Gebäude der Chirurgie. 1697.

ALBUCASIS. See ABULCASIS [936?-1013?]

ALBUS, SEBASTIAN. *See* ALBINUS, Sebastian [17th cent.]

ALCADINO [*fl.* 1191] De balneis Puteolanis. *In* Bartoli, S. Breve ragguaglio. 1667.

ALCHINDUS. *See* YĀʿKUB IBN ISḤĀK IBN ṢUB-BĀH, Abū Yūsuf, al-Kindī [*d. ca.* 873]

ALDES, THEODORUS, *pseud. See* SLADE, Matthew [1628-1689]

ALDINI, TOBIA. *See* CASTELLI, P. Exactissima descriptio. 1625.

ALDROVANDI, ULISSE [1522-1605?] De animalibus insectis libri septem . . . Bonon., Apud Clementem Ferronium, 1638.

[10], 767, [43] p.   illus.   36 cm.   **[180]**
Engraved title page.
Colophon: Bononiae, Typis Jo. Baptistae Ferronii, 1644.

—De piscibus libri V et De cetis lib. unus. Joannes Cornelius Uterverius . . . collegit. Hieronymus Tamburinus in lucem edidit . . . Bononiae, Apud Bellagambam, 1613.

[8], 372 (i.e. 732), [27] p.   illus.   37 cm.
                                          [181]
Engraved title page.
Colophon: Bononiae, Apud Joannem Baptistam Bellagambam, sumptibus Hieronymi Tamburini, 1612.

—[The same.] . . . Marc. Antonius Bernia in lucem restituit . . . Bononiae, Apud Nicolaum Thebaldinum, 1638.

[6], 732, [27] p.   illus.   36 cm.   **[182]**
Engraved title page.
Colophon: Bononiae, Typis Jo. Baptistae Ferronii, sumptibus Marci Antonii Berniae, 1661.

—De quadrupedibus digitatis viviparis libri tres et De quadrupedibus digitatis oviparis libri duo. Bartholomaeus Ambrosinus . . . collegit . . . Bonon., Apud Nicolaum Tebaldinum, sumptibus M. Antonii Berniae, 1645.

[4], 718, [16] p.   illus.   37 cm.   **[183]**
Engraved title page.
". . .De quadrupedibus digitatis oviparis. Libri III . . ." has special title page.

—De quadrupedibus solidipedibus volumen integrum. Joannes Cornelius Uterverius . . . collegit, & recensuit. Marcus Antonius Bernia in lucem restituit . . . Bononiae, Apud Nicolaii Thebaldinum, 1639.

[6], 495, [30] p.   illus.   37 cm.   **[184]**
Engraved title page.
Colophon: Bononiae, Typis Nicolai Tebaldini, sumptibus Marci Antonii Berniae, 1639.

—De reliquis animalibus exanguibus libri quatuor, post mortem ejus editi: nempe de mollibus, crustaceis, testaceis, et zoophytis . . . Bononiae, Typis Jo. Baptistae Ferronii, sumptibus Marci Antonii Berniae, 1642.

[1], 593, [27] p.   illus.   36 cm.   **[185]**
Engraved title page.
Colophone dated 1654.

—Dendrologiae naturalis scilicet arborum historiae libri duo. Sylva glandaria, acinosumque pomarium ubi eruditiones omnium generum una cum botanicis doctrinis ingenia quaecunque non parum juvant, et oblectant. Ovidius Montalbanus . . . opus . . . collegit . . . Hieronymus Bernia . . . in lucem editum dicavit. Bononiae, Typis Jo. Baptistae Ferronii, 1668 [1667]

[9], 660, [52] p.   illus.   37 cm.   **[186]**
Engraved title page.

—Het lof van den swaen. *In* Veeler wonderens wonderbaarelijck lof. 1664.

—Monstrorum historia. Cum Paralipomenis historiae omnium animalium. Bartholomaeus Ambrosinus . . . volumen composuit. Marcus Antonius Bernia in lucem edidit . . . Bononiae, Typis Nicolai Tebaldini, 1642.

2 parts in 1 v.   illus.   37 cm.   **[187]**
Engraved title page
Part [2] has special title page: Paralipomena accuratissima historiae omnium animalium, quae in voluminibus Aldrovandi desiderantur. Bartholomaeus Ambrosinus . . . collegit . . .

—Musaeum metallicum in libros IIII distributum. Bartholomaeus Ambrosinus . . . composuit . . . Marcus Antonius Bernia . . . in lucem edidit . . . [Bononiae, Typis Jo. Baptistae Ferronii, 1648]

[6], 979, [13] p. illus. 37 cm. **[188]**

Engraved title page.

Imperfect: sig. 401 and 404 wanting; supplied in photocopy from University of Michigan library.

—Ornithologiae; hoc est, De avibus historiae libri XII [-XX] . . . Bonon., Apud Nicolaum Tebaldinum, sumptibus Marci Antonii Berniae, 1637-46 [v. 1, 1646]

3 v. illus. 37 cm. **[189]**

Vol. 2 has date: 1645.

Engraved title pages.

Colophons: vol. 1: 1645; vol. 2: Bononiae, Typis Jo. Baptistae Ferronii, 1652; vol. 3: Bononiae, Typis Nicolae Tebaldini, 1640.

—Quadrupedum omnium bisulcorum historia. Joannes Cornelius Uterverius . . . colligere incaepit, Thomas Dempsterus baro a Muresk . . . perfecte absolvit. Marcus Antonius Bernia denuo in lucem edidit . . . Bonon., Apud Jo. Baptistae Ferronii, 1642.

[5], 1040, [12] p. illus. 37 cm. **[190]**

Engraved title page.

Colophon: Bononiae, Typis Jo. Baptistae Ferronii, impensis Marci Antonii Berniae, 1641.

Imperfect: p. 233-236 wanting; supplied in photocopy from University of Michigan library.

—Serpentum, et draconum historiae libri duo. Bartholomaeus Ambrosinus . . . opus concinnavit . . . Bononiae, Apud Clementem Ferronium, sumptibus M. Antonii Bernię, 1640.

[6], 427, [28] p. illus. 37 cm. **[191]**

Engraved title page.

—See Università di Bologna. Collegio de medicina. Antiodotarium Bononien. a Medicinae Collegio nuperrime auctum et emendatum. 1641, 1674 [and] Antidotarium Bononiense novissimum. 1674.

ALEMAND, Louis Augustin [1653?-1728] tr. See SANTORIO, S. Science de la transpiration; ou, Medecine statique. 1694.

—See Les secrets de la medecine des Chinois. 1671.

[**ALENCÉ**, Joachim, d', d. 1707?] Traitté de l'aiman. Divisé en deux parties. La prémiére contient les expériences; & la seconde les raisons que l'on en peut rendre. Par Mr. D***. Amsterdam, Henry Wetstein, 1687.

[20], 140, [8] p. plates. 16 cm. **[192]**

Added engraved title page.

—Traittez des barometres, thermométres, et notiométres, ou hygrométres. Par Mr. D***. Amsterdam, Henry Wetstein, 1688.

[12], 139, [4] p. plates. 16 cm. **[193]**

Added engraved title page, illustrated.

—[German tr.] Abhandlung dreyer so nothwendig- als nützlichen Instrumenten. Nemlich dess Barometri, Thermometri, und Notiometri oder Hygrometri . . . auss dem Frantzösichen ins Teutsche vorgetragen von D. M. H. C. J. Auff dess Herrn Ubersetzers Unkosten gedruckt. Mäyntz, Ludwig Bourgeat, 1688.

[8], 51 p. plates. 19 cm. **[194]**

—[The same.] Neu-erfundene mathematische Curiositäten enthaltend: die wunderbareste Würckungen der Natur und Kunst, worinnen vermittels drey sonderbaren Instrumenten l. die Schwere und Leichte, 2. die Truckene und Feuchte, 3. das Ab- und Zunehmen der Hitz und Kälte, der Lufft zu beobachten und zu erkennen seynd . . . Auss dem Frantzösischen ins Teutsch übersetzt . . . Mayntz, Ludwig Bourgeat, 1695.

[10], 51 p. plates. 18 cm. **[195]**

Added engraved title page reads: Tractatus de barometris thermometris et notionmetris vel higrometris. Anno 1688.

Translated by D. M. H. C. J.

A reissue of the 1688 edition with new title page and added engraved title page.

ALESSANDRI, Antonio d' [fl. ca. 1440] See SICILY. Protomedico. Constitutiones. 1657.

ALESSANDRI, Francesco degli [1529-1587] Apollo . . . omnem omnium usu receptorum tam simplicium, quam compositorum medicamentorum, materiam, naturam, vires, normam, & compositionem, radiis, ac fulgore suo, ita splendide irradians & illustrans, ut posthac omni librorum copia neglecta, sola hac regula contenti, omnes & medici, & pharmacopolae aegrorum saluti tutius consulere possint . . . Francofurti, Apud Johannem Spiessium, 1604.

[8], 732, [20] p. 20 cm. **[196]**

ALESSANDRINI, Giulio [1506-1590] See ALEXANDRINUS, Julius [1506-1590]

ALESSI, Alessandro [fl. 1627-1632] Consilia medica, et epitome pulsuum . . . In quibus methodus accurata cum praxi theorica conjungitur … Patavii, Apud Gasparem Crivellarium, 1627.

[20], 133, [10] p. 22 cm. [197]

—[The same.] … Addita sunt in hac 2. ed. ejusdem multae lineae, duo consilia, epitome urinarum, & post editionem menda potiora ad finem libri emendata. Patavii, Typis Pauli Frambotti, 1660.

[7], 119, [8] p. 22 cm. [198]

Bound with Thoner, A. Observationum medicinalium. 1651.

—Cratylus morborum. Sive de peculiarium corporis humani morborum appellationibus, essentia, & curatione libri tres … Patavii, Typis Pauli Frambotti, 1657.

[16], 300, [24] p. 23 cm. [199]

—De syrupo rosato solutivo libellus … Patavii, Apud Gasparem Crivellarium, 1630.

31 p. 16 cm. [200]

—Preservatione dalla peste e'historia della peste di Este … Di nuovo ristampata, è di molti errori emendata. Padova, Paolo Frambotto, 1660.

[4], 35, [1] p. 22 cm. [201]

Bound with Thoner, A. Observationum medicinalium. 1651.

ALESSIO PIEMONTESE. De' secreti del R. D. Alessio piemontese [pseud.? i.e. Girolamo Ruscelli?] Nuovamente ristampati, & con somma diligentia corretti. Prima [-terza] parte. Et di nuovo aggiontovi la quarta parte … Venetia, Pietro Miloco, 1620.

4 parts in 1 v. 15 cm. [202]

Imperfect: ll. 53 of part 1 mutilated.

Parts 2–4 have special title pages and imprints: part 2, Francesco Miloco, 1620; part 3, Michel Miloco, 1620; part 4, De' secreti … Ne' quali si contengono diversi medicamenti veri & approvati, tolti tutti da' principali auttori della medicina. Nuovamente dati in luce … Parte quarta, & ultima … 1619.

First published under title: Secreti del reverendo donno Alessio piemontese. For the description of the 1555 edition see Durling 106.

—[The same.] … Venetia, Heredi dell'Imberti, 1644.

4 parts in 1 v. 16 cm. [203]

Imperfect: Tavola della quarta parte multilated.

Parts 3–4 have special title pages.

A reprint of the 1620 Venice edition.

—[The same.] De' secreti del R. D. Alessio piemontese. Parti quattro. Nuovamente ristampati, e da molti errori ricorretti … Venetia, Valentino Mortali, 1666.

554, [37] p. 17 cm. [204]

—[The same.] … Venetia, Appresso Angelo Bodio, 1674.

554, [37] p. 17 cm. [205]

A reprint of the 1666 edition.

—[The same.] … Venetia, Biagio Maldura, 1683.

554, [34] p. 17 cm. [206]

Different setting of type.

—[Latin tr.] D. Alexii Pedemontani De secretis libri septem, a Joan. Jacobo Weckero … ex Italico sermone in Latinum conversi … Accessit ejusdem Weckeri opera, octavus de artificiosis vinis liber. Ed. 4. Basileae, Sumptibus Ludovici Künig, 1603.

361, [30] p. 16 cm. [207]

—[Dutch tr.] De sekreten vanden … Alexis Piemontois. Inhoudende seer excellente ende wel gheapprobeerde remedien, teghen veelderhande crancheden, wonden, ende andere accidenten: met de maniere van te distilleren, perfumeren, confitueren maken, te verwen, coleuren, ende gieten. Wt den Françoyse overgheset. Delft, Jacob Cornelissz. Amstelredam, Cornelis Claess, 1602.

260, [12] p.; 164, [10] p. 15 cm. [208]

Imperfect: pages 27–28 of part 2 wanting.

Part 2 has special title page: Dat tweede deel der sekreten vanden … Alexis van Piemont.

—[English tr.] The secrets of Alexis containing many excellent remedies against divers diseases, wounds, and other accidents. With the maner to make distillations, parfumes, confitures, dyings, colours, fusions, and meltings … Newly corr. and amended, and … enl. … London, Printed by William Stansby for Richard Meighen and Thomas Jones, 1615.

[6], 348, [14] ll. 18 cm. [209]

Imperfect: A1–4 (including title page), F1–8, I1–K8, 2F3–6, 2X6–2Z8 wanting; supplied in photocopy from the Henry E. Huntington Library; upper margins trimmed; mutilated.

STC 312.5.

"The second part [-third part] … now newly corr. and augmented by William Ward … 1614": ll. [118]–267; "The fourth part … translated … by Richard Androse … 1614.": ll. [268]–348. Items have special title pages. The fourth part includes "The fifth and laste parte of the secrets … ": ll. 295–348.

—[French tr.] Les secrets du … Alexis piemontois. Rev. & augm. d'une infinite de rares & admirables secrets. Lyon, Pierre Bailly, 1639.

675 (i.e. 711), [70] p. 17 cm. [210]

Contents the same, including the Livre de distillations and the Oecoiatrie by Christophe Landré, as in the edition published in

Paris in 1576, except that the woodcut illustrations of the Livre de distillations are here omitted.

—[The same.] Recueil de plusieurs secrets des médecines; par . . . Alexis piémontois & plusieurs autres auteurs. Divisé en sept parties. Appartenant au sr. Grassal, lieutenant de monsieur le premier chirurgien du roi, en la communauté des maîtres en chirurgie, à Saint-Flour. [n.p., 16--]

675 (i.e. 711), [70] p.   illus.   16 cm.   [211]

Imperfect: wants original title page, which has been replaced by one specially printed and bearing the name of the owner of the volume, and last two leaves, including the final leaf of the Table; some pages mutilated.

Contents as in the 1576 Paris edition, except that Plantin's note to the reader is here omitted, and the woodcut illustrations to the Livre de distillations are here different. The Oecoiatrie (p. 648-675) is by Christophe Landré.

Generally identical with the 1639 Lyons edition.

—[The same.] Les secrets du . . . Alexis piemontois. Rev. & augm. d'une infinité de rares & admirables secrets. Rouen, Martin de la Motte, 1642.

675 (i.e. 711), [70] p.   illus.   17 cm.   [212]

Different setting of type.

—[The same.] . . . Rouen, Jean Oursel, 1691.

713 (i.e. 711), [70] p.   17 cm.   [213]

Imperfect: p. 703-704 and p. [38-43] mutilated and mounted. Contents as in the 1639 Lyons edition without the author's preface.

—[The same.] . . . Rouen, Jean-Baptiste Besongne, 1699.

715 (i.e 711), [70] p.   17 cm.   [214]

Different setting of type.

—[German tr.] Mirabilia magna naturae; das ist, Wunder-, Künst-unndt Artzneybuch. Darinnen allerhand . . . Wunder-und Kunststück zu befinden, mit Beschreibung allerhand Farben . . . ingleichen von Pflantzung wunderlicher Gewächss unnd Blumen, auch wie man den Wein künstlich halten soll, dass er nicht verderbe . . . Beneben vielen Experimenten, dardurch der menschliche Cörper kan vor Unfall praeservirt, auch do er allbereit Mangelhafft ist, widerumb redintegrirt . . . werden. Das erste [-achte] Buch. Durch . . . Alexium Pedemontanum in welscher und lateinischer Sprache auffgezeichnet, hernach aber, durch D. Jacobum Wecker . . . in Teutsch transferirt. Jetzundt revidirt, und auffs newe . . . an Tag gegeben. Erffurdt, Bey und in Vorlegung Tobia Fritzschen, 1622.

4 parts in 1 v.   port.   20 cm.   [215]

Parts [2-4] have special title pages.

Books 1-7 were published previously (books 1-6 alone in 1569, reissued with the addition of book 7 in 1571) in Basel under title: Kunst Buch dess . . . Herren Alexii Pedemontani. Book 8 is the translator's Ein nutzliches Büchlein von . . . Wasseren, Ölen, unnd Weinen, which was originally published separately in Basel in 1569.

—Nützlich Artzney Buch. *In* Columella, L. J. M. Agricultur; oder, Ackerbaw. 1612.

"This is not a translation of Alessio, but a re-arrangement in three books, under different diseases. It is purely medical." Cf. Ferguson (B) no. 51.

—[Spanish tr.] Secretos. Del reverendo don Alexo. Piamontes. Traduzidos de lengua italiana en castellana, añadidos, y emendados en muchos lugares en esta ultima impression. 38 . . . Alcala, Por Maria Fernandez. A costa de Manuel Lopez, 1647.

[8], 280, [16] ll.   15 cm.   [216]

Imperfect: title page mutilated and backed.

Parts 2, 4 have special title pages.

—*See* VICARY, T. The English mans treasure. 1613, 1633, 1641 [and] The surgions directorie. 1651.

ALETHEUS, THEOPHILUS. *See* LYSER, Johann [1631-1684]

ALETHOPHANES, *archiater, pseud. See* BLONDEL, François [1609?-1682]

ALETHOPHANIS archiatri ad Jacobum Thevartum. 1655. *See* [BLONDEL, F.]

ALETOPHILUS, *Germanus. See* LYSER, Johann [1631-1684]

ALETOPHILUS, Janus Modestinus. Unvorgreiffliches Bedencken uber D. Conrad Horlachers Tractat Die höchstschädliche Würckung dess Aderlassens und Purgierens gennant, in welchem die in bemeltem Tractat angeführte Beweissgründe umbständlich überlegt und gründlich widerlegt; benebens auch, was in demselben wider D. Geuders Tractat: Heilsame medicinische Lebens-Mittel &c. genannt, geandet worden, unpartheyisch beantwortet wird . . . Franckfurt, Johann Görlin, 1691.

[2], 44 p.   16 cm.   [217]

Bound with Neu-vermehrtes . . . Aderlass-Büchlein. [ca. 1670]

ALEXANDER THE GREAT [B.C. 356-323] [Epistola Alexandri Macedonia]

331-349 p., part 1.   19 cm.   (*In* Morgenstern, Philipp, *ed.* and *tr.* Turba philosophorum. Basel, 1613)

Title from table of contents.   [218]

—[Expositio epistolae Alexandri regis]
245–249 p., vol. I.   17 cm.   (*In* Artis auriferae.
Basileae, 1610)   [219]
  Running title.

—*See* JĀBIR IBN ḤAĪYAN, al-Ṭarasūsī.
Gebri ... Summa perfectionis magisterii in sua
natura. 1682.

ALEXANDER, *of Aphrodisias*. De febribus. *In*
Fontaine, J. Jacobi Fontani ... Opera. 1612.

—Problemata. *In* Aristoteles. Aristotelis, aliorumque philosophorum, ac medicorum problemata. 1631.

—[English tr.] *In* Aristoteles. The problems of
Aristotle. 1670; 1684.

ALEXANDER TRALLIANUS [6th cent.] De
lumbricis. *In* Mercuriale, G. Tractatus varii de re
medica. 1618, 1623; Opuscula aurea, & selectiora. 1644.

—*See* ROLFINCK, W. Epitome methodi cognoscendi
& curandi particulares corporis affectus. 1655, 1675.

ALEXANDER, FRANCISCUS. *See* ALESSANDRI,
Francesco degli [1529–1587]

ALEXANDRINUS, JULIUS [1506–1590] *See*
SCHOLTZ, L. Consiliorum medicinalium ... liber
singularis. 1610.

ALEXANDRO, ANTONIUS DE. *See* ALESSANDRI,
Antonio d' [*fl. ca.* 1440]

ALEXIS PEDEMONTANUS. *See* ALESSIO
PIEMONTESE, *pseud.?*

ALEXIUS, ALEXANDER. *See* ALESSI, Alessandro
[*fl.* 1627–1632]

ALFERI, GIACINTO [*fl.* 1628–1646]. Opus de modo
consultandi, sive ut vulgus vocat collegiandi, in quo
non modo variae, vagęque medicae quaestiones,
verum omnium scientiarum nonnullae ad opus spectantes examinantur ... Fogiae, Ex typographia
Laurentii Valerii, 1646.
    [16], 195, [6] p.   25 cm.   [220]

ALFONSO X, *el Sabio, king of Castile and Leon*
[1221–1284] *ed.* and *tr. See* ARTEPHIUS. Alphonsi, regis
Castellae ... Liber philosophiae occultioris. [1660]

**ALFONSO Y DE LOS RUICES DE
FONTECHA**, JUAN. *See* ALONSO Y DE LOS RUYZES
DE FONTECHA, Juan [1560-1620]

ALFRED, *of Sarashel. See* ALFREDUS ANGLICUS,
philosopher, fl. ca. 1215.

ALFREDUS ANGLICUS, *philosopher, fl. ca.* 1215,
tr. See ARISTOTELES. Tractatulus ... de practica
lapidis philosophici. 1610.

ALGAER, LARS M. [*fl.* 1684] *respondent. See* SPOLE,
A., *praeses.* Disputatio physica de frigore. 1684.

ALHAMBRA, BALTASAR VICENTE DE. *See*
VICENTE DE ALHAMBRA, Baltasar.

ALHEM, JOSQUIN D'. *See* DALHEM, Josquin [*fl. ca.*
1573]

ALIBRAY, CHARLES VION D'. *See* DALIBRAY,
Charles Vion, *sieur de* [*ca.* 1600–*ca.* 1655]

ALIDOSI, GIOVANNI NICCOLÒ PASQUALI
[1570–1627] I dottori bolognesi di teologia, filosofia,
medicina, e d'arti liberali dall'anno 1000, per tutto
marzo del 1623 ... Bologna, Tebaldini, 1623.
    [28], 226 p.   21 cm.   [221]
  Engraved title page.

—Li dottori forestieri, che in Bologna hanno letto
teologia, filosofia, medicina, & arti liberali, con li rettori dello studio da gli anni 1000, fino per tutto maggio del 1623 ... Bologna, Nicolò Tebaldini, 1623.
    [8], 103 (i.e. 95) p.   21 cm.   [222]

ALIMONY arraign'd. 1654. *See* IVIE, *Sir* T.

ALISCHER, SEBASTIAN [*b. ca.* 1672] *respondent. See*
HOFFMANN, F. [1660-1742] *praeses.* Disputatio inauguralis medica sistens febris quartanae tutam ac
felicem curationem. 1696.

—*See* HOFFMANN, F. [1660-1742] Propempticon inaugurale de mechanica febrium doctrina Hippocratica. 1696.

ALITHOPHILUS. Alithophili Observationes ex-
temporaneae ad erecta a Carolo Drelincurtio ...
Libitinae, nec non famae suae trophaea, & c.
Amstelodami, Apud Petrum Gavium [1681?]
    84 p.   13 cm.   [223]
  Attributed to Bartholomaeus Franck by DG. BMC lists Jean
Farine as possible author.
  Bound with Drelincourt, C. Libitinae tropaea. 1680.

—*See* FLUDD, Robert [1574–1637]

ALIUS MEDICUS. *See* Animadversions on the
medicinal observations. 1674.

ALKINDUS, Jacobus. *See* Yā'kub ibn Ishāk ibn Subbāh, Abū Yūsuf, al-Kindī [*d. ca.* 873]

ALKOFER, Erasmus Sigmund [*fl.* 1699–1713] *praeses*. Trutina vacui . . . Jenae, Typis Gollnerianis [1699]

    34, [9] p. 19 cm.   **[224]**
    Diss.—Jena (J.C. Bleidner, *respondent)*

ALLACCI, Leone [1586–1669] *ed. See* Cardano, G. Opuscula medica. 1638.

ALLATIUS, Leo. *See* Allacci, Leone [1586–1669]

ALLEGORIAE sapientum: supra librum Turbae XXIX distinctiones.

    57–89 p., vol. 5. 20 cm.   (*In* Zetzner, Lazarus, *ed.* Theatrum chemicum. Argentorati, 1659–61)**[225]**
    Caption title.

ALLEMAND, Louis Augustin. *See* Alemand, Louis Augustin [1653?–1728]

ALLEN, Benjamin [1663–1738] The natural history of the chalybeat and purging waters of England, with their particular essays and uses. Among which are treated at large the apoplexy & hypochondriacism. To which are added, some observations on the bath waters of Somersetshire . . . London, S. Smith and B. Walford, 1699.

    [40], 185, [6] p. 18 cm.   **[226]**

[ALLESTREE, Richard, 1619–1681] A discourse concerning the period of humane life: whether mutable or immutable. The 2d ed., corr. By the author of The duty of man laid down in express words of scripture. London, Printed by F.R. for Enoch Wyer, 1677.

    [10], 134 p. 15 cm.   **[227]**

ALLIOT, François Fauste [*d.* 1700] *praeses*. Quaestio medica . . . An hyemali peripneumoniae venae sectio ἡγεμονιχον? [Parisiis, Apud Franciscum Muguet, 1691]

    4 p. 25 cm.   **[228]**
    Caption title.
    Diss.—Paris (M. Sauvalle, *respondent)*

ALLIOT, Jean Baptiste [*fl.* 1698] Traité du cancer, où l'on explique sa nature, & où l'on propose les moyens les plus sûrs pour le guerir methodiquement. Avec un examen du système & de la pratique de M.r Helvetius . . . Paris, François Muguet, 1698.

    [24], 168 p. 17 cm.   **[229]**

ALMELOVEEN, Theodoor Jansson van, 1657–1712. Bibliotheca promissa et latens. Huic subjunguntur Georgii Hieronymi Velschii de scriptis suis ineditis epistolae. Gaudae, Apud Justum ab Hoeve, 1688.

    [15], 160 p. 16 cm.   **[230]**
    Dedication dated 1692.

——Collectio monumentorum, rerumque maxime insignium, Belgii faederati . . . Carmina & caetera Belgica Latine reddita. Per Phileleutherum Timareten [pseud. i.e. T.J. van Almeloveen] Pars prima . . . Amstelodami, Apud viduam Josephi Brouning, ad Janum Bursae Borealem, 1684.

    [16], 458, [13] p. 18 cm.   **[231]**
    No more appears to have been published.

——Inventa nov-antiqua. Id est brevis enarratio ortus & progressus artis medicae; ac praecipue de inventis vulgo novis, aut nuperrime in ea repertis. Subjicitur ejusdem rerum inventarum onomasticon . . . Amstelaedami, Apud Janssonio-Waesbergios, 1684.

    [32], 249, [7] p.; [6], 85 p. 16 cm.   **[232]**
    Added engraved title page.
    In 2 parts. Part [2] has special title page.

——*ed. See* Celsus, A.C. De medicina libri octo. 1687; *See* Hippocrates, Ἀφορισμοί . . Aphorismi. 1685.

——*tr. See* Heide, A. de. Ontledinge des mossels. 1684.

ALONSO Y DE LOS RUYZES DE FONTECHA, Juan, [1560–1620] Diez previlegios para mugeres preñadas . . . Con un diccionario medico . . . Alcala de Henares, Luys Martynez Grande, 1606.

    [12], 230, [2] p.; 158 ll. 21 cm.   **[233]**
    Part [2] has caption title: Diccionario de los nombres de piedras, plantas, fructos, yervas, flores, enfermedades, causas, y accidentes.

ALÓS, Juan [*fl.* 1664–1694] De corde hominis disquisitio physiologico-anatomica . . . Barcinone, Ex typog. Antonii Ferrer, & Balthasaris Ferrer, per Jacobum Gascon, 1694.

    [27], 247 p. 22 cm.   **[234]**

——Pharmacopoea Cathalana; sive, Antidotarium Barcinonense restitutum, et reformatum . . . Barcinone, Ex typographia Antonii Ferrer & Balthasari Ferrer, 1686.

    [16], 256, [8] p. 30 cm.   **[235]**

ALPAGO, ANDREA [d. 1521] *ed.* and *tr. See* AVICEN-NA. Avicennae Arabum medicorum principis. 1608.

—*tr. See* WELSCH, G. H. Exercitatio de vena medinensi. 1674.

ALPHERIO, HYACINTHE DE. *See* ALFERI, Giacinto [*fl.* 1628-1646]

ALPHONSI regis Clavis sapientiae. *See* Artephius. Alphonsi, regis Castellae ... Liber philosophiae occultioris. [1660]

ALPINI, ALPINI [*d.* 1637] *ed. See* ALPINI, P. De plantis exoticis. 1627, 1629.

ALPINI, PROSPER [1553-1617] De balsamo dialogus. *In his*, De plantis Aegypti liber. 1639.

—[French tr.] *In* Orta, G. d'. Histoire des drogues. 1619.

—De medicina Aegyptiorum libri quatuor, & Jacobi Bontii ... De medicina Indorum. Editio ultima. Parisiis, Apud Nicolaum Redelichuysen, 1645.

    [8], 150, [25] ll. ; 39, [1] ll. illus. 22 cm.   **[236]**

Part [2] has half title.
Part [1] is a dialogue with Melchior Guilandinus.

—Another issue. 25cm.   **[237]**

The title page is a cancel (23 cm.) with variant imprint: Parisiis, Apud viduam Gulielmi Pelé, & Joannem Duval, 1646.

—[Italian tr.] Book 4, chapters 8-12 *In* Antidotario romano latino e volgare. 1624, 1635, 1639, 1675, 1678.

—De medicina methodica libri tredecim in quibus medendi ars methodica ... denuo restituitur, atque in medicorum commodum quadantenus ad medicinam dogmaticam conformatur ... Patavii, Apud Franciscum Bolzettam, ex typographia Laurentii Pasquati, 1611.

    [44], 424 p. 29 cm.   **[238]**

—De plantis Aegypti liber. Cum observationibus & notis Joannis Veslingii ... Accessit Alpini De balsamo liber. Editio altera emendatior. Patavii, Typis Pauli Frambotti, 1638-40 [v.1, 1640]

    3 v. in 1. illus. 23 cm.   **[239]**

De balsamo dialogus (v. [2]) has imprint: Patavii, Apud Paulum Frambottum, 1639.

Vesling's Observationes (v. [3]) has title: De plantis Aegyptiis observationes et notae ad Prosperum Alpinum, cum additamento aliarum ejusdem regionis. Patavii, Apud Paulum Frambottum, 1638.

Vol. 1 is a dialogue with Melchior Guilandinus.

—[Italian excerpts.] *In* Togni, M. Raccolta delle singolari qualità dell caffé, 1675.

—De plantis exoticis libri duo ... Opus completum, editum studio, ac opera Alpini Alpini ... Venetiis, Apud Jo. Guerilium, 1627.

    [16], 344 p. illus. 21 cm.   **[240]**

—[The same.] ... Apud Jo. Guerilium, 1629.

    [16], 344 p. illus. 21 cm.   **[241]**

—Copy 2. 20 cm.

Date altered by hand to MDCLVI.

—De praesagienda vita, et morte aegrotantium. Libri septem. In quibus ars tota Hippocratica praedicendi in aegrotis varios morborum eventus cum ex veterum medicorum dogmatis, tum ex longa accurataque observatione, nova methodo elucescit ... Venetiis, Apud haeredes Melchioris Sessae, 1601.

    [7], 163, [16], ll. 23 cm.   **[242]**

[The same.] ... Francofurti, Apud Jonam Rhodium, 1601.

    [16], 806, [31] p. 18 cm.   **[243]**

—*See* RAUWOLFF, L. A collection of curious travels & voyages. 1693.

ALQUIÉ, FRANÇOIS SAVINIEN D' [*fl.* 17th cent.] *See* KIRCHER, A. La Chine. 1670.

—*tr. See* HUARTE DE SAN JUAN, J. L'examen des esprits pour les sciences. 1672.

ALSACE. Conseil souverain. Arrest notable du Conseil souverain d'Alsace, en faveur des maistres chirurgiens de la ville de Colmar. Contre Pierre Taucher soy disant chirurgien de la ditte ville. Du 10. Maji 1680. [Brisac? 1680]

    12 p. 20 cm.   **[244]**

ALSAHARAVIUS. *See* ABULCASIS [936?-1013?]

ALSARIO DALLA CROCE, VINCENZO [1576?-1631?] Consilium de catharro curando ... Ravennae, Sumptibus heredum Petri Joanelli, 1611.

    [80] p. 21 cm.   **[245]**

Signature I is misbound.

—De epilepsia; seu, Comitiali morbo, lectionum Bononiensium libri tres; in quibus praeter magni illius morbi theoriam, hoc est definitionem, ejusque probationem, differentias, caussas, & signa, veterum quoque loca explanata ... reperiuntur ... Venetiis, Apud Danielem Zanettum, 1603.

    [8], 104 ll. 21 cm.   **[246]**

—De morbis capitis frequentioribus ... hoc est de catarrho, phrenitide, lethargo, & epilepsia, seu comitiali morbo, libri septem ... Romae, Apud Gulielmum Facciottum, 1617.

[16], 489 (i.e. 485), [39] p. 23 cm. **[247]**

—De quaesitis per epistolam in arte medica centuriae quatuor ... Vincentio Alsario Crucio ... auctore ... Venetiis, Apud Juntas, 1622.

[20], 442, [64] p. 33 cm. **[248]**

Errata: p. [63-64]

—Disquisitio generalis ad historiam foetus editi nonimestris quidem & organici, sed emortui, ac parvae adeo molis, seu corpulentiae, ut vix quadrimestris fuerit aestimatus. In adolescentula primipara tam ante, quam post partum integra sanitate fruente ... Romae, Typis Gulielmi Facciotti, 1627.

[9], 128 p. 22 cm. **[249]**

Imperfect: p. 1-2 wanting.

—Providenza metodica, per preservarsi dall'imminente peste. Discorso pratico, ove sono rimedii preservativi e curativi ancora, cavati co'lmezzo di scopi metodici dalla cirurgia, farmacia, e dieta ... Roma, Paolo Masotti, 1630.

[8], 179, [1] p. 22 cm. **[250]**

Imperfect: sig. Y6 wanting; supplied in photocopy from British Museum.

—Vesuvius ardens; sive, Exercitatio medico-physica ad Ρίγόπύρετον [sic], id est, motum & incendium Vesuvii montis ... Libris II. comprehensa ... Romae, Ex typographia Guilelmi Facciotti, 1632.

[8], 317, [3] p. 22 cm. **[251]**

ALSEM, Arnold van [fl. 1671] respondent. Disputatio medica inauguralis de humoribus ... Lugduni Batavorum, Apud viduam & heredes Joannis Elsevirii, 1671.

[32] p. 23 cm. **[252]**

Diss.—Leyden.

ALSLEBEN, Kaspar [fl.1648] respondent. See Sperling, J., praeses. Disputatio physica de capite humano. 1648.

ALSOO mijn heeren van den gherechte deser stadt Haerlem. 1636. See Haarlem. Ordinances, local laws, etc.

ALSTED, Johann Heinrich [1588-1638] Clavis artis Lullianae, et verae logices duos in libellos tributa. Id est, Solida dilucitatio Artis magnae,

generalis, et ultimae, quam Raymundus Lullius invenit ... edita in usum et gratiam eorum qui impendis delectantur compendiis, & confusionem sciolorum, qui juventutem fatigant dispendiis ... Accessit Novum speculum logices minime vulgaris. Argentorati, Sumptibus heredum Lazari Zetzneri, 1652.

[8], 150 p. illus. 19 cm. **[253]**

Rogent and Duràn 234.
Bound with copy 2 of Lull, R. Opera. 1651.

—See Lavinheta, B. de. Opera omnia. 1612.

ALTDORF. Academia. See Academia Aldorfiana.

ALTERMANN, Tobias [fl. 1688] respondent. See Leichner, E., praeses. Dissertatio inauguralis medica de chlorosi. 1688.

ALTHUS, Hendrik [fl. 1668-1669] respondent. Disputatio medica inauguralis de gravedine & catarrhis ... Lugduni Batavorum, Apud viduam & haeredes Joannis Elsevirii, 1669.

[16] p. 23 cm. **[254]**

Diss.—Leyden.

ALTMANN, Johann Caspar [fl. 1684] respondent. See Leichner, E., praeses. De mensium suppressione. 1684.

ALTOMARE, Donato Antonio [1506-1562] De mendendis humani corporis malis. In Salius Diversus, P. De febre pestilenti tractatus. 1656, 1681.

ALTWEIN, Johannes [fl. 1687] praeses. Disputatio inauguralis medica de febre quartana ... Erfordiae, Typis Groschianis [1687]

28, [4] p. 20 cm. **[255]**

Diss.—Erfurt (J. P. Farneck, respondent)

ÁLVAREZ, Miguel Sabuco y. See Sabuco y Álvarez, Miguel [fl. 1563-1590]

ALVAREZ MIRAVAL, Blas [fl. 1597-1598] Libro intitulado la conservacion de la salud del cuerpo y del alma, para el buen regimiento de la salud ... Salamanca, Andres Renaut, 1601.

[67], 480 ll. 21 cm. **[256]**

A reissue of the 1597 edition with new title page.

ALVETANUS, Cornelius [fl. 1565] De conficiendo divino elixire; sive, Lapide philosophico ...

815-821 p., vol. 5. (Same text repeated: 501-507 p., vol. 6) 20 cm. (*In* Zetzner, Lazarus, *ed.* Theatrum chemicum. Argentorati, 1659-61)   [**257**]

Caption title.

ALVISO, URBANO D' [*b.* 1618?] *See* PORZIO, L. A. In Hippocratis librum De veteri medicina ... paraphrasis. 1681.

AMABILE, GIOVANNI SISINIO [*fl.* 1615] De natura foetus disputatio ... Romae, Ex typographia Andreae Phaei, 1615.

147, [2] p.   15 cm.   [**258**]
Errata: p. [2]

AMAND, JEAN DE SAINT. *See* SAINT-AMAND, Jean de [13th cent.]

AMAT, JUAN CARLOS [1572-1642] Fructus medicinae, ex variis Galeni locis decerpti ... Nunc primum prodit in lucem. Lugduni, Sumptibus Ludovici Prost, haeredis Roville, 1623.

[24], 284, [16] p.   15 cm.   [**259**]

—[The same.] ... Ed. altera auctior, innumerisque locis correctior. Lugduni, Typis Hugonis Denoüally, 1681.

[24], 262, [14] p.   15 cm.   [**260**]

AMATO, CINTIO D' [17th cent.] Prattica nuova, et utilissima di tutto quello, ch'al diligente barbiero s'appartiene; cioè di cavar sangue, medicar ferite; & balsamar corpi humani ... Venetia, Appresso Gio. Battista Brigna, 1669.

[24], 88, [14] p.   illus.   21 cm.   [**261**]

—[The same.] Nuova et utilissima prattica di tutto quello ch'al diligente barbiero s'appartiene: divisa in due librii, ove si discorre del cavar sangue, medicar ferite, et balsamar corpi humani ... Per Tomaso Antonio Riccio ristampata. 3a. impresione ... Napoli, Appresso Geronimo Fasulo, 1671.

[10], 168, [10] p.   plates.   21 cm.   [**262**]
Engraved title page.

AMATUS LUSITANUS, 1511-1568. Curationum medicinalium centuriae septem, varia multiplicique rerum cognitione refertę & in hac ultima editione recognitae & valde correctę. Quibus praemissa est commentatio de introitu medici ad aegrotantem, deque crisi & diebus decretoriis ... Burdigalae, Ex typographia Gilberti Vernoy, 1620.

[37], 800 (i.e. 796), [19] p.   25 cm.   [**263**]

—Curationum medicinalium. Centuria quinta [-septima] Venetiis, Apud Franciscum Storti, 1653.

240; 344; 312 p.   15 cm.   [**264**]
Parts [2] and [3] have special title pages.

—Dialogo de las heridas de la cabeça. *In* Montemayor, C. Medicina y cirugia de vulneribus capitis. 1664.

—In Dioscoridis De medica materia enarrationes. *See* MATTIOLI, P. A. Opera quae extant omnia. 1674.

AMBROGINI, ANGELO, *of Monte Pulciano. See* POLIZIANO, Angelo [1454-1494]

AMBROSINI, BARTOLOMMEO [1588-1657] Paralipomena accuratissima historiae animalium. *See* ALDROVANDI, U. Monstrorum historia. 1642.

—*ed. See* ALDROVANDI, U. De quadrupedibus digitatis viviparis libri tres. 1645 [and] Musaeum metallicum. 1648 [and] Serpentum, et draconum historiae libri duo. 1640.

AMBROSINI, GIACINTO [1605-1671] Phytologiae; hoc est, De plantis partis primae tomus primus. In quo herbarum nostro seculo descriptarum, nomina, aequivoca, synonyma, ac etymologiae investigantur ... Bononiae, Sumptibus haeredum Evangelistae de Ducciis, 1666.

[13], 576, [68] p.   front., illus.   33 cm.
                                                          [**265**]
Imperfect: p. 321-328 wanting; supplied in manuscript.

AMELDUNG, JOHANN HEINRICH [*b.* 1673] *respondent. See* WEDEL, G. W., *praeses.* Dissertatio medica inauguralis de cholera. 1697.

—*See* CRAUSE, R. W. Propemticum inaugurale de difficultate in studio medico hodie emergente. 1697.

AMELUNG, HEINRICH CHRISTIAN [*fl.* 1690] Chymische Untersuchung von dem Unterscheid des philosoph. und mineralischen Antimonii wie auch des Mercurii Philosophorum & vulgaris ... Dresden, In Verlag Michael Günthers, Druckts Johann Riedel, 1690.

[12], 107 p.   14 cm.   [**266**]

AMELUNG, PETER [*fl.* 1607] Tractatus nobilis primus, in quo alchimiae seu chemicae, artis antiquissimae ... cum invento et progressio, obscuratio

& instauratio, tum dignitas, necessitas & utilitas, demonstratur ... Lipsiae, Michael Lantzënberger excudebat, sumtibus Jacobi Apelii, 1607.

 250 (i.e. 248) p. 15 cm.   **[267]**

AMERICUS, *pseud. See* METZGER, Georg Balthasar [*d.* 1687]

AMICO, DIOMEDE [*fl.* 1596] De morbis sporadibus opus novum ... in quo singulari cum facilitate, exactoque cum judicio ea omnia, quę ad illarum corporis humani affectionum diagnosticen, prognosticen, therapeuticen, prophylacticen, analepticen: item ad gerocomicen: denique ad tria medica instrumenta in universum pertinent ... explicantur. Omnia accurate nunc primum excusa ... Venetiis, Apud Jo. Antonium & Jacobum de Franciscis, 1605.

 [12], 200, [8] ll. 23 cm.   **[268]**

AMIRALES, DĒMĒTRIOS. *See* AMMIRALLOS, Dēmētrios [*fl.* 1687]

AMLING, JAKOB [*fl.* 1678-1694] *praeses.* Dissertatio inauguralis Galeno Hippocratica de affectione hypochondriaca ... Herbipoli, Typis Eliae Michaelis Zinck [1678]

 [1], 18 p. 20 cm.   **[269]**

 Diss—Würzburg (J. F. Haack, *respondent*)

—Theses inaugurales medicae de theoria et therapia famis caninae ... Herbipoli, Typ. haer. Zinck. typogr. per Martinum Richter [1694]

 [4], 19 p. 19 cm.   **[270]**

 Diss.—Würzburg (F. L. Moser, *respondent*)

AMMAN, GEORG CHRISTOPH [*fl.* 1655-1659] *respondent. See* RAABE, J. J., *praeses.* Exercitatio medica casum practicum exponens. 1656.

AMMAN, JOHANN. *See* AMMIANUS, Joannes [*fl.* 1667]

AMMAN, JOHANN CONRAD [1669-1724] Dissertatio de loquela qua non solum vox humana, & loquendi artificium ex originibus suis eruuntur: sed & traduntur media, quibus ii, qui ab incunabulis surdi & multi fuerunt, loquelam adipisci, quique difficulter loquuntur, vitia sua emendare possint ... Amstelaedami, Apud Joannem Wolters, 1700.

 [24], 120 p. table. 16 cm. **[271]**

—Surdus loquens, seu methodus qua, qui surdus natus est, loqui discere possit ... Amstelaedami, Apud Henricum Wetstenium, 1692.

 53, [1] p. 16 cm.   **[272]**

—[Dutch tr.] Surdus loquens; of, De doove sprekende. *In* Helmont, F. M. van, *baron.* Een Zeer korte afbeelding van het ware natuurlyke Hebreuwse A. B. C. welke te gelyk de wyse vertoont. 1697.

—[English tr.] The talking deaf man: or, A method proposed, whereby he who is born deaf, may learn to speak ... Imprinted at Amsterdam, by Henry Westein, 1692. And now done out of Latin into English, by D. F. M. D. [i.e. Daniel Foot] 1693. London, Printed for Tho. Howkins, 1694.

 [36], 93, [3] p. 15 cm.   **[273]**

—*respondent.* Disputatio inauguralis sistens aegrum pleuro-pneumonia laborantem ... Basileae, Literis Jacobi Bertschii [1687]

 [35] p. 20 cm.   **[274]**

 Diss. — Basel.

AMMANN, PAUL [1634-1691] Consilium de institutionum medicarum emendatione necessario suscipienda. Cui accessit I. Archaeus syncopticus, contra Leichnerum. II. Disputatio de resonitu. III. Resol. probl. Monspel: Vade, et occide Cain. Lipsiae, Impensis Joh. Heinichen [1693]

 [23], 673 (i.e. 681), [57] p. front. 14 cm.

              [275]

 The first work was previously published under title: Paraenesis ad discentes, occupata circa institutionum medicarum emendationem.

—Irenicum Numae Pompilii, cum Hippocrate, quo veterum medicorum & philosophorum hypotheses in Corpus juris civilis pariter, ac canonici, hactenus transsumtae, a praeconceptis opinionibus vindicantur mediatore D. P. A. ... Francofurti & Lipsiae, Sumptibus Authoris, 1689

 [15], 272, [16] p. 17 cm.   **[276]**

 Bound with his Praxis vulnerum lethalium ... 1690.

—Paraenesis ad discentes, occupata circa institutionum medicarum emendationem. Rudolstadii, Typis Freyschmidianis; impensis Joh. Barthol. Olearii, 1673.

 [22], 432, [47] p. 13 cm.   **[277]**

—Medicina critica; sive decisoria, centuria casuum medicinalium in concilio Facult. med. Lips. antehac resolutorum, comprehensa, nunc vero in physicorum, practicorum, studiosorum, chirurgorum aliorumque usum notabilem collecta, correcta, & variis discursibus aucta ... Erffurti, Litteris Joh.

Georgi Hertzi, impensis Joh. Bartholom. Ohleri, 1670.

[46], 490, [4] p.   19 cm.   [278]
Text mainly in German.

—[Latin tr.] Medicina critica, sive decisoria, centuria casuum medicinalium in concilio Facult. Lips. antehac resolutorum, comprehensa, & in physicorum, practicorum, studiosorum, chirurgorum, aliorumque usum notabilem primum collecta, ac variis discursibus aucta, nunc ab innumeris sphalmatis vindicata, & exterorum in gratiam, Latinitati donata, opera D. Christiani Francisci Paullini ... Stadae, Typis ac impensis Johann Fesselii, 1677.

[56], 612 (i.e. 582), [26] p.   20 cm.   [279]
A translation of his Medicina critica ... first published in German with similar Latin title.

—Another issue, with front., and new title page; imprint reads: Lipsiae, Apud Joh. Heinichen, 1693.
                                              [280]

—Oratio de autopsia medica. Lipsiae, Typis Johannes Wilhelmi Krügeri [ca. 1674]

[20] p.   19 cm.   [281]
Printed ca. 1660 according to DG. v. 4., col. 34; but J. W. Krüger printed in Leipzig from 1674 until 1708. Cf. Benzing (A) p. 273.

—Praxis vulnerum lethalium, sex decadibus historiarum rariorum, ut-plurimum traumaticarum, cum cribrationibus singularibus adornata ... Francofurti, Sumptibus Autoris, apud Johann Friedrich Gleditsch, 1690.

[35], 483, [32] p.   17 cm.   [282]
Added half title.
With this is bound *his* Irenicum Numae Pompilii, cum Hippocrate. 1689.

—D. Paulus Ammann ... pro-cancellarius. L. S. [Lipsiae, Literis Joh. Georg, 1680]

[8] p.   19 cm.   [283]
Program—Leipzig (with vita of C. J. Lange)

—Pro-cancellarius Facultatis Medicae in Academia Lipsiensi D. Paulus Ammann lecturis S. [Lipsiae, Literis Banckmannianis, 1689.]

[8] p.   19 cm.   [284]
Program—Leipzig (for J. C. Grimm)

—Supellex botanica, hoc est: Enumeratio plantarum, quae non solum in Horto medico Academiae Lipsiensis, sed etiam in aliis circa urbem viridariis, pratis ac sylvis &c. progerminare solent: cui brevis accessit ad materiam medicam in usum philiatrorum manuductio ... Lipsiae, Sumptibus Joh. Christ. Tarnovii, 1675.

[16], 137, [1] p.; [1], 193, [17] p.   17 cm. [285]

Dissertations—Leipzig

—*praeses.* De ardore ventriculi; sive, De soda diatribe ... Lipsiae, Johann Wittigau [1663]

[12] p.   18 cm.   [286]
J. Loss, *respondent.*

—Disputatio chirurgica, de resonitu, vel contrafissura cranii ... Lipsiae, Ex Officina Spöreliana [1674]

[20] p.   19 cm.   [287]
J. C. von Ettner, *respondent.*

—Disputatio inauguralis de palpitatione cordis ... Lipsiae, Literis Christiani Michaelis, 1680.

[24] p.   20 cm.   [288]
J. D. Schmoller, *respondent.*

—Disputatio inauguralis medica de spina ventosa ... Lipsiae, Literis Christiani Michaelis [1672]

[28] p.   19 cm.   [289]
T. Olitzsch, *respondent.*

—Disputatio inauguralis medica de suffocatione uterina ... Lipsiae, Typis Johan-Erici Hahnii [1668]

[16] p.   18 cm.   [290]
S. Eichler, *respondent*

—Disputatio medica de cancromammarum ... Lipsiae, Typis Johannis Georgii [1669]

[19] p.   19 cm.   [291]
J. C. Zuckmantel, *respondent.*

—Disputatio medica de phthisi ... Lipsiae, Typis Christiani Michaelis [1664]

[12] p.   19 cm.   [292]
M. Clemas, *respondent.*

—Disputationem inauguralem de haemorrhagia ... publico examini subjicit Daniel Friderici ... Lipsiae, Literis Christiani Michaelis [1667]

[32] p.   18 cm.   [293]
D. Friderici, *respondent.*

—Disputationem inauguralem de pleuritide vera ... publico examini subjicit M. Johann Bohn ... Lipsiae, Literis Ritzschianis [1666]

[32] p.   19 cm.   [294]
J. Bohn, *respondent.*

—Dissertatio inauguralis de remediis stomachicis ... Lipsiae, Literis Christiani Scholvini [1689]

[24] p.   20 cm.   [**295**]

J. C. Schamberg, *respondent.*

—Dissertatio medica inauguralis de mictione cruenta ... Lipsiae, Typis viduae Joh. Wittigau [1673]

[47] p.   20 cm.   [**296**]

J. Wolf, *respondent.*

—[The same.] ... [Jenae?] Recusa, prostat apud Joh. Jacob. Ehrtium [1686?]

[71] p.   21 cm.   [**297**]

Johann Jakob Ehrt worked in Jena between 1686 and 1694. Cf. Benzing (B).

J. Wolf, *respondent.*

—Dissertationem inauguralem de ictero ... sistit M. Johannes Wilhelmus Pauli ... Lipsiae, Literis Johann Georg [1681]

[36] p.   20 cm.   [**298**]

J. W. Pauli, *respondent.*

—Quaestio physica de caloris nativi natura ... Lipsiae, Typis Bauerianis [1657]

[23] p.   19 cm.   [**299**]

J. A. Kreutter, *respondent.*

—Theses medicae de lithiasi renum et vesicae ... Lipsiae, Typis Johannis Georgii, 1669.

[21] p.   19 cm.   [**300**]

D. Lungwiz, *respondent.*

—Theses physicae de auctione ... Lipsiae, Literis Bauerianis [1658]

[12] p.   20 cm.   [**301**]

J. L. Weissberger, *respondent.*

—Theses physicae de motu; sive, Circulatione sanguinis ... [Lipsiae] Typis Johannis Baueri [1659]

[16] p.   20 cm.   [**302**]

C. Beccer, *respondent.*

—Theses physicae de nutritione ... [Lipsiae] Literis Bauerianis [1657]

[12] p.   18 cm.   [**303**]

J. P. Klipper, *respondent.*

—*respondent.* See LANGE, C., *praeses.* Disputatio medica de ambustionibus. 1658; MICHAELIS, J., *praeses.* Disputatio inauguralis ... de paresi. 1660.

—*ed.* See FEDELE, F. Fortunati Fidelis ... De relationibus medicorum libri quatuor. 1674, 1679.

—*See* LEICHNER, E. De principiis medicis. 1675.

AMMIANUS, JOANNES [*fl.* 1667] ... Sonderbarer Tractat und grundlicher Bericht von der Pest. Worinnen begriffen, in was eigentlich deroselben Wäsen bestehe, von was Ursachen sie entstehe, worbei sie zu erkennen, und wie man sich durch göttliche Hilff nicht nur vor derselben bewahren, sondern auch wann man darmit behafftet, heilen könne ... Aus den berühmtesten Pest-Scribenten ... zusamen getragen ... und ... in das Teutsche übersetzet. Durch Joannem Ammianum med. doctorem Scaphusianum. Schaffhausen, Johann Caspar Suter, 1667.

[10], 168, [1] p.   17 cm.   [**304**]

Added engraved title page.

AMMIRALLOS, DĒMĒTRIOS [*fl.* 1687] *See* THULLIER, C. Lettre ... a ... Demetrius Ammirally 1693.

AMMON, KLEMENS [17th cent.] *engr. See* BOISSARD, J. J. Bibliotheca chalcographica. 1650–54.

AMODEO, JOANNES. *See* [CYNTHIUS, C.] Disputationes medicae de natura atque facultatibus ligni sancti. 1602.

AMPSING, JOHANNES ASSUERUS [1558–1642] Dissertatio iatromathematica. In qua de medicinae et astronomiae praestantia, deque utriusque indissolubili conjugio disseritur ... Ed. 2. Rostochi, Typis haeredum Richelianorum, impensis Johannis Hallervordii, 1629.

[1], 311, [7] p.   16 cm.   [**305**]

—Hectas affectionum capillos et pilos humani corporis infestantium. Rostochi, Typis & impensis Augustini Ferberi, 1623.

[6], 120 p.   16 cm.   [**306**]

—*praeses.* Disputatio de calculo ... Rostochii, Typis exscripsit Joachimus Pedanus [1617]

[87] p.   21 cm.   [**307**]

Diss.—Rostock (C. Smilovius, *respondent*)

De AMSTELDAMSCHE nyptan, of samenspraak tussen Belzebub en Lucifer ... [Amsterdam?] Gedrukt in de Brouwery van de Werelt [1678]

13 p.   16 cm.   [**308**]

Occasioned by the controversy between Andreas Boekelman and Bonaventura van Dortmont.

AMSTERDAM. Collegium Medicum. *See* Collegium MEDICUM, Amsterdam.

AMSTERDAM. Collegium Privatum. *See* COLLEGIUM PRIVATUM AMSTELODAMENSE.

AMSTERDAM. Ordinances, local laws, etc. Extract uyt het register van de willekeuren der Stadt Amstelredam, geteeckent met de letter m. ordonnantie ... aengaende de huysen, die met de peste ... besmet ... Amsterdam, Jan Banning, 1655.
    [10] p.   21 cm.   [309]
Dated 21 August 1655.

—Keure en ordonnantie, op het dragen en begraven van doden, binnen de Stad van Amsterdam, en de jurisdictie van dien. Amsterdam, Jan Rieuwertsz, 1696
    15 p.   20 cm.   [310]
Dated 10 Jan. 1696.

—*See* PHARMACOPOEA AMSTELREDAMENSIS. 1636, 1639?, 1659.

AMTHOR, KASPAR [16th-17th cent.] Noscomium infantile, et puerile; das ist, Kinder Lazaret, darinnen die vornembsten Anstösse der jungen Kinder erzehlet ... Schleusingen, Gedruckt durch Peter Schmiden, 1638.
    [46] p.   16 cm.   [311]
Bound with Charleton, W. Spiritus gorgonicus. 1650.

AMTHOR, KASPAR [*fl.* 1626] *respondent. See* SENNERT, D., *praeses.* Theses de catarrho. 1626.

AMTHOR, WOLFGANG HEINRICH [*fl.* 1656] *respondent. See* POSNER, C., *praeses.* De causarum generibus. 1656.

AMTHOR, WOLFGANG ULRICH [*fl.* 1628] *respondent. See* BRENDEL, Z. [1592-1638] *praeses.* Disputatio inauguralis de dysenteria. 1628.

AMWALD, GEORG. *See* WALD, Georg am [*fl.* 1580-1596]

AMY, HONORÉ L'. *See* LAMY, Honoré.

AMYES, JOHN. *See* AYMES, John.

ANASTASIUS. *See* HYGIEIA. 1628; Regimen sanitatis Salernitanum. De conservanda bona valetudine. 1607, 1619; Medicina Salernitana. 1605, 1611, 1612, 1622, 1624, 1628, 1638; Schola Salernitana. 1649, 1657, 1667, 1683,

L'ANATOMIE du corps humain, avec ses maladies. 1680, 1684-85. *See* [SAINT HILAIRE, *sieur de.*]

The ANATOMY of humane bodies epitomized. 1682. *See* [GIBSON, T.]

The ANATOMY of melancholy. 1621. *See* BURTON, R.

The ANATOMY of the humane body abridged. 1698. *See* KEILL, J.

L'ANCIENNE guerre des chevaliers. *See* [URALTER RITTER-KRIEG. French *tr.*] 1699.

Les ANCIENS et renommés autheurs de la medecine & chirurgie. 1634. *See* GUIDI, G. [*ca.* 1500-1569]

ANCILLON, PAUL [*fl.* 1688-1689] *respondent.* Disputatio medica de suppressione mensium ... Basileae, Typis Jacobi Bertschii [1689]
    [16] p.   20 cm.   [312]
Diss. — Basel.

—*See* HARDER, J. J., *praeses.* Exercitatio medica de chylificatione. 1688.

—*See* HARDER, J. J. Alexander Pfisterus. 1689.

[**ANDALA**, RUARD, 1665-1727] Uiterste verleegentheid van Doctor Balt. Bekker. Duidelijk aangeweesen door wederlegginge van alle sijne aanmerkingen ... Uitgegeeven door een discipel van der Heer J. vander Waeyen ... Franeker, Hans Gyzelaar, 1696.
    [8], 234, [6] p.   20 cm.   [313]
Linde 166.

ANDERNACUS, GUINTERIUS JOANNES. *See* GUINTERIUS, Joannes, Andernacus [1505-1574]

ANDERSON, GUILIELMUS [*fl.* 1657] *respondent.* Disputatio medica inauguralis, de dolore nephritico ... Ultrajecti, Ex officina Jacobi à Doeyenborgh, 1657.
    [12] p.   20 cm.   [314]
Diss. — Utrecht.

ANDERSON, PATRICK [*fl.* 1618-1635] *See* GRANA ANGELICA. 1679.

ANDLA, ANCHISES [*fl.* 1618-*ca.* 1644] *respondent. See* VORSTIUS, A.E., *praeses.* Disputatio medica de regio morbo. 1621.

ANDLO, Petrus ab. *See* Mansveld, Regner van [1639-1671]

ANDRÉ, François de. *See* Saint André, François de [*fl.* 1677-1725]

ANDRÉ, Nicolas. *See* Andry de Boisregard, Nicolas [1658-1742]

ANDREAE, Hermann [*fl.* 1660] *respondent*. De sulphure. *In* Rolfinck, W., *praeses*. Dissertationes chimicae sex de tartaro. 1660, 1679.

— *See* Rolfinck, W., *praeses*. Dissertatio medica inauguralis, de dolore colico. 1660.

ANDREAE, Johann David [*fl.* 1683] *respondent*. Dissertatio inauguralis medica de arthritide ... Argentorati, Typis Johannis Welperi [1683]

24 p.   20 cm.   [**315**]

Diss. — Strasbourg.

ANDREAE, Johannes Wilhelm [*fl.* 1668] *respondent*. *See* Schmid, J. Pulveris sympathetici, examen physicum. 1668.

ANDREAE, Tobias [1633-1685] *praeses*. Disputatio inauguralis medica de catharris ... [Francofurti ad Viadrum] Typis Friderici Eichornii, 1678.

[24] p.   19 cm.   [**316**]

Diss. — Frankfurt an der Oder (C. J. Lossau, *respondent*)

— Sacrosancta triade annuente trias exercitationum de mente et corpore ... Francofurti cis Viadrum, Typis haeredum Johannis Ernesti, 1679.

3 v.   19 cm.   [**317**]

Title from general title page.

Volume [1] has special title page with imprint: Typis Fridrici Eichornii.

Contents. — Exercitatio 1. De conjugio mentis et corporis ad Hipp. Aphor. VI. Sect. II. — Exercitatio 2. De cura mentis per corpus ad Hipp. Aphor. VI. Sect. II. — Exercitatio 3. De cura corporis per mentem ad Hipp. Aphor. VI. Sect. II.

At head of titles: Ad solius Dei gloriam exercitationum prima [-tertia & ult.]

Diss.-Frankfurt an der Oder (C. J. Brecht, *respondent*)

— *See* Bils, L. de. Responsio. 1669.

ANDREAS, Hyacinthus. *See* Andreu, Jacinto [*fl. ca.* 1651-*ca.* 1675]

ANDREAS, Olaus [*fl.* 1656] *respondent*. *See* Bartholin, T., *praeses*. Disputatio medica de variolis hujus anni epidemiis. 1656.

ANDREAS, Zacharias [*fl.* 1644] *respondent*. *See* Sebisch, M. [1578-1674?] *praeses*. Disputationes de dentibus quatuor. 1645.

ANDREU, Jacinto [*fl. ca.* 1651-*ca.* 1675] Practicae Gotholanorum, pro curandis humani corporis morbis, descriptae juxta medicinae rationalis leges ... antiquitatis luminaria Hippocrates, et Galenus tomus primus ... Aucthor ... Hyacinthus Andreas ... Barchinone, Ex typis Francisci Cormellas, per Vincentium Suria, 1678.

[19], 532, [28] p.   31 cm.   [**318**]

No more volumes published. Cf. Palau 12297.

ANDREWS, Richard. *See* Androse, Richard.

ANDREWS, William [*fl.* 1656-1683] Physical observations, for the year 1671. Monthly collected, from the most material disposition, of the coelestial bodies, in the same year. Wherein is clearly discovered those sundry diseases ... which will befal those persons who shall be taken sick, at ... times mentioned therein ... London, Printed by E. Crowch for Thomas Vere, 1671.

[36] p.   illus.   19 cm.   [**319**]

ANDRIOLI, Michelangelo [1672-1713] Domesticorum auxiliorum, et facile parabilium remediorum tractatus quinque ... Appendix prima ad Concilium veterum, & neotericorum de conservanda valetudine ... Venetiis, Apud Hieronymum Albriccium, 1698.

[20], 373 (i.e. 375) p.   24 cm.   [**320**]

— Enchyridium practicum medicum; seu, Ad manus libellus; atque appendix secunda ad Libellum de conservanda valetudine. In quo domestica, & usitatoria auxilia recentiorum. Pro universis morbis curandis exarantur. Sex particulis ... dissectum ... Venetiis, Apud Hieronymum Albriccium, 1700.

[12], 323 p.   24 cm.   [**321**]

— Ὑγινης concilium veterum, et neotericorum de conservanda valetudine seu de morborum causis procatharticis ... Lugduni, Apud Jo. de Lupisa, 1693.

48, 352 p.   24 cm.   [**322**]

ANDRIOT, François [*d.* 1704] *illus. See* Genga, B. Anatomia per uso et intelligenza del disegno. 1691.

ANDROMACHUS, *the elder*. Theriaca. *In* Charas, M. Histoire naturelle des animaux. 1668 [and]

Theriaque d'Andromacus. 1685; Tidicaeus, F. De theriaca et ejus multiplici utilitate. 1607.

— *See* BARTISCH, G. Warhafftige . . . Beschreibung. 1602; BONVINIUS, E. De theriaca liber. 1610.

— *as subject See* AD THERIACAE ANDROMACHI. 1642; CASTELLI, A. Dell'uso, et virtù della Theriaca di Andromaco il vecchio. 165–?

ANDROSE, RICHARD, *ed.* and *tr. See* ALESSIO PIEMONTESE, *pseud*.? The secrets. 1615.

ANDRY, NICOLAS. *See* ANDRY DE BOISREGARD, Nicolas [1658–1742]

ANDRY DE BOISREGARD, NICOLAS [1658–1742] De la génération des vers dans le corps de l'homme . . . Avec trois lettres écrites à l'auteur, sur le sujet des vers; les deux premieres d'Amsterdam par M. Nicolas Hartsoéker, & l'autre de Rome par M. Georges Baglivi. Paris, Laurent d'Houry, 1700.

    [64], 486, [5] p. plates. 17 cm.   **[323]**

    "Question . . . Sçavoir si le fréquent usage du tabac abrege la vie": p. 347–386, is the translation of the 1699 Paris dissertation published under title "Quaestio medica . . . An ex tabaci usu frequenti vitae summa brevior?" by Guy Crescent Fagon and Claude Berger.

ANGE DE SAINT JOSEPH, *Father*. *See* ANGELUS DE SANCTU JOSEPHO, *Father* [1636–1697]

ANGEL ANGELERES, BUENAVENTURA [*fl.* 1692] Real filosofia, vida de la salud temporal sabiduria sophica, testamento filomedico arcanos filochimicos hipocratica, galenica, lilibetanica. Parte segunda de la parte primera del regimiento general, prudente, fisico, y moral, brevedad, verdad, claridad en cada genero de catolica, y phisica sabiduria . . . Madrid, Mariana del Valle, 1692.

    [32], 272, 42, [18] p. 21 cm.   **[324]**

    Imperfect: wormholes throughout.

ANGELERES, FRAY BUENAVENTURA. *See* ANGEL ANGELERES, Buenaventura [*fl.* 1692]

ANGELI, ALESSANDRO DEGLI [1542–1620] *In* astrologos conjectores libri quinque . . . Nunc primum prodit in lucem . . . Lugduni, Sumptibus Horatii Cardon, 1615.

    [28], 351, [31] p. illus. 25 cm.   **[325]**

ANGELI, STEFANO DEGLI [1623–1697?] *See* BORELLI, G. A. De vi percussionis. 1686.

ANGELICO, MICHELANGELO [16th–17th cent.] *tr. See* GALENUS. L'antidotario. 1613.

ANGELINI, FACONDINO [*fl.* 1641] Methodus pro venae sectione eligenda . . . Patavii, Typis Joannis Baptistae Pasquati, MDCIXL [i.e. 1641]

    [8], 80 p. 19 cm.   **[326]**

ANGELIS, ALEXANDRE DE. *See* ANGELI, Alessandro degli [1542–1620]

ANGELOCRATOR, HENRICUS CHRISTIANUS [*fl.* 1695] *respondent.* Dissertatio inauguralis anatomico-medica. De glandulis mucilaginosis Haverianis . . . Marburgi Cattorum, Typis haered. Joh. Jodoci Kürsneri, 1695.

    20 p. 20 cm.   **[327]**

    Diss. — Marburg.

ANGELUCCI, TEODORO [*d. ca.* 1600] *See* GARZONI, T. L'hospidale de' pazzi incurabili. 1605, 1617.

ANGELUS DE SANCTU JOSEPHO, *Father* [1636–1697] *tr. See* Pharmacopoea Persica ex idiomate Persico in Latinum conversa. 1681.

ANGLUS, THOMAS. *See* WHITE, Thomas [1593–1676]

ANGERMANN, JOHANN [*fl.* 1673] Microscopium acidularum bruzensium philosophico-medicum; das ist, Aussführliche philosophisch, und medicinalische Beschreibung dess noch niemal in Druck gegebenen Sawr, oder Rässbrunnen zu Prutz, in . . . Tyrol. Was derselbe für Natur, Krafft und Würckung habe . . . Ynssprugg, Jacob Christoff Wagner, 1673.

    [22], 108 (i.e. 208), [10] p. 16 cm.   **[328]**

ANGO, PIERRE [1640–1694] L'optique divisée en trois livres ou l'on démontre d'une maniere aisée tout ce qui regarde. 1. la propagation & les proprietex de la lumiere. 2. La vision. 3. La figure & la disposition des verres qui servent à la perfectionner [sic] . . . Paris, Estienne Michallet, 1682.

    [8], 367, [1] p. illus. 16 cm.   **[329]**

ANGUILBERTUS, THEOBALDUS. *See* MENSA PHILOSOPHICA. 1602.

ANHALT, ELEONORA, *Fürstin von. See* ELEONORA, *consort of George I, landgrave of Hesse-Darmstadt* [1551 or 2–1618]

ANHALT, HEINRICH [*fl.* 1689–*ca.* 1697] *respondent.*
See GERDES, J. *praeses.* Ideam errantem ac furibundam, in hydrophobia conspicuam . . . publicae
eruditorum censurae ventilandam, exhibebit . . . H.
A. 1689.

—*See* GERDES, J. Programma, quo . . . ad dissertationem inauguralem . . . Henrici Anhalt . . . d. 21.
Aug. . . . ventilandam . . . invitat Johannes Gerdes
. . . decanus. 1690.

ANHORN VAN HARTWISS, BARTHOLOMAEUS
[1616–1700] Magiologia. Christliche Warnung für dem
Aberglauben unnd Zauberey: darinnen gehandlet
wird von dem Weissagen, Tagwellen und
Zeichendeuten, von dem Bund der Zauberer mit dem
Teufel . . . Basel, Johann Heinrich Meyer, 1674.

[32], 1107 (i.e. 1105), [70] p. 16 cm. [**330**]
Added engraved title page has title: Aberglauben und Zauberey.

ANIMADVERSIONS on the medicinal observations, of the Heidelberg, Palatinate, Dorchester practitioner of physick, Mr. Frederick Loss . . . by Alius
Medicus. London, William Willis, 1674.

[19], 123, [22] p. 16 cm. [**331**]
Epistle dedicatory signed T. B.
"Mr. Loss his letter to Alius Medicus": p. [1–16]; "Alius Medicus
his answer to Mr. Loss": p. [17–20]

ANNESI, NICOLO [17th cent.] Breve trattato delle
virtù, qualità operationi, et facoltà delli nobili, antichi, et pretiosi bagni di Bormio di Valtellina . . .
Bolgiano, Gerolamo Francesco Sibilla, 1691.

23 p. 21 cm. [**332**]

ANOMAEUS, JOANNES JOACHIMUS. *See*
ANOMOEUS, Johann Joachim [*fl.* 1608]

ANOMOEUS, JOHANN JOACHIM [*fl.* 1608] *respon-*
dent. See HORST, G. [1578–1636] *praeses.* Problematum
medicorum θεραπευτικων decades priores quinque.
1608; TANDLER, T., *praeses.* De melancholia ejusque
speciebus. 1608.

ANONYMI Tractatus varii de morbis. *See* TRAC-
TATUS VARII DE MORBIS. 1690.

ANONYMUS, CHRISTIANUS. *See* DICKINSON, E.
Edmund Dickinson . . . De chrysopoeia. 1687?

ANONYMUS, PHILOMUSUS. *See* CARRICHTER,
Bartholomäus [1507–1573]

ANONYMUS VON FELDTAW. Crollius
redivivus; das ist, Hermetischer Wunderbaum,

warinn zu sehen, wie die wunderbahre Werck Gottes von Liebhabern wahrer chymischer Artzney recht
zu verstehen und zu erkennen . . . Aus dem grossen
hermetischen Lustgarten zusammen getragen und in
sieben Büchlein abgetheilet . . . Franckfurt am
Mäyn, Hans Friederich Weiss, 1647.

83 p. illus. 24 cm. [**333**]
Paged by hand: 647–729.
First published in 1635 by Schönwetter; in 1647 published by
Weiss separately and as a part of Oswald Croll's Hemetischer pro-
bier Stein, the German version of the Basilica chymica. Cf. DG
vol. 5, col. 178.

ANOTHER collection of philosophical conferences
of the French virtuosi. 1665. *See* [RENAUDOT, E.]

ANSELMI, AURELIO [*fl.* 1605] Gerocomica. Sive,
De senum regimine. Opus non modo philosophis &
medicis gratum, sed omnibus hominibus utile . . .
Venetiis, Apud Franciscum Ciottum, 1606.

II, [17], 292 p. 21 cm. [**334**]
—Copy 2.
With this is bound Casaleno, G.A. Disputatio. Venetiis, 1605.

ANSORG, PHILIPPUS [*fl.* 1632] *respondent. See*
SEBISCH, M. [1578–1674?] *praeses.* Galeni Ars parva in
disputationes triginta resoluta. 1633.

An ANSWER to the pretended refutation of Dr.
Olyphant's [i.e. Charles Oliphant] defence. Edinburgh, Printed by J. W. for Thomas Carruthers,
1699.

14 p. 16 cm. [**335**]

ANTARVETUS, JOANNES, *pseud. See* RIOLAN,
Jean [1580–1657]

ANTERO MARIA DA SAN BONAVENTURA
[1620–1686] Li lazaretti della città, e riviere di Genova
del MDCLVII. Ne quali oltre á successi particolari
del contagio si narrano l'opere virtuose de quelli che
sacrificorno se stessi alla salute del prossimo, e si
danno le regole di ben governare un popolo flagellato
dalla peste . . . Genova, Pietro Giovanni Calenzani
e Francesco Meschini, 1658.

[16], 560, [32] p. 21 cm. [**336**]

ΑΝΘΟΛΟΓΊΑ; seu, Selecta quaedam poemata
Italorum qui Latine scripserunt . . . Londini, Impensis R. Green, & F. Hicks, bibliopolarum Can-
tabrigiensium, 1684.

[9], 216 p. 16 cm. [**337**]
First preliminary leaf (blank) wanting.
Supposedly edited by Thomas Power.

"Hieronymi Fracastorii Siphylis [sic], sive morbus Gallicus": p. 40-77. Includes also letters from Girolamo Fracastoro.

Published in 1740 under title: Selecta poemata Italorum.

Baumgartner—Fulton 16a.

ANTHONY, FRANCIS [1550-1623] The apologie, or defence of a verity heretofore published concerning a medicine called aurum potabile, that is, the pure substance of gold, prepared, and made potable and medicinable without corrosives, helpefully given for the health of man in most diseases . . . London, John Legatt, 1616.

[6], 126 p. 18 cm. [**338**]

STC 666.

—[Latin tr.] Panacea aurea sive tractatus duo de ipsius auro potabili, nunc primum in Germania ex Londinensi exemplari excusi, opera M. B. F. B. . . . Hamburgi, Ex Bibliopolio Frobeniano, 1618.

[16], 205 p. 17 cm. [**339**]

"Medicinae chymicae, et veri potabilis auri assertio . . . "; p. 1-57: "Apologia veritatis illucescentis, pro auro potabili . . .": p. 59-199.

—Aurum-potabile. *In* Collectanea chymica. 1684.

—*See* GWINNE, M. Aurum non aurum. 1613; RAWLIN, T. Admonitio pseudo-chymicis. 1610?

ANTHORA; das ist, Gifft-heil. 1677. *See* FELGENHAUER, P.

ANTHROPOLOGIE abstracted; or, The idea of humane nature reflected in briefe philosophicall, and anatomicall collections . . . London, Printed for Henry Herringman, 1655.

[7], 201 (i.e. 191) p. 18 cm. [**340**]

ANTICLAUDIANUS. *See* ALANUS, *Bp. of Auxerre* [d. 1212]

ANTIDOTARII Romani; seu, De modo componendi medicamenta quę sunt in usu . . . Mediolani, Apud Hieronymum Bordonum, 1607.

[16], 152 ll. 16 cm. [**341**]

Compiled by the Collegio dei medici at Rome.

Published in Rome in 1583 under the present title. Published in Venice in 1585 under title: Antidotarium Romanum. Later editions containing the Latin text with an Italian translation were published under title: Antidotario romano.

ANTIDOTARIO romano commentato dal dott. Pietro Castello. 1648. *See* CASTELLI, P.

ANTIDOTARIO romano latino e volgare. Tradotto da Ippolito Ceccarelli . . . Con l'aggiunta dell'elettione de' semplici, e prattica delle compositioni. E due trattati, uno de la teriaca romana, e ragione de suoi ingredienti. L'altro de la teriaca egittia . . . Roma, Ad istanza di Gio. Angelo Ruffinelli, stampato da Andrea Fei, 1624.

[24], 232 p. 22 cm. [**342**]

Compiled by the Collegio dei medici at Rome.

"Trattato de la teriaca egittia" (p. 179-191) is a translation of Prosper Alpini's De medicina Aegyptiorum, book 4, chapters 8-12.

"Ricette aggionte dall'autore" (p. 174-178), "Conditioni e regole appartenenti al buon spetiale" (p. 192-197) and "Sommario dell'elettione de semplici" (p. 197-232) are by Ippolito Ceccarelli.

—[The same.] . . . Aggiontovi in questa ultima impressione le avertenze, & osservationi appartenenti alla compositione de medicamenti del sig. Lodovico Settala . . . Milano, Giov. Battista Bidelli, 1635.

[19], 232; [8], 126 p. 23 cm. [**343**]

The first part ([19], 232 p.) is mainly a reprint of the 1624 edition.

"Avertenze et osservationi . . . tradotte dal nono libro delle osservatione del sig. Lodovico Settala . . . da Alessandro Tadino" ([8], 126 p. at end) has special title page with imprint: Milano, Stampa Ambrosiana, 1630.

—[The same.] . . . Con le annotationi del sig. Pietro Castelli . . . E nuova aggiunta di molte ricette ultimamente publicate dal Collegio de' medici di Roma . . . Roma, Appresso Pietro Antonio Facciotti, ad instanza di Pompilio Totti, 1639.

[20], 359, [1] p. 23 cm. [**344**]

Without L. Settala's "Avertenze et osservationi."

—[The same.] . . . In questa nova impressione accresciuto con l'aggiunta del Memoriale calendario per li spetiali, e lista rerum petendarum [di Pietro Castelli] . . . Roma, Gioseppe Corvo e Bartolomeo Lupardi, 1675.

[28], 363, 30, [3] p. 21 cm. [**345**]

"Memoriale per lo spetiale romano" and "Calendario" (30 p., with special title page) are by Pietro Castelli.

—[The same.] . . . Venetia, Cio. Francesco Valvasense, 1678.

[24], 335 p. 22 cm. [**346**]

"Memoriale per lo spetiale romano" and "Calendario" (p. [307]-332, with special title page) are by Pietro Castelli.

ANTIDOTARIUM Bononiense. 1641. *See* UNIVERSITÀ DI BOLOGNA. Collegio de medicina.

ANTIDOTARIUM Bononiense novissimum. 1674. *See* Università di Bologna. Collegio de medicina.

ANTIDOTARIUM Florentinum. *See* FEDELISSIMI, R. Enchiridion pharmaceuticum medicamentorum omnium. 1617.

ANTIDOTUM melancholiae; vel, Schola curiositatis, omnibus hypochondriacis & atrabili laborantibus, sive fratribus spleneticis & melancholicis, vulgo denen Miltzbrüdern, aperta . . . Francofurti, Impensis Joannis Bencardi, 1670.

[10], 199 p. 14 cm. [347]

Added engraved title page: Schola curiositatis; sive, Antidotum melancholiae joco serium.

ANTIGONUS OF CARYSTUS [3d cent. B.C.] Historiarum mirabilium collectanea. Joannes Meursius recensuit, & notas addidit. Lugduni Batavorum, Apud Isaacum Elzevirium, 1619.

[8], 210, [1] p. 19 cm. [348]

Contains the Greek text with the Latin translation by Gulielmus Xylander.

L'ANTIMOINE purifié sur la sellette. Paris, Nicolas Pepinglé, 1668.

[6], 53 p. 17 cm. [349]

ANTISCORBUTICK and catholick medicines. *In* Maynwaring, E. Morbus polyrhizos et polymorphaeus. 1666.

ANTOINE, Dominique [17th–18 cent.] Methode pour conserver la santé: suivant le cours des saisons, et des differens temperamens; et le moyen de les connoistre . . . Paris, Barthelemy Girin, 1699.

2 v. in 1. 17 cm. [350]

ANTON, Paul [1661–1730] *praeses.* Exercitationem historicam de circumcisione gentilium . . . subjiciunt M. Paulus Antonius, Z. L. praeses & respondens Godofredus Weissius . . . Lipsiae, Typis Christophori Güntheri [1682]

[32] p. 19 cm. [351]

Diss.—Leipzig (G. Weiss, *respondent*)

ANTONI, Sámuel [*fl.* 1694] *respondent. See* Schmid, J.A., *praeses.* Medicinam affectuum . . . proponent . . . S.A. 1694.

ANTONIUS, Paulus. *See* Anton, Paul [1661–1730]

ANTONIUS, Wilhelm [*d.* 1611] *ed. See* Mizauld, A. Centuriae IX. 1613.

ANTONIUS DE ABBATIA. *See* Abbatia, Antonius de.

ANTWERP. Ordinances, local laws, etc. Gheboden ende uyt-gheroepen by mijne heeren, den onderschouteth, borghermeesteren, schepenen, ende raedt der stadt van Antwerpen, op den 31. Julij, 1646 . . . [Antwerpen, 1646?]

[1] p. 28 cm. [352]

Signed at end: P. van Valckenissen.

—Gheboden ende uyt-gheroepen by mijne heeren, den schouteth, borgher-meesteren, schepenen, ende raedt der stadt van Antwerpen, op den 9. October, 1647 . . . [Antwerpen, 1647?]

[1] p. 28 cm. [353]

Signed at end: G. de Weerdt.

—Gheboden ende uyt-gheroepen by mijne heeren den schouteth, borgher-meesteren, schepenen, ende raedt der stadt van Antwerpen, op den 31 Julij 1668 . . . [Antwerpen, 1668?]

[1] p. 28 cm. [354]

Signed at end: A. van Valckenisse.

Text differs from other ordinance issued on the same day.

—Gheboden ende uyt-gheroepen by mijne heeren den schouteth, borgher-meesteren, schepenen, ende raedt der stadt van Antwerpen, op den 31. Julij 1668 . . . [Antwerpen, 1668?]

[1] p. 28 cm. [355]

Signed at end: A. van Valckenisse.

Text differs from other ordinance issued on the same day.

ANTWOORD op seker boekjen, rakende de genesinge van een hooft-wonde, voorgevallen binnen de stad Delet, en geintituleerd, Attestatie van de Faculteyt in de medicine binnen de stadt Leyden . . . [n. p.] 1687.

[8], 37, [3] p. 21 cm. [356]

Concerns controversy with Jan de Geus.

APARISIUS. *See* Parisius [*fl.* 1620]

APELLES, *pseud. See* Scheiner, Christoph, *Father* [1575–1650]

APFFELSTATT, Johann Konrad [*fl.* 1685–1686] *respondent.* Disputatio medica inauguralis de anorexia . . . Lugduni Batavorum, Apud Abrahamum Elzevier, 1686.

[8] p. 23 cm. [357]

Imperfect: title page and last leaf mutilated.
Diss.—Leyden.

—*See* Franck von Franckenau, G., *praeses.* Disputationem medicam ordinariam de coryza . . . proponet . . . J.K.A. 1685.

APHRODISAEUS, Alexander. *See* Alexander, *of Aphrodisias.*

APIN, JOHANN LUDWIG [1668–1703] Febris epidemicae, anno 1694. & 95. in Noricae ditionis oppido Herspruccensi & vicino tractu grassari deprehensae, tandemque petechialis redditae, historica relatio, in observationum semicenturiam digesta, praevioque discursu, morbi aetiologiam & curandi rationem novam, eam vero expeditissimam complexo, illustrata publicaeque nunc luci exposita ... Noribergae, Sumptibus Andreae Ottonis Swobaci, Literis Mauritii Hagen, 1697.

    [16], 312 (i.e. 310), [1] p.   17 cm.   [**358**]
Errata: [1] p. at end.

— respondent. See BRUNO, J. P., *praeses*. Aeolus microcosmo commodans & incommodans. 1687.

APOLLINARIS, QUINTUS, *pseud. See* RYFF, Walther Hermenius [*d.* 1548]

APOLLO mathematicus. 1695. *See* [EIZAT, Sir E.]

APOLOGIA pro Hippocratis et Galeni medicina. 1603. *See* [RIOLAN, J., 1580–1657]

APOMASAR. *See* AḤMAD IBN SĪRĪN [*fl.* 813–833]

APPEL, JOHANN DANIEL [*fl.* 1687] *respondent. See* LIMMER, C.P., *praeses*. Collegii Physici disputatorii disputatio duodecima. 1687.

APPEL, PETER [*fl.* 1674] *respondent. See* FRANCK VON FRANCKENAU, G., *praeses*. Disputationem inauguralem qua febris militum diaetetica, vulgo die bissher grassirende Hitzige Kranckheit ... pertractatur examinandam propono ... Petrus Appel. 1674.

APPENDIX bibliothecae medico philosophico philologicae. 1680. *See* FARNESIUS, G.T.

APPENDIX consilii antipodagrici specialis darinnen X consilia specialissima. 1625. *See* [PANSA, M.]

An APPENDIX to Solomon's prescription for the removal of the pestilence. 1667. *See* MEAD, M.

APPLAUSUS gratulatori honoribus ... Joh. Jacobi Schychzeri ... medicinae doctor rite designaretur. Erecti ab amicis et conterraneis. Lugduni Batavorum, Apud viduam & haeredes Johannis Elsevirii, 1669.

    [12] p.   23 cm.   [**359**]

APPONUS, PETRUS. *See* ABANO, Pietro d' [1250–1315?]

APPROBIRTE Land-und Feld-Apothecken; das ist, Allerhand innerliche und äusserliche Kranckheiten, sie entstehen bey dem Menschen zufälliger oder gewaltsamer Weise, ihrem Unterscheid nach, zu erkennen, und leicht und gewiss ... zu curiren, entweder Galenice oder Hermetice und magice. Nebst einen Anhang, zu welcher Zeit die Wund-Kräuter sollen eingesamlet werden ... Durch einen der Medicin Erfahrnen G. O. F. Franckfurt am Mayn, Philipp Fievet, 1690.

    115 p.   14 cm.   [**360**]
Bound with Loss, L. Chirurgisches Hand-Büchlein. [1682]

APROSIO, Angelico [1607–1681] La grillaia curiosita erudite. Di Scipio Clareano [pseud. i.e. Angelico Aprosio] Napoli, Novello de Bonis, 1668.

    [22], 584, [4] p.   16 cm.   [**361**]

A PUTEO, ZACCHARIAS [*fl.* 1611] Clavis medica rationalis spagyrica, et chyrurgica; quae in tractatu consultorio de stranguria, pruritu, & herpete exedente varia ... recludit praesidia ... Cui additur ... Consultatio responsiva Hieronymi Venerosii ... Venetiis, Apud typographum Leonis Aureati, 1612.

    [24], 306 p.; [15] p.; [40] p.; [72] p.   illus.   21 cm.   [**362**]
Errata: p. [69–72]
Part [2] has special title page: Hieronymi Venerosii ... Consultatio responsiva ... Venetiis, Ad officinam Leonis Aurati, 1611.
Part [3] has special title page: Officina chymica fornacium, vasorum, ac instrumentorum ad destillationem pertinentium, per Zacchariam a Puteo ... collecta. Venetiis, Ad bibliothecam Leonis Aurati, 1611.
The illustrations which form part [3] are reproductions of those originally published in Biringucci's Pirotechnia, in Venice, in 1540.

AQUA salsa dulcorata. 1683. *See* FITZGERALD, R.

AQUAPENDENTE, HIERONYMUS FABRICIUS AB. *See* FABRICIUS, Hieronymous, *ab Aquapendente* [*ca.* 1533–1619]

AQUENZA Y MOSSA, PEDRO [*fl.* 1696–1726] De sanguinis missione libri IV. contra Eraxistratei-Portiani dialogos IV. quibus accedunt fracmentum [sic] ad doctrinam de venae sectione pertinens, atque historia quaedam de veneni exhibiti suspitione ... Matriti, Typis Emmanuelis Ruiz, 1696.

    [24], 351, [15] p.   16 cm.   [**363**]

AQUILA, H., Thuringus, Doctrina singularis. *In* [COMBACH, L.] *ed.* and *tr.* Tractatus. 1647.

AQUIILANO, Sebastiano [*d.* 1543] De febre sanguinis. *In* Gatinaria, M. De medendis humani corporis malis practica. 1604.

AQUIN, Pierre d'. *See* Daquin, Pierre [*fl.* 1673–1696]

AQUINAS, Thomas, *Saint. See* Thomas Aquinas, *Saint* [1225?–1274]

AQUITANUS, Barnardus Georgius Londrada a Portu. *See* Penot, Bernard Georges [*d.* 1617?]

ARANTIUS, Julius Caesar. *See* Aranzi, Giulio Cesare [1530–1589]

ARANZI, Giulio Cesare [1530–1589] De humano foetu libellus. *In* Plazzoni, F. De partibus generationi inservientibus. 1664.

—In librum Hippocratis De vulneribus capitis commentarius. Cum Claudii Porralii annotationibus marginalibus. Lugduni Batavorum, Ex officina Joannis Maire, 1639.

179 p. 14 cm. [**364**]

"De contusis puerorum capitibus praetermissa ab Hip.": p. 172–179.
Includes Latin text of De capitis vulneribus.

—*See* Scholtz, L. Consiliorum medicinalium . . . liber singularis. 1610 [and] Epistolarum philosophicarum: medicinalium, ac chymicarum . . . volumen. 1610.

ARAS, Georgius [*fl.* 1666] Enchiridion hermetico medicum. In quo virtutes, doses, atque appropriationes omnium fere medicamentorum spagyricorum . . . describuntur . . . Venetiis, Apud Jo. Jacobum Hertz, 1666.

6, 100 p. 15 cm. [**365**]

ARBERIUS. La physique d'uzage; contenant avec Un discours géneral sur la médecine, La description du corps humain per Mr Arberius. Puis l'explication des maladies, & de leurs remédes, tirée des principes de la méchanique, & de la philosophie de Mr Descartes, par M^rs d'Orlix & Plempius . . . Paris, Pierre Aubouin, et Philippe d'Arbisse, 1664.

[10], 91 p.; [1], 73, [1] p. 15 cm. [**366**]

Part [1], has half title: Discours sur la medecine & sur les parties du corps humain composé en Latin par Mr Arberius, et traduit en françois par D. R. Part [2] has half title: Theses de Louvain, soutenues sous M^rs d'Orlix & Plempius [traduit par D. R.]

Attributed to Louis Henry Rouviére by BNC based on Barbier (p. 883, vol. 3) but Bouvet (p. 5) denies this attribution.

—*See* Nouveau cours de medecine. 1669, 1683.

ARCAEUS, Franciscus. *See* Arceo, Francisco [1494–1575]

ARCANA Petri Poterii . . . Inventa chymica. 1700. *See* [Ettner, J. C. von]

ARCANGELI, Lodovico [*fl.* 1616] *ed. See* Colle, G. De omnibus malignis, et pestilentibus affectionibus, & earum medela. 1616.

ARCANGELO ROMANO [*fl.* 17th cent.] De infirmitatibus humanae vitae, compendium medicinae, in quo declaratur quid sit unaquaeque infirmitas, unde proveniant ipsae infirmitates, quos effectus producant, & assignantur simplicia, & domestica, quae eis prosunt . . . Romae, Apud Franciscum Caballum, 1643.

[16], 192 p. 17 cm. [**367**]

With this is bound his Remedii semplici, e familiari. 1643.

—[The same.] . . . Cum nova aditione . . . Romae, Typis Manelphi Manelphii, 1648.

220 p. 15 cm. [**368**]

With this is bound his Remedii semplici, e familiari. 1648.

—Remedii semplici, e familiari, utili per l'infirmità dell' humana vita . . . Roma, Francesco Cavalli, 1643.

167, [1] p. 17 cm. [**369**]

Bound with his De infirmitatibus humanae vitae. 1643.

—[The same] . . . Raccolti insieme con nuova addittione . . . Roma, Manelfo Manelfi, 1648.

168, [8] p. 15 cm. [**370**]

Bound with his De infirmitatibus humanae vitae. 1648.

ARCANUM; or, The grand secret of Hermetick philosophy. 1650. *In* Dee, A. Fasciculus chemicus. 1650.

ARCANUM Hermeticae philosophiae opus. *In* Aubigné de la Fosse, N. Bibliotheca chemica. 1653; [Espagnet, J. d'] Enchiridion physicae restitutae. 1623, 1647.

ARCASIO, Francesco [*fl.* 1630] Discorso . . . sopra la preserva, et cura della contagione. Raccolto dalla dottrina, & esperienza di molti gravi autori . . . Tradotto in volgare da un amico . . . Genova, Giuseppe Pavoni, 1630.

36, [1] p. 15 cm. [**371**]

ARCEO, Francisco [1494-1575] De recta curandorum vulnerum ratione et aliis ejus artis praeceptis libri II . . . Ejusdem De febrium curandarum ratione. Amstelodami, Ex officina Petri vanden Berge, 1658.

[24], 311 p.   14 cm.   [*372*]

Added engraved title page.
Edited by Benedictus Arias Montanus.
With annotations by Alvaro Nuñez.

—[Dutch tr.] Kortbondige, ende rechte middel, en kunst; om allerhande zoorten van wonden op de kortste ende zeekerste manier te geneezen . . . in't Latijn beschreeven . . . Met aanteekeningen op een yeder hooftdeel verrijkt, ende overgezet door Jacobus Geusius . . . Leeuwarden, Yvo Takes Wielsma, 1667.

[24] 339, [2], 59, [3] p.   plate.   14 cm [*373*]

With annotations by Alvaro Nuñez.
"Wonderlijke ende uytneemende aanmerkingen van alderhande zoorten van wonden, ende der zelver geneezinge, uyt verscheyden van de vermaarste wondheelers te zaamen getrokken, ende in de Nederduytsche taale overgezet door Jacobus Geusius": [2], 59 p. at end has half title.

—*See* Héry, T. de. La methode curatoire de la maladie venerienne. 1634.

ARCERIUS, Sixtus [*ca.* 1570-1623] *ed.* and *tr. See* Galenus. [Selections, etc. Latin.] Ad artium liberalium studium capescendum oratio adhortaria. 1616.

ARCHANGELUS ROMANUS. *See* Arcangelo Romano [*fl.* 17th cent.]

ARCHANGELUS, Ludovicus. *See* Arcangeli, Lodovico [*fl.* 1616].

ARCHER, John [*fl.* 1660-1684] Every man his own doctor, compleated with an herbal: shewing first, how every one may know his own constitution and complection, by certain signs. Also the nature . . . of all foods . . . The second part shews the full knowledge and cure of the pox . . . The 2d ed., with additions . . . London, Printed for the author, 1673.

[15], 127, 143, [8] p.   17 cm.   [*374*]

"Three experiments and inventions of the authors . . .": p. [3-8] at end.
Part 2, and the Herbal have special title pages. The Herbal has imprint: Printed by E. C. for the author.

—Secrets disclosed, of consumptions; shewing, how to distinguish between the scurvy and venereal disease: also how to prevent and cure the fistula by chymical drops, without cutting . . . London, Printed for the author, 1684.

[6], 70, [2] p.   19 cm.   [*375*]

ARCHIMEDES, *pseud. See* Pitcairne, Archibald [1652-1713]

ARCHIOSPIDALE dell' incurabili di Roma. *See* Ospedale di San Giacomo in Augusta, Rome.

ARCIÑEGA, Francisco Vélez de. *See* Vélez de Arciniega, Francisco [*fl.* 1593-1613]

ARCIOSPEDALE di San Giacomo in Augusta. *See* Ospedale di San Giacomo in Augusta, Rome.

ARCISSEWSKI, Christophorus. *See* Arciszewski, Krzysztof [*fl.* 1643]

ARCISZEWSKI, Krzysztof [*fl.* 1643] *ed. See* Cnöffel, A. Epistola de podagra. 1643, 1644.

ARCULARIUS, Joannes Henricus [*fl.* 1632] *respondent. See* Sebisch, M. [1578-1674?] *praeses.* Galeni Ars parva in disputationes triginta resoluta. 1633.

ARDENSBACH, Wenceslas Maximilian [17th cent.] Armamentarium antiloimicum; das ist, Ein eingerichtes Pest-Zeüg-Hauss, in welchem unterschiedliche Waffen, den grausammen Menschen-Feind die Pest, zu vertilligen, sich zu verfechten auffbehalten werden . . . Ollmütz, Johann Joseph Kylian, 1679.

[6], 151 p.   13 cm.   [*376*]

ARDERNE, James [1636-1691] *See* Stubbs, H. A censure upon certain passages contained in the history of the Royall Society. 1671.

ARDIZZONE, Fabrizio [17th cent.] Ravivamento, o sia discorso dimostrativo . . . sopra l'essenza, caose, & effetti dell'acque minerali singolarmente del Monte di Corsena . . . Genova, Guiseppe Bottari, 1680.

[14], 180 (i.e. 160) p.   23 cm.   [*377*]

—Ricordi . . . intorno al preservarsi, e curarsi dalla peste . . . Genova, Gio: Maria Farroni, 1656.

[18], 136, [6] p.   21 cm.   [*378*]

Errata: p. [4-6] at end.

AREND, Johann Georg [*fl.* 1669-1675] *respondent* Disputatio medica inauguralis de cephalalgia . . .

Lugduni Batavorum, Apud viduam & heredes Johannis Elsevirii, 1675.

[14] p.   24 cm.   [379]

Diss.—Leyden.

ARENS, JOHANN ANTON [*fl.* 1698] *respondent. See* HEIMREICH, J., *praeses.* Dissertatio physica de chylificatione. 1698.

ARENS, JOHANN GEORG [*fl.* 1671] *respondent. See* SCHENCK, J. T., *praeses.* Trigam simplicium medicamentorum illustrem: fermentantium, sedativorum, et praecipitantium ... subjicit ... J. G. A. 1671.

ARETAEUS. Ἰατρικά. Aetiologica, simeiotica et therapeutica morborum acutorum & diuturnorum ... Graece & Latine conjunctim edita. Tribus MSS. codicibus, Veneto, Bavarico, Augustano collatis. Cum commentario, quo obscura doctrina de nominibus & parte affecta morborum singulorum cum suis signis perspicua methodo illustratur, auctore Georgio Henischio ... Augustae Vindelicorum, Sumptibus Georgii Willeri, apud Davidem Francum, 1603.

[20], 446, [16] p.   32 cm.   [380]

Latin translation by Giunio Paolo Grassi.

Where the text of Aretaeus is defective, the editor has inserted excerpts from Galen, Alexander Trallianus, and especially Paulus Aegineta.

—Libri septem. Nunc in primum e tenebris eruti. A Junio Paulo Crasso ... accuratissime in Latinum sermonem versi. Ed. novissima. Patavii, Typis Petri Mariae Frambotti, 1700.

[8], 280 p.   17 cm.   [381]

Reprint of the Venice edition of 1552. Contains the 4 books of the De causis et signis acutorum et diuturnorum morborum and 3 books of the De curatione acutorum et diuturnorum morborum, with chapters 12 and 13 only of the 2d book of the De curatione diuturnorum morborum; lacks the 5 additional chapters printed in the Paris edition of 1554.

—*See* ROLFINCK, W. Epitome methodi cognoscendi & curandi particulares corporis affectus. 1655, 1675.

ARGENTERIO, GIOVANNI [1513–1572] Opera nunquam excusa, jamdiu desiderata, ac e tenebris in lucem prodita. In duas partes distincta. Quarum prior commentarios in Hippocratis Aphorismorum primam, secundam, & quartam sectiones plus sex, & triginta annorum spatio elaboratos: altera vero De febribus tractatum singularem: & primi libri [GALENI] ad Glauconem praeclaras explanationes:

item De calidi significationibus, ac calido nativo doctissimum libellum complectitur ... Cum indice rerum, ac sententiarum insignium locupletissimo ... Venetiis, Apud Juntas, 1606.

2 v. in 1.   32 cm.   [382]

Vol. 2 has title: ... Operum nunquam excusorum ... pars altera. Each part is separately indexed.

The commentaries on Hippocrates' Aphorismi include the Latin text of books 1, 2, and 4 in Niccolò Leoniceno's version. The commentaries on Galen's De febribus ad Glauconem include an incomplete Latin text of book 1, and are followed by additional material on fever by Argenterio.

—Opera ... Quorum nonnulla jam ante excusa ... ab haeredibus ipsius reperta & in lucem prolata sunt. Omnia nunc pridem ex exemplari Veneto diligentius revisa, ex divisis quatuor partibus in unum volumen collecta, ac ab innumeris ... mendis emaculata ... Accessit ad haec Fabii Paulini ... in libros Artis medicinalis Galeni per tabulas oeconomia ... Hanoviae, Typis Wechelianis apud haeredes Claudii Marnii, 1610.

[23] p., 2598 col., [28] p.   37 cm.   [383]

Edited by Peter Uffenbach.

"In Claudii Galeni Pergameni, Artem medicinalem commentarii [I–III]" (col. 1–760) include the Greek text and Latin version of Galen's Ars medica. "In lib. I [II, IV] Aphoris[morum] Hippocr[atis] comment[arii]" (col. 761–1420) include the Greek text and Niccolò Leoniceno's Latin version. "Comment[arii] in libr. Gal. de febribus ad Glauconem" (col. 2321–2568) include a partial Greek text and Latin version of Galenus' De methodo medendi ad Glauconem.

—De urinis liber. Lipsiae, Johann Christ. Wohlfart, 1682.

92, [2] p.   16 cm.   [384]

—*See* HOFMANN, C. Rejectanea pathologica. 1639.

ARGENTIER, GIOVANNI. *See* ARGENTERIO, Giovanni [1513–1572]

ARGOLI, ANDREA [1570–1657] De diebus criticis et de aegrorum decubitu libri duo. Patavii, Apud Paulum Frambottum, 1639.

2 v. in 1.   illus.   22 cm.   [385]

Engraved title page.

With this is bound Zacchia, P. De mali hipochondriaci libri due. 1639.

—[The same.] Ab auctore denuo recogniti, ac altera parte auctiores, paeneque novi. Patavii, Apud Paulum Frambottum, 1652.

2 v. in 1.   21 cm.   [386]

Continuous pagination.

Vol. 2 dated 1651.

ARGONAUTA, *pseud. See* FEHR, Johann Michael [1610–1688]

ARGUMENTORUM ludicrorum et amoenitatum scriptores varii ... Lugduni Batavorum, Godefridus Basson, 1623.

[8], 318 (i.e. 320), 143 p.   15 cm.   **[387]**

In 1638 published under title: Dissertationum ludicrarum et amoenitatum, scriptores varii.

Includes Wilibald Pirckheimer's Laus podagrae.

ARIAS MONTANUS, BENEDICTUS [1527–1598] *ed. See* ARCEO, F. De recta curandorum vulnerum ratione. 1658.

ARIOSTO, FRANCESCO [*fl.* 1460] De oleo montis Zibinii, seu petroleo agri Mutinensis libellus ... editus ab Oligero Jacobaeo ... Nunc autem ad fidem codicis MS. ex bibliotheca Estensi recognitus, & recusus, adjecta ejusdem argumenti epistola Bernardini Ramazzini ... Mutinae, Typis Antonii Capponi, 1698.

[8], 67, [3], 35 p.   15 cm.   **[388]**

ARISLAEUS. *See* ARISLEUS.

ARISLAUS. *See* GRATAROLI, Guglielmo [1516–1568]

ARISLEUS. *See* Turba philosophorum. 1610, 1660; [German ed.] 1613.

ARISTHEUS. *See* ARISLEUS.

ARISTOTELES. Τὰ σωζόμενα. Operum Aristotelis ... nova editio, Graece & Latine ... Adscriptis ad oram libri ... emendationibus: in quibus plurimae nunc primum in lucem prodeunt, ex bibliotheca Isaaci Casauboni ... Accesserunt huic editioni Kyriaci Strozae Libri duo politicorum Graeco Latini ... Genevae, Apud Petrum de la Roviere, 1605 [1606]

2 v.   40 cm., 38 cm.   **[389]**

—[De anima. Greek] *In* Guarinoni, C. Sententiarum Aristotelis de anima seu mente humana interpretatio. 1601.

—[Latin tr.] *In* Universidade de Coimbra. Collegium Conimbricense Societatis Jesu. Commentarii Collegii Conimbricensis Societatis Jesu, in tres libros De anima Aristotelis. 1606.

—[The same, *as subject.*] *See* RINALDINI, C. Pagina. 1689.

—[De animalium historia. Greek and Latin] Περὶ ζώων ισγορίας ... Historia de animalibus, Julio Caesare Scaligero interprete, cum ejusdem commentariis. Philippus Jacobus Maussacus ... opus ... primus vulgavit & restituit, additis Prolegomenis & Animadversionibus. Accedit Fragmentum quod decimus historiarum inscribitur ... Tolosae, Apud Dominicum & Petrum Bosc [Apud Raymundum Colomerium] 1619.

[31], 1248, [23] p.   illus.   36 cm.   **[390]**

—[De coloribus. Latin.] *In* Joannes Actuarius De urinis libri VII. 1670; Willich, J. Exercitationes et probationes de urinis libri IV. 1688.

—[De generatione et corruptione. Latin.] In Universidade de Coimbra. Collegium Conimbricense Societatis Jesu. Commentarii Collegii Conimbricensis, e Societate Jesu, in duos libros De generatione & corruptione, Aristotelis. 1616.

—[The same, *as subject.*] Díaz de los Llanos, F. De generatione, et corruptione tractatus. 1699; Wangnereck, H., *praeses.* Conclusiones philosophicae ex libris De generatione [Aristotelis] 1628.

—[De lapide philosophico. Latin.] Tractatulus ... de practica lapidis philosophici ... [&] Avicenna De congelatione & conglutinatione lapidum.

232–245 p., vol. 1.   17 cm.   (In Artis auriferae. Basileae, 1610).   **[391]**

Caption title.

The second treatise is an Arabic alchemistic commentary appended in Arabic-Latin versions to the fourth book of the Meteorologica of Aristotle and published repeatedly as a work by Avicenna under titles: De mineralibus, and De congelatione et conglutinatione lapidum. The translation is by Alfredus Anglicus.

—[German tr.] Tractälein [sic] oder Büchlein von der Practica dess philosophischen Steines.

310–321 p., part 1.   19 cm.   (In Morgenstern, Philipp, *ed.* and *tr.* Turba philosophorum. Basel, 1613)   **[392]**

Caption title.

—[Metaphysica. Greek and Latin.] Commentarii Joannis Ludovici Havenreuteri ... In libros Metaphysicorum Aristotelis Stagiritae sex priores ... Francofurti, E collegio Musarum Paltheniano, 1604.

[16], 597, [2] p.   17 cm.   **[393]**

—[The same, *as subject.*] *See* MAGIRUS, J. Physiologiae peripateticae libri sex. 1610, 1616, 1618, 1619, 1638, 1642.

—[Parva naturalia.] *See* WANGNERECK, H. Conclusiones selectae ex Parvis naturalibus Aristotelis. 1628.

—[Physica. Bk. I. Greek, Latin, and French] *In* Cureau de la Chambre, M. Novae methodi pro explanandis Hippocrate & Aristotele specimen. 1655, 1662.

—[The same, *as subject*] *See* CASE, J. Lapis philosophicus. 1629.

—[Physiognomonica. Latin] Phisiognomia . . . ordine compositorio edita, ad facilitatem doctrinae. Commentariis illustrata . . . Studio & labore D. J. Fontani . . . Parisiis, Apud Joannem Paquet, 1611.
     171 (i.e. 163) p.   17 cm.   **[394]**

—[Problemata. Greek and Latin] *In* Guastavino, G. Commentarii in priores decem Aristotelis Problematum sectiones. 1608.

—[Latin tr.] Aristotelis, aliorumque philosophorum, ac medicorum problemata, ad varias quaestiones & philosophiam naturalem cognoscendas in primis utilia. Adjunctis Hippocratis . . . Aphorismorum libris septem . . . Duaci, Apud Gerardum Patte, 1631.
     237 p.   15 cm.   **[395]**
   Imperfect: p. 165-168 mutilated.
   "Marci Antonii Zimarae . . . Problematum liber unus": p. [93]-137; "Alexandri Aphrodisei super nonnullis physicis dubitationibus solutionum liber, Angelo Politiano interprete": p. 138-192; "Hippocratis Coi liber Aphorismorum, Jano Cornario . . . interprete": p. 193-237.

—[English tr.] The problems of Aristotle, with other philosophers and physitians. Wherein are contained, divers questions with their answers, touching the estate of mans body. London, Printed for W. K., 1670.
     [143] p.   16 cm.   **[396]**
   This translation first published in London in 1595.
   "Marcus Antonius Zimaras Sanctipertias his problems": p. [78-100]; "Alexander Aphrodiseus, his problems": p. [101-143]

—[The same.] . . . London, Printed for J. Wright and R. Chiswell, and sold by John Smith, 1684.
     [144] p.   16 cm.   **[397]**
   A reprint of the 1670 edition.

—[French tr.] Les problemes d'Aristote et autres philosophes et medecins, selon la composition du corps humain. Avec ceux de A. Zimara. Rouen, Nicolas Angot, 1618.
     152 (i.e. 142), [1] ll.   14 cm.   **[398]**

These translations by George de La Bouthière were previously published in Lyons in 1554, with the addition of his French version of the Problemata of Alexander of Aphrodisias.

—[The same.] Les problemes d'Aristote. Oeuvre fort agreable & utile aux chirurgiens; & à tous ceux qui veulent aprendre les admirables secrets de la nature. Rouen, Guillaume Machuel, 1683.
     240 (i.e. 238) p.   14 cm.   **[399]**
   "Les Problèmes de Marc-Antoine Zimara": p. 189-240.

—[German tr.] Problemata Aristotelis; das ist, Gründtliche Erörterung und Aufflösung mancherley zweiffelhafftiger Fragen, des hochberühmbten Aristotelis, und vieler anderer bewehrter Naturkündiger, fast nützlich und kurtzweilig, allerley fürgebrachte Fragen eigentlich und scheinbarlich zu entscheiden. Hamburg, In Verlegung M. Frobenii, 1604.
     [2], 190 p.   16 cm.   **[400]**
   Translation of the complete Problemata attributed to Aristotle, from the ancient Latin version which begins: Omnes homines.
   "Andere fast schöne nutzliche Fragstück, mit derselben Erklärung": p. 138-139.
   "Ausserlesene Fragestücke, Marci Anthonii Zimare": p. 140-190.
   With this is bound Albertus Magnus. Daruth der Fruwens ere Heimlicheit. 1613.

—[The same.] . . . Sammt einem Anhang . . . CIV. Fragstücken Marci Antonii Zimarae . . . Darbey sich dann auch befinden die Problemata Joh. Bodini, von denen Dingen, die am Himmel, in der Lufft, auff und in der Erden sich begeben und zugetragen. Alles in Frag und Antwort gestellt. Basel, Verlag Emanuel Königs und Söhnen, 1679.
     284 p.   17 cm.   **[401]**

—[Adaptations, etc. Italian] *In* Manfredi, G. Libro intitolato Il perche. 1607, 1613, 1667, 1668, 1678.

—[Secretum secretorum. Excerpts] *In* Stefani, G. In Aristotelis libellum [de conservatione sanitatis. 1637].

—*as subject. See* BASSO, S. Philosophiae naturalis adversus Aristotelem libri XII. 1621; BOURDELOT, P. Conversations de l'Academie. 1672; BUONAMICI, F. De alimento libri V. 1603 [colophon 1602]; CREMONINI, C. De calido innato, et semine. 1634; FRANZOSI, G. Tractatus apologeticus de semine pro Aristotele adversus Galenum. 1645; [GRAINDORGE, A.] In fictilem figuli exercitationem de principiis foetus. 1658; HOFMANN, C. De generatione hominis. 1629 [and] De usu lienis, cerebri et de ichoribus. 1639 [and] De usu lienis secundum Aristotelem. 1615 [and] Variarum lectionum lib. VI. 1619; LANCETTA, T. Raccolta medica. 1645; LICETI, F. De natura primo-movente libri duo. 1634; MÜLLER, V., *praeses.* Aristotelis De longitudine et brevitate vitae. 1617; PETIT, P. De motu animalium spontaneo liber unus. 1660; ROSS, A. ARCANA MICROCOSMI. 1651, 1652; SÁNCHEZ, F. Opera medica. 1636 [and] Tractatus philosophici: Quod nihil scitur. 1149 (i.e. 1649); SENNERT, D. De chymicorum cum Aristotelicis et Galenicis consensu ac dissensu liber. 1629, 1655; SEVERINO, M. A. Antiperipatias. 1655–1659; SILATAN, F. L'interprete de la nature. 1655; STEFANI, G. Hippocratis Coi theologia. 1638; UNIVERSIDADE DE COIMBRA. Collegium Conimbricense Societatis Jesu. In libros Ethicorum Aristotelis ad Nicomachum . . . disputationes. 1616.

ARISTOTELES, *alchemist.* Tractatus Aristotelis alchymistae ad Alexandrum Magnum, de lapide philosophico . . .

787–798 p., vol. 5. 20 cm. (*In* Zetzner, Lazarus, *ed.* Theatrum chemicum. Argentorati, 1659–61) [402]

Caption title.

ARISTOTELES master-piece. *See* ARISTOTLE, *pseud.*

ARISTOTLE. *See* ARISTOTELES.

ARISTOTLE, *pseud.* Aristoteles master-piece; or, The secrets of generation displayed in all the parts thereof . . . To which is added . . . the pictures of several monsterous births drawn to the life . . . London, J. How, 1684.

[1], 190, [11] p. front., illus. 15 cm. [403]
Imperfect: p. 65–72 and 101–102 mutilated.

—[The same.] . . . London, Printed, and sold at the Hand and Scepter near Temple-bar, 1692.

[7], 182 p. front., illus. 15 cm. [404]

ARIZZARRA, GIULIO CESARE, *tr. See* GUY DE CHAULIAC. Il maestro in chirurgia. 1697.

ARLENSIS DE SCUDALUPIS, PETRUS. *See* PETRUS ARLENSIS DE SCUDALUPIS.

ARLOTTI, POMPEO [*fl.* 1627] De tempore secandi venam in febribus intermittentibus opportuno. Opinio nova . . . Ubi quam plurima de sanguinis missione . . . proponuntur . . . Regii, Flaminio Bartholo, 1627.

[16], 99, [16] p. 23 cm. [405]
Errata: p. [16] at end.

ARMENGANDUS BLASII [*fl. ca.* 1280–1309] *tr. See* AVICENNA. Avicennae Arabum medicorum principis. 1608.

ARMIN, PHILIP [*fl.* 1650] *tr. See* GLISSON, F. A treatise of the rickets. 1668.

ARNALDUS DE VILLANOVA [*d.* 1313?] Omnia, quae exstant, opera chymica: videlicet, Thesaurus thesaurorum: seu Rosarius philosophorum . . . Lumen novum. Flos florum, & Speculum alchimiae . . . nunc primum ita conjunctim edita, opera & impensis Hieronymi Megiseri . . . Francofurti, Typis Joachimi Bratheringii, 1603.

120; 80 p. 16 cm. [406]
The Speculum alchimiae has special title page with imprint: Francofurti, Ex officina typographica Matthiae Beckeri, 1603.

—Consilium ad regem Aragonum de salubri hortensium usu. In Diocles Carystius. Aurea ad Antigonum regem epistola. 1607; Mizauld, A. Opusculorum pars prima [-secunda] 1607.

—Practica medica . . . Ein fürtreffliche Kunst lang zu leben. In zwey sonderbare Büchlein unterscheyden. Deren erstes ein bewerthes Mittel den menschlichen Leib bey erwünschter Gesundheit, auch ohne Verletzung der Sinne, Verstandts und Gedächtnuss biss auff das höchste Alter zu erhalten. Das ander wie alle des menschlichen Leibs Gebrechen, vom Haupt an biss auff die Fussohlen, zu sampt den viel und mancherley Fiebern, Pestilentz, hinfallenden Seuch, Podagra und sonderlich alle Kinder Kranckheiten zu curieren . . . Franckfurt, Bey Nicolao Steinio, 1619.

310 (i.e. 322), [12] p. 17 cm. [407]
Book 1 is a translation of the author's De conservanda juventute; book 2, a compilation from his medical works, especially the Breviarium practicae medicinae, translated from the Latin.

With this are bound: Albertus Magnus. Von Weiberen und Geburten der Kinder. 1659 —Müller, Balthasar. Ein neuer . . . Tractat von rechtem . . . Gebrauch . . . der . . . distilirten Wasser. 1664.

—Liber perfecti magisterii, qui lumen luminum nuncupatur . . . vocatur etiam flos florum . . . [&] Practica . . . ex libro dicto, Breviarius librorum alchemiae [&] De decoctione lapidis philosophorum, et de regimine ignis . . . [Argentorati, Sumptibus heredum Eberh. Zetzneri, 1659]

128–143 p., vol. 3.   20 cm.   (*In* Zetzner, Lazarus, *ed.* Theatrum chemicum. Argentorati, 1659–61)   [**408**]

Caption titles.

—Quaestiones . . . de arte transmutationis . . . [&] . . . [Novum] Testamentum . . .

151–165 p. and 175–185 p., vol. 3.   17 cm.   (*In* Artis auriferae. Basileae, 1610)   [**409**]

Caption and running titles.

—Regimiento de sanidad. *In* Johannes XXI, *Pope.* Libro de medicina llamado Thesoro de pobres. 1611.

—Rosarium philosophorum [&] . . . Novum lumen [&] . . . Flos florum ad regem Aragonum . . . [&] . . . Epistola super alchimia ad regem Neapolitanum.

253–326 p., vol. 2.   17 cm.   (*In* Artis auriferae. Basileae, 1610)   [**410**]

Caption titles.

—Schatz aller Schätze und das Rosarium der Philosophorum . . . [&] . . . Novum lumen [&] . . . Blum aller Blumen [an den König Aragonum geschrieben][&] Ein Brieff und Epistel . . . uber die Alchimiam, geschrieben an der newstetter König.

369–426 p., part 2.   19 cm.   (*In* Morgenstern, Philipp, *ed.* and *tr.* Turba philosophorum. Basel, 1613)   [**411**]

Caption title.

—Speculum alchmiae . . . [&] Carmen [&] . . . Quaestiones tam essentiales quam accidentales . . . ad Bonifacium Octavum. [Argentorati, Sumptibus heredum Eberh. Zetzneri, 1659]

515–553 p., vol. 4.   20 cm.   (*In* Zetzner, Lazarus, *ed.* Theatrum chemicum. Argentorati, 1659–61)   [**412**]

Caption titles.

—Le tresor des pauvres, auquel sont contenus plusieurs remedes, bruvages, oignements, emplastres, pillules, electuaires, preservatifs, & receptes contre toute sorte de maladies. Fait par maistre Arnoul de Ville-Nove, & autres docteurs en medecine. Paris, Nicolas Lescuyer, 1618.

392, [16] p.   14 cm.   [**413**]

Imperfect: pages 217–240 wanting.

A variant issue of the above is entered as a French translation of Johannes XXI. Thesaurus pauperum . . . in Bibl. Portug. v. 2, p. 338.

—[Excerpts] *In* DOLHOPFF, G. A., *comp.* Lapis animalis microcosmicus. 1681.

—, *ed. See* HYGIEIA. 1628; REGIMEN SANITATIS SALERNITANUM. De conservanda bona valetudine. 1607, 1619; MEDICINA SALERNITANA. 1605, 1611, 1612, 1622, 1624, 1628, 1638; REGIMEN SANITATIS SALERNI; or, The Schooll of Salernes regiment of health. 1617, 1634, 1649; SCHOLA SALERNITANA. 1625, 1649, 1657, 1667, 1672, 1683; [Dutch tr.]: 1658.

—, *tr. See* AVICENNA. Avicennae Arabum medicorum principis. 1608.

— *as subject. See* POPPE, J. Von der gifftigen epidemischen Hauptkranckheit. 1623.

ARNALDUS, *Novicomensis. See* ARNALDUS DE VILANOVA [*d.* 1313?]

ARNAU DE VILANOVA. *See* ARNALDUS DE VILLANOVA [*d.* 1313?]

ARNAUD DE VILLENEUVE. *See* ARNALDUS DE VILLANOVA [*d.* 1313?]

ARNAUD, E. R. [*fl.* 1650] Introduction a la chymie, ou la vraye physique . . . Lyon, Claude Post, 1655.

[40], 112 p.   18 cm.   [**414**]

ARNAULD, PIERRE, *sieur de la Chevallerie, ed.* and *tr.* Trois traitez de la philosophie naturelle non encore imprimez. Scavoir Le secret livre du . . . Artephius, traitant de l'art occulte & transmutation metallique, Latin François. Plus Les figures hierogliphiques de Nicolas Flamel . . . au Cimetiere des Innocens à Paris . . . avec l'explication d'icelles par iceluy Flamel. Ensemble, Le vray livre du docte Synesius . . . sur la mesme subject . . . traduit par P. Arnauld sieur de la Chevallerie Poiteuin . . . Paris, Guillaume Marette, 1612.

103 p.   illus., plate.   22 cm.   [**415**]

ARNAULD DE LA CHEVALLERIE, PIERRE. *See* ARNAULD, Pierre, *sieur de la Chevallerie.*

ARNISAEUS, FRIDERICUS [*fl.* 1623?] *respondent. See* WORM, O. [1588–1654] *praeses.* Disputatio medica de melancholia hypochondriaca. 1623?

ARNISAEUS, HENNING [*d.* 1636?] Disquisitiones de partus humani legitimis terminis. Ejusdemque observationes & controversiae anatomicae. Franco-furti, Apud Johannem Davidem Zunnerum, 1641.

    292 (i.e. 192) p.   13 cm.   **[416]**

—*praes.* Disputatio medica de apoplexia et epilepsia cognoscendis et curandis . . . Francofurti Marchionum, Literis Joannis Eichorn [1610]

    [28] p.   19 cm.   **[417]**
    Diss.—Frankfurt an der Oder (M. Gosky, *respondent*)

—Disputatio medica de lue venerea cognoscenda et curanda . . . Francofurti, Andreas Eichorn [1610]

    [28] p.   19 cm.   **[418]**
    Diss.—Frankfurt an der Oder (M. Gosky, *respondent*)

—Disputatio medica therapeutica. De praeserva-tione a peste . . . [Francofurti Marchionum] Typis Friderici Hartmanni [1611]

    [24] p.   18 cm.   **[419]**
    Imprint partly supplied from Jöcher, v. 1., p. 554.
    Diss.—Frankfurt an der Oder (J. Albinus, *respondent*)

—Observationes aliquot anatomicae: ex quibus controversiae multae medicae & physicae breviter deciduntur . . . Francofurti Marchionum, Typis ex-cusae per Joannem Eichorn, 1610.

    [24] p.   20 cm.   **[420]**
    Diss.—Frankfurt an der Oder (J. Freitag, *respondent*)

—Theses medicas de hydropum essentia et cura-tione . . . Helmaestadii, Typis haeredum Jacobi Lucii, 1617.

    [31] p.   19 cm.   **[421]**
    Diss.—Helmstedt (B. Oheim, *respondent*)

ARNOBIO, CLEANDRO [*fl.* 1602] Tesoro delle gioie trattato marviglioso. Nel quale si discorre pienamente delle virtù, & proprietà di tutte le gioie . . . balsami, cocco, e malecca. Et di tutte l'altre pietre più famose, & pregiate. Da diligenti scrittori antichi, moderni . . . sacri, & mondani . . . & medicinali . . . Raccolto, & ordinato per Cleandro Arnobio . . . Vinetia, Gio. Battista Ciotti, 1602.

    [8], 256 p.   16 cm.   **[422]**

—[The same.] . . . Padova, Pietro Paolo Tozzi, 1626.

    [24], 212, [1] p.   15 cm.   **[423]**

—[The same.] . . . Venetia, Francesco Ginami, 1662.

    [12], 212 p.   14 cm.   **[424]**

ARNOLD, ERNST. *See* ARNOLDI, Ernst [*fl.* 1677]

ARNOLD, GOTTFRIED [1665–1714] *praes.* Lo-tionem manuum, disquisitione historica ad factum Ponti Pilati recensitam . . . ad disputandum publice exhibet Bartholomaeus Bausnerus . . . Wittenbergae, Typis Matthaei Henckelii [1689]

    [20] p.   19 cm.   **[425]**
    Diss.—Wittenberg (B. Bausner, *respondent*)

ARNOLD, JOHANN MARTIN [*fl.* 1690] *respondent.* Disputatio medica inauguralis de dysenteria . . . [Altdorfii] Literis Henrici Meyeri [1690]

    [18] p.   20 cm.   **[426]**
    Diss.—Altdorf.

ARNOLD, SIMON JOHANN, *tr. See* PEARSON, J., *Bp. of Chester.* Expositio symboli apostolici. 1691.

ARNOLDI, ERNST [*fl.* 1677] *respondent. See* BLEN-DINGER, A. Dissertatio inauguralis medica. 1677.

ARNOLDT, JOHANN [*fl.* 1688] *respondent.* Dis-putatio medica inauguralis de vertigine . . . Altdorf-fii, Typis Henrici Meyeri [1688]

    [20] p.   20 cm.   **[427]**
    Diss.—Altdorf.

ARNOLDUS DE VILLA NOVA. *See* ARNALDUS DE VILLANOVA [*d.* 1313?]

ARNOLDUS, CORRADUS. *See* CORRADUS, Ar-noldus [*fl.* 1601]

ARNOUL, FRANÇOIS, *Father* [*fl. ca.* 1625] Traictez curieux, de medecine et chirurgie. Le premier con-tenant une doctrine generale, des fractures du crane . . . Le second est un tres excellent traicté, de la dissenterie, composé par Guillaume Fabri, medecin de Hilden. Le troisiéme les Revelations charitables, de plusieurs remedes souverains, contre les plus cruelles & perilleuses maladies qui puissent arriver au corps humain . . . Rouen, François Vaultier, 1673.

    3 parts in 1 v.   14 cm.   **[428]**
    Various pagings.
    Part [3] has special title page.

ARNOULD, FRANÇOIS. *See* ARNOUL, François, *Father* [*fl. ca.* 1625].

ARNOUTS, JOANNES [*fl.* 1670] *respondent.* Disputatio medica inauguralis positiones varias con-tinens . . . Lugduni Batavorum, Apud viduam & haeredes Joannis Elsevirii, 1670.

    [8] p.   23 cm.   **[429]**
    Diss.—Leyden.

AROMATARI, Giuseppe degli [1586-1660] Disputatio de rabie contagiosa cui praeposita est Epistola de generatione plantarum ex seminibus. Qua detegitur, in vocatis seminibus contineri plantas vere conformatas, ut dicunt, actu ... Venetiis, Apud Jacobum Sarcinam, 1625.

  [16], 96 p. 20 cm.   [**430**]

  The Disputatio and the Epistola have special title pages.

—[The same.] De rabie contagiosa ... discursus, cui epistola de plantarum ex seminibus generatione praeposita est, qua detegitur, in vocatis seminibus contineri plantas verè conformatas, ut dicunt, actu ... Francofurti, Apud Johannem Beyerum, 1626.

  72 p. 21 cm.   [**431**]

ARQUATI, Giovanni Francesco [*fl.* 1608] Medicus, reformatus, ob varias in medicina καταχρήσεις seu abusus ... Venetiis, Apud Petrum Cieram, 1618.

  [16], 116 p. 22 cm.   [**432**]

ARRAES, Duarte Madeira. *See* Madeira Arraiz, Duarte [*d.* 1652]

ARRAGONI, Rannutio. Della cura singolare del parto settimestre, e del fascino naturale de fanciulli ... Verona, Dominico Rossi [pref. 1663]

  [4], [9]-20, 9-33 p. 19 cm. [**433**]

  Imperfect: all before p. [5] wanting; part of text on title page blocked out.

ARRAGOS, Guillaume [1513-1610] *See* Scholtz, L. Epistolarum philosophicarum: medicinalium, ac chymicarum ... volumen. 1610.

ARRAIS, Amador [1530?-1600] Dialogos ... revistos, e acrescentados pelo mesmo autor nesta segunda impressão. Coimbra, Diogo Gomez Lovreyro, 1604.

  [22], 346 (i.e. 341) ll. 27 cm. [**434**]

ARRAIZ, Amador, *Bp. of Portalegre. See* Arrais, Amador [1530?-1600]

ARREST. 1680. *See* Alsace. Conseil Souverain.

ARREST de la Cour de Parlement. 1623. *See* France. Parlement (Paris)

ARREST de la Cour de Parlement de Toulouse. 1681. *See* France. Parlement (Toulouse)

ARREST de nosseigneurs du Parlement. [1698] *See* France. Parlement (Paris)

ARREST, portant reglement des chirurgiens privilegiez. [1668] *See* France. Conseil privé.

ARRIETA, Filippo de [*fl.* 1693] Raguaglio historico del contaggio occorso nella provincia di Bari negli anni 1690. 1691., e 1692 ... Napoli, Dom. Ant. Parrino, e Michele Luigi Mutii, 1694.

  [24], 413 (i.e. 412), [1] p. plates. 23 cm.

              [**435**]

ARS salutis sive institutio perfecte vivendi, tribus praeceptis comprehensa, menstruo Christianarum cogitationum, & affectuum circulo velut fomento conservanda & promovenda ... Passavii, Typis Georgii Höller, 1689.

  [12], 153, [2] p. 13 cm.   [**436**]

ARSONCINUS, Thomas. De jure alchymiae responsum. [Argentorati, Sumptibus heredum Eberh. Zetzneri, 1659]

  248-252 p., vol. 4. 20 cm. (*In* Zetzner, Lazarus, *ed.* Theatrum chemicum. Argentorati, 1659-61)

              [**437**]

  Caption title.

L'ART de saigner. 1686, 1689. *See* [Meurisse, H. E.]

ARTE DE' MEDICI E DEGLI SPEZIALI, Florence. *See* Ricettario Fiorentino. 1623, 1670, 1696.

ARTEFIUS *See* Artephius [12th cent.]

ARTEMIDORUS DALDIANUS. Artemidori Daldiani & Achmetis Sereimi f. Oneirocritica. Astrampsychi & Nicephori versus etiam oneirocritici. Nicolai Rigaltii ad Artemidorum notae. Lutetiae, Apud Marcum Orry, 1603.

  4 parts in 1 v. 24 cm.   [**438**]

  Various pagings. Greek and Latin text in parallel columns.

  With a Latin version of Artemidorus by J. Cornarius; of Ahmad, by J. Leunclavius; of Astrampsychus, by J. Opsopoeus, and of Nicephorus, by N. Rigaltius.

ARTEPHIUS [12th cent.] Clavis majoris sapientiae ...

  198-213 p., vol. 4. 20 cm. (*In* Zetzner, Lazarus, *ed.* Theatrum chemicum. Argentorati, 1659-61)

              [**439**]

  Caption title.

—Alphonsi, regis Castellae ... Liber philosophiae occultioris (praecipu metallorum) profundissimus, cui titulorum fecit: Clavis sapientiae ...

766-786 p., vol. 5. illus. 20 cm. (*In* Zetzner, Lazarus, *ed.* Theatrum chemicum. Argentorati, 1659-61) [**440**]

Caption title.

Translation of the Arabic work ascribed to Artephius.

—*See* ARNAULD, P. Trois traitez de la philosophie naturelle. 1612; SALMON, W. Medicina practica. 1692.

ARTHUSIUS, GUILIELMUS [*fl.* 1628-1630] *respondent. See* SEBISCH, M. [1578-1674?] *praeses.* Liber Galeni de differentiis morborum in theses contractus. 1630 [and] Libri sex Galeni De morborum differentiis. 1632.

ARTICLES concernants ce que les commissaires des quartiers doibuent faire en temps de soubçon de maladie contagieuse. 1631. *See* NANCY. Ordinances, local laws, etc.

ARTIS auriferae, quam chemiam vocant, volumina duo, quae continent Turbam philosophorum aliosque antiquiss. auctores ... Accessit noviter volumen tertium ... Basileae, Typis Conradi Waldkirchii, 1610.

3 v. in 1. illus. 17 cm. [**441**]

Contains 24 treatises of which 22 were previously published in Basel in 1572 under title: Auriferae artis.

Analyzed in part. For full contents see Ferguson (A) Vol. 1, p. 51-52.

—[German tr.] *See* MORGENSTERN, P. *ed.* and *tr.* Turba philosophorum. 1613.

ARTOCOPHINUS, HENRICUS. *See* BRODKORB, Heinrich [*fl.* 1620]

ARTOPÄUS, JOHANN DANIEL [*fl.* 1673] *praeses.* Dissertatio anti-Baroniana, num Alexander III. Fridericum Barbarossam calcaverit pedibus? ... Lipsiae, Literis Johann-Erici Hahnii, 1673.

[2], 22 p. 20 cm. [**442**]

Diss.—Leipzig (J. Fritzschen, *respondent*)

ARTORIUS, MARCUS. *See* STOCKHAMER, Franz [*fl.* 1677]

[**ARTUS**, THOMAS, *sieur d'Embry, b.* 1550?] Les hermaphrodites ... n.p. [1605]

[2], 235 p.; 191 p. illus. 14 cm. [**443**]

Part [2] has caption title: "Discours de Jacophile à Limne".

Date supplied from DBF, v. 3, p. 1219.

Imperfect: p. 105-6 of part 1 wanting.

ARVISET, ÉTIENNE [*fl.* 1577-1623] Consolation et resjouissance pour les malades, tristes, et affligez ... Derniere ed. rev. & augm. S. Omer, Charles Boscart, 1618.

[16], 604, [4] p. 15 cm. [**444**]

ASCLEPIADEA sacra, quibus in arte medica licentia privilegia & honores doctorales assumendi ... Andreae Rivino ... Lipsiae ... conferebatur; emblematicos & epigrammaticos a ... collegis & amicis ... illustrata. [Lipsiae] Excusa a Timotheo Ritzschio [1638]

[8] p. 29 cm. [**445**]

ASCOLI, SALADINO DI. *See* SALADINUS, Asculanus [*fl. ca.* 1430-1448]

ASELLIO, GASPARE [1581-1626] De lactibus, sive lacteis venis, quarto vasorum mesaraicorum genere novo invento ... dissertatio, qua sententię anatomicę multę, vel perperam receptę convelluntur vel parum perceptę illustrantur ... Mediolani, Apud Jo. Baptistam Bidellium, 1627.

[14], 79, [8] p. 4 fold. col. plates., port. 23 cm. [**446**]

Imperfect: port. wanting.

Engraved title page and portrait by Cesare Bassano; woodcut plates ascribed to Bassano or to Domenico Falcini. Cf. Choulant-Frank.

Dedicatory epistle signed: Alexander Tadinus, & Senator Septalius.

—[The same.] ... Lugduni Batavorum, Ex officina Johannis Maire, 1640.

[15], 104, [8] p. 4 plates. 20 cm. [**447**]

—De lactibus [&] Tabulae De venis lacteis. *In* Spiegel, A. van de. Opera quae extant, omnia. 1645.

—[The same, *as subject.*] *See* WALAEUS, J. Twee brieven van de bewegingen des chyls ende des bloeds. 1650.

—*See* VESLING, J. Syntagma anatomicum. 1666, 1677, 1696.

ASFALCK, GEORG FRIEDRICH [*fl.* 1608-1610] *respondent.* Themata medica de ratione administrandi cibum & potum in extra morbos ... Basileae, Typis Johannis Schroeteri, 1610.

[16] p. 20 cm. [**448**]

Diss.—Basel.

ASHMOLE, Elias [1617-1692] Theatrum chemicum Britannicum. Containing severall poeticall pieces of our famous English philosophers, who have written the Hermetique mysteries in their owne ancient language. Faithfully collected into one volume, with annotations thereon ... The first part. London, Printed by J. Grismond for Nath. Brooke, 1652.

[16], 486, [9] p. front. (port.), illus., plates. 19 cm. **[449]**

Imperfect: port., plates, and errata leaf p. [9] at end wanting, supplied in photocopy; p. [3-8] at end mutilated, supplied in photocopy.

No more published.

Includes the Ordinall of alchemie by Thomas Norton and the Compound of alchemie by George Ripley.

—, tr. See Dee, A. Fasciculus chemicus. 1650.

ASSEMBLÉE charitable à Paris. Bouillons et tysannes. Pour les pauvres gens quand ils sont malades. [Paris, 1677]

4 p. 25 cm. **[450]**

Caption title.

At head of title: Pauvres. Fait à Paris l'an 1677.

—Potages. [Pour les pauvres gens] [Paris? ca. 1677]

8 p. 24 cm. **[451]**

Caption title.

At head of title: Pauvres.

—Remedes. Pour les pauvres gens & leurs bestiaux, qui coustent peu. [Paris, 1677]

[8] p. 25 cm. **[452]**

Caption title.

At head of title: Pauvres. Fait à Paris l'an 1677.

ASSEMBLÉE générale du Clergé. See France. Assemblée générale du Clergé.

ASSENDELFT, Nicolaes van, tr. See Fabricius von Hilden, W. Aanmerkingen ... rakende de genees ende heelkonst. 1656; Harvey, W. Vande beweging van't hert. 1650; Walaeus, J. Twee brieven van de beweginge des chyls ende des bloeds. 1650.

ASSENDELFT, Simon [fl. 1668] respondent. Disputatio medica inauguralis de febre quadam epidemia ... Lugduni Batavorum, Apud viduam & haeredes Joannis Elsevirii, 1668.

[22] p. 23 cm. **[453]**

Diss.—Leyden.

ASSER, H. van [fl. 17th cent.] Myn Heer, alsoo Godt almachtigh eenige steden met de droevige sieckte van pestelentie ... ende wy noyt uur ofte tijdt verseeckert zijn ... soo hebbe ick ... seecker geschreven boecken geintutileert Medecijnboeck ... oock' eene van de selve aan uw. E. mededeel ende vereere ... hier mede met presentatie van mijn onderdanige dienst blijve ... [n. p., ca. 1650]

broadside. 30 x 21 cm. **[454]**

Signed by hand: H. van Asser.

ASSING, Johann [fl. 1613] respondent. See Michael, J. Εξεξασις physica. 1613.

ASSMANN, Friedrich Sigismund [fl. 1664] respondent. See Sebisch, M. [1578-1674? praeses. Disputatio solennis de constipatione alvi. 1664.

ASTARI, Biagio. De febribus. In Gatinaria, M. De mendendis humani corporis malis practica. 1604.

ASTARIUS, Blasius. See Astari, Biagio.

ASTELL, James [17th cent.] See [Starkey, G.] Liquor alchahest. 1675.

ASTORGA, Pedro Barea de. See Barea de Astorga. Pedro [b. ca 1630]

ASTRAMPSYCHUS. See Artemidorus Daldianus. Artemidori Daldiani & Achmetis Sereimi f. Oneirocritica. 1603.

ASTRONOMIA inferior; seu, Planetarum terrestrium motus & variatio.

507-510 p., vol. 6. 20 cm. (In Zetzner, Lazarus, ed. Theatrum chemicum. Argentorati, 1659-61] **[455]**

Caption title.

AT the council-chamber in Whitehall, Monday the 22th. of October, 1688. 1688. See Gt. Brit. Sovereign [1685-1688] (James II)

AT the Court at Whitehall the ninth of January 1683. 1683. See Gt. Brit. Privy Council.

ATHENAEOS OF NAUCRATIS. See Athenaeus.

ATHENAEUS. See Hofmann, C. Variarum lectionum lib. VI. 1619.

ATHENAEUS NAUCRATITA. See Athenaeus.

ATHENAIOS. See Athenaeus.

ATHENIUS, Gulielmus, ed. *See* Mercuriale, G. Consultationes. [1604–20], 1624–25 [and] Medicina practica. 1603, 1606, 1617, 1627.

ATKINS, William [*fl.* 1694] A discourse shewing the nature of the gout . . . Also helps for palsies, plurisies, cholick . . . With receipts and directions for the cure of the king's evil, and other diseases . . . London, Tho. Fabian, 1694.

[1], xvi, 128 p. front. (port.) 15 cm. [**456**]

AU bureau de l'Hôtel-Dieu . . . de Lyon. 1690? *See* Hôtel-dieu de Lyon.

AU bureau du Grand Hôtel-Dieu . . . de Lion. 1696? *See* Hôtel-Dieu de Lyon.

AUBERT, Jacques [*d. ca.* 1586] De metallorum ortu et causis. *See* Duchesne, J. Opera medica. 1614; Ad Jacobi Auberti . . . De ortu et causis metallorum. 1659; Drey medicinische Tractätlein. 1631; Traicté familier. 1630, 1639, 1648.

AUBERY, Jean [1569–1622] L'antidote d'amour. Avec un ample discours, contenant la nature & les causes d'iceluy, ensemble les remedes les plus singuliers pour se preserver & guerir des passions amoureuses . . . Delff, Arnold Bon, 1663.

253, [5] p. 14 cm. [**457**]
Added engraved title page.

—Les bains de Bourbon Lancy et Larchanbaud . . . Paris, Adrian Perier, 1604.

[8], 129 (i.e. 228), [3] ll. illus. 17 cm. [**458**]
Engraved title page.

AUBIGNAC, François Hédelin d', *Father* [1604–1676] Des satyres brutes, monstres et demons, de leur nature et adoration contre l'opinion de ceux qui ont estimé les satyres estre une espece d'hommes distincts & separez des adamicques . . . Paris, Nicolas Buon, 1627.

[23], 236 p. 17 cm. [**459**]

AUBIGNÉ, Nathan d'. *See* Aubigné de la Fosse, Nathan [1601–1669?]

AUBIGNÉ DE LA FOSSE, Nathan [1601–1669?] Carmen aureum. *In* Augurello, G.A. Chrysopoeia et Vellus aureum. [1650]

—, *ed.* Bibliotheca chemica contracta ex delectu & emendatione Nathanis Albinei . . . in gratiam & commodum artis chemicae studiosorum. Genevae,

Sumpt. Joannis Ant. & Samuelis de Tournes, 1653.
4 parts in 1 v. 17 cm. [**460**]
Various pagings.
Parts [2]–[4] have special title pages.
Contents—[pt.1] Augurello, G.A. Chrysopoeia, et Vellus aureum . . . Cum Nathanis Albinei . . . carmine aureo.—[pt.2] [Sendivogius, Michael] Novum lumen chemicum . . . cui accessit Tractatus de sulphure.—[pt.3] [Espagnet, Jean d'.] Enchiridion physicae restitutae.—[pt.4] Arcanum Hermeticae philosophiae opus.

AUBIN, Eustache d' [*fl.* 1634] *ed. See* Guidi, G. [*ca.* 1500–1569] Les anciens et renommés autheurs de la medecine & chirurgie. 1634.

[**AUBIN**, Nicolas, *b.* 1655?] Histoire des diables de Loudun; ou, De la possession des religieuses Ursulines, et de la condamnation & du suplice d'Urbain Grandier curé de la même ville. Amsterdam, Abraham Wolfgang, 1694.

[2], 473 (i.e. 471) p. 14 cm. [**461**]

AUBREY, John [1626–1697] Miscellanies, viz. I. Day-fatality. II. Local fatality. III. Ostensa. IV. Omens. V. Dreams . . . XXI. Second-sighted-persons . . . London, Edward Castle, 1696.

[6], 179 p. illus. 20 cm. [**462**]

AUBRI, Claude [17th cent.] Testis examinatus . . . by Vauclius Dathirius Bonglarus [pseud.] [London, 1688]

843–844 p. plate. 22 cm. [**463**]
Caption title.
Reprinted from the original edition published in Florence in 1658.

AUBRY, Jean d' [*d.* 1667] Le Triomphe de l'archée et la merveille du monde; ou, La medecine universelle et veritable pour toutes sortes de maladies les plus desesperées . . . 3 ed. Augmentée de l'apologie de l'autheur, contre certains docteurs en medecine . . . Et de plusieurs remercimens des cures & guerisons . . . Et de beaucoup de consultations faites & envoyées en diverses langues . . . Paris, L'autheur [166–]

[10], 176, [8] p.; 36 p.; 227 p. 24 cm. [**464**]
Date supplied from Carrère, v. 1., p. 244.
Imperfect: p. 145–227. wanting.

—[The same] . . . 4 ed. . . . Paris, L'autheur [166–]
[20], 36 p.; 227, [1] p.; 7–260, [8], 69–119 p. 24 cm. [**465**]
Date written by hand on title page: 1661, but cf. Carrère, v. 1., p. 224.

AUDA, Domenico [*fl.* 1652] Breve compendio di maravigliosi secreti rationali, cavati d'approvati autori praticati con felice successo nell'indispositioni & infermità corporali. Diviso in quattro libro. Nel primo si tratta de' secreti medicinali. Nel II. de secreti appartenenti à diverse cose. Nel III. de secreti chimici di varie sorti. Nel IIII. d'astrologia medicinale. Con un trattato bellissimo nel fine per conservarsi in sanità . . . Roma, Nella stamperia d'Ignatio de Lazari, a spese di Nicolò Germano, 1652.

  [22], 276, [1] p. 17 cm.   **[466]**

—[The same.] . . . In questa 2. impr. ampliato di nuovi secreti dall'autore. . .Roma, Francesco Alberto Tani, 1655.

  [29]. 303 p. tables. 17 cm. **[467]**
Added half title.

—[The same.] . . . In questa 4. impr. ricorretto, & ampliato di bellissimi secreti dall'istesso autore. Venetia, Per il Turrini, 1663.

  [16], 312 p. 15 cm.   **[468]**

[The same.] . . . 6. impr. . . . Torino, Gio. Sinibaldo, ad instanza di Giuseppe Vernoni, 1665.

  [16], 352 p. 17 cm.   **[469]**
Added half title.

—[The same.] . . . Con nuova aggionta dell'istesso autore. Venetia et Bassano, Il Remondini [*ca.* 1670]

  [20], 316 p. 15cm.   **[470]**

—[The same.] . . . Venetia, Li Zinni, 1673.

  [20], 316 p. 14 cm.   **[471]**
Different setting of type.

—[The same.] . . . Bologna, Gioseffo Longhi, 1673.
  [24], 336 p. 15 cm.   **[472]**

—[The same.] . . . Venetia, Giacomo Zini, 1676.
  [20], 316 p. 14 cm.   **[473]**
Imperfect: title page mutilated.
Different setting of type.

—[The same.] Pratica de' speciali che per modo di dialogo contiene gran parte anco di theorica . . . Con un trattato delle confettioni nostrane per uso di casa. Et una nuova aggiunta di segreti utilissimi . . . Venetia, Zaccaria Conzatti, 1678.

  328, [4] p. 14 cm.   **[474]**
The "Trattato delle confettioni nostrane . . ." (p. [263]–279) and the "Nuova aggiunta di secreti . . ." (p. [281]–332) have special title pages.

—[The same.] . . . Venetia, Zaccaria Conzatti, 1683.

  329, [4] p. 16 cm.   **[475]**
The "Trattato delle confettioni nostrane . . ." (p. [265]–283) and the "Nuova auggiunta di secreti . . ." (p. [282]–329) have special title pages.

—[The same.] Breve compendio di maravigliosi secreti approvati con felice successo nelle indispositioni corporali . . . Con nuova aggionta dell'istesso auttore.Venetia, Andrea Baroni, 1686.

  [20], 316 p. 14 cm.   **[476]**
Different setting of type.

—[The same.] Pratica de' spetiali, che per modo di dialogo contiene gran parte anco di theorica . . . Con un trattato delle confettioni nostrane per uso di casa; et una nuova aggiunta de secreti utilissimi. Venetia, Li Prodotti, 1696.

  329, [4] p. 15 cm.   **[477]**
Added half title.
Different setting of type.
The "Trattato delle confettioni nostrane . . ." (p. [265]–281) and the "Nuova aggiunta di secreti . . ." (p. [283]–329) have special title pages.

AUDRAN, Gérard [1640–1703] Les proportions du corps humain mesurées sur les plus belles figures de l'antiquité. Paris, Girard Audran, 1683.

  [7] p., 30 plates. 44 cm. **[478]**

AUFF- und zugemachte Schnupff Tabacks Büchse, neben einer lustigen Invention vom Taback-Trincken. Niesenburg [1694?]

  [24] p. 19 cm.   **[479]**
Bound with Pechlin, J. N. Theophilus Bibaculus. 1684.

AUGENIO, Illario [*fl.* 1604] *ed. See* Augenio, O. De febribus. 1604; 1605; 1607.

AUGENIO, Orazio [*ca.* 1527–1603] De febribus, febrium signis, symptomatibus, & prognostico libri septem, ab ipso authore ab anno 1568. usque ad 1572. singuli conscripti: nunc vero post ejus obitum ab Hilario Augenio . . . in lucem emissi . . . His septem libris, accesserunt postmodum alii tres ejusdem materiae, I. De curatione symptomatum febrium pestilentium. II. De febribus pestilentibus. III. De curatione variolarum ac morbillorum. Francofurti ad Moenum, Ex officina Matthiae Beckeri, sumptibus Jo. Theobaldi Schönwetteri, 1604.

  [11], 443, [11] p. 32 cm. **[480]**

—[The same.] ... Francofurti, Impensis haeredum Andr. Wecheli, Claudii Marnii, & haered. Joan. Aubrii, 1605.

[10], 443, [11] p.   34 cm.   **[481]**

Reissue of the 1604 ed. with new title page and preliminary pages reset.

—[The same.] ... Venetiis, Apud haeredem Damiani Zenarii, 1607.

[8], 305 (i.e. 304), [8] p.   34 cm.   **[482]**

Bound with his Epistolarum medicinalium tomi tertii libri duodecim. 1607.

—Epistolarum et consultationum medicinalium prioris tomi libri XII [-alterius tomi libri XII] ... Hac ed. 5 ab eodem authore recognitum, adauctum, & emendatum. Quibus accessere ejusdem authoris De hominis partu libri duo, nunc tertio editi ... Venetiis, Apud Damianum Zenarium, 1602.

2 v. in 1.   port.   34 cm.   **[483]**

De hominis partu (at end of vol. [2]) is identical in contents, except for the omission of the dedication, with the edition which was included as vol. [2] of his Epistolarum & consultationum medicinalium libri XXIIII, published in Frankfurt in 1597, with title: ... Quod homini certum non sit nascendi tempus: libri duo ... The addition to this with running title "Historia foetus petrificati" is Jean Ailleboust's Portentosum lithopaedion, with a note by Siméon de Provanchères, as published in Sens in 1582.

—Epistolarum medicinalium tomi tertii libri duodecim. In quibus non solum maximae difficultates ad medicinam & philosophiam pertinentes dilucidantur; sed etiam Alexandri Massariae Vicentini Additamentum apologeticum, & disputationem secundum Hippocratis & Galeni doctrinam funditus evertuntur. Nunc primum Venetiis in lucem editi ... Venetiis, Apud haeredem Damiani Zenarii, 1607.

[8], 341, [30] p.   34 cm.   **[484]**

With this is bound his De febribus. 1607.

—*See* MASSARIA, A. Disputationes duae. 1622.

AUGSBURG. Collegium Medicum. *See* COLLEGIUM MEDICUM AUGUSTANUM.

AUGSBURG. Ordinances, local laws, etc. *See* PHARMACOPOEIA AUGUSTANA. 1613, 1622, 1684, 1694.

AUGURELLO, GIOVANNI AURELIO [1454?–1537?] Chrysopoeia et Vellus aureum. Quorum illa emendatissima prodit: hoc vero nunc primum ex veteri manuscripto sub typos venit ... [Genevae, J. de Tournes, 1650?]

84 p.   16 cm.   **[485]**

Half title.

Imprint supplied from BMC.

Imperfect: p. 81–84 wanting.

"Nathanis Albinei D. M. Carmen aureum": p. 79–84.

—*In* Aubigné de la Fosse, N. Bibliotheca chemica. 1653.

—[Chrysopoeia carmine conscripta]

197–266 p., vol. 3.   20 cm.   (*In* Zetzner, Lazarus, *ed.* Theatrum chemicum. Argentorati, 1659–61)
[486]

Title from table of contents.

AUGUSTIN, CHRISTIAN [*fl.* 1620] *respondent.* Theses hasce medicas miscellaneas ex omnibus medicinae partibus desumptas ... proponit, Christianus Augustinus ... Basileae, Typis Johannis Schroeteri [1620]

[16] p.   23 cm.   **[487]**

Diss. — Basel.

AURELI, LODOVICO *Father* [*d.* 1637] *tr. See* FERRARI, G. B., *Father.* Flora. 1638.

AURELIAE occultae philosophorum. 1659. *See* BASILIUS VALENTINUS.

AURELIUS, ANSELMUS. *See* ANSELMI, Aurelio [*fl.* 1605]

AUREUS tractatus de philosophorum lapide. 1677. *See* [GRASSHOFF, J.]

AURIFABER, ANDREAS. *See* GOLDSCHMIDT, Andreas [1512–1559]

AURIFERAE artis [German] *ed. See* MORGENSTERN, P. *ed.* and *tr.* Turba philosophorum. 1613.

AURIFONTINA chymica. 1680. *See* HOUPREGHT, F. J., *comp.*

AURORA consurgens: quae dicitur aurea hora ...

119–158 p., vol. 1   17 cm.   (*In* Artis auriferae. Basileae, 1610)   **[488]**

Caption title.

—[German tr.] Aurora consurgens; oder, Auffstehende Morgenröhte, welche genandt wirdt aurea Hora, die guldene Zeit oder Stunde ...

141–199 p., part 1.   19 cm.   (*In* Morgenstern, Philipp, *ed.* and *tr.* Turba philosophorum. Basel, 1613)
[489]

Caption title.

AURUM potabile. *See* ADMONITO . . . De via ad aurum potabile. [1661]

AUSFELD, JOHAN CHRISTOPH [*fl.* 1681] *respondent. See* CRAUSE, R. W., *praeses.* Disputatio inauguralis medica de pleuritide. 1681

AUSSFELDT, CHRISTOPH [*fl.* 1645-1650] *respondent. See* MÖBIUS, G., *praeses.* Dissertatio medica de chylificatione. 1645.

AUSTRIA. Sovereign, 1658-1705 (Leopold I) . . . Neue Infections-Ordnung. Wie es insgemein auss dem Land in den Infections-Sachen zu halten. Hall in Sachsen, Gedruckt und verlegt von Carl Waltern [1680?]

48 p. 20 cm. [490]

AUSTRIACUS, JOANNES, *pseud. See* MAGIRUS, Johann [*d.* 1596]

AUSTRIUS, SEBASTIANUS [*d.* 1550] De infantium sive puerorum morborum & symptomatum dignotione. In Fonteyn, N. Nicolai Fontani Commentarius in Sebastianum Austrium . . . De puerorum morbis. 1642.

AUSTROPEDIUS, AGAPETUS KOZERUS, *tr. See* THURNEISSER ZUM THURN, L. Reise und Kriegs-Apotecken. 1602.

AUTUN, JACQUES DE. *See* CHEVANES, Jacques de [*ca.* 1608-1678]

[**AUVERGNE**, ANNE-MARIE D', 17th cent.] Secrets touchant la medecine. Paris, Michel Vaugon, Pierre Promé, 1668 (i.e. 1678)

[6], 280, [8] p. 15 cm. [491]

—Recueil de secrets touchant la medecine, éprouvez en quantité de maux qui arrivent au corps humain. En faveur des pauvres, par les soins de Mademoiselle D'Auvergne. Paris, Michel Vaugon, 1692.

468 (i.e. 460), [52] p. 17 cm. [492]

AUZOUT, ADRIEN [1622-1691] *See* PETTY, Sir W. Five essays in political arithmetick. 1687.

AVANZI, CARLO [*fl. ca.* 1630] *ed. See* FIERA, B. Coena notis illustrata a Carolo Avantio. 1649.

AVANZI, JACOPO [*fl.* 1649] *See* FIERA, B. Coena notis illustrata a Carolo Avantio. 1649.

AVELLINO, FRANCESCO [*fl. ca.* 1637] . . . Oratio in exornandis philosophiae, et medicinae laurea, Antonio Costa, et Nicolao Andrea Garufi, comitis don Petri Castelli Romani auditoribus. Messanae, Apud Paulum Bonacota, 1660.

7 p. 21 cm. [493]

Bound with Castelli, P. De abusu. 1659.

AVEN EZRA, ABRAHAM. *See* IBN EZRA, Abraham ben Meïr [1092-1167]

AVENARE, ABRAHAM. *See* IBN EZRA, Abraham ben Meïr [1092-1167]

AVENEEZRA, ABRAHAM. *See* IBN EZRA, Abraham ben Meïr [1092-1167]

AVENZOAR [*d. ca.* 1162] TAISÎR. *In* COLLE, G. De cognitu difficilibus in praxi ex libris Avenzoaris per sententias dilucidatas auctore Joanne Colle. 1628.

AVERHOULT, ANTOINE D'. *See* AVEROULT, Antoine d', *Father* [1553-1614]

AVEROULT, ANTOINE D', *Father* [1553-1614] Excellents remedes, ou preservatifs contre la peste & autre maladie contagieuse. Par lesquels l'on se pourra asseurément preserver & guarentir desdites maladies . . . Lyon, Claude Armand dit Alphonce, 1619.

16 p. 16 cm. [494]

AVERROËS [1126-1198] Averroeana: being a transcript of several letters from Averroes . . . to Metrodorus a young Grecian nobleman, student at Athens, in the years 1149, and 1150. Also several letters from Pythagoras to the King of India, together with his reception at the Indian court, and an account of his discourse with the King . . . To which is prefixt, a Latin letter by Monsieur Grinau, one of the messieurs du Port Royal . . . concerning the subject of these papers . . . The work having been long concealed, is now put into English for the benefit of mankind . . . London, T. Sowle, 1695.

[2], 162 p. 15 cm. [495]

The Latin dedicatory letter by Grinau is given in an English version also.

The letters are spurious.

AVERROËS, *the elder. See* AVERROËS [1126-1198]

AVICENNA [980?-1037] Avicennae Arabum medicorum principis. Ex Gerardi Cremonensis versione, & Andreae Alpagi Belunensis castigatione. A

Joanne Costço, & Joanne Paulo Mongio annotationibus jampridem illustratus. Nunc vero ab eodem Costaeo recognitus, & novis alicubi observationibus adauctus ... Vita ipsius Avicennae ex Sorsano Arabe ejus discipulo, a Nicolao Massa Latine scripta ... Additis nuper etiam librorum Canonis oeconomiis, necnon Tabulis isagogicis in universam medicinam ex arte, Humain [sic], idest Joannitii Arabis. Per Fabium Paulinum Utinensem ... Venetiis, Apud Juntas, 1608.

  3 v. in 1. illus. 35 cm.   [**496**]

 Added engraved title page, with title: Avicennae ... Canon medicinae ... Ejusdem De viribus cordis. [De] removendis nocumentis in regimine sanitatis. [De] syrupo acetoso ...

 "Tabulae isagogicae in universam medicinam ..." (v. l.) has special title page.

 Contents as in the 1595 ed.

 — ... Ad Hasen regem epistola de re recta [&] Declaratio lapidis physici ... filio suo Aboali [&] ... De congelatione et conglutinatione lapidum.

  863-887 p., vol. 4. 20 cm. (*In* Zetzner, Lazarus, *ed*. Theatrum chemicum. Argentorati, 1659-61)   [**497**]

 Caption titles.

 —[Canon. Liber I, fen. 1. Arabic and Latin] 1674. *In* Welsch, G. H. Exercitatio de vena medinensi. 1674.

 —[Latin tr.] ... Fen. I, lib. I. Canonis ... Vicentiae, Apud Franciscum Lenium, 1611.

  87 ll. 10 cm.   [**498**]

 Bound with Galenus. Ars medicinalis. 1606.

 —[The same.] Gerardo Cremonense iterprete ... Nova ed. castigatior. Patavii, Typis Pauli Frambotti, 1648.

  275 (i.e. 273), [5] p. 14 cm.   [**499**]

 Bound with Galenus. Ars medicinalis. 1642.

 —[The same.] ... Fen. I, lib. I. Canonis. Venetiis, Apud Turrinum, 1663.

  84 (i.e. 104) p. 11 cm. (Part [3] *in* Schola medica in qua Hippocratis, Galeni, Avicennaeque ... habentur fundamenta. Venetiis, 1663.) [**500**]

 —[The same.] Patavii, Apud Cadorinum, 1682.

  127 p. 11 cm. (Part [2] *in* Schola medica in qua Hippocratis, Galeni, Avicennaeque ... habentur fundamenta. Patavii, 1682-84.) [**501**]

 "Capita, sive puncta quae laureandis proponi solent in celeberrimis collegiis": p. 122-127.

—[The same.] *In* Ponce de Santa Cruz, A. [*d. ca.* 1650] Opuscula medica, et philosophica. 1624; Santorio, S. Commentaria in primam fen primi libri Canonis Avicennae. 1646; Opera omnia. 1660.

 —[The same.] *See* GARCIA CARRERO, P. Disputationes medicae super fen primam libri primi Avicenae. 1611.

 —[Canon, lib. I-II. Latin] *In* Cardano, G. Opera omnia. 1663.

 —[Canon. Liber I-II; Liber IV, fen. 1. Latin] Canon medicinae interprete & scholiaste Vopisco Fortunato Plempio. Tom. I [-Liber secundus] Librum primum & secundum Canonis exhibens, atque ex libro quarto tractatum De febribus. Lovanii, Typis ac sumptibus Hieronymi Nempaei, 1658.

  2 v. in 1. 33 cm.   [**502**]

 —[Canon. Liber II. Arabic and Latin]

  كتاب الثاني من ڤانون القانون لا بن سينا — ; id. est, Liber secundus De canone canonis a filio Sinâ studio sumptibus ac typis Arabicis Petri Kirsteni ... ex Asiatico & Africano Mss ... Arabice per partes editus, & ad verbum in Latinum Translatus, notisque ... illustratus. Breslae, 1609.

  [1], 8, [28], 9-132 p. 32 cm. [**503**]

 Engraved title page.

 —[Canon. Liber III.] *See* SALIUS DIVERSUS, P. In Avicenna librum tertium de morbis particularibus totius corporis. 1673.

 —[Canon. Liber IV, fen. 1. Latin] Quarti libri canonis fen prima de febribus. Nova ed. ceteris accuratior ... Patavii, Typis Matthaei Cador, 1659. [colophon 1660]

  [20], 334, [1] p. 17 cm.   [**504**]

 Added engraved title page, and half-title.

 Dedicatory epistle by Jo. Baptista Pasquati.

 —[The same.] *See* GARCIA CARRERO, P. Disputationes medicae, et commentaria in fen. primam libri quarti Avicinnae. 1628.

 —Canticum principis ... de medicina; seu, Breve perspicuum, & concinne digestum institutionum medicarum compendium. Cui adjecti Aphorismi medici Johannis Mesuaei ... Ex Arabico Latine reddita, ab Antonio Deusingio ... Accessit hujusce Oratio de felicitate sapientum. Groningae, Ex officina Joannis Nicolai, 1649.

  [24], 250 p. 14 cm.   [**505**]

"Antonii Deusingii Oratio panegyrica de felicitate sapientum": p. 194-250.

With this is bound (as issued?): Deusing, A. Synopsis medicinae universalis. 1649.

—De anima [Excerpts.] *In* Bacon, R. De arte chymiae scripta. 1603.

—De congelatione & conglutinatione lapidum. *In* Aristoteles. Tractatulus . . . de practica lapidis philosophici. 1610.

—[German tr.] Von der Congelirung und zusammen fügung [des Steins]

   322-330 p.   part I.   19 cm.   (*In* Morgenstern, Philipp, *ed.* and *tr.* Turba philosophorum. Basel, 1613)   [506]

   Title partly from table of contents.

—De mineralibus. *In* Aristoteles. Tractatulus . . . de practica lapidis philosophici. 1610.

—Abugalii filii Sinae . . . De morbis mentis tractatus, editus in specimen normae medicorum universae ex Arabico in Latinum de integro conversae & a barbarorum inscitia spurcitiaque vindicatae; interprete Petro Vatterio . . . Parisiis, Apud Interpretem, et apud Jo. Huart, 1659.

   [24], 216 p.   18 cm.   [507]

—De purgantibus vegetabilibus [Excerpts.] *In* Rolfinck, W. Liber de purgantibus vegetabilibus. 1667.

—Tractatulus [de alchimia] Istum librum dividam in octo capitula vel partes.

   260-280 p., vol. I.   17 cm.   (*In* Artis auriferae. Basileae, 1610)   [508]

   Title partly from table of contents.

—[German tr.] Tractatulus [von der Alchimia]

   351-378 p.,   part I.   19 cm. (*In* Morgenstern, Philipp, *ed.* and *tr.* Turba philosophorum. Basel, 1613)

   Title partly from table of contents.   [509]

—*as subject.* See BERTOCCI, A. Methodus curativa. 1608; CASTELLI, B. Lexicon medicum Graeco-Latinum. 1628, 1651, 1657, 1664, 1665, 1669, 1685. COLLE, G. Elucidarium chirurgicum commentaria. 1620. REYS TAVARES, M. dos. Controversias philosophicas, et medicas. 1667. SCARABICIO, S. De ortu ignis febriferi historia. 1655.

AVIGNON. **Ordinances, local laws, etc.** Reglement general pour la santé. Avignon, Jean Bramereau, 1629.

   33 p.   18 cm.   [510]

AVVERTIMENTI per sanare gl'infermi dal male contagioso. Con nota particolare de' veri medicamenti per suarire la peste, esperimentati in questi ultimi giorni nelle città di Terra Ferma . . . In Venetia, Ferrara, & in Bologna, Clemente Ferroni, 1630.

   [8] p.   20 cm.   [511]

AXT, JOHANN KONRAD [*fl.* 1669-1681] Abortus in morbis acutis lethalis; oder, Eine sehr nützliche und nothwendige Frage, ob einem christlichen Medico zugelassen sey, bey einer schwangern Frauen, welche an einer schweren Kranckheit darnieder lieget, die Frucht abzutreiben . . . Jena, Zufinden bey Joh. Bielcken, druckts Johann Nisius, 1681.

   72 p.   14 cm.   [512]

—Dialogus de partu septimestri, an nempe ille sit perfectus, vegetus et per consequens legitimus? Nunc primum in lucem editus . . . Jenae, Typis Gollnerianis, 1679.

   105 p.   13 cm.   [513]

—Tractatus de arboribus coniferis et pice conficienda, aliisque ex illis arboribus provenientibus . . . Jenae, Impensis Johannis Bielkii, 1679.

   [I], 131 (i.e. 129) p.   illus.   15 cm.   [514]

   Added engraved title page.
   "Epistola ad amicum de antimonio": p. 119-131.

— *respondent.* See MEIBOM, H., *praeses.* Disputatio medica inauguralis de paracentesi in hydrope. 1670; VOGLER, V. H., *praeses.* Dissertatio medica de pleuritide. 1669.

AYALA, GERÓNIMO DE [1632-1702] Principios de cirurgia utiles, y provechosos, para que puedan aprovecharse los principiantes en esta facultad. En esta ultima impression va añadido el Tratado de cirugia, sacado de la Cirugia universal, que escriviò el . . . Juan Fragoso, conforme se practica en el Hospital general de Madrid . . . Madrid, Lorenzo Garcia [1683?]

   [8], 225, [13] p.   20 cm.   [515]

   "Suma de la tassa" dated 1683.
   "Autoridades que se citan en este libro": p. [226-238]

—[The same.] . . . En esta ultima impression va añadido el libro intitulado Del parto humano, compuesto por . . . Francisco Nuñez . . . y el Tratado de cirugia, sacado de la Cirugia universal que [escri]vió el . . . Juan Fragoso, conforme se practica en el Hospital general de Madrid . . . Valencia, Vincente Cabrera, 1693.

[8], 317 (i.e. 319), [16] p. illus. 20 cm.
[516]

Erasures on title page; part of text worn through.

—, *ed. See* FRAGOSO, J. Tratado de cirugia. 1692.

AYCHOLZIUS, JOHANNES. *See* AICHHOLTZ, Johann [1520–1588]

AYLWIN, THOMAS [*b. ca.* 1641] *See* RYCKE, T., *praeses*. Disputatio medica inauguralis de nephritide. 1682.

AYMES, JOHN. A rich store-house, or treasury for the diseased. Wherein is discovered 69. rare secrets to cure most diseases: many of them never before in print . . . The 4th ed. London, Printed by E. Crowch, and sold by F. Coles, T. Vere, J. Wright and J. Clark, 1676.

[2], 22 p. illus. 15 cm.
[517]

Added half title.
Wing 4292A.

AYNSCOM, FRANÇOIS XAVIER, *Father* [1620–1660] Expositio ac deductio geometrica quadraturarum circuli, R. P. Gregorii a S. Vincentio . . . cui praemittitur liber de natura et affectionibus, rationum ac proportionum geometricarum. Antverpiae, Apud Jacobum Meursium, 1656.

[8], 182 p. illus. 32 cm.
[518]

Bound with Guericke, O. von. Experimenta nova . . . Magdeburgica. 1672.

AYRER, CHRISTOPH HEINRICH [*fl.* 1592–1607?] Regiment und Ordnung, wie man sich in den Seiten der epidemischen rothen Ruhr verhalten, und der Kranckheit durch Gottes Hülffe widerstehen möge . . . Leipzig [Gedruckt durch Jacobum Gaubisch, typis haeredum Zachariae Berwaldi, in Vorlegung Henningi Grossen, 1601]

[7], 41, p. 19 cm.
[519]

AYRER, IMMANUEL WILHELM [*fl.* 1670] *respondent. See* SCHENCK, J. T., *praeses*. Disputatio inauguralis medica de vermibus intestinorum. 1670.

AYRER, JOHANN CHRISTOPH [*fl.* 1621] *respondent.* Συζητησις medica de morbo Ungarico . . . [Basel, 1631]

[18] p. 20 cm.
[520]

Signatures R–S⁴, T¹. Detached from a collection of theses. Cf. Carrère, vol. I, p. 265.
Diss. — Basel, 1621.

AYRER, JOHANN CHRISTOPH [*fl.* 1677–1678] *respondent*. Disputatio medica inauguralis de palpitatione cordis . . . Altdorffii, Literis Henrici Meyeri [1678]

[4], 32 p. 20 cm.
[521]

Diss. — Altdorf.

—*See* HOFFMANN, J. M., *praeses*. Θεωρήματα ίατρικά de differentiis alimentorum et medicamentorum. 1677.

AYRER, JOHANN WILHELM [*fl.* 1687–1688] *respondent*. De scirrho hepatis . . . [Altdorfii] Literis Schönnerstaedtianis [1688]

[20] p. 20 cm.
[522]

Diss. — Altdorf.

—*See* HOFFMANN, J. M., *praeses*. Dissertatio medica publica de vena portae. 1687.

AYROLDUS, JOANNES PETRUS. *See* AIROLDI, Giovanni Pietro.

AZEUEDO, MOYSES SALOM DE. *See* AZEVEDO, Moyses Salom de [*fl. ca.* 1661]

AZEVEDO, MANOEL DE, *Father, d.* 1672. Correcão de abusos introduzidos contra o verdadeiro methodo da medicina. Em tres tratados . . . Lisboa, Diogo Soares de Bulhoens, 1668–80.

2 v. ([29], 467, [32] p.; [8], 278 p.) illus., plates. 19, 20 cm.
[523]

Vol. 2 has title: Correccam de abusos, introduzidos contra o verdadeiro methodo da medicina, & farol medicinal para medicos, cyrurgiones, & boticarios. II. parte em tres tratados . . . Lisboa, Na officina de Ioam da Costa, a custa de Martim Vaz Tagarro, 1680.

—[The same.] . . . Primeira parte [-II parte]. E novamente accrescentado com as instrucções de tomar a agoa de Inglaterra: & huma carta do contagio, que houve na Praça de Mazagão no anno de 1678. [2 ed.] Lisboa, Na officina de Manoel Lopes Ferreira, 1690–1705.

2 v. illus. 20 cm.
[524]

Imperfect: p. 211–212, vol. 1, mutilated.

"Instrucçoens a quem houver de usar da agoa de Fernam Mendes": p. 287-293; "Breve conta do contagio, que houve na Praça de Mazagaõ no anno de 1678 [de João da Costa de Barros]": p. 294-303; vol. 1.

AZEVEDO, Moyses Salom de [*fl. ca.* 1661]

Disputatio medica inauguralis de asthmate ... Lugduni Batavorum, Ex officina Danielis & Abrahami à Gaesbeeck, 5422 [i.e. 1661 or 2]

[8] p. 19 cm. **[525]**

Diss. — Leyden.

B

B****, *Monsr. See* Basnage, Henri, *sieur de Beauval* [1656-1710]

B*******, J., D. M. *See* Riolan, J. [1638?-1605?] Chirurgie. 1669.

B., C., *gent. See* A short-method of physick. 1659.

B., C. B., M. D. [*fl.* 1696] *See* Medicus legalis. 1696.

B., D. *See* Belin, Jean Albert [*ca.* 1610-1677]

B., D. *See* Bussotti, Dionigi, *Bp. of Borgo San Sepolcro* [*d.* 1654]

B., D. *See* A rich store-house, or treasury for the diseased. 1650.

B., D., *gent. See* Boate, Arnold [1606-1653]

B., D., *Medicinae Doctor. See* Tolet, F. Verhandlung von der Lithotomie. 1700.

B., E., *tr. See* Scultetus, J. [1595-1645] The chyrurgeons store-house. 1674.

B., H., *philochymicus* [*fl. ca.* 1685] *tr. See* Dickinson, E. De chrysopoeia. 1687?, Epistola ... ad Theodorum Mundanum. 1686.

B., I. *See* Bonamour, J. [*fl.* 17th cent.]

B., J. *See* B*******, J., D. M.

B., J. *See* Bate, John [*fl.* 1634]

B., J. *See* Bullokar, J. An English expositour.

B., J. *See* Bulwer, John [*fl.* 1644-1662]

B., M. B. F. [*fl.* 1618] *ed. See* Anthony, F. Panacea aurea. 1618.

B., R. *See* Boyle, *Hon.* Robert [1627-1691]

B., R. *See* A brief account of some choice & famous medicines. 1676.

B., R. [*fl. ca.* 1695] *tr. See* La Charrière, J. de. A treatise of chirurgical operations. 1695.

B., S. *See* Brunet, Claude [*fl.* 1686-1737]

B., S. D. *See* Saumaise, Claude de [1588-1653]

B., T. *See* Bonet, Théophile [1620-1689]

B., T. *See* Brewer, Thomas [*fl.* 1624]

B., T. *See* Browne, *Sir* Thomas [1605-1682]

B., T. *See* Brugis, Thomas [*fl.* 1640-1651]

B., T. [17th cent.] *See* Animadversions on the medicinal observations. 1674.

B., T., V. J. *See* Bartholin, Thomas [1616-1680]

B., Th. *See* Bedford, Thomas [*d.* 1635]

B., W. *See* Bolton, William.

B., W. *See* Boraston, William [*fl.* 1630-1633]

B., W. C. *See* Cooper, William [*fl.* 1669-1689]

BÅÅK, Olav Jan [*fl.* 1628] *respondent. See* Raicus, J. *praeses.* Tractatus de podagra medico-kimicus. 1621.

BABA, Francesco *ed. See* Mercuriale, G. Opuscula aurea, & selectiora. 1644.

BACCHINI, Benedetto, *Father* [1651-1721] *tr. See* Beddevole, D. Saggi d'anatomia. 1687, 1690.

BACCHINI, Bernardino. *See* Bacchini, Benedetto, *Father* [1651-1721]

BACCI, Andrea [1524-1600] De gemmis et lapidibus pretiosis, eorumque viribus & usu tractatus, Italica lingua conscriptus ... nunc vero non solum in Latinum sermonem conversus, verum etiam ... annotationibus & observationibus auctior redditus, a Wolfgango Gabelschovero ... Cui accessit disputatio, de generatione auri in locis subterraneis, illiusque temperamento. Francofurti, Ex officina Matthiae Beckeri, impensis Nicolai Steinii, 1603.

231, [22] p.   16 cm.   [526]

Errata: p. [22]

"... Joannis Langii ... epistola, an auri et argenti, & gemmarum, usus, in medicamentis & electuariis, & epithematis ac trageis, sit salutaris ...": p. 220-231.

— De thermis ... Libri septem ... In quo agitur de universa aquarum natura, deque earum differentiis omnibus, ac mistionibus cum terris, cum ignibus, cum metallis. De terrestris ignis natura nova tractatio: de fontibus, fluminibus, lacubus: de balneis totius orbis, & de methodo medendi per balneas. Deque lavationum, simul atque exercitationum institutis in admirandis thermis Romanorum. Demum ab ipso auctore recognitum, novis historiis locupletatum, ac plus mille locis illustratum, & auctum ... Romae, Ex tyopgraphia Jacobi Mascardi, 1622.

[8], 425 (i.e. 441), [18] p.   31 cm.   [527]

BACCINO, DOMENICO [*fl.* 17th cent.] Controversiae medicae dictatio ... Romae, Per Franciscum Monetam, 1664.

13 p.   21 cm.   [528]

BACERNI, GIOSEFFO [*fl.* 1659] Breve narratione de mirabili, e naturali effetti della potentissima, et arcana medicina del'oro potabile senza corrosivo ... Bologna, Francesco Maria Sarti, 1659.

186, [15] p.   plate, port.   21 cm.   [529]

BACHMANN, ANDREAS. *See* RIVINUS, Andreas [*ca.* 1601-1656]

BACHMANN, AUGUSTUS QUIRINUS. *See* RIVINUS, Augustus Quirinus [1652-1723]

BACHMAYER, WOLFGANG WILHELM [*fl.* 1695] *respondent.* Disputatio medica inauguralis de singultu ... Altdorffii, Literis Henrici Meyeri [1695]

20 p.   20 cm.   [530]

Diss. — Altdorf.

BACHMEISTER, MATTHAEUS. *See* BACMEISTER, Matthaeus [1580-1626]

BACHOFEN VON ECHT, JOHANN *See* ECHT, Johann, [1515?-*ca.* 1568]

BACHON, ROGERIUS. *See* BACON, Roger [1214?-1294]

BACHOT, ÉTIENNE [1608-1688] Apologie ou defense pour la saignée contre ses calomniateurs: avec une réponse au libelle intitulé Examen ou raisonnements sur l'usage de la saignée ... Paris, Sebastien et Gabriel Cramoisy, 1646.

[16], 180, [1] p.   17 cm.   [531]

Errata: p. [181]

— [The same.] ... 2 ed. Paris, Sebastien et Gabriel Cramoisy, 1648.

[16], 180, [1] p.   18 cm.   [532]

Imperfect: p. [11-16] and the errata leaf wanting.
A reissue of the 1646 edition.

— Vesperiae et pileus doctoralis, cum aliquot quaestionibus medicis in utramque partem agitatis, in scholis medicorum ann. MDCLXXIV. Novembris VIII. Decembris X. & XX. necnon VIII. Januarii anni sequentis ... Parisiis, Typis viduae Edmundi Martini, 1675.

[16], 148, [1] p.   17 cm.   [533]

Errata: p. [149]

Orations etc. written for the graduation of Nicolas de Jouvanci and Nicolas Raveau.

BACHOT, GASPARD [1550?-1630] Erreurs populaires touchant la medecine et regime de santé ... Oeuvre nouvelle, desirée de plusieurs, & promise par feu M. Laurens Joubert. Lyon, Barthelemy Vincent, 1626.

[128], 509 p.   17 cm   [534]

— Another issue, with title: Troisiesme des erreurs populaires ... Lyon, Pour la vefue de feu Thomas Souborn, 1626.

                                                         [535]

BACHOU, JEAN, *tr. See* BOODT, A. B. de. Le parfaict joaillier. 1644; [ESPAGNET, J. d'] La philosophie naturelle restablie en sa pureté, 1651.

BACHOV, GEORG HEINRICH [*b.* 1652] *respondent. See* CAMERARIUS, E. R., *praeses.* Dissertatio medica de anorexia. 1679; WEDEL, G. W., *praeses.* Dissertatio inauguralis medica, de apoplexia. 1680.

BACHOVEN VON ECHT, JOHANN. *See* ECHT, Johann [1515?-*ca.* 1568]

BACK, JACOBUS DE [1593 *or* 4-1658] Dissertatio de corde. *In* Harvey, W. De motu cordis. 1648, 1654, 1660, 1671; [English tr.] 1653, 1673.

— *as subject. See* BARTHOLIN, T. Opuscula nova anatomica. 1670.

BACKHAUSS, Augustin Severus [*b.* 1655] *respondent. See* Fasch, A. H., *praeses.* Dissertationem inauguralem de amore insano ... exponit. 1686.

—*as subject. See* Wedel, G. W. Propemticon inaugurale de fortuna medici. 1686.

BACKHUSIUS, Augustinus Severus. *See* Backhauss, Augustin Severus [*b.* 1655]

BACKMEISTER, Eberhard [*fl.* 1682–1683] *respondent. See* Camerarius, E.R., *praeses.* Dissertatio de vomitu gravidarum. 1682 [and] Historia cardialgiae sublatae. 1683.

BACKMEISTER, Matthias Dietrich [*fl.* 1695] *respondent.* Disputatio medica inauguralis de fistulis ... Lugduni Batavorum, Apud Abrahamum Elzevier, 1695.

    [20] p.   22 cm.   **[536]**
   Diss.—Leyden.

BACMEISTER, Johann [1563–1631] *praeses.* Disputatio inauguralis de peste ... Rostochii, Typis Joachimi Pedani, 1623.

    [76] p.   19 cm.   **[537]**
   Diss.—Rostock (A. Kirchof, *respondent.*

BACMEISTER, Johann [1624–1686] Programma, quo ... decanus Joannes Bacmeisterus ... ad inauguralem disputationis actum ... Georgii Dethardingii ... invitat. Rostochii, Typis Johannis Kilii, 1667.

    [8] p.   18 cm.   **[538]**
   Program—Rostock (with vita of G. Detharding)

BACMEISTER, Matthaeus [1580–1626] *ed. See* Joel, F. [1510–1579] Operum medicorum ... tomus primus [-sextus] 1616–1631, 1622–1652 [v. 1, 1652]

BACON, Francis, *viscount St. Albans* [1561–1626] Operum moralium et civilium tomus. Qui continet Historiam Regni Henrici Septimi ... Sermones fideles ... Tractatum de sapientia veterum. Dialogum de Bello Sacro. Et Novam Atlantidem. Ab ipso ... auctore ... Latinitate donatus. Cura & fide Guilielmi Rawley ... In hoc volumine, iterum excusi, includuntur Tractatus de augmentis scientiarum. Historia ventorum. Historia vitae & mortis. Cum privilegio. Londini, Excusum typis Edwardi Griffini, prostant apud Richardum Whitakerum, 1638.

   [12], 386 p.; [15], 475 p.   front. (port.)   29 cm.
                                [539]
   Each work has special title page.
   Gibson 196.
   STC 1109

—Opera omnia, quae extant philosophica, moralia, politica, historica ... In quibus complures alii tractatus ... comprehensi sunt. Hactenus nunquam conjunctim edita ... & ab innumeris mendis repurgata ... Francofurti ad Moenum, Impensis Joannis Baptistae Schonwetteri, typis Matthaei Kempferri, 1665–68.

   [18] p.   1324 columns, [29] p.   port.   36 cm.
                                  [540]
   Added half title.
   De sapientia veterum liber has special title page dated 1668, all other special title pages have date 1664.
   Gibson 235.

—Baconiana. Or, Certain genuine remains of Sr. Francis Bacon ... in arguments civil and moral, natural, medical, theological, and bibliographical; now the first time faithfully published. An account of these remains, and of all his ... other works, is given ... in a discourse ... London, Printed by J. D. for Richard Chiswell, 1679.

   [2] 104, [6], 270 p.   front. (port.)   19 cm.
                                  [541]
   In 7 parts. Each part—except part [2]—has special title page. "An account of all the Lord Bacon's works": p. 1–104, signed T. T. [i.e. Thomas Tension, *archbishop of Canterbury*]; "Characters of the Lord Bacon": p. [261]–270.
   Gibson 237b.

—Another issue, without imprimatur: sig. A4 blank.   18 cm.   **[542]**
   Gibson 237a.

—[Advancement of learning.] The two bookes of Francis Bacon. Of the proficience and advancement of learning, divine and humane ... London, Henrie Tomes, 1605.

   [1], 45 ll.; 118 (i.e. 121) ll.   19 cm.   **[543]**
   Errata wanting.
   Gibson 81.
   STC 1164.

—[De augmentis scientiarum.] [Opera ... tomus primus: qui continet De dignitate & augmentis scientiarum, libros IX ...] Londini, In officina Joannis Haviland, 1623.

   [19], 493, [1] p.   30 cm.   **[544]**

Date on second title page altered by hand from MDCXXIII to MDCXXIIII.

Imperfect: first title page wanting.

Published also under title De augmentis scientiarum.

Gibson 129b.

STC 1108.

—[The same.] De dignitate & augmentis scientiarum, libri IX ... Ed. nova ... Lugd. Batav., Apud Franciscum Moyardum & Adrianum Wijngaerde, 1645.

[18], 749 [70] p.   13 cm.   [545]

Added engraved title page reads: De augmentis scientiarum lib. IX.

Gibson 132.

—[The same.] De augmentis scientiarum lib. IX. Amstelaedami, Sumptibus Joannis Ravesteinii, 1662.

[20], 607, [67] p.   14 cm.   [546]

Gibson 135.

—[English retranslation] Of the advancement and proficience of learning; or, The partitions of sciences IX bookes ... Interpreted by Gilbert Wats ... Oxford, Printed by Leon. Lichfield, for Rob. Young, & Ed. Forrest, 1640.

[37], 60, [11], 477, [22] p.   front. (port.)   29 cm.

Engraved title page.   [547]

Gibson 141b.

STC 1167.3

—The essays; or, Counsels, civil & moral ... With a Table of the colours of good and evil, whereunto is added the Wisdome of the ancients. Enlarged ... and now more exactly published. London, Printed by Thomas Ratcliffe and Tho. Daniel, for Humphrey Robinson, 1668.

3 parts in 1 v.   front. (port.)   15 cm.   [548]

Part [3] has special title page: The Wisdome of the ancients. Written in Latine by ... Sir Francis Bacon ... Done into English by Sir Arthur Gorges ... London ... 1669.

Gibson 21b.

—[Historia ventorum.] Historia naturalis & experimentalis de ventis, &c. Lugd. Batavorum, Apud Franciscum Hackium, 1648.

[16], 232, [16] p.   13 cm.   [549]

Engraved title page.

"Aditus ad titulos in proximos quinque menses destinatos": p. 113–126.

"Historia naturalis, et experimentalis de forma calidi": p. [127]–189.

"De motus, sive virtutis activae variis speciebus": p. [190]–232.

Gibson 110a.

—[The same.] ... Amstelodami, Ex officina Elzeviriana, 1662.

[16], 232, [16] p.   14 cm.   [550]

Engraved title page.

Gibson III. Willems 1277. (Printed in Leyden by the widow and heirs of Jean Elsevier.)

Bound with *his* Novum organum scientiarum. 1660.

—Historia vitae & mortis. Sive, titulus secundus in Historia naturali & experimentali ad condendam philosophiam: quae est Instaurationes magnae pars tertia. Londini, In officina Jo. Haviland, impensis Matthaei Lownes, 1623.

[5], 454 (i.e. 458) p.   17 cm.   [551]

Gibson 147.

STC 1156.

—[The same.] ... Lugduni Batavorum, Ex officina Joannis Maire, 1636.

476, [71] p.   12 cm.   [552]

Gibson 148.

—[The same.] Historia vitae et mortis cum annotatioinb [sic] Barthol. Moseri ... noviter in lucem data ... Dilingae, Typis academ., 1645.

[12], 526, [52] p.   11 cm.   [553]

Engraved title page.

Gibson 150.

—[English tr.] The historie of life and death. With observations naturall and experimentall for the prolonging of life ... London, by I. Okes, for Humphrey Mosley, 1638.

[13], 323 p.   15 cm.   [554]

Added engraved title page.

Gibson 153.

STC 1157.

—[The same.] History naturall and experimentall, of life and death. Or, Of the prolongation of life. Written in Latine ... London, Printed by John Haviland for William Lee, and Humphrey Mosley, 1638.

[29], 395 (i.e. 435) p.   15 cm.   [555]

Edited by William Rawley.

Gibson 154.

STC 1158.

—[French tr.] Le medecin historial; ou, Le parfait regime de vivre, dans lequel est décrit la vertu de tous les animaux, des simples, plantes, racines, arbres, fruicts, des perles, pierres, pierreries, ioyaux, & de toutes sortes de metaux qui servent, & ont la propriété pour conserver la santé de l'homme . . . Par M. Baudoin. Paris, Chez la veufue G. Loyson, 1652.

[31], 508 (i.e. 506), [2] p.   18 cm.   **[556]**

Imperfect: first preliminary leaf (blank?) wanting.
Running title: Histoire de la vie, et de la mort.
Translated by Jean Baudoin.
Gibson 1551.

—[Novum organum.] Instauratio magna . . . Londini, Apud Joannem Billium, 1620.

[9], 360 (i.e. 352), 36, [1] p.   32 cm.   **[557]**

Engraved title page.
Running title: Novum organum.
Gibson 103b.
STC 1163.

—[The same.] Novum organum scientiarum. Ed. 2. Amstelaedami, Sumptibus Joannis Ravesteiny, 1660.

[23], 404 p.   14 cm.   **[558]**

Engraved title page.
Gibson 106.
With this is bound *his* Historia naturalis . . . de ventis. 1662.

—Sylva sylvarum; or, A naturall historie. In ten centuries . . . Published after the authors death by William Rawley . . . London, Printed by J. H. for William Lee, 1627.

2 parts in 1 v.   front.   (port.)   27 cm.

[559]

Part [2] has special title page: New Atlantis. A worke unfinished.
Imperfect: engraved title page wanting.
Gibson 171.
STC 1169.

—Sylva sylvarum; or, A natural history. In ten centuries. Whereunto is newly added the History naturall and experimentall of life and death; or, Of the prolongation of life . . . Published after the authors death, by William Rawley . . . Hereunto is now added an alphabetical table of the principall things contained in the ten centuries. The 7th ed. London, Printed for William Lee, and sold by Thomas Williams, 1658.

3 parts in 1 v.   front.   (port.)   28 cm. **[560]**

Added engraved title page.
Each part has special title page.
Contents. — [pt. 1] Sylva sylvarum: or, a Natural history. [Followed by: Articles of enquiry, touching metals and minerals . . . Newly put forth this yeare 1661. by the former publisher (with special title page dated 1662)] — [pt. 2] New Atlantis. A work unfinished. — [pt. 3] History natural and experimental, of life and death. Or, Of the prolongation of life.
Gibson 177b.

—[The same.] . . . The 8th ed., whereunto is added Articles of enquiry touching metals and minerals . . . London, Printed by J. F. and S. G. for William Lee, and are sold by Thomas Williams, 1664.

3 parts in 1 v.   front.   (port.)   29 cm. **[561]**

Added engraved title page.
Gibson 178.

—[The same.] . . . The 10th ed., in which is added . . . his . . . Novum organum . . . never before published in English. London, Printed by S. G. and B. Griffin for Thomas Lee, 1676.

3 parts in 1 v.   front.   (port.)   31 cm. **[562]**

Added engraved title page.
Part [2] has half title; part [3] and remaining treatises have special title pages.
Gibson 180.

—*as subject. See* Ross, A. Arcana microcosmi. 1652.

BACON, Petrus. *See* Dispensatorium chymicum. 1626.

BACON, Roger [1214?–1294] De arte chymiae scripta. Cui accesserunt opuscula alia ejusdem authoris. Francofurti, Typis Joannis Saurii, Sumptibus Joannis Theobaldi Schönvvetteri, 1603.

408 p.   14 cm.   **[563]**

Contents. — "Excerpta ex libro sexto scientiarum": p. 7–16. — "Excerpta de libro Avicennae": p. [17]–94. — "Breviarium de dono Dei": p. 95–264. — "Verbum abbreviatum de leone viridi": p. 264–284. — "Secretum secretorum naturae de laude lapidis philosophorum": p. 285–408.

—De alchemia libellus, cui titulum fecit, speculum alchemiae.

377–385 p., vol. 2.   20 cm.   (*In* Zetzner, Lazarus, *ed.* Theatrum chemicum. Argentorati 1659–61)

Caption title.   **[564]**

—[English tr.] Speculum alchymiae; The true glass of alchemy. *In* Collectanea chymica. 1684.

—*See* Basilius Valentinus. Triumph-Wagen Antimonii . . . 1676; Salmon, W. Medicina practica. 1692.

—De mirabili potestate artis & naturae . . . libellus.

327–346 p., vol. 2.   17 cm.   (*In* Artis auriferae. Basileae, 1610)   **[565]**

Caption title.

—[De retardandis senectutis accidentibus. English.] The cure of old age, and preservation of youth ... Translated out of Latin; with annotations, and an account of his life and writings. By Richard Browne ... Also A physical account of the tree of life, by Edw. Madeira Arrais. Translated likewise out of Latin by the same hand. London, Tho. Flesher and Edward Evets, 1683.

[40], 156 p; [5], 108, 7 p. 18 cm.   [566]

2 v. in 1. Each v. has special title page.
Translated from the abridgment published in 1590.

—Epistola fratris Rogerii Baconis, de secretis operibus artis et naturae, et de nullitate magiae. Opera Johannis Dee ... e pluribus exemplaribus castigata olim, et ad sensum integrum restituta ... Cum notis quibusdam partim ipsius Johannis Dee, partim edentis. [Argentorati, Sumptibus heredum Eberh. Zetzneri, 1660]

834-868 p., vol. 5. illus. 20 cm. (In Zetzner, Lazarus, ed. Theatrum chemicum. Argentorati, 1659-61)   [567]

Caption title.

—[English tr.] His discovery of the miracles of art, nature, and magick. Faithfully translated out of Dr Dees own copy, by T. M. and never before in English. London, Simon Miller, 1659.

[12], 51, [7] p. 14 cm.   [568]

—[French tr.] De l'admirable pouvoir et puissance de l'art & de nature, ou est traicté de la pierre philosophale. Traduit en françois par Jacques Girard de Tournus. Paris, Pierre Billaine, 1629.

63 (i.e. 64) p. 17 cm.   [569]

Contains Girard's letter to Charles Fontaine (p. 53-62).

—[German tr.] Von der wunderbahrlichen Gewalt der Kunst und der Natur.

426-455 p., part 2. 19 cm. (In Morgenstern, Philipp, ed. and tr. Turba philosophorum. Basel, 1613)   [570]

Caption title.

BACON, WILLIAM [17th cent.] A key to Helmont. See CASE, J. The wards of the Key to Helmont. 1682.

BACQUERE, BENEDICTUS DE [fl. 1673] Senum medicus, quaedam praescribens observanda, ut sine magnis molestiis aliquousque senectus protrahatur ... Coloniae Agrippinae, Sumptibus haeredum Joannis Widenfeldt, 1673.

[32], 285, [19] p. 17 cm.   [571]

BADEN, ANDREW [fl. 1683-1697] tr. See LE CLERC, D. The history of physick. 1699.

BADGER, JOHN [fl. 1693] The case between Doctor John Badger and the College of Physicians London: who ... in ... 1683, presented himself to the president and censors to be examined ... [London, 1693]

4 p. 21 cm.   [572]

Imprint supplied from Wing B383.

—See THE STATUTES OF THE COLLEDGE OF PHYSICIANS LONDON. 1693.

BADI, SEBASTIANO. See BALDI, Sebastiano [fl. 1650-1676].

BADILI, VALERIO [fl. 1603] Tractatus de secanda vena in pueris vel ante XIV. aetatis annum ... Veronae, Typis Tamianis, 1606.

[8], 103 p. 19 cm.   [573]

BADO, SEBASTIANO. See BALDI, Sebastiano [fl. 1650-1676]

BAERLE, KASPAR VAN [1584-1648] Methodus morum. In Groot, H. de. H. Grotii et aliorum dissertationes de studiis instituendis. 1645.

—Rerum per octennium in Brasilia et alibi gestarum, sub praefectura ... I. Mauritii Nassaviae &c. comitis, historia. Ed. 2. Cui accesserunt Gulielmi Pisonis ... Tractatus 1. De aeribus, aquis & locis in Brasilia. 2. De arundine sacchariferá. 3. De melle silvestri. 4. De radice altili mandihoca ... Clivis, Ex officina Tobiae Silberling, 1660.

[23], 664, [21] p. plates. (incl. port., maps) 16 cm.   [574]

Added engraved title page reads: Res Brasiliae ...

—See CORVINUS, J. A. Oratio in obitum ... D. Casparis Barlaei. 1648; REGIMEN SANITATIS SALERNITANUM. Schola Salernitana. 1649, 1657, 1667, 1683.

BAGATO, CAMMILLO. Breve discorso di fisonomia et un ... trattato della compiessione del corpo humano. Con una regola per cognietturare l'inclinatione, e costumi di ciascun temperamento ... Parma, Piacenza, Livorno, & Lucca, Per Jacint. Paci, 1659.

[12] p. 15 cm.   [575]

BAGGER, HANS, Bp. of Zeeland [1646-1693] See PAULLI, S. Commentarius de abusu tabaci. 1665;

WORM, W. Oratio in excessum ... Thomae Bartholini. 1681.

BAGGER, JOHANNES. *See* BAGGER, Hans, *Bp. of Zeeland* [1646-1693]

BAGLIONUS, TOMAS, *ed. See* MASSARIA, A. Libelli duo de pulsibus, & urinis. 1603.

BAGLIVI, GIORGIO [1668?-1707?] De fibra motrice et morbosa; nec non, De experimentis, ac morbis salivae, bilis, & sanguinis, ubi obiter de respiratione, & somno. De statice aeris, & liquidorum per observationes barometricas, & hydrostaticas ad usum respirationis explicata. De circulatione sanguinis in testudine, ejusdemque cordis anatome. Epistola ad Alexandrum Pascoli. Perusiae, Apud Constantinum, 1700.

[1], 58 p. front., illus. 22 cm. **[576]**
Bound with (as issued?) Pascoli, A. Il corpo-umano. 1700.

—De praxi medica ad priscam observandi rationem revocanda. Libri duo. Accedunt dissertationes novae. Romae, Typis Dominici Antonii Herculis, sumptibus Caesaretti, 1696.

[20], 259 p.; 119, [1] p. 17 cm. **[577]**
Imperfect: p. 47-48 (2d group of paging) wanting.
The Dissertationes novae have special title pages. Dissertatio 1 has title: De anatome, morsu, & effectibus tarantulae. Dissertatio 2 has title: De usu & abusu vesicantium. Dissertatio 3 has title: De observationibus anatomicis, & practicis varii argumenti.

—De praxi medica ad priscam observandi rationem revocanda, libri duo. Accedunt dissertationes novae: I. De anatome, morsu & effectibus tarantulae ... II. De usu & abusu vesicantium. III. Experimenta varia anatomico infusoria. IV. De circulatione sanguinis in rana. V. Historia morbi & sectionis cadaveris Marcelli Malpighii ... VI. Appendix de apoplexiis fere epidemicis ... Lugduni, Sumptibus Anisson & Joann. Posuel, 1699.

[16], 407 p. 20 cm. **[578]**

—Another issue, with new title page. Imprint reads: Lugduni, & veneunt Parisiis, Apud Joannem Anisson, 1699.

[16], 407 p. illus. 20 cm. **[579]**

—[The same.] ... Lugduni Batav., Apud Fredericum Haringium, 1700.

[20], 259, 119, [9] p. illus. 17 cm. **[580]**
De praxi medica incorrectly bound after Dissertationes novae.
The Dissertationes novae have special title pages dated 1699.
A reprint of the 1696 edition.

—*See* ANDRY DE BOISREGARD, N. De la génération des vers dans le corps de l'homme. 1700.

BAIER, JOHANN JACOB [*b.* 1664] *respondent. See* WALDSCHMIDT, J. J., *praeses.* Medicus Cartesianus. 1687.

—*See* WEDEL, G. W. Propempticon inaugurale de contractura daemoniaca. 1691.

BAIER, JOHANN JAKOB [1677-1735] *respondent. See* CRAUSE, R. W., *praeses.* Dissertatio medica inauguralis de capillis. 1700; HOFFMAN, F. [1660-1742] *praeses.* Dissertatio medica de necessaria salivae inspectione ad conservandam et restaurandam sanitatem. 1698; WEDEL, G. W., *praeses.* Dissertatio medica de ambra. 1698.

—*as subject. See* SLEVOGT, J. A. Facultatis Medicae decani Jo. Hadriani Slevogtii ... prolusio inauguralis, de exceptionibus medicis. 1700.

BAILEY, WALTER. *See* BAYLEY, Walter [1529-1593]

BAILLARD, EDME, *pseud. See* PRADE, Jean Le Royer, *sieur de* [*fl.* 1640-1685]

[**BAILLET**, ADRIEN, 1649-1706] La vie de Mr Descartes. Réduite en abregé. Paris, Guillaume de Luynes, La veuve de P. Boüillerot et Claude Cellier, 1692.

[18], 374, [2] p. 18 cm. **[581]**

BAILLON, GUILLAUME DE. *See* BAILLOU, Guillaume de [1538-1616].

BAILLOU, GUILLAUME DE [1538-1616] Commentarius in libellum Theophrasti De vertigine. Editore M. Jacobo Thevart ... Parisiis, Apud Jacobum Quesnel, 1640.

[4], 41, [3] p. 23 cm. **[582]**
Includes Greek and Latin text of Theophrastus's De vertigine.
Bound with (as issued?) *his* Epidemiorum et ephemeridum libri duo. 1640.

—Consiliorum medicinalium libri II. A Jacobo Thevart ... scholiis nonnullis illustrati, digesti ac in lucem primum editi. Tomus primus [-secundus] ... Adjecta est authoris vitae [ex libro Renati Moraei]. Parisiis, Apud Jacobum Quesnel, 1635-1636.

2 v. in 1. 22 cm. **[583]**
Vol. 2 dated 1636.

—[The same.] ... Tomus primus [-secundus; Liber III, et postremus]. Adjecta est authoris vitae [ex libro Renati Moraei]. Parisiis, Apud Jacobum Quesnel, 1635-1649.

3 v.   23 cm.   [584]

Vol. 2 dated 1649. Vol. 3 dated 1649 has title: Consiliorum medicinalium, liber III. et postremus. Item, Paradigmata et historiae morborum ob raritatem observatione dignissimae . . . The Liber paradigmatum has special title page dated 1649.

—De convulsionibus libellus. In quo solennis quaestio explicatur, cur sauciatis dextra capitis parte convulsio sanae partis contingat. Editore M. Jacobo Thevart . . . Parisiis, Apud Jacobum Quesnel, 1640.

[16], 51, [4] p.   23 cm.   [585]

—De virginum et mulierum morbis liber, in quo multa ad mentem Hippocratis explicantur, quae & ad cognoscendum & ad medendum pertinebunt. Studio . . . M. Jacobi Thevart . . . in lucem primum editus & scholiis aliquot locupletatus . . . Parisiis, Apud Jacobum Quesnel, 1643

[24], 269 (i.e. 251), [32] p.   port.   23 cm.
                                                   [586]

—Definitionum medicarum liber . . . Immo saepe data opera relicto ipsius disputationis filo loci Hippocratis & Galeni obscuri explicantur, ut commentarii adinstar esse possit. Studio & opera M. Jacobi Thevart . . . in lucem primum editus . . . Parisiis, Apud Jacobum Quesnel, 1639,

[19], 108, [8] p.   23 cm.   [587]

Bound with (as issued?) his Epidemiorum et ephemeridum libri duo. 1640.

—Epidemiorum et ephemeridum libri duo, studio & opera M. Jacobi Thevart . . . digesti . . . in lucem primum editi . . . Parisiis, Apud Jacobum Quesnel, 1640.

[19], 273, [18] p.   23 cm.   [588]

With this are bound (as issued?): his Definitionum medicarum liber. 1639; Commentarius in libellum Theophrasti De vertigine. 1640; De convulsionibus libellus. 1640.

—Opuscula medica, de arthritide, de calculo et de urinarum hypostasi. In quibus omnibus Galeni & veterum authoritas contra J. Fernelium defenditur. Item libellus vere aureus De rheumatismo & pleuritide dorsali . . . Editore M. Jacobo Thevart . . . Parisiis, Apud Jacobum Quesnel, 1643.

[16], 300 (i.e. 196), [27] p.   22 cm.   [589]

Liber De rheumatismo . . . has special title page, dated 1642.

—Pharos medicorum hoc est cautiones, animadversiones, et observationes practicae ex operibus, Gulielmi Ballonii . . . erutae, ordini practico traditae & libris decem comprehensae. Opera & sumptibus Theophili Boneti . . . Genevae, Apud Franciscum Miege, 1668.

[12], 695 p.   14 cm.   [590]

—[The same.] Labyrinthi medici extricati; sive, Methodus vitandorum errorum qui in praxi occurrunt, monstrantibus Gulielmo Ballonio & Lud. Septalio. Opera Theophili Boneti . . . Additus est ejusdem Septalii Tractatus de naevis. Genevae, Sumptibus Samuelis de Tournes, 1687.

[28], 733 (i.e. 735), [44] p.; 20, [3] p.   24 cm.
                                                   [591]

A reprint, with additions.

—[The same.] Filum ariadnaeum medicorum quo duce errores in praxi devitantur. Deductum ex operibus Gulielmi Ballonii . . . Opera Th. Boneti D. M. Genevae, Ex Typographia Duilleriana, 1688.

[12], 695 p.   15 cm.   [592]

A reissue, with new title page and preliminary material reset, of the Geneva 1668 edition, published under title Pharos medicorum hoc est Cautiones, animadversiones, et observationes practicae.

BAILLY, HEINRICH [fl. 1659-1662] respondent. Disputatio medica inauguralis de colica . . . Lugduni Batavorum, Ex officina Petri Didier, 1662.

[20] p.   23 cm.   [593]

Imperfect: p. [17-20] wanting.
Diss.—Leyden.

—See LINDEN, J. A. van der, praeses. Hippocrates de circuitu sanguinis, exercitatio V. 1660.

BAILLY, PIERRE [17th cent.] Questions naturelles et curieuses: contenans diverses opinions problematiques, recueillies de la medecine, touchant le regime de santé. Ou se voient plusieurs proverbes populaires . . . Paris, Pierre Bilaine, 1628.

[24], 733 (i.e. 725), [2] p.   [594]

Imperfect: pages 659-666 wanting.

—Les songes de phestion, paradoxes phisiologiques. Ensemble un dialogue De l'immortalité de l'ame & puissance de nature . . . Paris, Pierre Menard, 1634.

[15], 761, [38] p.   17 cm.   [595]

Errata: p. [38]
"De l' immortalité de l' ame" has special title page (p. [667])

BAILY, WALTER. See BAYLEY, Walter [1529-1593]

BAIRO, PIETRO [1468-1558] De medendis humani corporis malis enchiridion; quod vulgo veni mecum vocant: cui adjunximus ... Tractatum de peste. Francofurti, Apud Joannem Saurium, impensis Jacobi Fischeri, 1612.

[31], 859, [20] p. 13 cm. **[596]**
Dedication signed: Theodorus Zuingger.

—[The same.] ... Conimbricae, Apud Josephum Ferreyra, a custa de Manoel Carvalho, 1689.

[31], 773, [19] p. 16 cm. **[597]**

—[Italian tr.] Secreti medicinali ... Nei quali si contengono i rimedii, che si possono usar in tutte l' infermità, che vengono all'huomo, cominciando da capelli fino alla pianta de piedi ... Venetia, Nicolò Tebaldini, 1602.

[8], 262 ll. 16 cm. **[598]**
Translation by Giovanni Tatti, pseud. of Francesco Sansovino.

—[The same.] ... Venetia, Giorgio Valentini, 1629.

[8], 223 ll. 17 cm. **[599]**

BAJER, JOHANN JACOB [*fl.* 1687] *See* BAIER, Johann Jacob [*b.* 1664]

BAK, JACOB DE. *See* BACK, Jacobus de [1593 or 4-1658]

BAKER, GEORGE [1540-1600] The nature and propertie of quicksilver. *In* CLOWES, W. A profitable and necessarie booke of observations. 1637.

BAKER, ROBERT [17th cent.] Cursus osteologicus; being a compleat doctrine of the bones; according to the newest ... notions of anatomy ... To which is annexed by way of appendix, an excellent method of whitening, cleansing, preparing, and uniting the bones, to form a movable skeleton ... 2d ed. London, T. Leigh and D. Midwinter, 1699.

[10], 125, [1] p. plate. 17 cm. **[600]**

BALAMI, FERDINANDO [*fl.* 1514-*ca.* 1552] *tr. See* GALENUS. De ossibus. 1630, 1665.

BALASCON DE TARANTA. *See* VALESCO DE TARANTA [*fl.* 1382-1418]

BALBIAN, JOSSE VAN [*ca.* 1560-1616] [Tractatus septem de lapide philosophico]

649-698 p., vol. 3. 20 cm. (*In* Zetzner, Lazarus, *ed.* Theatrum chemicum. Argentorati, 1659-61) **[601]**
Title from table of contents.

—, *tr. See* ALANUS, *Bp. of Auxerre.* Dicta. 1659.

BALCIANELLI, GIOVANNI [*fl.* 1592-1603] Discorso contro l'abuso dell'antimonio preparato, o argento vivo sublimato, o del precipitato in medicine solutive ordinati ... Verona, Angelo Tamo, 1603.

30 p. 20 cm. **[602]**

BALDASSARRI, BALDASSARRE [*fl.* 1618] Ragioni, con le quali si dimostra, che il lapis lazuli si deve lavare, & non abbrucciare, per la confettione Alchermes de Mesue ... Ferrara, Stampa Camerale, 1618.

18 p. 21 cm. **[603]**

BALDE, JAKOB, *Father* [1604-1668] Medicinae gloria per satyras XXII. asserta ... Monachii, Sumptibus Joannis Wagneri, typis Lucae Straubii, 1651.

[8], 73 p. **[604]**

—Satyra contra abusum tabaci ... [Ingolstadii, Typis Ederianis excudebat, suis sumptibus Joannes Ostermayr, 1657]

[1], 31, [2] p. 16 cm. **[605]**

—[German tr.] Die truckene Trunkenheit. Eine aus ... Lateinischem gedeutschte Satyra oder Straff-Rede wider den Missbrauch des Tabaks. Samt einem Discurs von dem Nahmen, Ankunfft, Natur, Krafft und Würkung dieses Krauts. Nürnberg, Michael Endter, 1658.

[6], 256 p. front. 14 cm. **[606]**
A free translation by Sigmund von Birken. Cf. Arents, 265.

—Solatium podaricorum ... libri duo ... Monachii, Typis Lucae Straub, sumptibus Joannis Wagneri, 1661.

[24], 247 (i.e. 147), [1] p. front. 14 cm. **[607]**
"Solatii podagricorum pars II. Lusus satyricus sive fragmenta poëmatis ... Adversus Burghardum Sallium Gintrionem": p. [73]-247, has special title page.

BALDESI, ANTONIO [*fl.* 17th cent.] *ed. See* SEGNI, G. Questio de gangraenae et sphaceli diversa curatione ab ... Ant. Baldesio. 1613.

BALDEWEIN, CHRISTIAN ADOLPH. *See* BALDUIN, Christian Adolph [1632-1682]

BALDI, BALDO [*d.* 1645] De loco affecto in pleuritide disceptatio. Parisiis, Apud Sebastianum Cramoisy, 1640.

    121 (i.e. 117) p.   17 cm.   **[608]**
    With this is bound (as issued?): Moreau, René. Epistola exegetica. 1641.

—De loco affecto in pleuritide disceptationes. Ac Renati Moreau De eadem re Epistola exegetica. Romae, Typis Francisci Caballi, 1643.

    232 p.   17 cm.   **[609]**
    "Epistola exegetica de affecto loco in pleuritide. Ad . . . Baldum Baldium. Autore Renato Moreau": p. [65]-96 has special title page.
    "Baldo Baldi De loco affecto in pleuritide. Disceptatio secunda": p. 97-232 has caption title.

—Disquisitio iatro-physica ad textum 23. libri Hippocratis De aere, aquis, & locis; num in eo legi debeat χολωδέσωτατον, vel Θολωδέστατον, idest, biliosissimum, vel turbidissimum. In qua de calculorum causis, ac de aquae Tiberis bonitate strictim disseritur. Et quaestio de majori nunc, quam praeterito saeculo, calculosorum in urbe frequentia elucidatur. Romae, Ex typographia Ludovici Grignani, 1637.

    [12], 69, [3] p.   22 cm.   **[610]**

—Opobalsami orientalis in conficienda theriaca Romae abhibiti. Medicae propugnationes . . . Romae, Ex typographia Reverendae Camerae Apostolicae, 1640.

    69, [3] p.   23 cm.   **[611]**

—*See* COLLEGIO DEI MEDICI, Rome. Ordini. 1641.

—*as subject. See* PANUZZI, F., *ed.* Francesco Panuzzi . . . a i lettori. 1640.

BALDI, CAMILLO [1547?-1634] De humanarum propensionum ex temperamento praenotionibus, De naturalibus ex unguium inspectione pręsagiis, et De ratione cognoscendi mores, & qualitates scribentis ex ipsius Epistola missiva, nunc primum in Latinum sermonem prodiens tractatus tres . . . Bononiae, Typis HH. Evangelistae de Ducciis, 1664.

    [4], 251, [1] p.   22 cm.   **[612]**
    The second treatise edited by Hyppolito Scaffiliono is dated 1662; the third treatise is edited by Petrus Velius. Both have special title pages.

—De humanarum propensionum ex temperamento praenotionibus tractatus. Ex privatis Camilli Baldi . . . sermonibus; olim ab Hyppolito Scaffigliono . . . excerptus, & in lucem editus . . . Bononiae, Apud haeredes Joannis Rossii, 1629.

    [4], 141, [30] p.   21 cm.   **[613]**

—De naturali ex unguium inspectione praesagio comment. Ab eodem Hyppolito Scaffiliono . . . Ex ejusdem Camilli Baldi . . . sermonibus collectus ac typis mandatus . . . Bononiae, Apud haeredes Joannis Rossii, 1629.

    [6], 72, [8] p.   21 cm.   **[614]**

—In Physiognomica Aristotelis commentarii . . . Opus . . . Hieronymi Tamburini diligentia, & sumptibus nunc primum in lucem editum . . . Bononiae, Apud Sebastianum Bonomium, 1621.

    [16], 562, [20] p.   31 cm.   **[615]**
    Engraved title page.

BALDI, SEBASTIANO [*fl.* 1650-1676] Anastasis corticis Peruviae; seu, Chinae chinae defensio, Sebastiani Badi . . . Contra ventilationes Joannis Jacobi Chifletii, gemitusque Vopisci Fortunati Plemppii . . . Opus in tres libros distinctum, & ineis documentae medicinae, & philosophiae . . . Genuae, Typis Petri Joannis Calenzani, 1663.

    [39], 278 p.   25 cm.   **[616]**
    With this is bound (as issued?) *his* Phlebotomiae necessitas. 1663.

—Phlebotomiae necessitas, asserta a Sebastiano Bado, in variolis, morbillis, exanthematis, etiam apparentibus. Genuae, Typis Petri Joannis Calenzani, 1663.

    53, [19] p.   25 cm.   **[617]**
    Bound with (as issued?) *his* Anastasis corticis Peruviae. 1663.

—*See* LICETI, F. De motu sanguinis. 1647.

—*as subject. See* FELLINI, F. Apologemma jocosum. 1664.

BALDIT, MICHEL [*fl.* 1666] Speculum sacromedicum octogonum. In quo medicina octo ex angulis, veluti totidem fontibus a primo & in primum salientibus, sacra repraesentatur, Praefixa appendice gemina . . . Lugduni, Apud Danielem Gayet, 1666.

    363 p.   plate.   18 cm.   **[618]**
    Imperfect: p. 31-32 wanting.

BALDO, SEBASTIANO. *See* BALDI, Sebastiano [*fl.* 1650-1676].

BALDO DEGLI ABBATI, ANGELO. *See* ABATI, Baldo Angelo [16th cent.]

BALDOV, JOHANN [*ca.* 1604–1662] Disputatio physica de natura . . . Lipsiae, Typis Gregorii Ritzschii [1637]

    [20] p. 18 cm. **[619]**

Diss. pro loco—Leipzig.

BALDUCCI, VALERIO [16th–17th cent.] De putredine libri duo. Urbini, Apud Bartholomęum, & Simonem Ragusios, 1608.

    [14], 190 p. 22 cm. **[620]**

BALDUIN, PAUL FRIEDRICH [*fl.* 1694] *respondent.* See WEISS, S. Dissertatio physica de excrescentiis plantarum animatis. 1694.

    [58] p. 14 cm. **[621]**

Ferguson (A) lists a 58 p. edition of the same year published in Leipzig by Georg Heinrich Frommann.

BALDUIN, MICHAEL. See BOUDEWYNS, Michiel [1601–1681]

BALDUIN, PAUL FRIEDRICH [*fl.* 1694] *respondent.* See WEISS, S. Dissertatio physica de excrescentiis plantarum animatis. 1694.

BALDUS, BALDUS. See BALDI, Baldo, [d. 1645]

BALDUTIUS, VALERIUS. See BALDUCCI, Valerio, [16th–17th cent.]

BALEN, GYSBERT VAN [*fl.* 1699] *respondent.* Disputatio medica inauguralis de syncope . . . Lugduni Batavorum, Apud Abrahamum Elzevier, 1699.

    [15] p. 22 cm. **[622]**

Diss.—Leyden.

BALESCUS DE TARANTA. See VALESCO DE TARANTA [*fl.* 1382–1418]

BALESTRA, GIUSEPPE [d. 1657?] Gli accidenti più gravi del mal contagioso osservati nel lazzaretto all'Isola, con la specialitá de' medicamenti profittevoli, esperimentati per lo spatio di sette mesi . . . Roma, Francesco Moneta, 1657.

    [12], 75 p. 21 cm. **[623]**

BALEY, WALTER. See BAYLEY, Walter [1529–1593]

BALFOUR, *Sir* ANDREW [1630–1694] Letters written to a friend [i.e. Patrick Murray] . . . containing excellent directions and advices for travelling thro' France and Italy . . . Published from the author's original MS. Edinburgh, 1700.

    [12], x, 274 p. 16 cm. **[624]**

Edited by M. Balfour.

BALFOUR, M., *ed.* See BALFOUR, *Sir* A. Letters writen to a friend. 1700.

BALIANI, GIOVANNI BATISTA [1582–1666] Trattato della pestilenza . . . Savona, Gio. Tomaso Rossi, 1647.

    [4], 133, [6] p. 20 cm. **[625]**

—[The same.] . . . Stampato già l'anno M.DC. XLVII. et hora rivueduto, & ampliato dall'autore. Genova, Benedetto Guasco, 1653.

    [10], 198, [17] p. 21 cm. **[626]**

Dates altered by hand from MDCXLVII to MDCXCVII, and from MDCLIII to MDCXCVIII.

BALINGHEM, ANTOINE DE [1571–1630] Apresdinees et propos de table contre l'excez au boire, et au manger; pour vivre longuement, sainement, et sainctement, dialogisez entre un prince & sept scavants personnages . . . 2. ed., enrichie par l'autheur de plusieurs nouveaux discours, & de belles histoires. Avec Douze propositions pour passer plaisamment & honestement les jours des quaresmeaux . . . S. Omer, Charles Boscart, 1624.

    [24], 679 (i.e. 680) p. 16 cm. **[627]**

"Douze propositions . . . 3. ed." (p. [617]–679) has special title page, dated 1625.

BALLONIUS, GULIELMUS. See BAILLOU, Guillaume de [1538–1616]

BALNEUM Emsianum, das ist: Warhaffte Beschreibung dess hochfürlichen Schwebelbadts, unfehrn von Embs gelegen . . . Sampt einer Badordnung . . . Embs, Bey Bartholome Schnell, 1678.

    23 p. illus., plate. 16 cm. **[628]**

BALTZER, BARTHOLD [*fl.* 1676–1677] *respondent.* See SCHWELING, J. E., *praeses.* Bartholdus Baltzers . . . Dissertationem hydrographico-physicam de maribus . . . submittet. 1676.

BANC, JEAN [*fl.* 1605] La memoire renouvellee des merveilles des eaux naturelles. En faveur de nos nymphes françoises, & des malades qui ont recours à leurs emplois salutaires. Paris, Pierre Sevestre, 1605.

    [12], 140 ll. 18 cm. **[629]**

Imperfect: p. 96–97 mutilated.

3 treatises in 1 v. Treatise 2 has special title page: De l'usage et employ des eaux naturelles contre les maladies . . . Par Jean

Ban. Treatise 3 has special title page: La mémoire renouvellee . . .
Par Jean Ban.

—[The same.] La merveille des eaux naturelles,
sources et fontaines medicinales les plus celebres de
la France . . . Paris, Pierre Sevestre, 1606.

[8], 140, [4] ll. 17 cm. [630]

A reissue of the 1605 edition with new title page dated 1606 and
index added.

BANDI, et provisioni. *See* BOLOGNA. Ordinances,
local laws, etc.

BANDI, provigioni, et ordini. 1632. *See* MODENA.
Ordinances, local laws, etc.

BANDO contro a chl [sic] fraudolentemente
dispenserà l'orvietano de Francesco di Jacopo Sozzi.
See TUSCANY. Laws, statutes, etc.

BANDO et ordini sopra la conservatione della
sanità nello stato ecclesiastico. 1630. *See* CATHOLIC
CHURCH. Camera apostolica.

BANDO, et provisione. *See* BOLOGNA. Ordinances,
local laws, etc.

BANDO in occasione di peste. 1611, 1630. *See* REG-
GIO EMILIA (CITY) Ordinances, local laws, etc.

BANDO per causa di contagio. 1634. *See* MODENA.
Ordinances, local laws, etc.

BANDO per cause di contagio. 1656. *See* ROME
(CITY) ORDINANCES, local laws, etc.

BANDO per causa di peste. 1630, 1634. *See*
MODENA. Ordinances, local laws, etc.

BANDO per occasione di contagio. 1639. *See*
MODENA. Ordinances, local laws, etc.

BANDO per occasione di sospetto di peste. 1629.
See REGGIO EMILIA (CITY) ORDINANCES, local laws,
etc.

BANDO, provvisioni, et ordini per conservazione
della sanità. 1682. *See* MODENA (DUCHY) LAWS,
statutes, etc.

BANDO sopra la peste. 1611. *See* REGGIO EMILIA
(CITY) ORDINANCES, local laws, etc.

BANDO sopra le guardie delle marine per causa
di peste. 1690. *See* URBINO (DUCHY) ORDINANCES, local
laws, etc.

BANDO sopra quelli, che essercitano la medicina.
1680. *See* URBINO (DUCHY) ORDINANCES, local laws,
etc.

BANESIUS, FAUSTUS NAIRONUS. *See* NAIRONI, Antonio Fausto [1635 or 6-1707]

BANESTER, JOHN. *See* BANISTER, John,
[1540-1610]

BANHOLZER, JOHANN, *Father* [*fl.* 1682] *praeses.*
Oculus per quaestiones acroamaticas et exotericas explicatus . . . Dilingae, Typis Joannis Caspari Bencard, 1682.

[4], 35, [1] p. 23 cm. [631]

Diss.—Dillingen. (T. Götschl, respondent)

BANISTER, JOHN [1540-1610] The workes of . . .
Mr. John Banester; by him digested into five bookes.
His cure, 1. Of tumors. 2. Of wounds in generall and
particular. 3. Of ulcers. 4. Of fractures and luxations.
5. His Antidotary, being a storehouse of all sorts of
medicines belonging to the chyrurgians use. To
which is added a treatise for distilling of oyles of all
sorts, with a perfect order to prepare all minerals,
and to draw forth their oyles and salts, &c. London,
Thomas Harper, 1633.

3 v. in 1. 19 cm. [632]

Imperfect: vol. [1]: prelim. leaf (half title?) wanting; vol. [3]:
p. 13-28 wanting.

Vol. [1] has an unidentified stub between p. 272 and 273.

Books 1-4, comprising vol. [1], were previously published in London in 1585 under title: A compendious cyhrurgerie, gathered and
translated especially out of Wecker.

Book 5 (vol. [2]) has special title page: An antidotary chyrurgicall:
or, A storehouse of all sorts of medicines that commonly fall into
the chyrurgians use.

The appended treatise (vol. [3]) has special title page: A
storehouse of physicall and philosophicall secrets . . . Also issued
separately in the same year. The same work purporting to be "first
written in the German tongue by . . . Paraselsus [sic], and now
published in the English tongue, by John Hester," also appeared
in London in 1633 under title: The secrets of physick and
philosophy.

With this is bound *his* A treatise of chirurgerie. 1633.

—A treatise of chirurgerie: briefly comprehending
the generall and particular curation of ulcers. Collected out of severall famous authors, especially Antonius Calmeteus Vergesatus, and Johannes
Tagaltius . . . Herunto is annexed certaine experiments . . . truly tryed . . . London, Thomas
Harper, 1633.

[16], 166 p. 19 cm. [633]

Last leaf (blank?) wanting.

"A generall diet, necessarie to be observed in the curation of ulcers, taken out of Angerius Ferrerius": p. 97–110.

"A table of simples": p. 111–137.

Bound with *his* The workes. 1633.

BANISTER, RICHARD [1570?–1626] Breviary of the eyes. *See* GUILLEMEAU, J. A treatise of one hundred and thirteene diseases of the eyes. 1622.

BANZER, MARKUS [1592–1664] Fabrica receptarum, id est: Methodus brevis . . . in qua quae sint remediorum compositorum formae . . . planissime edocetur . . . Augustae Vindelicorum, Ex officina typographica Andreae Apergeri, sumptibus Sebastiani Mylii, 1622.

[30], 663, [6] p.   tables.   16 cm.   **[634]**

Errata: p. [669]

—*praeses.* Disputatio medica de incubo . . . Wittebergae, Typis Johannis Röhneri, 1651.

[16] p.   19 cm.   **[635]**

Diss.—Wittenberg (A. Wanckel, *respondent*)

BARASIN, LOUIS [*fl.* 1685] *respondent. See* POSTEL, N., *praeses.* Quaestio medica. 1685 [and] Factum. 1685.

BARBA, PEDRO [1590–1650] Breve, y clara resumpta, y tratado de la essencia, causas, prognostico, preservacion, y curacion de la peste . . . Madrid, Alonso de Paredes, 1648.

[2], 12 (i.e. 18) p.   20 cm.   **[636]**

—Vera praxis de curatione tertianae . . . [Lovanii? 1642?]

[26] p.   20 cm.   **[637]**

Bound with Plemp, V. F. Animadversio. 1642.

—*See* MOHY, H. Tertianae crisis. 1642?; PLEMP, V. F. Animadversio. 1642; SOERS, M. Stricturae in ceritum quemdam Eburonem inconditum blateronem controversiae de curanda tertiana inter D. D. Petrum Barbam et V. F. Plempium. 1642.

BARBARO, ERMOLAO [1453 *or* 4–1493] *See* PLINIUS SECUNDUS, C. Naturalis historiae, tomus primus [-tertius] 1668–1669.

BARBATO, BARTOLOMEO [*fl.* 1618–1640] Il contagio di Padova nell'anno M.DC.XXXI . . . Rovigo, Giacinto Bissuccio, 1640.

[8], 58, [3] p.   front.   31 cm.   **[638]**

Errata: p. [61]

BARBATO, GIROLAMO [17th cent.] De arthritide libri duo . . . Accessit De sanguine, & ejus sero exercitatio . . . Venetiis, Typis Valentini Mortali, 1665.

16, 123, [1] p.   front.   22 cm.   **[639]**

—De formatrice, conceptu, organizatione, & nutritione foetus in utero dissertatio anatomica. Patavii, Apud Bodium, 1676.

14, 144, [12] p.   plates.   23 cm.   **[640]**

—Dissertatio elegantissima de sanguine et ejus sero, in qua praeter varia lectu dignissima, Conringii, Lindeni & Barthol. circa sanguificationem opiniones, Stenoniana sanguinis dealbatio, Willisii succi nervorum vis, Regii transitus chyli ad lienem, Liceti nutritio embryonis, Warthoni & Charletonis lactis expositio, Harvei masculini Seminis retentio rejecta, Moebii spirituum animalium materia & alia clarissimorum neotericorum prolata . . . exponuntur. Parisiis, Apud Robertum de Ninville, 1667.

[8], 88 p.   15 cm.   **[641]**

—[The same.] . . . Francofurti ad Moen. Impensis Joh. Davidis Zunneri, literis Johannis Andreae, 1667.

[2], 82 p.   14 cm.   **[642]**

BARBE, SIMON [17th cent.] Le parfumeur françois, qui enseigne toutes les manieres de tirer les odeurs des fleurs; & à faire toutes sortes de compositions de parfums . . . Lyon, Thomas Amaulry, 1693.

[46], 132, [10] p.   15 cm.   **[643]**

BARBECK, FRIEDRICH GOTTFRIED [*d.* 1704?]

Dissertations—Duisburg

—*praeses.* Disputatio medica altera de veneno . . . Duisburgi ad Rhenum, Apud Franconem Sas, 1689.

20 p.   20 cm.   **[644]**

J. Sudecius, *respondent.*

—Disputatio medica de generatione animalium . . . Duisburgi ad Rhenum, Apud Franconem Sas, 1693.

[2], 30 p.   20 cm.   **[645]**

J. T. Schombart, *respondent.*

—Disputatio medica de generatione corporis humani . . . Duisburgi ad Rhenum, Typis Johannis Sas, 1695.

16 p.   20 cm.   **[646]**

S. à Bergh, *respondent.*

—Disputatio medica de vita . . . Duisburgi ad Rhenum, Apud Johannem Sas, 1694.

    32 p.   20 cm.   **[647]**

    P. H. Schmitz, *respondent*.

—Disputatio medico-philosophica de generatione hominis . . . Duisburgi ad Rhenum, Apud Johannem Sas, 1695.

    32 p.   20 cm.   **[648]**

    J. K. Melm, *respondent*.

—Dissertatio medica de febrium differentia ac natura . . . Duisburgi ad Rhenum, Typis Johannis Sas, 1696.

    [2], 28 (i.e. 38) p.   20 cm.   **[649]**

    B. H. Brauns, *respondent*.

BARBEIRAC, CAROLUS. *See* BARBEYRAC, Charles de [1629–1699]

BARBERINI, CARLO, *Cardinal* [1630–1704] *See* URBINO (DUCHY) Ordinances, local laws, etc. Bando sopra quelli, che essercitano la medicina. 1680.

BARBERINI, FRANCESCO, *Cardinal* [1597–1679] *See* CATHOLIC CHURCH. Camera apostolica. Bando et ordini sopra la conservatione della sanità nello stato ecclesiastico. 1630.

BARBETTE, PAUL [*ca.* 1623–1666] Opera omnia medica et chirurgica notis et observationibus nec non pluribus morborum historiis, & curationibus illustrata & aucta, cum appendice eorum quae in Praxi omissa vel concise nimia pertrectata fuerant. Opera et studio Joh. Jac. Mangeti . . . Genevae, Apud Johannem Ant. Chouët, 1682.

    [8], 273, [7], 174, 138, [39] p. plate. 22 cm.

                            [650]

Imperfect: plate wanting (referred to in the text, p. 42–43 (4th group))

The appendix mentioned in the title did not appear until the "editio novissima" appeared in 1688. Cf. editor's pref.

The Praxis, includes the notes of Frederik Dekkers. The other works, originally written in Dutch, are reprinted from the Latin edition first published by Gelder in Leyden in 1672.

—Another issue, with imprint date altered to 1683 and preliminary matters reset.   **[651]**

—[The same.] . . . Genevae, Sumptibus Joannis Antonii Chouët, 1688.

    [8], 332, [28], 542, [10] p. illus., plates. 21 cm.

                            [652]

Manget's appendix (referred to in the title of the 1682 edition, but not actually printed with it) first appeared in the present edition. Cf. editor's pref.

—[German tr.] Chirurgische, anatomische und medicinische Schrifften, als nemlich: 1. Von der Wundartzney. 2. Von der Entgliederung dess menschlichen Leibs, benebens deren Gebrauch in der Wund-Artzney. 3. Von der Beschreibung der Pest . . . 4. Sampt der Practick der Artzney . . . Auss dem Holländischen ins Teutsche übersetzet . . . Franckfurt am Mayn, In Verlegung Johann Peter Zubrodts und Joh. Baptistä Schönwetters seel. Erben, gedruckt bey Johann Andreä, 1673.

    [14], 544, [29] p. illus. 18 cm.   **[653]**

Added engraved title page has title: Medicin- undt chÿrurgische Schriefften.

—Medicinische, chirurgische und anatomische Schrifften, samt beygefügten schönen Bericht von der Pest und eigenen wie auch D. Joh. Frider. Deckers nothwendigen Anmerckungen nach den heutigen neuen Erfindungen in der Anatomie und Circulation des Geblütes eingerichtet und mit Zusatz vieler heilsamen Artzney-Mittel aus D. Joh. Jacob. Magnets [sic] und anderer hocherfahrnen Autoren auffs neue zum vierdtenmahl vermehret . . . heraus gegeben. Lübeck und Leipzig, Johann Wiedemeyer, 1700.

    2 v. in 1. plate 17 cm.   **[654]**

Vol. [2] has special title page only: . . . Arzney-Practick mit beygefügten Anmerckungen Friderici Deckers . . . und Jo. Jacob. Magneti [sic] . . . Auff Begehren aus dem Lateinischen in das Teutsche übersetzet und zum drittenmahl verbessert heraus gegeben.

Each volume has added engraved title page.

Vol. [1] has title: Chirurgische und medicinische Wercke; vol. [2] has title: Praxis medica.

—Chirurgie nae de hedendaeghse practijck beschreven . . . Amsterdam, Jacob Lescaille, 1655.

    [16], 211, [13], p. 16 cm.   **[655]**

Engraved title page.

—[The same.] . . . Amsterdam, Jacob Lescaille, 1662.

    [18], 219 p. illus. 16 cm.   **[656]**

Engraved title page.

Imperfect? first prelim. leaf wanting?

With this is bound *his* Pest-beschryving. 1662.

—[Latin tr.] Opera chirurgico-anatomica, ad circularem sanguinis motum, aliaque recentiorum inventa, accommodata. Accedit De peste tractatus, observationibus illustratus. Lugd. Batab., Ex officina Hackiana, 1672.

[12], 461, [31] p. illus. 15 cm. [657]

Added engraved title page has title: Chirurgia.

"Tractatus de peste" (p. [405-461]) has special title page.

Translations of the Chirurgie (including the third part, Anatomia practica) and of Pest-beschryving.

—[The same.] ... Lugd, Batav., Joh. à Gelder, 1672.

[24], 216, 221, [19] p. illus. 14 cm. [658]

Added engraved title page has title: Chirurgia Barbettiana.

Errata: p. [19] at end.

—[The same.] ... Patavii, Typis Petri Mariae Frambotti, 1678.

[22], 425, [21] p. illus. 15 cm. [659]

Added engraved title page has title: Chirurgia Barbettiana.

—[The same.] ... Bononiae, Typis HH. Joannis Recaldini, 1685.

[19], 462 (i.e. 466), [1] p. illus. 15 cm. [660]

—[The same.] Chirurgia, notis ac observationibus rarioribus illustrata secundum verae philosophiae fundamenta ac recentiorum inventa, opera Johannis Muis ... Accedit De peste tractatus, observationibus illustratus. Amstelaedami, Apud Joannem Wolters, 1693.

[24], 543 (i.e. 541),[35] p. illus. 14 cm. [661]

Added engraved title page.

The Latin translations of the two works are based upon the edition published by Gelder, Leyden in 1672.

—[English tr.] The chirurgical and anatomical works. ... Composed according to the doctrine of the circulation of the blood, and other new inventions of the moderns. Together with A treatise of the plague, illustrated with observations. Translated out of Low-Dutch into English. Lonon [sic] Printed by J. Darby, and sold by Moses Pitt, 1672.

[15], 342 (i.e. 346), 52, [16] p. illus. 18 cm. [662]

Added engraved title page has title: Chirurgery according to the moderne practice.

Imperfect: 4th and 5th prelim. leaves wanting; 1 leaf (Z4 (blank!)) at end of the Chirurgery, wanting.

A fold of unpaged leaves, signed (*), containing the author's preface to the Practical anatomy (pt. 3 of the Chirurgery) is inserted before p. 201.

Translations of Chirurgie (including the 3d part, Anatomia practica) and of Pest-beschryving (52 p., 3d group)

—[The same.] Thesaurus chirurgiae: the chirurgical & anatomical works ... Composed according to the doctrine of the circulation of the blood, and other new inventions of the moderns. Together with A treatise of the plague; illustrated with observations. Translated out of Low-Dutch into English. The 3d ed. To which is added The surgeon's chest, furnished both with instruments and medicines ... and to make it more compleat, is adjoyned a treatise of diseases that for the most part attend camps and fleets. Written in High-Dutch by Raymundus Mindererus. London, Printed, and sold by Moses Pitt, 1676.

3 v. in 1. illus., plates. 18 cm. [663]

Added engraved title page has title: Chirurgery according to the moderne practice.

Vols. [2-3] have imprints: London, Printed by W. Godbid, and sold by Moses Pitt, 1674.

Vol. [2] has title: Cista militaris; or, A military chest ... Written in Latin, by Gulielmus Fabritius Hildanus. Englished for publick benefit. Vol. [3] has title: Medicina militaris: or, A body of military medicines experimented. By Raymundus Mindererus ... Englished out of the High-Dutch.

—[The same.] ... The 4th ed. ... London, Printed for Henry Rhodes, 1687.

[14], 394 (i.e. 398), [14] p.; [3], 119, [8] p. illus., plates. 18 cm. [664]

Part [2] has two special title pages (both bound at the beginning of the text which is paged continuously) with imprint: London, Printed for Charles Shortgrave, 1686.

The titles read: Cista militaris; or, A military chest ... written in Latine, by Gulielmus Fabritius Hildanus. Englished for publick benefit; and Medicina militaris: or, A boby [sic] of military medicines experimented. By Raymundus Mindererus ... Englished out of High-Dutch.

—[French tr.] Oeuvres chirurgiques et anatomiques ... appropriées à la circulation du sang, et autres découvertes des modernes. Avec un Traité de la peste enrichi d'observations. Geneve, François Miege, 1674.

[26], 625, [26] p. plate. 16 cm. [665]

Imperfect: added engraved title page and plate wanting.

Translations of Chirurgie (including the third part, Anatomia practica) and of Pest-beschryving, based on the Latin versions published by Gelder, Leyden, 1672.

Errata: p. [26] at end.

—[The same.] ... Lyon, Jacques Faeton, 1680.

[23], 554 (i.e. 454), [22] p. plate. 15 cm. [666]

Added engraved title page has title: La chirurgie.

—[The same.] . . . Derniere éd. Lyon, & se vend a Paris, Chez Laurent d'Houry, 1687.

[26], 554 (i.e. 454), [22] p.   plate.   16 cm.

[667]

Added engraved title page has title: La chirurgie.
Different setting of type.

—[Italian tr.] Opera chirurgica anatomica conformata al moto circolare del sangue, & altre invenzioni de' più moderni. Aggiuntovi un Trattato della peste con varie osservazioni [sic] . . . Tradotta dalla fiaminga nella latina, e da questa nella nostra lingua volgare. Venetia, Nicolò Pezzana, 1682.

[12], 478 p.   plate.   15 cm.   [668]

Imperfect: title page mutilated, plate wanting.
Dedicatory epistle, signed: Gasparo Storti [the translator?]

—[The same.] . . . Bologna, Longhi, 1692.

[12], 563, [1] p.   plate.   15 cm.   [669]

Imperfect: plate wanting (referred to in the text, p. 73-74).
Without the dedicatory epistle.

—[The same.] . . . Venetia, Francesco Groppo, 1696.

[12], 452 p.   plate.   15 cm.   [670]

Imperfect: plate wanting.

—Pest-beschryving . . . Den. 3. druck, met historische aenmerckingen vermeerdert. Amsterdam, Jacob Lescaille, 1662.

60 + p.   16 cm.   [671]

Imperfect: all after p. 60 wanting.
Bound with *his* Chirurgie. 1662.

—Praxis Barbettiana. Amstelaedami, Apud Jacobum Lescaille, 1665.

[8], 95 p.   16 cm.   [672]

—[The same] . . . Cum notis & observationibus Frederici Deckers . . . Lugd. Batav., Sumptibus auctoris, prostant apud Gaasbekios, 1669.

[16], 248, [56] p.   14 cm.   [673]

Added engraved title page.

—Another issue. Five of the eight errors have been corrected at press, although the errata have not been omitted on p. [56] at end.   [674]

—[The same.] . . . Bononiae, Sumptibus Petronii de Ruinettis, 1675.

[8], 183, [1] p.   16 cm.   [675]

This edition lacks the "Index rerum & verborum" present in the Leyden edition.

—[The same.] . . . Patavii, Typis Petri Mariae Frambot., 1676.

[13], 253, [47] p.   15 cm.   [676]

Added engraved title page.

—[The same.] . . . Amstelodami, Apud Adrianum Gaasbequium, 1678.

[16], 248, [56] p.   15 cm.   [677]

Added engraved title page.
One of two different printings of this edition issued by the same publisher in 1678.
Reprinted from the 1669 Leyden edition, without the errata printed in that edition, although four of the eight errors are not corrected in the text. This printing has comma after "lector" on p. [7] and has no running title on p. [8].

—[The same.] . . . Amstelodami, Apud Adrianum Gaasbequium, 1678.

[16], 248, [56] p.   15 cm.   [678]

Added engraved title page.
One of two different printings of this edition issued by the same publisher in 1678.
Reprinted from the 1669 Leyden edition, without the errata printed in that edition, although two of the eight errors are not corrected in the text. This printing has period after "lector" on p. [7] and has running title "Praefatio" on p. [8].

—[The same.] . . . Patavii, Typis Petri Mariae Frambot., 1681.

[14], 249, [46] p.   14 cm.   [679]

Added engraved title page.

—[The same.] . . . Amstelaedami, Apud Joannem Wolters, 1693.

[16] 248, [56] p.   15 cm.   [680]

Added engraved title page.

—[English tr.] The practice of the most successful physitian Paul Barbette . . . with the notes and observations of Frederick Deckers . . . Faithfully rendered into English. London, Printed by T. R. for Henry Brome, 1675.

[15], 271, [1] p.   17 cm.   [681]

Added engraved title page has title: The practice of phisick of Dr Paul Barbette with Dr. Fr. Deckers notes.

[French tr.] La pratique de medecine . . . enrichie de quantité de notes, observations, & histoires medicales. Par Frederic Deckers. Et augmentée en dernier lieu de plusieurs maladies qui y avoient esté omises ou traitées trop briévement, avec des annotations tres-utiles pour la pratique. Par J. Jacob Manget D. Med. Le tout nouvellement . . . traduit en françois. Lyon, Jean Bapt. Guillimin, 1692.

2 v. illus. 16 cm. [682]

"Traité de la peste . . . illustré de diverses remarques & observations" with "Traité de la petite verole, & de la rougeole": v. 2, p. 218–408.

— respondent. See SEBISCH, M. [1578–1674?] praeses. Disputatio de variolis et morbillis prima [-sexta & ultima] 1642.

— See PEST-BESCHRIJVING. 1664.

— as subject. See BILS, L. DE. Kort bericht over de waarschouwinge. 1660 [and] Responsio. 1661; STENO, N., Bp. De musculis et glandulis observationum specimen. 1664, 1683; WALDSCHMIDT, J. J. Praxis medicinae rationalis succincta. 1690, 1691.

[BARBEYRAC, CHARLES DE, 1629–1699] Traités nouveaux de medecine, contenans les maladies de la poitrine, les maladies des femmes, & quelques autres maladies particulieres, selon les nouvelles opinions. Lyon, Jean Certe, 1684.

[512], 357 p. 16 cm. [683]

— [The same.] . . . 2 ed. Lyon, Jean Certe, 1688.
[12], 357 p. 16 cm. [684]
Different setting of type.

Le BARBIER medecin. 1672. See MICHAULT, J.

BARCA DE ASTORGA, PEDRO. See BAREA DE ASTORGA, PEDRO [b. ca. 1630]

BARCHUSEN, JOHANN CONRAD [1666–1723] Pharmacopoeus synopticus; seu, Synopsis pharmaceutica, plerasque medicaminum compositiones, ac formulas, eorumque dextram, tam chemicam, quam Galenicam conficiendi methodum exhibens; in medicinae & pharmaciae studiosorum usum conscripta . . . Francofurti ad Moenum, Sumptibus Friderici Knochii, 1690.

[5], 179 p. 13 cm. [685]

— [The same.] . . . 2 ed., correcta, cumque plurimis curiosis aucta . . . Cui loco mantissae accedunt duae tabulae . . . Trajecti ad Rhenum, Ex officina Francisci Halmae, 1696.

[15], 249, [7] p. 17 cm. [686]
Added engraved title page.

— Pyrosophia, succincte atque breviter iatrochemiam, rem metallicam et chrysopoeiam pervestigans. Opus medicis, physicis, chemicis, pharmacopoeis, metallicis &c. non inutile. Lugduni Batavorum, Impensis Cornelii Boutestein, 1698.

[16], 469, [1] p. plates. 20 cm. [687]

BARCLAY, WILLIAM [1570?–1630?] Judicium, de certamine G. Eglisemmii cum G. Buchanano, pro dignitate paraphraseos Psalmi CIIII . . . Adjecta sunt, Eglisemmii ipsum judicium, ut editum fuit Londini . . . 1619: et . . . ejusdem Psalmi elegans paraphrasis Thomae Rhaedi. Londini, Apud Georgium Eldum, 1620.

[16], 61 p. 15 cm. [688]

BARDI, GIROLAMO [1604?–1667] Medicus politico catholicus; seu, Medicinae sacrae tum cognoscendae, tum faciundae idea . . . Genuae, Typis Jo. Mariae Farroni, 1644.

[23], 387 (i.e. 367), [20] p. 17 cm. [689]
Added half title.
Errata: p. [20] at end.

BARDILI, GEORG [fl. ca. 1664] respondent. See BROTBECK, J. K., praeses. Progymnasmatis medici pars prima. 1664.

BARDILI, GEORG KONRAD [fl. 1647] respondent. See BARDILI, K., praeses. Disputatio inauguralis. 1647.

BARDILI, KARL [fl. 1621–1647] praeses. Disputatio inauguralis theorico-practica de apoplexia. In qua neglecta, & rejecta Hippocratis, Galeni, & medicorum tot seculis radicata opinione, hujus gravissimi, & formidabilis affectus vera causa ex fundamentis medicis demonstratur . . . Tubingae, Typis Philberti Brunnii, 1647.

[2], 38 p. 19 cm. [690]
Diss. — Tübingen (G. K. Bardili, respondent).

— respondent. Dissertatio inauguralis theoricopractica, de pestilentia . . . Argentorati, Typis Johannis Reppii, 1626.

[16] p. 19 cm. [691]
Imperfect: first line of text cropped off on sig. A4, recto and verso.
Diss. — Strasbourg.

BAREA DE ASTORGA, PEDRO [b. ca. 1630] ed. See HEREDIA P. M. de. Opera medica. 1665, 1673, 1690.

BARET, RENÉ, sieur de Rouvray. Traicté des chevaulx . . . Paris, Sebastien Piquet, 1645.

[8], 105, [2] p. 22 cm. [692]
Engraved title page.

BARGELLINI, Giulio [*fl.* 1617] Dissertationes philosophicae et medicae ... [Florentiae, Apud Cosmum Juntam, 1617]

[23] p.   19 cm.   **[693]**

Imperfect: lower margin of title page trimmed with loss of imprint.

BARGER, Vitus Ulrich [*fl.* 1631] *respondent. See* Sigfrid, J., *praeses.* Positiones physicae de principiis. 1631.

BARIC, Arnaud [1607–1668] Les rares secrets, ou remedes incomparables, universels, & particuliers, preservatifs & curatifs, contre la peste des hommes, & des animaux ... Tolose, François Boude, 1646.

120 p.   14 cm.   **[694]**

BARICELLI, Giulio Cesare [*b.* 1574] De hydronosa natura; sive, Sudore humani corporis libri quatuor. In quibus non solum de origine, differentiis & praesagio; verum atque de usu apparatu, et curatione sudorum disseritur ... Neapoli, Apud Lazarum Scoriggium, 1614.

[18], 428, [25] p.   19 cm.   **[695]**

Engraved title page.

Date altered by hand from 1614 and 1618.

—De lactis, seri, & butyri facultatibus, & usu, opuscula. Cum iucunda, tum utilia, cum pleraque praeter medicorum commumem multorum opinionem notatu digna examinantur. Accessit in fine de chymico butyro non inutilis conventus ... Neapoli, Apud Lazarum Scoriggium, 1623.

[40], 167 p.   21 cm.   **[696]**

Engraved title page.

—Hortulus genialis; sive, Rerum iucundarum, medicarum, & memorabilium compendium, in quo multa naturę arcana, multę rerum sympathiae, & antipathiae, & auctoris observationes reserantur ... Neapoli, Apud Scipionem Boninum, 1617.

418 (i.e. 420), [28] p.   10 cm.   **[697]**

Imperfect: leaves of index after sig. Ee8 wanting.

—[The same.] Hortulus genialis; sive, Arcanorum valde admirabilium tam in arte medica quam reliqua philosophia, compendium, curiosis naturae scrutatoribus lectu tam utile quam iucundum ... Coloniae, Matthaeus Smitz, 1620.

353, [19] p.   14 cm.   **[698]**

—[The same.] ... Huic accessit liber De esculentorum potulentorumque facultatibus, Arnaldo Preitagio [sic] ... auctore. Genevae, Apnd [sic] Philippum Albert, 1620.

[12], 339, [28] p.; 320, [8] p.   12 cm.   **[699]**

Part [2] "De esculentorum potulentorumque facultatibus" has separate title page and pagination. It is a Latin version of Baldassare Pisanelli's Trattato della natura de' cibi e del bere.

—*See* Canale, F. Officina medicinale. 1622.

BARIGAZZI, Jacopo. *See* Berengario, Jacopo [*ca.* 1460–1530]

BARIL, Jean [*fl.* 1653] Physiologia humana et pathologia per tabulas synopticas ex Hippocratis et Galeni genio. Accessit Diaeta sanorum generalis, cum Summa de sectis medicorum ... Cadomi, Ex typographia Joannis Guesnon, Sumptibus authoris, 1653.

[10], 135, [1] p.   plate.   29 cm.   **[700]**

BARISANO, Francesco Domenico [1633–1719] Magnus Hippocrates medico-moralis ad utramque corporum scilicet, atque animarum salutem per geminam ejusdem Aphorismorum expositionem accommodatus ... Augustae Taurinorum, Ex typographia Bartholomei Zappatae, 1682.

[18], 411, [6] p.   front. (port.), illus.   23 cm.   **[701]**

Errata: p. [417]

[**BARKER**, Sir Richard *fl.* 1662–1676] The great preservative of mankinde; or, The transcendent vertue of the true spirit of salt. Long look'd for, and now philosophically prepared and purified from all hurtfull or corroding qualities ... London, R. D., 1662.

[1], 5, 4 p.   19 cm.   **[702]**

"Directions for the use of the spirit of salt" (4 p.) has caption title.

BARKHAUSEN, Johann Conrad. *See* Barchusen, Johann Conrad [1666–1723]

BARLAEUS, Caspar. *See* Baerle, Kaspar van [1584–1648]

BARLES, Louis [17th cent.] Les nouvelles decouvertes sur les organes des femmes, servans à la generation. Ensemble leu composition, connexion, action, & usages ... Lyon, Esprit Vitalis, 1674.

[20], 209, [6] p.   plates.   14 cm.   **[703]**

Errata: p. [6] at end.

—[The same.] ... Lyon, Esprit Vitalis, 1679.

[18], 208, [5] p.   plates.   16 cm.   **[704]**

—Les nouvelles decouvertes sur les organes des hommes, servans à la generation. Ensemble leur composition, connexion, action, & usages ... Lyon, Esprit Vitalis, 1675.

[26], 160 p. plates. 15 cm. [705]

Imperfect: added engraved title page wanting.

—Les nouvelles découvertes sur toutes les parties principales de l'homme, et de la femme. Ensemble leur composition, connexion, action, & usages ... 3. ed. rev. & corr. ... Lyon, Esprit Vitalis, 1680.

2 parts in 1 v. front. (port.), plates. 16 cm. [706]

Added engraved title page.

Part 2 dated 1682 has title: Les nouvelles decouvertes sur toutes les parties principales infermées dans la capacité du bas ventre; ensemble leur composition, connexion, actions, & usages.

—Les nouvelles decouvertes sur toutes les parties principales enfermées dans la capacité du bas ventre. Ensemble leur composition, connexion, actions, & usages ... Lyon, Esprit Vitalis, 1673.

[40], 275 p. plates. (port.) 16 cm. [707]

Added engraved title page.

BARLET, ANNIBAL [*fl.* 1650] Le vray et methodique cours de la physique resolutive, vulgairement dite chymie. Represente par figures generales & particulieres. Pour connoistre la theotechnie ergocosmique, c'est à dire, l'art de Dieu, en l'ouvrage de l'univers ... Paris, N. Charles, 1653.

[8 +], 626, [10] p. plates. 24 cm. [708]

Imperfect: added engraved title page wanting.

BARNAUD, NICOLAS [*d.* 1605?] Brevis elucidatio, illius Arcani philosophorum ...

784-789 p., vol. 3. 20 cm. (*In* Zetzner, Lazarus, *ed.* Theatrum chemicum. Argentorati, 1659-61)

[709]

Caption title.

—[... Commentariolum in quoddam Epitaphium Bononiae studiorum, ante multa secula marmoreo lapidi insculptum] [&] [Processus chemici aliquot]

744-764 p., vol. 3. 20 cm. (*In* Zetzner, Lazarus, *ed.* Theatrum chemicum. Argentorati, 1659-61)

[710]

Titles supplied from table of contents.

—Quadrigae auriferae prima rota [-quarta rota] [&] [Auriga chemicus; sive, Theosophiae palmarium] [&] [De occulta philosophia] [&] [Dicta sapientum]

791-859 p., vol. 3. plate. 20 cm. (*In* Zetzner, Lazarus, *ed.* Theatrum chemicum., Argentorati, 1659-61)

[711]

—, *tr. See* LAMBSPRINGK. De lapide philosophico. 1659, 1677.

BARNER, JAKOB [1641-1686] Prodromus Sennerti novi; sive, Delineatio novi medicinae systematis, in quo quicquid a primis seculis in hunc usque diem de arte prodiit, Hippocratis, Galeni, Paracelsi, Helmontii, Sylvii, Willisii, &c. dogmata, ex principiis anatomico-chymicis examinantur. Augustae Vindelicorum, Sumptibus Theophili Göbelii, typis Johannis Schönigkii, 1674.

55, [5] p. 19 cm. [712]

—Spiritus vini sine acido; hoc est, In spiritu vini & oleis indistincte non esse acidum, nec ea propterea a spiritu urinae revera coagulari, demonstratio curiosa, cum modo conficiendi salia volatilia oleosa, eorumque usu. Lipsiae, Sumptibus Johannis Fritzschii, literis Joh. Eric Hahnii, 1675.

40 p. 16 cm. [713]

—*See* MACHIAVELLUS MEDICUS. 1698.

—*as subject. See* BECKE, D. von der. Barnerus leviter & amice castigatus. 1675; PORZ, J. D. Demonstratio brevis medico chyrurgica de tumoribus. 1679

BARNES, JOHN [*fl.* 1594-1621] *ed. See* BAYLEY, W. Two Treatises concerning the preservation of eiesight. 1616; VAUGHAN, W. Directions for health 1626, 1633.

BARNES, JOSHUA [1654-1712] Gerania: a new discovery of a little sort of people anciently discoursed of, called Pygmies. With a lively description of their stature, habit, manners, buildings, knowledge, and government, being very delightful and profitable ... London, Printed by W. G. for Obadiah Blagrave, 1675.

[7], 110 [10] p. front. 15 cm. [714]

BARNSTEIN, HEINRICH [1608-1660?] Tabacks Wunder Kunst, und Artzneymittel. Wo er seinen Nahmen her habe, und wie er mehr genennet werde, wie vielerley er sey, und wie er wachse, wo, wan und wie er gepflantzet, gewartet, gesamlet und zugerichtet werde, was er vor Tugenden und Eigenschafften an sich habe, wie, von welchen gesunden Leuten, vor welche Kranckheiten, und wann er nützlich gebrauchet werden könne ... vermehret und in Truck gegeben durch Johann. Balthasar Funcken ... Erffurt, Joh. Georg Hertz, 1677.

[46] p.   16 cm.   [715]

BARNSTORFF, BERNHARD [1645-1704] *respondent.* See DÖBEL, J. J., *praeses.* Disputatio medica inauguralis de morbo virgineo seu foedis virginum coloribus. 1670.

BARNSTORFF, EBERHARD [1672-1712] *respondent.* See HOFFMAN, F. [1660-1742] *praeses.* Disputatio inauguralis medica de amputatione membrorum sphacelatorum. 1696.

BARNSTORFF, ERNST [*fl.* 1668-1672] *respondent.* See TAPPE, J., *praeses.* Disputatio medica pathologica de comate et caro. 1668.

BARNUEVO ROCHA Y BENAVIDES, PEDRO DE PERALTA. *See* PERALTA BARNUEVO ROCHA Y BENAVIDES, Pedro de [1663-1743]

BARONIO, CESARE, *Cardinal* [1538-1607] Epistola ad Sacram Regiam Catholicam Majestatem de monarchia Sicula. Edita ex museo Joachimi Morsii. Lugduni Batavorum, Excudebat Jacobus Marci, 1619.

[8] p.   21 cm.   [716]

BARONIO, FRANCESCO [*d.* 1679] De corpore ejusque partibus, et membris tractatus novus ... in quo ... agitur, de corpore, tam vivo, quam mortuo, et quot modis sumatur, de irregularitate, de immunitate ecclesiastica, de homicidio ... Panormi, Sumptibus Augustini Bossio, 1664.

[8], 388, [35] p.   31 cm.   [717]

BARONIO, VINCENZIO [*fl.* 1634] De pleuripneumonia anno Domini MDCXXXIII. et aliis temporibus Flaminiam aliasque regiones populariter infestante, ac a nemine hactenus observata. Libri duo ... Forolivii, Apud Jo. Cimattium, 1636.

[24], 378, [48] p.   23 cm.   [718]

BAROZZI, JACOPO. *See* VIGNOLA, Giacomo Barozzio, *called* [1507-1573]

BARRA, PIERRE [17th cent.] Hippocrate, de la circulation du sang et des humeurs ... Imprimé à Lyon, & se vend a Paris, chez Laurent d'Houry, 1683.

[24], 349, [5] p.   16 cm.   [719]

Contains extracts in French from Hippocrates. The first two books (L'anatomie du coeur; La circulation du sang dans le coeur)

form an epitome of and commentary on the De corde. The third book (La circulation universelle) is concerned with various Hippocratic works.

—De veris terminis partus humani libri tres ex Hippocrate ... Accessit Historia mulieris Romanae jam ab annis quatuor gravidae, cum responsione vaticina ejusdem authoris, & explicatione responsionis. Lugduni, Sumpt. Christophori Fourmy, 1666.

[40], 101, [3] p.   18 cm.   [720]

In part a criticism of Jean de Peysonnel's De temporibus humani partus, juxta doctrinam Hippocratis, published in Lyons in 1665.

Contains extracts in Greek and Latin from various Hippocratic works, especially from the De septimestri partu.

—L'usage de la glace, de la neige et du froid ... Lyon, Antoine Cellier fils, 1675.

[16], 249, [21] p.   15 cm.   [721]

BARRALIS, BARTHÉLEMY, *tr. See* FACIO, S. Paradoxes de la peste. 1620.

BARRERA, OLIVA SABUCO DE NANTES. *See* SABUCO DE NANTES BARRERA, Oliva [1562-1622?]

BARRIOS, JUAN DE [*fl.* 1590-1610] Verdadera medicina, cirugia, y astrologia, en tres libros dividida ... Mexico, Fernando Balli, 1607.

3 parts. in 1 v.   port.   27 cm.   [722]

Title and imprint from the microfilm copy of Francisco Guerra. The original is presumably in the Wellcome Historical Medical Library, London.

At head of title: Jesus Maria.

Title page supplied in manuscript has title: De la verdadera cirugia, medicina y astrologia.

Running title: De la berdadera [SIC] medicina, astrologia, y cirugia. (Order of words varies)

Medina 232.

Imperfect: title page, colophon, and several leaves of preliminary matter and text in third part wanting; a number of leaves mutilated; closely trimmed, with loss of many signatures and catchwords. Badly numbered.

Binder's error: last treatise of book 3 precedes the first of this book.

BARROUGH, PHILIP [*fl.* 1590] The method of phisick, containing the causes, signes, and cures of inward diseases in mans body, from the head to the foote. Whereunto is added, the forme and rule of making remedies and medicines, which our physitions commonly use at this day, with the proportion, quantitie, and names of each medicine ... The 4th ed., corr. and amended. London, Richard Field, 1610.

[16], 477, [7], p.   19 cm.   [723]

STC 1512.

—[The same.] ... The 5th ed., corr. and amended. London, Richard Field, 1617.

[16], 477, [7] p. 19 cm. [**724**]

Different setting of type.
STC 1513.

—[The same.] ... The 6th ed. London, Richard Field, 1624.

[16], 477, [7] p. 18 cm. [**725**]

Imperfect: p. 183–186 wanting.
Different setting of type.
STC 1514.

—[The same.] ... The 7th ed. London, George Miller, 1634.

[16], 477, [7] p. 19 cm. [**726**]

Different setting of type.
STC 1515.

—[The same.] ... The 8th ed. London, George Miller, 1639.

[16], 477, [7] p. 20 cm. [**727**]

Different setting of type.
STC 1516.

—[The same.] ... London, Printed by Abraham Miller, and sold by John Blague and Samuel Howes, 1652.

[16], 477, [7] p. 19 cm. [**728**]

Different setting of type.

BARROW, Philip. *See* Barrough, Philip [*fl.* 1590]

BARTELMAEI, Jakob [*fl.* 1667] *respondent.* Disputatio medica inauguralis de lethargo ... Lugduni Batavorum, Apud viduam & haeredes Joannis Elsevirii, 1667.

[14] p. 23 cm. [**729**]

Diss.—Leyden.

BARTELS, Nikolaus Adolf [*fl.* 1659–1662] *respondent.* Disputatio medica inauguralis de phthisi ... Basileae, Typis Joh. Jacobi Deckeri [1662]

[16] p. 22 cm. [**730**]

Diss.—Basel.

—*respondent. See* Linden, J. A. van der, *praeses.* Hippocrates de circuitu sanguinis, exercitatio II. 1659.

BARTH, C. *See* Barth, Kaspar von [1587–1658]

BARTH, Gottfried [1650–1728] *respondent. See* Thomasius, J. [1622–1684] *praeses.* De barba. 1671, 1672.

BARTH, Jeremias [*fl.* 1603–1618] *See* Béguin, J. Tyrocinium chymicum. 1643, 1650, 1659, 1669.

—*respondent, See* Loss, W., *praeses.* Themata de calculorenum et vesicae. 1603.

BARTH, Kaspar von [1587–1658] *See* Kiranus, *King of Persia.* Moderante auxilio redemptoris supremi, Kirani Kiranides. 1638, 1681; [English tr.] 1685.

BARTH, Michael [*d.* 1584] *See* Scholtz, L. Epistolarum philosophicarum: medicinalium, ac chymicarum. 1610.

BARTHELMAEI, Jakob [*fl.* 1694] *respondent. See* Schaper, J. E., *praeses.* Dissertatio medica inauguralis de morbo arquato. 1714 (i.e. 1694).

—*as subject. See* Schaper, J. E. Programma quo Facultatis Medicae ... decanus ... ad disputationem inauguralem de morbo arquato a ... candidato Dn. Jacobo Barthelmaei ... habendam ... invitat. 1694.

BARTHIUS, Christian [*fl.* 17th cent.] *See* Farnesius, G. T. Appendix bibliothecae medico philosophico philologicae. 1680.

BARTHOLDUS PONTANUS A BRAITEN-BERG, Georgius. *See* Pontanus a Braitenberg, Georgius Bartholdus [*d.* 1616]

BARTHOLETUS, Fabritius. *See* Bartoletti, Fabrizio [1576–1630]

BARTHOLIN, Caspar [1585–1629] Opuscula quatuor singularia: I. De unicornu ejusque affinibus & succedaneis. II. De lapide nephritico, & amuletis praecipuis. III. De pygmaeis. IV. Consilium de studio medico inchoando, continuando & absolvendo ... Hafniae, Georgius Hantzschius, 1628.

4 parts in 1. 16 cm. [**731**]

Opuscula I–II have half titles; III–IV special title pages. All have separate foliation.

—Anatomicae institutiones corporis humani utriusque sexus historiam & declarationem exhibentes cum plurimis novis observationibus & opinionibus nec non illustriorum quae in anthropologia occurrunt, controversiarum decisionibus ... [Vitebergae] Apud Bechtoldum Raaben, 1611.

[16], 603 (i.e. 493), [69] p. 17 cm. [**732**]

—[The same.] ... Argentorati, Conradus Scher, 1626.

[24], 417, [47] p. 14 cm. [**733**]

—[The same.] Institutiones anatomicae, corporis humani utriusque sexus, historiam & declarationem exhibentes, cum plurimis novis observationibus opinionibus & controversiarum occurrentium decisionibus ... Ed. nova corr. & locupletata. Goslariae, Typis Nicolai Dunckeri, impensis Johannis Hallervordii Rostochiensis, 1632.

[16], 482 (i.e. 462), [62] p.   17 cm.   **[734]**

With this is bound *his* Controversiae anatomicae. 1631.

—[The same.] Institutiones anatomicae, novis recentiorum opinionibus & observationibus, quarum innumerae hactenus editae non sunt, figurisque auctae ab auctoris filio Thoma Bartholino. Lug. Batavorum, Apud Franciscum Hackium, 1641.

[20], 408, [12], 409-496, [44] p.   illus., plates. 19 cm.   **[735]**

Imperfect: original engraved title page wanting; engraved title page from another copy inserted.

"Epistola [-Altera epistola] Johannis Walaei de motu sanguinis ...": p. 385-408, [1-12]

—[The same.] ... Lug. Batavorum, Apud Franciscum Hackium, 1645.

[16], 442 (i.e. 432), [2], 443-488, [24] p.   illus., plates, port.   19 cm.   **[736]**

"Johannis Walaei Epistolae duae de motu chyli et sanguinis ad Thomam Bartholinum ... Editio quarta": p. [1-2], 443-488, with half title.

—[French tr.] Institutions anatomiques ... augm. & entrichies pour la seconde fois, tant des opinions & observations nouvelles des modernes, dont la plus grande partie n'a jamais esté mise en lumiere, que de plusieurs figures en taille douce, par Thomas Bartholin ... fils de l'autheur, et traduictes en françois par Abr. du Prat ... Paris, Mathurin Henault et Jean Henault, 1647.

[16], 656, [38] p.   illus., plates, port.   21 cm.   **[737]**

Added engraved title page.
"Deux lettres de Monsieur Jean Walaeus du mouvement du chyle et du sang. A Mr. Thomas Bartholin": p. [589]-656, has half title.

—[Adaptations] *See* BARTHOLIN, T. Anatomia. 1651, 1655, 1660, 1663, 1666, 1669, 1674, 1677, 1684, 1686; [Dutch tr.] 1653, 1656, 1658, 1688; [English tr.] 1665, 1668; [German tr.] 1677.

—[Anatomicae institutiones, *as subject*] *See* RIOLAN, J. [1580-1657] Opera anatomica vetera. 1650 [and] Opuscula anatomica nova. 1649.

—Astrologia; seu, De stellarum natura, affectionibus, & effectionibus. Exercitatio ... Ed. 6. correctior mendosa tertia & melior. [Vitebergae] Apud Bechtoldum Raab, 1616.

[24], 260, [25] p.   13 cm.   **[738]**

Previously published as the author's dissertation, Wittemberg, 1606; Wilhelm Gros, respondent.

—Consilium. *In* Conring, H. In universam artem medicam singulasque ejus partes introductio. 1687.

—Controversiae anatomicae, & affines nobiliores ac rariores. Goslariae, Typis Nicolai Dunckeri, impensis Johannis Hallervordii Rostochiensis, 1631.

[2], 615, [7] p.   17 cm.   **[739]**

Bound with *his* Institutiones anatomicae. 1632.

—De aere pestilenti corrigendo consilium. Hafniae, Apud Salomonem Sartorium, 1619.

[30] p.   17 cm.   **[740]**

Published also as part [2] of *his* Syntagma medicum, 1624.

—De terra, aere et igni institutio physica succincta: cum praemissa elementorum theoria generali. Gryphiswaldii, Typis Johannis Albini, apud Joh. Hallervordeum, 1624.

[114] p.   13 cm.   **[741]**

—Enchiridion metaphysicam. *In* Magirus, J. Physiologiae peripateticae libri sex. 1610, 1616, 1618, 1619, 1638, 1642.

—Enchiridion physicum ex priscis & recentioribus philosophis accurate concinnatum, & controversiis naturalibus potissimis, utilissimisque, illustratum ... Argentinae, Sumptibus Eberhardi Zetzneri, 1625.

[12], 865 (i.e. 857), [71] p.   14 cm.   **[742]**

—Syntagma medicum & chirurgicum de cauteriis praesertim potestate agentibus seu ruptoriis, olim in Academia Patavina nationi Germanicae praelectum, nunc ... revisum, auctum, arcanisque cauteriis usu probatissimis locupletatum & publici juris factum. Accessit ejusdem autoris De aëre pestilenti corrigendo consilium medicum ... Hafniae, Impensis Salomonis Sartorii, 1624.

[14], 140 p.; [4], 30 p.   20 cm.   **[743]**

Imperfect: p. [9-14]. 1-2; [1-4], 1-30 wanting; supplied in photocopy from the British Museum.

De aere pestilenti (ed. 2. auctior) has special title page and separate paging.

—*See* LE BOË, F. de. Opera medica. 1679, 1680, 1681, 1693, 1695, 1697, 1698.

BARTHOLIN, Caspar [1655-1738] De ductu salivali hactenus non descripto observatio anatomica. Hafniae, Typis Joh. Phil. Bockenhoffer, sumptibus Christiani Hauboldt & Johannis Liebe, 1684.

[6], 16, [2] p.   plate.   18 cm.   **[744]**

—[The same.] ... Ultrajecti, Apud Franciscum Halma, 1685.

[6]-27, [6] p.   plate.   17 cm.   **[745]**

Additional title page at end has caption: Editio secunda.

—De inauribus veterum syntagma. Accedit Mantissa ex Thomae Bartholini miscellaneis medicis de annulis narium. Amstelodami, Sumptibus J. Henrici Wetstenii, 1676.

[16], 148 p.; [1], 17, [9] p.   illus., plate.   14 cm.
[746]

Part [2] has half title: Mantissa ex Thomae Bartholini miscellaneis medicis De morbis biblicis, cap. XIX. de annulis narium.

—De nervorum usu in motu musculorum epistola. *In* Jacobaeus, H. De ranis observationes. 1676, 1682.

—De ovariis mulierum et generationis historia epistola anatomica ... Cui jam accessit alia ejusdem argumenti. Amstelaedami, Sumptibus J. Henr. Wetstenii, 1678.

69, [2] p.   14 cm.   **[747]**

—[The same.] *In* Cellier, A. *ed.* Opuscula nova anatomica. 1680.

—De respiratione animalium disputatio ... Hafniae, Literis viduae Joh. Phil. Bockenhoffer [1700]

12 p.   20 cm.   **[748]**

—De secretione humorum in corpore animato disputatio ... Hafniae, Johan Philip Bockenhoffer [1696]

15, [1] p.   20 cm.   **[749]**

—De tibiis veterum, et earum antiquo usu libri tres. Ed. altera, figuris auctior. Amstelaedami, Apud J. Henr. Wetstenium 1679.

[24], 415, [5] p.   illus., plates, port.   13 cm.
[750]

Added engraved title page.

—De via alimentorium & chyli in corpore humano disputatio ... Hafniae, Literis viduae Joh. Phil. Bockenhoffer [1700]

15, [1] p.   20 cm.   **[751]**

—De vita & nutritione animalium disputatio ... Hafniae, Literis Johan. Philip. Bockenhoffer [1697]

20 p.   19 cm.   **[752]**

—Diaphragmatis structura nova. Accessit methodus praeparandi viscera per injectiones liquorum, & descriptio instrumenti, quol mediante peraguntur ... Parisiis, Apud Ludovicum Billaine, 1676.

[16], 138 p.   plates, port.   19 cm.   **[753]**

Added half title.
Imperfect: portrait wanting.

—[The same.] ... Parisiis, Apud Renatum Guignard, 1682.

[18], 138 p.   front (port.), plates.   18 cm.
[754]

A reissue of the 1676 edition with new title page.
Imperfect: plate 3 wanting; other plates misbound at end of Jacobeus' De ranis.
With this is bound Jacobaeus, H. De ranis observationes. Parisiis, 1682.

—Exercitationes miscellaneae varii argumenti imprimis anatomici. Lugd. Batav., Ex Officina Hackiana, 1675.

[24], 151, [7] p.   illus.   17 cm.   **[755]**

—Expositio veteris in puerperio ritus ex arca sepulchrali antiqua desumpti. Romae, Excudebat Mascardus, sumptibus Benedicti Carrarae, 1677.

63 p.   plate.   18 cm.   **[756]**

"Thomae Bartholini de puerperio veteri ad filium Casparum Bartholinum epistola": p. 55-63.

—Speciminis philosophiae naturalis novissimis rationibus & experimentis illustratae disputatio quinta ... Hafniae, Literis Johannis Philippi Bockenhoffer [1692]

[2], 89-100, [2] p.   19 cm.   **[757]**

Caption title: Caput decimum tertium. De globo terraqueo.

—Thesium philosophicarum disputatio prima ... Hafniae, Literis Joh. Phil. Bockenhoffer [1696]

8 p.   19 cm.   **[758]**

Dissertations — Copenhagen

—*praeses.* De cordis structura & motu disquisitio ... Hafniae, Typis viduae Georgii Godiani [1678]

20 p.   20 cm.   **[759]**

G. N. Seerup, *respondent.*

—De olfactus organo disquisitio anatomica ... Hafniae, Literis Cornificii Luft [1679]

20 p. 19 cm. [760]
G. N. Seerup, *respondent.*

—Disputatio inauguralis medico anatomica de formatione et nutritione foetus in utero . . . Hafniae, Typis Joh. Phil. Bockenhoffer, 1687.
24 p. 19 cm. [761]
D. M. M Grotius à Deswig, *respondent.*

—Dissertatio inauguralis chirurgicomedica de meliceria Celsi sive synovia, Germ. Gliedwasser . . . [Hafniae] Joh. Phil. Bockenhoffer [1695]
[2], 20, [2] p. 18 cm. [762]
R. Wagner, *respondent.*

—Dissertatio inauguralis de diaeta jejunantium . . . Hafniae, Literis Johannis Philippi Bockenhoffer [1693]
[2], 21 p. 20 cm. [763]
A. Kahle, *respondent.*

—Dissertatio inauguralis medica de ascite hydrope . . . Hafniae, Literis Joh. Jac. Bornheinrich [1699]
[2], 22 p. 22 cm. [764]
·D. Máday, *respondent.*

—Dissertatio medica inauguralis de cruditate ventriculi; sive, Fermentatione alimentorum laesa . . . Hafniae, Literis Joh. Phil. Bockenhoffer [1685]
23 p. 19 cm. [765]
Day and year of the presentation written on title page by contemporary hand.
P. Schwendi, *respondent.*

—Dissertatio medica inauguralis de pleuritide atque peripneumonia . . . Hafniae, Literis viduae Joh. Phil. Bockenhoffer [1700]
[6], 18, [6] p. 19 cm. [766]
J. de Buchwald, *respondent.*

—Dissertatio medica inauguralis de spina ventosa . . . Hafniae, Imprimebat Joh. Jac. Bornheinrich [1695]
[30] p. 20 cm. [767]
C. Hemmer, *respondent.*

—Exercitatio anatomica de corporis humani oeconomia . . . Hafniae, Typis viduae Georgii Gödiani [1678]
22 p. 19 cm. [768]
M. Severini, *respondent.*

—Positiones anatomicae . . . Hafniae, Typis viduae Georgii Gödiani [1678]

20 p. 18 cm. [769]
H. Nicolai, *respondent.*

—*ed. See* BARTHOLIN, T. Antiquitatum veteris puerperii synopsis. 1676 [and] De armillis veterum schedion. 1676 [and] De unicornu observationes novae. 1678.

BARTHOLIN, CASPAR THOMESEN. *See* BARTHOLIN, Caspar [1655-1738]

BARTHOLIN, RASMUS [1625-1698] De naturae mirabilibus quaestiones academicae. Hafniae, Sumptibus Petri Hauboldi, literis Georgii Gödiani, 1674.
[8], 200 p. plate. 20 cm. [770]

—De poris corporum et consuetudine quaestiones academicae. [n.p.] Prostant apud Joannem Blaeu & Danielem Paulli, 1666.
[8], 94 (i.e. 96) p. 16 cm. (Part [2] *In* Bartholin, Thomas. De hepatis exautorati desperata causa. Hafniae, 1666) [771]

—Erasmius Bartholinus . . . Facultatis Medicae decanus, L. S. [Hafniae, 1684]
[8] p. 20 cm. [772]
Program - Copenhagen (for G. Hannaeus)

—*See* BARTHOLIN, T. De nivis usu medico observationes variae. 1661.

BARTHOLIN, THOMAS [1616-1680] Opuscula nova anatomica, de lacteis thoracicis et lymphaticis vasis. Uno volumine comprehensa . . . Hafniae Sumtib. Danielis Paulli, praelo Aegidii Vogelii, 1670.
[16], 726 p. plates. 18 cm. [773]
11 treatises in 1 v. Each has special title page.
Contents.—pt. [1] De lacteis thoracicis in homine brutisque nuperrime observatis historia anatomica.—pt. [2] Vasa lymphatica, nuper Hafniae in animantibus inventa, et hepatis exsequiae.—pt. [3] Dubia anatomica de lacteis thoracicis, & an hepatis funus immutet medendi methodum.—pt. [4] Vasa lymphatica, in homine nuper inventa.—pt. [5] Defensio vasorum lacteorum et lymphaticorum. Adversus Joh. Riolanum.—pt. [6] De lacteis venis sententia cl. v. Guilielmi Harvei expensa.—pt. [7] Spicilegium I. ex vasis lymphaticis, ubi cl. v. Glissonii & Pecqueti Sententiae expeduntur.—pt. [8] Spicilegium II. ex vasis lymphaticis ubi cl. v. Backii, Cattierii, Le Noble, Tardii, Whartoni, Charletoni, Bilsii &c. sententiae examinantur.—pt. [9] Responsio de experimentis anatomicis Bilsianis & difficili hepatis resurrectione.—pt. [10] Dissertatio anatomica de hepate defuncto novis Bilsianorum observationibus opposita.—pt. [11] De hepatis exautorati desperata causa, cum praecipuis eruditae Europae medicis concertatio.

—Anatomia, ex Caspari Bartholini parentis Institutionibus, ominiumque recentiorum & propriis observationibus tertium ad sanguinis circulationem reformata. Cum iconibus novis accuratissimis. Lugd. Batav., Apud Franciscum Hackium, 1651.

[16], 576, [13] p. illus., plates, port. 20 cm.
[**774**]

Imperfect: p. 65–66, 85–86, 123–124 and 191–192 wanting.
Added engraved title page has title: Anatomia reformata.
"Johannis Walaei Epistolae duae de motu chyli et sanguinis ad Thomam Bartholinum . . . Editio quinta": p. [529]–576.

—[The same.] . . . Accessit huic postremae editioni Th. Bartholini appendix De lacteis thoracicis & [De] vasis lymphaticis. Hagae-Comitis, Ex typographia Adriani Vlacq, 1655.

[16], 592, [13] p. illus., plates, port. 20 cm.
[**775**]

—[The same.] . . . Hagae-Comitis, Ex typographia Adriani Vlacq, 1660.

[16], 592, [13] p. illus., plates, port. 20 cm.
[**776**]

Imperfect: 8th prelim. leaf with port. on verso wanting.
Added engraved title page, dated 1655 has title: Anatomia reformata.
Different setting of type.

—[The same.] . . . Hagae-Comitis, Ex typographia Adriani Vlacq, 1663.

[16], 592, [15] p. illus., plates, port. 19 cm.
[**777**]

Added engraved title page, dated 1655 has title: Anatomia reformata.
"[Joh. Walaei] Epistola prima [et altera] de motu chyli et sanguinis ad Thomam Bartholinum . . . Editio septima": p. [529]–576.
Different setting of type.

—[The same.] . . . Hagae-Comitis, Ex typographia Adriani Vlacq, 1666.

[16], 594, [14] p. illus., plates, port. 21 cm.
[**778**]

—[The same.] . . . Amstelodami, Sumptibus Sebastiani Combi & Joannis Lanou, 1669.

[16], 594, [14] p. illus., plates, port. 21 cm.
[**779**]

Imperfect: added engraved title page and 8th prelim. leaf with port. on verso wanting.
Different setting of type.

—[The same.] . . . Lugd. Batav. & Roterod., Ex Officina Hackiana, 1669.

[12], 592, [11] p. illus., plates, port. 21 cm.
[**780**]

"Joh. Walaei Epistola prima [et altera] de motu chyli et sanguinis: ad Thomam Bartholinum": p. [529]–576; "[Th. Bartholinus] De lacteis thoracicis": p. 577–587; "[Th. Bartholinus] De vasis lymphaticis": p. 587–592.

—[The same.] Anatome ex omnium veterum recentiorumque observationibus imprimis Institutionibus b. m. parentis Caspari Bartholini, ad circulationem Harveianam, et vasa lymphatica quartum renovata . . . Lugduni Batavorum, Ex Officina Hackiana, 1673 [i.e. 1674]

[30], 807, [16] p. illus., plates, port. 20 cm.
[**781**]

Imperfect: plate facing p. 206 wanting.
Added engraved title page has title: Anatomia Bartholiniana. Lugd. Batav., Ex Officina Hackiana, 1674.
"Johannis Walaei Epistolae duae: de motu chyli, et sanguinis: ad Thomam Bartholinum . . . Editio decima": p. [759]–804.

—[The same.] . . . Lugduni. Joan. Ant. Huguetan, & soc., 1677.

[30], 807, [18] p. illus., plates, port. 19 cm.
[**782**]

Imperfect: port. wanting.

—[The same.] . . . Lugduni, Sumpt. Marci & Joan. Henrici Huguetan, 1684.

[30], 805, [19] p. illus., plates, port. 19 cm.
[**783**]

Imperfect: port. and plates facing p. 122 and 748 wanting.
Added engraved title page has title: Anatomia Bartholiniana. Lugd., Sumpt. Jo. Ant. Huguetan, 1677.

—[The same.] . . . Lugduni Batavorum, Apud Jacobum Hackium, 1686.

[30], 806, [16] p. illus., plates, port. 20 cm.
[**784**]

Imperfect: plate facing p. 748 wanting.

—[Dutch tr.] Anatomia: ofte, Ontledinge des menschelijcken lichaems . . . onlanghs uyt sijn vaders, als oock vele nieuwe schrijvers, en eyghene ondervindinghe in 't Latijn t'samen ghestelt. Hier zijn by gevoeght twee brieven van Joh. Walaeus, raeckende de bewegynge des gijls ende bloets. Als mede, een kort verhael, van een nieuw ghevonden wegh des gijls naer het herte . . . In de Nederduytsche spraeck overgeset door Mr. Thomas Staffard . . . Leyden, By Françoys Hackes, 1653.

[16], 701 (i.e. 703) p. illus., plates, port. 21 cm.
[**785**]

Added engraved title page.

—[The same.] . . . Dordrecht, Jacobus Savry, 1656.

[16], 573 p.. plates, port. 16 cm.   [**786**]

— [The same.] . . . Den 2. druck door den selven oversien ende doorgaens vermeerdert; daer-en-boven met een beschrijvinge vande nieuw gevonden water-vaten. 's Graven-Hage, Adriaen Vlack, 1658.

[16], 774 (i.e. 776), [8] p. illus., plates, port. 21 cm.   [**787**]
Imperfect: plates facing p. 460 and 676 mutilated.

— [The same.] . . . Den 3. druck . . . Amsteldam, Johannes van Someren, 1669.

[16], 685, [3] p. illus., plates, port. 19 cm.   [**788**]
Imperfect: added engraved title page, and 8th prelim. leaf (poem on recto, port. on verso) wanting; all except port. supplied in photocopy from the British Museum.

— [The same.] Ontledinge volgens den omloop des bloeds en nieuw gevondene watervaten. In het Latijn beschreven . . . Vertaald door A. H. S. V. P. D. M. D. Amsterdam, By de wed. van Johannes van Someren, en Abraham van Someren, 1688.

[8], 769, [3] p. illus., plates. port. 21 cm.   [**789**]
Added engraved title page reads: Anatomia; ofte, Ontledinge des menschelyken lichaams.
"Twe brieven, rakende de beweging des gyls, en des bloeds, door Johannes Walaeus": p. [711]-754; — "Kort verhaal van een nieuw-gevonden weg des gyls na het hert. Nu eerst in 't licht gebragt, en uyt de Latijnse tale t'samen-gesteld, en overgeset door Mr. Thomas Stafford": p. [759]-766.

— [English tr.] Anatomy; made from the precepts of his father, and from the observations of all modern anatomists; together with his own . . . In four books and four manuals . . . Published by Nich. Culpeper . . . and Abdiah Cole . . . London, Peter Cole, 1665.

[14], 169, 301-377 p. illus., plates. 27 cm.   [**790**]
Imperfect: p. 37-40 wanting; p. 75-76 mutilated.
"Two epistles of Johannes Walaeus concerning the motion of the chyle and the blood": p. 358-377.
With this are bound: Riolan, J. A sure guide. 1665; Culpeper, N. Pharmacopoeia Londinensis. 1665.

— [The same.] . . . London, John Streater, 1668.
[8], 169, 301-328, 333-377 p. illus., plates. 29 cm.   [**791**]

— [German tr.] Neu-verbesserte künstliche Zer-legung dess menschlichen Leibes, in vier absonder-liche Bücher eingetheilet . . . Denen noch über das Johannis Walaei zwey Send-Schreiben von der

Bewegung dess Milch-Safftes und Gebluts beygefüget sind. Alles aus der alten und neuen Anatomicorum merckwürdigen Beobachtungen, sonderlich seines sel. Herrn Vatters Caspari Bartholini Institutionibus . . . Nunmehr . . . aus der lateinischen in die teutsche Sparche übersetzet durch Eliam Wallnern . . . Nürn-berg, In Verlegung Johann Hofmanns, gedruckt bey Andrea Knortzen, 1677.

[40], 903 (i.e. 901), [25] p. front. (port.), illus., plates. 20 cm.   [**792**]
Added engraved title page has title: Anatomia Bartholiniana.

— Anatomicae vindiciae Cl. V. Casparo Hof-manno . . . aliisque oppositae. Accedunt ejusdem Animadversiones in anatomica Hoffmanni. Hafniae, Typis Melch. Martzan, 1648.

[8], 136, [12] p. 23 cm.   [**793**]
With this is bound: Bogdan, M. Insidiae structae Cl. V. Thomae Bartholini . . . Vasis lymphaticis. 1654.

— Antiquitatum veteris puerperii synopsis a filio Casparo Bartholino commentario illustrata. Cum Thomae Bartholini ad filium epistola. Amstelodami, Sumptibus J. Henrici Wetstenii, 1676.

[28], 179, [5] p. illus., plates. 14 cm. [**794**]

— Carmina varii argumenti. Hafniae, Apud Danielem Paulli, literis Henrici Gödiani, 1669.

[6], 239, [9] p. 16 cm.   [**795**]

— Cista medica Hafniensis, variis consiliis, cura-tionibus, casibus rarioribus, vitis medicorum Haf-niensium, aliisque ad rem medicam, anatomicam, botanicam & chymicam spectantibus referta. Accedit ejusdem Domus anatomica brevissime descripta. Hafniae, Typis Matthiae Godicchenii, impensis Petri Hauboldi, 1662.

[19], 645, [7] p.; 62, [1] p. front., illus. 16 cm.   [**796**]
Added engraved title page.
Part [2] has special title page with imprint: Hafniae, Literis Henrici Gödiani, sumptibus P. Hauboldi, 1662.

— De anatome practica, ex cadaveribus morbosis adornanda, consilium, cum operum autoris hactenus editorum catalogo. Hafniae, Sumptibus Petri Hauboldi, literis Georgii Gödiani, 1674.

[4], 48 p. 19 cm.   [**797**]

— De angina puerorum Campaniae Siciliaeque epidemica exercitationes. Accedit De laryngotomia cl. v. Renati Moreau . . . epistola. Lutetiae Parisiorum, Apud Olivarium de Varennes, 1646.

[20], 140 p. 15 cm. **[798]**

Imperfect: p. 135–136 mutilated.

—De armillis veterum schedion. Accessit Olai Wormii De aureo cornu Danico ad Licetum responsio. Ed. nov., figuris aeneis illustrata. Amstelodami, Sumptibus J. Henrici Wetstenii, 1676.

[16], 114, [14] p.; 40 p. illus., plates. 14 cm. **[799]**

Added engraved title page.
Edited by Caspar Bartholin.

—De bibliothecae incendio dissertatio ad filios. Hafniae, Typis Matthiae Godicchenii, sumptibus Petri Haubold, 1670.

114, [14] p. 16 cm. **[800]**

—De cometa consilium medicum cum monstrorum nuper in Dania natorum historia ... Hafniae, Apud Matthiam Godicchenium, sumptibus Petr. Haubold, 1665.

154, [6] p. 17 cm. **[801]**

"Th. Bartholini Synopsis consilii de abscessu coeli, seu cometa. Ad ... Stanislaum Lubienieszky de Lubienietz": p. 150–154.

—De cruce Christi hypomnemata IV. I. De sedili medio. II. De vino myrrhato. III. De corona spinea. IV. De sudore sanguineo. Amstelodami, Sumptibus Andreae Frisii, 1670.

290, [22] p. illus. 14 cm. **[802]**

"Bartoldi Nihusii De cruce epistola ad Thomam Bartholinum": [197]–261, has half title.

—De flagrorum usu medico epistola. *In* Meibom, J. H. De usu flagrorum. 1670.

—De flammula cordis epistola cum Jacobi Holsti ... ejusdem argumenti dissertatione. Accessit De carnibus lucentibus Danielis Puerarii responsio. Hafniae, Apud Danielem Paulli, Literis Henrici Gödiani [1667]

136 p. 16 cm. **[803]**

"Jacobi Holsti De flammula cordis dissertatio" (p. [15]–115) has special title page.

—De hepatis exautorati desperata causa, cum praecipuis eruditae Europae medicis concertatio. Accessere: Erasmi Bartholini De poris corporum & consuetudine quaestiones academicae. Hafniae, Praelo Henrici Gödiani [1666].

[10], 146, [5] p.; [8], 94 (i.e. 96) p. 16 cm. **[804]**

2 parts in 1 v. Each part has special title page with imprint: Prostat [prostant] apud Joannem Blaeu & Danielem Paulli. Title page of part [2] has date 1666.

With this is bound Mayow, J. Tractatus duo. 1671.

—De insolitis partus humani viis dissertatio nova. Accedunt ... Johannis Veslingi ... de pullitie Aegyptiorum & aliae ejusdem observationes anatomicae & epistolae medicae posthumae. Hafniae, Typis Matthiae Godicchenii, sumptibus Petri Haubold, 1664.

[8], 248 p.; [8], 248 p. 15 cm. **[805]**

Part [2] has special title page: Joannis Veslingi ... observationes anatomicae & epistolae medicae ex schedis posthumis selectae & editae a Th. Bartholino.

Bound with *his* Historiarum anatomicarum rariorum centuria I–VI. 1654–61.

—De lacteis thoracicis, in homine brutisque nuperrime observatis, historia anatomica. Parisiis, Apud viduam Mathurini du Puis, 1653.

69 p.; 32, [1] p.; 36 p. 18 cm. **[806]**

Part [2] has special title page: Vasa lymphatica, nuper Hafniae in animantibus inventa, et hepatis exsequiae. Part [3] has special title page: Dubia anatomica de lacteis thoracicis, et an hepatis funus immutet medendi methodum.

Bound with (as issued?) Riolan, J. Opuscula nova anatomica. 1653.

—De lacteis thoracicis. *In* Hemsterhuis, S. Messis aurea triennalis. 1654, 1659; Munierus, J. A. *ed.* De venis tam lacteis thoracicis. 1654.

—De latere Christi aperto. Dissertatio. Lipsiae, Impensis Johan. Christian-Wohlfartii, typis Johan. Coleri, 1685.

[16], 144 p. 17 cm. **[807]**

Bound with *his* De morbis biblicis. 1672.

—De luce animalium libri III. admirandis historiis rationibusque novis referti. Lugd. Batav. Ex officina Francisci Hackii, 1647.

[12], 396, [8] p. 17 cm. **[808]**

—De luce hominum & brutorum libri III. Novis rationibus, & raris historiis secundum illustrati. Hafniae, Typis Matthiae Godicchenii, Impensis Petri Hauboldi, 1669.

[24], 531, [45] p.; 82, [22] p. illus. 16 cm. **[809]**

Half title reads: Thomas Bartholini De luce hominum & brutorum; & Conradi Gesneri De lunariis.

Part [2] has special title page with title: Conradi Gesneri ... De raris & admirandis herbis, quae, sive quod noctu luceant, sive alias ob causas, lunariae nominantur, & obiter de aliis etiam rebus, quae in tenebris lucent, commentariolus. Ed. 2 emendatior. Cum iconibus quibusdam herbarum novis.

—De medicina Danorum domestica dissertationes X. cum ejusdem vindiciis & additamentis. Hafniae, Typis Matthiae Godicchenii, sumptibus Petri Haubold, 1666.

[16], 527, [1] p. 16 cm. [810]

—De medicis poetis dissertatio. Hafniae, Prostat apud Danielem Paulli, Literis Henrici Gödiani, 1669.

[4], 149, [7] p. 16 cm. [811]

—De morbis biblicis miscellanea medica. Ed. 2. correctior. Francofurti, Ex bibliopolio Hafniensi Danielis Paulli [pref. 1672]

[8], 100, [2] p. 17 cm. [812]

With this are bound *his* De sanguine vetito. 1676; *his* Paralytici N. T. medico . . . commentario illustrati. 1662; *his* De latere Christi aperto . . . 1685.

—[The same.] . . . Ed. 3. correctior . . . 1692.

[8], 119, [1] p. 16 cm. [813]

—[The same.] . . . Ed. 3. correctior . . . 1697.

[8], 119, [1] p. 17 cm. [814]

Different setting of type.

—De nivis usu medico observationes variae. Accessit D. Erasmi Bartholini De figura nivis dissertatio; cum operum authoris catalogo. Hafniae, Typis Matthiae Godicchii, sumptibus Petri Haubold, 1661.

3 parts in 1 v. plate. 16 cm. [815]

Parts [2] and [3] have special title pages.

—De peregrinatione ad cognatum suum Theodorum Fuiren juniorem Dn. de Windingaard &c. Danicae juventutis florem propempticon. Hafniae, Literis Georgii Gödiani, 1674.

30 p. 20 cm. [816]

—De peregrinatione medica . . . Hafniae, Literis Christiani Weringii, sumpt. Danielis Paulli, 1674.

73, [3] p. 20 cm. [817]

—De pulmonum substantia & motu diatribe . . . Accedunt . . . Marcelli Malpighii De pulmonibus observationes anatomicae. Hafniae, Typis Henrici Gödiani, prostant apud P. Hauboldum, 1663.

[8], 107 [i.e. 127], [9] p. plate. 16 cm. [818]

—[The same.] *In* Malpighi, M. Opera omina. 1687.

—De sanguine vetito disquisitio medica, cum Cl. Salmasii judicio. Francofurti, Ex officina Hafniensi Petri Hauboldi, 1673.

[8], 104 p. 18 cm. [819]

—Christiani Theophili [pseud. i.e. Thomas Bartholin] De sanguine vetito disquisitio uberior, pro Th. Bartholino. Accessit ejusdem Bartholini De sanguinis abusu disputatio. Francofurti, Ex officina Hafniensi Petri Hauboldi, typis Johann-Georgii Drulmanni, 1676.

[8], 150 p. 17 cm. [820]

Bound with *his* De morbis biblicis. [1672]

—De transplantatione morborum.

528-531 p. 21 cm. (*In* Theatrum sympatheticum auctum. Norimbergae, 1662) [821]

Caption title.

—[The same.] *In* Grube, H. De arcanis medicorum non arcanis commentatio. 1673.

—De unicornu observationes novae. 2 ed. auctiores & emendatiores editae a filio Casparo Bartholino. Amstelaedami, Apud J. Henr. Wetstenium, 1678.

[16], 381, [15] p. illus., plate. 14 cm. [822]

Added engraved title page.

—De visitatione officinarum pharmaceuticarum programma. Hafniae, Apud Danielem Paulli, 1672.

16 p. 19 cm. [823]

Imperfect: p. 15-16 mutilated.

— . . . Programma III. Hafniae, Apud Danielem Paulii, 1674.

20 p. 19 cm. [824]

— . . . Programma IV. Hafniae, Typis Matthiae Godicchenii, 1675.

12 p. 19 cm. [825]

— . . . Programma V. Hafniae, Typis Matthiae Godicchenii, 1676.

16 p. 19 cm. [826]

Imperfect: p. 15-16 mutilated.

—Defensio vasorum lacteorum et lymphaticorum adversus Joannem Riolanum . . . Accedit . . . Gulielmi Harvei De venis lacteis sententia expensa ab eodem Th. Bartholino. Hafniae, Typis haeredum Melchioris Martzanis, & sumptibus Georgii Holst. 1655.

[8], 195 p. 19 cm. [827]

—Dissertatio anatomica de hepate defuncto novis Bilsianorum observationibus opposita. Hafniae, Excudebat Christian. Wering, sumptibus Petri Hauboldi, 1661.

    84 p. 17 cm.   **[828]**

—Dissertatio prima [-secunda] de theriaca in officina Christophori Heerford . . . 1. Febr. 1671 dispensata. Hafniae, Literis Matthiae Godicchenii,sumptibus Petri Hauboldi [1671]

    40 p.; 40 p. 18 cm.   **[829]**

Part [2] has special title page with title: Dissertatio secunda de theriaca in officina Joh. Gothofredi Becker . . . dispensata.

—Dubia anatomica de lacteis thoracicis. *In his* De lacteis thoracicis. 1653.

—Epistola de simplicibus medicamentis inquilinis cognoscendis. *In* Grube, H. Commentarius de modo simplicium medicamentorum facultates cognoscendi. 1669.

—Epistolarum medicinalium a doctis vel ad doctos scriptarum, centuria I. & II. [-centuria IV] . . . Hafniae, Typis Matthiae Godicchenii, impensis Petri Haubold, 1663-1667.

    3 v. in 2. illus. 16 cm.   **[830]**

—Historiarum anatomicarum rariorum centuria I et II. [-III, IV. Ejusdem cura accessere Observationes anatomicae . . . Petri Pawi; -V, VI. Accessit . . . Joannis Rhodii Mantissa anatomica] Hafniae, Typis Academicis Martzani sumptibus Petri Hauboldt, 1654-61.

    3 v. in 2. illus., plates. 17, 15 cm. **[831]**

Vol. 1 has engraved title page with the author's portrait.

Vol. 2 has imprint: Hafniae, Typis Petri Hakii, sumptibus Petri Haubold, 1657. Vol. 3 has title . . . Historiarum anatomicarum & medicarum rariorum centuria . . . Hafniae, Typis Henrici Gödiani, sumptibus Petri Hauboldi, 1661.

With this is bound *his* De insolitis partus humani viis dissertatio. 1664.

—Another issue. (Centuria III–VI only.)

    2 v. 16 cm.   **[832]**

Variant state (dedicatory epistle and index of Centuria III–IV in different setting of type; title page mutilated).

—Historiarum anatomicarum rariorum centuria I et II. Amstelodami, Apud Joannem Henrici, 1654.

    [16], 326, [9] p. illus., port., plates. 16 cm.   **[833]**

Engraved title page with the author's portrait.

—[The same.] . . . Hagae Comitum, Ex typographia Adriani Vlacq, 1654.

    [16], 314, [6] p. illus., port., plates. 15 cm.   **[834]**

Engraved title page with the author's portrait.
Imperfect: p. [15–16] wanting.
Vol. 2, containing Centuria III–IV, was published in 1657.

—[The same.] . . . centuria II. In Collectanea de diuturna graviditate. 1662.

—[Dutch tr.] Twee hondert getal van Thomas Bartholyns seltsame ondervindigen ofte geschiedenissen, omtrent de anatomia ofte onteldinge . . . Overgeset door L. V. B. Dordrecht, Jacobus Savry, 1657.

    [6], 275, [5] p. illus., plates, port. 16 cm.   **[835]**

—[Letters] *In* Borro, G. F. Epistolae duae. 1669.

—Orationes varii argumenti. Hafniae, Sumtibus Danielis Paulli, prostantque Francofurti apud Gothofridum Herbert [pref. 1668]

    [12], 384 p. 16 cm.   **[836]**

—Paralytici N. T. medico & philologico commentario illustrati. Ed. 2. Basileae, Apud Joannem König, 1662.

    [4], 105 p. 17 cm.   **[837]**

Bound with *his* De morbis biblicis. 1672.

—[The same.] . . . Ed. 3. Lipsiae, Sumptibus Joh. Christian. Wohlfartii, typis Johan.Coleri, 1685.

    [4], 103, [1] p. 16 cm.   **[838]**

—Quaestiones nuptiales . . . nuptiis . . . Petri Schumacheri . . . consecratae. Hafniae, Literis Henrici Gödiani, 1670.

    [4], 53, [3] p. 19 cm.   **[839]**

—Responsio de experimentis anatomicis Bilsianis et difficili hepatis resurrectione . . . Hafniae, Apud Petrum Haubold, 1661.

    40 p. 16 cm.   **[840]**

—Vasa lymphatica, nuper Hafniae in animantibus inventa, et hepatis exsequiae. *In his* De lacteis thoracicis. 1653; Munierus, J. A. *ed.* De venis tam lacteis thoracicis. 1654.

—[The same, *as subject.*] *See* BOGDAN, M. Insidiae structae Cl. V. Thomae Bartholini . . . Vasis lymphaticis. 1654; *See* RUDBECK, O. Insidiae structae Olai Rudbeckii. 1654;

—Vasorum lymphaticorum historia nova. *In* Hemsterhuis, S. Messis aurea triennalis. 1654, 1659.

—Ad secundum N. T. paralyticum omnium ordinum auditores opposituros pro disputatione ordinaria . . . respondente Jano. Joh. Wandalino . . . invitat . . . Hafniae, Praelo Martzaniano [1649]

[1], 15-30 p. illus. 18 cm.   [841]

Signatures []¹, C-D⁴.
Program—Copenhagen (for J. J. Wandalin)

Dissertations — Copenhagen

—*praeses.* Collegii Anatomici disputatio quinta de epate et bilis receptaculis . . . Hafniae, Typis Melchioris Martzan, 1650.

[16] p. 18 cm.   [842]

I. Leganger, *respondent*

—Cygni anatome ejusque cantus . . . Hafniae, Praelo Lamprechtiano [1650]

[30] p. plate. 18 cm.   [843]

J. J. Bewerlinus, *respondent.*

—De lacteis thoracicis in homine brutisque nuperrime observatis, historia anatomica . . . Hafniae, Typis Melchioris Martzan, 1652.

71 p. illus. 20 cm.   [844]

M. Lyser, *respondent.*

—De usu thoracis partiumque ineo contentarum dissertatio anatomica . . . Hafniae, Literis Georgii Lamprechtii [1657]

[24] p. 18 cm.   [845]

W. Oderus, *respondent.*

—Disputatio medica de variolis hujus anni epidemiis . . . Hafniae, Literis Petri Morsingii [1656]

[12] p. 20 cm.   [846]

O. Andreas, *respondent.*

—Disputatio medica inauguralis de gutta seu morbo articulari . . . Hafniae, Literis Henrici Gödiani, 1664.

[2], 30 (i.e. 28), [1] p. 20 cm.   [847]

C. Kölichen, *respondent.*

—Spicilegium ex vasis lymphaticis, ubi . . . Glissonii & Pecqueti sententiae expenduntur . . . Hafniae, Literis Petri Morsingii [1655]

[32] p. 19 cm.   [848]

J. C. Stolbergk, *respondent.*

—Spicilegium secundum ex vasis lymphaticis. Ubi Cl. V. Backii, Cattierii, Le Noble, Tardii, Whar-

toni, Charletoni, Bilsii &c. sententiae examinantur . . . Hafniae, Literis viduae Petri Morsingii [1660]

[3], 47, [1] p. 18 cm.   [849]

F. Hammericus, *respondent.*

—Tertium N. T. paralyticum . . . publice proponet . . . Wilhelmo Wormio . . . Hafniae, Ex officina Melch. Martzan [1653]

[1], 31-54, [1] p. illus. 20 cm.   [850]

W. Worm, *respondent.*

—, *ed. and tr. See* COLIN, S. Declaratio fraudum et errorum apud pharmacopoeos commissorum. 1667, 1671.

—, *ed.* Acta medica & philosophica Hafniensia ann. 1671 [-1679]. Cum aeneis figuris. Hafniae, Sumptibus Petri Haubold, Typis Georgii Gödiani, 1673-1680.

5 v. in 3. illus., plates. 19 cm.   [851]

Each volume, except v. 4 has special title page.
Imperfect: first 2 leaves of index wanting in vol. 5; supplied in photocopy from John Crerar Library.

—, *ed. See* BARTHOLIN, C. [1585-1629] Institutiones anatomicae. 1641, 1645, [French tr.] 1647; PAUW, P. Observationes anatomicae selectiores. 1656; RODE, J. De acia dissertatio ad Cornelii Celsi mentem. 1672 [and] Antiquitates philosophicae, medicae & chirurgicae. 1691; VESLING, J. Observationes anatomicae & epistolae medicae ex schedis posthumis selectae & editae a Th. Bartholino. 1664.

—, *tr. See* CORNARO, L. Et edrue lesnets gafn oc nytte. 1681.

—*See* BARTHOLIN, C. [1655-1738] De inauribus veterum syntagma. 1676 [and] Expositio veteris in puerperio ritus ex arca sepulchrali antiqua desumpti. 1677; DEUSING, A. Exercitationes physico-anatomicae de nutrimento animalium ultimo. 1661; HOBOKEN, N. Anatomia secundinae vitulinae. 1675; LYSER, M. Culter anatomicus. 1665, 1679; PECQUET, J. New anatomical experiments. 1653; SEGER, G. Dissertatio anatomica. 1658 [and] Triumphus et querimonia cordis. 1661; SEVERINO, M. A. Therapeuta Neapolitanus. 1653; VESLING, J. Syntagma anatomicum. 1666, 1677, 1696.

—*as subject. See* BILS, L. de. Brief . . . aan Th. Bartholijn. 1661; HERFELT, H. G. Philosophicum hominis, de corporis humani machina. 1687; MAJOR, J. D. Consideratio physiologica. 1669? MØINICHEN,

H. Observationes medico-chirurgicae. 1688; RIOLAN, J. [1580-1657] Opuscula nova anatomica. 1653; RODE, J. Mantissa anatomica ad Thomam Bartholinum. 1661; SPIEGEL, A. van de. Opera quae extant, omnia. 1645; STEPHANUS, N. Castigatio epistolae maledicae. 1661; WALAEUS, J. Epistolae duae. 1647; WANDAL, H. Vindiciae libertatis Christianae circa sanguinem escarium. 1678; WORM, W. Oratio in excessum ... Thomae Bartholini. 1681; ZAS, N. Epistola apologetica ad magnum Th. Bartholinum. 1661.

BARTHOLOMAEI, Hieronymus Matthias [*fl.* 1687] *respondent. See* WEDEL, G. W., *praeses.* Disputatio medica de aegra dysenteria laborante. 1687.

BARTHOLOMAEI, JOHANN [*fl.* 1648-1651] *praeses.* Dissertatio physica de pandiculatione ... [Lipsiae] Typis heredum Timothei Hönii [1648]

[23] p. 19 cm. **[852]**

Diss.—Leipzig (M. Bartholomaei, *respondent*)

BARTHOLOMAEI, JOHANN CHRISTIAN [*fl.* 1690] *respondent. See* SCHMID, J. A., *praeses.* Surdus de sono judicans. 1690.

BARTHOLOMAEI, MICHAEL [*fl.* 1648] *respondent. See* BARTHOLOMAEI, J., *praeses.* Dissertatio physica de pandiculatione. 1648.

BARTHOLOMAEUS ANGLICUS [13th cent.] De genuinis rerum coelestium, terrestrium et inferarum proprietatibus, libri XVIII. Opus incomparabile theologis, jureconsultis, medicis, omniumque disciplinarum & artium alumnis, utilissimum futurum. Cui accessit liber XIX. De variarum rerum accidentibus. Jam nunc nova specie, novaque plane forma renatum, & ab immundis mendis ad amussim repurgatum, adjunctoque indice ... Procurante D. Georgio Bartholdo Pontano a Braitenbert ... Francofurti, Apud Wolfgangum Richterum, impensis Nicolai Steinii, 1601.

[16], 1261, [17] p. 18 cm. **[853]**

BARTHOLOMAEUS DE MONTAGNANA. *See* MONTAGNANA, Bartolomeo.

BARTHOLOMÄUS, CHRISTOPH. *See* MERCLIN, Christoph Bartholomäus [*fl.* 1610]

BARTHOLOMEW THE ENGLISHMAN. *See* BARTHOLOMAEUS ANGLICUS [13th cent.]

BARTISCH, GEORG [1535-*ca.* 1607?] Augen-Dienst; oder, Kurtz und deutlich verfasster Bericht von allen und jeden in-und äusserlichen Mängeln ... de Augen ... Nunmehr zum andernmal an den Tag gelegt. Sultzbach, In Verlegung Georg Scheurers in Nürnberg, gedruckt bey Abraham Lichtenthaler, 1686.

[42], 426, [16] p. plates. 20 cm. **[854]**

Added engraved title page.

—Warhafftige, eigentliche und ausführliche Beschreibung der vielfeltigen Krafft, Tugend, Wirkung und Nutzbarkeit des ... Confects oder Latwergen des grossen Theriacks Andromachi ... [n. p.] 1602.

[44] p. port. 20 cm. **[855]**

Imperfect: wormholes throughout.

With this is bound: Leemann, B. Instrumentum instrumentorum. 1604.

BARTOLETTI, FABRIZIO [1576-1630] Anatomica humani microcosmi descriptio. Per theses disposita ex ... Anphiteatro Pisano proposita ... Bononiae, Typis Sebastiani Bonomii, 1619.

[3], 31 p. plates. 36 cm. **[856]**

—Encyclopaedia hermetico-dogmatica; sive, Orbis doctrinarum medicarum physiologiae, hygiinae pathologiae, simioticae, et therapeuticae ... Bononiae, Apud Sebastianum Bonomium [1619]

[16], 321, [27] p. 23 cm. **[857]**

Engraved title page.

—Methodus in dyspnoeam; seu, De respirationibus libri IV. Cum synopsibus. Quibus quintus pro colophone accessit de curationibus ex dogmaticorum et hermeticorum poenu depromptis. Opus ... anno MDCXXVIII publicis lectionibus explicatum ... Bononiae, Per heredes Evangelistae Dozzae, typis Nicolai Tebaldini, 1633.

[12], 561 (i.e. 559), [22] p. plate, tables. 23 cm. **[858]**

Engraved title page.

Dedicatory epistle of printers dated 1638.

BARTOLI, DANIELLO, *Father* [1608-1685] Del ghiaccio e della coagulatione trattati ... Roma, Varese, 1681.

[8], 230, [8] p. 23 cm. **[859]**

—[The same.] ... Bologna, Gio. Recaldini, 1682.

[8], 230, [8] p. 21 cm. **[860]**

A reprint of the 1681 ed.

—Del suono de' tremori armonici e dell'udito . . . Bologna, Pietro Bottelli, 1680.

[12], 330 p.   illus.   21 cm.   [861]

BARTOLI, Sebastiano [1629-1676] Breve ragguaglio de' bagni di Pozzuolo dispersi . . . Napoli, Roncagliolo, 1667.

[16], 9-76 p.   20 cm.   [862]

Includes "Le antichita di Pozzuolo . . . descritte da Ferrante Loffredo" (p. 9-36) and excerpts from the Chroniche di Napoli, attributed to Giovanni Villani, and from the poem De balneis Puteolanis, variously ascribed to Alcadino, Eustazio da Matera, and Petrus de Ebulo.

—Nuncius Parnassius. *In* Celeberr. virorum apologiae pro R. D. Carolo Musitano. 1700.

—Thermologia Aragonia; sive, Historia naturalis thermarum in occidentali Campaniae ora inter Pausilippum, & Misenum scatentium, jam aevi injuria deperditarum, & Petri Antonii ab Argonia studio ac munificentia restitutarum . . . opus posthuman recensitum a Michaele Blancardo . . . Tomus primus. Neap., Novelli de Bonis, 1679.

2 v.   17 cm.   [863]

Vol. 2 wanting.

BARTOLUCCI, Giovanni Battista [*fl.* 1636] Sommario sopra le virtù del bagno dell'acqua bianca di Nocera nell'Umbria . . . Perugia, Angelo Bartoli, 1636.

30 p.   20 cm.   [864]

Bound with Camilli, A. Del bagno di Nocera nell'Umbria. 1627.

BARTSCH, Benjamin [*fl.* 1684] *respondent. See* Mirus, A. E., *praeses.* Erotema physicum an & quomodo sol calefaciat? 1684.

BARTSCH, Jakob [1600-1633] Exercitationum medicinalium ex Fernelio octava: De signis, eorumq. differentiis. Quam ex ejusdem Semiotice, seu Therapeutices lib. II. capp. 13 . . . inclusam . . . prioribus adjecit . . . M. Jacobus Bartschius . . . Argentorati, Typis Hollandi Findleri, 1624.

[24] p.   19 cm.   [865]

—Exercitationum medicinalium ex Fernelio nona, De indicationibus, seu medendi ratione in genere. Quam ex ejusdem Therapeuticis seu methodi medendi lib. I. . . . inclusam . . . prioribus adjecit . . . M. Jacobus Bartschius . . . Argentorati, Typis Hollandi Findleri, 1624.

[24] p.   19 cm.   [866]

—Exercitationum medicinalium ex Fernelio decima et ultima, De medicamentis eorumq. facultatibus et compositione. Quam ex ejusdem Therapeutices seu methodi medendi libr. IV. capp. 8 . . . inclusam . . . typis exscribi curavit M. Jacobus Bartschius . . . Argentinae, Typis Hollandi Findleri, 1624.

[24] p.   19 cm.   [867]

—, *respondent.* Inaugurales theses Hippocraticae Greaco-Latin, ex libris Hippocr. De morbis, juxta 5. medicinae partes ita collectae . . . Argentorati, Typis Pauli Ledertz, 1630.

[16] p.   18 cm.   [868]

Text in Greek and Latin.
Diss. —Strasbourg.

—*See* Saltzmann, J. R. [1573-1656] *praeses.* Exercitationum medicinalium ex Fernelio tertia: De abdominis. 1622 [and] . . . quinta: De capitis. 1623 [and] . . . septima: De symptomatis. 1624; Sebisch, M. [1578-1674?] *praeses.* Exercitationes medicae. 1639 [and] Exercitationum medicinalium ex Fernelio prima [-secunda] 1622 [and] . . . sexta. 1623.

BARTSCH, Johann Philipp [*fl.* 1623] *respondent. See* Ager, N. Disputatio physica de visu. 1623.

BARUH ENRIQUES, Semuel. *See* Henriques, Semuel Baruh [*fl.* 1674]

BASILIUS VALENTINUS. Von dem grossen Stein der Uhralten, daran so viel tausend Meister anfangs der Welt hero gemacht haben. Neben angehängten Tractätlein . . . Jetzo von newen . . . ans Liecht gebracht. Strassburg, In Verlegung Caspari Dietzels, 1651.

[8], 156, [4] p.   illus.   17 cm.   [869]

Includes also: Die zwölff Schlüssel, dadurch die Thüren zu dem Uhralten Stein unser Vorfahren eröffnet; De microcosmo; oder, Von der kleinen Welt; Von der grossen Heimlichkeit der Welt, und ihrer Artzney; Von der Meisterschafft der sieben Planeten.

—The last will and testament of Basil Valentine . . . To which is added two treatises the first declaring his manual operations. The second shewing things natural and supernatural . . . London, Printed by S. G. and B. G. for Edward Brewster, 1671.

[24], 534 p.   illus.   17 cm.   [870]

Imperfect: p. 313-342 wanting.

5 parts in 1 v. Each part has a special title page dated 1670.
Partly translated and corrected by J. W.

"A practick treatise together with the XII. keys and appendix of the great stone of the ancient philosophers": p. [211]-367; ". . . His treatise concerning the microcosme, or the little world, which is mans body . . .": p. [383]-414.

—Les douze clefs de philosophie de . . . Basile Valentin . . . traictant de la vraye medecine metalique. Plus L'azoth; ou, Le moyen de faire l'or caché des philosophes. Traduction francoise. Paris, Pierre Moët, 1660.

    167 (i.e. 176) p.; 196 p. illus. 17 cm. **[871]**

Part [2] has special title page dated 1659.

Translated from the German (Die zwölff Schlüssel, dadurch die Thüren zu dem Uhralten Stein unser Vorfahren eröffnet) and Latin (Practica, cum duodecim clavibus et appendice, de magno lapide antiquorum sapientum) Cf. Preface (p. 10) by David Lagneau.

With this is bound (as issued) Bernardus Trevirensis. Traicté de la nature de l'oeuf des philosophes. 1659.

—[Aureliae occultae philosophorum partes duae]
    462-512 p., vol. 4. illus. 20 cm. (*In* Zetzner, Lazarus, *ed.* Theatrum chemicum. Argentorati, 1659-61) **[872]**

Title from table of contents.

Ascribed by some to Basilius Valentinus. Cf. Ferguson (A) Vol. 1, p. 57.

—Haliographia de praeparatione, usu, ac virtutibus omnium salium, mineralium, animalium, & vegetabilium, ex manuscriptis, & originalibus . . . collecta . . . Bononiae [Typis Nicolai Tebaldini] 1644.
    [16], 102, [1] p. 16 cm. **[873]**

Added engraved title page.

—[The same.] *In* Suchten, A. von. Of the secrets of antimony. 1670.

—Practica. *In* Maier, M. Tripus aureus. 1618, 1677.

—Triumph-Wagen Antimonii . . . Allen, so den Grund der uhralten Medicin suchen, auch zu der hermetischen Philosophie Beliebnis tragen, zu gut publiciret, und samt noch sieben andern . . . Tractätlein an den Tag gegeben durch Johann Thölden . . . Nürnberg, In Verlegung Johann Hoffmanns, gedruckt von Johann Christoph Lochnern, 1676.
    [15], 467, [21] p. front. 17 cm. **[874]**

Includes also Roger Bacon's De oleo stibii tractatus, oder Von der Tinctur; Johannes Isaaci, Hollandus' Opus saturni, oder Philosophische Betrachtung des Bleyes; and Georg Fedro von Rodach's Practica lapidis philosophici, oder Vom Stein der Weisen.

Bound with Suchten, A. von. Mysteria gemina antimonii. 1675.

—[Latin tr.] Theodori Kerckringii . . . Commentarius in Currum triumphalem antimonii Basilii Valentini, a se Latinitate donatum. Amstelodami, Sumptibus Andreae Frisii, 1671.
    [24], 342, [17] p. front. 14 cm. **[875]**

Kerckring's commentary is printed as notes accompanying his translation of Basilius Valentinus's Triumph Wagen Antimonii.

—[The same.] . . . Amstelaedami, Apud Henricum Wetstenium, 1685.
    [20], 342, [17] p. front. 14 cm. **[876]**

Different setting of type.

—[English tr.] The triumphant chariot of antimony; being a conscientious discovery of the many reall transcedent excellencies included in that minerall . . . Faithfully Englished . . . By J[ohn H[arding] Oxon. London, Printed for Thomas Bruster, 1660.
    [6], 175 p. 1 illus. 15 cm. **[877]**

Imperfect: first preliminary leaf (blank?) wanting.

—Another issue, with imprint: London, Printed for W.S. and sold by Samuel Thomson, 1661.
    [878]

—[The same.] Triumphant chariot of antimony, with annotations of Theodore Kirkringius, M.D. With The true book of the learned Synesius a Greek abbot taken out of the emperour's library, concerning the philosopher's stone. London, Dorman Newman, 1678.
    [16], 176 p. 4 plates. 20 cm. **[879]**

The true book . . . has special title page.

—Von den natürlichen unnd übernatürlichen Dingen. Auch von der ersten Tinctur, Wurtzel und Geiste der Metallen und Mineralien, wie dieselbe entpfangen, aussgekochet, geboren, verendert und vermehret werden. Trewlich eröffnet durch Fratrem Basilium Valentinum . . . Und nunmehr aus seiner eigenen Handschrifft in Druck publiciret, durch Johan Thölden . . . Leipzig, In Vorlegung Jacob Apels [Gedruckt zu Eissleben bey Jacob Gaubisch] 1603.
    [9], 124, [2] p. 16 cm. **[880]**

—[Latin tr.] Tractatus chymico-philosophicus de rebus naturalibus & supernaturalibus metallorum & mineralium. Francofurti ad Moenum, Sumptibus Jacobi Gothofredi Seylet, 1676.
    64 p. 16 cm. **[881]**

—[Excerpts] *In* Dolhopff, G. A., *comp.* Lapis animalis microcosmicus. 1681 [and] Lapis vegetabilis. 1681.

—*See* MEISNER, L. Gemma gemmarum alchimistarum. 1608; REINHART, H. C. Der gülden Gesundbrunnen. 1611; SALA, A. Processus ... de auro potabili. 1630.

BASNAGE, HENRI, *sieur de Beauval* [1656–1710] Histoire des ouvrages des sçavans, par Monsr. B**** docteur en droit. Mois de septembre 1687 [-juin 1709] Rotterdam, Reinier Leers, 1687–1709.

24 v. 14 cm. [882]

Incomplete: vols. 2–24 wanting.

In addition to collective title pages for the volumes, many numbers have special title pages. The dates given in imprints of the special title pages vary in some cases from date of original month of issue.

BASSANO, Cesare [*b.* 1584] *illus. See* ASELLIO, G. De lactibus. 1627; 1640.

BASSO, SEBASTIAN [16th cent.] Philosophiae naturalis adversus Aristotelem libri XII. in quibus abstrusa veterum physiologia restaurantur, & Aristotelis errores solidis rationibus refelluntur ... Genevae, Apud Petrum de la Roviere, 1621.

[40], 701, [29] p. 18 cm. [883]

Errata: p. [29] at end.

[BASTON, SAMUEL, *fl.* 1695] Baston's case vindicated: or, A brief account of some evil practices of the present Commissioners for Sick and Wounded ... London, 1695.

[4], 55 p. 20 cm. [884]

BASTON'S case vindicated. 1695. *See* [BASTON, S.]

BATE, GEORGE [1608–1669] Pharmacopoeia Bateana. In qua, octingenta circiter pharmaca ... e praxi Georgii Batei ... excerpta, ordine alphabetico concise exhibentur ... Huic accessit Orthotonia medicorum observata: annexa item est ... Tabula posologica ... Cura Ja[mes] Shipton ... Londini, Impensis Sam. Smith, 1688.

[11], 130, 12, 16, [3] p. illus. 17 cm. [885]

Errata: p. [3] at end.

—[The same.] ... Ed. altera a priori locupletior ... Huic accesserunt Arcana Goddardiana ... item ... Orthotonia medicorum observata: insuper & Tabula posologica ... Cura J[ames] S[hipton] ... Londini, Impensis Sam. Smith, 1691.

[11], 192, 16, 12, 16, [28] p. illus. 16 cm.

[886]

—[The same.] ... Ed. 3. cum Appendice ex autographo eximii authoris nunc primum desumpta. Londini, Sam. Smith & Benj. Walford, 1700.

[8], 286 (i.e. 290), [2] p. 17 cm. [887]

The preface to the Appendix signed: T. Fuller.

—[Dutch tr.] Pharmacopoea Batheana. Ofte den apotheek van ... Georgius Bath ... Uitgegeven door ... Jac. Shipton ... Amsterdam, Jan ten Hoorn, 1698.

[14], 242, [3] p. 14 cm. [888]

Added engraved title page.

—[English tr.] Pharmacopoeia Bateana; or, Bate's Dispensatory. Translated from the 2 ed. of the Latin copy, published by Mr. James Shipton. Containing his choice ... recipe's ... the Arcana Goddardiana and their recipe's intersperst in their proper places, which are almost all wanting in the Latin copy ... To which are added in this English edition, Goddard's drops, Russel's pouder and the emplastrum febrifugum ... By William Salmon ... London, S. Smith and B. Walford, 1694.

[16], 965, [19] p. plate. 18 cm. [889]

—[The same.] ... Translated from the last ed. of the Latin copy ... The 2d ed. with emendations ... By William Salmon, M. D. London, S. Smith and B. Walford, 1700.

[16], 747, [13] p. plate. 20 cm. [890]

—*See* GLISSON, F. De rachitide. 1650, 1660, 1671, 1682; [English tr.] 1668.

BATE, JOHN [*fl.* 1634] The mysteries of nature and art. In foure severall parts. The first of water works. The second of fire works. The third of drawing, washing, limming, painting, and engraving. The fourth of sundry experiments. The 2d ed.; with many additions unto every part ... [London] Printed for Ralph Mabb, 1635.

[9], 288, [16] p. front. (port.), illus., plates. 19 cm. [891]

Imperfect: title page trimmed and mounted. Sig. Y3-4 and Z1 wanting.

Treatises 2–4 have special title pages with imprint: London, Printed by Thomas Harper for Ralph Mab, 1635.

—[The same.] The mysteries of nature and art in four severall parts. The first of water-works. The second of fire-works. The third of drawing, colouring, limming, paynting, graving, and etching. The fourth

of experiments . . . London, By R. Bishop for Andrew Crook, 1654.

[3], 221, [15] p.   illus.   20 cm.   [892]

Added title pages: The 3d ed., with many additions.
Treatises 2–4 have special title pages.

BATEN, CAREL [*fl.* 1569-1609?] Handboek der
cirurgijen: waer in veel exquisite ende secrete remedien, teghens alle wtwendighe ghebreken, zo wel int
generale als int particuliere verhaelt staen . . .
Schiedam, By Adiaen Corneliss voor Jaspar Troyens,
1606.

408, [24] p.   illus.   17 cm.   [893]

"Sommige Aphorismi van Hippocrates, die tot de conste der
chirurgijen behooren": p. [5-6]

—[The same.] . . . Waer by gevoeght is Hippocrates Vande wonden in't hooft. Als mede
Guilhelmus Fabrisius Hildanus Vande verbrantheydt, daer in by na alle accidenten, ofte toe-vallen
der selber klaerlijck vertoont worden. Amstelredam,
Hendrick Laurentsz, 1634.

336, [20], 71, [7], 61 p.   illus. port.   15 cm.

[894]

"Hippocrates Van die wonden des hoofts, nu eerst uytten Latyne
overgheset in't Nederduyrsch [sic], door M. Peter Haslardus . . .
Met een korte verklaringe door den selven P. Hasslardus" (71, [7]
p., 3d and 4th groups of paging) has colophon: Amstelredam,
Ghedruckt by Johannes Jaquet . . . 1634.
"Guilhelmus Fabricius Hildanus, Van de verbranthent door olye,
heet water, gloeyende yser, puspoeder, blixem, etc." (61 p. at end)
is a translation of his De combustionibus, quae oleo et aqua fer-
vidis, ferro candente, pulvere tormentario, fulmine et quavis alia
materia ignita fiunt.

—[The same.] . . . Amsterdam, Johannes van
Ravesteyn, 1653.

336, [20], 71, [7], 61 p.   illus.   16 cm.   [895]

Different setting of type.

—Secreet-boeck van vele diversche en heerlicke
consten in veelderleye materien, met weel remedien
teghen de innerlijcke en uytterlijcke gebreken der
menschen. Wt Latijnsche, Francoische, Hoogh-
duytsche ende Nederduytsche autheuren vergadert
. . . Verrijckt met verscheyden secreten van wijnen,
verwen ende schrijf-konsten. Haerlem, Thomas Fonteyn, 1650.

490 (i.e. 492) p.; [2], 73, [4] p.   14 cm. [896]

"Aenhanghsel van verscheyden sonderlinge secreten . . ." has
special title page dated 1651.

—[The same.] . . . Amsterdam, Jan Wilting, 1656.
573, [3] p.   14 cm.   [897]

—[The same.] . . . Amsterdam, I. I. Schipper,
1661.

573, [3] p.   15 cm.   [898]

Different setting of type.

—, *tr. See* PARÉ, A. De chirurgie. 1615, 1636, 1649,
1655; WIRSUNG, C. Medecyn boec. 1601, 1605, 1616,
1627.

BATESON, T., *tr. See* SCHRÖDER, J. Ζωολογια;
or, The history of animals as they are useful to
physick and chirurgery. 1650.

BATH, GEORGE. *See* BATE, George [1608-1669]

Le **BATIMENT** des receptes; ou, Les vertus et
proprietés de plusieurs beaux secrets, utiles tant pour
la beauté, que pour la santé du corps. Corrigés &
augmentés de nouveau. Comme aussi des remedes
pour la guerison des bestiaux. Et divisés en trois parties. Avec les secrets des arts, & pour les pierreries.
De la boutique de Jacques Lions. A Lton [i.e. Lyon]
Louis Servant [1693]

156, [24] p.   15 cm.   [899]

BATT, CAREL. *See* BATEN, Carel [*fl.* 1569-1609?]

BATTIER, DANIEL [*fl.* 1676-1679] *respondent.* Consultatio medica περι της μυδριάσεως . . . Basileae,
Typis Joh. Rodolphi Genathii [1679]

[12] p.   22 cm.   [900]

Diss. — Basel.

—*See* BAUHIN, J. K., *praeses.* Theses has medicas
de asthmate . . . subjicit M. D. B. [1676]

BATTIER, SAMUEL [1667-1744] *respondent.* Dissertatio de generatione hominis . . . Basileae, Typis
Jacobi Werenfelsii [1690]

[24] p.   20 cm.   [901]

Diss. — Basel.

BATTUS, KAREL. *See* BATEN, Carel [*fl.*
1569-1609?]

BATTUS, LEVINUS [1545-1591] *See* SMET, H.
Miscellanea . . . medica. 1661.

BAUCINETUS, GULIELMUS. *See* BAUCYNET,
Guillaume [*fl.* 1604]

BAUCYNET, Guillaume [*fl.* 1604] *See* HARVET,
I. Animadversiones 1604.

BAUDERON, BRICE [*ca.* 1540-1623] Paraphrase
sur la pharmacopoee. Divisee en deux livres . . .

Rev., corr., & augm. par l'autheur . . . Rouen, Nicolas L'Oyselet, 1612.

[23], 721, [20] p. 15 cm.   [902]

First published in 1588.

—[The same.] . . . Ensemble un Traicté des eaux distillées, qu' un apothicaire doit tenir en sa boutique, faict par Laurens Catelan . . . Dernière éd. Rouen, Martin de la Motte, 1627.

[14], 524 (i.e. 516), [12], 31 p. 18 cm.   [903]

"Traicté des eaux distillées . . . par Laurens Catelan": 31 p. at end has special title page.

Edited by Gratien Bauderon.

—[The same.] Pharmacopee divisee en deux livres, avec une ample paraphrase de M. Brice Bauderon . . . Ensemble les additions de feu M. Gratian Bauderon . . . Derniere ed., augm. par ledict M. Brice Bauderon de plusieurs medicamens, & des vertus & facultés cy-devant omises, de tous les remedes simples ou composés y contenus. Avec correction parfaicte des compositions, paraphrases & additions. Lyon, La vefue de Claude Rigaud & Philippe Borde, 1640.

[20], 526, [18], 32 p. 17 cm.   [904]

"Traicté des eaux distillées . . . par Laurens Catelan": 32 p. at end.

—[The same.] Pharmacopee de Bauderon. Rev., corr. & augm. de plusieurs compositions necessaires: & des facultez de chaque composition. Avec un Traicté des plus usitez & celebres medicamens chimiques. Par G. Sauvageon . . . Rouen, Clement Malassis, 1644.

[16], 704, [64], 77 (i.e. 79), [8] p. 17 cm.
                                                    [905]

Imperfect: p. 323–334 wanting.

"Traicté chimique . . . par G. Sauvageon" (77 p.) has special title page.

"Traicté des eaux distillées . . . par Laurens Catelan": p. [19]–[64] (3d group of paging)

—[The same.] . . . Paris, Jean Jost, 1650.

[16], 512, [16], 32, [4] 97, [10] p. 17 cm.
                                                    [906]

Imperfect: p. 431–432 wanting.

"Traicté des eaux distillées . . . par Laurens Catelan": 32 p. (4th group of paging)

"Traité chymique . . . par G. Sauvageon": [4], 97 p. at end, has special title page.

—[The same.] . . . Lyon, Claude La Riviere, 1655.

[16], 785 (i.e. 783), [19], 51, [4], 97 [9] p. 17 cm.
                                                    [907]

"Traicté des eaux distillées . . . par Laurens Catelan": 51 p. (4th group of paging)

"Traité chimique . . . par G. Sauvageon" ([4], 97, [9] p. at end) has special title page dated 1656.

—[The same.] La pharmacopée de Bauderon, a laquelle, outre les corrections & augmentations de toutes les precedentes editions, sont adjoustées de nouveau . . . Par François Verny . . . Lyon, Barthelemy Riviere, 1663.

[16], 408 p.; 294, [12] p. 23 cm.   [908]

Added half title.

The "Second livre" includes Gratien Bauderon's Appendix ad pharmacopoeam, Laurent Catelan's Traicté des eaux distillées, and Guillaume Sauvageon's Traicté chymique.

—[The same.] . . . Avec la réponse à l'apologie de Mr. Jean Zwelfer . . . & un examen des ingrediens de la confection d'alkermes qu'il a inventée & décrite dans sa Pharmacopée royale. Par François Verny . . . Derniere éd. Lyon, Jean Girin & Barthelemy Riviere, 1672.

[16], 534, 415, [16] p. 24 cm.   [909]

Added half title.

—[The same.] . . . Nouv. ed., rev. & exactement corr. de quantité de fautes qui s'etoient glissées dans les autres editions. Lyon, Guillaume Chaunod & Cesar Chappuis, 1681.

[16], 785 (i.e. 783), [19], 51, [4], 97, [9] p. 18 cm.
                                                    [910]

"Traité chymique . . . par G. Sauvageon": ([4], 97, [9] p. at end) has special title page.

"Traicté des eaux distillées . . . par Laurens Catelan": 51 p. (4th group of paging)

—[Latin tr.] Pharmacopoea, cui adjecta sunt paraphrasis et miscendorum medicamentorum modus. Primum Gallice scripta . . . nunc vero a . . . Philemone Hollando . . . in Latinum sermonem conversa. Huic accedunt Joannis Du Boys . . . Observationes in methodum miscendorum medicamentorum topicorum, [c. Londini, Typis Edwardi Griffini, sumptibus Richardi Whitakeri, 1639.

[8], 293 (i.e. 297), [24], 121, [8] p. 29 cm.
                                                    [911]

STC 1592.

The Pharmacopoea edited by Henry Holland, the Observationes by Thomas Johnson.

"Tractatus de aquis destillatis . . . per Laurentium Catellanum": p. 277–293.

—Praxis in duos tractatus distincta. In priore agitur de febribus essentialibus tam simplicibus quam compositis, confusis, erraticis, malignis ac pestiferis, & symptomaticis in genere, & in specie curandis. In posteriore de symptomatis & morbis internis a capite ad pedes usque. Lutetiae Parisiorum, Sumptibus Nicolai Buon, 1620.

[39], 849 (i.e. 889), [13] p.   port.   25 cm.
[912]

—[English tr.] The expert phisician: learnedly treating of all agues and feavers. Whether simple or compound. Shewing their different nature, causes, signes, and cure ... translated into English by B[enjamin] W[ells] ... London, Printed by R. I. for John Hancock, 1657.

[13], 160 p.   15 cm.   [913]

Imperfect: p. 131-2 wanting; supplied in photocopy from Library of Congress.

—See FONTEYN, N. Institutiones pharmaceuticae. 1633.

BAUDERON, GRATIEN [1583-1615] *ed. See* BAUDERON, B. Paraphrase sur la pharmacopee. 1627, 1640.

BAUDIS, JOACHIM [*fl.* 1570-1598] Zwey Tractätlein von der Pest, deroselben Praeservation und Curation. Lignitz, Gedruckt durch Nicolaum Schneider, 1613.

[88] p.   illus.   20 cm.   [914]

Published from manuscripts in possession of the author's son-in-law, J. B. Reiman, who signed the dedication.

—See SCHOLTZ, L. Consiliorum medicinalium ... liber singularis. 1610.

BAUDIS, JOHANN GOTTLOB [*b.* 1663] *respondent. See* CRAUSE, R. W., *praeses.* Dissertatio medica inauguralis de varis. 1697.

—See CRAUSE, R. W. Propemticum inaugurale de calendario valetudinariorum perpetuo. 1697.

BAUDISS, LEONHART [*fl.* 1607-1608] *See* KNOBLOCH, T., *praeses.* Disputationes anatomicae. 1608, 1612.

BAUDOIN, JEAN [1590?-1650] *tr. See* BACON, F., *viscount St. Albans.* Le medecin historial. 1652.

BAUER, GEORG. *See* AGRICOLA, Georg [1494-1555]

[**BAUGIER**, EDME, *b.* 1644] Traité des eaux minerales d'Attancourt en Champagne. Avec quelques observations sur les eaux minerales de Sermaise. Chaalons, Edme Seneuze, 1696.

[42], 44, [8] p.   15 cm.   [915]

BAUHIN, CASPAR. *See* BAUHIN, Kaspar [1560-1624]

BAUHIN, FRIEDRICH [*fl.* 1675-1678] *respondent.* Theses ... περι Χορδάψου ... Basileae, Typis Jo. Rodolphi Genathi [1678]

[8] p.   20 cm.   [916]

Diss.—Basel.

—*See* BAUHIN, J. K., *praeses.* Theses has medicas de cholera ... submittit [1675]

BAUHIN, HIERONYMUS [1637-1667] *praeses.* Assertiones medicae de catarrho ... Basileae, Typis Johan. Jacobi Deckeri [1665]

[20] p.   20 cm.   [917]

Diss.—Basel (J. J. Staehelin, *respondent*)

—*praeses.* De spiritibus theses ... [Basileae] Georgius Deckerus [1660]

[8] p.   19 cm.   [918]

Diss.—Basel (J. J. Bauhin, *respondent*)

—*praeses.* Disputatio medica de tertiana intermittente exquisita ... Basileae, Typis Johan. Jacobi Deckeri [1666]

[16] p.   20 cm.   [919]

Diss.—Basel (J. H. Hegner, *respondent*)

— *praeses.* Theses ... de diaeta sanorum ... Basileae, Typis Joh. Jac. Deckeri [1666]

[16] p.   22 cm.   [920]

Diss.—Basel (J. H. Ott, *respondent*)

—, *ed. See* THEODORUS, J. Neuw vollkommentlich Kreuterbuch. 1664.

BAUHIN, JOHANN [1541-1613] De aquis medicatis nova methodus libris quatuor comprehensa. Agitur in iis de fontibus celebribus, thermis, balneis universae Europae, & potissimum Ducatus Wirtembergici ... Item De variis fossilibus stirpibus & insectis ... Montisbeligardi, Apud Jacobum Foillet, 1612.

[42], 291 p.   plates.   21 cm.   [921]

Contains the first 3 books.

—[Historia novi et admirabilis balneique Bollensis. German.] Ein new Badbuch, und historische Beschreibung, von der wunderbaren Krafft und Würckung, des Wunder Brunnen und heilsamen

Bads zu Boll . . . im Hertzogthumb Würtemberg . . . Ins Deutsch gebracht, durch M. David Förter . . . Stutgart, Getruckt durch Marx Fürstern, 1602

4 v. in 1. illus. 21 cm. [922]

Vol. 4 has title: Badbuch . . . das vierdte Buch. Von den Steinen unnd metallischen Sachen . . . auch von allerhand Erdgewechsen, Vögeln, Gewürm und andern Thierlein . . . zum theil in der Nähe herumb gefunden . . .

—Historia plantarum universalis, nova, et absolutissima cum consensu et dissensu circa eas. Auctoribus Joh. Bauhino . . . et Joh. Hen. Cherlero . . . quam recensuit & auxit Dominicus Chabraeus . . . Juris vero publici fecit, Franciscus Lud. a Graffenried . . . Ebroduni, 1650-1651.

3 v. illus. 39 cm. [923]

Each volume has added engraved title page and half title.

—*See* GOCKEL, E. Enchiridion medico-practicum de peste. 1669.

BAUHIN, JOHANN JAKOB [*fl.* 1660-1662] *respondent.* Διάσκεψιν hancce διαιτητικην . . . exhibet Joannes Jacobus Bauhinus. [Basileae] Proelo Joan. Jacobi Deckeri [1661]

[15] p. 20 cm. [924]

Diss.—Basel.

—*respondent.* Theses . . . de calculo renum . . . Basileae, Typis Joh. Jacobi Deckeri [1662]

[8] p. 20 cm. [925]

Diss.—Basel.

—*See* BAUHIN, H., *praeses.* De spiritibus theses. 1660.

BAUHIN, JOHANN KASPAR [1606-1685] *praeses.*

Dissertations — Basel

—Consultatio medica de angina . . . Basileae, Typis Joh. Jacobi Deckeri [1667]

[12] p. 19 cm. [926]

J. von Muralt, *respondent.*

—Dissertationem hancce de epilepsia . . . offert Joh. Georgius Mangoldt . . . Basileae, Apud Jacobum Werenfelsium [1672]

[10] p. 17 cm. [927]

J. G. Mangoldt, *respondent.*

—Historiam venaesectionis . . . in publicum eruditorum examen offert . . . anni a jubilaeo secundo secundi almae universitatis patriae Jacobus

Rothius . . . Basileae, Typis Joh. Jacobi Deckeri [1662]

[16] p. 20 cm. [928]

J. Roth, *respondent.*

—Theses de humoribus . . . Athenis Rauracis, Typis Georgii Deckeri, 1660.

[28] p. 20 cm. [929]

S. Eglinger, *respondent.*

—Theses has medicas de asthmate . . . subjicit M. Daniel Battier. Basileae, Typis Jo. Jacobi Deckeri [1676]

[11] p. 20 cm. [930]

D. Battier, *respondent.*

—Theses has medicas de cholera . . . submittit Fridericus Bauhinus . . . Basileae, Proelo Jo. Jacobi Deckeri [1675]

[8] p. 20 cm. [931]

F. Bauhin, *respondent.*

—Theses medicae de veneni natura . . . Basileae, Typis Georgii Deckeri, 1659.

[8] p. 18 cm. [932]

H. J. Ziegler, *respondent.*

—, *ed. See* BAUHIN, K. Vivae imagines. 1640.

—*See* ZWINGER, T. Oratio panegyrica in obitum . . . Jo. Caspari Bauhini. 1687.

BAUHIN, JOHANN KASPAR [*b.* 1632] *respondent. See* STUPANUS, E., *praeses.* Signorum medicorum doctrina. 1649.

BAUHIN, JOHANN KASPAR [*fl.* 1685-1687] *respondent.* Dissertatio medica inauguralis de auditus laesione . . . Basileae, Typis Jacobi Bertschii [1687]

[12] p. 20 cm. [933]

Diss.—Basel.

—*See* EGLINGER, N., *praeses.* Positionum botanico anatomicarum centuria. 1685.

BAUHIN, KASPAR [1560-1624] Animadversiones in Historiam generalem plantarum Lugduni editam. Item Catalogus plantarum circiter quadringentarum eo in opere bis terve positarum . . . Francoforti, Excudebat Melchior Hartmann, impensis Nicolai Bassaei, 1601.

95 p. 21 cm. [934]

The Historia generalis plantarum, which was published anonymously in Lyons in 1586-87, was the work of Jacques Dalechamps.

Bound with Mercado, L. De mulierum affectionibus. 1602.

—Catalogus plantarum circa Basileam sponte nascentium cum earundem synmonymiis & locis in quibus reperiuntur . . . Basileae, Typis Johan. Jacobi Genathii, 1622.

113, [15] p.   18 cm.   [935]

—De compositione medicamentorum: sive, Medicamentorum componendorum ratio & methodus, in praelectionib. pub. proposita. Offenbachii Ysenburgicorum, Typis Conradi Nebenii, impensis heredum Nicolai Bassaei, 1610.

[10], 294 p.   18 cm.   [936]

—[De corporis humani fabrica.] Institutiones anatomicae corporis virilis et muliebris historiam exhibentes . . . Hippocrat. Aristotel. Galeni auctoritat. illustratae & novis inventis plurimis auctae. Additis novis aliquot figuris & indice. [Lugduni] Apud Joannem Le Preux, 1604.

[16], 237, [26] p.   illus.   17 cm.   [937]

Published in its original form in 1590 under title: De corporis humani fabrica. A revised version was published in 1597 under title: Anatomica corporis virilis et muliebris historia.

—[The same.] . . . Ed. 4. Basileae, Apud Joann. Schroeter, 1609.

[15], 260, [51] p.   6 illus.   17 cm.   [938]

"Tabulae venarum, arteriarum, nervorum, musculorum et ossium" and "Icones aliquot ex libro naturae, praeter communem anatomicorum senteniam, desumptae": p. [261-303]

—[The same.] Institutiones anatomicae Hippoc. Aristot. Galeni auctorita. illustratae, hac editione quinta & postrema ab auctore emaculatae, & auctae. Francofurti, Apud Paulum Jacobi, impensis Jo. Theodor. de Bry, 1616.

[16], 260, [41] p.   port., 5 tables.   17 cm.   [939]

Reprinted with a few changes in the text from the 4th ed. 1609. The 5 folded tables, revisions of those in the original edition of 1590, were not in the 1609 edition. The illustrations in the 1609 edition are omitted in this edition.

"Tabulae ossium, musculorum, venarum et arteriarum nervorum": p. [261-291]

—De hermaphroditorum monstrosorumque partuum natura, ex theologorum, jureconsultorum, medicorum, philosophorum, & rabbinorum sententia libri duo hactenus non editi: plane philologici, infinitis exemplis illustrati . . . Oppenheimii, Typis Hieronymi Galleri, aere Johan-Theodori de Bry, 1614.

36, 594, [1] p.   illus., plate, port., table.   17 cm.   [940]

Title within engraved border has additional imprint: Francofurti, Excudebat Mathaeus Becker impensis Jo. Theo. & Jo. Israel de Bry, frat., 1600.

Imperfect: plate for p. 588 wanting; fig. 4 not printed (p. 580 blank except for caption and catchword).

—[The same.] . . . Francofurti, Apud Matthaeum Merianum, 1629.

36, 572 p.   table.   17 cm.   [941]

A reprint without the section of illustrations at end.

—De homine oratio . . . Athenis Rauracis, Apud Jo. Jacobum Genathium [1614]

39 p.   19 cm.   [942]

—De lapidis bezaar orient. et occident. cervini item et Germanici ortu, natura, differentiis, veroque usu ex veterum & recentiorum placitis liber hactenus non editus. Basileae, Apud Conr. Waldkirch., 1613.

[24], 288 (i.e. 290), [8] p.   plates.   16 cm.
                                                                 [943]

Leaf inserted after p. 78 with caption: Joachimus Camerarius in suo horto medico. Verso blank.

"Πίναξ eorum quorum opera usi sumus": p. [10-17]

—[The same.] . . . Priore editione auctior. Basileae, Sumptibus Ludovici Regis, 1625.

[24], 294, [9] p.   illus.   17 cm.   [944]

—Hygiae et panaceae parente . . . Casparus Bauhinus . . . agonothetes ab . . . Medic. Acad. Basil. collegio rite lectus & dictus viris genere virtute eruditione philosoph. et medica in . . . Germaniae academ. comparata & privat. & public. examinib. & disput. comprob. conspicuis D. M. Philippo Webero . . . Johanni Creutzmanno . . . Georgio Titschardo . . . Michaeli Seidelio . . . Martino Scheffero . . . summos in arte medica titulos . . . in brabeuter. acad. collaturus . . . Basileae Rauracorum, Typis Johannis Schroeteri, 1610.

broadside. 39 × 21 cm.   [945]

Bound with Weber, P. Problematum medicorum triades tres. 1610.

—Πίναξ theatri botanici; sive, Index in Theophrasti Dioscoridis et botanicorum qui a seculo scripserunt opera, plantarum circiter sex millium ab ipsis exhibitarum nomina cum earundem synonymiis & differentiis methodice secundum genera & species proponens. Opus XL. annorum summopere expetitum ad autoris autographum recensitum. Basileae, Impensis Joannis Regis, 1671.

[24], 518, [21] p.   26 cm.   [946]

Errata: p. [21] at end.

A considerably revised, enlarged and altered form of the author's Phytopinax. Cf. Burckhardt, p. 113.

"Nomina authorum quorum opera usi sumus": p. [11-17]

"Appendix. Aliquot plantarum descriptiones adponere lubet": p. 516-518.

With this is bound *his* Πρόδρομος theatri botanici. 1671.

—Πρόδρομος theatri botanici, in quo plantae supra sexcentae ab ipso primum descriptae cum plurimis figuris proponuntur. Ed. alt. emendatior. Basileae, Impensis Joannis Regis, 1671.

    [4], 160, [12] p. illus. 26 cm.   **[947]**

Bound with *his* Πίναξ theatri botanici. 1671.

—Theatrum anatomicum, novis figuris aeneis illustratum et in lucem emissum opera & sumptibus Theodori de Brÿ p. m. relictae viduae & filiorum Joannis Theodori & Joannis Israelis de Brÿ. Francofurti at [sic] Moenum, Typis Matthaei Beckeri, 1605.

    [16], 1314 (i.e. 1308), [46] p. illus., port. 19 cm.
    [948]

Engraved title page.

Imperfect: page 213-214 (including plate 24 of bk. 1) wanting; plate 16 of bk. 3 not printed (page is blank)

With this is bound *his* Appendix ad Theatrum anatomicum. 1600 [i.e. 1605]

—[The same.] Theatrum anatomicum ... infinitis locis auctum, ad morbos accommodatum & ab erroribus ab authore repurgatum, observationibus & figuris aliquot novis aeneis illustratum, opera sumptibusque Johan. Theodori de Bry. [Francofurti] 1621.

    [14], 664 (i.e. 662), [16] p. 24 cm.   **[949]**

Imperfect: portrait of author cut out of title page.

Issued without the illustrations of the edition of 1605; they were published separately, in 1620, under title: Vivae imagines partium corporis humani.

With this is bound *his* Vivae imagines partium corporis humani. 1620.

—[The same.] *See* RIOLAN, J. [1580-1657] Opuscula anatomica nova. 1649 [and] Opera anatomica vetera. 1650.

—Appendix ad Theatrum anatomicum ...; sive, Explicatio characterum omnium qui figuris totius operis additi fuere, quae seorsim compingi debet. Francofurti, Excudebat Mathaeus Becker impensis Jo. Theo. & Jo. Israel de Brÿ, 1600 [i.e. 1605]

    [8], 197, [1] p. port. 19 cm.   **[950]**

Imperfect: sign. n⁴ (last leaf, blank?) wanting.

Engraved title page.

Author's portrait, dated 1605, on the verso of title page.

Bound with *his* Theatrum anatomicum. 1605.

—Vivae imagines partium corporis humani aeneis formis expressae & ex Theatro anatomico ... desumptae, opera sumptibusque Johan. Theodori de Bry. [Francofurti] 1620.

    265, [21] p. illus. 24 cm.   **[951]**

Imperfect: upper third of title page, with portrait of the author, cut away.

The plates are those of the author's Theatrum anatomicum, previously published in Frankfort, 1605. They are here issued in corrected form and with 10 new plates; and are intended for separate use or to accompany the unillustrated edition of the text published the following year, 1621. Cf. Preface.

Bound with *his* Theatrum anatomicum. 1621.

—[The same.] ... Opera ... Matthaei Meriani. [Francofurti] 1640.

    265, 22, [1] p. illus., port. 23 cm.   **[952]**

A reprint of the 1620 edition with new preface by Johann Kaspar Bauhin.

—*praeses*. Assertiones medicae de catarrho, brancho & coryza morbis plerunque connexis ... Athenis Rauracorum, Typis Johannis Schroeteri, 1610.

    [24] p. 20 cm.   **[953]**

Diss.—Basel (J. Schaller, *respondent*)

With this is bound Stupanus, J. N. Gratiosi medicorum Basiliens. 1610.

—*praeses*. Praeludia anatomica ... Atheneis Rauracis, 1601.

    [32] p. 22 cm.   **[954]**

Diss.—Basel (P. Hoechstetter, *respondent*)

— *ed. See* FERNEL, J. Pharmacia. 1605; MATTIOLI, P. A. Opera quae extant omnia. 1674; THEODORUS, J. Neuw vollkommentlich Kreuterbuch. 1613, 1625, 1664.

—*See* CROOKE, H. Μιϰϱοϰοσμογϱαψία. A description of the body of man. 1615, 1618, 1631, 1651; Histoire des plantes de l'Europe. 1680, 1689; JONCQUET, D. Hortus. 1659; MERCURIALE, G. De morbis muliebribus. 1601, 1618; ROUSSET, F. Exsectio foetus vivi ex matre viva sine alterutrius vitae periculo. 1601; STRUTHIUS, J. Ars sphygmica. 1602.

—*as subject. See* RAY, J. Stirpium Europaearum extra Britannias nascentium sylloge. 1694.

BAULOT, JACQUES. *See* BEAULIEU, Frère Jacques de [1651-1714]

BAUMANN, JOHANN [*fl.* 1600-1601] *ed. See* MASSARIA, A. Practica medica. 1601.

BAUMANN, JOHANN NICOLAUS [*fl.* 1622-1629] *respondent.* Dissertatio inauguralis de tabaci virtutibus usu et abusu . . . Basileae, Impensis Johan. Jacobi Genathii [1629]

31 p. 20 cm. [**955**]

Diss. — Basel.

— *See* HORST, G. [1578-1636] 'Εξετάσεων παθολογικων. 1629 [and] Prognosis febrium. 1622; SEBISCH, M. [1578-1674?] *praeses.* Exercitationes medicae. 1639.

BAUMBACH, JOHANN LUDWIG a [*fl.* 1682] *respondent. See* KAHLER, J., *praeses.* Dissertatio catoptrica. 1682.

BAUMGARTER, TOBIAS [*fl.* 1660] *respondent.* Disputatio inauguralis de vulneribus capitis . . . Basileae, Typis Georgii Deckeri [1660]

[16] p. 19 cm. [**956**]

Diss. — Basel.

BAURMEISTER, WILHELM HEINRICH [*fl.* 1696] *respondent. See* ALBINUS, B. Dissertatio inauguralis medica, de pleuritide vera. 1696.

BAUSCH, JOHANN LORENZ [1605-1665] Schediasma posthumum de coeruleo & chrysocolla . . . Jenae, Impensis Viti Jacobi Trescher, typis Johannis Nisii, 1668.

[8], 168 p. 16 cm. [**957**]

— Schediasmata bina curiosa de lapide haematite et aetite, ad mentem Academiae naturae curiosorum congesta. Lipsiae, Impensis Viti Jacobi Trescheri, typis Johannis-Erici Hahnii, 1665.

[4], 164 p.; [8], 79 p. plates. 19 cm. [**958**]

Part [2] has special title page.

— *See* FEHR, J. M. Anchora sacra. 1666?

BAUSNER, BARTHOLOMAEUS [1629-1682] De consenu partium humani corporis, libri. III . . . Amstelodami, Apud Joaunem Ravesteynium, 1556 [colophon 1656]

[23], 185, [1] p. plates. 16 cm. [**959**]

BAUSNER, BARTHOLOMAEUS [*fl.* 1689] *respondent. See* ARNOLD, G., *praeses.* Lotionem manuum . . . exhibet. [1689]

BAUTSCHNER, EZECHIEL. Kurtzer Raht, wie sich der gemeine Mann, und arme Leute, in Sterbensläufften verhalten, auch . . . mit geringen,

und fast überal bekommenden Mitteln, helffen möge . . . Dem gemeinen Mann . . . zu Nutz, auf das neue in den Druck verfertigen lassen . . . vermehret, und verbessert. Nürnberg, In Verlegung Michael Endters, 1653.

[1], 85 p. 16 cm. [**960**]

BAUTZ, JOHANN ADAM [*fl.* 1688] *See* KLEIN, F. Convivium lacteum pro podagricis animo desolatis. 1688.

BAUZNER, BARTHOLOMAEUS. *See* BAUSNER, Bartholomaeus [1629-1682]

BAXTER, RICHARD [1615-1691] *See* LONG, T. A review of Mr. Richard Baxter's life. 1697.

BAYER, GEORG [*fl.* 1625] *respondent. See* SCHALLER, W., *praeses.* Sesquicenturia positionum medicarum de arthritide. 1625.

BAYERISCHE Kranckheit beneben Geschwulst dess Magens an welcher I. Fürstl. Durchl. in Bayern Todtkranck, und hart darnieder liegen, zusampt derselben Chur; das ist, Ein medicinisches Bedencken, dass dem Hertzogen in Beyern Maximiliano die Pfaltz zu restituiren, dieselbe nicht seinem eygenen Herrn vorzuenthalten, viel nützlicher und rathsamer seye . . . durch hocherfahrne parnassische Medicos gestellt . . . Prag, Hans Patz, 1632.

[8] p. 20 cm. [**961**]

BAYFIELD, ROBERT [1629-1670] Enchiridion medicum: containing the causes, signs, and cures of all those diseases, that do chiefly affect the body of man . . . Whereunto is added a treatise, De facultatibus medicamentorum compositorum, & dosibus . . . London, Printed by E. Tyler for Joseph Cranford, 1655.

[32], 431, [2] p. front. (port.) 18 cm. [**962**]

Errata: p. [433]

— Exercitationes anatomicae, in varias regiones humani corporis, partium structuram atque usum ostendentes . . . Ed. 2. Londini, 1668.

2 v. in 1. [**963**]

— Τῆς ἰατρικῆς καρπος; or, A treatise de morborum capitis essentiis & prognosticis. Adorned with above three hundred choice and rare observations . . . London, Printed by D. Maxwel, and are to be sold by Richard Tomlins, 1663.

[23], 190, [1] p. front. (port.) 17 cm. [**964**]

Imprimatur bound before frontispiece.

—Tractatus de tumoribus praeter naturam; or, A treatise of preternatural tumors: divided into four sections, and adorned with many choice and rare observations . . . London, William Nowell, 1662.

242, [9] p.   15 cm.   [965]

Imperfect: p. 227-8 wanting; supplied in photocopy from College of Physicians of Philadelphia library.

Errata: p. [251]

BAYLE, FRANÇOIS [1622-1709] Discours sur l'experience et la raison, dans lequel on montre la nécessité de les joindre dans la physique, dans la medecine, & dans la chirurgie . . . Paris, Thomas Moette, 1675.

[14], 97, [3] p.   15 cm.   [966]

"Réponse de monsieur l'abbé Bourdelot, a monsieur Bayle": p. 81-97.

—Dissertationes medicae tres. I. De causis fluxus menstrui mulierum. II. De sympathia variarum corporis partium cum utero. III. De usus lactis ad tabidos reficiendos, & de immediato corporis alimento. In quibus receptae communiter circa subjectam materiam, veterum ac recentiorum opiniones erroneae refelluntur, & verae morborum ac symptomatum causae assignantur & demonstrantur . . . Tolosae, J. Pech, 1670.

[16], 128 p.   21 cm.   [967]

Date altered by hand from 1670 to 1680.

—[The same.] . . . Hagae-Comitis, Apud Petrum Hagium, 1678.

[18], 98 p.   14 cm.   [968]

—Dissertationes physicae in quibus principia proprietatum in mistis, oeconomia corporum in plantis & animalibus . . . demonstrantur . . . Hagae-Comitis, Apud Petrum Hagium, 1678.

[14], 208, [3] p.   plate.   14 cm.   [969]

—Histoire anatomique d'une grossesse de 25. ans; avec la recherche des causes de ce, qu'on a observé de considerable, tant dans le corps de la mere, que dans celuy de l'enfant, qui a esté trouvé hors de la matrice attaché à l'epiploon . . . Toulouse, B. Guillemette, 1678.

[4], 71 p.   plate.   14 cm.   [970]

—Institutiones physicae ad usum scholarum accomodatae . . . Tolosae, Apud J. Paulum Douladoure, 1700.

2 v. in 1.   plates.   24 cm.   [971]

Last leaf of vol. 2 (blank?) wanting.

[—] Problemata physica et medica. In quibus varii veterum & recentiorum errores deteguntur . . . Dissertationes physicae, in quibus principia proprietatum in mistis. Oeconomia corporum in plantis & animalibus . . . demonstrantur . . . [n. p.] 1677.

[22], 180 p.; [13], 192 p.   plates.   16 cm.

[972]

Part [2], Dissertationes physicae . . . has special title page with imprint: Tolosae, Ex officina Guillelmi Ludov. Colomeri & Hieronimi Poysuel.

—[The same.] . . . Hagae-Comitis, Apud Petrum Hagium, 1678.

[8], 197, [11] p.   plate.   14 cm.   [973]

—Tractatus de apoplexia: in quo hujus affectionis causa penitius inquiritur & curatio exponitur. Ex doctrina Hippocratis . . . Tolosae, B. Guillemette, 1677.

[11], 33, 125, [6] p.   15 cm.   [974]

—[The same.] . . . Ed. 2 emendatior. Hagae-Comitis, Apud Petrum Hagium, 1678.

[48], 137, [5] p.   14 cm.   [975]

—*tr. See* CORDEMOY, L. G. de. A discourse written to a learned frier. 1670.

—*See* [LUFNEU, J.] Ein Send-Schreiben. 1700.

BAYLE, PIERRE [1647-1706] Dictionaire historique et critique . . . Tome premier [-second] . . . Rotterdam, Reinier Leers, 1697.

2 v.   39 cm.   [976]

Each volume has continuous pagination, but each is divided in two parts with special title pages for the second parts.

BAYLEY, FRANCIS [*fl.* 1688] *respondent.* Disputatio medica inauguralis de phthisi . . . Lugduni Batavorum, Apud Abrahamum Elzevier, 1688.

[24] p.   21 cm.   [977]

Diss.—Leyden.

BAYLEY, WALTER [1529-1593] Two treatises concerning the preservation of eie-sight. The first written by Doctor Baily . . . the other collected out of those two famous phisicions Fernelius and Riolanus. Oxford [i.e. London] Printed by Joseph Barnes, for John Barnes, 1616.

[6], 62 p.   14 cm.   [978]

Imperfect: title page trimmed, with loss of publisher's name and date.

Imprint supplied from film of the copy in the British Museum.

"The whole book, with the possible exception of the title page, was printed in London." Cf. Madan (v. 1, p. 105, and Imprints, no. 34, p. 297).

The second work, "A treatise of the principall diseases of the eyes" (p. 25-62) is apparently extracted in part from the Ars bene medendi of Jean Riolan, the elder. The compiler is unknown, although Wood (v. 1, p. 586) states that "both [treatises] now go under the name of Bailey."

STC 1196.

Bound with Bright, T. A treatise wherein is declared the sufficiencie of English medicines. 1615.

—[The same.] *In* Vaughan, W. Directions for health. 1626, 1633.

BAYLIE, WALTER. *See* BAYLEY, Walter [1529-1593]

BAYNON, ELIAS. *See* BEYNON, Elias [*fl.* 1665]

BAYRUS, PETRUS. *See* BAIRO, Pietro [1468-1558]

BEANTWORTUNG eines Anonymi Anmerkungen . . . über das Alter des vierhundert-jährigen Friderici Gualdi. *See* COMMUNICATION einer vortrefflichen chymischen Medicin. 1700.

BEARN [FRANCE] Relations envoyées a Monsieur Pelisson . . . qui distribuë les remedes de la part du Roy par Monsieur le primier President du Parlement de Pau . . . Contenant diverses cures extraordinaires . . . Du 14. Novembre, 1679 & 26. Aoust 1680. [n. p.] 1680.

    3 p. 24 cm.   **[979]**
    Caption title.

BEAULIEU, FRÈRE JACQUES DE [1651-1714] *See* MÉRY, J. Observations. 1700..

BEAUMONT, SIMON VAN [1641-1726] *See* [KIGGELAER, F.] Horti Beaumontiani exoticarum plantarum catalogus. 1690.

BEAUVAL, JACQUES BOUCHER. *See* BOUCHER DE BEAUVAL, Jean [*fl.* 1673]

BECCER, CHRISTOPH [*fl.* 1659-1661] *respondent. See* AMMANN, P., *praeses*. Theses physicae de motu. 1659; LANGE, C., *praeses*. Exercitationem medicam de cancro in genere . . . publice proponit Christophorus Beccerus. 1661.

BECCIUS, GEORGIUS THEODORUS [*fl.* 1700] *respondent. See* STÜBNER, A. G., *praeses*. Ex historia et scientia naturali de animalibus noctu videntibus. 1700.

BECHER, JOHANN JOACHIM [1635-1682] Actorum laboratorii chymici Monacensis; seu, Physicae subterraneae libri duo, quorum prior profundam subterraneorum genesin, nec non admirandam globi terr-aeque-aërei super & subterranei fabricam,

posterior specialem subterraneorum naturam, resolutionem in partes partiumque proprietates exponit, accesserunt sub finem mille hypotheses seu mixtiones chymicae . . . Francofurti, Imp. Joh. Davidis Zunneri, 1669.

    [38], 633, [7] p. 17 cm.   **[980]**
    Added engraved title page reads: Mille hypotheses chymicae de subterraneis. 1668.
    Running title: Physicae subterraneae lib. I.

—Experimentum chymicum novum, quo artificialis & instantanea metallorum generatio & transmutatio ad oculum demonstratur. Loco supplementi in physicam suam subterraneam et responsi ad D. Rolfincii Schedas de non entitate mercurii corporum . . . Francofurti, Sumptibus Joh. Davidis Zunneri, typis Henrici Friesii, 1671.

    172 p. 17 cm.   **[981]**
    First supplement to *his* Actorum laboratorii chymici Monacensis; seu, Physicae subterraneae libri duo, first published in 1669.

—Institutiones chimicae prodromae, id est . . . Oedipus chimicus obscuriorum terminorum & principiorum chimicorum, mysteria aperiens & resolvens . . . Amstelodami, Apud Elizeum Weyerstraten, 1664.

    [14], 202, [7] p. plate. 14 cm.   **[982]**
    Added engraved title page reads: Oedipus chimicus.

—[German tr.] Oedipus chymicus; oder, Chymischer Rätseldeuter, worinnen derer verdunckelten chymischen Wortsätze Urhebungen und Geheimnissen offenbahret und aufgelöset werden . . . ins Teutsch übersetzet . . . [n. p.] 1680.

    [156], [4] p. 18 cm.   **[983]**

—Medicinische Schatz-Kammer, darinnen zu finden, wie man die Kinder-Kranckheiten . . . curiren kan. Aus . . . hinterlassenen raren Manuscripts . . . zusammen getragen von H. I. I. Leipzig, In Verlegung Christoff Hülsens, 1700.

    [7], 464, [8] p.; 128 p. 17 cm.   **[984]**
    Added engraved title page.
    Imperfect: sig. a1 of last group of paging wanting.
    Signature a2 has caption title: Ein köstlich Kinder-Pulver.
    Bound with Mynsicht, A. von. Medicinisch-chymische Schatz- und Rüst-Kammer. 1695.

—Parnassus medicinalis illustratus. Oder: Ein neues, und dergestalt, vormahln noch nie gesehenes Thier- Kräuter- und Berg-Buch, sampt der Salernischen Schul, cum commentario Arnoldi Villanovani, und den Praesagiis vitae & mortis, Hippocratis Coi; auch gründlichem Bericht von Destilliren, Purgiren, Schwitzen, Schrepffen und Aderlassen. Alles in hoch-teutscher Sprach, so wol in Ligatâ als Prosâ ... in vier Theilen beschrieben ... Ulm, In Verlegung Johann Görlins, 1663.

    4 parts in 1. v. illus. 34 cm.   [985]

Added engraved title page.

Each part has special title page, dated 1662.

"Pars quarta, Schola Salernitana ... " contains also "Diocles Carystius ...schreibet dem Antigono ..." a translation of the Epistola de secunda valetudine tuenda (p. 128-130); "Etliche Reguln von Erhaltung der Gesundheit ... durch Joannem Katzchium ... auffs new übersehen und verbessert," a translation of his De gubernanda sanitate, which includes extracts from Hippocrates and Galen (p. 133-145); and "Hippocratis Zeichen dess Lebens und Tods [i.e. the Prognostica] ... von J. J. Becher ... ins Teutsch zum erstenmal übersetzet" (p. 154-162).

— Tripus hermeticus fatidicus, pandens oracula chymica, seu I. Laboratorium portatile cum methodo vere spagyrice ... Accessit ... II. Magnorum duorum productorum nitri & salis textura & anatomia ... adjunctum est III. Alphabetum minerale ... His accessit Concordantia mercurii lunae ... Francofurti ad Moenum, Sumptibus Johannis Georgii Schiele, 1689.

    186, [11] p. illus., plates. 18 cm.   [986]

Added engraved title page.

—, ed. See SENNERT, D. Aphorismi ex institutionibus medicis Sennerti. 1663.

BECHMANN, ANDREAS [*fl.* 1687] *respondent. See* WEDEL, G. W., *praeses.* Disputatio inauguralis medica de peripneumonia. 1687.

BECHMANN, JOHANN VOLKMAR [1624-1689] *praeses.* De coitu damnato ... Jenae, Literis Nisianis [1684].

    [4], 40, [4] p. 19 cm.   [987]

Diss. — Jena (J. W. Steltzner, *respondent*)

BECHMANN, WILHELM [*fl.* 1685-1687] *respondent. See* STURM, J. C., *praeses.* Diducendi alias uberius argumenti de plantarum animaliumque generatione ...exhibent ... G. B. 1687.

BECHT, JOHANN GEORG [*fl.* 1677-1680] *respondent.* Disputatio inauguralis medica de syncope ... Giessae, Ex Chalcographeo Academ. Kargeriano, 1680.

    [2], 34 p. 20 cm.   [988]

Original imprint date altered by hand. May read 1680.

Diss. — Giessen.

BECIUS, JOHAN [*d.* 1694] *respondent.* Disputatio medica inauguralis de praegnantium pica ... Lugduni Batavorum, Apud Johannem Meyer, 1653.

    [8] p. 23 cm.   [989]

Diss. — Leyden.

BECK, ADAM HEINRICH [*fl.* 1683] *respondent.* Disputatio medica inauguralis de dysenteria rohte Ruhr ... Marburgi Cattorum, Typis Johannis Henrici Stockenii [1683]

    27 p. 19 cm.   [990]

Diss. — Marburg.

BECK, JOHANN ANTON [*fl.* 1674-1679] *respondent.* Disputatio inauguralis medica, aegrum asthmate scorbutico laborantem exhibens ... Giessae, Imprimebat Joh. Eberh. Petri [1679]

    16 p. 18 cm.   [991]

Diss. — Giessen.

— *See* TEICHMEYER, H. T., *praeses.* Dissertatio inauguralis medica de hydrope ascite. 1674.

BECK, JOHANN RUDOLF [*fl.* 1680] *respondent.* Disputatio inauguralis medica de gonorhoea virulenta ... Basileae, Typis Jacobi Werenfelsii [1680]

    [12] p. 19 cm.   [992]

Diss. — Basel.

BECKE, DAVID VON DER [1648-1684] Barnerus leviter & amice castigatus ... Hamburgi, Ex officina Gothofredi Schultzen, 1675.

    64 p. 15 cm.   [993]

— Dissertatio anatomico-practica de procidentia uteri ab erroribus clar. Joannis Garmeri ... vindicata ... Hamburgi, Ex officina Petri Grooten, 1683.

    [2], 106 p. plates. 17 cm.   [994]

Includes contributions by Johann Garmers, Job van Meekren, and Hendrick van Roonhuyse.

— Epistola ad ... Joelem Langelottum ... qua salis tartari, aliorumque salium fixorum, ab omnibus philo-chymicis ac curiosis medicis, hactenus adeo desiderata volatilisatio, ex principiis ac causis ... demonstratur. Hamburgi, Ex officina Gothofredi Schultzen; & Amsterodami, Apud Joannem Janssonium à Waesberge, 1672.

    32 p. 16 cm.   [995]

— Experimenta et meditationes, circa naturalium rerum principia. Quibus quae circa fixi & alcalisati salis, ante calcinationem in misto praeexistentiam, ac causas volatilisationis, obscura aut dubia esse poterant, clare solvuntur ... Hamburgi, Ex officina Gothofredi Schultzen, 1674.

[16], 335, [1] p.   16 cm.   **[996]**
Added engraved title page.

—[The same.] ... Ed. 2. priori auctior. Hamburgi, Apud Gotofredum Schultzen, 1684.

[14], 423, [41] p.   illus.   17 cm.   **[997]**
Added engraved title page.

—[The same.] ... Ed. 3. prioribus auctior. Amburgi, & Ferrariae, Typis Bernardini Pomatelli, 1688.

[12], 516 p.   illus.   15 cm.   **[998]**
"Additamenta et notae ...": p. [377]-496.

BECKER, ADRIAN [*fl.* 1661] *respondent.* Disputatio medica inauguralis de pleuritide ... Lugduni Batavorum, Typographia Severini Matthiae, 1661.

20 p.   19 cm.   **[999]**
Imperfect: title vignette excised.
Diss. — Leyden.

BECKER, DANIEL. *See* BECKHER, Daniel.

BECKER, DANIEL CHRISTOPH. *See* BECKHER, Daniel Christoph [1658-1691].

BECKER, GOTTLIEB [*fl.* 1673-1675] *respondent. See* SCHNEIDER, K. V., *praeses.* Lapidem bezoar ... submittit ... G. B. 1673.

BECKER, JAKOB [*fl.* 1642-1644] *respondent. See* SEBISCH, M. [1578-1674?] *praeses.* Disputatio de variolis et morbillis prima [-sexta & ultima] 1642 [and] Disputationes de dentibus quatuor. 1645 [and] Disputationes de respiratione tres. 1643.

BECKER, JOHANN [*fl.* 1660] Dissertationem meteorologicam de grandine ... submittunt M. Johannes Becker ... & respondens Gottfridus Reiche ... [Lipsiae] E Chalcographeo Coleriano [1660]

[16] p.   20 cm.   **[1000]**
Diss. — Leipzig (G. Reiche, *respondent*)

BECKER, JOHANN GOTTFRIED [1639-1711] *See* BARTHOLIN, T. Dissertatio prima [-secunda] de theriaca. 1671.

BECKER, SIMON ANDREAS [*fl.* 1676-1678] *respondent. See* CRAUSE, R. W., *praeses.* Disputatio inauguralis medica de angina. 1678; FASCH, A. H., *praeses.* Dissertationem de myrrha ... submittet S.A.B. 1676; WEDEL, G. W., *praeses.* Aegrum singultu

ex febri maligna laborantem ... publice examinandum proponit S. A. B. 1676.

BECKERS, JAKOB [*fl.* 1669] *respondent.* Disputatio medica inauguralis de alimentorum fastidio ... Lugduni Batavorum, Apud viduam & haeredes Joannis Elsevirii, 1669.

[12] p.   23 cm.   **[1001]**
Diss. — Leyden.

BECKERS, NICOLAUS WILHELM [*d.* 1705] Florilegium Hippocraticum et Galenicum praecipua tam theorica, quam practica Hippocratis, ac Galeni dogmata continens; lucubrationibus immensis ex eorum voluminibus sententiose concinnatum ... Viennae Austriae, Typis Leopoldi Voigt, 1677.

[18], 879, [48] p.   17 cm.   **[1002]**
Added engraved title page dated 1674.
Contains selections from the work of Hippocrates and Galen.

—[The same.] ... Viennae Austriae, Typis Leopoldi Voigt, 1688.

[18], 879, [48] p.   16 cm.   **[1003]**
Added engraved title page dated 1674.
A reissue of the 1677 edition. The 8 preliminary leaves are of a different setting of type.

BECKHER, DANIEL [1594-1655] De cultrivoro Prussiaco observatio & curatio singularis decade positionum, variis rariorum observationum historiis refertarum, illustrata ... Regiomonti, Typis Laurentii Segebadii, 1636.

[12], 79, [1] p.   18 cm.   **[1004]**

—[The same.] Cultrivori Prussiaci curatio singularis ... Tertiae huic editioni accesserunt testimonia serenis. Poloniae regis, & Reip. Regiomontanae: similesque aliquot ad mirandae curationes ... Lugduni Batavorum, Ex officina Joannis Maire, 1640.

[12], 129, [7] p.   plate.   15 cm.   **[1005]**

—[Dutch tr.] Een besondere genesinge van den Prussiaenschen mes-inslicker ... By desen derden druck sijn de getuygenissen, van den ... Coninck van Polen ... gevoeght ... Uyt het Latyn vertaelt door Thomas Staffard ... Leyden, Cornelis Banheyningh, 1649.

[47], 189 p.   plate.   13 cm.   **[1006]**

—[German tr.] Historische Beschreibung des Preussischen Messerschluckers, wie er nicht allein durch einen Schnitt des Messers befreyet ... sondern

... sich auch biss anhero frisch und gesund befindet ... Königsberg, In Verlegung Peter Hendels und gedruckt durch Johann Reusnern, 1643.

[142] p. plate. 19 cm.   [1007]

Added engraved title page has title: Historische Relation dess Preüsischen Messerschlückers.

—De unguento armario.

514-526 p. 21 cm. (*In* Theatrum sympatheticum auctum. Norimbergae, 1662) [1008]

Caption title.

—Historia morbi Academici Regiomontani; seu, Febris malignae epidemiae civibus academicis inprimis communis electoralis mensae convictoribus funestae cum indolis & causarum ejusdem explicatione ... consensu ... facultatis medicae in Academia Regiomontana consignata ... Regiomonti, Typis & sumptibus Joh. Reusneri, 1649.

[80] p. 19 cm.   [1009]

—Spagyria microcosmi, tradens medicinam, e corpore hominis tum vivo; tum extincto docte eruendam, scite praeparandam, & dextre propinandam ... Rostochii, Litteris & impensis Augustini Ferberi, 1622.

[23], 188 (i.e. 190), [1] p. 14 cm.   [1010]

Errata: p. [1] at end.

—[The same.] Medicus microcosmus; seu, Spagyria microcosmi triplo auctior & correctior, exhibens medicinam corpore hominis tum vivo, tum extincto docte eruendam, scite praeparandam & dextre propinandam ... Lugduni Batavorum, Ex officina Jacobi Marci, 1633.

[16], 170, [6] p. 20 cm.   [1011]

—[The same.] ... Ed. nova triplo auctior & correctior. Londini, Prostant apud Jo. Martin, Ja. Allestry & Tho. Dicas, 1660.

[32], 304, [23] p. 14 cm.   [1012]

—*praeses.* Disputatio physica de lachrymis ... Regiomonti, Typis Laurenti Segebadii, 1634.

[16 +] p. 16 cm.   [1013]

Imperfect; all after p. [16] wanting.

Diss. — Königsberg (J. Michaelis, *respondent*)

—*See* Loth, G. Kurtze Relation. 1635.

BECKHER, Daniel [1627-1670] *praeses.* Disputatio medica de epilepsia ... Regiomonti Borussorum, Typis excud. Pasch. Mensenius & Josua Segebad, 1661.

[12] p. 19 cm.   [1014]

Diss. — Königsberg (F. Lepner, *respondent*)

—Disputatio medica de intestinorum vermibus ... Regiomonti, Typis Friderici Reusneri [*ca.* 1666]

[20] p. 18 cm.   [1015]

Diss. — Königsberg (C. Nitzschke, *respondent*)

—Disputatio medica de medicamentis purgantibus, eorumque facultatibus in genere ... Regiomonti, Typis excus. per Pasch. Mesenium & Josuam Segebadium [1662]

[16] p. 18 cm.   [1016]

Diss. — Königsberg (J. Wollitz, *respondent*)

—Dissertatio medica de opio ... Regiomonti, Typis Johannis Reusneri [1652]

[28] p. 18 cm.   [1017]

Diss. — Königsberg (G. Seger, *respondent*)

—*respondent.* Disputatio inauguralis medica de pestilentia ... Argentorati, Typis Eberhardi Welperi, 1652.

[28] p. 18 cm.   [1018]

Diss. — Strassbourg.

BECKHER, Daniel Christoph [1658-1691] *praeses.* Disputatio medica de salubri potu calidae ... Regiomonti, Typ. Friderici. Reusneri [1686]

[32] p. 20 cm.   [1019]

Dis. — Königsberg (C. a Lohen, *respondent*)

—*respondent.* Disputatio medica inauguralis, de respiratione ... Trajecti ad Rhenum, Ex officina Johannis Ribbii, 1684.

[18] p. 22 cm.   [1020]

Diss. — Utrecht.

BECKKER, Adrian *See* Becker, Adrian [*fl.* 1661]

BECMANN, Johann Christoph [1641-1717] *praeses.* Dissertatio de prodigiis sanguinis ... Francofurti ad Viadrum, Excudit Christophorus Zeitlerus [1676]

[1], 48, [2] p. 18 cm.   [1021]

Diss. — Frankfurt an der Oder (J. E. Starck, *respondent*)

BECTE, David von der. *See* Becke, David von der [1648-1684]

BECUDE, Frans [*fl.* 1670] *respondent.* Disputatio medica inauguralis de menstruorum suppressione

. . . Lugduni Batavorum, Apud viduam & haeredes Joannis Elsevirii, 1670.

[12] p. 23 cm. [1022]

Diss. — Leyden.

[**BEDDEVOLE**, DOMINIQUE, 1657–*ca.* 1693] Essais d'anatomie, où l'on explique clairement la construction des organes & leurs opérations méchaniques selon les nouvelles hypotheses. Par *** docteur en médecine [i.e. Dominique Beddevole]. Leide, Pierre vander Aa, 1686.

[II], 189 p. 14 cm. [1023]

Added engraved title page.

—[The same.] . . . 3. ed. rev. & corr. Leide, Jordan Luchtmans, 1699.

195 (i.e. 193) p. illus. 13 cm. [1024]

Imperfect: p. 185–6 mutilated.

—[English tr.] Essayes of anatomy in which the construction of the organs and their mechanical operations, are clearly explained according to the new hypotheses. By **** Dr. in medicine . . . Edinburgh, George Mosman, 1691.

[13], 184 p. 15 cm. [1025]

Translated by J. Scougall.

—[The same.] . . . The 2d ed. London, Walter Kettilby, 1696.

[14], 142, [2] p. 16 cm. [1026]

—[Italian tr.] Saggi d'anatomia, ne quali chiaramente si spiega la struttura degli organi del corpo animato, el le loro operationi mecaniche secondo l'hipotesi nuove di *** dottore in medicina, tradotti dalla francese, nella lingua italiana dagli autori del Giornale de letterati di Parma . . . Parma, Giuseppe dall' Oglio, & Ippolito Rosati, 1687.

[24], 266 p. 15 cm. [1027]

The translation is presumably largely due to Benedetto Bacchini, editor of the Giornale de'letterati di Parma. Cf. Melzi v. 3, p. 6.

—[The same.] . . . Milano, A spese di Aluise Pavin, 1690.

[16], 271 p. 15 cm. [1028]

—*respondent.* Disputatio inauguralis medica de epilepsia . . . Basileae, Typis Jacobi Bertshii [1681]

[16] p. 19 cm. [1029]

Diss. — Basel.

BEDENCKEN und Unterricht, wie man sich . . . vor der Pest, zeitlich vorsehen und bawahren, oder

. . . curiren soll . . . Gestellet durch die ordinarios Medicos der Städte Nürnberg, Regensburg und Ulm, samt einem Unterricht, wie sich die Geistlichen, item Balbierer, Bader . . . verhalten sollen. Franckurt am Mayn, Adolph Hartman, 1680.

144 p. 14 cm. [1030]

BEDFORD, THOMAS [*d.* 1635] A true and certaine relation of a strange-birth, which was borne at Stonehouse in the parish of Plimmouth, the 20. of October 1635. Together with the notes of a sermon, preached . . . in the church of Plimmouth, at the interring of the sayd birth. By Th[omas] B[edford] B. D. Pr. Pl. London, Printed by Anne Griffin, for Anne Bowler. 1635.

[2], 22 p. illus. 18 cm. [1031]

STC 1791.

BEE, John [*fl.* 1669] *respondent.* Disputatio medica inauguralis de epilepsia . . . Lugduni Batavorum, Apud viduam & haeredes Joannis Elsevirii, 1669.

[15] p. 23 cm. [1032]

Diss. — Leyden.

BEER, GEORG ALEXANDER [*fl.* 1672] *respondent. See* KIRCHMAJER, T., *praeses.* Schediasma physicum de viribus mirandis toniconsoni. 1672.

BEER, JOHANN ABRAHAM [*fl.* 1696] *See* RIVINUS, A. Q. L. S. D. Facultatis Medicae . . . procancellarius, Augustus Quirinus Rivinus. 1696.

—*respondent. See* ORTLOB, J. F., *praeses.* Disputatio inauguralis de pleuritide. 1696 [and] Exercitatio medico–chirurgica. 1696.

BEER, LEONHARD. *See* URSIN, Leonhard [1618–1664]

BEERBALCK, CHRISTIAN FRIEDRICH [*fl.* 1687–1688] *respondent. See* LIMMER, C. P., *praeses.* Collegii Physici disputatorii disputatio decima tertia. 1687 [and] Disputatio medico–physica de partu legitimo. 1688; WEDEL, G. W., *praeses.* Disputatio medica de venae sectione rite adhibenda. 1675.

BEEST, ARNOLD FRANS VAN [*fl.* 1689] *respondent.* Disputatio medica inauguralis, de phthisi . . . Trajecti ad Rhenum, Ex officina Francisci Halma, 1689.

10, [2] p. 22 cm. [1033]

Diss. — Utrecht.

BEEVERWYCK, JOHAN VAN. *See* BEVERWIJCK, Jan van [1594–1647]

BÉGUIN, JEAN [*fl.* 1608–*ca.* 1612] Novum lumen ad Tyrocinium chymicum ex auctographo Joannis Beguini denuo recognitum . . . Coloniae Agrippinae, Apud Antonium Boëtzerum, 1625.

 385, [II] p. plate. 14 cm.   [**1034**]

Imperfect: wormholes throughout.

Michael Sendivogius's Novum lumen chymicum (p. 8–66) is followed by three books of Tyrocinium chymicum by Jean Béguin.

—Tyrocinium chymicum . . . Antehac a . . . d. Christophoro Gluctradt [pseud. i.e. Johann Hartmann], & d. Jeremia Barthio . . . notis elegantibus illustratum, formulisque medicamentorum optimis & secretis locupletatum. Nunc vero a Jo. Georgio Pelshofero . . . notis & medicamentorum formulis in unum systema redactis . . . Venetiis, Apud Baleonium, 1643.

 [56], 480, [43] p. illus., table. 16 cm.
                                        [**1035**]

—[The same.] . . . Wittebergae, Impensis Andreae Hartmanni, typis Johannis Röhneri, 1650

 [80], 480, [43] p. illus., table. 17 cm.
                                        [**1036**]

Different setting of type.

—[The same.] . . . Genevae, Excudebat Blasius Le Melais, 1659.

 [80], 480, [43] p. illus., table. 17 cm.
                                        [**1037**]

Added engraved title page has date: 1660.
Different setting of type.

—[The same.] Tyrocinium chymicum, commentariis illustratum a Gerardo Blasio . . . Amstelodami, Apud Aegidium Valkenier, & Casparum Commelinum, 1659.

 [12], 405 (i.e. 403), [24] p. table. 14 cm.
                                        [**1038**]

Added engraved title page.
Errata: p. [23–24]

—[The same.] . . . Ed. 2. Priori locupletior & emendatior. Amstelodami, Apud Casparum Commelinum, 1669.

 [36], 314 (i.e. 332), [8] p. table. 14 cm.
                                        [**1039**]

Added engraved title page.

—[The same.] Tyrocinium chymicium . . . antehac a . . . D. Christophoro Gluctradt [psued. i.e. Johann Hartmann], et D. Jeremia Barthio . . . notis . . . illustratum, formulisque medicamentorum optimis, & secretis locupletatum. Nunc vero a Jo.

Georgio Pelshofero . . . utriusque notis & medicamentorum formulis in unum systema redactis . . . Venetiis, Apud Baleonium, 1669.

 [40], 360, [24] p. illus., table. 17 cm.
                                        [**1040**]

—[French tr.] Les elemens de chymie . . . Paris, Mathieu le Maistre, 1615.

 [16], 290, [2] p. table. 17 cm.   [**1041**]

—[The same.] . . . Reveus, notez, expliquez, & augmentez par I. L. D. R. B. IC. E. M. . . . Paris, Mathieu le Maistre, 1620.

 [15], 398, [50] p. illus. 18 cm.   [**1042**]

The initials stand for Jean Lucas du Roi, Baccal. Juris C. et Med. Cf. Ferguson (A), vol. 1, p. 94.

—[The same.] . . . Rouen, Jean Boullay, 1627.

 [15], 432, [48] p. illus. 17 cm.   [**1043**]

—[The same.] . . . En ceste derniere edition ont esté adjoustées plusieurs explications obmises aux precedentes impressions, & plusieurs preparations de remedes tirés de la derniere edition latine. Lyon, Pierre Rigaud & Estienne Michalet, 1658.

 [15], 384, [47] p. illus., plate. 17 cm.
                                        [**1044**]

—[The same.] . . . Lyon, André Olyer, 1665.

 [15], 384, [47] p. illus., plate. 17 cm.
                                        [**1045**]

Different setting of type.

BÉGUIN, JEAN [*fl.* 1608–*ca.* 1612] Tyrocinium chymicum. *In* Müller, Philipp. Miracula & mysteria chymico-medica. 1614, 1616, 1623, 1656.

—*See* BILLICH, A. G. Thessalus in chymicis redivivus. 1640; HARTMANN, J. Opera omnia medico-chymica. 1684, 1694.

BEHEMB, MARTIN. *See* BEHM, Martin [1557–1622]

BEHM, FRIEDRICH [*fl.* 1691] *ed.* and *tr. See* GREEF, V. Tuba D. Vincentii. 1692.

BEHM, MARTIN [1557–1622] Die drey grossen Landtplagen, Krieg, Tewrung, Pestilentz, welche jetzundt vor der Welt Ende, in vollem Schwang gehen. Den frommen Kindern Gottes, welchen bey dieser kümmerlichen Zeit hertzlich bange ist, zu Lehr und Trost: den sichern Weltkindern aber zur Warnung und Schrecken. In XXIII. Predigten erkleret . . . Wittenberg, Gedruckt durch Lorentz Seuberlich, in

Verlegung Samuel Seelfisch, 1601.

[12], 203, [1] ll. 19 cm. [1046]

BEHRENS, ANDREAS [*fl.* 1656] *respondent. See* CONRING, H., *praeses.* Disputatio medica de calculo renum et vesicae. 1672; MEIBOM, H., *praeses.* Disputatio medica inauguralis de leniorum medicamentorum eximio usu. 1692 [and] Dissertatio medica de aquae calidae potu. 1689.

BEHRENS, GEORG HENNING [1662-1712] *praeses.* Dissertatio inauguralis medica de lue Pannonica, vulgo dicta die Haupt-oder ungarische Kranckheit ... Erfurt, Typis Johann-Henrici Groschii [1687]

[48] p. 19 cm. [1047]

Diss. — Erfurt (J. E. Jacobi, *respondent*)

BEHRENS, JULIUS GEORG [*fl.* 1657-1659] *respondent. See* CONRING, H., *praeses.* Disputatio medica inauguralis de scorbuto. 1659.

BEHRENS, KONRAD BARTHOLD [1660-1736] *respondent. See* MEIBOM, H., *praeses.* Disputatio inauguralis de suffocatione hysterica. 1684.

BEHRNAUER, GOTTLOB [*fl.* 1692] *praeses.* Dissertationem inauguralem, de morbis archaelibus ... exhibet praeses Gottlob Behrnauer ... respondente Johanne Petro Diselio ... Erfurti, Charactere Kindlebiano [1692]

32 p. 20 cm. [1048]

Diss. — Erfurt (J. P. Diselius, *respondent*)

BEIER, ARNOLD FRIEDRICH [*b.* 1673] *See* CRAUSE, R. W. Prompempticum inaugurale de efficaci influxu astrorum in corpus humanum. 1697.

—*respondent. See* SLEVOGT, J. A., *praeses.* Aegram ex lochiorum retentione graviter decumbentem ... exhibebit A. F. B. 1697.

BEIER, GOTTFRIED [*fl.* 1669-1674] *praeses.* Dissertatio academica, unicum problema, circa arteriotomiam occurens, continens ... Jenae, Literis Johannis Wertheri [1673]

20 p. 20 cm. [1049]

Diss. — Jena (A. Werner, *respondent*)

—Erotematum medicorum de peste, decades quatuor ... Jenae, Ex molybdographia Wertheri [1674]

[24] p. 19 cm. [1050]

Diss. — Jena (D. Valder, *respondent*)

—*respondent. See* FRIDERICI, J. A., *praeses.* Aloen publicae florae cultorum censurae exponit. 1670.

BEIER, JOHANN HARTMANN. *See* BEYER, Johann Hartmann [1563-1625]

BEILFUSS, JAKOB [*fl.* 1668] Wolgemeinetes Bedencken, was von der Astrologia oder von der, aus dem Positu des Gestirns geschöpffeten Weissagung zuhalten? ... Alten Stetin, Gedruckt bey Michael Höpfnern, 1688.

60 p. 21 cm. [1051]

BEINTEMA VAN PEIMA *pseud. See* WORB, Johan Ignaz [*b.* 1666]

BEKESTEYN, JOANNES [*fl.* 1692] *respondent.* Disputatio medica inauguralis, de dyspepsia ... Trajecti ad Rhenum, Ex officina Francisci Halma, 1692.

II, [1] p. 22 cm. [1052]

Diss. — Utrecht.

BEKKER, BALTHASAR [1634-1698] Aanmerkinge op de handelingen der twee laatste Noordhollandsche synoden, in de sake van B. Bekker, ten opsighte van sijn boek genaamd De betoverde weereld ... Enkhuisen [1692?]

16 p. 21 cm. [1053]

Caption title.
Contains author's signature at end.
Linde 52.

—Brief ... aan den ... prinsse Hendrik Kasimyr ... Over de opdraght voor het boek van den Heer J. vander Waeyen, tegens hem uitgegeven. Amsterdam, Daniel vanden Dalen, 1693.

24 p. 19 cm. [1054]

Imperfect: all after p. 8 wanting.
Linde 158.

—Brief ... aan ... Joannes Aalstius ... ende D. Paulus Steenwinkel ... over derselver zedige aanmerkingen op een deel des tweeden boex van sijn werk genaamd De betoverde weereld. Amsterdam, Daniel vanden Dalen, 1693.

II p. 21 cm. [1055]

Linde 72.

[—De betoverde weereld. English.] The world bewitch'd; or, An examination of the common opinions concerning spirits ... Divided into IV parts ... Vol. I. Translated from the French copy ... [London] R. Baldwin, 1695.

[81], 264 p. 17 cm. [1056]

Imperfect: sig. A1 (blank?) wanting; half title, and lower quarter of title page also wanting but supplied in photocopy.
No more published.
Linde 28.

— [French tr.] Le monde enchanté; ou, Examen des communs sentimens touchant les esprits, leur nature, leur pouvoir, leur administration, & leurs opérations. Et touchant les éfets [sic] que les hommes sont capables de produire par leur communication & leur vertu. Divisé en quatre parties . . . Traduit du hollandois. Amsterdam, Pierre Rotterdam, 1694.

    4 v. front. (port.), plates. 15 cm. **[1057]**
    Linde 24.

— [German tr.] Die bezauberte Welt; oder, Eine gründliche Untersuchung des allgemeinen Aberglaubens, betreffend, die Art und das Vermögen . . . des Satans und der bösen Geister über den Menschen . . . in 4 Büchern . . . Aus dem Holländischen nach der letzten vom Authore vermehrten Edition . . . in die teutsche Sprache übersetzet. Amsterdam, Daniel von Dahlen, 1693.

    1 v. plate. 21 cm. **[1058]**
    Various pagings.
    Linde 25.

— Engelsch verhaal van ontdekte tovery . . . Amsterdam, Daniel van den Dalen, 1689.

    24 p. 21 cm. **[1059]**
    Linde 13.

— Balthazar Bekkers En insonderheyd syner voedsterlingen onkunde, onbescheidentheyd en dwaalingen . . . ontdekt door een discipel van de Heer J. vander Waeyen . . . Franeker, Hans Gyzelaar, 1696.

    [4], 107 p. 19 cm. **[1060]**
    Linde 165.

— Kort bericht van Balthasar Bekker . . . aangaande alle de schriften, welke over sijn boek De betoverde weereld enen tijd lang heen en weder verwisseld zijn. 2. druk . . . vermeerderd. Amsterdam, Daniel vanden Dalen [1692?]

    80 p. 21 cm. **[1061]**
    Linde 76a.

— Kort en waarachtig verhaal van 't gebeurde tsederd den 31 Mey 1691. tot den 21. Aug. 1692. in den kerkenraad en classis van Amsterdam, en de synode van Noord-Holland. In de sake van Balthasar Bekker . . . over sijn boek genaamd De betoverde weereld. Amsterdam, Daniel vanden Dalen, 1692.

    32 p. 21 cm. **[1062]**
    Linde 47a.
    Signatures: A–D⁴.

— Naakt verhaal van alle de kerkelike handelingen, voorgevallen in den kerkenraad en de classis van Amsterdam, alsmede in de synoden van Noordholland, tsdert den 31. May 1691. tot den 21. Aug. 1692 . . . Amsterdam, Daniel vanden Dalen, 1692.

    [12], 80, 40, 78 p. 21 cm. **[1063]**
    Linde 50.

— Nodige bedenkingen op de niewe beweegingen, onlangs verwekt door den circulairen brief en andere middelen, tegen den auteur van 't boek De betoverde weereld . . . Amsterdam, Daniel vanden Dalen [1692?]

    [2], 62, [1] p. 21 cm. **[1064]**
    Errata: p. [63]
    Linde 42.

— Ondersoek en antwoord . . . op 't request door de gedeputeerden der Noordhollandsche synode tot Edam, in den herfst des jaars 1691. ingegeven aan de ed. gr. mog. heeren staten van Holland en West Friesland tegen sijn boek De betoverde weereld . . . Amsterdam, Daniel vanden Dalen, 1693.

    [4], 98 p. 21 cm. **[1065]**
    Linde 53.

— Viervoudige beantwoordinge van beswaarnissen, voorgesteld aan Balthasar Bekker . . . over sijn boek, genaamd De betoverde weereld . . . Amsterdam, Daniel van den Dalen, 1692.

    [14], 74, 108, [2], 16 p. 21 cm. **[1066]**
    Contains author's signature after Voorrede.
    Imperfect: 16 p. wanting.
    Errata: p. [109–110]
    Linde 49.

— *See* AARDIGE DUYVELARY [1691?]; [ANDALA, R.] Uiterste verleegentheid van Doctor Balt. Bekker. 1696; [COSTER, F.] De gebannen duyvel weder geroepen. 1691?; HOOGHT, E. van der. Omstandig bericht. 1693; P[ost] S[criptum] of, na-courier, van de Tweede missive aen Dr. Balthasar Bekker. 1692; [SCHUTS, J.] De betoverde Bekker. 1691? [and] Missive, aen D. Balthazar Bekker. 1692 [and] Tweede missive aen d'Heer Balthasar Bekker, 1692; VERVOLG van de Aardige duyvelary. 1691.

BEKKER, CHRISTOPH [*fl.* 1684] *respondent. See* WEDEL, G. W., *praeses.* Exercitatio medica, sistens aegrum vulnere capitis laborantem. 1684.

BELDEREN, JOANNES ARNOLDUS. *See* CORVINUS, Johannes Arnoldi [*ca.* 1582-1650]

BELEBAT, JACQUES ROLAND, *sieur de*. *See* ROLAND, Jacques, *sieur de Belebat* [*fl.* 1625-1630]

BELIAS, JOHANNIS. *See* BELYE, John.

[**BELIN**, JEAN ALBERT, *ca.* 1610-1677] La poudre de sympathie justifiee . . . Paris, Pierre de Bresche, 1658.

    [16], 88 (i.e. 86) p.   14 cm.   **[1067]**
    Dedicatory epistle signed: D. B.

BELISSON, PAUL. *See* PELLISSON-FONTANIER, Paul. 1624-1693

BELLAMY, EDWARD [*fl.* 1698] *tr. See* HUARTE DE SAN JUAN, J. Examen de ingenios; or, The tryal of wits. 1698.

BELLARMINO, ROBERTO FRANCESCO ROMOLO, *Saint* [1542-1621] De scriptoribus ecclesiasticis liber unus. Cum adjunctis indicibus undecim, & brevi Chronologia ab orbe condito usque ad annum M.DC.XII. Romae, Ex typographia Bartholomaei Zannetti, 1613.

    258, [14], 37 p.   23 cm.   **[1068]**
    Imperfect: last leaf (blank?) wanting.

BELLEAU, REMY [1527?-1577] Dictamen metrificum de bello Huguenotico. *In* Martin, L. L'Eschole de Salerne. 1650, 166-?, 1664, 1697.

BELLI, CONSTANTINO [*fl.* 1672-1677] *tr. See* I MEDICI ALLA CENSURA. 1678, 1683.

BELLI, ONORIO [*d.* 1604] *See* L'ÉCLUSE, C. de. Caroli Clusii . . . Rariorum plantarum historia. 1601.

BELLIÈRE, CLAUDE DE LA. *See* LA BELLIÈRE, Claude de, *sieur de la Niolle* [*fl.* 1663-1664]

BELLINI, LORENZO [1643-1704] De urinis et pulsibus de missione sanguinis de febribus de morbis capitis, et pectoris . . . Bononiae, Ex typographia Antonii Pisarii, 1683.

    [20] 606 (i.e 608) p.   24 cm.   **[1069]**

—[The same.] . . . Cum praefatione Johannis Bohnii . . . Francofurti, Sumptibus Johannis Grossii typis Christiani Scholvini, 1685.

    [32], 688, [32] p.   21 cm.   **[1070]**
    With this is bound Wedel, G. W. Exercitationum medico-philologicarum decades duae. 1686.

—[The same.] . . . Ed. 2. priori correctior. Francofurti et Lipsiae, Sumptibus Johannis Grosii, viduae & haered.; Cizae, Charactere Huchonis, 1698.

    [32], 688, [32] p.   23 cm.   **[1071]**

—Exercitatio anatomica . . . de structura et usu renum . . . Florentiae, Ex typographia sub signo Stellae, 1662.

    28 p.   plates.   24 cm.   **[1072]**

—Exercitatio anatomica de structura & usu renum. Cui renum monstrosorum exempla, ex medicorum celebrium scriptis addidit Gerardus Blasius . . . Amstelodami, Sumptibus Andreae Frisii, 1665.

    132 p.   plates.   14 cm.   **[1073]**
    "Appendix ad tractatum de renibus": p. [97]-132.

—Gustus organum . . . novissime deprehensum; praemissis ad faciliorem intelligentiam quibusdam de saporibus . . . Bononiae, Typis Pisarrianis, 1665.

    [16], 247, [1] p.   13 cm.   **[1074]**

—Opuscula aliquot ad Archibaldum Pitcarnium . . . Pistorii, Ex nova officina Stephani Gatti, 1695.

    [20], 215, [3] p.   plates.   24 cm.   **[1075]**
    Contents: "Motus cordis intra et extra uterum": p. 1-114. —"De motu bilis, et liquidorum omnium per corpora animalium . . .": p. 115-142. —"De fermentis, et glandulis rursus": p. 143-162. —"De missione sanguinis": p. 163-187. —"De contractione naturali, et villo contractili": p. 188-215.

—[The same.] Opuscula aliquot, ad Archibaldum Pitcarnium . . . in quibus praecipue agitur de motu cordis in & extra uterum, ovo, ovi aere & respiratione. De motu bilis & liquidorum omnium per corpora animalium. De fermentis & glandulis, &c. Lugduni Batavorum, Apud Cornelium Boutesteyn, 1696.

    [20], 261 (i.e. 251), [3] p.   plates.   20 cm.
                                [1076]
    "De missione sanguinis": p. 200-228; "De contractione naturali et villo contractili": p. 229-261.
    Imperfect: wormholes on p. 75-94.

—*See* VESLING, J. Syntagma anatomicum. 1666, 1677, 1696.

—*as subject. See* CAMERARIUS, E. Dissertationes tres. 1694; SCHELHAMMER, G. C. Ad . . . Georgium Wolfgangum Wedelium epistola. 1690.

BELLINZANI, LODOVICO [*fl.* 1647-1648] Il mercurio estinto resuscitato. Discorso apologetico . . . nel quale si prova con ragioni, & autorità di più accreditati scrittori l'untione dell'argento vivo esser rimedio efficacissimo, non solo al morbo gallico, mà ancora à diversi altri mali ... Roma, Francesco Cavalli, 1648.

[16], 24 p. 19 cm. [1077]

BELLON, Peter, *tr. See* Le Fèvre, N. A discourse. 1664.

BELLONIUS, Petrus. *See* Belon, Pierre [1517?-1564]

BELLOSTE, Augustin [1654-1730] Le chirurgien d'hôpital, enseignant une maniere douce & facile de guerir promptement toutes sortes de playes. Avec un moyen d'éviter l'exfoliation des os, & une plaque nouvellement inventée pour le pansement des trépans ... Paris, Laurent d'Houry, 1696.

[40], 367, [1] p. illus. 17 cm. [1078]

BELLUNENSIS, Andreas. *See* Alpago, Andrea [d. 1521]

BELLUS, Honorius. *See* Belli, Onorio [d. 1604]

BELON, Peter. *See* Bellon, Peter.

BELON, Pierre [1517?-1564] *See* Gesner, K. Historiae animalium liber primus [-liber V]. 1617-1621 [v. 1, 1620]; L'écluse, C. de. Caroli ... Clusii ... Exoticorum libri decem. 1605; Rauwolff, L. A collection of curious travels & voyages. 1693.

BÉLOSTE, Augustin. *See* Belloste, Augustin [1654-1730]

BELOT, Jean [*fl.* 1618] Les oeuvres ... Contenant la chiromence, physionomie, l'art de memoyre de Raymond Lulle; traicté des divinations, augures & songes; les sciences steganographiques, paulines, armadelles & lullistes; l'art de doctement prescher & haranguer, &c. Derniere ed. rev. corr. & augm. ... Rouen, Jacques Caillouë, 1640.

[16], 432 p.; [4], 138, [2] p. illus., plates, port. 17 cm. [1079]

In 3 sections. Section 2 (p. [255]-432) has half-title: La seconde partie, ou second livre auquel et traité de la physionomie metoposcopie, & oneïrocratie. Section [3] ([4], 138 p. at end) has special title page: L'oeuvre des oeuvres; ou, Le plus parfaict des sciences steganographiques, paulines, armadelles, & lullistes.

—Copy 2.
Imperfect: p. 417-418 wanting.

With this is bound Moult, T. G. Propheties perpetuelles. Paris, 1741.

—[The same.] ... Lyon, Claude la Riviere, 1654.

[16], 343 p.; [4], 117, [1] p. illus., plates, port. 17 cm. [1080]

—Familieres instructions pour apprendre les sciences de chiromance & physionomie ... Avec un traicté des divinations, augures, & songes ... Paris, Nicolas Bourdin, 1624.

14, [2], 432 p. illus., plates, port. 17 cm. [1081]

In 2 sections. Section 2 (p. [255]-432) has half title: La seconde partie, ou second livre auquel est traité de la physionomie, metoposcopie, & oneïrocratie. The date has been altered by hand from MDCXXIII to MDCXXIIII.

"Que c'est que la memoire artificielle, ou l'art de Raymond Lulle": p. 415-432.

BELOW, Jacob Christian [*fl.* 1682-1685] *respondent. See* Leichner, E., *praeses.* Dissertatio inauguralis, casum matronae hypochondriacae exhibens. 1685; Loss, J., *praeses.* De glandulis in genere. 1682.

BELOW, Karl Fredrik [*fl.* 1698-1699] *respondent. See* Schaper, J. E., *praeses.* Dissertatio de digitis manus dextrae. 1698 [and] Dissertatio solennis medica. 1699.

BELTRANO, Ottavio [17th cent.] *ed. See* Benincasa, R. Almanacco perpetuo. 1665.

BELYE, John. Tractatus duo chemici. *In* [Combach, L.] *ed. and tr.* Tractatus. 1647.

BEN, Johann [*fl.* 1683] *respondent.* Disputatio medica inauguralis de suffocatione hypochondriaca ... Lugduni Batavorum, Apud Abrahamum Elzevier, 1683.

[20] p. 22 cm. [1082]
Diss. — Leyden.

BEN-ADAM. *See* Floretus A Bethabor. Traum-Gesicht. 1682.

BEN SHEM-TOB, Abraham. *See* Abraham ben Shem-tob [13th cent.]

BENANCIO, Lisset. *See* Colin, Sébastien [1519?-1578?]

BENAVENTE, Juan de Quiñones de. *See* Quiñones, Juan de [d. ca. 1650]

BENAVIDES, PEDRO DE PERALTA BARNUEVO ROCHA Y. *See* PERALTA BARNUEVO ROCHA Y BENAVIDES, Pedro de [1663-1743]

BENCIO, UGONE. *See* BENZI, Ugo [1376-1439]

BENDINELLI, VINCENZO [*fl.* 1618-1630] Parere della pietra Lazuli. Per la Confettione Alchermes, di Gio. Mesue ... Lucca, Appresso Ottaviano Guidoboni, e Baldassari del Giudice, 1618.
[23] p.   21 cm.   **[1083]**

—Thesoro preservativo contro la peste ... Pistoia, Pier' Antonio Fortunati, 1630.
[12], 59, [1] p.   21 cm.   **[1084]**

BENEDETTI, ALESSANDRO [*fl.* 1512] Collectiones medicinae. In Hippocrates. Aphorismi, Latin. 1663.

—*See* DODOENS, R. Medicinalium observationum exempla rara. 1621.

BENEDETTI, GIULIO CESARE [*d.* 1656] Consultationum medicinalium opus utile, jucundum, necessarium, medicorum principum tutela, dogmatum varietate, et ordinata morborum omnium curatione ... Venetiis, Apud Bertanos, 1650.
[16], 422, [17] p.   23 cm.   **[1085]**
Engraved title page.

—De pepasmo seu coctione quaestiones ad mentem Hippocratis ... Aquilae, Ex typographia Francisci Marine, 1636.
[12], 9-171, [9] p.   18 cm.   **[1086]**
Engraved title page.

—Epistolarum medicinalium libri decem recondita Hippocratis doctrina singularique eruditione referti ... Romae, Apud Andream Phaeum, sumptibus Bertanorum, 1649.
[16], 9-56, 615, [28] p.   port.   23 cm.
[1087]

—Tutelaris columna in qua statuitur pleuritidem fieri dum una pulmonis ala afficitur rationum, Hippocratisque stabilita tutela ... Romae, Typis Dominici Marciani, 1644.
[16], 262 p.   17 cm.   **[1088]**

BENEDICTUS, ALEXANDER. *See* BENEDETTI, Alessandro [*d.* 1512]

BENEDICTUS, CHRISTOPHORUS. *See* BENNET, Christopher [1617-1655]

BENEDICTUS, JULIUS CAESAR. *See* BENEDETTI, Giulio Cesare [*d.* 1656]

BENEDICTUS, LIBERIUS. Liber aureus de principiis naturae & artis; das ist: Ein güldenes Büchlein, so da beschreibet wie die Metallen in den Klüfften der Erden, durch die Natur in iren Mineren geboren, unnd darauss die Wissenschafft der Primae Materiae, oder Lapidis Philosophorum erlernet und durch Kunst möge guberniret werden ... Franckfurt am Mayn, In Verlegung Lucae Jennisii, 1630.
160 p.   16 cm.   **[1089]**

BENEVENIUS, ANTONIUS. *See* BENIVIENI, Antonio [1443-1502]

BENGE, JOHANN MELCHIOR. *See* GENGE, Johann Melchior [*fl.* 1684-1687]

BENINCASA, RUTILIO [1555-*ca.* 1626] Almanacco perpetuo di Rutilio Benincasa Cosentino, illustrato, e diviso in cinque parti, da Ottavio Beltrano ... Opera molto necessaria ... ad astrologi, fisonomici, medici, fisici, chirurgi ... Venetia, Combi, & La Noù, 1665.
[16], 516 (i.e. 518), [4] p.; 142 (i.e. 144) p.   illus.   17 cm.   **[1090]**
Part [2] has special title page: Quinta parte dell'Almanaco perpetuo fisico trattato. D'aritmetica ove con facilità s'insegna il vero modo d'apprenderla da se medesimo in breve tempo, con suoi essempii, e demostrationi chiari, & intelligibili. Diviso in cinque opuscoli ... di Ottavo Beltrano ...

BENIVIENI, ANTONIO [1443-1502] De abditis nonnullis ac mirandis morborum et sanationum causis. *In* Dodoens, R. Medicinalium observationum exempla rara. 1621.

BENNET, CHRISTOPHER [1617-1655] Tabidorum theatrum: sive, Pthisios, atrophiae, & hecticae xenodochium. Authore Christophero Benedicto ... Londini, Typis Tho. Newcomb, impensis Sam. Thompson, 1656.
[22], 187, [5] p.   illus., port., plates.   16 cm.
[1091]
Imperfect: port. wanting.
Edited by Martin Lluelyn.
Includes *his* Theatri tabidorum vestibulum first published separately in 1654.

—[The same.] ... Francofurti, Sumpt. Georgii Fickwirtti, typis Aegidii Vogelii, 1665.
[22], 208, [6] p.   illus.   14 cm.   **[1092]**

—*ed. See* MOFFETT, T. Healths improvement. 1655.

BENOICT, ALBERT [*fl.* 1674] *respondent*. Dissertatio inauguralis de dysenteria . . . Basileae, Excudebat Joh. Rodolphus Genathius [1674]

[12] p.   19 cm.   [**1093**]

Diss. — Basel.

BENOORDEN, GERARD [*fl.* 1686] *respondent*. Disputatio medica inauguralis de febribus . . . Trajecti ad Rhenum, Ex officina Francisci Halma, 1691.

13, [7] p.   18 cm.   [**1094**]

Diss. — Utrecht, 1686.

The date of the dissertation is given as 1686, and the pagination as 13 p. in BMC.

BENSHEIM, ERNEST [*fl.* 1699] Tractatus de hydrope, in quo simul ostenditur vera veri medici cognitio, & quinam medici in curandis morbis & ad officia archiatrica admittendi, quinam vero rejiciendi; omnia brevissime descripta . . . Lipsiae, Typis Joh. Christoph. Brandenburgeri, 1699.

48 p.   22 cm.   [**1095**]

— [The same.] . . . 1700.   [**1096**]

A reissue of the 1699 edition with date changed to 1700.

BENTIUS, HUGO. *See* BENZI, Ugo [1376-1439]

BENTIVOGLIO, IPPOLITO D'ARAGONA, *marchese* [*d.* 1685] Antidoto politico contro la peste; overo, Ordini da tenersi nella città in occasione di contagio . . . Ferrara, Nella Stampa camerale, 1680.

[9], 196 p.   28 cm.   [**1097**]

BENTLEY, RICHARD [1662-1742] The folly and unreasonableness of atheism demonstrated from the advantage and pleasure of a religious life, the faculties of humane souls, the structure of animate bodies, & the origin and frame of the world: in eight sermons . . . The 4th ed. corr. London, Printed by J. H. for H. Mortlock, 1699.

[4], 280 p.   21 cm.   [**1098**]

— *See* WOOTON, W. Reflections upon ancient and modern learning. 1697.

BENTZIUS, ADOLPHUS CHRISTOPHORUS. *See* BENZ, Adolph Christoph [*fl.* 1690-*ca.* 1715]

BENTZON, NICOLAUS [*fl.* 1637-1638] *praeses*. Theoria iatrica affectuum septentrionales cumprimis divexantium . . . Basileae, Ex officina typographica Georgii Deckeri [1638]

[23] p.   22 cm.   [**1099**]

Diss. — Basel (J. F. Zwinger, *respondent*)

BENZ, ADOLPH CHRISTOPH [*fl.* 1690-*ca.* 1715] *respondent*. Disputatio medica inauguralis de pituita vitrea insipida . . . Altdorffii, Typis Henrici Meyeri [1690]

28 p.   20 cm.   [**1100**]

Diss. — Altdorf.

BENZ, JOHANN GEORG [*fl.* 1699] *respondent*. Disputatio inauguralis medica mulierem dolore capitis periodico cum abscessu laborantem exhibens . . . [Altdorffii] Typis Henrici Meyeri [1699]

20 p.   20 cm.   [**1101**]

Diss. — Altdorf.

BENZI, UGO [1376-1439] Regole della sanità et della natura de cibi . . . Con le annotationi di Gio. Lodovico Bertaudo . . . Opera utile, ornata di varie storie, et arricchita d'un trattato nuovo della ebbrietà, & dell'abuso del tabaco. Torino, Gli heredi di Gio. Domenico Tarino, 1618.

[32], 850 (i.e. 800) p.   13 cm.   [**1102**]

Published in Milan in 1481 under title: Trattato circa la conservazione della sanità.

— [The same.] . . . Et nuovamente in questa seconda impressione aggiontovi alle medeme materie i trattati di Baldasar Pisanelli, e sue historie naturali; & annotationi del medico Galina. Torino, Gli heredi di Gio. Domenico Tarino, 1620.

[32], 898 (i.e. 798), [1] p.   18 cm.   [**1103**]

Contains large selections from Pisanelli's Trattato de' cibi . . . Ridotto in un assai bell'ordine . . . dal sig. Franc. Gallina, published in Carmagnola in 1589.

BERCKELMAN, WERNER [*fl.* 1656] *respondent. See* CONRING, H., *praeses*. Disputatione medica de inflammatione hepatis. 1656.

BERCKHOFF, JOHANN GEORG [*fl.* 1673] *respondent. See* GRUVE, M., *praeses*. Disputatio physica de origine animae humanae. 1673.

BERCKHUYS, ANTON [*fl.* 1652] *respondent. See* DEUSING, A., *praeses*. Disputationum anatomicarum quinta. 1652 [and] Idea doctrinae de febribus. 1655.

BERENCLON, BERNARDUS MARTINUS DE [*fl.* 1689-1695] Bernardus Martinus de Berenclon . . . Methodum usualem, sicuti a superioribus fuit injunctum servabit, & I. a corde exordium sumens, veluti a natura ordinatum thermametron, ut inde examinetur fetmentationis vitalis, sanguinisque distributionis in omnes corporis partes paradoxon . . . [Patavii, Typis Petri Mariae Frambotti, 1689]

[7] p.   23 cm.   [1104]

At head of title: Anno 1689. 1690.

Issued without title page; title from beginning of text.

BERENGARIO, JACOPO [*ca.* 1460–1530] De fractura cranii liber aureus. Hactenus desideratus. Ed. nova, ab innumeris mendis vindicata. Lugduni Batavorum, Ex officina Joannis Maire, 1629.

[6], 321, [3] p.   illus.   16 cm.   [1105]

—Μιϰϱοϰοσμογϱαφία; or, A description of the body of man: being a practical anatomy shewing the manner of anatomizing from part to part; the like hath not been set forth in the English tongue . . . Done into English by H. Jackson . . . London, Livewell Chapman, 1664.

[14], 376 p.   front., plates.   15 cm.   [1106]

Imperfect: frontispiece wanting; sig. A3-4, p. 99–112 also wanting but supplied in photocopy.

BÉRENGER, N. [*fl.* 1694-1701] Celandre; ou, Traité nouveau des décentes [sic] de leurs differentes especes, & de leur parfaite guérison. Avec un autre Traité des maux de ventre, ou maladies intestinales, & des moyens de les guérir . . . Paris, Laurent d'Houry, 1695.

[16], 380, [35], 24 p.   17 cm.   [1107]

"Des proprietez, vertus, & usages de plusieurs rares & excellens remedes experimentez": p. 1-24 at end.

BERENS, FRANZ CHRISTOPH [*fl.* 1663-1667] respondent. See JENICHEN, G., praeses. Disputatio physica, de fulmine. 1663.

BEREVELT, ABRAHAM [*fl.* 1698] respondent. Disputatio philosophica inauguralis de immortalitate mentis humanae . . . Lugduni Batavorum, Apud Abrahammum Elzevier, 1698.

[26] p.   24 cm.   [1108]

Diss.—Leyden.

BERG, JOHANN [*fl.* 1657] praeses. Disputatio psychologica prior de πoῦ adaequato animae hominis, dum informat . . . [Lipsiae] Typis Johannis Wittigau [1657]

[16] p.   20 cm.   [1109]

Diss.—Leipzig (J. A. Scheffer, *respondent*)

BERG, PAUL [*fl.* 1620] respondent. De apoplexia . . . Lugduni Batavorum, Ex officina Jacobi Marci. 1620.

[8] p.   21 cm.   [1110]

Diss. — Leyden.

BERGAMO. **Collegio dei medici.** See COLLEGIO DEI MEDICI, Bergamo.

BERGEN, JOHANN GEORG VON [1672-1738] respondent. See ALBINUS, B. Dissertatio inauguralis medica, de abortu. 1697.

BERGEN, PAULUS VON. See BERG, Paul [*fl.* 1620]

BERGER, CLAUDE [1679-1712] respondent. See ANDRY DE BOISREGARD, N. De la génération des vers dans le corps de l'homme. 1700; FAGON, G.C. Quaestio medica. 1699.

BERGER, JOANNES BENEDICTUS [1589-1626] See ROTHENBURG OB DER TAUBER. Ordinances, local laws, etc. Ernstliche, trewhertzige Ordtnung. 1625.

BERGER, JOHANN GOTTFRIED VON [1659-1736] Lectori benevoli S. D. eundemque ad anatoman publicam cadaveris foeminei . . . invitat D. Jo. Gothofredus Berger . . . decanus. Wittenbergae, Typis Martini Schultzii [1689]

[12] p.   20 cm.   [1111]

—Lectori benevolo S. P. D. eundemque ad anatomen publicam cadaveris feminei . . . invitat, Jo. Gothofredus Berger . . . Vitembergae, Ex Officina Kreusigiana [1698]

[14] p.   19 cm.   [1112]

—Nobilissimis medicinae & scientiae naturalis cultoribus S. F. Q. D. et ad praelectiones publicas de foetu humano, eosdem humanissime invitat Jo. Gothofredus Berger . . . Wittenbergae, Typis Martini Schultzii [1688]

[8] p.   20 cm.   [1113]

—Rector . . . Jo. Gothofredus Berger . . . civibus academicis salutem plurimam dicit, fructusque et beneficia Christi resurgentis ex animo apprecatur. [Wittebergae, 1694]

[8] p.   20 cm.   [1114]

—Dissertationem medicam de mania . . . sistit Johannes Gothofredus Bergerus . . . respondente Friderico Gothofredo Glück . . . Lipsiae, Literis Johannis Georgii [1685]

[20] p.   20 cm.   [1115]

Diss. pro loco—Leipzig (F. G. Glück, *respondent*)

—Ordinis medici in Academia Vitembergensi decanus . . . Jo. Gothofredus Berger . . . lectori benevolo S. P. D. eundemque ad dissertationem inauguralem de hydrope ab ... Dn. Henrico Emanuele Rüel ... publice defendendam ... invitat. [Witebergae] Literis Kreusigianis [1693]

[12] p. 19 cm. [1116]

Program—Wittenberg (for H. E. Rüel)

—Ordinis medici in Academia Vitembergensi decanus ... Jo. Gothofredus Berger ... lectori benevolo S. P. D. eundemque ad dissertationem inauguralem de morbis senum ab autore ... Paullo Hofmanno ... publice habendam ... [Wittenbergae] Typis Christiani Schrödteri [1693]

[16] p. 20 cm. [1117]

Program—Wittenberg (for P. Hofmann)

Dissertation—Leipzig

—praeses. Disputationem de chylo ... submittit M. Johannes Jacobus Fickius ... Lipsiae, Literis Johannis Georgi, 1686.

[24] p. 20 cm. [1118]

J. J. Fick, respondent.

Dissertations—Wittenberg

—praeses. De succi nutricii per nervos tansitu ... Vitembergae, Typis Christiani Schrödteri [1695]

48 p. 20 cm. [1119]

G. A. Agricola, respondent.

—Dissertatio inauguralis de morbis oculorum ... Vitembergae, Typis Christiani Kreusigii [1698]

54 p. 19 cm. [1120]

C. J. Fahr, respondent.

—Dissertatio medica inauguralis de odoratu, ejusque praecipuis laesionibus, coryza, polypo & ozaena ... Vitembergae, Prelo Christiani Kreusigii [1698]

[62] p. 19 cm. [1121]

E. G. Bergmann, respondent.

—Dissertatio solennis de febribus malignis ... Vitembergae, Prelo Christiani Kreusigii [1696]

[35] p. 19 cm. [1122]

J. C. Wolff, respondent.

—Dissertatio solennis de haemorrhoidibus ultra modum profusis et caecis ... Vitembergae, Typis Christ, Fincelii, 1700.

52 p. 20 cm. [1123]

C.G. Riz, respondent.

—Dissertatio solennis de inflammatione ... Vitembergae, Typis Christiani Schrödteri [1695]

32, [4] p. 20 cm. [1124]

J. J. Marchand, respondent.

—Dissertatio solennis de tympanite ... Witembergae, Typis Johannis Michaelis Goderitschii, 1700.

[1], 34 p. 20 cm. [1125]

J. C. Stisser, respondent.

—Dissertationem inauguralem de ischuria ... p. p. Joachimus Gottlieb Lehmann ... Wittebergae, Typis Johannis Michaelis Goderitschii [1691]

[40] p. 20 cm. [1126]

J. G. Lehmann, respondent.

—Dissertationem inauguralem de leienteria ... p. p. M. Gothofredus Rothe ... Vitembergae, Typis Martini Schulzii [1691]

28 p. 20 cm. [1127]

G. Rothe, respondent.

—Dissertationem inauguralem de metalorum solutione ... p. p. Johannes Katsch ... Wittebergae, Excudebat Martinus Schultze [1689]

[24] p. 20 cm. [1128]

J. Katsch, respondent.

—Dissertationem inauguralem de suppressione catameniorum, sive fluxus menstrui ... exhibet Johannes Simeon Reinhard ... Wittenbergae, Typis Martini Schultzii [1692]

36 p. 20 cm. [1129]

J. S. Reinhard, respondent.

—Dissertationem solennem de difficultate respirandi ... p. p. Nathanael Heer ... Witembergae, Literis Goderitschianis [1700]

56 p. 19 cm. [1130]

Imperfect: lower margin of title page trimmed.

N. Heer, respondent.

—Exercitationem inauguralem de animi deliquiis ... p. p. M. Gothofredus Thomasius ... Vitembergae, Typis Martini Schultzii [1689]

30, [2] p. 18 cm. [1131]

G. Thomasius, respondent.

—Exercitationem inauguralem de epilepsia ... p. p. Christianus Etzlerus ... Wittenbergae, Charact. Matthaei Henckelii [1690]

[28] p. 20 cm. [1132]

C. Etzler, respondent.

—Exercitationem inauguralem de morbis senum ... p. p. Paulus Hofmann ... Vitembergae, Typis Christiani Schrödteri [1693]

28 p.   20 cm.   [**1133**]

P. Hofmann, *respondent.*

—Exercitationem inauguralem de polypo cordis ... p. p. Jo. Raphael Pretten ... Wittenbergae, Typis C. Fincelii [1689]

38 (i.e. 36) p.   19 cm.   [**1134**]

J. R. Pretten, *respondent.*

—Inauguralem disputationem de angina ... submittit M. Christianus Ludovicus Welsch ... Wittebergae, Typis Martini Schultzii [1691]

[24] p.   18 cm.   [**1135**]

C. L. Welsch, *respondent.*

—Positiones physiologicas de homine ... p. p. ... Augustus Christianus Pauli ... Wittebergae, Typis Martini Schultzii [1691]

[48] p.   18 cm.   [**1136**]

A. C. Pauli, *respondent.*

—*respondent. See* FASCH, A. H., *praeses.* Dissertatio inauguralis de circulatione lymphae. 1682.

BERGER PETER [*fl.* 1697] *respondent. See* GREULINCK, J. H., *praeses.* De multiplicatione hominis. 1697.

BERGGOLD, GOTTLOB [*fl.* 1694–1697]. *See* BOHN, J. Lectori Benevolo D. Johannes Bohn ... Salutem! 1695.

—*respondent. See* BOHN, J., *praeses.* Dissertatio chirurgica. 1694; LANGE, C. J., *praeses.* Disputatio medica inauguralis de hydrope. 1695.

BERGH, SAMUEL à [*fl.* 1695–1696] *respondent. See* BARBECK, F. G. *praeses.* Disputatio medica de generatione corporis humani. 1695.

BERGH-val; ofte, Wederlegginge van Michiel de Montaigne. *See* BEVERWIJCK, J. van. Lof der medicine. 1641, 1647.

BERGHE, ROBERT VAN DEN. *See* MONTANUS, Robert [*fl.* 1624–1632]

BERGHE, THOMAS VAN DEN [1615–1685] Qualitas loimodea; sive, Pestis Brugana anni M. DC. LXVI. Hippocratico-Hermetice discussa per Thomas Montanum ... Opus pro hac praesenti peste anni M. DC. LXIX. praeservanda & curanda utilis-

simum ... Brugis Flandrorum, Apud Lucam Kerchovium, 1669.

[16], 184, [14] p.   20 cm.   [**1137**]

BERGMAN, HEINRICH SALOMON [*fl.* 1617] *respondent. See* MEIBOM, H., *praeses.* Exercitatio medica de bubonibus. 1671.

BERGMANN, ERNST GOTTLOB [*fl.* 1696–1698] *respondent. See* BERGER, J. G. von, *praeses.* Dissertatio medica inauguralis. 1698; SCHACHER, P. G., *praeses.* Hominis loquelam ... exponit. 1696.

BERGMANN, GOTTFRIED [*fl.* 1682] *respondent. See* VESTI, J., *praeses.* Disputatio medica, de diarrhoea. 1682.

BERGMILLER, THOMAS [*fl.* 1694] *ed. See* FRISCH, G. Anatomia alchymiae. 1695.

BERICHT und Ordnung wie man sich in den jetzo anfelligen bösen Fiebern ... verwahren und curiren sol. Durch die Medicos der Stadt Görlitz zu Wolfarth ihres geliebten Vater Landes gestellet. Görlitz, Gedruckt durch Johann Rhambaw, 1613.

[23] p.   19 cm.   [**1138**]

BERINGUCCI, CARLO. *See* BIRINGUCCI, Carlo [*d.* 1648]

BERLU, JOHN JACOB. The treasury of drugs unlock'd; or, A full and true description of all sorts of drugs, and chymical preparations, sold by drugists ... London, John Harris and Tho. Howkins, 1690.

[5], 125 (i.e. 147), [14] p.   15 cm.   [**1139**]

BERNAGIE, PIETER [1656–1699] Antwoord ... op de brief, van Kornelis Botekoe ... Amsterdam, Jan Bouman, 1682.

[4], 96 p.   16 cm.   [**1140**]

—Brief ... aan Kornelis Bontekoe ... Amsterdam, Jan Bouman, 1682.

85, [1] p.   16 cm.   [**1141**]

—*See* BONTEKOE, C. Antwoord. 1682.

BERNARD, *of Treves. See* BERNARDUS TREVIRENSIS [14th cent.]

BERNARD DE GORDON [*fl. ca.* 1283–*ca.* 1308] Lilium medicinae ἑπτάφυλλον tractatus nimirum septem foliis sive particulis, accuratissimam omnium morborum ... curationem complectens. Cui accesserunt Tractatus de methodo curandi affectus praeter nat. De regimine acutorum, De prognosticis, urinis & pulsibus, una cum Decem tabulis pharmacorum Remacli Limburgensis. Omnia ... nunc vero per Petrum Uffenbachium ... revisa a quam plurimis mendis corr., & multis annotatiunculis adaucta. Francofurti, Apud Lucam Jennis, 1617.

[31], 170 (i.e. 1172), [27] p.   18 cm.   **[1142]**

Based on the edition published in Lyons in 1550 (cf. editor's dedication, p. [9–10]) not on the more complete edition of 1574.

BERNARD, Francis [1627–1698] A catalogue of the library of the late learned Dr. Francis Bernard, fellow of the College of Physicians, and physician to S. Bartholomew's Hospital. Being a large collection of the best theological, historical, philological, medicinal and mathematical authors, in the Greek, Latin, Italian, Spanish, French, German, Dutch and English tongues, in all volumes, which will be sold by auction at the doctor's late dwelling house in Little Britain, the sale to begin on Tuesday, Octob. 4, 1698 ... [London, 1698]

192, 151, 88, 19 p.   19 cm.   **[1143]**

Contains autograph of Harvey Williams Cushing.

BERNARDI, Florio [17th cent.] L'ignoranza convinta, l'inganno, e la menzogna scoperta al sole della veritá ... Cosmopoli [i.e. Venice?] Filotimo Buonpensieri, 1669.

368 (i.e. 366), [2], 29 p.   17 cm.   **[1144]**

A reply to the Confutazione della diatriba, publicata da Florio, detto Bernardi, sotto nome di Scipione Obez, inglese, del dott. Giovanni Cesare Manfroncini [Manfroccini pseud. i.e. Francesco Cameroni or Cecilio Follio or Fuoli?] published in July 1668. Cf. p. [5] and Melzi, v. 2, p. 154, and Passano's supplement, p. 195, 235–6.

—See Claudini, G. C. Responsionum, et consultationum medicinalium tomus unicus. 1646.

BERNARDINIS, Aegidius de [fl. 1680] Institutionum medicinalium ad tyrones opusculum in quinque partes divisum ... Romae, Sumpt. Tinassii, 1680.

[24], 267 p.   15 cm.   **[1145]**

Imperfect: p. 3–4 mutilated; wormholes on p. 259–268.

BERNARDUS TREVIRENSIS [14th cent.] [De chemico miraculo, quod lapidem philosophiae appellant]

683–709 p., vol. 1.   20 cm.   (*In* Zetzner, Lazarus, *ed.* Theatrum chemicum. Argentorati, 1659–61)   **[1146]**

Title from table of contents.
Running title: De alchemia liber.

—Bernardi Trevirensis [responsio] ad Thomam de Bononia [de mineralibus, & elixiris compositione, Roberti Vallensis tabulis illustrata]

38–68 p., vol. 2.   17 cm.   (*In* Artis auriferae. Basileae, 1610)   **[1147]**

Caption title.
Running title: De transmutatione metallorum.
Title partly from table of contents.

—[German ed.] Ein Antwort Bernhardi Trevirensis, an Thomam von Bononia [von den Mineralen, unnd zusammensetzung oder zurichtung dess Elixirs, erkläret unnd aussgelegt mit den Tafeln Roberti Vallensis]

46–93 p., part 2.   19 cm.   (*In* Morgenstern, Philipp, *ed.* and *tr.* Turba philosophorum. Basel, 1613)   **[1148]**

Title partly from table of contents.

[—] Le texte d'alchymie, et le songe-verd. Paris, Laurent d'Houry, 1695.

115, [2] p.   illus.   17 cm.   **[1149]**

—Traicté de la nature de l'oeuf des philosophes ... Paris [Pierre Moët] 1659.

63 p.   17 cm.   **[1150]**

Bound (as issued) with Basilius Valentinus. Les douze clefs de philosophie. 1660.

—See Collectanea chymica. 1684; [Combach, L.] *ed.* and *tr.* Tractatus. 1647; Houpreght, J. F., *comp.* Aurifontina chymica. 1680.

BERNARDUS TREVISANUS. *See* Bernardus Trevirensis [14th cent.]

BERNDT, Christian [*fl.* 1695–1696] *respondent. See* Vater, C., *praeses.* De transpiratione insensibili corporis humani. 1695 [and] Inauguralis dissertatio medica de contracturis. 1696.

BERNER, Gottlieb Ephraim [*fl.* 1696–ca. 1738] *respondent. See* Hoffmann, F. [1660–1742] *praeses.* Dissertatio medica inauguralis, exhibens salis volatilis genesin, usum. 1696.

BERNHARD, *Prince of Saxony* [1649–1706] *See* Saxony. Laws, statutes, etc. Nothwendig-und nützlicher Unterricht. 1682.

BERNHARD VON TARVIS. *See* BERNARDUS TREVIRENSIS [14th cent.]

BERNHARDI, GREGOR [*fl.* 1662-1663] *respondent.* De χλωροσει ... Altdorffii, Aere Goebeliano [1663] [4], 32 p. 18 cm. **[1151]**
Diss. — Altdorf.

BERNHARDI DE BERNITZ, MARTIN. *See* BERNITZ, Martin Bernhard [*fl.* 1651]

BERNHARDUS, *a Doma. See* DEUSING, A. Vindiciae foetus. 1664; HISTORIA FOETUS MUSSIPONTANI. 1669; SINIBALDI, G. B. Geneanthropeiae. 1669

BERNHARDUS TREVISANUS. *See* BERNARDUS TREVIRENSIS [14th cent.]

BERNIA, JERONIMO [*fl.* 1664] *ed. See* ALDROVANDI, U. Dendrologiae naturalis ... libri duo. 1668; GRIMALDI, F. M. Physico-mathesis de lumine. 1665.

BERNIA, MARCO ANTONIO [*fl.* 1638-1661] *ed. See* ALDROVANDI, U. De piscibus libri V. 1638 [and] De quadrupedibus solidipedibus volumen integrum. 1639 [and] Monstrorum historia. 1642 [and] Musaeum metallicum. 1648 [and] Quadrupedum omnium bisulcorum historia. 1642.

BERNIER, CHRISTOPHE [*fl.* 1645] Questions anatomiques, recueillies de divers autheurs. Divisées en quatre parties ... Paris, Louys Julian, 1645. [12], 240 p. 17 cm. **[1152]**

—[The same.] ... Paris, Claude le Groult, 1648. [12], 240 p. 17 cm. **[1153]**
Imperfect: sig. a3-4 wanting.

BERNIER, FRANÇOIS [1620-1688] Excerpta e laboratorio Ceylonico. *In* Schröder, J. Pharmacopoea Schrödero-Hoffmanniana illustrata et aucta. 1687.

—Excerpta e pharmacopoea Persica. *In* Schröder, J. Pharmacopoea Schrödero-Hoffmanniana illustrata et aucta. 1687.

—*See* GASSENDI, P. Abregé de la philosophie de Gassendi. 1678.

BERNIER, JEAN [1622-1698] Essais de medecine où il est traité de l'histoire de la medecine et des medecins. Du devoir des medecins à l'égard des malades, & de celui des malades à l'égard des medecins ... Paris, Chez Simon Langronne [De l'imprimerie d'Antoine Lambin] 1689. [8], 559, cxxxvi, [8] p. 26 cm. **[1154]**

—[The same.] Histoire cronologique de la medecine, et des medecins, ou il est traité de l'origine, du progrés, & de tout ce qui apartient à cette science. Du devoir des medecins à l'égard des malades. Et celuy des malades à l'égard des medecins ... 2. ed. Rev. corr. & abregée en quelques endroits. Paris, Chez Laurent d'Houry, Simon Langronne, et Michel Brunet [De l'imprimerie de Christophe Journel] 1695. [8], 315, cxxxvi, [8] p. 25 cm. **[1155]**

BERNINCK, ARNOLD [*fl.* 1665] *respondent. See* FRENZEL, S. F., *praeses.* Serpentem ... publicae eruditorum contemplationi sistit ... A. B. 1665.

BERNITZ, MARTIN BERNHARD [*fl.* 1651] *See* SCHRÖDER, J. Pharmacopoea Schrödero-Hoffmanniana illustrata et aucta. 1687.

BERNOULLI, JAKOB [1654-1705] Dissertatio de gravitate aetheris. Amstelaedami, Apud Henr. Wetstenium, 1683. [14], 269, [3] p. plates. 15 cm. **[1156]**

BERNOULLI, JOHANN [1667-1748] Mathematical disquisitions concerning muscular motion. *In* Browne, J. Myographia nova. 1698.

—*respondent.* Dissertatio inauguralis physico-anatomica de motu musculorum ... Basileae, Typis Johann. Conradi à Mechel [1694] [20] p. illus. 19 cm. **[1157]**
Diss. — Basel.

BERTALDI, GIOVANNI LODOVICO [*d.* 1625] Medicamentorum apparatus, in quo remediorum omnium compositorum non usualium modo, sed praecipuorum etiam magistralium, vires, durationes, doses, ac formulae, cum universa utendi methodo, disertissime enodantur ... Adjectis ... plerisque remediis, quae nunquam antea typis evulgata peculiariter in tota Pedemontana regione usurpantur ... Taurini, Ex officina FF. de Cavaleriis, 1612. [56], 973 (i.e. 873), [5] p. 22 cm. **[1158]**
Two more parts were published in 1614. Cf. BNC, v. II, col. 1156.

—, *ed. See* BENZI, U. Regole della sanità. 1618, 1620.

BERTAUDO, GIOVANNI LODOVICO. *See* BERTALDI, Giovanni Lodovico [*d.* 1625]

BERTHEMIN, Dominique, *sieur de Pont* [*b.* 1580] Discours des eaux chaudes, et bains de plombieres divisez en deux traictez . . . Nancy, Jacob Garnich, 1615.

[8], 167 (i.e. 166) ll.   16 cm.   **[1159]**

BERTHIOLI, Antonio [*fl. ca.* 1585] *See* Ferrari, G., *ed.* Idea theriacae. 1601.

BERTHOLOMEUS. *See* Bartholomaeus Anglicus [13th cent.]

BERTI, Giovanni Battista [*fl.* 1616] Discorso sopra il bere fresco, nel quale si prova con autorità di medici, filosofi, poeti, & oratori, che il bere fresco con la neve è sano al corpo humano . . . Roma, Giacomo Mascardi, 1616.

[4], 48 p.   21 cm.   **[1160]**

BERTINI, Antonio Francesco [1658-1726] La medicina difesa dalle calunnie degli uomini volgari, e dalle opposizioni de' dotti, divisa in due dialoghi . . . Lucca, Per i Marescandoli, 1699.

[14], xx, 153 (i.e. 353), [3] p.   26 cm.   **[1161]**
Errata: p. [2-3] at end.

—Risposta apologetica . . . al discorso familiare di Teofilo Pamio [pseud. i.e. Giovanni Andrea Moniglia] contro l'autore della Medicina difesa . . . In Cosmopoli [i.e. Firenze] Per Giorgio della Piazza, 1700.

[14], 139 p.   24 cm.   **[1162]**
Imprint partly supplied from Melzi v. 3, p. 135.

—*See* Monte-Mellini, N. Problema. 1700.

BERTOCCI, Alfonso [*fl.* 1556] Methodus curativa generalis et compendiaria: ex Hippocratis, Galeni, Avicennae & Montani placitis, in medicinae studiosorum gratiam descripta; auctoribus . . . Alphonso Bertotio . . . et Ioanne Cratone de Craffth-heim . . . Accesserunt Ideae doctrinae Hippocraticae: I. De generatione pituitae. II. De melancholico humore. III. De coctione & praeparatione humorum. IV. De victus ratione. Autore Joan. Bapt. Montano. Francofurti, Apud Joannem Saurium, impensis Nicolai Steinii, 1608.

[7], 140 p.; [11], 108 (i.e. 110) p.   17 cm.
                                        [1163]
The first work, by Bertocci, was originally published in Venice in 1556 under title: Methodus generalis & compendiaria ex Hippocratis, Galeni et Avicennae placitis deprompta. It was also published under title: Therapeutica.

The second work, by Johann Crato von Krafftheim, has special title page: Methodus Θεραπευτική, ex sententia Galeni et Joannis Baptistae Montani. This, with Crato's edition of the four works by Monte, was first published in Basel in 1555.

BERTOLLOTTI, Alfonso [*fl.* 1629] *See* Reggio Emilia (City) Ordinances, local laws, etc. Bando per occasione di sospetto di peste. 1629.

BERTOLOTTI, Antonio [17th cent.] Le pregiate virtù del composto contro veleno, come risagallo, arsenico, solimato, & ogni morsicatura di qualsivoglia animal velenoso, & infirmità simili . . . Bologna, Antonio Pisarri [16--]

broadside, 22 x 17 cm.   **[1164]**
Antonio Pisarri printed in Bologna during the first part of the 17th century. Cf. Sorbelli, p. 152.

BERTOTIUS, Alphonsus. *See* Bertocci, Alfonso [*fl.* 1556]

BERTRAM, Christian [*fl.* 1623] *respondent.* Disputatio medica inauguralis de phthisi . . . Lipsiae, Ex Officina Bavarica, 1623.

[16] p.   19 cm.   **[1165]**
Diss. — Leipzig.

BERTRAM, Jeremias [*fl.* 1641] *respondent. See* Schneider, K. V., *praeses.* Disputatio medica inauguralis . . . de fluxu alvi colliquativo. 1641.

BERTRAND [*fl.* 1683] Reflexions nouvelles sur l'acide et sur l'alcali: où apres avoir demonstré que ces deux sels ne peuvent pas être les principes des mixtes, on fait voir le veritable usage qu'on en peut faire dans la physique & dans la medecine . . . Lyon, Thomas Amaulry, 1683.

[20], 359 p.   16 cm.   **[1166]**
Criticizes Otto Tachenius's Hippocrates chymicus.

BERTRAND, Gabriel [*fl.* 1613-1638] Les veritez anatomiques et chirurgicales, des organes de la respiration, & des artificieux moiens dont la nature se sert pour la preparation de l'air, observation nouvelle du mouvement de la poictrine, ensemble la methode de bien & deüëment faire toutes les ouvertures, & contre ouvertures de la poitrine, tant en la curation des playes, que pour evacuer les matieres estrangeres contenuës en icelle . . . Paris, Jean Jost, 1639.

[18], 175 p.   17 cm.   **[1167]**
"Paraphrase du Serment d'Hippocrate": p. [17-18]
Bound with Marque, J. de. Methodique introduction à la chirurgie. 1641.

—[The same.] *In* Gelée, T. L'anatomie francoise. 1656, 1668, 1671.

BERTUCCI, GIOVANNI BATTISTA. *See* CALESTANI, G. Delle osservationi ... parte prima [-seconda] 1606, 1639, 1655, 1673.

BERTUCH, JOHANN MICHAEL [*fl.* 1681–1684] *respondent. See* FASCH, A. H., *praeses.* Dissertatio anatomica de ovario mulierum. 1681 [and] Sterilitas. 1684; WEDEL, G. W., *praeses.* Exercitatio medica, sistens aegrum mictu cruento laborantem. 1683.

BESANÇON, CHARLES. *See* BEZANÇON, Germain de [*fl.* 1676]

BESANÇON, FRANCE. *Diocese.* Reglemens de la conduite des hôpitaux du diocese de Besançon, et des religieuses qui y servent les pauvres & les malades. Besancon, François Loüis Rigoine, 1697.

129, [3] p.   14 cm.   **[1168]**

BESARD, JEAN-BAPTISTE [*b. ca.* 1576] Antrum philosophicum, in quo pleraque arcana physica, quae ad vulgatiores humani corporis affectus curandos attinent ... ad experimenti legem breviter ... revelantur. Quibus ... diversa medicamenta tam e mineralibus, quam vegetabilibus conficiendi modus immediate subjicitur. Atque huic, tractatus de rebus quae humano corpori eximiam, & venustam formam inducunt. De variis mineralium, et metallorum praeparat. Deque plurimis experimentis ... breves ... annectuntur. [Augustae Vindelicorum, Imprimebat David Franck, impensis authoris, 1617]

[23], 248 p.   illus.   20 cm.   **[1169]**

BESCHREIBUNG des mineralischen Brunnen. 1609. *See* WOLFF, H.

BESLER, MICHAEL RUPERT [1607–1661] Observatio anatom.-medica singularis, mulieris cujusdam ... tres filios naturalis magnitudinis viventes enixae ... [Nuremberg, 1644]

[2], 25 p.   plate.   19 cm.   **[1170]**
Imperfect: plate wanting.
Imprint supplied from BMC.

—*respondent. See* SEBISCH, M. [1578–1674?] *praeses.* Exercitationes medicae. 1639.

BESSER, GOTTFRIED [*fl.* 1663–1666] *respondent.* Dissertationem inauguralem medicam de hydrope ascite ... publice ventilandam praelet Godofredus

Besser ... Lugduni Batavorum, Ex officina Petri & Cornelii Hackii, 1666.

[15] p.   24 cm.   **[1171]**
Diss. — Leyden.

BESSER, SEBASTIAN [*fl.* 1675] *respondent. See* GRÜBEL, C., *praeses.* De salutatione. 1675.

BESSON, JACQUES [16th cent.] *See* LIBAVIUS, A. [*d.* 1616] Praxis alchymiae. 1604.

[**BETBEDER**, PIERRE DE, *fl. ca.* 1665] Observations de medecine, contenant la guerison de plusieurs maladies considerables. Avec la maniere de bien preparer & administrer les remedes, dont l'auteur s'est servi en ces occasions. Paris, Hilaire Foucault, 1689.

[20], 283, [7] p.   17 cm.   **[1172]**

—Questions nouvelles sur la sanguification & circulation du sang. Ensemble, un Traité des vaisseaux lymphées ou lymphatiques, découverts depuis peu ... Paris, Jean d'Houry, 1666.

[16], 152 p.   16 cm.   **[1173]**

BETERA, FELICIANO [1534–1610] De cunctis humani corporis affectibus. Maligna scilicet, & delecteria qualitate. De febribus malignis, et pestilentibus: de morbo Gallico, venefico, malignitate, feritate, cacurgia, veneno ... Quae in duodecim libris resolvitur ... Brixiae, Apud Franciscum Thebaldinum, 1629.

726, [9] p.   32 cm.   **[1174]**
Colophon: Brixiae, Apud Ploycretum Turlinum, 1601.
Caption title reads: Noctium Brixianarum, de igne pestilenti ... Liber primus [p. 3]
Running title: De igne pestilenti.
Imperfect: title page mutilated.

—Enarrationes in morborum malignitatem ... Brixiae, Apud Sabbios, 1611.

[12], 144 p.   32 cm.   **[1175]**

BETHABOR, FLORETUS A. *See* FLORETUS A BETHABOR.

BETTEN, HEINRICH [*fl.* 1687] *respondent.* Disputatio medica inauguralis, de pica ... Trajecti ad Rhenum, Ex officina Francisci Halma, 1687.

10, [2] p.   22 cm.   **[1176]**
Diss. — Utrecht.

BETTS, JOHN [*d.* 1695] De ortu et natura sanguinis ... Londini, Ex officina E. T. vaeneuntque apud Gulielmum Grantham, 1669

[37], 325, [1] p. 18 cm. **[1177]**

Errata: p. [1] at end.

"Anatomia Thomae Parri annum centesimum quinquagesimum secundum & novem menses agentis. Cum ... Guliellmi Harvaei aliorumque adstantium medicorum regiorum observationibus": p. [317]-325.

Keynes (D), no. 49.

—*See* THOMSON, G. Αἱματιασις; or, The true way of preserving the bloud in its integrity. 1670.

BETULIUS, SIGMUND. *See* BIRKEN, Sigmund von [1626-1681]

BEUGHEM, CORNELIUS à [*fl.* 1678-1710] Bibliographia mathematica et artificiosa novissima perpetuo continuanda, seu Conspectus primus. Catalogi librorum mathematicorum sc. arithmeticorum, geometricorum, astronomicorum, geographicorum ... Quotquot currente hoc semiseculo ... aut novi, emendatiores & auctiores typis prodierunt ... Amstelodami, apud Janssonio-Waesbergios, 1688.

[14], 526 p. 13 cm. **[1178]**

No more appears to have been published.

—Bibliographia medica & physica novissima: perpetuo continuanda; sive, Conspectus primus catalogi librorum medicorum chymicorum, anatomicorum, chyrurgicorum, botanicorum ut & physicorum, &c. quotquot currente hoc semisaeculo, id est ab anno ... 1651 (inclusive) per universam Europam, in quavis lingua ... aut novi aut emendatiores & auctiores typis prodierunt. Undique acquisitis subsidiis adornata & adornanda ... Amstelaedami, Apud Janssonio-Waesbergios, 1681.

[8], 503 p. 14 cm. **[1179]**

No more appears to have been published.

—Incunabula typographiae; sive, Catalogus librorum scriptorumque proximis ab inventione typographiae annis, usque ad annum Christi M.D. inclusive, in quavis lingua editorum; opusculum saepius expetitum, notisque historicis, chronologicis & criticis intermixtum accurante ... Amstelodami, apud Joannem Wolters, 1688.

[12], 191 p. 13 cm. **[1180]**

—Syllabus recens exploratorum in re medica physica & chymica, prout in miscellaneis medico-physicis naturae curiosorum Germaniae, Galliae, Daniae & Belgii sparsim extant, in ordinem redactus & juxta indicem harmonice adornatus ... Amstelodami, Apud Janssonio-Waesbergios, 1696.

[44], 316 p. 14 cm. **[1181]**

BEUKEN, PIETER [*fl.* 1683] *respondent.* Disputatio medica inauguralis de chlorosi ... Lugduni Batavorum, Apud Abrahamum Elzevier, 1683.

[12] p. 22 cm. **[1182]**

Diss.—Leyden.

BEUTEL, JOHANN [*fl.* 1616] *respondent.* De phthisi positiones ... Basileae, Typis Joh. Jacobi Genathii [1616]

[19] p. 19 cm. **[1183]**

Diss.—Basel.

BEUTLER, JOHANN BENJAMIN [*fl.* 1685] *respondent. See* ALBERTI, V. Dissertatio physica. 1685

BEUTLER, JOHANN WILHELM [*fl.* 1680] *respondent. See* WALDSCHMIDT, J. J., *praeses.* Disputatio medica de glandulae pinealis statu naturali & praeternaturali. 1680.

BEUTTEL, JOHANN GEORG [*d.* 1709] *respondent.* Dissertatio medica inauguralis de bile sana et aegra ... Basileae, Typis Emanuelis & Joh. Georgii König [1687]

[44] p. 19 cm. **[1184]**

Diss.—Basel.

—*See* HOFFMANN, J. M., *praeses.* Disputatio medica publica de medicamentis martialibus. 1685.

BEUTTEL, JOHANN KASPAR [*fl.* 1643] *respondent. See* SEBISCH, M. [1578-1674] *praeses.* Disputationes de respiratione tres. 1643.

BEVERLAND, ADRIAAN [1654?-1712] De fornicatione cavenda admonitio; sive, Adhortatio ad pudicitiam et castitatem. Ed nova & ab autore correcta. Juxta exemplar Londinense. 1698.

109 p. 15 cm. **[1185]**

Not in STC(B).

BEVEROVICIUS, JOHANNES. *See* BEVERWIJCK, Jan van [1594-1647]

BEVERS, ANDREAS [*fl.* 1662] *respondent.* Disputatio medica inauguralis, de epilepsia ... Ultrajecti, Ex officina Jacobi à Doeyenburch, 1662.

[10] p. 19 cm. **[1186]**

Diss.—Utrecht.

BEVERWIJCK, Jan Van [1594-1647] Alle de wercken soo in de medecyne als chirurgye . . . [Utrecht, Harman Specht, 1651]

    7 parts in 1 v. illus., port. 25 cm. **[1187]**

Title from general half title.

Imperfect: sig. (1) 1 wanting.

Contents. — [1] Schat der gesontheyt. — [2] Schat der ongesontheydt. — [3] Lof der medicine, ofte genees-konste. — [4] Inleydinge tot de Hollandtsche genees-middelen. — [5] Steen-stuck. — [6] Heelkonste, ofte derde deel van de genees-konste. — [7] Vervolgh van de heel-konste. Items [1], [4-7] have special title pages. Others have half titles. Item [1] was printed by H. Specht in Utrecht, items [4-7] have imprint: Amsterdam, 1651.

Poems in parts [1-2] are by Jacob Cats.

    — [The same.] . . . Amsterdam, Jan Jacobz Schipper [1656]

    6 parts in 1 v. illus. 26 cm. **[1188]**

Engraved title page.

Each part has special title page.

Contents: pt. [1] Schat der gesontheydt. — pt. [2] Schat der ongesontheydt. — pt. [3] Inleydinge tot de Hollandtsche geneesmiddelen. — pt. [4] Steen-stuck. — pt. [5] Heel-konste. — [6] Vervolgh van de heel-Konste.

    — [The same.] . . . 1660. **[1189]**

Items have special title pages. Items [1] and [5] are dated 1660, the others 1656.

    — [The same.] Wercken der genees-konste, bestaende in den Schat der gesontheyt, Schat der ongesontheyt, Heel-konste; mitsgaders eenige tractaten daer onder begrepen, en oock verscheyde stucken, die ten deele na des autheurs overlijden, ten deele uyt sijn Latijnsche wercken overgeset, en nu eerst daer by gevoegt zijn. Alles . . . van nieus overzien . . . vermeerdert en verbetert . . . Verçiert met historien, kopere platen, als oock vermeerdert met verssen van den . . . Jacob Cats . . . Amsterdam, Jan Jacobsz. Schipper, 1664.

    3 parts in 1 v. illus. 24 cm. **[1190]**

Added engraved title page reads: Alle de wercken, zo in de medecyne als chirurgie.

Each part has special title page dated 1663.

Contents: pt. [1] Schat der gesontehyt [sic]. — pt. [2] Schat der ongesontheydt. Including: Inleydinge tot de Hollantsche geneesmiddelen; Lof der gichte, uyt het Latijn van Hieronymus Cardanus vertaelt; Lof der genees-konste, and Wederlegginge van Michiel de Montaigne, over . . . der genees-konste. — pt. [3] Heelkonste, Including: Aenhangsel van verscheyde brieven van geleerde heeren aen desen autheur . . . Als oock een Tracteat van pocken ende maselen, door Dr. Willem Swinnas . . . Mitsgaders een toe gift van 't Geschil des hayrs, door . . . Plempium.

    — [The same.] . . . Amsterdam, By de weduwe van J. J. Schipper, 1672.

    3 parts in 1 v. illus. 24 cm. **[1191]**

Each part has special title page; part 3 dated 1671.

    — De calculo renum & vesicae liber singularis. Cum epistolis & consultationibus magnorum virorum. Lugd. Batav., Ex Officina Elseviriorum, 1638.

    [16], 305, [15] p. 13 cm. **[1192]**

    — Epistolica quaestio de vitae termino, fatali, an mobili? Cum doctorum responsis. Dordrechti, Excudebat Henricus Essaeus, impensis Joannis Maire, 1634.

    [20], 424 p. 16 cm. **[1193]**

    — [The same.] . . . 2 ed. triplo auctior. Lugduni Batavorum, Ex officina Joannis Maire, 1636.

    [18], 488, [8] p.; [20], 152 p. 20 cm. **[1194]**

"Pars altera, ante hac nunquam edita" (p. [183]-488) has special half title. "Pars tertia, et ultima, nunc primum edita. Seorsim accedit . . . Annae Mariae a Schurman de eodem argumento epistola, totius disputationis terminus. Item ejusdem argumenti alia, a Joanne Elichmanno, M. D. ex mente & monimentis Arabum & Persarum contexta" has special title page dated 1639.

    — [The same.] . . . 3 ed. auctior & emendatior. Lugduni Batavorum, Ex officina Johannis Maire, 1651.

    [8], 488, [8] p.; [20], 152 p. 20 cm. **[1195]**

A reprint of the 1636-1639 ed. Pars tertia is of the original typesetting.

    — Epistolicae quaestiones, cum doctorum responsis. Accedit ejusdem, nec non Erasmi, Cardani, Melanchthonis, Medicinae encomium. Roterodami, Sumptibus Arnoldi Leers, 1644.

    [15], 112 (i.e. 250) p.; 140 p. illus. 16 cm. **[1196]**

3 parts in 1 v.

Part [2] has special title page: Joh. Beverovicii. Medicinae encomium. Part [3] (p. [81]-140) has special title page: Encomia medicinae; Des. Erasmi Roterodami, Hieronymi Cardani, Philippi Melanchthonis.

The Epistolicae include (p. 118-149) letters on the circulation of the blood by René Descartes.

    — [The same.] DD. virorum epistolae et responsa, tum medica, tum philosophica. Quibus ob materiae affinitatem adduntur Encomia medicinae, nec non pulveris sympathetici, compositio accuratissima . . . Roterodami, Excudebat Rudolphus a Nuyssel, 1665.

    [8], 112 (i.e. 250) p.; [6], 15-140 (i.e. 138) p. illus. 15 cm. **[1197]**

Part [2] has special title page: Encomia medicinae. Johannis Beverovicii, Des. Erasmi Roterodami, Hieronymi Cardani, nec non Philippi Melanchthoni.

Imperfect: Sig. * 1 before title page wanting.

—Exercitatio in Hippocratis aphorismum de calculo ad N. V. Claudium Salmasium ... Accedunt ejusdem argumenti doctorum epistolae. Lugd. Batavorum, Ex Officina Elseviriorum, 1641.

285 p.   13 cm.   **[1198]**

—Heel-konste; ofte, Derde deel van de Genees-konste, om de uytwendige gebreken te heelen. Dordrecht, Gedruckt by Hendrick van Esch, voor Pieter Looymans ende Maerten de Bot, 1645.

[44], 487 (i.e. 477), [7] p.   illus.   16 cm.
                                   [1199]

Added engraved title page.

With this is bound Plemp, V. F. Verhandeling der spieren. Dordrecht, 1645.

—[The same.] ... Hier achter is by-gevoeght het vierde deel, verhandelende wonden, gehartheyt, oirspronck van bus-poeder, ende geschut, kout-vyer, ontleden, ende gebroke beenderen ... Ende met nieuwe ... platen verçiert ... Dordrecht, Jacob Braat, 1651.

[28], 514, [18] p.   illus.   16 cm.   **[1200]**

"Vervolgh van de heel-konste, verhandelende wonden, gehartheyt ... ende gebroke beenderen" has special title page (p. [329]).

—Idea medicinae veterum ... Lugd. Batav. Ex officina Elseviriorum, 1637.

[8], 390, [10] p.   16 cm.   **[1201]**

—Lof der medicine; ofte, Genees-konste. [Dordrecht? 1641]

152 p.   16 cm.   **[1202]**

Includes (p. [35]-152) Bergh-val; ofte, Wederlegginge van Michiel de Montaigne, tegens de nootsakelickheyt der genees-konste.

Bound with (as issued?) his Schat der ongesontheyt. Dordrecht, 1642.

—[The same.] Lof der genees-konste, Wederlegginge van Montaigne over de nootsakelickheydt van de selve ... Dordrecht, Jacob Braat, 1647.

115, [5] p.   17 cm.   **[1203]**

Bound with (as issued?) his Schat der ongesontheyt. Dordrecht, 1647.

—Schat der gesontheyt. Met verssen verçiert door ... Jacob Cats ... [Dordrecht] Voor Mathias Havius, by Hendrick van Esch, 1637.

[16], 507, [5] p.; 175 p.   illus.   15 cm.   **[1204]**

Colophon dated 1636.

Part [1] (p. [73]-507) and part [2] (175 p.) have special title pages.

—[The same.] ... Tweede druck ... Merckelick vermeedert ... Dordrecht, Voor Matthias Havius, gedruckt by Hendrick van Esch, 1638.

[16], 778 (i.e. 780) p.   illus.   16 cm.   **[1205]**

Added engraved title page.

Eerste [Tweede] deel have special title pages. Tweede deel has imprint: Dordrecht, Gedruckt by Hendrick van Esch, 1637.

—[German tr.] Schatz der Gesundheit; das ist, Kurtzer Begrif der algemeinen Bewahrkunst ... Aus dem Niederdeutschen ... übergetragen ... durch Filip von Zesen. Amsterdam, Bei Johan Blauen, 1671.

[8], 258, [10] p.; [8], 381, [11] p.   illus.   33 cm.
                                   [1206]

Part [2] has half title: Schatz der Ungesundheit ...

"... Lob der Gicht, aus des Hieronimus Kardanus Lateinischem verhochdeutschet": p. 245-255 (part [1]).

Imperfect: p. 273-276 of part [2] wanting; supplied in photocopy from the Wellcome Medical Library.

—Schat der ongesontheyt; ofte, Genees-konste van de sieckten. Verçiert met historyen, ende kopere platen; als oock met verssen van ... Jacob Cats ... Dordrecht, Jasper Gorissz, 1642.

[32], 632 p.   illus.   16 cm.   **[1207]**

Special title page of Eerste deel has imprint: Dordrecht, Hendrick van Esch, 1641. Special title page of Tweede deel has imprint: Dordrecht, Hendrick van Esch, 1642.

With this is bound (as issued?) his Lof der medicine. [Dordrecht? 1641]

—[The same.] ... Dordrecht, Jacob Braat, 1647.

[30], 693, [1] p.   illus., port.   17 cm.   **[1208]**

Eerste [-Derde] deel have special title pages.

With this is bound (as issued?) his Lof der genees-konste. Dordrecht, 1647.

—[The same.] ... Neerstelijck op nieuws by den autheur oversien en gecorrigeert, ende tusschen beyde vergroot: mit sgaders met meer kopere platen als voor desen gedruckt. Het tweede deel. Dordrecht, Jacob Braat, 1649.

[17], 553, [5] p.   illus., front.   16 cm.   **[1209]**

Text differs from Jacob Catt's editions of 1642 and 1647.

"Lof der gichte, uyt het Latijn van Hieronymus Cardanus, vertaelt": p. 523-540.

—Steen-stuck. Aen-wysende, den oorspronck, teykenen 't voor komende genesinge van steen ende graveel alsmede het II. deel. Wesende brieven van meest alle de treffelijckste geneesmeesteren deser eeuwe beroerende deselve materie. Dordrecht, Leendert van Heck, 1649.

[7], 337 p. illus., port. 13 cm. **[1210]**
Added engraved title page.

—*See* SAUMAISE, C. de. Interpretatio Hippocratei aphorismi LXIX. sectione IV. de calculo. 1640.

BEVERWYCK, JOHAN VAN. *See* BEVERWIJCK, Jan van [1594-1647]

BEVILAQUA, ANTONIUS. Tractatus specialis de curatione febrium malignarum, quem singulari cura, & lucubratione in multorum utilitatem & salutem elaborare, & in publicam lucem emittere voluit ... Graecii, Apud haeredes Widmanstadii, 1682.

[8], 57, [2] p. 20 cm. **[1211]**
Errata: p. [59]

BEWARE of pick-purses. 1605. *See* [OBERNDÖRFER, J.]

BEWERLINUS, JOHANNES JACOBUS [*fl.* 1650-1651] *respondent. See* BARTHOLIN, T., *praeses.* Cygni anatome ejusque cantus. 1650.

BEX, ABRAHAM [*fl.* 1680] *respondent.* Disputatio medica inauguralis de melancholia ... Ultrajecti, Ex officina Francisci Halma, 1680.

[16] p. 20 cm. **[1212]**
Diss. — Utrecht.

BEY, JEAN LE. *See* LE BEY, Jean.

BEYER, GEORG [1665-1714] Bey hochansehnlicher Beerdigung der ... Frauen Annen Sabinen gebohrnen Schüssin, des ... Herrn Christian Wolffs Medicinae Doct ... Ehe-Liebsten, welche den 28. Septembr. 1693. in ihren Erlöser entschlaffen, und den 1. Octobr. zu ihrer Ruhestätte ins Paulinum gebracht worden, solte dem ... Hn. Wittber ... sein schuldiges Beyleid in Eyl bezeigen Georg Beyer ... Leipzig, Johann Heinrich Richter [1693]

[4] p. 31 cm. **[1213]**

BEYER, JAN [*fl.* 1669] *respondent.* Disputatio medica inauguralis de febre hectica ... Lugduni Batavorum, Apud viduam & haeredes Joannis Elsevirii, 1669.

[26] p. 23 cm. **[1214]**
Diss. — Leyden.

BEYER, JOANNES [*fl.* 1647] *ed. See* SALA, A. Opera medico-chymica. 1647.

BEYER, JOHANN FRIEDRICH [*fl.* 1685-1687] *respondent.* Theses medicae inaugurales casum de pleuritide examinantes ... Lugduni Batavorum, Apud Abrahamum Elzevier, 1687.

[16] p. 19 cm. **[1215]**
Diss. — Leyden.

—*See* VATER, C., *praeses.* Motum sanguinis per venam portae ... exponet J.F.B. 1685.

BEYER, JOHANN HARTMANN [1563-1625] *ed. See* CAPIVACCIO, G. Medendi methodus universalis tabulis comprehensa. 1606 [and] Opera omnia. 1603, 1617; FABRICIUS, H., *ab Aquapendente.* Pentateuchos cheirurgicum. 1604; MERCADO, L. Opera omnia. 1608 [and] Operum tomus primus [-quintus] 1614-1620; VALESCO DE TARANTA. Philonium pharmaceuticum et chirurgicum, de medendis omnibus ... humani corporis affectibus a Valesco de Taranta. 1680.

BEYER, PHILIPP HEINRICH [*fl.* 1666-1669] *respondent.* Disputatio inauguralis medica de rabie seu hydrophobia ... Gissae, Literis Kargerianis [1669]

[2], 31, [3] p. 19 cm. **[1216]**
Diss. — Giessen.

BEYNON, ELIAS, *the younger. See* BEYNON, Elias [*fl.* 1665]

BEYNON, ELIAS [*fl.* 1665] Barmhertziger Samariter; oder, Freund brüderlicher Rath, vor allerhand Kranchkheiten und Gebrechen dess menschlichen Leibs, dieselbigen mit geringen verachteten Mitteln und Artzneien ... zu heilen ... Und in besondere zwey Theile, mit einen nützlichen Anhange etzlicher Regeln von Erhaltung guter Gesundheit, eingetheilet ... Anjetzo zum vierten Mahle gedruckt. [n. p.] 1670.

[5], 362 (i.e. 365), [12] p. illus. 14 cm. **[1217]**
"Dess Barmhertzigen Samariters anderer Theil" has special title page (p. [114]).

—Der neuvermehrte und barmhertzige Samariter; oder, Freund-brüderlicher Rath, allerhand Kranckheiten und Gebrechen des Menschlichen Leibes ... zu heilen ... Mit Anhang, guter Haussmittel, für schwangere, gebährende Frauen, und kleine Kinder ... [n. p.] 1677.

[5], 85, [6] p. illus. 16 cm. **[1218]**

—Barmhertziger Samariter; oder, Freundbrüderlicher Rath, allerhand Kranckheiten und Gebrechen des menschlichen Leibs ... zu heilen ... Auch einem sehr nutzlichen Unterricht vor die Hebammen in allen zustossenden Fällen. Nebst einem neuen Anhang von der Pest ... Anjetzo aufs neu übersehen, und von vielen Druck-fehlern gereiniget. Sultzbach, Abraham Lichtenthaler, 1685.

[8], 7–330 (i.e. 332), [12], 108 p.   14 cm.

[1219]

Added engraved title page.

"Des Barmhertzigen Samariters anderer Theil" has special title page (p. [119]).

"Anthora, das ist: Gifft-heil, oder Beschreibung des Giffts der Pestilentz ... durch P[aul] F[elgenhauer]": p. [53]–108 at end, has special title page.

— Barmhertziger Samariter; oder Freundbruderlicher Raht, allerhand Kranckheiten und Gebrechen des menschlichen Leibs ... zu hailen, mit geringen und verachteten Mitteln und Artzneyen ... Neben einem neuen Anhange eines sehr nutzlichen Underrichts vor die Heb-Ammen in allen zustossenden Fällen ... Basel, Johann Conrad von Mechel, 1686.

[3], 360, [8] p.   15 cm.   [1220]

Added engraved title page.

Imperfect: p. 333–334 mutilated.

"Des Barmhertzigen Samariters anderer Theil" has special title page (p. [111]). "Kurtzer und nutzlicher Underricht vor die Heb-Ammen" (p. [313]–360) also has special title page.

— Barmhertziger Samariter, oder: Freundbrüderlicher Raht, allerhand Kranckheiten und Gebrechen dess menschlichen Leibs ... zu heilen ... Auch einem sehr nutzlichen Unterricht vor die Hebammen in allen zustossenden Fällen, nebst einem neuen Anhang von der Pest ... Nürnberg, Johann Hoffmann, 1696.

[1], 346, 49, [11] p.; 58 p.   14 cm.

[1221]

Added engraved title page.

"Dess barmhertzigen Samariters anderer Theil" has special title page dated 1695 (p. [127]).

Part [2] has special title page: Kurtzer und nützlicher Unterricht für die Hebammen. Part [3] has special title page: Anthora; das ist, Gifft-heil, oder: Beschreibung dess Giffts der Pestilentz ... geschrieben durch P[aul] F[elgenhauer]

— [The same.] ... Nürnberg, Verlegts Johann Hoffmanns seel, Wittib, und Engelbert Streck, 1700.

[1222]

— [Danish tr.] Barmhjertige Samaritan; eller, Broderlig-kjerligheds raad for allehaande legemlige siugdomme oc strøbelige tilfalde i mennisken baade

... at hielpe ... Til fleeres beste paa Danske udsat. Kiøbenhafn, Hos Daniel Paulli, 1682.

[7], 224, [8] p.; [16] p.   front.   16 cm.

[1223]

Added engraved title page.

"En kort underviiszning at forekomme oc curere den grasserende blod-soet, for fattige oc rige ... forfattet aff Facultate medica. Kiøbenhaffn, Hos Daniel Paulli, 1677" [16] p. at end has special title page.

— [The same.] ... Kiøbenhafn, Hos Johann Jost Erytropilo, 1696.

[7], 224, [24] p.   front.   16 cm.   [1224]

Imperfect: sig. A1–4 wanting; supplied in photocopy. Different setting of type.

— [French tr.] Le samaritain charitable; ou, Advis et conseil salutaire pour la guerison de toutes maladies, playes & ulceres du corps humain ... Traduit d'allemand en françois par Louys Franc. Geneve, Jean Herman Widerhold [1673]

[15], 96 p.; [7], 144, [6] p.   18 cm.   [1225]

Part 2 has special title page: Suite du samaritain charitable. Seconde partie.

Part 2 was published separately also with a title page of different setting of type.

Imperfect: p. 49–64 of part 2 wanting, bound in instead is p. 49–69 of Jacob de Constant de Rebecque's La chirurgien charitable.

Bound with La medecine domestique. 1673.

— Suite du Samaritain charitable, où il se trouve toutes sortes de medicaments & remedes éprouvés par diverses personnes qui s'en sont tres-bien trouvées ... Le tout fait en faveur des pauvres bourgeois & paysans, lesquels dans la necessité n'ont pas le moyen d'avoir un medecin expert, & faire la despense pour avoir des remedes chers & precieux ... Traduit d'alleman en françois par Louys Franc ... Geneve, Jean Herman Widerholdt, 1673.

[7], 144, [6] p.   17 cm.   [1226]

Issued also (with a title page of different setting of type) as part [2] of Beynon, E. Le samaritain charitable. [1673]

Bound with Constant de Rebecque, J. de. Le chirurgien charitable. 1673.

BEZA, JOHANN ADAM [*fl.* 1659–1660] *respondent. See* SEBISCH, J. A., *praeses.* Disputatio medica de syncope. 1659; SEBISCH, M. [1578–1674?] *praeses.* Disputatio solennis de variis medicae artis curationis problematibus. 1660.

BEZA, THEODORUS. *See* BÈZE, Théodore de [1519–1605]

BEZANÇON, GERMAIN DE [*fl.* 1676] Les medecins a la censure; ou, Entretiens sur la medecine . . . Paris, Louis Gontier, 1677.

    [12], 370, [1] p. 16 cm.   **[1227]**

[—] La medecine pretendüe reformée, ou l'examen d'un traité des fievres imprimé à Utrecht, & composé par un auteur hollandois, qui pretend renverser toutes les opinions des medecins anciens & modernes . . . Paris, L. d'Houry, 1683.

    165, [3] p. 16 cm.   **[1228]**

BÈZE, THÉODORE DE [1519-1605] De pestis contagio & fuga dissertatio. Accessit Andreae Riveti ejusdem argumenti epistola; in qua & mos, cadavera mortuorum in templis sepeliendi, redarguitur. Lugd. Batav., Ex Officina Elseviriorum, 1636.

    [12], 154, [1] p. 13 cm.   **[1229]**

Edited by Adolph Vorstius.

"Andrë Riveti Epistola . . .": p. 61-129.

"Illustria aliquot . . . exempla, per quae pestis vis effera & contagiosa, a nonnullis in dubium vocata, confirmatur" (p. [130]-154) added by the printer. (Cf. p. [130])

Errata: p. [154]

  —*See* Variorum tractatus theologici de peste. 1655.

BEZOLD, NIKOLAUS CHRISTOPH [*b.* 1675] *See* SLEVOGT, J. A. Decani Facultatis Medicae Jo. Hadriani Slevogtii . . . invitatio publica ad dissertationem inauguralem de ulceribus crurum antiquis. 1699.

  — *respondent. See* CRAUSE, R. W., *praes.* Dissertatio inauguralis medica de ulceribus crurum antiquis. 1699; WEDEL, G. W., *praes.* Lemmata medica. 1699.

BIANA, JUAN DE. *See* VIANA MENTESANO, Juan de [*fl.* 1636-1649]

BIANCHI, PAOLO EMILIO [*fl. ca.* 1620] De partu hominis liber. Omnibus non medicis modo, sed etiam jurisperitis admodum utilis, & necessarius. In quo praeter omnium opinionem rationibus admodum validis, & auctoritatibus ostenditur, quod sexto mense partus vitae superstes esse potest, & naturalis . . . Papiae, Jo. Baptista Rubeus, 1621.

    [8], 116 p. 22 cm.   **[1230]**

BIARD, GABRIELE [*fl.* 1633] *praeses.* Quaestio medica . . . An imbecillitati ventriculi quae vis roborantia? Ed. 2. [Paris? 1647]

    2 p. 24 cm.   **[1231]**

Caption title.

Diss.—Paris, 1633 (J. Pietre, *respondent*)

BIBLE. O. T. Psalm XCI. *German. Paraphrase.* 1633. Cunrad. Der XCI. Psalm, neben noch einem Gebethe umd gnädige Abwendung gegenwärtiger Pest, poëtisch gesetzet von Christian Cunraden. Breslaw, Georg Baumann, 1633.

    [7] p. 18 cm.   **[1232]**

BIBLIOTHECA chalcographica. *See* BOISSARD, J. J.

BIBLIOTHECA exotica; sive, Catalogus officinalis librorum peregrinis linguis usualibus scriptorum. 1610. *See* [DRAUD, G.]

BIBLIOTHECA medico-philosophico-philologica. 1677. *See* STOCKHAMER, F.

La BIBLIOTHEQUE des acoucheurs [sic] et des sages-femmes. Contenant le Traité des maladies des femmes grosses, & de celles nouvellement acouchées. Par M. Mauriceau . . . La pratique des acouchemens soûtenuë d'un grand nombre d'observations. Par Paul Portal . . . Avec une Dissertation curieuse sur la generation, & la nutrition de fétus dan la matrice suivant l'opinion des modernes. [Geneve, Jacques Dentant, 1693]

    3 parts in 1 v. illus., plates. 23 cm.

                        [1233]

Engraved title page.

Mauriceau's Traité has special title page dated 1693 and added engraved title page (illustrated) dated 1682. Portal's La pratique des acouchemens has half title. The Dissertation sur la generation des animaux has caption title.

BICAISE, HONORÉ [*b.* 1590] Discours des causes, effects tant physics que moraux, preservatif general & individuel de la peste . . . Par M. H. Bicays . . . Aix, Jean Roize, 1630.

    [8], 132 p. 13 cm.   **[1234]**

  —*Comp. See* HIPPOCRATES. [Selections, etc. Latin] Manuale medicorum. 1637, 1659, 1660.

BICAISE, MICHEL [17th cent.] La maniere de regler la santé par ce qui nous environne, par ce que nous recevons, et par les exercices, ou par la gymnastique moderne . . . Aix, Charles David, 1669.

    [11], 337, [3] p. 18 cm.   **[1235]**

BICKER, JOHANN [*fl.* 1608-1611] Hermes redivivus, declarans hygieinam, de sanitate vel bona valetudine hominis conservanda. In qua omnia ex antiquae sapientiae fontibus, Hippocrate, Galeno, aliisque Graecis & Arabibus atque Latinis deducuntur, cum chymiatrorum principiis & Paracelsi dogmatibus veris conjunguntur & methodice describuntur. Giessae, Impensis Casparis Chemlini & Antonii Humm, 1612.

    [29], 480 (i.e. 482) p. 16 cm.   **[1236]**
Imperfect: p. 479-480 wanting.

—[The same.] ... Hanoviae, Impensis Conradi Eifridi, 1620.

    [29], 480 (i.e. 482) p. 16 cm.   **[1237]**
A reissue of the 1612 Giessen edition with new title page and preliminary matter reset.

BIDLOO, GODEFRIED. *See* BIDLOO, Govard [1649-1713]

BIDLOO, GOVARD [1649-1713] Anatomia humani corporis centum & quinque tabulis, per artificiosiss. G. de Lairesse ad vivum delineatis, demonstrata ... Amstelodami, Sumptibus viduae Joannis à Someren, haeredum Joannis à Dyk. Henrici & viduae Theodori Boom, 1685.

    [138] p. port., plates. 53 cm.   **[1238]**
Added engraved title page.
Imperfect: portrait wanting.

—[Dutch tr.] Ontleding des menschelyken lichaams ... uitgebeeld, naar het leeven, in honderd en vyf aftekeningen, door de Heer Gerard de Lairesse ... Amsterdam, By de weduwe van Joannes van Dyk, Hendrik en de weduwe van Dirk Boom, 1690.

    [138] p. port., plates. 53 cm.   **[1239]**
Added engraved title page.

—Brief ... aan Antony van Leeuwenhoek, wegens de dieren, welke men zomtyds in de lever der schaapen en andere beesten vind. Delft, Henrik van Kroonevelt, 1698.

    [1], 34 p. illus., plate. 21 cm.   **[1240]**
Bound with vol. 6 of Leeuwenhoek, A. van. Ondekte onsigtbaarheeden. 1694-1718.

—Dissertatio de antiquitate anatomes, habita in auditorio magno, cum anatomicam professorus, in alma Academia Batava inauguraretur. Anno MDCXCIV octavo iduum Martii. Lugduni Batavorum, Apud Abrahamum Elzevier, 1694.

    [6], 26, [10], p. 39 cm.   **[1241]**

—Gulielmus Cowper, criminis literarii citatus, coram tribunali ... Societatis Britanno-regiae [sic] ... Lugduni Batavorum, Apud Jordanum Luchtmans, 1700.

    [1], 54 p. plates. 24 cm.   **[1242]**

—Oratio, in funere viri clarissimi Pauli Hermanni ... Ed. alt. Lugduni Batavorum, Apud Abrahamum Elzevier, 1695.

    [4], 28 p. 24 cm.   **[1243]**

—Vindiciae quarundam delineationum anatomicarum, contra ineptas animadversiones Fred. Ruyschii ... Lugd. Batavorum, Apud Jordanum Luchtmans, 1697.

    [1], 60 p. illus., plates. 22 cm.   **[1244]**

—*praeses.* Disputatio medica inauguralis de chlorosi, sive morbo virgineo ... Lugduni Batavorum, Apud Abrahamum Elzevier, 1696.

    [16] p. 23 cm.   **[1245]**
Diss.—Leyden (P. Maton, *respondent*)

—*See* RUYSCH, F. Responsio ad Godefridi Bidloi libellum. 1697; STEENEVELT, C. a. Dissertatio, de ulcere verminoso. 1697.

BIDLOO, JOHANNES [*fl.* 1666] *respondent.* Disputatio medica inauguralis de peste ... Lugduni Batavorum, Ex officina Petri & Cornelii Hackii, 1666.

    [23] p. 24 cm.   **[1246]**
Diss.—Leyden.

BIECHLING, JOHANN [*fl.* 1692] *respondent.* Disputatio medica inauguralis de variolis ... Lugduni Batavorum, Apud Abrahamum Elzevier, 1692.

    [16] p. 21 cm.   **[1247]**
Diss.—Leyden.

BIENDISANT, CLAUDE [*fl.* 1666-1647] *praeses.* Quaestio medica ... An pleuritidi saphenae sectio? [Parisiis, Ex typographia Francisci Muguet, 1674]

    4 p. 25 cm.   **[1248]**
Caption title.
Diss.—Paris (F. Afforty, *respondent*)

BIERLING, CASPER GOTTLIEB [*d.* 1693] Adversariorum curiosorum centuria prima, cum annexis scholiis & appendice variorum, tam chimicorum quam aliorum medicamentorum. Jenae, Sumptibus Johannis Lüderwald, typis Samuelis Krebsii, 1679.

    [8], 261, [3] p.; 188, [16] p. 21 cm.   **[1249]**
Part [2] has half title: Appendix variorum, tam chimicorum, tam aliorum medicamentorum.

—Thesaurus theoretico-practicus, continens praesertim observationes & curationes medicas salutares de praecipuis corporis humani affectibus aliisque rebus medicis ac physicis curiosis, consignatas, & Joh. Michaelis ... arcanis, euporistis, uti & aliis notis proficuis modernae praxi congruis, nec non scholiis instructas atque illustratas ... atque propter inopinatam autoris mortem praefixa praefatio Jacobi Wolff ... [Jenae, Literis Krebsianis] Sumptibus haeredum Johannis Lüderwaldi, 1695.

[1], 8, 1236, [23] p.   front.   20 cm.   [1250]

—[The same.] Medicus theoretico-practicus ostendens observationes & curationes medicas salutares de praecipuis corporis humani affectibus aliisque rebus medicis ac physicis curiosis ad mentem Helmontii, Willisii, Sylvii, aliorumque neotericorum scriptorum, eorumque praestantissimorum ... [Jenae, Literis Krebsianis] Sumptibus autoris [sic] 1697.

[8], 1236, [23] p.   20 cm.   [1251]

A reissue of the 1695 edition of his Thesaurus Theoretico-practicus, substituting new preliminary matter for the original preface by Jacob Wolf.

—Problema pharmaceutico-medicum an in nostra Magdeburgensi peste medicamenta ἄνω καὶ κάτω evacuantia, tuto ... adhibita fuerint, necne ... Helmstadi, Typis Conradi Erichii, apud Johannem Lüderwald, 1684.

32 (i.e. 47) p.   20 cm.   [1252]

BIERLING, Caspar Theophil. See Bierling, Casper Gottlieb [d. 1693]

BIERLING, Johann Georg [fl. 1679] respondent. See Müller J., [fl. 1672-1679] praeses. Disputatio physica de corporum defunctorum operationibus. 1679.

BIERMANN, Martin [fl. 1588-1594] See Tandler, T. Dissertationes physicae-medicae. 1613.

BIESTER, Johann Peter [b. 1669] See Wedel, G. W. Propemticon inaugurale de physiologia exidii sodomorum et statuae salis. 1692.

—, respondent. See Wedel, G. W., praeses. Dissertatio medica de notis gravidarum. 1690 [and] Dissertatio medica inauguralis de natura et usu acidorum. 1692.

BIESTER, Peter [fl. 1659-1664] respondent. Disputatio medica inauguralis de phthisi ...

Lugduni Batavorum, Apud Gualterum de Haes, 1664.

[20] p.   19 cm.   [1253]

Diss.—Leyden.

BIFFI, Giovanni Ambrogio, tr. See Porta, G. B. della. Della Fisionomia dell'huomo. 1644, 1668.

BIGGS, Noah. Mataeotechnia medicinae praxeωs. The vanity of the craft of physick; or, A new dispensatory. Wherein is dissected the errors, ignorance, impostures and supinities of the schools, in their main pillars of purges, blood-letting, fontanels or issues, and diet, &c. and the particular medicines of the shops. With an humble motion for the reformation of the universities, and the whole landscap of physick, and discovering the terra incognita of chymistrie. To the Parliament of England ... London, Giles Calvert, 1651.

[31], 232 p.   19 cm.   [1254]

BILBERG, Johan [1646-1717] praeses. Specimen cogitationum de magnetismis rerum ... Stockholmiae, Excudebat Nicolaus Wankijf, 1683.

[43] p.   20 cm.   [1255]

Diss.—Stockholm (E. E. Odhelius, respondent)

BILGER, Johann Friedrich [1625-1708] Kurtze Beschreibung von Ursprung, Gelegenheit und Würckung, auch nutzlichen Gebrauch, dess in der Herrschafft Röttemberg ligenden heylsamen Bade, die Aw oder Burgeckh genannt ... Augspurg, Gedruckt bey Johann Schultes, 1653.

[6] p.   20 cm.   [1256]

—respondent. Disputatio inauguralis medica de lithiasi renum et vesicae ... Altdorphi, Typis Scherffianis [1645]

[16] p.   19 cm.   [1257]

Diss.—Altdorf.

BILGER, Philipp Friedrich [fl. 1698-1700] respondent. See Camerarius, R. J., praeses. De calculis renum et vesicae. 1698 [and] Dissertatio inauguralis de colore sanguinis. 1700.

BILITZER, Christopher [fl. 1607-1611] See Horst, G. [1578-1636] Dissertatio de natura amoris. 1611; Knobloch, T., praeses. Disputationes anatomicae. 1608, 1612.

BILLICH, Anton Günther [1598-1640] Anatome fermentacionis Platonicae. In Conring, H. De sanguinis generatione, et motu naturali. 1646.

—De tribus chymicorum principiis et quincta essentia exercitatio ... Bremae, Apud Thomam Villerianum, 1621.

[8], 69, [1] p. 16 cm.   [1258]

Bound with Follinus, H. Amuletum Antonianum. 1618.

—Observationum ac paradoxorum chymiatricorum libri duo: quorum unus medicamentorum chymicorum praeparationem: alter eorundem usum succincte perspicueque explicat. Lugduni Batavorum, Ex officina Joannis Maire, 1631.

173, [1] p. 20 cm.   [1259]

Engraved title page.
Imperfect: Sig. B1 wanting.

—Thessalus in chymicis redivivus; id est, De vanitate medicinae chymicae, Hermeticae, seu spagiricae dissertatio fundamentalis; ex ipsismet artis chymicaeproceribus Quercetano, Beguino Crollio, &c. deducta ... accessit Anatomia fermentationis Platonicae apodictica & paradoxologa ... Francofurti ad Moenum, Impensis Johannis Beyeri, typis Casparis Rötelii, 1640.

[16], 318 p. 17 cm.   [1260]

BILS, Lodewijk de [1623?-1669] Aan alle ware liefhebbers der anatomie. Rotterdam, Joannes Naeranus, 1659.

6 p. 20 cm.   [1261]

Bound with (as issued?) *his* Kopye van zekere ampele acte. 1659.

—[The same.] *In* Horne, J. van. Waerschouwinge, aen alle lieff-hebbers der anatomie. 1660.

—Brief ... aan Th. Bartholijn ... Rotterdam, Joannes Naeranus, 1661.

13 p. 19 cm.   [1262]

—Epistolica dissertatio, qua verus hepatis circa chylum, & pariter ductus chiliferi hactenus dicti usus, docetur. Roterodami, Typis Joannis Naerani, 1659.

6 p. plate. 20 cm.   [1263]

—Exemplar fusioris codicilli ... in quo agitur de vera humani corporis anatomia. Roterodami, Typis Joannis Naerani, 1659.

8 p. 20 cm.   [1264]

—Kopye van zekere ampele acte van Jr. Louijs de Bils ... rakende de wetenschap van de oprechte anatomije des menselijken lichaams. Rotterdam, Joannes Naeranus, 1659.

8 p. 20 cm.   [1265]

With this is bound (as issued?) *his* Aan alle ware liefhebbers der anatomie. 1659.

—Kort bericht over de waarschouwinge van de Heer ... Joan van Horne ... als mede een antwoord op de aanmerkingen van de Heer Paulus Barbette ... op d'anatomische schriften van ... Lodewijk de Bils ... Rotterdam, Joannes Naeranus, 1660.

42 p. plate. 19 cm.   [1266]

—Omnibus verae anatomes studiosis. Roterodami, Apud Joannem Naeranum, 1660.

[4] p. 20 cm.   [1267]

—Responsio ad admonitiones D^i. Johannis ab Horne ... ut & ad animadversiones D^i. Pauli Barbette ... in academia Bilsiana. Interprete G. Buenio. Roterodami, Ex officina Arnoldi Leers, 1661.

80 p. plate. 20 cm.   [1268]

"Ludovici de Bils ... ad Th. Bartholinum ... epistola": p. 33-39.
"Antonii Deusingii ... appendix exercitationum: in qua de admiranda anatome ... Ludovici de Bils"; p. 40-77.
Bound with *his* Specimina anatomica. 1661.

—Responsio ... ad literas ad ipsum datas & nuper transmissas a ... Tobia Andreae ... qua ostenditur verus usus vasorum hactenus pro lymphaticis habitorum ... Cum adjecta delineatione suorum actorum anatomicorum; nec non brevi ac compendiosa historia eorum, quae spectant artem ac scientiam condiendi balsamo singulari ac methodo nulli hactenus communi humana cadavera. Roterodami, Ex officina Arnoldi Leers, 1669.

46 p. 20 cm.   [1269]

—Specimina anatomica, cum clariss. doctissimorumque virorum epistolis aliquot & testimoniis. Interprete G. Buenio ... Roterodami, Ex officina Arnoldi Leers, 1661.

27 p. plates. 20 cm.   [1270]

Descriptions by F. de Raedt, A. Parent, and L. Jordaen, of dissections carried out by L. de Bils.
With this are bound (as issued?): Zas, N. Epistola apologetica. 1661; *his* Responsio ad admonitiones D^i. Johannis ab Horne. 1661.

—Waarachtig gebruik der tot noch toe gemeende gijlbuis, beneffens de verrijzenis der lever, voorheen zoo lichtvaardig in't graf gestooten ... Briefsgewijze bekend gemaakt aan ... L. Jordaan. Rotterdam, Joannes Naeranus, 1658.

11 p. plate. 20 cm.   [1271]

—Waerachtig vertoog der handelinge van de anatomie ... Rotterdam, Arnout Leers, 1668.

62 p. 17 cm. [1272]

Bound with Blasius, G. Ontleeding des menschelyken lichaems. 1675.

—*See* DEUSING, A. Erercitationes [sic] physico-anatomicae, de nutrimenti in corpore elaboratione. 1660; PAULLI, J. H. Anatomiae Bilsianae anatome. 1665; STEPHANUS, N. Castigatio epistolae maledicae. 1661; ZAS, N. Epistola apologetica ad magnum Th. Bartholinum. 1661.

—*as subject. See* BARTHOLIN, T. Dissertatio anatomica de hepate defuncto novis Bilsianorum observationibus opposita. 1661 [and] Responsio de experimentis anatomicis Bilsianis et difficili hepatis resurrectione. 1661; GUTSCHOVEN, G. van. Description de cinq corps embaûmez et anatomisez. 1662?; PARENT, A. Anatomisch vertoon ven het ghehoor by ... Louys de Bils. 1655; PAULLI, J. H., *praeses.* Anatome anatomiae Bilsianae. 1663; RAEDT, F. de Anatomische beschrijvinge van een wanschepsel. 1659; SORBIÈRE, S. Extraict d'un discours ... touchant l'estat des sciençes en Hollande. 166-?; STENO, N., *Bp.* Observationes anatomicae. 1662, 1680; ZAS, N. Brief. 1661 [and] Den dauw der dieren. 1660.

BIMET, CLAUDE [*fl.* 1663] Quatrains anatomiques des os et des muscles du corps humain: ensemble un discours de la circulation du sang ... Lyon, Marc-Antoine Gaudet, 1664.

[12], 94 p. 17 cm. [1273]

BIMIUS, LEONARDUS J. [17th cent.] Pestis ad vivum delineata et curata ... Leodici Eburonum, Apud Guilielmum Henricum Streel, 1671.

[8], 71 p. 15 cm. [1274]

Imperfect: wormholes on first 4 leaves.

BIMIUS, PAULUS HIERONYMUS. *See* BIUMI, Paolo Girolamo [*d.* 1731]

BINDER, CHRISTOPH [1575-1616] Αἰτιολογικὸν theologicum, de causis pestis: methodo analytica explicatis. Ubi animadvertet lector in ipsa διεξόδω, & rejectione causarum ignorantiae, tractari quaestiones: an morbi in genere, & pestis in specie, fieri possint, vel fiant? Vel I. Daemonum operatione, & insidiis? II. Astrorum motu, influentia, configuratione? III. Fatali lege, & immutabili necessitate? IV.

Casu & fortuito ... Tubingae, Typis Theodorici Werlini, Sumptibus Johannis Berneri, 1611.

[1], 106 p. 15 cm. [1275]

BINDI, GIOVANNI BATISTA [*fl. ca.* 1656] Loemographiae Centumcellensis; sive, De historia pestis contagiosae, quae anno intercalari MDCLVI. in ecclesiastica ditione primum civitatem veterem invasit, & inde in pontificiarum triremium ducem fuit illata, libri quinque ... Romae, Typis Varesii, 1658.

[19], 190, [16] p. 24 cm. [1276]

BINET, ÉSTIENNE [*d. ca.* 1628] *ed. See* COURTIN G. Leçons anatomiques et chirurgicales. 1612, 1656.

BINET, ÉTIENNE, *Father* [1569-1639] Essay des merveilles de nature, et des plus nobles artifices ... Par René François [pseud.] 8. ed., corr. & augm ... Rouen, Jean Osmont, 1631.

[16], 607 p. illus. 17 cm. [1277]

BINETEAU, JULIEN [*fl.* 1650-1656] La seignee reformee, ses abus, son mauvais & trop frequent usage corrigé par quantité de raisons naturelles, & d'autoritez d'Hipocrate, & de Galen ... Lafleche, Par Gervais Laboe, et se vend a Paris, chez Jean Hesnault, 1656.

[24], 211 p. 14 cm. [1278]

BINNART, MARTIN [17th cent.] Biglotton amplificatum; sive, Dictionarium Teutonico-Latinum novum ... Hac editione mendis quam plurimis expurgatum, dictionibusque non paucis locupletatum. Amstelodami, Ex officina Abrahami a Someren, 1688.

[536] p. 19 cm. [1279]

BINNINGER, JOHANN NIKOLAUS [*b.* 1628] Observationum et curationum medicinalium, centuriae quinque ... Montbelgardi, Apud authorem, typis Hyppianis, 1673.

[16], 622, [22] p. port. 18 cm. [1280]

—*respondent. See* STUPANUS, E., *praeses.* Signorum medicorum doctrina. 1649.

BIONDO, MICHELANGELO [1497-1565] *See* UFFENBACH, P. Thesaurus chirurgicae. 1610.

BIRD, JOHN [*fl.* 1660] Ostenta Carolina; or, The late calamities of England with the authors of them. The great happiness and happy government of K. Charles II ensuing miraculously foreshewn by the finger of God in two ... diseases, the rekets and kings-evil ... London, Printed for Fra. Sowle, and sold by Robert Harrison, 1661.

[8], 91 p.   91 p.   19 cm.   [**1281**]

Pages 49-56 (sheet H) in duplicate.

BIRINGUCCI, CARLO [*d.* 1648] L'assistente christiano ... Si dimostrano gli effetti della buona assistenza, è si scuoprono gl'inganni, & errori, che giornalmente succedono nelle case dove sono ammalati, Aggiuntovi la Cura spirituale dell'anima per qualunque infermo. Roma, Per li HH. del Corbelletti, 1655.

[24], 288 p.   16 cm.   [**1282**]

Added engraved title page.

BIRINGUCCIO, VANNOCCIO [1480-1539?] *See* A PUTEO, Z. Clavis medica rationalis spagyrica. 1612.

BIRKEN, SIGMUND VON [1626-1681] *tr. See* BALDE, J., *Father.* Die truckene Trunkenheit. 1658.

BIRNBAUM, ABRAHAM [1612-1695] *respondent. See* ROLFINCK, W., *praeses.* Disputatio inauguralis de catarrho. 1637.

BIRNBAUM, GOTTFRIED SIGMUND [*fl.* 1671-1674] respondent. *See* ALBERTI V. De sternutatione. 1671; BOHN, J., *praeses.* Dissertatio physiologico-pathologica de lactis defectu. 1674.

BIRR, MARTIN [*fl.* 1648-1649] *respondent. See* BRUNN, J. J. von, *praeses.* Disputatio medica de humoribus. 1648; STUPANUS, E., *praeses.* Signorum medicorum doctrina. 1649.

BIRRIUS, MARTINUS [*b. ca.* 1625] *See* [PHILALETHES, E.] Tres tractatus de metallorum transmutatione. 1668.

BISCACCIANTI DA FONTE, LELIO [*d.* 1643] Laelii a Fonte Eugubini ... consultationes medicinales ... Ejusdem disputationes duae ... una de modo visionis; altera de vesicantium usu ... Venetiis, Apud Joannem Guerilium, 1609.

[40], 458, [2] p.   34 cm.   [**1283**]

—[The same.] ... Nunc primum in Germania editae. Francofurti ad Moenum, Impensis Rulandior, typis Matthiae Beckeri, 1609.

[16], 942, [95] p.   19 cm.   [**1284**]

BISCIOLA, PAOLO [*b.* 1555] Relatione verissima del progresso della peste di Milano. Qual principio'

nel mese d'agosto 1576 e segui sino al mese di maggio 1577 ... Dove si raccontano tutte le provisioni fatte da ... Cardinal Borromemo, & di sua eccellenza, senato, & signori deputati sopra la sanità. Dove si può imparare, il vero modo d'un perfetto pastore amator del suo gregge: e come un principe deve governar una città, nel tempo di peste, cosa molto utile. Con un raguaglio, del seguito della sua liberatione per sino alli 20. di luglio 1577. Bologna, Per Carlo Malisardi, ad instanza di Sebastiano Balestra, 1630.

[4], 30, [2] p.   20 cm.   [**1285**]

"Relatione d'alcuni casi occorsi in Venetia al tempo della peste l'anno 1576 e 1577": p. 17-30.

BISCOP, JAN [*fl.* 1662] *respondent.* Disputatio medica inauguralis de motu cordis & palpitatione ejus ... Lugduni Batavorum, Apud Franciscum Moyart, 1662.

[16] p.   21 cm.   [**1286**]

Diss. — Leyden.

BITISKIUS, FRIEDRICH, *ed. See* PARACELSUS. Opera omnia medico-chemico-chirurgica. 1658.

BITTERKRAUT, JOHANN CHRISTOPH [*fl.* 1670-1677] Wehmühtige Klag-Thränen der löblichen höchst-betrangten Artzney-Kunst, durch welche der betrübte elende Stand dieser edlen Wissenschafft ... vorgestellet wird ... [Nuremberg] Gedruckt und verlegt durch Michael und Johann Friderich Endter, 1677.

[32], 660, [37] p.   20 cm.   [**1287**]

Added engraved title page.

Imperfect: p. [37] (errata) mutilated.

Imprint partly supplied from Zedler, vol. 3. col. 1993.

—*ed.* and *tr. See* MYL, A. van der. Merchkwürdiger Discurss von dem Ursprung der Thier. 1670.

BIUMI, PAOLO GIROLAMO [*d.* 1731] *See* HIPPOCRATES. Prognostica. Adaptationa, etc. Latin. 1696.

BIX, JOHANN ULRICH [*fl.* 1673-1677] *respondent. See* MAPP, M., *praeses.* Tractationis medicae du potu calido. 1673.

BLACKBURNE, RICHARD [*b.* 1652] Vitae Hobbianae auctarium. *In* Thomae Hobbes Angli Malmesburiensis philosophi vita. 1682.

BLACKLOW, THOMAS. *See* WHITE, Thomas [1593-1676]

BLADIN, Pierre [*fl.* 1612–1613] *respondent. See* Stupanus, J. N., *praeses.* Exercitatio physico-medica. 1612.

BLAES, Abraham. *See* Blasius, Abrahamus [*b.* 1650]

BLAES, Gerard. *See* Blasius, Gerardus [1626?–1692?]

BLAGRAVE, Joseph [1610–1682] Astrological practice of physick discovering, the true way to cure all kinds of diseases . . . Being performed by such herbs and plants which grow within our own nation . . . Also, a discovery of some notable phylosophical secrets . . . London, Printed by S. G. and B. G. for Obad. Blagrave, 1671.

[24], 187 (i.e. 154), [4] p.   illus.   17 cm.
[**1288**]

—[The same.] . . . London, Obadiah Blagrave, 1689.

[16], 139, [5] p.   illus.   18 cm.   [**1289**]

—Supplement or enlargement, the Mr. Nich. Culpeppers English physitian. Containing a description of the form, names, place, time, coelestial government, and virtues, of all such medicinal plants as grow in England, and are omitted to his book . . . To which is annexed, a new tract for the cure of wounds made by gun-shot . . . London, Obadiah Blagrave, 1674.

[4], 237, [15], 46 p.   18 cm.   [**1290**]

—Another issue, dated 1677.   [**1291**]

Imperfect: p. 45–46 of "A new tract for the cure of wounds made by gun-shot" wanting.

Bound with Culpeper, N. The English physitian enlarged. 1681.

BLANCARD, Stephen. *See* Blankaart, Steven [1650–1702]

BLANCARDI, Michele [*fl.* 1678] *ed. See* Bartoli, S. Thermologia Aragonia. 1679.

BLANCARDUS, Nicolaus. *See* Blankaart, Nikolaas [1624–1703]

BLANCKAERT, Nicolaas. *See* Blankaart, Nikolaas [1624–1703]

BLANCKAERT, Steven. *See* Blankaart, Steven [1650–1702]

BLANCKEN, Gerardus. Catalogus antiquarum et novarum rerum ex longe dissitis terrarum oris congestis, quarum visendarum copia Lugduni in Batavis in anatomica publica, curiosis spectatoribus datur . . . Lugduni Batavorum, Typis Huberti vander Boxe, 1700.

14, [2] p.   20 cm.   [**1292**]

—*See* [Voorn, J.] Catalogus antiquarum et novarum rerum. 1690?

BLANCQUEBYL, Johannes [*fl.* 1689] *respondent.* Disputatio medica inauguralis, de dolore colico . . . Trajecti ad Rhenum, Ex officina Francisci Halma, 1689.

24, [2] p.   22 cm.   [**1293**]

Diss.—Utrecht.

BLANCUS, Paulus Emilius. *See* Bianchi, Paolo Emilio [*fl. ca.* 1620]

BLANK, Georg Jakob [*fl.* 1674] *See* Pechlin, J. N. Facultatis Medicae h. t. decanus Johannes Nicolaus Pechlin . . . officiose invitat. 1674.

—*respondent. See* Pechlin, J. N., *praeses.* Disputatio medica inauguralis de vulneribus sclopetorum in genere. 1674.

BLANKAART, Nikolaas [1624–1703] *See* Academia Franekerana. Acclamationes, ad . . . D. Nicolaum Blancardcum. 1670.

—*ed.* and *tr. See* Harpocration, V. Λ'εξιχὸν τῶν δέχα ῥητόϱων . . . Lexicon decem oratorum. 1683.

BLANKAART, Steven [1650–1702] Anatomia practica rationalis; sive, Rariorum cadaverum morbis denatorum anatomica inspectio. Accedit item Tractatus novus de circulatione sanguinis per tubulos, deque eorum valvulis &c. [4 ed.] Amstelodami, Ex officina Corn. Blancardi, 1688.

[23], 321, [12] p.   14 cm.   [**1294**]

Added engraved title page.

—Collectanea medico-physica; oft, Hollands Jaar-Register der genees- en natuur-kundige Aanmerkingen van gantsch Europa &c. Beginnende met het jaar 1680[–1688]. Door eigen ondervinding en gemeen-making van verscheide heeren en liefhebbers . . . Amsterdam, Johan ten Hoorn, 1680–1688.

3 v. in 1.   tables, port., plates.   16 cm.

[**1295**]

—[German tr.] Collectanea medico-physica; oder, Holländisch Jahr-Register, sonderbahrer Anmerckungen, die so wol in der Artzney-Kunst, als Wissenschaft der Natur in gantz Europa vorgefallen. Angefangen mit dem Jahr 1680[–1681]. Theils aus selbst eigener Erfindung, theils aus Communication unterschiedener Herren und Liebhaber zusammen getragen durch Stephanum Blankart ... Aus dem Holländischen in das Hoch-Teutsche übersetzet durch T. P. M. C. G. L. Leipzig, Verlegts Moritz George Weidmann, 1690.

2 v. in 1.   plates.   18 cm.   [1296]

—Het gast-huis der zieken, bestaande in verscheide medicinale gevallen in practyk, alle volgens de redeneringe der philosophie opgelost ... Nevens een Aanhangsel van verscheide medicinale consultatien, door brieven geschreven, rakende de praktyk der medicyne. Voorgevallen en uitgegeven door S[teven] B[lankaart]. Amsterdam, Timotheus ten Hoorn, 1690.

[8], 407 p.   16 cm.   [1297]

With this is bound *his* Nauwkeurige verhandelinge van de scheur-buik. 1684.

—De Kartesiaanse Academie; ofte, Institutie der medicyne, Behelsende de gansche medicyne ... Amsterdam, Johannes ten Hoorn, 1683.

[16], 440, [36] p.   plates.   16 cm.   [1298]

—[The same.] ... 2. druk. Amsterdam, Jan ten Hoorn, 1691.

[8], 438, [26] p.   plates.   16 cm.   [1299]

Imperfect: plate 7 wanting.
A corrected reprint of the 1683 edition.

—[German tr.] Cartesianische Academie; oder, Grund-Lehre der Artzney-Kunst, worinnen die völlige Artzney-Lehre, wie solche in Wissenschafft der Gesundheut und deren Erhaltung, auch in Erkäntnüss der Kranckheiten und ihrer Heilung bestehet, auf den natur-gemässen Gründen des weltberühmten Cartesii aufgeführet wird ... Anjetzo aus dem Niederländischen ins Hochdeutsche übersetzet. Zum andern Mahl aufgelegt. Leipzig, Verlegts Johann Friedrich Gleditsch, 1693.

[8], 408, 428, [60] p.   illus., plates.   17 cm.   [1300]

—Lexicon medicum, Graeco-Latinum, in quo termini totius artis medicae, secundum neotericorum placita, definiuntur vel circumscribuntur. Graecae item voces ex origine sua deducuntur, & Belgica nomina, si quae fuerint, adjunguntur. Amstelodami, Ex officina Johannis ten Hoorn, 1679.

[14], 318 (i.e. 314), [4] p.   front. (port.)   17 cm.   [1301]

—[The same.] ... Graeca item vocabula ex originibus suis deducuntur ... Nunc vero tertia fere parte auctum & pluribus in locis emendatum. Belgicis quoque prioris editionis nominibus Germanica ... in hac sunt substituta. Jenae, Literis Müllerianis, 1683.

[2], 505, [4] p.   17 cm.   [1302]

Errata: p. [509]
With this is bound: Johnson, W. Lexicon chymicum. 1678.

—[The same.] ... Lexicon novum medicum Graeco-Latinum, caeteris editionibus longe perfectissimum. In hoc enim totius artis medicae termini, in anatomia, chirurgia, pharmacia, chymia secundum neotericorum placita dilucide & vere exponuntur & definiuntur. Graecae quoque voces ex origine sua deducuntur; hisce praeterea adjungitur Belgica, Germanica, Gallica & Anglica interpretatio ... Lugduni Batavorum, Apud Cornelium Boutesteyn, Jordaanum Luchtmans, 1690.

[14], 661 (i.e. 639), [141] p.   front. (port), tables.   20 cm.   [1303]

—[English tr.] A physical dictionary; in which, all the terms relating either to anatomy, chirurgery, pharmacy, or chymistry, are very accurately explain'd ... London, Printed by J. D. and sold by Samuel Crouch and John Gellibrand, 1684.

[8], 302 (i.e. 304) p.   18 cm.   [1304]

—[The same.] The physical dictionary. Wherein the terms of anatomy, the names and causes of diseases, chyrurgical instruments and their use; are accurately describ'd. Also the names and virtues of medicinal plants, minerals, stones, gums, salts, earths, &c. and the method of choosing the best drugs ... The 2d ed., with the addition of above a thousand terms of art, and their explanation ... London, S. Crouch, 1693.

[4], 113 (i.e. 213), [3] p.   18 cm.   [1305]

—Nauwkeurige verhandelinge van de scheur-buik en des selfs toevallen. Als ook een naakt vertoog wegens de fermentatie oft innerlijke beweginge der lighamen, meest op de gronden van Des-Cartes gebouwt ... Amsterdam, Jan Ten Hoorn, 1684.

[8], 226 (i.e. 224) p.; [1], 158, [21] p.   plates.   16
cm.   [1306]
Part [2] has half title.
Bound with *his* Het gast-huis der zieken. 1690.

—[German tr.] Gründliche Beschreibung vom
Scharbock und dessen Zufällen. Nebenst einem
ausführlichen Bericht von der Fermentation oder in-
wendigen Bewegung der Cörper, meistens auf den
Grund Renatus des Cartes gerichtet . . . Ins
Hochdeutsche gesetzet von D. J. S. Leipzig, Verlegts
Joh. Friedrich Gleditsch, 1690.
    [16], 439 (i.e. 441) p.   plates,   17 cm.   [1307]
Bound with (as issued?) *his* Accurate Abhandlung von dem
Podagra. 1690.

—[The same.] . . . Die 2. Aufl. Leipzig, Verlegts
Johann Friedrich Gleditsch, 1693.
    [16], 436 (i.e. 433) p.   plates.   17 cm.   [1308]

—Den Neder-landschen Herbarius; ofte, Kruid-
boek der voornaamste kruiden, tot de medicyne,
spys-bereidingen en konstwerken dienstig . . .
Amsterdam, Jan ten Hoorn, 1698.
    [8], 621, [27] p.   plates.   17 cm.   [1309]
Added engraved title page.

—De nieuw hervorm de anatomie; ofte, Ontleding
des menschen lichaams. Gebouwd op de waaragtigste
en naaukeurigste ondervindingen deser eeuw. Zijnde
met een groot getal kunstige platen verçiert. Als ook
een Verhandelinge van het balsemen der lichamen.
Noit voor desen dusdanig bekent gemaakt . . .
Amsterdam, Jan ten Hoorn, 1686.
    [14], 611, [13] p.   plates.   20 cm.   [1310]
Added engraved title page.
Imperfect: sig. *8 (portrait?) wanting.

—[The same.] . . . Amsterdam, Jan ten Hoorn,
1696.
    [14], 761, [20] p.   plates, port.   20 cm.
                                                   [1311]
Added engraved title page.

—[Latin tr.] Anatomia reformata; sive, Concinna
corporis humani. Dissectio, ad neotericorum mentem
adornata, plurimisque tabulis chalcographicis illustrata. Accedit ejusdem authoris De balsamatione,
nova methodus, a nemine antehac hoc modo descripta. Lugduni Batavorum, Apud Cornelium Boutesteyn, Jordanum Luchtmans, 1687.
    [14], 319 p.; 288, [7] p.   front.   (port.), plates.
20 cm.   [1312]

Added engraved title page, illustrated.
Imperfect: plate XXVIII in second part wanting.

—Another issue. 1688. With publishers' names in
imprint reversed. Added engraved title page has date:
1687.
                                                   [1313]
Imperfect: p. 295-298 wanting.

—[The same.] . . . Ed. nov. plurimis recens in-
ventis, tabulisque novis emendatior ac locupletior . . .
Lugduni Batavorum, Apud Cornelium Boutestein,
Jordanum Luchtmans, 1695.
    [14], 759 (i.e. 769), [14] p.   port., plates.   19 cm.
                                                   [1314]
Added engraved title page.
Imperfect: port. wanting; supplied in photocopy from variant
copy.

—Another issue, with publishers' names in imprint
reversed.   [1315]

—[German tr.] Neue und besondere Manier alle
verstorbene Cörper, mit wenig Unkosten, dergestalt
zu balsamiren, dass solche in etlichen hundert Jahren
nicht verwesern, noch Farbe und Gestalt verlieren
können. Wie denn auch dabey communiciret
werden, unterschiedliche Recepten, köstliche
wolriechende Poma Ambrae oder Bysamknöpff,
Rauch-Kertz- und Küchlein und wolriechende
Seiffen-Kugeln zu machen . . . Aus Holländ: in unser
Mutter-Sprach übersetzet von G. A. M. Hannover
und Wolffenbüttel, Verlegts Gottfried Freytag, 1697.
    104 p.   17 cm.   [1316]
The Neue und besondere Manier . . . zu balsamieren, is extracted from his De nieuw hervormde anatomie.

—Nieuw lichtende praktyk der medicynen,
gefondeert op de gronden van de deftighste autheuren
deses tijdts: nevens De hedendaagse chymia, als ook
De Nederlantsche apothekers winkel . . . Amsterdam, Jan Claesz. ten Hoorn, 1678.
    3 parts in 1 v.   16 cm.   [1317]
Added engraved title page.
Each part has special title page.

—[The same.] Nieuw-ligtende praktyk der
medicinen, waar in getoond werd, dat alle ziekten
een verdiktheid des bloeds en sappen zyn, en alleen
uit suur, sout, en slym voortkomen. Hier nevens een
verehandelinge van De hedensdaagse chymie, in
welke over des selfs bereidingen nauwkeurig

geredeneert werd . . . Den 4. druk merkelijk verm. en verb. Amsterdam, Jan ten Hoorn, 1690.

[8], 515, [5] p.; 138, [6] p.   illus., table.   17 cm.   [1318]

Added engraved title page.
Part [2] has half title.

—[The same.] . . . Den 5. druk merkelyk verm. en verb. Amsterdam, Jan ten Hoorn, 1696.

[8], 512, [7] p.; 126 (i.e. 128), [8] p.   illus., table.   17 cm.   [1319]

—[German tr.]Neuscheinende Praxis der Medicinae, worinn angewiesen wird, dass alle Krankheiten eine Verdikkung des Bluts und der Säffte sind, und bloss von Sauer and Schleim entstehen . . . Auffs neue gedrukt und abgetheilet in drey Theile . . . Aus der Holländ . . . übersetzet von G. H. W. Med. Doct. Hannover und Wolffenbüttel, Gottfried Freytag, 1700.

[1], 766 p.   front.   17 cm.   [1320]

[—De nieuwe hedensdaagse stof-scheiding oft chymia. German.] Die neue heutiges Tages gebräuchliche Scheide-Kunst; oder, Chimia nach den Gründen des fürtreflichen Cartesii und des Alcali und Acidi eingerichtet . . . Hannover und Wolffenbüttel, Gottlieb Heinrich Grentz, 1689.

179, [1] p.   illus.   17 cm.   [1321]

—[The same.] . . . Hannover und Wolffenbüttel, Gottfried Freytag, 1697.

179, [11] p.   illus.   17 cm.   [1322]

—Nieuwe konst-kamer der chirurgie; ofte, Heelkonst. Gefondeert op nieuwer gronden als oyt voor desen . . . Amsterdam, Johannes ten Hoorn, 1680.

[8], 388 (i.e. 402), 4 p.   17 cm.   [1323]

Added engraved title page.

—[German tr.] Newe Kunst-Kammer der Chirurgie; oder Heilkunst. Worinnen die auff gewissen und wahrhafftigen Gründen gebawete Chirurgie auffgestellet und von den Instrumenten . . . operationen . . . gehandelt wird. Aus der niederländischen in die hock-teutsche Sprache übersetzet . . . Hannover und Hildesheim, Verlegts Gottlieb Heinrich Grentz, 1688.

[14], 607 (i.e. 597), [11] p.   17 cm.   [1324]

Added engraved title page.

—Praxeos medicae idea nova. In qua origo omnium morborum ex acido, humorum incrassatione, atque eorundem obstructione, verissimis & rationi

congruentissimis fundamentis esse ostenditur. Amstelodami, Ex officina Joannis ten Hoorn, 1685.

[16], 170, [6] p.   plates.   16 cm.   [1325]

Includes considerable portions of the text of *his* De Kartesiaanse academie; ofte, Institutie de medicyne.

—[Schou-burg der rupsen, wormen, ma'den, en vliegende dierkens daar uit voortkomende. German.] Schau-Platz der Raupen, Würmer, Maden und fliegenden Thiergen welche daraus erzeuget werden, durch eigene Untersuchung zussamen gebracht . . . Aus dem Niederländischen ins Hochteutsche übersetzt durch Johann Christian Rodochs . . . Leipzig, In Verlegung Joh. Friedrich Gleditschen, 1690.

[15], 178, [6] p.   plates.   17 cm.   [1326]

Added engraved title page.

—Theatrum chimicum; ofte, Geopende deure der chymische verborgentheden . . . Met een vervolg over de chymische verborgentheden aangaande de verandering en verbetering der metalen en gesteenten. Door . . . K. Digby. Amsterdam, 1693.

[16], 490 (i.e. 398), [22] p.; 170, [6] p.   front., plates.   17 cm.   [1327]

Imperfect: title page mutilated.
Part [2] has half title: Vervolg van het Theatrum chymicum . . . door Kenelmus Digby.

—[German tr.] Theatrum chimicum; oder, Eröffneter Schau-Platz und Thür zu den Heimligkeiten in der Scheide-Kunst. Nebenst einer Vermehrung wie die geringen Metallen und gemeinen Steine zu verbessern sind, durch Kenelm. Digby. Leipzig, Thomas Fritsch, 1700.

[7], 472, [48] p.; 155, [5] p.   front., plates.   18 cm.   [1328]

Part [2] has special title page: Vermehrung des Theatri Chimici . . . durch Kenelmus Digby.

—Venus belegert en ontset; oft, Verhandelinge van de pokken, en des selfs toevallen, met een grondige en zekere genesinge. Steunende meest op de gronden van Cartesius . . . Item, een nauwkeurige beschryvinge der pokken door de heeren F. Sylvius, T. Sydenham, en J. Wierus. Amsterdam, Timotheus ten Hoorn, 1684.

[8], 522, [14] p.   17 cm.   [1329]

Added engraved title page dated 1685.

—[The same.] . . . Item, een nauwkeurige beschryvinge der pokken, door heeren F. Sylvius, T. Sydenham, J. Wierus, en A. Everaars. 2. druk, een derden verm. en verb. Amsterdam, Timotheus ten Hoorn, 1688.

[8], 456, [6] p.   plates.   16 cm.   [**1330**]

Added engraved title page, illustrated, with date; 1685.

—[The same.] Venus belegert en ontset. Zynde een verhandelinge van de pokken, en des selfs toevallen, van druipers, chankers, klapooren, Spaanse kragen, sand-klooten, cordeé uitwasschen, enz. Met een zekere en grondige genezinge. Steunende op de Cartesiaanse philosophie, en het sondigende suur en sout . . . Item een nauwkeurige beschryvinge der pokken, door . . . Sylvius, Sydenham, Wierus en Everaarts. Amsterdam, Timotheus ten Hoorn, 1696.

[8], 492 (i.e. 502), [8] p.   plates.   16 cm.

Added engraved title page.   [**1331**]

—[French tr.] Traité de la verole, gonorrhee, chancres, bubes venereens, & de leurs accidens, avec une guerison veritable & solide . . . Traduit par Guillaume Willis. Amsterdam, Corneille Blankard, 1688.

[8], 241 (i.e. 243), [5] p.   17 cm.   [**1332**]

—[German tr.] Die belägert-und entsetzte Venus, das ist; Chirurgische Abhandlung der sogenanten frantzossen, auch spanischen Pocken-Kranckheit, Drüpper, Sjankert, Klap-Ohren, &c. und andern sich dabey findenden Zufällen; worinnen derselben, vornemlich auf des weltbekanten Cartesii Gründe, befestigte sichere und unfehlbare Cur vollkömmlich angewiesen wird . . . Nebst . . . Fr. Sylvii, Th. Sydenham, Joh. Wieri und Ant. Everaars . . . Beschreibungen dieses Ubels. Aus dem Niederländischen . . . in unsere hochdeutsche Sprach übersetzet. Leipzig, Verlegts Joh. Friedrich Gleditsch, 1689.

[7], 544, [7] p.   plates.   17 cm.   [**1333**]

Added engraved title page.

Translated by Wachendorf. Cf. Proksch, v. 1, p. 26.

—[Excerpts. English.] *In* A new method of curing the French-pox. 1690

—**Verhandelinge** van de coffee. *In* Bontekoe, C. Gebruik en misbruik van de thee. 1686.

—[**Verhandelinge** van de operatien ofte werkingen der medicamenten in's menschen lighaam. German.] Von Würckungen derer Artzneyen in dem menschlichen Leibe, zeigende die wahre Ursach von deren unterschiedlichen Würckungen. Wie auch ein

Entwurff von einer neuen Pharmacie, nach der heutigen Arth Artzneyen zu verschreiben . . . Vorgestellet und aus dem Niederländischen ins Hochteutsche übergesetzet von Johann Christian Rodochs, D. Leipzig, Verlegts Joh. Friedrich Gleditsch, 1690.

[16], 360, [8] p.   17 cm.   [**1334**]

Bound with (as issued?) *his* Accurate Abhandlung von dem Podagra. 1690.

—Verhandelinge van het podagra en vliegende jicht; waar in des zelfs ware oorzaak en zekere genezingen werden voorgestelt. Als ook een korte beschrijvinge van de krachten des melks . . . Item de Chineese en Japanse wijse om door het branden van moxa en het steken met een goude naald, alle ziekten en voornamelijk het podagra te genesen. Door . . . W. ten Rhyne . . . Amsterdam, Jan ten Hoorn, 1684.

[16], 301, [19] p.   15 cm.   [**1335**]

Added engraved title page.

"Beschrijvinge van Philipp. Jac. Sachs à Lewenheimb, achtende dat de melk een troost der podagristen is": p. [175]–200, has half title.

—[German tr.] Accurate Abhandlung von dem Podagra und der lauffenden Gicht, worinnen deren wahre Ursachen und gewisse Cur gründlich vorgestellet, auch die herrlichen Kräfften der Milch . . . beschrieben werden . . . Nebst des Herrn Wilhelm ten Rhyne . . . curieuser Beschreibung, wie die Chinesen und Japaner Vermittelst des Moxa-Brennens und guldenen Nadel-Stechens alle Kranckheiten, insonderheit aber das Podagra gewiss curiren. Aus der niederteutschen in die hochteutsche Sprache übersetzet. Leipzig, Verlegts Joh. Fried. Gleditsch, Druckts Christoph Fleischer, 1690.

[11], 351, [21] p.   17 cm.   [**1336**]

"Herrn Philipp. Jac. Sachs von Lewenheimb Beschreibung der Milch; worinnen dargethan wird, dass solche der Podagristen bester Trost sey": p. [207]–236.

With this are bound (as issued?): *his* Gründliche Beschreibung vom Scharbock. 1690; *his* von Würckungen derer Artzneyen in dem menschlichen Leibe. 1690.

—[The same.] . . . [Leipzig] Joh. Fried. Gleditsch, 1692.

[11], 351, [21] p.   17 cm.   [**1337**]

Different setting of type.

—Verhandelinge van de opvoedinge en ziekten der kinderen. Vertoonende op wat wyse de kinderen gezond konnen blyven, en ziek zijnde, bequamelyk konnen herstelt werden . . . Amsterdam, Hieronymus Sweerts, 1684.

[8], 332, [19] p.   plates.   16 cm.   **[1338]**
Added engraved title page.

—*respondent. See* MATTHAEUS, P., *praeses.* Disputatio medica de hydrope ascite. 1674.

—*ed. See* LANCIILLOTTI, C. De brandende salamander. 1680.

—*tr. See* SANTORIO, S. De ontdekte doorwaassem-ing des menschen lichaams. 1684.

—*See* STERRE, D. van der. Verhandeling der genees-en heel-konstige practyk der medicynen. 1687.

—*as subject. See* STERRE, D. van der. Tractatus novus de generatione ex ovo. 1687; VERHEYEN, P. Corporis humani anatomia. 1697, 1699.

BLAS, GEORG [*fl.* 1691] *respondent. See* WEINHART, F. K., *praeses.* Thesaurus sanitatis. 1691.

BLASII, ARMENGANDUS. *See* ARMENGANDUS BLASII [*fl. ca.* 1280–1309]

BLASIUS, ABRAHAMUS [*b.* 1650] *tr. See* MEEKREN, J. van. Observationes medico-chirurgicae. 1682.

BLASIUS, Gerardus [1626?–1692?] Anatome animalium, terrestrium variorum, volatilium, aquatilium, serpentum, insectorum, ovorumque, structuram naturalem ... proponens ... Amstelodami, Sumptibus viduae Joannis a Someren, Henrici & viduae Theodori Boom, 1681.

[8], 494, [2] p.   illus., plates.   27 cm.
                                              [1339]
Added engraved title page.

—Anatome contracta, in gratiam discipulorum conscripta, et edita. Amstelodami, Apud Gerbrandum Schagen, 1666.

[8], 281, [22] p.   14 cm.   **[1340]**
Added engraved title page.

—Anatome medullae spinalis, et nervorum inde provenientium. Amstelodami, Apud Casparum Commelinum, 1666.

74, [2] p.   plates.   14 cm.   **[1341]**
With this is bound Collegium privatum Amstelodamense. Observations. 1667 [–1673]

—Commentaria in Syntagma anatomicum Joannis Veslingii. *In* Vesling, J. Syntagma anatomicum. 1659, 1666, 1677, 1696; [Dutch tr.] 1661; [German tr.] 1676.

—Impetus Jacobii Primirosii ... in Vop. Fort. Plempium ... retusus a Gerardo Leon. Blasio ... Amstelodami, Sumptibus Joannis Ravesteynii, 1659.

[8], 219, [2] p.   21 cm.   **[1342]**
Errata: p. [12]

—Institutionum medicarum compendium, disputationibus XII in illustri Amstel. Athenaeo publice ventilatis, absolutum ... Amstelodami, Apud Petrum vanden Bergh, 1667.

[8], 147, [1] p.   14 cm.   **[1343]**
Added engraved title page.
Imperfect: added engraved title page wanting.

—Medicina curatoria, methodo nova in gratiam discipulorum conscripta. Amstelodami, Apud Henricum & Theodorum Boom, 1680.

[12], 351, [19] p.   17 cm.   **[1344]**

—Medicina universa; hygieines & therapeutices fundamenta methodo nova brevissime exhibens. Amstelodami, Apud Petrum vanden Berge, 1665.

[16], 464, [16] p.   21 cm.   **[1345]**
"Catalogus eorum quaee opera mea edita sunt": p. [16] at end.

—Miscellanea anatomica, hominis, brutorumque variorum, fabricam diversam magna parte exhibentia. Amstelodami, Apud Casparum Commelinum, 1673.

[16], 309, [11] p.   plates.   16 cm.   **[1346]**
Added engraved title page reads: Anatome hominis, brutorumque variorum.

—[The same.] Zootomiae; seu, Anatomes variorum aniimalium pars prima ... Amstelodami, Apud Abrahamum Wolfgang, 1676.

87 (i.e. 79), [1], 292, [4] p.   illus., plates.   16 cm.   **[1347]**
Added engraved title page dated 1677 reads: Zootomia, seu, Anatome hominis, brutorumque variorum.
With this is bound *his* Observationes medicae rariores. 1677.

—[Dutch ed.] Ontleeding des menschelyken lichaems, beschreeven en in verscheydene figuren afgebeelt ... Amsterdam, Abraham Wolfgangh, 1675.

[16], 204, [34] p.   illus.   17 cm.   **[1348]**
Imperfect: added engraved title page wanting.
With this are bound: Reverhorst, Maurits van. Dissertatio ... de motu bilis. 1696; Bils, L. de. Waerachtig vertoog der handelinge van de anatomie. 1668; Korte verhandelinge ... der wanschepsels. Amsterdam, 1703; Palfijn, Jan. Anatomycke of ontleedkundige beschryving. Ghendt, 1703.

—Observata anatomica in homine, simia, equo, vitulo, ove ... variisque animalibus aliis. Accedunt extraordinaria in homine reperta praxin medicam aeque ac anatomen illustrantia. Lugd. Batav. & Amstelod., Apud Gaasbeeck, 1674.

[6], 141, [11] p. illus. 18 cm. [1349]

Added engraved title page.

—Observationes medicae rariores. Accedit monstri triplicis historia. Amstelodami, Apud Abrahamum Wolfgang, 1677.

[8], 120 p.; [4], 71, [1] p. plates. 16 cm.

[1350]

Part [2] contains: "Historia infantis monstrosi a ... Michaele Heiland ... anno 1676": p. [1]-54.
—Historia agni monstrosi [and] Historia vituli monstrosi a ... Mauritio Hoffmanno": p. [55]-[72]
Bound with *his* Zootomiae. 1676.

—Pest-geneesing en bewaaring voor deselve ... Amsterdam, Evert Nieuwenhof, 1663.

35, [4] p. 16 cm. [1351]

Bound with Puthman, Evert. Puthmans manuael; oft, Cleyn pest-boecxken. 1603.

Dissertations—Amsterdam.

—*praeses.* Disputatio medica de peste, prior. Quae de praeservatione ... Amstelodami, Apud Joannem Ravesteinium, 1663.

[12] p. 18 cm. [1352]

C. de Vogel, *respondent.*

—Disputatio medica de peste, posterior. Quae de curatione ... Amstelodami, Apud Joannem Ravesteinium, 1663.

[12] p. 18 cm. [1353]

Imperfect: lower margin of title page trimmed including date of printing.
C. de Vogel, *respondent.*

—Exercitatio anatomica de intestinis ... Amstelodami, Apud Joannem Ravesteinium, 1663.

[12] p. 19 cm. [1354]

P. Boddens, *respondent.*

—Exercitationum medicarum de humoribus prima, de chylo ... Amstelodami, Apud Joannem Ravesteinium, 1661.

[12] p. 19 cm. [1355]

W. A. Senguerd, *respondent.*

—Exercitationum medicarum de humoribus secunda, de sanguine prior ... Amstelodami, Apud Joannem Ravesteinium, 1662.

[8] p. 19 cm. [1356]

W. A. Senguerd, *respondent.*

—Exercitationum medicarum de humoribus tertia, de sanguine posterior ... Amstelodami, Apud Joannem Ravesteinium, 1662.

[8] p. 19 cm. [1357]

W. A. Senguerd, *respondent.*

—Exercitium anatomicum de pulmone ... Amstelodami, Apud Joannem Ravesteinium, 1662.

[8] p. 19 cm. [1358]

C. de Vogel, *respondent.*

—, *ed. See* BÉGUIN, J. Tyrocinium chymicum. 1659, 1669; MOREL, P. Methodus praescribendi formulas remediorum. 1659, 1665, 1680; MÜLLER, Philipp. Miracula chymica et mysteria medica libris quinque enucleata. 1659; POLVERINO, G. G. Medicina practica. 1649; WILLIS, T. Opera omnia. 1682, 1694.

—*See* BELLINI, L. Exercitatio anatomica. 1665.

—*as subject. See* BONTEKOE, C. Notae provocatoriae in corollaria. 1682; LICETI, F. De monstris. 1665, 1668;

BLASIUS, GERARDUS LEONARDI. *See* BLASIUS, Gerardus [1626?-1692?]

BLAUSCHMIED, CHRISTIAN. *See* PFAUTZ, C., *praeses.* Dissertatio historico-physica. 1664.

BLAWEN, ANDREAS DE. Epistola ... ad Petrum Andream Matthiolium in qua agitur de multiplici auri potabilis parandi ratione. [Argentorati, Sumptib. haeredum Eberhardi Zetzneri, 1661]

458-470 p., vol. 6. 20 cm. (*In* Zetzner, Lazarus, *ed.* Theatrum chemicum. Argentorati, 1659-61) [1359]

Caption title.

—*See* ORTHELIUS. Discursus ... de ... epistola Andreae de Blawen. 1659.

BLEGNY, NICOLAS DE [1642?-1722] L'art de guerir les hernies; contenant plusieurs observations curieuses & nouvelles, & un grand nombre de remedes ... pour la guerison des tumeurs ... Avec la construction, l'usage ... des brayers & des pessaires à ressort, inventez par l'autheur ... Paris, L'autheur, 1676.

[36], 270, [29] p. illus. 16 cm. [1360]

—[The same.] L'art de guerir les hernies, ou descentes, de toutes especes dans les deux sexes. Avec le remede du roy, les bandages de la manufacture royale, & divers autres remedes experimentez ... 3. éd. corr. & augm. par l'autheur. Paris, La veuve Jean d'Houry et Laurent d'Houry, 1688.

[24], 297, [38] p. plate. 16 cm.   [**1361**]

"Avis touchant l'infirmerie des voyageurs": p. 28–38

—[The same.] ... Nouvelle ed. corr. & augm. par l'auteur. Paris, Laurent d'Houry, 1693.

[24], 297, [38] p. plate. 16 cm.   [**1362**]

A reissue of the 1688 edition with new title page.

—[L'art de guerir les maladies veneriennes.] Observations curieuses et nouvelles, sur l'art de guerir la maladie venerienne, ou grosse verolle. Et les accidens qu'elle produit ... les effects du mercure, & de ses autres remedes ... Paris, L'autheur, 1674.

[22], 366, [6] p. 15 cm.   [**1363**]

—[The same.] L'art de guerir les maladies veneriennes, expliqué par les principes de la nature & des méchaniques ... 2. éd. corr. & augmentée par l'autheur. Paris, L'autheur et Jean d'Houry, 1677–1678.

2 v. illus. 16 cm.   [**1364**]

Vol. 3 was published in 1679. Cf. BNC, vol. 14, col. 118.

—[The same.] ... 3 éd. corr. par l'autheur ... Paris, Estienne Michallet, 1683.

3 v. in 1. illus. 17 cm.   [**1365**]

—[The same.] ... 3. éd. ... Suivant la copie imprimé à Paris. La Haye, Pierre Hagen, 1683.

3 v. in 1. illus. 14 cm.   [**1366**]

Different setting of type.

—[The same.] ... 4. éd. corr. par l'autheur. Lyon, Antoine Briasson, 1692.

[16], 468 (i.e. 466), [22] p. illus. 16 cm.   [**1367**]

—[The same.] ... 4. éd. corr. par l'autheur. Lyon, Jacques Lyons, 1693.

[16], 468 (i.e. 466), [22] p. illus. 15 cm.   [**1368**]

—[The same.] ... 4. éd. ... Suivant la copie imprimée à Paris. Amsterdam, Abraham de Hoogenhuysen, 1696.

3 v. in 1. illus. 14 cm.   [**1369**]

Tome 2: 3. ed., dated 1696.

"Quatrième partie": tome 3, p. 121–178.

—[The same.] ... 5. éd. rev. & corr. Suivant la copie de Paris. La Haye, Henry van Bulderen, 1696.

3 v. in 1. illus. 15 cm.   [**1370**]

Imperfect: title page and p. 1–2 of vol. 1 mutilated.

—[English tr.] New and curious observations on the art of curing the venereal disease. And the accidents that it produces in all its degrees, explicated by natural and mechanical principles, with the motions, actions and effects of mercury, and its other remedies ... Written in French ... Englished by Walter Harris ... London, Tho. Dring and Tho. Burrel, 1676.

[32], 182, [2] p. 17 cm.   [**1371**]

—Le bon usage du thé du caffé et du chocolat pour la preservation & pour la guerison des maladies ... Paris, Estienne Michallet, 1687.

[24], 358 (i.e. 356), [4] p. front., illus. 16 cm.
     [**1372**]

—La découverte de l'admirable remede anglois, pour la guerison des fiévres, au moyen de laquelle chacun pourra se procurer la facilité de guerir à tres-peu de frais ... Paris, Claude Blageart et Laurent d'Houry, 1680.

92, [2] p. 14 cm.   [**1373**]

Bound with *his* Histoire anathomique d'un enfant. 1679.

—La doctrine des raports de chirurgie, fondé sur les maximes d'usage & sur la disposition des nouvelles ordonnances ... Lyon, Thomas Amaulry, 1684.

[24], 272 p. 16 cm.   [**1374**]

—Histoire anathomique d'un enfant, qui a demeuré vingt-cinq ans dans le ventre de sa mere. Avec des reflexions qui en expliquent tous les phenomenes ... Paris, Laurent d'Hourry, 1679.

43, [1] p. plate. 14 cm.   [**1375**]

With this are bound *his*: La découverte de l'admirable remede anglois, pour la guerison des fiévres. 1680; Spon, Jacob. Observations sur les fievres et les febrifuges. 1681; and Sur les stryges de Russie. [16–-?]

—[Les nouvelles descouvertes sur toutes les parties de la médecine. Latin.] Zodiacus medico-gallicus; sive, Miscellaneorum medico physicorum Gallicorum, titulo recens in re medica exploratorum, unoquoque mense Parisiis Latine prodeuntium annus primus [-annus quintus] sçilicet M. DC. LXXIX [-M. DC. LXXXIII] ... Genevae, Sumptibus Leonardi Chouët, 1680-1685.

5 v. in 2. illus., plates. 23 cm.   [1376]
Translated by Théophile Bonet.

—[German tr.] Monatliche neueröffnete Anmerckungen, über alle Theile der Artzney-Kunts zusammen gebracht im Jahr 1679[-1682] ... Aus dem Frantzösischen ins Teutsche übersetzet durch J[ohann] L[ange] M. C. Hamburg, Auff Gottfried Schultzens Kosten, Merseburg, Druckts Caspar Forberger, 1680-1683.
4 parts in 1 v. illus., plates. 17 cm. [1377]
Parts [2-4] have special title pages.

—Le remede anglois pour la guerison des fievres ... avec les observations de Monsieur le premier medecin de Sa Majesté, sur la composition, les vertus, & l'usage de ce remede ... Paris, Chez l'autheur et la veufve d'Antoine Padeloup, 1682.
152 p. illus. 16 cm.   [1378]

—[The same.] ... Paris, Estienne Michallet, 1683.
119 p. illus. 16 cm.   [1379]
With this is bound Fouquet, Marie (de Maupeou) vicomtesse de Vaux. Recueil de remedes. 1683.

—[Latin tr.] In [Nigrisoli, F. M.] ed. Febris china chinae expugnata. 1687, 1700.

—Secrets concernant la beauté et la santé ... Paris, Laurent d'Houry et la veuve de feu Denis Nion, 1688-1689.
2 v. 19 cm.   [1380]

—See MASSARD, J. Traité des panacées. 1681; [Dutch tr.] 1687; SPON, J. Observations sur les fievres et les febrifuges. 1681; TALBOR, Sir R. The English remedy. 1682.

BLEIDNER, JOHANN CHRISTIAN [fl. 1699] respondent. See ALKOFER, E. S. Trutina vacui. 1699.

BLENDINGER, ABRAHAM [fl. 1677] Dissertatio inauguralis medica, de cancro ... Erfurti, Typis Johann Georg Hertzii [1677]
[16] p. 19 cm.   [1381]
Diss.—Erfurt (E. Arnoldi, respondent)

BLEZINUS, JOANNES [fl. 1608] ed. See SCHYRON, J. Methodi medendi. 1609, 1623.

BLOCHWITZ, JOHANNES [fl. 1631] ed. See BLOCHWITZ, M. Anatomia sambuci. 1631, 1650.

BLOCHWITZ, MARTIN [fl. 1624-1626] Anatomia sambuci, quae non solum sambucum & hujusdem

medicamenta singulatim delineat, verum quoque plurimorum affectuum, ex una fere sola sambuco curationes breves, rationibus, exemplis, historiis & medicamentis specificis non paucis illustratas simul exhibet ... Lipsiae, Sumptibus Gothofredi Grosi, 1631.
[22], 281, [6] p. 13 cm.   [1382]
Edited by Johannes Blochwitz.

—[The same.] ... Lipsiae, Sumptibus Gothofredi Grosi, 1631.
[32], 298, [6] p. 14 cm.   [1383]
Bound with Grüling, P. Florilegium chymicum. 1631.

—[The same.] ... Londini, Typis Johannis Field sumptibus Octaviani Pulleyn, 1650.
[22], 281, [6] p. 13 cm.   [1384]

—[English tr.] Anatomia sambuci; or, The anatomie of the elder. Cutting out of it, plain, approved, and specifick remedies for most and chiefest maladies; confirmed and cleared by reason, experience, and history ... Translated for the advancement of our language and medicines [by Christopher Irvine] London, Tho. Heath, 1655.
[12], 203 (i.e. 201) p. 15 cm.   [1385]

—[The same.] ... London, Printed for Tho. Sawbridge, and to be sold by H. Brome, 1670.
[12], 230 (i.e. 228) p. 15 cm.   [1386]
Imperfect: title page and p. [7]-[12] wanting; supplied in photocopy from the John Crerar Library.

—[The same.] ... London, H. Brome and Tho. Sawbridge, 1677.
[16], 230 (i.e. 228) p. 15 cm.   [1387]
A reprint with the addition of the translator's dedication, signed: C. de Iryngio

BLOCK, JOHANN [b. 1651] respondent. See FASCH, A. H., praeses. Dissertationem medicam inauguralem de peste ... subjicit ... J. B. 1681; WEDEL, G. W. praeses. Dissertatio medica, aegrum haemorrhagia narium laborantem sistens. 1679.

BLOEMAERT, GODEFRID [fl. 1657] Disputatio medica inauguralis, de ascite ... Ultrajecti, Pro Adriano à Dam, 1657.
[8] p. 20 cm.   [1388]
Diss.—Utrecht.

BLOM, CORNELIS VAN [fl. 1683] respondent. Disputatio medica inauguralis de abortu ...

Lugduni Batavorum, Apud Abrahamum Elzevier, 1683.

[12] p.   22 cm.   [1389]
Diss.—Leyden.

BLOME, RICHARD [*d.* 1705] *ed.* and *tr. See* LE GRAND, A. An entire body of philosphy. 1694.

BLOMMART, ANTON [*fl.* 1681] *respondent. See* FRANCK VON FRANCKENAU, G., *praes.* Disputatio inauguralis medica exhibens casum viri colica labornatis. 1681.

[**BLONDEL**, FRANÇOIS, 1609?–1682] Alethophanis archiatri [pseud., i.e. François Blondel] ad Jacobum Thevartum ex-medicum Parisiensem & R. M. hoc est reum manifestarium violati sacramenti nec non corruptae artis. Epistola. Cui accessit stibii Pithoegia, & pro auctario Pithoegia vindicata . . . Eleutheris [Paris?] Typis Notoriis, 1655.

[2], 34 (i.e. 35), [1], 12, 16 p.   22 cm.   [1390]
With this is bound: Prolusiones apologeticae approbatorum stibii, adversus authorem libelli infandi, qui inscribitur Pithoegia. 1654.

—, *ed. See* HIPPOCRATES. [Collected works. Greek and Latin] Hippocratis Coi, et Claudii Galeni . . . Opera. 1679.

—*See* UNIVERSITÉ DE PARIS. Faculté de médecine. Statuta facultatis medicinae Parisiensis. 1660.

—*as subject. See* THÉVART, J. Defense [-Deuxiéme defense] de la Faculté de medecine de Paris. 1668.

BLONDEL, FRANÇOIS [1613–1703] Lettres . . . au sieur Jaques Didier . . . touchant les eaux minerales chaudes d'Aix & de Borcet; et au sieur Jean Gaen . . . Bruxelles, Jean Mommart, 1662.

[8], 109, [3] p.   13 cm.   [1391]

—Thermarum Aquisgranensium et Porcetanarum descriptio. Congruorum quoque ac salubrium usuum balneationis & potationis elucidatio. Accedunt Probae thermarum Aquisgranensium. Trajecti ad Mosam, Apud Jacobum de Preys, 1685.

[24], 208, [11] p.   plates.   15 cm.   [1392]
Added engraved title page.
Bound with copy 2 of Cottereau Du Clos, S. Observationes super aquis mineralibus . . . Galliae. 1685.

—Thermarum Aquisgranensium, et Porcetanarum elucidatio, & thaumaturgia. Sive admirabilis earumdem natura, & admirabiliores sanationes;

quas producunt in usibus balneationis potationis . . . Ed. 3. . . . prioribus auct. & emend. Aquisgrani, Sumptibus authoris, typis Joannis Henrici Clemens, 1688.

[28], 160, [8] p.   illus., plates, port.   20 cm.   [1393]
Added engraved title page.

—*See* DIDIER, J. Lettre. 1661.

BLONDEL, JAMES AUGUSTUS [*ca.* 1666–1734] *respondent.* Disputatio medica inauguralis de crisibus . . . Lugduni Batavorum, Apud Abrahamum Elzevier, 1692.

[16] p.   21 cm.   [1394]
Diss.—Leyden.

BLONDUS, MICHAEL ANGELUS. *See* BIONDO, Michelangelo [1497–1565]

BLOTENBURG, CORNELIUS à [*fl.* 1699] *respondent.* Dissertatio medica inauguralis de partu difficili . . . Lugduni Batavorum, Apud Abrahamum Elzevier, 1699.

[22] p.   22 cm.   [1395]
Diss.—Leyden.

BLOUNT, *Sir* HENRY [1602–1682] *See* RUMSEY, W. Organon salutis. 1657, 1659, 1664.

BLOUNT, THOMAS [1618–1679] Glossographia; or, A dictionary, interpreting the hard words of whatsoever language, now used in our refined English tongue; with etymologies, definitions, and historical observations on the same. Also the terms of divinity, law, musick, physick, mathematicks, war, heraldry, and other arts and sciences explicated . . . 4th ed., with many additions. By T[homas] B[lount] of the Inner-Temple, esq. [London] Printed by Tho. Newcomb, sold by Robert Boulter, 1674.

[16], 706, [1] p.   18 cm.   [1396]
Errata: p. [707]

BLUM, EMANUEL [*fl.* 1671] *respondent. See* ETTMÜLLER M., *praes.* Disputatio medica de dolore hypochondriaco. 1683 [and] Exercitium medicum de dolore hypochondriaco, vulgo sed falso putato splenetico . . . submittit. 1671.

BLUM, MORITZ [*fl.* 1619–1625] *praes.* Centuria positionum medicarum de melancholia hypochondriaca . . . Wittebergae, Excusa typis Johannis Gormanni [1625]

[23] p. 19 cm. [1397]

Diss. — Wittenberg (J.A. Steininger, *respondent*).

— Decas problematum medicorum ... Wittebergae, Ex officina typographica Johannis Gormanni, 1624.

[24] p. 19 cm. [1398]

Diss. — Wittenberg (G. Wolff, *respondent*).

— Positiones medicae de imbecillitate ventriculi ... Wittebergae, Prelo Johannis Gormanni, 1624.

[32] p. 19 cm. [1399]

Diss. — Wittenberg (U. Lucae, *respondent*).

— *respondent. See* NYMANN G., *praeses.* Disputatio medica de apoplexia. 1619.

BLUMBERG, GOTTFRIED WILLIAM [*b.* 1662] *respondent. See* WEDEL, G. W., *praeses.* Venus medica et morbifera. 1688.

— *See* CRAUSE R.W., Rudolfus Wilhelmus Crasius ... lectori benevolo salutem. 1688.

BLUME, CHRISTIAN ULRICH [*fl.* 1682–1683] *respondent. See* ENGELBRECHT, G., *praeses.* Discursum juridicum de peste. 1683.

BLUME, JOHANN HENRICH [*fl.* 1699] *respondent. See* SCHRADER, F., *praeses.* Dissertatio medica inauguralis de senectutis praesidiis. 1699.

BLUMENTROST, JOHANN DEODATUS [1676–1756] *respondent. See* GOTTSCHED, J., *praeses.* Exercitatio practica, sistens medicum castrensem exercitui Moscovitarum praefectum. 1700.

BLUMENTROST, LORENZ [*fl.* 1648] *respondent. See* ROLFINCK, W., *praeses.* Disputatio inauguralis de scorbuto. 1648.

BLUMIGK, JOHANN [*fl.* 1688] *respondent.* Disputatio medica inauguralis de febribus ... Lugduni Batavorum, Apud viduam & haeredes Joannis Elsevierii, 1668.

[15] p. 23 cm. [1400]

Diss. — Leyden.

BLUNDEVILLE, THOMAS [*d.* 1605] The fower chiefyst offices belongyng to horsemanshippe. *See* MARKHAM, G. Markhams maister-peece. 1636, 1643, [i.e. 1644], 1651, 1694 [i.e. 1695]

BLYENBURCH, CORNELIS [*fl.* 1682] *respondent.* Disputatio physica de sapore ... Lugduni

Batavorum, Apud Abrahamum Elzevier, 1682.

[8] p. 20 cm. [1401]

Diss. — Leyden.

BOATE, ARNOLD [1606–1653] Observationes medicae, de affectibus omissis ... Londini, Excudebat Tho. Newcomb pro Tho. Whitaker, 1649.

[54] p. 16 cm. [1402]

— [The same.] ... Secundum editae cum praefatione Henrici Meibomii. Helmestadii, Typis & sumptibus Henningi Mulleri, 1664.

[16], 36 p. 19 cm. [1403]

— [The same.] ... *In* Borel, P. Historiarum et observationum medicophysicarum centuriae IV. 1676.

— *See* MØINICHEN, H. Observationes medico-chirurgicae. 1688; PLAT, *Sir* H. The jewel house of art and nature. 1653.

BOCANGELINO, NICOLAO [*d. ca.* 1622] De febribus morbisque malignis et pestilentia necnon de earum causis, praesagiis, curatione, & praeservatione ... Madriti, Apud Ludovicum Sanchez, 1604.

[4], 251 (i.e. 253), [26] p. 21 cm. [1404]

BOCCONE, PAOLO [1633–1704] D. Sylvii Bocconis ... Curiöse Anmerckungen uber ein und ander natürliche Dinge. Aus seinem noch nie im Druck gewesenen Museo, experimentali-physico zusammen gezogen, und im Durchreisen durch Teutschland, zum Andencken seiner in teutscher Sprach zum Druck hinterlassen. Franckfurt und Leipzig, In Verlegung Michael Rohrlachs seel. Wittib und Erben, 1697.

[20], 501, [3] p. illus., plates, port. 14 cm. [1405]

Colophon: Jena, Gedruckt bey Paul Ehrichen.
Imperfect: portrait wanting.

— Icones & descriptiones rariorum plantarum Siciliae, Melitae, Galliae, & Italiae. Quarum unaquaeque proprio charactere signata, ab aliis ejusdem classis facile distinguitur ... [Oxonii], E Theatro Sheldoniano, 1674.

[10], 96, [7] p. illus. 24 cm. [1406]

Edited by Robert Morison.

— Museo di fisica e di esperienze variato, e decorato di osservazioni naturali, note medicinali, e ragionamenti secondo i principii de' moderni ...

Venetia, Per Jo. Baptistam Zuccato, 1697.
  [8], 319 p.   front. (port.), illus., plates.   24 cm.
                                                        [**1407**]
  Imperfect: p. 203-206 wanting.

—Museo di piante rare della Sicilia, Malta, Corsica, Italia, Piemonte, e Germania ... Con l'Appendix ad libros de plantis Andreae Caesalpini, e varie osservazioni curiose con sue figure in rame ... Venetia, Per Jo. Baptista Zuccato, 1697.
  [8], 196 p.   front., plates.   24 cm.   [**1408**]

—Osservazioni naturali ove si contengono materie medico-fisiche, e di botanica, produzioni naturali, fosfori diversi, fuochi sotterranei d'Italia, & altre curiosità ... Bologna, Per li Manolessi, 1684.
  [14], 400, [10] p.   plates.   15 cm.   [**1409**]

—See RAY, J. Stirpium Europaearum extra Britannias nascentium sylloge. 1694.

BOCCONI, SILVIO. See BOCCONE, Paolo [1633-1704]

BOCHART, SAMUEL [1599-1667] See WÖRGER, F. Triga dissertationum sacrarum. 1679.

BOCHMAN, JOHANN [*fl.* 1607] *respondent.* Disputatio medica de ephialte ... Basileae Rauracorum, In typographeio Jani Exertier, 1607.
  [8] p.   20 cm.   [**1410**]
  Diss.—Basel.

BOCKSHAMMER, DANIEL SIGISMUND [*fl.* 1697] *respondent. See* VESTI, J., *praeses.* Dissertatio medica inauguralis, proponens casum aegri ascitici. 1697.

BODAEUS, EGBERTUS [*fl.* 1644] *ed. See* THEOPHASTUS. De historia plantarum libri decem, Graece & Latine. 1644.

BODAEUS, JOHANNES [*d.* 1636] *See* THEOPHRASTUS. De historia plantarum libri decem, Graece & Latine. 1644.

BODDENS, PETER [*fl.* 1663] *respondent. See* BLASIUS, G., *praeses.* Exercitatio anatomica de intestinis. 1663.

BODE, HEINRICH VON [1652-1720] *praeses.* Disputatio inauguralis juridica de juribus infirmorum seu aegrotorum singularibus ... Rinthelii, Typis G. C. Wächters [1693]
  [4], 36 p.   20 cm.   [**1411**]
  Diss.—Rinteln (J. L. Wetzel, *respondent*)

BODENSTEIN, ADAM VON [1528-1577] Bericht von der Kranckheit Podagra, welche etwan der Cyprian genennet wird. Dem beygefügt, gebürliche Wartung der Krancken, sonderlich deren, so mit dem schmertzhaften Podagra, Pestilentz, oder andern Kranckheiten behafftet seyn. Item Kurtze Beschreibung und Nutz der Kräuter, so den 12. himmlischen Zeichen in ihrer Eigenschafft und Wirckung sich vergleichen. Vor disem durch D. Adam von Bodenstein, und D. Gualtherum Ryff an Tag geben ... Amberg, Michael Forster, 1611.
  2 v.   16 cm.   [**1412**]
  "Gebührliche Wartung der Krancken" (p. [41]-117, vol. 1) has special title page.
  Vol. 2 has special title page: Kurtze Beschreibung und Nutz der Kräter.

BODIKERUS, JOHANNES. *See* BÖDIKER, Johann [1641-1695]

BODIN, HEINRICH. *See* BODE, Heinrich von [1652-1720]

BODIN, JEAN [1530-1596] De magorum daemonomania; seu, De testando lamiarum ac magorum cum Satana commercio, libri IV. Recens recogniti, et multis in locis a mendis repurgati. Accessit ejusdem Opinionum Joannis Wieri confutatio ... Francofurti, Typis Wolffgangi Richteri, impensis omnium haeredum Nicolai Bassaei, 1603.
  557 p.   17 cm.   [**1413**]
  "Determinatio Parisiis facta per almam Facultatem theologicam ... M. CCC. XCVII. super quibusdam superstitionibus noviter exortis": p. 33-40.
  Apparently a reprint of the 1581 Basel edition.
  The translator is identified as Franciscus Junius (i.e. François Du Jon) in J. M. Quérard's Les supercheries littéraires dévoilées, 2. éd. t. 3, column 1244.

—[German tr.] *In* Aristoteles. Problemata. 1679.

BODINUS, HENRICUS. *See* BODE, Heinrich von [1652-1720]

BOË, FRANCISCUS DE LE. *See* LE BOË, Frans de [1614-1672].

BOÈCE DE BOODT, ANSELM. *See* BOODT, Anselm Boèce de [1550?-1632]

BOECHER, MARTIN [*fl.* 1604-1605] *respondent. See* SENNERT, D., *praeses.* De febribus disputatio VIII. & ultima, de febre hectica ... 1605 [and] De differentiis morborum, disputatio prima. 1605 [and] De differentiis morborum disputatio altera. 1605.

BÖCHM, János Ephraim [*fl.* 1683] *respondent. See* VATER, C., *praeses.* Examen sulphuris vitriolo anodyni. 1683.

BOECKELMANN, ANDRIES. *See* BOEKELMAN, Andreas [*fl.* 1677]

[**BOECKELMANN**, Johann Friedrich, 1633?-1681] Medicus Romanus servus sexaginta solidis aestimatus; sive, Tractatus de veterum medicorum nominibus functionibus & vili conditione . . . 2 ed. Lugduni Batavorum, 1681.
     [1], 55 p.   14 cm.   **[1414]**
     Attributed to Andries Boeckelman by Wellcome, vol. 2, p. 186.

BÖCKLER, GEORG ANDREAS [*fl. ca.* 1644-1698] Der nützlichen Hauss -und Feld-Schule, erster [-zweyter] Theil in welchem ausführlich enthalten, wie man ein Land-Feld-Guth und Meyerey mit aller Zugehöre . . . mit Nutzen anordnen solle: worbey dann auch zugleich eine zur Hausshaltung auf dem Lande nützliche Hauss-Artzney für Menschen und Viehe . . . mit sonderbarem Fleiss colligirt . . . Franckfurt und Leipzig, In Verlegung Joh. Adam Merckels, 1699.
     2 v.   front., illus., plates.   21 cm.   **[1415]**
     Imperfect: all pages wanting in vol. 2 after p. 1592.

BÖDIKER, JOHANN [1641-1695] Treur-klacht, en eer-galm, van . . . Cornelis Bontekoe . . . In een lijck-en afscheyt-reden voor gesteld, en in druck uytgegeven van Johannes Bodikerus. Uyt het hooghduyts vertaelt. Waer by noch gevoeght sijn eenige soo Latynse als Duytse lofen lijk-gedichten, ter eeren van den selven, by verscheyde persoonen gemaeckt. 's Gravenhage, Pieter Hagen, 1685.
     64 p.   16 cm.   **[1416]**
     Bound with Bontekoe, C. Tractaat van het excellenste kruyd thee. 1685.

BÖHEIM, MARTIN. *See* BEHM, Martin [1557-1622]

BÖHM, MARTIN. *See* BEHM, Martin [1557-1622]

BÖHM, TOBIAS [*fl.* 1607-1614] *respondent.* Disputatio de angina . . . Basileae, Typis Joh. Jacobi Genathii [1614]
     [8] p.   22 cm.   **[1417]**
     Diss. — Basel.

     —*See* KNOBLOCH, T., *praeses.* Disputationes anatomicae. 1608, 1612.

BÖHME, JOHANN GOTTFRIED [*fl.* 1673] *respondent. See* RIVINUS, Q. S. F. Schediasma de noctu lucentibus. 1673.

BÖKEL, WILHELM [*fl.* 1607] Kurtzer Bericht, und einfeltige Unterweisung, wie man sich in diesen jetzigen gefehrlichen Zeiten, der jetzt einreissenden Pest verhalten, wie man sich praeservirn, und so einer damit befallen, ördentlicher Weise zur Cur schreiten sol. Wobey allen Balbierern und Wundartzten gründliche Anleitung unnd allerhand bewehrte Experiment vorgeschrieben seyn . . . Helmstadt, Gedruckt durch Jacobum Lucium, 1607.
     [56] p.   20 cm.   **[1418]**

BOEKELMAN, ANDREAS [*fl.* 1677] De onschult of zamenspraak tusschen de geesten van imandt en niemandt; over de droevige pellegrimagie van Lysbet Jantz van Ravesway. [n. p.] Gedrukt tot Buyk-sloot, voor den aucteur Mr. Andries Boeckelman [1678]
     48 p.   16 cm.   **[1419]**

     —Nader vertoog . . . waer in aengewesen worden de quade proceduren van . . . Bonaventura van Dortmont, en des selfs onkunde, aengaende het afhalen van een doode vrucht, en der selver toevallen . . . Amsterdam, Pieter van den Berge, 1677.
     84 p.   16 cm.   **[1420]**

     —Nootwendig bericht . . . aengaende het afhalen van een doode vrucht. Amsterdam, Jan Rieuwertsz, 1677.
     24 p.   16 cm.   **[1421]**

     —Notariale insinuatie van Mr. Andries Boeckelman, en protestatie van Bonaventura van Dortmont . . . tegen deselve. Amsterdam, Hieronymus Sweerts, 1677.
     14 p.   16 cm.   **[1422]**

     —Wederlegging van Dr. Bonaventura van Dortmonts Antwoort, op het nootwendig bericht . . . aengaende het af-halen van een doode vrucht . . . Amsterdam, Jan Rieuwertsz, 1677.
     56 p.   16 cm.   **[1423]**

     —*See* AANMERKINGEN. 1677; AEN DEN EEDELEN COCCEAANSCHEN DOCTER. [1677]; DE AMSTELDAMSCHE NYPTANG. 1678; DE KOECKOECXZANGH. 1677; DE TWEEDE ONSCHULT. 1678; DORTMONT, B. van. Aennemingh van de presentatie, van Mr. Andries Boekelman. 1677 [and] Antwoort, op het nootwendigh bericht, van Mr. Andries Boekelman. 1677 [and]

Nootwendigh bericht. 1677 [and] Verklaring over de aen-neming van de presentatie van Mr. Andries Boekelman. 1677; EXTRAORDINARE AMSTERDAMSCHE MAENDAEGSCHE COURANT. 1678; KOECKOECX NAAR SANG. 1677; REGISTER DER BOECKJENS. [1677-1678]; SCHOPPEN IS TROEF. 1678; SENTIMENTS D'UN VOYAGEUR SUR PLUSIEURS LIBELLES DE CE TEMPS. 1677; STAETKUNDIGE BEDENCKING, over het verschil tusschen den Heer Bonaventura Dortmond. 1677; STRIJCK OP DEN BRUY EEN SESJEN. 1677; EEN WOORTJE IN TRANSITU. 1678.

BOENIGK, GOTTFRIED [*fl.* 1689] *respondent. See* SCHAMBERG, J. C., *praeses.* Disputatio physica de gustu ex recentiorum philosophorum hypothesi explicato. 1689.

BOERHAAVE, MARKUS [*fl.* 1695] *respondent.* Disputatio medica inauguralis, continens medicinae miscellanea themata ... Harderovici, Apud Albertum Sas, 1695.
[16] p. 25 cm. [1424]
Diss. — Harderwijk.

BOERHAVEN, MARCUS. *See* BOERHAAVE, Markus [*fl.* 1695]

BOERIO, LUCHINO [*ca.* 1521-*ca.* 1590] Trattato delli buboni, e carboni pestilenti, con le loro cause, segni, e curationi. Composto ... ad instanza delli ... Conservatori della sanità, della ... Republica di Genova, di nuovo ristampato. Genova, Giuseppe Pavoni, 1630.
64 p. 15 cm. [1425]

BÖRINGER, JOHANN KONRAD [*fl.* 1623] *respondent. See* AGER, N. Decas quaestionum. 1623.

BOESIUS, DANIEL. *See* BOESS, Daniel [*fl.* 1683-1687]

BOESS, DANIEL [*fl.* 1683-1687] *praeses.* Dissertatio medica, exhibens aegrum febri quartana intermittente laborantem ... Jenae, Literis Krebsianis [1687]
15, [1] p. 20 cm. [1426]
Diss. — Jena (A. Rosa, *respondent*)

— Specimen pathologico-therapeuticum de plica ... Jenae, Stanno G. H. Mülleri [1687]
[8] p. 19 cm. [1427]
Diss. — Jena (J. P. Pilling, *respondent*)

— *respondent. See* FASCH, A. H., *praeses.* Disputatio inauguralis medica de epilepsia. 1686; SAND, G.,

praeses. Disputatio academica de areae generibus. 1683.

BOETIUS DE BOOT, ANSELMUS. *See* BOODT, Anselm Boèce de [1550?-1632]

BOEZO, HEINRICH [1615-1689] *respondent. See* MICHAELIS, J., *praeses.* Disputatio medica inauguralis de pica. 1638.

BOGDAN, MARTIN [1631-1682] Insidiae structae Cl. V. Thomae Bartholini ... Vasis lymphaticis ab Olao Rudbekio ... in suis Ductibus hepaticis, & vasis glandularum serosis Arosiae editis, detectae a Martino Bogdan ... Francofurti, Apud Petrum Hauboldum [pref. 1654]
[44] p. 23 cm. [1428]
Bound with Bartholin, T. Anatomicae vindiciae Cl. V. Casparo Hofmanno ... aliisque oppositae. 1648.

— *In* Rudbeck, O. Insidiae structae Olai Rudbeckii, 1654.

— *respondent.* Tractatus de recidiva morborum ... Basileae, Typis Georgii Deckeri [1659]
[32] p. 19 cm. [1429]
Diss. — Basel.

— *See* LYSER, M. Culter anatomicus. 1665, 1679; SIMEO SETHUS. Σύνταγμα κατὰ στοιχείων περὶ τροφων δυνάμεων. 1658.

BOGIDAM, MARTIN. *See* BOGDAN, Martin [1631-1682]

BOGNER, ABRAHAM [*fl.* 1607] *See* KNOBLOCH, T., *praeses.* Disputationes anatomicae. 1608, 1612.

BOGNER, MICHAEL. *See* TOXITES, Michael [1515-1581]

BOHEMUS, CHRISTIAN [*fl.* 1650-1651] *respondent. See* POMARIUS, S., *praeses.* De modo visionis disputatio tertia. 1650.

BOHEMUS, MARTINUS. *See* BEHM, Martin [1557-1622]

BOHEMUS, TOBIAS. *See* BÖHM, Tobias [*fl.* 1607-1614]

BOHN, JOHANN [1640-1718] Circulus anatomico-physiologicus; seu, Oeconomia corporis animalis, hoc est, cogitata, functionum animalium potissimarum formalitatem & causas concernentia ... Lipsiae,

Sumtibus Joh. Friedrich Gleditsch, typis Christophori Fleischeri, 1686.

[8], 479, [25] p. 20 cm.   [1430]

—[The same.] ... Lipsiae, Apud Thomam Dritsch, 1697.

[6], 478, [20] p. 20 cm.   [1431]

—De renunciatione vulnerum; seu, Vulnerum lethalium examen, exponens horum formalitatem & causas, tam in genere, quam in specie ac per singulas corporis partes. Lipsiae, Sumtibus Joh. Frid. Gleditsch, typis Christophori Fleischeri, 1689.

[8], 400, [8] p. 17 cm.   [1432]

—Dissertationes chymico-physicae, quibus accedunt ejusdem tractatus, De aeris in sublunaria influxu, et De alcali et acidi insufficientia. Lipsiae, Apud J. Thomam Fritsch, 1696.

[16], 554, [22] p. 16 cm.   [1433]

—Disputatio medica, de cholera ... Lipsiae, Literis Ritzschianis [1666]

[18] p. 20 cm.   [1434]

Imperfect: p. [3-4] mutilated.
Diss. pro loco — Leipzig (G. A. Grobius, *respondent*)

Programs — Leipzig

—D. Johannes Bohn ... p. t. procancellarius L. S. [Lipsiae, Typis Johannis Erici Hahnii, 1673]

[8] p. 22 cm.   [1435]

For diss. of J. S. Wider.

—Facultatis Medicae in Academia Lipsiensi p. t. pro-cancellarius, D. Johannes Bohn ... L. S. D. [Lipsiae, Literis Christoph, Fleischeri, 1694]

[12] p. 19 cm.   [1436]

For diss. of C. G. Finger.

—Facultatis Medicae in Academia Lipsiensi p. t. pro-cancellarius, D. Johannes Bohn ... L. S. D. [Lipsiae, Typis Christoph, Fleischeri, 1694]

[12] p. 21 cm.   [1437]

For diss. of Samuel Veiel.

—Facultatis Medicae in Academia Lipsiensi p. t. procancellarius D. Johannes Bohn ... L. S. D. [Lipsiae, Literis Fleischerianis, 1700]

[12] p. 19 cm.   [1438]

For diss. of C. H. Erndl.

—Lectori benevolo D. Johannes Bohn ... Facultatis Medicae in Academia Lipsiensi p. t. procancellarius. Salutem! [Lipsiae, Literis Joh. Heinrici Richteri, 1695]

[12] p. 19 cm.   [1439]

For diss. of G. Berggold.

—Lectori benevolo Facultatis Medicae in Academia Lipsiensi p. t. procancellarius, D. Johannes Bohn ... S. D. [Lipsiae, Literis Goezianis, 1696]

[8] p. 19 cm.   [1440]

For diss. of H. H. Helcher.

—Lectori benevolo Facultatis Medicae in Academia Lipsiensi p. t. pro-cancellarius D. Johannes Bohn, P. P. salutem! [Lipsiae, 1697]

[8] p. 19 cm.   [1441]

For diss. of M. E. Ettmüller.

—Lectori salutem Facultatis Medicae in Academia Lipsiensi p. t. procancellarius, D. Johannes Bohn ... [Lipsiae, Typis Joh. Heinrici Richteri, 1696]

[12] p. 19 cm.   [1442]

For diss. of J. A. Kirch.

Dissertations — Leipzig

—*praeses*. Dissertationes chymico-physicae, chymiae finem, instrumenta & operationes frequentiores explicantes ... Quibus accessit ejusdem tractatus, olim editus, De aeris in sublunaria influxu. Lipsiae, Sumptibus Joh. Friderici Gleditschii, literis Christiani Gözii. 1685.

[256] p.; [36] p. 21 cm.   [1443]

Part [1] contains 15 theses originally published between 1680 and 1685. Part [2] has special title page. (Respondents: J. W. Pauli, no. 1; E. G. Heyse, no. 2; J. C. Taubenheim, no. 3; G. Thomasius, no. 4; C. L. Helvetius, no. 5; C. G. Schmalkalden, no. 6; H. Siegfried, no. 7; J. F. Ortlob, no. 8; D. K. Jeltsch, no. 9; E. E. Odhelius, no. 10; J. A. Kiesewetter, no. 11; J. A. Seyler, no. 12; K. F. Luther, no. 13; D. Kinner, no. 14; A. Geissler, no. 15).

Bound with Harder, J. J. Apiarium observationibus medicis centum. 1687.

—Exercitationum physiologicarum prima, de appetitu ... [-decima tertia, de urinae secretione] ... Lipsiae, Typis Joh. Georg [1674?]

[104] p. 19 cm.   [1444]

Contains 13 Leipzig dissertations originally published between 1668 and 1674. Cf. Heffter. vol. 2, part 1, items 631-643. (Respondents: J. A. Hermann, no. 1; A. de Nepita, no. 2; E. Nitschke, no. 3; A. Klaunig, no. 4; J. Wolf, no. 5; C. Stempel, no. 6; H. Warnatius, no. 7; C. Wolff, no. 8; G. Schmidt, no. 9; J. E. Oldenborch, no. 10; J. A. Limprecht, no. 11; G. Heintke, no. 12; K. Oehmb, no. 13).

—De medici officio dissertatio prima ... Lipsiae, Literis Fleischerianis [1697]

[32] p. 19 cm.   [1445]

J.C. Lehmann, *respondent*.

—De medici officio dissertatio secunda . . . Lipsiae, Literis Fleischerianis [1697]

[40] p.   20 cm.   [**1446**]

J. Brasche, *respondent.*

—De medici officio dissertatio quarta . . . Lipsiae, Literis Fleischerianis [1699]

[28] p.   19 cm.   [**1447**]

C. F. Richter, *respondent.*

De medici officio dissertatio quinta . . . Lipsiae, Literis Fleischerianis [1700]

[36] p.   19 cm.   [**1448**]

G. F. Jäschke, *respondent.*

—Disputatio inauguralis de cephalalgia . . . Lipsiae, Literis Joh. Georg [1680]

[16] p.   18 cm.   [**1449**]

C. J. Lange, *respondent.*

—Disputatio physiologica de duumviratu hypochondriorum . . . Lipsiae, Stanno Banckmanniano [1689]

[30] p.   20 cm.   [**1450**]

J. G. Lehmann, *respondent.*

—Disputatio therapeutica de symptomate urgente . . . Lipsiae, Excudebat Christoph. Fleischerus [1697]

[28] p.   20 cm.   [**1451**]

J. A. Wedel, *respondent.*

—Dissertatio chirurgica de trepanationis difficultatibus . . . Lipsiae, Joh. Heinrici Richteri [1694]

[38] p.   19 cm.   [**1452**]

G. Berggold, *respondent.*

—Dissertatio medica de atrophia in genere . . . Lipsiae, Typis Krügerianis [1688]

[27] p.   20 cm.   [**1453**]

J. T. Meisner, *respondent.*

—Dissertatio medica de catarrhis . . . Lipsiae, Literis Johann Erici Hahnii [1675]

[20] p.   20 cm.   [**1454**]

K. Oehmb, *respondent.*

—Dissertatio medica de dyspnoea . . . Lipsiae, Typis Andreae Balli [1686]

[30] p.   20 cm.   [**1455**]

K. Stisser, *respondent.*

—Dissertatio medica de inflammatione . . . Lipsiae, Literis Wittigavianis [1686]

[20] p.   19 cm.   [**1456**]

B. Müller, *respondent.*

—Dissertatio medica de polypo narium . . . Lipsiae, Literis Johann-Erici Hahnii [1672]

[16] p.   18 cm.   [**1457**]

J. E. Jahn, *respondent.*

—Dissertatio medica inauguralis de haemorrhoidibus caecis . . . Lipsiae, Typis Christoph. Fleischeri [1694]

[32] p.   19 cm.   [**1458**]

J. J. Hering, *respondent.*

Dissertatio physiologico-pathologica de lactis defectu . . . Lipsiae, Literis Johann-Erici Hahnii [1674]

[20] p.   20 cm.   [**1459**]

G. S. Birnbaum, *respondent.*

Dissertationem de variolis, hactenus in patria grassatis . . . subjicit Andreas Buxbaum . . . Lipsiae, Typis Eliae Fiebig [1679]

28, [1] p.   20 cm.   [**1460**]

A. Buxbaum, *respondent.*

—Dissertationem inauguralem de angina . . . examini exponit M. Fridericus Wilhelmus Klose . . . [Lipsiae] Typis Goezianis [1696]

[38] p.   20 cm.   [**1461**]

F. W. Klose, *respondent.*

—Dissertationem inauguralem de singultu . . . exponet M. Michael Ernst Ettmüller . . . Lipsiae, Literis Joh. Georg [1697]

[38] p.   20 cm.   [**1462**]

M. E. Ettmüller, *respondent.*

—Dissertationem inauguralem de torminibus colicis . . . publice ventilandam . . . sistit Johann Caspar Grimm . . . Lipsiae, Typis Christiani Banckmanni [1689]

[32] p.   19 cm.   [**1463**]

J. C. Grimm, *respondent.*

—Dissertationem medicam de haemorrhagia . . . submittet . . . Pancratius Wolff . . . Lipsiae, Litteris Johann-Erici Hahnii [1674]

[12] p.   19 cm.   [**1464**]

P. Wolff, *respondent.*

—Dissertationem medicam de vomitu . . . publicae disquisitioni exhibet Johannes Simeon Reinhard . . . Lipsiae, Literis Johannis Georgii [1688]

[24] p.   19 cm.   [**1465**]

J. S. Reinhard, *respondent.*

—Dissertationum chymico-physicarum quarta de aëre ... Lipsiae, Literis Johann. Wilhelmi Krügeri [1683]

[18] p.   19 cm.   [1466]

G. Thomasius, *respondent.*

—Dissertationum chymico-physicarum sexta de menstruis ... Lipsiae, Literis Johann. Wilhelmi Krügeri [1683]

[18] p.   19 cm.   [1467]

G. Günther, *respondent.*

—Dissertationum chymico-physicarum septima de comminutione atque attenuatione ... Lipsiae, Literis Christophori Fleischeri [1683]

[18] p.   19 cm.   [1468]

H. Siegfried, *respondent.*

—Dissertationum chymico-physicarum duodecima de calcinatione ... Lipsiae, Typis Krügerianis [1685]

[18] p.   19 cm.   [1469]

J. A. Seyler, *respondent.*

—Dissertationum chymico-physicarum decima quarta de solutione et inspissatione ... Lipsiae, Typis Krügerianis [1685]

[18] p.   19 cm.   [1470]

D. Kinner, *respondent.*

Exercitatio academica physiologica de cordis motu ... [Lipsiae] Typis Christiani Goezii [1690]

[24] p.   19 cm.   [1471]

J. Forrest, *respondent.*

Exercitatio physiologica de menstruo universali animali ... Lipsiae, Typis haered. Ballii [1687]

[20] p.   19 cm.   [1472]

J. A. Kirchhoff, *respondent.*

Specimen primum medicinae forensis ... Lipsiae, Stanno Backmanniano [1690]

[32] p.   19 cm.   [1473]

J. G. Rudolph, *respondent.*

Specimen tertium medicinae forensis ... Lipsiae, Stanno Banckmanniano [1692]

[40] p.   20 cm.   [1474]

E. Langermann, *respondent.*

—*respondent. See* AMMANN, P. Disputationem inauguralem de pleuritide vera ... subjicit. 1666; THOMASIUS, J. [1622-1684] *praeses.* Disputatio physica de putredine. 1660.

—*See* BELLINI, L. De urinis et pulsibus. 1685, 1698; FABRICIUS, H., ab Aquapendente. Opera omnia anatomica & physiologica. 1687.

—*as subject. See* CAMERARIUS, E. Dissertationes tres. 1694.

[BOILEAU, JACQUES, 1635-1716] Historia flagellantium de recto et perverso flagrorum usu apud Christianos, ex antiquis scripturae, patrum, pontificum, conciliorum, & scriptorum profanorum monumentis cum cura & fide expressa. Parisiis, Apud Joannem Anisson, 1700.

[20], 341, [19] p.   17 cm.   [1475]

Imperfect: sig. a2 wanting.

BOIM, MICHAŁ. *See* BOYM, Michał Piotr [1612-1659]

BOIREL, ANTOINE [1621-*ca.* 1702] Traité des playes de teste ... Alencon, Martin de la Motte & la veuve Malassis [1677]

[16], 367 (i.e. 369) p.   15 cm.   [1476]

BOISREGARD, NICOLAS ANDRY DE. *See* ANDRY DE BOISREGARD, Nicolas [1658-1742]

BOISSARD, JEAN JACQUES [1528-1602] Bibliotheca chalcographica illustrium virtute atque eruditione in tota Europa, clarissimorum virorum theologorum, jurisconsultorum, medicorum, historicorum ... collectore Iano Iacobo Boissardo ... sculptore Jan. Theod. de Bry ... Francofurti [Heidelbergae] Impensis Johannis Ammonii [1650-54]

5 v. in 1.   ports.   21 cm.   [1477]

The first volume contains the plates of the author's Icones virorum illustrium.

The second to fifth volume (each with special title page) are designated as "pars vi–ix" of the Bibliotheca, and also "continuatio prima–quarta" of the Icones.

Portraits of "pars vi" engraved by Sebastian Furck; those of "pars vii–viii" by Clemens Ammon; several portraits of "pars ix" signed: Heim F.

Without text except list of names at the beginning of each volume, and a distich below each portrait (with some exceptions in "pars vii").

BOISSON, JACOB DU. *See* BUISSON, Jacob du.

BOKELIUS, GUILIELMUS. *See* BÖKEL, Wilhelm [*fl.* 1607]

BOKENHAM, Henry [*fl.* 1655] *respondent.* Disputatio medica inauguralis, de arthritide ... Trajecti ad Rhenum, Typis Theodori ab Ackersdijck & Gisberti à Zijill, 1655.

[8] p.   20 cm.   [**1478**]

Diss. — Utrecht.

BOLLINGER, Ulrich [*fl.* 1609] *See* Croll, O. Basilica chymica. 1609, 1622?, 1631.

BOLLMANN, Justus Friedrich [*fl.* 1659] *respondent. See* Rolfinck, W., *praeses.* Discursus medicus de vertiginis διαγνωσει. 1659.

BOLNEST, Edward [*fl.* 1665-1672] Aurora chymica; or, A rational way of preparing animals, vegetables, and minerals, for a physical use; by which preparations they are made most efficacious, safe, pleasant medicines for the preservation and restoration of the life of man ... London, Printed by Tho. Ratcliffe, and Nat. Thompson, for John Starkey, 1672.

[16], 146 (i.e. 142), [2] p.   17 cm.   [**1479**]

—[Latin tr.] Aurora chymica; sive, Rationalis methodus praeparandi animalia, vegetabilia & mineralia ad usum medicum ... Hamburgii, Impensis Johannis Naumanni & Georgii Wolffii, 1675.

[10], 134 p.   17 cm.   [**1480**]

Translated by Johann Lange. Cf. Biog. méd., v. 2, p. 356-7.

—Medicina instaurata; or, A brief account of the true grounds and principles of the art of physick ... Whereto is added, a ... discourse, as a light to the true preparation of animal and vegetable arcana's. Together with a discovery of the true subject of the philosophick mineral mercury, and that from the authorities of the most famous of philosophers ... Also an epistolary discourse upon the whole by the author of Medela medicinae [i.e. Marchamont Nedham] London, John Starkey, 1665.

[31], 151 p.   15 cm.   [**1481**]

BOLOGNA, Giovanni Stefano. Discorso famigliare, e succinto intorno alle febbri fondato sopra le ragioni fisiche notomiche, col metodo facile, e ragionevole per medicarle, à cui s'aggiugne un picciol ragionamentano Dell' ipocondria e suoi accidenti. Colla cura stabilita senza gran apparecchio de medicamenti ... [Vienna] Appresso gli heredi del Viviani, 1684.

[12], 294, [5] p.   16 cm.   [**1482**]

BOLOGNA. Compagnia de gli maestri spetiali medicinalisti. *See* Università di Bologna. Collegio de medicina. Conventioni fra l'accelentiss. Collegio de medici. 1606 [and] Gl'indirizzi dell'arte dello spetiale medicinalista. 1658?

BOLOGNA. Ordinances, local laws, etc. Bandi, et provisioni, sopra quelli, che senza auttorità, & licenza dell'eccellentissimo Collegio di Medicina di Bologna ordinano, danno, & applicano medicamenti, overo essercitano alcuna parte di medicina. Et ordini da osservarsi da' barbieri, & speciali nel loro essercitio ... Bologna, Vittorio Benacci, 1617.

12 p.   22 cm.   [**1483**]

—Bando, et provisione sopra quelli, che senza autorità, & licenza dell'eccellentiss. Collegio di Medicina danno, ordinano, vendono, & applicano medicamenti in alcun modo. Et moderatione rinovata sopra li speciali, & barbieri ... Bologna, Vittorio Benacci, 1604.

[16] p.   22 cm.   [**1484**]

—Raccolta di tutti li bandi, ordini, e provisioni fatte per la città di Bologna in tempo di contagio imminente, e presente, li anni 1628, 1629, 1630, & 1631 ... Bologna, Girolamo Donini, 1631.

[8], 208 (i.e. 206) p.   21 cm.   [**1485**]

Compiled by Girolamo Donini.

BOLOGNA. Università. *See* Università di Bologna.

BOLOGNA. Università. Collegio de medicina. *See* Università di Bologna. Collegio de medicina.

BOLOGNINI, Angelo [*fl.* 1506-1517]. *See* Uffenbach, P. Thesaurus chirurgicae. 1610.

BOLTON, William. In laurum Apollini dicatam.[Latin and English] *In* Willis, T. A plain and easie method. 1691.

BOLZETTA, Attilio [1589-1635] Attilii Bulgetii ... De affectionibus cordis tractatus in tres libros divisus. Quibus accessit De morbis venenatis, venenisque tractatus generalis ... Patavii, Apud Joannem Baptistam Pasquati, 1657.

[8], 143, [1] p.   20 cm.   [**1486**]

De morbis venenatis has special title page.
Edited by Francesco Panizzola.

BOMPART, Marcellin Hercule [1594-1648] Miser homo, penicillo medico-physico Marcellini

Bompartii . . . Ed. 2. Parisiis, Apud Nicolaum Boisset, 1650.

[4], 12 p.   27 cm.   [1487]

—Nouveau chasse peste . . . Paris, Philippes Gaultier, 1630.

[16], 178, [13] p.   18 cm.   [1488]

—, *ed.* and *tr. See* HIPPOCRATES. [Epistolae. French tr.] La conference et entreveuë d'Hippocrate et de Democrite. 1632.

BON, JEAN LE. *See* LE BON, Jean [*d.* 1583?]

BONACCIUOLI, LUIGI [*d. ca.* 1540] *See* PINEAU, S. De integritatis & corruptionis virginum notis. 1639, 1640, 1641, 1650, 1663, 1690.

BONACCORSI, BARTOLOMMEO [*fl.* 1618–*ca.* 1650] De humano sero . . . [Bononiae, Typis Jo. Baptistae Ferronii] 1650.

[8], 96, [23] p.   21 cm.   [1489]

Engraved title page.
Running title: De urinis Bonacursii.

—Della natura de polsi . . . [Bologna, Giacomo Monti, 1647]

274 p.   21 cm.   [1490]

Engraved title page.

—Praesidiorum descriptiones adversus pestiferam luem . . . A Fr. Gabriele Melletio . . . in lucem editae. Bononiae, Ex typographia Clementis Ferronii, 1630.

51, [1] p.   20 cm.   [1491]

BONACIOLUS, LUDOVICUS. *See* BONACCIUOLI, Luigi [*d. ca.* 1540]

BONACIUOLI, LODOVICO. *See* BONACCIUOLI, Luigi [*d. ca.* 1540]

BONACURSIUS, BARTOLOMMEO. *See* BONACCORSI, Bartolommeo [*fl.* 1618–*ca.* 1650]

BONAFEDE, GIACOMO [*fl.* 1699] Unicomistica chirurgia opera breve . . . nella quale si tratta delli disetti de capelli, deformita cutanee, ferite, ulcere, e fratture . . . Todi, Vincenso Galassi, 1699.

[18], 287 p.   14 cm.   [1492]

First preliminary leaf (blank?) wanting.

BONALDI, PIETRO ANTONIO. Discorso rationale

contra la presente epidemia pestilente . . . Trevigi, Aurelio Righettini, 1631.

[16] p.   21 cm.   [1493]

BONAMICO, FRANCISCUS. *See* BUONAMICI, Francisco [*d.* 1604]

BONAMOUR, J. [*fl.* 17th cent.] *ed. See* VARANDA, J. de. Traité des maladies des femmes. 1666.

BONANNI, FILIPPO. *See* BUONANNI, Filippo [1638–1725]

BONATIOLUS, LUDOVICUS. *See* BONACCIUOLI, Luigi [*d. ca.* 1540]

BONAVENTURA, *Saint, Cardinal* [1221–1274] Medicamen spirituale contra pestem, constans quinque psalmis B. Virginis, ex Psalterio S. Bonaventurae cum litaniis & aliis oratiunculis ad eandem ac SS. patronos tempore pestis ad B. Virginem Mariam. Monachii, Typis Sebastiani Rauch, 1671.

[4], 20 p.   10 cm.   [1494]

—Psalterium. *See* Geistliche Artzney in Zeit der Pest. [16——?]

BONAVENTURA, FEDERICO [1555–1602] De partus octomestris natura, adversus vulgatam opinionem . . . libri decem. Opus . . . in Germania jam primum visum . . . correcte editum. In quo absolutissima de humani partus natura cognitio traditur; nimirum de conceptione, articulatione, maturitate, de partuum numero, pariendique terminis ac temporibus; utrum ante septimum mensem, ac post decimum undecimique initium, partus naturaliter edi possit. De septimestri, nonomestri, decimestri, undecimestrique partu, deque veris horum omnium causis plenissime, Aristotle duce, disputatur . . . Adjecta est ejusdem auctoris compendiosa de eodem partu disceptatio . . . Francoforti, Typis Melchioris Hartmanni, impensis Nicolai Bassaei, 1601.

[28], 704, [54] p.   tables.   35 cm.   [1495]

The "Compendiosa disceptatio" mentioned on the title page does not seem to have been included.

Previously published in 1600 in Urbino under title: De natura partus octomestris adversus vulgatam opinionem libri decem.

BONAVERA, DOMINICO MARIA. *See* BONAVERI, Domenico [*b. ca.* 1640]

BONAVERI, DOMENICO [*b. ca.* 1640] *ed. See* [VESALIUS, A.] Notomie de Titiano *ca.* 1670.

BONCKENBURGH, PIETER [*fl.* 1667] *respondent.* Disputatio chirurgico-medica inauguralis de phlegmone . . . Lugduni Batavorum, Apud viduam & haeredes Joannis Elsevirii, 1667.

[II] p.   23 cm.   **[1496]**

Diss. — Leyden.

BONCLARUS, VAUCLIUS DATHIRIUS, *pseud. See* AUBRI, Claude [17th cent.]

BONCORE, TOMMASO [*fl.* 1622] De populari, horribili, ac pestilenti gutturis, annexarumque partium affectione nobilissimam urbem Neapolim, ac totum fere regnum vexante consilium . . . Neapoli, Ex typographia Lazari Scorrigii, 1622.

131, [1] p.   illus.   20 cm.   **[1497]**

BONDT, JAKOB DE [1592-1631] De medicina Indorum lib. IV. 1. Notae in Garçiam ab Orta. 2. De diaeta sanorum. 3. Meth. medendi Indica. 4. Observationes e cadaveribus. Lugduni Batav., Apud Franciscum Hackium, 1642.

[6], 212, [4] p.   12 cm.   **[1498]**

Engraved title page.

The Notae of the 1st book pertain to Garcia de Orta's Coloquios dos simples, e drogas he cousas medicinais da India.

— [The same.] *In* Alpini, P. De medicina Aegyptiorum. 1645.

— Historiae naturalis & medicae Indiae orientalis libri sex. *In* Piso, W. De Indiae utriusque re naturali et medica libri quatuordecim. 1658.

— Oost-Indische warande, vervatende de leef-konst ende genees-konst daer gebruyckelijck . . . Getrocken uyt de Latijnsche schriften van Jacob Bont . . . Onse lants-luyden vrymoedigh medegedeelt, ende verrijckt door N. Zas. Hier achter is bygevoeght de Chirurgijns scheeps-kist. Amsterdam, Jan Claesz. ten Hoorn, 1673.

2 v.   14 cm.   **[1499]**

Added engraved title page.

"Aenteyckeningen op de historie der speceryen, aerd-en-boom-gewassen, dieren, ende der andere Indianse vremdigheden van Garcias ab Orta": p. 139-196, vol. 1.

Vol. 2 has title page: Chirurgyns scheepps-kist zijnde een catalogus ofte lijste der medicamenten . . . door J. v. B. [i.e. Johannes Verbrugge]

— Oost-en West-Indische warande. Vervattende aldaar de leef-en genees-konst. Met een verhaal van de speceryen, boom-en aard-gewassen, dieren &c. in Oost-en West Indien voorvallende. Door Jacobus

Bontius, Gulielmus Piso, en Georgius Markgraef . . . Hier nevens is bygevoegt De nieuw verbetende chirurgijns scheep-kist. Amsterdam, Jan ten Hoorn, 1694.

[8], 304, [7] p.; 96 p.   16 cm.   **[1500]**

Added engraved title page dated 1693.

"Aenteykeningen op de historie der speceryen, aerd-en-boom gewassen, dieren, ende der andere Indianse vremdigheden van Garcias ab Orta": p. 123-171.

Part [2] has special title page dated 1693: De nieuwe verbeterde chirurgyns scheeps-kist, sijnde een catalogus oft lijste der medicamenten . . . door J. Verbrugge . . .

BONENBERG, NIKOLAUS [*fl.* 1666-1667] *respondent. See* GRÜZMANN, D., *praeses.* Dissertatio academica. 1667.

BONET, JEAN [*fl.* 17th cent.] *See* [JAMET, N. P.] Traité de la circulation des esprits animaux. 1682.

BONET, JUAN PABLO [1579-1633] Reduction de las letras, y arte para enseñar a ablar los mudos . . . Madrid, Francisco Abarca de Angulo, 1620.

[26], 308, [6] p.   plates.   21 cm.   **[1501]**

Engraved title page.

"Tratado de las cifras": p. 280-288. "Tratado de la lengua griega": p. 289-304.

Two tables of Greek abbreviations at end.

BONET, PABLO JUAN. *See* BONET, Juan Pablo [1579-1633]

BONET, THÉOPHILE [1620-1689] *ed.* Corps de medecine et de chirurgie. Contenant la maniere de guerir toutes les maladies . . . Avec toutes les operations de chirurgie. Et les cures des tumeurs contre nature, des playes, des ulceres, des fractures & dislocations. Le tout extraict des plus celebres practiciens, tant anciens que modernes. Par T[héophile] B[onet] . . . Geneve, Jean Anthoine Choüet, 1679.

4 v.   plates.   23 cm.   **[1502]**

Imperfect: plates mutilated in vol. 1.

Vol. 2. translated by Théophile Bonet. Cf. Barbier, vol. 3, col. 597.

Contents. — [v. 1] De la medecine efficace; ou, La maniere de guerir les plus grandes . . . maladies . . . Par Marc Aurele Severin. — [v. 2] Observations chirurgiques de Guillaume Fabri de Hilden. — [v. 3] Observations et histoires chirurgiques tirées des oeuvres de quatre excellens medecins (i.e. Pieter van Foreest, Felix Platter, Balthasar Timaeus von Güldenklee, Pietro de Marchetti — [v. 4] Observations et histoires chirurgiques tirées des oeuvres latines des plus renommés practiciens de ce temps.

"Introduction methodique a la chirurgie. Par Jean Van Horn": p. [7-30] vol. 1.

—Medicina septentrionalis collatitia; sive, Rei medicae, nuperis annis a medicis Anglis, Germanis & Danis emissae, sylloge & syntaxis. Exhibens observationes medicas, in quibus nova, abdita, admirabilia et monstrosa exempla adducuntur ... Genevae, Sumptibus Leonardi Chouët & socii, 1684-1687.

2 v. plates. 36 cm.   [1503]

—Another issue, dated 1686.   [1504]

—Mercurius compitalitius; sive, Index medico-practicus per decisiones, cautiones ... & observationes in singulis affectibus praeter naturam et praesidiis medicis ... ex probatissimis practicis ... depromptas veram et tutam medendi viam ostendens. Accessit appendix de medici munere ... Genevae, Sumptibus Leonardi Chouët, & socii, 1682.

[24], 987, [15] p. 37 cm.   [1505]

—[English tr.] A guide to the practical physician: shewing from the most approved authors, both ancient and modern, the truest and safest way of curing all diseases ... whether by medicine, surgery, or diet. Lately published in Latin ... and now rendred into English ... To which is added, an appendix concerning the office of a physician by the same author. London, Thomas Flesher, 1684.

[10], 868 (i.e. 785), [4] p. 35 cm.   [1506]

—Observations et histoires chirurgiques tirées des oeuvres latines des plus renommés practiciens de ce temps, par un docteur medecin, et comprises en douze centuries ... Geneve, Pierre Chouët, 1670.

[63], 664, [47] p. 23 cm.   [1507]

Published in 1679 as vol. 4 of his Corps de medecine et de chirurgie.

—Polyalthes; sive, Thesaurus medico-practicus ex quibuslibet rei medicae scriptoribus congestus, pathologiam veterem et novam exhibens ... In quo ... Johannis Jonstoni Syntagma explicatur. Tomus primus [-tertius] ... Genevae, Sumptibus Leonardi Chouët, & socii, 1691-1693.

3 v. port. 36 cm.   [1508]

—Another issue, dated 1694.
3 v. in 2.   [1509]

—Sepulchretum; sive, Anatomia practica, ex cadaveribus morbo denatis, proponens historias et observationes omnium pene humani corporis effectuum ... Tomus primus [-secundus] ... Genevae, Sumptibus Leonardi Chouët, 1679.

[40], 1706, [1] p. port. 35 cm.   [1510]

Errata: p. [1707]

Contains 4 books with a special title page for tomus secundus inserted before book 3.

—[The same.] ... Ed. alt., quam novis commentariis et observationibus ... illustravit, ac tertia ad minimum parte auctiorem fecit Johannes Jacobus Mangetus ... Tomus primus [-tertius] Genevae, Sumptibus Cramer & Perachon, 1700.

3 v. port. 37 cm.   [1511]

Contains 4 books.

—, ed. See BAILLOU, G. de. Filum ariadnaeum medicorum. 1688 [and] Labyrinthi medici extricati. 1687 [and] Pharos medicorum. 1668; FERNEL, J. Universa medicina. 1679; HARTMANN, J. Praxis chymiatrica. 1682.

—, tr. See BLEGNY, N. de. Zodiacus medico-gallicus. 1680-1685; FABRICIUS VON HILDEN, W. Observations chirurgiques. 1669; MAYERNE, Sir T. T. de. Medicinal councels. 1677; ROHAULT J. Tractatus physicus. 1682.

—See MAYERNE, Sir T. T. de. Tractatus de arthritide. 1676.

BONET Y PUEYO, JOSÉ DE RIVILLA. See RIVILLA BONET Y PUEYO, José de.

BONEVAAL, JAN VAN [*fl.* 1647] respondent. Disputatio medica inauguralis de paralysi ... Lugd. Bat., Apud Franciscum Moyardum, 1647.

[8] p. 22 cm.   [1512]

Diss.—Leyden.

BONFANTE, BARTOLOMEO. See MONTI, D. Modo di adoperare il pretioso oglio de filosofi. [16--]

BONGARS, JACQUES [1554-1612] Jacobi Bongarsii et Georgii Michaelis Lingelshemii epistolae. Argentorati, Ex officina Josiae Staedelii, 1660.

[8], 349 p. 14 cm.   [1513]

Imperfect: p. 313-336 wanting.

Bound with Ficino, M. Libri III de vita. 1647.

BONGLARUS, VAUCLIUS DATHIRIUS, *pseud.* See AUBRI, Claude [17th cent.]

BONHAM, THOMAS [*d.* 1629?] The chyrurgians closet; or, An antidotarie chyrurgicall. Furnished with varietie and choyce of: apophlegms, balmes, baths, caps ... unguents, and waters. The greatest part ... scatteredly set downe in sundry bookes and papers; by ... Thomas Bonham ... and now drawne into method, and forme, by Edward Poeton ... London, Printed by George Miller, for Edward Brewster, 1630.

[8], 359, [27] p. 19 cm. [**1514**]

Errata: p. [27]

STC 3279.

—*See* PARKINSON, J. Theatrum botanicum. 1640.

Le BON-HEUR de la vie. 1666. *See* DALICOURT, P.

BONI, JACOPO ANTONIO [*d.* 1587] *See* GALENUS. Opera ex octava [-nona] Juntarum editione. 1609, 1625.

BONI, PIETRO ANTONIO, *of Ferrara.* Margarita pretiosa novella correctissima exhibens introductionem in artem chemiae integram ...

507-713 p., vol. 5. 20 cm. (*In* Zetzner, Lazarus, *ed.* Theatrum chemicum. Argentorati, 1659-61) [**1515**]

Caption title.

BONIFACIO, GIOVANNI [1547-1635] L'arte de' cenni con la quale formandosi favella visible, si tratta muta eloquenza, che non è altro che un facondo silentio. Divisa in due parti. Nella prima si tratta de icenni, che da noi con le membra del nostro corpo sono fatti ... Nella seconda si dimostra come di questa cognitione tutte l'arti liberali, e mecaniche si prevagliano ... Vicenza, Francesco Grossi, 1616.

[20], 623, [1] p. 21 cm. [**1516**]

BONILLA SAMANIEGO, ANTONIO DE [*fl.* 1664] Exercitacion medica, phylosophica, sobre la essencia de el morbo gallico. Por D. Antonio de Bonilla Samaniego ... Escrita á el ... Sebastian de Cubas ... Cordoba, Andres Carillo de Paniagua, 1664.

[4], 20 ll. 20 cm. [**1517**]

BONINUS, PLINIUS. *See* CIRCAMUNDUS, J.B. Consultatio de hydrargyrio. 1618.

BONNART, Jean [*d.* 1638] Methode pour bien seigner, utile à tous chirurgiens ... Paris, Hierosme de la Fonteine, 1628.

[6], 85, [2] p. 17 cm. [**1518**]

—La semaine des medicaments, observée és chef-d'oeuvres des maistres barbiers, chirurgiens de Paris. Où est sommairement traicté des vertus, proprietez, & usages des plantes, mineraux, animaux, des par-

ties & excremens d'iceux, avec le moyen de s'en servir ... Paris, Rollin Baraignes, 1629.

[52], 446 p. 18 cm. [**1519**]

Date altered by hand from MDCXXIX to MDCLXXIX.

BONNE-MAISON, ALONSO DE [*fl.* 1678] *respondent.* Disputatio medica inauguralis, de melancholia hypochondriaca ... Lugduni Batavorum, Apud viduam & heredes Joannis Elsevirii, 1678.

[19] p. 22 cm. [**1520**]

Diss. — Layden.

BONNET, CLAUDE [*fl.* 1654] *ed. See* SENNERT, D. Epitome universam Dan. Sennerti doctrinam ... complectens. 1655, 1660 [and] Operum in quinque tomos divisorum. 1666 [and] Operum in sex tomos divisorum tomus primus [-sextus] 1676.

BONNET, PIERRE [1638-1708] Oratio habita in scholis medicorum 19. Novembris 1679 ... Parisiis, Ex officina Christophori Ballard, 1679.

64 p. 15 cm. [**1521**]

Caption-title: Oratio. De methodo docendi.

BONNET, THÉOPHILE. *See* BONET, THÉOPHILE [1620-1689]

BONNET-BOURDELOT, PIERRE. *See* BONNET, Pierre [1638-1708]

BONOMO, GIOVANNI COSIMO [1663-1696] Osservazioni intorno a' pellicelli del corpo umano fatte dal dottor Gio. Cosimo Bonomo, e da lui con altre osservazioni scritte in una lettera all'illustriss. sig. Francesco Redi. Firenze, Piero Matini, 1687.

[1], 16 p. plate. 24 cm. [**1522**]

BONTEKOE, CORNELIS [1640?-1685] Alle de philosophische, medicinale en chymische werken ... behelsende een afwerp der ongefondeerde medicyne ... Neffens den opbouw van een ware philosophie, medicyne en chymie ... Eerste deel [-tweede deel] Amsterdam, Jan ten Hoorn, 1689.

[56], 355 p.; 402 (i.e. 406) p. port. 23 cm. [**1523**]

"Kort verhaal van het leven en de dood van den heer Corn. Bontekoe": p. [49-54]

—Antwoord ... aan de schryvers van de brief onder de naam van Pieter Bernagie M. D. uytgegaan ... Amsterdam, Jan Bouman, 1682.

63 p. 16 cm. [**1524**]

—[Fragmenta, dienende tot een onderwijs van de beweginge, en vyandschap of liever vrindschap van het acidum met het alcali. German.] Grund-Sätze der Medicin; oder, Die Lehre vom Alcali und Acido durch Würckung der Fermentation und Effervescentz ... Ins Hochteutsche übergesetzet durch H. H. Franckfurt und Leipzig, In Verlegung Philip Gottfried Saurmans, 1691.

[8], 168 p. 16 cm.   [1525]

—Gerbruik en mis-bruik van de thee, mitsgaders een verhandelinge wegens de deugden en kragten van de tabak. Door Cornelis Bontekoe ... Hier nevens een Verhandelinge van de coffee ... Door Stephanus Blankaart ... s' Gravenhage, Pieter Hagen. Amsterdam, Jan ten Hoorn, 1686.

[16], 192 p. 16 cm.   [1526]

—Korte verhandeling van 's menschen leven, gesondheid, siekte, en dood, begrepen in een drie ledige reden, I. over 't lighaam en sijne werkingen in gesondheid; II. over de siekte en desselfs oorsaken; III. over de middelen, om het leven en de gesondheid te bewaren en te verlengen ... Synde een korte vervulling van 't Niew gebouw der chirurgie, van 't Tractaat van thee, van de Reden over de koortzen ... Als mede Drie verhandelingen, I. Over de natuur. II. Over de bevinding. III. Over de sekerheit in de genees en heel-kunde ... 's Gravenhage, Pieter Hagen, 1684.

[124], 409, [13] p.; [4], 76 p. 16 cm. [1527]
Part [2] (Drie verhandelingen) has special title page dated 1685.

—[French tr.] Nouveaux elemens de medecine; ou, Reflexions physiques sur les divers états de l'homme. Divisées en trois parties. La premiere traite du corps humain & de ses operations. La seconde, des maladies, de la mort, & de leurs causes. Et la troisiéme, des moïens de prolonger la vie & de conserver la santé ... Nouvellement traduit en françois par un maître chirurgien [i.e. Jean Devaux]. Paris, Laurent d'Houry, 1698.

2 v. 17 cm.   [1528]

Vol. [2] has title: Suite des nouveaux elemens de medecine ou troisiéme partie des reflexions physiques sur les moïens de prolonger la vie, & de conserver la santé. Avec trois petits traitez ajoûtez.

"Discours physique, sur les proprietez de la sauge, & sur le reste des plantes aromatiques ... Par M. Hunault ..." at end of v. 2 has half title.

—[German tr.] Kurtze Abhandlung von dem menschlichen Leben, Gesundheit, Kranckheit, und Tod, in drey ... Theilen verfasset. Davon das I. Unterricht giebet von dem Leibe, und desselben zur Gesundheit dienlichen Verrichtungen. II. Von der Kranckheit, und derselben Ursachen. III. Von denen Mitteln, das Leben und die Gesundheit zu unterhalten und zu verlängern ... Wobey noch angehänget Drey kleine Tractätlein, I. Von der Natur. II. Von der Experienz oder Erfahrung. III. Von der Gewissheit der Medicin oder Heil-Kunst. Erstlich in holländischer Sprache beschrieben ... Anitzo aber in die hoch-teutsche Sprache versetzet [by R. J. H.] Budissin, In Verlegung Friedrich Arnst, Druckts Andreas Richter, 1686.

[1], 553, [7] p. front. (port.) 17 cm. [1529]
With this is bound (as issued?) [Dufour, P. S.] Drey neue curieuse Tractätgen. 1686.

—Een nieuw bewys van d'onvermijdelijke noodsakelijkheid en grootste nuttigheid van een algemene twyfeling, nevens De reden, tegens alle redelose ... al redenerende betwist-redent ... Nevens Een brief aan Jan Frederik Swetsertje ... Amsterdam, Jan ten Hoorn, 1685.

[1], 117 p.; [1], 33 p.; 24 p. 16 cm. [1530]
Parts [2-3] have half titles.
Bound with his Tractaat van het excellenste kruyd thee. 1685.

—[Nieuw gebouw van de chirurgie oof heel-konst stuks-gewiise op-getimert. German.] Neues Gebäude der Chirurgie, worinnen der alten Theoria, Anatomie und Lehre von Geschwülsten, Wunden, Geschwüren, Aderlassen, Purgieren, Repelliren ... Defendiren und vielen andern Mitteln abgebrochen, auch in einer ... Vorrede dargethan, warum die Artzney-und Heil-Kunst bisshero zu keiner grössern Perfection gelanget? ... Nebst des Herrn Autoris Lebens-Lauff ... in die hochteutsche Sprache übergesetzet und mit vielen ... Anmerckungen vermehret von Johanne Petro Albrecht ... Franckfurth und Leipzig, Verlegts Gottfried Freytag, 1697.

[43], 956 p. front. (port.) 17 cm. [1531]

—Notae provocatoriae in corollaria, quae disputationi suae de ictero opposuerat ... Gerardus Blasius ... Amstelodami, Typis Johannis ten Hoorn, 1682.

[7], 69 p. 16 cm.   [1532]

—Reden over de koortzen; door welke aangewesen word, dat de gemene theorie en praktijk valsch, schadelijk en moordadig is. 4. druk, vermeerderd . . . Met een Provocatie aan alle doctoren, chirurgijns, apothekers en in't besonder aan die van de stad Amsterdam. 's Gravenhage, Pieter Haagen, 1682.

[32], 101, [13] p.   16 cm.   **[1533]**

—[French tr.] Traitée des fiévres, où l'auteur découvre l'erreur des medecins anciens & modernes, tant en leur theorie que dans leur pratique. Utrecht, Jean Ribbius, 1682.

94 p.   16 cm.   **[1534]**

—Tractaat van het excellenste kruyd thee: 't welk vertoond het regte gebruyk, en de groote kragten van 't selve in gesondheyd, en siekten: benevens Een kort discours op het leven, de siekte, en de dood: mitsgaders op de medicijne van dese tijd . . . 2. druk vermeerdert, en vergroot met byvoegine van noch twee korte verhandelingen, I. Van de coffi; II. Van de chocolate, mitsgaders van Een apologie van den autheur tegens sijne lasteraars. 's Gravenhage, Pieter Hagen, 1679.

[31], 367 (i.e. 341) p.   16 cm.   **[1535]**
Items have special title pages.

—[The same.] . . . 3. druk vermeerdert . . . 's Gravenhage, Pieter Hagen, 1685.

[55], 343 p.   16 cm.   **[1536]**
Added engraved title page.
Items have special title pages.
"De lof van koffi . . . aan den Heer Johan van Duverden van Voord": p. [37-53]
With this are bound *his* Een nieuw bewys. 1685; Bödiker, Johann. Treur-klacht, en eer-galm, van . . . Cornelis Bontekoe. 1685.

—*See* BERNAGIE, P. Antwoord . . . op de brief, van Kornelis Bontekoe. 1682 [and] Brief . . . aan Kornelis Bontekoe. 1682; BÖDIKER, J. Treur-klacht. 1685; GEHEMA, J. A. a. De morbo vulgo dicto plica Polonica. 1683; OVERKAMP, H. Nieuw gebouw der chirurgie of heel-konst. 1682; [German tr.] 1689, 1692 [and] Reden. 1685.

BONTEKOE, PAULUS [*fl.* 1666-1667] *respondent.* Disputatio medica inauguralis de alimentorum in ventriculi alteratione . . . Lugduni Batavorum, Apud vidaum & haeredes Joannis Elsevirii [1667]

[19] p.   19 cm.   **[1537]**
Diss. — Leyden.

BONTIUS, JACOBUS. *See* BONDT, Jakob de [1592-1631]

BONUS, JACOBUS ANTONIUS. *See* BONI, Jacopo Antonio [*d.* 1587]

BONUS, JOSEPHUS MORENU. *See* MORENU BONUS, Joseph [*fl.* 1669]

BONUS, PETRUS. *See* BONI, Pietro Antonio, *of Ferrara.*

BONUS OF FERRARA. *See* BONI, Pietro Antonio, *of Ferrara.*

BONVINIUS, ELIAS [*d.* 1612] De theriaca liber, quo de theriacae descriptione, ingredientium delectu, quantitate, praeparatione, ipsius denique antidoti compositione, ex Andromachi senioris mente agitur. Vratislaviae, Typis Georgii Bauman, 1610.

[1], 239 (i.e. 229) p.   16 cm.   **[1538]**

BOODT, ANSELM BOÈCE DE [1550?-1632] Gemmarum et lapidum historia, qua non solum ortus, natura, vis & precium, sed etiam modus quo ex iis, olea, salia, tincturae, essentiae, arcana & magisteria arte chymica confici possint, ostenditur . . . Hanoviae, Typis Wechelianis, apud Claudium Marnium & heredes Joannis Aubrii, 1609.

[20], 294 (i.e. 288), [16] p.   illus., tables.   23 cm.   **[1539]**

—[The same.] . . . Nunc vero recensuit, a mendis repurgavit, commentariis, & pluribus, melioribusque figuris illustravit . . . Adrianus Toll . . . Lugduni Batavorum, Ex officina Joannis Maire, 1636.

[8], 576, [21] p.   illus., tables.   18 cm.   **[1540]**

—[French tr.] Le parfaict joaillier; ou, Histoire des peirreries: où sont amplement descrites leur naissance, iuste prix, moyen de les cognoistre, & se garder des contrefaites, facultez medecinales, & proprietez curieuses. Composé par Anselme Boece de Boot . . . et de nouveau enrichi de belles annotations, indices & figures, par André Toll . . . Lyon, Jean-Antoine Huguetan, 1644.

[32], 746, [34] p.   illus., tables.   18 cm.
                                    [1541]
Translated by Jean Bachou.

BOONACKER, WILLEM [*fl.* 1665] *respondent.* Disputatio medica inauguralis, de palpitatione cordis . . . Ultrajecti, Ex officina Johannis à Renswou, 1665.

10, [1] p.   20 cm.   **[1542]**
Diss. — Utrecht.

BOOT, ANSELMUS BOETIUS DE. *See* BOODT, Anselm Boèce de [1550?-1632]

BOOT, ARNOLD. *See* BOATE, Arnold [1606-1653]

BOOTH, RICHARD, *ed. See* FIORAVANTI, L. A discourse upon chyrurgery. 1626.

BOPP, GEORG [*fl.* 1650] Trifons Adlholzianus antipodagricus, das ist: Historische unnd medicinalische Hydrographia oder Wasser Beschreibung, dess . . . Wildtbadts Adelholzen, im . . . Obern Bayrn gelegen. Darinnen allerley Krancken . . . wunderbarliche Hülff erlangt haben, und gesund worden . . . München, Getruckt durch Nicolaum Henricum, 1650.

    [2], 132 (i.e. 134) p.   plate.   19 cm.   [**1543**]

"Additio": p. 117-132.

—[The same.] . . . München, Gedruckt durch Johann Jäcklin, 1666.

    116 (i.e. 117) p.   plate.   20 cm.   [**1544**]

A reprint of the 1650 edition without the Additio.

BORASTON, WILLIAM [*fl.* 1630-1633] *See* VICARY, T. The English mans treasure. 1633, 1641.

BORBÓN, FELIPE [*fl.* 1686] Medicina domestica, necessaria a los pobres, y familiar a los ricos. Transcrita del medico caritativo con algunos remedios, de otros autores. Con escolios en las materias, y afectos que se tratan, assi chirurgicos, como medicos . . . Zaragoça, Domingo Gascon, 1686.

    [24] 356, [4] p.   20 cm.   [**1545**]

BORBONI, MATTEO [*ca.* 1600-*ca.* 1669] Teatro anatomico di Bologna . . . del qual teatro il disegno presente danno . . . Matteo Borboni, e Lorenzo Tinti . . . [Bologna? 1668?]

    [1] p.   4 plates.   41 cm.   [**1546**]

Caption title.

BORCH, OLUF [1626-1690] Conspectus scriptorum chemicorum illustriorum, libellus posthumus cui praefixa historia vitae ipsius ab ipso conscripta. Havniae, Sumptibus Samuelis Germanni, 1697.

    [12], 48 p.   20 cm.   [**1547**]

—De ortu, et progressu chemicae, dissertatio. Hafniae, Typis Matthiae Godicchenii, sumptibus Petri Haubold, 1668.

    [12], 150, [1] p.   20 cm.   [**1548**]

Errata: p. [151]

—De usu plantarum indigenarum in medicina, et sub finem, de clysso plantarum & theé specifico, enchiridion. Hafniae, Literis & impensis Joh. Phil. Bockenhoffer, 1688.

    [8], 104 p.   15 cm.   [**1549**]

—Dissertatio de lapidum generatione in macro, & microcosmo. Cui accessit Additio . . . Joseph Lanzoni . . . Ferrariae, Typis Hyeronimi Filoni, 1687.

    [7], 76, [11] p.   14 cm.   [**1550**]

—Dissertatio de somno et somniferis,· maxime papavereis, quam . . . publice . . . tuebuntur . . . Dithlevius Jani Lucoppidanus [and others] Praeside Olao Borrichio. Hafniae, Typis viduae Cornificii Luft, 1680.

    [1], 48, [2] p.   19 cm.   [**1551**]

—[The same.] De somno et somniferis maxime papavereis dissertatio. Hafniae & Francofurti, Prostat apud Danielem Paulli, typis Aegidii Vogelii, 1681.

    38 p.   19 cm.   [**1552**]

—Another issue, with new title page, and imprint: Hafniae & Francofurti, Prostat apud Danielem Paulli, 1682.

    38 p.   21 cm.   [**1553**]

—[The same.] . . . Hafniae, Apud Danielem Paulli, 1683.

    40 p.   20 cm.   [**1554**]

—[Docimastice metallica clare & compendario tradita. German.] Metallische Probier-Kunst deutlich und kurtz beschrieben. Verteutscht durch Georgium Kus. Kopenhaven, Bei Daniel Paulli, 1680.

    74 (i.e. 72) p.   17 cm.   [**1555**]

—Hermetis, Aegyptiorum, et chemicorum sapientia ab Hermanni Conringii animadversionibus vindicata . . . Hafniae, Sumptibus Petri Hauboldi, 1674.

    [12], 448, [8] p.   plate.   20 cm.   [**1556**]

—Lingua pharmacopoeorum; sive, De accurata vocabulorum in pharmacopoliis usitatorum pronunciatione. Hafniae, Typis Matthiae Godicchenii, sumptibus Petri Hauboldi, 1670.

    [49] ll.   19 cm.   [**1557**]

Dissertations — Copenhagen

—*praeses.* Disputatio medica de ictero . . . Hafniae, Typis Matthiae Goddicchenii [1677]

[14] p. 19 cm. **[1558]**
L. Christiani, *respondent.*

—Disputatio medica inauguralis de ascite ... Hafniae, Literis viduae Cornificii Lufe [1682]
[16] p. 18 cm. **[1559]**
G. Kus, *respondent.*

—Disputatio medica inauguralis de phthisi ... Hafniae, Typis Johan. Adolph. Bexman, 1688.
[12] p. 20 cm. **[1560]**
N. Erici, *respondent.*

—Dissertatio medica de alimentorum cursu, eorumque in chylum, sanguinem & corporis humani substantiam mutatione ... Hafniae, Literis Georgii Gödiani, 1676.
[12] p. 19 cm. **[1561]**
J. Jürgens, *respondent.*

—Dissertatio medica inauguralis de apoplexia ... Hafniae, Literis Christiani Weringii [1676]
[32] p. 19 cm. **[1562]**
J. Michaelis, *respondent.*

—Dissertatio medica inauguralis de morbis soporosis comate somnolento, lethargo, caro & apoplexia ex intemperie sangvinis crassa & frigida oriundis ... Hafniae, Literis Joh. Philippi Bockenhoffer [1683]
26, [1] p. 19 cm. **[1563]**
F. Reenberg, *respondent.*

—Dissertationem hanc inauguralem de malo hypochondriaco ... submittit Paulus Brand ... Hafniae, Typis Matthiae Georgii F. Godicchenius [1676]
[48] p. illus. 19 cm. **[1564]**
"Simonis Paulli Epistolaris gratulatio ad Paulum Brandium": p. [39-44]
P. Brand, *respondent.*

—*ed. See* DEUSING, A. Deusingius heautontimorumenos. 1661.

—*See* CONRING, H. De Hermetica medicina libri duo. 1669; DEUSING, A. Resurrectio hepatis asserta. 1662; SINIBALDI, G. B. Geneanthropeiae. 1669.

BORCHT, PIETER, VAN DER [*fl.* 1686] *respondent.* Disputatio medica inauguralis de dysenteria ... Lugduni Batavorum, Apud Abrahamum Elzevier, 1686.
[8] p. 18 cm. **[1565]**
Diss.—Leyden.

BORDEGATO, MATTEO [*d.* 1689] Themata dissertationum logicarum, quas habiturus est in lib. secundum posteriorum resolutiorum Aristotelis ... [Patavii, Typis Petri Mariae Frambotti, *ca.* 1688]
[6] p. 23 cm. **[1566]**
The senior Matteo Bordegato was professor of logic at Padova from 1685 until his death. Cf. Facciolati, part III, p. 304, and Papadopoli, vol. I, p. 187.
Caption title.

BOREL, PIERRE [*ca.* 1620-1671] Bibliotheca chimica, seu, Catalogus librorum philosophicorum hermeticorum in quo quatuor millia circiter, authorum chimicorum, vel de transmutatione metallorum, re minerali, & arcanis, tam manuscriptorum, quam in lucem editorum, cum eorum editionibus, usque ad annum 1653, continentur. Cum ejusdem bibliothecae appendice, & corollario ... Parisiis, Apud Carolum Du Mesnil et Thomam Jolly, 1654.
[12], 276 p. 15 cm. **[1567]**

— De curationibus sympatheticis.
526-528 p. 21 cm. (*In* Theatrum sympatheticum auctum. Norimbergae, 1662) **[1568]**
Caption title.

—De vero telescopii inventore, cum brevi omnium conspiciliorum historia ... Accessit etiam centuria Observationum microcospicarum [sic] Hagae–Comitum, Ex typographia Adriani Vlacq, 1655.
[12], 67 p.; 63 p.; 45, [4] p. illus., plate, ports. 19 cm. **[1569]**
Part [3] has special title page dated 1656.

—Historiarum, et observationum medico-physicarum, centura prima [-secunda] In qua, non solum, multa utilia, sed & rara, stupenda ac inaudita continentur. Castris, Apud Arnaldum Colomerium, 1653.
[24], 240 p. illus. 16 cm. **[1570]**
Centuria secunda (p. 113), has special title page.

—Historiarum, et observationum medico-physicarum, centuriae IV. In quibus non solum multa utilia, sed & rara, stupenda ac inaudita continentur. Accesserunt D. Isaaci Cattieri ... Observationes medicinales rarae, Dom. Borello communicatae: et Renati Cartesii vita eodem P. Borello authore. Quae omnia nunc primum in lucem prodeunt. Parisiis, Apud Joannem Billaine et viduam Mathurini Dupuis, 1656.

[16], 184 (i.e. 384) p.; 77, [1] p.; [4], 59, [1] p.   illus., plate.   18 cm.   **[1571]**

Parts [2-3] have special title pages.

—Another issue, with the imprint date altered on the general title page to 1657.   **[1572]**

—[The same.] . . . Francofurti, Apud Laur. Sigismund. Cörnerum, 1670.

[16], 352, [30] p.; 86 p.; 55 p.   illus.   16 cm.   **[1573]**

Added engraved title page.

Parts [2-3] have special title pages.

—[The same.] . . . Nunc autem aliunde ob argumenti similitudinem accedunt Joh. Rhodii Observationes, Arnoldi Bootii De affectibus omissis tractatus & Petri Matthaei Rossii Consultationes & observationes selectae. Francofurti & Lipsiae, Apud Laur. Sigism. Cörnerum, 1676.

6 parts in 1 v.   illus.   17 cm.   **[1574]**

Added engraved title page.

Parts [2-3] and [5-6] have half titles. Part [4] has special title page.

—Hortus; seu, Armamentarium simplicium, mineralium, plantarum & animalium, ad artem medicam utilium. Cum brevi et accurata . . . eorum etymologia, descriptione, loco, temperie & viribus . . . Castris, Apud Bernardum Barcoudanum, 1666.

[8], 384, [4] p.   17 cm.   **[1575]**

BOREL, Pierre [1620?-1689] *See* Gassendi, P. Viri illustris Nicolai Claudii Fabricii de Peiresc . . . vita. 1655.

BORELLI, Alfonso. *See* Borelli, Giovanni Alfonso [1608-1679].

BORELLI, Giovanni Alfonso, [1608-1679] De vi percussionis, et motionibus naturalibus a gravitate pendentibus; sive, Introductiones & illustrationes physico-mathematicae apprime necessariae ad opus ejus intelligendum De motu animalium una cum ejusdem auctoris responsionibus in animadversiones . . . Stephani de Angelis ad librum De vi percussionis. Ed. prima Belgica . . . correctior & auctior . . . Accurante J. Broen . . . Lugduni Batavorum, Apud Petrum vander Aa, 1686.

[16], 262, [22] p.; [4], 360, [32] p.   tables.   20 cm.   **[1576]**

Added engraved title page: . . . Atrium physico-mathematicum apertum ad aedificium ejus magnificum De motu animalium . . .

Each part has special title page.

—De motionibus naturalibus a gravitate pendentibus, liber . . . Regio Julio, In officina Dominici Ferri, 1670.

[8], 566, [5] p.   illus.   24 cm.   **[1577]**

Added half title.

With this is bound *his* Historia et meteorologia incendii Aetnaei. 1670.

—De motu animalium . . . opus posthumum. Romae, Ex typographia Angeli Bernabo, 1680.

[12], 376, [11] p.; [4], 520 p.   plates.   22 cm.   **[1578]**

Pars altera has special title page dated 1681.

Edited by Carolus Joannes a Jesu.

—[The same.] De motu animalium pars prima [-pars altera] . . . Ed. altera. Correctior & emendatior. Lugduni in Batavis, Apud Cornelium Boutesteyn, Danielem a Gaesbeeck, Johannem de Vivie & Petrum vander Aa, 1685.

[16], 280 (i.e. 274), [17] p.; [4], 365, [15] p.   plates.   22 cm.   **[1579]**

Added engraved title page.

Part 2 has special title page.

—Another issue, with imprint: Lugduni in Batavis, Apud Johannem de Vivie, Cornelium Boutesteyn, Danielem a Gaesbeeck, & Petrum vander Aa, 1685.   **[1580]**

—De vi percussionis liber . . . Bononiae, Ex typographia Jacobi Montii, 1667.

[12], 300, 30, [2] p.   tables.   22 cm.   **[1581]**

—Delle cagioni delle febbri maligne della Sicilia. Negli anni 1647 e 1648 . . . Cosenza, Gio. Battista Rosso, 1649.

[4], 218, [2] p.   illus.   21 cm.   **[1582]**

Errata: p. [219-220]

—Historia, et meteorologia incendii Aetnaei anni 1669 . . . accessit responsio ad censuras Rev. P. Honorati Fabri contra librum auctoris De vi percussionis. Regio Julio, In officina Dominici Ferri, 1670.

[11], 162, [1] p.   plate, illus.   24 cm.   **[1583]**

Added half title.

Errata: p. [163]

Bound with *his* De motionibus naturalibus. 1670.

—[Vitae Renati Cartesii. English] Summary or compendium, of the life of the most famous philosopher Renatus Descartes. Written originally in Latin by Peter Borellus . . . to which is also added an epitome of his life by Marcus Zurius Boxhornius

... London, Printed by E. Okes, for George Palmer, 1670.   **[1584]**

—*See* [VERDUC, J. B.] Nouvelle osteologie. 1689.

—*as subject. See* LA SCALA, D. Phlebotomia damnata. 1696; STURM, J. C. Epistola ... ad Joh. Georgium Volckamerum. 1684.

BORELLUS, PETRUS. *See* BOREL, Pierre [*ca.* 1620-1671]

BORGARUCCI, BORGARUCCIO [*fl.* 1570-1578] *ed. See* FALLOPPIO, G. Secreti. 1618, 1650, 1687; ROSTINIO, P. Compendio di tutta la cirugia. 1607, 1677.

BORGHERUCCI, BORGHERUCCIO. *See* BORGARUCCI, Borgaruccio [*fl.* 1570-1578]

BORGHESE. *See* URBIGERUS, Baro.

BORLASE, EDMUND [*d.* 1682] The reduction of Ireland to the crown of England. With the governours since the conquest by King Henry II. Anno MCLXXII. With some passages in their government. A brief account of the rebellion Anno Dom. MDCXLI. Also the original of the Universitie of Dublin, and the Colledge of Physicians ... London, Printed by Andr. Clarke for Robert Clavel, 1675.
    [49] 284 p. illus. 18 cm.   **[1585]**

BORNEMANN, ANTON PHILLIPP [*fl.* 1699] *respondent. See* HOFFMANN, F. [1660-1742] *praeses.* Dissertatione physico-medica inaugurali affectus hereditarios. 1699.

BORNETTUS, DUNCANUS. *See* BURNET, Duncan [16th-17th cent.]

BORRÁS, GULIELMO SALVADOR. *See* SALVADOR BORRÁS, Guillermo.

BORRICHIUS, OLAUS. *See* BORCH, Oluf [1626-1690]

BORRO, GIUSEPPE FRANCESCO [1627-1695] Epistolae duae. I. De cerebri ortu & usu medico. II. De artificio oculorum humores restituendi. Ad Th.Bartholinum. Hafniae, Prostant apud Danielem Paulli, 1669.
    [4], 68 p. illus. 20 cm.   **[1586]**
Contains also two letters by Thomas Bartholin addressed to G. F. Borro.

—Specimina quinque chimiae Hyppocraticae ... Coloniae, 1664.
    [1], 56 p. 21 cm.   **[1587]**

—*See* MAJOR, J. D. Consideratio physiologica. 1669?

BORROMEO, ALESSANDRO [1625-1708] Grandes materias ingenia parva non sustinent, & in ipso conatu ultra vires ausa, succumbunt; quantoque majus fuerit quod dicendum est, tanto magis obruitur qui magnitudinem rerum verbis non potest explicare ... [Patavii? ca. 1685]
    [7] p. 23 cm.   **[1588]**
Issued without title page; title from beginning of text.

—Preclara res est, quae ex opere, quod quis didicit, proficiscitur oratio. Medicina altissimi donum, res sacra, sacris tradenda viris, sapientiae soror, ac contubernalis, traducenda est ad sapientiam, & hanc oportet transferre ad medicinam, ut inde sapiens medicus ab Hippocrate Deo aequalis habeatur ... [Patavii? ca. 1688]
    3 p. 23 cm.   **[1589]**
Issued without title page; title from beginning of text.

—Quoniam lumen est Deus illustrans omnia, omnia eodem perfundit, cuicumque etenim, quae perficiant, contigunt ... [Patavii, Apud Cadorinum, 1689
    7 p. 23 cm.   **[1590]**
Issued without title page; title from beginning of text.

—Regium cor, cono, ac pineae nuci haud absimile, iram nutriens, thoracem induens, disquisitioni nostrae datur, quod utique defatigabit mentis, vel purgatissimae, dilucidissimaeque aciem cujuscumque conantis rite lustrare ea quae de eodem appollinei viri, sacri perscrutatores abditissimorum naturae latentissimae mysteriorum, effatu digna, scituque necessaria pronunciarint, & evulgaverint ... [Patavii, 1687]
    [4] p. 23 cm.   **[1591]**
Issued without title page; title from beginning of text.

BORROMEO, CARLO, *Saint. See* CARLO BORROMEO *Saint* [1538-1584]

BORTEL, GOMER VAN [1660-1724] *tr. See* PORTAL, P. De practyk der vroed' meesters, en vroed' vrouwen. 1690.

BOSCH, GERARD VAN DEN. *See* HAFACKER, G. Leer om leer, voor Petrus van den Bosch. 1678.

BOSCH, GUILLAUME VAN DEN. *See* BOSSCHE, Guillaume van den [*fl.* 1638]

BOSCH, JACOB [*fl.* 1697] *respondent.* Disputatio medica inauguralis de diabete ... Trajecti ad Rhenum, Ex officina Francisci Halma, 1697.

     [12] [3] p.   22 cm.   [**1592**]
     Diss. — Utrecht.

BOSCH, PIETER VAN DEN. Antwoort ... op de toegift van Dr. Johan Baptista Lamsweerde, begrepen in sijn geluk-wensching. Amsterdam, Anthoni Lescailje, 1678.

     29 p.   16 cm.   [**1593**]

— *See* HAFACKER, G. Leer om leer, voor Petrus van den Bosch. 1678.

BOSCHI, IPPOLITO [*ca.* 1540-1612] De curandis vulneribus capitis brevis methodus ... Ferrariae, Apud Victorium Baldinum, 1609.

     48 p.   21 cm.   [**1594**]

— Diario overo breve trattato del modo, che si deve tenere per conservarsi sano ne' tempi contagiosi composto per Hippolito Bosco ... Modena, Per Giulian Cassiani, 1630.

     12 p.   20 cm.   [**1595**]

BOSCO, FRANCESCO DAL [*d.* 1640] La prattica dell' infermiero ... nella quale con osservationi fondate nell'uso di moltissimi anni s'addottrina l'assistente, e caritativo infermiere per ben conoscere, e ne' casi repentini applicar li rimedii proportionati a' mali dei suoi infermi ... Verona, Gio. Battista Merlo, 1664.

     [8], 384, [23] p.   20 cm.   [**1596**]
     Errata: p. [23]

— [The same.] ... Venetia, Gio. Giacomo Hertz, 1669.

     [40], 460, [4] p.   16 cm.   [**1597**]

— [The same.] ... Di nuovo ristampato ... Milano, Gioseffo Marelli, 1670.

     [28], 366, [1] p.   15 cm.   [**1598**]

— [The same.] ... Bologna, Gioseffo Longhi, 1677.
     [36], 396 p.   15 cm.   [**1599**]

— [The same.] ... Venetia, Per il prodocimo, 1687.

     [36], 396 p.   14 cm.   [**1600**]

Imperfect: p. 299-302 wanting.
Different setting of type.

— [The same.] ... Milano, Giuseppe Marelli, 1693.

     [28], 366, [1] p.   15 cm.   [**1601**]
     A reprint of the 1670 edition.

BOSELLI, FRANCESCO [1620-1680] Amaltheum medico-politicum, (theatri medici praeludia) tres in apparatus digestum, doctrinae varietate. Tum laureandis, cum medicis, tum caeteris sapientiae mystis non minus conferens, quam jucundum. Antenorea in Academia ab anno 1631 usque adhuc medicinae professorum encomiis pro Corollario addita elogiorum heroum publica in ejus bibliotheca expictorum descriptione ... Patavii, Typis heredum Pauli Frambotti, 1665.

     [40], 734 (i.e. 736), [32] p.   22 cm.   [**1602**]

BOSSCHE, GUILLAUME VAN DEN [*fl.* 1638] Historia medica, in qua libris IV. animalium natura, et eorum medica utilitas exacte & luculenter tractantur ... Bruxellae, Typis Joannis Mommarti, 1639.

     [16], 422 (i.e. 434), [20] p.   illus.   21 cm.
                                      [**1603**]

BOSSEN, JOHANN HEINRICH [*fl.* 1650] *respondent.* *See* CONRING, H., *praeses.* Disputatio medica de hydrope ascite. 1650.

BOSSERT, JOHANN ANDREAS [*fl.* 1658-1660] *respondent. See* MÖBIUS, G., *praeses.* Institutionum medicarum disputatio decima quarta de usu partium genitalium in foeminis. 1658; SCHENCK, J. T., *praeses.* Dissertatio inauguralis medica περι της ανορεξιας. 1660.

BOSZ, HENRICUS. *See* BUSZ, Henricus.

BOTALLO, LEONARDO [*d.* 1587] Opera omnia medica & chirurgica. Hac postrema editione a mendis repurgata, methodice disposita, paragraphis distincta, notis marginalibus, & authorum testimoniis aucta, hinc inde annotationibus illustrata, prodeunt e musaeo Joannis van Horne ... Lugduni Batavorum, Ex officina Danielis & Abrahami a Gaasbeeck, 1660.

     [16], 800, [24] p.   plates.   17 cm.   [**1604**]
     Added engraved title page.
     The same works were published in Lyons in 1565 under title: Commentarioli duo ... Caetera ...

—De curatione per sanguinis missionem: liber. De incidendae venae, cutis scarificandae, & hirudinum affigendarum modo . . . Postrema auctoris cura ita recognitus, & multis disputationibus ac examplis auctus, ut novum plane opus dici possit. Editio novissima. Lugduni, Sumptibus Michaelis Duhan, 1655.

[16], 217 (i.e. 219) p.   illus.   18 cm.   **[1605]**

A reprint (with the addition of a new dedication by the publisher) of the edition published in Antwerp in 1583.

—Zwey chirurgische Bücher: handlende, das I. Von der Frantzosen-Kranckheit, und ihrer Cur. Das II. Von den Schuss-Wunden, und wie dieselben zu heilen. Mit zweyen Registern . . . versehen, und allen Wund-Aertzten zu grossen Nutzen, aus der lateinischen in die teutsche Sprach übersetzet. Samt einem Anhang einer kurtzen Kriegs-Wund-Artzney. Nürnberg, Johann Daniel Tauber, 1676.

3 parts in I v.   plates.   17 cm.   **[1606]**

Added engraved title page has title: Schuss-Wunden und Frantzosen-Cur verteutscht.

Part 2 has special title page: . . . Zweytes Buch, von den Schuss-Wunden. Vol. [3], the "Anhang," has special title page: Kurtze Kriegs-Wund-Artzney; oder, Die Kunst Schuss- und Kugel-Wunden zu heylen, beschrieben von Leonard Tassin.

Translations of Botallo's Luis venereae curandae ratio and De curandis vulneribus sclopetorum, and of Tassin's Chirurgie militaire.

BOTELHO, FERNÃO MARECOS [*fl.* 1604] *See* PORTUGAL. Sovereigns, etc. [1598–1621] (Philip II). Regimento dos medicos e boticarios. 1604.

BOTERO, GIOVANNI [*ca.* 1533–1617] *See* GUALDO, P. Vita Joannis Vincentii Pinelli. 1607.

BOTHIÈRE, GEORGE DE LA. *See* LA BOUTHIÈRE, George de [16th cent.]

BOTHIUS, JOHANN CHRISTIAN [*fl.* 1700] *respondent. See* SPERLING, P. G., *praeses.* Dissertatio solennis de vermibus in primis viis. 1700.

BOTTARELLI, GIOVANNI [*fl.* 1688] De bagni di San Casciano . . . Firenze, Vincenzio Vangelisti [1688].

308 (i.e. 310) p.   plates.   14 cm.   **[1607]**

BOTTER, HENDRIK [*fl.* 1600–1607] *ed. See* VESALIUS, A. De humani corporis fabrica librorum epitome. 1600 [i.e. 1601] [and] Anatomia. 1617.

BOTTHIUS, GEORG HEINRICH [*fl.* 1619] *respon-*

dent. See STEPHAN, S., *praeses.* Disputatio medica de cerebri natura. 1619.

BOTTI, GIUSEPPE [17th cent.] Cecità illuminata; cioè, Breve compendio della formazione, e struttura dell'occhio, e delle sue parti constituenti; d'onde si mostra come si formi la visione, con l'assegnazione de mali dell'occhio, e le loro cause, col modo di guarirle per mezzo del salutifero estratto di varie essenze . . . Parma, Giuseppe Rossetti, 1698.

63, [1] p.   16 cm.   **[1608]**

Engraved coat of arms of dedicatee: p. [1]

BOTTONI, ALBERTINO [*d.* 1596?] *See* SCHOLTZ, L. Consiliorum medicinalium . . . liber singularis. 1610.

BOUCHARD, JEAN JACQUES [1606–1641?] *See* GASSENDI, P. Viri illustris Nicolai Claudii Fabricii de Peiresc . . . vita. 1655.

BOUCHER DE BEAUVAL, JEAN [*fl.* 1673] Traité de la populaire colique bilieuse de Poitou . . . La Rochelle, Toussaints de Goüy, 1673.

[20], 77, [3] p.; 28 p.; [24] p. 18 cm.

[1609]

Part [2] contains several pieces concerning Boucher de Beauval. Part [3] has caption title: Abbregé historique & chronologique de la ville de la Rochelle.

BOUDENS, GEORGE [*fl.* 1691] *respondent.* Disputatio medica inauguralis de scorbuto . . . Lugduni Batavorum, Apud Abrahamum Elzevier, 1691.

[16] p.   22 cm.   **[1610]**

Diss. — Leyden.

BOUDEWYNS, MICHIEL [1601–1681] Dienstich ende ghenuchelijck tyt-verdryf voor siecken, om ghesont te worden, en voor ghesonde om niet sieck te zijn: handelende van alle die menschen de welcke in een sieck-huys van noode sijn . . . Door M[ichiel] B[oudewyns] medic. Antverp. Antwerpen, Fransoys Fickaert, 1654.

[24], 467, [1] p.   16 cm.   **[1611]**

—Another issue, pages 465-[468] reset.   **[1612]**

—Ventilabrum medico-theologicum quo omnes casus, tum medicos, cum aegros, aliosque concernentes eventilantur . . . Antverpiae, Apud Cornelium Woons, 1666.

[24], 454, [42] p.   21 cm.   **[1613]**

Added engraved title page.

BOUILLONS et tysannes. Pour les pauvres gens. *See* ASSEMBLÉE CHARITABLE À PARIS.

BOULENCOURT. *See* LE JEUNE DE BOULENCOURT.

BOULENE, JEAN MARCEL DE. *See* MARCEL, Jean.

BOULTON, RICHARD [*fl.* 1697-1724] An examination of Mr. John Colbatch his books, viz. I. Novum lumen chirurgicum. II. Essay of alkalies and acids. III. An appendix to that essay. IV. A treatise of the gout. V. The doctrin of acids further asserted, &c. VI. A relation of a person bitten by a viper &c. To which is added An answer to Dr. Leigh's remarks on a Treatise concerning the heat of the blood. Together with remarks on Dr. Leigh's book intituled Exercitationes quinque printed at a private press in Oxford, without the license of the university. As also a short view of Dr. Leighs Reply to Mr. Colbatch ... London, Tho. Bennet, 1699.

[17], 291 (i.e. 301), [1] p. 18 cm.   [**1614**]

—A treatise of the reason of muscular motion; or The efficient causes of the contraction of a muscle. Wherein most of the phaenomena about muscular motion are explained ... London, A. and J. Churchill, 1697.

[10], 116, [5] p. 14 cm.   [**1615**]

—*ed. See* BOYLE, *Hon.* R. The works. 1699-1700.

BOULTON, SAMUEL [*fl.* 1656] Medicina magica tamen physica: magical, but natural physick; or, A methodical tractate of diastatical physick. Containing the general cures of all infirmities: and of the most radical, fixed, and malignant diseases belonging not only to the body of man, but to all other animal and domestic creatures whatsoever, and that by way of transplantation. With a description of a most excellent cordial out of gold ... London, Printed by T. C. for N. Brook, 1656.

[8], 195 (i.e. 197), [3] p. 15 cm.   [**1616**]

BOUNEUS, PETRUS. *See* BOWNE, Peter [1575-1624?]

BOURDELOT, PIERRE [*fl.* 1633] *ed. See* FABRICIUS, H., *ab Aquapendente.* Medicina practica. 1634.

BOURDELOT, PIERRE [1610-1684 *or* 5] Conversations de l'Academie de ... Bourdelot, contenant diverses recherches, observations, experiences, & raisonnemens de physique, medecine, chymie, &

mathematique. Le tout recueilly par le S^r Le Gallois. Et le parallele de la physique d'Aristote & de celle de Mons. Des Cartes, leu dans ladite academie. Paris, Thomas Moette, 1672.

[10], 76, 350, [8] p. 16 cm.   [**1617**]

—[Excerpts.] In Response a un censeur. 1672.

—Recherches et observations sur les viperes ... répondant à une lettre qu'il a receüe de Mr Redi ... Paris, Claude Barbin, 1671.

79 (i.e. 69) p. 16 cm.   [**1618**]

"Coppie de la lettre de Monsieur Des Trapieres, à Monsieur l'abbé Bourdelot": p. 70-79.

—*See* BAYLE, F. Discours sur l'experience et la raison. 1675.

—*as subject. See* REDI, F. Experimenta circa res diversas naturales. 1675 [and] Lettera ... sopra alcune opposizioni fatte alle sue Osservazioni intorno alle vipere. 1670, 1685 [and] Osservazioni intorno alle vipere. 1687.

BOURDON, AMÉ [1636 *or* 8-1706] Nouvelle description anatomique de toutes les parties du corps humain, & de leurs usages, avec le cours de toutes les humeurs. Sur le principe de la circulation, & conformément aux nouvelles découvertes. Le tout représenté au naturel sur plusieurs grandes tables ... Paris, Jacques Langlois, M. DC. LXXVIX [i.e. 1679?]

[34], 510 (i.e. 508), [4] p. plate. 16 cm.   [**1619**]

Approbations dated 1676 and 1678.
"Achevé d'imprimer pour la premiere fois le quinziéme novembre mil six cens soixante dix-huit": p.[34]
The text is designed to accompany a folio volume containing eight plates published in 1678 under title: Nouvelles tables anatomiques.

—[The same.] ... 2 ed. rev. corr. & augm. ... Paris, Laurent d'Houry, 1683.

[24], 504 p. 16 cm.   [**1620**]

—[The same.] ... 3 ed. rev. augm.... Paris, Laurent d'Houry, 1687.

[24], 534 (i.e. 532) p. 16 cm.   [**1621**]

—Nouvelles tables anatomiques, ou sont représentés au naturel toutes les parties du corps humain ... On y à [sic] joint un petit livre qui en fait la description et en explique clairement les usages ... Combray, L'autheur. Paris, Laurens d'Houry, 1678.

8 (i.e. 16) p.   plates.   55 cm.   [1622]
The plates are designed to accompany Bourdon's Nouvelle description anatomique de toutes les parties du corps humain.

BOURGDIEU, CHARLES VALOIS du. *See* DU-BOURGDIEU, Carolus Valesius.

BOURGEOIS, LOUISE. *See* BOURSIER, Louise (Bourgeois) [1563-1636]

BOURGEOIS, TOUSSAINT. Divers secrets. *In* PORTA, G. B. della. La magie naturelle. 1678.

BOURSIER, LOUISE (Bourgeois) [1563-1636]
Fidelle relation de l'accouchement, maladie & ouverture du corps de feu Madame. [Paris? 1627]
       21 p.   16 cm.   [1623]
Caption title.
Also published under title: Apologie contre le Rapport des médecins.
"Rapport de l'ouverture du corps de feu Madame": p. 19-21.

—[German tr.] Schutzrede, oder Verantwortung Frawen Loysa Burgeois, genannt Burcier ... zu Rettung ihrer Ehren wieder den Bericht etlicher Medicorum und Wund-Artzte zu Pariss in offnen Truck aussgesprenget, anlangendt den Todt einer hohen fürstlichen Weibsperson in Franckreich. Auss dem Frantzösischen ins Teutsch ubergesetzt. Franckfurt, Matthaeus Merian, 1629.
       14 p.   20 cm.   [1624]
"Bericht was sich bey Eröffnung dess todten Cörpers der verstorbenen Fürstin und Frawen befunden": p. 13-14.
Bound with Mercurio, G. La commare. 1652.

—Observations diverses sur la sterilité, perte de fruict, foecondité, accouchements, et maladies des femmes, et enfants nouveaux naiz. Amplement traittees, et heureusement practiqueés par L. Bourgeois dite Boursier ... Paris, A. Saugrain, 1609.
       [12], 121 (i.e. 120), [3] ll.   port.   18 cm.
                                             [1625]
Engraved title page.
Imperfect? Sig. a2 wanting?

—[The same.] ... Paris, A[braham] Saugrain, 1617.
       2 v. in 1.   ports.   18 cm.   [1626]
Vol. 1 has engraved title page.
Vol. 2 includes observations which were also published under title "Récit véritable de la naissance de messeigneurs et dames les enfans de France" (p. 112-197), and "Introduction [sic] à ma fille" (p. [199]-251)

—[The same.] ... Paris, Melchior Mondiere, 1626.
       3 v. in 1.   ports.   18 cm.   [1627]
Vol. 1 has engraved title page.
Imperfect: last leaf (table of contents) mutilated.
"Recit veritable de la naissance de messeigneurs et dames les enfans de France": v. 2, p. [109]-196. "Instruction à ma fille": v. 2, p. 197-251.

—[The same.] ... Rouen, La veufve Thomas Daré, 1626.
       2 v. in 1.   port.   18 cm.   [1628]
Vol. 2 has special title page.
A reprint of the 1617 edition.

—[The same.] ... Paris, Melchior Mondiere, 1642-44.
       3 v. in 1.   ports.   17 cm.   [1629]
Vol. 1 has engraved title page.
A reprint of the 1626 Paris edition.
With this is bound *his* Recueil des secrets. 1635.

—[The same.] ... Paris, Henry Ruffin, 1642.
       [20], 158, [5] p.   ports.   17 cm. [1630]
Engraved title page.
Imperfect? Sig. a2 wanting?
A reprint of the 1609 edition without the "Privilege du roy."

—[The same.] ... Paris, Jean Dehoury [1652]
       3 v. in 1.   ports.   17 cm.   [1631]
Vol. 1 has engraved title page.
Vols. 2-3 have special title pages with imprint: Paris, Henry Ruffin ... M. DC. LII.
"Recit veritable de la naissance de messeigneurs et dames les enfans de France": v. 2, p. [91]-149.
"Instruction à ma fille": v. 2, p. 150-184.
With this is bound *his* Recueil des secrets. 1653.

—Recueil des secrets, de Louyse Bourgeois dite Boursier ... auquel sont contenues ses plus rares experiences pour diverses maladies, principalement des femmes, avec leurs embellissemens. Paris, Melchior Mondiere, 1635.
       [12], 226, [1] p.   port.   17 cm.   [1632]
Bound with *his* Observations diverses. 1642-44.

—[The same.] ... Paris, Jean Dehoury, 1653.
       [17], 151 p.   17 cm.   [1633]
Bound with *his* Observations diverses. [1652]

—[Dutch tr.] Verscheyde aenmerckingen, nopende de onvruchtbaerheyt, misvallen, vrugtbaerheyt, kinderbaren, siecten der vrouwen, ende de geboorte der kinderen. Beschreven door Louyse

Bourgoise . . . Nu nieuwelijcx uyt het François int' Nederduyts vertaelt. Delf, Aernold Bon, 1658.

2 v. in 1. 16 cm. **[1634]**

A third volume of observations, which appeared in the original work, and a portion of vol. 2 (Récit véritable de la naissance de messeigneurs et dames les enfans de France) are omitted in this translation.

"Inleydinge aen mijn doghter": v. 2, p. 62–88.

— [German tr.] Hebammen Buch, darinn von Fruchtbarkeit und Unfruchtbarkeit der Weiber, zeitigen und unzeitigen Geburt, Zustand der Frucht in und ausserhalb Mutterleib, zufälligen Kranckheiten so wol der Kindbetterin als dess Kindes . . . weitläufftig gehandelt wird. Erstmals durch Fraw Louyse Bourgeois . . . in frantzösischer Sprach beschrieben. Hernach aber . . . in die teutsche Sprach . . . ubersetzt und nach der Fraw Urheberin corr. und verm. Exemplar wider von newem auffgelegt . . . Hanaw, In Verlegung Matthaei Merian [1628–48]

4 parts in 1 v. illus., port. 20 cm. **[1635]**

Imprint of special title pages varies: part 2: Zum 2. Mahl getruckt, corr. und verm. Franckfurt, Bey Erasmo Kempffern, in Verlegung Matthaei Merian, 1628; part 3: Franckfurt am Mayn, Bey Philips Fievet, in Verlegung Matthaei Merian, 1648; part 4: Franckfurt am Mayn, Bey Matthaeo Merian, 1644.

Parts 1–2 and 4 are a translation of Observations diverses sur la sterilité, perte de fruict, foecondité, accouchements, et maladies des femmes, et enfants nouveaux naiz. Part 3 is derived chiefly from Pineau's Opusculum physiologum et anatomicum.

"Anhang der dreyen Theilen dieses Hebammen Buchs: darinnen alles das jenig, was in denselben anatomischer unnd natürlicher Weiss angezeigt und gemeldet, mit eylff . . . Kupfferstücken oder Tafel vor Augen gestellt wird . . . durch Johannem Theodorum de Bry": part 3, p. [47]–67.

Bound with Mercurio, G. La commare. 1652.

— [The same.] . . . Hanaw, In Verlegung Matthaei Merian 1644–52

4 parts in 1 v. illus., port. 21 cm. **[1636]**

Imprint varies: part 2: Zum 3. Mahl getruckt, corr. und verm. Hanaw, Bey Johann Aubry, in Verlegung Matthaei Merian, 1652; part 3: Franckfurt am Mayn. Bey Philips Fievet, in Verlegung Matthaei Merian, 1648; part 4: Franckfurt am Mayn, Bey Matthaeo Merian, 1644.

— See The compleat midwife's practice enlarged. 1663, 1697, 1698.

BOUTEROUE, MICHEL [*fl.* 1609–*ca.* 1623] Pyretologia. Divisa in duos libros: quorum primus universalia febrium signa prognostica continet. Alter uniuscujusque febris diagnosium, prognosim, & therapeiam complectitur . . . Parisiis, Apud Joannem Laquehay, 1623.

[15], 416, [18] p. 18 cm. **[1637]**

Errata: p. 17–18

BOUTHEROVE, MICHEL. *See* BOUTEROUE, Michel [*fl.* 1609–*ca.* 1623]

BOUTHIÈRE, GEORGE DE LA. *See* LA BOUTHIÈRE, George de [16th cent.]

BOUVIER, SAMUEL [*fl.* 1670] *respondent.* Disputatio medica inauguralis de affectibus nonnullis infantium . . . Lugduni Batavorum, Apud viduam & haeredes Joannis Elsevirii, 1670.

[15] p. 23 cm. **[1638]**

Diss. — Leyden.

— *See* JUBILIUM VOTIVUM 1670.

BOUWER, JOHANNES [*fl.* 1688] *respondent.* Disputatio medica inauguralis, de affectione hypochondriaca . . . Trajecti ad Rhenum, Ex officina Francisci Halma, 1688.

8 p. 22 cm. **[1639]**

Diss. — Utrecht.

BOVET RICHARD [*b. ca.* 1641] Pandaemonium; or, The devil's cloyster. Being a further blow to modern Sadduceism, proving the existence of witches and spirits . . . With an account of the lives and transactions of several notorious witches. Also a collection of several authentick relations of strange apparations of daemons and spectres . . . London, J. Walthoe, 1684.

[11], 239 p. front. 15 cm. **[1640]**

BOVIE, JOHANNES [*fl.* 1696] *respondent. See* SENGUERDIUS, W., *praeses.* Exercitium experimentale duodecimum. 1696.

BOVIO, GIACINTO [*fl. ca.* 1660–1673] *comp.* Flores medicinales; seu, Sententiae, authoritates, & rationes ex Hippocrates, Galeno, Avicenna, & allis summis authoribus . . . collectae. Opus in quatuor libris partitum: cui additur brevis tractatus De virtute, & usu theriacae, ac De aloe, & De diffinitionibus morborum, & symptomatum . . . Venetiis, Apud Franciscum Salerni & Joannem Cagnolini, 1668.

574 (i.e. 576), [24] p. 15 cm. **[1641]**

BOVIO, TOMMASO. *See* BOVIO, Zefiriele Tommaso [1521–1609]

BOVIO, ZEFIRIELE TOMMASO [1521–1609] Opere contra medici putaticii rationali . . . Padova, Pietro Paolo Tozzi, 1626.

5 parts in 1 v. 15 cm. **[1642]**

Engraved title page.

Each part has special title page and separate paging.

Contents.—Fulmine contro de' medici putatitii rationali.—Flagello de' medici rationali.—Risposta ad un certo libro contra medici rationali [di] Claudio Gelli.—Melampigo.—Dialogo de gl'inganni d'alcuni malvaggi speciali, di Gio. Antonio Lodetto.

—Opere ... cioè, Flagello, Fulmine, & Melampigo, contro de' medici putatitii rationali. Con la Risposta dell'eccell. dottor Claudio Gelli. In quest'ultima impressione ricorrette, e migliorate ... Venetia, Francesco Baba, 1626.

[14], 351 p.; [4], 51 p. 15 cm. **[1643]**

Part [2] has special title page.

A similar collection to the 1626 Padova edition, without the last work.

—[The same.] ... Venetia, Steffano Curti, 1676.

598 (i.e. 596) p. 17 cm. **[1644]**

The publisher's dedication and the index are omitted.

—Flagello contro de' medici communi, detti rationali ... nel quale non solo si scuoprono molti errori di quelli: mà s'insegna ancora il modo di emendargli, & correggerli. Di nuovo rev. corr., & dal proprio auttore ampliato ... Verona, Francesco dalle Donne, 1601.

[8], 56 p. 21 cm. **[1645]**

—Copy 2. 22 cm.

With this is bound *his* Il fulmine contro de' medici putatitii rationali. 1602.

—[The same.] Flagello de' medici rationali ... Milano, Gio. Batt. Bid[elli] 1617.

109 (i.e. 89), [1] p. 15 cm. **[1646]**

Bound with *his* Fulmine contro de' medici putatitii rationali. 1617.

—[The same.] ... Padova, P. P. Tozzi, 1626.

90], [1] p. 15 cm. **[1647]**

With this are bound: *his* Melampigo. 1676.—Gelli, Claudio. Risposta ... ad un certo libro contra medici rationali. 1626.—Lodetti, G. A. Dialogo de gl'inganni d'alcuni malvaggi speciali. 1626.

—Another issue.

90, [1] p., part [2] (*In his* Opere contra medici putaticii rationali. Padova, 1626.) **[1648]**

—[The same.] *See* GELLI, C. Risposta ... ad un certo libro contra medici rationali. 1617, 1626.

—Il fulmine contro de' medici putatitii rationali ... nel quale non solo si scuoprono molti errori di quelli; mà s'insegna ancora il modo di emendargli,

& correggerli. Di nuovo revisto, corretto, & dal proprio auttore ampliato ... Verona, Francesco dalle Donne, 1602.

[8], 176 p. 22 cm. **[1649]**

Colophon dated 1601.

The author's original dedication of the edition of 1592 has been replaced by a dedication from the publisher, dated Verona, 25 February 1602.

Bound with copy 2 of *his* Flagello contro de' medici communi, detti rationali. 1601.

—[The same.] ... Milano, Gio. Batt. Bidelli, 1617.

[11], 269, [5] p. 15 cm. **[1650]**

With this are bound: Gelli, Claudio. Risposta ... ad un certo libro contra medici rationali. 1617.—Bovio, Z. T. Melampigo. 1617.—Bovio, Z. T. Flagello de' medici rationali. 1617.

—Melampigo; overo, Confusione de' medici sofisti, che s'intitolano rationali, et del dottor Claudio Geli, & suoi complici nuovi Passali, & Achemoni ... Milano, Gio. Batt. Bidelli, 1617.

163 p. 15 cm. **[1651]**

"Hyppocratis libellus. De medicorum astrologia [i.e. Imbrasius, of Ephesus. Prognostica de decubitu] ... a Petro de Abbano in Latinum traductus": p. 146-162.

Bound with *his* Fulmine contro de' medici putatitii rationali. 1617.

—[The same.] ... Padova, Pietro Paolo Tozzi, 1626.

162 p. 15 cm. **[1652]**

Bound with *his* Flagello de' medici rationali. 1626.

—Another issue.

162 p. part [4] (*In his* Opere contra medici putaticii rationali. Padova, 1626.) **[1653]**

BOVIUS, HYACINTHUS. *See* BOVIO, Giacinto [*fl. ca.* 1660-1673]

BOWNE, Peter [1575-1624?] Pseudo-medicorum anatomia. In qua maxima improborum et indoctorum turba sub Dio enudatur, quos aut subdola pietatis pelle velatos, aut insolenti scientiae fumo seu fuco obductos, vel irreligio mera, vel rapax avaritia omnes ultra impudentes ad medicinae praxin egit praecipites ... Londini, Excudebat Aug. Matheus, 1624.

[35] p. 19 cm. **[1654]**

Signatures: [A]¹, A⁴, B², C⁴, c¹, a⁴, b².

STC 3442.4

BOXBART, THEODOR [*fl.* 1675] *respondent.* Disputatio medica inauguralis de variolis ... Basileae, Typis Jacobi Werenfelsii [1675]

[12] p.   20 cm.   [**1655**]
Diss. — Basel.

BOXBARTER, Antonius [*fl.* 1626] *respondent. See* Charstadius, V., *praeses.* Disputationum medicarum sexta de causis morborum. 1626; Disputationum medicarum ultima de pharmacia. 1626; Sebisch, M. [1578-1674?] *praeses.* Exercitationes medicae. 1639.

BOXHORN, Marcus Zuerius [*d.* 1653] *ed. See* Joostens, P. De alea libri duo. 1642.

— *See* Borel, P. A summary or compendium, of the life of the most famous philosopher Renatus Descartes. 1670.

BOYLE, *Hon.* Robert [1627-1691] Collected works are placed first; other works are arranged according to Fulton(A).

— Opera omnia, nunc primum in unum corpus redacta ... accurate recognita, & a mendis repurgata ... Venetiis, Sumptibus Jo. Jacobi Hertz, 1697.
     3 v.   port., plates, illus.   24 cm.   [**1656**]
Imperfect: p. 371-2 of vol. 2 mutilated.
Fulton(A) 242. (Variant state: date of vol. 1: M. DC. XCVI. changed in red type to M. DC. XCVI.I)

— The works ... epitomiz'd ... By Richard Boulton ... London, J. Phillips and J. Taylor, 1699-1700.
     4 v.   front. (port.), plates.   20 cm. [**1657**]
Vol. 4 has imprint: London, Thomas Bennet and John Wyat, 1700.
Imperfect: plate 5 of vol. 1 wanting; supplied in photocopy from Library of Congress.
"A general idea of the epitomy of the works of Robert Boyle, Esq. To which are added general heads for the natural history of a country. By R. Boulton": p. [1]-22 at end of vol. 4.
Fulton(A) 243.

— Opera varia, quorum posthac exstat catalogus ... Genevae, Apud Samuelem de Tournes, 1677.
     1 v.   plates.   23 cm.   [**1658**]
Various pagings.
Fulton(A) 246.
With this are bound *his*: Cogitationes de S. Scripturae stylo. 1680; Tractatus, in quibus continentur suspiciones de latentibus quibusdam qualitatibus aeris. 1679; Experimentorum novorum physico-mechanicorum continuatio secunda. 1682.

— New experiments physico-mechanicall, touching the spring of the air, and its effects, (made, for the most part, in a new pneumatical engine) ... Oxford, Printed by H. Hall for Tho. Robinson, 1660.
     [32], 399 (i.e. 389), [1] p.   plate.   17 cm.
                                        [**1659**]

Added half title.
Fulton(A) 13.

— New experiments physico-mechanical, touching the air. The 2d. ed. Whereunto is added A defence of the authors explication of the experiments, against the objections of Franciscus Linus, and, Thomas Hobbes. [Oxford, H. Hall for Tho. Robinson, 1662]
     3 parts in 1 v.   plates.   20 cm.   [**1660**]
Half title.
Incomplete: part [1] wanting.
Imperfect: plate following p. 50 of part 2 wanting.
Part [2] has special title page: A defence of the doctrine touching the spring and weight of the air ... against the objections of Franciscus Linus ... London, F. G. for Thomas Robinson, 1662.
Part [3] has special title page: An examen of Mr. T. Hobbes his Dialogus physicus ... London, F. G. for Thomas Robinson, 1662.
Fulton(A) 14.

— [The same.] ... The 3d ed. ... [London, Printed by Miles Flesher for Richard Davis, 1682]
     3 parts in 1 v.   plates.   22 cm.   [**1661**]
Half title.
Each part has special title page.
Fulton(A) 15.

— A continuation of new experiments physico-mechanical, touching the spring and weight of the air, and their effects. The I. part ... Whereto is annext a short discourse of the atmospheres of consistent bodies ... Oxford, Printed by Henry Hall for Richard Davis, 1669.
     [21], 198, [11] p.   plates.   21 cm.   [**1662**]
Fulton(A) 16.
With this is bound *his* A continuation of new experiments physico-mechanical ... The second part. 1682.

— Experimentorum novorum physico-mechanicorum continuatio secunda. In qua experimenta varia tum in aere compresso, tum in factitio, instituta, circa ignem, animalia, &c. una cum descriptione machinarum continentur ... Genevae, Apud Samuelem de Tournes, 1682.
     [8], 130, [2] p.   plates.   23 cm.   [**1663**]
Fulton(A) 17.
Bound with *his* Opera varia. 1677.

— A continuation of new experiments physico-mechanical touching the spring and weight of the air, and their effects. The second part ... London, Printed by Miles Flesher for Richard Davis, Oxford, 1682.
     [16], 198, [9] p.   plates.   21 cm.   [**1664**]
Fulton(A) 18.

Bound with *his* A continuation of new experiments physico-mechanical ... The I. part. 1669.

—Nova experimenta physico-mechanica de vi aëris elastica et ejusdem effectibus. Accessit Defensio adversus objectiones Franc. Lini ... Roterodami, Apud Arnoldum Leers, 1669.

    2 parts in 1 v. plates. 14 cm.   **[1665]**
Various pagings.
Engraved general title page. Each part has special title page.
Fulton(A) 22.

—Certain physiological essays, written at distant times, and on several occasions ... London, Henry Herringman, 1661.

    [4], 105, [11], 107–249 p. 21 cm.   **[1666]**
Fulton(A) 25.

—[The same.] ... The 2d ed. Wherein some of the tracts are enlarged by experiments, and the work is increased by the addition of a discourse about the Absolute rest in bodies. London, Henry Herringman [1668]–1669.

    [7], 292 p.; [3], 30 p. 22 cm.   **[1667]**
Part [2] has half title.
Fulton(A) 26.

—Tentamina quaedam physiologica diversis temporibus & occasionibus conscripta ... cum ejusdem Historia fluiditatis et firmitatis. Ex Anglico in Latinum sermonem translata. Amstelodami, Apud Danielem Elzevirium, 1667.

    [7], 424 p. 15 cm.   **[1668]**
Fulton(A) 29.

—[The same.] ... Ed. nova prioribus corr. Londini, Impensis H. Herringman, 1668.

    [4], 101, [9], 148, [1] p. 21 cm.   **[1669]**
Imperfect: sig. o4 of part [1] (blank) wanting; p. 75–76 of part [2] mutilated.
Part [2] has special title page.
Errata: p. [149]
Fulton(A) 30.

—[The same.] ... Accessit de novo tractatus De absoluta quiete in corporibus ... Genevae, Apud Samuelem de Tournes, 1680.

    [4], 60, [6], 94, 18 p. 22 cm.   **[1670]**
Fulton(A) 32A.

—The sceptical chymist; or, Chymico-physical doubts & paradoxes, touching the experiments whereby vulgar spagirists are wont to endeavour to evince their salt, sulphur and mercury, to be the true

principles of things. To which in this edition are subjoyn'd divers Experiments and notes about the producibleness of chymical principles. Oxford, Printed by Henry Hall for Ric. Davis, and B. Took, 1680 [i.e. 1679]

    [20], 440 p.; [27], 268 p. 18 cm.   **[1671]**
Part [2] has special title page.
Fulton(A) 34. (Actually printed in 1679)

—Chymista scepticus vel dubia et paradoxa chymico-physica, circa spagyricorum principia, vulgo dicta hypostatica, prout proponi & propugnari solent a turba alchymistarum. Cui pars praemittitur alterius cujusdam dissertationis ad idem argumentum spectans ... Ed. secunda priori emendatior. Rotterodami, Ex officina Arnoldi Leers, 1668.

    [28], 392 p. 14 cm.   **[1672]**
Added engraved title page.
Fulton(A) 38.

—[The same.] ... Genevae, Apud Samuelem de Tournes, 1680.

    [12], 148 p. 22 cm.   **[1673]**
Fulton(A) 39A.

—Experimenta et notae circa producibilitatem chymicorum principiorum. Quae sunt totidem partes appendicis ad scepticum chymicum ... Genevae, Apud Samuelem de Tournes, 1693.

    [12], 92 p. 22 cm.   **[1674]**
"Editoris monitum" signed J. M.
Part [2] of *his* Chymista scepticus, vel, dubia et paradoxa chymico-physica ... Coloniae Allobrogum, 1680.
Fulton(A) 40.

—Cogitationes de S. Scripturae stylo ... Genevae, Apud Samuelem de Tournes, 1680.

    [15], 87 p. 23 cm.   **[1675]**
Fulton(A) 48.
Bound with *his* Opera varia. Genevae, 1677.

—Some considerations touching the usefulnesse of experimental naturall phylosophy ... Oxford, Printed by Hen. Hall for Ric. Davis, 1663.

    2 parts in 1 v. illus. 21 cm.   **[1676]**
Imperfect: label title and general half title pages wanting.
Part 1 has half title; part 2 has special title page and half title.
"An appendix to the first section of the second part" has half title.
Fulton(A) 50.

—[The same.] ... A 2d ed. (since the first published June 1663). Oxford, Printed by Hen. Hall, for Ri. Davis, 1664.

[15], 126 (i.e. 124), [4] p.; 416 (i.e. 400), [17] p.   illus.   22 cm.   [**1677**]

Fulton(A) 52.

With this is bound *his* Some considerations touching the usefulnesse of experimental natural philosophy. 1671.

—[The same.] . . . The second tome containing later section of the second part. Oxford, Printed by Henry Hall, for Ric. Davis, 1671.

I v.   22 cm.   [**1678**]

The six essays are separately paged, each with half title.
Fulton(A) 53.

Bound with *his* Some considerations touching the usefulnesse of experimental natural philosophy. 1664.

—Experiments and considerations touching colours. First occasionally written, among some other essays, to a friend; and now suffer'd to come abroad as the beginning of an experimental history of colours . . . London, Henry Herringman, 1664.

[40], 423 p.   plate.   17 cm.   [**1679**]

"A short account of some observations made by Mr. Boyle": p. [389]-423, has special title page.
Fulton(A) 57.

—Experimenta et considerationes de coloribus, primum ex occasione, inter alias quasdam diatribas, ad amicum scripta, nunc vero in lucem prodire passa, ceu initium historiae experimentalis de coloribus . . . Amstelodami, Apud Gerbrandum Schagen, 1667.

[23], 371, [21] p.   15 cm.   [**1680**]

"Brevis enarratio quarundam observationum, factarum a . . . Roberto Boyle de adamante in tenebris lucente": p. [341]-371, has special title page.
Fulton(A) 60.

—[The same.] . . . Genevae, Apud Samuelem de Tournes, 1677.

[20], 168, [8] p.   22 cm.   [**1681**]

"Brevis enarratio quarundam observationum, factarum a . . . Roberto Boyle de adamante in tenebris lucente": p. [153]-167, has half title.
Fulton(A) 62A.

—[The same.] . . . Genevae, Apud Samuelem de Tournes, 1680.

[20], 168, [8] p.   plates.   22 cm.   [**1682**]

Different setting of type.
Fulton(A) 63A.

—New experiments and observations touching cold; or, An experimental history of cold, begun. To which are added An examen of antiperistasis, and An examen of Mr. Hobs's doctrine about cold . . . Whereunto is annexed An account of freezing,

brought in to the Royal Society, by . . . Dr. C. Merret . . . London, Printed for John Crook, 1665.

I v.   plates.   18 cm.   [**1683**]

Various pagings.
Errata: p. [55].
Both plates bound before p. 1.
"An advertisement to the readers . . ." bound at end.
Fulton(A) 70.

—[The same.] . . . Together with An appendix, containing some promiscuous experiments and observations relating to the precedent history of cold . . . London, Richard Davis, 1683.

I v.   21 cm.   [**1684**]

Various pagings.
Imperfect: plates wanting.
Fulton(A) 71.

—Paradoxa hydrostatica novis experimentis (maximam partem physicis ac facilibus) evicta . . . Nuper ex Anglico sermone in Latinum versa. Roterodami, Ex officina Arnoldi Leers, 1670.

[46], 240, [2] p.   illus., plates.   14 cm.
                                                      [**1685**]

Fulton(A) 74.

—The origine of formes and qualities, (according to the corpuscular philosophy,) illustrated by considerations and experiments, (written formerly by way of notes upon an Essay about nitre) . . . Oxford, Printed by H. Hall for Ric. Davis, 1666.

[54], 433, [1] p.   15 cm.   [**1686**]

Fulton(A) 77.

—[The same.] . . . The 2d ed. augmented by a discourse of subordinate formes . . . Oxford, Printed by H. Hall for Ric. Davis, 1667.

[34], 363 (i.e. 365) p.   19 cm.   [**1687**]

Fulton(A) 78.

—Origo formarum et qualitatum juxta philosophiam corpuscularem considerationibus & experimentis illustrata. (Ad modum annotationum in tentamen circa nitrum primitus conscripta) . . . Genevae, Apud Samuelem de Tournes, 1688.

[32], 147 p.   23 cm.   [**1688**]

Fulton(A) 82A.

—Tractatus de qualitatibus rerum cosmicis. De suspicionibus cosmicis. De temperie regionum submarinarum. De temperie regionum sub-terranearum. De fundo maris. Una cum praemissa Introductione ad historiam qualitatum particularium. Quibus in hac editione Latina accessere tractatus tres, Observationes de salsedine maris. Dissertatio de motu intestino particularum in quiescentibus solidis. Nova experimenta pneumonia respirationem spectantia ... Londini, Impensis Ric. Davis, 1672.

[1], 271, [1] p.   14 cm.   [1689]
Fulton(A) 88.
With this is bound *his* Tractatus ... Ubi 1. Mira aeris ... rarefactio detecta. 1670.

—Introductio ad historiam qualitatum particularium. Cui subnectuntur Tractatus de cosmicis rerum qualitatibus. De cosmicis suspicionibus. De temperie subterranearum regionum. De temperie submarinarum regionum. De fundo maris ... Genevae, Apud Samuelem de Tournes, 1680.

[7], 18, 12, 12, 20, 9, 8 (i.e. 7) p.   23 cm.   [1690]
The "Introductio ad historiam qualitatum particularium" ([1], 18 p.) and "Tractatus tres; de temperie subterranearum regionum, de temperie submarinarum regionum, et de fundo maris" (20, 9, 8 p.) have half titles.
Fulton(A) 90.

—Tractatus ... Ubi 1. Mira aeris ... rarefactio detecta. 2. Observata nova circa durationem virtutis elasticae aeris expansi. 3. Experimenta nova de condensatione aeris, solo frigore facta; ejusque compressione sine machinis. 4. Ejusdem quantitatis aeris rarefacti & compressi mire discrepans extensio. Londini, Impensis Henrici Herringman, 1670.

[8], 53 p.   14 cm.   [1691]
Fulton(A) 91.
Bound with *his* Tractatus de qualitatibus rerum cosmicis. 1672.

—An essay about the origine & virtues of gems ... London, Printed by William Godbid, and are sold by Moses Pitt, 1672.

[15], 185 (i.e. 184) p.   17 cm.   [1692]
Fulton(A) 96.

—Exercitatio de origine & viribus gemmarum. In qua proponuntur & historice illustrantur conjecturae quaedam circa materiae gemmarum consistentiam, necnon subjecta, quibus praecipuae earum vires inhaerent ... Londini, Typis Gulielmi Godbid, & venales prostant apud Mosem Pitt, 1673.

[13], 143 (i.e. 150), [6] p.   14 cm.   [1693]
Fulton(A) 97.

—[The same.] Specimen de gemmarum origine & virtutibus. In quo proponuntur & historice illustrantur quaedam conjecturae circa consistentiam materiae lapidum pretiosorum, & subjecta, in quibus

eorum praecipuae virtutes consistunt ... Genevae, Apud Samuelem de Tournes, 1680.

[6], 58 p.   23 cm.   [1694]
Fulton(A) 100A.

—Tracts ... containing new experiments, touching the relation betwixt flame and air. And about explosions. An hydrostatical discourse occasion'd by some objections of Dr. Henry More ... To which is annex't, An hydrostatical letter ... New experiments, of the postive or relative levity of bodies under water; of the air's spring on bodies under water; about the differing pressure of heavy solids and fluids. London, Richard Davis, 1672.

1 v.   18 cm.   [1695]
Various pagings.
Fulton(A) 101. (Sheets (*) and (**) bound after sheet [A].

—Essays of the strange subtilty, determinate nature, great efficacy of effluviums. To which are annext New experiments to make fire and flame ponderable: together with A discovery of the perviousness of glass ... London, Printed by W[illiam] G[odbid] for M[oses] Pitt, 1673.

[7], 69, [1], 47, 74, [9], 85, [6] p.   18 cm.
                                             [1696]
Fulton(A) 106.

—Exercitationes de atmosphaeris corporum consistentium; deque mira subtilitate, determinata natura, & insigni vi effluviorum. Subjunctis Experimentis novis, ostendentibus, posse partes ignis & flammae reddi stabiles ponderabilesque. Una cum detecta penetrabilitate vitri a ponderabilibus partibus flammae ... Ex Anglico in Latinum sermonem versae ... Londini, Typis Guil. Godbid, impensis Mosis Pitt, 1673.

2 parts in 1 v.   13 cm.   [1697]
Various pagings.
Each part has special title page.
Fulton(A) 108.

—[The same.] ... Lugd. Batav. Ex officina Felicis Lopez, 1676.

312 p.   14 cm.   [1698]
Fulton(A) 110A.

—Tracts consisting of observations about the saltness of the sea: an account of a statical hygroscope ... with an appendix about the force of the air's moisture: a fragment about the natural and preternatural state of bodies ... To all which is premis'd a sceptical dialogue about the positive or privative nature of cold . . . London, Printed by E. Flesher for R. Davis in Oxford, 1674.

9 parts in 1 v.   18 cm.   **[1699]**

Each part has separate pagination, parts [2-7] have half titles and parts [8-9] have special title pages.

Fulton(A) 113.

—Observations de salsedine maris . . . Coloniae Allobrogum, Apud Samuelem de Tournes, 1686.

23 p.   22 cm.   **[1700]**

Fulton(A) 115A.

—The excellency of theology, compar'd with natural philosophy, (as both are objects of men's study.) . . . by T. H. R[obert] B[oyle] E. . . . To which are annex'd some occasional thoughts About the excellency and grounds of the mechanical hypothesis . . . London, Printed by T. N. for Henry Herringman, 1671.

[29], 232, [1] p.; [4], 40 (i.e. 41), [1] p.   17 cm.   **[1701]**

Errata: p. [233] and [42]

The special title page of part [2] is a cancel.

Fulton(A) 116.

—Tractatus. In quibus continentur, I. Suspiciones de latentibus quibusdam qualitatibus aeris; una cum appendice De magnetibus coeletsibus, nonnullisque argumentis aliis. II. Animadversiones in D. Hobbesii Problemata de vacuo. III. Dissertatio De causa attractionis per suctionem . . . Ex Anglico in Latinum sermonem versi. Londini, Typis Gulielmi Godbid, impensis Mosis Pitt, 1676.

5 parts in 1 v.   14 cm.   **[1702]**

Parts [2-5] have special title pages.

Fulton(A) 120.

—[The same.] . . . Genevae, Apud Samuelem de Tournes, 1679.

[4], 87 p.   23 cm.   **[1703]**

Fulton(A) 121.

Bound with *his* Opera varia. 1677.

—Experiments, notes &c. about the mechanical origine or production of divers particular qualities: among which is inserted a discourse Of the imperfection of the chymist's doctrine of qualities; together with some Reflections upon the hypothesis of alcali and acidum . . . London, Printed by E. Flesher, for R. Davis in Oxford, 1676.

11 parts in 1 v.   18 cm.   **[1704]**

The essays are separately paged, each with special title page dated 1675. Part [10]: Experiments and notes about the mechanical production of magnetism, has date 1676.

Fulton(A) 124.

—[Mechanical qualities (Tastes & odours) French] Experiences sur les saveurs et sur les odeurs. *In* [Grew, N.] Recueil d'experiences et observations sur le combat, qui procede du mélange des corps. 1679.

Fulton(A) 130.

—[The same.] Sur les saveurs et sur les odeurs. *In* Grew, N. Anatomie des plantes. 1685.

Fulton(A) 131.

—Noctiluca aeria; sive, Nova quaedam phaenomena in substantiae factitiae sive artificialis, sponte lucidae, productione observata . . . Atque Experimenta nova & observata facta in glacialem noctilucam. Quibus adjicitur Paradoxon chymicum . . . Genevae, Apud Samuelem de Tournes, 1693.

108 p.   23 cm.   **[1705]**

The "Experimenta nova" and the "Paradoxon chymicum" have half titles.

Fulton(A) 142.

—Die lufftige Noctiluca; oder, Etliche neue Phoenomena, sampt einer Anleitung allerhand Phosphoros und selbstscheinende Wesen zu zubereiten . . . In Hochteutsch überzetzet durch J[ohann] L[ange] M[edicinae] C[andidatum] Hamburg, Auff Gottfried Schultzens Kosten, 1682.

[1], 88 (i.e. 90) p.   17 cm.   **[1706]**

Fulton(A) 143.

—A discourse of things above reason. Inquiring whether a philosopher should admit there are any such. By a fellow of the Royal Society. To which are annexed . . . some Advices about judging of things said to transcend reason. Written by a fellow of the same society. London, Printed by E. T. and R. H. for Jonathan Robinson, 1681.

[4], 94 p.; 100 p.   17 cm.   **[1707]**

The Advices (100 p.) has caption title.

Fulton(A) 145.

—Memoirs for the natural history of humane blood, especially the spirit of that liquor . . . London, Samuel Smith, 1683/4.

[16], 289, [7] p.   15 cm.   **[1708]**

Fulton(A) 146.

—Apparatus ad historiam naturalem sanguinis humani, ac spiritus praecipue ejusdem liquoris . . .

Pars I [-IV]. Ex Anglico sermone in Latinum traducebat D. A. M. D. ... Londini, Impensis Samuelis Smith, 1684.

[19], 179, 55 p.   15 cm.   [**1709**]
Fulton(A) 146B.

— [The same.] ... Genevae, Apud Samuelem de Tournes, 1685.

[8], 91 p.   21 cm.   [**1710**]
Fulton(A) 147.

— [The same.] ... Coloniae Allobrogum, Apud Samuelem de Tournes, 1686.

[8], 91 p.   24 cm.   [**1711**]
Fulton(A) 148A.

— Experiments and considerations about the porosity of bodies, in two essays ... London, Sam. Smith, 1684.

[4], 145 p.   18 cm.   [**1712**]
Fulton(A) 149

— Tentamen porologicum; sive, Ad porositatem corporum tum animalium, tum solidorum detegendam ... Genevae, Apud Samuelem de Tournes, 1686.

[6], 46 p.   22 cm.   [**1713**]
Imperfect: sig. +4 (blank) and F4 (blank) wanting.
Translator's preface signed: D.A.M.D.
Fulton(A) 151.

— Short memoirs for the natural experimental history of mineral waters. Addressed by way of letter to a friend ... London, Samuel Smith, 1684/5.

[18], 112, [13] p.   17 cm.   [**1714**]
Date altered by hand to 1686.
Fulton(A) 159.

— An essay of the great effects of even languid and unheeded motion. Whereunto is annexed An experimental discourse of some little observed causes of the insalubrity and salubrity of the air and its effects. London, Printed by M. Flesher, for Richard Davis, 1685.

[8], 123 p.; [8], 96 p.   17 cm.   [**1715**]
Imperfect: part [2] wanting.
Fulton(A) 163.

— [The same.] ... London, Sam. Smith, 1690.
[9], 158 p.; [7], 113 (i.e. 139) p.   18 cm. [**1716**]
Part [2] has special title page with imprint: London, Printed by M. Flesher, for Richard Davis, 1685.
Fulton(A) 165.

— Of the reconcileableness of specifick medicines to the corpuscular philosophy. To which is annexed a discourse about the advantages of The use of simple medicines ... London, Sam. Smith, 1685.

[14], 225 (i.e. 227), 13 p.   18 cm.   [**1717**]
Fulton(A) 166. (A variant issue with different half-title to "Simple medicines" (p. 137): AN/INVITATION/ To the Use of/SIMPLE MEDICINES./ By the Honourable/ ROBERT BOYLE Fellow of the /Royal Society.)

— De specificorum remediorum cum corpusculari philosophia concordia. Cui accessit dissertatio de varia simplicium medicamentorum utilitate, usuque ex Anglico in Latinum sermonem traducebat. D. A. M. D. ... Londini, Impensis Sam. Smith, 1686.

[12], 180 p.   14 cm.   [**1718**]
Fulton(A) 167.

— [The same.] ... Genevae, Apud Samuelem de Tournes, 1687.

[8], 64 p.   23 cm.   [**1719**]
Fulton(A) 168.

— Nouveau traité de Monsieur Boyle ... sur la convenance des remedes specifiques avec la philosophie des corpuscules, & sur l'usage & les proprietez des medicamens simples. De la traduction de Mr Rostagny ... Lyon, Jean Certe, 1689.

[22], 360, [9] p.   15 cm.   [**1720**]
Fulton(A) 169A.

— A free enquiry into the vulgarly receiv'd notion of nature; made in an essay, address'd to a friend. By R[obert] B[oyle] ... London, Printed by H. Clark, for John Taylor, 1685/6.

[26], 412, [2] p.   18 cm.   [**1721**]
Fulton(A) 170.

— Tractatus de ipsa natura, sive libera in receptam naturae notionem disquisito ad amicum ... Genevae, Apud Samuelem de Tournes, 1688.

[15], 111 p.   22 cm.   [**1722**]
Translator's preface signed: D. A. M. D.
Fulton(A) 172.

— Medicinal experiments; or, A collection of choice remedies, for the most part simple, and easily prepared ... London, Sam. Smith, 1692.

[11], 11, 88 p.; [2], 17 p.   15 cm.   [**1723**]
"The latter five decads being a second part": p. [47]-88; "A catalogue of the philosophical books and tracts written by the Honourable Robert Boyle Esq. ...": p. [1]-17 at end, have special title pages.
Fulton(A) 179.

—[The same.] . . . The first and second volumes [–The third and last volume] . . . The 3d ed. London, Samuel Smith, and B. Walford, 1696.

[24], 154 p.; [24], 95 p.   front. (port.) 16 cm.
[1724]

Vols. 1 and 2 are paged continuously, v. 2 with half-title only (p. [47]).

Vol. 3 has title page with imprint: London, J. Taylor, 1694. Imperfect: portrait wanting.

Fulton(A) 181.

—Medicinische Experimente; oder, Hundert zusammengetragene auserlesene Artzney-Mittel, welche meistentheils schlecht und leicht zu verfertigen . . . aussm [sic] Englischen ins Teutsche übersetzet. Leipzig, Johann Friedrich Gleditsch, 1692.

78, [10] p.   14 cm.
[1725]

Fulton(A) 185B.

—A disquisition about the final causes of natural things: wherein it is inquir'd, whether, and (if at all) with what cautions, a naturalist should admit them? . . . To which are subjoyn'd, by way of appendix Some uncommon observations about vitiated sight . . . London, Printed by H. C. for John Taylor, 1688.

[16], 274, [6] p.
[1726]

Some uncommon observations about vitiated sight (p. [239]–274) has special title page.

Fulton(A) 186.

Medicina hydrostatica; or, Hydrostaticks applyed to the materia medica. Shewing, how by the weight that divers bodies, us'd in physick, have in water; one may discover whether they be genuine or adulterate. To which is subjoyn'd A previous hydrostatical way of estimating ores . . . London, Samuel Smith, 1690.

[23], 217, [7] p.; [2], 14 p.   front. 17 cm.
[1727]

Half title: Experiments and observations, relating to the materia medica. Tome I.

Part [2] has special title page: A catalogue of the philosophical books and tracts, written by the Honourable Robert Boyle Esq. . . .

Imperfect: sig. A2 (the half title) wanting.

Fulton(A) 189.

—Medicina hydrostatica; sive, Hydrostatica materiae medicae applicata: ubi ostenditur variorum corporum a medicis in remedia adhibitorum pondere in aqua, quaenam eorum genuina sint, quaenam vero adulterata. Accessit Praevia methodus hydrostatica explorandi mineras . . . Genevae, Apud Samuelem de Tournes, 1693.

[12], 66 (i.e. 64), [4] p.   22 cm.
[1728]

Fulton(A) 190.

—Experimenta & observatione physicae: wherein are briefly treated of several subjects relating to natural philosophy in an experimental way. To which is added, a small collection of Strange reports . . . London, John Taylor and John Wyat, 1691.

[26], 158 p.; [1], 28, [2] p.   17 cm.
[1729]

Part [2] has half title: Strange reports, in II. parts. Imperfect: p. 101–102 mutilated.

Fulton(A) 193. (Title slightly varies.)

—The general history of the air . . . London, Awnsham and John Churchill, 1692.

xii, 259, [1] p.   20 cm.
[1730]

Fulton(A) 194.

—General heads for the natural history of a country, great or small; drawn out for the use of travellers and navigators . . . To which is added, other directions for navigators . . . by another hand. London, John Taylor and S. Holford, 1692.

[4], 134 (i.e. 138), [2] p.   17 cm.
[1731]

Fulton(A) 195.

—Nova experimenta pneumatica respirationem spectantia . . . Coloniae Allobrogum, Apud Samuelem de Tournes, 1686.

47 p.   plates.   23 cm.
[1732]

Fulton(A) 222C.

—See Burnet, G., Bp. of Salisbury. A sermon. 1692; Fitzgerald, R. Salt-water sweetned. 1683; [Latin tr.] 1683; Perrault, F. The devill of Mascon. 1658; Vallerius, N. Tentamina physico-chymica. 1699.

—as subject. See Camerarius, E. Dissertationes tres. 1694; Ettmüller, M. praeses, Abstrusum respirationis humanae negotium. 1676; Greatrakes, V. A brief account of Mr Valentine Greatraks. 1666; Hooke, R. Lectures and collections. 1678; Mullins, J. Some observations made upon the Cylonian plant. 1695; [Peachie, John] Some observations made upon the Bermudas berries. 1694 [and] Some observations made upon the herb cassiny. 1695; Some observations made upon the Russia seed. 1694; Saint André, F. de. Entretiens sur l'acide et sur l'alkali. 1677, 1680; Stubbs, H. The miraculous conformist. 1666.

BOYM, Michał Piotr [1612–1659] Clavis medica ad Chinarum doctrinam de pulsibus . . . Hujus operis ultra viginti annos jam sepulti fragmenta, hinc

inde dispersa, collegit & ... in lucem Europaeam
produxit ... Andreas Cleyerus ... [Nürnberg] 1686.

144 p.   illus., plates.   21 cm.   [**1733**]

A reprint of the 1685 edition in Miscellanea curiosa ...
Academiae Naturae Curiosorum, Dec. II, 4, Nürnberg, 1686,
Anhang, p. 1-144. Cf. NDB, v. 3, p. 290-1.

[—] *tr.* Specimen medicinae Sinicae; sive,
Opuscula medica ad mentem Sinensium, continens
I. De pulsibus libros quatuor e Sinico translatos. II.
Tractatus de pulsibus ab erudito Europaeo collectos.
III. Fragmentum operis medici ibidem ab erudito
Europaeo conscripti. IV. Excerpta literis eruditi
Europaei in China. V. Schemata ad meliorem
praecedentium intelligentiam. VI. De indiciis mor-
borum ex linguae coloribus & affectionibus ...
Edidit Andreas Cleyer ... Francofurti, Sumptibus
Joannis Petri Zubrodt, 1682.

[4], 48 p.; 99 p.; 16 p.; 54 p.   illus., charts,
plates.   21 cm.   [**1734**]

"Auctoris Vam Xó Hó pulsibus explanatis medendi regula": p.
[1]-24; "Medicamenta simplicia, quae a Chinensibus ad usum
medicum adhibentur": p. [25]-54 last group of paging.

These translations from the Chinese were made by Michał
Boym, and published (with Boym's name omitted) by Andreas
Cleyer. Several of the works are by Vám Xó Hó (i.e. Wang Shu-
ho) Cf. NUC, vol. 64, p. 221.

—Another issue, last plate re-engraved.   [**1735**]

Imperfect: outer margins of charts on signatures n and o
trimmed.

—*See* LES SECRETS DE LA MEDECINE DES CHINOIS.
1671.

BOYS, JEAN DU. *See* DU BOYS, Jean.

BOYVIN DU VAUROÜY, HENRY DE [*b.* 1623]
tr. See ADAMANTIUS. La physionomie. 1635.

BRA, HENDRIK VAN [1554-1622] Catalogus
medicamentorum simplicium & facile pararbilium
adversus epilepsiam, et quomodo iis utendum sit
brevis institutio ... Arnhemi, Apud Johannem
Johannis, 1605.

[16], 115 p.   15 cm.   [**1736**]

—De curandis venenis, per medicamenta simplicia
& facile parabilia, libri duo ... Leovardiae, Typis
Abrahami Radaei, Apud Johannem Starterum, 1616.

[24], 360 p.   16 cm.   [**1737**]

—Copy 2.

With this is bound Schneeberger, Anton. Catalogus medicamentorum simplicium & facile parabilium pestilentiae veneno adver-
santium. 1616.

—, *ed. See* SCHNEEBERGER, A. Catalogus medicamentorum simplicium. 1605, 1616.

—*as subject. See* GOCKEL, E. Enchiridion medico-
practicum de peste. 1669.

BRAAMSZ, MENZO [*fl.* 1669] *respondent.*
Disputatio medica inauguralis de lochiorum fluxu
aucto ... Lugduni Batavorum, Apud viduam &
haeredes Joannis Elsevirii, 1669.

[9] p.   23 cm.   [**1738**]

Diss. — Leyden.

BRACCESCHI, GIOVANNI. *See* BRACESCO,
Giovanni [*b. ca.* 1481]

BRACESCO, GIOVANNI [*b. ca* 1481] De alchemia,
dialogi duo nunquam ante hac conjunctim sic editi,
correcti, & emaculati. Praemittuntur propositiones
centum viginti novem idem argumentum compendiosa brevitate complectentes ... Hamburgi, Apud
Johannem Naumannum & Georgium Wolffium,
1673.

[16], 272 p.   17 cm.   [**1739**]

—Dialogus primus, veram et genuinam librorum
Gebri sententiam explicans (p. [1]-152) was first
published in Venice in 1544 under title: La espositione di Geber. Lignum vitae (p. [153]-272, with
special title page) was first published in Rome in 1542
under title: Il legno della vita. These Latin versions
by Guglielmo Grataroli were included in the
translator's compilation "Verae alchemiae ... doctrina certusque methodus" published in Basel in 1561.

The prefatory "propositiones" are headed: Expositio librorum Gebri et Raimundi, ex Tuscanico
idiomate traducta ... incerto authore.

—Il legno della vita. *In* Lull, R. Testamentum.
1663?

BRACHELIUS, HIEREMIAS THRIVERUS. *See*
DRYVERE, Jérémie de [1504-1554]

BRACHI, JACOPO [*d.* 1737] Pensieri fisicomedici
circa gli animali, che muoiono, e ne' recipienti vacui
d'aria, e ne' ripieni d'arie fattitie, elevate da diversi
misti per mezzo della fermentatione ... Venetia, Andrea Poletti, 1685.

76, [2] p.   18 cm.   [**1740**]

BRADWELL, STEPHEN [*fl.* 1594-1636] Helps for
suddain accidents endangering life. By which those
that live farre from physitions or chirurgions may

happily preserve the life of a poore friend or neighbour, till such a man may be had to perfect the cure. Collected out of the best authors for the generall good ... London, Printed by Thomas Purfoot for T. S. and sold by Henry Overton, 1633.

[16], 127 p.   15 cm.   **[1741]**

STC 3535.

—Physick for the sicknesse, commonly called the plague. With all the particular signes and symptoms, whereof the most are too ignorant. Collected, out of the choycest authors, and confirmed with good experience ... London, Benjamin Fisher, 1636.

[7], 53 p.   19 cm.   **[1742]**

STC 3536.

With this is bound: Gt. Brit. Privy council. Orders thought meet by His Maiestie. 1625.

—A watch-man for the pest. Teaching the true rules of preservation from the pestilent contagion, at this time fearefully over-flowing this famous cittie of London. Collected out of the best authors, mixed with auncient experience, and moulded into a new and most plaine method ... London, Printed by John Dawson for George Vincent, 1625.

[4], 57, [2] p.   19 cm.   **[1743]**

STC 3537.

With this is bound Garencières, Théophile de. A mite cast into the treasury of the ... city of London. 1665.

BRADY, ROBERT [1627?-1700] *See* SYDENHAM, T. Epistolae responsoriae duae. 1680, 1683.

BRAEDIUS, HUBERT [*fl.* 1646] *respondent.* Disputatio medica inauguralis de empyemate ... Lugduni Batavorum, Apud Davidem Lopez de Haro, 1646.

[8] p.   19 cm.   **[1744]**

Diss. — Leyden.

BRAITENBERG, GEORGIUS BARTHOLDUS PONTANUS A. *See* PONTANUS A BRAITENBERG, Georgius Bartholdus [*d.* 1616]

BRANCHI, ANTON GIUSEPPE. *See* BERTINI, Anton Francesco [1658-1726]

BRANCO, JOÃO RODRIGUEZ DE CASTELLO. *See* AMATUS LUSITANUS [1511-1568]

BRAND, GEORG FRIEDRICH. Consilium medicum; oder, Kurtze Unterrichtung, wie man sich bey dieser gefährlichen herumb schwebenden Pest praeserviren und curiren soll ... Cöthen, Gedruckt von Michael Röelen, 1681.

[24] p.   19 cm.   **[1745]**

BRAND, PAUL [*d.* 1687] Dissertatio de ovo humano ... Hafniae, Typis Matthiae Georgii F. Godicchenii, 1677.

[8] p.   18 cm.   **[1746]**

—*respondent. See* BORCH, O., *praeses.* Dissertationem hanc inauguralem de malo hypochondriaco ... submittit. 1676; WILLE, J. V., *praeses.* Synopsis tractatus de morbis castrensibus internis. 1676.

BRAND, PHILIPP HEINRICH. *See* BRANDT, Philipp Heinrich [*fl.* 1699-1700]

BRANDAU, MATTHÄUS ERBEN VON. *See* ERBEN VON BRANDAU, Matthias [*fl.* 17th cent.]

BRANDEN, GEORG FRIEDERICH. *See* BRAND, Georg Friedrich.

BRANDENBURG (Electorate) Laws, statutes, etc. Revidirte Ordnung, wie es in des durchleuchtigsten Fürsten und Herrn, Herrn Christian Ernsts, Marggrafens zu Brandenburg, zu Magdeburg, in Preussen ... Land und Fürstenthum by künfftig sich ereignender Pestilentz-Seuche, (davor aber der allerhöchste Gott in Gnaden männiglich behüten wolle) in einem und andern gehalten werden solle. Bayreuth, Johann Gebhard, 1680.

16 p.   19 cm.   **[1747]**

BRANDENBURG (Province) Laws, statutes, etc. *See* DISPENSATORIUM BRANDENBURGICUM. 1698.

BRANDMÜLLER, DANIEL [*fl.* 1699] *respondent. See* ZWINGER, T., *praeses.* Dissertatio academica de vita hominis sani. 1699.

BRANDMYLLERUS, DANIEL. *See* BRANDMÜLLER, Daniel [*fl.* 1699]

BRANDT, BONAVENTURA [*fl.* 1686] *respondent. See* WORM, O. [*fl.* 1686] *praeses.* De harmonia sensuum. 1686.

BRANDT, PHILIPP HEINRICH [*fl.* 1699-1700] *respondent.* Disputatio inauguralis medico-chirurgica de gangraena ... Altdorf, Literis Henrici Meyeri, 1700.

16 p.   18 cm.   **[1748]**

Diss. — Altdorf.

—*See* BRUNO, J. P., *praes.* Dissertatio medica de epilepsia puerili. 1699.

BRANT, GUALTHERUS. *See* BRUELE, Gualtherus.

BRASAVOLA, ANTONIO MUSA [1500-1555] Examen omnium loch. *In* Rostinio, P. Trattato di mal francese. 1623.

—, *tr. See* HIPPOCRATES. Aphorismorum … sectiones septem. 1610 [i.e. 1611] 1622, 1623, 1646, 1649, 1663, 1674, 1684; LATIOSO, A. *In* Hippocratis Aphorismos … commentarii. 1667.

—*See* GALENUS. Opera ex octava [-nona] Juntarum editione. 1609, 1625; HIPPOCRATES. [Selected works, Greek and Latin] Aphorismi Graece, & Latine, una cum Prognosticis. 1607, 1627.

BRASAVOLA, GIROLAMO [1628-1709] *See* CONGRESSO MEDICO ROMANO. Congressus Medico-Romanus habitus in aedibus D. Hieronymi Brasavoli. 1682.

BRASCH, GEORG [*fl.* 1680] *respondent. See* PECHLIN, J. N., *praeses.* Disputatio medica inauguralis de haemorrhagia narium. 1680.

BRASCHE, JOHANN [1671-1720] *respondent. See* BOHN, J., *praeses.* De medici officio dissertatio secunda. 1697; WEDEL, G. W., *praeses.* Dissertatio medica inauguralis de inflammatione renum. 1697.

BRAUEL, JOHANNES PHILIPPUS. *See* GRAUEL, Johann Philipp [*fl.* 1675]

BRAUN, CHRISTIAN FRIEDRICH [*fl.* 1676] *respondent. See* MÜLLER, J. [*fl.* 1672-1679] *praeses.* Disputatio physica de tarantula. 1676.

BRAUN, JEREMIAS JACOB [*fl.* 1685] *respondent. See* VESTI, J., *praeses.* Disputatio inauguralis medica de suffocatione hysterica. 1685.

BRAUN, JOHANN [*fl.* 1676] *respondent. See* LAUTERBACH, W. A., *praeses.* Positiones juridicae de domiciliis pauperum, von Hospitälen. 1676.

BRAUN, JOHANN [*fl.* 1681] *respondent.* Dissertatio medica inauguralis de gutta rosacea … Argentorati, Literis Joh. Friderici Spoor [1681]

[2], 30 p. 19 cm.   **[1749]**

Diss. — Strasbourg.

BRAUN, NICOLAS [*d.* 1639] Kurtzer und eygentlicher Bericht, von der Curation der rohten Ruhr, oder Dysenteriae, so jetziger Zeit in der Stat Marpurg eingerissen, wie sich hierin Gesunde und Krancke zu verhalten … Marpurg, Gedruckt durch Nicolaum Hampelium, 1629.

29 p. 17 cm.   **[1750]**

—*See* THEODORUS, J. Neuw vollkommentlich Kreuterbuch. 1613, 1625, 1664.

BRAUN, SALOMON [*fl.* 1665-1672] *respondent. See* METZGER, G. B., *praeses.* Febris maligna petechialis. 1665.

BRAUN, SALOMON [*fl.* 1688-1690] *respondent. See* CAMERARIUS, E. R., *praeses.* Dissertatio medica inauguralis, de casu. 1690 [and] Expositio medico-chirurgica. 1688.

BRAUNS, BERNARD HEINRICH [*fl.* 1696] *respondent. See* BARBECK, F. G., *praeses.* Dissertatio medica de febrium differentia ac natura. 1696.

BRAUNSCHWEIG, HIERONYMUS. *See* BRUNSCHWIG, Hieronymus [*ca.* 1450-*ca.* 1512]

BRAUNSCHWEIG-LÜNEBURG, GEORG WILHELM, *Herzog von. See* GEORG WILHELM, Herzog von Braunschweig-Lüneburg [1624-1705]

BRAVO DE SOBREMONTE RAMIREZ, GASPAR [1603-1683] Resolutiones medicae in quatuor partes tributae, quarum I. Physiologiae universae. II. Pathologiae. III. Febrium theoriae ac curationis. IV. & ultima, sanguinis missionis, purgationis, ac de sudore controversias proponit, excutit, ac dirimit … Lugduni, Sumpt. Philippi Borde, Laurentii Arnaud, & Claudii Rigaud, 1654.

[43], 594, [53] p. front. (port.) 36 cm.
                                            [1751]

—[The same.] Resolutionum, & consultationum medicarum. Tertia editio. In sex partes distributa … quarum I. Physiologiae. II. Pathologiae. III. Febrium theoriae, ac curationis. IV. Sanguinis missionis, purgationis, & de sudore. V. Sanguinis circulationis, & ipsa praesupposita, artis sphygmicae theoriae, e Galeni mente, ac prognosis recidivae naturae, quorumdam eunuchorum potentiae controversias proponit, excutit, ac dirimit. In VI. Selectas aliquas observationes, & consultationes medicas proponit. Lugduni, Sumptib. Philippi Borde et Laurentii Arnaud, 1662.

[52], 756, [62] p. (port.) 36 cm.   **[1752]**

—[The same.] Resolutionum et consultationum medicarum editio post tres Gallicas quarta in Germania. Tribus tomis distincta, ac in septem partes distributa ... [Coloniae Agrippinae] Sumptibus Joannis Wilhelmi Friessem, 1674.

3 v.   21 cm.   **[1753]**

Each vol. has added engraved title page.

BRAVO RAMIREZ, Gaspar. *See* Bravo de Sobremonte Ramirez, Gaspar [1603-1683]

BRAYER, Nicolas [*fl.* 1670-1671] *praeses.* Quaestio medica ... An quae hydrargyro non cedit syphilis, hidroticis percuranda? [Parisiis, Ex typographia Francisci Muguet, 1670]

4 p.   24 cm.   **[1754]**

Caption title.

Diss.—Paris (C. Puylon, *respondent*)

BRAZIUS, Conradus Wilhelmus [*fl.* 1659] *respondent. See* Kirchmayer, G. K., *praeses.* Ex physicis disputationem publicam de sale ... sistet. 1659.

BREBIS, Johann Friedrich [*fl.* 1695] *respondent. See* Vesti, J., *praeses.* Disputationem inauguralem medicam de pollinctura ... submittit J. F. B. 1695.

BREBISS, Johann Georg [*fl.* 1694] *respondent. See* Stahl, G. E., *praeses.* Disputatio inauguralis medica de mensium muliebrium fluxu. 1694 [and] Propemticum inaugurale, de commotione sanguinis translatoria. 1694.

BRECHAEUS, Joannes. *See* Brèche, Jean [*ca.* 1514–*ca.* 1583]

BRÈCHE, Jean [*ca.* 1514–*ca.* 1583] *ed.* and *tr. See* Hippocrates. Les Aphorismes. 1605, 1606, 162-?, 1627, 1628, 1646, 1660, 1671.

BRECHT, Clemens Joseph [*fl.* 1679] *respondent. See* Andreae, T. Sacrosancta triade annuente trias exercitationum de mente et corpore. 1679.

BRECHTFELD, Johann Heinrich [*d.* 1699] *respondent. See* Conring, H., *praeses.* Disputatio medica inauguralis de morbo hypochondriaco. 1662; Vogler, V. H., *praeses.* Disputatio medica de venenis. 1661.

BREHM, Johann Salomon [*fl.* 1684-1688] *respondent. See* Vesti, J., *praeses.* Inaugurales de hydrocephalo theses. 1688.

BREHME, Johann Salomo. *See* Brehm, Johann Salomon [*fl.* 1684-1688]

BREITERT, Johann Friedrich [*fl.* 1689] *respondent. See* Wedel, G. W., *praeses.* Disputatio medica de contagio et morbis contagiosis. 1689.

BREITINGER, Johann Jacob [1575-1645] *See* Von der Pestilentz. 1629.

—[**BREM**, Wolfgang Sigismund, *fl.* 1651-1658] Nutzliche, bewehrte und an vilen öffters probierte Hauss-Mittel, für schwangere und gebährende Frawen. Item: Für die klaine Kinder. Deren Anligen, Schwachheit, und Gefährligkeit, in grossen Nöthen, mit ringem Unkosten wol zugebrauchen. Allen ehrsamen Matronen und Frawen, zu sonderbahren Ehren und Nutzen an Tag gegeben ... Ingolstat, Gedruckt bey Johann Ostermayr, 1665.

[1], 44, [2] p.   16 cm.   **[1755]**

Bound with Schöenfeld, P. J. Tractatus brevis de hieronosologia. 1675.

BREMER, Elias Georg [*b.* 1664] *respondent. See* Crause, R. W., *praeses.* Dissertatio inauguralis medica de nymphomania. 1691; Wedel, G. W. Propempticon inaugurale de balsamatione corporum in genere. 1691.

BREMER, William [*fl. ca.* 1586] *ed. See* Vicary, T. The English mans treasure. 1613, 1633, 1641 [and] The surgions directorie. 1651.

BRENDEL, Adam [*d.* 1719] *praeses.* De Homero medico ... Vitembergae, Ex officina Christiani Schrödteri [1700]

[24] p.   20 cm.   **[1756]**

Diss.—Wittenberg (J. G. Oertel, *respondent*)

—*praeses.* Dissertationem medicam de catalepsi ... exponet ... Urbanus Gothofredus Bucher ... Vitembergae, Ex Officina Goderitschiana [1700]

[32] p.   20 cm.   **[1757]**

Diss.—Wittenberg (U. G. Bucher, *respondent*)

—Another issue. Page [2] is blank.   **[1758]**

BRENDEL, Johann Philipp [*fl.* 1595-1615] *respondent. See* Varus, A., *praeses.* Theses medicae de febri maligna. 1605.

—, *ed.* and *tr.* Consilia medica, celeberrimorum quorundam Germaniae medicorum. Collecta et partim etiam ex idiomate Germanico conversa ...

utilitatis publicae caussa nunc primum edita ...
Francofurti, Ex Bibliopolio Paltheniano, 1615.

    [8], 412 p.   21 cm.   [1759]

    Bound with copy 2 of Petraeus, H. Nosologia harmonica. 1615.

BRENDEL, Zacharias [1553-1626] *praeses.* De
pleuritide themata medica ... Jenae, Typis Tobiae
Steinmanni, 1604.

    [16] p.   19 cm.   [1760]

—, *ed. See* Eugalenus, S. De scorbuto morbo liber.
1623 [i.e. 1624?], 1658.

BRENDEL, Zacharias [1592-1638] Chymia in artis formam redacta et publicis praelectionibus
philiatris in Academia Jenensi communicata ...
Jenae, Typis viduae Weidnerianae, impensis Johan.
Reiffenbergeri, 1630.

    [23], 218, [30] p.   13 cm.   [1761]

—[The same.] ... Chimia in artis formam redacta
... disquisitio curata de famosissima praeparatione
auri potabilis instituitur. Ed. 2 corr., & auct ... consilio Werneri Rolfinck ... iterum luci tradita, cum
ejusdem praefatione. Jenae, Sumtibus Johannis Reiffenbergeri, 1641.

    [16], 175, [16] p.   16 cm.   [1762]

    With this are bound: Kerner, A. Tetras chymiatrica. 1618. —
Sala, Angelo. Processus ... de auro potabili. 1630.

—[The same.] ... Lugduni Batavorum, Ex officina Arnoldi Doude, 1671.

    167, [13] p.   13 cm.   [1763]

    Added engraved title page dated 1672.

—*praeses.* Disputatio inauguralis de dysenteria ...
Jenae, Typis Weidnerianis, 1628.

    [20] p.   19 cm.   [1764]

    Diss.—Jena (W. U. Amthor, *respondent*)

BRENNER, Sebastian. *See* Prenner, Sebastian.

BRENTA, Andrea [ca. 1460-ca. 1485] Variae
philosophorum sententiae perveniendi ad lapidem
benedictum ...

    333-363 p., vol. 4.   20 cm.   (*In* Zetzner, Laza-
rus, *ed.* Theatrum chemicum. Argentorati, 1659-61)
                                  [1765]

    Caption title.

BRENTZIUS, Andreas. *See* Brenta, Andrea [ca.
1460-ca. 1485]

BRENZIO, Andrea. *See* Brenta, Andrea [ca.
1460-ca. 1485]

BRENZONI, Ottavio [*fl.* 1610-1628] Brevis logica
... Veronae, Apud Angelum Tamum, 1628.

    [8], 102, [1] p.   20 cm.   [1766]

    Bound with *his* Sermo de causis atque natura pestis. 1610.

—Sermo de causis, atque natura pestis, et cura ...
Veronae, Typis Tamianis, 1610.

    64 (i.e. 74), [1] p.   20 cm.   [1767]

    With this is bound *his* Brevis logica. 1628.

BREREWOOD, Edward [1656?-1613] Tractatus
quidam logici de praedicabilibus et praedicamentis
... In lucem editi: per T[homas] S[ixesmith] ... Ed.
3. in qua accesserunt duo ejusdem authoris insignes
tractatus; prior de meteoris, posterior de oculo ...
Oxoniae, Excudebat Guilielmus Turner, & vaeneunt
apud Hen. Cripps, Ed. Forrest, Hen. Curteyne, &
Joh. Willimot, 1637.

    [31], 431 p.; [3], 105, [3], 26 p.   tables, illus.   17
cm.   [1768]

    Part [2] has special title page: Tractatus duo, quorum primus
est de meteoris. Secundus, de oculo.
    STC 3630.

BRESCIA. Academia Philoexoticorum. *See* Accademia dei filesotici, Brescia.

BRESMAL, Jean-François [ca. 1660-1724] La circulation des eaux; ou, L'hydrographie des minerales
d'Aix et de Spa ... Liege, Christian Bronckart [1699]

    3 parts in 1 v.   16 cm.   [1769]

    Parts 2 and 3 have special title pages dated 1700.
    Date supplied from Eloy, v. 1, p. 446.

BREST, Pieter [*fl.* 1684] *respondent.* Disputatio
medica inauguralis de paralysi ... Lugduni
Batavorum, Apud Abrahamum Elzevier, 1684.

    [13] p.   22 cm.   [1770]
    Diss.—Leyden.

BRETAG, Andreas [*fl.* 1697] *respondent. See*
Lehmann, J. C., *praeses.* Disputationem physicam de
transmutationibus corporum extraordinariis ... Joh.
Christianus Lehmann ... et ... Andreas Bretag ...
exponent. 1697.

BREVE & succinctum theoreticae philosophiae
theatrum. *See* Schweitzer, J. H. Compendium
physicae Aristotelico-Cartesianae. 1695.

BREVE instruttione per preservarsi dal contagio pestilente. 1630. *See* COLLEGIO DEI MEDICI, Lucca.

BREVIS ad materiam medicam in usum philiatrorum manuductio. Lipsiae, Literis Christiani Michaelis [1675?]

[1], 193, [13 +] p.   15 cm.   **[1771]**
Imperfect: all after p. [13] wanting.
Bound with copy 2 of Welsch, Gottfried. Rationale vulnerum lethalium judicium. 1662.

BREVIS excursus in battologiam Quercetani. 1604. *See* [RIOLAN, J., 1580–1657]

BREWER, JÁNOS [*fl.* 1661–1664] *respondent. See* SCHNEIDER, K. V., *praeses.* Disputatio medica de arthritide. 1663 [and] Disputationem inauguralem de ictero flavo . . . publice habebit J. B. 1664.

[**BREWER**, THOMAS, *fl.* 1624] A dialogue betwixt a citizen, and a poore countrey-man and his wife, in the countrey, where the citizen remaineth now in this time of sicknesse. Written by him in the countrey, who sent the coppie to a friend in London. Being both pittifull and pleasant. London, By R. Oulton for H. Gosson, 1636.

[22] p.   illus.   19 cm.   **[1772]**
First preliminary leaf wanting.
STC 3717.7.

BREYER, LUDWIG FRIEDRICH [*fl.* 1688–1698] *respondent. See* CAMERARIUS, R. J., *praeses.* Dissertatio inauguralis medica de potu aquarum ardentium. 1698.

BREYNE, JAN FILIP [1680–1764] *respondent. See* DEKKERS, F., *praeses.* Dissertatio botanico-medica. 1700.

BREYNIUS, JOANNES PHILIPPUS. *See* BREYNE, Jan Filip [1680–1764]

BRIAN, THOMAS [*fl.* 1637] The pisse-prophet; or, Certaine pisse-pot lectures. Wherein are newly discovered the old fallacies, deceit, and jugling of the pisse-pot science, used by all those . . . who pretend knowledge of diseases, by the urine . . . London, Printed by E. P. for R. Thrale, 1637.

[10], 108, [1] p.   16 cm.   **[1773]**
STC 3723.

— [German tr.] Der englische Wahrsager aus dem Urin; oder, Gewisse Wahrsagungen aus dem Wasser-Blase . . . In englischer Sprache beschrieben,

anjetzo aber ins Teutsche übersetzet von Johann Reinhard Stolberg, M. C. Hamburg, Gottfried Liebezeit, 1693.

[14], 167 p.; [10], 107 p.   17 cm.   **[1774]**
Imperfect: sig.):(8 wanting; Vorrede of part [2] bound between p. 72 and 73.
Part [2] has special title page: Urin-Büchlein . . . Bericht, wie man die Kranckheiten an seinem Leibe gewiss erkennen sol. Sampt des . . . Herrn Apollinaris [pseud., i.e. Walther Hermenius Ryff] Tractälein vom Urin und Pulss . . . in Druck verfertiget durch Theodorum Majum . . . 1663 (i.e. 1693)

BRICCIUS, CHRISTIANUS [*fl.* 1651] *respondent. See* SEBISCH, M. [1578–1674?] *praeses.* Galeni quinque priores libri. 1651.

BRIDEWELL Hospital, London. *See* LONDON. Corporation. Court of Common Council. The order of the hospitalls of K. Henry the viijth. [Not before 1690]

BRIDLER, ANDREAS [*fl.* 1677] *See* STOCKHAMER, F. Bibliotheca medico-philosophico-philologica. 1677.

A BRIEF account of some choice & famous medicines: together with their virtues and operations in the body. Oxford, Leonard Lichfield. 1676.

[8], 29, [1] p.   **[1775]**
Errata: p. [1] at end.
Preface signed: R. B.

A BRIEFE discourse of the hypostasis, or substance of the water of Spaw; containing in small quantity many pots of that minerall water. Verie profitable for such patients, as cannot repaire in person to those fountaines, as by perusing this discourse, it will plainly appeare. Translated out of French into English, by G. T. This above saide hypostasis, or substance of the water of Spaw, is to be sold by Doctor Hieronimus Seminus, Italian, dwelling in S. Paules Alley, in Red-crosse-street. [London, W. Jaggard, 1612?]

[1], 11 p.   19 cm.   **[1776]**
Partly based on Des fontaines acides de la forest d'Ardenne, et principalement de celle qui se trouva à Spa, par M. Gilbert Lymborh [pseud., i.e. Gilbert Fusch, called also Gilbertus Philaretus] Anvers, 1559.
STC 22975.

BRIES, DANIEL DE [*fl.* 1686] *respondent.* Disputatio medica inauguralis, continens praecipuas ex omnibus medicinae partibus desumptas quaestiones . . . Lugduni Batavorum, Apud Abrahamum Elzevier, 1686.

[8] p. 22 cm.   [**1777**]
Diss.—Leyden.

BRIGANTI, ANNIBALE [*d.* 1582] *tr. See* ORTA, G.
d'. Dell'historia de i semplici aromati. 1605, 1616.

BRIGEL, JOHANN MATTHIAS [*fl.* 1685-1689]
respondent. See CAMERARIUS, E. R., *praeses.* Dissertatio
medica de clysmatibus. 1688 [and] Dissert.
medico-chirurgica inauguralis, de ulceribus antiquis.
1689; MÖGLING, J. L. [*fl.* 1662-1685] *praeses.*
Exercitatio physica de inferno naturali. 1685.

BRIGGS, WILLIAM [*ca.* 1650-1704] Nova visionis
theoria, Regiae Societati Londin. proposita . . . Ed.
altera. Londini, Typis J.P. impensis Sam Simpson,
bibliopol. Cantabrig. & prostant venales apud Sam.
Smith. Londin., 1685.
[16], 80 p. plates. 17 cm.   [**1778**]
"Epistola D. Isaaci Newtoni . . . ad authorem conscripta":
p. [3]-[6]
Contains two treatises, previously published in English. The first
(Nova visionis theoria, p. 1-34) was expounded before the Royal
Society in 1681 and printed in the Philosophical collections edited
by Robert Hooke, no. 6, 1682. The second (Continuatio theoriae
praecedentis, p. 35-80) was printed in the Philosophical transactions
of the Royal Society, no. 146, 1683.
Bound with (as issued) *his* Ophthalmo-graphia. 1685.

—Ophthalmo-graphia; sive, Oculi ejusque partium descriptio anatomica . . . Cantabrigiae, Excudebat Joan. Hayes, impensis Jon. Hart, 1676.
[24], 80, [7] p. plates. 16 cm.   [**1779**]

—[The same.] . . . Cui accessit Nova visionis
theoria, Regiae Societati Londin. proposita . . . Ed.
altera. Londini, Typis J. P. impensis Sam. Simpson,
et prostant venales apud Sam. Smith. Londin., 1685
[24], 80, [7] p.; [16], 80 p. plates. 17 cm.
[**1780**]
Imperfect: dedicatory epistle (p. [3]-[6]) of the Ophthalmo-
graphia wanting.
With this is bound (as issued) *his* Nova visionis theoria. 1685.

—[The same.] Ophthalmo-graphia; sive, Oculi
ejusque partium descriptio anatomica; nec non,
ejusdem Nova visionis theoria, Regiae Societati Londinensi proposita. Lugd. Batavor., Apud Petrum
vander Aa, 1686.
312, [12] p. plates. 14 cm.   [**1781**]
Added engraved title page.

—Ophthalmographia; sive, Oculi ejusque partium
descriptio anatomica . . . Ed. 2, ab auctore recognita.

Londini, Typis M. C. impensis Ricardi Green,
bibliopolae Cantabrigiensis, 1687.
[24], 80, [7] p. illus. 17 cm.   [**1782**]
A reprint of the first edition, Cambridge, 1676.

—*See* VIEUSSENS, R. Réponse . . . a trois lettres . . .
du sieur Chirac. 1698.

BRIGHT, TIMOTHY [1551?-1615] A treatise of
melancholy. Containing the causes thereof, and
reasons of the strange effects it worketh in our minds
and bodies: with the physicke cure, and spirituall
consolation for such as have thereto adjoyned afflicted
conscience. The difference betwixt it, and
melancholy, with divers philosophicall discourses
touching actions, and affections of soule, spirit, and
body . . . Newly corr. and amended. London,
William Stansby, 1613.
[22], 347 p. 16 cm.   [**1783**]
STC 3749.
Keynes(E) 16.

[—] A treatise, wherein is declared the sufficiencie
of English medicines, for cure of all diseases, cured
with medicines. Whereunto is added A collection of
medicines growing (for the most part) within our
English climat, approved and experimented against
the jaundise, dropsie, stone, falling-sicknesse,
pestilence. London, Printed by H. L[ownes] for Tho.
Man, 1615.
[11], 127 p. 14 cm.   [**1784**]
STC 3752.
Keynes(E) 3.
Erratum at end.
With this are bound: Bayley, W. Two treatises concerning the
preservation of eie-sight. 1616; Cary, Walter. [A breefe treatise,
called Careys farewell to physicke . . . with The hammer for the
stone] London, 1597.

BRIGNOLE SALE, ANTONIO GIULIO, *marchese di
Groppoli* [1605-1665] Copia di lettera d'incerto inviata
al . . . Anton Giulio Brignole ove pienamente si
discorre intorno alle vere cause della peste che regna
in Genova, & in alcune parti d'Italia ed intorno a'
veri rimedii contro d'essa . . . Genova, Gio. Maria
Farroni [1657]
23 p. 19 cm.   [**1785**]

BRION, STEPHAN [*fl.* 1682] *respondent. See* KLEIN,
F., *praeses.* Stephanus Brion . . . dissertationem
inauguralem de catarrho . . . subibit [sic]. 1682.

BRISBANE, Matthew [*d.* 1699] Disputatio medica inauguralis, de catalepsi ... Ultrajecti, Ex officina Theodori ab Ackersdyck [1661?]

[20] p. 19 cm. **[1786]**

Imperfect: lower margin of title page trimmed, affecting imprint date.

Brisbane graduated M. D. at Utrecht in 1661. Cf. Comrie, vol. 1, p. 278.

Diss.—Utrecht.

BRISBAR, Joannes Maximilianus [*fl.* 1699] *respondent. See* Deidier, A., *proponent.* Quaestio medica eaque physiologica de motu musculari. 1699.

BRISSEAU, Pierre [1626-1717] Traité des mouvemens simpatiques. Avec une explication de ceux qui arrivent dans le vertige, l'epilepsie, l'affection hypocondriaque, & la passion hysterique ... Mons, Erneste de la Roche, 1692.

[8], 149, [5] p. 15 cm. **[1787]**

BRISSOT, Pierre [1478-1522] Apologetica disceptatio, in qua docetur per quae loca sanguis mitti debeat in viscerum inflammationibus praesertim in pleuritide. Ed. nova, Renato Moreau ... illustrata, qui διάλεξιν De missione sanguinis in pleuritide subjunxit ... Parisiis, Apud Abrahamum Pacard, 1622.

2 v. in 1. illus. 18 cm. **[1788]**

Vol. [2] has special title page only: De missione sanguinis in pleuritide ... Adjuncta est Pet. Brissoti ... vita. Auctore Renato Moreau.

With this is bound Fontaine, J. Methodus generalis et specialis cognoscendi & curandi morbos. 1612.

BRITISH Merlin. *See* Riders (1677.) British Merlin. 1677.

BRODKORB, Heinrich [*fl.* 1620] Prodromus mysteriorum naturae mysteriosissimorum, emissus: omnibus omnium scientiarum ... cultoribus summe necessarius ... et aurora medicinae universalis consurgens; veluti digito, fiduciae regula, demonstrata, ab Henrico Artocophino ... Stetini, Typis Samuelis Kelneri, 1620.

37, 169 (i.e. 168), [47] p. illus., port. 19 cm. **[1789]**

"Sequntur anagrammata & epigrammata in symbolum, Duce Jehovah. Et in nomen ... Dn. Henrici Artocophini ...": p. [5-47]

BRODTBECKIUS, Johannes Conrad. *See* Brotbeck, Johann Konrad [1620-1677]

BRÖCKING, Johann [*fl.* 1620] *respondent. See* Steffek a Kolodieg, S., *praeses.* Pentas medica miscella. 1620.

BROEKHUIZEN, Benjamin van [*d. ca.* 1686] Dissertatio recitata in illust. Sylva-Ducensi Athenaeo ... Sylva-Ducis, Apud Stephanum du Mont [1677]

[17] p. 19 cm. **[1790]**

Imperfect: upper margins trimmed.

—Oeconomia corporis animalis; sive, Cogitationes succinctae, de mente, corpore, et utriusque conjunctione, juxta methodum philosophiae Cartesianae deductae. Noviomagi, Typis Regneri Smetii, 1672.

[20], 361, [20] p. 15 cm. **[1791]**

—[The same.] Amstelaedami, Apud Henricum Wetsteinium, 1683.

[17], 641 (i.e. 639), [22] p. 21 cm. **[1792]**

Added engraved title page.

BROEKHUIZEN, Daniel van [*fl.* 16th cent.] Secreta alchimiae magnalia D. Thomae Aquinatis, de corporibus supercoelestibus, & quod in rebus inferioribus inveniantur, quoque modo extrahantur: de lapide minerali, animali, & plantali. Item thesaurus alchimiae ... Accessit et Joannis de Rupescissa Liber lucis, ac Raymundi Lullii opus ... quod inscribitur Clavicula & apertorium in quo omnia quae in opere alchimiae requiruntur, venuste declarantur ... opera Danielis Brouchuisii ... Cum praefatione D. Joannis Heurnii. Ed. 3. Lugduni Batavorum, Ex officina Thomae Basson, 1602.

71 p. 16 cm. **[1793]**

BROEN, Johann [*fl.* 1678-ca. 1695] Animadversiones medicae, theoretico practicae in Henrici Regii Praxin medicam, quibus editio prior, Observationum ... D. Theod. Craanen ... emendatur & repurgatur. Lugd. Batavorum, Apud C. Boutestein, J. Lugtmans et Joannem du Vivie, 1695.

[8], 709, [17] p. 21 cm. **[1794]**

—Exercitatio physico-medica. De duplici bile veterum ... Lugduni Batavorum, Apud Johannem Prins, 1685.

[32], 249, [66] p. 14 cm. **[1795]**

Added engraved title page.

—*respondent.* Disputatio medica inauguralis de somno & somnifero opio ... Lugduni Batavorum, Apud Abrahamum Elzevier, 1683.

[16] p.   22 cm.   **[1796]**

Diss. — Leyden.

—*respondent. See* CRAANEN, T., *praeses.* Disputatio medica de phthisi s. tabe vera. 1682 [and] Disputatio medica de palpitatione cordis. 1681.

—, *ed. See* BORELLI, G. A. De vi percussionis. 1686.

BROGNOLI, CANDIDO [1607-1677] Alexicacon; hoc est, Opus de maleficiis, ac morbis maleficis. Duobus tomus distributum ... Venetiis, Typis Jo. Baptistae Catanei, 1668.

2 v. in 1.   illus.   33 cm.   **[1797]**

Added engraved title page and half titles.
Vol. 1 has added special title page.

BROMFIELD, M. A brief discovery of the true causes, symptoms and effects of that most reigning disease the scurvie ... Whereunto is added a short account of those incomparable and most highly approved diaphoretique, diuretique, and cathartique pills, called pilulae in omnes morbos; or, pills against all diseases ... Prepared and set forth for the publike benefit, by M. Bromfield, approved physician ... [n. p., 1672]

[8] p.   18 cm.   **[1798]**

Wing B4884H.

BRONCHORST, HENRICUS VAN [*fl.* 1687] *respondent.* Disputatio medica inauguralis de apoplexia ... Lugduni Batavorum, Apud Abrahamum Elzevier, 1687.

[28] p.   18 cm.   **[1799]**

Diss. — Leyden.

BRONCKHORST, JOHANNES [*fl.* 1687] *respondent.* Disputatio medica inauguralis, de doloribus ... Trajecti ad Rhenum, Ex officina Francisci Halma, 1687.

8 p.   22 cm.   **[1800]**

Diss. — Utrecht.

BRONDOLO, FILIPPO [*fl.* 1639] *See* MANTUA, Italy (City). Ordinances, local laws, etc. Il maestrato della sanità certificati noi dalli signori della sanità di Genova, Bologna, & Modona. 1639.

BRONZERIO, GIOVANNI GIROLAMO [1577-1630] De innato calido et naturali spiritu disputatio ... In qua pro rei veritate Galeni doctrina passim

explicatur, defenditur. [Patavii, Apud Petrum Paulum Tozzium, 1626]

[8], 88 p.   25 cm.   **[1801]**

BROOKE, HUMPHREY [1617-1693] Ὑγιεινη; or, A conservatory of health. Comprized in a plain and practicall discourse upon the six particulars necessary to mans life, viz. 1. Aire. 2. Meat and drink. 3. Motion and rest. 4. Sleep and wakefulness. 5. The excrements. 6. The passions of the mind. With the discussion of divers questions pertinent thereunto. Compiled and published for the prevention of sickness, and prolongation of life ... London, Printed by R. W. for G. Whittington, 1650.

[32], 256 p.   13 cm.   **[1802]**

BROSSE, GUY DE LA. *See* LA BROSSE, GUY DE [1586?-1641]

BROSSE, JOSEPH DE LA. *See* ANGELUS DE SANCTU JOSEPHO, *Father* [1636-1697]

BROSSGEBAUER,   PHILIPPUS.   *See* GROSSGEBAUER, Philipp [1653-1711]

BROTBECK, DAVID [*fl.* 1689-1693] *respondent. See* CAMERARIUS, E. R., *praeses.* Anatome hydropicae. 1691; Positiones chirurgicae de fractura cum vulnere. 1693 [and] Schematismi colorum, infuso ligni nephritici propriorum. 1689.

BROTBECK, JOHANN KONRAD [1620-1677]

Dissertations — Tübingen

—*praeses.* Commentarius medicus in historiam Galeni, de peste ... Tubingae, Literis Kernerianis, 1661.

[16] p.   19 cm.   **[1803]**

The Galenic fragment here allegedly excerpted from *his* De cucurbitula & scarificatione ... chap. 20, actually corresponds to a passage in the spurious compilation printed in Kühn under title De venae sectione. Cf. Kühn, vol. XIX, p. 524.

B. Ehrhart, *respondent.*

—Disputatio medica de hydrope ascite ... Tubingae, Typis Johann-Henrici Reisii, 1676.

16 p.   19 cm.   **[1804]**

J. Hafenreffer, *respondent.*

—Dissertatio medica de pica seu malacia ... Tubingae, Typis Johann-Henrici Reisii, 1676.

16 p.   20 cm.   **[1805]**

J. S. Müller, *respondent.*

—Disputatio medica de sanguine menstruo . . . Tubingae, Typis Johann-Henrici Reisii, 1676.

　　12 p.　19 cm.　　　　　　　　　　[1806]

　　J. P. Caspar, *respondent.*

—Progymnasmatis medici pars prima, Historiae Galeni ex libr. 10 meth. med. cap. 3. de febre ardente analysin exhibens . . . Tubingae, Typis Johann-Henrici Reisi, 1664.

　　[28] p.　19 cm.　　　　　　　　　　[1807]

　　G. Bardili, *respondent.*

—Scrutinium pepasmi sive disquisitio physico-medica de coctione materiae febrilis . . . Tubingae, Typis Johann-Henrici Reisii, 1671.

　　16 p.　19 cm.　　　　　　　　　　[1808]

　　J. L. Schlapperitius, *respondent.*

BROTBEQIUS, DAVID. *See* BROTBECK, David [*fl.* 1689-1693]

BROTBEQUIUS, JOHANNES CONRAD. *See* BROTBECK, Johann Konrad [1620-1677]

BROUCHUISIUS, DANIEL. *See* BROEKHUIZEN, Daniel van [*fl.* 16th cent.]

BROUN, ANDREW. *See* BROWN, Andrew [*fl.* 1687-1691]

BROUNCKER, WILLIAM, *2d Viscount* [1620 *or* 21-1684] *See* WALLIS, J. A defence of the Royal Society. 1678.

BROUWER, JOHANNES [*fl.* 1684] *respondent.* Disputatio medica inauguralis, de angina . . . Ultrajecti, Typis Appelarianis, 1684.

　　[19] p.　22 cm.　　　　　　　　　　[1809]

　　Diss. — Utrecht.

BROUWERS, NICOLAUS [*fl.* 1666] *respondent.* Disputatio medica inauguralis, de ictero . . . Trajecti ad Rhenum, Ex officina Anthonii Smytegelt, 1666.

　　[15] p.　20 cm.　　　　　　　　　　[1810]

　　Diss. — Utrecht.

BROWALLIUS, GEORG [*fl.* 1687-1688] *respondent.* *See* DROSSANDER, A., *praeses.* De sale volatili disputatio chymico physica. 1687.

BROWN, *See* also BROWNE.

BROWN, ANDREW [*fl.* 1687-1691] The epilogue to the five papers lately past betwixt the two physicians Dr. O. [i.e. Charles Oliphant] and Dr. E. [i.e. Sir Edward Eizat] containing some remarks . . . concerning that debate, and the usefulness of vomiting and purging in fevers . . . Edinburgh, John Reid, 1699.

　　40 p.　15 cm.　　　　　　　　　　[1811]

—A vindicatory schedule, concerning the new cure of fevers: containing a disquisition . . . of the new . . . method of cureing continual fevers, first invented and delivered, by . . . Tho. Sydenham . . . With an Appendix of Sanctorius his Medicina statica, for clearing the doctrine of insensible perspiration, whereupon that hypothesis is founded . . . Edinburgh, Printed by John Reid, sold be [sic] John Mackie, 1691.

　　[48], 211 p.　plate.　15 cm.　　　　[1812]

—*See* In speculo teipsum contemplare Dr. Black. 1692.

BROWNE, EDWARD [1644-1708] An account of several travels through a great part of Germany: in four journeys . . . Wherein the mines, baths, and other curiosities of those parts are treated of . . . London, Benj. Tooke, 1677.

　　[4], 179, [1] p.　plates.　21 cm.　　[1813]

—A brief account of some travels in Hungaria, Servia, Bulgaria, Macedonia, Thessaly . . . As also some observations on the gold, silver, copper, quicksilver mines, baths, and mineral waters in those parts . . . London, Printed by T. R. for Benj. Tooke, 1673.

　　[10], 144, [3] p.　illus., plates.　20 cm.　[1814]

　　Errata: p. [147]

　　First preliminary leaf (blank) wanting.

—[The same.] . . . 2d ed. with many additions . . . London, Benj. Tooke, 1685.

　　[3], 222, [6] p.　plates.　33 cm.　　[1815]

—[Dutch tr.] Naukeurige en gedenkwaardige reysen . . . door Nederland, Duytsland, Hongaryen, Servien, Bulgarien, Macedonien, Thessalien, Oostenrijk, Stiermark, Carinthien, Carniole, en Friuli, enz . . . Uit het Engels vertaelt door . . . Jacob Leeuw . . . Amsterdam, Jan ten Hoorn, 1682.

　　[8], 87, 159, 128, [8] p.　plates.　21 cm.　[1816]

　　Added engraved title page.

BROWNE, JOHN [1642-*ca.* 1702] Adenochoiradelogia; or, An anatomick-chirurgical treatise of glandules & strumaes, or Kings-Evil-swellings. Together with the royal gift of healing, or cure thereof by contact or imposition of hands, performed for above 640 years by our Kings of England, continued with their admirable effects, and miraculous events; and concluded with many wonderful examples of cures by their sacred touch ... London, Printed by Tho. Newcomb for Sam. Lowndes, 1684.

3 parts in 1 v. fronts. (port.) 19 cm. **[1817]**
Imperfect: 2 engraved frontispieces wanting.

Each part has special title page. Part [1] has title: Adenographia; or, An exact anatomical treatise of the glandules. Part [2] has title: Chaeradelogia; or, An exact discourse of strumaes, or Kings-Evil-swellings. Part [3] has title: Charisma Basilicon; or, The royal gift of healing strumaes, or Kings-Evil.

—A compleat discourse of wounds both in general and particular: whereunto are added the severall fractures of the skull, with their variety of figures. As also a treatise of gunshot-wounds in general. Collected and reduced into a new method ... London, Printed by E. Flesher for William Jacob, 1678.

[8], 349, [3] p. 20 cm. **[1818]**

—A compleat treatise of preternatural tumours, both general and particular, as they appear in humane body from head to foot. To which also are added many excellent and modern historical observations ... Collected from the learned labours both of ancient and modern physicians and chirurgions ... London, Printed by S. R. for R. Clavel, 1678.

[16], 395, [4] p. front. (port.) illus., plates. 19 cm. **[1819]**
Imperfect: p. [2-3] at end wanting; supplied in photocopy from New York Academy of Medicine library.

—A compleat treatise of the muscles, as they appear in humane body, and arise in dissection; with diverse anatomical observations not yet discover'd ... [London] Printed by Tho. Newcombe for the author, 1681.

[31], 213 (i.e. 237) p. front. (port.), plates. 35 cm. **[1820]**
The description of the muscles is based on William Molins' Μυσκοτομια, and the plates on Guilio Casserio's Tabula anatomicae.

—Another issue, with new title page ... London, Printed for Dorman Newman, 1683.

[31], 213 (i.e. 237) p. front. (port.), plates. 32 cm. **[1821]**

—[The same.] ... Myographia nova; or, A graphical description of all the muscles in humane body, as they arise in dissection: distributed into six lectures ... Together, with an accurate and concise

discourse of the heart, and its use; as also of the circulation of the blood, and the parts of which the sanguinary mass is made and framed. Written by ... Dr. Lower ... London, Printed by Tho. Milbourn for the author, 1697.

[41], 109 p. front. (port.), plates. 33 cm. **[1822]**

—[The same.] ... Together with a philosophical and mathematical account of the mechanism of muscular motion, and an accurate ... discourse of the heart and its use, with the circulation of the blood, &c. ... London, Printed by Tho. Milbourn for the author, 1698.

[9], viii, [20], x, 9-186 p. front. (port.), illus., plates. 33 cm. **[1823]**
"A treatise of muscular dissection. A letter ... By Dr. Connor ...": p. i-x. —"Mathematical disquisitions concerning muscular motion; communicated in the Lypswick Transactions by John Bernoullius ...": p. 171-176. —"An appendix of the heart ... Written by ... Dr. Lower ...": p. 177-183.

—Another issue, setting of type partly differs ... London, Printed by Tho. Milbourn for the author, 1698.

[45], x, 98, 171-176, 99-109 p. front. (port.), plates. 32 cm. **[1824]**

—[Latin tr.] Myographia nova; sive, Musculorum omnium (in corpore humano hactenus repertorum) ... descriptio, in sex praelectiones distributa ... Londini, Excudebat Joannes Redmayne, 1684.

[13], 88 (i.e. 90), [8] p. front. (port.), illus., plates. 35 cm. **[1825]**
"Syllabus ... Caroli Scarburgii ... De universis corporis humani musculis ..." is inserted on a folded sheet after sheet C.

—[The same.] ... Lugduni Batavorum, Apud Jacobum Mouckee, 1687.

[10], 56, [4] p. plates. 35 cm. **[1826]**
Added engraved title page.

—[The same.] ... Amstelaedami, Apud Joannem Wolters, 1694.

[16], 90, [3] p. illus., plates. 37 cm. **[1827]**

BROWNE, JOSEPH [*fl.* 1700-1721] *ed. See* MAYERNE, *Sir* T. T. de. Opera medica. 1700.

BROWNE, RICHARD [*fl.* 1674-1694] Prosodia pharmacopaeorum; or, The apothecary's prosody. Shewing the exact quantities, in the pronunciation of the names of animals, vegetables, minerals and medicines, and of all other words made use of in pharmacy ... London, Benj. Billingsley, 1685.

[32], 237 p.   18 cm.   **[1828]**

—*See* BACON, R. The cure of old age. 1683.

BROWNE, *Sir* THOMAS [1605–1682] The works ... Containing I. Enquiries into vulgar and common errors. II. Religio medici: with Annotations and Observations upon it. III. Hydriotaphia; or, Urn-burial: together with The garden of Cyrus. IV. Certain miscellany tracts ... London, Tho. Basset, Ric. Chiswell, Tho. Sawbridge, Charles Mearn, Charles Brome, 1686.

1 v.   front. (port.), illus.   34 cm.   **[1829]**

Various pagings.
Items have special title pages. The Religio medici is dated 1685.
Keynes(B) 201.

—Certain miscellany tracts ... London, Charles Mearn, 1683.

[9], 215, [6] p.   front. (port.)   18 cm.   **[1830]**

Edited by Thomas Tenison.
Keynes(B) 127.

—Another issue, with imprint: London, Printed for Charles Mearne, and are to be sold by Henry Bonwick, 1684.   **[1831]**

Imperfect: front. wanting.
Keynes(B) 128.

—Hydriotaphia urne-buriall; or, A discourse of the sepulchrall urnes lately found in Norfolk. Together with The garden of Cyrus, or The quincunciall, lozenge, or net-work plantations of the ancients, artificially, naturally, mystically considered. With sundry observations ... London, Hen. Brome, 1658.

[13], 102 (i.e. 202), [5] p.   plates, illus.   16 cm.   **[1832]**

Errata pasted to p. [2] at end.
Imperfect: engraved plate of urns wanting; supplied in photocopy from Osler Library, McGill University.
The Garden of Cyrus has special title page (p. [87])
Keynes(B) 93.

—Nature's cabinet unlock'd. Wherein is discovered the natural causes of metals, stones, precious earths, juyces, humors, and spirits, the nature of plants in general ... Together with a description of the individual parts and species of all animate bodies ... By Tho. Brown D. of physick. London, Edw. Farnham, 1657.

[6], 331, [2] p.   15 cm.   **[1833]**

Keynes(B) 189. ("This ... work ... is not in any way worthy of Sir Thomas Browne with whose name it was falsely associated. The true author ... is not known.")

—Pseudodoxia epidemica; or, Enquiries into very many received tenents, and commonly presumed truths ... London, Printed by T. H. for Edward Dod, 1646.

[19], 386 p.   28 cm.   **[1834]**

Keynes(B) 73.

—[The same.] ... The 2d ed. corr. and much enl. ... Together with some marginall observations ... London, Printed by A. Miller, for Edw. Dod and Nath. Ekins, 1650.

[16], 329, [10] p.   28 cm.   **[1835]**

Keynes(B) 74.

—[The same.] ... The 4th ed. with marginal observations ... Whereunto are now added two discourses the one of Urn-burial, or Sepulchrall urns, lately found in Norfolk. The other of the Garden of Cyrus, or Network plantations of the antients ... London, Printed for Edward Dod. and are to be sould by Andrew Crook, 1658.

2 parts in 1 v.   plates, illus.   23 cm.   **[1836]**

Various pagings.
Hydriotaphia urne-buriall and The garden of Cyrus are bound before Pseudodoxia epidemica and have special title pages.
Hydriotaphia urne-buriall has imprint: London, Hen. Brome, 1658.
Imperfect: sig. 5 π 1–2 and sig 5D4 wanting.
Keynes(B) 76, 94.

—[The same.] ... The 5th ed. ... London, Edward Dod, 1669.

[15], 414 (i.e. 418), 16 p.; [8], 70 p.   front. (port.), plates, illus.   22 cm.   **[1837]**

Hydriotaphia, urn-burial has special title page with imprint: London, Henry Brome, 1669. The garden of Cyrus has special title page dated 1668.
Keynes(B) 78, 96.

—[The same.] ... Together with the Religio medici ... The 6th and last ed. corr. and enl. ... Together with many more marginal observations ... London, Printed by J. R. for Nath. Ekins, 1672.

[23], 440, [11] p.; [8], 144 p.   front. (port.)   23 cm.   **[1838]**

Religio medici, the 7th ed., Annotations upon Religio medici, and Observations upon Religio medici, by Sr. Kenelm Digby, the 5th ed. have special title pages, with imprints: London, Andrew Crook, 1672.
The Urn-burial and The garden of Cyrus are not present in this edition.
Keynes(B) 79, 10.

—[German tr.] Pseudodoxia epidemica, das ist: Untersuchung derer Irrthümer, so bey dem gemeinen Mann, und sonst hin und wieder im Schwange gehen ... Mit Beyfügung ... eines Werkes wider die gemeinen Irrthümer von der Bewegung natürlicher Dinge; ingleichen Herrn D. Henrici Mori von unkörperlichen Dingen in der Welt, wider Cartesium ... Alles ... aus dem Englischen und Lateinischen ... in die reine hochteutsche Sprach übersetzt, mit ungemeinen Anmerkungen erläutert ... durch Christian Peganium, in Teutsch Rautner genannt ... Franckfurt und Leipzig, In Christoff Riegels Verlag, 1680.

[8], 987, [20] p. illus., plates. 21 cm.[**1839**]
Keynes(B) 86.

—Religio medici. [London] Andrew Crooke, 1642.
[1], 190 p. 15 cm.   [**1840**]
Signatures: [ ]¹, A–M⁸.
Engraved title page.
Keynes(B) 1. (The first unauthorized edition)

—[The same.] Religio medici. [London] Andrew Crooke, 1642.
[1], 159 p. 15 cm.   [**1841**]
Signatures: [ ]¹, A–K⁸.
Engraved title page.
Keynes(B) 2. (The second unauthorized edition)

—[The same.] A true and full copy of that which was most imperfectly and surreptitiously printed before under the name of: Religio medici. [London] Andrew Crooke, 1643.
[18], 183 (i.e. 185) p. 15 cm.   [**1842**]
Engraved title page.
Keynes(B) 3

—[The same.] ... [London] Andrew Crooke, 1645.
[16], 174 p. 15 cm.   [**1843**]
Engraved title page.
Keynes(B) 5.
With this is bound Digby, Sir K. Observations upon Religio medici. 1644.

—[The same.] ... The 4th ed. corr. and amended. With Annotations never before published, upon all the obscure passages therein [by Thomas Keck] London, Printed by E. Cotes for Andrew Crook, 1656.
[17], 297, [5], p. 15 cm.   [**1844**]
Added engraved title page.
Annotations upon Religio medici has special title page.

The author of the Annotations is stated by Wilkin to have been Thomas Keck. Cf. Wilkin, v. 2, p. 297–8.
Keynes(B) 6.

—[The same.] ... Also, Observations by Sir Kenelm Digby, now newly added. London, Printed by Tho. Milbourn for Andrew Crook, 1659.
2 parts in 1 v. 15 cm.   [**1845**]
Added engraved title page dated 1660.
Annotations upon Religio medici has special title page. Part [2] has special title page: Observations upon Religio medici. Occasionally written by Sr Kenelm Digby ... The 3d ed. corr. and enl. London, Printed by A. M. for L. C. and are to be sold by Andrew Crook, 1659.
Keynes(B) 8.

—[The same.] ... The 7th ed. corr. and amended. With Annotations never before published, upon all the obscure passages therein [by Thomas Keck] Also Observations by Sir Kenelm Digby, now newly added. London, R. Scot, T. Basset, J. Wright, R. Chiswell, 1678.
[15], 371 (i.e. 381), [3] p. 16 cm.   [**1846**]
Added engraved title page.
Annotations upon Religio medici has special title page dated 1677. Observations upon Religio medici ... The 5th ed. corr. and enl. has special title page.
Keynes(B) 11.

—[The same.] ... The 8th ed. corr. and amended ... London, R. Scot, T. Basset, J. Wright, R. Chiswell, 1682.
[15], 371 (i.e. 381), [3] p. 17 cm.   [**1847**]
Added engraved title page.
Annotations upon Religio medici, and Observations upon Religio medici ... The 6th ed. ... have special title pages.
Keynes(B) 12.
Imperfect: added engraved title page wanting.

—[Latin tr.] Religio medici. Juxta exemp. Lug. Batavor., [Paris] 1644.
174 (i.e. 244), [3] p. 15 cm.   [**1848**]
Engraved title page.
"Lectori" (signatures ãiii, ãiiiv, ãv, and one leaf unsigned) bound at end.
Translated into Latin by John Merryweather.
Keynes(B) 60. (A pirated edition printed at Paris. Cf. p. 8.)

—[The same.] Religio medici cum annotationibus. Argentorati, Sumptibus Friderici Spoor, 1652.
[16], 440, [40] p. 16 cm.   [**1849**]
Engraved title page.
The Praefatio signed by the author of the annotations: L. N. M. E. M. The initials are believed to stand for Levinus Nicolas Moltkenius, Eques Misniensis.
Keynes (B) 63.

—[The same.] . . . 1665.

[16], 440, [40] p.   17 cm.   [1850]

Engraved title page.
A reprint.
Keynes(B) 64.

—[The same.] . . . Argentorati, Sumpt. Jo. Friderici Spoor & Reinh. Waechtler, 1677.

[16], 440, [40] p.   16 cm.   [1851]

Engraved title page.
A reprint.
Keynes(B) 65.

—[The same.] *See* Digby, *Sir* K. Observations upon Religio medici. 1643, 1644.

—[French tr.] La religion du medecin; c'est à dire, Description necessaire par Thomas Brown . . . touchant son opinion accordante avec le pur service divin d'Angleterre. [n. p.] 1668.

[24], 360 p.   14 cm.   [1852]

Added engraved title page.
A translation from the Dutch edition of 1665, sometimes attributed to Nicolas Le Fèvre. According to Willems (no. 1784) printed by Blaeu in Amsterdam. La Haye has also been suggested as place of imprint. Cf. Keynes, loc. cit.
Keynes(B) 71.

—*See* Pechlin, J. N. Jani Philadelphi [pseud.] Consultatio desultoria de optima Christianorum secta. 1588.

—*as subject. See* Ross, A. Arcana microcosmi. 1651, 1652 [and] Medicus medicatus. 1645.

BRUCAEUS, Heinrich [1530 or 31-1593] De scorbuto. *In* Brunner, B. De scorbuto tractatus duo. 1658.

—*See* Smet, H. Miscellanea . . . medica. 1661.

BRUCKMANN, Hendrik Crato [*fl.* 1695] *respondent.* Dissertationem inauguralem de scorbuto . . . examini subjicit Hendricus Crato Bruckmann . . . Duisburgi ad Rhenum, Typis Johannis Sas, 1695.

24 p.   20 cm.   [1853]

Diss.—Duisburg.

BRUCKNER, Ernestus Christianus. *See* Brückner, Ernst Christian [*fl.* 1693]

BRUCOEUS, Henri. *See* Brucaeus, Heinrich [1530 *or* 31-1593]

BRÜBELING, Franciscus Henricus. *See* Grübeling, Franz Heinrich [*fl.* 1699-1701]

BRÜCKNER, Ernst Christian [*fl.* 1693] *respondent.* Disputatio medica inauguralis de hemicrania . . . Lugduni Batavorum, Apud Abrahamum Elzevier, 1693.

[35] p.   22 cm.   [1854]

Diss.—Leyden.

BRÜCKNER, Johann. *See* Pontanus, Johannes [*d.* 1572]

BRÜGGEN, Johann Konrad à [*fl.* 1658] *respondent.* Cataclysmus microcosmi; id est, Disputatio medica inauguralis, hydropem asciten, infestum vitae humanae hostem in natali suo solo cum suis parentibus & fructibus palam exhibens . . . Giessae, Apud Chemlinianos, 1658.

[8], 36 p.   19 cm.   [1855]

Diss.—Giessen.

BRUELE, Gualtherus. Praxis medicinae theorica et empirica . . . In qua eruditiss. dilucidissimaque ratione morborum internorum cognito, eorundemque curatio traditur . . . Venetiis, Apud Societatem Venetam, 1602.

[8], 194, [2] ll.   17 cm.   [1856]

—[The same.] Praxis medicinae theorica et empirica familiarissima . . . In qua pulcherrima dilucidissimaque ratione morborum internorum cognitio, eorundemque curatio traditur. [Lugduni Batavorum] Ex officina Plantiniana Raphelengii, 1612.

[12], 421, [7] p.   17 cm.   [1857]

Imprint partly supplied from Carrere, v. 2, p. 144.

—[The same.] . . . Genevae, Apud Jacobum Chouët, 1628.

[16], 476 (i.e. 478), [2] p.   16 cm.   [1858]

Original place of printing "Aurelianae" blocked out.

—[The same.] . . . Lugduni Batavorum, Ex officina Joannis Maire, 1628.

[12], 421, [7] p.   16 cm.   [1859]

[The same.] . . . Accedit Petri Paschalis De febribus. Lugduni Batavorum, Ex officina Joannis Maire, 1647.

[16], 423, [9] p.; 181, [1] p.   17 cm.   [1860]

Part [2] has special title page dated 1631.

—[English tr.] Praxis medicinae; or, The physicians practice: wherein are contained inward diseases from the head to the foote: explayning the nature of each disease, with the part affected: and also the signes, causes, and prognostiques, and likewise what temperature of the ayre is most requisite for the patients abode, with direction for the diet he ought to observe, together with experimentall cures for every disease ... London, Printed by John Norton for William Sheares, 1632.

[4], 407 (i.e. 411), [4] p.   19 cm.   [**1861**]
STC 3929.

—[The same.] ... The 2d ed. newly corr. and amended. London, Printed by John Norton for Wiliam Sheares, 1639.

[4] 407 (i.e. 411), [4] p.   18 cm.   [**1862**]
Different setting of type.
STC 3930.

—[The same.] ... The 3d ed. newly corr. and amended ... London, Printed by R. Cotes for William Sheares, 1648.

[4], 407 (i.e. 411), [4] p.   19 cm.   [**1863**]
Different setting of type.

BRÜNING, BERTHOLD MAGNUS [*fl.* 1671] *respondent. See* KERN, J., *praeses.* De Witteberga dissertationem historicam ... submittit B. M. B. 1671.

BRÜSCHMANN, GREGOR [*fl.* 1677] *respondent. See* MÜLLER, J. [*fl.* 1672-1679] *praeses.* Disputatio physica de notis & figuris infantum. 1677, 1681.

BRUGGEMAYR, MARTIN MAXIMILIANUS. *See* PRUGGMAYR, Martin Maximilian [*fl.* 1687]

BRUGHIUS, ADAM. *See* BRUXIUS, Adam [*fl.* 1604-1630]

BRUGIS, THOMAS [*fl.* 1640-1651] The marrow of physicke; or, A learned discourse of the severall parts of mans body. Being a medicamentary teaching the maner and way of making ... oiles, unguents, sirrups ... pilles, &c. ... And also an addition of divers experimented medicines, which may serve against any disease that shall happen to the body. Together with some rare receipts for beauties, and the newest and best way of preserving and conserving: with divers other secrets never before published. Collected ... by ... T[homas] B[rugis] ... London, Richard Hearne, 1640.

[15], 88 p.; 175, [22] p.   illus., plate.   20 cm.
[**1864**]
STC 3931.

—[The same.] ... London, Printed by T. H. and M. H. and are to be sold by Thomas Whittaker, 1648.
[15], 88, 175, [22] p.   illus., plate.   19 cm.
[**1865**]
A reissue of the 1640 edition with new title page.

—Vade mecum; or, A companion for a chyrurgion. Fitted for times of peace or war. Briefly shewing the use of every instrument necessary, and the vertues and qualities of such medicines as are ordinarily used, with the way to make them ... Together with the manner of making reports ... The 2d ed. corr. with the addition of a treatise concerning bleeding at the nose ... London, Printed by T. H. for Tho. Williams, 1653.

[29], 237, [1] p.   front. (port.)   15 cm.
[**1866**]

—[The same.] ... The 4th ed. corr. with the addition of directions, for vomiting and purging ... London, Printed by E. C. for Tho. Williams, 1665.
[33], 263, [1] p.   front. (port.)   15 cm.
[**1867**]
Imperfect: front. and sig. A12 wanting.

—[The same.] ... The 5th ed. corr. with the addition of directions, for vomiting and purging ... London, Printed by E. C. for Tho. Williams, 1670.
[32], 263, [1] p.   front. (port.)   14 cm.
[**1868**]
A reprint.

—[The same.] ... The 7th ed. amended and augmented. With an institution of physic, and seven new treatises, viz. of tumor, wounds, ulcers, fractures, dislocations, lues-venerea, anatomy. By Ellis Prat M.D. London, Thomas Flesher, 1681.
[48], 407 p.   front. (port.)   15 cm.   [**1869**]

—[The same.] ... Being amended, and augmented with an institution of phisic, and seven new treatises, viz. of tumors, wounds, ulcers, fractures, dislocations, lues-venerea, anatomy. By Ellis Prat, M.D. The 7th ed. London, Printed for B. T. and T. S. and sold by Randal Taylor, 1689.
[47], 407 p.   front. (port.)   15 cm.   [**1870**]
Apparently reprinted from the 1681 edition.

—[The same.] ... Being amended, and augmented with an institution of physick, and seven new treatises ... Whereto is also added, (by way of supplement) another new discourse called Chirurgus methodicus; or, The young chirurgion's conductor through the labyrinth of the most difficult cures occuring in this whole art, and whereby he is distinguished from empyricks and quack salvers. By Ellis Prat, M. D. The 7th ed. London, Printed for B. T. and T. S. and sold by Fr. Hubbert, 1689.

[49], 407 p.; [8], 78 p.   front. (port.)   15 cm.
[1871]

Part [2] has special title page: Chirurgus methodicus . . . Being a supplement to Brugi's Vade mecum. By E. Pratt, M. D. London, T. Sawbridge, 1689.

BRUINSTEEN, Herman [*fl.* 1674] *respondent.* Disputatio medica inauguralis de inflammatione . . . Lugduni Batavorum, Apud viduam & heredes Johannis Elsevirii, 1674.

[36] p.   22 cm.   [1872]
Diss. — Leyden.

BRUMMET, Christoph. *See* Grummet, Christoph [*fl. ca.* 1677]

BRUNACCI, Gaudenzio [1631–1668] De cina; seu, Pulvere ad febres sytagma physiologicum . . . Venetiis, Apud Nicolaum Pezzana, 1661.

150 p.   16 cm.   [1873]

BRUNCK, Franz Anton [*fl.* 1697] *respondent.* Disputatio medica inauguralis de catarrhis in genere . . . Basileae, Typis Johannis Brandmülleri [1697]

[14] p.   19 cm.   [1874]
Diss. — Basel.

BRUNDEL, Georgius. *See* Grundel, György [*b.* 1659]

BRUNE, Jean de la. *See* La Brune, Jean de [*b. ca.* 1660]

BRUNE, Matthias de [*fl.* 1631?] *respondent. See* Burgersdijck, F. P., *praeses.* Collegium physicum. 1642.

BRUNER, Balthasar. *See* Brunner, Balthasar [1533–1604]

BRUNET, Claude [*fl.* 1686–1737] Le progrès de la medecine, contenant un recueil de tout ce qui s'observe d'utile à la pratique: avec un jugement de tous les ouvrages qui ont rapport à la théorie de cette science. Paris, Laurent d'Hourry, 1695.

[20], 242 p.; [1], 66 p.   plates.   17 cm.
[1875]

Part [2] has half title: Nouvelle lettre de M. Malpighi, sur la structure des glandes conglobées; avec un Discours sur l'utilité du microscope. [Par Verduc le fils.]

—Le progrès de la medecine, contenant un recueil de tout ce qui s'observe de singulier par raport à sa théorie & à sa pratique: avec un jugement sur toute sorte d'ouvrages de physique: et de nouvelles [sic] explications des principaux phénomênes de la nature. Pour l'année 1697 . . . Paris, Laurent d'Houry, 1698.

[4], 160, [2] p.; 37 p.   plates.   17 cm. [1876]
"Recit exact d'une grossesse extraordinaire. Observée à l'Hotel-Dieu de Paris": 37 p.
With this is bound *his* Le progrès de la medecine. Journal singulier pour l'année 1698. 1699.

—Another issue, with imprint: Paris, Barthelemy Girin, 1698.   [1877]
Imperfect: plate facing p. 45, and p. 1–37 at end wanting. Table bound after title page.

—Le progrès de la medecine. Journal singulier pour l'année 1698. Où l'on examine le sentiment de M. Mery . . . sur la circulation du sang dans le foetus par le trou ovalaire. Paris, Laurent d'Houry, 1699.

[3], 80 p.; 47, [1] p.; 91, [1] p.   plates.   17 cm.
[1878]

Contains contributions by Paul Buissière, Peter Silvestre and Philipp Verheyen.
Bound with *his* Le progrès de la medecine. 1698.

—Supplement du volume des Journaux de Médecine de l'année M. DC. LXXXVI; ou, Nouvelles conjectures sur les organes des sens où l'on propose un nouveau sistéme d'optique, avec une théorie particuliere du mouvement. Par le S. B[runet] Paris, Daniel Horthemels, 1687.

285, [19] p.   plates.   16 cm.   [1879]
Imperfect? Copy listed in BNC has 312 pages.
A reissue of the fourth part of Journal de medecine (1686) with new title page and p. 3 reset.

BRUNI, Paulo Francisco. *See* Giorgi, M. Phlebotomia liberata. 1697.

BRUNN, Johann Conrad von. *See* Brunner, Johann Conrad [1653–1727]

BRUNN, Johann Jakob von [1591–1660] *praeses.* De humoribus corporis humani conclusiones . . . Basileae, Typis Joh. Jacobi Genathii, 1619.

[16] p.   18 cm.   [1880]
Diss. — Basel (J. L. Chmieleck a Chmielnick, *respondent*)

—De morborum causis in genere . . . Basileae, Typis Joan. Jacobi Genathii [1617]

    [8] p.   21 cm.   **[1881]**

Diss.—Basel (H. Matthias, *respondent*)

—Disputatio medica de humoribus . . . Basileae, Typis Georgii Deckeri, 1648.

    [16] p.   18 cm.   **[1882]**

Diss.—Basel (M. Birr, *respondent*)

—Manuductio ad consultationem medicam recte instituendam . . . Basileae, Typis Johan. Jacobi Genathii [1634]

    [27] p.   20 cm.   **[1883]**

Diss.—Basel (S. Schöneberg, *respondent*)

—, *ed. See* MOREL, P. Formulae remediorum studio & opera Jo. Jacob à Brunn. 1647, 1657; [English tr.] 1657.

BRUNN VON HAMMERSTEIN, JOHANN CONRAD. *See* BRUNNER, Johann Conrad [1653–1727]

BRUNNER, BALTHASAR [1533–1604] Consilia medica summo studio collecta & revisa a Laurentio Hofmano . . . Hallae-Saxonum, Typis Petrus Faber, impensis Joachimi Krusicken, 1617.

    [31], 421, [11] p.   plates.   20 cm.   **[1884]**

—De scorbuto tractatus duo . . . Hagae Comitis, Ex typographia Adriani Vlacq, 1658.

    72 p.   16 cm.   **[1885]**

"De scorbuto propositiones, de quibus disputatum est publice Rostochii sub . . . Henrico Brucaeo . . .": p. [51]–72 has special title page.

Bound with (as issued?) copy 2 of Eugalenus, S. De morbo scorbuto liber. 1658.

BRUNNER, CHRISTOPH [*fl.* 1616–1618] *respondent. See* WOLF, M., *praeses.* Disputationum acroamaticarum quinta de natura et discrimine physici ac mathematici. 1618.

BRUNNER, ISAAC [*fl.* 1617] *respondent. See* MÜLLER, V., *praeses.* Aristotelis De longitudine et brevitate vitae. 1617.

BRUNNER, JOHANN CONRAD [1653–1727] Experimenta nova circa pancreas. Accedit Diatribe de lympha & genuino pancreatis usu . . . Amstelaedami, Apud Henr. Wetstenium, 1683.

    [16], 168, [8] p.   front., plates.   17 cm.

                              [1886]

Imperfect: front. wanting.

"Joh. Conradi Peyeri Schediasma, de pancreate et ejus usu, ad Joh. Conradum Brunnerum . . .": p. [149]–158. —"Joh. Conr. Brunneri Responsum ad Schediasma de pancreate et ejus usu, ad Joh. Conradum Peyerum . . .": p. [159]–168.

With this is bound Pechlin, J. N. Jani Leoniceni Veronensis [pseud.] Metamorphosis. 1672.

—*praeses.* Exercitatio anatomica de glandula pituitaria . . . Heidelbergae, Typis Joh. David. Bergmanni [1688]

    26 (i.e. 32) p.   18 cm.   **[1887]**

Diss.—Heidelberg (F. S. Vorster, *respondent*)

—[Exercitatio anatomico-medica de glandulis in intestino duodeno hominis detectis, quam respondente Georgio Friderico Franco . . . proponit in Brabeuterio Universitatis . . . M DC XXC VII. Primum habita Heidelbergae, nunc recusa Schwobaci, C. E. Buchta, 1688.

    24 p.   plate.   20 cm.   **[1888]**

Diss.—Heidelberg, 1687 (G. F. Franck von Franckenau, *respondent*)

—Festo seculari Heidelbergensis Academiae tertio . . . panaceas . . . examini apponet Gottfried Hennicke . . . Heidelbergae, Excudebat Joh. David. Bergmann. Walterian haeres [1686]

    20 p.   20 cm.   **[1889]**

Diss.—Heidelberg (G. Hennicke, *respondent*)

—*respondent.* Foetum monstrosum et bicipitem dissertatione hac inaugurali . . . sistit Joh. Conradus Brunnerus . . . Argentorati, Typis Johannis Welperi, 1672.

    [6], 42 p.   plate.   20 cm.   **[1890]**

Diss.—Strasbourg.

BRUNNMANN, ANDREAS [*fl.* 1623] *respondent. See* LOTH, G., *praeses.* De urinis disputatio II. de urinarum judicio. 1623.

BRUNNZELL, JOHANN CHRISTOPH [*fl.* 1688] *respondent.* Disputatio medica inauguralis, de lienteria . . . Trajecti ad Rhenum, Ex officina Francisci Halma, 1688.

    14, [2] p.   22 cm.   **[1891]**

Diss.—Utrecht.

BRUNO, FRIEDRICH JAKOB [*fl.* 1683–1690] *respondent.* Dissertationem solennem de catarrho suffocativo . . . p. p. Fridericus Jacobus Bruno . . . [Altdorffii] Typis Henrici Meyeri [1690]

[1], 22 p.   20 cm.   [**1892**]
Diss. — Altdorf.

— *See* HOFFMANN, J. M., *praeses*. De glandulis renalibus exercitationem anatomico-medicam ... subjicit ... F. J. B. 1683

BRUNO, GEORGE [*fl.* 1616] *respondent. See* VORSTIUS, A. E., *praeses.* Disputatio medica de crisibus et diebus decretoriis. 1616.

BRUNO, JAKOB PANCRAZ [1629-1709] Dogmata medicinae generalia, in ordinem noviter redacta, a rebus extraneis depurata, & ad vera, recentiorum praesertim, principia accomodata. Norimbergae, Sumtibus Michaelis & Johan. Friderici Endterorum, 1670.

[34], 802, [29] p.   port.   17 cm.   [**1893**]
Added engraved title page.

Dissertations — Altdorf

—*praeses.* Aeolus microcosmo commodans & incommodans; sive, Disquisitio physico-pathologica de flatibus ... Altdorfii, Literis Henrici Meyeri [1687]
[1], 16, [2] p.   20 cm.   [**1894**]
J. L. Apin, *respondent.*

— Αἱματοζυμωσιολογία; hoc est, De fermentatione sanguinis diatribe medica ... [Altdorffii] Literis Georgii Hagen, 1663.
[32] p.   19 cm.   [**1895**]
J. K. Wider, *respondent.*

— Cholegraphia; h. e. Dissertatio physico-pathologica de bile ... Altdorfii, Literis Henrici Meyeri [1694]
36 p.   20 cm.   [**1896**]
J. M. Funk, *respondent.*

— Disputatio physiologica de transpiratione insensibili ... Altdorffii, Typis Henrici Meyeri [1680]
28 p.   21 cm.   [**1897**]
L. Miller, *respondent.*

— Disputationem medicam de medicamentis ex homine qua vivo qua mortuo desumtis ductu Schroederiano tractatis ... submittit ... Johannes Paulus Wurffbain ... Altdorffii, Typis Henrici Meyeri [1677]
[2], 38 p.   19 cm.   [**1898**]
J. P. Wurfbain, *respondent.*

— Disquisitionem medicam de medicamentorum facultatibus ... examini subjicit Georgius Reitmeyer

... Altdorffii, Typis viduae Joh. Leonhardi Winterbergeri [1670]
24 p.   19 cm.   [**1899**]
G. Reitmeyer, *respondent.*

— Dissertatio medica de epilepsia puerili ... Altdorffii, Typis Henrici Meyeri [1699]
[2], 30 p.   21 cm.   [**1900**]
P. H. Brandt, *respondent.*

— Λιγνυογραφια; h. e. De fuliginibus humanis dissertatio physio-pathologica ... [Altdorffii] Literis Henrici Meyeri [1688]
16 p.   20 cm.   [**1901**]
E. Kupitz, *respondent.*

— Remorae ac impedimenta purgationis exercitationibus aliquot ex scriptis Hippocratis detecta, perque vera artis medicae principia confirmata, quarum primam de natura purgantium nocua ... publice ventilandam offert ... Joh. Christophorus Maier ... [Altdorffii] Ex officina Henrici Meyeri [1672]
[4], 24 p.   20 cm.   [**1902**]
J. C. Maier, *respondent.*

— *respondent. See* HOFFMANN, M., *praeses.* Disputatio medica de tumoribus. 1649.

—, *ed. See* CASTELLI, B. Castellus renovatus; hoc est, Lexicon medicum. 1682, 1688, 1700; JESSEN, J. von. De sanguine. 1668.

BRUNO, NICOLAS. *See* BRAUN, Nicolas [*d.* 1639]

BRUNSCHWIG, HIERONYMUS [*ca.* 1450–*ca.* 1512] Kleines Destillierbuch. *In* Dioscorides, Pedanius, of Anazarbos. Kräuterbuch. 1610.

BRUNSWICK (DUCHY). Kurtzer, doch gründlicher Rath-und Unterricht, wie man sich ... bey diesen ... Zeiten, in welchen nicht allein die gifftig anstekkende Krankheiten und ... Flekk-Fieber ... sondern auch die pestilentzische Fieber und Peste ... sich ... verspüren lassen ... bewahren Könne ... Neben einem Anhang von der rothen Ruhr, diesem Fürstenthum Braunschweig und Lüneburg, in specie der Stadt Braunschweig ... zu ... Zuflucht und Gebrauch ... publiciret. Braunschweig, Durch Christoff-Freidrich Zilligern, 1680.
87 p.   21 cm.   [**1903**]

— Kurtzer Unterricht, wie man sich für der giftigen anklebenden Seuche der Pestilentz ...

bewahren ... solle: auf Verordnung und Befehl der hohen Landes-Fürstlichen Obrigkeit, aufgesetzet. Wolffenbüttel, Gedruckt bey Paul Weissen, 1680.

[20] p.   18 cm.   [1904]

—Nohtwendiger Unterricht, wie der gifftigen anklebenden Seuche der Pestilentz ... vorzubauen und dieselbe zu curiren sey, auff Anordnung und Befehl der hohen Landes-Fürstl. Obrigkeit. Vor diesem Anno 1657 auffgesetzt, und jetzo revidiret, und in vielem geendert worden. Zell, Gedruckt bey Andreas Holwein, 1680.

[32] p.   20 cm.   [1905]

—, **Laws, Statutes, etc.** Georg Wilhelms, Hertzogen zu Braunschweig und Lüneburg, etc. ... Verordnunge: wornach man sich bey ereugender Pest, und andern dergleichen anklebenden Seuchen, zu achten. Zelle, Andreas Holwein, 1680.

[16] p.   21 cm.   [1906]

BRUNSWICK-LÜNEBURG, GEORG WILHELM, *Duke of. See* GEORG WILHELM, *Herzog von Braunschweig-Lüneburg* [1624-1705]

BRUSASCHI, JOANNES JACOBUS. *See* BRUSASCO, Giovanni Giacomo [*fl.* 1693]

BRUSASCO, GIOVANNI GIACOMO [*fl.* 1693] Delius bilinguis; sive, Disceptationes problematicae medicinales ... Romae, Typis Dominici Ant. Herculis, 1693.

[1], xvi, 262, [1] p.   front.   17 cm.   [1907]

BRUSCHIUS, FRANCISCUS. *See* BRUSCO, Francesco, *count* [*fl.* 1623]

BRUSCO, FRANCESCO, *count* [*fl.* 1623] Promachomachia jatrochymica. In qua chymiatriae praestantia adversus mysochymicum pugnando propugnatur ... A comite Francisco Bruschio ... in suae existimationis defensionem ędita ... Mantuae, Apud Aurelium, & Ludovicum Osannam fratres, 1623.

II, 341 p.   29 cm.   [1908]

BRUSSELS. Collegium Medicum. *See* COLLEGIE DER MEDECYNE, Brussels.

BRUXIUS, ADAM [*fl.* 1604-1630] Pilulae sine quibus esse non vult Adamus Bruxius D.   Bericht, von einer newen und sonderlichen Art Pillen vor hartleibige, und dann auch andere Manns-und

Weibs Personen, die sich schwerer Kranckheiten befahren ... Leipzig, In Verlegung Zachar. Schur. S. Erben und Matt. Götzen, Gedruckt by Gregorio Ritzschen, 1631.

66 p.   13 cm.   [1909]

—*respondent.* De melancholia hypochondriaca positiones una cum adnexis corollariis ... Basileae, Typis Conradi Waldkirchii, 1604.

[28] p.   21 cm.   [1910]
Diss. — Basel.

BRUYER, JOANNES. *See* BRUYERIN, Jean Baptiste [*fl.* 1530-1560]

BRUYERIN, JEAN BAPTISTE [*fl.* 1530-1560] Dipnosophia seu sitologia. Esculenta et poculenta, quae cuivis nationi, homini, sexui, sanis, aegris, senibus, juvenibus, idonea vel minus, usu probata complectens omnia ... Revisa, emaculata, duplicique indice locupletata, ab Othone Gasmanno E. S. Francofurti, Ex Officina Paltheniana, 1606.

[16], 863, [21] p.   17 cm.   [1911]
Dedicatory epistle by Peter Uffenbach.
The main text is a reissue of the edition published by the same press in 1600 under title: De re cibaria.

—[The same.] Cibus medicus; sive, De re cibaria libri XXII omnium ciborum genera, omnium gentium moribus, et usu probata, complectentes. Norimbergae, Apud Johann. Andream et Wolffgangi Endteri Jun. haeredes, 1659.

[16], 863 p.   17 cm.   [1912]
A reissue, with reprinted preliminaries.

BRUYERY, elk zijn gelt weer, of samen-spraek tusschen den Ouden Hillebrant en Steene Roelandt. Haerlem, Jan Winter [1677]

31 p.   16 cm.   [1913]

BRUYN, JOHANNES DE [1620-1675] Epistola ad ... Isaacum Vossium, ubi judicium fertur super ipsius libro De natura et proprietate lucis, & simul Cartesii doctrina defenditur ... Amstelodami, Apud Ludovicum & Danielem Elzevirios, 1663.

68 p.   illus.   20 cm.   [1914]

—*praes.* Disputatio physica de alitura foetus in utero ... Ultrajecti, Ex officina Meinardi a Dreunen, 1670.

[10] p.   25 cm.   [1915]
Diss. — Utrecht (J. Munniks, *respondent*)

—*praes.* Disputationis physicae de alitura pars sexta ... Trajecti ad Rhenum, Typis Gisberti a Zijll & Theodori ab Ackersdijck, 1660.

[8] p.   21 cm.   [1916]

Diss.—Utrecht (C. Melder, *respondent*)

—*praes.* Disputatio physica, qua rationes pro formis substantialibus adferri solitae expenduntur ... Trajecti ad Rhenum, Typis Gisberti a Zijll, & Theodori ab Ackersdijck, 1557 [i.e. 1657]

[12] p.   19 cm.   [1917]

Diss.—Utrecht (H. Quellenburgh, *respondent*)

BRY, JOHANN THEODOR DE [1561-1623?] *ed. See* BAUHIN, K. Theatrum anatomicum. 1621 [and] Vivae imagines. 1620.

—,*engr. See* BOISSARD, J. J. Bibliotheca chalcographica. 1650-54.

—*See* BOURSIER, L. (Bourgeois). Hebammen Buch. 1628-48, 1644-52.

BRY, THEODOR DE [1528-1598] *ed. See* BAUHIN, K. Theatrum anatomicum. 1605.

BSCHERER, DANIEL [1656-1718] *respondent. See* FRANCK VON FRANCKENAU, G., *praeses.* Ἀτπμογραφα microcosmica. 1681.

BUBBEN, FRANZ [*fl.* 1652] *respondent.* De nephritide ... Basileae, Typis Georgii Deckeri [1652]

[15] p.   20 cm.   [1918]

Diss.—Basel.

BUCH, JOHANN WOLFFGANG [*fl.* 1651] *respondent. See* HOPP, J., *praeses.* Catarrhus suffocativus disputationis thesibus resolutus. 1651.

BUCHANAN, GEORGE [1506-1582] *See* BARCLAY, W. Judicium. 1620.

BUCHER, URBAN GOTTFRIED [*fl.* 1700-*ca.* 1722] *respondent. See* BRENDEL, A., *praeses.* Dissertationem medicam de catalepsi ... exponet ... 1700.

BUCHWALD, JOHANNES DE [1658-1738] *respondent. See* BARTHOLIN, C. [1655-1738], *praeses.* Dissertatio medica inauguralis de pleuritide atque peripneumonia. 1700.

BUCHWALT, JOHANNES DE. *See* BUCHWALD, Johannes de [1658-1738]

BUCKISIUS, CHRISTIANUS [*fl.* 1649-1651] *respondent. See* SEBISCH, M. [1578-1674?] *praeses.* Galeni quinque priores libri. 1651.

BUCRETIUS, DANIEL [*d.* 1631] *respondent. See* HOFMANN, C., *praeses.* Theses de hepate. 1621.

—, *ed. See* SPIEGEL, A. van de. De humani corporis fabrica libri decem. 1627, 1632 [and] Opera quae extant, omnia. 1645.

—*See* CASSERIO, G. Julii Casserii Placentini Tabulae anatomicae LXXIIX. 1627, 1632; [German tr.] *ed.* 1656; 1683.

BUDAEUS, GOTTLIEB [1664-1734] *respondent. See* VATER, C., *praeses.* Naturam et curam memoriae ... exhibet ... G. B. 1686; WEDEL, G. W., *praeses.* Disputatio medica inauguralis de palpitatione cordis. 1690.

BUDAEUS, THEOPHILUS. *See* BUDAEUS, Gottlieb [1664-1734]

BÜCHELMANN, JOHANN SEBASTIAN [*b.* 1675] *respondent. See* SLEVOGT, J. A., *praeses.* Rhonchum infantis. 1699; WEDEL, G. W. Propempticum inaugurale de ramo aureo Virgilii. 1699.

BÜCHING, GOTTFRIED [*fl.* 1695-1703] *respondent. See* SCHMID, J. A., *praeses.* Geomantia, olim pulveri inscripta. 1695.

BÜCKING, JOHANN JUSTUS [*fl.* 1675] *respondent. See* FASCH, A. H., *praeses.* Consultatio medica practica proponens aegrotum arthritico-nephriticum. 1675; WEDEL, G. W., *praeses.* Aegrum pollutione nocturna laborantem ... examini exponet ... J. J. B. 1675.

BÜHREN, DAVID FRIEDRICH [*fl.* 1691-1698] Disputatio inauguralis medica sistens aegram suffocatione uterina laborantem ... Erfurti, Charactere Kindlebiano [1698]

36 p.   19 cm.   [1919]

Diss.—Erfurt.

BUELIUS, LUDOVICUS GOTHOFREDUS [*fl.* 1680-1682] *respondent. See* WALDSCHMIDT, J. J., *praeses.* Disputatio medica, de mania vulgo die Tobsucht oder Wahnwitzigkeit. 1680 [and] Exercitationem medicam de acidulis ... exponit ... L. G. B. 1682.

BUENA-MAISON, ALONSO DE. *See* BONNE-MAISON, Alonso de [*fl.* 1678]

BÜNGER, Johann [*fl.* 1672] *respondent. See* Kirch-major, T., *praeses.* Διασκεψις physica. 1672.

BUENIUS, Gideon [*fl.* 1658] *tr. See* Bils, L. de. Responsio. 1661 [and] Specimina anatomica. 1661.

BÜRGER, Rudolf Gottfried [*fl.* 1664] *respondent. See* Pihringer, K., *praeses.* Disputatio physica de monstro. 1664.

BÜRLEIN, Jakob [*fl.* 1661-1664] *respondent.* De foeminis ex suppressione mensium barbatis disputatio medica inauguralis ... [Altdorfii] Typis viduae Johannis Göbelii [1664]

    21, [3] p. 19 cm.   **[1920]**
  Diss. — Altdorf.

   — *See* Nicolai, C., *praeses.* Disputatio medica, de pernicioso Paracelsistarum hoplochrismate. 1662.

BÜRLINUS, Jacobus. *See* Bürlein, Jakob [*fl.* 1661-1664]

BÜSCH, Georg Engelbert [*fl.* 1698] *respondent. See* Schmid, J. A., *praeses.* Mulier orthodoxa. 1698.

BUGGS, John [*fl.* 1633] *respondent.* Disputatio medica inauguralis de pleuritide vera & exquisita ... Lugduni Batavorum, Ex officina Wilhelmi Christiani, 1633.

    [15] p. 18 cm.   **[1921]**
  Diss. — Leyden.

BUGIUS, Jacobus [*fl.* 1663] *respondent. See* Frenzel, S. F., *praeses.* Disputatio publica prima, de anima. 1663.

BUISSIÈRE, Paul [*d.* 1739] *See* [Brunet, C.] Le progrès de la medecine. 1699.

BUISSON, Jacob du, *tr. See* Diemerbroeck, I. van. Traktaat vande peste. 1672.

BUKKY, Christian [1676-1705] *respondent.* Disputatio medica inauguralis, de medicina stercoraria ... Trajecti ad Rhenum, Ex officina Guilielmi vande Water, 1700.

    16 p. 23 cm.   **[1922]**
  Diss. — Utrecht.

   —*See* Rivinus, A. Q., *praeses.* Medicum inculpatum ... sistit ... C. B. 1699.

BULETUS, Gulielmus [*fl.* 1610] *respondent. See* Stupanus, J. N., *praeses.* Σημειωτices particularis cap. I. De affectibus. 1610.

   —*See* Stupanus, J. N. Gratiosi medicorum Basiliens. Collegii decreto. 1610.

BULGETI, Attilio. *See* Bolzetta, Attilio [1589-1635]

BULGEZIO, Attilio. *See* Bozetta, Attilio [1589-1635]

BULLART, Jacques Ignace, *ed. See* Bullart, I. Academie des sciences et des arts. 1682.

BULICHIUS, Albertus [*fl. ca.* 1609] *respondent.* Disputatio de ascitis natura et curatione ... Basileae, Typis Johannis Schroteri, 1609.

    [12] p. 20 cm.   **[1923]**
  Diss. — Basel.

BULLART, Isaac [1599-1672] Academie des sciences et des arts, contenant les vies, & les eloges historiques des hommes illustres, qui ont excellé en ces professions depuis environ quatre siécles parmy diverses nations de l'Europe: avec ... plusieurs inscriptions funebres, exactement recueillies de leurs tombeaux ... Paris, Loüis Bilaine, 1682.

    2 v. ports. 34 cm.   **[1924]**
  Imperfect: first preliminary leaves (blank?) of both volumes wanting.
  The Epistre dedicatoire is signed by Jacques Ignace Bullart, the editor.

BULLMANN, Benedict [*fl.* 1697] *respondent. See* Pauli, J. W., *praeses.* Disputatio inauguralis medica de dolore capitis. 1697.

BULLOKAR, John [*fl.* 1622] An English expositour; or, Compleat dictionary; teaching the interpretation of the hardest words, and most useful terms of art used in our language. First set forth by J[ohn] B[ullokar] D^r of physik ... and now the 5th time rev., corr., and very much augm. with several additions ... by a lover of the arts. Cambridge Hayes, 1676.

    [284] p. 16 cm.   **[1925]**

BULTYNCK, Abraham [*fl.* 1669] *respondent.* Disputatio medica inauguralis de epilepsia ... Lugduni Batavorum, Apud viduam & haeredes Joannis Elsevirii, 1669.

    [34] p. 23 cm.   **[1926]**
  Diss. — Leyden.

BULWER, John [*fl.* 1644-1662] Anthropometamorphosis: man transform'd; or, The artificial changeling. Historically presented, in the mad and cruel gallantry, foolish bravery, ridiculous beauty, filthy finenesse, and loathsome lovelinesse of most nations, fashioning & altering their bodies from the mould intended by nature. With a vindication of the regular beauty and honesty of nature. And An appendix of the pedigree of the English gallant. By J[ohn] B[ulwer] ... London, J. Hardesty, 1650.

[26], 263, [43] p.   front. (port.), plate.   15 cm.
[1927]

— [The same.] ... London, William Hunt, 1653.
[52], 528, [28] p.   front., port., illus., plates.   19 cm.   **[1928]**
Imperfect: front. and port. wanting.

— Chirologia; or, The naturall language of the hand. Composed of the speaking motions, and discoursing gestures thereof. Whereunto is added Chironomia; or, The art of manuall rhetoricke. Consisting of the naturall expressions, digested by art in the hand, as the chiefest instrument of eloquence, by historicall manifesto's, exemplified out of the authentique registers of common life, and civill conversation ... By J[ohn] B[ulwer] ... London, Printed by Tho. Harper and are to be sold by R. Whitaker, 1644.

2 parts in 1 v.   front., plates.   17 cm. **[1929]**
Part [2] has special title page and front.

— [The same.] ... London, Printed by T. H. and are to be sold by Fran. Tyton, 1648.
2 parts in 1 v.   front., plates.   18 cm. **[1930]**
Part [2] has special title page and front.
A reissue of the 1644 edition with new title page.

— Pathomyotomia; or, A dissection of the significative muscles of the affections of the minde. Being an essay to a new method of observing the most important movings of the muscles of the head, as they are the neerest and immediate organs of the voluntarie or impetuous motions of the mind. With the proposall of a new nomenclature of the muscles. By J[ohn] B[ulwer] ... London, Printed by W. W. for Humphrey Moseley, 1649.

[36], 240 p.   15 cm.   **[1931]**
Bound with *his* Philocophus. 1648.

— Philocophus; or, The deafe and dumbe mans friend. Exhibiting the philosophicall verity of that subtile art, which may inable one with an observant eie, to heare what any man speaks by the moving

of his lips ... By J[ohn] B[ulwer] ... London, Humphrey Mosely, 1648.

[38], 191 p.   15 cm.   **[1932]**
Added engraved title page.
With this is bound *his* Pathomyotomia. 1649.

BUMALDI, Giovanni Antonio, *pseud. See* Montalbani, Ovidio [1601-1671]

BUNCK, Christian. *See* Buncken, Christian [*d.* 1659]

BUNCKEN, Christian [*d.* 1659] Speculum optimi et perfecti medici, ex conditionibus in studioso artis medicae, in tyrone medico ad praxin jam accessuro, in medico ad aegrum praesentem jam adhibitio, requisitis inaugurali oratione exhibitum ... Gissae, Typis Josephi Dieterici Hampelii, 1651.

60 p.   20 cm.   **[1933]**

— *respondent. See* Schelhammer, C., *praes.* Disputationem medicam de febre ardente ... publice exponit ... C.B. 1646.

BUONACCIOLI, Lodovico. *See* Bonacciuoli, Luigi [*d. ca.* 1540]

BUONACCORSI, Bartolommeo. *See* Bonaccorsi, Bartolommeo [*fl.* 1618-*ca.* 1650]

BUONAMICI, Francisco [*d.* 1604] De alimento libri V. ubi multę medicorum sententię delibantur, & cum Aristotele conferuntur. Complura etiam problemata in eodem argumento notantur, & quibusdam ex Greca lectione pristinus nitor restituitur ... Florentiae, Apud Bartholomęum Sermartellium Juniorem, 1603 [colophon 1602]

[23], 759, [26] p.   plates.   22 cm.   **[1934]**

BUONANNI, Filippo [1638-1725] Observationes circa viventia, quae in rebus non viventibus reperiuntur. Cum Micrographia curiosa; sive, Rerum minutissimarum observationibus, quae ope microscopii recognitae ad vivum exprimuntur. His accesserunt aliquot animalium testaceorum icones non antea in lucem editae ... Romae, Typis Dominici Antonii Herculis, 1691 [i.e. 1692]

[1], xx, 342, [1] p.; 106, [1] p.   front., illus., plates.   23 cm.   **[1935]**
Frontispiece dated 1692.
"Pars secunda; seu, Supplementum recreationis mentis et oculi in observatione testaceorum quorum aliqua exprimuntur non antea in lucem edita": p. [308]-335 has engraved half title; "Micrographia curiosa ...": p. 1-103 at end has caption title.

—Ricreatione dell'occhio e della mente nell'osservation' delle chiocciole . . . Roma, Varese, 1681.

[17], 384, [16] p. front., illus., plates. 24 cm.

[1936]

—[Latin tr.] Recreatio mentis, et oculi in observatione animalium testaceorum . . . Italico sermone primum proposita . . . nunc . . . Latine oblata centum additis testaceorum iconibus . . . Romae, Ex typographia Varesii, 1684.

[16], 270, [8] p. illus., plates. 24 cm.

[1937]

—See MARSIGLI, A. F. Relazione del ritrovamento dell"nova di chiocciole. 1695.

BUONAVENTURA, FEDERICO. See BONAVENTURA, Federico [1555-1602]

BURBAUM, ANDREAS. See BUXBAUM, Andreas [d. 1730]

BURCARDUS, JOHANNES RUDOLPHUS. See BURCKHARDT, Johann Rudolph [1637-1687]

BURCHARD, CHRISTOPH MARTIN [1680-1742] respondent. See SCHELHAMMER, G. C. Exercitationum medicarum quinta continens theses selectas de principio motus animali. 1700.

BURCHARD, JOHANN HEINRICH. See BURCKHARD, Johann Heinrich [1676-1738]

BURCHARD, VALENTIN JOHANN [fl. 1700] respondent. See VESTI, J., praeses. Disputatio inauguralis medica de motu sanguinis. 1700.

BURCHARDI, MICHAEL BALTHASAR [fl. 1670] respondent. See FRIDERICI, J. A., praeses. Dissertatio inauguralis medica de mola. 1670.

BURCKARD, CHRISTOPH [fl. 1700] respondent. See WETTSTEIN, J. R., praeses. Disputatio theologica de circumcisione. 1700.

BURCKHARD, JOHANN HEINRICH [1676-1738] respondent. Disputatio inauguralis medica de respiratione integra et laesa . . . [Altdorffii] 1697.

[20] p. 20 cm. [1938]

Diss.—Altdorf.

—See STURM, J. C., praeses. Dissertatio physica de elephante. 1696.

BURCKHARD, JOHANN KONRAD [fl. 1603] respondent. See ROOMEN, A. van, praeses. Disputatio anatomica de partibus corporis nutritioni dicatis. 1603.

BURCKHARDI, CHRISTOPH MARTIN. See BURCHARD, Christoph Martin [1680-1742]

BURCKHARDT, JOHANN RUDOLPH [1637-1687] praeses. Exercitatio medica de dysenteria . . . Basileae, Typis Georgi Deckeri, 1660.

[15] p. 19 cm. [1939]

Diss.—Basel (F. von Juvalta, respondent)

BURDEGATUS, MATTHAEUS. See BORDEGATO, Matteo [d. 1689]

BURDO, JOSEPHUS JUSTUS, pseud. See SCALIGER, Joseph Juste [1540-1609]

BUREAU D'ADRESSE, Paris. Conférences. See CONFERENCES DU BUREAU D'ADRESSE, Paris.

BURG, JOHANN [fl. 1674] respondent. See WEDEL, G. W., praeses. Visum . . . physiologice examinandum . . . disquisitioni sistet . . . J. B. 1674.

BURGAUER, JOHANN [1600-1635] respondent. Disputatio medica de ruminatione humana . . . Basileae, Typis Johan. Jacobi Genathii [1626]

[28] p. 19 cm. [1940]

Diss.—Basel.

BURGAUER, JOHANN [fl. 1685-1686] respondent. Disputatio medica inauguralis de pleuritide ejusque causis . . . Basileae, Typis Jacobi Bertschii [1686]

[16] p. 20 cm. [1941]

Diss.—Basel.

—See HARDER, J. J., praeses. Dissertatio anatomico-practica. 1685.

BURGER, JAKOB [fl. 1694] respondent. Disputatio medica inauguralis de sanguine . . . Lugduni Batavorum, Apud Abrahamum Elzevier, 1694.

[22] p. 21 cm. [1942]

Diss.—Leyden.

BURGERSDICIUS, FRANCO. See BURGERSDIJCK, Franco Petri [1590-1635]

BURGERSDIJCK, FRANCO PETRI [1590-1635] praeses. Collegium physicum, disputationibus XXXII. absolutum; totam naturalem philosophiam compendiose proponens . . . Ed. 2., autoris manu aucta. Lugd. Batavorum, Ex officina Elziviriorum, 1642.

[4], 353, [3] p.   14 cm.   **[1943]**

Includes 34 Leyden dissertations by 19 authors. This collection was first published in 1632; the present edition has a publishers' preface dated 1637. Respondents: D. Schelkens, no. 1, 14; F. Abbama, no. 2, 18, 31; J. Eduard, no. 3, 19; A. Wiltens, no. 4, 20, 28; G. Neodorpius, no. 5, 17; M. de Brune, no. 6, 11; D. à Sonnevelt, no. 7, 15, 23; D. de Haro, no. 8; S. Carlier, no. 9, 13; N. Forestus, no. 10; C. Schalken, no. 12, 29; L. Thorer, no. 16, 21; T. Velthuis, no. 22; A. Roylandus, no. 24, 30; A. Paludano, no. 25; L. P. Rolandus, no. 26, 27; W. Praetorius, no. 32; A. Hereboort, no. 33; J. Weuelichoven, no. 34.

BURGGRAFIUS, JOANNES PHILIPPUS. *See* BURGGRAVE, Johann Philipp [1673-1746]

BURGGRAV, JOHANN ERNST [*fl.* 1600-1629] Achilles πανοπλος redivivus; seu, Panoplia physicovulcania [qua] in praelio φιλοπλος in hostem educitur sacer et inviolabilis. Cui praemissa est Marcelli Vranckheim ... Ἐπικρισις σοχαστικη ad Achilem πανυπεροπλομαχον. Amsterodami, Apud Hendricum Laurentium [1612]

130, [3] p.   19 cm.   **[1944]**

Engraved title page.

—Biolychnium; seu, Lucerna, cum vita ejus, cui accensa est Mystice, vivens jugiter; cum morte ejusdem expirans; omnesque affectus graviores prodens. Huic accessit Cura morborum magnetica ex Theophr. Parac. Mumia: itemque omnium venenorum Alexipharmacum. Auctiora & emendatiora omnia ... Franekerae, Ex officina Ulderici Dominici Balck, 1611.

176 (i.e 184) p.   16 cm.   **[1945]**

"Cura morborum magnetica, qua vera Theophrasti Mumia significatur": p. 129-149.

—De oleis variis arte chymica destillatis. *In* Hartmann, J. Praxis chimiatrica. 1634,1639,1682.

—Introductio in vitalem philosophiam. Cui cohaeret omnium morborum astralium & materialium; seu morborum omnium, elementatorum & haereditariorum ex libro naturae, codice philosophicae & medicae veritatis, additis veterum placitis, Hippocratis, Galeni, Celsi, aliorum, explicatio atque curatio. In speciali explicatione morborum agitur de curationum mysteriis, indicationum compendiis, remediorum arcanis. Et primum Galeni & aliorum veterum medicamenta proferentur deinde Paracelsi, Turnheuseri, Quercetani aliorumque

neotericorum philosophorum experientia demonstratur, medicamenta omnium morborum ex anatomia & arte signata, tam simplicia, quam composita ostendendo. Francofurti, Typis Hartm. Palthenii, sumtibus Joh. Th. de Bry, & Joh. Ammonii, 1623.

[8], 166 p.   21 cm.   **[1946]**

"Tractatus alter, de causis et curatione morborum omnium ...": p. [45]-166, has special title page with imprint: Francofurti, Aere Joh. Theodori de Bry & Joannis Ammonii, 1623.

—[The same.] ... Ed. postrema. Hanoviae, Sumptibus Johann. Ammonii, 1643.

[8], 166 p.   19 cm.   **[1947]**

A reissue of the 1623 edition with new title page.
With this is bound Rhenanus, J. Solis e puteo emergentis. 1613.

—Lampadem vitae & mortis omniumque graviorum in microcosmo παθῶν indicem; hoc est, Biolychnium sive lucernam; cum vita ejus, cui accensa est mystice, viventem jugiter; cum morte ejusdem expirantem; omnesque affectus graviores prodentem. Antehac ... studio J[ohannis] E[rnesti] B[urgravii] ... traditam: nunc, dilucidiori stylo, se expositurum intimat G. F. MDCS. Lugd. Batav., Apud Arnoudum Doude, 1678.

72 p.   plates.   13 cm.   **[1948]**

Added engraved title page dated: 1679.
Published in 1611 as part of Biolychniun; seu, Lucerna.

—Tractat von der ungarischene Hauptschwachheit, auch andern epidemischen gifftigen Fiebern ... sampt deren praeservatifs und curatifs Mitteln. Widerumb publicirt ... Franckfurt am Mayn, Getruckt bey Caspar Röteln, in Verlegung Wilhelm Fitzers, 1627.

110 p.   20 cm.   **[1949]**

—[The same.] ... Widerumb publicirt ... Franckfurt am Mayn, Getruckt bey Caspar Röteln, in Verlegung Johann Beyers, 1640.

110 p.   20 cm.   **[1950]**

A reissue of the 1627 edition with new title page.

—ed. *See* CLODIUS, B. Officina chymica. 1620.

BURGGRAVE, JOHANN PHILIPP [1673-1746] *respondent.* Dissertatio inauguralis physico-medica de malo sinensi aureo ... Lugduni Batavorum, Apud Abrahamum Elzevier, 1694.

[24] p.   22 cm.   **[1951]**

Diss. — Leyden.

BURGIS, Thomas. *See* Brugis, Thomas [*fl.* 1640-1651]

BURGH, Anton van der [*fl.* 1684] *respondent.* Disputatio medica inauguralis de pica ... Lugduni Batavorum, Apud Abrahamum Elzevier, 1684.

    [II] p. 22 cm. **[1952]**
Diss.—Leyden.

BURGO, Giovanni Battista de [17th cent.] Hydraulica; osia, Trattato dell'aque minerali del Massino, S. Mauritio, Favera, Scultz, e Bormio, con la guerra della Valtellina del 1618. sin' al 1638., & altre curiosita ... Milano, Agnelli, 1689.

    [12], 428 p. 15 cm. **[1953]**
Imperfect: p. 1-2 mutilated.

BURGOS, Alonso de [*fl.* 1640] Methodo curativo, y uso de la nieve. En que se declara, y prueva la obligacion que tienen los medicos de dar a los purgados agua de nieve, con las condiciones y requisitos que se dirà ... Cordova, Andres Carrillo. 1640.

    [8], 176 ll. 21 cm. **[1954]**
Imperfect: ll. 173-176 wanting; supplied in manuscript.

BURGOWERUS, Johannes. *See* Burgauer, Johann [*fl.* 1685-1686]

BURGUNDUS, Johannes [*fl.* 1627] *ed.* and *tr. See* Wirsung, Medicyn-boeck. 1627.

BURING, Johann [*fl.* 1684] *respondent.* Disputatio medica inauguralis de influxu facultatum animae; de causis & curatione methodica stuporis ac paralyseos ... Lugduni Batavorum, Apud Abrahamum Elzevier, 1684.

    [23] p. 22 cm. **[1955]**
Diss.—Leyden.

BURLACE, Edmund. *See* Borlase, Edmund [*d.* 1682]

BURNET, Duncan [16th-17th cent.] Iatrochymicus; sive, De praeparatione et compositione medicamentorum chymicorum artificiosa, tractatus ... Studio ac opera Joannis Danielis Mylii ... Francofurti, Typis Nicolai Hoffmanni, sumptibus Lucae Jennis, 1616.

    [12], 115 p. cm. **[1956]**

—[The same.] ... Ed. alt. ... Francofurti ad Moenum, Typis Erasmi Kempfferi, sumptibus Lucae Jennis, 1621.

    [8], III p. 20 cm. **[1957]**

BURNET, Gilbert, *Bp. of Salisbury* [1643-1715] A sermon preached at the funeral of the Honourable Robert Boyle; at St. Martins in the Fields, January 7. 1691/2. ... London, Ric. Chiswell and John Taylor, 1692.

    40 p. 21 cm. **[1958]**
Fulton(A) 300.

BURNET, *Sir* Thomas [1632?-1715?] Thesaurus medicinae practicae, ex praestantissimorum tum veterum tum recentiorum medicorum observationibus, consultationibus, consiliis & epistolis, summa diligentia collectus ordineque alphabetico dispositus ... Londini, Excudebat G. R. pro R. Boulter, & prostant apud R. Brown, J. Carnes & J. Mason, 1673.

    [32], 933 (i.e. 931), [9] p. 20 cm. **[1959]**
Edited by William Burnet.

—[The same.] ... a Daniele Puerario ... auctus observationibus selectissimis ... Genevae, Joh. Herm. Widerhold, 1678.

    2 v. 15 cm. **[1960]**
Vol. 1 has added engraved title page.

—[The same.] ... Venetiis, Typis Gasparis Storti, 1687.

    2 v. 16 cm. **[1961]**
Vol. 1 has added engraved title page.

—*ed. See* Hippocrates. [Selected works. Adaptations, etc. Latin.] Hippocrates contractus. 1685, 1686.

BURNET, William, *ed. See* Burnet, *Sir* T. Thesaurus medicinae practicae. 1673.

BURRHUS, Franciscus Josephus. *See* Borro, Giuseppe Francesco [1627-1695]

BURSER, Joachim [1583-1639] De febri epidemia; seu, Petechiali probe agnoscenda & curanda ... commentatio philosophico-medica. Locupletata variis animadversionibus in opiniones hucusque receptas, circa pathologica quaedam tam geralia, quam specialia, ad illustrationem & confirmationem veritatis in arte medica. Lipsiae, Impensis haeredum Thomae Schüreri, excudebat Fridericus Lanckisch, 1621.

    [16], 109, [2] p. 16 cm. **[1962]**

—*praeses.* Assertiones medicae de phlegmone renum & vesicae, cum nonnullis medico-physicis paradoxis ... Basileae, Typis Joh. Jacobi Genathii [1615]

[12] p. 20 cm. **[1963]**
Diss.—Basel (P. Wagner, *respondent)*

—*See* STROBELBERGER, J. S. Epistolaris concertatio super variis ... quaestionibus. 1625.

BURTHOGGE, RICHARD [1638?–*ca.* 1700] An essay upon reason, and the nature of spirits ... London, John Dunton, 1694.
[4], 280 p. illus. 18 cm. **[1964]**

—Of the soul of the world; and of particular souls. In a letter to Mr. Lock, occasioned by Mr. Keil's reflections upon an essay lately published concerning reason. By the author of that essay ... London, Daniel Brown, 1699.
46, [2] p. 19 cm. **[1965]**

—*respondent.* Disputatio medica inauguralis de lithiasi et calculo ... Lugduni Batavorum, Apud Philippum de Cro-Y, 1662.
[12] p. 24 cm. **[1966]**
Diss. — Leyden.

BURTON, ROBERT [1577–1640] The anatomy of melancholy, what it is. With all the kindes, causes, symptomes, prognostickes, and severall cures of it. In three maine partitions ... Philosophically, medically, historically, opened and cut up. By Democritus Junior [pseud., i.e. Robert Burton] ... Oxford, Printed by John Lichfield and James Short, for Henry Cripps, 1621.
[3], 72 (i.e. 76), [8], 783, [8] p. 20 cm. **[1967]**
Errata: p. [8] at end.
STC 4159.

—[The same] ... The 2d ed., corr. and augm. by the author ... Oxford, Printed by John Lichfield and James Short, for Henry Cripps, 1624.
[3], 64, [4], 557 (i.e. 579) p. 30 cm. **[1968]**
STC 4160.

— [The same] ... The 4th ed., corr. and augm. by the author ... Oxford, Printed for Henry Cripps [by John Lichfield] 1632.
[13], 78, [2], 722, [10] p. 29 cm. **[1969]**
Engraved title page.
STC 4162.

—[The same.] ... The 5th ed. corr. and augm. by the author ... Oxford, Printed for Henry Cripps, 1638.
[10], 78, [6], 723 (i.e. 727), 9 p. 29 cm.
[1970]

Engraved title page.
Imperfect: short title on p. [1] pasted over with blank sheet.
STC 4163.

—[The same.] ... The 7th ed., corr. and augm. by the author ... London, for John Garvay [1660]
[10], 78, [6], 723, [9] p. 30 cm. **[1971]**
Engraved title page.
Colophon: London, Printed for Henry Cripps, and are to bee sold by him and by Elisha Wallis, 1660.
Imprint covered with slip cancel, mutilated, affecting date.

—[The same.] ... The 8th ed. corr. and augm. by the author ... London, Printed [by R.W.] for Peter Parker, 1676.
[8], 46, [6], 434, [10] p. 34 cm. **[1972]**
Engraved title page.

BURWELL, THOMAS [1626–1702] *See* [PEACHIE, John] Some observations made upon the herb called perigua. 1694 [and] ... the Mexico seeds. 1695 [and] ... the serpent stones. 1694

BUSAEUS, JOANNES. *See* BUYS, Jan [1547–1611]

BUSCH, HENDRIK VAN DEN [1644–1682] *respondent.* Disputatio medica inauguralis de delirio ... Lugduni Batavorum, Apud viduam & haeredes Joannis Elsevirii, 1668.
[20] p. 18 cm. **[1973]**
Diss. — Leyden.

—*See* LAURUS BATAVA IN HONOREM ... Henrici à Busch. 1668.

BUSCHMAN, PETER [*fl.* 1678] *respondent.* Disputatio medica inauguralis de haemoptoë, sive sanguinis sputo ... Lugduni Batavorum, Apud viduam & heredes Johannis Elsevirii, 1678.
[11] p. 22 cm. **[1974]**
Diss. — Leyden.

BUSCOFIUS, HERMANN. *See* BUSSCHOF, Hermann [17th cent.]

BUSÉE, JEAN. *See* BUYS, Jan [1547–1611]

BUSSCHOF, HERMANN [17th cent.] [Net podagra mets gaders desselfs geneezinge. English.] Two treatises, the one medical, of the gout, and its nature more narrowly search'd into than hitherto; together with a new way of discharging the same ... By Herman Busschof Senior ... The other partly chirurgical, partly medical, containing some observations and practices relating both to some extraordinary cases of women in travel; and to some other uncommon cases of diseases in both sexes. By Henry van Roonhuyse ... Englished out of Dutch by a careful hand. London, Printed by H. C. and sold by Moses Pitt, 1676.

[14], 136 p.; [6], 208, [4] p. plate. 18 cm.

[1975]

Added engraved title page: A new way of curing the gout.

Part [2] has special title page and running title: Medico-chirurgical observations.

Imperfect: added engraved title page wanting. Plate in part [2] wanting; supplied in photocopy from British Museum.

— [German tr.] Das genau untersuchte, und auserfundene Podagra, vermittelst selbst sicher-eigenen Genäsung, und erlösenden Hülff Mittels ... Niederländisch beschrieben, und anjetzo ins Deutsch überzetzet von einem aus dem Collegio Naturae Curiosorum. Bresslau, In Verlegung Esaiae Fellgibels, 1677.

[1], 135 p. 14 cm.   [1976]

BUSSIÈRE, Paul. See Buissière, Paul [d. 1739]

BUSSIUS, Theodor [fl. 1659] respondent. See Möbius, G., praeses. Disputatio inauguralis medica de epilepsia. 1659.

BUSSOTTI, Dionigi, Bp. of Borgo San Sepolcro [d. 1654] See Soldi, J. Antidotario per il tempo di peste. 1630.

BUSZ, Henricus, respondent. See Deusing, A., praeses. Synopsis medicinae universalis. 1649.

BUTIN, Jean [d. 1584] See Hippocrates. Aphorismi et Prognostica. 1625.

BUTIUS, Vincentius. See Buzio, Vincenzio [16th-17th cent.]

BUTLER, John B. D. Ἁγιαστρολογία; or, The most sacred and divine science of astrology. 1. Asserted, in three propositions; shewing the excellency and great benefit thereof, where it is rightly understood, and religiously observed. 2. Vindicated, against the calumnies of the Reverend Dr. More, in his 'Explanation of the grand mysterie of godliness'. 3. Excused, concerning pacts with evil spirits, as not guilty in humble considerations upon the ... discourse upon that subject, by the Right Reverend ... Joseph sometimes Lord Bishop of Norwich. By J[ohn] B[utler] B.D. ... London, Printed for the author, and sold by William Bromwich, 1680.

[41], 91, [2] p.; [11], 128 p. 19 cm.   [1977]

Each part has special title page.
Dedicatory epistle signed: John Butler.

BUXBAUM, Andreas [d. 1730] Catechesis medica, per modum dialogi proposita, ex qua in medica arte initiandi artis principia, neotericorum hypothesibus accommodata, facili negotio addiscere possunt ... Martisburgi, Impensis Christiani Forbergeri, typis Christiani Gottschickii, 1695.

[280] p. 16 cm.   [1978]

— respondent. See Bohn, J., praeses. Dissertationem de variolis ... subjicit ... A. B. 1679; Vesti, J., praeses. Disputatio inauguralis medica de ventriculi inflatione. 1686.

BUXBAUM, Libmann [fl. 1697] respondent. Disputatio medica inauguralis de hydrope ... Lugduni Batavorum, Apud Abrahamum Elzevier, 1697.

[32] p. 23 cm.   [1979]

Diss. — Leyden.

BUYS, Jan [1547-1611] Πανάριον; hoc est, Arca medica variis divinae Scripturae priscorumque patrum antidotis adversus animi morbos instructa, et in gratiam confessariorum concionatorum, et religiosa vitae cultorum edita a Joanne Busaeo ... Moguntiae, Apud Joannem Albinum, 1608.

[16], 604, [24] p. 26 cm.   [1980]

Engraved title page.

BUYES, Jan [fl. 1685] respondent. Disputatio medica inauguralis de atrophia ... Lugduni Batavorum, Apud Abrahamum Elzevier, 1685.

[16] p. 22 cm.   [1981]

Diss. — Leyden.

BUZIO, Vincenzio [16th-17th cent.] De calido, frigido, ac temperato antiquorum potu et quo modo calida in delitiis uterentur ... Romae, Ex typographia Vitalis Mascardi, 1653.

[8], 69, [12] p. front. (port.) 20 cm.

[1982]

BYFIELD, T. See Byfield, Timothy.

BYFIELD, Timothy. The artificial spaw; or, Mineral-waters to drink: imitating the German spaw-water in its delightful and medicinal operations on humane bodies, &c. ... London, Printed by James Rawlins for the author and sold by Matthew Keinton, 1684.

[7], 70 p. 14 cm.   [1983]

—A short discourse of the rise nature, and management of the small-pox, and all putrid fevers ... Together with a philosophical account of an excellent remedy for these and many other diseases ... London, John Harris, 1695.

[1], 26 p.   20 cm.   [1984]

BYFIELDE, J. *See* Byfield, Timothy.

BYLER, Lucas [*fl.* 1618] *respondent*. De ictero flavo theses ... Basileae, Typis Johan. Jacobi Genathii [1618]

[8] p.   18 cm.   [1985]
Diss. — Basel.

BYWAART, Gerard [*fl.* 1683] *respondent*. Disputatio medica inauguralis de asthmate ... Lugduni Batavorum, Apud Abrahamum Elzevier, 1683.

[16] p.   22 cm.   [1986]
Diss. — Leyden.

C

C. *Dr. See* Cable, Daniel.

C., A. D. P. *See* Le medecin reformé; Response au Medecin reformé.

C., B. *See* Ciccolini, Barnaba [*fl.* 1674–ca. 1696]

C., D. F. *See* Du Four de La Crespelière.

C., D. L. *pseud. See* Pinsonnat, François.

C., G., *gent., practicioner in phisicke. See* Dariot, C. Dariotus redivivus: or, A briefe introduction conducing to the judgement of the stars. 1653; A treatise of mathematicall physick. 1653.

C., G., *tr. See* Weidenfeld, J. S. von. Four books ... concerning the secrets of the adepts. 1685.

C., G. C. L. *See* Leclerc, Charles Gabriel [1644–1700?]

C., H. H. S. I. *See* Waldschmidt, J. J. Vade mecum Waldschmidianum. 1696.

C***, I***, *tr. See* Cordemoy, L. G. de. Tractatus physici duo. 1679.

C., J. *See* Casteleyn, Johannes [ca. 1612–1665]

C., J., D. *See* Crull, Jodocus [*d.* 1713?]

C., J., *M. D. See* Crull, Jodocus [*d.* 1713?]

C., J., M. D. R. *See* Crull, Jodocus [*d.* 1713?]

C., J. G. R. M. *See* Synopsis doctrinae ac medicinae volnerum. 1690.

C., J. H. *See* Cardilucius, Johannes Hiskias [17th cent.]

C., J. L. M. *See* Lange, Johann [*fl.* 1667–1696]

C., L. L. M. *See* Le manuel du chirurgien d' armée. 1686, 1693.

C., N., *tr. See* Fabricius von Hilden, W. Lithotomia vesicae. 1640.

C., P. *See* Chamberlen, Peter [1601–1683]

C., P. D. *esq. See* Cardonnel, Pierre de [*d.* 1667]

C., P.M.T.*Ph. See* T., P. M. [*fl.* 1688]

C., R. *See* The compleat midwife's practice enlarged. 1663, 1697, 1698.

C., R., *chymist. See* Clark, R. [*fl.* 1687]

C., R., *Esquire. See* Carew, Richard [1555–1620]

C., T. *See* Cocke, Thomas [*fl.* 1675]

C., W. *See* Calebius, Willem; Cooper, William [*fl.* 1669–1689]

C.B.B.D. *See* B., C. B., *M. D.* [*fl.* 1696]

C.B.B.M.D. *See* B., C. B., *M. D.* [*fl.* 1696]

C. C. *See* Carneau, Étienne [1610–1671]

C. W., *M.S. See* Cockburn, William [1669–1739]

CABALA chemica. *See* Physica naturalis rotunda visionis chemicae cabalisticae. 1661.

CABALLETUS, Papirius [*fl.* 1605] Peripatetica medicaque placita ... Genuae, Apud Josephum Pavonium, 1605.

39 p.   21 cm.   [1987]

CABALLUS, FRANCISCUS. *See* CAVALLO, Francesco [*d.* 1540]

CABEI, NICOLÒ, *Father* [1586-1650] Philosophia magnetica in qua magnetis natura penitus explicatur, et omnium quae hoc lapide cernuntur causae propriae afferuntur: nova etiam pyxis construitur, quae propriam poli elevationem, cum suo meridiano, ubique demonstrat ... Ferrariȩ, apud Franciscum Succium, 1629.

[16], 412, [12] p. illus., diagrs. 33 cm.**[1988]**
Engraved title page.
Imperfect: p. [9-12] at end mutilated.
Concerns William Gilbert's views on magnetism.

CABIAS, JEAN BAPTISTE DE [*fl.* 1622] Les merveilles des bains d'Aix en Savoye ... Lyon, Jacques Roussin, 1623.

208, [8] p. 17 cm. **[1989]**

CABLE, DANIEL, *tr. See* SUCHTEN, A. von. Of the secrets of antimony. 1670.

CABOTIN, A. Commentaire en vers sur les Aphorismes d'Hypocrate. Par le sieur Cabotin, advocat en Parlement. Paris, Guillaume Sassier et Jacques Talon, 1665.

[12], 160 p. 16 cm. **[1990]**
Covers book I only. Includes Niccolò Leoniceno's Latin version.

CABREVIL, BARTHÉLEMY. *See* CABROL, Barthélemy [*b.* 1529].

CABRIADA, JUAN DE [*fl.* 1679-1688] *See* TIXEDAS, C. Verdad defendida. 1688.

CABROL, BARTHÉLEMY [*b.* 1529] Alphabet anatomic, auquel est contenue l'explication exacte des parties du corps humain: reduites en tables selon l'ordre de dissection ordinaire: avec l'osteologie, et plusieurs observations particulieres. Derniere ed. rev. & corr. par l'auteur, & augm. de plusieurs observations ... [Lyon] Pierre & Jacques Chouët, 1624.

[16], 110 p. 24 cm. **[1991]**
First published in Tournon, in 1594.

—[Latin tr.] Ἀλφαβητον ἀνατομικον; hoc est, Anatomes elenchus accuratissimus, omnes humani corporis partes, ea qua solent secari methodo, delineans. Accessere osteologia, observationesque medicis juxta ac chirurgis perutiles ... Genevae, Apud Jacobum Chouet, 1604.

144 p. 24 cm. **[1992]**

With this is bound Pardoux, B. Bartholomaei Perdulcis ... In Jac. Sylvii anatomen et in lib. Hippocratis De natura humana commentarii. 1643.

—[Dutch tr.] Het anatomiicke A. B. C. dat is; Een seer bondigh onderricht vande anatomie alle de partijen des menschelijcken lichaems ... Hier by zijn ghevoecht de osteologia, dat is de beschrijvinge der beenderen ... Verduyscht door Dr. Casparum Nollens. 's Graven-Haghe, By de weduwe ende erfghenamen van wijlen Hillebrant Jacobssz van Wouw, 1630.

[1], 67 ll. 21 cm. **[1993]**
Bound with (as issued?) Fabricius, Hieronymus, *ab Aquapendente*. De chirurgicale operatien. 1630.

—Ontleeding des menschelycken lichaems. Eertijts in't Latijn beschreven ... Nu verduytscht en met by-voechselen als oock figuren verrijckt. Door V[opiscus] F[ortunatus] P[lempius] Amsterdam, By Cornelis van Breugel voor Hendrick Laurentsz, 1633.

[16], 262 p. illus., plates. 32 cm. **[1994]**
Added engraved title page.

—[The same.] ... Amsterdam, By Gillis Joosten voor Hendrick Laurents, 1648.

[16], 262 p. illus., plates. 32 cm. **[1995]**
Added engraved title page dated: 1633.
A reprint of the 1633 ed.

CABROL, BARTHÉLEMY [*b.* 1529] [Selections] *In* Jasolino, G. Collegium anatomicum. 1668.

—*See* VOLCKAMER, J. G. [1616-1693] Collegium anatomicum. 1654.

CACHET, CHRISTOPHE [1572-1624] Controversiae theoricae, practicae, in primam Aphorismorum Hippocratis sectionem. Opus in duas partes divisum ... in quo quaecunque ad venae sectionem, purgationem, & probam victus rationem pertinent, non minus accurate, quam acute ac eleganter in utramque partem disputantur ac enodantur ... Pars prima. Tulli, Apud Sebastianum Philippe, 1612.

[32], 799 (i.e. 792), [4] p. 18 cm. **[1996]**
No second part was published. Cf. BMC, vol. 104 (1961) col. 244.
Includes Greek and Latin text of aphorisms 1-12.

—Exercitationes equestres in epigrammatum centurias sex distinctae. Quarum prima, & quarta de virtute, & moribus. Secunda de Deo, & divis. Tertia de fide, & religione. Quinta miscellanea continet. Sexta circa res medicas occupatur. His accesserunt elegiae duae, prima de morte & passione

Christi. Altera de assumptione Deiparae Virginis. Nanceii, Typis Anthonii Charlot, sumptibus Claudii Ludovici, 1622.

[8], 234 p.   17 cm.   **[1997]**

CADEMAN, AUGUST [*fl.* 1632] *respondent. See* MULLER, J. *praeses.* Ανθρωποψυχολογίας διάσκεψις secunda de corpore ejusque partibus similaribus. 1632.

CADEMAN, Sir THOMAS [1590?–1651] *ed. See* MAYERNE, Sir T. T. de. The distiller of London. 1639, 1652.

—*See* HONORIBUS DOCTORALIBUS MERITISSIMIS . . . Dn. Thomae Cademani Angli. 1620.

CAELIUS, ANTONINUS. *See* CELI, Antonino [*fl. ca.* 1618]

CAELNATUS, THEOPHILUS. *See* CELNATUS, Theophilus.

CAESALPINUS, ANDREAS. *See* CESALPINO, Andrea [1519–1603]

CAESAR, JOACHIM [*fl.* 1612] *tr. See* HUARTE DE SAN JUAN, J. Scrutinium ingeniorum. 1637.

CAESAR, JOHANN CHRISTOPH [*fl.* 1677–1680] *respondent. See* RIVINUS, A. Q., *praeses.* Disputatio medica, in qua agrestis vitae sanitas . . . exhibetur. 1677.

CAESAREO-LEOPOLDINA Naturae Curiosorum Academia. *See* ACADEMIA NATURAE CURIOSORUM.

CAESATUS, ANTONIUS [*fl. ca.* 1657] Antonii Caesati physici Viglevamensis, ac in eadem civitate medicinam facientis Tyrocinium medicum huic addita sunt epidemicae febris anno 1657. Viglevani grassantis brevis descriptio, malignisque in febribus epilogistica prognostica . . . Mediolani, Ex typographia Ambrosii Ramellati, 1659.

[18], 186, [3] p.   22 cm.   **[1998]**

CAESIUS, FEDERICUS. *See* CESI, Federico, *duca di Acquasparta* [1585–1630]

CAESIUS, PHILIPPUS. *See* ZESEN, Philipp von [1619–1689].

CAGNATI, MARSILIO [1543–1612] De morte caussa partus medica quidem disputatio, sed forensibus

negotiis tractandis necessaria . . . Romae, Apud Aloysium Zannettum, 1602.

59, [1] p.   21 cm.   **[1999]**
"Marsilii Cagnati De ligno sancto prima [-altera] disputatio": p. 33–59.

—De sanitate tuenda. Libri duo. Primus de continentia, alter de arte gymnastica . . . Patavii, Apud Franciscum Bolzettam, ex typographia Laurentii Pasquati, 1605.

[18], 196 ll.   20 cm.   **[2000]**

—In Aphor. Hyppoc. XXII sectionis primae Germana quamvis nova expositio. *In* Cleti, E. Dilucidatio in Aphor. 22. primae sect. pro defensione interpretationis Marsilii Cagnati. 1621; Manelfi, G. Responsio brevis ad annotationes Prosperi Martiani. 1621.

—*See* FERRARI, G. B., *Father.* In funere Marsilii Cagnati medici praestantissimi laudatio Joannis Baptistae Ferrarii . . . Habita . . . 1612; MARZIANI, P. Apologeticus liber. 1617.

CAHAGNESIUS, JACOBUS. *See* CAHAIGNES, Jacques de [1548–1612?].

CAHAIGNES, JACQUES DE [1548–1612?] Brevis facilisque methodus curandorum capitis affectuum . . . Cadomi, Apud Petrum Poisson, 1618.

[10], 338, [1], p.   16 cm.   **[2001]**
Errata: p. [339]
With this is bound *his* Brevis facilisque methodus curandarum febrium. 1616.

—Brevis facilisque methodus curandarum febrium . . . Cadomi, Apud Petrum Poisson, 1616.

[20], 153, [1] p.   16 cm.   **[2002]**
Bound with *his* Brevis facilisque methodus curandorum capitis affectuum. 1618.

CAILLE, ANDRÉ [1515–1580?] *tr. See* DUBOIS, J. La pharmacopee. 1604; MIZAULD, A. Le jardin medecinal. 1605.

CAIMO, POMPEIO [1568–1631] De calido innato libri tres. In quibus non solum ejus natura explicatur, sed solida etiam medicorum in hoc argumento doctrina ostenditur, & Galenica praecipue a neotericorum objectionibus vindicatur . . . Venetiis, Apud Hieronymum Piutum, 1626.

[12], 455 p.   19 cm.   **[2003]**

—De febrium putridarum indicationibus juxta Galeni methodum colligendis, & adimplendis. Libri duo ... Patavii, Apud Petrum Paulum Tozium, 1628.

[8], 265, [1] p.   21 cm.   [2004]

CAIUS, BERNARDINUS [*fl.* 1596–1612] Disputatio ... de vesicantium usu ... Venetiis, Apud Evangelistam Deuchinum, 1606.

[12], 87 p.   24 cm.   [2005]

— *See* OBIZZI, I. Apologia. 1612.

CALAFATTI, GIORGIO. *See* CALAPHATES, Georgius [1652–1726]

CALAPHATES, GEORGIUS [1652–1726] Trattato sopra la peste nel quale dottrinalmente si dimostra l'essenza di questo male: si propongono, e si dicchiarano li segni, e le cause, dalle quali hà la sua origine ... Venetia, Gio. Giacomo Hertz, 1682.

[16], 269 p.   18 cm.   [2006]

CALART, JEAN-BAPTISTE. *See* POSTEL, N. Factum. 1685.

CALCAGNINI, CELIO [1479–1541] Het lof des vloos. *In* Veeler wonderens wonderbaarelijck lof. 1664.

— *tr. See* JOANNES ACTUARIUS. De urinis libri VII. 1670; WILLICH, J. Exercitationes et probationes de urinis libri IV. 1688.

CALCAR, JAN STEPHAN VON [1499–*ca.* 1546] *See* [VESALIUS, A.] Notomie di Titiano. *ca.* 1670.

CALCEOLARIUS, FRANCISCUS. *See* CALZOLARI, Francesco [*fl.* 1622]

CALCKHOFF, JOHANN CHRISTIAN. *See* KALCKHOFF, Johann Christian [*fl.* 1674–1678]

CALDERA, CASPAR. *See* CALDERA DE HEREDIA, Gaspar [*b.* 1591]

CALDERA DE HEREDIA, GASPAR [*b.* 1591] Tribunal, medicum, magicum, et politicum. Pars prima [-altera] Lugduni Batavorum, Apud Johannem Elsevirium, 1658.

[12], 534, [21] p.; 194, 21 p.   35 cm.   [2007]

Imperfect: wormholes throughout; p. 139–142 wrongly imposed. Part 2 has special title page.

— Tribunalis medici illustrationes et observationes practicae. Accessit liber aureus de facile parabilibus ... Antverpiae, Apud Jacobum Meursium, 1663.

[28], 354, [32] p.   34 cm.   [2008]

— *See* ORTIZ DE LA LAGUNA, G. Responde al doctor Simon Ramos ... a un papel que embiò contra el doctor Caldera. 1634.

CALDESI, GIOVANNI BATTISTA. Osservazioni anatomiche di Giovanni Caldesi Aretino intorno alle tartarughe marittime, d'aqua dolce, e terrestri. Scritte in una lettera all'illustriss. sig. Francesco Redi. Firenze, Piero Matini, 1687.

[3], 91, [9] p.   plates.   25 cm.   [2009]

CALEBIUS, WILLEM, *tr. See* DELLON, G. Naauwkeurig verhaal van een reyse door Indien gedaen. 1687, 1688.

CALENI, PAUL JULIUS [*fl.* 1656] *respondent. See* MÖBIUS, G., *praeses.* Dissertatio inauguralis medica de pleuritide. 1656.

CALEPINO, AMBROGIO [1435–1511] Dictionarium octo linguarum. In quo primis & praecipuis dictionibus Latinis, Hebraeas, Graecas, Gallicas, Italicas, Germanicas, Hispanicas, nunc Anglicas dictiones ... addidimus ... Ult. ed. Parisiis, Apud viduam Guillelmi Chaudieri, 1606.

[2], 729 ll.   41 cm.   [2010]

Original date changed to 1606.

CALESTANI, GIROLAMO [1510–1572] Delle osservationi ... parte prima [-seconda] ... [Con due tavola ... di M. Gio. Battista Bertuccio] ... Venetia, Agostino Angelieri, 1606.

2 v. in 1   21 cm.   [2011]

Contents. — pt. 1 Osservationi nelli semplici. — pt. 2. Nella quale s'insegna di comporre gl'antidoti, e medicamenti, che più si costumano nell'Italia à uso della medicina.

— [The same.] ... Nuovamenta ... ricorretta, & ampliata ... Venetia, Ghirardo Imberti, 1639.

[2012]

— [The same.] ... Venetia, I Giunti, 1655.

[2013]

— [The same.] ... Venetia, Nicolò Pezzana, 1673.

[2014]

CALID, *filius Jazichius. See* KHĀLID IBN YAZĪD, al-Umawi.

CALISIUS, ADAM [*fl.* 1650–1651] Dissertatio de aere, quam ... Philosophorum Collegio in Academia Lipsiansi P. P. M. Adam Calisius ... & Martinus Seidemann ... Lipsiae, Literis Hönianis, 1651.

[16] p.   19 cm.   [2015]

Diss. — Leipzig.

—*See* Pufendorff, E., *praeses*. De igne nativo disquisitio. 1650.

CALLARD DE LA DUQUERIE, Jean Baptiste [1620-1718] Lexicon medicum etymologicum; sive, Tria etymologiarum millia quas in scholis publicis medicinae alumnos ita postulantes edocuit ... Cadomi, Apud Joannem Briard, 1691.

[14], 372 p.   15 cm.   [2016]

—[The same.] Cadomi, & prostat Parisiis, Apud Stephanum Michallet, 1692.

[14], 372 p.   15 cm.   [2017]

A reissue of the 1691 edition with new title page.

CALLY, Pierre [1630-1709] Primum philosophiae perficiendae rudimentum, anthropologia; sive, Tractatio de homine ... Cadomi, Apud Joannem Cavelier, 1683.

[4], 294, [5] p.   23 cm.   [2018]

CALMETTE, François de la. *See* La Calmette, François de [*fl.* 1684]

CALMETUS, Antonius. *See* Chaumette, Antoine, [16th cent.]

CALVISIUS, Sethus [1639-1698] Theses physicae de sermone ... publicae proponit M. Sethus Calvisius, Jun. ... respondente Christophoro Vogelio ... Lipsiae, Praelo Coleriano [1660]

[20] p.   19 cm.   [2019]

Imperfect: p. [3-4] wanting.
Diss.—Leipzig (C. Vogel, respondent)

CALVO, Fernando [16th-17th cent.] Libro de albeiteria en el qual se trata del cavallo, mulo, y jumento, y de sus miembros, y calidades, y de todas sus enfermedades, con la causas, señales, y remedios de cada una dellas ... y un nuevo arte de herrar en octavas. Va repartido en quatro libros ... Nuevamente corr., y enmend. en esta 6. impr. ... Madrid, Por Andres Garcia de la Iglesia, acosta de Gabriel de Leon ... 1675.

[6], 383 p.   30 cm.   [2020]

Imperfect: p. 185-186 and p. 209-212 wanting; p. 353-386 mounted with loss of text; title page mutilated, affecting imprint date. Date supplied from Palau, 40537a.

CALVO, Juan [*fl.* 1568-*ca.* 1580] Primera y segunda parte de la cirugia universal, y particular del cuerpo humano, quae trata de las cosas naturales, no naturales ... y del antidotario, en el qual se trata de la facultad de todos los medicamentos ... segun

Galeno en el libro quarto y quinto de la facultad de los simples, con otros tratados ... Uno De anotomia, y otro De morbo gallico del mismo autor, con otro De fracturas, y dislocaciones, por el ... Andres de Tamayo ... Corr., y enmend. en esta ult. impr. Valencia, Los herederos de Chrysostomo Garriz, por Bernardo Noguès, acosta de Benito Durànd ... 1647.

[8], 618, [3] p.   29 cm.   [2021]

—[The same.] ... Madrid, Antonio Gonçalez de Reyes [1674]

[8], 690 (i.e. 590), [2] p.   31 cm.   [2022]

Imprint partly supplied from Palau 40554a.

—[The same.] ... Valencia, Jayme de Bordazar, 1690.

[8], 690 (i.e. 590), [1] p.   32 cm.   [2023]

Different setting of type.

—*See* Courtin, G. Les oeuvres anatomiques et chirurgicales. 1656.

CALVOLI, Giovanni Cinelli. *See* Cinelli Calvoli, Giovanni [1625-1706]

CALZOLARI, Francesco [*fl.* 1622] *See* Ceruti, B. Musaeum Franc. Calceolarii jun. ... a Benedicto Ceruto ... incaeptum, et ab Andrea Chiocco ... luculenter descriptum. 1622.

CAMAFFI, Luca Antonio [*d.* 1641] Reggimento per viver sano ne i tempi caldi ... Perugia, Nella Stampa Augusta, 1610.

256, [14] p.   16 cm.   [2024]

CAMEL, Friedrich [*fl.* 1700-1702] *respondent. See* Hoffmann, F. [1660-1672] *praeses*. Dissertatio medica de pulverum sternutatoriorum vero usu. 1700.

CAMERARIUS, Elias [1673-1734] Dissertationes tres, exhibentes I. Spirituum animalium statum naturalem, et p. n. occasione experimenti Bellino-Bohniani. II. Spiritum D. Boylii fumantem obviaque circa ipsum phaenomena. III. Usum et abusum potuum thee et caffe in his regionibus. Praefatio quaedam de Nuckianis Mercurii injectionibus continet. Tubingae, Impensis Philiberti Brunnii, typis Joh. Conradi Reisii, 1694.

[16], 62 p.; 48 p.; 62 p.   17 cm.   [2025]

—*praeses*. Quaestionem casuistarum medico-legalem, an liceat medico pro salute matris abortum procurare? Nec utilem esse, nec necessariam, ostendet . . . Samuel Herzog . . . Tubingae, Literis Joh. Conradi Eitelii, 1697.

15 p.   19 cm.   [2026]

Diss. — Tübingen (S. Herzog, *respondent*)

CAMERARIUS, ELIAS RUDOLF [1641–1695]

Dissertations — Tübingen

—*praeses.* Anatome hydropicae, cum scholiis . . . Tubingae, Typis Martini Rommeii, 1691.

20 p.   19 cm.   [2027]

D. Brotbeck, *respondent.*

—Disputatio inauguralis medica, cur epilepsia hodie inter nos tam frequens sit? . . . Tubingae, Excudit Gregorius Kerner, 1680.

[28] p.   20 cm.   [2028]

J. J. Schmidlin, *respondent.*

—Disputatio inauguralis medica de febre tertiana maligna . . . Tubingae, Typis Martini Rommeii, 1692.

24 p.   18 cm.   [2029]

J. D. Mauchart, *respondent.*

—Disputatio inauguralis medica de ictero . . . Tubingae, Typis Johann-Henrici Reisii [1679]

16 p.   19 cm.   [2030]

J. B. Mögling, *respondent.*

—Disputatio inauguralis medica de mictione pultacea . . . Tubingae, Typis Johann-Henrici Reisii, 1683.

[2], 32 p.   18 cm.   [2031]

G. F. Cellius, *respondent.*

—Disputatio inauguralis medica de vomitu aquae ex gula, vulgo: Hertz-oder Gallen-Wasser . . . Tubingae, Typis viduae Johann-Henrici Reisii, 1686.

16 p.   20 cm.   [2032]

M. F. Geuder, *respondent.*

—Disputatio medica de ozaena . . . Tubingae, Typis Martini Rommeii, 1692.

11 p.   20 cm.   [2033]

G. F. Metzger, *respondent.*

—Disquisitio inauguralis medica de phrenitide . . . Tubingae, Typis Johann-Henrici Reisii, 1684.

24 p.   21 cm.   [2034]

G. N. Weinlin, *respondent.*

—Disquisitio medica inauguralis de phlogosibus vagis cum scorbuto . . . Tubingae, Typis Johann-Henrici Reisii [1684]

16 p.   19 cm.   [2035]

P. F. Jäger, *respondent.*

—Disquisitio medica quale signum in morbis praebeat urina . . . Tubingae, Typis Johann-Henrici Reisii, 1680.

16 p.   19 cm.   [2036]

G. F. Cellius, *respondent.*

—Dissertatio de vomitu gravidarum . . . [Tubingae] Literis Gregorii Kerneri, 1682.

16 p.   18 cm.   [2037]

E. Backmeister, *respondent.*

—Dissertatio inauguralis medica de febre intermittente anomala . . . Tubingae, Johann-Conradi Reisii, 1692.

24 p.   19 cm.   [2038]

J. H. Gsell, *respondent.*

—Dissertatio medica de acidularum usu externo . . . Tubingae, Literis Heinianis [1677]

39 p.   20 cm.   [2039]

J. C. Cellarius, *respondent.*

—Dissertatio medica de anorexia . . . Tubingae, Typis Joachimi Heinii, 1679.

[1], 28, [2] p.   20 cm.   [2040]

G. H. Bachov, *respondent.*

—Dissertatio medica de clysmatibus . . . Tubingae, Literis Rommeianis, 1688.

32 p.   20 cm.   [2041]

J. M. Brigel, *respondent.*

—Dissertatio medica de febribus in genere . . . Tubingae, Johann-Conradi Reisii, 1692.

[1], 18 p.   20 cm.   [2042]

J. H. Gsell, *respondent.*

—Dissertatio medica inauguralis, de casu, in quo menses P. N. emanentes per menagoga ciendi non sunt . . . Tubingae, Typis Martini Rommeii, 1690.

[1], 20 p.   19 cm.   [2043]

S. Braun, *respondent.*

—Dissertatio medica inauguralis, de glandulis p. n. patulis . . . Tubingae, Typis Martini Rommeii [1689]

[1], 14 p.   19 cm.   [2044]

E. J. Albeckh, *respondent.*

—Dissertatio medica inauguralis de palpitatione cordis . . . Tubingae, Typis Martini Rommeii, 1681.

[2], 30 p.　21 cm.　　　　**[2045]**
J. K. Remmelin, *respondent.*

—Dissertatio medica inauguralis. In qua obex curationis morborum tam frequens quam gravis, occasione Hippocrat. Aph. 52. S. 2 monstratur ... Tubingae, Typis Georg Henrici Reisii, senioris, 1691.
　32 p.　20 cm.　　　　**[2046]**
J. G. Glocken, *respondent.*

—Dissertatio medica posterior, de cichorio ... Tubingae, Typis Martini Rommeii, 1691.
　[2], 15-29, [3] p.　22 cm.　　　　**[2047]**
W. F. Hölderlin, *respondent.*

—Dissertatio medica prior de coryza sicca ... Tubingae, Typis Martini Rommeii [1688]
　[1], 16 p.　20 cm.　　　　**[2048]**
J. C. Hummel, *respondent.*

—Dissertatio medica prior [-posterior] de tenesmo ... Tubingae, Typis viduae Martini Rommeii [1693]
　23 (i.e. 43) p.　21 cm.　　　　**[2049]**
Dissertatio medica posterior has special title page (p. [25])
S. Caspar, *respondent.*

—Dissert. medico-chirurgica inauguralis, de ulceribus antiquis ... Tubingae, Typis Martini Rommeii [1689]
　[1], 28 p.　20 cm.　　　　**[2050]**
J. M. Brigel, *respondent.*

—Expositio medica casus de aegritudine animi ... Tubingae, Typis Martini Romeii, 1688.
　[2], 24 p.　20 cm.　　　　**[2051]**
E. J. Albeckh, *respondent.*

—Expositio medico-chirurgica casus de polypo narium aquoso ... Tubingae, Literis Rommeianis, 1688.
　[1], 28 p.　20 cm.　　　　**[2052]**
S. Braun, *respondent.*

—Another issue.
　[4], 28 p.　19 cm.
Dedications added.　　　　**[2053]**

—Historia anatomica renum et vesicae ... Tubingae, Typis Johann-Henrici Reisii, 1683.
　[1], 22 p.　19 cm.　　　　**[2054]**
G. N. Weinlin, *respondent.*

—Historia cardialgiae sublatae ... Tubingae, Typis Gregorii Kerneri [1683]

16 p.　18 cm.　　　　**[2055]**
E. Backmeister, *respondent.*

—Historiam pleuritidis et abscessus pectoris cum succedente colica spasmodica et gutta serena, & in eam commentarium ... submittit Johan-Samuel Knisel ... Tubingae, Typis Martini Rommeii [1690]
　24 p.　21 cm.　　　　**[2056]**
J. S. Knisel, *respondent.*

—Indicatio symptomatum ... Tubingae, Typis viduae Johann-Henrici Reisi, 1686.
　[2] 46 p.　20 cm.　　　　**[2057]**
A. Planer, *respondent.*

—Modus subitaneae refectionis enucleatus ... Tubingae, Literis Kernerianis [1683]
　[16] p.　21 cm.　　　　**[2058]**
P. F. Jäger, *respondent.*

—Positiones chirurgicae de fractura cum vulnere ... Tubingae, Typis Johann-Conradi Reisii, 1693.
　[1], 8 p.　19 cm.　　　　**[2059]**
D. Brotbeck, *respondent.*

—Positiones has medicas publico ... submittit examini Ferdinandus Gottlieb Schmeltz ... Tubingae, Typis Georg-Henrici Reisii, 1690.
　24 p.　20 cm.　　　　**[2060]**
F. G. Schmeltz, *respondent.*

—Tensio cordis, lipothymiae causa, occasione experimenti pneumatici exposita ... Tubingae, Typis Martini Rommeii [1686]
　[4], 24 p.　19 cm.　　　　**[2061]**
R. J. Camerarius, *respondent.*

—Theses medicae de catalepsi epileptica ... Tubingae, Typis Martini Rommeii, 1690.
　[8] p.　20 cm.　　　　**[2062]**
J. G. Glock, *respondent.*

—Theses medicae de tremore a cessante scabie ... Tubingae, Typis Martini Rommeii, 1688.
　8 p.　19 cm.　　　　**[2063]**
F. G. Schmeltz, *respondent.*

Valetudinarii senilis lineas speciales ... examini subjicit ... Theodorus Carolus ... Tubingae, Literis Kernerianis [1684]
　[4], 52 p.　23 cm.　　　　**[2064]**
Imperfect: p. [3-4] and 1-14 wanting.
T. Carolus, *respondent.*

— *respondent. See* METZGER, G. B., *praeses.* Dissertatio medica inauguralis de acidulis. 1663.

— *See* EBERHARD-KARLS-UNIVERSITÄT, Tübingen. Rector Academiae Tubingensis lect. ben. sal. 1695.

CAMERARIUS, JOACHIM [1500-1574] *tr. See* REGIMEN SANITATIS SALERNITANUM. Schola Salernitana. 1649, 1657, 1667, 1683.

— *See* HYGIEIA 1628; REGIMEN SANITATIS SALERNITANUM. De conservanda bona valetudine. 1607, 1619; REGIMEN SANITATIS SALERNITANUM. Medicina Salernitana. 1605, 1611, 1612, 1622, 1624, 1628, 1638.

CAMERARIUS, JOACHIM [1534-1598] [De recta ratione praeservandi a pestis contagio. German.] Unterricht von der Pest. [Breslau? 1626?]

[60] p. 18 cm. [2065]

Cancel half leaf pasted over lower part of p. [40] (sig. E₄) "Vorrede" by the unnamed translator (p. [3-15]) is dated from Breslau, Jan. 20, 1626.

Translation of Camerarius' De recta et necessaria ratione, praeservandi a pestis contagio, and of its two appendices: Constitutiones, leges, et edicta quaedam, tempore pestis ano Christi 1576 & 1577 publice Venetiis & alibi proposita, and Ratio expurgandum rerum infectarum.

— Symbolorum et emblematum centuriae tres. I. Ex herbis & stirpibus. II. Ex animalibus quadrupedibus. III. Ex volatilibus & insectis. Ed. 2., auctior & accuratior. Accessit noviter Centuria IV. Ex aquatilibus & reptilibus. Cum figuris aeneis. [Lipsiae] Typis Voegelinianis, 1605.

4 parts in 1 v. illus. 21 cm. [2066]

Each Centuria has special engraved title page (dated 1590 [i.e. 1593] 1595, 1596, and 1604, respectively) and separate pagination.

Edited by Ludwig Camerarius, who has supplied a general dedicatory epistle, dated 31 Jan. 1605, a general note to the reader, a note at the end of Centuria 3, and a special dedicatory epistle for Centuria 4.

The engravings are by Johann Sibmacher.

— *ed. See* MATTIOLI, P. A. Kreutterbuch. 1611, 1626, 1678.

CAMERARIUS, JOHANN RUDOLF [*b.* 1588] Sylloges memorabilium medicinae et mirabilium naturae arcanorum, centuriae IV . . . Augustae Trebocorum, Sumptibus Eberhardi Zetzneri, Typis Johannes Reppius, 1624.

[47], 288 p. 14 cm. [2067]

Bound with copy 2 of Du Laurens, A. Discursus philosophicus et medicus. 1620.

— Sylloges memorabilium medicinae et mirabilium naturae arcanorum, centuriae duodecim . . . Argentorati, Sumptibus Eberhardi Zetzneri, 1630.

9 v. in 1. 14 cm. [2068]

Centuriae V-XII are separately paged with special title pages variously dated 1626-1628 and 1630.

— Sylloges memorabilium medicinae et mirabilium naturae arcanorum centuriae sedecim . . . Argentorati, Sumptibus Eberhardi Zetzneri, 1652.

3 v. 13, 14 & 12 cm. [2069]

Contents: v. 1. Centuriae I-VIII. v. 2. Centuriae VIII (repeated)-XII. v. 3. Centuriae XIII-XVI.

Centuriae V-XII have special title pages variously dated 1626-1630. Centuriae I-IV, and XIII-XVI are continuously paged.

— Sylloges memorabilium medicinae et mirabilium naturae arcanorum centuriae XX . . . Ed. alt. emendata, & quatuor centuriis postumis aucta . . . Tubingae, Sumptibus Joh. Georg. Cottae, typis Martini Rommeii, 1683.

[20], 1662, [95] p. 19 cm. [2070]

CAMERARIUS, LUDWIG [1573-1651] *ed. See* CAMERARIUS, J. [1534-1598] Symbolorum et emblematum centuriae tres. 1605.

CAMERARIUS, RUDOLF JAKOB [1665-1721]

Dissertations — Tübingen

— *praeses.* Continuatio tentaminum circa lignum nephriticum . . . Tubingae, Typis Martini Rommeii, 1690.

8 p. 19 cm. [2071]

J. E. Wagner, *respondent.*

De calculis renum et vesicae . . . Tubingae, Ex typographeio Georg-Henrici Reisii, 1698.

[2], 30 p. 19 cm. [2072]

P. F. Bilger, *respondent.*

— De colica paretico-epileptica . . . Tubingae, Literis Joh. Conradi Eitelii, 1698.

[24] p. 19 cm. [2073]

S. Herzog, *respondent.*

— De convenientia plantarum in fructificatione et viribus . . . Tubingae, Typis Joh. Conradi Reisii, 1699.

16 p. 20 cm. [2074]

G. F. Gmelin, *respondent.*

— De diabete hypochondriacorum periodico . . . Tubingae, Aere Georg-Henrici Reisii, 1696.

28 p.   19 cm.   [2075]

C. A. Megerlin, *respondent.*

—De panacea mercuriali ... Tubingae, Ex typographeo Georg-Henrici Reisii, 1700.

12 p.   20 cm.   [2076]

J. Caspar, *respondent.*

—Dissertatio inauguralis de colore sanguinis e vena secta missi florido ... Tubingae, Ex typographio Georg-Henrici Reisii, 1700.

[2], 34 p.   19 cm.   [2077]

P. F. Bilger, *respondent.*

—Dissertatio inauguralis medica de potu aquarum ardentium ... Tubingae, Typis Johann-Conradi Reisii, 1698.

24 p.   19 cm.   [2078]

L. F. Breyer, *respondent.*

—Dissertatio physica de elementis ... Tubingae, Typis Georg-Henrici Reisii, senioris, 1692.

20 p.   19 cm.   [2079]

J. K. Raith, *respondent.*

—Schematismi colorum, infuso ligni nephritici propriorum ... Tubingae, Typis Martini Rommeii, 1689.

16 p.   20 cm.   [2080]

D. Brotbeck, *respondent.*

—*respondent. See* CAMERARIUS, E. R., *praeses.* Tensio cordis, lipothymiae causa, occasione experimenti pneumatici exposita. 1686.

CAMERONI, FRANCESCO [17th cent.] *See* BERNARDI, F. L'ignoranza convinta. 1669.

CAMILLI, ALESSANDRO [*fl.* 1638-1646] *ed. See* CAMILLI, Annibale. Del bagno di Nocera. 1638, 1646, 1660.

CAMILLI, ANNIBALE [*fl.* 1601-1627] Del bagno di Nocera nell'Umbria, detto acqua santa, overo acqua bianca. Trattato dove si dechiara la miniera, la virtu, e l'uso, di tal acqua ... Perugia, Vincentio Colombara erede d'Andrea Bresciano, 1601.

24 p.   21 cm.   [2081]

—[The same.] ... Perugia, Marco Naccarini, 1614.

48 p.   illus.   21 cm.   [2082]

—[The same.] ... Perugia, Angelo Bartoli, 1627.

46, [2] p.   illus.   20 cm.   [2083]

With this are bound: Descrittione di molte virtù della terra medicinale del bagno di Nocera. 1638; Bartolucci, G. B. Sommario sopra le virtù del bagno dell'acqua bianca di Nocera nell'Umbria. 1636.

—[The same.] ... Aggiuntavi in questa 4. impr. la virtù della terra di cette bagno nuovamente ritrovata ... Perugia, Angelo Bartoli, 1638.

47 p.   illus.   22 cm.   [2084]

Edited by Alessandro Camilli.

—[The same.] ... Perugia, Appresso gli heredi di Pietro Tomassi & Sebastiano Zecchini, 1646.

47 p.   illus.   22 cm.   [2085]

A reprint.

—[The same.] ... 6. impr. ... Perugia, Sebastiano Zecchini, 1660.

47 p.   illus.   21 cm.   [2086]

A reprint with new dedicatory epistle.

CAMILLI, CAMILLO [*d.* 1615] *tr. See* HUARTE DE SAN JUAN, J. Examen de ingenios. The examination of mens wits. 1604, 1616.

CAMILLUS THOMAIUS. *See* TOMAI, Camillo [*d.* 1549]

CAMP, M. Ja. Co. vande, *tr. See* RULAND, M. [1532-1602] Empirica. 1660.

CAMPANELLA, TOMMASO [1568-1639] Astrologicorum libri VII. In quibus astrologia omni superstitione Arabum, & Judaeorum eliminata physiologice tractatur, secundum S. Scripturas, & doctrinam S. Thomae, & Alberti, & summorum theologorum; ita ut absque suspicione mala in Ecclesia Dei multa cum utilitate possint. Francofurti, 1630.

[8], 232, [6] p.; 24 p.   illus., tables.   24 cm.

[2087]

—De sensu rerum et magia, libri quatuor, pars mirabilis occultae philosophiae, ubi demonstratur, mundum esse Dei vivam statuam, beneque cognoscentem ... Tobias Adami recensuit, et nunc primum evulgavit. Francofurti, Apud Egenolphum Emmelium, impensis Godefridi Tampachii, 1620.

[15], 371 p.   22 cm.   [2088]

—[The same.] De sensu rerum, et magia. Libros quatuor ... Correctos et defensos a stupidorum incolarum mundi calumniis per argumenta & testimonia divinorum codicum, naturae, sc. ac scripturae, eorumdemque interpretum, scilicet, theologorum & philosophorum, exceptis atheis. Jure potissimo dedicat consecratque. Parisiis, Apud Dionysium Bechet, 1637.

[16], 92 p.; 229 p. 23 cm. [2089]

"Thomae Campanellae ... defensio libri sui De sensu rerum": p. 1–92.

—Medicinalium, juxta propria principia, libri septem ... Lugduni, Ex officina Joannis Pillehotte, sumptibus Joannis Caffin & Francisci Plaignard, 1635.

[26], 690, [1] p. 23 cm. [2090]

Edited by Jacques Gaffarel.

CAMPDOMERCUS, JOHANNES JACOBUS [*fl.* 1693-1696] Epistola anatomica, problematica quarta, ad ... Fredericum Ruyschium ... de glandulis, fibris, cellulisque lienalibus ... Amstelaedami, Apud Joannem Wolters, 1696.

16 p. illus. 22 cm. [2091]

"Frederici Ruyschii responsio ...": p. 6–12.

CAMPEGIUS, JOANNES BRUYERINUS. *See* BRUYERIN, Jean Baptiste [*fl.* 1530-1560]

CAMPEN, CHRISTOFFEL VAN [*d. ca.* 1696] Collectanea therapeutica, de pleuritide et apoplexia. In quibus ad mentem veterum medicorum disseritur, de clysterium, purgantium, vomitoriorum ... topicorum, usu & abusu. Subjicitur ejusdem Exercitationum medicinalium decas I ... [-decas X] ... Bredae, Typis Cornelii Seldenslach, 1691.

176 p. 16 cm. [2092]

—Another issue. Imprint date altered from M.DC.LXXXXI. to M.DC.LXXXXII. [2093]

—*respondent.* Disputatio medica inauguralis de calculo renum ... Lugduni Batavorum, Apud viduam & haeredes Joannis Elsevierii, 1668.

[11] p. 23 cm. [2094]

Diss. — Leyden.

CAMPI, BALDASSAR [*d. ca.* 1653] Baldassari, e Michel Campi al sig. Antonio Manfredi ... In dilucidotione, e confermatione maggiore di alcune cose state da noi dette nella risposta al sig. Gaspari medico in Roma. Pisa, Francesco delle Dote, 1641.

12 p. 22 cm. [2095]

—Nuovo discorso col quale si dimostra qual sia il vero mitridato ... Con un breve capitolo del vero Aspalato. Di Baldassar e Michel Campi ... Lucca, Ottaviano Guidoboni, 1623.

[8], 60 p. 21 cm. [2096]

—Parere sopra il balsamo di Baldassar, e Michel Campi ... Lucca, Pellegrino Bidelli, 1639.

19 p. 22 cm. [2097]

CAMPI, MICHELE [*fl.* 1623-*ca.* 1660] *See* CAMPI, B. Baldassari, e Michel Campi 1641 [and] Nuovo discorso. 1623 [and] Parere. 1639.

CAMPO, BALTHAZAR. *See* CAMPI, Baldassar [*d. ca.* 1653]

CAMPO, MICHEL. *See* CAMPI, Michele [*fl.* 1623-*ca.* 1660]

CAMPOLONGO, EMILIO [1550-1604] Σημειωτικη; seu, Nova cognoscendi morbos methodus, ad analyseos Capivaccianae normam, ab Aemylio Campolongo ... expressa; nunc primum vero per Johannem Jessenium a Jessen, recte discentium & medentium usui, publicata. Wittebergae, Typis Laurentii Seuberlichii, 1601.

[8], 97 ll. 17 cm. [2098]

—*See* FABRICIUS, H., *ab Aquapendente.* Medicina practica. 1634.

CAMPOLONGO, OTTAVIO [*fl.* 1614] Considerationi ... intorno alla theriaca. Ove si scoprono secondo l'opinionè di Galeno, & d'altri celebri scrittori, molti gravissimi errori fin'hora commessi da coloro, che la compongono ... Venetia, Gio. Battista Bertoni, 1614.

23 ll. 18 cm. [2099]

With this is bound Mostravero, A. Risposta alle Considerationi d'Ottavio Campolongo. 1614 [i.e. 1615]

—*See* MOSTRAVERO, A. Risposta alle Considerationi d'Ottavio Campolongo. 1614 [i.e. 1615]

CAMPY, DAVID DE PLANIS. *See* PLANIS CAMPY, David de [*b.* 1589]

CAMPY, PIERRE DE PLANIS. *See* PLANIS CAMPY, Pierre de.

CANADELLE, MOYSE [16th-17th cent.] Petit traicte et familier de la peste. Contenant la description, les symptomes, & effects d'icelle, avec la methode, & remedes y requis, tant preservatifs que curatifs ... Rev. augm. et corr. de nouveau, par l'autheur. Geneve, Estienne Gamonet, 1615.

[10], 68 p.   16 cm.   **[2100]**

CANALE, FLORIANO [*fl.* 1612] De' secreti universali raccolti et sperimentati [sic] ... trattati nove. Ne' quali si hanno rimedii per tutte le infermità de' corpi humani, come anco de cavalli, bovi, & cani. Con molti secreti appertinenti all'arte chemica, agricoltura & caccie ... Brescia, Bartolomeo Fontana, 1613.

[24], 269 p.   illus.   16 cm.   **[2101]**

—[The same.] ... Venetia, Pietro Bertano, 1613.

[16], 266 p.   15 cm.   **[2102]**

—[The same.] Officina medicinale ... trattati nove. Ne' quali si hanno rimedii per tutte le infermità de' corpi humani, come anco de cavalli, bovi, & cani. Con molti secreti appartinenti all'arte chemica, agricoltura, & caccie ... Con l'aggiunta d'alcuni secreti curiosi scielti dall'horto geniale di Giulio Cesare Baricello ... Brescia, Bartolomeo Fontana, 1622.

[16], 288 p.   illus.   16 cm.   **[2103]**

—[The same.] De' secreti universali raccolti, et esperimentati ... Trattati nove. Ne' quali si hanno rimedii per tutte l'infermità de' corpi humani. Come anco de' cavalli, bovi, & cani. Con molti secreti appartenenti all'arte chemica, agricoltura, & caccie ... Venetia, Ghirardo Imberti, 1640.

[16], 304 p.   17 cm.   **[2104]**

CANAPPE, JEAN [*b.* 1495] *tr.* See GALENUS. [De simplicium medicamentorum facultatibus. French.] Deux livres des simples de Galien. 1610 [and] [Selected works. French.] Les six principaux livres de la methode therapeutique. 1605.

CANDELE, JACOB LE [*fl.* 1671] *respondent.* Disputatio medica inauguralis de atrophia ... Lugduni Batavorum, Apud viduam & heredes Joannis Elsevirii, 1671.

[16] p.   23 cm.   **[2105]**

Diss.—Leyden.

CANEPARI, PIETRO MARIA. *See* CANEPARI, Pietro Martire [*fl.* 1618]

CANEPARI, PIETRO MARTIRE [*fl.* 1618] De atramentis cujuscunque generis. Opus sane novum, hactenus a nemine promulgatum. In sex descriptiones digestum ... Londini, Excudebat J. M., impensis Jo. Martin, Ja. Alestry, Tho. Dicas, 1660.

[16], 568 p.   20 cm.   **[2106]**

CANEPARIUS, PETRUS ANTONIUS. *See* CANEPARI, Pietro Martire [*fl.* 1618]

CANEVARI, DEMETRIO [1559-1625] De primis rerum natura factarum principiis commentarius; in quo quaecunque ad corporum naturalium ortus, & interitus cognitionem desiderari possunt ... explicantur. Huic accessit commentarius alter, in quo quidquid de corporum natura factorum principiis generatim jam perquisitum, discussumque est ... Genuae, Apud Josephum Pavonem, 1626.

[12], 178 p.   33 cm.   **[2107]**

—Copy 2.   31 cm.

With this is bound *his* Ars medica. 1626.

—Morborum omnium qui corpus humanum affligunt ut decet, & ex arte curandorum accurata, & plenissima methodus ... Venetiis, Apud Robertum Meiettum, 1605.

[12], 350, [3] p.   15 cm.   **[2108]**

—[The same.] Ars medica; seu, Curandorum morborum, affectuumue praeter naturam, qui corpus humanum affligunt accurata, absolutaque methodus. Accessit Febrium curandarum exercitatio ... Genuae, Apud Josephum Pavonem, 1626 [colophon 1627]

[13], 326, [1] p.   31 cm.   **[2109]**

Bound with copy 2 of *his* De primis rerum natura factarum principiis commentarius. 1626.

CANGE, CHARLES DU FRESNE, *sieur du. See* DU CANGE, Charles Du Fresne, *sieur* [1610-1688]

CANGEMIUS DE TERRANOVA, FRANCISCUS. *See* TERRANOVA, Francesco di, *Father* [*fl.* 1658]

CANONHERIUS, PETRUS ANDREAS. *See* CANONIERI, Pietro Andrea [*d.* 1639]

CANONIERI, PIETRO ANDREA [*d.* 1639] De curiosa doctrina libri quinque ... Florentiae, Apud Volcmarium Timan, 1607.

347, [5] p.   16 cm.   **[2110]**

—Discorso del vino . . . Firenze, Volcmar Timan, 1605.

    22 p. 22 cm.   [2111]

—In septem aphorismorum Hippocratis libros, medicae, politicae, morales, ac theologicae interpretationes . . . Antverpiae, Apud Petrum & Joannem Belleros, 1617-18.

    3 v. in 2. 23 cm.   [2112]
    Includes Latin text of the Aphorismi.

CANTELMO, *Cardinal* [*fl.* 1590] *See* URBINO (DUCHY) Ordinances, local laws, etc. Bando sopra le guardie delle marine per causa di peste. 1690.

CANTEREL, ROBERT. L'Aesculape francois hymne. Par R[obert] C[anterel] P[ontoysien] R. N. Paris, Jean Libert, 1614.

    19 p. 16 cm.   [2113]
    A poem in honor of "Mr. Tournier . . . medecin & docteur en la . . . Faculté de Paris" (i.e. Jean Tournier?)

CANYVET, JEAN. *See* GANIVET, Jean [*fl.* 1431-1434]

CAPACCIO, GIULIO CESARE [*ca.* 1550-1631] Puteolana historia a Julio Caesare Capacio Neapolitanae urbis a secretis et cive conscripta. Accessit ejusdem De balneis libellus. Neapoli, Excudebat Constantinus Vitalis, 1604.

    [16], 208 p.; 88 p. illus. 24 cm.   [2114]

—La vera antichita di Pozzuolo . . . Ove con l'historia di tutte le cose del contorno, si narrano la bellezza de Posilipo, l'origine della città di Pozzuolo, Baia, Miseno, Cuma, Ischia riti, costumi . . . e quanto appartiene alle cose naturali di terme, bagni, e di tutte le miniere . . . Napoli, Gio. Giacomo Carlino e Costantino Vitale, 1607.

    [39], 386, [1] p. illus. 17 cm.   [2115]

—[The same.] . . . Roma, Filippo de' Rossi, 1652.
    [38], 384 p. illus., plates. 16 cm.   [2116]

CAPAULIS, HERCULES à [*fl.* 1665] *respondent.* Disputatio medica inauguralis de melancholia hypochondriaca . . . Lugduni Batavorum, Ex officina Petri & Cornelii Hackii, 1665.

    [16] p. 20 cm.   [2117]
    Diss.—Leyden.

CAPELLA, GALEAZZO FLAVIO [1487-1537] *See* PUTEANUS, E. Historiae Medicaeae libri duo. 1634.

CAPELLE, BERNHARD CHRISTIAN [*fl.* 1668-1670] *respondent.* Disputatio medica inauguralis de mammarum inflammatione . . . Lugduni Batavorum, Apud viduam & haeredes Joannis Elsevirii, 1670.

    [16] p. 23 cm.   [2118]
    Diss.—Leyden.

—*See* TRUMPH, J. G., *praeses.* Dissertatio medica de salivatione mercuriali. 1668.

CAPELLUTI, ROLANDO [*b. ca.* 1430] Tractatus Rolandi Capelluti . . . Parmensis de curatione pestiferorum apostematum . . . prodit ex bibliotheca Hermanni Conringii . . . Francofurti ad Moenum, Sumptibus Johannis Davidis Zunneri, 1642.

    29 p. 16 cm.   [2119]

—[The same.] *In* Salmuth, P. Observationum medicarum centuriae tres posthumae. 1648.

CAPITANI, GIUSEPPE TESTORI DE. *See* TESTORI DE CAPITANI, Giuseppe.

CAPITOULS de Toulouse. *See* TOULOUSE (CITY). Capitouls.

CAPIVACCIO, GIROLAMO [1523-1589] Medicina practica; sive, Methodus cognoscendorum, & curandorum omnium corporis humani affectuum; nunc denuo edita, & in multis juxta germanas authoris lectiones, & potissimum circa febres adaucta, atque omni diligentia absoluta. Cui adjecta sunt & reliqua, quae adhuc extant, ejusdem . . . opera omnia quae postremo in hac 3. ed. duobus tractatibus; altero quidem De foetus formatione, reliquo vero De pulsibus, nec non Expositione in primum librum Aphorismorum Hippocratis; ac De arte collegiandi, & Modo interrogandi aegros locupletata sunt, industria, ac labore Boncii Leonis . . . Venetiis, Apud haeredes Melchioris Sessae, 1601.

    [29], 175 ll.; 301 (i.e. 310) p.; [2], 12, 175 p. 32 cm.   [2120]

    Part [3] has special title page: Tractatus; de foetus formatione. Published in 1594 under title: Practica medicina.
    The first two parts are reprinted page for page from the Sessa edition of 1598.

—Opera omnia, quinque section. comprehensa, quarum I. Physiologica, II. Pathologica, III. Therapeutica, IV. Mista, V. Extranea, qua editione, tum Capivaccii plurima typis hactenus nondum vulgata in lucem proferuntur: tum depravatissimi Gallorum atque Italorum codices penitus abolentur.

Cura Johannis Hartmanni Bayeri . . . Francofurti, E Paltheniana, curante Jona Rhodio, 1603.

[20], 1051, [15] p. port. 36 cm.   [2121]
"Enarratio sectionis primae Aphorismorum Hippocratis" (p. 305-456) includes Latin text of Hippocrates.
With this is bound *his* Medendi methodus universalis. 1606.

—[The same.] . . . Hac sexta, et novissima editione ejusdem auctoris Consilia jam diu desiderata, ac alia plurima, typis hactenus nondum in lucem edita: nunc autem castigatissima in publicum . . . prolata . . . Venetiis, Apud Sessas, 1617.

[30], 910 p. 32 cm.   [2122]
Imperfect: printer's device excised from title page.
"Enarratio sectionis primae Aphorismorum Hippocratis" (p. 266-395) includes Latin text of Hippocrates.
A reprint of the 1603 Frankfurt edition edited by J. H. Beyer.

—De pulsibus tractatus. *In* Struthius, J. Ars sphygmica. 1602.

—De recta cauteriorum administratione. *In* Crato von Krafftheim, J. Consiliorum & epistolarum medicinalium . . . liber. 1620, 1671.

—Medendi methodus universalis tabulis comprehensa. In usum medicorum tum theoricorum, tum practicorum. Francofurti, E Collegio Musarum Paltheniano, 1606.

63 p. 36 cm.   [2123]

Edited by Johann Hartmann Beyer.
Bound with *his* Opera omnia. 1603.

—Practica medicina. *See* MÜNSTER, J. Discussio eorum quae ab Abrahamo Schopffio . . . scripta sunt. 1603.

—Tractatus: de foetus formatione, De pulsibus, Expositio in primum librum Aphorismorum Hippoc., De arte collegiandi, & De modo interrogandi aegros . . . Venetiis, Apud haeredes Melchioris Sessae, 1601.

[2], 12, 175 p., part 3. 32 cm. [In his Medicina practica . . . Cui adjecta sunt & reliqua, quae adhuc extant . . . opera omnia. Venetiis, 1601.   [2124]
"Expositio in primum librum Aphorismorum Hippocr." (p. [23]-164) includes Latin text of Hippocrates.

—*See* CAMPOLONGO, E. Σημειωτικη. 1601; SCHOLTZ, L. Consiliorum medicinalium . . . liber singularis. 1610 [and] Epistolarum philosophicarum: medicinalium, ac chymicarum . . . volumen. 1610.

CAPO DI VACCA, GIROLAMO. *See* CAPIVACCIO, Girolamo [1523-1589]

CAPOA, CESARE DI. *See* CAPOA, L. di. Lezioni intorno alla natura delle mofete. 1683.

CAPOA, LIONARDO DI [1617-1695] Lezioni intorno alla natura delle mofete . . . Napoli, Salvatore Castaldo, 1683.
[16], 179 (i.e. 176), [15] p. 22 cm.   [2125]
With a dedicatory epistle by Cesare di Capoa.

—Parere . . . divisato in otto ragionamenti, ne' quali partitamente narrandosi l'origine, e'l progresso della medicina, chiaramente l'incertezza della medesima si fa manifesta. Napoli, Antonio Bulifon, 1681.
[8], 658, [22] p. 26 cm.   [2126]

—[The same.] . . . 2. impr. Napoli, Giacomo Raillard, 1689.
2 parts in 1 v. 23 cm.   [2127]
Part [2] has special title page: Ragionamenti . . . intorno alla incertezza de' medicamenti.

—[The same.] . . . 3. impr. . . . Napoli, Giacomo Raillard, 1695.
2 parts in 1 v. 23 cm.   [2128]
Part [2] has special title page.

—[English tr.] The uncertainty of the art of physick, together with an account of the innumerable abuses practised by the professors of that art . . . Also divers contests between the Greeks and Arabians concerning its authors . . . Made English by J[ohn] L[ancaster] Gent. London, Printed by Fr. Clark for Thomas Malthus, 1684.
[9], 102 p. 15 cm.   [2129]
Imperfect: translator's dedicatory letter to Robert Boyle (sig. A?) wanting; supplied in photocopy.
Translation of Parere . . . Ragionamento primo.

[—] [The same.] The conclave of physicians, the second part; further detecting their intrigues, frauds and plots against their patients. London, William Bonbridge, 1684.
[9], 102 p. 15 cm.   [2130]
Another issue of The uncertainty of the art of physick, printed by Fr. Clark in the same year, with new title page.

—*See* CORNELIO, T. Progymnasmata physica. 1663, 1688.

CAPON, John. The new booke of Mr. John Capons wits, dedicated to all witty folkes. [n. p., 16 — ?]

4 p. 16 cm. [2131]

Bound with In speculo teipsum contemplare Dr. Black. Edinburgh, 1692.

CAPPELLA, Giovanni Antonio [*fl.* 1646] De hydrophobia; seu, De pavore aquae in rabie problema perdifficillimum . . . Neapoli, Matthaeus Nuccius, 1646.

[12], 87, [1] p. 21 cm. [2132]

CAPPOCCI, Francesco [*fl.* 1686] Artis medicae praxeos de morbis mulierum . . . Vicetiae, Typis Jo. Bernii, 1686.

[8], 270 p. 22 cm. [2133]
"De medicamentis usualibus": p. [183]-270.

CAPRA, Galeazzo Flavio. *See* Capella, Galeazzo Flavio [1487-1537]

CAPRILI, Pio Enea [*d.* 1593] Libri duo. Quorum primus est de febribus putridis in genere; alter in specie. In quibus praeter exactissimam harum febrium doctrinam, quamplures etiam Hippocratis, Galeni, & aliorum auctorum controversiae, locique difficiles explicantur . . . Ed. alt. emend. Patavii, Typis & impensis Pauli Frambotti, 1643.

[56], 328 p. 22 cm. [2134]

CAPUA, Leonardo da. *See* Capoa, Lionardo di [1617-1695]

CARACCIOLO, Pasqual [16th cent.] La gloria del cavallo, opera . . . divisa in dieci libri: ne' quali, oltre gli ordini appartenenti alla cavalleria, si descrivono tutti i particolari, che sono necessarii nell'allevare, custodire, maneggiare, & curar cavalli . . . Di nuova ricorretta, a ristampata: & . . . aggiuntevi le postille, e tre libri di Gio. Antonio Cito . . . ne' quali si tratta delle infirmita, che 'avvengono al cavallo, & al bue, co' rimedii di esse . . . Venetia, Bernardo Giunti, Gio. Battista Ciotti, & compagni, 1608.

[68], 969, [1] p.; [8], 136 p. 20 cm. [2135]
Part [2] has special title page: Del conoscere le infermita, che avvengono al cavallo et la bue, co' rimedii à ciascheduna di esse di Gio. Antonio Cito . . . libri tre . . .

CARANTA, Giacomo [*fl.* 1623] Decadum medicophysicarum liber primus [-secundus] de natura auri arte facti, & num sit pharmacum cordiale . . . Saviliani, Apud Christophorum Strabellam, 1623.

[40], 288, [2] p. 21 cm. [2136]
". . . Liber secundus de morsu canis rabidi . . .": p. 121-231; ". . . Liber unicus de natura visionis . . .": p. [233]-288, have special title pages.

—Viri nati cum uno teste tantum, & alterius sine testibus scroto prorsus vacuo, num ad generationem sint idonei. Judicium. Cunei, Apud Christophorum Strabellam, 1624.

38, [2] p. 21 cm. [2137]

CARANZA, Alfonso a. *See* Carranza, Alonso [*fl.* 1628-1636]

CARAVAJAL, Juan [*fl.* 1621] *See* Rossell, J. F. Ad sex libros Galeni De differentiis. 1627.

CARBASIUS, Thomas [*fl.* 1608-1610] *See* Platter, F. [1536-1614] Felix Platerus . . . decreto. 1610.

CARCANO, Francesco [*ca.* 1500-1580] Dell'arte del strucciero con il modo di conoscere, e medicare falconi, astori, e sparavieri, e tutti gli uccelli di rapina . . . Milano, Filippo Ghisolfi, 1645.

82, [2] p. illus. 15 cm. [2138]

CARCEUS, Márton [*fl.* 1670-1671] Index materiae medicae; seu, Medicamentorum, in Francisci de Le Boe Sylvii, Praxeos medicae libri primo, tam in formulis, quam extra ipsas laudatorum . . . Lugduni-Batavorum, Apud viduam Joh. Carpenterii, 1671.

[96] p. 14 cm. [2139]
Bound with Le Boë, F. de. Praxeos medicae idea nova liber primus. 1671.

—*See* Le Boë, F. de. Praxeos medicae idea nova liber primus. 1671, 1672.

CARCEUS DE KARCZAGH-UJSZÁLLÁSA, Martinus. *See* Carceus, Márton [*fl.* 1670-1671]

CARDALUCIUS, Johannes Hiskias. *See* Cardilucius, Johannes Hiskias [17th cent.]

CARDAN, Jerome. *See* Cardano, Girolamo [1501-1576]

CARDANO, Girolamo [1501-1576] Opera omnia: tam hactenus excusa, hic tamen aucta & emendata; quam nunquam alias visa, ac primum ex auctoris ipsius autographis eruta: cura Caroli Sponii . . . Tomus primus [-decimus] . . . Lugduni, Sumptibus Joannis Antonii Huguetan et Marci Antonii Ravaud, 1663.

10 v. port., illus. 36 cm. [2140]

"Vita Cardani . . . Per Gabrielem Naudaeum": p. [15–26], vol. i.; "In primam primi Hasen commentariorum liber primus [-secundus]": p. 462–567, vol. 9, includes text of Avicenna in Latin.

Hippocratic commentaries, including the Latin texts: Commentaria in librum De alimento, vol. 7, p. 356–515; Commentariorum in librum De aëre, aquis et locis libri VIII, Commentariorum in Aphorismos libri VII, Commentariorum in Prognosticon libri IV, vol. 8 ([4], 806 p.); In librum De septimestri partu commentarius, vol. 9, p. 1–47.

—Contradicentium medicorum libri duo, quorum primus centum & octo, alter vero totidem disputationes continet. Addita praeterea ejusdem autoris De sarza parilia, De cina radice, ejusque usu, cum Consilio pro dolore vago. Accessere itidem Jacobi Peletarii Contradictiones ex Lacuna desumptae, cum ejusdem Axiomatibus . . . Marpurgi, Typis Pauli Egenolphi, 1607.

    [32], 1134 p. 16 cm.   **[2141]**

—De propria vita liber . . . Adjecto hac 2. ed. De praeceptis ad filios libello. Amstelaedami, Apud Joannem Ravesteinium, 1654.

    [70], 288 p. 14 cm.   **[2142]**

Colophon: Goudae, Typis Guilielmi vander Hoeve, 1654.
"Gabrielis Naudaei de Cardano judicium": p. [6–66]
With this are bound: Roraio, G. Quod animalia bruta ratione utantur melius homine. 1654.—Pereira, B. De magia. 1612.

—De subtilitate libri XXI. Jam postremo, ab authore plusquam mille locis illustrati, nonnullis etiam cum additionibus. Addita insuper Apologia adversus calumniatorem, qua vis horum librorum aperitur . . . Basileae, Per Sebastianum Henricpetri [1611]

    [80], 1148, [4] p. illus., port. 18 cm. **[2143]**

—De utilitate ex adversis capienda libri IV. Franikerae, Excudit Idzardus Balck, 1648.

    [20], 879, [20] p. 16 cm.   **[2144]**

Engraved title page.
Edited by Johannes Antonides van der Linden.

—[The same.] . . . Amstelodami, Apud Joannem Ravesteinium, 1672.

    [32], 870, [10] p. 17 cm.   **[2145]**

Engraved title page.

—De venenis libri tres. Patavii, Apud Paulum Frambottum, 1653.

    [8], 132, [11] p. illus. 23 cm.   **[2146]**

—In Aphorismos Hippocratis commentaria luculentissima cum Graeco textu. Accedit ejusdem

—De providentia temporum liber. Pavia, Apud Paulum Frambottum, 1653.

    [8], 634, [70] p. illus. 24 cm.   **[2147]**

Edited by Paulus Frambottus.
Includes Greek and Latin text of Hippocrates' Aphorismi.

—Metoposcopia libris tredecim, et octingentis faciei humanae eiconibus complexa. Cui accessit Melampodis De naevis corporis tractatus, Graece & Latine nunc primum editus. Interprete Claudio Martino Laurenderio . . . Lutetiae Parisiorum, Apud Thomam Jolly, 1658.

    [8], viii, 225, [2] p. illus. 34 cm. **[2148]**

—[French tr.] La metoposcopie . . . Comprise en treize livres, et huit cens figures de la face humaine. A laquelle a esté adjousté, le traicté Des marques naturelles du corps, par Melampus . . . Le tout traduit en françois, par . . . C. M. De Laurendiere . . . Paris, Thomas Jolly, 1658.

    [8], viii, 225, [2] p. illus. 34 cm. **[2149]**

—[German tr.] In Höchstfürtreflichtes chiromantisch- und physiognomisches Klee-Blat. 1695.

—Opuscula medica senilia in quatuor libros tributa, quorum I. De dentibus. II. De rationali curandi ratione. III. De facultatibus medicamentorum, praecipue purgantium. IV. De morbo regio. Omnia nunc primum ex MS. Bibliothecae Romanae in lucem data . . . Lugduni, Sumptibus Laurenti Durand, 1638.

    [32], 531, [18] p. 18 cm.   **[2150]**

Edited by Leone Allacci.

—Podagrae encomium. In Lösel, J. De podagra tractatus. 1639; Admiranda rerum admirabilium encomia. 1666, 1677.

—[Dutch tr.] Lof voor 't podagra. In Veeler wonderens wonderbaarelijck lof. 1664.

—Proxeneta; seu, De prudentia civili liber; recens in lucem protractus, vel e tenebris erutus. Lugd. Bat., Ex Officina Elzeviriana, 1627.

    [24], 767 p. 13 cm.   **[2151]**

Engraved title page.

—[Excerpts.] In Lancetta, T. Raccolta medica. 1645.

—, tr. See BEVERWIJCK, J. van. Schat der ongesontheyt. 1649.

—*See* BEVERWIJCK, J. van. DD. virorum epistolae et responsa. 1665 [and] Epistolicae quaestiones, cum doctorum responsis. 1644 [and] Schatz der Gesundheit. 1671 [and] Wercken der genees-konste. 1664, 1672.

—*as subject. See* SCALIGER, J. C. Exotericarum exercitationum liber XV de subtilitate. 1620.

CARDELLINO, VITTORE. De origine foetus libri duo. In quibus praeter caetera luculentis Graecorum auctoritatibus calidum a calore dirimitur ... Vincentiae, Apud haeredes Dominici Amadei, 1628.

131, [3] p. 25 cm. [2152]

CARDILUCIUS, JOHANNES HISKIAS [17th cent.] Cunei ad duros morborum nodos; oder, Keile zu den harten Knorren der Kranckheiten. Das ist: wie man auss den Metallen und Mineralien solche Essentzen könne zurichten, da man mit einer einigen allerhand wiederspenstige, und von Kräutern uncurirliche Suchten bändigen kan ... Auch wie dergleichen Panacea auss mehr als einem Subjecto, und auf was Weise solche zu machen ... [n. p.] 1670.

[10], 81 p. 18 cm. [2153]

With this is bound Carrichter, G. Kräuter-und Artzney-Buchs. 1670.

—Heilsame Artzney-Kräffte des nürnbergischen Wild-Bades, wie nemlich solche herfliessen von einer darinn enthaltenen roten solarischen und weissen lunarischen Mineral-Tinctur, und nach solcher tragenden zweyfachen Signatur dienlich seyn zu den fürnemsten Gebresten des Geblüts, und der weissen Leibs-Safftigkeit, nebst dessen rechtem Gebrauch und mitlauffenden andern kräfftigen Artzneyen ... Nürnberg, In Verlegung Wolfgang Moritz Endters und Johann Andreae Endters seel. Söhne, 1681.

[24], 124, [7] p. 14 cm. [2154]

—Historische Exempel, was auf die meisten Cometen von Christi Geburt hero erfolget, woraus erhellet, dass nicht ohne Ursach in dem Cardilucianischen Pest-Tractätlein unter die Ursachen der Pest auch die Cometen geachtet worden. Nebst einem Discours über den zu End des 1680sten Jahrs erschienenen sehr langgeschweiften Cometen. Bey anitziger zweyten Edition erwehnten Tractätleins zu einem zweyten Anhange desselben mit beygefüget von dessen Authore. Nürnberg, In Verlegung Wolfgang Moritz Endters und Johann Andreae Endter s. Söhne, 1681.

140 p. 14 cm. [2155]

Bound with (as issued?) *his* Tractat von der leidigen Seuche der Pestilentz. 1681.

—Kurtz verfasseter Bericht, von der jetzigen grassirenden ansteckenden und tödtlichen Lager-Seuche, oder Ungerischen Flecken-und Pedecken-Sucht, welche fast bey allen Kriegs-Zügen unter den Soldaten entstehet ... Nebst einem umständlichen Tractat von der Rothen Ruhr ... Nürnberg, In Verlegung Wolffgang Moritz Endters, 1684.

[24], 215 p. 15 cm. [2156]

—Tractat von der leidigen Seuche der Pestilentz ... Aus eigener bey persönlicher Gegenwart in infectis locis, nemlich An. 1663. bis 64. in Holland, und Anno 1666. bis 67. am Reinstrom genommenen Observation ... publiciret ... Nürnberg, In Verlegung Wolffgang Moritz Endters, und Johann Andreae Endters sel. Söhnen, 1679.

[14], 90 p. 14 cm. [2157]

—[The same.] ... Anitzo ... vermehret und zum Andernmahl ausgefertiget ... Nürnberg, In Verlegung Wolffgang Moritz Endters und Johann Andreae Endters sel. Söhne, 1681.

[26], 105 p. 14 cm. [2158]

With this are bound (as issued?) *his:* Anhang über das ... Tractätlein von der Pestilentz. 1681; *his* Extract aus Johann Hiskiae Cardilucii ... Tractat und dessen Anhang von der Pestilentz. [1680]; *his* Historische exempel. 1681.

—Appendix; oder, Anhang uber das ... Cardilucianische Tractätlein, von der Pestilentz, darinn die jenige Sachen in gedachtem Tractätlein, welche unverschuldeter Massen von etlichen haben wollen zweifflich gemacht werden, hierinn unwidersprechlich noch mit mehrem erwiesen, und weiter unterschiedliche ... Dinge treulich communiciret werden ... Nürnberg, In Verlegung Wolffgang Moritz Endters und Johann Andreae Endters sel. Söhnen, 1679.

121, [10] p. 14 cm. [2159]

Includes an answer to Johann Paul Wurfbain concerning his letter on the same subject.

—Anhang über das ... Cardilucianische Tractätlein, von der Pestilentz, darinn die jenige Sachen in gedachtem Tractätlein, welche unverschuldeter Massen, von etlichen haben wollen zweifflich gemacht werden, hierinn unwidersprechlich noch mit mehrem erwiesen ... und itzo in dieser zweyten Edition abermahl mit mercklicher Vermehr- und

Verbesserung ausgefertiget worden, nebst angehengter gründlichen Antwort auf Herrn D. Wurffbeins wider ged. Pest-Tractätlein geschriebene Epistel. Durch Joh. Hiskiam Cardilucium ... Nürnberg, In Verlegung Wolffgang Moritz Endters und Johann Andreae Endters sel. Söhne, 1681.

131, [22] p. 14 cm. [2160]

Bound with (as issued?) *his* Tractat von der leidigen Seuche der Pestilentz. 1681.

—Extract aus ... Tractat und dessen Anhang von der Pestilentz, darinnen die Natur, Kenzeichen, Praeservirung und Cur, derselben auffs gründlichste und gewisseste zu sehen ... Berlin, Verlegts Rupertus Völcker [1680?]

[72] p. 14 cm. [2161]

Preface dated 1680.
Bound with (as issued?) *his* Tractat von der leidigen Seuche der Pestilentz. 1681.

—Zodiacus medicus. *In* Hartmann, J. Officina sanitatis. 1677.

—*ed.* and *tr.* Neuaufgerichtete Stadt- und Land-Apotheke. Darinn zuforderst vorgetragen werden die ... Artzney-Schrifften dess deutschen Hippocratis nemlich dess ... Herrn Carrichters ... nebenst beygefügtem deutschen Alphabet der Kranckheiten ... samt angehengtem Tractat von Bereitigung einer Panaceae oder universal-Artzney. Da denn über diss bey itziger neuren oder zweyten Edition noch darzu kommt ein vollständiges Diaet-Buch ... Alles ... verfasset, und aufs neue mit vieler Vermehr- und Verbesserung zum Druck verordnet von Johanne Hiskia Cardilucio ... Nürnberg, In Verlegung Wolfgang Moritz Endters und Johann Andreae Endters seligen Erben, 1673-80 [v. 1, 1677]

5 v. front., illus. 18 cm. [2162]

Imperfect: title page and all after sig. 2Y7 (Turbit in index) of v. [5] wanting.
Vols. 3-4 have added engraved title pages. Vols. 2-4 (1st ed.?) lack edition statement.
Vol. 2 has title: Neuer Stadt- und Land-Apothecken zweyter Tomus, darinn dess obristen Medici und Naturalisten Hippocratis Coi, seine ... Aphorismi oder artzneyische Erfahrungs-Sprüche verhochteutschet ... Mit angehengtem Compendio Medicinae Hippocratico, darinn die itztübliche Praxis der Artzney-Kunst, durch gedachte Aphorismos, und hinwieder solche Aphorismi durch itzige Praxin medicam illustrirt ... werden ... Nebenst Untermeng- und Beyfügung vieler geheimen Experimenten ... Nürnberg, In Verlegung Johann Andreae und Wolfgang Endters dess Jüngern seel. Erben, 1673. Includes "Aphorismorum Hippocratis liber primus [-octavus] Das erste [-achte] Buch der

Erfahrungs-Sprüche Hippocratis" (p. 1-406) in Latin (mainly following Niccolò Leoniceno's version) and in German (translated by Cardilucius).
Vol. 3 has title: Ehren-Krone der Artzney; oder Der neuen Stadt- und Land-Apothecken dritter und fürnemster Tomus ... Nürnberg, 1674.
Vol. 4 has title: Artzneyische Wasser- und Signatur-Kunst; oder, Beschreibung der fürnehmsten teutschen Saur- und Gesundheit-Brunnen ... Gestellet zu einem vierdten Tomo, Der Stadt- und Land-Apotheken ... Nürnberg, 1680.
Vol. [5] is described in the editor's Vorrede as a new "Anbau oder Anhang ... über den ersten und andern Tomum." Includes "D. Barthol. Carrichters Bericht, von den vier Materien der vier Geister" (p. 1-48)—"Clavis; oder, Schlüssel über den Carrichterischen Tractat von den vier Materien ... von Joh. Hiskia Cardilucio" (p. 49-483)—"Hippocratis ... Prognosticorum libri tres. Das ist: Hippocratis ... Drey Bücher von den Vorherverkündigungen ... aus dem Griechischen verhochdeutschet, und über alle Aussprüche dess Authoris, helle deutliche Ausleg- und Erklärung gestellet: von Joh. Hisk. Cardilucio" (p. [484]-704) in Latin and German, with commentary in German.

—*See* Croll, O. Königlicher chymischer und artzneyischer Palast. 1684.

—, *ed.* Magnalia medico-chymica; oder, Die höchste Artzney-und Feuerkünstige Geheimnisse, wie nemlich mit dem Circulato majori & minori oder dem Universal aceto mercuriali, und spiritu vini tartarisato die herrlichsten Artzneyen zum langen Leben und Heilung der unheilsamen Kranckheiten zu machen; zwar aus Paracelsi Handschrift schon im vorigen Seculo ausgangen ... itzo aber aufs neue verhochdeutschet, und ... erläutert, nebenst beygefügtem Hauptschlüssel aller Hermetischen Schrifften ... publiciret von Johanne Hiskia Cardilucio ... Nürnberg, In Verlegung Wolffgang Moritz Endters und Johann Andreae Endters sel. Erben, 1676.

[48], 409, [30] p.; 32 p. illus. 17 cm.

[2163]

The authorship of the first 2 books is attributed to Joannes de Rupescissa.
Contains (p. [297]-399) Eirenaeus Philalethes' Introitus apertus. Cardilucius' supplement (32 p. at end) corrects errors in the Latin edition from the English edition which he has consulted. Half title to this section reads: Appendix Introitus aperti ad occlusum regis palatium ... Zum Druck befördert durch J. H. C.
Sudhoff 405.

—*See* Le Fèvre, N. Neuvemehrter chymischer Handleiter. 1685; Wurfbain, J. P. Epistola. 1679?

—, *tr. See* [Philalethes, E.] Der vortreffliche Tractat. 1676.

CARDONNEL, Pierre de [*d. 1667*] *tr. See* Le Fèvre, N. A compleat body of chymistry. 1664, 1670.

CARDOSO, Fernando of Celorico. *See* Cardoso, Isaac [*ca. 1604–1680*]

CARDOSO, Fernando Rodriguez [*d. 1608*] Tractatus absolutissimus … de sex rebus non naturalibus, primum quidem ab autore ipso editus, nunc vero … vitiis emendatus … annotatiunculis in margine illustratus … in lucem denuo emissus per Petrum Uffenbachium … Francofurti ad Moenum, Typis Pauli Jacobi, impensis Jacobi de Zetter, 1620.

[16], 389, [10] p.   21 cm.   **[2164]**

CARDOSO, Isaac [*ca. 1604–1680*] Philosophia libera in septem libros distributa: in quibus omnia, quę ad philosophum naturalem spectant, methodice colliguntur, & accurate disputantur … Venetiis, Bertanorum sumptibus, 1673.

[16], 758, [20] p.   34 cm.   **[2165]**

CARDOSO, Isaac Fernando. *See* Cardoso, Isaac [*ca. 1604–1680*]

CARDOSO DE SEQUEIRA, Gaspar [16th–17th cent.] Thesouro de prudentes, novamente tirado alus … Contem em si quatro livros, cuja relaçao vay, no seguinte prologo. Coimbra, Nicolao Carualho, 1612.

[8], 218 ll.   illus.   20 cm.   **[2166]**

CARDULLO, Giovanni Domenico [*fl. 1637*] Teriaca d'Andromaco composta publicamente in Messina … Ove tutti li semplici di quest'antidoto sotillmente s'esaminano, si dichiarano, e s'approvano. Messina, La vedoua di Gio. Francesco Bianco, 1637.

[8], 64 p.   21 cm.   **[2167]**

CARE, Henry [*1646–1688*] *tr. See* Sennert, D. Practical physick. 1679.

CARELLI, Vincenzo [*fl. 1646*] De auri essentia, et ejus facultate in medendis, ac sanandis morbis compendium … Venetia, Sub signo Minervae, 1646.

76 p.   17 cm.   **[2168]**

CARERA, Antonio Pricivallo [*fl. 1652*] Le confusioni de medici. Opera di Rafaello Carrara [pseud.] … Nella quale si scuoprono gl'errori, & gl'inganni de medici. Milano, Gio. Pietro Cardi, 1652.

[8], 191 p.   23 cm.   **[2169]**

—*See* Peruca, R. Apologia. 1655.

CAREW, Richard [*1555–1620*] *tr. See* Huarte de San Juan, J. Examen de ingenios. The examination of mens wits. 1604, 1616.

CAREY, Henry, *2nd Earl of Monmouth. See* Monmouth, Henry, *2nd Earl of* [*1596–1661*]

CARIE, Walter. *See* Cary, Walter [*fl. 1580–1611*]

CARITA, Peter [*fl. 1698*] *respondent. See* Winther, J. G., *praeses.* Dissertat. inauguralem medicam de rabie … subjicit … P. C. 1698.

CARL, Johann Samuel [*1676–1757*] *respondent. See* Hoffmann, F. [*1660–1742*] *praeses.* Analysin chymico-medicam reguli antimonii medicinalis … exponet. 1698.

CARLIER, Samuel [*fl. 1631?*] *respondent. See* Burgersdijck, F. P. *praeses.* Collegium physicum. 1642.

CARLO, *called* Il gran villano. Compendio di avvertimenti per conservarsi sani, con alcuni segreti medicinali. Col trattato della fisonomia dell' huomo, e della donna, e sua condizione, & alcuni rimedi de' mali, che vengono a' cavalli, & a' bovi. Dato in luce da me Carlo detto il gran villano … Firenze, Vincenzio Vangelisti, 1678.

24 p.   15 cm.   **[2170]**

CARLO BORROMEO, *Saint* [*1538–1584*] De cura pestilentiae. *In* Catholic Church. Province of Milan. Constitutiones, et decreta sex provincialium synodorum Mediolanensium. 1603.

—[Italian tr.] Della cura della peste. Instruttione di S. Carlo, cardinal di Santa Prassede, & arcivescovo di Milano. Registrata nel quinto suo concilio provinciale, già stampata in latino, hora tradotta nella volgar lingua. Vicenza, Francesco Grossi, 1630.

[4], 75 p.   20 cm.   **[2171]**

—*See* Bisciola, P. Relatione verissima del progresso della peste di Milano. 1630.

CARMENI, Daniele [*fl. 1621–1642*] De medendi methodo libri sex … Bononię, Typis Nicolai Thebaldini, 1636.

[12], 350, [26] p.   30 cm.   **[2172]**
Engraved title page.

CARMINA gratulatoria, in honorem ... D. Johannis Lubberti ... cum in Academia Lugd. Bat. post habitam honorifice de podagra & lue venerea disputationem publicam 7. Aprilis 1655. med. doct. renuntiaretur. Lugduni Batavorum, Apud Johannem Elsevirium, 1655.

[12] p.   22 cm.   [2173]

Bound with Lubbert, J. Disputatio medica. 1655.

CARNEAU, Célestin. See Carneau, Étienne [1610-1671]

CARNEAU, Étienne [1610-1671] La stimmimachie; ou, Le grand combat des medecins modernes touchant l'usage de l'antimoine. Poëme historicomique, dedié a messieurs les medecins de la Faculté de Paris. Par le sieur C[élestin] C[arneau] Paris, Jean Paslé, 1656.

[16], 131, [1] p.   17 cm.   [2174]

CARNEVALE, Giovanni Battista [fl. 1620] De epidemico strangulatorio affectu, in Neapolitanam urbem grassante, & per regna Neapolis, & Siciliae vagante ... Neapoli, Apud Scipionem Bonium, 1620.

[16], 135 p.   21 cm.   [2175]

CAROCCI, Francesco. See Falcinelli, B. Apologia. 1646.

CAROLUS JOANNES A JESU [1640-1686] ed. See Borelli, G. A. De motu animalium. 1680, 1685.

CAROLUS, Jean [fl. 1671] respondent. See Le Boë, F. de, praeses. Disputatio medica de venae-sectione. 1671.

CAROLUS, Theodor [fl. 1683-1684] respondent. See Camerarius, E. R., praeses. Valetudinarii senilis lineas speciales ... subjicit. 1684.

CARON, Ludovicus. See Garon, Louis [ca. 1580-ca. 1636]

CARON, Philippe [1690] respondent. See Hodencq, M. de. Quaestio medica. 1690.

CARPI, Jacopo. See Berengario, Jacopo [ca. 1460-1530]

CARPINETO, Tarquinio [d. 1616] De gutta; sive, Juncturarum dolore quem arthritim dicunt ... Patavii, Apud Franciscum Bolzettam, 1609.

[4], 38 ll.   20 cm.   [2176]

CARPZOV, Samuel [fl. 1680] respondent. See Riemer, J., praeses. Duella mulierum. 1680.

CARQUET, Isaac. See Cattier, Isaac [fl. 1637-1665]

CARR, Richard [1651-1706] Epistolae medicinales variis occasionibus conscriptae ... Londini, Impensis Stafford Anson, 1691.

[12], 200, [6] p.   16 cm.   [2177]

CARR, William [fl. ca. 1655-1657] tr. See Rivière, L. The universal body of physick. 1657.

CARRANZA, Alonso [fl. 1628-1636] Diatriba. Super primore temporum doctrina, in libris Pat. Dionys. Petavii, novissime prostantibus, contenta ... Madridii, Ex typographia Francisci Martinez, 1628.

68 p.   29 cm.   [2178]

Bound with (as issued) his Disputatio. 1628.

—Disputatio de vera humani partus naturalis et legitimi de signatione ... In qua de hominis conceptu: animatione: efformatione ... et superfoetato agitur ... Madridii, Auctoris impensis, ex typographia Francisci Martinez, 1628.

[62], 684, [68] p.   port.   29 cm.   [2179]

Added engraved title page.

With this is bound (as issued) his Diatriba. 1628.

—Tractatus novus ... de partu naturali et legitimo: ubi controversiae juridicae, philologicae, philosophicae, medicae discutiuntur, ad fori usum & praxim. De partus conceptione, formatione ... Cui propter argumenti similitudinem, additae sunt Duae exercitationes Caroli Annibalis Fabroti antecessoris aqui-sextiensis, de tempore humani partus, & de numero puerperii. Item ejusdem Alphonsi a Carranza Diatriba, super prima temporum doctrina, adversus Dionysium Petavium, ubi agitur de anno Hebraeorum, Aegyptiorum, Graecorum, Romanorum. Genevae, Sumptib. Joann. de Tournes et Jacobi de la Pierre, 1629.

[59], 734, [54] p.; 31 p.; 78 p.   24 cm. [2180]

Part [2] and [3] have special title pages.

—[The same.] Tractatus juridicus & practicus de partu ... Cum Diatriba ejusdem, super primore temporum doctrina, in libris Pat. Dionysii Petavii, novissime prostantibus, contenta: ubi agitur de anno Hebraeorum, Aegyptiorum, Graecorum, & Romanorum. Additae insuper Caroli Annibalis

Fabroti ... Exercitationes duae: 1a. de tempore humani partus, 2a de numero puerperii. Coloniae, Sumptibus Joannis de Tournes & Jacobi de la Pierre, 1629.

[59], 734, [54] p.; 31 p.; 78 p.   24 cm.   [2181]

Part [2] and [3] have special title pages with imprint: Genevae ... Reissue of Tractatus novus ... de partu naturali et legitimo ... Genevae, 1629, with new title page.

—[The same.] ... Coloniae Allobrogum, Ex typographia Jacobi Stoer, 1630.

[60], 734, [54] p.; 31 p.; 78 p.   24 cm.   [2182]

Part [2] and [3] have half-titles.
Different setting of type.

CARRARA, Rafaello, *pseud. See* Carera, Antonio Pricivallo [*fl.* 1652]

CARRERO, Pedro Garcia. *See* Garcia Carrero, Pedro [16th–17th cent.]

CARRETTO, Nicolas Cevoli, *marquis del. See* Cevoli, Nicola, *marquis del Carretto* [*fl.* 1696]

CARRICHTER, Bartholomäus [1507–1573] Horn dess Heyls menschlicher Blödigkeit; oder, Gross Kräuter Buch ... Darinn die Kräuter dess Teutschlands ... beschrieben ... Hier ist zu Ende beygefügt das menschliche Kräuter-Bild, nach denen zwölff himmlischen Zeichen und vier elementarischen Complexionen auff die innerliche und äusserliche Glieder dess menschlichen Leibes gerichtet: zusammen getragen auss obgedachten Auctoris Schrifften von Theophilo Krafften ... Franckfurt am Mayn, In Verlegung Thomae Matthiae Götzens sel. Erben, 1673.

[35], 374, [15] p.   fold. ll., illus. 21 cm.   [2183]

Imperfect: folded leaf of text inserted before sig. b3, wanting.
Edited by Michael Toxites.

—Kräuter und Artzeneybuchs erster [-dritter] Theil, in welchem begriffen; unter welchem Zeichen Zodiaci, auch in welchem Gradu ein jedes Kraut stehe; wie dieselben im menschlichen Leibe, und zu allen Schäden zu bereiten, auch zu welcher Zeit sie zu colligieren seyn. Darbey ein gründlicher Bericht, Clavis oder Schlüssel über gedachtes Kräuter und Artzneybüchlein ... Nürnberg, Gedruckt und verlegt durch Jeremiam Dümler, 1652.

3 parts in 1 v.   17 cm.   [2184]

Various pagings. Each part has special title page. Part 3 has title and imprint: ... Kräuter unnd Artzeneybuchs dritter unnd letzter Theil, genande Der Teutschen Speisskammer ... Nürnberg, Getruckt und verlegt durch Simon Halbmayern, 1631. Also published separately with same imprint under title: ... Tractat der Teutschen Speisskammer genannt ... Cf. BMC, vol. 32 (1941) col. 991.
Edited by Michael Toxites.

—Kräuter-und Artzney-Buchs dritter und letzter Theil, genandt Der Teutschen Speisskammer; das ist, Kurtze Beschreibung dess jenigen, was bey den Teutschen, so wohl die tägliche Nahrung der Gesunden, als die Auffenthaltung krancker Menschen betreffend, in gemeinem Gebrauch ist ... [n. p.] 1670.

[10], 256, [16] p.   18 cm.   [2185]

Bound with Cardilucius, J. H. Cunei ad duros morborum nodos. 1670.

—[Von gründtlicher Heylung der zauberischen Schäden. Latin.] *In* Mercklin, G. A. Sylloge physicomedicinalium casuum incantationi vulgo adscribi solitorum. 1698.

—*See* Cardilucius, J. H., *ed.* and *tr.* Neuaufgerichtete Stadt- und Land-Apotheke. 1673–80.

CARRIÓN, Manuel Ramírez de. *See* Ramírez de Carrión, Manuel [1584–1650]

CARRONUS, Jacob, *ed. See* Gesner, K. Historiae animalium liber primus [-liber V] 1617–1621 [v. 1, 1620]

CARSTEN, Karl Gottlieb [*b.* 1664] *respondent. See* Wedel, G. W., *praeses.* Disputatio inauguralis medica de bulimo. 1691.

—*See* Crause, R. W. Collegii Medici decanus ... Rudolfus Guilielmus Crausius ... lectori benevolo S. P. D. 1691.

CARTA que escrivio un medico Christiano, que estava curando en Antiberi, à un cardenal de Roma, sobre la bebida del cahuè, ò cafè. [n. p., not before 1617]

4 p.   33 cm.   [2186]

The unidentified author quotes Prosper Alpini's De medicina Aegyptiorum (1591) and mentions Alimech, ambassador of sultan Mustafa. (Mustafa I (?), 1617–18, 1622–23)

CARTE, Renato delle. *See* Descartes, René [1596–1650]

CARTESIUS, Renatus. *See* Descartes, René [1596–1650]

CARVINUS, Joannes [*fl.* 1558] De sanguine dialogi VII, omnibus medicinam cum honore & aegrorum usu facturis lectu pernecessarii. Hanoviae, Typis Wechelianis, apud Claudium Marnium & haeredes Joan. Aubrii, 1605.

24, 258, [1] p.   illus.   14 cm.   **[2187]**
A reprint of the 1562 edition.

CARY, Walter [*fl.* 1580-1611] Caries farewell to physicke. First published in the yeere 1587. and now, in 1611. reviewed and augmented. The VI. ed., with a speciall caveat to the reader ... London, Companie of Stationers, 1611.

[8], 88 (i.e. 86) p.   15 cm.   **[2188]**
"The hammer for the stone: so named, for that it sheweth the most excellent remedie that ever was knowne for the same: devised by Walter Carie ... London, Humfrey Lownes, 1611" (p. [65]-88) has special title page.
STC 4732.

CARYSTIUS, Diocles. *See* Diocles Carystius.

CARYSTUS, Antigonus of. *See* Antigonus, of Carystus [3d cent. B.C.]

CASALENO, Giovanni Antonio [*fl.* 1605] Disputatio. De secanda vena in pleuritide revulsionis gratia, adversus medicos Francavillenses. Venetiis, Apud Jo. Baptistam Ciottum, 1605.

124 (i.e. 130), [2] p.   21 cm.   **[2189]**
Edited by Lucio Scarano.
Bound with copy 2 of Anselmi, A. Gerocomica. 1606.

CASAUBON, Isaac [1559-1614] *ed. See* Aristoteles. Τὰ σωζόμενα. Operum ... nova editio. 1605 [1606]

—*tr. See* Theophrastus. Θεοφράστον ... ᾽άπαντα. Theophrasti ... Graece & Latine opera omnia. 1613.

—*See* Celsus, A. C. De medicina libri octo. 1687.

—*as subject. See* [Thorius, R.] Medici Londinensis eximii epistola. 1619.

CASAUBON, Meric [1599-1671] A treatise concerning enthusiasme, as it is an effect of nature; but is mistaken by many for either divine inspiration, or diabolicall possession ... 2d ed. rev. and enl. London, Printed by Roger Daniel and sold by Thomas Johnson, 1656.

[15], 297, [4] p.   17 cm.   **[2190]**

CASE, John [*d.* 1600] Lapis philosophicus; seu,

Commentarius in octo lib. phys. Aristot. in quo arcana physiologiae examinantur ... Oxoniae, Excudebat Johannes Lichfield, 1629.

[26], 869, [16] p.   21 cm.   **[2191]**
STC 4757.5.

CASE, John [*fl.* 1680-1700] Compendium anatomicum nova methodo institutum ... Amstelodami, Apud Georgium Gallet, 1696.

[13], 121 (i.e. 193), [1] p.   front., plates.   14 cm.   **[2192]**
With this is bound: Malpighi, M. Epistolae anatomicae. 1669.

—Ἐξηγητὴς Ἰατρικός; or The medical expositor, in an alphabetical order. With the division of man's body, into its several parts; with their various names, and the diseases they are subject to: in Latin, Greek and English ... London, J. Dawks, 1698.

[15], 186 p.   front. (port.)   14 cm.   **[2193]**

—The wards of the Key to Helmont proved unfit for the lock; or, The principles of Mr. William Bacon examined and refuted, and the honour and value of true chymistry asserted ... London, Printed for the author and sold by John Smith, 1682.

[4], 24 p.   illus.   18 cm.   **[2194]**

The **CASE** of divorce and re-marriage thereupon discussed. 1673. *See* [Wolseley, *Sir* C.]

CASELIUS, Johannes [1533-1613] *See* Luchten, A. Oratio Adami Luchtenii. 1611.

CASEMBROOT, Gysbert Hendrik [*fl.* 1696] *respondent.* Disputatio philosophica inauguralis de aestu marino ... Lugduni Batavorum, Apud Abrahammum Elzevier, 1696.

[24] p.   22 cm.   **[2195]**
Diss.—Leyden.

CASERTA, Francesco Antonio [16th-17th cent.] Tractationes duae ad medicinae praxim pertinentes. Altera de natura, & usu aquarum potabilium, tum in sanis, tum in aegris corporibus. Alia de natura, & usu vinorum, tum in sanis, tum in aegrotis ... Aquae potum podagricis, & arthriticis esse infestum, vini vero potum esse utilem, veris Hyppocratis, & Galeni auctoritatibus, ac verissimis ronibus demonstratur ... Neapoli, Ex typographia Secundini Roncalioli, 1623.

[7], 104 p.; [8], 174 p.   22 cm.   **[2196]**
Part [2] has special title page: Tractatio de natura, et usu vinorum.

CASMANN, OTTO [*d.* 1607] Nucleus mysteriorum naturae, enucleatus laboribus aliquando scholasticis ex solertissimorum ac sagacissimorum seculi nostri interpretum naturae scriptis, methodiceque digestus . . . Hamburgi, Ex Bibliopolio Frobeniano, 1605.

[12], 419 p.   17 cm.   **[2197]**

Imperfect: p. [1-12] wanting: supplied in photocopy from British Museum.

— *ed.* See BRUYERIN, J. B. Dipnosophia seu sitologia. 1606.

CASOLANI, PROTO. *See* CASULANUS, Prothus [*fl.* 1610-*ca.* 1621].

CASONI, GUIDO [1575-1640] *See* GARZONI, T. L'hospidale de' pazzi incurabili. 1605, 1617.

CASPAR, JOHANN [*fl.* 1700] *respondent. See* CAMERARIUS, R. J., *praeses.* De panacea mercuriali. 1700.

CASPAR, JOHANN PHILIPP [*fl.* 1676-1679] *respondent. See* BROTBECK, J. K., *praeses.* Disputatio medica de sanguine menstruo. 1676.

CASPAR, SAMUEL [*fl.* 1693-1733] *respondent. See* CAMERARIUS, E. R., *praeses.* Dissertatio medica prior [-posterior] de tenesmo. 1693.

CASPARI, JOHANN BALTHASAR [*fl.* 1668] *respondent.* Disputatio medica inauguralis de pleuritide vera . . . Lugduni Batavorum, Apud viduam & haeredes Joannis Elsevirii, 1668.

[16] p.   23 cm.   **[2198]**

Diss. — Leyden.

CASSERIO, GIULIO [1561?-1616] De vocis auditusque organis historia anatomica singulari fide methodo ac industria concinnata tractatibus duobus explicata ac variis iconibus aere excusis illustrata . . . [Ferrariae, 1601]

[60], 191, [1], 126, [1] p.   illus., 2 ports.   41 cm.
                                    [2199]

Colophon (p. [127] at end): Ferrariae, Excudebat Victorius Baldinus . . . sumptibus Unitorum Patavii, 1600.
Colophon on p. [192] dated 1601.
Engraved title page.
Engravings by Josias Murer. Cf. Choulant-Frank. p. 223.

— Pentaestheseion; hoc est, De quinque sensibus liber, organorum fabricam variis iconibus fideliter aere incisis illustratam, nec non actionem et usum, discursu anatomico & philosophico accurate explicata

continens . . . Venetiis, Apud Nicolaum Misserinum [1609]

[8], 346, [17] p.   illus.   40 cm.   **[2200]**

Errata: p. [17]

— [The same.] . . . Jam primum in Germania visus . . . Francofurti, Sumptibus haeredum Nicolai Bassaei, 1610.

[12], 355, [15] p.   illus.   32 cm.   **[2201]**

Reissued in 1612 by Johann Bassée under title: Nova anatomia.

— Julii Casserii Placentini . . . Tabulae anatomicae LXXIIX . . . Daniel Bucretius . . . XX quæ deerant supplevit et omnium explicationes addidit. Venetiis [Apud Evangelistam Deuchinum] 1627.

[4], 97 ll.   illus.   42 cm.   **[2202]**

Engraved title page.
Bound with Spiegel, A. van de. De humani corporis fabrica libri decem. 1627.

— [The same.] . . . Francofurti, Impensis & coelo Matthaei Meriani, 1632.

221 p.   illus.   23 cm.   **[2203]**

Presumably designed to accompany Bucretius' edition of Adriaan van de Spiegel's De humani corporis fabrica.
With this are bound: Oddi, O. degli. Expositio, in librum Artis medicinalis Galeni. 1607. — Terilli, D. De vesicantibus. 1607.

— [The same.] *In* Spiegel, A. van de. Opera quae extant, omnia. 1645; Browne, J. A compleat treatise of the muscles. 1681, 1683, 1697, 1698; [Latin tr.] 1684, 1687, 1694.

— [German tr.] Julii Casserii Placentini Anatomische Tafeln, mit denselben welche Daniel Bucretius hinzugethan, und aller beygefügten Erklärung; zu Nutz und Ehren der Wund-Artzte . . . Auff Anordnung D. Simonis Paulli . . . für diesem ins Deutsche übergesetzet, nun aber allererst an den Tag gegeben, nebenst einer lateinischen Zugabe, in sich begreiffend die Einführung der Anatomey-Kunst, und derer offentlichen Ubung, auff der . . . Königlichen Academien Kopenhagen. Franckfurt am Mayn, In Verlegung Thomae Matthiae Götzen, 1656.

[48], 218 p.; 18, [1] p.; 94 p.   illus., plates, port.   21 cm.   **[2204]**

Imperfect: four leaves between title page and sig. (a)³ [Aufftrag-Schrifft . . .] wanting.
Added engraved title page: Jul. Cas. Placentini Anatomische Tafeln verdeütschet. Sim. Paulli.
Part [2] has special title page: Herrn Adriani Spigelii . . . Büchlein von der Frucht in Mutter-Leibe; oder, Ander Theil, derer von Simone Paulli . . . verdeutscheten Anatomia.

Part [3] has general title page: Appendix.

Contents: De anatomiae origine, praestantia, et utilitate, syntagma; auctore Simone Paulli ... conscriptum & editum anno 1643, ed. 2. corr. (p. [3]-28). Oratio introductoria, in Regia Haffniensi Academia ... habita a Simone Paulli ... cum Galenum De ossibus, ad Sceleton, publice in Collegio Finckiano esset interpretaturus; edita anno 1641 (p. [29]-59). Simonis Paulli ... Programma ad ornatissimos Dn. studiosos in incluta Regia Hafniensi Academia commorantes; affixum ... Anno 1644 (p. [61]-66). ... Theatrum Anatomicum, Hafniae noviter extructum, rege ... Christiano quarto ... anno 1644 [Scribebat ... Michaël Kirstenius] (p. [67]-79). Programma ... Simon Paulli ... S. P. D. (p. [80]-86). Michaelis Kirstenii ... Epigrammata: quae in Regio Haffniensi Theatro anatomico leguntur (p. [91]-94). Items have special or half title pages.

Part [1] is the translation of Casserio's Tabulae anatomicae ... and part [2] of Spiegel's De formato foetu.

— [The same.] Julii Casserii Placentini, und Danielis Bucretii Anatomische Tafeln, zusambt deroselben nothwendigen ... Erklärung ... In die teutsche Sprache übersetzet, und nebest einer lateinischen, die Einführung und Offentliche Ubung der Anatomi-Kunst in sich begreiffender Zugabe, angeordnet und aussgefertiget von Simone Paulii ... Franckfurt am Mayn, Georg Heinrich Oehrling, 1683.

[44], 218 p.; 18, [1] p.; 94 p.   illus., plates.   22 cm.   **[2205]**

A reissue of the 1656 edition with new title page and some pages reset. First item of part [3] has new title page: Simonis Paulli ... De anatomiae ortu, progressu, praestantia, et utilitate, diatribe ... Francofurti, Sumptibus Georgii Henrici Oehrlingii, 1683.

CASSIODORUS SENATOR, Flavius Magnus Aurelius [*ca.* 487 — *ca.* 580] Formula comitis archiatrorum, commentario illustrata a Joanne Henrico Meibomio. Helmestadii, Typis & sumptibus Henningi Mulleri, 1668.

[8], 86 (i.e. 88) p.   20 cm.   **[2206]**

The Formula comitis archiatrorum is the 19th chapter of book 6 of the author's Variae lib. XII.

Edited by Heinrich Meibom.

CASSIUS PARMENSIS, *pseud. See* TELESIO, Antonio [1482-1533?]

CASSIUS, Andreas [1645-*ca.* 1700] De triumviratu intestinali cum suis effervescentiis, repetita disputatio. Cui accessit Epistola amici ad amicum quae praecedens disputatio examinatur. Neomagi, Apud Nicolaum Placidum, 1669.

[1], 70 (i.e. 68) p.   13 cm.   **[2207]**

"... Exerpta e thesibus inauguralibus De arthritide ... Joannis de Raei ...": p. 66-70.

— *respondent. See* MAJOR, J. D., *praeses.* Dissertationem medicam de febre artificiali ... pro virili tueri conabitur Andreas Cassius. 1666.

CASTAGNE, Gabriel de. *See* CASTAIGNE, Gabriel de, *Father* [*ca.* 1562-*ca.* 1630]

CASTAGNO, Pietro. See CASTAÑO, Pedro [16th-17th cent.]

CASTAIGNE, Gabriel de, *Father* [*ca.* 1562-*ca.* 1630] Les oeuvres ... tant medicinales que chymiques, divisées en quatre principaux traitez. I. Le paradis terrestre. II. Le grand miracle de la nature metallique. III. L'or potable. IV. Le thresor philosophique de la medecine metallique. 2. ed. A quoy sont adjoustez les Aphorismes Basiliens, & la Methode particuliere pour bien faire le merveilleux onguent appellé Manus Dei ... Paris, Jean d'Hourry, 1661.

4 parts in 1 v.   18 cm.   **[2208]**

Various pagings.

Part [2] has special title page dated 1660 and contains the "Oeuvre philosophique de Jean Saunier. Faite en l'an 1432. le 7 May." Part [3]: L'or potable ... has special title page dated 1660 and includes Le tresor philosophique de la medecine metallique, and Aphorismes Basiliens. Part [4] has special title page: Methode particuliere ... 1660.

Edited by Jean Baptiste de La Noue.

— L'or potable qui guarit de tous maux ... Par ... Gabriel de Castagne ... Paris, Charles Sevestre, 1611.

104 p.; 38, [1] p.   17 cm.   **[2209]**

Part [2] has caption title: Le tresor philosophique de la medecine metallique. Traduit d'italien en françois par ... Gabriel de Castagne.

CASTALIONE, S. *See* CORTILIO, Sebastiano.

CASTANAEUS, Maturinus [*fl.* 1692] *praeses.* Pathologia generalis; seu, Dissertatio in genere de affectibus animae ... Hafniae, Literis Joh. Phil. Bockenhoffer [1692]

[6], 30 p.   20 cm.   **[2210]**

Diss. — Copenhagen (D. Mathesius, *respondent*)

CASTAÑO, Pedro [16th-17th cent.] Reggimento contra peste del ... Pietro Castagno ... per conservare li sani, & curare gl'infermi. Con il modo d'usare il composto, over'oglio contro peste, & veleni, che si fà ogn'anno per l'illustrissima communità di Ferrara ... Ferrara, Francesco Suzzi [*ca.* 1620]

[8] p.   23 cm.   **[2211]**

Imprint partly supplied from Palau 47545.

CASTEL, Jacobus du. *See* Du Castel, Jean [*fl.* 1668]

CASTELEYN, Johannes [*ca.* 1612-1665] *tr. See* De wonderlijcke en wel geoeffende genees en heelmeester. 1663; Digby, *Sir* K. D'eminente oratie. 1661; Papin, N. Theatrum sympateticum. 1662.

CASTELLAN, Pierre. *See* Castellanus, Petrus [1585-1632]

CASTELLANI, Giovanni Maria [1585-1655] [Phylacterium, seu sanguinis missione. German.] Ausführliche und nothwendige Verzeichniss, wie auch sehr nützliche Anmerckung, aller und jeder gewöhnlichen Adern, sie seyn gleich Blut-Flüss-oder Lufft-Adern, wie die Namen haben, wie solche sollen und mögen geschlagen werden ... Erstlich in lateinischer Sprach beschrieben von Johann Castellano ... anjetzo aber verteutscht, und vermehrt durch einen Liebhaber derselben. Nürnberg, Johann Hoffmann, 1665.

70 p. 13 cm. [**2212**]
Translated by Lazarus von Heyden.

—[Italian tr.] Filactirion della flebotomia, et arteriotomia ... con l'aggiunta di un trattato, nel quale parimente s'insegna il vero modo d'applicar le ventose, ò coppe ... Tradotta novamente in volgare da Domenico Piccinetti ... Viterbo, Pietro & Agostino Discepoli, 1619.

44 p. plates. 23 cm. [**2213**]

CASTELLANUS, Johannes. *See* Castellani, Giovanni Maria [1585-1655]

CASTELLANUS, Petrus [1585-1632] Κρεωφαγία; sive, De esu carnium libri IV ... Antverpiae, Ex officina Hieronymi Verdussii, 1626.

[8], 296 p. 18 cm. [**2214**]

—Vitae illustrium medicorum qui toto orbe, ad haec usque tempora floruerunt ... Antverpiae, Apud Guilielmum a Tongris, 1618.

255, [8] p. 16 cm. [**2215**]

CASTELLI, Alessandro. Dell'uso, et virtù della theriaca di Andromaco il vecchio. Composta, et dispensata per noi Alessandro, e Pietro Giorgio Castelli ... Venetia, Ferretti [165-?]

7 p. 20 cm. [**2216**]
Probably printed by Ognibene, Giambatista, or Giacomo Ferretti, listed as active in Venice in 1651, 1658, & 1680 respectively. Cf. Brown, p. 404.

CASTELLI, Bartolomeo [*d. ca.* 1607] Lexicon medicum, Graeco Latinum ... Ex Hippocrate, et Galeno desumptum ... Venetiis, Apud Nicolaum Polum, & Franciscum Bolzettam, 1607.

[16], 388, [19] p. 16 cm. [**2217**]
A reprint of the 1598 Messina edition with a new dedicatory epistle by the publisher.
"Praecipuarum Arabicarum vocum, ad artem medicam facientium ... series": p. [389-407]

—[The same.] ... Venetiis, Apud Georgium Valentinum & Franciscum Bolzettam, 1626.

[16], 349, [18] p. 17 cm. [**2218**]
A reprint of the 1607 edition with a new dedicatory epistle by the publisher.

—[The same.] Lexicon medicum Graeco-Latinum, compendiosiss. a Bartholomaeo Castello ... inchoatum: nunc vero ... opera & studio Emmanuelis Stupani ... ex Hippocr. Galen. Avicenn. & complurium aliorum summe celebrium medicorum monumentis auctum, illustratum, & perfectum. Basileae, Impensis Joh. Jacobi Genathi, 1628.

[12], 382 (i.e. 372) p. 18 cm. [**2219**]

—[The same.] Lexicon medicum, Graeco Latinum ... Ex Hippocrate, et Galeno desumptum ... Venetiis, Apud Jo. Baptistae Cestari & Franciscum Bolzettam, 1642.

[8], 348, [20] p. 18 cm. [**2220**]

—[The same.] ... Editio postrema, sedulo recognita, & quamplurimis mendis expurgata. Rotterodami, Sumptibus Arnoldi Leers, 1644.

[1], 351, [18] p. 16 cm. [**2221**]

—[The same.] Lexicon medicum Graeco-Latinum, a Bartholomaeo Castello ... inchoatum. Nunc vero ... opera et studio Adriani Ravesteinii ... ex Hippocr. Galen. Avicenn. atque aliorum celeberrimorum medicorum monumentis, tertia ... parte auctius, & innumeris ... mendis, expurgatum, ac perfectum. Roterodami, Apud Arnoldum Leers, 1651.

[16], 517, [18] p. 17 cm. [**2222**]

—[The same.] ... Roterodami, Apud Arnoldum Leers, 1657.

[16], 517, [18] p. 16 cm. [**2223**]

—[The same.] ... Venetiis, Apud Paulum Balleonium, 1664.

[10], 481, [19] p. 17 cm. [**2224**]

—[The same.] . . . Roterodami, Apud Arnoldum Leers, 1665.

[16], 517, [18] p.   16 cm.   [2225]

—[The same.] . . . Tolosae, Apud Bernardum Dupuy, 1669.

[8], 619, [25] p.   16 cm.   [2226]

—[The same.] . . . Patavii, Apud Cadorinum, 1685.

[24], 557, [2] p.   17 cm.   [2227]

—Castellus renovatus; hoc est, Lexicon medicum, quondam a Barth. Castello . . . inchoatum, per alios postmodo continuatum, nunc vero . . . correctum, & innumerabilium pene vocabulorum accessione amplificatum cura & studio Jacobi Pancratii Brunonis . . . Norimbergae, Sumtibus Johan. Danielis Tauberi, imprimebat Christian-Sigismundus Frobergius, 1682.

[19], 1208, [1] p.; [2], 46 p.   front. (port.)   22 cm.   [2228]

Added engraved title page.

Part [2] has half title: Mantissa nomenclaturae medicae hexaglottae, vocabula Latina ordine alphabetico cum annexis Arabicis, Hebraeis, Graecis, Gallicis & Italicis proponentis, cura & studio Jacobi Pancratii Brunonis.

—[The same.] Amaltheum Castello-Brunonianum; sive, Lexicon medicum . . . Norimbergae, Sumtibus Johannis Danielis Tauberi, literis Henrici Meyeri, 1688.

[19], 939 p.   front. (port.)   21 cm.   [2229]

Added engraved title page.

—[The same.] . . . Accesserunt . . . Joannis Rhodii . . . additiones . . . Patavii, Sumptibus Jacobi de Cadorinis, 1700.

[16], 827 p.   25 cm.   [2230]

CASTELLI, JEAN FRANÇOIS. *See* CASTELLI, Alessandro.

CASTELLI, JOHANN. *See* CASTELLUS, Joannes [*fl.* 1608]

CASTELLI, PIETRO [*ca.* 1590-1661] Antidotario romano commentato dal dott. Pietro Castello . . . Que s'apporta il primo autore di ciascheduna compositione, si fa la collatione con l'altre ricette . . . Cosenza, Gio. Battista Russo, 1648.

[19], 384 p.   illus.   30 cm.   [2231]

Contains the text of the Antidotarii Romani, compiled by the Collegio de'medici at Rome.

With this is bound *his* Memoriale per lo speziale romano. 1638.

—Balsamum examinatum . . . Messanae, Typis viduę Jo. Francisci Bianco, 1640.

[8], 63 (i.e. 167) p.   port., plate.   22 cm.   [2232]

Engraved title page.

Half title on p. [3] reads: . . . Opobalsamum examinatum, defensum, judicatum, absolutum, & laudatum.

Running title: Petri Castelli. Opobalsamum.

—Breve ortographia . . . Tradotta in volgare, e data alle stampe dal . . . Gio. Pietro Corvino Castello . . . Messina, Paolo Bonacota, 1659.

48 p.   16 cm.   [2233]

Bound with *his* De abusu circa dierum criticorum enumerationem. 1642.

—Breve ricordo dell'elettione, qualita, et virtu dello spirito, et oglio acido di vitriolo . . . Nel quale s'insegna con l'autorità di molti medici, & chimici eccellentissimi il vero modo d'adoprare questi salutiferi medicamenti in più di 170 infirmità . . . Roma, Giacomo Mascardi, 1621.

30 p.   21 cm.   [2234]

—Chrysopos, cujus nomina, essentia, usus, & dosis facili methodo traduntur. Quem sequitur: Problema de lacte in virginibus, experimentis, auctoritatibus, & rationibus explanatum. Messanae, Apud viduam Joannis Francisci Bianco, 1638.

[8], 54 p.   22 cm.   [2235]

—De abusu circa dierum criticorum enumerationem . . . Messanae, Apud viduam de Bianco, 1642.

[32], 158, [7] p.   16 cm.   [2236]

Caption title on p. 1 reads: De abusu circa dierum criticorum enumerationem contra Hippocratis, et Galeni usum.

With this are bound: *his* De abusu phlebotomiae. 1628; *his* Breve ortographia. 1659. Corvino, G. De diatartari iulapii temperamento. 1645.

—De abusu exhibitionis medicamenti purgantis in octavo die . . . Messanae, Apud Paulum Bonacota, 1659.

[8], 42 p.   21 cm.   [2237]

Added half title reads: Abusus octavae diei.

With this are bound: *his* Illustrissimis senatoribus . . . Petrus Castellus . . . foelicitatem. [1648]; Avellino, F. Oratio. 1660.

—De abusu phlebotomiae . . . Romae, Typis Francisci Corbeletti, 1628.

[24], 96 p.   16 cm.   [2238]

Imperfect: sig. b1-4 of index misbound.

Bound with *his* De abusu circa dierum criticorum enumerationem. 1642.

—De febre tritaeophya. Cosenzae, Apud Jo. Bapt. Russum, 1648.

37 p. 15 cm. [2239]

—De optimo medico. *In* Conring, H. In universam artem medicam singulasque ejus partes introductio. 1687.

—De visitatione aegrotantium. Pro suis auditoribus, & discipulis ad praxim instruendis. Romae, Apud Jacob. Mascardum, 1630.

130 p. 13 cm. [2240]

—Discorso della differenza tra gli semplici freschi, et i secchi, con il modo di seccarli . . . Roma, Giacomo Mascardi, 1629.

48 p. 21 cm. [2241]

—Discorso della duratione de medicamenti tanto semplici, quanto composti . . . Roma, Giacomo Mascardi, 1621.

[8], 68 p. 22 cm. [2242]

—Discorso dell'eletuario rosato di Mesue, nel quale si raggiona delle rose, che entrano in detto eletuario, e della scammonea . . . Roma, Giacomo Mascardi, 1633.

21 p. 21 cm. [2243]

—Epistola . . . ad . . . Joannem Manelphum, et Aetium Cletum . . . In qua agitur nomine hellebori simpliciter prolato, tum apud Hippocratem, tum alios auctores intelligendum album, & ab hoc purgatas a Melampode Proeti regis Argivorum furentes filias, atque ab Anticyreo sanatum Herculem insanientem. Romae, Ex typographia Jacobi Mascardi, 1622.

28 p. 22 cm. [2244]

—Epistola secunda de helleboro . . . In qua confirmantur ea, quae in alia Epistola de helleboro allata fuere. Romae, Typis Jacobi Mascardi, 1622.

48 p. 22 cm. [2245]

—Epistolae medicinales . . . Romae, Typis Jacobi Mascardi, 1626.

[12], 252, [8] p. 22 cm. [2246]

[—] Exactissima descriptio rariorum quarundam plantarum, quę continentur Romę in Horto Farnesiano: Tobia Aldino Cesenate auctore . . . Romae, Typis Jacobi Mascardi, 1625.

[12], 100, [8] p. illus. 36 cm. [2247]

Engraved title page.

The printer's preface indicates that the author chose to publish the work under the name of another, and the laudatory poem (p. [5-6]) apparently divulges the author's name as Petrus Castellus. Castelli is considered the author by Mazzuchelli (v. 1, p. 386-7).

—Hortus Messanensis. Messanae, Typis viduae Joannis Francisci Bianco, 1640.

[20], 51 p. plates. 21 cm. [2248]

Added engraved title page.

—De hyaena odorifera εξετάσις . . . figuris aeneis adornata. Editio nova auctior. Francofurti, Apud Hermannum a Sande, 1668.

79, [5] p. plates. 14 cm. [2249]

Published in 1638 under title Hyaena odorifera. Cf. BMC.

—Illustrissimis senatoribus . . . Petrus Castellus Romanus foelicitatem. [Messanae, Apud haeredes Petri Breae, 1648]

31 p. 21 cm. [2250]

Caption title: Praeservatio corporum sanorum ab imminenti lue ex aeris intemperie hoc anno 1648.

Bound with *his* De abusu exhibitionis medicamenti purgantis in octavo die. 1659.

—Memoriale per lo speziale romano. Nel quale si pone il tempo in Roma consueto, di raccogliere, e seccare le radici, l'erbe, i fiori, i frutti, & i semi necessarii per le spetiarie . . . Messina, Vedova di Gio. Francesco Bianco, 1638.

27 p. 30 cm. [2251]

Bound with *his* Antidotario romano. 1648.

—Opobalsamum triumphans. [Messina? 1640?]
[6], 44 (i.e. 54) p. 22 cm. [2252]

Engraved title page.

Concerns controversy with Antonio Manfredi and Vincenzio Panutio.

—Optimus medicus in quo conditiones perfectissimi medici exponuntur. Messanae, Apud vidua Jo. Franc. Bianco, 1637.

[8], 32 p. 21 cm. [2253]

—[Selections] *In* Antidotario romano latino, e volgare. 1639, 1675, 1678.

—, *ed. See* ANTIDOTARIO ROMANO LATINO, E VOLGARE. 1639, 1675, 1678.

—*See* AVELLINO, F. Oratio in exornandis philosophiae. 1660; SEVERINO, M. A. Seilo-phlebotome castigata. 1654.

—*as subject. See* PITTORE, P. Opobalsami Romani censura. 1642; VERBEZIUS, D. Pro Raymundi Mindereri ... disquisitione iatrochymica de chalcantho. 1626.

CASTELLI, PIETRO GIORGIO. *See* CASTELLI, A. Dell'uso, et virtù della theriaca di Andromaco il vecchio. 165–?

CASTELLINI, GIACOMO. *See* CASTELLINI, Giovanni [*fl.* 1613–1646]

CASTELLINI, GIOVANNI [*fl.* 1613–1646] De dura cerebri vestiente meninge. Tractatus apologeticus. Venetiis, Typis Francisci Valuesensis, 1646.

    63, [1] p. 16 cm.   [**2254**]

Imperfect: text on p. 14–15 wanting.

Poem of 4 pages in honor of Castellini inserted between p. 6 and 7 with caption title: Del sig. Francesco Rovai, all'autore. Canzone.

—, *ed. See* SEGNI, G. Questio de gangraenae et sphaceli diversa curatione ab ... Ant. Baldesio. 1613.

CASTELLINI, LUDOVICO, *tr. See* FOUQUET, M. (de Maupeou) *vicomtesse de Vaux*. I rimedii di madama Fochetti. 1683, 1685, *ca.* 1688, 1693, 1697.

CASTELLO, PEDRO VASCO [*fl.* 1616] Exercitationes medicinales, ad omnes thoracis affectus, decem tractatibus absolutae ... Quibus perquam multae novae difficultates medicae, ac physicae, tam theoricae quam practicae, discutiuntur, & pene innumera Hippocratis, Galeni, aliorumque medicinae procerum loca pugnantia conciliantur, difficilia explanantur, & ad usus medicos reducuntur ... Tolosae, Apud Raymundum Colomerium, 1616.

    [44], 986, [33] p. 23 cm.   [**2255**]

—Another issue, with imprint: Tolosae, Sumptibus Joannis Petri Charlot, 1616.

                             [**2256**]

CASTELLO BRANCO, JOÃO RODRIGUES DE. *See* AMATUS LUSITANUS [1511–1568]

CASTELLUS, JOANNES [*fl.* 1608] Tractatus de peste, nec non de ipsius causis, signis, praesagiis, curatione & praeservatione. Ex doctissimorum phylosophorum ac medicorum scriptis collectus ... Augustae Vindelicorum, Excudebat Christophorus Mangus, 1608.

    [5], 187, [8] p. 17 cm.   [**2257**]

CASTELLUS, PETRUS. *See* CASTELLANUS, Petrus [1585–1632]

CASTELLUS, PHILOTHEUS, *pseud. See* CASTRO, Benedict de [*ca.* 1597–1684]

CASTIGLIONE, BRANDA FRANCESCO [*d.* 1712] *See* COLLEGIO DEI FISICI, Milan. Prospectus pharmaceuticus. 1668.

CASTIGLIONE, GIOVANNI ONORATO [*d.* 1679] *See* COLLEGIO DEI FISICI, Milan. Prospectus pharmaceuticus. 1668 [and] Prospectus pharmaceutici ed. 2. 1698.

CASTIGLIONE, PIETRO MARIA [1594–1629] Admiranda naturalia ad renum calculos curandos. Mediolani, Ex apotheca Gratiadei Ferioli, 1622.

    222, [1] p. port. 16 cm.   [**2258**]

Imperfect: 217–220 mutilated.

CASTILLO, JOANNES, *Seguntini chirurgi. See* CASTILLO, Juan de [*fl.* 1683]

CASTILLO, JUAN DE [*fl.* 1683] Tractatus quo continentur summe necessaria tàm de anatome, quàm de vulneribus, & ulceribus, tàm in genere, quàm in particulari, ac pro locorum differentia, tùm rationibus, tùm authoritatibus gravissimorum virorum illustratus ... Matriti, Apud Dominicum Garcia Morras, 1683.

    [34], 348 p. 29 cm.   [**2259**]

Includes extracts from Galenus.

CASTILLO, JUAN DEL [*fl.* 1608] Pharmacopoea. Universa medicamenta in officinis pharmaceuticis usitata complectens, & explicans. Autore Joanne Castello ... Gadibus, Apud Joannem de Borja, 1622.

    [6], 335 (i.e. 331) ll. 20 cm.   [**2260**]

Imperfect: title page and ll. 325 wanting; supplied in photocopy from British Museum.

CASTLE, GEORGE [1635?–1673] The chymical Galenist: a treatise, wherein the practise of the ancients is reconcil'd to the new discoveries in the theory of physick ... In which are some reflections upon a book, intituled, Medela medicinae ... London, Printed by Sarah Griffin for Henry Twyford and Timothy Twyford, 1667.

    [15], 196, [12] p. 17 cm.   [**2261**]

The Medela medicinae ... by Marchamont Nedham was published in 1665.

CASTRENSIS. *See* CASTELLI, Pietro [*ca.* 1590–1661]

CASTRENSIS, ROBERTUS. *See* ROBERT OF CHESTER [*fl.* 1141-1150]

CASTRILLO, HERNANDO [1586-1667] Magia natural; o, Ciencia de filosofia oculta ... Primera parte, donde se trata de los secretos que pertenecen a las partes de la tierra. Trigueros, Diego Perez Estupiñan, 1649.

[19], 224 ll.   19 cm.   **[2262]**

No more appears to have been published.

CASTRO, ANDRÉS. *See* CASTRO, Andrés Antonio de [*d.* 1642]

CASTRO, ANDRÉS ANTONIO DE [*d.* 1642] De febrium curatione libri tres quibus accessere duo alii libelli de simplicium medicamentorum facultatibus; & alter de qualitatibus alimentorum, quae humani corporis nutritioni sunt apta ... Villaviçosae, Apud Emmanuelem [Carballeo, 1636?]

[12], 271, [13] ll.   29 cm.   **[2263]**

Imperfect: title page mutilated, affecting imprint. Imprint partly supplied from Palau 48610.

CASTRO, BARUCH NEHEMIAS. *See* CASTRO, Benedicto de [*ca.* 1597—1684]

CASTRO, BENEDICTO DE [*ca.* 1597-1684] Monomachia; sive, Certamen medicum, quo verus in febre synocho putrida cum cruris inflammatione medendi usus per venae sectionem in brachio demonstratur, praeposterus autem ejus abusus per sanguinis missionem in pede, tanquam perniciosus improbatur. Hamburgi, Typis Jacobi Rebenlini, 1647.

[16], 88 p.   20 cm.   **[2264]**

—*respondent. See* VORSTIUS, A. E., *praeses.* Disputatio medica de apoplexia. 1621.

CASTRO, ESTEVÃO RODRIGUES DE [1559-1637?] Commentarius in Hippocratis Coi, libellum De alimento, in quo multiplici didascalia variae controversiae in utramque partem disputantur, et argumentorum funibus, authorumque securibus Satyro cornua ligantur, confringuntur. Opus in quatuor sectiones divisum quarum priores duae in hoc volumine continentur ... Florentiae, Typographia Sermartelliana, 1635-39.

3 vols. in 1.   35 cm.   **[2265]**

Sections 1-2 paged continuously, sect. 2 with caption title only. Sect. 3 has special title page: Commentarii in librum Hippocratis Coi De alimanto ... Sectio tertia. Florentiae, Excussum in

Typographia Pignonium, 1637 [colophon 1638]. Sect. 4, edited and published in 1639 by the author's son Francisco de Castro has special title page with imprint: Florentiae, Typis novis Amatoris Massae, & soc., 1639.

Includes the Latin text of De alimento, in Janus Cornarius' version.

—Compendio d'avvertimenti per preservazione, e curazione della peste ... Firenze, Gio. Batista Landini, 1630.

117 p.   15 cm.   **[2266]**

—Il curioso nel quale in dialogo si discorre del male di peste ... Pisa, Francesco Tanagli, 1631.

76 p.   20 cm.   **[2267]**

—De asitia tractatus. Florentiae, Apud Zenobium Pignonium, 1630.

101, [1] p.   17 cm.   **[2268]**

—[The same.] *See* LICETI, F. De feriis altricis animae nemeseticae disputationes. 1631.

—De meteoris microcosmi libri quatuor ... Florentiae, Apud Juntas, 1621.

[12], 229, [17] p.   31 cm.   **[2269]**

—Expositiones in aliquos Hippocratis aegrotos ... Auctore Stephano Roderico Castrense ... Venetiis, Apud Franciscum Brogiollum, 1656.

136 p. 17 cm. (Part [2] in his Variae exercitationes medicae ... Accesserunt ... Expositiones in aliquos Hippocratis aegrotos. Venetiis, 1656.)   **[2270]**

Edited by the author's son Francisco de Castro.
"Auctoris elogium": p. 6-10.
Includes Latin text of 9 case histories from book 1 of Hippocrates' Epidemiorum libri.

—Medicae consultationes ... Florentiae, Typis Amatoris Masse, & Laurentii de Landis, 1644.

[8], 147 p.   21 cm.   **[2271]**

—Posthuma Stephani Roderici Castrensis ... varietas a Francisco ejus filio in lucem edita. Florentiae, Typis Amatoris Massae, & socii, 1639.

4, 110, [1] p.   21 cm.   **[2272]**

—Quae ex quibus opusculum in quatuor libros divisum, medicinae studiosis valde utile, & recondita doctrina refertum ... Florentiae, Apud Petrum Cecconcellium, 1627.

[20], 360 (i.e. 358) p.   15 cm.   **[2273]**

—[The same.] Quae ex quibus. Opusculum vere aureum, ac praecipua prognoseos mysteria reserans. Lugduni, Apud Joan. Caffin, 1645.

[16], 278, [2] p.   15 cm.   **[2274]**

—Syntaxis praedictionum medicarum . . . Accessit triplex ejusdem authoris elucubratio. I. De chyrurgicis administrationibus. II. De potu refrigerato. III. De animalibus microcosmi. Lugduni, Sumpt. Phil. Borde, Laur. Arnaud et Cl. Rigaud, 1661.

[12], 452, [14] p.   23 cm.   **[2275]**

Edited by Francisco de Castro.

—Copy 2.

With this is bound *his* Tractatus de natura muliebri. 1668.

—Tractatus de complexu morborum studio, & diligentia, Valerii Nervii . . . Florentiae, Apud Zenobium Pignonium, 1624.

250, [2] p.   16 cm.   **[2276]**

Imperfect: text of p. 11-12 wanting; duplicate of p. 25-26 printed instead.

—Tractatus de natura muliebri; seu, Disputationes ac lectiones Pisanae. Nunc primum in lucem editus. Francofurti, Apud Hermannum a Sande, 1668.

[4], 132, [2] p.   front. (port.), plate.   20 cm.   **[2277]**

Edited by Francisco de Castro.

Bound with copy 2 of *his* Syntaxis praedictionum medicarum. 1661.

—Tractatus de sero lactis. Florentiae, Ex Typographia Sermartelliana, 1631.

76 p.   18 cm.   **[2278]**

—[The same.] *See* SERVI, P. Persii Trevi [*pseud.*] Ad librum de sero lactis Stephani Roderici Lusitani declamationes. 1634.

—Variae exercitationes medicae . . . privatae lectiones, Stephani Roderici Castrensis . . . His accesserunt in hac secunda editione Expositiones in aliquos Hippocratis aegrotos . . . Venetiis, Apud Franciscum Brogiollum, 1656.

[12], 223, [1] p.; 136 p.   17 cm.   **[2279]**

Added half title: Opuscula duo, videlicet Variae exercitationes medicae, et Expositiones in aliquos aegrotos Hippocratis.

Part [2] has special title page.

Edited by Francisco de Castro.

With this are bound: Wepfer, J. J. Observationes anatomicae. 1658. — Kolhans, T. Litterae . . . de spiritu animali. 1658.

CASTRO, ESTEVÃO RODRIGUES DE [1559-1637?] *See* [LICETI, F.] Verveceidos libri duo. 1636.

CASTRO, EZECHIELE DI. *See* CASTRO, Pedro de [1603-*ca.* 1657]

CASTRO, FRANCISCO DE [*fl.* 1638] *ed. See* CASTRO, E. R. de. Expositiones in aliquos Hippocratis aegrotos. 1656 [and] Syntaxis praedictionum medicarum. 1661 [and] Tractatus de natura muliebri. 1668 [and] Variae exercitationes medicae . . . privatae lectiones, Stephani Roderici Castrensis. 1656.

—*See* CASTRO, E. R. de. Commentarius in Hippocratis Coi, libellum De alimento. 1635-39.

—*as subject. See* CASTRO, E. R. de. Posthuma Stephani Roderici Castrensis . . . varietas. 1639.

CASTRO, MOSES OROBIUS A. *See* OROBIO À CASTRO, Moses [*fl.* 1678]

CASTRO, PEDRO DE [1603-*ca.* 1657] Bibliotheca medici eruditi . . . Patavii, Typis Jo. Baptistae Pasquati, 1654.

[11], 78, [24] p.   14 cm.   **[2280]**

—Il colostro. *In* Mercurio G. La commare . . . dell' Scipion Mercurii. 1642, 1645, 1680, 1686.

—Febris maligna puncticularis aphorismis delineata. Norimbergae, Ex officina Endterorum jun., 1652.

[11], 2-269, [8] p.   14 cm.   **[2281]**

Interleaved.

—[The same.] . . . Patavii, Typis Jacobi de Cadorinis, 1685.

[12], 148, [8] p.   14 cm.   **[2282]**

—Ignis lambens; historia medica, prolusio physica, rarum pulchrescentis naturae specimen . . . Aloysio Georgio Divi Marci procuratori . . . d. Ezechiel de Castro . . . Veronae, Apud Franciscum Rubeum, 1642.

[24], 198 p.   18 cm.   **[2283]**

—Pestis Neapolitana, Romana, et Genuensis annorum 1656. & 1657 . . . Veronae, Typis Rubeanis, 1657.

[24], 263 p.   15 cm.   **[2284]**

Added engraved title page.

—, *ed. See* PONCE DE SANTA CRUZ, A. [*d. ca.* 1650] De impedimentis magnorum auxiliorum in morborum curatione. 1652.

—*See* VALLES, F. de. Imber aureus. 1661.

CASTRO, RODRIGO DE [1541-1627] De universa mulierum medicina . . . Pars prima theorica [-pars secunda] . . . In quibus cuncta, quae ad mulieris naturam, anatomen, semen, menstruum, conceptum, uteri gestationem, foetus formationem, & hominis ortum attinent . . . explicantur . . . Hamburgi, In Officina Frobeniana, typis Philippi de Ohr, 1603.

2 parts in 1 v. illus. 32 cm. [2285]

Part 2 has special title page: . . . Pars secunda, sive praxis . . . in quibus mulierum morbi universi . . . traduntur . . . Additis insuper singulis fere capitibus ejusdem authoris scholiis . . . quibus pleraque Hippocratis & Galeni difficilima loca universaque fere ars medica illustratur.

—[The same.] De universa muliebrium morborum medicina . . . 2. ed. auct. et emend. Hamburgi, Ex Bibliopolio Frobeniano, 1617.

2 parts in 1 v. illus., table. 20 cm. [2286]

—[The same.] . . . 3. ed. auct. et emend. Hamburgi, Ex Bibliopolio Frobbeniano, 1628.

2 parts in 1 v. illus., table. 21 cm. [2287]

—[The same.] . . . Venetiis, Apud Paulum Baleonium, 1644.

[52], 598, [40] p. illus., plate. 23 cm. [2288]

Special title page bound after p. 598.

—[The same.] . . . 4. ed. auct. et emend. Hamburgi, Apud Zachariam Hertelium, 1662.

2 parts in 1 v. illus., plate. 20 cm. [2289]

With this is bound (as issued?) *his* Medicus politicus. 1662.

—[The same.] . . . 5. ed., auct. et emend. Coloniae Agrippinae, Sumptibus Servatii Noethen, 1689.

2 parts in 1 v. illus., plate. 21 cm. [2290]

—Medicus-politicus; sive, De officiis medico-politicis tractatus, quatuor distinctus libris: in quibus non solum bonorum medicorum mores ac virtutes exprimuntur, malorum vero fraudes & imposturae deteguntur . . . Hamburgi, Ex Bibliopolio Frobeniano, 1614.

[8], 277, [17] p. 20 cm. [2291]

—[The same.] . . . Hamburgi, Ex bibliopolio Zachariae Hertelii, 1662.

[8], 277, [17] p. 20 cm. [2292]

A reprint, nearly page for page like the 1614 Froben edition. Bound with (as issued?) *his* De universa muliebrium morborum medicina. 1662.

CASTRO Y AGUILA, TOMÁS DE [17th cent.] Remedios espirituales, y temporales, para preservar la republica de peste: y conseguir otros buenos sucessos en paz, y guerra . . . Antequera, Vicente Alvarez de Mariz, 1649.

60 (i.e. 64) ll. 20 cm. [2293]

CASULANUS, PROTHUS [*fl.* 1610-*ca.* 1621] De lingua qua maximum est morborum acutorum signum. Opus, in re medica, novi argumenti . . . Coloniae Agrippinae, Apud Matthaeum Smitz, 1626.

[16], 148 p. 15 cm. [2294]

CATALOGUE de toutes les principales raretez qui se montre sur la chambre de rarite dans la ville de Boislducque. 1700. *See* 's HERTOGENBOSCH, Netherlands. Rare Kamer.

A CATALOGUE of books continued, printed, and published at London. 1676. *See* TERM CATALOGUES.

A CATALOGUE of the library of . . . Francis Bernard. 1698. *See* BERNARD, F.

CATALOGUS antiquarum et novarum rerum ex longe dissitis terrarum oris. [1690?] *See* [VOORN, J.]

CATALOGUS et valor medicamentorum in officinis pharmaceüticis Stockholmiensibus prostantium. [1698?] *See* COLLEGIUM MEDICUM, Stockholm.

CATALOGUS & valor medicamentorum simplicium & compositorum in officinis Hafniensibus prostantium. 1672. *See* COPENHAGEN. Ordinances, local laws, etc.

CATALOGUS medicamentorum. *See* STAPHORST, N. Officina chymica Londinensis. 1685.

CATANIA, FRANCESCO [*ca.* 1598-*ca.* 1688] Quaestio de medicamento purgante. [Panormi, Ex Typographia Petri de Isola, 1648]

24, 291 p. 21 cm. [2295]

Engraved title page.
Imperfect: p. 257-291 misbound after p. 8.

CATANUTO, Nicola [*fl. ca.* 1658] Catanense dispensatorium; sive, Antidotarium ea continens medicamenta, quae apud nostros medicos usitatiora habentur ... Catanae, Ex typographia Josephi Bisagni, 1666.

[18], 300, [14] p. front. 18 cm. **[2296]**

CATARROJA, Juan Bautista. *See* Insa, A. J. Officina medicamentorum. 1601 [colophon: 1603], 1698.

CATE, Theodoor ten [*fl.* 1694] *respondent.* Disputatio medica inauguralis de diarrhoea ... Lugduni Batavorum, Apud Abrahamum Elzevier, 1694.

[28] p. 22 cm. **[2297]**
Diss. — Leyden.

CATELAN, Laurent [*ca.* 1568-1647] Discours et demonstration des ingrediens de la confection d'alkermes reformee ... contre les discours faicts par le Sr. Jacques Fontaine ... Lyon, Jaques Mallet, 1614.

316 p. 15 cm. **[2298]**

—Preservatifs contre la contagion, recueillis des ordonnances faites pendant ce temps. Par messieurs les professeurs en l'Université de Medecine de Montpellier. Ensemble l'usage des provisions medicales qu'on peut garder aux champs dans de layettes lors qu'on est esloigné des bonnes villes ... Montpellier, Jean Pech, 1629.

27 p.; 12 p. 15 cm. **[2299]**
Part [2] has special title page: Vertus, proprietez et usage des provisions medicales contenues en cette layette.

—[Traicté de l'origine, vertus, proprietez et usage de la pierre bezoar. German.] Ein newer historischer und medicinischer Tractat vom Bezoar Stein ... Ins Teutsch ubergesetzt. Franckfurt am Mayn, In Velegung Lucae Jennisii, 1627.

[66] p. 16 cm. **[2300]**
Translated by Georg Faber. Cf. Jöcher, vol. 1, col. 1768.

—Traicté des eaux distillées. *In* Bauderon, B. Paraphrase sur la pharmacopee. 1627 [and] Pharmacopee divisee en deux livres. 1640 [and] Pharmacopee de Bauderon, 1644, 1650, 1655, 1663, 1672, 1681. [Latin tr.] 1639.

—*See* Strobelberger, J. S. Tractatus novus. 1620.

CATHOLIC CHURCH. Camera apostolica. Bando et ordini sopra la conservatione della sanità nello stato ecclesiastico ... Ravenna, Pietro de' Paoli e Gio Battista Giovanelli, 1630.

broadside. 121 x 53 cm. **[2301]**
Includes text of original edict issued in Rome, signed by Cardinal Francesco Barberini.

—**Congregatio Sacrorum Rituum.** Congregatione Sacrorum Rituum ... Beatificationis, & canonizationis ... Turibii Alphonsi Mogrobesii archiepiscopi Limani. Positio super dubio. An ex pluribus deductis pro miraculis in processibus constet de sex in vita, & decem post obitum, in casu, & ad effectum de quo agitur. Romae, Ex typographia Rev. Camerae Apostolicae, 1675.

1 v. 32 cm. **[2302]**
Various pagings.

—**Pope,** 1471-1484 (Sixtus IV) *Variis quamquam* (14 Dec. 1471) Sixtus Papa IV. Ad perpetuam rei memoriam. [Romae? 1675?]

4 p. 22 cm. **[2303]**
Concerns the Collegio dei medici in Rome.

—**Pope,** 1523-1534 (Clemens VII) *In supremae dignitatis* (8 Sept. 1531). Clementis Papae VII. Bulla de protomedici & Collegii Medicorum urbis jurisdictione, & facultatibus. Romae, Ex typographia Rev. Camerae Apost., 1627.

[24] p. 22 cm. **[2304]**

—**Pope,** 1550-1555 (Julius III) *Meritis devotionis* (21 Apr. 1553). Julius Papa III. Meritis devotionis vestrae, erga Nos, & Romanam ecclesiam inducumur, ut petitionibus vestris quantum cum Deo possumus favorabiliter annuamus. [Romae, Ex typographia Rev. Cam. Apost., 1674]

5 p. 22 cm. **[2305]**
Caption title.
Text dated 1583 (i.e. 1553)
Imperfect: outer margins mutilated.
Concerns the Collegio dei medici in Rome.

—**Pope,** 1559-1565 (Pius IV) *Motu proprio* (12 Sept. 1562). Pius Papa IV. Confirmatio privilegiorum Collegii Medicorum urbis. [Romae? 1675?]

8 p. 22 cm. **[2306]**
Caption title.

—**Pope,** 1566-1572 (Pius V) *Romanus pontifex* (12 Aug. 1570). Pius Papa V. Ad perpetuam rei memoriam. [Romae, Ex typographia Reverendae Camerae Apostolicae, 1675]

[7] p.   22 cm.   [2307]

Caption title.
Concerns the Collegio dei medici in Rome.

—**Pope**, 1572-1585 (Gregorius XIII) *Cum officio* (1 July, 1575) *See* COLLEGIO DEI MEDICI, Rome. Motus proprius confirmationis concordiae. 1675.

—*In Apostolico dignitatis* (1 Nov. 1576). Gregorius Papa XIII ad perpetuam rei memoriam. [Romae, Ex typographia R. Cam. Apost. 1675]

[6] p.   22 cm.   [2308]

Caption title.
Concerns the Collegio dei medici in Rome.

—**Pope**, 1593-1603 (Clemens VIII) *Quo viri* (10 Nov. 1593). Clemens Papa Octavus ad perpetuam rei memoriam. [Romae? 1675?]

[6] p.   22 cm.   [2309]

Caption title.
Concerns the Collegio dei medici in Rome.

—**Pope**, 1623-1644 (Urbano VIII) *Artis medicae* (4 Dec. 1641) *See* COLLEGIO DEI MEDICI, Rome. Statuta Collegii DD. almae urbis medicorum. 1642.

—**Pope**, 1670-1676 (Clemens X) *Cum nos alias* (12 Nov. 1674). Clemens PP. X. Ad perpetuam rei memoriam. [Romae, Ex typographia Reverendae Cam. Apost., 1675]

[8] p.   22 cm.   [2310]

Caption title.
Concerns the Collegio dei medici in Rome.

—**Province of Milan**. *Concilio provinciale*, 1565-1582. Constitutiones, et decreta sex provincialium synodorum Mediolanensium. Quas . . . Carolus Borrhomaeus . . . habuit. Ab anno . . . MDLXV . . . ad annum MDLXXII [i.e. 1582] . . . Hoc volumine, sex libris distincto . . . contexta. Per . . . Dominicum Zucchinettum . . . Tractatus De cura pestilentiae: inter decreta concilii quinti provincialis inserto separatim post ipsum indicem collocato. Brixiae, Apud Societatem Brixiensem, 1603.

[16], 897 (i.e. 955), [204], 84, [15] p. plate. 22 cm.   [2311]

CATS, JACOB [1577-1660] *See* BEVERWIJCK, J. van. Alle de wercken soo in de medecyne als chirurgye. 1651, 1656 [and] Schat der gesontheyt. 1637, 1638, 1642, 1647 [and] Wercken der genees-konste. 1664, 1672.

CATTIER, ISAAC [*fl.* 1637-1665] Divers traictez, a scavoir, De la nature des bains de Bourbon, & des abus qui se commettent à present en la boisson de ces eaux; avec une instruction pour s'en servir utilement. De la macreuse. De la poudre de sympathie. Response à Monsieur Papin . . . touchant la poudre de sympathie, en laquelle est traicté de l'esprit universel, & des proprietez de l'ayman. Paris, Pierre David, 1651.

3 v. in 1.   17 cm.   [2312]

Imperfect: Title page of v. [2] wanting?
The 3 works in the first two volumes were issued together in 1650 under titles: De la nature des bains de Bourbon, and De la macreuse et De la poudre de sympathie. The two works in v. [2] were apparently also issued separately in 1650 and in 1651 respectively.
Vol. [3], Response a Monsieur Papin, has special title page with imprint: Paris, Imprimerie d'Edme Martin, 1651.
Bound between v. [2] and v. [3] are two works by Nicolas Papin: De pulvere sympathico dissertatio. 1650; and La poudre de sympathie, deffendue contre les objections de Mr Cattier. 1651.

—De la poudre de sympathie. *See* PAPIN, N. La poudre de sympathie, deffendue contre les objections de Mr Cattier. 1651.

—Dissertatio de rheumatismo. In qua non solum hujus affectionis natura, & curatio exacte proponuntur: sed & praeterea . . . quaedam de natura doloris intricatissima perspicue enodantur, novisque observationibus illustrantur. Parisiis, Apud viduam Petit, 1653.

[16], 153, [1] p.   17 cm.   [2313]

—Observationes medicinales. *In* Borel, P. Historiarum, et observationum medicophysicarum, centuriae IV. 1656, 1657, 1670, 1676.

[—] Seconde apologie de l'université en medecine de Montpellier. Répondant aux Curieuses recherches des universitez de Paris & de Montpellier; faites par un vieil docteur medecin de Paris. Envoyée à Monsieur Riolan, professeur anatomique, par un jeune docteur en medecine de Montpellier . . . Paris, Jean Piot, 1653.

[8], 248, [2] p.   22 cm.   [2314]

Jean Riolan's Curieuses recherches sur les escholes en medecine de Paris et de Montpelier had appeared anonymously in Paris in 1651.
Errata: p. [249-250]

—*See* LE GIVRE, P. Le secret des eaux minerales acides. 1667; [Latin tr.] 1682.

—*as subject.* See BARTHOLIN, T. Opuscula nova anatomica. 1670; GUILLEMEAU, C. Cani miuro; sive, Curto fustis. 1654.

CAUFAPÉ, ANICET [17th cent.] Nouvelle explication de la gangrene, proposée et demandée par Messieurs de l'Academie de Paris dans leur Journal du mois de fevrier de l'année presente . . . Toulouse, Jean Boude, 1681.

[8], 112 p.   18 cm.   [2315]

—Nouvelle explication des fievres et de la gangrene. Avec une methode paticuliere pour les guerir, & une dissertation singuliere sur leurs causes . . . sur l'acide & sur l'alkali, sur le quiquina, & les autres febrifuges . . . Toulouse, Pierre Salabert, 1687.

[28], 424 p.; 124, [28] p.   16 cm.   [2316]

Part 2 has caption title: Nouvelle explication des crises et de la gangrene.

—Observations singulieres sur le frequent usage de la saignée, sur le dereglement de la circulation du sang, & sur une methode pour la prolongation de la vie . . . Toulouse, Pierre Salabert, 1691.

[12], 99 p.; [8], 200, [4] p.   15 cm.   [2317]

Part [2] has special title page: Methode singuliere, pour prolonger la vie . . . avec un Traité de la nature des alimens.

CAUFUNGER, GEORG [*fl.* 1603] *ed. See* MAGIRUS, J. Anthropologia. 1603.

CAULIACO, GUIDO DE. *See* GUY DE CHAULIAC [*ca.* 1300-1368]

CAULIER, PIERRE [*fl.* 1652] *respondent. See* LINDEN, J. A. van der, *praeses.* Mulieris colicae historia. 1652.

CAUSE, DE. *See* CAUX, David de [*fl.* 1670-1674]

CAUSINO, NICOLO. *See* CAUSSIN, Nicolas [1583-1651]

CAUSSIN, NICOLAS [1583-1651] Effemeride astrologica, et historica . . . Tradotta dalla lingua latina nell'italiana. Bologna, Carlo Zenero, 1652.

[23], 477 p.   tables.   14 cm.   [2318]

Added half title.

CAUX, DAVID DE [*fl.* 1670-1674] Varia philosophica et medica. De atomis. De circulari sanguinis motu. Adversus Pyrrhonios. De generatione hominis. De usu lienis. De causa motus pulmonum in ispiratione. Anatomica quaedam. Rothomagi, Apud Jacobum Lucas, 1674.

8, [3], 239 p.   15 cm.   [2319]

CAUX, N. DE. *See* CAUX, David de [*fl.* 1670-1674]

CAVALIER, PIERRE. *See* CAULIER, Pierre [*fl.* 1652]

CAVALLARA, GIOVANNI BATTISTA [*fl.* 1586] De morbo epidemiali, qui Nolam, & Campaniam universam vexavit curativus, & praeservativus. Discursus. Neapoli, Apud Jo. Jacobum Carlinum, 1602.

[8], 92, [4] p.   22 cm.   [2320]

CAVALLO, FRANCESCO [*d.* 1540] De animali thirio. *In* Cermisone, A. Consillia medicinalia. 1604.

CAVENDISH, MARGARET, *duchess of Newcastle. See* NEWCASTLE, Margaret (Lucas) Cavendish, *duchess of* [1624?-1674]

CAVILLARD, JOSEPH. *See* COUILLARD, Joseph [*d.* 1660]

CAVLERIUS, PETRUS. *See* CAULIER, Pierre [*fl.* 1652]

CECCARELLI, IPPOLITO [Selections] *In* Antidotario romano latino e volgare. 1624, 1635, 1639, 1675, 1678.

CECCHINI, MARIO [*fl.* 1684] Elenchus lectionum, et ostensionum anatomicarum. Quibus per D. Marium Cecchinum . . . humani corporis systemma anatomicum ostendetur. In theatro anatomico archixendochii S. Jacobi incurabilium . . . Romae, Typis Michaelis Erculis, 1684.

24 p.   23 cm.   [2321]

CELEBERR. virorum apologiae pro R. D. Carolo Musitano adversus Petrum Antonium de Martino . . . qui Trutinam medicam anno 1688 . . . editam, qua Harveana sanguinis circulatio aliaeque recentiorum medicorum sententiae statuminantur, temere, & inepte impugnare ausus est. Kruswick, Apud Petrum Antonium Martellum, 1700.

196, [10] p.   24 cm.   [2322]

"Nuncius Parnassius, seu, Epistola ex Parnasso a Sebastiano Bartholo ad . . . Carolum Musitanum" [by Giuseppe Prisco]: p. [41]-[104]; "Martinus in Trutina; sive, Apologetica per dialogos disquisitio . . . authore Jo. Andrea Lizzano": p. [105]-196. Items have special title pages.

Bound with vol. 2 of Musitano, C. Opera medica chymicopractica. 1700.

CELI, ANTONINO [*fl. ca.* 1618] Antonini Caelii . . . Introductio universalis ad medicam facultatem; ac Brevis methodus curandi particulares praeter naturam corporis humani affectus: necnon De pulsibus tractatio: quibus additur Commentarius in primum librum Aphorismorum Hippocratis. Messanae, Ex typographia Petri Breae, 1618.

    [8], 214, [2] p.   table.   20 cm.   [2323]

    "Commentarius in primum librum Aphorismorum Hippocratis" (p. 103-214) includes Latin text of Hippocrates in Niccolò Leoniceno's version.

CELLARIUS, CHRISTOPH [1638-1707] *praeses.* Origines et antiquitates medicas . . . ad disputandum proponit . . . Salomo Cellarius . . . Halae Magdeburgicae, Litteris Chr. Henckelii [1696]

    [20] p.   20 cm.   [2324]

    Diss.—Halle (S. Cellarius, *respondent*)

CELLARIUS, FRIEDRICH [*fl.* 1686] *respondent. See* MEIBOM, H., *praeses.* Disputatio medica de hernia. 1686.

CELLARIUS, GEORG FRIEDRICH [*fl.* 1677] *respondent. See* FASCH, A. H., *praeses.* Respirationis laesiones hypochondriaco-scorbuticas . . . exponit . . . G. F. C. . . . 1677.

CELLARIUS, HEINRICH [*fl.* 17th cent.] Kurtzer Bericht vom Scharbock. Halberstadt, Johann Erasmus Hynitzsch, 1675.

    72 p.   14 cm.   [2325]

    Bound with Viel-vergröster und hellerpolirter Schorbocks-Spiegel. 1659.

—Die vermeinete Mutterbeschwerung . . . Halberstadt, Joh. Erasmus Hynitzsch, 1677.

    [46], 367 p.   14 cm.   [2326]

CELLARIUS, HEINRICH [*fl.* 1671] *respondent. See* ROLFINCK, W., *praeses.* Dissertationem hanc inauguralem de affectu hypochondriaco . . . submittit . . . H.C. 1671.

CELLARIUS, JEREMIAS CUNRADUS [*fl.* 1677-1679] *respondent. See* CAMERARIUS, E. R., *praeses.* Dissertatio medica de acidularum usu externo. 1677; METZGER, G. B., *praeses.* De aneurysmate. 1679.

CELLARIUS, JUSTUS [*fl.* 1674-1682] *praeses.* Exercitatio academica de natura panis . . . Helmestadii, Typis Henrici Davidis Mulleri [1676]

    [32] p.   20 cm.   [2327]

    Diss.—Helmstedt (F. Schrader, *respondent*)

CELLARIUS, SALOMO [1676-1700] *respondent. See* CELLARIUS, C., *praeses.* Origines et antiquitates

medicas. 1696; HOFFMANN, F. [1660-1742] *praeses.* Dissertatio inauguralis physico-medica de natura morborum medicatrice mechanica. 1699.

CELLARIUS, THEODOR [*fl.* 1665] *praeses.* Disputatio physica de tactu . . . Tubingae, Ex Officina Reisiana [1665]

    12 p.   19 cm.   [2328]

    Diss.—Tübingen (J. J. Roth, *respondent*)

CELLEOR, ELIZABETH. *See* CELLIER, Elizabeth [*fl.* 1680-1688]

CELLIER, ANTOINE [*fl.* 1680] *ed.* Opuscula nova anatomica, Thomae Petruccii, Casparis Bartholini, et Joannis Verle. Lugduni, Apud Antonium Cellier filium, 1680.

    [10], 179, [1] p.   plates.   15 cm.   [2329]

    Contents: [1] Petrucci, Tomasso. Spigilegium anatomicum. [2] Bartholin, Caspar. De ovariis mulierum & generatione historia. [3] Verle, Giovanni Battista. Anatomia artificialis oculi humani.

CELLIER, ELIZABETH [*fl.* 1680-1688] To Dr. ------ an answer to his queries, concerning the colledg of midwives. [London, 1688]

    8 p.   20 cm.   [2330]

    Caption title.

    Imprint supplied from BMC.

CELLIUS, GEORG FRIEDRICH [*fl.* 1680-1683] *respondent. See* CAMERARIUS, E. R., *praeses.* Disputatio inauguralis medica de mictione pultacea. 1683 [and] Disquisitio medica quale signum in morbis praebeat urina. 1680.

CELNATUS, THEOPHILUS. *See* MAIER, M. Themis aurea. 1656.

CELSUS, AULUS CORNELIUS. De re medica libri octo. Item, Q. Sereni Liber de medicina. Q. Rhemmii Fannii Palaemonis De ponderibus & mensuris liber. Vindiciani carmen. Omnia ex diversorum codicum diligentissima collatione castigata, additis ad marginem variis lectionibus. [Lugduni] Apud Joannem Tornaesium, 1608.

    [32], 575, [1] p.   12 cm.   [2331]

    "Vindiciano attributum carmen" (p. 573-575) attributed to Vindicianus appears in editions of the De medicamentis liber by Marcellus Empiricus, and is to be attributed to that author.

    A reprint of the edition of 1587.

—[The same.] . . . Genevae, Sumptibus Johannis de Tournes, 1625.

    [31], 671 p.   13 cm.   [2332]

    "Vindiciano attributum carmen" (p. 669-671).

—De medicina libri octo, ex recognitione Joh. Antonidae vander Linden ... Lugduni Batav., Apud Johannem Elsevirium, 1657.

[24], 558, [2] p. 14 cm. [2333]

Added engraved title page.

Errata: p. [559-560]

— [The same.] ... Ed. 2. Lugduni Batavorum, Apud Salomonem Wagenaer, 1665.

[24], 592, [8] p. 13 cm. [2334]

—De medicina libri octo, brevioribus Rob. Constantini, Is. Casauboni aliorumque scholiis ac locis parallelis illustrati. Cura & studio Th. J. ab Almeloveen, M.D. Amstelaedami, Apud Joannem Wolters, 1687.

[48], 574, [25] p. illus., port. 16 cm.

[2335]

Added engraved title page.

"Aurelii Cornelii Celsi vita a ... Joanne Rhodio conscripta": p. [25-38]; "Libri quorum J. A. van der Linden usus fuit in hoc opere recognoscendo": p. [39-42]; "Indiculus editionum Celsi in folio; Testimonia et elogia de Celso": p. [43-48]; "Breviora variorum auctorum in Celsi libros scholia": p. 559-574.

Revised and expanded from Linden's edition of 1657.

—De re medica liber octavus. Ejus priora quatuor capita commentariis illustrata a Petro Paaw. Lugduni Batavorum, Apud Jodocum a Colster, 1616.

[2], 128 p. illus. 20 cm. (*In* Pauw, Pieter. Succenturiatus anatomicus ... Additae in aliquot capita libri VIII C. Celsi explicationes. Lugduni Batavorum, 1616.) [2336]

—[Selections] *In* Hippocrates. [Aphorismi, Greek and Latin.] Aphorismi et Prognostica. 1625 [and] Ἀφορισμοί. 1685 [and] [Aphorismi. Latin.] Tripus medicinae. 1681; Rossi, G. Annotationes in libros octo Cornelii Celsi De re medica. 1616.

—, *tr. See* LATIOSO, A. In Hippocratis Aphorismos ... commentarii. 1667.

—*See* DALECHAMPS, J. Chirurgie françoise. 1610; GALENUS. [De ossibus ad tirones. Greek and Latin.] De ossibus. 1665; HIPPOCRATES. [Selected works. Greek and Latin.] Aphorismi Graeco-Latini. 1631.

—*as subject. See* CHIFFLET, J. J. Acia Cornelii Celsi propriae significationi restituta. 1633; RODE, J. Antiquitates philosophicae, medicae & chirurgicae. 1691 [and] De acia dissertatio ad Cornelii Celsi mentem. 1639, 1672.

CENTORIO DEGLI HORTENSII, ASCANIO [16th cent.] I cinque libri de gli avvertimenti, ordini, gride, et editti: fatti, et osservati in Milano, ne' tempi sospetosi della peste; de gli anni MDLXXVI. & LXXVII. con molti avvedimenti utili, e necessari à tutte le città d'Europa, che cadessero in simili infortunii, e calamità ... Milano, Filippo Ghisolfi, ad instanza, & spese di Gio. Battista Bidelli, 1631.

[24], 380 p. 23 cm. [2337]

Includes (p. 323-329) an account of the plague in Latin by Cesare Rincio, later republished by Joachim Camerarius in his Synopsis commentariorum de peste, Norimbergae 1583, under title: Disputatio de peste Mediolanensi.

CENTURIA rariorum problematum historicomedico-physicorum. [Francofurti? 1690?]

136 (i.e. 154) p. 20 cm. [2338]

Imprint supplied from BMC.

CERASTUS CORNANUS, CORNELIUS. *See* CRUFENAS, Cariollinus Tevetio. Themata medica de beanorum. 1651?

CERF, PETRUS LE. *See* LE CERF, Pierre Théodore [*fl.* 1682-1694]

CERIMONIE nuzziali di tutte le nationi del mondo. 1685. *See* [GAYA, L. de]

CERMISONE, ANTONIO [*d.* 1441] Consilia medicinalia contra omnes fere aegritudines a capite usque ad pedes, una cum Francisci Caballi tractatu De animali thirio ... Francofurti, Prodeunt ex Collegio musarum Paltheniano, 1604.

[1], 156, [3] p. 34 cm. [2339]

Bound (as issued?) with Montagnana, B. Selectiorum operum ... Montagnanae. 1604.

CERTAIN necessary directions. 1636, 1665. *See* ROYAL COLLEGE OF PHYSICIANS, London.

CERTAIN orders thought meet to be put in execution against the infection of the plague. 1641. *See* GT. BRIT. LAWS, STATUTES, etc.

A CERTAINE relation of the hogfaced gentlewoman called Mistris Tannakin Skinker, who was borne at Wirkham ... Who was bewitched in her mothers wombe in the yeare 1618 ... Also relating the cause, as it is since conceived, how her mother came so bewitched. London, Printed by J. O[kes] and are to be sold by F. Grove, 1640.

[16], p. 24 cm. [2340]

STC 22627.

CERTAINE statutes especially selected, and commanded by His Majestie. 1630. *See* Gt. Brit. Laws, statutes, etc.

CERUTI, Benedetto [*d.* 1620] Musaeum Franc. Calceolarii jun. . . . a Benedicto Ceruto . . . incaeptum, et ab Andrea Chiocco . . . luculenter descriptum, & perfectum. In quo multa ad naturalem, moralemque philosophiam spectantia, non pauca ad rem medicam pertinentia erudite proponuntur, & explicantur . . . [Veronae, Apud Angelum Tamum, 1622]

    [50], 746 p. illus., plate. 31 cm.   [2341]
Engraved title page.

CERVI, Annibale [*d.* 1701] *See* Ramazzini, B. Exercitatio iatropologetica. 1679.

CESALPINO, Andrea [1519-1603] Artis medicae, liber VII [-VIII] de morbis ventris. Romae, Ex typographia Aloysii Zannetti, 1603.

    455 p. 15 cm.   [2342]
"... Artis medicae liber octavus de genitalium morbis": p. 229-455.
Artis medicae pars prima, de morbis universalibus (lib. 1-3) and Artis medicae pars II. de morbis internarum partium (lib. 4-6) . . . were published in 1602 by Zannetti. Cf. BNC, vol. 25, col. 869.

—[The same.] Κάτοπτρον; sive, Speculum artis medicae Hippocraticum: spectandos, dignoscendos curandosque exhibens universos, tum universales tum particulares, totius corporis humani morbos . . . Antea quidem Romae excusum, nunc vero castigatius editum. Francoforti, Typis Matthiae Beckeri, impensis Lazari Zetzneri, 1605.

    [16], 663 p. 17 cm.   [2343]
Running title: Artis medicae liber primus [-VIII]

—[The same.] Praxis universae artis medicae, generalium aeque, ac particularium humani corporis praeter naturam affectuum dignotionem, juditium & curam omnium uberrime complectens, summo labore, et studio concinnata, & unum recenter in volumen conjecta . . . Tarvisii, Sumptibus Roberti Meietti, 1606.

    [16], 715 p. 15 cm.   [2344]

—[The same.] Κάτοπτρον; sive, Speculum artis medicae Hippocraticum . . . Argentorati, Impensis Georgii Andreae Dolhopfii & Joh. Eberhardi Zetzneri, 1670.

    [16], 663 p. 16 cm.   [2345]
The main text is a reissue of the 1605 edition.

—De metallicis libri tres . . . Noribergae, Recusi, curante Conrado Agricola [Ex officina Katharinae, viduae Alexandri Theodorici] 1602.

    [15], 222, [1] p. 21 cm.   [2346]
Errata: p. [223]
Edited by Philip Scherb.
Bound with Nehemias, A. Methodus medendi universalis. 1604.

—*See* Boccone, P. Museo di piante rare della Sicilia, Malta, Corsica, Italia, Piemonte, e Germania. 1697.

CESARELLI, Hippolito. *See* Ceccarelli, Ippolito.

CESI, Federico, *duca di Acquasparta* [1585-1630] *See* Hernández, F. Rerum medicarum Novae Hispaniae thesaurus. 1628, 1651.

CEVOLI, Nicola, *marquis del Carretto* [*fl.* 17th cent.] *See* Le souverain a donné la science aux hommes. 1696?

CHABODIE, David [*d. ca.* 1640] Le petit monde ou sont representantees au vrai les plus belles parties de l'homme . . . Paris, Daniel Guillemot et Ethiene Roland, 1604.

    [8], 128 p.; 86 (i.e. 90), [8] ll. front., illus. 18 cm.   [2347]
Engraved title page.
Imperfect: front. wanting; verso of sig. [Avii] and recto of [Aviii] at end blank, possibly wanting text.

CHABRAEUS, Dominicus. *See* Chabrey, Dominique [1610-1669]

CHABREY, Dominique [1610-1669] Stirpium icones et sciagraphia, cum scriptorum circa eas consensu et dissensu, ac caeteris plaerisque omnibus quae de plantarum natura . . . usu & virtutibus, scitu necessaria . . . Genevae, Typis Phil. Gamoneti & Jac. de la Pierre, 1666.

    [10], 661, [28] p. illus. 38 cm.   [2348]
Added engraved title page.

—[The same.] Stirpium icones et sciagraphia cum omnibus, quae de plantarum natura . . . usu & virtutibus, scitu nacessaria, quibus accessit scriptorum circa eas consensus, & dissensus . . . Genevae, Apud Joannem Anthonium Chouët, 1677.

    [8], 661, [28] p. illus. 35 cm.   [2349]
A reissue of the 1666 edition with new title page.

—*respondent. See* Sebisch, M. [1578-1674?] *praeses.* Examen vulnerum singularum humani corporis partium. 1639 [and] Galeni Ars parva in disputationes triginta resoluta. 1633 [and] Prodromi examinis vulnerum singularum humani corporis partium. 1632.

—, ed. See BAUHIN, J. Historia plantarum universalis. 1650-1651.

CHACÓN, DIONISIO DAZA. See DAZA CHACÓN, Dionisio [1510–ca. 1596]

CHAILLOU, JACQUES [ca. 1636-1720] Recherches de l'origine et du mouvement du sang, du coeur, et de ses vaisseaux; du lait, des fiévres intermittentes & des humeurs ... Paris, Jean Couterot, 1675.

    [24], 407 p.   16 cm.   **[2350]**
With this is bound *his* Traite du mouvement des humeurs. 1678.

—[The same.] ... Nouvelle ed. corr. par l'auteur. Paris, Jean Couterot & Loüis Guerin, 1687.

    [16], 416 p.   15 cm.   **[2351]**

Colophon: Paris, De l'imprimerie d'Antoine Lambin, 1687.

—[The same.] ... Paris, Laurent d'Houry, 1699.
    [16], 416 p.   15 cm.   **[2352]**
Colophon: Paris, De l'imprimerie d' Antoine Lambin, 1687.
Reissue of the 1687 edition with a new title page.

—Traite du mouvement des humeurs, dans les plus ordinaires émotions des hommes ... Paris, Jean Couterot, 1678.

    69, [3] p.   16 cm.   **[2353]**
Bound with *his* Recherches de l'origine et du mouvement du sang. 1675.

CHALES, CLAUDE FRANÇOIS MILLIET DE, *Father* [1621-1678] Cursus seu mundus mathematicus. Tomus primus [-quartus] ... Ed. alt. ex manuscriptis authoris aucta & emendata, opera & studio R. P. Amati Varcin ... Lugduni. Apud Anissonios, Joan. Posuel & Claud. Rigaud, 1690.

    4 v.   illus., tables.   36 cm.   **[2354]**
"Oratio habita in funere R. P. Claudii Francisci Milliet Dechales ... a ... Hyacinto Ferrerio ... 28 Martii 1678": vol. 1, 4 p. following preface.
Contents.—vol. 1: De progressu matheseos et illustribus mathematicis.—Euclidis Elementorum libri XIII.; Elementorum Euclidis aut potius Hypsiclis Alexandrini liber decimus quartus.—Theodosii Elementa sphaerica.—De sectionibus conicis.—Arithmetica.—Trigonometria.—Algebra.—Hypotheseon Cartesianarum refutatio.—vol. 2: Geometri practica.—Mechanica.—Statica.—Geographia.—De magnete.—Architectonica civilis.—Ars tignaria.—De lapidum sectione.—vol. 3: Architectura militaris.—Hydrostatica.—De fontibus naturalibus, & fluminibus.—De machinis hydraulicis.—Ars navigandi.—Optica.—Perspectiva.—Catoprica.—Dioptrica.—vol. 4: Musica.—Pyrotechnia.—De astrolabiis.—Gnomonica.—

Astronomia.—Astrologia.—Appendix ad astronomiam: De meteoris.—Kalendarium.

CHĀLID IBN JAZĪD IBN MU'ĀWĪJA. *See* KHĀLID IBN YAZĪD, al-Umawî.

CHALLINOR, MRS. *See* WOOLLEY, Hannah [*fl.* 1670]

CHALMETEUS, ANTONIUS. *See* CHAUMETTE, Antoine [16th cent.]

CHALOPIN, JACQUES. Remedes preservatifs, et curatifs, de la peste avec la maniere de faire l'opiat. Paris, Pierre Chevalier [ca. 1610]

    54 p.   17 cm.   **[2355]**
Engraved title page.
Pierre Chevalier was active in Paris between 1602 and 1622.

CHAMBERLAIN, HUGH, *the elder*. *See* CHAMBERLEN, Hugh [*b.* ca. 1630]

CHAMBERLAIN, PETER. *See* CHAMBERLEN, Peter [1601-1683]

[CHAMBERLAYNE, JOHN, 1666-1723] *comp.* Schatzkammer rarer und neuer Curiositäten, in den aller-wunderbahresten Würckungen der Natur und Kunst, darinnen ... Geheimnüsse, bewehrte Artzneyen, Wissenschafften und Kunst-Stücke zu finden ... Der dritte Druck, jetzo mit dem dritten Theil von vielen chymischen Experimenten ... vermehret. Deme angehenget ist ein Tractat, Naturgemässer Beschreibung der Coffee, Thee, Chocolate Tabacks ... Hamburg, Auff Gottfried Schultzens Kosten, 1689.

    [8], 592, [24] p.   front.   17 cm.   **[2356]**
"Naturgemässe Beschreibung der Coffee, Thee, Chocolate und Tabacks, in vier unterschiedlichen Abtheilungen, mit einem Tracktätlein, von Hollunder-und Wachholder-Beeren ... Wie auch den Weg die Mumme zu bereiten ... Auss der englischen in die hochteutsche Sprache übersetset, durch J[ohann] L[ange] M[edicinae] C[andidatum]": p. [561]-589.
Partly based on P. S. Dufour's Traitez nouveaux. Cf. Mueller, p. 43.

—, *tr. See* DURANTE, C. A treasure of health. 1686, 1689.

CHAMBERLEN, HUGH [*b. ca.* 1630] A few queries relating to the practice of physick, with remarks upon some of them. Modestly proposed to the serious consideration of mankind, in order to their information how their lives and healths ... may be better preserved ... London, T. Soule, 1694.

    [10], 122 p.   15 cm.   **[2357]**

By the elder Hugh Chamberlen; erroneously attributed to his son of the same name by Munk. Cf. Aveling, p. 152.

"A proposal for the better securing of health, intended in the year, 1689, and still ready to be humbly offered to the consideration of the Honourable Houses of Parliament": p. 95-110. "An appendix to the Queries": p. III-122.

—, *tr. See* MAURICEAU, F. The accomplisht midwife. 1673, 1697.

—*See* CHAMBERLEN, P. Dr. Chamberlain's midwifes practice. 1665; THE COMPLEAT MIDWIFE'S PRACTICE ENLARGED. 1663, 1697, 1698.

CHAMBERLEN, HUGH [1664-1728] *See* CHAMBERLEN, H. [*b. ca.* 1630] A few queries relating to the practice of physick. 1694.

CHAMBERLEN, PETER [1601-1683] Dr. Chamberlain's midwifes practice; or, A guide for women in that high concern of conception, breeding, and nursing children. In a plain method, containing the anatomy of the parts of generation: forming the child in the womb: what hinders and causes conception: of miscarriages: and directions in labour, lying-inne, and nursing children ... London, Thomas Rooks, 1665.

[16], 288 p.   plate.   16 cm.   [**2358**]

Dedicatory epistle signed: P. C.
Attributed also to the elder Hugh Chamberlen. Cf. Carrere, vol. 2, p. 458.

—A vindication of publick artificiall baths & bath-stoves from the objections and scandalls obtruded on them, by those that do not, or will not know their great benefit to the publick. By way of answer to some Fellowes of our Colledge of Physitians in London and others ... London, 1648.

[1], 6 p.   19 cm.   [**2359**]

CHAMBÉRY. Academie chimique. *See* ACADEMIE CHIMIQUE, Chambéry.

CHAMBRE, MARIN CUREAU DE LA. *See* CUREAU DE LA CHAMBRE, Marin [1593 or 4-1669]

CHAMPIER, JEAN BAPTISTE BRUYERIN. *See* BRUYERIN, Jean Baptiste [*fl.* 1530-1560]

CHANDELIER, JAN SIX VAN. *See* SIX VAN CHANDELIER, Johan [*b.* 1612]

CHANDLER, JOHN [*fl.* 1662] *tr. See* HELMONT, J. B. van. Oriatrike; or, Physick refined. 1662.

CHANUEL, CLAUDE [*fl.* 1609] Le chasse-verole des petits enfans ... Lyon, Barthelemy Vincent, 1610.

[24], 195 (i.e. 193), [10] p.   port.   15 cm.   [**2360**]

CHAPEAUVILLE, JEAN [1551-1617] Tractatus de necessitate et modo ministrandi sacramenta tempore pestis ... Coloniae, Apud Petrum Cholinum, 1625.

547 (i.e. 574), [25] p.   [**2361**]

CHAPITRE singulier tiré de Guidon. *See* ABEILLE, S. L'anatomie de la teste. 1689.

CHAPMAN, HENRY [*fl.* 1673] Thermae redivivae: the city of Bath described: with some observations on those soveraign waters, both as to the bathing in, and drinking of them, now so much in use ... London, Printed for the author, and are to be sold by Jonathan Edwin, 1673.

[6], 17 p.   19 cm.   [**2362**]

CHAPPUYS, GABRIEL [1546-1611] *tr. See* HUARTE DE SAN JUAN, J. Examen des esprits propres et naiz aux sciences. 1602, 1608, 1619.

The CHARACTER of a compleat physician, or naturalist. *See* [MEE, Dr.]

CHARAS, MOYSE [1618-1698] Opera tribus tomis distincta: I. Pharmacopoea regia Galenica. II. Pharmacopoea regia chymica. III. Tractatus de theriaca & Tractatus de vipera. [Genevae, Sumptibus Joannis Ludovici Du-Four, 1684]

3 v. in 1.   front. (port.), plates.   25 cm.   [**2363**]

A reissue of the 2 volumes published in 1683 by Du-Four in Geneva under title: ... Pharmacopoea regia Galenica et chymica ... Tomus primus [-secundus] with the addition of Pharmacopoeae pars quarta, title pages reset, and added engraved title page.

Vol. 3 has added engraved title page: Theriaca Andromachi conscribente Mose Charas, and title page: Operum tomus tertius, continens Historiam naturalem animalium, plantarum et mineralium, Theriacae Andromachi compositionem ingredientium; cum Experimentis circa viperam, addita serie novorum experimentorum.

—Histoire naturelle des animaux, des plantes, & des mineraux qui entrent dans la composition de la theriaque d'Andromachus. Dispensee et achevee publiquement à Paris ... Avec les reformations & les observations de l'auteur ... Paris, Olivier de Varennes, 1668.

[28], 310, [9], 12 p.   16 cm.   [**2364**]

Added engraved title page: Theriaque d'Andromachus.

—[The same.] Theriaque d'Andromacus, avec une description particuliere des plantes, des animaux & des mineraux employez à cette grande composition, et les reformations & observations necessaires ... Nouvelle ed., rev. & augm. Paris, Laurent d'Houry, 1685.

[14], 305, [7], 12 p.   16 cm.   [2365]
Added engraved title page.

—Nouvelles experiences sur la vipere, ou l'on verra une description exacte de toutes ses parties, la source de son venin, ses divers effects, et les remedes exquis que les artistes peuvent tirer de la vipere, tant pour la guerison de ses morsures, que pour celle de plusieurs autres maladies ... Paris, L'auteur et Olivier de Varennes, 1669.

[14], 200 p.; [1], [201]-278 p.; 201-218, [6] p. plates.   19 cm.   [2366]
Added engraved title page.
Duplicate of added engraved title page, inserted after p. 200.
Imperfect: plates opposite p. 58, 59 and 61 wanting.
"Suite des nouvelles experiences sur la vipere, avec une dissertation sur son venin, pour servir de replique à une lettre que Monsieur François Redi ... écrite à Messieurs Bourdelot & Morus, imprimée à Florence en l'année 1670. Par Moyse Charas ... [colophon]: Cette Suitte d'experiences a esté achevée d'imprimer le 4 Aoust 1671": p. [201]-278; "Echiosophium ... [at end]: Pangebat M. Charas ... M.DC.LXIX": p. 201-218.

—Another issue, dated 1670 without duplicate of added engraved title page.   [2367]

—[The same.] ... Avec une Suite des nouvelles experiences sur la vipere, et une dissertation sur son venin, pour servir de replique à une lettre que Monsieur François Redi ... a écrite à Messieurs Bourdelot & Morus, imprimée à Florence en l'année 1670 ... Paris, Chez l'auteur, Jean d'Houry, Olivier de Varennes, Thomas Moette, 1672.

[14], 200 p.; [4], [201]-278 p.; 201-245, [6] p. plates.   19 cm.   [2368]
Added engraved title page.
Suite des nouvelles experiences sur la vipere ... has special title page.
A reissue, with additions, of the 1669 edition.

—[The same.] ... 2. ed. rev. & augm. par l'auteur. Paris, Laurent d'Houry, 1694.

[12], 367, [24] p.   plates.   20 cm.   [2369]
Added engraved title page.
"Suite des nouvelles experiences sur la vipere, avec une dissertation sur son venin, pour servir de replique à une lettre que Monsieur François Redi ... a écrite à Messieurs Bourdelot & Morus, imprimée à Florence en l'année 1670 ...": p. [207]-282 has

half title; "Supplement d'experiences sur la vipere ...": p. 282-319; "Echiosophium": p. 321-340.

—[English tr.] New experiments upon vipers. Containing also an exact description of all the parts of a viper, the seat of its poyson, and the several effects thereof, together with the exquisite remedies, that by the skilful may be drawn from vipers, as well for the cure of their bitings, as for that of other maladies. Originally written in French ... Now rendered English ... London, Printed by T. N. for J. Martyn, 1670.

[16], 223 p.   plates.   18 cm.   [2370]
Added engraved title page.

—Pharmacopée royale galenique et chymique ... Paris, L'auteur, 1676.

[14], 1060, [34] p.   front., plates.   25 cm.   [2371]

—[The same.] ... 2. ed. Rev., & corr. par l'auteur. Avec des additions considerables sur les plus curieuses matieres. Tome premier [-second] Paris, Laurent d'Houry, 1681.

2 v.   plates.   20 cm.   [2372]

—[The same.] ... 3. ed., rev. corr. & augm. par l'auteur. Paris, Chez l'auteur, 1681.

[8], 454 p.; 328, [24] p.   plates.   24 cm.   [2373]

—[The same.] ... Nouvelle ed. Rev., corr., & augm., par l'auteur. Tome premier. Lyon, Anisson & Posuel, 1693.

2 parts in 1 v.   front., plates.   24 cm.   [2374]
Part [2] has half title: Pharmacopée royale chymique.
Imperfect: p. 71-72 of part 1 mutilated.

—[Latin tr.] Pharmacopoea regia, Galenica et chymica, Gallice ab authore conscripta, jam vero Latinitate donata. Tomus primus [-secundus] Genevae, Sumptibus Joannis Ludovici Du-Four, 1683.

2 v. in 1.   plates.   25 cm.   [2375]

—[English tr.] The royal pharmacopoea, Galenical and chymical, according to the practice of the ... physitians of France ... London, John Starkey, and Moses Pitt, 1678.

[8], 272, 245, [15] p.   plates.   33 cm.   [2376]
Imperfect: the first leaf of "The index for the chymical part" interchanged with the first leaf of "The index for the Galenick part."

CHARLES BORROMEO, *Saint. See* CARLO BORROMEO, *Saint* [1538-1584]

CHARLES XI, *King of Sweden* [1655-1697] *See* SWEDEN. Laws, statutes, etc. 1699.

CHARLES XII, *King of Sweden* [1682-1718] *See* SWEDEN. Laws, statutes, etc. 1699.

CHARLETON, WALTER [1619-1707] The darknes of atheism dispelled by the light of nature. A physico-theologicall treatise ... London, Printed by J. F. for William Lee, 1652.

    [50], 355 p. port. 21 cm.   **[2377]**
Imperfect: port. wanting.

    —De scorbuto liber singularis ... Lugduni Batavorum, Apud Felicem Lopez, 1672.

    288 p. 13 cm.   **[2378]**

    [—] The Ephesian and Cimmerian matrons, two notable examples of the power of love and wit ... [London] In the Savoy, Henry Herringman, 1668.

    [11], 80 p.; [25], 77, [5] p. front. 17 cm.
                              [2379]
Imprint partly supplied from Wing, 3670.
Part [2] has special title page: The Cimmerian matron, to which is added, The mysteries and miracles of love. By P. M. Gent.
The Cimmerian matron is based on the Comus of Erycius Puteanus. Cf. BMC.

    —Exercitationes pathologicae, in quibus morborum pene omnium natura, generatio, & caussae, ex novis anatomicorum inventis sedulo inquiruntur ... Londini, Typis Tho. Newcomb, prostant autem venales apud Joh. Martin, Jac. Allestry, & Tho. Dicas, 1661.

    [24], 208 p. 20 cm.   **[2380]**

    —[The same.] ... Bononiae, Sumptibus Petronii de Ruinettis, 1675.

    [3], 237, [1] p. 16 cm.   **[2381]**

    —Inquisitiones medico-physicae, de causis catameniorum, sive fluxus menstrui; nec non uteri rheumatismo, sive fluore albo. In qua etiam nervose probatur sanguinem in animali fermentescere nunquam ... Lugd. Batavorum, Apud Petrum vander Aa, 1686.

    [8], 204 p. 14 cm.   **[2382]**
With this is bound *his* Exercitationes physico-anatomicae, de oeconomia animali. 1678.

    —Natural history of nutrition, life, and voluntary motion. Containing all the new discoveries of anatomist's, and most probable opinions of physicians, concerning the oeconomie of human nature; methodically delivered in exercitations physico-anatomical ... London, Henry Herringman, 1659.

    [18], 210 (i.e. 208), [13] p. illus. 23 cm.
                              [2383]

    —[Latin tr.] Exercitationes physico-anatomicae, de oeconomia animali, novis in medicina hypothesibus superstructa, & mechanice explicata ... Ed. 2., priori multo correctior. Amstelaedami, Apud Joannem Ravesteynium, 1659.

    [20], 243, [1] p. illus. 14 cm.   **[2384]**
Latin edition first published in London in 1659 under title: Oeconomia animalis, novis in medicina hypothesibus superstructa et mechanice explicata.

    —[The same.] Oeconomia animalis, novis in medicina hypothesibus superstructa & mechanice explicata. Accessere ejusdem Dissertatio epistolica, de ortu animae humanae; & Consilium hygiasticum ... Ed. 3. Londini, Ex officina Rogeri Danielis, 1666.

    [23], 302 (i.e. 312) p. illus. 15 cm. **[2385]**

    —[The same.] ... Ed. 4. Londini, Ex officina Johannis Redmayne, prostant venales apud Johannem Creed, Cantab., 1669.

    [23], 302 (i.e. 312) p. illus. 16 cm. **[2386]**
Different setting of type.
Another title page (2d prelim. leaf) differs in typographical ornament and in imprint: Londini, Ex officina Johannis Redmayne, anno, 1669.

    —[The same.] Exercitationes physico-anatomicae, de oeconomia animali novis in medicina hypothesibus superstructa, & mechanice explicata ... Ed. 2., priori multo correctior. Lugd. Batav., Apud Petrum de Graef, & Jacobum Moukee, 1678.

    [20], 243 (i.e. 291), [1] p. illus. 14 cm.
                              [2387]
Bound with *his* Inquisitiones medico-physicae, de causis catameniorum. 1686.

    —Another issue, with imprint: Lugd. Batav., Apud Jacobum Moukee, & Petrum de Graef, 1678.

    [12], 243 (i.e. 291), [1], 31 p. illus. 15 cm.
                              [2388]
The preliminaries are of a different setting of type.
"Dissertatio epistolica de ortu animae humanae. Ut et Consilium hygiasticum" (31 p. at end) has special title page with imprint: Lugd. Batav., Apud Jacobum Moukee, 1678.
With this is bound: Hoghelande, C. van. Cogitationes. 1676.

    —[The same.] Exercitationes de oeconomia animali novis in medicina hypothesibus superstructa,

& mechanice explicata. Quibus accessere Guilielmi Cole ... De secretione animali cogitata, ad hanc oeconomiam praecipue spectantia. Ed. novissima, prioribus emendatior & correctior. Hagae-Comitum, Apud Arnoldum Leers, 1681.

[16], 262, [1] p.; [12], 159, [2] p.   illus.   14 cm.
[2389]

Part [2] has special title page.

— Enquiries into human nature, in VI. anatomic praelections in the new theatre of the Royal Colledge of Physicians in London ... London, Printed by M. White for Robert Boulter, 1680.

[41], 544 (i.e. 326), [4] p.   port., illus., plate.   21 cm.
[2390]

Imperfect: port. wanting.

An extensively rewritten edition of the Natural history of nutrition. Cf. H. Rolleston in Bulletin of the History of Medicine, vol. 8 (1940) p. 413.

[—] Natural history of the passions ... [London] In the Savoy, Printed by T. N. for James Magnes, 1674.

[47], 188 p.   19 cm.   [2391]

This work has been mistakenly described as "based on 'De l'usage des passions' by J.F. Senault." (BMC) There is no textual similarity between the two. Cf. R. A. Hunter in Journal of the History of Medicine, vol. 13 (1958) p. 87-92.

— Onomasticon zoicon, plerorumque animalium differentias & nomina propria pluribus linguis exponens. Cui accedunt Mantissa anatomica; et quaedam De variis fossilium generibus ... Londini, Apud Jacobum Allestry, 1668.

[20], 309, [34] p.   plates.   20 cm.   [2392]

Bound with Spiegel, A. van de. De lumbrico lato liber. 1618.

—[The same.] Exercitationes de differentiis & nominibus animalium. Quibus accedunt Mantissa anatomica, et quaedam De variis fossilium generibus, deque differentiis & nominibus colorum ... Ed. 2., duplo fere auctior priori ... Oxoniae, E Theatro Sheldoniano, 1677.

[20], 119 p.; [1], 78, [19] p.; 106 p.   illus., plates.   31 cm.   [2393]

— Physiologia Epicuro-Gassendo-Charltoniana; or, A fabrick of science natural, upon the hypothesis of atoms, founded by Epicurus, repaired by Petrus Gassendus, augmented by Walter Charleton ... The first part ... London, Printed by Tho. Newcomb, for Thomas Heath, 1654.

[30], 475, [3] p.   illus.   31 cm.   [2394]

— Spiritus gorgonicus, vi sua saxipara exutus; sive, De causis, signis, & sanatione lithiaseωs, diatriba ... Lugd. Batav. Ex Officina Elseviriorum, 1650.

[12], 242 p.   16 cm.   [2395]

With this are bound: Ferriolus, B. A. Morbosi ventriculi infelix hactenus tentata cura. 1668; Amthor, K. Noscomium infantile. 1638; Universitas Regia Hafniensis. Facultas medica. Kurtzer Unterricht vom Blut- oder Hoffgang. 1652.

— Three anatomic lectures, concerning 1. the motion of the bloud through the veins and arteries; 2. the organic structure of the heart; 3. the efficient causes of the hearts pulsation: read on the 19, 20, and 21 days of March 1682/3 in the anatomic theatre of His Majesties Royal College of Physicians in London ... London, Walter Kettilby, 1683.

[5], 105, [6] p.   illus., plates.   22 cm.   [2396]

[—] Two discourses. I. Concerning the different wits of men ... II. The mysterie of vintners, or a discourse concerning the various sicknesses of wines ... London, R. W. for William Whitwood, 1669.

[14], 230 p.   19 cm.   [2397]

Imperfect: sig. A1 wanting?

Each Discourse has special title page.

"Some obervations concerning the ordering of wines. By Dr. Merret": p. 201-230.

—[The same.] ... The 2d ed. enl. London, F. L. for William Whitwood, 1675.

[16], 235 (i.e. 237), [1] p.   17 cm.   [2398]

Imperfect: sig. A1 wanting?

Each Discourse has special title page.

—[The same.] Two discourses. The first, concerning the different wits of men. The second ... concerning the various sicknesses of wines ... To which is added in this 3d ed. the art and mystery of vintners ... London, Will Whitwood, 1692.

[8], 183, [12] p.   15 cm.   [2399]

The second and third discourses have special title pages.

—, tr. See HELMONT, J. B. van. Deliramenta catarrhi. 1650 [and] A ternary of paradoxes. 1650.

—See MAYERNE, Sir T. T. de. Praxeos Mayernianae. 1690, 1691.

—as subject. See BARTHOLIN, T. Opuscula nova anatomica. 1670; LA SCALA, D. Phlebotomia damnata. 1696.

CHARRIÈRE, JOSEPH DE LA. See LA CHARRIÈRE, Joseph de [17th-18th cent.]

CHARSTADIUS, Valerius [*fl.* 1623–*ca.* 1627]
Synopsis universae medicinae dogmaticae. Brevi &
perspicua methodo in duodecim disputationibus
adumbrata. Argentorati, Typis Eberhardi Welperi,
1634.

[1], 309 (i.e. 297) p.   table.   15 cm.   **[2400]**

Dissertations — Strasbourg

—*praeses.* Disputationum medicarum prima de
constitutione medicinae . . . Argentorati, Typis
Rihelianis, 1626.

[12] p.   20 cm.   **[2401]**
J. W. Fabricius, *respondent.*

—Disputationum medicarum secunda de sanitate
ejusque subjecto . . . Argentorati, Typis Rihelianis,
1626.

[12] p.   20 cm.   **[2402]**
Signatures: [B₄], C⁴, D¹.
J. G. Halbmayer, *respondent.*

—Disputationum medicarum tertia de animae
facultatibus et earum functionibus . . . Argentorati,
Typis Rihelianis, 1626.

[12] p.   20 cm.   **[2403]**
J. Tesserar, *respondent.*

—Disputationum medicarum quarta de diaeta . . .
Argentorati, Typis Rihelianis, 1626.

[12] p.   20 cm.   **[2404]**
Signatures: [A]¹, G⁴, H¹.
J. W. Lorich, *respondent.*

—Disputationum medicarum quinta de morbo . . .
Argentorati, Typis Rihelianis, 1626.

[12] p.   20 cm.   **[2405]**
Signatures: [A]¹, I⁴, K¹.
G. K. Prediger, *respondent.*

—Disputationum medicarum sexta de causis morborum . . . Argentorati, Typis Rihelianis, 1626.

[13] p.   20 cm.   **[2406]**
Signatures: [K₄], L⁴, M¹.
A. Boxbarter, *respondent.*

—Disputationum medicarum septima de symptomatibus, eorundemque differentiis et causis . . .
Argentorati, Typis Rihelianis, 1626.

[12] p.   20 cm.   **[2407]**
Signatures: [M₄], N⁴, O¹.
J. J. Seubertus, *respondent.*

—Disputationum medicarum octava de signis
diagnosticis et prognosticis . . . Argentorati, Typis
Rihelianis, 1626.

[12] p.   20 cm.   **[2408]**
Signatures: [A]¹, P⁴, Q¹.
J. Tesserar, *respondent.*

—Disputationum medicarum nona de urina et
pulsu . . . Argentorati, Typis Rihelianis, 1626.

[12] p.   20 cm.   **[2409]**
Signatures: [A]¹, R⁴, S¹.
J. W. Lorich, *respondent.*

—Disputationum medicarum decima de methodo
medendi in genere . . . Argentorati, Typis Rihelianis,
1626.

[12] p.   20 cm.   **[2410]**
P. Hiltmann, *respondent.*

—Disputationum medicarum undecima de
methodo medendi in specie . . . Argentorati, Typis
Rihelianis, 1626.

[12] p.   20 cm.   **[2411]**
Signatures: [A]¹, X⁴, Y¹.
G. K. Prediger, *respondent.*

—Disputationum medicarum duodecima de
chirurgia . . . Argentorati, Typis Rihelianis, 1626.

[14] p.   20 cm.   **[2412]**
J. Tesserar, *respondent.*

—Disputationum medicarum ultima de pharmacia
. . . Argentorati, Typis Rihelianis, 1626.

[15] p.   20 cm.   **[2413]**
Signatures: B⁴-C⁴.
A. Boxbarter, *respondent.*

—*respondent.* See Sebisch, M. [1578–1674?] *praeses.*
Disputatio de voce hominis. 1623 [and] Exercitationes
medicae. 1639.

CHARTERIUS, Renatus. *See* Chartier, René
[1572–1654]

CHARTIER, Jean [1610–1662] La science du
plomb sacré des sages; ou, De l'antimoine, où sont
décrites ses rares & particulieres vertus, puissances,
& qualitez . . . Paris, J. de Senlecque et François le
Cointe, 1651.

[4], 56 p.   25 cm.   **[2414]**

—[Latin tr.] Scientia plumbi sacri sapientium; seu,
Cognitio rararum & singularium virtutum
potestatum & qualitatum antimonii . . . [Argentorati,
Sumptib. haeredum Eberhardi Zetzneri 1661]

569-599 p., vol. 6.   20 cm.   (*In* Zetzner,
Lazarus, *ed.* Theatrum chemicum. Argentorati,
1659-61)   **[2415]**
Caption title.

—, *tr. See* PALLADIUS IATROSOPHISTA. De febribus concisa synopsis. 1646.

CHARTIER, RENÉ [1572–1654] *ed. See* HOULLIER, J. Commentarius in Jacobi Hollerii . . . librum De morbis internis. 1611 [and] De morbis internis liber. 1611 [and] Omnia opera practica. 1623, 1635, 1664; PARDOUX, B. Bartholomaei Perdulcis . . . Universa medicina. 1630, 1650.

—*See* HIPPOCRATES. [Collected works. Greek and Latin] Hippocratis Coi, et Claudii Galeni . . . Opera. 1679.

CHASTEAU-BRIAND, BRETAGNE. Hospital general. 1680. *See* CHAURAND, H., *Father.*

CHASTEL, PIERRE. *See* CASTELLANUS, Petrus [1585–1632]

CHASTELAIN, JEAN [*d.* 1715] Quaestiones medicae duodecim ab . . . Michaele de Chicoyneau [et al.] . . . propositae . . . pro regia professione vacante . . . per obitum . . . Petri Benoist . . . quas . . . propugnabit . . . Joannes Chastelain. Monspelii, Apud Danielem Pech, 1668.

    23 p.   22 cm.   **[2416]**
    Thèse de concours—Montpellier.

—Traité des convulsions et des mouvemens convulsifs, qu'on appelle à present vapeurs . . . A Lyon & se vend a Paris, J. Anisson, 1691.

    [10], 288 p.   15 cm.   **[2417]**

—*See* SORACI, P. Reponse a la lettre ecrite par Mr. Chatelain. 1699.

CHASTELAIN, PIERRE [*d.* 1711] Quaestiones medico-chymico-practicae duodecim ab . . . Michaele Chicoyneau [et al.] . . . propositae . . . pro regia chymiae professione vacante per obitum . . . Arnaldi Fonsorbe . . . quas propugnabit . . . Petrus Chastelain . . . Monspelii, Apud Honoratum Pech, 1697.

    36 p.   22 cm.   **[2418]**
    Thèse de concours—Montpellier.

CHASTRE, RENÉ DE LA. *See* LA CHASTRE, René de.

CHATEL, PIERRE. *See* CASTELLANUS, Petrus [1585–1632]

CHÂTRE, RENÉ DE LA. *See* LA CHASTRE, René de.

CHAULIAC, GUY DE. *See* GUY DE CHAULIAC [*ca.* 1300–1368]

CHAUME, DE LA. *See* LA CHAUME, de [*fl.* 1679]

CHAUMETTE, ANTOINE [16th cent.] [Enchiridion chirurgicum. Dutch.] Handt-boeck der chirurgie, soo de algemeyne als bysondere middelen teghens de uytwendighe ghebreken seer kortelijck vervattende. Waer by gekomen is een wel besochte maniere om de Spaensche pocken te ghenesen . . . In onse Nederlandtsche tale over-gheset door Gysbert Coets . . . Hier by zijn noch ghevoecht eenighe aphorismi; ofte kort-bondige spreucken uyt Hippocrate, den chirurgijnen dienstijck wesende . . . Arnhem, Jan Jacobsz., 1640.

    [15], 488, [8] p.   15 cm.   **[2419]**
    Translation of Enchiridion chirurgicum, as first published in five books in Paris in 1560.
    Selected aphorisms of Hippocrates in Dutch translation: p. 475–488.

—[French tr.] Le parfaict chirurgien; ou, Recueil general de ce qu'il doit scavoir, contenant les remedes tant universels, que particuliers des maladies externes. Avec une methode tres-approuvée pour guerir la verolle: ensemble un excellent traicté des fievres . . . Nouvelle traduction, augm. d'Observations amples & necessaires sur chacun chapitre, par M. Jean Vigier . . . Plus un recueil de consultations chirurgicales non encor imprimées. Paris, Cardin Besongne, 1628.

    4 parts in 1 v.   17 cm.   **[2420]**
    Imperfect: all after p.32 of part [4] wanting.
    Translation of Enchiridion chirurgicum, with two supplements entitled La suite de l'Enchiridion (part [2]) and Observations necessaires sur l'Enchiridion (part [3]) each of which has a special title page bearing the imprint date 1627.
    Part [4] has special title page: Guillaume Ader . . . De la methode de consulter les maladies chirurgicales.

—[Excerpts. English.] *In* Banister, J. A treatise of chirurgerie. 1633; Enchiridion practicum medico-chirurgicum. 1621, 1627, 1644; Fernel, J. Universa medicina. 1679.

CHAURAND, HONORÉ, *Father* [1615–1697] Chasteau-Briand, Bretagne. Hospital general. Extrait de la lettre du . . . Chaurand missionaire jesuite . . . qui établit les hospitaux generaux en Bretagne . . . Le 17. Octobre 1680. [n. p.] 1680.

    4 p.   24 cm.   **[2421]**
    Caption title.

CHAUVIN, PIERRE [*fl.* 1689] *ed. See* ETTMÜLLER, M. Operum omnium medico-phisicorum. 1690.

CHEAPE and good husbandry for the well-ordering of all beasts. 1631, 1660.

CHEIRAGOGIA Heliana de auro philosophico nec dum cognito. 1612, 1659. *See* [Eglinus Iconius, R.]

CHEMIA rationalis rationibus philosophicis, observationibus medicis, debitis dosibus, &c. illustrata ... Accedit Praxis chymiatrica rationalis, demonstrans qua in re singularum partium consistat operatio, per quam causam tollatur, & per quaenam remedia ... possit restitui ... Auctore P. T. Med. Doct. Lugd. Batav., Apud Jacobum Mocquee, 1687.

     2 parts in 1 v.   21 cm.   **[2422]**

     Part [2] has special title page.

     —[The same.] ... Lugd. Batav., Apud Fredericum Haaring, 1690.

     2 parts in 1 v.   21 cm.   **[2423]**

     Part [2] has special title page.
     A reissue of the 1687 edition with new title pages.

Le **CHEMIN** frayé et infaillible aux accouchemens, qui servira de flambeau aux sages-femmes, pour les éclairer en leurs operations, cachées dans les plus obscures cavernes de la matrice ... Lille, François Fievet, 1689.

     [10], 74, [3] p.   plates.   19 cm.   **[2424]**

     Added engraved title page.
     Dedicatory letter signed: M. C. I.

CHEMINEAU, AMBROS NICOLAS [*fl.* 1692-1705] *respondent. See* THOMASSEAU, J., *praeses.* Quaestio medica ... An vivat miserè, qui vivit medicè? 1693.

CHEMNITIUS. *See* CHEMNITZ.

CHEMNITZ, FRANZ [*b.* 1609] *respondent.* Disputatio medica inauguralis de dysenteria ... Argentorati, Typis Johannis Reppii, 1631.

     [11] p.   19 cm.   **[2425]**

     Diss. — Strasbourg.

CHEMNITZ, SAMUEL [*fl.* 1672-1677] *respondent. See* CRAUSE, R. W., *praeses.* Specimen hoc inaugurale medico-chirurgicum de extractione foetus mortui ex utero materno ... discutiendum proponit ... S. C. 1677; FRIDERICI, J. A., *praeses.* Dissertationem medicam de atrophia ... examini sistit ... S.C. 1672; WEDEL, G. W., *praeses.* Dissertatio medica, sistens aegrum hydropicum. 1674.

CHENA, PIETRO DELLA [*fl.* 1638] Le rare, e gran virtu del balsamo, e quint'essenza, che si cava dal rosmarino ... Roma, 1638.

     [16] p.   15 cm.   **[2426]**

CHERLER, JOHANN HEINRICH [*ca.* 1570-*ca.* 1610] *See* BAUHIN, J. Historia plantarum universalis. 1650-1651.

CHÉRUBIN D'ORLÉANS, *Father* [1613-1697] La dioptrique oculaire; ou, La theorique, la positive, et la mechanique, de l'oculaire dioptrique en toutes ses especes ... Paris, Thomas Jolly & Simon Benard, 1671.

     [48], 419, [30] p.   plates.   37 cm.   **[2427]**

     Colophon: Paris, Jean Cusson, 1670.
     Added engraved title page.

     —Dissertation en laquelle sont resolvës quelques difficultez pretenduës au sujet de l'invention du binocle, & de quelques autres contenües dans les livres de la vision parfaite ... [n. p., not before 1681]

     72 p.   17 cm.   **[2428]**

     Author's copy.
     Bound with this are p. 363-432 of *his* Effets de la force de la contiguité des corps, printed in Paris in 1688 or 1689.

     —La vision parfaite; ou, Le concours des deux axes de la vision en un seul point de l'objet ... Paris, Sebastien Mabre-Cramoisy, 1677-81.

     2 v. in 1.   illus., plates.   36 cm.   **[2429]**

     Added engraved title page.
     Vol. 2 has title: La vision parfaite; ou, La veue distincte par le concours des deux axes en un seul point de l'objet ... Paris, Edme Couterot, 1681.

     —[Latin tr.] De visione perfecta; sive, De amborum visionis axium concursu in eodem objecti puncto ... Parisiis, Apud Sebastianum Mabre-Cramoisy, 1678.

     [28], 176, [18] p.   front., plates.   37 cm.

                                   [2430]

     Vol. 1 only.

     —*See* HOOKE, R. Lectures and collections. 1678.

CHESNE, JOSEPH DU. *See* DUCHESNE, Joseph [*ca.* 1544-1609]

CHESNEAU, NICOLAS [*ca.* 1601-*ca.* 1680] Observationum ... libri quinque. Quibus accessit Ordo remediorum alphabeticus ad omnes fere morbos conscriptus. Sicut & Epitome de natura & viribus luti,

& aquarum Barbotanensium. Parisiis, Apud Fredericum Leonard, 1672.

[16], 652, [12] p.   19 cm.   [2431]

— La pharmacie theorique, nouvellement recueillie de divers autheurs . . . Paris, Frederic Leonard, 1660.

[6], 252, [8] p.   24 cm.   [2432]

— *See* SCHNEIDER, K. V., *praeses*. Disputationem medicam . . . contra ineptam opinionem Nicolai Chesneau, de spasmorum subjecto . . . habebit Georgius Himselius. 1676.

CHESSEL, JOHANN. *See* CASELIUS, Johannes [1533–1613]

CHEVALIER DE HASTEVILLE. *See* HASTEVILLE, de.

CHEVANES, JACQUES DE [*ca.* 1608–1678] L'incredulité sçavante, et la credulité ignorante: au sujet des magiciens et des sorciers, auecque la response à un livre intitulé Apologie pour tous les grands personnages, qui ont esté faussement soupçonnés de magie. Par le P. Jaques d'Autun [pseud., i.e. Jacques de Chevanes] . . . Lyon, Jean Molin, 1671.

[40], 1108, [24] p.   23 cm.   [2433]

CHEVILLARD, FRANÇOIS [*d.* 1678] Le petit tout dans lequel l'homme aura la connoissance de soy-mesme par l'intelligence de ses propres causes scavoir, de Dieu, comme cause efficiente, Du corps, comme cause materielle. De l'ame, comme cause formelle. De la beatitude, comme cause finale . . . Divisé en III. parties et en IV. tomes . . . Premiere [-troisieme] partie . . . Paris, Michel Vaugon, 1664.

3 v. in 1.   tables.   26 cm.   [2434]

"Suite de la seconde partie du Petit tout, ou de la connoissance de l'homme par ses causes, où il est parlé de la maladie, & de la medecine": p. 367–501, vol. 2.

CHEWT, ANTHONY. *See* CHUTE, Anthony [*d.* 1595?]

CHIARAMONTE, GIROLAMO [*fl.* 1619–*ca.* 1633] Osservationi, e breve discorso del contagioso mal di canna. Che cosa sia questo male, & da che proceda, & come, & non che si debbia curare . . . Napoli, Secondino Roncagliolo, 1637.

24 p.   22 cm.   [2435]

— Trattato dell'ammirabil facolta, et effetti della polvere, ò elixir vitae . . . In che provasi concludentemente esser questa sola polvere, vero, &

sicurissimo rimedio contro qualunque spetie di febre, & di ogni male . . . Firenze, Zanobi Pignoni, 1620.

[3], 135 (i.e. 139) p.   22 cm.   [2436]

"Relatione dell'isperienze publicamente fatte della polvere, ò elixir vitae. Da Geronimo Chiaramonte . . . nell'hospitale di Santa Maria Nuova di Firenze": p. [17]–42; "Relatione dell'isperienze publicamente fatte della polvere, seu elixir vitae. Da Geronimo Chiaramonte . . . nel sacr'hospitale della Santissima Annuzziata di Napoli": p. [43]–62; "Informationi vere, et autentiche prese per la gran corte della Vicaria di Napoli. De gli effetti, & isperienze fatte della polvere, o vero elixir vitae . . .": p. [63]–135. Items have special title pages.

— Trattato . . . delle polveri, bianca, e cinericia dette elixir vite. Medicamento mirabile per mantenere in ogni tempo il corpo sano, & ben disposto à tutte, operationi naturali, senza, sospetto di nocumento alcuno, & contra qualsivoglia febre . . . Genova, Giuseppe Pavoni, MCDXXVIII [colophon; 1628]

380, [32] p.   22 cm.   [2437]

Imperfect: p. 113–128 wanting.
Contains 9 tracts, 2 of which were published in 1620 under title: Trattato dell'ammirabil facolta, et effetti della polvere, ò elixir vitae. Items have special title pages; lower part of item 7 is cut off.

CHIARAMONTI, SCIPIONE [1565–1652] De conjectandis cujusque moribus et latitantibus animi affectibus σημειωτικὴ moralis, seu de signis Scipionis Claramontii . . . Venetiis, Ex officina Marci Ginammi, 1625.

[20], 448 p.   23 cm.   [2438]

CHIAVENNA, GIACOMO ANTONIO [*fl.* 1648] Clavis Clavennae aperiens naturae thesaurum, ejusque gemmas depromens: vires scilicet plantarum in generali earundem Historia ex Dalecampio potissimum sumpta a Gulielmo Rovillio Lugduni semel edita, sparsim descriptas . . . Elaborata, per Jacobum Antonium Clavennam . . . Cum indicibus 1. Plantarum . . . 2. Plantarum cum morbis. 3. Morborum, & ex his multorum adhuc sub Graeco vocabulo cum definitionibus, ex Jo. Gorrço . . . 4. Morborum cum plantis . . . Tarvisii, Ex typographia Hieronymi Righettini, 1648.

[12], 1062, [216] p.   front., port.   34 cm.
                    [2439]

Errata: p. [213–216]
Imperfect: sheet C of index wanting.

CHICOT, JEAN [*fl.* 1656] Epistolae et dissertationes medicae. De anno & anni tempestatibus. De purgandi ratione. De rheumatismo. De variolarum & morbillorum ortu, causis & curatione. De dolore.

De somno & vigilia. De melancholia morbo. Accessit Manuductio ad medicinam faciendam. Parisiis, Apud Carolum du Mesnil, 1656.

[12], 354, [1] p.   22 cm.   [2440]

Errata: p. [355]
Added engraved title page.

—[The same.] Posteriores cogitationes; seu, Epistolarum & dissertationum medicarum. Ed. 3 auct. & emend. Parisiis, Apud Emmanuelem Langlois, 1669.

[12], 242, [1] p.; 22 p.   19 cm.   [2441]

Errata: p. [243]
"De cholera morbo epistola . . .": p. 229-242; "De asthmate; seu, Suspirioso anhelitu dissertatio . . .": p. 1-22 at end.

CHICOYNEAU, MICHEL [ca. 1626–1701] proponent. See CHASTELAIN, J. Quaestiones medicae duodecim. 1668; Chastelain, P. Quaestiones medico-chymico-practicae duodecim. 1697; DEIDIER, A. Quaestiones medico-chymico-practicae duodecim. 1697; FABRE, J. Quaestiones medico-chymico-practicae duodecim. 1697; GAUTERON, A. Quaestiones medico-chymico-practicae duodecim. 1697; PICHON, P. Quaestiones medicae duodecim. 1673; RICOME, L. Quaestiones medico-chymico-practicae duodecim. 1696; RIDEUX, P. Quaestiones medico-chymico-practicae duodecim. 1697; RIVIÈRE, G. Quaestiones medico-chymico-practicae duodecim. 1696.

CHIFFLET, JEAN [d. ca. 1610] Singulares tam ex curationibus, quam cadaverum sectionibus observationes. Parisiis, Apud Joannem Richer, 1612.

[8], 52 ll.   18 cm.   [2442]

Edited by Jean Jacques Chifflet.

CHIFFLET, JEAN JACQUES [1588–1660] Acia Cornelii Celsi propriae significationi restituta: Alphonsus Nuñez . . . defensus . . . Antverpiae, Ex Officina Plantiniana Balthasaris Moreti, 1633.

22 p.   24 cm.   [2443]

—Daedalmatum libri duo priores. Parisiis, Apud Joannem Richer, 1611.

[4], 61, [2] ll.   17 cm.   [2444]

—De morte praecellentis viri D. Francisci de Paz . . . epistola ad . . . D. Joannem Gallego de la Serna . . . Antverpiae, Ex officina Plantiniana Balthasaris Moreti, 1640.

11 p.   23 cm.   [2445]

—Pulvis febrifugus orbis Americani . . . [Antwerp] 1653.

45 p.   18 cm.   [2446]

—[The same.] In Fabri, H. Pulvis Peruvianus. 1655.

—, ed. See CHIFFLET, J. Singulares tam ex curationibus, quam cadaverum sectionibus observationes. 1612.

—See BALDI, S. Anastasis corticis Peruviae. 1663.

CHILIANI, BALTHASAR [1636–1712] respondent. See MÖBIUS, G., praeses. Dissertatio medica inauguralis de epilepsia. 1664.

CHILMEAD, EDMUND [1610–1654] tr. See FERRAND, J. Ἐρωτομανία; or, A treatise discoursing of the essence . . . of love. 1640.

CHILMEAD, EDWARD. See CHILMEAD, Edmund [1610–1654]

CHIOCCO, ANDREA [d. 1624] Commentarius quaestionum quarundam de febre mali moris, & de morbis epidemicis. Item Disputatio de sectione venae in obstructione ex humorum qualitate . . . Venetiis, Apud Jo. Baptistam Ciottum, 1604.

36 p.   21 cm.   [2447]

—De Collegii Veronensis illustribus medicis, et philosophis, qui vel scribendo, vel publice profitendo Collegium, patriam, & bonas literas illustrarunt, ex quorum moribus, & institutis, praeceptisve perfecta optimi medici idea colligi potest . . . Veronae, Typis Angeli Tami, 1623.

[16], 171, [1] p.   22 cm.   [2448]

—See CERUTI, B. Musaeum Franc. Calceolarii jun. . . . a Benedicto Ceruto . . . incaeptum, et ab Andrea Chiocco . . . luculenter descriptum. 1622.

CHIODINI, GIULIO CESARE. See CLAUDINI, Giulio Cesare [d. 1618]

CHIRAC, PIERRE [1650–1732] De motu cordis adversaria analytica. Monspelii, Apud Joannem Martel, 1698.

[16], 344 p.; [2], 34 p.   plate.   15 cm. [2449]

"Appendix . . . Caput XI. De motu cordis & auricularum illius": p. [1]-34 at end.
Text of Appendix is identical with caput II of "Tractatus duo. Primus. De remotis et proximis mixti principiis in ordine ad corpus humanum spectatis" II by Raymond Vieussens published in 1688.

—praeses. Dissertatio academica . . . An incubo ferrum rubiginosum . . . [Montispessulani, Apud Gabrielem & Honoratum Pech 1692]

[12], 138, [10] illus. 16 cm.   **[2450]**

Diss.—Montpelier (J. B. de Rosnel, *respondent*)

—*See* SIDOBRE, A., *respondent*. Almae medicorum Monspeliensium Academiae hoc primum specimen. 1694; VIEUSSENS, R. Réponse ... a trois lettres ... du sieur Chirac. 1698.

CHIRCHER, ATANASIO. *See* KIRCHER, Athanasius [1602–1680]

CHMIELECIUS, JOHANN LUCAS. *See* CHMIELECK A CHMIELNICK, Johann Lucas [d. 1662]

CHMIELECK A CHMIELNICK, JOHANN LUCAS [d. 1662] *respondent. See* BRUNN, J. J. von, *praeses.* De humoribus corporis humani. 1619.

CHOICE and profitable secrets both physicall, and chirurgical. 1658. *See* [WOOD, O.]

CHOLIUS, CASPAR [*fl.* 1605] *respondent. See* SENNERT, D., *praeses.* De symptomatum caussis disputatio quarta. 1605.

CHORTALASSAEUS. *See* GRASSHOFF, Johann [d. 1623]

CHOUET, SAMUEL [*fl.* 1657] *ed. See* HIPPOCRATES. [Collected works. Greek and Latin] Τὰ εὑρισκόμενα. 1657, 1662.

CHRADER, JUSTUS. *See* SCHRADER, Justus [b. 1646]

CHRISAEUS, BARTHOLOMAEUS. *See* CHRYSAEUS, Bartholomaeus [*fl.* 1582]

CHRISAORIO, LORENZO, *tr. See* VIGO, G. de. La prattica universale in cirugia. 1605.

CHRISTEN, WOLFGANG [1633–1712] *ed.* and *tr. See* MARTINUS, J. Etliche Gewissens-Fragen von der Pestilentz. 1668.

CHRISTIANI, DIDERICUS [*fl.* 1691] *respondent. See* ALBINUS, B. Dissertatio medica de pica. 1691.

CHRISTIANI, FRIEDRICH [*fl.* 1663] *respondent. See* HABERMAN, K., *praeses.* Discursus physicus. 1663.

CHRISTIANI, JOHANN WILHELM [*fl.* 1686] *respondent. See* FRANCK VON FRANCKENAU, G., *praeses.* Disputatio medica inauguralis qua casum, dysuria ad stranguriam vergente laborantis, resolutum ... exhibet. 1686.

CHRISTIANI, LAURENTIUS [*fl.* 1677] *respondent. See* BORCH, O., *praeses.* Disputatio medica de ictero. 1677.

CHRISTIANUS. *See* ANONYMUS CHRISTIANUS, *pseud.*

CHRISTIANUS, WOLFFGANGUS. *See* CHRISTEN, Wolfgang [1633–1712]

CHRISTLICHER Bericht ... von den Heb-Ammen. *See* VÖLTER, C. Neu eröffnete Heb-Ammen-Schuhl. 1679.

CHRISTOPHORUS GEORGIUS DE HONESTIS. *See* HONESTIS, Christophorus de [d. 1392]

CHRISTOPHORUS PARISIENSIS [13th cent.] [... Elucidarius seu artis transmutatoriae summa major cum Appendice.]

195–293 p., vol. 6. 20 cm. (*In* Zetzner, Lazarus, *ed.* Theatrum chemicum. Argentorati, 1659–61)   **[2451]**

Title from table of contents.

CHRIST'S Hospital, London. A psalm of thanksgiving, to be sung by the children of Christ's-Hospital ... in Easter holy-days ... 1678 ... A true report of the great number of poor children, and other poor people, maintained in the several hospitals, under the pious care of the Lord Mayor ... of the city of London, the year last past ... London, William Godbid, 1678.

broadside. 47 x 35 cm.   **[2452]**

—*See* LONDON. Corporation. Court of Common Council. The order of the hospitalls of K. Henry the viijth. [Not before 1690]

CHROŚCIEJOWSKI, JAN HIERONIM [*fl.* 1583–1612] *ed. See* MERCURIALE, G. De morbis puerorum. 1601, 1615.

CHROSCZIEYOIOSKIUS, JOHANNES. *See* CHROŚCIEJOWSKI, Jan Hieronim [*fl.* 1583–1612]

CHROSIEWSKI, JAN HIERONIM. *See* CHROŚCIEJOWSKI, Jan Hieronim [*fl.* 1583–1612]

CHROUET, WARNER. Dissertatio medico-physica de trium oculi humorum aliarumque ejus partium origine, natura, & formatione mechanice explicata ... Leodii, Apud Guilielmum Henricum Streel, 1688.

38, [1] p. 16 cm. [2453]

A criticism of the views of Anton Nuck.

Bound with Goodschalk, D. Prodromus de ossium tum generatione, tum corruptione interna. 1691.

—[The same.] ... Ed. 2. Cui accedunt Solutiones apologeticae, ad objectiones & difficultates clarissimi Professoris Nuck ... Leodii, Apud Guilielmum Henricum Streel, 1691.

32 p. 16 cm. [2454]

—[The same.] See NUCK, A. Defensio ductuum aquosorum. 1691.

CHRYSAEUS, BARTHOLOMAEUS [*fl.* 1582] *See* SCHOLTZ, L. Epistolarum philosophicarum: medicinalium, ac chymicarum ... volumen. 1610.

CHRYSOPOEIA, et Vellus aureum. *In* Aubigné de la Fosse, N. Bibliotheca chemica. 1653.

CHÜDEN, JOHANN JOACHIM [*fl.* 1694] *respondent.* See ALBINUS, B. Dissertatio solennis medica, de febre. 1694; FRANCK VON FRANCKENAU, G., *praeses.* De morbo Q. Enii poetae. 1694.

CHUNO, PHILIPP HEINRICH [*fl.* 1676-1679] *respondent.* Disputatio inauguralis medica de apoplexia ... Marpurgi Cattorum, Typis Salomonis Schadewitzii, 1677.

26 p. 20 cm. [2455]

Diss. — Marburg.

—*See* WALDSCHMIDT, J. J., *praeses.* Monita medica circa opii et opiatorum usum vulgo Schlaff-Tränck. 1679.

CHURCH OF ENGLAND. Liturgy and ritual. A forme of prayer, necessary to bee used in these dangerous times, of warre and pestilence, for the safety and preservation of His Majesty and his realmes ... London, Bonham Norton and John Bill, 1626.

[86] p. 20 cm. [2456]

STC 16366.

—A form of common prayer with thanksgiving to God, for asswaging the late contagion and pestilence, to be used on Tuesday the 20th of this instant November, in the cities of London and Westminster ... [London] In the Savoy, Assigns of John Bill and Christopher Barker, 1666.

[28] p. 19 cm. [2457]

[**CHUTE,** ANTHONY, *d.* 1595?] Een korte beschrijvinge van het wonderlijcke kruyt tobacco, komende uyt verre ende vreemde landen, het welcke zeer bequaem ende nut is teghen veel gebreken des hoofts, der mage, ende andere leden des lichaems, dienende principalijck de zee-varende lieden ... Obergeset uyt 't Engels. Rotterdam, Joris Pauwelsz, 1623.

[48] p. illus. 14 cm. [2458]

CHYMICA vannus. *See* RECONDITORIUM ac reclusorium opulentiae sapientiaeque numinis mundi magni. 1666.

CHYMICAL, medicinal, and chyrurgical addresses: made to Samuel Hartlib, Esquire ... London, Printed by G. Dawson for Giles Calvert, 1655.

[7], 181 (i.e. 159), [24] p. 15 cm. [2459]

Contains contributions by Gerard de Malynes, Gabriel Plattes, Théophraste Renaudot, and George Ripley.

CHYMISCHE Artzney- und Werck-Schul. *See* GLASER, C. Novum laboratorium medico-chymicum. 1677.

CHYTRAEUS, NATHAN [1543-1598] Epistola satyrica contra pestem. Rostochii, Literis Joachimi Pedanii, 1624.

[12] p. 18 cm. [2460]

CIANI, TOMMASO [*d.* 1630] *See* MURATORI, F. Scelta. 1630.

CIAPPI, MARCO ANTONIO [*fl.* 1577-1601] Regola da preservarsi in sanita ne' tempi de suspetto di peste ... Con altri avertimenti, & segreti aprovati ... Roma, Luigi Zannetti, 1601.

[48] p. 20 cm. [2461]

CICCARELLI, IPPOLITO. *See* CECCARELLI, Ippolito.

CICCOLINI, BARNABA [*fl.* 1674-*ca.* 1696] Brevis disceptatio de morbo epidemico, anni M.DC.LXXIII. & M.DC.LXXIV ... Maceratae, Ex typographia Josephi Piccini, 1674.

12 p. 19 cm. [2462]

—Via brevis ad veram naturalis phylosophiae, et medicinae scientiam perducens ... Contra atomistarum dogmata. Duobus diversis libris, Latino, & vulgari idiomate pro universali usu, facili dialogo clarius demonstrata. Liber primus [-Libro secondo] Romae, Typis Dominici Ant. Herculis, 1696.

[14], 424 p. 15 cm. [2463]

Libro secondo has half title (p. [59]): La filosofia e medicina, antica, e moderna. Opposta all'antica, e moderna filosofia, e medicina degli atomi.

CICERO, MARCUS TULLIUS. *See* PAËPP, J. Vita M. Tullii Ciceronis. 1618.

CIERMANS, JEAN, *Father* [1602-1648] Disciplinae mathematicae traditae anno institutae Societatis Jesu seculari . . . [Lovanii, Apud Everardum de Witte, 1640]

[216] p. illus. 29 cm. [2464]

Engraved title page.

CIGALINI, MARCO [17th cent.] *ed. See* CIGALINI, P. In Aphor. Hippocratis lib. primum et secundum lectiones. 1653.

CIGALINI, PAOLO [*d.* 1598] De C. Plinii Secundi patria. *In* Plinius Secundus, C. Naturalis historiae, tomus primus [-tertius] 1668-1669.

—In Aphor. Hippocratis lib. primum et secundum lectiones. Quibus accesserunt Tabula de plenitudine, Tractatus de diebus decretoriis, Consultatio de victus ratione pro praeservatione oculi ab obscuritate. Novocomi, Ex officina impressoria Nicolai Caprani, 1653.

[35], 314 (i.e. 316) p. 35 cm. [2465]

Includes Latin text of books 1-2 of the Aphorismi in Niccolò Leoniceno's version.

Edited by Marco Cigliani.

CIGNOZZI, GIUSEPPE [1652-1730] *ed.* and *tr. See* HIPPOCRATES. De ulceribus. 1690.

CINELLI, CALVOLI, GIOVANNI [1625-1706] *See* FALCINELLI, B. Apologia. 1646.

CIRCAMUNDUS, JOANNES BAPTISTA. Consultatio de hydrargyrio . . . Maceratae, Apud Petrum Salvionum, 1618.

38, [1] p. 19 cm. [2466]

"Consultatio de hydrargyrio. Facta ab . . . Plinio Bonino . . .": p. 17-33.

CIRCAMUNDUS, PAULUS. See CIRCAMUNDUS, Joannes Baptista.

CITESIUS, FRANCISCUS. *See* CITOIS, François [*ca.* 1572-1652]

CITO, GIOVANNI ANTONIO [*fl.* 1585] *See* CARACCIOLO, P. La gloria del cavallo. 1608.

CITOIS, FRANÇOIS [*ca.* 1572-1652] . . . Opuscula medica. Parisiis, Apud Sebastianum Cramoisy, 1639.

[15], 302, [1] p. 24 cm. [2467]

Errata: p. [303]

—Abstinens confolentanea, cui obiter annexa est pro Juberto apologia . . . Augustoriti Pictonum, Ex officina Joannis Blancheti, 1602.

[10], 78, [3] p. 14 cm. [2468]

—Advis sur la nature de la peste, et sur les moyens de s'en preserver et guerir . . . Paris, 1640.

[359]-449 p. 17 cm. [2469]

—De novo et populari apud pictones dolore colico bilioso diatriba . . . Augustoriti Pictonum, Apud Antonium Mesnier, 1616.

[15], 104 p. 14 cm. [2470]

CIUCCI, ANTONIO FILIPPO [*fl.* 1679-1681] Filo d'Arianna; o, Vero fedelissima scorta alli esercenti di chirurgia, per uscire dal laberinto delle relazioni, e ricognizioni di varii morbi, e morti. Con un capitolo addiettivo della quiddità della peste, e la dichiarazione del sito delle parti, & alcune figure anatomiche; al quale si aggiunge un breve trattato della circulazione del sangue . . . Macerata, Giuseppe Piccini, 1681.

216 p.; [84] p. front., illus. 15 cm. [2471]

Part [2] has special title page: Breve discorso intorno al moto delli humori, quali nutriscono il corpo, detto volgarmente circulazione del sangue.

—[The same.] . . . Macerata, Giuseppe Piccini, 1682.

216 p.; [108] p. front., illus. 15 cm. [2472]

Special title page of part [2] is dated 1681.

Reissue of the 1681 edition, with the addition of verses and a letter by the publisher.

—[The same.] . . . Macerata, Per Gio. Battista, e Girolamo Sassi, 1689.

333, [2] p. port., illus. 14 cm. [2473]

Special title page of part [2] is dated 1685.

—Promptuarium chirurgicum in quo agitur de morbis, qui indigent manuali operatione artis chirurgiae praemissa serie auctorum, & locorum, in quibus ipsi agunt de quaesita materia . . . Maceratae, Typis Josephi Piccini, 1680.

[14], 198, [4] p. front., plates. 20 cm.

[2474]

"Promptuarii chirurgici pars secunda in qua reperies annotationes quamplurimas non parum utiles chirurgiae exercentibus ... 1679" (p. [131]-198) has special title page.

CLAMER, KASPAR GÜNTHER [*fl.* 1668] *respondent.* Disputatio medica inauguralis de peste ... Lugduni Batavorum, Apud viduam & haeredes Joannis Elsevirii, 1668.

    [19] p. 23 cm.   **[2475]**
Diss. — Leyden.

CLARAMONS, SCIPIO. *See* CHIARAMONTI, Scipione [1565-1652]

CLARAMONTIUS, CAROLUS. *See* CLAROMONTIUS, Carolus [*fl. ca.* 1671]

CLARAMONTIUS, SCIPIO. *See* CHIARAMONTI, Scipione [1565-1652]

CLARIER DE LONGVAL, FRANÇOIS DE, *tr. See* GARZONI, T. L'hospital des fols incurables. 1620.

CLARK, R. [*fl.* 1687] Vermiculars destroyed, with an historical account of worms: collected from the best authors ... And experiments proved by that admirable invention of the microscope ... By R. C[lark] chymist ... London, Printed by J. Wilkins, for the author [1691?]

    30 p. plate, illus. 21 cm.   **[2476]**
Wing C4485.

CLARKE, WILLIAM [1640?-1684] The natural history of nitre; or, A philosophical discourse of the nature, generation, place, and artificial extraction of nitre, with its vertues and uses ... London, Printed by E. Okes for Nathaniel Brook, 1670.

    [15], 93 p. 17 cm.   **[2477]**

—[Latin ed.] Naturalis historia nitri; sive, Discursus philosophicus de natura, generatione, loco & artificiaii extractione nitri, ejusque virtutibus & usibus ... Francofurti & Hamburgi, Impensis Joannis Naumanni & Georgii Wolffii, 1675.

    79 p. 17 cm.   **[2478]**
Bound with copy 2 of Fedele, F. De relationibus medicorum libri quatour. 1674.

CLAROMONTIUS, CAROLUS [*fl. ca.* 1671] De aere, locis, & aquis terrae Angliae; deque morbis Anglorum vernaculis. Cum observationibus ratiocinatione & curandi methodo illustratis. Londini, Typis Thomae Roycroft, & impensis Johannis Martyn, 1672.

    [48], 180 p. 13 cm.   **[2479]**

Imperfect: sig. 2 wanting.
"Observationes medicae. Cambro-Britannicae" (p. [75]-180) has half title.

CLASEN, NATHAN [*fl.* 1609] *respondent.* Theses medicae de nephritico dolore ... Athenis Rauracorum, Typis Johannis Schroeteri, 1609.

    [8] p. 20 cm.   **[2480]**
Diss. — Basel.

CLAUDER, CHRISTIAN ERNST [*fl.* 1671-1674] *respondent. See* FRIDERICI, J. A., *praeses.* Disputatio medica de ventriculo. 1671; WEDEL, G. W., *praeses.* Disputatio inauguralis de arthritide vaga scorbutica. 1674.

CLAUDER, FRIEDRICH WILHELM [*b.* 1654] *respondent. See* WEDEL, G. W., *praeses.* Disputationem inauguralem de bubone pestilenti ... subjicit F. W. C. 1681.

CLAUDER, GABRIEL [1633-1691] Ad ... Doct. Marcum Ruych ... De observatione practico-anatomica mirabili. Epistola. Patavii, Typis Sebastiani Sardi [1661]

    [14] p. 19 cm.   **[2481]**

—Dissertatio de tinctura universali (vulgo lapis philosophorum dicta) ... Altenburgi, Apud Godofredum Richterum, 1678.

    [12], 272, [24] p. 20 cm.   **[2482]**

—Inventum cinnabarinum; hoc est, Dissertatio de cinnabari nativa Hungarica, longa circulatione in majorem efficaciam fixata et exaltata ... Jenae, Sumtibus Johannis Bielkii, 1684.

    [4], 68 p. 20 cm.   **[2483]**

—Methodus balsamandi corpora humana, aliaque majora sine evisceratione et sectione hucusque solita ... Adnexa item est methodus parandi varias essentias atque spiritus chymicos extemporanee, sine igne aut destillatione ... Altenburgi, Apud Godofredum Richterum, 1679.

    [16], 216, [11] p. 21 cm.   **[2484]**

—*respondent. See* MICHAELIS, J., *praeses.* Disputationem de phthisi ... subjicit ... G. C. 1658 [and] Disputationem inauguralem de philtris ... subjicit ... G. C. 1661; MÖBIUS, G., *praeses.* Institutionum medicarum disputatio decima de usu hepatis et bilis. 1654.

CLAUDER, ISRAEL [*fl.* 1650] *respondent. See* SAGITTARIUS, C., *praeses.* De sale philologemata. 1650.

CLAUDER, JOHANN CHRISTIAN [*fl.* 1689-1694] *respondent. See* WEDEL, G. W., *praeses.* Dissertatio medica inauguralis de dulcium natura. 1694 [and] Dissertatio medica, physiologiam pulsus exhibens. 1689.

CLAUDINI, FRANCESCO [*fl.* 1619] *ed. See* CLAUDINI, G. C. [*d.* 1618] De ingressu ad infirmos. 1619, 1627 [and] Empyrica rationalis libris VI. 1653.

CLAUDINI, GIULIO CESARE [*d.* 1618] De ingressu ad infirmos libri duo. In quibus medici omne ex tempore medicinam facturi munus, sive per se curet, sive cum aliis de curando consultet, accuratissime, tanquam in tabula delineatum, continetur. Accessit Appendix. De remediis generosioribus . . . Adjecta est coronidis loco Quaestio philosophico-medica de sede principum facultatum. Bononiae, Apud Jo. Baptistam Bellagambam, Sumptibus Hieronymi Tamburini, 1612.

    8, [8], 228, [32], 5-20 p.   25 cm.   **[2485]**

—[The same.] . . . Basileae, Sumptibus Joan. Jacobi Genathii, 1617.

    [18], 529, [49], 36 p.   17 cm.   **[2486]**

—[The same.] . . . Adjectus est coronidis loco Tractatus de catarrho. Quae omnia cum ab ipso auctore dum viveret copiosissime aucta, & studiosissime recognita fuerint, nunc secundo opera, & studio Francisci Claudini . . . edita sunt. Bononiae, Apud Sebastianum Bonomium, Sumptibus Hieronymi Tamburini, 1619.

    [38], 258 (i.e. 260), 40 p.   21 cm.   **[2487]**

—[The same.] . . . Hanoviae, Typis Wechelianis, apud Claudium Marnium & haeredes Joann. Aubrii, 1627.

    [38], 362 (i.e. 364), [8] p.   table.   21 cm.   **[2488]**

    "Julii Caesaris Claudini . . . Tractatus de crisibus, et diebus criticis": p. 295-[370]

—[The same.] . . . Venetiis, Apud Donatum Pasquardum agentem P. P. Tozzii, 1628.

    [50], 258 (i.e. 260), 40, 90, [13] p.   table.   22 cm.   **[2489]**

    Engraved title page.
    Added half-title: Julii Caesaris Claudini De ingressu ad infirmos libri duo. De sede facultatum principum. De catarro tractatus, De crisibus et diebus criticis.
    "Julii Caesaris Claudini . . . Ad tractatum suum De ingressu ad infirmos Appendix de remediis generosioribus": p. 166-238.

—[The same.] . . . Quibus adjectus est coronidis loco De catarrho, nec non De crisibus, & diebus criticis ejusdem auctoris tractatus. Venetiis, Apud Bertanos, 1647.

    [28], 225, [1], 35 (i.e. 36), 62 p.   table.   26 cm.   **[2490]**

—[The same.] . . . Venetiis, Apud Bertanos, 1663.

    [32], 324 p.   tables.   22 cm.   **[2491]**

—[The same.] Opuscula. I. Libri duo de ingressu ad infirmos, in quibus omne munus medici, ex tempore medicinal facturi, sive curet per se, sive cum aliis de curando consultet, accuratissime tanquam in tabula delineatum continetur. II. Appendix de remediis generosioribus. III. Quaestio philosophico-medica de sede principum facultatum. IV. Tractatus de catarrho. V. De crisibus & diebus criticis . . . Francofurti ad Moenum, Sumptib. Alberti Ottonis Fabri, Typis Joh. Dieterici Friedgen, 1676.

    [2], 256 p., 257-318 ll., 319-842, [46] p.   table.   17 cm.   **[2492]**

    Imperfect: p. [23-24] of indexes wanting.

—[The same.] De ingressu ad infirmos, libri duo. De sede facultatum principum. De catarrho tractatus. De crisibus, et diebus criticis. Omnia multo, quam antea, emendatiora. Venetiis, Apud Aloysium Pavinum, 1690.

    [36], 238 (i.e. 246), 61, [7] p.   table.   24 cm.   **[2493]**

    "Julii Caesaris Claudini . . . ad tractatum suum De ingressu ad infirmos, Appendix de remediis generosioribus": p. 134-194.

—Empyrica rationalis libris VI. absoluta, et in duo volumina divisa, in quorum alio universi corporis humani affectus, penes totum, & partes; in altero vero penes speciem, individuum, atque aetates, causas manifestas, reconditasque sive practicis omnibus noti, aut prolapsi, sive novi, & peregrini, rationabiliter, & absolutissime curantur. Per olim Franciscum auctoris filium . . . in typos parata, nunc primum a Julio Caesare Claudino juniore . . . publicae utilitati commissa, cui ut faciliori negotio medicinam facientes, quicquid in opere continetur, inveniant, praeter annotationes in margine, geminus accessit index Jo. Caroli Matthesilani . . . Bononiae, Typis Jacobi Montii, 1653.

    2 v.   port.   35 cm.   **[2494]**

    Added engraved title page and half title.

Vol. 1 has Approbationes on recto of 6th prelim. leaf. Last leaf of final signature is blank.

—Another issue.   **[2495]**

Added engraved title page.

Vol. 1 has letter from Hieronymus Bardi to Giovanni Carlo Mattesillani on recto of 6th prelim. leaf. Last leaf of final signature contains Approbationes on recto and Registrum on verso.

—Responsionum, et consultationum medicinalium tomus unicus in duas sectiones partitus, in quarum prima Responsiones, in altera Consultationes continentur ... Venetiis, Apud Hieronymum Tamburinum 1607.

[36], 154, 367 p.   33 cm.   **[2496]**

—[The same.] ... Francofurti, Sumptibus Lazari Zetzneri, 1607.

[31], 970, [30] p.   19 cm.   **[2497]**

—[The same.] ... Nunc accurate recognitus, & ab omnibus erroribus ea, qua fieri potuit diligentia repurgatus ... Hanoviae, Typis Wechelianis, apud Claudium Marnium & haeredes Joann. Aubrii, 1628.

[32], 602 p.   21 cm.   **[2498]**

—Another issue, with imprint: Augustae Taurinorum, Apud HH. Jo. Dominici Tarini, 1628.

         [2499]

—[The same.] Additur brevis exercitatio De ultimo corporis alimento cum aliquot digressiunculis. Auctore Florio Bernardo ... Venetiis, Apud Bertanos, 1646.

[32], 602 (i.e. 600), 19 p.   24 cm.   **[2500]**

—Tractatus de crisibus et diebus criticis; in quo cum de caeteris omnibus, quae ad horum pertinent cognitionem, tum de causis praecipue, accurate juxta, & ordine disseritur ... Bononiae, Ex typographia Bartholomaei Cochii, 1612.

[4], 62, [10] p.   29 cm.   **[2501]**

—[The same.] ... Basileae, Sumptibus Joan. Jacobi Genathii, 1620.   **[2502]**

—*See* LAUTENBACH, J., *ed.* Consilia medicinalia. 1605, 1660.

—*as subject. See* OBIZZI, I. Iatrastronomicon varios tractatus medicos. 1618.

CLAUDINI, GIULIO CESARE [*fl.* 1653?] *ed. See* CLAUDINI, G. C. [*d.* 1618] Empyrica rationalis libris VI. 1653.

CLAUS, PAUL [*fl.* 1603] *respondent. See* HORST, G. [1578-1636] *respondent.* Σκεψις. 1606, 1608.

CLAUSINGIUS, HENRICUS. *See* KLAUSING, Heinrich [1675-1745]

CLAVE, ÉTIENNE DE [*fl.* 1624-*ca.* 1635] Nouvelle lumiere philosophique des vrais principes et elemens de nature, & qualité d'iceux ... Paris, Olivier de Varennes, 1641.

[12], 493 (i.e. 515), [5] p.   17 cm.   **[2503]**

—Paradoxes; ou, Traittez philosophiques des pierres et pierreries, contre l'opinion vulgaire. Ausquels sont demonstrez la matiere, la cause efficiente externe, la semence, la generation, la definition, & la nutrition d'icelles ... Paris, La veufue Pierre Chevalier, 1635.

[24], 492, [1] p. plate. 18 cm.   **[2504]**

Errata: p. [493]

CLAVELL, ROBERT [*d.* 1711] *ed. See* TERM CATALOGUES. A catalogue of books continued, printed, and published at London. 1676.

CLAVENNA, JACOBUS ANTONIUS. *See* CHIAVENNA, Giacomo Antonio [*fl.* 1648]

CLAVERIA, JOSEPH ZAMORA. *See* ZAMORA Y CLAVERÍA, José [*b.* 1622]

CLAVES, GASTON LE DOUX, *known as* Gaston de [*b. ca.* 1530] Apologia chrysopoeiae et argyropoeiae, adversus Thomam Erastum ... Authore Gastone Dulcone sive Claveo ... Cum ... opere ... De triplici auri et argenti praeparatione. Ursellis, Cornelius Sutorius, 1602.

[16], 267, [1] p.   17 cm.   **[2505]**

Edited by Bernard Georges Penot.

—[Apologia chrysopoeiae & argyropoeiae adversus Thomam Erastum, in qua disputatur & docetur, an, quid & quomodo sit chrysopoeia & argyropoeia.] 6-80 p., vol. 2. 20 cm. (*In* Zetzner, Lazarus, *ed.* Theatrum chemicum. Argentorati, 1659-61)

Title from table of contents.   **[2506]**

—De triplici praeparatione auri et argenti [&] De recta et vera ratione progignendi lapidis philosophici, seusalis argentifici et aurifici ... [&] Canones seu regulae decem, de lapide philosophico ...

372-416 p., vol. 4. 20 cm. (*In* Zetzner, Lazarus, *ed.* Theatrum chemicum. Argentorati, 1659-61)   **[2507]**

Caption titles.

—Philosophia chymica tribus tractatibus comprehensa ... Opus ... nunc primum integrum in lucem editum ... Lugduni [Jean Vignon?] 1612.

[15], 151, 94 p.   16 cm.   [2508]

Printed in Geneva by Jean Vignon? The device on the title page (reproduced in P. Heitz, Genfer Buchdrucker- und Verlegerzeichen, no. 51, as used by Jean Crespin) was used by Eustache Vignon and his successors, including Jean Vignon, in the early 17th cent.

"Cum Bernardi G. Penoti ... epistola, praefatione, & marginalibus annotationibus."

Contents.—Apologia chrysopoeiae & argyropoeiae adversus Doct. Thomam Erastum.—De triplici praeparatione auri & argenti.—De ratione progignendi lapidis philosophici, seu salis argentifici & aurifici.—Canones decem, totius operis basim constituentes.

Bound with Follinus, H. Amuletum Antonianum. 1618.

—[German tr.] Claveus Germanicus; das ist, Ein köstlichess Büchlein von dem Stein der Weisen ... auss dem Latein ins Teutsch versetzt, durch einen Liebhaber der uhralten ... Kunst Chymiae. Hall in Sachsen, Gedruckt bey Peter Schmidt, in Verlegung Joachimi Krusicken, 1617.

[16], 398 p.   16 cm.   [2509]

—See DICTIONAIRE HERMETIQUE. 1695.

CLAVEUS, GASTON. See CLAVES, Gaston Le Doux, known as Gaston de [b. ca. 1530]

CLAYTON, Dr. of Wakefield. See FLOYER, Sir J. An enquiry into the right use and abuses of the hot, cold, and temperate baths in England. 1697.

CLEMAS, MATTHÄUS [1640 or 44-1702] praeses. Disputatio physica de putredine ... Lipsiae, Literis Christiani Michaelis [1666]

[12] p.   20 cm.   [2510]

Diss.—Leipzig (A. Fidler, respondent)

—respondent. See AMMANN, P., praeses. Disputatio medica de phthisi. 1664; HELWIG, C. Dissertationem chirurgicam de vulneribus cum fracturis & luxationibus sive conjunctis eorum praecipuis & symptomatibus ... submittit M. M. C. 1674.

—as subject. See HELWIG, C. Programma quo ad inauguralem de vulneribus disputationem, quam ... Matthaeus Clemasius ... habebit ... invitat. 1674.

CLEMENS, CYNTHIUS. See CYNTHIUS, Clemens [fl. 1601]

CLEMENS Papa Octavus ad perpetuam rei memoriam. 1675? See CATHOLIC CHURCH. Pope, 1593-1603 (Clemens VIII)

CLEMENS PP. X. Ad perpetuam rei memoriam. 1675. See CATHOLIC CHURCH. Pope, 1670-1676 (Clemens X)

CLÉMENT, GUILLAUME [fl. 1637-1672] Sententiae principum medicorum, in tres libros divisae. Hyppocratis sententiae. Lib. I. Galeni sententiae. Lib. II. Illustrium quorumdam medicorum sententiae. Lib. III. Morborum prognosis methodus generalis, Guillielmi Clementis ... Lib. IV. Observationes rarae ejusdem. Lib. V. Avenione, Typis Antonii Duperier, 1672.

[12], 468, [35] p.   15 cm.   [2511]

Clément's Morborum prognosis methodus generalis has special title page (p. 305).

"Sententiae poetarum, ad animorum relaxationem & recreationem collectae": p. 456-465.

Errata: p. [35]

CLEMENTIS Papae VII. Bulla de protomedici & Collegii Medicorum urbis jurisdictione, & facultatibus. 1627. See CATHOLIC CHURCH. Pope, 1523-1534 (Clemens VII)

CLEMENTIUS, PETRUS [fl. 1658] respondent. Disputatio medica inauguralis de leucophlegmatia ... Lugduni Batavorum, Ex typographia Severini Matthiae, 1658.

[7] p.   24 cm.   [2512]

Diss. — Leyden.

CLENCH, ANDREW [d. 1692] See HARRISON, H. The last words of a dying penitent. 1692.

CLEOPHAS, MICHAEL [fl. 1657-1664] respondent. See SENNERT, M., praeses. Disputatio medica inauguralis de suppressione mensium. 1664.

CLERICUS, JOANNES. See LE CLERC, Jean [1657-1736]

CLERICUS, STEPHANUS. See LE CLERC, Étienne [1599-1676]

CLERMONT, CHARLES. See CLAROMONTIUS, Carolus [fl. ca. 1671]

CLERSELIER, CLAUDE [1614-1684] ed. See DESCARTES, R. L'homme ... et un traitté De la formation du foetus. 1664, 1677, 1680 [and] Lettres. 1663, 1667.

—, *tr. See* DESCARTES, R. Les meditations metaphysiques. 1647.

—*See* DESCARTES, R. Les passions de l'ame. 1649 [and] Tractatus De homine, et De formatione foetus. 1677, 1686, 1692; [Dutch tr.] 1695.

CLETI, EZIO [*fl.* 1621] Dilucidatio in Aphor. 22. primae sect. pro defensione interpretationis Marsilii Cagnati. Nuper edita per Philandrnm [sic] Colutium . . . Romae, Apud haeredem Bartholomaei Zannetti, 1621.

[8], 88 p.   17 cm.   [2513]

—*See* CASTELLI, P. Epistola. 1622; MARZIANI, P. Apologeticus liber. 1617; VERBEZIUS, D. Pro Raymundi Mindereri . . . disquisitione iatrochymica de chalcantho. 1626.

CLEYBURGH, PIETER VAN [*fl.* 1689] *respondent. See* LUYTS, J., *praeses.* Exercitatio philosophica. 1689.

CLEYER, ANDREAS [1634–1697 *or* 8] *ed. See* BOYM, M. P. Clavis medica ad Chinarum doctrinam de pulsibus. 1686 [and] Specimen medicinae Sinicae. 1682.

CLINCH, Dr. *See* CLENCH, Andrew [*d.* 1692]

CLODIUS, BALDUINUS. Officina Chymica. Das ist: Künstliche Spagyrischen Zuzubereitung der animalischen, vegetabilischen, metallischen und mineralischen Medicamenten . . . Sampt beygefügtem Consilio, wie man sich in pestilentzischen Läufften verhalten soll. Jetzo publiciert und an Tag geben durch J[ohann] E[rnst] B[urggrav] . . . Oppenheim, Getruckt bey Hieronymo Gallern, in Vorlegung Johann Theodor de Bry, 1620.

[8], 189, [7] p.   20 cm.   [2514]

CLODIUS, BARTHOLOMAEUS. *See* CLODIUS, Balduinus.

CLOKE, THOMAS [*fl.* 1675] *respondent.* Disputatio medica inauguralis de atrophia . . . Lugduni Batavorum, Apud viduam & haeredes Johannis Elsevirii, 1675.

[16] p.   21 cm.   [2515]
Diss. — Leyden.

CLOOTHACK, MARK [*fl.* 1687] *respondent.* Disputatio medica inauguralis de catalepsi . . . Lugduni Batavorum, Apud Abrahamum Elzevier, 1687.

[16] p.   20 cm.   [2516]
Diss. — Leyden.

A CLOSET for ladies and gentlewomen. Or, The art of preserving, conserving, and candying. With the manner how to make divers kindes of sirups, and all kinde of banqueting stuffes. Also divers soveraigne medicines and salves for sundry diseases. London, John Haviland, 1632.

[192] p.   13 cm.   [2517]
STC 5438.

CLOSIUS, PAULUS [*fl.* 1577–1582] *See* SCHOLTZ, L. Epistolarum philosophicarum: medicinalium, ac chimicarum . . . volumen. 1610.

CLOSIUS, SIGISMUNDUS [*fl.* 1644–1647] *respondent. See* SEBISCH, M. [1578–1674?] *praeses.* Disputationes de dentibus quatuor. 1645 [and] Galeni quinque priores libri. 1651.

CLOSIUS, SIGISMUNDUS [*fl.* 1697] *respondent. See* WEDEL, G. W., *praeses.* Dissertatio medica inauguralis de spiritu vini. 1697.

CLOTZ, JOHANN ANTON [*fl.* 1662–1664] *respondent. See* ROLFINCK, W., *praeses.* Commentarius in Hippocratis primum libri Aphorismum. 1662.

CLOUCQUIUS, ANDREAS [*fl.* 1610] *ed. See* [MEURS, J. van, 1579–1639] Illustrium Hollandiae & Westfrisiae ordinum alma Academia Leidensis. 1614.

CLOWES, WILLIAM [1544–1604] A profitable and necessarie booke of observations, for all those that are burned with the flame of gun-powder . . . With an addition of most approved remedies . . . Last of all is adjoyned a short treatise, for the cure of lues venerea . . . heretofore by me collected: and now againe newly corrected and augmented in the year . . . 1596 . . . The 3d ed. London, Printed by M. Dawson, and are to be sold by Benjamin Allen and Peter Cole, 1637.

[4], 229 (i.e. 225), [3] p.   illus.   20 cm.
                    [2518]
"A briefe and necessary treatise, touching the cure of the disease now usually called lues venerea . . .": p. [145]-224, with special title page; "The nature and propertie of quicksilver, by G. Baker . . .": p. 226-229.
STC 5445.7.

—A right frutefull and approved treatise, for the artificiall cure of that malady called in Latin struma, and in English the evill . . . London, Edward Allde, 1602.

[8], 68, [2] p.   18 cm.   [2519]
Imperfect: upper margin of title page and The epistle to the reader multilated.
STC 5446.

CLUSIUS, CAROLUS. *See* L'ÉCLUSE, Charles de [1526-1609]

CLUTIUS, AUGERIUS. *See* CLUYT, Outger [*fl.* 1627-*ca.* 1636]

CLUYT, OUTGER [*fl.* 1627-*ca.* 1636] Augerii Clutii M. D. Opuscula duo singularia. I. De nuce medica. II. De hemerobio sive ephemero insecto, & majali verme. Amsterodami, Typis Jacobi Charpentier, 1634.

[38], 103, [3] p.   illus., plate.   21 cm. [2520]

CNEUFFEL, ANDREAS. *See* CNÖFFEL, Andreas [*d.* 1658]

CNÖFFEL, ANDREAS [*d.* 1658] Epistola de podagra curata per Doctorem Andream Cneuffelium. Amstelredami, Apud Johannem Blaeu, 1643.

118 p.   14 cm.   [2521]
Edited by Krzysztof Arciszewski.

—[The same.] . . . Gorlicii, Impensis Conradi Wörneri, Excud. Martinus Hermannus, 1644.

118 p.   13 cm.   [2522]
A reprint of the Amsterdam 1643 edition.

—Exercitatio, qua . . . Augustini Corrade D. calumnias & curationem in febribus acutis perstringit; & suam solide medicaturis huic epidemia nostrae Europeae & pestilentiali, simul & publicae experientiae commendat . . . Exscripta typis ex Alethiopoli commodatis, 1654.

[80] p.   20 cm.   [2523]

—*See* SCHRÖDER, J. Pharmacopoea Schrödero-Hoffmanniana illustrata et aucta. 1687.

CNOPFF, JOHANN JAKOB [1660-1739] *respondent.* Dissertatio medica inauguralis de pica . . . [Altdorffii] Literis Henrici Meyeri [1687]

32 p.   20 cm.   [2524]
Diss. — Altdorf.

—*See* HOFFMANN, J. M., *praeses.* De odoramentis et suffimentis dissertatio medica publica. 1686.

CNUPPIUS, JOHANN RUDOLF [*fl.* 1667] *respondent.*

See VOIGT, G., *praeses.* Disputatio physica prima de stillicidio sanguinis. 1667.

CNUTIUS, JUSTUS [*fl.* 1600-*ca.* 1608] Compendium universae medicinae juxta doctrinam Hippocratis, & Galeni . . . Vicentiae, Apud Petrum Bertellium, 1608.

152, [6] p.   17 cm.   [2525]

—[The same.] . . . Patavii, Apud Cadorinum, 1679.

[10], 144, [4] p.   17 cm.   [2526]
Imperfect: sig. a2-4 wanting?

CNYRIM, JOHANN NIKOLAUS [*fl.* 1686] *respondent.* *See* WALDSCHMIDT, J. J., *praeses.* Disputatio inauguralis physico-hydroscopica. 1686.

COBERUS, THOBIAS. *See* KOBER, Tobias [*ca.* 1570-*ca.* 1612]

COCCEJUS, JOHANNES [1603-1669] Oratio in V. C. Johannis Antonidae van der Linden . . . funere dicta II Martii A. M.DC.LXIV. Lugduni Batavorum, Ex officina Danielis & Abrahami à Gaesbeeck, 1664.

[36] p.   20 cm.   [2527]

COCCI, ALESSANDRO [1634-1707] *See* MARINIS, D. Dissertatio philosophico-medica. 1678.

COCHEIM, JOHANN HEINRICH [*fl.* 1625] Ein philosophisch und chymischer Tractat: genandt: Errantium in rectam & planam viam reductio. Das ist: Beständiger . . . Bericht von der wahren universal Materia, dess grossen universal Steins der Weisen . . . Angehengt, ein . . . Arbeit, die sich monatlich auff ein merckliche Gradation zur gläntzenden Apollinis Kron in der Diana erstrecken thut . . . Strassburg, In Verlegung Eberhardi Zetzners, 1626.

[16], 118, [1] p.   16 cm.   [2528]

COCHON DU PUY, JEAN [1674-1757] Histoire d'une enflûre du bas ventre tres-particuliere, qui confirme la nouvelle opinion de la generation de l'homme par les oeufs, & qui êtablît un nouveau genre de maladies des femmes . . . La Rochelle, Pierre Mesnier, et se vend a Paris chez Laurent d'Houry [1698]

46 p.   plate.   16 cm.   [2529]

—Quaestiones medicas . . . [Rupellae, Apud Petrum Mesnier, 1698]

14 p.   22 cm.   [2530]

"Quaestio prima. Est-ne unicum et simplex vitale principium?": p. 4-9; "Quaestio secunda. An medicus a morte liberet?": p. 9-15.

COCK, THOMAS. *See* COCKE, Thomas [*fl.* 1675]

COCK VAN KERCKWIJK, CHRISTOPHORUS [*d.* 1678] Pest-basiliscus, en verduysterde liefde in des werelts laten avondt-stondt; met een by-gevoeghde Ontmaskerde pest-mom, of klare ... beschrijvinge der pestilentie ... Hertogenbosch, Stephanus du Mont, 1668.

[24], 136 p.; [8], 45, [25] p.   plates.   20 cm. **[2531]**

Part [2] has special title page.

COCKBURN, WILLIAM [1669-1739] Oeconomia corporis animalis ... Londini, Excudebat F. Leach, impensis Hugonis Newman, 1695.

[9], 137 (i.e. 141) p.   19 cm. **[2532]**

—[The same.] ... Juxta editionem Londinensem, de'anno 1695 recusa. Augustae Vindelicorum, Impensis Kronigeri & haeredum Goebelii, 1696.

[12], 190, [1] p.   14 cm. **[2533]**

— , *tr. See* HARRIS, W. An exact enquiry into, and cure of the acute diseases of infants. 1693.

COCKE, THOMAS [*fl.* 1675] Υτιεινή; or, A plain and practical discourse upon the first of the six non-naturals, viz. air: with cautionary rules and directions for the preservation of people in this time of sickness ... London, Printed by E. C. for Philem. Stephens Sen., Philem Stephens Jun., Peter Dring, Joseph Leigh, 1665.

[12], 23, [5] p.   20 cm. **[2534]**
Errata: p. [28]

—Kitchin-physick; or, Advice to the poor, by way of dialogue betwixt Philanthropos, physician, Eugenius, apothecary, Lazarus patient. With rules and directions, how to prevent sickness, and cure diseases by diet ... as also, for the better enabling of nurses ... London, 1675.

[6], 87 p.; [1], 68 p.   plate.   14 cm. **[2535]**
Imperfect: p. 53-68 of part [2] wanting.
Part [2] has special title page: Miscelanea medica; or, A supplement to Kitchin-physick; to which is added, a short discourse on stoving and bathing: with some transient and occasional notes on Dr. George Thompsons Γαληνο-μεμψις.

—[The same.] ... London, Printed for the author, and are to be sold by T. Basset, 1676.

[4], 87 p.; [8], 68 (i.e. 70) p.   plate.   15 cm. **[2536]**

The special title page of part [2] is dated 1675. In part [2] inserted after p. 24 is another special title page: A practical and short discourse of stoving and bathing ... London, Printed for the author, and sold by T. Basset, 1676.

A reissue of the 1675 edition with new title pages; without Cocke's signed Epistle dedicatory before part [1] and with a new Epistola dedicatoria signed T. C. before part [2]

COCLES, BARTOLOMMEO DELLA ROCCA, *known as* [1467-1504] [Physiognomiae & chiromantiae compendium. French.] Enseignemens de physionomie et chiromancie. Monstrans par le regard du visage, signes de la face & lignes de la main, les moeurs & complexions des hommes ... Paris, Denys Bechet, 1638.

[222] p.   illus.   17 cm. **[2537]**
Signatures: A-O^8 (last leaf blank)
"La parfaite et absolue raison de la chiromancie, par André Corve ou Corbeau": p. [35-222]
French versions were also published under 2 other titles: Le compendium et brief enseignement de physiognomie et chyromancie (Paris, 1546) and La physiognomie naturelle, et la chiromance (Rouen, 1698)
The same version of the Chiromantia by Corvus was published in Paris in 1578 under title: Excellente chiromancie.

COCLITE, BARTOLOMMEO DELLA ROCCA, *known as. See* COCLES, Bartolommeo della Rocca, *known as* [1467-1504]

COCQ, JOANNES DE [1639-1721] *respondent.* Disputatio medica, inauguralis, de hydrope ... Lugduni Batavorum, Ex officina Salamonis Wagenaer, 1661.

[12] p.   20 cm. **[2538]**
Diss.—Leyden.

COCQUIS, PIETER [*fl.* 1688] *respondent.* Disputatio medica inauguralis, continens selectiores quasdam positiones medicas ... Lugduni Batavorum, Apud Abrahamum Elzevier, 1688.

[12] p.   23 cm. **[2539]**
Diss.—Leyden.

CODDYN, MATTHIAS [*fl.* 1683] *respondent.* Disputatio medica inauguralis de lienteria una cum succorum in corpore humano separatione ... Lugduni Batavorum, Apud Abrahammum Elzevier, 1683.

[16] p.   22 cm. **[2540]**
Diss.—Leyden.

CODEX medicamentarius; seu, Pharmacopoea Tolosana ... in lucem edita ... Pontio Francisco Purpan ... Tolosae, Apud Arnaldum Colomerium, 1648.

[12], 116 p.   20 cm.   [2541]

Approved by the Faculté de médecine de Toulouse.

CODRONCHI, BATTISTA. *See* CODRONCHI, Giovanni Battista [1547-1628]

CODRONCHI, GIOVANNI BATTISTA [1547-1628] Commentarius de annis climactericis, ac ratione vitandi eorum pericula, vitamque producendi ... Bononiae, Typis Bartholomaei Cochii, 1620.

[16], 174, [2] p.   15 cm.   [2542]

Errata: [2] p.

— [The same.] ... De annis climactericis necnon de ratione vitandi eorum pericula, itemque de modis vitam producendi ... commentarius ... Coloniae, Sumptibus Matthaei Smitz, 1623.

[8], 168 p.   15 cm. cm.   [2543]

— De Christiana ac tuta medendi ratione libri duo. Opus medicis praecipue, itemque aegrotis, & ministris, atque etiam sacerdotibus ad confitendum admissis utilissimum ... Quod opus alias editum nuperrime fuit ab auctore emendatum ... Bononiae, Typis Clementis Ferronii, 1629.

[16], 167, [16] p.   21 cm.   [2544]

— De morbis, qui Imolae, et alibi communiter hoc anno M.DCII. vagati sunt, commentariolum, in quo potissimum de lumbricis tractatur, et de morbo novo prolapsu scilicet mucronatae cartilaginis libellus ... Bononiae, Apud Jo. Baptistam Bellagambam, impensis Simeonis Parlaschae, 1603.

62 p.   20 cm.   [2545]

"De morbo novo ...": p. [43]-62 has special title page.

— De morbis veneficis, ac veneficiis. Libri quattuor. In quibus non solum certis rationibus veneficia dari demonstratur, sed eorum species, caussae, signa, & effectus nova methodo aperiuntur. Postremo de eorum curatione ac praeservatione exacte tractatus, veraque nova, & experta remedia proponuntur ... Opus ... ab auctore emendatum, ac ... auctum ... Mediolani, Apud Jo. Bapt. Bidellium, 1618.

[30], 248, [29] p.   16 cm.   [2546]

Imperfect: title page mutilated.

— De rabie, hydrophobia communiter dicta, libro duo. De sale absynthii libellus. De iis, qui aqua im-

merguntur, opusculum: et De elleboro commentarius. Francofurti, Typis Matthiae Beckeri, impensis haeredum Nicolai Bassaei, 1610.

471 p.   16 cm.   [2547]

CODRONCUS, BAPTISTA. *See* CODRONCHI, Giovanni Battista [1547-1628]

COEGELEN À DORTMONT, JAN LODEWIJK [*fl.* 1692] *respondent.* Disputatio medica inauguralis de phthisi ... Lugduni Batavorum, Apud Abrahamum Elzevier, 1692.

[43] p.   21 cm.   [2548]

Diss. — Leyden.

CÖLER, JOHANNES ACHATIUS [*fl.* 1685] *respondent.* *See* STURM, J. C., *praeses.* Primaria gravium leviumque phaenomena ad principia causasque suas reducens exercitatio. 1685.

COELI, ANTONINUS. *See* CELI, ANTONINO [*fl. ca.* 1618]

CÖLLER, HEINRICH [*fl.* 1658] *respondent.* Disquisitio iatrosophica inauguralis, morbum sacrum veluti ignotum in rep. medica humani corporis hospitem, vulgata medicorum de eodem dogmata, refellendo, ac veram illius essentiam itemque sedem genuinam, sicut & locum corporis affectum ex novis principiis pathologicis declarando, in scenam introducens ... Gissae Cattorum, Typis Josephi Dieterici Hampelii, 1658.

[8], 46 p.   19 cm.   [2549]

Diss. — Giessen.

CÖRNER, BALTHASAR [*fl.* 1626-1627] *respondent. See* JANUS, J., *praeses.* Dissertatio medica de morbis haereditariis. 1627; SENNERT, D., *praeses.* Exercitatio medica de vigiliis nimiis. 1626.

COETS, GYSBERT [*fl.* 1640] *tr. See* CHAUMETTE, A. Handt-boeck der chirurgie. 1640.

COFONE. *See* COPHO.

COGAN, THOMAS [1545?-1607] The haven of health, chiefly made for the comfort of students, and consequently for all those that have a care of their health, amplified upon five words of Hippocrates, written Epid. 6 labour, meat, drinke, sleepe, Venus ... Corr. and augm. Hereunto is added a preservation from the pestilence: with a short censure of the late sicknesse at Oxford ... London, Printed by Melch. Bradwood for John Norton, 1612.

[16], 275 p.   19 cm.   [2550]

Imperfect: last leaf mutilated.
STC 5483.

—[The same.] ... The 4th ed., corr. and amended. London, Printed by Anne Griffin, for Roger Ball, 1636.

[16], 321, [22] p.   19 cm.   [2551]

STC 5484.

COHAUSEN, Johann Heinrich [1665-1750] Tentaminum physico-medicorum curiosa decas de vita humana theoretice et practice per pharmaciam prolonganda ... Cosfeldiae, Sumptibus authoris, typis Joann. Barth. Steinii, 1699.

[28], 187, [1] p.   18 cm.   [2552]

COIMBRA. Universidade. Faculdade de Medicina. *See* Universidade de Coimbra. Faculdade de Medicina.

COITER, Volcher [1534-1576] Tractatus anatomicus de ossibus infantis. *In* Eyssonius, H. Tractatus anatomicus. 1659.

COLANTONIO, Giuseppe [*fl.* 1657] Raguaglio della peste scuoperta nella città di Riete li 25. Ottobre 1656 ... Roma, Gl ' heredi del Mancini, 1658.

[10], 67, [1] p.   24 cm.   [2553]

Added engraved title page.

COLBATCH, *Sir* John [1670-1728] Four treatises of physick and chirurgery: viz. I. A physico-medical essay concerning alkaly and acid. II. Farther considerations by way of Appendix to the said essay. III. Novum lumen chirurgicum, or a new light of chirurgery. IV. Novum lumen chirurgicum vindicatum, or the new light of chirurgery vindicated from many unjust aspersions ... The 2d ed. corr. and enlarged. London, Printed by J. D. for Daniel Brown, 1698.

xxiii, [1], 122 p.; 86 p.; xxxii (i.e. xxx), 143 p.   18 cm.   [2554]

Each work has special title page.

—A collection of tracts, chirurgical and medical; viz. I. A new light of chirurgery ... II. The new light of chirurgery vindicated ... III. A physico-medical essay concerning alkaly and acid ... IV. Further considerations concerning alkaly and acid ... V. A treatise of the gout ... VI. The doctrin of acids in the cure of diseases further asserted ... VII. A relation of a sudden and extraordinary cure of a person

bitten by a viper, by the means of acids ... London, Dan. Brown, 1700.

[4], 568, [15] p.   20 cm.   [2555]

Half title (p. [1]): Dr. Colbatch's works.
Each work has special title page dated 1699, except work II, which has date 1698.

—The doctrine of acids in the cure of diseases farther asserted: being an answer to some objections raised against it by Dr. F. Tuthill ... In which are contained somethings relating to the history of blood ... To which is added an exact account of The case of Edmund Turner Esq. ... London, Dan. Brown and Abel Roper, 1689 [i.e. 1698]

xvi, 128 p.   18 cm.   [2556]

—Another issue, dated 1698.   [2557]

—Novum lumen chirurgicum vindicatum; or, The new light of chirurgery vindicated from the many unjust aspersions of some unknown calumniators. With the addition of some few experiments made this winter in England ... London, D. Brown, 1695.

[13], 46, [1] p.   17 cm.   [2558]

—A physico medical essay, concerning alkaly and acid, so far as they have relation to the cause or cure of distempers; wherein is endeavoured to be proved, that acids are not ... the cause of all or most distempers; but that alkalies are. Together with an account of some distempers ... as also a short digression, concerning specifick remedies ... London, Dan. Browne, 1696.

[29], 147 (i.e. 137), [1] p.   16 cm.   [2559]

Dedicatory letter bound after p. 142 (i.e. p. 132)
With this is bound *his* Some farther considerations concerning alkaly and acid. 1696.

—A relation of a very sudden and extraordinary cure of a person bitten by a viper, by the means of acids. Together with some Remarks upon Dr. Tuthill's vindication of his objections against the doctrine of acids ... London, Dan. Brown, Abel Roper and Tho. Leigh, 1698.

[12], 116 p.   18 cm.   [2560]

—Some farther considerations concerning alkaly and acid, by way of appendix to a late essay. Wherein the terms are made clear, and the natures of them both more fully explained: together with an answer to the objections that have been raised against some things contained in the essay ... London, Dan. Brown, 1696.

[12], 100 p. 16 cm. [2561]
Bound with *his* A physico medical essay, concerning alkaly and acid. 1696.

—A treatise of the gout: wherein both its cause and cure are demonstrably made appear. To which are added, some medicinal observations concerning the cure of fevers, &c. by the means of acids ... London, Printed for Daniel Brown and Roger Clavel, 1697.
xxxii (i.e. xxx), 143 p. 17 cm. [2562]

—*See* BOULTON, R. An examination of Mr. John Colbatch his books. 1699; EMES, T. A dialogue between alkali and acid. 1698, 1699; NOVUM LUMEN CHIRURGICUM EXTINCTUM. 1695.

COLBE, JOACHIM [*d.* 1657] *respondent.* Theses de phthisi... Basileae, Typis Joh. Jacobi Genathii [1614]
[8] p. 22 cm. [2563]
Diss. — Basel.

—*See* SENNERT, D. Practicae medicinae. 1636-54.

COLBIUS, JOACHIMUS JOHANNES. *See* KOLB, Joachim Johann [*fl.* 1682]

COLBIUS, THEODORUS [*fl.* 1659] *respondent. See* LINDEN, J. A. van der., *praeses.* Hippocrates de circuitu sanguinis, exercitatio I. 1659.

COLE, ABDIAH [1610?-1670?] *tr. See* RIVIÈRE, L. The practice of physick. 1655, 1658-61, 1672, 1678; RULAND, M. [1532-1602] Experimental physick. 1662; SENNERT, D. Two treatises. 1660.

—*See* BARTHOLIN, T. Anatomia. 1665, 1668; CULPEPER, N. Pharmacopoeia Londinensis. 1661; JONSTONUS, J. The idea of practical physick. 1661; PLATTER, F. [1536-1614] A golden practice of physick. 1662.

COLE, WILLIAM [1635-1716] De febribus ac De secretione animali. *In* Morton, R. Opera medica. 1696, 1697, 1699.

—De secretione animali ... Oxon., E Theatro Sheldoniano, 1674.
[19], 275 (i.e. 279) p. 16 cm. [2564]

—Novae hypotheseos, ad explicanda febrium intermittentium symptomata et typos excogitatae hypotyposis. Una cum aetiologia remediorum; speciatim vero de curatione per corticem Peruvianum. Accessit Dissertatiuncula de intestinorum

motu peristaltico ... Londini, D. Browne & S. Smith, 1693.
[39], 266 p.; [1], 17 p. port. 18 cm. [2565]
Imperfect: port. wanting.
Part [2] has special title page.

— [The same.] ... Lipsiae, Sumpt. Joh. Jacobi Winckleri, 1695.
[23], 278 (i.e. 248) p.; 16, [12] p. 17 cm.
[2566]
Part [2] has half title page.

—[The same.] ... Genevae, Sumptibus Cramer & Perachon, 1696.
[12], 95 (i.e. 103), [5] p. 22 cm. [2567]

—[The same.] ... Amstelodami, Apud Georgium Gallet, 1698.
[32], 143 p. 20 cm. [2568]
Running title: De febribus intermittentibus.
Bound with Lister, M. Octo exercitationes medicinales. 1698.

—A physico-medical essay concerning the late frequency of apoplexies. Together with a general method of their prevention, and cure. In a letter to a physitian ... Oxford, Printed at the Theater, 1689.
[2], 196 p. 18 cm. [2569]
Addressed to Samuel Kimberley.

—Tractatus de secretione animali. Genevae, Sumptibus Cramer & Perachon, 1696.
[8], 72 p. 22 cm. [2570]

—[The same.] ... Ed. ult. Amstelodami, Apud Georgium Gallet, 1698.
[16], 93 p. 20 cm. [2571]
Bound with Lister, M. Octo exercitationes medicinales. 1698.

—*See* CHARLETON, W. Exercitationes de oeconomia animali. 1681.

—*as subject. See* SYDENHAM, T. Dissertatio epistolaris ad ... Guilielmum Cole 1682, 1684.

COLER, CHRISTIAN [*fl.* 1651] *respondent. See* WOLFF, A., *praeses.* De quatuor anni temporibus dissertationem philosophicam ... P. P. ... C. C. 1651.

COLER, JACOB [*fl.* 1604-1608] *respondent. See* SENNERT, D., *praeses.* De methodo medendi disputatio VII, de morbi tempore purgationi apto. 1604.

COLER, JOHANN [*d.* 1639] Oeconomia ruralis et domestica darinn das gantz Ampt aller trewes Hauss-Vätter, Hauss-Mütter, beständiges und allgemeines

Hauss-Buch, vom Hausshalten, Wein-Acker-Gärten-Blumen and Feld-Baw, begrieffen ... Sampt beygefügter einer experimentalischer Hauss-Apotecken und kurtzer Wundartzney-Kunst ... Jetzo ... corrigirt, vermehret und verbessert, in zwey Theil abgetheilet ... Mayntz, Durch Nicolaum Heyl, 1645.

     2 parts in 1 v.   illus.   34 cm.   **[2572]**
    Added engraved title page.
    Part 2 has special title page dated 1651.
    "Traumbuch Apomasaris": 57 p. at end of part 2.

COLER, JOHANN ACHATIUS [*fl.* 1688-1698] *praeses.* Ex mechanicis de vesica, tanquam potentia mechanica considerata, ejusdemque usu in explicando animalium membrorum per musculos motu ... disputabit ... Coburgi, Literis Joh. Nic. Monachi, 1698.

     [16] p.   illus.   18 cm.   **[2573]**
    Diss.—Coburg (C. H. Richter, *respondent*)

COLER, JOHANN JEREMIAS [*fl.* 1699-1704] *respondent. See* STAHL, G. E., *praeses.* Dissertatio medica de sangvisugarum utilitate. 1699.

COLER, MARTIN CLEMENS [*fl.* 1654-*ca.* 1668] *praeses.* Exercitatio physica de formis materialibus ... Wittebergae, Typis haered. Johannis Haken [1654]

     [20] p.   19 cm.   **[2574]**
    Diss.—Wittenberg (M. Meicherner, *respondent*)

COLER, THEOPHIL [1618-1685] *respondent. See* LANCKISCH, F. von., *praeses.* Δεκας Θεωρηματων φυσικων de calico innato in genere. 1641.

COLES, WILLIAM [1626-1662] Adam in Eden; or, Natures paradise. The history of plants, fruits, herbs and flowers. With their several names, whether Greek, Latin or English ... London, Printed by J. Streater, for Nathaniel Brooke, 1657.

     [20], 144, 75-78, 145-165, 116-396 (i.e. 392), 66, 551-629, [24] p.   29 cm.   **[2575]**

COLEVELT, NIKOLAAS [*fl.* 1664] *respondent.* Disputatio medica inauguralis de plethora ... Lugduni Batavorum, Ex officina Jacobi Voorn, 1664.

     [16] p.   24 cm.   **[2576]**
    Diss.—Leyden.

COLIN, ANTOINE [*fl.* 1600-1602] *tr. See* ORTA, G. d'. Histoire des drogues. 1602.

COLIN, SÉBASTIEN [1519?-1578?] Declaratio fraudum et errorum apud pharmacopoeos commis-

sorum. Authore Lisseto Benancio [pseud.] Latinitate donata & edita ex museo Thomae Bartholini. Accessit ejusdem argumenti Dialogus Joh. Antonii Lodetti. Francofurti, Apud Justum Rächerum, 1667.

     159, [1] p.   16 cm.   **[2577]**
    "Dialogus de fraudibus pharmacopoeorum nonnullorum authore Joh. Antonio Lodetto ... Latinitate donatus & editus ex museo Thomae Bartholini" (p. [99]-159) has half title.

—[The same.] ... Ed. 2. Francofurti, Apud Justum Rächerum, 1671.   **[2578]**
    A reprint of the 1667 edition.

COLLADON, THÉODORE [*d. ca.* 1636] Adversaria, seu, commentarii medicinales critici dialytici ... Ubi varii & multiplices neotericorum ... errores aperiuntur ... ac pristina, genuinaque antiquorum doctrina ... restituitur. Coloniae Allobrogum, Typis Jacobi Stoer, 1615.

     2 v. in 1.   17 cm.   **[2579]**

COLLE, GIOVANNI [1558-1631] Cosmitor medicaeus triplex, in quo exercitatio totius artis medicae ... consultationes medicinales, et quaestiones practicae enucleatae proponuntur ... Venetiis, Apud Baretium Baretium, 1621.

     [52], 322, [1] p.   33 cm.   **[2580]**
    Colophon dated 1620.

—De cognitu difficilibus in praxi ex libello Hippocratis De insomniis, et ex libris Avenzoaris per commentaria, & sententias dilucidatas, auctore Joanne Colle ... Venetiis, Apud Evangelistam Deuchinum, 1628.

     [28], 123, [1] p.; 180 [i.e. 172), [17] p.   26 cm.   **[2581]**
    Part [1] has caption title: Commentaria in librum Hippocratis De insomniis. (Includes the Hippocratic text.)
    Part [2] has special title page: De cognitu difficilibus in praxi ex libris Avenzoaris per sententias dilucidatas. (Includes Latin text of "sententiae" adapted from Taisīr of Avenzoar.)
    Errata: part [1], p. [124]; part [2], leaf at end.

—De omnibus malignis, et pestilentibus affectionibus, & earum medela. Tomi duo ... In quibus universa praxis morborum, symptomatum universalium ... expenditur ... Immo diligenter cuncta Hipp. Gal Graecorum, & Arabum loca de acutis, & malignis, pestilentibus ... dilucidantur ... Additi sunt etiam libelli non amplius in lucem editi Dionisii, Titiani, Viventii, Bernardi, Bartholomei, Danielis, Avantii, Giorgii Colle Bellonensium de variis malignis, pestilentibns [sic] ... ab anno 1340. usque ad annum 1547. Cum locupletissima tabula notabilium ... Jacobi Magalloti ... atque accurata correctione ... Ludovici Archangeli ... Pisauri, Ex typographia Hieronymi Concordiae, 1616.

2 v. in 1.   32 cm.   [2582]

—[The same.] Medicina practica; sive, Methodus cognoscendorum, & curandorum omnium affectuum malignorum, & pestilentium ... Pisauri, Sumptibus Roberti Meietti, 1617.

2 v. in 1.   33 cm.   [2583]

Imperfect: title page of vol. 2 wanting.
A reissue with new title page.

—Elucidarium chirurgicum, commentaria in librum quartum fen quartam Avicennae cum tractatibus chirurgicis ex Hippocrate, Galeno, Graecis, et Arabibus ... Venetiis, Apud Evangelistam Deuchinum, 1620.

[26], 3-160 p.   31 cm.   [2584]

—Monumenta sinoptica de peste curanda, & praeservanda cum dilucidatione locorum Hipp., Aris., Gal., Rasis, Avic., antiquorum Arabum, & Gręcorum ... Patavii, Apud Gasparem Crivellarium, 1631.

[108] p.   20 cm.   [2585]

Imperfect: sig. N4 wanting?

COLLECTANEA chymica; A collection of ten several treatises in chymistry, concerning the liquor alkahest, the mercury of philosophers, and other curiosities worthy the perusal ... London, William Cooper, 1684.

[6], 193, [4] p.; 32 p.; 16 p.   15 cm.   [2586]

Contents. —[1] The secret of the immortal liquor called alkahest, or ignis-aqua. By Eireneaus Philalethes ... has added title page in Latin, and text in English and Latin. —[2] The practice of lights; or, An excellent and ancient treatise of the philosophers stone. — [3] Praecipiolum; or, The immature-mineral-electrum ... By Jo. Bapt. Van-Helmont. —[4] Aurum-potabile; or, The receit of Dr. Fr. Antoine ... —[5] A treatise of Bernard earl of Trevisan, of the philosophers stone. —[6] The bosome-book of Sir George Ripley ... —[7] Speculum alchymiae; The true glass of alchemy ... By Roger Bacon. —[8] The admirable efficacy ... of true oyl, which is made of sulphur-vive, set on fire, and called ... oyl of sulphur per campanam ... [by] George Starkey ... —[9] Sundry new, and artificial remedies against famine ... by Sir Hugh Platt ... —[10] The tomb of Semiramis hermetically sealed ...

Items have special title pages dated 1683.
"George Starkey's pill vindicated ...": 16 p. at end.

COLLECTANEA chimica curiosa. 1693. *See* THOM, J. D., *ed.*

COLLECTANEA chymica Leidensia Maetsiana & Maregraviana. 1696. *See* [MORLEY, C. L.]

COLLECTANEA chymica Leydensia. 1696, 1700. *See* MORLEY, C. L., *ed.*

COLLECTANEA de diuturna graviditate ... Amstelodami, Apud Petrum van den Berge, 1662.

[6], 3-60, [2], 3-27 p., 30-31 ll.   illus.   14 cm.   [2587]

Portentosum lithopaedion has special title page dated 1622 [i.e. 1662?]

Contents. —Portentosum lithopaedion, sive Embryum petrefactum urbis Senonensis a Joan. Albosio de istius indurationis causis. —Simeonis Provancherii Opinio de iisdem. —Thomae Bartholinii Historia centesima, centuriae secundae, de eodem foetu. — Ostentum Dolanum, seu Historia mirabilis infantis in ventre a morte matris reperti post annos sexdecim et amplius graviditatis [per Franciscum Bernardum Schnorf] —Arnoldi Senguerdi Discursus de ostento Dolano. —Observatio singularis Mussipontani foetus extra uterum, in abdomine retenti, tandemque lapidescentis [per Antonium Deusingium]

Bound with part 2 of Harvey, W. Exercitationes anatomicae, de motu cordis. 1671.

COLLECTANEA medico-physica. 1680-1688, 1690. *See* BLANKAART, S.

COLLEGE AND CORPORATION OF SURGEONS OF EDINBURGH. *See* ROYAL COLLEGE OF SURGEONS OF EDINBURGH.

COLLÈGE DE DIJON. *See* COLLÈGE DES MÉDECINS, Dijon.

COLLÈGE DE MÉDECINE, Lyons. *See* COLLÈGE DES MÉDECINS, Lyons.

COLLÈGE DES MAÎTRES CHIRURGIENS JURÉS DE PARIS. Traicté de la peste, avec les remedes certains & approuvez pour s'en preserver & garantir; nouvellement faict ... 2. ed., rev. & augm. Paris, Nicolas Buon, 1606.

48 p.   16 cm.   [2588]

COLLÈGE DES MÉDECINS, Dijon. Dissertation sur les fievres pourprées; ou, La veritable methode pour traiter ceux qui en sont malades. Par les medecins agregés au College de Dijon. Avec la Réponse de messieurs de la Faculté de Medecine de Paris. Dijon, J. Ressayre, 1685.

59 p.   14 cm.   [2589]

COLLÈGE DES MÉDECINS, Lyons. *See* PHARMACOPOEA LUGDUNENSIS. 1627.

COLLEGE MÉDICAL DE BRUXELLES. *See* COLLEGIE DER MEDECYNE, Brussels.

COLLEGE OF PHYSICIANS IN LONDON. *See* ROYAL COLLEGE OF PHYSICIANS, London.

COLLEGIE DER MEDECYNE, Brussels. Collegie der Medecyne, op-gericht door den magistraet der stadt Brussel. Brussel, Martinus van Bossuyt, 1650.

[4], 70, [4] p.   21 cm.   **[2590]**

With this is bound *its* Noodighe op-rech-tinghe van't Collegie der Medecyne. Brussel, 1660.

—[Latin ed.] Statuta Collegii Medici Bruxellensis, ab amplissimo Senatu sancita, a Roberto Fervacquio ... Latine edita ... Bruxellae, Ex officina Joannis Mommarti, 1650.

[12], 71, [5] p.   20 cm.   **[2591]**

—Noodighe op-rechtinghe van't Collegie der Medecyne, opentlyck bewesen aen d'in-woonders der stadt van Brussel ... Brussel, Guilliam Scheybels, 1660.

[6], 101, [1] p.   21 cm.   **[2592]**

Bound with *its* Collegie der Medecyne. 1650.

—*See* PHARMACOPOEA AUCTIOR. 1671.

COLLEGIO D'ARTE E MEDICINA, Bologna. *See* UNIVERSITÀ DI BOLOGNA. Collegio di medicina.

COLLEGIO DE' FISICI DI ROMA. *See* COLLEGIO DEI MEDICI, Rome.

COLLEGIO DE' MEDICI, Bologna. *See* UNIVERSITÀ DI BOLOGNA. Collegio di medicina.

COLLEGIO DE' MEDICI DI FIRENZE. *See* ARTE DE' MEDICI E DEGLI SPEZIALI, Florence.

COLLEGIO DE' MEDICI DI ROMA. *See* COLLEGIO DEI MEDICI, Rome.

COLLEGIO DE' SPETIALI DI ROMA. *See* COLLEGIO DEGLI SPEZIALI, Rome.

COLLEGIO DEGLI SPEZIALI, Naples. Parere dell'almo Collegio de Spetiali di Napoli sopra l'opobalsamo mandatoli dalli signori consoli del Collegio de' Spetiali di Roma. Con un picciolo Trattato dell'opobalsamo orientale di Gioseppe Donzelli ... Napoli, Francesco Savio, 1640.

[8] p.   22 cm.   **[2593]**

COLLEGIO DEGLI SPEZIALI, Rome. Summa statutorum, facultatum, privilegiorum, & jurisdictionis aromatariorum a summis pontificibus concess. confirmat, & amplia. Noviter à spectabili Collegio Aromatariorum urbis in unum collecta. Romae, Ex typographia Reverendae Camerae Apostolicae, 1693.

[1], 100 p.   22 cm.   **[2594]**

—*See* COLLEGIO DEI MEDICI, Rome. Motus proprius confirmationis concordiae. 1675; COLLEGIO DEGLI SPEZIALI, Naples. Parere dell'almo Collegio de spetiali di Napoli. 1640.

COLLEGIO DEI FILOSOFI E MEDICI, Turin. Statuta vetera, et nova sacri venerandique Collegii D. D. phylosophorum, et medicorum augustae civitatis Taurini, in hac secunda impressione novis additionibus, ac explanationibus illustrata. Taurini, Apud Jo. Jacobum Rustis, 1664 (i.e. 1665).

82, [1] p.   24 cm.   **[2595]**

"Sequitur eorundem statutorum novissima confirmatio ... [&] Eorundem statutorum cum novissimis additionibus ... &c. publicatio, acceptatio, & ad effectum deductio: cum serie status collegii, penes tres ordines residentium; prout anno 1665. die prima Aprilis dispositum invenitur": p.LXV-LXXII, inserted in duplicate between p. 64 and 65.

COLLEGIO DEI FISICI, Milan. Decreta Collegii physicorum Mediolanensium. Mediolani, Apud Jo. Baptistam, & Julium Caesarem Malatestam, 1645.

[1], 42, [3] p.   22 cm.   **[2596]**

With this are bound (as issued?): *its* Ven. Collegii physicorum Mediolanensium antiquitas. [1645?]; Ferdinand III, Emperor of Germany. Privilegium. 1653.

—Prospectus pharmaceuticus, sub quo Antidotarium Mediolanense spectandum proponitur ... Collegii ... physicorum dictae civitatis spetiali ordine demandatum Joanni Honorato Castillioneo ... Quibus accessere tractatus De extractis, salibus, spiritibus, fucis, ac de metallorum ... natura, & cognitione. Mediolani, Apud Joannem Baptistam Ferrarium, 1668.

[24], 438, [1] p.; [6], 102, [1] p.   front.   32 cm.   **[2597]**

Part [2] has special title page: Brandae Francisci Castillionei ... De spiritibus, extractis, salibus, fucis, ac de metallorum ... simpliciumue origine, natura, & cognitione.

—Prospectus pharmaceutici ed. 2, sub quo Antodotarium Mediolanense Galeno-chimicum ...

Collegii . . . physicorum dictae civitatis ordine olim demandatum Joanni Honorato Castillioneo . . . nunc vero Brandae Francisci Castillionei . . . studio, & labore noviter emendatum, auctum, & in tres partes divisum; quarum prima complectitur regulas, & tempora pharmacopolis aptiora ad disponenda ea, quae ad eorum officinas conferunt, cum exacta ponderum, ac mensurarum usualium designatione . . . Secunda, Mantissam chimicam spagiricam Nicolai de Lemmery . . . e Gallico in Italicum traductam . . . Tertia, Tractatus de tinctura coralliorum, alkaest, & auro potabile . . . Mediolani, Ex typographia Caroli Josephi Quinti, 1698.

[44], 484 p.; [34], 216 p.; 118 p. front., plate. 30 cm.   [2598]

Pages [1-2] (blank) of part 3 wanting.
Parts 2 and 3 have special title pages.
Part 2 has running title: Corso di chimica.

—Ven. Collegii physicorum Mediolanensium antiquitas. Privilegia, statuta, & ordinationes in compendium redacta. [Mediolani? 1645?]

34 (i.e. 42) p. 22 cm.   [2599]

Caption title.
Bound with (as issued?) its Decreta. [1645]

—See SELVATICO, G. B. Collegii Mediolanensium medicorum origo. 1607.

COLLEGIO DEI MEDICI, Bergamo. La farmacopea o'antidotario dell'eccellentissimo Collegio de' signori medici di Bergomo, nel quale si contiene il modo di comporre i medicamenti hoggidì più usitati nelle speciarie. Tradotto dalla latina nella volgar lingua per D. Tito Sanpellegrino . . . Venetia, Nicolò Moretti, 1597. Bergamo, Per li fratelli Rossi, 1680.

[22], 84, 47 [1] ll. 30 cm.   [2600]

A reprint, with additional preliminary matter, of the 1597 ed.

COLLEGIO DEI MEDICI, Lucca. Breve instruttione per preservarsi dal contagio pestilente. Fatta d'ordine del Collegio de medici di Lucca l'anno 1630. Lucca, Ottaviano Guidoboni, 1630.

22 p. 20 cm.   [2601]

—[The same.] . . . Di nuovo ristampato. Genova, Giuseppe Pavoni, 1630.

31, [1] p. 17 cm.   [2602]

—See PEZZINI, S. Del modo di purgare le case e robbe infette. 1631.

COLLEGIO DEI MEDICI, Modena. *See*

MODENA. Ordinances, local laws, etc. Tassa delle robbe medicinali. 1677.

COLLEGIO DEI MEDICI, Rome. Motus proprius confirmationis concordiae. Inter Collegium Physicorum, & Collegium Aromatariorium urbis, & eorumdem Collegiorum jurisdictionis. Romae, Ex typographia Reverendae Camerae Apostolicae, 1675.

[8] p. 22 cm.   [2603]

Caption title on p. [2] reads: Gregorius Papa XIII. Ad perpetuam rei memoriam.

—Ordini da osservarsi nella visita generale delli Spetia[li] & altri dal vice-protomedico, & suoi ministri per tutto lo stato e[ccle]siastico mediatè, & immediatè soggetto alla santa Se[de] Apostolica. Roma, Nella Stamperia della Reverenda Camera Apo[sto]lica, 1641.

broadside. 38 x 24.   [2604]

Signed: Dominicus Guidarellus, Bernardinus Messorius, Baldus Baldus.
Imperfect: mutilated.
Bound with its Statuta Collegii. DD almae urbis medicorum. 1642.

—Statuta Collegii DD. almae urbis medicorum ex antiquis Romanorum pontificum bullis congesta, & hactenus per Sedem Apostolicam recognita, & innovata. Demum a sanctiss. D. N. Urbano Papa VIII confirmata. Romae, Ex typographia Rev. Cam. Apost., 1642.

100 p. 21 cm.   [2605]

"Nomina, et cognomina DD. Collegii Romani Medicorum, quorum memoria extat . . ." (p. 89-96) has caption title.
With this is bound its Ordini. 1641.

—Statuta Collegii DD. almae urbis medicorum ex antiquis Romanorum Pontificum bullis congesta, & hactenus per Sedem Apostolicam recognita, & innovata. Mox ab Urbano Octavo confirmata, eorumdemque statutorum in apostolicis litteris inserctione corroborata, & novis auctariis amplificata. Romae, Ex typographia Rev. Cam. Apost., 1676.

[16], 116 p. 22 cm.   [2606]

"Nomina, et cognomina DD. Collegii Romani Medicorum, quorum memoria extat . . ." (p. 105-116) has caption title.

—See ANTIDOTARII ROMANI. 1607; ANTIDOTARIO ROMANO LATINO E VOLGARE. 1624, 1635, 1639, 1675, 1678; CASTELLI, P. Antidotario romano. 1648.

—*as subject. See* CATHOLIC CHURCH. *Pope,* 1471-1484 (Sixtus IV). Sixtus Papa IV. Ad perpetuam rei memoriam. 1675? [and] *Pope,* 1523-1534 (Clemens VII)

Clementis Papae VII. Bulla de protomedici & Collegii Medicorum urbis jurisdictione, & facultatibus. 1627 [and] *Pope*, 1550–1555 (Julius III). Julius Papa III. Meritis devotionis vestrae. 1674 [and] *Pope*, 1559–1565 (Pius IV), Pius Papa IV. Confirmatio privilegiorum Collegii Medicorum urbis. 1675? [and] *Pope*, 1566–1572 (Pius V). Pius Papa V. Ad perpetuam rei memoriam. 1675 [and] *Pope*, 1572–1585 (Gregorius XIII). Gregorius Papa XIII ad perpetuam rei memoriam. 1675 [and] *Pope*, 1593–1603 (Clemens VIII). Clemens Papa Octavus ad perpetuam rei memoriam. 1675? [and] *Pope*, 1670–1676 (Clemens X). Clemens PP. X. Ad perpetuam rei memoriam. 1675.

COLLEGIUM AROMATARIORUM. *See* Collegio degli speziali, Rome.

COLLEGIUM MEDICORUM, Bergamo. *See* Collegio dei medici, Bergamo.

COLLEGIUM MEDICORUM, Bologna. *See* Università di Bologna. Collegio di medicina.

COLLEGIUM MEDICORUM LUGDUNENSIUM. *See* Collège des médecins, Lyons.

COLLEGIUM MEDICORUM, Rome. *See* Collegio dei medici, Rome.

COLLEGIUM MEDICUM, Amsterdam. *See* Pharmacopoea Belgica. 1659; Pharmacopoeia Amstelredamensis. 1636, 1639?, 1659.

COLLEGIUM MEDICUM, Augsburg. *See* Collegium medicum Augustanum.

COLLEGIUM MEDICUM AUGUSTANUM. *See* Pharmacopoeia augustana. 1613, 1622, 1643, 1684, 1694; Schroeck, L. Hygea Augustana. 1682.

COLLEGIUM MEDICUM BRUXELLENSE. *See* Collegie der Medecyne, Brussels.

COLLEGIUM MEDICUM ELECTORALE, Berlin. *See* Dispensatorium Brandenburgicum. 1698.

COLLEGIUM MEDICUM, Haarlem. *See* Pharmacopoea Harlemensis senatus auctoritate munita. 1693.

COLLEGIUM MEDICUM, Hague. *See* Pharmacopoea Hagiensis communi Collegii Medici ejusdem loci opera adornata. 1659.

COLLEGIUM MEDICUM NORIMBERGENSE. *See* Kollegium der Aerzte, Nuremberg.

COLLEGIUM MEDICUM PHARMACEUTICUM, Haarlem. *See* Collegium Medicum, Haarlem.

COLLEGIUM MEDICUM, Ratisbon. *See* Kollegium der Aerzte, Regensburg.

COLLEGIUM MEDICUM, Regensburg. *See* Kollegium der Aerzte, Regensburg.

COLLEGIUM MEDICUM, Stockholm. Catalogus et valor medicamentorum in officinis pharmaceüticis Stockholmiensibus prostantium. Apothecare-taxa, uppå alla de medicamenter och wahror, som på apotheken i Stockholm finnes til sahlu. Apotheker-Taxt, aller Medicamenten undt Wahren, welche in denen stockholmischen Apotheken zu finden seyn. [Stockholmiae, 1698?] [8], 96, [27] p. 21 cm. [2607]

Bound with Sweden. Laws, statutes, etc. Kongl. May:tz i nader uthgifne sidste medicinal-ordningar. 1699.

—*See* Pharmacopoeia Holmiensis. 1686.

COLLEGIUM MEDICUM ZU WITTENBERG. *See* Universität Wittenberg. Medizinische Fakultät.

COLLEGIUM NATURAE CURIOSORUM. *See* Academia Naturae Curiosorum.

COLLEGIUM PHILOSOPHORUM ET MEDICORUM, Bologna. *See* Università di Bologna. Collegio di medicina.

COLLEGIUM PHISICORUM, Rome. *See* Collegio dei medici, Rome.

COLLEGIUM PHYSICORUM, Milan. *See* Collegio dei fisici, Milan.

COLLEGIUM PRIVATUM AMSTELODAMENSE. Observationes anatomicae selectiores Collegii Privati Amstelodamensis . . . Amstelodami, Apud Casparum Commelinum, 1667[-1673] 45 p.; 53 p. illus., plates. 14 cm. [2608]

Part [2] has special title page: Observationum anatomicarum . . . pars altera . . . 1673.

Bound with Blasius, G. Anatome medullae spinalis. 1666.

COLLEGIUM ROMANORUM MEDICORUM. *See* Collegio dei medici, Rome.

COLLESSON, Jean. Idea perfecta philosophiae Hermeticae; seu, Abbreviatio theoriae & praxeos lapidis philosophici observationibus ... aucta ...

143-162 p., vol. 6. 20 cm. (*In* Zetzner, Lazarus, ed. Theatrum chemicum. Argentorati, 1659-61)   **[2609]**

Caption title.
Translation of part 1 of L'idée parfaicte.

COLLINS, Samuel [1618-1710] A systeme of anatomy, treating of the body of man, beasts, birds, fish, insects, and plants. Illustrated with many schemes ... engraven in seventy four ... plates. And after every part of man's body hath been anatomically described, its diseases, cases, and cures are concisely exhibited ... [London] In the Savoy, Thomas Newcomb, 1685.

2 v. ([18], lvi, [13], 678 p.; [6], 679-1263, [191] p.) front., port., illus. 39 cm.   **[2610]**

Imperfect: p. 21-24, 51-54, 673-676 of vol. 1 wanting, supplied in photocopy from Library of Congress; p.[17-18] of The epistle dedicatory mutilated.

COLLINUS, Gasparus [16th cent.] *See* Simmler, J. Vallesiae et Alpium descriptio 1633.

COLLUMBUS, Realdus. *See* Colombo, Realdo [*ca.* 1515-1559]

COLMENERO, Antoine. *See* Colmenero de Ledesma, Antonio [16th-17th cent.]

COLMENERO, José [17th cent.] Reprobacion del pernicioso abuso de los polvos de la corteza de el quarango, o china china ... A que se junta un provechosissimo manifiesto de las muchas virtudes de las salutiferas, y sulphureas aguas de los baños de Ledesma ... Salamanca, Eugenio Antonio Garcia, 1697.

[18], 198 p.; [8], 80, [3] p. plate. 21 cm.   **[2611]**

Part [2] has special title page: Tratado maravilloso, y utilissimo de las enfermedades, que se curan con las salutiferas aguas de los bānos de la villa de Ledesma.

—*See* Muñoz y Peralta, J. Escrutinio phisico medico de un peregrino especifico de las calenturas intermitentes. 1699.

COLMENERO DE LEDESMA, Antonio [16th-17th cent.] [Curioso tratado de la naturaleza y calidad de chocolate. Latin.] Chocolata inda. Opusculum de qualitate & natura chocolatae ...

Hispanico antehac idiomate editum: nunc vero curante Marco Aurelio Severino ... in Latinum translatum. Norimbergae, Typis Wolfgangi Enderi, 1644.

[20], 73, [6] p. plate. 13 cm.   **[2612]**

Errata: p. [79]
Edited by Johann Georg Volckamer.
With this is bound (as issued?) Volckamer, J. G. Opobalsami orientalis. 1644.

—[French tr.] Du chocolate discours curieux, divisé en quatre parties ... Traduit d'espagnol en françois sur l'impression faite à Madrid l'an 1631. & esclaircy de quelques annotations. Par René Moreau ... Plus est adjousté un dialogue touchant le mesme chocolate ... Paris, Sebastien Cramoisy, 1643.

[8], 59 p. 21 cm.   **[2613]**

"Du chocolate. Dialogue entre un medecin, un indien, & un bourgeois. Composé par Barthelemy Marradon ... imprimé à Seville l'an 1618. Tourné à present de l'Espagnol, & accommodé à la françoise": p. [45]-59.

—[Italian tr.] Della cioccolata ... Tradotto ... con aggiunta d'alcune Annotationi da Alessandro Vitrioli ... Roma, Nella stamparia della R. C. A., 1667.

94 (i.e. 96) p. 15 cm.   **[2614]**

—[The same.] ... Venetia, Per il Valvasense, 1678.

80 p. 15 cm.   **[2615]**

—*See* [Dufour, P. S.] De l'usage du caphé, du thé, et du chocolate. 1671 [and] Tractatus novi de potu caphe, de Chinensium the, et de chocolata. 1685, 1699.

COLOGNE. Ordinances, local laws, etc. *See* Pharmacopoea, sive dispensatorum Coloniense. 1628.

COLOMBANI, Astolfo. *See* Columbani, Alfonso.

COLOMBINA, Gasparo [*d.* 1650] Il bomprovifaccia, per sani, & amalati ... Padova, Pietro Paolo Tozzi, 1621.

[31], 335 (i.e. 367) p. illus. 17 cm.   **[2616]**

COLOMBO, Matteo Realdo. *See* Colombo, Realdo [*ca.* 1515-1559]

COLOMBO, Michele [*d.* 1600] *ed. See* Mercuriale, G. Consultationes. [1604-20], 1624-25 [and] De morbis muliebribus. 1601, 1618 [and] Tractatus: De compositione medicamentorum. 1601.

—, *tr. See* VALVERDE, J. de. Anatome corporis humani. 1589 [colophon 1607]

COLOMBO, REALDO [*ca.* 1515–1559] [De re anatomica libri XV. German.] Anatomia; das ist, Sinnreiche, künstliche, begründte Auffschneidung, Theilung, unnd Zerlegung eines vollkommenen menschlichen Leibs und Cörpers . . . Erstlichen . . . in Latein begriffen . . . anjetzo aber . . . vermehrt, zumal in die teutsche . . . Spraach ubersetzt. Mit angefügter analogischer Zugaab darinn Sceleta bruta, oder Beschreibung . . . der Bein Cörper underschiedlicher Thier begriffen . . . durch Johannem Andream Schenckium . . . Franckfort am Mayn, Gedruckt durch Matthiam Becker, in Verlegung Theodori de Bry seligen Wittib, sampt zweyer Söhnen, 1609.

[7], 274 (i.e. 294) p. illus., table 32 cm.

[**2617**]

Anatomia and Sceleta bruta have special title pages dated 1608.

—*See* Sánchez, F. Opera medica. 1636.

COLOMESIUS, PÀULUS. *See* COLOMIÈS, Paul [1638–1692]

COLOMIÈS, PAUL [1638–1692] *See* VOSSIUS, I. Observationum ad Pomp. Melam appendix. 1686.

COLONNA, EGIDIO [1247?–1316] De humani corporis formatione . . . Nova hac impressione repurgatum ac multo magis illustratum per . . . Angelum Vancium . . . Arimini, Apud Jo. Symbenium, 1626.

[8], 166, [2] p. 21 cm. [**2618**]

COLONNA, FABIO [1567–1650] Minus cognitarum rariorumque nostro coelo orientium stirpium εκφρασις . . . Item de aquatilibus aliisque nonnullis animalibus libellus . . . Romae, Apud Jacobum Mascardum, 1616.

[8], 340 p.; [12], 99 p.; lxxiii, [7] p. illus., port. 23 cm. [**2619**]

Engraved title page.

Part 2 has special engraved title page. Part [3] has caption title: Aquatilium, et terrestrium aliquot animalium, aliaquarumque naturalium rerum observationes.

With this is bound (between part 1 and 2) *his* Purpura. 1616.

—Purpura; hoc est, De purpura ab animali testaceo fusa, de hoc ipso animali, aliisque rarioribus testaceis . . . Romae, Apud Jacobum Mascardum, 1616.

[8], 42 p. illus. 23 cm. [**2620**]

Engraved title page.

"De glossopetris dissertatio": p. 31–39.

Bound (between part 1 and 2) with *his* Minus cognitarum rariorumque nostro coelo orientium stirpium εκφρασις. 1616.

—*See* HERNÁNDEZ, F. Rerum medicarum Novae Hispaniae thesaurus. 1628, 1651; RAY, J. Stirpium Europaearum extra Britannias nascentium sylloge. 1694.

COLSON, LANCELOT [*fl.* 1660–1676] Philosophia maturata: an exact piece of philosophy, containing the practick and operative part thereof in gaining the philosophers stone . . . Whereunto is added, a work compiled by St. Dunstan, concerning the philosophers stone, and the experiments of Rumelius and preparations of Angelo Sala . . . London, G. Sawbridge, 1668.

[10], 142 p. 13 cm. [**2621**]

COLTELLINI, AGOSTINO [1613–1693] *See* RECTORIUS, L. De lapidis renum, ac vesicae affectus curatione. 1666.

COLTON, THOMAS. *See* COULTON, Thomas [*d.* 1731]

COLUMBA, GERARDO [16th–17th cent.] Disputationum medicarum de febris pestilentis cognitione et curatione, libri duo . . . Nunc primum . . . castigati, & . . . in Germania editi . . . Accessit tractatus singularis Nicolai Macchelli . . . De morbo Gallico, ejusque curatione. Francofurti, Apud heredes Romani Beati, Georgium Beatum & Joannem Ludovicum Bitschium, 1601.

[21], 278, [17] p.; 61, [7] p. 19 cm. [**2622**]

Part [2] has special title page.

—, *ed. See* MACCHELLI, N. Tractatus methodicus. 1608.

COLUMBANI, ANFONSO. *See* CRISTINI, B., ed. Pratica medicinale. 1680–1681.

COLUMBUS, MATTHAEUS REALDUS. *See* COLOMBO, Realdo [*ca.* 1515–1559]

COLUMBUS, MICHAEL. *See* COLOMBO, Michele [d. 1600]

COLUMELLA, LUCIUS JUNIUS MODERATUS. Agricultur; oder, Ackerbaw. Der beyden hocherfahrnen und weitberühmbten Römer, L. Columellae

& Palladii. Worinnen aussführlich gehandelt wird von allerley Feldtbaw, an Getreidig, Wein, und sonsten allerley Früchten und Kräutern ... Item: wie man allerley Leibes Beschwerung ... curiren sol, beneben einem aussführlichen Bericht von Praeservirung, und Cur der Pest, durch ... A. Pedemontanum vormahls in welscher Sprach publiciret.Frommen Haussvätern und Haussmüttern, zu sonderlicher Nachrichtung auss lateinischer Sprach ... verdeutschet, auch mit neuen Additionen und nothwendigen Bericht vom Urin, und Serti Platonicis Artzneybuch, von Vogeln ... Thieren vermehret, durch Theodorum Majum ... Magdeburgk, Bey Johan Francken, 1612.

      I v. illus. 32 cm.   [2623]

     Various pagings.
     Colophon: Magdeburgk, Gedruckt bey Mertin Rauschern, in Verlegung Johan Francken, 1612.
     Imperfect: p. 97-98 and p. 107-108 of part [1] wanting; p. 149-150 of part [3] mutilated.
     Part [3] has caption title: Nützlich Artzney Buch, des ... Alexii Pedemontani [pseud.? i.e. Girolamo Ruscelli?] nach allerhandt Leibes Kranckheiten ... zu curiren ... In Deutsch gebracht ... durch Johannem Jacobum Weckerum ... Part [4] has caption title: Urin Büchlin ... Sampt einem nützlichen Tractätlin, vom Urin und Pulss des ... Herrn Apollinaris [pseud. i.e. Walther Hermann Ryff] sehr Nützlich zu lesen. Jetzo auffs new beschrieben ... durch Theodorum Majum.

COLUMNA, AEGIDIUS DE. *See* COLONNA, Egidio [1247?-1316]

COLUTIUS, FRANCISCUS. *See* COLUZIO, Francesco [*fl.* 1619]

COLUTIUS, PHILANDER [*fl.* 1621] *ed. See* CLETI, E. Dilucidatio in Aphor. 22. primae sect. pro defensione interpretationis Marsilii Cagnati. 1621.

COLUZIO, FRANCESCO [*fl.* 1619] De querelis nephriticis ex renum calculo, libri tres. In quorum tertio tractatur de aqua Tyberina calculum generante, nova methodo, prout sequens pagina demonstrabit. Romae, Apud Bartholomaeum Zannettum, 1619.

      [16], 339, [42] p. 16 cm.   [2624]

     — [The same.] ... In quatuor libros divisus, ac Romanis praelectionibus locupletatus ... Romae, Typis Alexandri Zannetti, 1624.

      [12], 321, [27] p. 23 cm.   [2625]

[**COMBACH**, LUDWIG, 1590-1657] *ed.* and *tr.* Tractatus aliquot chemici singulares summum philoso-

phorum arcanum continentes. 1. Liber de principiis naturae, & artis chemicae, incerti authoris. 2. Johannis Belye ... tractatulus novus, & alius Bernhardi Comitis Trevirensis, ex Gallico versus. Cum fragmentis Eduardi Kellaei, H. Aquilae Thuringi, & Joh. Isaaci Hollandi. 3. Fratris Ferrarii tractatus integer, hactenus fere suppressus, & in principio & fine plus quam dimidia parte mutilatus. 4. Johannis Daustenii Angli Rosarium. Opuscula partim nondum in lucem producta ... Geismariae, Typis Salomonis Schadewitz, Sumptibus Sebaldi Köhlers, 1647.

      15, [1], 56 p.; 38 p.; 84 p.; 110 p. 16 cm.
                                      [2626]

     Each part has special title page.
     "Visio ejusdem Johannis Daustenii ...": p. 101-110.

     —, *tr. See* HESTEAU, C., *sieur de Nuisement.* Tractatus de vero sale secreto philosophorum. 1671; SALA, A. Tractatus duo. 1649.

     —*See* SALA, A. Opera omnia medico chymica. 1682.

COMBE, JEAN DE. Hydrologie; ou, Discours des eaux; contenant les moyens de cognoistre parfaitement les qualités des fontaines chaudes, tant ocultes que manifestes, & l'adresse d'en user avec methode, & particulierement de celles de Greaux ... Aix, Estienne David, 1645.

      [16], 420 p. 18 cm.   [2627]

COMENTZIUS, JOHANNES JACOBUS [*fl.* 1646] *respondent. See* SEBISCH, M. [1578-1674?] *praeses.* Galeni quinque priores libri. 1651.

The **COMFORTS** of divine love. 1700. *See* GILPIN, R.

COMI, PIETRO [*fl.* 1692] *ed. See* RAGAZZINA, F. F. La medicina posta all'essame nel tribunale della verità. 1693.

COMIERS, CLAUDE [*d.* 1693] La medecine universelle; ou, L'art de se conserver en santé, & de prolonger sa vie ... Paris, et se vend a Bruxelles, chez Jean Leonard, 1687.

      [4], 44 p. 15 cm.   [2628]

     —[The same.] ... Nouv. ed. augm. d'une Réponse du même auteur aux reflexions & doutes d'un anonime, sur l'âge de quatre cens ans de Louis Galdo ... Bruxelles, Jean Leonard, 1688.

      71 p. 14 cm.   [2629]

COMITIBUS, Ludovicus. *See* Conti, Lodovico [17th cent.]

COMMELIN, Caspar [1667–1731] *See* Commelin, J. Horti medici Amstelodamensis. 1697–1701.

COMMELIN, Johannes [1629–1692] Horti medici Amstelodamensis rariorum tam Orientalis, quam Occidentalis Indiae, aliarumque peregrinarum plantarum magno studio ac labore, sumptibus civitatis Amstelodamensis, longa annorum serie collectarum, descriptio et icones ad vivum aeri incisae ... Opus posthumum. Latinitate donatum ... a Frederico Ruyschio ... & Francisco Kiggelario ... Amstelodami, Apud P. & J. Blaeu, nec non Abrahamum a Someren, 1697–1701.

    2 v. plates. 41 cm.   **[2630]**
  Each volume has added engraved title page, and added title page in Dutch: Beschryvinge en curieuse afbeeldingen van rare vreemde ... gewassen vertoont in den Amsterdamsche Kruyd-hof.
  In Latin and Dutch.

  —See Ray, J. Stirpium Europaearum extra Britannias nascentium sylloge. 1694.

COMMENTARII Collegii Conimbricensis, e Societate Jesu, in duos libros De generatione & corruptione, Aristotelis. 1616. *See* Universidade de Coimbra. Collegium Conimbricense Societatis Jesu.

COMMENTARII Collegii Conimbricensis Societatis Jesu, in tres libros De anima Aristotelis. 1606. *See* Universidade de Coimbra. Collegium Conimbricense Societatis Jesu.

COMMENTARIORUM alchymiae ... pars prima. *See* Libavius, A. [*d.* 1616] Alchymia. 1606.

COMMENTATIO de pharmaco catholico. *See* [Monte-Snyder, J. de]; Reconditorium ac reclusorium opulentiae sapientiaeque numinis mundi magni. 1666.

COMMERSTEIN, Johannes [*fl.* 1645] *respondent.* Disputatio medica inauguralis de epilepsia ... Lugduni Batavorum, Apud Philippum de Croï, 1645.

    [14] p. 22 cm.   **[2631]**
  Diss. — Leyden.

COMMIERS, Claude. *See* Comiers, Claude [d. 1693]

COMMISSION for Sick and Wounded. *See* Gt. Brit. Admiralty. Commission for Sick and Wounded.

A COMMISSION with instructions and directions, granted by his Maiestie. 1618. *See* Gt. Brit. Sovereign [1603–1625] (James I)

COMMUNICATION einer vortrefflichen chymischen Medicin, Krafft welcher nechst Gott und guter Diät der berühmte venetianische Edelmann Fridericus Gualdus, sein Leben auff 400, Jahr zu diesen unsern Zeiten conservirt, und kürtzlich noch Anno 1668. zu Venedig zu sehen gewesen, aus ... englisch- und italiänischen Manuscripts ... in die deutsche Sprache übersetzet ... Augsburg, In die Leipziger Jubilate-Mess an Lorentz Kroniger und Göbels Erben, 1700.

    [58], 297 p. front. (port.) 13 cm.   **[2632]**
  Imperfect: p. 95–96 wanting. Error in printing: pages 194–215 (sheet i) wrongly imposed.
  "Beantwortung eines Anonymi Anmerckungen und Zweiffels-Einwürffen über das Alter des vierhundert-jährigen Friderici Gualdi": p. [1]–94; "Die durch Artzneyen vermehrte Schwachheiten der Natur, von einem ... Engelländer entdecket, welcher auch dafür hält, dass nicht so viel Leute stürben wann man weniger Artzneyen gebrauchte": p. [97]–297. Items have half title pages.
  Colonia 1694 edition published under title: La critica della morte.

COMMUNICATION des Sympathetischen-Steins. 1700. *See* Lienbeck, H.

COMPANY of Parish Clerks of London. *See* London. Company of Parish Clerks.

COMPÉRAT, B. *See* Gourmelen, É. Les oeuvres chirurgicales. 1647.

The COMPLEAT cook. *See* The queens closet opened. 1658, 1675, 1683.

The **COMPLEAT** midwife's practice enlarged, in the most weighty and high concernments of the birth of man ... From the experience of ... Sir Theodore Mayern, Dr. Chamberlain, Mr. Nich. Culpeper ... With instructions of the Queen of France's midwife [i.e. Louise (Bourgeois) Boursier] ... The 3d ed. enl., with the addition of Sir Theodore Mayern's Rare secrets in midwifry, with the approbation of ... R.C. J.D. M.S. T.B. W.C. M.H. ... [London] Nath. Brook, 1663.

    [21], 321, [22] p. plates. 17 cm.   **[2633]**
  "Rare secrets brought to light. Which for many years were locked up in the brest of ... Sir Theodore Mayern ..." (p. [277]–321) has special title page.

  —[The same.] ... The 5th ed. corr., and much enl., by J[ohn] P[echey] ... London, R. Bentley, H. Rhodes, J. Philips, and J. Taylor, 1697.

[16], 351, [1] p.   plates.   18 cm.   **[2634]**

—[The same.] ... The 5th ed. corr., and much enl., by John Pechey ... London, H. Rhodes, J. Philips, J. Taylor, K. Bentley, 1698.

[16], 351, [1] p.   plates.   18 cm.   **[2635]**

Imperfect: p. 75-6 wanting; p. 351-[352] mutilated.

A reissue of the 1697 edition with new title page.

The **COMPLEAT** servant-maid; or, The young maidens tutor. Directing them how they may fit, and qualifie themselves for any of these employments ... Wherennto [sic] is added a Supplement containing the choicest receipts, and rarest secrets in physick and chyrurgery ... 3d ed. corr. and amended. London, T. Passinger, 1683.

178, [2] p.   15 cm.   **[2636]**

Imperfect: added engraved title page, or sig. A2 wanting; p. 23-6, 47-8, 121-2 wanting.

Sometimes attributed to Hannah Woolley.

Bound with Beauties treasury. London, 1705.

The **COMPLETE** jockey. See MARKHAM, G. Markham's master-piece revived. 1694 [i.e. 1695]

Le **COMTE** de Gabalis. 1675? See VILLARS, N. P. H. de Montefaucon.

The **CONCLAVE** of physicians. 1684. See [CAPOA, L. di]

CONDE, JOANNES BAPTISTA DE [d. 1653] See HIPPOCRATES. [Adaptations, etc. Latin.] Aphorismi. 1647, 1669.

CONDE, PEDRO GARCIA. See GARCÍA CONDE, Pedro [fl. 1681-1685]

CONDEESYANUS, HERMANNUS, pseud. See GRASSHOFF, Johann [d. 1623]

CONDESERVE. See TOLEDO, Gondisalvus [fl. 1496-1508]

CONERDING, CHRISTIAN ARNOLD [fl. 1671] respondent. See MEIBOM, H., praeses. Exercitatio medica de chylificatione. 1671.

CONERDING, HERMANN [fl. 1616] See GOLDAST, M. Paradoxon de honore medicorum. 1620.

CONERDING, HERMANN [fl. 1639-1642] respondent. See CONRING, H., praeses. Disputatio medica de epilepsia. 1642 [and] Disputatio philosophica ac medica de aquis. 1680.

La **CONFERENCE** et entreveuë d'Hippocrate et de Democrite. 1632. See HIPPOCRATES. Epistolae.

CONFERENCES DU BUREAU D'ADRESSE, Paris. A question. Why dead bodies bleed in the presence of their murtherers. Being one of those questions handled in the weekly conferences of Monsieur Renaudots Bureau d'Addresses, at Paris. Translated into English ... London, Printed by R[ichard] B[ishop] for Jasper Emery, 1640.

[1], 10 p.   19 cm.   **[2637]**

Signatures: C$^{1-4}$, C$^{1-2}$.

At head of title: Numb. 5.

STC 20884.

CONGREGATIONE SACRORUM RITUUM ... Beatificationis, & canonizationis ... Turibii Alphonsi Mogrobesii. 1675. See CATHOLIC CHURCH. Congregatio Sacrorum Rituum.

CONGRESSO MEDICO ROMANO. Catalogo del Congresso Medico Romano, ove sono descritti i nomi degli autori, e le materie da loro trattate ogni lunedi. Dal 10. giorno di marzo 1681. sino all' 8. di giugno 1682 ... Roma, Felice Cesaretti, 1682.

16 p.   21 cm.   **[2638]**

With this is bound its Congressus Medico-Romanus habitus in aedibus D. Hieronymi Brasavoli. 1682.

—Congressus Medico-Romanus habitus in aedibus D. Hieronymi Brasavoli die lunae 21. septembris 1682. Romae, Ex typographia Christophori Dragondelli, 1682.

47 p.   21 cm.   **[2639]**

Bound with its Catalogo del Congresso Medico Romano. 1682.

CONINCK, GUILJELMUS [fl. 1676] respondent. Disputatio medica inauguralis de palpitatione cordis ... Lugduni Batavorum, Apud viduam & haeredes Johannis Elsevirii, 1676.

[8] p.   22 cm.   **[2640]**

Diss. — Leyden.

CONNOR, BERNARD [1666?-1698] Evangelium medici; seu, Medicina mystica; de suspensis naturae legibus, sive de miraculis; reliquisque ἐν τοις βιβλίος memoratis, quae medicae indagini subjici possunt ... Londini, Sumptibus Richardi Wellinton, Henrici Nelme & Samuelis Briscoe, 1697.

1 v.   18 cm.   **[2641]**

Various pagings.

Includes with separate pagination a series of epistles: De secretione animali. — Novum oeconomiae animalis exemplar. — Nova tabula oeconomiae animalis.

— [The same.] . . . Amstelaedami, Apud Joannem Wolters, 1699.

[16], 193, [10] p. 17 cm.   [2642]

". . . Tentamen suum epistolare de secretione animali . . .": p. 157–176; ". . . Novum suum oeconomiae animalis exemplar exhibet": p. 181–184; "Nova tabula oeconomia animalis . . .": p. 185–193.

— The history of Poland, in several letters to persons of quality . . . With several letters relating to physick . . . Publish'd by the care and assistance of Mr. Savage. London, Printed by J. D. for Dan. Brown, A. Roper [and T. Leigh] 1698.

2 v. front. (ports.), plates. 20 cm.   [2643]

— A treatise of muscular dissection. *In* Browne, J. Myographia nova. 1698.

— Ζωōθανāσιον θαυμαστόν; seu, Mirabilis viventium interitus in Charonea Neapolitana crypta. Dissertatio physica . . . Coloniae Agrippinae, Typis Laurentii Kronigger, prostant Venetiis apud Jo. Jacobum Hertz, 1694.

68 p. illus. 13 cm.   [2644]

"Novissiumum Vesuvii montis incendium . . ." p. [49]–66.
Imperfect: upper margin of title page trimmed.

CONRAD, HEINRICH FRIEDRICH [*fl.* 1686] *respondent. See* CRAUSE, R. W., *praeses.* Disputatio inauguralis, sistens theses medico chimicas de principiis & transmutatione metallorum. 1686.

CONRAD, ISRAEL. *See* CONRADT, Israel [*fl.* 1659–1670]

CONRADI, ANDREAS PETER [*fl.* 1685–1714] *respondent. See* SCHRADER, F., *praeses.* Disputatio medica inauguralis de venae sectionis usu et abusu in febribus. 1686.

CONRADI, ELIAS [*fl.* 1662] *praeses.* Ex physicis de aere . . . Wittebergae, Ex officina Johannis Haken, 1662.

[16] p. 19 cm.   [2645]

Diss. — Wittenberg (J. C. Laurentius, *respondent*)

CONRADT, ISRAEL [*fl.* 1659–1670] Dissertatio medico-physica de frigoris natura et effectibus. [Gedani] Typis & sumptibus Monasterii Olivensis S. Ord. Cist., 1677.

[22], 204 p. 15 cm.   [2646]

Bound with Martini, H. Anteambulo medicus. 1668.

— *respondent.* Disputatio medica de febribus . . . Lugduni Batavorum, Ex officina Salomonis Wagenaer, 1659.

[24] p. 19 cm.   [2647]

Diss. — Leyden.

CONRING, HERMANN [1606–1681] De calido innato; sive, Igne animali liber unus. Helmestadii, Impensis Martini Richteri, excudit Henningus Mullerus, 1647.

[8], 263, [33] p. 20 cm.   [2648]

". . . De calido innato disputatio, publicae habita X. Novembr. M D C XXVII. Lugduni Batavorum": p. [8–33]

— De Germanicorum corporum habitus antiqui ac novi causis dissertatio. Helmestadii, Ex officina Henningi Mulleri, impensis Martini Richteri, 1645.

[124] p. 29 cm.   [2649]

— De Hermetica Aegyptiorum vetere et Paracelsicorum nova medicina liber unus. Quo simul in Hermetis Trismegisti omnia, ac universam cum Aegyptiorum tum chemicorum doctrinam animadversitur. Helmestadii, Typis Henningi Mulleri, sumptibus Martini Richteri, 1648.

[8], 404, [16] p. 19 cm.   [2650]

— De Hermetica medicina libri duo. Quorum primus agit de medicina, pariterque de omni sapientia veterum Aegyptiorum: altero non tantum Paracelsi, sed etiam chemicorum, Paracelsi laudatorum aliorumque, potissimum quidem medicina omnis, simul vero & reliqua universa doctrina examinatur. Ed. 2 . . . emend. & auct. Helmestadii, Typis & sumptibus Henningi Mulleri, 1669.

[22], 447, [63] p. 20 cm.   [2651]

"Hermanni Conringii Apologeticus adversus calumnias & insectationes Olai Borrichii": p. [419]–447.

— De morborum remediis magicis & unguento armario.

613–623 p. 21 cm. (*In* Theatrum sympatheticum auctum. Norimbergae, 1662)   [2652]

Caption title.

— De sanguinis generatione et motu naturali opus novum . . . Helmestadii, Sumtibus Jeremiae Rixneri, excudit Henningus Mullerus, 1643.

[16], 365, [5] p. 18 cm.   [2653]

Imperfect: upper margins of p. [367–370] trimmed.

—De sanguinis generatione, et motu naturali. Accedunt ejusdem, et Antonii Guntheri Billichii, De fermentatione libri duo. Lugd-Bat., Apud Franciscum Hackium, Amsterod, Apud Ludovicum Elzevirium, 1646.

[16], 626 p. 16 cm. [2654]

"Antonii Guntheri Billichii ... Anatome fermentationis Platonicae": p. [463]-546, with half title; —"Hermanni Conringii ... De fermentatione exercitationes, ad Antonii Guntheri Billichii ... Anatomen fermentationis Platonicae": p. [547]-622; —"Danielis Sennerti ad Antonii Guntheri Billichii, epistola": p. 623-626.

—Exercitatio physiologica de lacte. *In* Deusing A. De motu cordis. 1655.

—In universam artem medicam singulasque ejus partes introductio ex publicis ejus praecipue lectionibus olim concinnata nunc vero additamentis necessariis aucta continuata ad nostra tempora praecipuorum scriptorum serie. Accesserunt Johannis Rhodii, aliorumque ... consimilis argumenti commentationes. Cura ac studio Guntheri Christophori Schelhammeri ... Helmestadii, Typis & sumptibus Georg-Wolfgangi Hammii, 1687.

[26], 424, [24] p.; 153 (i.e. 163) p. 19 cm.
[2655]

Part [2] has half title page: Introductionis in artem medicam pars posterior ... It contains "Casp. Bartholini ... De studio medico inchoando, continuando, & absolvendo, pro accurato & supra vulgus futuro medico consilium breve atque extemporaneum. Hafniae olim excudebat, anno nimirum 1628. Georgius Hantzch": p. [5]-16; —"Petri Castelli ... Optimus medicus in quo conditiones perfectissimi medici exponuntur. Ad Messanensis editionis ubi 1637. prodiit exemplar": p. [17]-68; —"Joannis Antonides van der Linden Manuductio ad medicinam. Lovanii secundum edita a ... Vopisco Fortunato Plempio ... Typis Coenestenii, 1639": p. [69]-128; —"Johannis Rhodii Introductio ad medicinam paulo accuratiorem et bibliotheca medica ex manuscripto nunc primum edita": p. [129]-156. —Items have half titles.

Dissertations — Helmstedt

—*praeses*. Commentariolum in Cl. Galeni lib. XIII meth. med. de ratione curandi inflammationes cum delineatione novae methodi generalis, secundum quam omnium affectuum tam internorum quam externorum curatio feliciter absolvi potest ... Helmestadii, Excudebat Henningus Mullerus, 1663.

[2], 100 p. 18 cm. [2656]
J. M. Reinesius, *respondent.*

—De lacte exercitatio physiologica, quam ... anno M D CXLIX ... publice examinandam proponit Valentinus Henricus Voglerus. Helmestadii,

Typis Henrici Davidis Mulleri, 1678.
[31] p. 20 cm. [2657]
V. H. Vogler, *respondent.*

—De vertigine disputatio medica ... Helmestadi, Typis Henningi Mulleri, 1650.
[62] p. 19 cm. [2658]
V. H. Vogler, *respondent.*

—Disputatio de sale, nitro, et alumine ... Helmaestadii, Ex officina Jacobi Lucii, 1639.
[44] p. 19 cm. [2659]
H. Jordan, *respondent.*

—Disputatio inauguralis medica de peste ... [Helmestadii] In Typographeo Calixtino excuderunt Joh. Georg. Täger & Martinus Vogel, 1659.
[52] p. 18 cm. [2660]
T. Matthaeus, *respondent.*

—[The same.] Disputatio inauguralis medica de peste quam ... proponit Theophilus Matthaeus ... anno CIƆ IƆ C LIX. Helmestadii, Typis Henrici Davidis Mulleri, 1678.
[52] p. 20 cm. [2661]
T. Matthaeus, *respondent.*

—Disputatio medica de apoplexiae natura causis et curatione ... Helmaestadii, Ex officina Henningi Mulleri, 1640.
[32] p. 20 cm. [2662]
A. Probst, *respondent.*

—Disputatio medica de calculo renum et vesicae, quam ... ad diem Martii A. CIƆ IƆ C LVI publice examinandam proponit Andreas Behrens ... Helmestadii, Typis Henningi Mulleri, 1672.
[36] p. 20 cm. [2663]
A. Behrens, *respondent.*

—Disputatio medica de epilepsia ... Helmaestadii, Henningus Mullerus, 1642.
[39] p. 20 cm. [2664]
H. Conerding, *respondent.*

—Disputatio medica de epilepsia ... Helmestadii, Typis Henningi Mulleri, 1656.
[56] p. 19 cm. [2665]
A. W. Friese, *respondent.*

—Disputatio medica de hydrope ascite ... Helmestadii, Typis Henningi Mulleri, 1650.
[68] p. 19 cm. [2666]
J. H. Bossen, *respondent.*

—Disputatio medica de palpitatione cordis ... Helmestadii, Typis Henningi Mulleri, 1643.

    [28] p.   19 cm.   **[2667]**

    G. Huhn, *respondent.*

—Disputatio medica de paralysi ... Helmestadii, Ex officina Henningi Mulleri, 1644.

    [92] p.   20 cm.   **[2668]**

    H. Jordan, *respondent.*

—Disputatio medica de scorbuto ... quam publico examini subjicit Leonhardus Krüger ... ad d. 10 Novembr. 1638. Helmestadii, Typis Henningi Mülleri, 1671.

    [19] p.   19 cm.   **[2669]**

    L. Krüger, *respondent.*

—Disputatio medica de variolis et morbilis ... Helmaestadii, Typis Henningi Mülleri, 1641.

    [55] p.   19 cm.   **[2670]**

    H. Corbeius, *respondent.*

—Disputatio medica inauguralis de febre maligna vulgo dicta Ungarica ... Helmestadii, Typis Henningi Mulleri, 1668.

    [36] p.   20 cm.   **[2671]**

    H. K. Stisser, *respondent.*

—Disputatio medica inauguralis de haemoptysi ... Helmestadii, Typis Henrici Davidis Mulleri, 1676.

    [24] p.   19 cm.   **[2672]**

    M. Homeyer, *respondent.*

—Disputatio medica inauguralis de morbo hypochondriaco ... Helmestadii, Typis Henningi Mulleri, 1662.

    [80] p.   18 cm.   **[2673]**

    J. H. Brechtfeld, *respondent.*

—Disputatio medica inauguralis de peripneumonia ... Helmestadi, Ex officina Henningi Mulleri, 1644.

    [31] p.   19 cm.   **[2674]**

    G. Huhn, *respondent.*

—Disputatio medica inauguralis de peripneumonia ... Helmestadii, Typis Henrici Davidis Mulleri, 1676.

    [24] p.   20 cm.   **[2675]**

    J. A. Papke, *respondent.*

—Disputatio medica inauguralis de phrenitide ... Helmestadii, Ex officina Henningi Mulleri, 1645.

    [39] p.   19 cm.   **[2676]**

    H. Corbeius, *respondent.*

—Disputatio medica inauguralis de pleuritide opposita potissimum novis sententiis Johannis Baptistae ab Helmont ... Helmestadii, Typis Henningi Mulleri, 1654.

    [58] p.   19 cm.   **[2677]**

    J. Röseler, *respondent.*

—Disputatio medica inauguralis de podagra ... Helmestadii, Typis Henningi Mulleri, 1659.

    [20] p.   18 cm.   **[2678]**

    J. H. Hasselt, *respondent.*

—[The same.] Disputatio medica inauguralis de podagra quam ... publico examini subjicit Joannes Henricus Hasselt ... anno M D C LIX ... Helmestadii, Typis Henrici Davidis Mulleri, 1678.

    [22] p.   19 cm.   **[2679]**

    Diss. 1659. J. H. Hasselt, *respondent.*

—Disputatio medica inauguralis de scorbuto ... Helmestadii, Ex officina Henningi Mulleri, 1644.

    [35] p.   19 cm.   **[2680]**

    L. Giesler, *respondent.*

—Disputatio medica inauguralis de scorbuto ... Helmestadii, In typographeo Calixtino excudebant Martinus Vogel & Joh. Georg Täger, 1659.

    [28] p.   19 cm.   **[2681]**

    J. G. Behrens, *respondent.*

—Disputatio philosophica ac medica de aquis quam ... publico examini subjicit Hermannus Conerdingius ... anno M D C XXXIX ... Helmaestadii, Typis Henrici Davidis Mülleri, 1680.

    [40] p.   19 cm.   **[2682]**

    H. Conerding, *respondent.*

—Disputatio philosophica ac medica de terris ... proponit ... anno MDCXXXIIX ... Helmestadii, Typis Henrici Davidis Mülleri, 1678.

    [31] p.   19 cm.   **[2683]**

    A. Probst, *respondent.*

—Disputatio physiologica de vita et morte ... Helmestadii, Ex officina Henningi Mulleri, 1645.

    [40] p.   20 cm.   **[2684]**

    H. Eberhart, *respondent.*

—Disputatio medica de inflammatione hepatis . . . Helmestadii, Typis Henningi Mulleri, 1656.

[36] p. 18 cm.   [2685]

W. Berckelman, *respondent.*

—Disquisitionem de venae sectione . . . publice examinandam proponet Johan Garmers . . . Helmestadii, Typis Henningi Mulleri, 1651.

[48] p. 19 cm.   [2686]

J. Garmers, *respondent.*

—Dissertationem inauguralem de diabete . . . proponet . . . Augustus Quirin. Rivinus . . . Helmestadii, Typis Henrici Davidis Mulleri [1676]

[16] p. 20 cm.   [2687]

A. Q. Rivinus, *respondent.*

—Exercitatio philologico-medica, de incubatione in fanis deorum medicinae causa olim facta . . . Helmestadii, Typis Henningi Mulleri, 1659.

[40] p. 21 cm.   [2688]

H. Meibom, *respondent.*

—, *ed. See* CAPELLUTI, R. Tractatus. 1642; FEYENS, T. Thomae Fieni . . . Libri chirurgici XII. 1649 [and] Zwölff Bücher von der Wund-Arzney-Kunst. 1675; SALMUTH, P. Observationum medicarum centuriae tres posthumae. 1648.

—*See* JORDAN, H. De eo quod divinum aut supernaturale est in morbis humani corporis. 1651.

—*as subject. See* BORCH, O. Hermetis, Aegyptiorum, et chemicorum sapientia. 1674.

CONSENTINUS, THOMAS CORNELIUS. *See* CORNELIO, Tommaso [1614-1686]

CONSIDERATIEN en motiven dienende ter decisie ter ende ten voordeele van Dr. Joh. Baptista van Lamzweerde. 1677. *See* LAMSWEERDE, J. B. van.

CONSILIUM conjugii; seu, De massa solis & lunae . . .

429-507 p., vol. 5. 20 cm. (*In* Zetzner, Lazarus, *ed.* Theatrum chemicum. Argentorati, 1659-61)   [2689]

CONSILIUM contra diarrhoeam. *See* POTIER, P. Insignes curationes. 1625.

CONSTANT, JACQUES. *See* CONSTANT DE REBEQUE, Jacob de [1635-1730]

CONSTANT, PIERRE [*fl. ca.* 1626] *ed.* and *tr. See* RIOLAN, J. [1580-1657] Les oeuvres anatomiques. 1628-29.

CONSTANT DE REBECQUE, JACOB DE [1635-1730] L'apoticaire françois charitable, qui donne une parfaite connoissance de la matiere medecinale, de toutes les operations de pharmacie, tant Galenique que chymique, & des formules des medicaments tant internes qu'externes . . . Lyon, Jean Certe, 1683.

[14], 543 p. 19 cm.   [2690]

—Le chirurgien charitable comprenant le droit usage des principales operations & des principaux remedes de chirurgie. Et le moyen de s'en servir dans la cure particuliere des maladies exterieures du corps humain, comme tumeurs, playes, ulceres, fractures & dislocations . . . Geneve, Jean Herman Widerhold, 1673.

[8], 200, [1] p. 17 cm.   [2691]

Published also as part [3] of La medecine domestique. Geneve, 1673.

With this is bound Beynon, E. Suitte du Samaritain charitable. 1673.

—[The same.] Le chirurgien françois charitable. Comprenant le droit usage des principales operations & des principaux remedes de chirurgie, et le moyen de s'en servir dans la cure particuliere des maladies exterieures du corps humain . . . Lyon, Jean Certe, 1683.

[18], 339, [1] p. 18 cm.   [2692]

—Le medecin charitable, dans lequel par forme d'indice alphabetique . . . sont contenues les reigles & maximes . . . du gouvernement de la santé, et la curation des maladies . . . du corps humain . . .

35 p., part [4] 18 cm. (*In* La medecine domestique. Geneve, Jean Herman Widerhold, 1673)   [2693]

An index for Le gouvernement de la santé, L'apothiquaire charitable and Le chirurgien charitable.

—Le medecin françois charitable. Qui donne les signes & la curation des maladies internes qui attaquent le corps humain. Avec un Traité de la peste . . . Lyon, Jean Certe, 1683.

[16], 620 p. 18 cm.   [2694]

—Medicinae Helvetiorum prodromus; sive, Pharmacopoeae Helvetiorum specimen. Genevae, Typis Antonius Emery, 1677.

[29], 212 p. 15 cm.   [2695]

—[The same.] Atrium medicinae Helvetiorum, seu eorundem pharmacopoeae promptuarium; Observationesque medicae rarissimae ac selectissimae ... Genevae, Apud Samuelem de Tournes, 1690.

[47], 346 p.; 205, [23] p. illus. 15 cm. **[2696]**

Part [2] has special title page.

—, tr. See LÉMERY, N. Cursus chymicus. 1681.

CONSTANTIN, ANTOINE [d. 1616] Opus medicae prognoseos, in quo omnium quae possunt in aegris animadverti symptomatum in omnibus morbis, causae & eventus copiose & luculenter exponuntur. Omnia a Galeno, Hollerio, Dureto & Jacotio, fidelissimis summi Hippocratis interpretibus deprompta; & ... digesta ... Lugduni, Apud Claudium Morillon, 1613.

[16], 358, [40] p. 18 cm. **[2697]**

CONSTANTIN, ROBERT [ca. 1530-1605] ed. See SCALIGER, J. C. In librum De insomniis Hippocratis commentarius auctus nunc & recognitus. 1659.

—See CELSUS, A. C. De medicina libri octo. 1687; THEOPHRASTUS. De historia plantarum libri decem, Graece & Latine. 1644.

CONSTANTINOPOLITANUS, MANLIUS. See MANLIUS, Arnold [d. 1607]

CONSTITUTIONES, et decreta sex provincialium synodorum Mediolanensium. 1603. See CATHOLIC CHURCH. Province of Milan.

CONSTITUTIONES ... Regii Protomedicatus officii ... Siciliae Regni. See SICILY, Protomedico. Constitutiones. 1657.

CONSULTA de medici per preservarsi da mali correnti nella città di Napoli fatta per ordine di quei Deputati per la sanità, e ristampata in Roma. [Napoli, Egidio Longo, 1656. Roma, Nella stamperia della Rev. Cam. Apost. 1656]

[4] p. 27 cm. **[2698]**

Caption title.

CONTALGENI, OSTILIO, pseud. See COLTELLINI, Agostino [1613-1693]

CONTANT, JACQUES [fl. 1570] Les oeuvres de Jacques et Paul Contant pere et fils ... Divisées en cinq traictez. I. Les commentaires sur Dioscoride.

2. Le second Eden. 3. Exagoge mirabilium naturae e Gazophylacio. 4. Synopsis plantarum cum ethymologiis. 5. Le jardin & cabinet poëtique ... Poictiers, Julian Thoreau, & la vefue d'Antoine Mesnier, 1628.

4 parts in 1 v. illus., plates. 35 cm. **[2699]**

Parts [1-2] and [4] have engraved special title pages.

Pritzel 1850.

CONTANT, PAUL [ca. 1570-1632] See CONTANT, J. Les oeuvres. 1628.

CONTARENUS, GASPARUS. See CONTARINI, Gasparo, Cardinal [1484-1542]

CONTARINI, GASPARO, Cardinal [1484-1542] De elementis eorumque mixtionibus. Lib. V. Ed. 5 ... Lugduni Batavorum, Ex officina Justi Livii, 1633.

[16], 264 p. illus. 13 cm. **[2700]**

With this is bound Hermann, D. Manuale anatomicum. 1630.

CONTE, HEINRICH JAKOB [fl. 1693] respondent. Disputatio medica inauguralis de hydrope in genere ... Duisburgi ad Rhenum, Apud Franconem Sas, 1693.

44 p. 20 cm. **[2701]**

Diss. — Duisburg.

CONTI, LODOVICO [17th cent.] Clara fidelisque admonitoria disceptatio practicae manualis experimento veraciter comprobata. De duobus artis, & naturae miraculis: hoc est de liquore alchaest; nec non lapide philosophico, atque amborum materia, operandi ratione ... de sale quoque Tartari volatili ... Auctore Ludovico de Comitibus ... Francofurti, Apud Hermannum a Sande, 1664.

[20], 116 p. front. 15 cm. **[2702]**

Added engraved title page.

—[French tr.] Discours philosophiques sur les deux merveilles de l'art et de la nature, ou traité de la liqueur de l'alchaest, & de la medecine universelle ... Et de la voye qu'il faut tenir pour faire le sel de tartre volatil. Composez en latin, par Monsieur Des Comtes ... et mis en françois, par Robert Preud'homme ... 2. ed., rev. corr. Paris, Jean d'Houry, 1678.

195, [9] p. 16 cm. **[2703]**

CONTI, LUIGI DE. See CONTI, Lodovico [17th cent.]

CONTOLI, Giovanni Battista [*fl.* 1697-1702] Breve instruzione medica sopra il glutine, ò colla, che si genera ne' corpi umani, e suoi effetti di pietra, e gotta. Esaminati per la cura dell'una, e dell' altra . . . Roma, Il Bernabò, 1697.

[10], 19 p.   plate.   22 cm.   [**2704**]

—De lapidibus podagra, et chiragra in humano corpore productis . . . Auctore Jo. Baptista Contulo . . . Romae, Bernabò, 1699.

[8], 123 p.; [16] p.; 28 p.   illus., plates.   26 cm.
[**2705**]

Part [2] has half title: Auctoris epistolae ad amicos, containing 4 letters dated 1701-2.

Part [3] has caption title: Breve instruzione sopra il glutine, ò colla, che si genera ne' corpi umani, e suoi effetti di pietra, e gotta.

CONTROVERSIA medica. 1652? *See* [Valverde de Horozco, D. de]

CONTULO, Giovambattista. *See* Contoli, Giovanni Battista [*fl.* 1697-1702]

CONVENTIONI fra Collegio de'medici et Compagnia delli speciali medicinalisti di Bologna. *See* Università di Bologna. Collegio de medicina. Conventioni fra l'accelentiss. Collegio de medici. 1606.

CONYGIUS, Antimus, *pseud. See* Fabri, Honoré [1606-1688]

COOK, James. *See* Cooke, James [1614-1694?]

COOKE, James [1614-1694?] Mellificium chirurgiae; or, The marrow of many good authours, wherein is briefly and faithfully handled the art of chyrurgery, in its foure parts, with all the severall diseases unto them belonging . . . As also an appendix, wherein is methodically set down, the cure of these affects usually happening at sea, and in campe . . . And lastly, an addition of severall magistrall receipts . . . London, Samuel Cartwright, 1648.

[23], 478 (i.e. 454) p.   15 cm.   [**2706**]

—[The same.] . . . To which is added new Institutions, physical and chirurgical; Hyppocrates Aphorismes . . . at the end of which you have several approved receipts . . . London, Printed by T. R. for John Sherley, 1662.

[35], 351, 509 p.   15 cm.   [**2707**]

—[The same.] . . . To which is now added Anatomy, illustrated with twelve brass cuts, and also The marrow of physick: both in the newest way . . .

London, Printed by J. D. for Benj. Shirley, 1676.
[38], 872 (i.e. 864) p.   front. (port.), plates.   18 cm.   [**2708**]

Imperfect: port. wanting.
"Institutions": p. 1-84.
"Hippocrates; his Aphorisms, in classical order with com.": p. 85-175.

—[The same.] . . . An anatomical treatise. Institutions of physick, with Hippocrates's Aphorisms largely commented upon. The marrow of physick, shewing the causes, signs and cures of most diseases incident to humane bodies. Choice experienced receits for the cure of several distempers. The 4th ed., enl. with many additions, and purged from many faults that escaped in the former impressions. Illustrated in its several parts with twelve brass cuts . . . London, Printed by T. Hodgkin, for William Marshall, 1685.

[16], 616 (i.e. 608), [11] p.   front. (port.), plates.
20 cm.   [**2709**]

Imperfect: port. wanting.

—[The same.] . . . With the anatomy of human bodies according to the most modern anatomists; illustrated with many anatomical observations. Institutions of physick, with Hippocrates's Aphorisms largely commented upon. The marrow of physick, shewing the causes, signs and cures of most diseases incident to human bodies. Choice experienced receits for the cure of several distempers. The 4th ed., enl., with many additions . . . Rev., corr. and purged from many faults that escaped in the former editions . . . by Tho. Gibson . . . London, W. Marshall, 1693.

[16], 616 (i.e. 608), [11] p.   front. (port.), plates.
20 cm.   [**2710**]

Imperfect: plate facing p. 165 wanting.
Reissue of the 1685 edition. The title page and final leaf are cancels.

—Supplementum chirurgiae; or, The supplement to The marrow of chyrurgerie. Wherein is contained fevers, simple and componnd [sic], pestilential, and not, rickets, small pox and measles, with their definitions, causes, signes, prognosticks, and cures . . . As also The military chest, containing all necessary medicaments, fit for sea, or land-service . . . London, John Sherley, 1655.

[10], 431 p.   15 cm.   [**2711**]

—, *tr. See* Hall, J. Select observations on English bodies. 1657, 1679, 1683.

COOPER, ROBERT [*d.* 1733] *See* [WALKER, O.] Propositions concerning optic-glasses. 1679.

COOPER, WILLIAM [1666-1709] *See* COWPER, William [1666-1709]

COOPER, William [*fl.* 1669-1689] A catalogue of chymicall books. In three parts. In the first and second parts are contained such chymical books as have been written originally, or translated into English: with a large account of their titles, several editions and volumes. Likewise in the third part is contained a collection of such things published in the Philosophical transactions of the Royal Society (for ten years together) as pertain to chymistry, or the study of nature by art in the animal, vegetal, and mineral kingdoms ... London, 1675-88.

    [139] p.   17 cm.   **[2712]**

   "The continuation or appendix to the second part of The catalogue of chymical books, printed with The philosophical epitaph, being either corrections, rectifications, or additions to the editions of the old books; and a continuation of such new books as have been printed since the year 1675. to this present year 1688": p. [67-116]

   — The philosophical epitaph of W[illiam] C[ooper] esquire, for a memento mori on his tomb-stone ... Also, A brief of the golden calf (the worlds idol) ... by Jo. Fr. Helvetius and, The golden ass well managed ... Written by Jo. Rod. Glauber. With Jehior [Aurora sapientiae,] or, The day-dawning or light of wisdom, containing the three principles or original of all things; whereby are discovered the great and many mysteries in God, nature, and the elements, hitherto hid, not revealed. All published by W[illiam] C[ooper] esquire. With A catalogue of chymical books. London, Printed by T. R. and N. T. for William Cooper, 1673-75.

    1 v.   illus., plates.   18 cm.   **[2713]**

   Various pagings.

   Signatures: A^{10}, B-O^{8}, *^{4}, P-R^{4}, A-G^{4}.

   Imperfect: added engraved title page wanting.

   Contains four treatises, each with an undated title page, and "A catalogue of chemical books. In three parts ... collected by Will. Cooper" with special title page dated 1675.

   —, *tr. See* HELVETIUS, J. F. The golden calf. 1670.

   —*See* HOUPREGHT, J. F., *comp.* Aurifontina chymica. 1680; PAGET, N. Bibliotheca medica. 1681.

COORNHERT, CORNELIS GERARD [*fl.* 1651] *respondent.* Disputatio medica inauguralis de catharro

in genere ... Lugduni Batavorum, Ex officina Wilhelmi Christiani Boxii, 1651.

    [8] p.   22 cm.   **[2714]**

   Diss. — Leyden.

COPENHAGEN. Ordinances, local laws, etc. Catalogus & valor medicamentorum simplicium & compositorum in officinis Hafniensibus prostantium. Apotecker Taxt ... Apothecker Taxa ... Hafniae, Prostant apud Petr. Haubold, Literis Georgii Godiani, 1672.

    [32], 125, [2] p.   20 cm.   **[2715]**

   Text in Latin, Danish and German.

   "Forordning om medicis oc apotecker etc. Constitutiones regiae de medicis & pharmacopoeis &c. Königliche Verordnung angehend die Medicos und Apothecker etc." (p. [9-32]) has special title page.

COPENHAGEN. Universitet. Medicinsk Facultet. *See* UNIVERSITAS REGIA HAFNIENSIS. Facultas medica.

COPHO. *See* MESUË [924 *or* 5-1015] Opera. 1602, 1623.

COPP, GUILLAUME. *See* COPUS, Gulielmus [*ca.* 1460-1532]

COPPENOLL, ANTON à [*fl.* 1663-1667] *respondent.* Disputatio medica inauguralis de motu bilis ejusque laesione de ictero ... Lugduni Batavorum, Apud viduam & haeredes Joannis Elsevirii, 1667.

    [16] p.   24 cm.   **[2716]**

   Diss. — Leyden.

COPPER, JACOB [*fl.* 1682] *tr. See* DESCARTES, R. De verhandeling van den mensch, en de makinge van de vrugt in 's moeders lichaam. 1695.

COPPONAY DE GRIMALDY, DENIS DE [*ca.* 1623-1717] Etablissement du laboratoire de S. A. R. et de son Academie chymique avec le combat de la medecine Galenique, contre elle fait dans la sale de l'auguste senat de Savoye. Ou la chymique mal traitée par la Galenique, & sans misericorde, est contrainte, malgré elle, de se deffendre ... [Chambéry?] L'auteur, 1684.

    429 p.   15 cm.   **[2717]**

   —*See* MAUBEC, D. de, *sieur de Copponay.* Vertus et usage de la medecine universelle. Not before 1678.

COPPONAY DE MAUBEC, DENIS. *See* MAUBEC, Denys de, *sieur de Copponay.*

COPUS, GULIELMUS [*ca.* 1460-1532] *tr. See* GALENUS. [Selected works. Latin] Αιτιολογιχη χαι παθολογιχη; sive, De morborum et symptomatum differentiis, et causis, libri sex. 1624 [and] Francisci Vallesii ... Commentaria illustria, in Cl. Galeni Pergameni libros. 1645; HIPPOCRATES. [Aphorismi. Latin] 1622, 1649, 1663, 1684 [and] [Prognostica. Latin] 1611, 1674.

COPY van twee gheschriften, ghevonden binnen 's Hertoghenbosch den 17en. Septemb. anno 1629 ... Waer van den eenen is, een presartief voor gheschut, kruyt ende loot: ende tweede, een remedie teghen de pest. [n. p.] 1629.

[7] p.   19 cm.   **[2718]**

CORBEAU, ANDRÉ. *See* CORVUS, Andreas.

CORBEEL, KAREL [*fl.* 1661] *respondent.* Disputatio medica inauguralis de inflammatione ... Lugduni Batavorum, Apud Georgium vander Dorp, 1661.

[12] p.   24 cm.   **[2719]**
Diss. — Leyden.

CORBEIUS, HERMANNUS [*fl.* 1620-1646] Gynaeceium ... sive, De cognoscendis, praecavendis, curandisque praecipuis mulierum affectibus, libri duo ... Adjecta est in calce quaestio ... De vulneribus lethalibus & non lethalibus, &c. Francofurti, Sumptibus haered. D. Palthenii, 1620.

[24], 376 p.   16 cm.   **[2720]**
"De vulneribus lethalibus et sanabilibus, oratio panegyrica ... Typis Hartmanni Palthenii ...": p. [315]-376, has special title page.

—*respondent. See* CONRING, H., *praeses.* Disputatio medica de variolis et morbilis. 1641 [and] Disputatio medica inauguralis de phrenitide. 1645.

—, *ed. See* CORBEIUS, T. Enumeratio morborum. 1661.

CORBEIUS, THEODORUS [*fl.* 1603-1615] Enumeratio morborum et affectuum omnium praeter naturam, qui corpus humanum invadere solent, ex veterum Graecorum, Latinorum, Arabumque fontibus, ac recentiorum limpidissimis rivulis exhausta, & compendiosa, facili, accurata, & perspicua methodo disposita ... Opera & studio Hermanni Corbeii ... Noribergae, Sumptibus Johann. Andreae Endteri & Wolfgangi junioris haeredum, 1661.

[41], 564 p.   17 cm.   **[2721]**

—*respondent. See* ELLENBERGER, H., *praeses.* Disputatio medica, de pleuritide. 1603.

CORBERUS, HERMANNUS FRIDERICUS. *See* KÖRBER, Hermann Friedrich [*fl.* 1674-1677]

CORBISERIUS, JOANNES BERNARDINUS, *ed. See* POLVERINO, G. G. De curandis, juxta hodiernum usum, singulis humani corporis morbis. 1629, 1643.

CORBYE, ANTOINE DE. Les fleurs de chirurgie, cueillies és livres des plus excellents autheurs qui ayent escrit d'icelle, tant anciens que modernes ... Paris, Jean Gesselin, 1641.

[4], 265, [3] p.   17 cm.   **[2722]**

—[The same.] Tolose, Pierre Bosc, 1642.

[4], 265, [3] p.   18 cm.   **[2723]**
Different setting of type.

CORDEMOY, GÉRAUD DE. *See* CORDEMOY, Louis Géraud de [1626-1684]

CORDEMOY, LOUIS GÉRAUD DE [1626-1684] A discourse written to a learned frier [i.e. Gabriel Cossart] by M. Des Fourneillis [pseud., i.e. Louis Géraud de Cordemoy] shewing, that the systeme of M. Descartes, and particularly his opinion concerning brutes, does contain nothing dangerous; and that all he hath written of both, seems to have been taken out of the first chapter of Genesis. To which is annexed the systeme general of the same Cartesian philosophy. By Francis Bayle ... Englished out of French. London, Moses Pitt, 1670.

139, [3] p.   15 cm.   **[2724]**
"The general systeme of the Cartesian philosophy" has special title page (p. [63]).

—Tractatus physici duo I. De corporis et mentis distinctione. II. De loquela. Latine versi a I.***. C.***. Genevae, Apud Joannem Pictetum, 1679.

[20], 180 p.; [12], 114, [6] p.   14 cm.   **[2725]**
Translation of Le discernement du corps et de l'âme, and Discours physique de la parole.

CORDES, WICHMANN [*fl.* 1691] *respondent. See* ALBERTI, H. C. Disquisitio inauguralis medica. 1691.

CORDO, SIMON À. *See* SIMON GENUENSIS.

CORDUS, EURICIUS [1484-1535] Opera poetica quotquot exstant, antehac ab auctore, nunc vero postquam diu a multis desiderata fuere, denuo luci data cura Henrici Meibomii . . . qui & vitam Cordi praefixit. Helmaestadii, Excudebat Jacobus Lucius, sumptibus Samuelis Bremi, 1614.

[40], 531, [16] p.   17 cm.   **[2726]**

CORDUS, VALERIUS [1515-1544] Dispensatorium; sive, Pharmacorum conficiendorum ratio. Cum Petri Coudenbergii, & Matthiae Lobelii scholiis, emendationibus, & auctariis. Accessit hac editione, praeter Guilielmi Rondeletii De theriaca tractatum, emendatiorem; & Formulas selectiorum pharmacorum, quorum post Val. Cordum usus passim receptus est, auctiores; alius Fr. Dissaldei ejusdem argumenti libellus. Lugduni Batavorum, Ex officina Joannis Maire, 1627.

661, [11] p. illus. 14 cm.   **[2727]**
"Appendix ex scriptis D. Jacobi Silvii [i.e. Jacques Dubois] . . . pro instructione pharmacopolarum": p. 398-422, 456-464.
Previously published under title Pharmacorum conficiendorum ratio (1548) and Pharmacorum omnium (1592)

—[The same.] . . . Novissime alia nonnulla hactenus nondum edita calci libri adjecta sunt. Lugduni Batavorum, Ex officina Joannis Maire, 1651 [1652]

[1], 749, [15] p. illus. 15 cm.   **[2728]**
Added engraved title page, illustrated, dated: 1652.
"Venenorum eorumdemque antidotorum seu Alexipharmacorum": p. 681-688. "Francisci Joelis De generali methodo medendi, & remediis usitatioribus liber": p. 689-749.

—[Dutch ed.] Den leytsman ende onderwijser der medicijnen; oft, Ordentlijcke uytdeylinghe ende bereyding-boeck vande medicamenten. Over al degelijcr vande medicamende apothekers onder den naem van Val. Cordi Dispensatorium bekent, ontfanghen ende ghebruyckt. Met de verclaringhen van M. P. Coudenberch en van Matthias de L'Obel. Nu van nieus hersien en . . . verbetert, ende verrijckt . . . Door P. T. . . . Amsterdam, Hendrick Laurentsz, 1632.

[16], 489, [15] p. 16 cm.   **[2729]**
"Register oft ghedachtenis boecxken van dagelijcksehe apothekers wercken . . . door Matthias de L'Obel": p. 10-18. "Van de succedaneis van M. de L'Obel": p. 18-56. "Aenhanck uyt den schriften van D. Jacob Silvius [i.e. Jacques Dubois] . . . tot onderwysinghe van den apothekers": p. 456-489.

—[The same.] . . . Nu van nieuws over-sien, ende van veel fauten verbertert . . . Door P. T. . . . Rotterdam, Pieter van Waesberge, 1656.

[16], 489, [17] p. 16 cm.   **[2730]**

—See DISPENSATORIUM PHARMACORUM OMNIUM. 1666; SCHOLTZ, L. Epistolarum philosophicarum. 1610.

CORFINIUS, SIMON [*fl.* 1667-1669] *respondent. See* THOMASIUS, J. [1622-1684] *praeses.* Exercitatio philosophica de morte in undis. 1667.

CORIA, FRANCISCO NUÑEZ DE [16th cent.] *See* NUÑEZ, Francisco [16th cent.]

CORIOLANI, CRISTOFORO [*b. ca.* 1540] *See* MERCURIALE, G. De arte gymnastica. 1601, 1672.

CORNACCHINI, MARCO [*d.* 1621] Methodus in pulverem. *In* Hartmann, J. Praxis chymiatrica. 1639, 1682.

—Methodus qua omnes humani corporis affectiones ab humoribus copia, vel qualitate peccantibus genitae, tuto, cito, et jucunde curantur . . . Florentiae, Apud Petrum Cecconcellium, 1619.

[16], 92, [12] p. table. 23 cm.   **[2731]**
Dedicatory epistle dated 1620.

—[The same.] . . . Ed. corr. & auct. Florentiae, Apud Petrum Cecconcellium, 1620 [colophon 1619]

[32], 156, [15] p. tables. 21 cm.   **[2732]**

—[The same.] . . . Francofurti, Impensis Johan. Theobaldi Schönwetteri, 1628.

146, [19] p. tables. 17 cm.   **[2733]**
With this is bound Hafenreffer, S. Πανδοχείον αἰολόδερμον. 1630.

—, ed. See CORNACCHINI, T. Tabulae medicae. 1605, 1609; MERCURIALE, G. Commentarii eruditissimi, in Hippocratis Coï Prognostica 1602.

—See MYLIUS, J. D. Pharmacopoeae spagyricae. 1628.

CORNACCHINI, ORAZIO [*d.* 1608] *ed. See* CORNACCHINI, T. Tabulae medicae. 1605, 1609.

CORNACCHINI, TOMMASO [*d. ca.* 1604] Tabulae medicae. In quibus ea fere omnia, quae a principibus medicis Graecis, Arabibus, & Latinis de curationis apparatu, capitis, ac thoracis morbis, febribus, pulsibus, urinis scripta sparsim reperiuntur, methodo adeo absoluta collecta sunt . . . Opus . . . in lucem editum a Marco, & Horatio ff. Additae sunt ejusdem auctoris in tabulas plerasque adnotationes. Insertae praeterea tabulae triginta, quas in patris opere desideratas Marcus f. . . . supplevit . . . Patavii, Ex officina Petri Pauli Tozzii [typis Laurentii Pasquati] 1605.

> [12], 368 p.   tables.   37 cm.   [2734]

—[The same.] Medicina practica rationalis, et empirica, tabulis CLXII. comprehensa ... Addita sunt authoris non modo in plerasque tabulas scholia; verum etiam duo tractatus ... nempe de pulsibus, & urinis ... Opus ... a Marco ... & ab Horatio ff. prolatum e tenebris, auctumque, & limatum ... Patavii, Ex officina Petri Pauli Tozzii, Venetiis, Sumptibus Joannis Guerilii, 1609.

> [12], 368 p.   tables.   36 cm.   [2735]
>
> Colophon: Patavii, Ex officina Petri Pauli Tozzii, typis Laurentii Pasquati, 1605.
>
> A reissue with new title page of the 1605 edition.

CORNACE, MATTEO. *See* CORNAX, Mathias [*d.* 1564]

CORNAND DE LA CROSE, JEAN DE [*d. ca.* 1705] *See* MEMOIRS FOR THE INGENIOUS. 1693.

CORNANUS, CORNELIUS CERASTUS, *pseud. See* CERASTUS CORNANUS, Cornelius, *pseud.*

CORNARIUS, DIOMEDES [*ca.* 1535-1600] *See* SCHOLTZ, L. Consiliorum medicinalium ... liber singularis. 1610.

CORNARIUS, JANUS [1500-1558] *tr. See* ARISTOTELES. Aristotelis, aliorumque philosophorum, ac medicorum problemata. 1631; ARTEMIDORUS DALDIANUS. Artemidori Daldiani & Achmetis Sereimi f. Oneirocritica. 1603; CASTRO, E. R. de. Commentarius in Hippocratis Coi, libellum De alimento. 1635-39; GALENUS. De ossibus Graece & Latine. 1665; HIPPOCRATES. Aphorismi [Greek and Latin] Ἀφορισμοί. 1675? [and] Aphorismi [Latin] 1633 [and] [Collected works. Greek and Latin] Opera omnia. 1665 [and] [Collected works. Latin] Opera. 1610, 1619, 1679 [and] De locis in homine. 1638; HYGIEIA. 1628; MARTIN, J. Praelectiones in librum Hippocratis ... De aere, aquis, et locis. 1646, 1655; MILLO, G. Naturae morbos decernentis arcanum opus. 1654; PARMA, I. Praxis chirurgica. 1608; REGIMEN SANITATIS SALERNITANUM. Medicina Salernitam. 1605, 1611, 1612, 1622, 1624, 1628, 1638 [and] Schola Salernitana. 1649, 1657, 1667, 1683; SALIUS DIVERSUS, P. Commentaria in Hippocratis libros quatuor De morbis. 1602, 1612, 1646; SINAPI, M. A. Absurda vera. 1697; STEFANI, G. In Hippocratis Coi Legem commentarius. 1637 [and]

In Hippocratis Coi libellum De virginum morbis commentarius. 1635.

CORNARIUS, JEREMIAS [*fl.* 1595-1606?] Fori medici adumbratio, et ex parte quidem, quae officinarum visitationem, assistentium atque externorum, ut Hippocr. vocat, directionem maxime spectat, in synopsi facta ... Coburgi, Typis Caspari Bertschii, 1607.

> [8] p.   tables.   31 cm.   [2736]
>
> Signatures: [A²], B³. (A1 and B4 (blank?) wanting.)

CORNARO, LUIGI [1475-1566] Discorsi della vita sobria ... Ne' quali con l'essempio di se stesso dimostra con quai mezzi possa l'huomo conservarsi sano insin'al'ultima vecchiezza. Nuovamente ristampati ... Venetia, Marc'Antonio Brogiollo, 1620.

> 80 p.   17 cm.   [2737]

—[The same.] ... Milano, Gio. Battista Bidelli, 1627.

> 90 p.   17 cm.   [2738]

—[The same.] *In* Regimen sanitatis Salernitanum. Scola Salernitana. 1630, 1662, 1666, 1677.

—[Latin tr.] Tractatus de vitae sobriae commodis. *In* Lessius, L. Hygiasticon. 1613, 1623, 1688.

—[Danish tr.] Et edrue lesnets gafn oc nytte ... Af det italianske sprock udsat af en hvers tienistberede. Kiøbenhafn, Daniel Paulli, 1681.

> 64 p.   16 cm.   [2739]
>
> Translated by Thomas Bartholin.

—[Dutch tr.] Handeling van de nuttigheden van't sober leven. *In* Lessius, L. De schat der soberheit. 1681.

—[English tr.] A treatise of temperance and sobrietie. *In* Lessius, L. Hygiasticon. 1634 [and] The temperate man. 1678.

—[French tr.] Trois discours nouveaux et curieux. *In* Lessius, L. Le vray regime de vivre. 1646.

—[German tr.] Tractat von Nutzbarkeiten eines mässigen Lebens. *In* Lessius, L. Kunst lang zu leben. 1697.

CORNAX, MATHIAS [*d.* 1564] Historia gestationis foetus mortui per annos plus quatuor. In Rousset, F. Exsectio foetus vivi ex matre viva sine alterutrius vitae periculo. 1601.

—*See* Dodoens, R. Medicinalium observationum exempla rara. 1621.

CORNEJO, Alonso. *See* López Cornejo, Alonso [*fl.* 1699]

CORNEJO, Alonso López. *See* López Cornejo, Alonso [*fl.* 1699]

CORNELIANUM dolium. 1638. *See* [Randolph, T.]

CORNELIO, Tommaso [1614-1686] Progymnasmata physica ... Venetiis, Typis haeredum Fran.^ci Baba, 1663.

    [16], 192, [8] p.   illus.   23 cm.   **[2740]**
Added engraved title page.
"Leonardus a Capua lectori": p. [7-8]

—[The same.] ... His accessere ejusdem authoris opera quaedam posthuma numquam antehac edita. Neapoli, Ex typographia Jacobi Raillard, 1688.

    [16], 502 p.; [14], 119 p.   port., illus.   18 cm.
                                   [2741]
Added engraved title page.
"Leonardus a Capua lectori": p. [11-15]

CORNICE, Flavio. Il lazzaretto, overo della peste di Flavio Cornicii da Santo Gemmino ... Roma, Ignatio de' Lazari, 1657.

    [6], 118, [2] p.   16 cm.   **[2742]**

CORNICIUS, Flavio. *See* Cornice, Flavio.

CORRADE, Augustinus [*fl.* 1653] *See* Cnöffel, A. Exercitatio. 1654.

CORRADINI, Augustinus. *See* Corrade, Augustinus [*fl.* 1653]

CORRADUS, Arnoldus [*fl.* 1601] *See* [Cynthius, C.] Disputationes medicae de natura atque facultatibus ligni sancti. 1602.

CORSELLIS, James [*b. ca.* 1633] Disputatio medica inauguralis, de phthisi ... Lugduni Batavorum, Ex officina Francisci Moyaert, 1659.

    [8] p.   19 cm.   **[2743]**
Diss.—Leyden.

CORSINI, Accursio [1549-1630] Apologetico della Caccia. Ove dopò narrati i vitii da molti scrittori rimproverati alla caccia, e cacciatori, scopronsi le virtù di lei, e'l modo d'usarla per conseguir'ottimo

temperamento di complessione, quadratura di corpo, continua sanità, fortezza, ed agilita militare ... e longa vita ... Bergamo, Valerio Ventura, 1626.

    [31], 654, [2] p.   22 cm.   **[2744]**

CORT bericht, tot voor-cominge ende genesinge vande peste. 1636. *See* Utrecht. Ordinances, local laws, etc.

CORTE, Hieronymus. Summa medendi methodus, in qua de phlebotomia, medicis cucurbitulis, hirudinibus, eorumdemque recto usu accuratissime agitur ... Venetiis, Apud haeredes Joannis de Salis, 1638.

    [16], 112, [8] p.   25 cm.   **[2745]**

CORTÉS, Jerónimo [*fl.* 1600] Phisonomia y varios secretos de naturaleza. Contiene cinco tratados ... todos revistos y mejorados en esta 3. imp. ... Barcelona, Lorenço Déu, 1629.

    [4], 107, [1] ll.   16 cm.   **[2746]**

CORTESE, Isabella [16th cent.] I secreti ... ne' quali si contengono cose minerali, & medicinali, artificiose, & alchimiche, et molte dell'arte profumatoria, appartenenti a ogni gran signora. Con altri ... secreti aggiunti. Di nuovo ristampati & ... corretti ... Venetia, Nicolò Tebaldini, 1603.

    [16], 206 p.   illus.   16 cm.   **[2747]**

—[The same.] Venetia, Lucio Spineda, 1619.

    [16], 206 p.   illus.   15 cm.   **[2748]**
Different setting of type.

—[The same.] Secreti varii ... ne' quali si contengono cose minerali, medicinali, profumi, belletti, artifitii, & alchimia. Con altre belle curiosità aggiunte ... Venetia, Antonio Tivanni, 1677.

    [24], 204 p.   15 cm.   **[2749]**

CORTESI, Giovanni Battista [1553 *or* 4-1634] In universam chirurgiam absoluta institutio. In qua tumorum omnium praeter naturam, ulcerum, vulnerum, fracturarumque ossium, ac eorundem luxationum exacta cognitio, facilisque curatio habetur ... Messanae, Apud haeredes Petri Breae, 1633.

    [22], 228 (i.e. 328), [31] p.   19 cm.   **[2750]**
Imperfect: leaves after p. [22] wanting?

—Miscellaneorum medicinalium decades denae, in quibus pulcherrima ac utilissima quaeque ad anatomen, chirurgiam, et totius fere medicinae theoriam, et praxim spectantia sparsim ... continentur ... Messanae, Ex typographia Petri Breae, sumptibus Raynaldi Reinae, 1625.

[41], 833, [17] p. illus., port. 33 cm. [2751]
Engraved title page.
Decade 3 concerns the surgical methods of Gaspare Tagliacozzi.

—Tractatus de vulneribus capitis, in quo omnia, quae ad cognitionem, curationemque laesionum calvariae attinent, accurate considerantur, et singula, quae ab Hippocrate tradita sunt in libro Περι τῶν τραυμάτωμ τῆς κεφαλῆς uberrimis commentariis illustrantur ... Adjecti sunt in calce duo tractatuli: alter de contusione calvariae in pueris: alter de eorumdem hydrocephalo ... Messanae, Typis Petri Breae, 1632.

[16], 341, [28], 31, [8] p. illus. 22 cm. [2752]
Includes Greek and Latin text of Hippocrates' De capitis vulneribus.
"Species humanorum capitum": p. [9-15] (first group of paging.)

CORTHNUMMIUS, Justus. *See* Cortnumm, Justus [*ca.* 1624-1675]

CORTHUM, Joachim [*fl.* 1659] *respondent. See* Thomasius J. [1622-1684] *praeses.* De visu talparum discursus physicus. 1671.

CORTI, Matteo [1475-1542] *See* Scholtz, L. Consiliorum medicinalium ... liber singularis. 1610.

CORTIAL, Jean Joseph. *See* Courtial, Jean Joseph [*fl.* 1684-1704]

CORTILIO, Sebastiano. *See* Marquarp, J. Practica medicinalis. 1610.

CORTNUMM, Justus [*ca.* 1624-1675] De morbo attonito liber unus ad Hippocraticam sanguinis in corpore humano periodum exaratus, in quo medici vulgares e veterno exitantur, & ad accuratiorem morborum investigationem Hippocratisque lectionem adhortantur ... Lipsiae, Sumptibus Georgii Heinrici Frommanni, 1677.

[22], 406, [31] p. front. (port.) 21 cm. [2753]
Added engraved title page, illustrated.
With this is bound Tiling, M. Dissertatio medica de dysenteria. 1677.

—[The same.] Nova, utilis ac curiosa apoplexiam; seu, Morbum attonitum curandi methodus, una cum observationibus lectu dignis, quibus medici vulgares

e veterno excitabuntur. Autore J[ustus] C[onradus] M[ichaelis] D. [pseud.] Hildesiae, Apud Christianum Denhardum, 1685.

[16], 406, [31] p. 21 cm. [2754]
A reprint with new title page; p. 1-2 reset, and some preliminary matter omitted.

—*respondent.* Disputatio medica inauguralis, de morbo attonito ... Lugduni Batavorum, Apud Johannem Elsevirium, 1661.

[8] p. 19 cm. [2755]
Diss.—Leyden.

CORUM, Andrieu. *See* Corvus, Andreas.

CORVE, André. *See* Corvus, Andreas.

CORVINO, Giovanni Pietro [*fl. ca.* 1644] De diatartari electuarii temperamento, qualitatibus, usu, & dosi. dilucidatio. Messanae, Typis haered. Petri Breç, 1644.

[10], 42, [3] p. tables. 15 cm. [2756]

—De diatartari iulapii temperamento, qualitatibus, usu, & dosi enarratio. Messanae, Typis haer. Petri Breae, 1645.

14 p. 16 cm. [2757]
Bound with Castelli, P. De abusu circa dierum criticorum enumerationem. 1642.

—, *ed.* and *tr. See* Castelli, P. Breve ortographia. 1659.

CORVINUS, Joachim Andreas [*fl.* 1663] *respondent. See* Schwendendörffer, G. T., *praeses.* Pervigilium philologico juridicum medicorum anatomen jure divino-humano licitam...defendet...J. A. C. 1690.

CORVINUS, Johannes Arnoldi [*ca.* 1582-1650] Oratio in obitum ... D. Casparis Barlaei ... recitata in auditorio statim a funere 18. Januarii 1648. Amstelodami, Apud Cornelium Janssonium, 1648.

16 p. 29 cm. [2758]

—*See* Theophrastus. De historia plantarum libri decem, Graece & Latine. 1644.

CORVUS, Andreas. Chiromantia. *In* Cocles, Bartolommeo della Rocca, known as. Enseignemens de physionomie et chiromancie 1638.

CORYLI, Samuel [*fl.* 1693-*ca.* 1726] *praeses.* Disputationem physicam de corylo Jacobi, ex Genes. XXX. vers. 37, 38, 39 ... Facultatis philosophicae indultu in alma Salana publicae philosophorum disquisitioni defendendam proponent . . . praeses M. Samuel Coryli alias Nitschmann . . . & respondens Christoph. Henric. Wentzel . . . Jenae, Typis Pauli Ehrichii [1698]

22, [2] p.   20 cm.   **[2759]**

Diss.—Jena (C. H. Wentzel, *respondent*)

COSCANUS, Oswald [*ca.* 1581-1637] *praeses.* Disputationis physicae de substantia corporea mobili a substantia spirituali separata pars altera . . . Ingolstadii, Ex typographeo Gregorii Haenlin [1619]

[1], 14 p.   19 cm.   **[2760]**

Diss. — Ingolstadt (B. Wolff, *respondent*)

COSCHWICIUS, Daniel. *See* Koschwitz, Daniel [*fl.* 1611-1616]

COSCHWICIUS, Godofredus [*fl.* 1645] *respondent. See* Sebisch, M. [1578-1674?] *praeses.* Disputatio de naturalibus facultatibus prima [-octava & ultima] 1644 [i.e. 1645]

COSCHWITIUS, Georgius Daniel. *See* Koschwitz, George Daniel [*fl.* 1693]

COSCHWITZ, Georg Daniel [1679-1729] *respondent. See* Stahl, G. E., *praeses.* Dissertatio inauguralis medica practica sistens aegrum haemoptysi periodica laborantem. 1699 [and] Dissertatio medica de motibus humorum spasmodicis. 1697.

—*See* Stahl, G. E. Propempticon inaugurale de sterilitate foeminarum per aetatem. 1699.

COSCHWITZ, Georg David. *See* Coschwitz, Georg Daniel [1679-1729]

COSMAS, *Saint. See* Mangin, P. Neo-panacea. 1684.

COSMOPOLITA. *See* Everaerts, Anthony [*d.* 1679]

COSMOPOLITAE [*pseud.*] Historia naturalis. 1686. *See* Everaerts, A.

COSMOPOLITE. *See* Sendivogius, Michael [1566-1636]

COSPI, Ferdinando [*fl.* 1677] *See* Legati, L. Museo Cospiano. 1677.

COSSART, Gabriel [1615-1674] *See* Cordemoy, L. G. de. A discourse written to a learned frier. 1670.

COSSON, Pieter [*fl.* 1669] *respondent.* Disputatio medica inauguralis de ileo . . . Lugduni Batavorum, Apud viduam & haeredes Joannis Elsevirii, 1669.

[12] p.   23 cm.   **[2761]**

Diss. — Leyden.

COSTA, Antonino [*fl.* 17th cent.] *See* Avellino, F. Oratio in exornandis philosophiae. 1660.

COSTA, Christovam da [*ca.* 1540-1599] Tractado de las drogas y medicinas de las Indias Orientales. French. *In* Orta, G. d'. Histoire des drogues. 1602, 1619.

—*See* L'Écluse, C. de. Caroli Clusii . . . Exoticorum libri decem. 1605.

COSTA, João da [*fl.* 1679] Breve conta do contagio. *In* Azevedo, M. de. *Father.* Correcçam de abusos. 1690.

COSTA, Josephus à. *See* Acosta, José de [*ca.* 1539-1600]

COSTA, Romanus a [*fl. ca.* 1620] *ed. See* Varanda, J. de. De morbis mulierum lib. III. 1620 [and] Tractatus therapeuticus primus de morbis ventriculi. 1620.

COSTA DE BARROS, João da. *See* Costa, João da [*fl.* 1679]

COSTAEUS, Joannes. *See* Costeo, Giovanni [*d.* 1603]

COSTANSONIUS, *ed. See* Regimen sanitatis Salernitanum. Schola Salernitana. 1625, 1672.

COSTEO, Giovanni [*d.* 1603] De facili medicina per seri, & lactis usum, libri tres . . . Papiae, Apud Petrum Bartolum, 1604.

[14], 121 p.   23 cm.   **[2762]**

The text is a reissue of his De lactis, serique natura, et in medicina usu, published in 1595.

—De humani conceptus formatione, ac partus tempore . . . Papiae, Apud Petrum Bartolum, 1604.

[8], 48 p.   22 cm.   **[2763]**

A reissue of the 1596 edition with new title page and dedicatory epistle.

—Tractatus de potu in morbis in quo de aquis, vino, omnique factitio potu in universum, ac de privato in singulis morborum generibus eorum usu plene disseritur . . . Papiae, Ex officina Jo. Baptistae Vismarae, 1604.

[30], 376, [98] p.   21 cm.   [**2764**]

Colophon: Ticini, Apud Petrum Bartolum.

COSTEO, Giovanni [*d.* 1603] *ed. See* Avicenna. Avicennae Arabum medicorum principis. 1608.

—*See* Mesuë [924 *or* 5-1015] Opera. 1602, 1623.

COSTER, Florens [*d.* 1703] De gebannen duyvel weder geroepen; ofte, Het vonnis van Doctor Bekker over den duyvel gevelt, in revisie gebraght. [n. p., 1691?]

[1], 37 p.   20 cm.   [**2765**]

Linde 87.

COSTER VON ROSENBERG, Johannes. *See* Küster, Johann [1614 *or* 15-1685]

COSTERUS, Johannes. *See* Küster, Johann [1614 *or* 15-1685]

COSTO, Tommaso [*ca.* 1560-*ca.* 1630] Il piacevolissimo fuggilozio . . . libri VIII. Ne'quali si contengono, malitie delle femine, e trascuragini de' mariti. Sciocchezze di diversi. Detti arguti. Fatti piacevoli, e ridicoli. Malvagità punite. Inganni maravigliosi. Detti notabili. Fatti notabili, & essemplati. In Venetia, Per il Ginammi, 1663.

180, 48 p.   14 cm.   [**2766**]

Previously published under title: Il fugilozio.

COTELERIUS, Joannes Baptista. *See* Cotelier, Jean Baptiste [1629-1686]

COTELIER, Jean Baptiste [1629-1686] *See* Sorbière, S. Sorberiana. 1694.

COTREAU DU CLOS, Samuel. *See* Cottereau Du Clos, Samuel [1598-1685]

COTTA, John [1575?-1650?] A short discoverie of the unobserved dangers of severall sorts of ignorant and unconsiderate practisers of physicke in England: profitable not onely for the deceived multitude, and easie for their meane capacities, but raising reformed and more advised thoughts in the best understandings: with direction for the safest election of a physition in necessitie . . . London, William Jones and Richard Botle, 1612.

[8], 135, [1] p.   18 cm.   [**2767**]

STC 5833.

—The triall of witch-craft, shewing the true and right methode of the discovery: with a confutation of erroneous wayes . . . London, Printed by George Purslowe for Samuel Rand, 1616.

[8], 128, [1] p.   18 cm.   [**2768**]

Errata: p. [129] wanting.

Imperfect: lower margin of title page and outer margins of several pages trimmed.

STC 5836.

COTTA, Georg Samuel [*b.* 1663] *respondent. See* Crause, R. W., *praeses.* Dissertatio inauguralis medica, aegrum chylificatione laesa hypochondriaca laborantem exhibens. 1689.

—*See* Wedel, G. W. Propempticon inaugurale de pane quotidiano. 1689.

COTTA, Jeremias [*fl.* 1677] *respondent. See* Franck von Franckenau, G., *praeses.* Specimen inaugurale quo medicus monstrosus . . . proponitur . . . examinandus a J. C. 1677.

COTTEREAU DU CLOS, Samuel [1598-1685] Observations sur les eaux minerales de plusieurs provinces de France, faites en l'Academie royale des sciences en l'année 1670. & 1671. Par le sieur Du Clos . . . [Paris] Imprimerie royale, 1675.

203, [7] p.   illus.   16 cm.   [**2769**]

—[Latin tr.] Dom. Du Clos . . . Observationes super aquis mineralibus diversarum provinciarum Galliae, in Academia Scientiarum Regia in annis 1670 & 1671 factae, et ejusdem Dissertatio super principiis mixtorum naturalium habita anno 1677. Lugd. Batav. Apud Petrum Vander Aa, 1685.

[3], 204, [5] p.   14 cm.   [**2770**]

Added engraved title page.

The Dissertatio has special title page.

—Copy 2.   15 cm.

With this is bound Blondel, F. Thermarum Aquisgranensium descriptio. 1685.

—[English tr.] Observations on the mineral waters of France, made in the Royal Academy of the Sciences, by the sieur Du Clos . . . Now made English. London, Henry Faithorne and John Kersey, 1684.

[4], 125, [7] p.   illus.   16 cm.   [**2771**]

Added engraved title page.

COTTEY, John. *See* Cotta, John [1575?-1650?]

COTTON, Charles [1630-1687] *tr. See* Du Vair, G. The morall philosophy of the Stoicks. 1664.

COTUGNUS, Jacobus. Liber de abusu venae sectionis, & quando, & quibus in morbis, & qua ratione ea aperiri deceat, satis quidem docte disseritur, et fusissime demonstratur. In cujus fine etiam est adjecta solemnis illa, & satis utilis, & necessaria scitu Quaestio ejusdem auctoris. An in diarrhea possit secari vena, & medicamentum exhiberi ad medicos Hostunienses. Pauli Martinelli ... opera, & studio in lucem editus. Romae, Expensis Joannis Martinelli, apud Stephanum Paulinum, 1604.

59 p. 20 cm. [2772]

COUCH, Robert. Praxis catholica; or, The countryman's universal remedy: wherein is plainly and briefly laid down the nature, matter, manner, place and cure of most diseases, incident to the body of man; not hitherto discovered ... Now published with divers useful additions ... by Chr. Pack ... London, Robert Harford, 1680.

[48], 165, [3] p. 14 cm. [2773]

COUDEMBERG, Pierre. *See* Coudenberg, Pierre [1520?-1594?]

COUDENBERG, Pierre [1520?-1594?] *ed. See* Cordus, V. Dispensatorium. 1627, 1651, [1652]; [Dutch ed.] 1632, 1656.

COUILLARD, Joseph [d. 1660] Le chirurgien operateur; ou, Traicté methodique des principales operations en chirurgie ... 2. ed. rev., augm. ... de plus, demy-centurie d'Observations iatrochirurgiques, pleines de remarques curieuses, & evenemens singuliers. Lyon, Pierre Ravaud, 1639-40 [part [1], 1640]

[28], 256 p.; 122, [47] p. 17 cm. [2774]
Part [2] has special title page dated 1639.

COULEIUS, Abrahamus. *See* Cowley, Abraham [1618-1667]

COULTON, Thomas [d. 1731] *respondent.* Disputatio medica inauguralis de chylosi vitiata ... Lugduni Batavorum, Apud Abrahamum Elzevier, 1691.

[23] p. 23 cm. [2775]
Diss. — Leyden.

The **COUNTRY-MAN'S** care for his ... cattle. *See* Markham, G. Markham's master-piece revived. 1694 [i.e. 1695]

The **COUNTRY-MANS** physician. Where is shew'd by a most plain and easie manner, how those that live far from cities ... may be able of themselves, by the help of this book, to cure most diseases happening to the body of man ... London, Richard Chiswel, 1680.

[15], 94 p. 16 cm. [2776]

COURCELLES, Étienne de [1586-1659] *tr. See* Descartes, R. Specimina philosophiae. 1644.

COURRADE, Augustin. L'hydre feminine, combative par la nymphe Pougoise; ou, Traité des maladies des femmes gueries par les eaux de Pougues ... Nevers, Jean Millot, 1634.

8, 196 p.; 23 p. 17 cm. [2777]
Part [2] has half title: Questions problematiques touchant l'usage des eaux de Pougues.

COURTIAL, Jean Joseph [*fl.* 1684-1704] Entretien sur l'usage de la rate et du foïe ... Toulouse, D. Desclassan, 1684.

[8], 29 (i.e. 92) p. 15 cm. [2778]

—, *tr. See* Juanini, J. B. Dissertation physique. 1685.

COURTIN, Germain [d. 1597] Leçons anatomiques et chirurgicales ... Dictées a ses escholiers estudiants en chirurgie, depuis l'année mil cinq cens septante huit, jusques à l'année mil cinq cens octante & sept. Recueillies, colligées, et corrigées ... par Estienne Binet ... Paris, François Jacquin, 1612.

[16], 779, [12] p. 37 cm. [2779]
"Commentaire sur le Chapitre singulier de Guy de Cauliac": p. 1-20; includes the text.

—[The same.] Les oeuvres anatomiques et chirurgicales ... traictant amplement de l'anatomie du corps humain, de la generation de l'homme, & de toutes les maladies externes ... avec leur guérison. Le tout rangé, divisé, noté & reduit en forme de commentaries, sur la Chirurgie de M. Guidon de Cauliac, par Estienne Binet ... Rev. & augm. en cette derniere ed. du Traicté des ulceres de Jean Calve ... Rouen, François Vaultier et Louys du Mesnil, 1656.

[16], 850, [12] p. 37 cm. [2780]
Juan Calvo's tract is translated by Brice Gay.

—, *ed. See* Guillemeau, J. Les oeuvres de chirurgie. 1612, 1649.

—, *tr. See* GOURMELEN, É. Le guide des chirurgiens. 1619 [and] Les oeuvres chirurgicales. 1647.

COURVAL, THOMAS SONNET, *sieur de. See* SONNET, Thomas, *sieur de Courval* [1557-1627?]

COURVAL-SONNET, THOMAS DE. *See* SONNET, Thomas, *sieur de Courval* [1577-1627?]

COURVÉE, JEAN CLAUDE DE LA. *See* LA COURVÉE, Jean Claude de [*ca.* 1615–*ca.* 1664]

COUSIN, JEAN [*fl. ca.* 1671] Novum asthma novis signis novam causam arguentibus novissime detectum ... Parisiis, Apud Joannem Bapt. Coignard, 1673.

     [12], 130 p.   15 cm.   **[2781]**

COUSIN, JEHAN [*ca.* 1522–*ca.* 1594] La vraye science de la pourtraicture descrite et demontrëe ... Representant par une facile instruction plusieurs plans & figures de toutes les parties separées du corps humain ... Paris, Guillaume Le Bé, 1676.

     40 ll.   illus.   19 x 26 cm.   **[2782]**

     Added engraved title page: Livre de pourtraicture.

COUSINOT, JACQUES, *the younger. See* DUPUIS, G. De occultis pharmacorum purgantium facultatib. 1654.

COUSTURIER, ETIENNE [*fl.* 1682] Traité des eaux minerales de Bourges ... Bourges, Jean Toubeau, 1683.

     [14], 96 p.   15 cm.   **[2783]**

COVARRUBIAS, FRANCISCO DE VALLES. *See* VALLES, Francisco de [1524-1592]

COVILLARD, JOSEPH. *See* COUILLARD, Joseph [*d.* 1660]

COWLEY, ABRAHAM [1618-1667] Poemata Latina. In quibus continentur, sex libri plantarum, viz. duo herbarum, duo florum, duo sylvarum. Et unus miscellaneorum ... Londini, Typis T. Roycroft, impensis Jo. Martyn, 1668.

     [34], 420 (i.e. 416) p.   front. (port.)   19 cm.   **[2784]**

     Edited with an introduction by Thomas Sprat, Bishop of Rochester.

—[The same.] ... Ed. 2 ... Londini, Typis M. Clark, impensis Jo. Martyn, 1678.

     [25], 343, [13] p.   front. (port.)   17 cm.

                                  [2785]

COWPER, SPENCER [1669-1728] *defendant.* The tryal of Spencer Cowper, Esq., John Marson, Ellis Stevens, and William Rogers, Gent., upon an indictment for the murther of Mrs. Sarah Stout ... July 18. 1699 ... With the opinions of the eminent physicians and chyrurgeons ... concerning drowned bodies ... London, Printed, and are to be sold by booksellers of London and Westminster, 1699.

     38 p.   32 cm.   **[2786]**

COWPER, WILLIAM [1666-1709] The anatomy of humane bodies, with figures drawn after the life by some of the best masters ... and ... engraven in one hundred and fourteen copper plates ... containing many new anatomical discoveries ... To which is added an introduction explaining the animal oeconomy ... Oxford, Printed at the Theater, for Sam. Smith and Benj. Walford, London, 1698.

     [71] ll.   front. (port.), plates.   58 cm. **[2787]**

     Added engraved title page.

     Cowper's new English text, with Gérard de Lairesse's plates previously published in Govard Bidloo's Anatomia.

— Myotomia reformata; or, A new administration of all the muscles of humane bodies; wherein the true uses of the muscles are explained, the errors of former anatomists concerning them confuted, and several muscles not hitherto taken notice of described, to which are subjoin'd, a Graphical description of the bones; and other anatomical observations ... London, Sam. Smith and Benj. Walford, 1694.

     [22], 280 p.   plates.   20 cm.   **[2788]**

— *See* BIDLOO, G. Gulielmus Cowper, criminis literarii citatus, coram tribunali ... Societatis Britanno-regiae. 1700; RIDLEY, H. The anatomy of the brain. 1695.

COXE, DANIEL [*d.* 1730] *See* [COXE, T.] A discourse, wherein the interest of the patient ... is ... debated. 1669.

— *as subject. See* MACKAILE, M. The diversitie of salts and spirits mantained. 1683.

[**COXE**, THOMAS, 1615-1685] A discourse, wherein the interest of the patient in reference to physick and physicians is soberly debated, many abuses of the apothecaries in the preparing their medicines are detected, and their unfitness for practice discovered. Together with the reasons and advantages of physicians preparing their own medicines ... London, Printed for Richard Chiswel, 1669.

[19], 333 (i.e. 269), [1] p.   16 cm.   [2789]

"Errata": [1] p. at end.
Variously attributed to T. Coxe and Daniel Coxe. Cf. BMC. Thomas Coxe is suggested as author by Munk.

— Another issue. Imprint changed to: London, Printed for C. R., 1669.   [2790]

CRAANEN, THEODORUS [1620-1688 *or* 90] Opera omnia. Nunc demum conjunctim edita tomus alter continens Observationes, quibus emendatur & illustratur Henrici Regii. Praxis medica, medicationum exemplis demonstrata. Antverpiae, Apud Joannem Baptistam Verdussen, 1689.

[7], 773 p.   21 cm.   [2791]

Imperfect: Title vignette excised.
This 2D volume of Opera omnia is a reissue (with new title page and without the Privilegie on p. [8]) of the Observationes published by Petrus van der Aa in the same year in Leyden.
Contains the text of Henricus Regius' Praxis medica.

— Observationes excerptae ex praelectionibus publicis, privatisque collegiis ... Theodori Craanen ... quibus emendatur & illustratur V. Institutionum liber Danielis Sennerti, De auxiliorum materia. Auctore P. V. D. med. doct. Lugd. Batav., Apud Jacobum Mouque, 1687.

[8], 210, [68] p.   14 cm.   [2792]

Includes the abridged text of Sennert's Institutionum medicinae, liber quintus, pars I. De medicamentis seu auxiliorum materia.

— Observationes, quibus emendatur & illustratur Henrici Regii. Praxis medica, medicationum exemplis demonstrata ... Lugduni Batavorum, Apud Petrum vander Aa, 1689.

[8], 773 p.   21 cm.   [2793]

Contains the text of Henricus Regius' Praxis medica.

— Oeconomia animalis ad circulationem sanguinis breviter delineata. In duas partes distributa. Item Generatio hominis ex legibus mechanicis. Omnium quaestionum in hoc libro ex sanioris philosophiae principiis solutarum elenchum, si quis desiderat, calcem cujusque tractatus adeat. Goudae, Ex officina Guilhelmi vander Hoeve, 1685.

1 v.   16 cm.   [2794]

Various pagings.

— Tractatus physico-medicus de homine, in quo status ejus tam naturalis, quam praeternaturalis, quoad theoriam rationalem mechanice demonstratur. Edente Theodoro Schoon ... Lugduni Batavorum, Apud Petrum vander Aa, 1689.

[16], 765, [51] p.   plates.   20 cm.   [2795]

Dissertations — Leyden

—*praeses.* Disputatio medica de calculo renum & vesicae ... Lugduni Batavorum, Apud viduam & heredes Johannis Elsevirii, 1676.

[20] p.   19 cm.   [2796]

Z. Regius, *respondent.*

—Disputatio medica de epilepsia, quam ... publico examini submittet Bernhardus Albinus ... anno M DC LXXVI. Francofurti ad Viadrum, Literis Christophori Zeitleri, de novo impressa anno 1690.

[12] p.   19 cm.   [2797]

B. Albinus, *respondent.*

—Disputatio medica de hydrope ... Lugduni Batavorum, Apud viduam & heredes Johannis Elsevirii, 1676.

[12] p.   22 cm.   [2798]

J. van Eysden, *respondent.*

—Disputatio medica de palpitatione cordis ... Lugduni Batavorum, Apud Abrahamum Elzevier, 1681.

[11] p.   22 cm.   [2799]

J. Broen, *respondent.*

—Disputatio medica de phthisi s. tabe vera ... Lugduni Batavorum, Apud Abrahamum Elzevier, 1682.

[12] p.   20 cm.   [2800]

J. Broen, *respondent.*

—Disputatio medico-chymica exhibens medicamenti veterum universalis, recentiorumque particularium verum in medicina usum ... Lugduni Batavorum, Apud viduam & heredes Johannis Elsevirii, 1679.

[16] p.   20 cm.   [2801]

J. Crull, *respondent.*

—*as subject. See* BROEN, J. Animadversiones medicae. 1695; DISSERTATIO PHYSICO-MEDICA, DE FEBRIBUS. 1688; GREBNER, D. von. Medicina vetus restituta. 1695; STERRE, D. van der. Tractatus novus de generatione ex ovo. 1687.

CRAFFTHEIM, JOHANN CRATO VON. *See* CRATO VON KRAFFTHEIM [1519-1585]

CRAMER, CASPAR [1648-1682]

Dissertations — Erfurt

—*praeses*. Archeus faber febrium intermittentium ... Erfurti, Typis Kirschianis [1679]

    [23] p. 19 cm.   **[2802]**

    L. F. Jacobi, *respondent.*

—Dissertatio inauguralis medica de inundatione microcosmi ... Erfurti, Literis Kirschianis [1682]

    [15] p. 20 cm.   **[2803]**

    A. Kazungius, *respondent.*

—Dissertatio medica inauguralis de vertigine ... Erfurti, Literis Kirschianis [1681]

    [32] p. 20 cm.   **[2804]**

    J. H. Zihn, *respondent.*

—Specimen inaugurale de spiritu mundi Nitneriano ... subjicit Gotthelff Andreas Unzerus ... Erphordiae, Typis Kirschianis [1680]

    [16] p. 20 cm.   **[2805]**

    G. A. Unzer, *respondent.*

—*respondent*. Dissertationem de transmutatione metallorum ... pro licentia ... in arte medica ... doctoralia rite capessendi Caspar Cramer ... respondente Johanne Christiano Calckhoff ... submittet ... Erfurti, Literis Kirschianis [1675]

    [28] p. 19 cm.   **[2806]**

CRAMER, FRIEDRICH [*fl.* 1675] *respondent. See* LEICHNER, F., *praeses.* Dissertationem de podagra ... submittet F. C. 1675.

CRAMER, GABRIEL [1641-1724] *respondent. See* SEBISCH, J. A., *praeses.* Theses anatomicae miscellaneae. 1663.

CRAMER, JOHANN ANDREAS [*fl.* 1688-1690] *respondent.* Dissertatio medica inauguralis de glandulis uterinis ... Lugduni Batavorum, Apud Abrahamum Elzevier, 1690.

    [16] p. 22 cm.   **[2807]**

    Diss. — Leyden.

—*See* WEDEL, G. W., *praeses.* Disputatio medica de tussi. 1688.

CRAMER, JOHANN ANDREAS [*fl.* 1697] *respondent.* Dissertatio inauguralis medica de nephralgia ... Basileae, Literis Jacobi Bertschii, 1697.

    [32] p. 19 cm.   **[2808]**

    Diss. — Basel.

CRAMER, JOHANNES BARTHOLOMAEUS [*fl.* 1681-1682] *respondent.* Disputatio inauguralis medica aegrum pleuritide laborantem exhibens ... Altdorffii, Literis Henrici Meyeri [1682]

    28 p. 20 cm.   **[2809]**

    Diss. — Altdorf.

—*See* HOFFMANN, J. M., *praeses.* Disputatio medica aegrum asthmate laborantem exhibens. 1681.

CRAMER, MELCHIOR CONRAD [*fl.* 1695] *respondent. See* HOFFMANN, J. M., *praeses.* Disputatio medica publica de ὑδροκεφάλω. 1695.

CRAMER, PÁL [*fl.* 1614] *respondent.* De colico dolore & illius symptomate paresi, quae vulgo dicitur contractura ... themata ... Basileae, Typis Joh. Jacobi Genathii, 1614.

    [8] p. 20 cm.   **[2810]**

    Diss. — Basel.

CRANZ, FRIEDRICH MAGNUS [*fl.* 1682] *respondent.* Disputatio inauguralis medica, de cardialgia ... Gissae, Ex chalcographeo Academ. Kargeriano [1682]

    28 p. 19 cm.   **[2811]**

    Diss. — Giessen.

CRASSEUS, JOANNES. *See* GRASSHOFF, Johann [*d.* 1623]

CRASSO, GIULIO PAOLO. *See* GRASSI, Giunio Paolo [*d.* 1574]

CRASSUS, JUNIUS PAULUS. *See* GRASSI, Giunio Paolo [*d.* 1574]

CRASSUS, PAULUS. *See* GRASSI, Paolo [1562-1622]

CRATES, *of Thebes* [Letters. Greek and Latin] *In* Lubin, E., *ed.* and *tr.* Epistolae Hippocratis, Democriti, Heracliti. 1601.

CRATO, JOHANN. *See* CRATO VON KRAFFTHEIM, Johann [1519-1585]

CRATO VON KRAFFTHEIM, JOHANN [1519-1585] Consiliorum & epistolarum medicinalium ... liber primus [-septimus] Studio & labore Laurentii Scholzii ... Francofurti, In officina Danielis ac

Davidis Aubriorum & Clementis Schleichii, 1609–1620 [v. 1., 1620]

7 v. in 5.   17 cm.   [2812]

Vols. 2–3 have imprint: Hanoviae, Typis Wechelianis, apud Claudium Marnium & heredes Joan. Aubrii, both dated 1609; vols. 4 and 6–7 have imprint: Hanoviae, Typis Wechelianis apud haeredes Joh. Aubrii, dated 1614, 1611, 1611 respectively; vol. 5 has imprint: Hanoviae, Typis Wechelianis, impensis Danielis ac Davidis Aubriorum & Clementis Schleichii, 1619.

Partial contents.—v. 1. Capivaccio, Girolamo. De recta cauteriorum administratione.—v. 3. Crato, J. Μιχροτεχνή, seu parva ars medicinalis, nunc primum studio & industria Laurentii Scholzii ... in lucem editus (with special title page)—v. 4. Goldschmidt, Andreas. Succini historia.—Hermann, Daniel. De rana et lacerta succino Prussiaco insitis.—Crato, J. Commentarius de vera praecavendi et curandi febrem pestilentem contagiosam ratione ... Germanico idiomate conscriptus. Nunc in Latinum ex postrema ... authoris recognitione conversus ... studio & opera Martini Weinrichii.

—[The same.] Consiliorum et epistolarum medicinalium libri septem. Studio & labore Laurentii Scholzii ... Liber primus [-secundus; Liber sextus (i.e. quintus -sextus)] cui accessit ejusdem autoris Introductio ad artem medicam ... Francofurti, Sumptibus Johannis Petri Zubrodt, 1671.

7 v.   17, 18 cm.   [2813]

Vols. 3–4 and 7 wanting.

—Methodus therapeutike. *In* Bertocci A. Methodus curativa. 1608.

—Ordnung der Praeservation: wie man sich zur Zeit der Infection vorwahren, auch Bericht wie die rechte Pestilentia erkandt und curirt werden sol: mit einer Lehre von dem Vorsorg der Geschwieren ... Bresslaw, Gedruckt durch Georgium Bawman, 1613.

[79] p.   19 cm.   [2814]

—*See* SCHOLTZ, L. Consiliorum medicinalium ... liber singularis. 1610 [and] Epistolarum philosophicarum. 1610.

CRATZMANN, GEORG HILMAR [*fl.* 1650] *respondent. See* SEBISCH, M. [1578–1674?] *praeses.* Disputatio de morbis contagiosis et contagio. 1650.

CRAUEL, GEORG ERNEST [*fl.* 1682–1685] *respondent. See* SCHRADER, F., *praeses.* Exercitatio medica de cognoscendis medicamentorum facultatibus. 1685.

CRAUEL, STATIUS HENRICUS. *See* CRAVELIUS, Statius Henricus [*fl.* 1649–*ca.* 1657]

CRAUSE, RUDOLF WILHELM [1642–1718]

Programs—Jena

—Collegii Medici decanus ... Rudolfus Guilielmus Crausius ... lectori benevolo S. P. D. Jenae, Literis Krebsianis, 1691.

8 p.   20 cm.   [2815]

With vita of K. G. Carsten.

—Decanus ... Collegii Medici Rudolfus Guilielmus Crausius ... lectori benevolo S. P. D. Jenae, Literis Krebsianis [1694]

8 p.   20 cm.   [2816]

With vita of C. Hagedorn.

—Decanus Collegii Medici Rudolfus Wilhelmus Crausius ... Lectori benevolo salutem plurimam. Jenae, Typis Krebsianis [1689]

8 p.   19 cm.   [2817]

With vita of J. C. Schröter.

—Rudolffus Wilhelmus Kraus ... Facult. Med. ... decanus. L. B. S. [Jenae] Litteris Nisianis [1682]

[8] p.   20 cm.   [2818]

With vita of D. Kanitz.

—Rudolffus Wilhelmus Krauss ... Collegii Medici decanus lectori benevolo S. P. D. [Jenae, 1683]

[8] p.   20 cm.   [2819]

With vita of G. E. Thill.

—Rudolfus Wilhelmus Crausius ... lectori benevolo salutem. Jenae, Literis Krebsianis [1688]

[8] p.   20 cm.   [2820]

With vita of G. W. Blumberg.

—Rudolfus Wilhelmus Crausius ... Facult. Med. ... decanus lectori benevolo salutem. Jenae, Literis Krebsianis [1688]

8 p.   20 cm.   [2821]

With vita of F. J. Erich.

—Rudolfus Wilhelmus Krauss ... Facult. Medic. ... decanus, lectori benevolo S. P. D. [Jenae, 1682]

[8] p.   20 cm.   [2822]

With vita of F. Käaseberg.

—Propemticum inaugurale de calendario valetudinariorum perpetuo. I. Jenae, Litteris Krebsianis [1697]

[8] p.   21 cm.   [2823]

With vita of J. G. Siber.

—Propemticum inaugurale de calendario valetudinariorum perpetuo. II. Jenae, Typis Christophori Krebsii [1697]

[8] p. 20 cm.   **[2824]**

With vita of J. G. Baudis.

—Propemticum inaugurale de difficultate in studio medico hodie emergente. Jenae, Literis Krebsianis [1697]

[8] p. 20 cm.   **[2825]**

With vita of J. H. Ameldung.

—Propemticum inaugurale de eo an, et quomodo aurora ut musis, ita quoque sanitati amica sit? Jenae, Literis Krebsianis [1697]

[8] p. 21 cm.   **[2826]**

With vita of J. W. S. Eck.

—Propemticum inaugurale de mathesi medico maxime necessaria. Jenae, Literis Krebsianis [1697]

[8] p. 20 cm.   **[2827]**

With vita of E. Leupold.

—Propempticum inaugurale de efficaci influxu astrorum in corpus humanum. Jenae, Literis Krebsianis [1697]

[8] p. 19 cm.   **[2828]**

With vita of A. F. Beier.

—Propempticum inaugurale de meteoris microcosmi. Jenae, Typis Christophori Krebsii [1699]

[8] p. 20 cm.   **[2829]**

With vita of J. G. Sondershausen.

—Propempticum inaugurale de temerario quorundam simplicium remediorum, apriscis commendatorum, contemtu. Jenae, Typis Christophori Krebsii [1700]

[8] p. 20 cm.   **[2830]**

With vita of C. Wedel.

Dissertations — Jena

—*praeses*. De opisthotono dissertationem inauguralem . . . submittit Fridr. Guilielm. de Rhoda . . . Jenae, Litteris Nisianis [1696]

18, [2] p. 20 cm.   **[2831]**

F. W. von Rhoda, *respondent*.

—Diatribe inauguralis medica . . . de fonticulis . . . Jenae, Typis Müllerianis [1675]

[44] p. 20 cm.   **[2832]**

J. P. Struve, *respondent*.

—Disputatio inauguralis de fermentatione in sanguine non existente . . . Jenae, Literis Krebsianis [1682]

[24] p. 19 cm.   **[2833]**

C. Knaut, *respondent*.

—Disputatio inauguralis de morbis mammarum . . . Jenae, Litteris Krebsianis [1689]

[4], 28 p. 20 cm.   **[2834]**

J. J. Fick, *respondent*.

—Disputatio inauguralis medica de alvi fluxu . . . Jenae, Literis Bauhoferianis, 1674.

[16] p. 18 cm.   **[2835]**

M. Frick, *respondent*.

—Disputatio inauguralis medica de angina . . . Jenae, Typis Samuelis Krebsii [1678]

[42] p. 20 cm.   **[2836]**

S. A. Becker, *respondent*.

—Disputatio inauguralis medica de apoplexia . . . Jenae, Litteris Krebsianis [1689]

40 p. 20 cm.   **[2837]**

J. Glosemeyer, *respondent*.

—Disputatio inauguralis medica de atrophia . . . [Jena] Literis Nisianis [1683]

20 p. 20 cm.   **[2838]**

C. Zschürner, *respondent*.

—Disputatio inauguralis medica de contractura . . . Jenae, Literis Krebsianis [1687].

24, 8 p. 21 cm.   **[2839]**

A. Rosa, *respondent*.

With this is bound (as issued) Wedel, G. W. Propempticon inaugurale de naturae ministro medico. 1687.

—Disputatio inauguralis medica de febre hectica . . . Jenae, Litteris Müllerianis [1695]

24 p. 19 cm.   **[2840]**

J. A. Eggert, *respondent*.

—Disputatio inauguralis medica de febre quotidiana intermittente . . . Jenae, Litteris Krebsianis [1692]

16 p. 19 cm.   **[2841]**

J. Schomburg, *respondent*.

—Disputatio inauguralis medica de fulmine tactis . . . Jenae, Litteris Krebsianis [1694]

32 p. 20 cm.   **[2842]**

A. G. Koehler, *respondent*.

—Disputatio inauguralis medica de hernia scroti a prolapsu intestini orta ... [Jenae] Literis Müllerianis [1675]
[20] p.   19 cm.   [2843]
J. Stechan, *respondent.*

—Disputatio inauguralis medica de ischuria ... Jenae, Literis Krebsianis [1686]
24 p.   20 cm.   [2844]
J. M. Ehrlich, *respondent.*

—Disputatio inauguralis medica de odontalgia ... Jenae, Typis Nisianis [1681]
[32] p.   19 cm.   [2845]
N. C. Heden, *respondent.*

—Disputatio inauguralis medica de phrenitide ... Jenae, Litteris Krebsianis [1689]
28 p.   20 cm.   [2846]
C. Pezold, *respondent.*

—Disputatio inauguralis medica de pleuritide ... Jenae, Literis Wertherianis [1681]
[40] p.   19 cm.   [2847]
J. C. Ausfeld, *respondent.*

—Disputatio inauguralis medica de scirrho lienis ... Jenae, Litteris Krebsianis [1694]
23, [1] p.   20 cm.   [2848]
P. Schlegel, *respondent.*

—Disputatio inauguralis medica de tinnitu aurium ... Jenae, Literis Krebsianis [1694]
23, [5] p.   20 cm.   [2849]
J. J. Volland, *respondent.*

—Disputatio inauguralis medica de ulceribus uteri ... Jenae, Literis Krebsianis [1690]
32 p.   20 cm.   [2850]
D. C. Schrön, *respondent.*

—Disputatio inauguralis medica de vulneribus per se lethalibus ... Jenae, Literis Krebsianis [1684]
32 p.   20 cm.   [2851]
J. C. Ursin, *respondent.*

—Disputatio inauguralis medica, exhibens aegrum bulimicum ... Jenae, Literis Krebsianis [1695]
24 p.   19 cm.   [2852]
J. C. Struve, *respondent.*

—Disputatio inauguralis, sistens theses medico chimicas de principiis & transmutatione metallorum ... Jenae, Literis Krebsianis [1686]

[16] p.   19 cm.   [2853]
H. F. Conrad, *respondent.*

—Disputatio medica de sphacelo ... Jenae, Literis Müllerianis [1678]
[28] p.   19 cm.   [2854]
H. J. Schmidt, *respondent.*

—Disputatio medica inauguralis de delirio in genere ... Jenâe, Literis Krebsianis [1686]
16 p.   21 cm.   [2855]
J. C. Cummius, *respondent.*

—Disputatio medica inauguralis de diabete ... Jenae, Litteris Krebsianis [1692]
32 p.   20 cm.   [2856]
J. Müller, *respondent.*

—Disputatio medica inauguralis de lumbricis ... Jenae, Literis Krebsianis [1685]
20 p.   20 cm.   [2857]
J. G. Glytz, *respondent.*

—Disputatio medica inauguralis de palpitatione cordis ... [Jenae] Typis Krebsianis [1684]
[20] p.   20 cm.   [2858]
P. Hille, *respondent.*

—Disputatio medica inauguralis de potu frigido ... Jenae, Literis Gollnerianis [1697]
[36] p.   19 cm.   [2859]
E. C. Wolff, *respondent.*

—Disputatio medica inauguralis de spasmo cynico ... Jenae, Typis Johannis Nisii [1677]
20 p.   20 cm.   [2860]
J. K. Heinlein, *respondent.*

—Disputationem de hypercatharsi ... proponit Petrus Edelmann ... Jenae, Literis Wertherianis [1681]
[32] p.   19 cm.   [2861]
P. Edelmann, *respondent.*

—Disputationem inauguralem, de morbis spirituum in genere ... proponit Georgius David Walther ... [Jenae] Literis Krebsianis [1688]
32 p.   19 cm.   [2862]
G. D. Walther, *respondent.*

—Disputationem inauguralem medicam de febre quartana intermittente ... subjiciet Johannes

Adamus Schott ... Jenae, Typis Samuelis Krebsii [1678]

39, [1] p.   20 cm.   [2863]

J. A. Schott, *respondent.*

—Dissertatio inauguralis medica, aegrum chylificatione laesa hypochondriaca laborantem exhibens ... Jenae, Literis Krebsianis [1689]

[1], 22 p.   20 cm.   [2864]

G. S. Cotta, *respondent.*

—Dissertatio inauguralis medica de abscessu ... Jenae, Typis Krebsianis [1690]

[1], 22 p.   20 cm.   [2865]

J. L. Hechtel, *respondent.*

—Dissertatio inauguralis medica de appetitu ventriculi depravato, in pica et malacia ... Jenae, Literis Christophori Krebsii [1698]

27, [1] p.   21 cm.   [2866]

T. Dehne, *respondent.*

—Dissertatio inauguralis medica de febre quartana intermittente ... Jenae, Literis Krebsianis [1694]

11, [1] p.   19 cm.   [2867]

M. Kauliz, *respondent.*

—Dissertatio inauguralis medica de nymphomania ... Jenae, Literis Krebsianis, 1691.

29, [3] p.   19 cm.   [2868]

E. G. Bremer, *respondent.*

—Dissertatio inauguralis medica de phthisi; seu, Exulceratione pulmonum cum febri hectica ... Jenae, Literis Krebsianis [1700]

24 p.   19 cm.   [2869]

P. C. Schmidt, *respondent.*

—Dissertatio inauguralis medica de signaturis vegetabilium ... Jenae, Typis Pauli Ehrichii [1697]

23 p.   20 cm.   [2870]

G. H. Rosenberg, *respondent.*

—Dissertatio inauguralis medica de strumis ... Jenae, Literis Krebsianis [1687]

28 p.   20 cm.   [2871]

J. M. Heinsius, *respondent.*

—Dissertatio inauguralis medica de tabe ... Jenae, Typis Krebsianis [1681]

[36] p.   18 cm.   [2872]

J. L. Dressler, *respondent.*

—Dissertatio inauguralis medica de ulceribus crurum antiquis, vulgo von alten offenen Schenckeln ... Jenae, Literis Christophori Krebsii [1699]

20 (i.e. 21), [3] p.   20 cm.   [2873]

N. C. Bezold, *respondent.*

—Dissertatio inauguralis medica de vertigine ... Jenae, Literis Krebsianis [1690]

29, [3] p.   fold. ll.   19 cm.   [2874]

J. C. Schuster, *respondent.*

—Dissertatio inauguralis medico-chirurgica de hirudinibus ... Jenae, Literis Mullerianis [1695]

28 p.   18 cm.   [2875]

J. L. Kamper, *respondent.*

—Dissertatio inauguralis medico-chirurgica de sclopetorum vulneribus, vulgo Schuss-Wunden ... Jenae, Literis Mullerianis [1695]

[4], 16 p.   19 cm.   [2876]

L. C. Guckelin, *respondent.*

—Dissertatio medica de carminativis ... Jenae, Literis Krebsianis [1699]

27, [5] p.   20 cm.   [2877]

J. G. Sondershausen, *respondent.*

—Dissertatio medica inauguralis de abortu ... Jenae, Litteris Nisianis [1697]

40 p.   20 cm.   [2878]

R. Genaspe, *respondent.*

—Dissertatio medica inauguralis de cachexia ... Jenae, Typis Samuelis Krebsii [1677]

[24] p.   19 cm.   [2879]

T. Mauricius, *respondent.*

—Dissertatio medica inauguralis de capillis ... Jenae, Typis Pauli Ehrichii [1700]

31 p.   20 cm.   [2880]

J. J. Baier, *respondent.*

—Dissertatio medica inauguralis de cordis palpitatione ... Jenae, Typis Joh. Jacobi Bauhoferi, 1672.

[24] p.   19 cm.   [2881]

J. J. Wittwer, *respondent.*

—Dissertatio medica inauguralis de memoria ejusque remediorum natura, usu, et abusu ... Jenae, Litteris Mullerianis [1696]

46 (i.e. 40) p.   20 cm.   [2882]

C. J. Wolff, *respondent.*

—Dissertatio medica inauguralis de tussi ... Jenae, Literis Nisianis [1678]
    [36] p.   20 cm.   [2883]
    M. Herford, *respondent.*

—Dissertatio medica inauguralis de varis ... Jenae, Typis Christophori Krebsii [1697]
    16 p.   20 cm.   [2884]
    G. Baudis, *respondent.*

—Dissertationem medicam inauguralem de incubo ... submittit Daniel Christophorus Meineke ... Jenae, Typis viduae Samuelis Krebsii [1683]
    [28] p.   20 cm.   [2885]
    D. C. Meineke, *respondent.*

—Mars salutifer omnigenum morborum debellator ... Jenae, Literis Johannis Nisii [1672]
    [40] p.   19 cm.   [2886]
    A. S. Scholtz, *respondent.*

—Specimen hoc inaugurale medico-chirurgicum de extractione foetus mortui ex utero materno ... discutiendum proponit Samuel Chemnitius ... Jenae, Litteris Krebsianis, 1677.
    [24] p.   20 cm.   [2887]
    S. Chemnitz, *respondent.*

—Theses medicae inaugurales, quas ... examini exponit M. Joan. Heimreich ... Jenae, Literis Krebsianis [1700]
    [8] p.   20 cm.   [2888]
    J. Heimreich, *respondent.*

CRAUSE, RUDOLF WILHELM [1642–1718] *See* WEDEL, G. W., *praeses.* Disputationem inauguralem de bubone pestilenti ... subjicit F.W.C. 1681.

CRAUSE DE MELLINGEN. *See* CRAUSE, Rudolf Wilhelm [1642–1718]

CRAVELIUS, GEORGIUS ERNESTUS. *See* CRAUEL, Georg Ernest [*fl.* 1682–1685]

CRAVELIUS, JOHANN [*fl.* 1613] *respondent. See* SIEGFRIED, J., *praeses.* Themata de melancholia ejusque curatione. 1613.

CRAVELIUS, STATIUS HENRICUS [*fl.* 1649–*ca.* 1657] Kurtze Anweisung wie man sich gegen die grassirende Seuche der Pestilentz mit göttlicher Hülffe verwahren und davon curiren könne ... Osteroda, Barthold Fuhrman, 1681.
    50, [6] p.   20 cm.   [2889]

—, *respondent. See* MÖBIUS, G., *praeses.* De natura et usu clysterum saluberrimo. 1649; SCHELHAMMER, C., *praeses.* Dissertatio medica inauguralis de colicodolore. 1651.

CREGUT, FREIDRICH CHRISTIAN [1675–1758] *respondent.* Aegritudines infantum ac puerorum ... Basileae, Typis Jacobi Bertschii [1696]
    [2], 76 p.   18 cm.   [2890]
    Diss. — Basel.

CRELL, JACOB [16th cent.] *ed. See* REGIMEN SANITATIS SALERNITANUM. Schola Salernitana. 1625, 1672.

CRELL, LUDWIG CHRISTIAN [1671–1733] *praeses.* Disputationem historico-physicam de locustis, non sine prodigio in Germania nuper conspectis ... publice habebunt ... Johannes Fridericus Hauptvogel ... Lipsiae, Literis Colerianis [1693]
    [28] p.   19 cm.   [2891]
    Diss. — Leipzig (J. F. Hauptvogel, *respondent*)

CREMA, LIBERALIS [*fl.* 1626] *ed. See* SPIEGEL, A. van de. De formato foetu liber singularis. 1626, 1631.

CREMER, JOHANN DAVID [*fl.* 1687] *respondent. See* LIMMER, C. P., *praeses.* Collegii physici disputatorii disputatio nona. 1687.

CREMER, JOHN [14th cent.] Testamentum. *In* Maier, M. Tripus aureus. 1618, 1677.

CREMONENSIS, GERARDUS. *See* GERARDUS CREMONENSIS [1113 *or* 14–1187]

CREMONINI, CESARE [1550–1631] De calido innato, et semine, pro Aristotele adversus Galenum. Lugd. Batavorum, Ex Officina Elseviriana, 1634.
    384 p.   12 cm.   [2892]
    "Galeni De semine libri duo Joanne Bernardo Feliciano interprete": p. 120–384.

—Oratio habita in creatione serenissimi Venetiarum principis Leonardi Donati nomine almae Universitatis Patavinae D D. philosophorum ac medicorum ... Venetiis et Patavii, Ex typographia Laurentii Pasquati, 1606.
    [12] p.   22 cm.   [2893]

—Tractatus tres. Primus est de sensibus externis. Secundus de sensibus internis. Tertius de facultate appetitiva. Opuscula haec revidit Troylus Lancetta

. . . & adnotationes confecit in margine. Venetiis, Apud Guerilios, 1644.

    248 p.   22 cm.   **[2894]**

—[Excerpts.] *See* LANCETTA, T. Raccolta medica. 1645.

CRESCENTIIS, PETRUS DE. *See* CRESCENZI, Pietro de [*ca.* 1230–1321]

CRESCENTIUS, PIERO. *See* CRESCENZI, Pietro de [*ca.* 1230–1321]

CRESCENZI, PIETRO DE [*ca.* 1230–1321] [De agricultura. German.] New Feldt und Ackerbaw, darinen . . . in xv. Bücher beschrieben ist, jedes Landgut . . . bey rechter Zeit auffs beste bestellen, und mit aller hand Feldarbeit recht versorgen . . . soll. Mehr, wie und an welchem Ort . . . Weinwachs zu zeugen . . . sey. Ferners, wie . . . allerley Vierfüssigs . . . auff einem Meyerhoff . . . zu ziehen und auffzubringen, dem Krancken aber mit zeitiger Hülff zuvorkommen. Dessgleichen, wie das Gesinde bey guter Gesundtheit zuerhalten, in Kranckheit aber ohne besuchen der Apotecken, vermittelst guter Haussartzneyen, von Kräutern und gebrännten Wassern schleunig Curiren . . . In unser teusche Sprach an Tag gebracht, auch mit andern vielen . . . Sachen und nützlichen Lehren . . . von newen gemehrt worden. Strassburg, In Verlegung Lazari Zetzners, 1602.

    [10], 646, [24] p.   illus.   34 cm.   **[2895]**

—[Italian tr.] Trattato dell'agricoltura . . . compilato . . . in latino, e diviso in dodici libri . . . già traslatato nella favella Fiorentina, e di nuovo rivisto, e riscontro con testi a penna dallo' Nferigno academico della Crusca [pseud., i.e. Bastiano de Rossi] Firenze, Cosimo Giunti, 1605.

    [8], 576, [12] p.   22 cm.   **[2896]**

CRESCENZIO, FRANCESCO [*fl.* 1575] De morbis epidemiis qui Panormi vagabantur anno M.D.LXXV. seu, De peste, ejusque natura, & praecautione, tractatus a Francisco Crescentio . . . Nunc vero impressus cura, et pietate Francisci Crescentii authoris filii . . . Panormi, Apud Joannem Baptistam Maringum, 1624.

    [39], 190 p.   table.   21 cm.   **[2897]**

CRESCENZIO, FRANCESCO [*d.* 1624?] *ed. See* CRESCENZIO, F. [*fl.* 1575] De morbis epidemiis qui Panormi vagabantur anno M.D.LXXV. 1624.

CRESCIENTIO, PIERO. *See* CRESCENZI, Pietro de [*ca.* 1230–1321]

CRESPELIÈRE, DU FOUR DE LA. *See* DU FOUR DE LA CRESPELIÈRE.

CRESSIUS, SEBASTIANUS. *See* KRESS, Sebastian [*fl.* 1682]

CRETZSCHMAR, GEORG [*fl.* 1663] *respondent. See* HEILAND, M., *praeses.* Theses inaugurales medicas de lue venerea. 1663.

CREUTZING, KASPAR [*fl.* 1686] *respondent. See* MÜLLER, Peter, *praeses.* Dissertatio de jocalibus vom Weiber-Schmuck. 1686.

CREUTZMAN, JOHANN [*fl.* 1610] *respondent.* Disputatio medica de oppilatione hepatis et lienis . . . Basileae, Typis Joan. Jacobi Genathi, 1610.

    [8] p.   20 cm.   **[2898]**
Diss. — Basel.

—*See* BAUHIN, K. Hygiae et panaceae parente . . . Casparus Bauhinus. 1610.

CREUTZMANN, CHRISTIAN ERNST [*fl.* 1679] *respondent. See* SENNERT, M., *praeses.* Disputatio medica de syncope. 1679.

CREUZAUER, JOHANN CHRISTOPHOR [*fl.* 1636] *respondent. See* SEBISCH, M. [1578–1674?] *praeses.* Exercitationes medicae. 1639.

CRINIUS, GISBERTUS [*fl.* 1676] *respondent.* Disputatio medica inauguralis, de asthmate . . . Ultrajecti, Ex officina Guilielmi Clerck, 1676.

    [11] p.   20 cm.   **[2899]**
Diss. — Utrecht.

CRISTINI, BERNARDINO, *ed.* Arcana Lazari Riverii . . . nusquam in lucem edita. Cum Institutionibus medicis, & regulis, consultationibus, & observationibus P. F. Bernardini Christini . . . quibus accesserunt Centuriae quinque curationum morborum, Tractatus de lue . . . De febre pestilentiali . . . et Astrologicus ad medicinam pertinens. Venetiis, Typis Bartholomaei Tramontini, 1676.

    [20], 198 (i.e. 184) p.; [12], 132 p.; [8], 78 p. 24 cm.   **[2900]**

    Part [2] has special title page: Observationum medicarum curationum insignium centuriae quinque.

    Part [3] has special title page: De lue . . . De febre pestilentiali. De regulis astrologicis ad medicinam spectantium. Arcana Lazari Riverii.

    Attributed to Bernardino Cristini. Cf. Carrère, vol. 2, p. 528.

—[The same.] ... Venetiis, Typis Joannis La Nou & sociorum, 1696.

[16], 476 (i.e. 376) p.   23 cm.   **[2901]**

—[Excerpts.] Arcana Lazari Riverii ... Ultrajecti, Ex officina Joannis Ribbii, 1680.

115, [4] p.   14 cm.   **[2902]**

—Pratica medicinale, & osservationi del ... padre F. Bernardino Christini ... Tradotta di latino ... e data in luce da Giuseppe Testori de Capitani. Divisa in trè libri ... Venetia, Angelo Bodio, 1680–1681.

3 v. in 2.   port.   23 cm.   **[2903]**

"Discorso dell'efficacissime virtu' del calice chimico chiamato regem medicamentorum purgantium omnium sublunarium. Estratto da diversi autori dal ... Astolfo Colombani ...": 16 p. at end of vol. 3.

CRISTOFORO DEGLI ONESTI. *See* HONESTIS, Christophorus de [*d.* 1392]

La CRITICA della morte; overo, L'apologia della vita, e le ricette dell'arte, ch'accrescono i languori della natura. Tradotta dall'inglese ... Colonia, 1694.

[8], 290 p.   front. (port.)   15 cm.   **[2904]**

Augsburg 1700 edition published under title: Communication einer vortrefflichen chymischen Medicin.

CRIVELLATI, CESARE [*fl.* 1596–1602] Trattato della cura d'amore. Nel quale si scuopre la sua natura, le cagioni, la parte afferta l'humor peccante, i segni, il pronostico, & finalmente cura ... Roma, Per Paolo Martinelli, appresso Domenico Gigliotti, 1602.

201, [3] p.   14 cm.   **[2905]**

CROCCAEUS, ADRIANUS [*fl.* 1688] *respondent.* Disputatio medica inauguralis de diarrhaea ... Trajecti ad Rhenum, Ex officina Francisci Halma, 1688.

11, [5] p.   22 cm.   **[2906]**

Diss. — Utrecht.

CROCE, GIOVANNI ANDREA DELLA [1514–1575] [Chirurgiae libri septem. German.] Officina aurea; das ist, Guldene Werckstatt der Chirurgy oder Wundt Artzney, von allen Gliedtmassen dess gantzen menschlichen Leibs und derselbigen eusserlichen Gebrechen. Als ... Geschwülsten, Wunden, Geschwärn, Frantzosen, Beinbrüchen, Verrenckungen ... Artzneyen und allen nothwendigen Instrumenten gantz conterfärisch vorgestellt ... Aus dem Italienischen ... in ... hoch teutsche Sprach

versetzt durch Petrum Uffenbachium ... Franckfort am Meyn, Getruckt bey Johann Saurn, in Verlegung Jonae Rhodii, 1607.

[20], 716, [9] p.   illus.   34 cm.   **[2907]**

—[Italian tr.] Cirugia universale e perfetta di tutte le parti pertinenti all'ottimo chirurgo ... Nellaquale si contiene la theorica, & prattica di ciò, che può essere nella cirugia necessario ... Aggiuntovi di nuovo in quest'ultima impressione, oltre li dissegni di tutti gl'istromenti antichi, & moderni in tal arte necessarii, le figure de cauterii, & anatomia ... Venetia, Roberto Meglietti, 1605.

[10], 319 ll.   illus.   31 cm.   **[2908]**

In 7 books, with the fourth book of La chirurgia, by Jean Tagault added as book 4; and with De la materia chirurgica, by Jacques Houllier, added as book 6.

"Esamina da farsi da leprosi, d'incerto auttore" (ll. 279^{v}–280^{r}) is a translation of the anonymous Examen leprosorum published in Otto Brunfel's Neotericorum aliquot medicorum ... introductiones, Strassburg 1533.

—[The same.] ... Venetia, Nicolò Pezzana, 1661.

[16], 540 p.   illus.   36 cm.   **[2909]**

Imperfect: p. 539–540 mutilated.

Contents as in the 1605 edition.

—[Chirurgiae libri septem, libri V–VII. Italian.] *In* Vigo, G. de. La prattica universale in cirugia. 1605, 1622, 1639, 1647, 1669, 1685.

CROCE, GIULIO CESARE [1550–1609] Il vero et pretioso thesoro di sanità nel quale si contengono secreti mirabilissimi, & sopranaturali, per sanare quanti mali possono venire alle persone, & stroppiar quanti sani si trovano al mondo. Opera del dottor Gratiano Scattolone [pseud., i.e. Giulio Cesare Croce?] [Verona, Bartolomeo Merlo, 1630?]

[8] p.   16 cm.   **[2910]**

Imperfect: outer margins trimmed.

In verse.

Bartolomeo Merlo was active in Verona in 1619 and 1630–31. Cf. Cinelli Calvoli, vol. 2 p. 215, and Wellcome.

CROCIUS, CHRISTIAN FRIEDRICH [1623–1673] *praeses.* Disputatio medica de empyemate ... Marburgi Cattorum, Typis Salomonis Schadewitzii, 1662.

[20] p.   19 cm.   **[2911]**

Diss. — Marburg (J. von der Lahr, *respondent*)

—Exercitatio medica ... Marburgi Cattorum, Typis Salomonis Schadewitzii, 1669.

24 p.   19 cm.   **[2912]**

Imperfect: p. 9-18 wanting.
Diss. — Marburg (J. K. Wolff, *respondent*)

CROESER, HERMAN [*d.* 1574] *tr. See* NAVARRO, J. B. Commentarii ad libros Galeni De differentiis febrium. 1651.

CROLL, JOHANN LORENZ [1641-1709] *praeses.* Dissertatio academica prima, de esu carnium humanarum ejusque moralitate ... Heidelbergae, Literis Samuelis Ammonii [1682]

16 p. 18 cm. **[2913]**

Diss. — Heidelberg (L. H. Stumpf, *respondent*)

CROLL, OSWALD [*ca.* 1560-1609] Basilica chymica, continens philosophicam propria laborum experientia confirmatam descriptionem & usum remediorum chymicorum selectissimorum è lumine gratiae & naturae desumptorum. In fine additus est autoris ejusdem Tractatus novus de signaturis rerum internis. [Francofurti, Apud Claud. Marnium & heredes Joannis Aubrii, 1609]

3 parts in 1 v. illus. 22 cm. **[2914]**

Engraved title page. Each part has half title.
Contents: pt. [1] Praefatio admonitoria ad lectorem candidum, in qua, juxta medicinae chymicae comprobatam praestantiam, & hominis microcosmi excellentem dignitatem a paucissimis observatam, de utriusque philosophiae gratiae scilicet & naturae mysteriis profundissimis ac reconditissimis agitur. — Basilica chymica. — pt. [2] Tractatus de signaturis internis rerum, seu, De vera et viva anatomia majoris & minoris mundi. — pt. [3] Elegia de vera antiqua philosophica medicina, scripta a M. Ulrico Bollingero. — Encomium Wetterae Athenarum Hassiae, scriptum ab M. Ulrico Bollingero.

—[The same.] ... Francofurti, Impensis Godefridi Tampachii [1622?]

3 parts in 1 v. illus. 23 cm. **[2915]**

Privilege dated 1622.
Engraved title page. Each part has half title.

—[The same.] ... Genevae, Apud Philippum Albertum, 1631.

1 v. illus. 18 cm. **[2916]**

Various pagings.
Contents. — [1] De vera antiqua philosophica medicina elegia. Ad Osvaldum Crollium ... [by] M. Ulrici Bollingeri. — [2] Encomium Wetterae Athenarum Hassiae, scriptum ab M. Ulrico Bollingero. — [3] Praefatio admonitoria ad lectorem candidum ... [4] Basilica chymica. — [5] Tractatus de signaturis internis rerum; seu, De vera & viva anatomia majoris & minoris mundi. Items 2, 3 & 5 have half titles.

—Basilica chymica, pluribus selectis & secretissimis propria manuali experientia approbatis descriptionibus, & usu remediorum chymicorum selectissimorum aucta a Joan. Hartmanno ... Edita a Johanne Michaelis ... et Georg. Everhardo Hartmanno ... Genevae, Sumptibus Petri Chouët, 1635.

3 parts in 1 v. illus. 18 cm. **[2917]**

Each part has half title page.
Contents. — pt. [1] Basilica chymica. — pt. [2] Tractatus de signaturis internis rerum, seu, De vera & viva anatomia majoris & minoris mundi. — pt. [3] Praefatio admonitoria.

—[The same.] ... Genevae, Apud Petrum Chouët, 1643. **[2918]**

—[The same.] ... Genevae, Apud Samuelem Chouët, 1658. **[2919]**

—[English tr.] Bazilica chymica, & Praxis chymiatricae; or, Royal and practical chymistry in three treatises. Wherein all those excellent medicines and chymical preparations are fully discovered, from whence all our modern chymists have drawn their choicest remedies ... Augm. and inl. by John Hartman. To which is added his Treatise of signatures of internal things ... As also The practice of chymistry of John Hartman M. D. augm. and inl. by his son [i.e. G. E. Hartmann] All ... Englished by a lover of chymistry. London, John Starkey and Thomas Passinger, 1670.

3 parts in 1 v. illus. 30 cm. **[2920]**

Each part has special title page. Part [2] has date 1669.

—[French tr.] La royalle chymie ... traduitte en francois par J. Marcel de Boulene. Lyons, Pierre Drobet, 1627.

3 parts in 1 v. illus. 19 cm. **[2921]**

Engraved title page.
Each part has half title.
Contents. — pt. [1] Preface admonitoire, contenant les mysteres tres-profonds & plus rares de la philosophie tant naturelle que de la grace, touchant l'excellence de la medecine chymique & grandeur du microcosme. — pt. [2] La royale chymie. — pt. [3] Traicté des signatures, ou, Vraye et vive anatomie du grand & petit monde. Each part has half title page.

—[The same.] ... Rouen, Jean Osmont, 1634. [4], 3-460, [62] p.; 126, [31] p. illus. 17 cm. **[2922]**

—[German tr.] Königlicher chymischer und artzneyischer Palast, vorin über dass weltberühmte Buch genant Basilica chymica: eine durch alle Capitel des gantzen Wercks vollständige Vermehr- und Erläuterung gestellet, und diejenige hohe Secreta, als

Laudanum Mercuriale, und andere, welche bisher in allen Exemplarien gedachter Basilicae Crolliano Hartmannianae ausgelassen worden, aus des Authoris Manuscript treulich ersetzt werden ... publiciret von Joh. Hiskia Cardilucio ... Nürnberg, In Verlegung Christoph Riegels, 1684.

IOIO, [22] p. front., illus. 17 cm. [2923]
Imperfect: frontispiece wanting.
Translated and commentated upon by J. H. Cardilucius.

—[Selections.] In Ziegler, A. Pharmacopoea spagyrica. 1628.

—Philosophy reformed & improved in four profound tractates. The I. Discovering the great and deep mysteries of nature: by ... Osw. Crollius. The other III. Discovering the wonderfull mysteries of the creation, by Paracelsus: being his Philosophy to the Athenians. Both made English by H. Pinnell ... London, Printed by M. S. for Lodowick Lloyd, 1657.

[21], 226 p.; [2], 70 p. front. (port.) 18 cm. [2924]
Part I is a translation of Croll's Praefatio admonitoria, from his Basilica chemica, first published in Franckfurt in 1608.
Part 2 has special title page: Three books of philosophy written to the Athenians: by ... Paracelsus ... Done into English ... By a young seeker of truth and holines.
Sudhoff 378.

—See BILLICH, A. G. Thessalus in chymicis redivivus. 1640; HARTMANN, J. Opera omnia medico-chymica. 1684, 1694; IRVINE, C. Medicina magnetica. 1656.

—as subject. See LIBAVIUS, A. [d. 1616] Appendix necessaria Syntagmatis arcanorum chymicorum. 1615.

CROLLIUS redivivus. 1647. See ANONYMUS VON FELDTAW.

CROMWELL, SAMUEL [fl. 1682] respondent. Disputatio medica inauguralis de tumoribus in genere ... Lugduni Batavorum, Apud Abrahamum Elzevier, 1682.

[24] p. 22 cm. [2925]
Diss. — Leyden.

CRONBUSCH, GEORG SIGMUND. See CRONPUSCH, Georg Sigismund [b. 1670]

CRONPUSCH, GEORG SIGISMUND [b. 1670] respondent. See FINGER, C. G., praeses. Dissertatio physica de quotidiano corporis humani decremento.

1694; VESTI, J., praeses. Dissertatio inauguralis medica, exhibens casum de doloribus vehementissimis partum praegredientibus. 1696.

—as subject. See EYSEL, J. P. Decanus Facultatis Medicae ... lectorem ... invitat. 1696.

CROOKE, HELKIAH [1576-1648] Μικροκοσμογραφία. A description of the body of man. Together-with the controversies thereto belonging. Collected and translated out of the best authors of anatomy, especially out of Gasper Bauhinus and Andreas Laurentius ... [London] William Jaggard, 1615.

[21], IIII (i.e. 1001), [1] p. illus. 35 cm. [2926]
STC 6062.
Imperfect: p. [1] at end wanting.

—[The same.] ... [London] W. Jaggard, 1618.
[18], IIII (i.e. 1001), [1] p. illus. 34 cm. [2927]
STC 6062.4.
A reissue of the 1615 edition with new title page and dedicatory epistle reset. "The contents of severall bookes" and the poems following it are not present in this copy.
Imperfect: p. 623-624 wanting; supplied in photocopy from National Library of Medicine's copy published in 1615.

—[The same.] ... The 2d ed. corr. and enl. London, Printed by Thomas and Richard Cotes, and are to be sold by Michael Sparke, 1631.
[29], 1012 (i.e. 1004) p.; [1], 60, [3] p. illus. 34 cm. [2928]
Added engraved title page.
Imperfect: sig. f3 (errata) and f4 (blank) wanting.
"An explanation of the fashion and use of three and fifty instruments of chirurgery. Gathered out of Ambrosius Pareus ... and done into English ... by H[elkiah] C[rooke]" ([2], 60, [5] p. at end) has special title page with imprint: London, Printed for Michael Sparke, 1631.
STC 6063.

—[The same.] ... London, Printed by R. C. and sold by John Clarke, 1651.
[27], 766 p. 35 cm. [2929]
Engraved title page.

[—] Σωματογραφια ανθρωπινη; or A description of the body of man ... [London] W. Jaggard, 1616.
[4], 154 (i.e. 153), [1] ll. illus. 18 cm. [2930]
Imperfect: first preliminary leaf (blank?) wanting.
STC 20782.
Extracted by Alexander Read from Crooke's Μικροκοσμογραφια.

—[The same.] ... With The practice of chirurgery, and the use of three and fifty instruments ... [London] Printed by Tho. Cotes, and sold by Michael Sparke, 1634.

[4], 154 (i.e. 153) ll.; [5], 117, [1] p. illus. 20 cm. **[2931]**

Imperfect: sig. A1 (half title?) wanting.

STC 20783.

Part [2] has special title page: An explanation of the fashion and use of three and fifty instruments of chirurgery. Gathered out of Ambrosius Pareus ... and done into English ... by H[elkiah] C[rooke] London, Michael Sparke, 1634.

[**CROONE**, WILLIAM, 1633-1684] De ratione motus musculorum ... Londini, Excudebat J. Hayes, prostant venales apud S. Thomson, 1664.

[1], 34 p. plate. 22 cm. **[2932]**

—[The same.] ... Ed. 2 priori emendatior. Amstelodami, Apud Casparum Commelinum, 1667.

34 p. plates. 14 cm. **[2933]**

Bound with (as issued?) Willis, T. Cerebri anatome. 1667.

—[The same.] In Willis, T. Cerebri anatome. 1664, 1666 [and] Opera medica & physica. 1676 [and] Opera omnia. 1676, 1680, 1681, 1694, 1695.

CROONEN, THEODORUS. See CRAANEN, Theodorus [1620-1688 or 90]

CROONENBURGH, WILLEM [*fl.* 1669] *respondent.* Disputatio medica inauguralis de diarrhaea ... Lugduni Batavorum, Apud viduam & haeredes Joannis Elsevirii, 1669.

[8] p. 23 cm. **[2934]**

Diss. — Leyden.

CROQUERUS, JOHANNES, *ed.* See RONDELET, G. Opera omnia medica. 1620, 1628, 1685.

CROQUERUS, PAULUS [*fl.* 1616-1643] See FABRICIUS VON HILDEN, W. Consilium. 1629 [and] Opera. 1646, 1682 [and] Wund-Artzney, gantzes Werck. 1652.

CROQUIERIUS, PAULUS. See CROQUERUS, Paulus [*fl.* 1616-1643]

CROSE, J. DE LA. See CORNAND DE LA CROSE, Jean de [*d. ca.* 1705]

CRUCE, JOANNES ANDREAS A. See CROCE, Giovanni Andrea della [1514-1575]

CRUCIUS, VINCENTIUS ALSARIUS. See ALSARIO DALLA CROCE, Vincenzo [1576?-1631?]

CRÜGENER, MICHAEL [*fl.* 1648-1679] Chymischer Früling; das ist, Sonderbares medicochymisches Tractätlein. 1. Von Gold und Silber. 2. Zien und Bley. 3. Eisen, Kupffer und Schwefel. 4. Mercurio und Antimonio. 5. Corallen. 6. Von Perlen, derer Mutter, Krebss- und Persskensteinen, Muscheln und Schneckenhäusslein. 7. Agt- und Pirnstein. 8. Menschenbeinen und Hirschhorn. Darinnen insonderheit kürtzlich und treufleissig dargethan wird, welches nicht allein irrige Meynungen, und falsche Processe aus obbemelten Dingen Artzneyen zu bereiten sondern auch im Gegentheil, richtige, kurtze, und wahre Processe, mit sonderbahren Hand griffen, auch beygefügten Gebrauch und Nutz, gewiesen werden ... Dresden, Getruckt bey Wolff. Seyfferten ... 1648.

[8], 205, [19] p. 20 cm. **[2935]**

Imperfect: publisher's name is not legible.

—XXV. medicinisch-historische Episteln; oder: Auffgezeichnete Curen, so durch Göttlichen Segen, mit Hülff der edlen Artzney Materia perlata wunderbarer Weise verrichtet ... durch L. Michael Krügenern ... Regenspurg, Paulus Dalnsteiner, 1679.

[23], 88 p. front., illus. 17 cm. **[2936]**

With this are bound: *his* Materia perlata. 1676; *his* Continuation seiner medicinischen Episteln. 1680.

—Continuation seiner medicinischen Episteln ... Regenspurg, Paulus Dalnsteiner, 1680.

[2], 72 (i.e. 78) p. 17 cm. **[2937]**

Bound with *his* XXV. medicinisch-historische Episteln. 1679.

—Michaelis Grügeneri ... Materia perlata. Dressden, In Verlag des Authoris, Druckts Paul August Hamann, 1675.

[2], 61, [1] p. 17 cm. **[2938]**

—[The same.] ... Edle und bewehrte Artzeney, wider Malum hypochondriacum, Miltz-Kranckheit, oder windige Melancholey genannt ... Regenspurg, Paulus Dalnsteiner, 1676.

[2], 46 p. 17 cm. **[2939]**

Bound with *his* XXV. medicinisch-historische Episteln. 1679.

CRÜGER, ANDREAS LORENZ [*fl.* 1665] *respondent.* See SULTZBERGER, S. R., *praeses.* Disputatio medica inauguralis de ictero flavo. 1665.

CRÜGER, BARTHOLOMÄUS [*fl.* 1610]

Dissertations — Wittenberg

—*praeses.* Disputatio medica prima de morbo morbique essentia in genere ... Wittebergae, Ex officina typographica Andreae Rüdingers, 1610.

[8] p. 18 cm.   **[2940]**

A. Schmitner, *respondent.*

—Disputatio medica secunda de summis primisque generibus morborum eorumque differentiis essentialibus ... Wittebergae, Ex officina typographica Andreae Rüdingers, 1610.

[8] p. 17 cm.   **[2941]**

G. Tisenius, *respondent.*

—Disputatio medica tertia de differentiis morborum accidentalibus seu secundariis ... Wittebergae, Ex officina typographica Andreae Rüdingers, 1610.

[8] p. 18 cm.   **[2942]**

G. Eberlin, *respondent.*

—Disputatio medica quarta de causis morborum in genere et specie ... Wittebergae, Ex officina typographica Andreae Rüdingers, 1610.

[8] p. 17 cm.   **[2943]**

F. Monavius, *respondent.*

—Disputatio medica quinta de symptomatum generibus, differentiis & causis ... Wittebergae, Ex officina typographica Andreae Rüdingers, 1610.

[8] p. 17 cm.   **[2944]**

J. Curtius, *respondent.*

—Disputatio medica sexta de signis eorumque primariis differentiis ... Wittebergae, Ex officina typographica Andreae Rüdingers, 1610.

[8] p. 18 cm.   **[2945]**

E. Fischer, *respondent.*

—Disputatio medica septima de crisibus et diebus judicatoriis in morbis ... Wittebergae, Ex officina typographica Andreae Rüdingers, 1610.

[8] p. 18 cm.   **[2946]**

C. B. Merclin, *respondent.*

CRÜGER, JOHANN BARTHOLOMÄUS [1608–1638] *respondent. See* HEINICK, A., *praeses.* Exercitium physicum de oscitatione. 1627.

CRUFENAS, CARIOLLINUS TEVETIO. Themata medica de beanorum, archibeanorum, beanulorum & cornutorum quorumcunque affectibus & curantine [sic] Ad quae praesidente ... Cornelio Cerasto Cornano [pseud.] ... respondebit Cariollinus Tevetio Crufenas [pseud.] Cornanae [Cornet sur Saulcy?] Typis Wolphgangi Blass ins Horn [1626?]

[24] p. illus. 20 cm.   **[2947]**

Burlesque dissertation.

CRUG, THEODOR CHRISTOPH [1655–1720 *or* 21] *respondent.* De morbis chronicis ex acido vitioso disquisitionem ... exponit Theodorus Christophorus Crugius ... Marburgi Cattorum, Typis Salomonis Schadewitzii [1676]

[3], 28 p. 18 cm.   **[2948]**

Diss. — Marburg.

CRUGER, BARTHOLOMÄUS. *See* CRÜGER, Bartholomäus [*fl.* 1610]

CRUGIUS, THEODORUS CHRISTOPHORUS. *See* CRUG, Theodor Christoph [1655–1720 *or* 21]

CRULL, JODOCUS [*d.* 1713?] *respondent. See* CRAANEN, T., *praeses.* Disputatio medico-chymica. 1679.

CRUSERIUS, HERMANNUS. *See* CROESER, Herman [*d.* 1574]

CRUSIUS, BENJAMIN [*fl.* 1642] *respondent. See* LINEMANN, A., *praeses.* Exercitatio philosophica. 1642.

CRUSIUS, CHRISTIAN [*fl.* 1665–1669] *respondent. See* SULTZBERGER, S. R., *praeses.* Dissertatio medica inaugurales de abortu. 1669.

CRUSIUS, DAVID [1589–1640] Theatrum morborum Hermetico-Hippocraticum; seu, Methodica morborum, et curationis eorundem dispositio ... Erfurti, Typis Nicolai Schmuckii, impensis Johannis Episcop, 1615–16.

2 v. in 1. table. 16 cm.   **[2949]**

Imperfect: leaf before p. 1 (vol. 2) wanting.

Vol. [2] has imprint: Typis Mechlerianis, 1616.

CRUSIUS, JEREMIAS [*fl.* 1657] *respondent. See* SCHENCK, J. T., *praeses.* Disputatio medico-chirurgica de fonticulis. 1657.

CRUSIUS, MARTIN [*fl.* 1618] *respondent. See* SCHALLER, W., *praeses.* Positionum medicarum semicenturia de syncope. 1618.

CRUSIUS, MICHAEL [*fl.* 1609] *respondent.* Theses medicae inaugurales de palpitatione cordis ... Basileae, Typis Johannis Schroeteri, 1609.

[8] p. 20 cm. [**2950**]

Diss. — Basel.

CRUZ, ANTONIO DE [16th-17th cent.] Recopilaçam de cirurgia ... acrescentada nesta setima impressam pello D. Francisco Soares Feyo, & pello ... Antonio Gonçalves ... Lisboa, Antonio Craesbeeck, 669 [i.e. 1669]

[4], 359, [9] p. illus. 20 cm. [**2951**]

"Tratado do scurbuto a que o vulgo chama mal de loanda pello Doctor Francisco Soares Feyo ...": p. [297]-344, with special title page; "Tratado da gonorrea pello ... Antonio Gonçalves ...": p. 345-359.

CUBAS, SEBASTIAN DE [*fl.* 1664] *See* BONILLA SAMANIEGO, A. de. Exercitacion medica. 1664.

CUFF, HENRY. *See* CUFFE, Henry [1563-1601]

CUFFE, HENRY [1563-1601] The differences of the ages of mans life: together with the originall causes, progresse, and end thereof ... London, Printed by B. A[lsop] and T. F. for Lawrence Chapman, 1633.

[15], 135 (i.e. 133) p. 15 cm. [**2952**]

STC 6104.

CUJACIUS, ISAACUS [*fl.* 1652] Medicina peregrinantium, nunquam antehac edita ... Bremae, Typis Bertholdi di Villiers, 1651.

[12], 120 p. 14 cm. [**2953**]

With this is bound *his* Uromantia. 1652.

—Uromantia; seu, Urocriterium, in quo perfecta urinarum cognitio ad morborum diagnosin continetur ... Bremae, Typis Bertholdi de Villiers, 1652.

[4], 100, [3] p. 14 cm. [**2954**]

Bound with *his* Medicina peregrinantium. 1651.

CUJACIUS, JACOBUS. *See* CUJAS, Jacques [1522-1590]

CUJAS, JACQUES [1522-1590] *ed.* and *tr.* Ἐπιστολαι Ελληνικαι ἀμοιβαιαι; hoc est, Epistolae Graecanicae mutuae, antiquorum rhetorum, oratorum, philosophorum, medicorum, theologorum, regum, ac imperatorum aliorumque praestantissimorum virorum a Jacobo Cujacio ... Latinitate donatae. Aureliae Allobrogum, Sumptibus Caldorianae Societatis, 1606.

[4], 458 p. 35 cm. [**2955**]

Imperfect: sig. pp8 (blank?) wanting.
In Greek and Latin.

CUJAUS, JACOBUS. *See* CUJAS, Jacques [1522-1590]

CULMANN, JOHANN [*fl.* 1554] *ed. See* HIPPOCRATES. [Collected works. Latin] Opera. 1610, 1619, 1679.

—*See* HYGIEIA. 1628; REGIMEN SANITATIS SALERNITANUM. Medicina Salernitana. 1605, 1611, 1612, 1622, 1624, 1628, 1638 [and] Schola Salernitana. 1649, 1657, 1667, 1683.

CULPEPER, NICHOLAS [1616-1654] Arts masterpiece; or, The beautifying part of physick. Whereby all defects of nature in both sexes are amended, age renewed, youth continued and all imperfections fairly remedied. With many the most approved physical experiments, so far discovered, that every man may be his own apothecary. Never before extant, though long since promised by Mr. Nic. Culpeper, but now published by B. T. Doctor in Physick. London, Nath. Brook, 1660.

[17], 140, [1] p. front. 14 cm. [**2956**]

The dedicatory epistle signed: L.D.
Attributed also to Johann Jacob Wecker. Cf. Wing (1951) W1234.

—A directory for midwives; or, A guide for women, in their conception, bearing, and suckling their children ... London, Peter Cole, 1651.

[33], 217 (i.e. 219), [23] p. front. (port.), illus., plates. 14 cm. [**2957**]

—[The same.] ... London, Printed, 1652.

[17], 120, [8] p. port. (front.), illus. 15 cm. [**2958**]

Not in Wing.

—[The same.] ... Newly corr. ... London, Printed by John Streater, and sold by George Sawbridge, 1671.

2 parts in 1 v. illus., plates. 15 cm. [**2959**]

Imperfect: p. 117-118 of part 1 wanting.
Part 1 has running title: Culpepers Midwife enlarged; part 2 has special title page. Caption title reads: The fourth book of practical physick. Of womens diseases.

—[The same.] ... London, George Sawbridge, 1675-76.

2 parts in 1 v. illus. 16 cm. [**2960**]

—[The same.] . . . London, George Sawbridge, 1681.

2 parts in 1 v. illus. 16 cm.						[2961]

—[The same.] . . . London, Printed, and sold by most booksellers in London and Westminster, 1700.

[8], 374, [1] p. illus. 16 cm.						[2962]

An extra title page at end has imprint: London, J. and A. Churchill, 1701.

—The English physician; or, An astrologo-physical discourse of the vulgar herbs of this nation . . . London, Printed for the benefit of the Commonwealth of England, 1652.

[25], 266 (i.e. 276), [11] p.	front. (port.) 14 cm.						[2963]

—The English physitian enlarged: with three hundred, sixty, and nine medicines made of English herbs that were not in any impression until this . . . Being an astrologo-physical discourse of the vulgar herbs of this nation . . . London, Peter Cole, 1653.

[20], 398 (i.e. 288), [16] p. illus. 18 cm.						[2964]

—[The same.] . . . London, Peter Cole, 1656.
[24], 398 (i.e. 288), [16] p. illus. 18 cm.						[2965]

Portrait mounted.
Different setting of type.

—[The same.] . . . London, Peter Cole, 1661.
[24], 398 (i.e. 288), [16] p. illus. 18 cm.						[2966]

Different setting of type.

—[The same.] . . . London, John Streater, 1669.
[13], 285, [17] p. 18 cm.						[2967]

—[The same.] . . . London, John Streater, 1671.
[13], 285, [18] p. 18 cm.						[2968]

A reissue of the 1669 edition with new title page.

—[The same.] . . . London, George Sawbridge, 1674.
[13], 285, [18] p. 18 cm.						[2969]

Different setting of type.

—[The same.] . . . London, George Sawbridge, 1681.
[13], 285, [18] p. port. 18 cm.						[2970]

Different setting of type.
With this is bound: Blagrave, J. Supplement; or, Enlargement to Mr. Nich. Culpeper's English physician. 1677.

—[The same.] . . . London, Printed for Hannah Sawbridge, sold by Tho. Malthus, 1683.

[13], 285, [18] p. 18 cm.						[2971]

Imperfect: wormholes throughout.
Different setting of type.

—[The same.] . . . London, A. and J. Churchill, 1695.

[12], 284, [16] p. 18 cm.						[2972]

—[The same.] . . . London, A. and J. Churchill, 1698.

[12], 284, [16] p. 18 cm.						[2973]

Different setting of type.

—[The same.] *See* BLAGRAVE, J. Supplement . . . to . . . Culpepers English physitian. 1674, 1677.

—Last legacy: left and bequeathed to his dearest wife, for the publicke good, being the choicest and most profitable of those secrets which while he lived were lockt up in his breast, and resolved never to be publisht till after his death. Containing sundry admirable experiences in severall sciences, more especially, in chyrurgery, and physick . . . [London] N. Brooke, 1656.

1 v. front. (port.) 17 cm.						[2974]

Various pagings.
Imperfect: p. 17 mutilated.
Contents: — [1] Of head-ach in general . . . — [2] Febrilia; or, A treatise of feavers in general (Includes: A treatise of the pestilence) — [3] Composita; or, A synopsis of the chiefest compositions in use now with Galenists. — [4] Aphorismes . . . — [5] Select aphorismes . . . — [6] Select medicinal aphorismes . . . Items [2–6] have special title pages dated 1656. Items [3–6] have imprints: London, Printed by T. C. for Nath. Brook.

—[The same.] . . . [London] N. Brooke, 1657.
1 v. front. (port.) 17 cm.						[2975]

Various pagings.
A reprint of the 1656 edition.

—[The same.] . . . The 4th impression; whereunto is added 200 choyce receipts, lately found . . . London, Printed by Tho. Ratcliffe for Nath. Brooke, Ben. Billingsley and Obadiah Blagrave, 1668.

[9], 276 (i.e. 274), [12] p. front. (port.) 17 cm.						[2976]

Contents: — [1] Of headach in general . . . —[2] Febrilia; or, A treatise of feavers in general. — [3] A treatise of the pestilence . . . — [4] Composita; or, A synopsis of the chiefest compositions now in use with our physicians . . . — [5] Aphorisms . . . [6] Select aphorisms . . . [7] Select medicinal aphorismes and receipts . . . [8] Rare secrets in physick and chirurgery . . . Items [2–8] have special title pages. Item [2] has imprint: London, 1667. Items [3–8] have imprints: London, Printed for N. Brook, and sold by Obadiah Blagrave ... 1667.

—[The same.] ... The 5th impression; whereunto is added an exact ... treatise of anatomy of the reins and bladder, brain and nerves of all parts of the body, never published before ... London, Nath. Brooke, 1676.

[9], 276 (i.e. 274), [13] p.; [1], 60, [5] p.   front. (port.)   18 cm.   [2977]

Part [1] is a reprint of the 1668 edition. Part [2] contains: "Opus physicum. A new exact & perfect treatise of the anatomy of the reins & bladder ...": p. [1]-7; — "The anatomy of the brain & nerves together with the marrow of the back ...": p. [9]-50; — "The eyes anatomized ...": p. [51]-60. Items have special title pages.

—[The same.] ... The 6th impression ... London, Obadiah Blagrave, 1685.

[9], 276 (i.e. 274), [13] p.; [1], 60, [18] p.   front. (port.)   18 cm.   [2978]

A reprint of the 1676 edition.

—A physicall directory; or, A translation of the London dispensatory made by the Colledge of Physicians in London. Being that book by which all apothicaries are strictly commanded to make all their physick with many hundred additions which the reader may find in every page marked with this letter A ... London, Peter Cole, 1649.

[19], 345 (i.e. 315), [28] p.   front.   (port.)   20 cm.   [2979]

—[The same.] A physical directory; or, A translation of the Dispensatory made by the Colledge of Physitians of London, and by them imposed upon all the apothecaries of England to make up their medicines by. Whereunto is added, the vertues of the simples, and compounds ... 2d ed. much enl. ... London, Peter Cole, 1650.

[10], 242 (i.e. 212), [19] p.   front. (port.)   28 cm.   [2980]

—[The same.] ... And in this 3d ed. is added A key to Galen's method of physick ... London, Peter Cole, 1651.

[12], 184, [18] p.   front. (port.)   28 cm.   [2981]

—[The same.] Pharmacopoeia Londinensis: or, The London dispensatory further adorned by the studies and collections of the fellows, now living of the said colledg. Wherein you may find, 1. The vertues, qualities, and properties of every simple ... 7.

In this impression the Latin name of every one of the compounds is printed, and in what page of the new folio Latin book they are to be found ... London, Peter Cole, 1653.

[12], 186 (i.e. 162), [2], 301-325, [15] p.   front. (port.)   28 cm.   [2982]

Imperfect: front. (port.) wanting; supplied in photocopy from the Yale Medical Library.

Inserted before title page is a photocopy of another title page from a copy in the Yale Medical Library with same imprint and title: Pharmacopoeia Londinensis: or, The London dispensatory further adorned by the studies and collections of the fellows, now living of the said colledg. Whereunto is added, 1. The vertues, qualities, and properties of every simple ... 6. What is added to the book by the translator, is of a different letter from that which was made by the colledg. By Nich. Culpeper ...

—[The same.] ... London, A Well-wisher to the Common-wealth of England, 1654.

[16], 3-386, [20] p.   port.   15 cm.   [2983]

—[The same.] ... 6th ed. ... London, Peter Cole, 1659.

[27], 377 (i.e. 299), [33] p.   18 cm.   [2984]

"A key to Galen's method of physick" has special title page dated 1658, and same running title.

—Another issue? 1659?

[14 +], 377 (i.e. 299), [29 +] p.   18 cm.   [2985]

Imperfect: all pages before sig. A1, and p. [25-33] at end wanting. Title and imprint supplied from the 1659 6th edition; contains same text in different setting of type.

"A key to Galen's method of physick" has special title page dated 1658, and running title: The 46. book of the physitians library, being a key to Galen and Hippocrates, their method of physick.

—[The same.] ... In this impression ... there is added, to the compounds, many vertues ... By divers learned ... doctors of physick ... and, by Abdiah Cole ... London, Peter and Edward Cole, 1661.

[14], 38, 101-229, [27] p.   29 cm.   [2986]

—[The same.] ... London, Peter Cole, 1665.

[14], 229 (i.e. 167), [27] p.   illus., plates.   29 cm.   [2987]

Bound with Bartholin, T. Anatomy. 1665.

—[The same.] ... London, Printed by John Streater, and sold by George Sawbridge, 1669.

[24], 305, [37] p.   18 cm.   [2988]

Contents as in the 1659 edition.

—[The same.] ... London, Printed by John Streater, and sold by George Sawbridge, 1672.

[24], 305 [37] p.   18 cm.   [2989]
Different setting of type.

—[The same.] . . . London, George Sawbridge,
1675.
[24], 305 [37] p.   18 cm.   [2990]
Different setting of type.

—[The same.] . . . London, George Sawbridge,
1679.
[24], 269 (i.e. 305), [37] p.   18 cm.   [2991]
Imperfect: 3d-8th prelim. leaves, p. 221-222, 241-242 wanting;
p. 221-222 supplied in photocopy from the Yale Medical Library.

—[The same.] . . . London, Hanna Sawbridge,
1683.
[24], 269 (i.e. 305), [37] p.   18 cm.   [2992]
Different setting of type.

—[The same.] . . . London, Awnsham and John
Churchill, 1695.
[24], 269 (i.e. 305), [37] p.   18 cm.   [2993]
Different setting of type.

—School of physick; or, The experimental practice of the whole art. Wherein are contained all inward diseases from the head to the foot, with their
. . . cures . . . The narrative of the authors life is
prefixed, with his nativity calculated, together with
the testimony of his late wife . . . and others . . . London, N. Brook, 1659.
[54], 361 (i.e. 461), [27] p.   front. (port.), illus.
17 cm.   [2994]
Imperfect: p. 167-170 wanting.
Partial contents: School of physick; or, The English
apothecary.—Fragmenta aurea.—The chyrurgeons guide.—The
treasury of life.—The expert lapidary.—Doctor Diets directory.—
Doctor Reason and Doctor Experience consulted with.—Chymical
institutions.—Items have special title pages.

—[The same.] . . . The 2d. ed. London, Printed
for O[badiah] B[lagrave] and R. H. and sold by
Robert Clavel, 1678.
[54], 361 (i.e. 461), [19] p.   front. (port.), illus.
18 cm.   [2995]
Contents as in the 1659 ed. Eight of the treatises have special
title pages dated 1677.

—[The same.] . . . The 3d ed. corr. London, R.
Bently, J. Phillips, H. Rhodes and J. Taylor, 1696.
[45], 313, [12] p.   front. (port.), illus.   17 cm.
                                              [2996]

—Semeiotica Uranica; Or, An astrological judgment of diseases from the decumbiture of the sick;

1. From Aven Ezra by way of introduction. 2. From
Noel Duret by way of direction. Wherein is layd
down, the way and manner of finding out the cause,
change and end of a disease . . . To which is added
The signs of life or death by the body of the sick party
according to the judgment of Hippocrates . . . London, Nathaniell Brookes, 1651.
[22], 190, [1] p.   front. (port.), illus., plates.
14 cm.   [2997]
Imperfect: front. (port.) and plates wanting.

—[The same.] Astrologicall judgment of diseases
from the decumbiture of the sick much enlarged . . .
Whereunto is added, a table of logisticall logarithmes,
to finde the exact time of the crisis. Hermes Trismegistus upon the first decumbiture of the sick . . . with
a compendious treatise of urine . . . London, Nath.
Brookes, 1655.
[23], 174 (i.e. 232) p.   front. (port.), illus.,
plates.   16 cm.   [2998]
Imperfect? Sig. M apparently skipped in signing.
"Urinalia; or, A treatise of the crisis hapning to the urine" has
special title page.

—[The same.] Semeiotica Uranica; or, An
astrological judgement of diseases from the decumbiture of the sick, much enlarged . . . The 3d ed. London, Nath. Brooke, 1658.
[15], 224 (i.e. 234), [12] p.   front. (port.), illus.,
plates.   17 cm.   [2999]

—Two books of physick: viz. I. Medicaments for
the poor; or, Physick for the common people . . . First
written in Latin by . . . John Prevotius . . .
Translated into English and somthing added, by
Nich. Culpeper . . . II. Health for the rich and poor,
by diet without physick. By Nich. Culpeper . . . Also
Culpepers ghost, is hereunto added; being a book of
truth, wit, and mirth. London, Peter Cole, 1656.
[22], 388 (i.e. 288) p.; [6], 41 p.; [8], 16 p.
17 cm.   [3000]
Each part has special title page.
Imperfect: sig. B (The contents; To the reader, and Mris.
Culpepers testimony) misbound before Mr. Culpeper's ghost; sig.
A (t. p. of Health for the rich and poor, and To the reader) misbound after the text of that treatise.

—, comp. See RULAND, M. [1532-1602] Experimental physick. 1662.

—, ed. See [MOREL, P.] The expert doctors dispensatory. 1657.

—, *ed.* and *tr. See* GALENUS. Galens art of physick. 1652.

—, *tr. See* JONSTONUS, J. The idea of practical physick. 1657, 1661; PARTLIZ, S. A new method of physick. 1654; RIOLAN, J. [1580–1657] A sure guide. 1657, 1665, 1671; RIVIÈRE, L. The practice of physick. 1655, 1658–61, 1672, 1678; SENNERT, D. Practical physick. 1679 [and] Two treatises. 1660; VESLING, J. The anatomy of the body of man. 1653, 1677.

—*See* BARTHOLIN, T. Anatomia. 1665, 1668; [GADBURY, J.] Philastrogus knavery epitomized. 1652; PLATTER, F. [1536–1614] A golden practice of physick. 1662; [PREVOST, J.] Medicaments for the poor. 1662, 1670.

—*as subject. See* THE COMPLEAT MIDWIFE'S PRACTICE ENLARGED. 1663, 1697, 1698; MACKAILE, M. Moffetwell. 1664.

CULPEPER revived from the grave. 1655. *See* PHILARETES, T. T. S.

CUMANUS, MARCELLUS. Curationes et observationes medicae. Nunc primum editae e bibliotheca Georgi Hieronymi Velschii, c. ejusdem notis.

[25]–89, [12] p., part [1] 20 cm. (*In* Welsch, Georg Hieronymus. Sylloge curationum. Aug. Vindel., 1667)   **[3001]**
Half title.

—Another issue, dated 1668.   **[3002]**

CUMMIUS, ALHARDUS HERMANNUS [*fl.* 1664] *respondent. See* ROLFINCK, W., *praeses.* Disputationem hanc inauguralem de partu difficili . . . ventilandam dabit A. H. C. 1664; *See* SCHENCK, J. T., *praeses.* Dissertatio medica de conceptione. 1664.

CUMMIUS, JOHANNES CHILIANUS [*b.* 1663] *respondent. See* CRAUSE, R. W., *praeses.* Disputatio medica inauguralis de delirio in genere. 1686.

—*See* WEDEL, G. W. Propempticon inaugurale de hyperico mystico. 1686.

CUNAEUS. *See* KEIL, Andreas von [*fl.* 1665–1688]

CUNELIUS, GEORGE [*d.* 1595] De dracunculis. *In* Welsch, G. H. Exercitatio de vena medinensi. 1674.

CUNEUS. *See* KEIL, Andreas von [*fl.* 1665–1688]

CUNISIUS, MICHAEL FRIEDRICH [*b.* 1671] *respon-*

dent. See SLEVOGT, J. A., *praeses.* Disputatio inauguralis de torminibus infantium. 1695.

—*See* SLEVOGT, J. A. Decani Facultatis Medicae Jo. Hadriani Slevogtii . . . prolusio inauguralis qua ostenditur nucem methel Avicennae esse daturam modernorum. 1695.

CUNITIUS, HENRICUS. *See* CUNITZ, Heinrich [*fl.* 1599–1625]

CUNITZ, HEINRICH [*fl.* 1599–1625] Kurtzer und trewer Bericht von zweyen spiritualischen und hochbewerten newen Gifft Artzneyen; nemblich; einem astralischen bezoärtischen Gifft Extract: und gleichem Gifft Saltz . . . Sambt einem astralischen kurtzen Rahtschlag: wie Arme und Reiche dieser Pestilentz Seuch . . . nützlich begegnen soll . . . [Lignitz, 1625]

[100] p.   19 cm.   **[3003]**

—, *respondent. See* MÖLLER, S., *praeses.* Themata de dysenteria. 1607.

CUNRAD, CHRISTIAN [1608–1671] *tr. See* BIBLE. O. T. Psalm XCI. 1633.

CUNRAD, CHRISTOPH [1671–1709] *praeses.* Dissertatio medica de colica flatulenta . . . Regiomonti, Typis Teusnerianis [1698]

24 p.   20 cm.   **[3004]**
Diss.—Königsberg (D. P. Vasmar, *respondent*)

CUNRADI, CASPAR [1571–1633] Prosopographiae melicae, millenarius I [-millenar. III] In quo virorum doctrina & virtute clarissimorum vita ac fama singulis distichis utcunque delineatur . . . Francofurti, Typis Antonii Hummii, impensis Martini Gnisen & Davidis Molleri, 1615–1621.

3 v. in 1.   17 cm.   **[3005]**
Vol. 3 has imprint: Hanoviae, Sumptibus Conradi Eifridi, 1621.

CUPIUS, JOHANNES, *tr. See* DUCHESNE, J. Spagririca. 1608.

CURÄUS, JOACHIM [1532–1573] *See* SCHOLTZ, L. Consiliorum medicinalium . . . liber singularis. 1610.

CURBO SEMMEDO, JUAN. *See* CURVO SEMMEDO, João [1635–1719]

CUREAU DE LA CHAMBRE, MARIN [1593 *or* 4–1669] L'art de connoistre les hommes. Premiere partie. Où sont contenus les discours preliminaires qui servent d'introduction à cette science ... Paris, P. Rocolet, 1659.

[16], 471, [1] p.   26 cm.   [3006]

Date altered by hand from M. DC. LIX. to M. DC. L X.

—[The same.] ... Amsterdam, Jacques Le Jeune, 1660.

[12], 278, [7] p.   14 cm.   [3007]

Engraved title page.

Imperfect: first preliminary leaf wanting.

—[The same.] ... Paris, P. Rocolet, 1661.

[8], 432, 10 p.   14 cm.   [3008]

—[English tr.] The art how to know men ... Rendred into English by John Davies ... London, Printed by T. R. for Thomas Dring, 1665.

[30], 330, [14] p.   17 cm.   [3009]

—[German tr.] Die Kunst und Art die Menschen zu erkennen ... in frantzösischer Sprach beschrieben und anjetzo ... in die Teutsche übersetzt. Franckfurt, Johann Georg Schiele, 1668.

[27], 498 p.   14 cm.   [3010]

Added engraved title page.

Last leaf (blank?) wanting.

—[Italian tr.] L'arte del conoscere gli uomini ... Transportata della lingua francese nell'italiana ... Venezia, Alvise Pavino, 1700

[24], 387, [9] p.   15 cm.   [3011]

Added engraved title page.

—Les characteres des passions ... Paris, Jacques d'Allin, 1663.

5 v.   16 cm.   [3012]

Vols. 2-4 are of the corrected second edition.

—Discours de l'amitié et de la haine qui se trouvent entre les animaux ... Paris, Claude Barbin, 1667.

[6], 248, [2] p.   19 cm.   [3013]

First preliminary leaf (blank?) wanting.

—Discours sur les principes de la chiromance ... Paris, P. Rocolet, 1653.

150, [1] p.   22 cm.   [3014]

Errata: p. [1]

—[English tr.] A discourse on the principles of chiromancy ... Englished by a person of quality. London, Printed by Tho. Newcomb, and sold by Tho. Basset, 1658.

[6], 93 p.   13 cm.   [3015]

First preliminary leaf (blank) wanting.

—Nouvelles conjectures sur la digestion ... Paris, Pierre Rocolet, 1636.

[32], 164 p.   [3016]

—Nouvelles observations et conjectures sur l'iris ... Paris, Pierre Rocolet, 1650.

[6], 340, [5] p.   illus.   25 cm.   [3017]

—[The same.] ... Paris, Jacques d'Allin, 1662.

[6], 340, [5] p.   illus.   24 cm.   [3018]

A reissue of the 1650 edition with new title page.

—Novae methodi pro explanandis Hippocrate & Aristotele specimen ... Parisiis, P. Rocolet, 1655.

[27], 158, 69 (i.e. 71) p.; [6], 43, [2] p.   25 cm.   [3019]

Errata: p. [2] at end.

Greek and Latin text of book 2 of Hippocrates' Aphorismi with commentary in Latin; Greek, Latin, and French text of book 1 of Aristotle's Physica.

—[The same.] ... Parisiis, Apud Jacobum d'Allin, 1662.

[21], 158 p.; 69 (i.e. 71), [6], 43, [2] p.   24 cm.   [3020]

Errata: p. [2] at end.

A reissue of the 1655 edition with new title page and without the author's dedicatory epistle.

—Le systeme de l'ame ... Paris, Jacques d'Allin, 1665.

[44], 554 p.   illus.   16 cm.   [3021]

—Traité de la connoissance des animaux, où tout ce qui a esté dict pour, & contre le raisonnement des bestes, est examiné ... Paris, Pierre Rocolet, 1648 [De l'imprimerie de Jacques Langlois, 1648]

[8], 30, [10], 390 (i.e. 388) p.; 80 p.   23 cm.   [3022]

Date on title page altered by hand from M.DC.XLVII to M.DC.XLVIII.

80 p. at end has caption title: Quelle est la connoissance des bestes, et jusques où elle peut aller.

—[The same.] ... Paris, Jacques d'Allin, 1662 [De l'imprimerie de Jacques Langlois, 1648]

[8], 30, [10], 390 (i.e. 388) p.   25 cm.   [3023]

A reissue of the 1648 edition with new title page and without the final tract.

—[The same.] ... Paris, Jacques d'Allin, 1664.

[56], 438, [2] p.   16 cm.   [3024]

—[English tr.] A discourse of the knowledg of beasts, wherein all that hath been said for, and against their ratiocination, is examined ... Translated into English by a person of quality. London, Printed by Tho. Newcomb for Humphrey Mosele, 1657.

[8], 304, 20 p. 17 cm. [3025]

CUREUS, Joachim. *See* Curäus, Joachim [1532-1573]

CURIE, Wilhelm [*fl.* 1699] *respondent.* Dissertatio medica inauguralis de insensibili transpiratione ... Basileae, Literis Jacobi Bertschii [1699]

[11] p. 22 cm. [3026]

Diss. — Basel.

CURIEUSE, neue, seltene, leichte, wohlfeile, gewisse, bewährte, nützliche, nöthige, ergötzliche und verwunderungswürdige Hauss-Apotheck, wie man durch seine eigene bey sich habende Mittel, als dem Blut, Urin, Hinter- und Ohren-Dreck, Speichel und andern natürlichen geringen Mitteln, seine Gesundheit erhalten ... könne ... Von einem Liebhaber der Medicin. Franckfurth am Mayn, In Verlegung Friedrich Knochens, Druckts Johannes Köllner, 1700.

[16], 395, [59] p. 17 cm. [3027]

CURIEUSES recherches sur les escholes en medecine de Paris. 1651. *See* Riolan, J. [1580-1657]

CURIO, Johannes [*d.* 1561] *ed. See* Hygieia. 1628; Regimen sanitatis Salernitanum. De conservanda bona valetudine. 1607, 1619 [and] Medicina Salernitana. 1605, 1611, 1612, 1622, 1624, 1628, 1638, [and] Schola Salernitanta. 1649, 1657, 1667, 1672, 1683.

CURIONE, Celio Augustino [1538-1567] *See* Valeriano Bolzani, G. P. Hieroglyphica. 1631. 1678.

Die CURIOSE Medicin. *See* [Tschirnhaus, E. W. von]

CURTAUDUS, Simeon [*d.* 1665?] *See* Guillemeau, C. Cani miuro; sive, Curto fustis. 1654.

CURTIUS, Alexander Carolus [*fl.* 1662-*ca.* 1665] *respondent.* Disputatio medica inauguralis, de calculo renum ac vesicae ... Lugduni Batavorum, Apud viduam & haeredes Johannes Elsevirii, 1662.

[8] p. 20 cm. [3028]

Diss. — Leyden.

CURTIUS, Joachim [*ca.* 1585-1642] *respondent. See* Crüger, B., *praeses.* Disputatio medica quinta. 1610.

CURTIUS, Matthaeus. *See* Corti, Matteo [1475-1542]

CURTIUS, Nicolaus [*d.* 1576] De medicamentis lenientibus. *In* Jessen, J. von. Adversus pestem consilium ... disputatione. 1614 [1615]

CURVO SEMMEDO, João [1635-1719] Polyanthea medicinal. Noticias galenicas, e chymicas, repartidas em tres tratados ... Lisboa, Miguel Deslandes, 1697.

[50 +], 844 p. plate, port. 31 cm. [3029]

Imperfect: plate, port., and last preliminary leaf (blank?) wanting.

—Tratado da peste ... Lisboa, João Galraõ, 1680.

[8], 54 p. 19 cm. [3030]

CURZIO, Matteo. *See* Corti, Matteo [1475-1542]

CUSAC, Louis [*fl.* 1682-1692] Reflexions sur la theorie et la pratique d'Hippocrate et de Galien. Avec la methode de guerir les malades, par les voyes de la transpiration & de l'evacuation ... Paris, L'auteur, et la veuve de Claude Thiboust et Pierre Exclassan, 1692.

[48], 284, [23] p. 16 cm. [3031]

—[The same.] ... 2. éd. Paris. L'auteur, et la veuve de Claude Thiboust et Pierre Esclassan, 1693.

[40], 284, [23] p. 15 cm. [3032]

A reissue of the 1692 edition with new title page.

—Traité de la transpiration des humeurs, qui sont les causes des maladies. Ou, La methode de guerir les malades sans le triste secours de la frequente saignée ... Paris, L'autheur, Laurent d'Houry, 1682.

[24], 276, [12] p. plates. 16 cm. [3033]

[CUSANI, Roberto, *fl.* 17th cent.] Il Galenista confuso; overo, L'arte convinta d'impostura nell'uso del salasso. Opera tradotta dal francese ... Venetia, Gian Giacomo Hertz, 1697.

[8], 180, [1] p. 18 cm. [3034]

The translator's dedicatory epistle signed: N. N.

Not translated from the French, but written in Italian by Roberto Cusani. Cf. Melzi, vol. 1, p. 436.

CUSINOTUS, Jacobus. *See* Cousinot, Jacques, *the younger.*

CUTENIUS, Matthias [*fl.* 1619] *respondent.* Themata physica de vita & morte ... Lipsiae, Excudebat Laurentius Cober, 1619.

[15] p.   19 cm.   **[3035]**
Diss.—Leipzig (P. Wilhelm, *respondent*)

CUTILLO, Lorenzo [*fl.* 1642] *ed.* and *tr. See* Mancini, J. Practica visitandi infirmos. 1642.

CUYPER, Jan Hendrik [*fl.* 1699] *respondent.* Dissertatio medica inauguralis de apoplexia ... Lugduni Batavorum, Apud Abrahamum Elzevier, 1699.

[16] p.   22 cm.   **[3036]**
Imperfect: wormholes throughout.
Diss.—Leyden.

[**CYNTHIUS,** Clemens, *fl.* 1601] Disputationes medicae de natura atque facultatibus ligni sancti nuper ut fuerunt aliqui ex Hollandia Romam delati ... Romae, Ex typographia Dominici Liliotti, 1602.

55 p.   22 cm.   **[3037]**
"Doctoris Sextilii Piccolominaei ad Corradum Arnoldum epistola in qua probat lignum Corradi esse veram, & optimam speciem ligni sancti": p. 7-11; "Doctoris Cynthii Clementis epistola apologetica ad Joannem Amodeum ...": p. [21]-55.

CYPRIAN, Abraham [*ca.* 1655-*ca.* 1730] Epistola historiam exhibens foetus humani post XXI. menses ex uteri tuba, matre salva ac superstite, excisi ... Lugduni Batavorum, Apud Jordanum Luchtmans, 1700.

[1], 94 p.   plates.   17 cm.   **[3038]**

CYPRIAN, Johann [1642-1723] *praeses.* Dissertatio physica de hominis definitione ... Lipsiae, Typis viduae Spörelianae, 1682.

[20] p.   19 cm.   **[3039]**
Diss.Leipzig (M. Goebel, *respondent*)

CYPRIANUS, Saint, Bp. of Carthage [De mortalitate. German] *In* Martinus, J. Etliche Gewissens-Fragen von der Pestilentz. 1668.

CYRANUS, *King of Persia. See* Kiranus, *King of Persia.*

CYRIAQUE DE MANGIN, Clément. *See* Henrion, Denis [*d. ca.* 1640]

CYSAT, Renward [1545-1614] *See* Nutzlicher unnd kurtzer Bericht, Regiment und Ordnung. 1611.

D

*** *Doctéur en Médecine. See* Beddevole, Dominique [1657-*ca.* 1693]

***** *Dr. in Medicine. See* Beddevole, Dominique [1657-*ca.* 1693]

*** *Dottore in Medicina. See* Beddevole, Dominique [1657-*ca.* 1693]

D***, M^r. *See* Alencé, Joachim d' [*d.* 1707?]

D*****, A. *See* Dilly, Antoine.

D., A. *See* Traité de la longue vie. 1698.

D., A.H.S.V.P.D.M., *tr. See* Bartholin, T. Anatomia. 1688.

D., C. *See* Dati, Carlo Roberto [1619-1675]

D., C.B.B.M. *See* B., C.B., *M.D.* [*fl.* 1696]

D., C.W. [*fl.* 1680] *See* Leipziger Pest-Schade. 1681.

D., G. *See* Dunn, George [*fl.* 17th cent.]

D., I.A.M. *See* A., I., M.D.

D., I. A. P. G. S. P. *See* Paëpp., Johann [*d.* 1613]

D., I.L., *ed.* and *tr. See* Hippocrates. Les Aphorismes. 1666.

D., J. *See* Davies, John [1625-1693]

D., J. *gent. See* A memorial for the learned. 1686.

D., J.C.M. *See* Cortnumm, Justus [*ca.* 1624-1675]

D., J.M.C. *See* Crull, Jodocus [*d.* 1713?]

D., J.P.W. *See* Wurfbain, Johann Paul [1655-1711]

D., L. *See* Culpeper, N. Arts master-piece. 1660.

D., M. J. [*fl.* 1659] *See* Glauber, J. R. Opera chymica. 1658-59.

D., N., *B. P., tr. See* Sennert, D. The institutions or fundamentals ... of physick and chirurgery. 1656?

D., N.E.D.E.D.F.M. *See* Félis, D. [*fl.* 1622-1645]

D., P. *See* DALICOURT, Pierre [*fl.* 1666–1668]

D., P., *tr.* *See* DAELMANS, G. Die neu abgefaste Heyl-Kunst, auff den Grund Alcali und Acidi erbauet. 1694.

D., P. V., *medical doctor.* *See* CRAANEN, T. Observationes. 1687.

D., R.G.M. *See* GOCLENIUS, Rudolph [1572–1621]

D., T. *See* [DUGARD, S.] The marriages of cousin Germans. 1673.

D., W. *See* DUGARD, William [1606–1662]

D., W., *nobilis Scoti Doctoris Med.* *See* DAVISON, William [*ca.* 1593–*ca.* 1669]

D. A. M. D. *See* A., D. [*fl. ca.* 1685]

D. B., *gent.* *See* BOATE, Arnold [1606–1653]

D. B. S. *See* BUSSOTTI, Dionigi, *Bp. of Borgo San Sepolcro* [*d.* 1654]

D. F. C. *See* DU FOUR DE LA CRESPELIÈRE.

D.H.P.E.M. *See* HENRION, Denis [*d. ca.* 1640]

D.L.C. *See* PINSONNAT, François.

D. L. C. D. M. *See* LE CLERC, Daniel [1652–1728]

D. M. H. C. J. [*fl.* 1688] *tr.* *See* ALENCÉ, J. d'. Abhandlung dreyer ... Instrumenten. 1688 [and] Neu-erfundene mathematische Curiositäten. 1695.

DAÇA DE VALDES, BENITO. *See* DAZA DE VALDÉS, Benito [*fl.* 17th cent.]

DACHSELT, MICHAEL [*fl.* 1662] *respondent.* *See* POSNER, C., *praeses.* Diatribe physica de virunculis metallicis. 1662.

DACIER, ANDRÉ [1651–1722] *ed.* and *tr.* *See* HIPPOCRATES. [Collected works. French] Les oeuvres. 1697.

DA COSTA, CHRISTOPHORUS. *See* COSTA, Christovam da [*ca.* 1540–1599]

DAEL, SIMON THEODOR VAN [*fl.* 1698] *respondent.* Disputatio physico-medica inauguralis de coloribus tanquam signis morborum ... Trajecti ad Rhenum, Ex officina Francisci Halma, 1698.

15, [5] p.   19 cm.   **[3040]**
Diss.—Utrecht.

DAELMANS, GILLES [*fl. ca.* 1689] De nieuwhervormde genees-konst, gebouwt op de gronden van het alcali en acidum ... Amsterdam, Jan ten Hoorn, 1687.

[20], 164, [8] p.   16 cm.   **[3041]**

—[German tr.] Die neu abgefaste Heyl-Kunst, auff den Grund Alcali und Acidi erbauet ... Anitzo in unsere hochteutsche Sprache übersetzet durch J. B. M. & P. D. ... Franckfurt an der Oder, Johann Völcker, 1694.

[28], 196 p.   17 cm.   **[3042]**

DAGERAAD; ofte, Nieuwe opkomst der geneeskonst, in verborgen grond-regulen der nature. 1660. *See* ORTUS medicinae. [Dutch. Extracts.]

DAHLEN, LUDWIG PHILIPP VON [*fl.* 1680] *respondent.* Disputatio inauguralis medica de syncope ... Duisburgi ad Rhenum, Apud Franconem Sas, 1680.

20 p.   20 cm.   **[3043]**
Diss.—Duisburg.

DAHLSTIERNA, GUNNO [1661–1709] *praeses.* Ηλεκτρον. Dissertatione historico-physica ... tuebitur ... Andreas Eurelius ... Lipsiae, Literis Joh. Georg [1687]

[28] p.   19 cm.   **[3044]**
Diss.—Leipzig (A. Eurelius, *respondent*)

DAILLÉ, JEAN [1594–1670] Joannis Dallaei De jejuniis, et quadragesima liber. Daventriae, Typis Johannis Columbii, 1654.

[16], 776 p.   15 cm.   **[3045]**

DAILLY, PIERRE. *See* AILLY, Pierre d' [*ca.* 1620–1684]

DALE, ANTONIUS VAN [1638–1708] De oraculis ethnicorum dissertationes duae: quarum prior de ipsorum duratione ac defectu, posterior de eorundem auctoribus. Accedit et schediasma De consecrationibus ethnicis. Amstelaedami, Apud Henricum & viduam Theodori Boom, 1683.

[30], 510, [15] p.   plate.   17 cm.   **[3046]**
Added engraved title page.

DALE, SAMUEL [1659?–1739] Pharmacologia; seu, Manuductio ad materiam medicam, in qua medicamenta officinalia simplicia, hoc est mineralia, vegetabilia, animalia earumque partes in medicina officinis usitata, in methodum naturalem digesta succincte & accurate describuntur . . . Londini, Sumptibus Sam. Smith & Benj. Walford, 1693.

[57], 656, [4] p.   17 cm.   [3047]

DALECHAMPS, Claude, tr. See Galenus. [De usu partium. French.] De l'usage des parties du corps humain. 1608.

DALECHAMPS, Jacques [1513-1588] Chirurgie françoise, recueillie par M. Jacques Dalechamps . . . avec plusieurs figures des instrumens necessaires pour l' operation manuelle: et depuis augmentee d'autres annotations sur tous les chapitres. Ensemble de quelques Traictez des operations de chirurgie, facilitees & esclaircies par M. Jean Girault . . . Paris, Olivier de Varennes, 1610.

[20], 664, [28] p.   illus.   23 cm.   [3048]
"Epitome du discours faict par monsieur Riolan . . . sur la fistule du fondement, avec la figure de l' instrument par luy inventé pour tel effet . . .": p. 657-662.
Contains also a French translation of Paulus Aegineta, De chirurgia (book 6 of his De re medica) with extensive commentary by the author, based largely on the writings of Abulcasis, Aetius of Amida, Avicenna, Celsus and Hippocrates.

—Histoire generale des plantes, contenant XVIII. livres . . . Sortie latine de la bibliotheque de Me Jaques Dalechamps, puis faite françoise par Me Jean des Moulins . . . Ou sont . . . descriptes infinies plantes . . . leurs especes . . . & vertus convenables à la medecine . . . Ensemble les tables des noms en diverses langues. Tome premier [-second] Lyon, Chez les heritiers Guillaume Roville, 1615.

2 v.   illus.   38 cm.   [3049]

—[The same.] . . . Dernier ed. rev., corr., & augm. . . . Lyon, Philip. Borde, Laur. Arnaud, & Cl. Rigaud, 1653.

2 v.   illus.   39 cm.   [3050]

See Bauhin, K. Animadversiones in Historiam generalem plantarum. 1601; Chiavenna, G. A. Clavis Clavennae aperiens naturae thesaurum. 1648; Plinius Secundus, C. Naturalis historiae, tomus primus [-tertius] 1668-1669.

DALGARNO, George [1626?-1687] Didascalocophus; or, The deaf and dumb mans tutor, to which is added a Discourse of the nature and number of double consonants . . . Oxford, At the Theater, 1680.

[10], 136 (i.e. 132) p.   plate.   16 cm.   [3051]

DALHEIM, Josquin. See Dalhem, Josquin [fl. ca. 1573]

DALHEM, Josquin [fl. ca. 1573] ed. and tr. See Paracelsus. La grand chirurgie 1603, 1608.

DALIBRAY, Charles Vion, sieur de [ca. 1600-ca. 1655] See Huarte de San Juan, J. L'examen des esprits pour les sciences. 1661, 1668.

[**DALICOURT,** Pierre, fl. 1666-1668] Le bonheur de la vie; ou, Le secret de la santé, contenu en divers preceptes tirez des meilleurs livres qui en ont traitté. Paris, 1666.

[34], 94, [2] p.   port.   15 cm.   [3052]

—[The same.] Le secret de retarder la viellesse; ou, L'art de rajeûnir, & de conserver la santé, selon les maximes des plus celebres autheurs de la medecine. Paris, La veuve Gervais Alliot & Gilles Alliot, 1668.

[36], 94, [2] p.   port.   15 cm.   [3053]
A reissue of the Paris 1666 edition under new title.

DALLA CROCE, Giovanni Andrea. See Croce, Giovanni Andrea della [1514-1575]

DALLAEUS, Joannes. See Daillé, Jean [1594-1670]

DALLA FABRA, Luigi. See Fabra, Luigi dalla [1655-1723]

DALLA TORRE, Giorgio. See Torre, Giorgio dalla [1607-1688]

DALQUIÉ, François Savinien. See Alquié, François Savinien d' [fl. 17th cent.]

DALRYMPLE, Sir James, 1st Viscount Stair [1619-1695] Physiologia nova experimentalis in qua, generales notiones Aristotelis, Epicuri, & Cartesii supplentur: errores deteguntur & emendantur . . . Authore D. de Stair . . . Nuper Latinitate donata . . . Lugduni-Batavorum, Apud Cornelium Boutesteyn, 1686.

[12], 632, [4] p.   plates.   20 cm.   [3054]
Added engraved title page.

DAM, Christian Wilhelm [fl. 1683] respondent. See Thile, J., praeses. Disputatio medica de purgatorio actu. 1683.

DAMA, Bernhardus a. See Bernhardus, a Doma.

DAMASCENUS, Joannes [*d.*857] *See* Mesuë [*d.* 857]

DAMHOUDER, Joost [1507-1581] Practycke in criminele saecken ... Nut en proffytelyck, voor alle souvereins, baillius borgemeesters ende schepenen ... Item hier is noch by ghevoecht d'Ordinantie op t'stuck van de criminele justitie in des Nederlanden. Rotterdam, Jan van Waesberghe de Jonge, 1628.

 [18], 366 p.; 102 p. illus. 19 cm. **[3055]**

Engraved title page.
Part [2] has special title page.

DAMIANUS, *Saint. See* Mangin, P. Neo-panacea. 1684.

DAMMENHAN, Johann [*fl.* 1640] *respondent. See* Schlegel, P. M., *praeses.* Disputatio medica inauguralis, de ascite. 1640.

DA MONTE, Giovanni Battista. *See* Monte, Giovanni Battista da [1498-1551]

DANCKERTS, Cornelis [1561-1634] *tr. See* [Remmelin, J.] Pinax microcosmographicus. 1645, 1660.

DANCKWERTH, Christian Gottfried [*d.* 1687] Es wird gefraget: ob das Podagra zu curiren sey? Und ob zwart mit nein fast von jederman auss eingebildeten Ungrunde der Unmögligkeit, und schmertzlichen Zeugniss so vieler Patienten dennoch mit ja auss gewissen Vernufft-Gründen und unwiedersprechlicher Experientz beantwortet, auch erwiesen, und dargethan von Christian Gottfried Danckwarten ... Alten Stettin, In Verlegung des Autoris, gedruckt by Daniel Starcken, 1683.

 [3], 72 p. 19 cm. **[3056]**

DANESI, Giovanni. *See* Dantzius, Joannes [*d.* 1546]

DANIEL, *the prophet. See* [Schuts, J.] Missive, aen D. Balthazar Bekker. 1692 [and] Tweede missive aen d'Heer Balthasar Bekker. 1692.

DANIELIS, Johannes [*fl.* 1617] *respondent. See* Raida, B., *praeses.* Disputatio medica de apoplexia. 1617.

DANIUS, Donatus [*fl.* 1616] *respondent. See* Vorstius, A. E., *praeses.* Theses medicae de natura morbi. 1616.

DANTI, Ignazio [1537-1586] *ed. See* Vignola, Giacomo Barozzio, *called.* Le due regole della pro-

spettiva pratica di M. Jacomo Barozzi da Vignola. 1644.

DANTZIUS, Joannes [*d.* 1546] *tr. See* Dioscorides, Pedanius, of Anazarbos. Kräuterbuch. 1610.

DANZ VON AST, Johann. *See* Dantzius, Joannes [*d.* 1546]

DANZIUS, Joannes. *See* Dantzius, Joannes [*d.* 1546]

DAPPER, Olfert [1636-1689] *tr. See* Digby, Sir K. Dissertatio de plantarum vegetatione. 1663.

DAQUIN, Pierre [*fl.* 1673-1696] *praeses.* Quaestio medica ... An in apoplexia, praemissa venae sectione, feliciter purgatio? [Parisiis, Apud Franciscum Muguet, 1696]

 4 p. 24 cm. **[3057]**

Caption title.
Diss.—Paris (C. Dufresne, *respondent*)

DA QUINTIANO, Antonio. *See* Quintiano, Antonio da [*fl.* 1668]

DARES, Johann Christian [*fl.* 1695] *respondent. See* Limmaer, C. P., *praeses.* Disputatio physica extraordinaria de sensibus internis. 1695.

DARIOT, Claude [1533-1594] Dariotus redivivus: or, A briefe introduction conducing to the judgement of the stars. Wherein the whole art of judiciall astrologie is briefly and plainly delivered ... Written at first by Claudius Dariott, at present much inlarged ... by N[athaniel] S[park] Also hereunto is added A briefe treatise of mathematical phisick. Written by G. C. Together with divers observations both of agriculture and navigation ... by N. S. London, Andrew Kemb, 1653.

 [10], 303, [4] p. front., illus., plates, tables. 19 cm. **[3058]**

Contents.—An introduction to the judgement of the stars.—A treatise of mathematicall physick ... by G. C.—A proportionall table, for more ready and facile expediting the aequation of the planets.—A tract concerning the weather, or change of the aire ... By N. S. Items (except the first) have special title pages.

—Die gulden Arch, Schatz, und Kunst-kammer, in drey Theil underscheiden. Im ersten werden ausführlich verhandlet drey Gespräch von spargirischer Preparation und Zubereitung der Artzneyen ... Im andern und letsten Theil hat der ... Leser vieler als der fürnembsten ausserlesenisten Philosophorum, Medicorum und Spargicorum

Geschrifften und Bücher ... Durch M. Claudium Dariotum ... in frantzösischer Sprach beschrieben. Nun aber ... ins Teutsch ... ubergesetzt, durch I. A. M. D. ... Basel, In Verlegung des Authorn, 1614.

3 parts in 1 v.   illus.   22 cm.   [3059]

Parts II. and III. are reprinted from the second volume of Trissmosinus' Aureum vellus published at Basel in 1604. The whole work appeared afterwards in 1708 under the title Eröffnete Geheimnisse des Steins der Weisen. The work purports to have been written in French, but it is not mentioned by Dariot's biographers. Cf. Ferguson (A) Vol. 1, p. 198.

—, *ed.* and *tr.* See PARACELSUS. La grand chirurgie. 1603, 1608.

DARMANSON, JEAN M. [*fl.* 1680–1691] La beste degradée en machine, divisé [sic] en deux discours ... Amsterdam, L'autheur, 1691.

[22], 93 p.   17 cm.   [3060]

DARNEDDENI, ANDREAS [*fl.* 1681] *respondent.* Disputatio medica inauguralis de ileo exemplo illustrata ... Basileae, Typis Jacobi Bertschii [1681]

[18] p.   20 cm.   [3061]

Diss.—Basel.

DASSEVAEL, PIETER [*fl.* 1662] *respondent.* Disputatio medica inauguralis de dysenteria ... Trajecti ad Rhenum, Apud Theodorum ab Ackersdyck, 1662.

[8] p.   21 cm.   [3062]

Diss.—Utrecht.

DASTIN, JOHN [*fl.* 1320] Visio. *In* [COMBACH, L.] *ed.* and *tr.* Tractatus. 1647.

DATI, CARLO ROBERTO [1619–1675] *See* REDI, F. Experienze intorno alla generazione degl'insetti. 1668, 1674, 1687, 1688; [Latin tr.] 1671.

DAUSTIN, JOHN. *See* DASTIN, John [*fl.* 1320]

DAVACH DE LA RIVIÈRE, JEAN [*fl.* 1696] Le miroir des urines. Par lesquelles on voit & connoît les differens temperamens, les humeurs dominantes, les sieges & les causes des maladies ... Paris, L'auteur, la veuve Cochart, Louis Josse, 1696.

[20], 337, [3] p.   15 cm.   [3063]

—[The same.] ... 2 ed., rev. & corr. ... & augm. ... Paris, Guillaume de Luyne et Nicolas Gosselin, 1700.

[24], 341, [18] p.   16 cm.   [3064]

—Le tresor de la medecine. Contenant l'anatomie ou division des parties du corps humain, les maladies ausquelles elles sont sujettes, le regime de vivre, les remedes specifiques, & la vertu des simples pour les guerir ... la circulation du sang, les nouvelles & dernieres decouvertes, avec des observations sur l'erreur des anciens, & un traité des maladies veneriennes ... Tome premier [-second] ... Paris, L'auteur et Barthelemy Girin, 1697.

2 v.   plates.   20 cm.   [3065]

DAVIDSON, WILLIAM. *See* DAVISON, William [*ca.* 1593–*ca.* 1669]

DAVIES, JOHN [1625–1693] *tr.* See CUREAU DE LA CHAMBRE, M. The art how to know men. 1665; NAUDÉ, G. The history of magick by way of apology. 1657; RENAUDOT, E. Another collection of philosophical conferences of the French virtuosi. 1665; SANTORIO, S. Medicina statica. 1676.

DAVIES, ROBERT. *See* GERARD, J. The herball; or, Generall historie of plantes. 1633, 1636.

DAVIN, ANTOINE. Tres singulier traité de la generale et particuliere preservation, & de la vraye & asseurée curation de la peste ... Grenoble, Richard Cocson, 1629.

154, [4] p.   17 cm.   [3066]

DAVISON, WILLIAM [*ca.* 1593–*ca.* 1669] Commentariorum in ... Petri Severini Dani [i.e. Peder Sørensen] Ideam medicinae philosophicae, propediem prodituum prodromus. In quo Platonicae doctrinae explicantur fundamenta, super quae Hippocrates, Paracelsus & Severinus: nec non ex antithesi, Aristoteles & Galenus sua stabilivere dogmata. Sub finem authoris doctrina, febrium exemplo, in praxim reducitur ... Hagae-Comitis, Ex typographia Adriani Vlacq, 1660.

[8], 708 p.   plates, table.   21 cm.   [3067]

—Philosophia pyrotechnica ... Seu, curriculus chymiatricus nobilissima illa & exoptatissima medicinae parte pyrotechnica instructus ... Parisiis, Apud Joannem Bessin, 1635.

[13], 208, [24], 209–393 p.; [21], 42 p.; [4], 178, [2] p.   illus., plates.   17 cm.   [3068]

Errata: p. [179–180]

"Pars tertia curriculi chymici de vocabulis chymicae operationi inservientibus. Ex curriculo W. D. ... 1633" and "Pars quarta curriculi chymici operationes chymicas multo faciliori methodo, tenuiori sumptu ... perficere docens ... 1633" have special title pages (2d and 3d group of pagination).

— [The same.] ... Parisiis, Apud Joannem Bessin, 1642.

[12], 487 p.; 272 p. illus., plates. 17 cm.

[3069]

"Pars tertia ... 1640" (p. [1]–38) and "Pars quarta ... 1640" (p. [39]–272 at end) have special title pages.

D'AYGLUN, Henry de Rochas, *sieur. See* Rochas, Henry de [*fl.* 1619–1648]

DAZA CHACÓN, Dionisio [1510 – *ca.* 1596] Pratica, y teorica de cirugia en romance, y en latin ... Dionisio Daça Chacon ... Va enmendada en esta ultima impression de los yerros que tenian las passadas 149. Valencia, En casa de los herederos de Chrysostomo Garriz, por Bernardo Nogues, 1650.

[8], 574 p. 30 cm. [3070]

Imperfect: sig. ¶ 2–3 wrongly imposed; sig. [¶] 5–6 wanting? All leaves after sig. Aaa5 wanting. Wormholes on several pages. Part 2 wanting.

DAZA DE VALDÉS, Benito [*fl.* 17th cent.] Uso de los antoios para todo genero de vistas: En que se enseña a conocer los grados que a cada uno le faltan de su vista, y los que tienen qualesquier antojos. Y assi mismo a que tiempo se an de usar, y como se pediran en ausencia, con ostros avisos importantes, a la utilidad y conservacion de la vista ... Sevilla, Diego Perez, 1623.

[12], 99 ll. port., illus. 21 cm. [3071]

"Romance de la aparicion de nuestra Señora de la Fuensanta en la ciudad de Cordova. Compuesto por un amigo del autor": ll. [6–9]

DE aquae usu medico in febribus. 1684. *See* [Moniglia, G. A.]

DE betoverde bekker. 1691? *See* [Schuts, J.]

DE calculo humano. *See* Lister, M. Conchyliorum bivalvium utriusque aquae exercitatio anatomica tertia. 1696.

DE conservanda bona valetudine. 1607, 1619. *See* Regimen sanitatis Salernitanum.

DE cura pestilentiae. *See* Catholic Church. Province of Milan. Constitutiones, et decreta sex provincialium synodorum Mediolanensium. 1603.

DE gebannen duyvel weder geroepen. 1691? *See* [Coster, F.]

DE gravidarum, parientium et puerperarum affectibus & morbis. *See* Rummel, J. P. Opuscula chymico-magico-medica. 1635.

DE inquirenda veritate libri sex. 1690. *See* Malebranche, N.

DE la guerison des fievres par le quinquina. 1680, 1681, 1688. *See* [Monginot, F., *the younger*]

DE la transformation metallique. *See* La metallique transformation. 1618.

DE la verdadera cirugia, medicina y astrologia. 1607. *See* Barrios, J. de.

DE l'egalité des deux sexes. 1676. *See* [Poulain de la Barre, F.]

DE l'usage du caphé, du thé, et du chocolate. 1671. *See* [Dufour, P. S.]

DE magni lapidis. 1613. *See* Zetzner, L., *ed.*

DE medicamentis universalibus dissertatio. *See* Dickinson, E. Edmund Dickinson ... De chrysopoeia. 1687?

DE medicina Brasiliensi. *See* Piso, W. Historia naturalis Brasiliae. 1648.

DE naturae aliquot arcanis, sympathiis et antipathiis, insignibusque medicamentis libelli duo aurei ... Bosphori, Apud Christophorum Justinum, 1622.

[1], 252, [17] p. 14 cm. [3072]

DE occulta ... curatione ... tractatus. *See* Schmuck, M. De occulta magico-magnetica morborum quorundam curatione naturali, tractatus. 1636?, 1649.

DE onschult of zamenspraak tusschen de geesten van imandt en niemandt. 1678. *See* Boekelman, A.

DE pest, naaukeurig onderzocht. *See* Pestbeschrijving. 1664.

DE ratione motus musculorum. 1664. *See* [Croone, W.]

DE remediis expertis liber [German] *See* [Stephanus Magnetes] Experiment Buch. 1623.

DE variolis. *See* Lister, M. Exercitatio anatomica altera. 1695.

DE viribus & usu auri & argenti, debite praeparati; das ist, Vom Nutz und Gebrauch der wahren Gold- und Silber Artzneyen, als die aus einer metallischen Form in ein würckliche Medicin gebührend und rechtmässig gebracht. Auss etlichen Autoribus, wie auch eigner Erfahrung zusammen getragen durch J. de B. Amsterdam, Aus Kosten Wilhelm Welmsonii und Leipzig by Joh. Herbord Klossen, 1699.

[46] p.   14 cm.   [3073]
Bound with Polemann, J. Novum lumen medicum. 1699.

DEANE, EDMUND [1572?-1640] Spadacrene Anglica; or, The English spaw-fountaine. Being a briefe treatise of the acide, or tart fountaine in the forest of Knaresborow, in the West-Riding of Yorkshire. As also a relation of other medicinall waters in the said forest ... London, Printed for John Grismand and sold by Richard Foster, 1626.

[4], 32 p.   20 cm.   [3074]
STC 6441.

— [The same.] Spadacrene Anglica, the English spaw; or, The glory of Knaresborough, springing from severall famous fountains there adjacent, called the vitrioll, sulphurous, and dropping wells, and also other minerall waters. Their nature, physicall use, situation, and many admirable cures being exactly exprest in the subsequent treatise of ... Dr. Dean, and the sedulous observations of ... Michael Stanhope ... Wherein it is proved ... that the vitrioline fountain is equall (and not inferiour) to the Germane spaw ... Published (with other additions) by John Taylor, apothecary in York. [York] Tho. Broad, 1649.

[6], 39 p.   18 cm.   [3075]
Dedication signed: John Taylor.
"A relation of certain particular cures" (p. 28-39) was extracted by John Taylor from Stanhope's Newes out of York-shire (London, 1626) and Cures without care (London, 1632)

—, ed. See NORTON, S. Mercurius redivivus. 1630 [and] Metamorphosis lapidum ignobilium in gemmas quasdam pretiosas. 1630 [and] Saturnus saturatus dissolutus. 1630 [and] Venus vitriolata. 1630.

DE B., J. See B., J. de

DE BOYVIN DU VAUROÜY, Henry. See BOYVIN DU VAUROÜY, Henry de [b. 1623]

DEBOZE, FRANÇOIS [fl. 1671-1683] tr. See RIVIÈRE,

L. Les observations de medecine de Lazare Riviere. 1680, 1688, 1694 [and] La pratique de medecine. 1682; SCULTETUS, J. [1595-1645] L'arcenal de chirurgie. 1672, 1674, 1675.

DECANI, JÁNOS [d. 1717] respondent. See FALCK, N. De discursu brutorum ex physicis. 1688.

DECANUS communitatis studii bonarum artium et philosophiae in Academia Lipsiensi ad auscultandam orationem, qua gratiosi medici adversus obtrectatores defenduntur, lectorem benevolum ... invitat. 1661. See UNIVERSITÄT LEIPZIG.

DECHANI, JOHANNES. See DECANI, J. [d. 1717]

DECKERS, FREDERICUS. See DEKKERS, Frederik [1648-1720]

DECLARATION du roy. 1672, 1673, 1680, 1695, 1696, 1698, 1699, 1700. See FRANCE. Sovereigns, etc. [1643-1715] (Louis XIV)

DECRETA Collegii physicorum Mediolanensium. 1645. See COLLEGIO DEI FISICI, Milan.

DECRETUM almae Universitatis Parisiensis. 1626. See UNIVERSITÉ DE PARIS.

DEDU, N. De l'ame des plantes. In Grew, N. Anatomie des plantes. 1685.

DEE, Arthur [1579-1651] Fasciculus chemicus, abstrusae Hermeticae scientiae, ingressum, progressum, coronidem, verbis apertissimis explicans ... Parisiis, Apud Nicolaum de la Vigne, 1631.

[19], 172 p.   14 cm.   [3076]

— [English tr.] Fasciculus chemicus; or, Chymical collections. Expressing the ingress, progress, and egress, of the secret Hermetick science, out of the choisest and most famous authors ... Whereunto is added, the Arcanum; or, Grand secret of Hermetick philosophy. Both made English by James Hasolle [pseud. i.e. Elias Ashmole] ... London, Printed by J. Flesher for Richard Mynne, 1650.

[52], 268 p.   front., illus.   14 cm.   [3077]
"Arcanum; or, The grand secret of Hermetick philosophy ... The work of a concealed author [i.e. Jean d'Espagnet] ... The 3d ed. amended and enl." (p. [155]-268) has special title page.

DEE, JOHN [1527-1608] Monas hieroglyphica ... mathematice, magice, cabalistice, anagogiceque, explicata ...

192–215 p., vol. 2 illus. 20 cm. (*In* Zetzner, Lazarus, *ed.* Theatrum chemicum. Argentorati, 1659–61)   [3078]

Caption title.

—, *ed. See* BACON, R. Epistola ... de secretis operibus artis et naturae. [1660]

A DEFENCE of tabacco. 1602. *See* [MARBECKE, R.]

DE FOUR, DAVID. *See* FOUR, David de [*fl.* 1675]

DEGEN, NIKOLAUS [*fl.* 1687] *respondent. See* LIMMER, C. P., *praeses.* Disputatio physica extraordinaria de natura & essentia mentis humanae. 1687.

DEGENHARD, JOHANN [*fl.* 1605–1609] *respondent. See* HORST, G. [1578–1636] *praeses.* Tractatus de scorbuto. 1609; SENNERT, D., *praeses.* De symptomatum caussis disputatio secunda. 1605.

DEGRAVERE, JULIUS. Thesaurus remediorum. A treasury of choice medicines internall and externall ... Whereunto is added, Diagnostic signs to know the temperament and constitution of each body; with a physicall dyet and select counsels for each complexion ... The 2d impression, rev., corr., and enl. ... by ... E. M. Doctor in Physick. London, Printed by G. P. [Sold by Samuel Thomson, Robert Horn, Thomas Basset, George Joyce] 1662.

[1], 46 p. 19 cm.   [3079]

DE GRAY, THOMAS. *See* DE LA GREY, Thomas.

DEHN ROTFELSER, JAKOB FRIEDRICH [*fl.* 1680] Dissertationis [sic] inauguralis chymico-medica de experimentorum chymicorum quorundam regni mineralis iniqua explicatione et applicatione ... Erfurti, Literis Groschianis [1680]

[32] p. 19 cm.   [3080]

Diss.—Erfurt (C. W. Förster, *respondent*)

DEHNE, TOBIAS [*b.* 1672] *respondent. See* CRAUSE, R. W., *praeses.* Dissertatio inauguralis medica de appetitu ventriculi depravato, in pica et malacia. 1698.

—*See* WEDEL, G. W. Propempticon inaugurale de nummis Gothicis. 1698.

DEICHMAN, WILHELM [*fl.* 1630–1631] *respondent. See* MAJUS, T., *praeses.* Disputatio medica de catarrheumatismo. 1630.

DEICHMANN, PETER [*fl.* 1695] *respondent. See* JACOBAEUS, H., *praeses.* Dissertatio medica inaguralis de febri lipyria. 1695.

DEIDIER, ANTOINE [*d.* 1746] Quaestiones medicochymico-practicae duodecim ab ... Michaele Chicoyneau [et al.] ... propositae ... pro regia chymiae professione vacante per obitum ... Arnaldi Fonsorbe ... Monspelii, Apud Honoratum Pech, 1697.

24 p. 22 cm.   [3081]

Thèse de concours—Montpellier.

—*proponent.* Quaestio medica eaque physiologica de motu musculari ... sub hac verborum serie an naturalis musculorum contractio Willisianam supponat explosionem? ... Monspelii, Apud Honoratum Pech, 1699.

[5], 9 p. 22 cm.   [3082]

Diss.—Montpellier (J. M. Brisbar, *respondent*)

DEISSLER, JOHANN PHILIPP [*fl.* 1660] *respondent. See* RAABE, J. J., *praeses.* Exercitatio medica theoricopractica. 1660.

DEKKERS, FREDERIK [1648–1720] Exercitationes medicae practicae circa medendi methodum observationibus illustratae ... Lugd. Bat. & Amst. Apud Danielem, Abrahamum & Adrianum à Gaesbeek, 1673.

[14], 693, [106] p. front. (port.) 16 cm.
                                                    [3083]

Added engraved title page.

—[The same.] Exercitationes practicae circa medendi methodum, auctoritate, ratione, observationibusve plurimis confirmatae ac figuris illustratae ... Ed. alt. priori duplo auctior. Lugduni Batavorum, Apud Cornelium Boutesteyn, Jordanum Luchtmans, 1694.

[16], 722, [29] p. plates. 21 cm.   [3084]

Added engraved title page, illustrated.
Errata: p. [29]
With this is bound Berger, J. von. De thermis Carolinis commentatio. 1709.

—*praeses.* Disputatio medica de epilepsia adultorum et insultibus infantum epilepticis ... Lugduni Batavorum, Apud Abrahamum Elzevier, 1697.

[24] p. 19 cm.   [3085]

Diss.—Leyden (J. Schmid, *respondent*)

—Disputatio medica de morbis soporosis ... Lugduni Batavorum, Apud Abrahamum Elzevier, MDC XCIXI (i.e. 1699).

[16] p. 22 cm. [3086]

Diss.—Leyden (A. Woesthoven, *respondent*)

—Dissertatio botanico-medica, de radice gin-sem, seu nisi, et chrysanthemo bidente Zeylanico acmella dicto ... Lugduni Batavorum, Apud Abrahamum Elzevier, 1700.

19, [1] p. plate. 21 cm. [3087]

Diss.—Leyden (J. F. Breyne, *respondent*)

DEKKERS, Frederik [1648-1720] *ed. See* BARBETTE, P. Medicinische, chirurgische und anatomische Schrifften. 1700 [and] Opera omnia medica et chirurgica. 1682, 1683, 1688 [and] Praxis Barbettiana. 1669, 1675, 1676, 1678, 1681, 1693; [English tr.] 1675; [French tr.] 1692.

DEKKERS, HUBERT [*fl.* 1694] *respondent.* Disputatio medica inauguralis de syncope ... Lugduni Batavorum, Apud Abrahamum Elzevier, 1694.

[24] p. 24 cm. [3088]

Diss.—Leyden.

DELABRE, JEAN CLAUDE [*fl.* 1681] *praeses.* Quaestio medica ... Suntne diuretica hycropis praecipua remedia? Parisiis, Apud Franciscum Muguet [1681]

4 p. 24 cm. [3088a]

Caption title.
Diss.—Paris (G.-E. Emmerez, *respondent*)

DE LA COUR, sieur. *See* PINSONNAT, F.

DE LA GREY, THOMAS. The compleat horseman, and expert ferrier. In two books. The first, shewing the best manner of breeding good horses ... The second, directing the most exact and approved manner how to know and cure all maladies and diseases in horses ... By Thomas de Grey ... The 3d ed. corr. with some additions. London, Printed by J. L. for Humphrey Moseley, 1656.

[31], 631 (i.e. 627), [12] p. front., illus. 19 cm. [3089]

—[The same.] ... The 4th ed. corr. with some additions. London, Printed by E. C. and A. C. for Samuel Lowndes, 1670.

[33], 583 (i.e. 554) p. illus. 21 cm. [3090]

Imperfect: front., or sig. A2 wanting?

—[The same.] ... The 5th ed. corr. with some additions. London, Printed by J. R. and R. H. for Samuel Lowndes, 1684.

[26], 224, 253, [7] p. illus. 20 cm. [3091]

DE LA PIERRE, PETRUS. *See* PETERS, Petrus [*fl.* 1679]

DELASSUS, RAYMUNDUS [*fl.* 17th cent.] *See* SÁNCHEZ, F. Opera medica. 1636.

DE LA VILLE. *See* LA VILLE, de [*fl.* 1677]

DELCAMPE. L'art de monter a cheval. Ou il est demonstré la belle methode de se pouvoir rendre bon homme de cheval. Ensemble les remedes les plus efficaces pour les maladies des chevaux ... Paris, Jacques Le Gras, 1658.

[16], 64, 264 (i.e. 380) p. plates. 17 cm. [3092]

Imperfect: leaves between sig. + Dviii and sig. A1 wanting.

DE L'ÉCLUSE, CHARLES. *See* L'ÉCLUSE, Charles de [1526-1609]

DE LEIVA Y AGUILAR, Francisco. *See* LEIVA Y AGUILAR, Francisco de.

DE LEÓN, FRANCISCO. *See* LEÓN, Francisco de [*fl.* 17th cent.]

DE LEÓN PINELO, ANTONIO RODRÍGUEZ. *See* LEÓN PINELO, Antonio Rodríguez de [*d.* 1660]

DE LERA GIL DE MURO, MATIAS. *See* LERA GIL DE MURO, MATÍAS DE [*fl.* 1657]

DELESCURE. *See* FOUQUET, M. (*de Maupeou*) *vicomtesse de Vaux.* Recueil de receptes. 1676 [and] Les remedes charitables. 1681, 1682, 1696; [Italian tr.] 1683, 1685, *ca.* 1688, 1693, 1697.

DE L'ISLE, GULIELMUS. *See* INSULANUS MENAPIUS, Gulielmus [*d.* 1556]

DELL' huomo indiviso, e nel suo tutto considerato. *See* SCARLATTINI, O. L'huomo, e sue parti figurato. 1683.

DELLA FABRA, LUIGI. *See* FABRA, Luigi dalla [1655-1723]

DELLA PORTA, GIOVANNI BATTISTA. *See* PORTA, Giovanni Battista della [1535?-1615]

DELLA TORRE, BARTOLOMEO. *See* TORRE, Bartolomeo della [*fl.* 1599-1602]

DELLON, C. *See* DELLON, Gabriel [*b. ca.* 1649]

DELLON, CHARLES. *See* DELLON, Gabriel [*b. ca.* 1649]

DELLON, GABRIEL [*b. ca.* 1649] Relation d'un voyage des Indes orientales ... Paris, Claude Barbin, 1685.

    3 parts in 1 v. 14 cm.   **[3094]**

    Parts [2] and [3] have special title pages. That to part 3 reads: Traité des maladies particulières aux pays orientaux, et dans la route, et de leurs remedes. Par M. C. D. D. E. M. [i.e. Gabriel Dellon]

  —[The same.] Nouvelle relation d'un voyage fait aux Indes orientales contenant la description des isles de Bourbon & de Madagascar, de Surate, de la côte de Malabar, de Calicut, de Tanor, de Goa, &c. Avec l'histoire des plantes & des animaux qu'on y trouve, & un Traité des maladies particulieres aux pays orientaux & dans la route, & de leurs remedes ... Amsterdam, Paul Marret, 1699.

    [15], 319 p. front., plates. 16 cm. **[3095]**

  —[Dutch tr.] Naauwkeurig verhaal van een reyse door Indien gedaen, en in 't Fransch beschreeven ... Waer by gevoegd is een Tractaat van de bysondere Ziekten, welke in d'Oostersche landen vallen, nevens derselver genees-middelen ... En vertaald door Willem Calebius. Utrecht, Johannes Ribbius, 1687.

    [4], 175 (i.e. 139), [8] p.; 19, [1] p. 19 cm.
    Part [2] has special title page. **[3096]**

  —[The same.] Aanmerkenswaardige reyse door Indien ... Amsterdam, Jan Karstens, Joannes Bloom, en Joannes Lantsmeer, 1688.

    [4], 175 (i.e. 139), [8] p.; 19, [1] p. 21 cm.
    Part [2] has special title page. **[3097]**
    A reissue with a new title page of the 1687 Utrecht edition.

DELORME, CHARLES [1584–1678] Πτελεινοδαφνεῖαι. Hoc est, Caroli Delorme Laureae Apollinares a prima ad supremam. Sive, Enneas quaestionum medicarum, pro baccal. tu licentia et doctoratu. His accesserunt varia ενδοξα, αμφιδοξα, ποράδοξα ... Parisiis, Apud Adrianum Beys, 1608.

    3 parts in 1 v. 17 cm.   **[3098]**

    Engraved title page.
    Part 2 has special title page.
    Imperfect: part containing [8], 14 p. wanting.
    Waller 2345.

  —*See* SAINT-MARTIN, M. de. Moiens faciles et éprouvés. 1682, 1683.

DELPHINUS, HIERONYMUS [*fl.* 1685] Eunuchi conjugium die Capaunen-Heyrath, hoc est scripta & judicia varia de conjugio inter eunuchum & virginem juvenculam anno M.DC.LXVI. contracto, t. t. a quibusdam supremis theologorum collegiis petita, postea hinc inde collecta ... Halae, Apud Melchiorem Oelschlägeln [1685]

    [8], 190 p. 20 cm.   **[3099]**

    Preface dated 1685.
    M. Oelschlegel died around 1643. Cf. Benzing (A.) p. 166.

DEL RIO, MARTIN ANTOINE [1551–1608] Disquisitionum magicarum libri sex ... Tomus primus [-tertius] Nunc secundis curis auctior longe, additionibus multis passim insertis: correctior quoque mendis sublatis. Moguntiae, Apud Joannem Albinum, 1603.

    3 .v. in 1. 32 cm.   **[3100]**
    Vol. 2 and 3 have half titles.

  —[The same.] ... Quibus continetur accurata curiosarum artium, et vanarum superstitionum confutatio, utilis theologis, jurisconsultis, medicis, philologis ... Moguntiae, Sumptibus Petri Henningii, 1617.

    [24], 1070 p. 25 cm.   **[3101]**

  —[The same.] ... Prodit opus ultimis curis longe accuratius ac castigatius ... Coloniae Agrippinae, Sumptibus Hermanni Demen, 1679.

    [16], 1221, [48] p. 23 cm.   **[3102]**
    Engraved title page.

  —Another issue. 22 cm.   **[3103]**
    Engraved title page lacks artist's signature; signature and catchword of sig. **2 have been omitted.

DEMOCRITUS [Letters. Greek and Latin.] *In* Lubin, E., *ed.* and *tr.* Epistolae Hippocratis, Democriti, Heracliti. 1601.

  —[French tr.] *See* HIPPOCRATES. [Epistolae. French. 1632.]

  —*See* ZACAIRE, D. Opusculum philosophiae naturalis metallorum. 1659.

DEMOCRITUS JUNIOR. *See* BURTON, Robert [1577–1640]

DEMPSTER, Thomas [1579?-1625] *See* Aldrovandi, U. Quadrupedum omnium bisulcorum historia. 1642.

DEN cleynen herbarius. 1602? 1637, 1660, 1683. *See* Jacobs, H.

DENAIS, Petrus. *See* Denaisius, Petrus [1560-1610]

DENAISIUS, Petrus [1560-1610] Apologia meri imperii, inclyto senatui civitatis spirensis in camerales competentis: ejusdemque anticrisis ad disputationem a Petro Denaisio ... contra praedictum senatum institutam, nec ita pridem in lucem emissam. Spirae Nemetum, Apud haeredes Bernhardi Albini, 1601.

    [8], 231 p. 21 cm.   **[3104]**

Bound with Guarinoni, C. De natura humana sermones. 1601.

DE NAYS, Petrus. *See* Denaisius, Petrus [1560-1610]

DENCKER, Mark Heinrich [*fl.* 1699] *respondent.* *See* Slevogt, J. A., *praes.* De crepatura viscerum. 1699.

DE NEPITA, Antonio. *See* Nepita, Antonio de [*fl.* 1668]

DENIS, J. *See* Denis, Jean Baptiste [*d.* 1704]

DENIS, Jean Baptiste [*d.* 1704] Lettre écrite a Monsieur **** par J. Denis ... Touchant une folie inveterée, qui a esté guérie depuis peu par la transfusion du sang. [Paris, Jean Cusson, 1668]

    12 p. 24 cm.   **[3105]**

Caption title.

—Recueil des memoires et conferences qui ont esté presentées a Monseigneur le Dauphin pendant l'année M.DC.LXXII [-MDCLXXIV] ... Paris, Frederic Leonard, 1672[-74]

    [8], 328 p. illus., plates. 25 cm.   **[3106]**

Made up of 12 Mémoires and 14 Conferences dated from Feb. 1, 1672 to Feb. 1, 1674.

Incomplete: the 3d plate, and all after p. 288 (Conferences 12-14) wanting.

—*See* Acton, G. Physical reflections. 1668.

DENISOT, Gérard [1521-1595] *See* Hippocrates. Aphorismi. [Adaptations, etc. Greek and Latin.] 1634.

DENISOT, Jacques [*fl.* 1634] *ed.* *See* Hippocrates. Aphorismi. Adaptations, etc. Greek and Latin. 1634.

DENIUS, Cornelius. *See* Matman, Rudolph [1566-1612]

DENSOV, Andreas [*fl.* 1629-1631] *respondent. See* Luden, L., *praes.* Disputatio physiologica de motu. 1631.

DENYAU, Alexander Michael [*fl.* 1681-1703] *praeses.* Quaestio medica ... An oculi sint pathematum idola? [Parisiis, Apud Franciscum Muguet, 1700]

    4 p. 24 cm.   **[3107]**

Caption title.
Diss. — Paris (C. Trichard, *respondent*)

DEODATUS, Alexandrus. Valetudinarium, seu, observationum, curationum, & consiliorum medicinalium satura. Lugduni Batav., Ex offic. Johan. Elsevier, 1660.

    [16], 402, [2] p. 14 cm.   **[3108]**

DEODATUS, Claudius [*fl.* 1603-1628] Pantheum hygiasticum Hippocratico-hermeticum, de hominis vita, ad centum et viginti annos salubriter producenda libris tribus distinctum ... politico-historica, & medico-spagyrica narratione exornatum ... Bruntruti, Excudebat Wilhelmus Darbellay, 1628.

    3 v. in 1. 24 cm.   **[3109]**

Imperfect: added engraved title page dated 1629 wanting?

DE PILES, Roger. *See* Piles, Roger de [1635-1709]

DEPPEE, Johann Jodocus [*fl.* 1697] *respondent.* Disputatio medica inauguralis, de febri maligna ... Erfordiae, Typis Joh. Heinr. Groschii [1697]

    24 p. 20 cm.   **[3110]**

Diss. — Erfurt.

DE PUT, Errijk. *See* Puteanus, Erycius [1574-1646]

DEREMITA DONATO. *See* Eremita, Donato d' [*fl.* 1624]

DERHAM, Samuel [1655-1689] Hydrologia philosophica; or, An account of Ilmington waters in Warwick-shire; with directions for the drinking of the same. Together with some experimental observations touching the original of compound bodies ... Oxford, Printed by Leon. Lichfield, for John Howell, 1685.

    [23], 162, [3] p. 18 cm.   **[3111]**

DE ROY, Henricus. *See* Regius, Henricus [1598-1679]

DES ... Herrn Johann Ernstens, Hertzogs zu Sachsen ... Anordnung. 1680. *See* SAXONY. Laws, statutes, etc.

DES BERGERIES, JACOB GIRARD. *See* GIRARD DES BERGERIES, Jean-Jacob [1614-1681]

DESCARTES, RENÉ [1596-1650] Opera philosophica. Ed. ult. Ab auctore recognita. [Amstelodami, Apud Johannem Jansonium juniorem, 1656]
3 v. in 1.   front. (port.), illus.   22 cm.**[3112]**
Contents. — Principia philosophiae. — Specimina philosophiae; seu, Dissertatio de methodo. — Passiones animae.

— Opera philosophica, quibus continentur Meditationes de prima philosophia, Principia philosophiae, Dissertationes de methodo, dioptrice, meteora, & tractatus De passionibus animae. His accessit nova hac editione Tractatus de homine et formatione foetus, cum notis Ludovici de la Forge, authoris vita, et in fine de quibusdam argumentis annotationes ... Francofurt ad Moenum, Sumptibus Friderici Knochii, 1692.
5 parts in 1 v.   illus.   22 cm.   **[3113]**
Each part has special title page.

[—] Discours de la methode pour bien conduire sa raison, & chercher la verité dans les sciences. Plus la dioptrique. Les meteores. Et la geometrie. Qui sont des essais de cette methode. Leyde, Jan Maire, 1637.
78, [1], 413, [34] p.   illus.   21 cm.   **[3114]**

— [The same.] ... Rev., & corr. en cette derniere ed. Paris, Theodore Girard, 1668.
[4], 413, [31] p.   illus.   23 cm.   **[3115]**
"La geometrie" is not included in this edition.

— [Latin tr.] Specimina philosophiae; seu, Dissertatio de methodo recte regendae rationis, & veritatis in scientiis investigandae: Dioptrice, et Meteora. Ex Gallico translata, & ab auctore perlecta variisque in locis emendata. Amstelodami, Apud Ludovicum Elzevirium, 1644.
[16], 331 p.   illus.   21 cm.   **[3116]**
Translated by Étienne de Courcelles.

— L'homme ... et un traitté De la formation du foetus du mesme autheur. Avec les Remarques de Louys de La Forge ... sur la Traitté d l'homme de René Descartes ... Paris, Charles Angot, 1664.
[70], 448, [8] p.   illus.   25 cm.   **[3117]**

"Version de la preface que Monsieur Schuyl a mise au devant de la version latine qu'il a faite du Traitté de l'homme de René Descartes": p. 409-448.
Edited by Claude Clerselier.

— [The same.] ... A quoy l'on a ajouté Le monde, ou Traité de la lumiere, du mesme autheur. 2. éd., rev. & corr. Paris, Theodore Girard, 1677.
[64], 511, [9] p.   illus.   25 cm.   **[3118]**

— [The same.] Les traitez de L'homme et de La formation du foetus, composez par Mr. Descartes, & mis au jour depuis sa mort, par Mr. Clerselier, Avec les Remarques de Louys de La Forge ... sur le Traité de l'homme du même auteur, & sur les figures par lui inventées. Amsterdam, Guillaume Le Jeûne, 1680.
[52], 276, [4] p.   illus.   21 cm.   **[3119]**

— [Latin tr.] De homine figuris et Latinitate donatus a Florentio Schuyl ... Lugduni Batavorum, Apud Franciscum Moyardum & Petrum Leffen, 1662.
[36], 121 (i.e. 123), [1] p.   illus.   22 cm.
                                            [3120]

— [The same.] ... Lugduni Batavorum, Ex Officina Hackiana, 1664.
[40], 121 (i.e. 123), [1] p.   illus.   21 cm.
                                            [3121]
With this are bound *his*: Musicae compendium. 1656; Tractatus de formatione foetus. 1672.

— Tractatus de formatione foetus, Gallice primum editus, nunc autem Latinitate fruens. Lugd. Batav. & Amstelod., Apud Danielem, Abrahamum & Adrianum à Gaesbeeck, 1672.
[6], 50 p.   21 cm.   **[3122]**
Bound with *his* De homine. 1664.

— Tractatus De homine, et De formatione foetus, quorum prior notis perpetuis Ludovici de La Forge ... illustratur. Amstelodami, Apud Danielem Elsevirium, 1677.
[76], 239 p.   illus.   20 cm.   **[3123]**
"Claudii Clerselier praefatio, Gallicae editioni praefixa, & in Latinum conversa": p. [5]-[70]

— [The same.] ... Amstelodami, Ex Typographia Blaviana, sumptibus Societatis, 1686.
[78], 239 p.   illus.   21 cm.   **[3124]**

— [The same.] ... Ed. nov. auct. & emend. ... Francofurti ad Moenum, Sumptibus Friderici Knochii, 1692.

[36], 188 p. illus. 23 cm. [3125]

Bound with (as issued) *his* Passiones animae. 1692.

—[Dutch tr.] De verhandeling van den mensch, en de makinge van de vrugt in 's moeders lichaam, t'zamengestelt door Renatus Des-Cartes, en na zijn dood in 't ligt gegeven door Clerzelier, met de aanteikeningen van Ludowyk de la Forge ... Uit het Latijn en Frans, in 't Nederduirs overgezet door Jacob Copper ... Leiden, Frederik Haaring, 1695.

[56], 236, 53 (i.e. 52), [28] p. illus. 20 cm.

[3126]

"Overzetting van de voor-reden die de Hr. Schuil heeft laten gaan voor de Latijnsche overzetting die hy gemaakt heeft van de Verhandeling van den mensch van R. Des-Cartes": p.[1]–[19] at end.

—Lettres ... Où sont expliquées plusieurs belles difficultez touchant ses autres ouvrages. Tome 2. Paris, Henry Le Gras, 1659.

[24], 564, [2] p. illus. 23 cm. [3127]

—Lettres ... Où sont traittées plusieurs belles questions touchant la morale, physique, medecine, & les mathematiques. Nouv. ed. Tome 1. Rev. et augm. Paris, Theodore Girard, 1663.

[24], 540 p. illus. 23 cm. [3128]

Edited by Claude Clerselier.

—[The same.] ... Paris, Charles Angot, 1666–67 [v. 1, 1667]

3 v. illus. 24 cm. [3129]

Vol. 2 dated 1666 has title: Lettres ... où sont expliquées plusieurs belles difficultez touchant ses autres ouvrages. Vol. 3 has title: Lettres ... où il répond à plusieurs difficultez qui luy ont esté proposées sur la dioptrique, la geometrie, & sur plusieurs autres sujets.

—[Latin ed.] Epistolae, partim ab auctore Latino sermone conscriptae, partim ex Gallico translatae ... Par prima [-secunda] Londini, Impensis Joh. Dunmore & Octaviani Pulleyn, 1668.

[8], 368 p.; [4], 404, [4] p. illus. 21 cm.

[3130]

Part 2 has special title page.

Part 2 is a reissue of part 2 of the edition published by Daniel Elzevir at Amsterdam, 1668. Cf. BMC.

—[The same. Selections.] *In* Beverwijk, J. van. D. D. virorum epistolae et responsa. 1665 [and] Epistolicae quaestiones, cum doctorum responsis. 1644.

—Meditationes de prima philosophia, in quibus Dei existentia, & animae humanae a corpore distinctio, demonstrantur. His adjunctae sunt variae objectiones doctorum virorum in istas de Deo & anima demonstrationes; cum responsionibus authoris. 3. ed. ... auct. & emend. Amstelodami, Apud Ludovicum Elzevirium, 1650.

[12], 191 p.; 164, 88 p. 21 cm. [3131]

Part [2] has special title page: Appendix, continens objectiones quintas & septimas in Renati Des-Cartes Meditationes ... cum ejusdem ad illas responsionibus & duabus epistolis, una ad Patrem Dinet ... altera ad D. Gisbertum Voetivum ... 1649. The Epistola ... ad ... Gisbertum Voetivum (88 p. at end) has half title.

—[French tr.] Les meditations metaphysiques ... touchant la premiere philosophie, dans lesquelles l'existence de Dieu, & la distinction réelle entre l'ame & le corps de l'homme, sont demonstrées. Traduites du latin de l'auteur par M le D. D. L. N. S. [i.e. Louis Charles d'Albert Luynes]. Et les objections faites contre ces Meditations par diverses personnes ... avec les résponses de l'auteur. Traduites par Mr C. L. R. [i.e. Claude Clerselier]. Paris, La veuve Jean Camusat, et Pierre le Petit, 1647.

[16], 606, [1] p. 24 cm.

[3132]

Without the Appendix.

—Le monde de Mr. Descartes; ou, Le traité de la lumiere, et des autres principaux objets des sens. Avec un Discours du mouvement local, & un autre Des fiévres ... Paris, Theodore Girad, 1664.

[16], 260 p.; 31 p.; 30 p. illus. 16 cm.

[3133]

Preface signed by the editor: D. R., i.e. Henry Louis de Rouvière.

—Musicae compendium. Amstelodami, Apud Joannem Janssonium Juniorem, 1656.

[4], 34 p. illus. 21 cm. [3134]

Bound with *his* De homine. 1664.

—Les passions de l'ame ... Paris, Henry Le Gras, 1649.

[47], 286 p. 16 cm. [3135]

Prefixed are two letters (by Picot? by Clerselier?) addressed to the author, with his answers.

—[Latin tr.] Passiones animae per Renatum Des Cartes: Gallice ab ipso conscriptae, nunc autem in exterorum gratiam Latina civitate donatae ab H[enry] D[esmarets] M. ... Amstelodami, Apud Ludovicum Elzevirium, 1650.

[56], 242, [13] p. 13 cm. [3136]

—[The same.] . . . Amstelodami, Ex typographia Blaviana, 1685.

[24], 92, [4] p.   21 cm.   [3137]

—[The same.] . . . Ed. nov. auct. & emend. . . . Francofurti ad Moenum, Sumptibus Frederici Knochii, 1692.

[24], 74, [6] p.   23 cm.   [3138]

With this is bound (as issued) *his* Tractatus De homine, et De formatione foetus. 1692.

—[English tr.] The passions of the soule in three books . . . Translated out of French . . . London, Printed for A. C. sold by J. Martin and J. Ridley, 1650.

[30], 173 p.   15 cm.   [3139]

—Vitae Renati Cartesii. *See* BOREL, P. Historiarum, et observationum medicophysicarum centuriae IV. 1656, 1657, 1670, 1676 [and] A summary or compendium, of the life of the most famous philosopher Renatus Descartes. 1670.

—*See* BLANKAART, S. Venus belegert en ontset. 1684, 1688, 1696; [French tr.] 1688; [German tr.] 1689; REGIUS, H. Medicinae libri IV. 1657, 1668.

—*as subject. See* ARBERIUS. La physique d'uzage. 1664; [BAILLET, A.] La vie de Mʳ Des-Cartes. 1692; BLANKAART, S. Cartesianische Academie. 1693 [and] De Kartesiaanse Academie. 1683, 1691 [and] Nauwkeurige verhandelinge van de scheur-buik en des selfs toevallen. 1684; [German tr.] 1690, 1693 [and] Die neue heutiges Tages gebräuchliche Scheide-Kunst. 1689, 1697; BOURDELOT, P. Conversations de l'Academie. 1672; BRUYN, J. de. Epistola ad . . . Isaacum Vossium. 1663; DESMARETS, S. De abusu philosophiae Cartesianae. 1670 [and] Indiculus. 1671 [and] Samuelis Maresii Clypeus orthodoxiae. 1671 [and] Vindiciae dissertationis . . . De abusu philosophiae Cartesianae. 1670; DOLÄUS, J. Encyclopaedia chirurgica rationalis. 1689, 1690, 1695 [and] Encyclopaedia, medicinae theoretico-practicae. 1684, 1686, 1688, 1690, 1691 [and] Opera omnia. 1695 [and] Systema medicinale, a compleat system of physick. 1686; CORDEMOY, L. G. de. A discourse written to a learned frier. 1670; GEULINCX, A. Annotata praecurrentia ad Renati Cartesii Principia. 1690; HERFELT, H. G. Philosophicum hominis, de corporis humani machina. 1687. LA FORGE, L. de. Traitté de l'esprit de l'homme. 1666, 1670; [Latin tr.] 1669, 1673, 1688; LE GRAND, A. An entire body of philosophy.

1694; MANSVELD, R. van. Animadversiones. 1671 [and] Specimen confutationis dissertationis. 1670 [and] Specimina bombomachiae Samuelis Maresii. 1672; Nouveau cours de medicine. 1669, 1683; OVERKAMP, H. Alle de medicinale . . . werken. 1694 [and] Nieuw gebouw der chirurgie of heel-konst. 1682; [German tr.] 1689, 1692 [and] Oeconomia animalis. 1690; PLEMP, V. F. Fundamenta medicinae ad scholae acribologiam aptata. 1654; REGIUS, H. Fundamenta physices. 1646, 1654, 1661.

DESCRITTIONE di molte virtù della terra medicinale del bagno di Nocera. Nuovamente ritrovata, & esperimentata con i segni per conoscere la megliore, affinche ogn'uno possa servirsi d'essa. Perugia, Angelo Bartoli, 1638.

Broadside. 28 x 19 cm.   [3140]

Reprinted in Annibale Camilli's Del bagno di Nocera. Perugia, 1646. p. 46-47.

Bound with Camilli, A. Del bagno di Nocera nell' Umbria. 1627.

DESCAZALS, JACQUES [*fl.* 1700] *respondent. See* HOFFMANN, F. [1600-1742] *praeses.* Dissertatio inauguralis medica de opiatorum nova eaque mechanica operandi ratione. 1700.

DES COMTES. *See* CONTI, Lodovico [17th cent.]

DESCRIPTION anatomique de divers animaux dissequez dans l'Academie royale des sciences. 1682. *See* [PERRAULT, C.]

DESCRIPTION anatomique d'un cameleon. 1669. *See* [PERRAULT, C.]

The **DESCRIPTION** and use of the double horizontall dyall. *See* [LEURECHON, J.] Mathematicall recreations. 1653.

DESCRIPTION generale de l'hostel royal des Invalides établi par Louis le Grand. 1683. *See* [LE JEUNE DE BOULENCOURT]

DESFOURNELLES. *See* CORDEMOY, Louis Géraud de [1626-1684]

DESGORRIS, JEAN. *See* GORRIS, Jean de [*fl.* 1572-1622]

DESHAIES-GENDRON, CLAUDE [*ca.* 1663-1750] Recherches sur la nature et la guerison des cancers. Paris, André Cramoisy, 1700.

[12], 155, [1] p.   17 cm.   [3141]

DES INNOCENS, Guillaume [*d. ca.* 1610] Osteologie; ou, Histoire generalle des os du corps humain . . . Bourdeaus, Par Simon Millanges, 1604.

[24], 543, [17] p.   18 cm.   [**3142**]

DESLER, Michael [*fl.* 1657] *respondent. See* Frimel, J., *praeses.* Disputationem physicam de aqua . . . publice sistunt . . . 1657.

DESMARETS, Henri, *tr. See* Descartes, R. Passiones animae. 1650, 1685, 1692.

DESMARETS, Samuel [1599–1673] Samuelis Maresii Clypeus orthodoxiae; sive, Vindiciarum suarum priorum pro sua dissertatione De abusu philosophiae Cartesianae in rebus theologicis & fidei, oppositarum cujusdam personati Petri ab Andlo [pseud. i.e. Regner van Mansveld] . . . convicioso & famoso specimini, vindiciae posteriores, ejusdem, tenebrionis heterodoxi novis Animadversionibus injuriosis & insulsis, refutandis destinatae. Groningae, Apud Tierck Everts, 1671.

[4], 80 p.   20 cm.   [**3143**]

—Samuelis Maresii De abusu philosophiae Cartesianae, surrepente & vitando in rebus theologicis & fidei, dissertatio theologica. Groningae, Apud Tierck Everts [Typis Henrici Cornelii Roosingh] 1670.

[12], 115, [1] p.   20 cm.   [**3144**]

—Indiculus praecipuarum controversiarum theologicarum, quas D. Samueli Maresio, insistenti receptis hactenus inter reformatos sententiis, ultro movit . . . Christ. Wittichius . . . tam in suis reprehensionibus continuis per plures annos repetitis & dictatis ad illius systema, quam in grandi suo opere nupero illis propugnandis destinatio, quod inscripsit Theologiam pacificam . . . Groningae, Typis Remberti Huysman, 1671.

[28], 55 p.   20 cm.   [**3145**]

—Samuelis Maresii Vindiciae dissertationis suae nuperae, De abusu philosophiae Cartesianae surrepente in rebus theologicis et fidei; oppositae ejus ineptissimae confutationi quae recens prodiit sub fictitio nomine Petri ab Andlo [pseud. i.e. Regner van Mansveld] . . . Groningae, Apud Tierck Everts [Typis Henrici Roosingh] 1670.

67, [1] p.   20 cm.   [**3146**]

—*See* Mansveld, R. van. Animadversiones. 1671 [and] Specimen confutationis dissertationis. 1670

[and] Specimina bombomachiae Samuelis Maresii. 1672.

DES MARETZ, Samuel Nicolaus [*fl.* 1688] *respondent.* Disputatio medica inauguralis de peripneumonia vera . . . Lugduni Batavorum, Apud Abrahamum Elzevier, 1688.

[32] p.   21 cm.   [**3147**]

Diss. — Leyden.

DESMOULINS, Jean [1530–1620?] *tr. See* Dalechamps, J. Histoire generale des plantes. 1615, 1653.

Den DESOLATEN boedel der medicinje deses tijds: Uytgesproocken van een Doctor over 't pesthuys, en een Apotheeker in 't gasthuys . . . 2. druck merckelijk verm., en van veel fauten verb. Amsterdam, Pieter Schijn [1677]

31 p.; 14 p.   16 cm.   [**3148**]

Part [2] has special title page.

—[The same.] Amsterdam, Pieter Schijn [1677?]

29 p.; 14 p.   15 cm.   [**3149**]

DESPOTICO CALATHINO, *See* Panaroli, Domenico [1587–1657]

DESPOTINUS, Gaspar [*fl.* 1613] Hirci mulctra. De sanguinis missione in quadam febre quotidiana continua, disceptatio medica. Cantabrigiae, Excudebat Cantrellus Legg, 1613.

[4], 52 p.   19 cm.   [**3150**]

STC 6786.

DESPRES, Jason. *See* Pratensis, Jason [1486–1558]

DES PREZ, Jacques [*fl.* 1677–1695] *praeses.* Quaestio medica . . . An praecavendis morbis ex humorum viscida congerie oriundis, balneum tepidum ex aqua dulci? [Parisiis, Apud Franciscum Muguet, 1691]

4 p.   25 cm.   [**3151**]

Caption title.

Diss. — Paris (P. de Toullieu, *respondent*)

—*respondent. See* Thomasseau, J., *praeses.* Quaestio medica . . . Est-ne uterus pars ad vitam necessaria? 1677.

DESROY, Henry. *See* Regius, Henricus [1598–1679]

DESS Raths zu Dressden Ordnung. 1680. *See*
DRESDEN. Rat. Ordinances, local laws, etc.

DESSE [*fl.* 1690] Traité de la veritable connoissance des fiévres continuës, intermittentes,
pourprées, pestilentielles & de la peste ... Et quelques observations necessaires sur l'usage de la
saignée, des purgatifs ... avec un traité des flux de
ventre ... Paris, Robert Pepie, 1691.

    [12], 308, [16] p.   17 cm.   **[3152]**

DES TRAPIÈRES [17th cent.] *See* BOURDELOT, P.
Recherches et observations sur les viperes. 1671.

DESVIOS de la naturaleza. 1695. *See* RIVILLA
BONET Y PUEYO, J. de.

A DETECTION of some faults in unskillful physitians. *See* Recorde, R. The urinal of physick. 1651,
1665.

DETHARDING, GEORG [*b.* 1645] *See* BACMEISTER,
J. Programma. 1667.

DETHARDING, GEORG [1671–1747] *praeses.* Exercitatio anatomico-physiologica de fontanella infantum ... [Altdorffii] Literis Kohlesianis [1695]

    16 p.   20 cm.   **[3153]**
    Diss.—Altdorf (U. S. Nimptsch, *respondent*)

—*respondent.* Disputatio medica inauguralis de
calculis microcosmi ... [Altdorffii] Typis Kohlesianis
[1693]

    31 p.   20 cm.   **[3154]**
    Diss.—Altdorf.

DEUBLINGER, DIETRICH OTTO [*fl.* 1688] *praeses.*
Exercitatio philosophica de signis vultus & frontis
humanae, utrum ex iis affectiones atque inclina-
tiones, moresve hominum dignosci valeant? ...
[Regiomonti] Typis Reusnerianis [1688]

    [8] p.   19 cm.   **[3155]**
    Diss.—Königsberg (G. Frölich, *respondent*)

DEUSING, ANTON [1612–1666] Anatome parvorum
naturalium; seu, Exercitationes anatomicae ac
physiologicae, de partibus humani corporis conser-
vationi specierum inservientibus. Groningae, Ex officina Johannis Sas, 1651.

    [8], 139, [1] p. 20 cm.   **[3156]**

—Consideratio physico anatomica foetus
Mussipontani, extra uterum, in abdomine detenti,
tandemque lapidescentis. *In* Historia foetus
Mussipontani. 1669; Sinibaldi, G. B. Geneanthropeiae, 1669.

—De anima humana dissertationes philosophicae.
Quibus adjectae ejusdem Familiares & amicae disquisitiones epistolares, habitae cum ... Joanne
Santeno ... de origine formarum naturalium, &
animae humanae substantia. Accessit Spongia adversus cavillationes quasdam, sub selecta disputatione
philosophico-theologica, in animae humanae
substantiam egestas. Hardervici, Ex officina Nicolai
à Wieringen, 1645.

    [12], 296 p. 19 cm.   **[3157]**

—De motu cordis et sanguinis itemque De lacte
ac nutrimento foetus in utero, dissertationes.
Publicae ventilationi submissae in ... Groningae &
Omlandiae Academia. Accessere disquisitiones &
dissertationes variae ... Groningae, Apud Franciscum Bronckhorst, 1655.

    [42], 719, [1] p. 14 cm.   **[3158]**
    "Objectiones ... Joannis Andreae Schmitz ... adversus disser-
tationem A. Deusingii De lacte": p. 442–446; — "Joh. Antonidae
van der Linden ... Dissertatio de lacte": p. 557–584; — "Hermanni
Conringii ... Exercitatio physiologica de lacte": p. 585–621.

—Deusingius heautontimorumenos; sive, Episto-
lae selectae eruditorum ... Ex autographis edente
Benedicto Blottesandaeo [pseud. i.e. Oluf Borch]
Hamburgi, Typis Nicolai Molybdii, 1661.

    [10], 48 p. 20 cm.   **[3159]**

—Disquisitio anti-Sylviana de motu cordis et
arteriarum. Qua ... Francisci Sylvii [i.e. Frans de
Le Boë] ... ineptiae & nugae ad libellam veritatis
expenduntur, excutiuntur, ac refutantur. Groningae,
Typis Francisci Bronchorstii, 1663.

    [12], 204 p. 13 cm.   **[3160]**
    Bound with copy 2 of *his* Sylva-caedua cadens. 1664.

—Disquisitio gemina de peste prior an contagiosa
pestis sit? Altera an vitanda? Et quomodo illaesa
charitate? Publice habitae in Academia Groningae
& Omlandiae, 11. & 12. Sept. 1656. Groningae, Typis
Francisci Bronchorstii, 1656.

    xviii, 93 p. 15 cm.   **[3161]**
    Issued also as part [2] of *his* Tractatus de peste. Groningae, 1658.

—Dissertatio de morborum quorundam
superstitiosa origine & curatione: speciatim de morbo Man-Slacht vulgo dicto: itemque De lycanthropia.
Nec non De surdis ab ortu; mutisque ac illorum
cognitione: ubi & De ratione et loquela brutorum

animantium. Groningae, Typis Johannis Cöllen, 1656.

227 p. 14 cm. [3162]

—Exercitationes de motu animalium ubi de motu musculorum & respiratione; itemque De sensuum functionibus ubi & de appetitu sensitivo, et affectibus. Groningae, Typis Francisci Bronchorstii, 1661.

[14], 319 p. 13 cm. [3163]

—Erercitationes [sic] physico-anatomicae, de nutrimenti in corpore elaboratione. Ubi De chylificatione, & chyli motu; sanguificatione; depuratione alimenti; itemque spiritibus. Quibus adjecta Appendix, in qua examini ac judicio aliorum subjiciuntur varia de chyli motu, & nutrimenti in corpore elaboratione, nec non De admiranda anatome ... Ludovici de Bils. Groningae, Typis Francisci Bronchorsti, 1660.

[10], 368 p. 13 cm. [3164]

—Exercitationes physico-anatomicae de nutrimento animalium ultimo. Ubi De sanguinis usu, ac Commento nutritii succi per nervos influentis. Accessit Dissertatio epistolica de hepatis officio, ad ... Thomam Bartholinum ... Groningae, Typis Francisci Bronchorstii, 1661.

[12], 257 (i.e. 357) p. 14 cm. [3165]
—Copy 2.
With this is bound (as issued?) *his* Appendix ad Dissertationem de hepatis officio. 1661.

—Appendix ad Dissertationem de hepatis officio; seu, Vinciciae hepatis redivivi, leni correctione tangentes sequiorem interpretationem ... J. van Horne ... Groningae, Typis Francisci Bronchorstii, 1661.

40 p. 14 cm. [3166]
Bound with (as issued?) copy 2 of *his* Exercitationes physico-anatomicae de nutrimento animalium ultimo. 1661.

—Fasciculus dissertationum selectarum, ab autore collectarum ac recognitarum: cum auctario ... Groningae, Typis Johannis Cölleni, 1660.

27, [1], 644 p. 14 cm. [3167]
—Copy 2.
With this are bound: Schoock, M. Tractatus de butyro. 1664. — Santorio, S. De statica medicina. 1664.

—Foetus Mussipontani, extra uterum in abdomine geniti, secundinae detectae: quibus multa naturae admiranda & abstrusa in lucem eruuntur. Accessit Historia partus infelicis: quo gemellorum ex utero

in abdominis cavum elapsorum, ossa sensim, multis annis post, per abdomen ipsum in lucem prodierunt ... Groningae, Typis Joannis Draper, 1662.

312, [2 +] p. 14 cm. [3168]
Imperfect: all pages after p. [314] wanting.
With this is bound Eyssonius, H. Dissertatio medica de foetu lapidefacto. 1661.

—[The same. Excerpts.] *In* Historia foetus Musipontani. 1669; Sinibaldi, G. B. Geneanthropeiae. 1669.

—Genesis microcosmi; seu, De generatione foetus in utero dissertatio. Accesserunt Curae secundae de generatione & nutritione ... Amstelodami, Apud Petrum van den Berge, 1665.

[20], 332, [1] p. 14 cm. [3169]
Errata: p. [333]

—Historia foetus extra uterum in abdomine geniti, ibidemque per sex prope lustra detenti, ac tandem lapidescentis: consideratione physico-anatomica illustrata ... Groningae, Typis Johannis Cölleni, 1661.

166, [1] p. 14 cm. [3170]

—Idea fabricae corporis humani; seu, Institutiones anatomicae ad circulationem sanguinis, aliaque recentiorum inventa, accommodatae. Groningae, Typis Francisci Bronchorstii, 1659.

[24], 552 p. 14 cm. [3171]
Imperfect: title page mutilated.

—In Sylvam echo; seu, Sylvius heautontimoroumenos. Cum appendice De bilis & hepatis usu: itemque Exercitatione utrum medicina sit scientia, an ars; Sylvianae vitilitigationi opposita. Groningae, Typis Johannis Cölleni, 1663.

470 p. 13 cm. [3172]
Concerns controversy with Sylvius, i.e. Frans de Le Boë.

—Oratio panegyrica de felicitate sapientium. *In* Avicenna. Canticum principis ... de medicina. 1649.

—Resurrectio hepatis asserta; contra socium larvatum Vincentium Slegelium, sub personati Blottesandaei [pseud. i.e. Oluf Borch] cohorte furiosa signiferum. Accessit Disquisitio ulterior, de chyli motu atque officio hepatis ... Groningae, Typis Francisci Bronchorstii, 1662.

[48], 336 p. 15 cm. [3173]

—Sylva-caedua cadens; seu, Disquisitiones anti-Sylvianae de alimenti assumpti elaboratione &

distributione. Quarum Iª. De alimentorum fermentatione in ventriculo. IIª. De chyli a faecibus alvinis secretione ... IIIª. De chyli mutatione in sanguinem; ac circulari sanguinis motu. Praemissa est Praefatio causas Sylviani in Deusingium furoris nude repraesentans; simulque Sylvium injuriosum aggressorem evidenter demonstrans. Groningae, Typis Francisci Bronchorstii, 1664.

[56], 272 p. 13 cm. [3174]

Concerns controversy with Franciscus Sylvius i.e. Frans de Le Boë.

— Copy 2.

With this is bound *his* Disquisitio anti-Sylviana de motu cordis. 1663.

— Sylva-caedua jacens; seu, Disquisitiones anti-sylvianae ulteriores. Quarum I. De spirituum animalium genesi, motu, & usu. II. De usu lienis & glandularum. Addita est Dissertatio de natura. Groningae, Typis Johannis Cöllenii, 1665.

[16], 367, [1] p. 14 cm. [3175]

Concerns controversy with Sylvius, i.e. Frans de Le Boë.

— Sympathetici pulveris examen: quo superstitiosa ac fraudibus cacodaemonis implicita vulnerum et ulcerum curatio in distans, per rationis trutinam, ad ipsas naturae leges expenditur; subversis curae sympatheticae fundamentis, ab illustriss. Comite Digbaeo, nec non D. D. Papinio, & Mohyo, positis ... Groningae, Typis Johannis Cöllenii, 1662.

[12], 660 p. 14 cm. [3176]

The works by Digby, Papin and Mohy had been printed in Nuremberg in 1660 in a collection entitled Theatrum sympatheticum.

— Tractatus de peste publice expositus in Academia Groningae & Omlandiae sub anni 1656 fine, et sequentis initio. Additae sunt ejusdem Disquisitiones de pestis contagio & devitatione. Groningae, Typis F. Bronchorstii, 1658.

[20], 459, [1] p.; xviii, 93 p. 14 cm. [3177]

Part [2] has special title page: Disquisitio gemina de peste prior an contagiosa pestis sit? ... 1656.

— Twee diepzinnige en heilzame onderzoekingen nopende de pest, waer van de eerste handelt of de pest ook bersmettelijk zy? De tweede of? en op wat wijze de zelve, zonder evenwel de liefde tot zijnen evennaesten te krenken, te schuwen zy? ... Amsterdam, Abraham Witteling, 1664.

63, [1] p. 16 cm. [3178]

Bound with (as issued?) Pest-beschrijving. 1664.

— Vindiciae foetus extra uterum geniti ... fasciculo dissertationum selectarum comprehensorum, De unicornu, lapide bezaar, manna ... ut & aliquarum Elegantiarum philologicarum examen ... Groningae, Typis Johannis Cöllenii, 1664.

[20], 362, [1] p. 13 cm. [3179]

"... Vindiciae aliorum quorundam suorum scriptorum, de unicornu, lapide bezar, manna ... contra ejusdem Bernhardi a Dom a furiosos insultus" (p. 213-314) has half title.

"... Elegantiarum philologicarum examen; seu, Calonum caterva disjecta: cujus antesignanus Antonius Rosinus personatus" (p. 315-362) has half title.

Errata: p. [1] at end.

Bound with Plazzoni, F. De partibus generationi inservientibus. 1664.

— Vindiciae foetus extra uterum geniti. Contra tenebrionem Bernhardum a Doma. *In* Historia foetus Mussipontani. 1669; Sinibaldi, G. B. Geneanthropeiae. 1669.

Dissertations — Groningen

— *praeses*. Idea doctrinae de febribus breviter, perspicue, ac methodice proposita, publicaeque ventilationi submissa, in ... Academia Groningae & Omlandiae ... Groningae, Typis viduae Edzardi Agricolae, 1655.

[19], 288 p. table. 14 cm. [3180]

Contains 10 Groningen dissertations by 3 respondents: A. Berckhuys, N. Prickius, M. Truyck.

— Synopsis medicinae universalis, seu Compendium institutionum medicarum. Publicis disputationibus exhibitum ac ventilatum in provinciali Groningae & Omlandiae Academia ... Groningae, Typis Joannis Nicolai, 1649.

[24], 508, [3] p. 14 cm. [3181]

Contains 24 Groningen dissertations by 6 authors: H. Busz, E. Engelen, J. Groene-Wolt, J. Sicman, D. Stoll, H. J. Wuysthaus.

Bound with (as issued?) Avicenna. Canticum principis ... de medicina. 1649.

— Disputationum anatomicarum tertia, de membranis in genere, ac speciatim de membrana carnosa, ac musculorum propria ... [Groningae? 1652?]

[8] p. 18 cm. [3182]

Signature: C⁴.

Caption title.

Imperfect:? Title page and all after p. [8] wanting?

M. Truyck, *respondent*.

— Disputationum anatomicarum quarta, de peritonaeo, omento, mesenterio, & pancreate ... Groningae, Ex officina Edzardi Agricolae, 1652.

[10] p. 19 cm.   [**3183**]
Signatures: [A]¹, D⁴.
M. Truyck, *respondent*.

—Disputationum anatomicarum quinta, de ventriculo, oesophago, & intestinis . . . Groningae, Ex
officina Edzardi Agricolae, 1652.
[12] p. 18 cm.   [**3184**]
Signature: [A]¹, E⁴, F¹.
A. Berckhuys, *respondent*.

—Disputationum anatomicarum octava, de par-
tibus genitalibus utrique sexui communibus . . .
Groningae, Typis Edzardi Agricolae, 1652.
[12] p. 18 cm.   [**3185**]
Signatures: [A]¹, I⁴, K¹.
S. Fridenrychius, *respondent*.

—Disputationum anatomicarum nona, de partibus
genitalibus itrivis sexui propriis . . . Groningae,
Typis Edzardi Agricolae, 1652.
[15] p. 19 cm.   [**3186**]
Signatures: K⁴, L⁴.
J. C. Agricola, *respondent*.

— , tr. See AVICENNA. Canticum principis . . . de
medicina. 1649.

—See COLLECTANEA DE DIUTURNA GRAVIDITATE.
1662; PEST-BESCHRIJVING. 1664; STRAUSS, L. Resolutio
casus Mussipontani foetus extra uterum in abdomine
retenti. 1662.

—as subject. See DIGBY, Sir K. Demonstratio im-
mortalitatis animae rationalis. 1664; LE BOË, F. de
Disputationum medicarum decas. 1674; RALL, G. F.
De generatione animalium. 1669; STENO, N., Bp.
Observationes anatomicae. 1662, 1680.

DEUTGEN, JOHANN THEODOR [*fl.* 1697] *respondent. See* WEDEL, G. W., *praeses*. Exercitationum
pathologico-therapeuticarum disputatio X de laesionibus motus. 1697.

**DEUTSCHE AKADEMIE DER NATUR-
FORSCHER LEOPOLDINA.** *See* ACADEMIA
NATURAE CURIOSORUM.

DEUX traitez nouveaux sur la philosophie
naturelle, contenant Le tombeau de Semiramis
nouvellement ouvert aux sages, et La refutation de
l'anonyme Pantaleon [pseud. i.e. Franz Gassmann],

soy disant disciple d'Hermes. Paris, Laurent
d'Houry, 1689.
84 p. 15 cm.   [**3187**]

DE VAUCOULEURS, MATTHAEUS MAHEULT.
See MAHEULT, Mathieu [1630-1700]

[**DEVAUX,** JEAN, 1649-1729] Le medecin de soi-
meme; ou, L'art de se conserver la santé par l'instinct.
Leyde, Chez de Graef, pour l'autheur, 1682.
[14], 294 p. plate. 14 cm.   [**3188**]

[—] [The same.] . . . 3. ed. Leyde, Claude Jordan, 1687.
[6], 280 p. 15 cm.   [**3189**]

[—] [The same.] . . . La Haye, Meyndert Uytwerf, 1699.
[II], 316, [4] p. front. 14 cm.   [**3190**]

—, tr. See BONTEKOE, C. Nouveaux elemens de
medecine. 1698.

—See [PINSONNAT, F.] Regime de santé. 1686.

DEVILLE, JEAN BAPTISTE. *See* HISTOIRE DES
PLANTES DE L'EUROPE. 1680, 1689.

DEVILLE, NICOLAS. *See* HISTOIRE DES PLANTES
DE L'EUROPE. 1680, 1689.

DE VITO, JOANNES. *See* VITO, Giovanni de [*fl.*
1602]

DEXBACH, AEGIDIUS [*fl.* 1665] *respondent*. Disputatio inauguralis medica de affectione hypochondriaca . . . Basileae, Typis Joh. Jacobi Deckeri [1665]
[8] p. 20 cm.   [**3191**]
Diss. — Basel.

DEXBACH, JOHANN GEORG [*fl.* 1696-1700]
respondent. See NEBEL, D., *praeses*. Exercitationum
anatomicarum prima. 1696.

DEZIUS, ZACHRIAS [*fl.* 1669] *respondent. See*
JENICHEN, G. F., *praeses*. Disputatio physica de
genesimantia. 1699.

A DIALOGUE between an East-Indian . . . and
a French gentleman. *See* TRYON, T.

A DIALOGUE between Philiater and Momus,
concerning a late scandalous pamphlet called The
conclave of physicians . . . London, Walter Kettilby,
1686.
[I], 226 p. 17 cm.   [**3192**]

A DIALOGUE betwixt a citizen, and a poore countrey-man. 1636. *See* BREWER, T.

DIALOGUES de la santé. 1683, 1684. *See* [FRÉMONT D'ABLANCOURT, N.]

DIAZ, FRANCISCO [*ca.* 1510-1590] Tratado nuevamente impresso, de todas las enfermedades de los riñones, vexiga, y carnosidades de la verga, y urina, y de su cura, dividido en tres libros ... Madrid, Carlos Sanches, 1643.

    [4], 11-194, [10] p. illus. 29 cm.   **[3193]**

Signatures: [2R]⁵, 2S-3E⁸, 3F², 3G¹.
Identical in contents with the edition published in 1588.
Palau y Dulcet 72124a.

DIAZ, FROILÁN. *See* DÍAZ DE LOS LLANOS, Froilán [*d.* 1709]

DÍAZ DE LOS LLANOS, FROILÁN [*d.* 1709] De generatione, et corruptione tractatus per quaestiones, et articulos divisus juxta mentem ang. doct. D. Thom. in duos libros Arist. De ortu, & interitu. Authore ... Fr. Froylano Diaz de Llanos ... Vallis Oleti, Ex typographia regia Josephi de Rueda, 1699.

    [16], 392, [4] p. 21 cm.   **[3194]**

DI CAPUA, LEONARDO. *See* CAPOA, Lionardo di [1617-1695]

DICELIUS, JOHANN SEBASTIAN [*fl.* 1670] *respondent. See* HARTMANN, M., *praeses.* Magni Hippocratis Coi Aphorismi VI sectionis VI. 1670.

DICKENSON, EDMUND. *See* DICKINSON, Edmund [1624-1707]

DICKINSON, EDMUND [1624-1707] ... De chrysopoeia; sive, De quintessentia philosophorum. Juxta exemplar Oxoniense editio hoc exemplari longe castigator. Accessit ob argumenti analogiam Anonymi Christiani De medicamentis universalibus dissertatio [n. p.] [1687?]

    [4], 183 p.; 56 p. 17 cm.   **[3195]**

"Theodori Mundani responsa Gallice scripta sed Latine reddita per ... H. B. philochymicum": p. 117-183.
Part [1] published in Oxford in 1686 under title: Epistola ... ad Theodorum Mundanum ... De quintessentia philosophorum et de vera physiologia. Part [2] has half title.

—Epistola ... ad Theodorum Mundanum ... De quintessentia philosophorum et de vera physiologia. Una cum questionibus aliquot de secreta materia physica. His accedunt Mundani responsa. Oxoniae, E Theatro Sheldoniano, nec non Londini in vico dicto Little Britaine, 1686.

    [3], 224 p. 21 cm.   **[3196]**

"Theodori Mundani responsa Gallice scripta sed Latine reddita per ... H. B. philochymicum": p. 145-224.

DICTIONAIRE hermetique, contenant l'explication des termes, fables, enigmes, emblemes & manieres de parler des vrais philosophes. Accompagné de deux traitez singuliers ... Par un amateur de la science. Paris, Laurent D'Houry, 1695.

    [12], 216 p.; 119 p. 16 cm.   **[3197]**

The Dictionaire hermetique has been variously ascribed to William Salmon and Nicolas Salomon.
Part [2] has special title page: Traité philosophique de la triple preparation de l'or et de l'argent. Par Gaston le Doux, dit De Claves. This is followed by another tract by the same author: De la droite et vraie maniere de produire la pierre philosophique.

DICTIONARIUM octo linguarum. 1606. *See* CALEPINO, A.

DICTIONNAIRE etymologique de mots grecs. *In* Thévenin, F. Les oeuvres. 1658, 1669, 1691.

DIDIER. *See* DIDIER, Jacques [*fl.* 1653-1661]

DIDIER, JACQUES [*fl.* 1653-1661] Lettre de Monsieur Didier docteur en medecine, & surintendant des eaux mineralles d'Aix la Chapelle & de Borcet. A Monsieur Blondel ... Touchant les vertus & les proprietés desdites eaux, & à quelles maladies elles sont profitables tant par les bains, que principalement par la boisson d'icelles ... Sedan, François Chayer, 1661.

    72 p. 15 cm.   **[3198]**

—Refutation de la doctrine nouvelle du sieur Helmont touchant les fievres. ... Sedan, François Chayer, 1653.

    [7], 374 p. 16 cm.   **[3199]**

—*See* BLONDEL, F. Lettres ... au sieur Jaques Didier ... touchant les eaux minerales chaudes d'Aix & de Borcet. 1662.

DIEMERBROECK, IJSBRAND VAN [1609-1674] Opera omnia, anatomica et medica partim jam antea excusa, sed plurimis locis ab ipso auctore emend. & aucta, partim nondum edita. Nunc simul collecta, & diligenter recognita, per Timannum de Diemerbroeck ... Ultrajecti, Apud Meinardum a Dreunen, & Guilielmum a Walcheren, 1685.

3 parts in 1 v.   plates, port.   34 cm. [**3200**]
Added engraved title page.

—[The same.] . . . Patavii, Ex typographia Petri Mariae Frambotti, 1688.
  2 v.   illus., plates.   24 cm.   [**3201**]
Added engraved title page.
Vol. 2 wanting.

—[The same.] . . . Genevae, Apud Samuelem de Tournes, 1688.
  2 v.   front. (port.), plates.   23 cm.   [**3202**]
Vol. 2 has added engraved title page, dated 1687.

—Anatome corporis humani, plurimis novis inventis instructa, variisque observationibus & paradoxis, cum medicis, tum physiologicis adornata . . . Ultrajecti, Sumptibus & typis Meinardi à Dreunen, 1672.
  [24], 963, [9] p.   plates.   21 cm.   [**3203**]
Added engraved title page.
Imperfect: plates 1, 5, 8, and 10 wanting.

—[The same.] Ed. novissima innumeris naevis quibus aliae scatent sedulo repurgata, & multis figuris aeneis de novo emendatis ditata. Genevae, Apud Samuelem de Tournes, 1679.
  [20], 844, [8] p.   plates.   23 cm.   [**3204**]
Added engraved title page.

—[The same.] . . . Ed. nova . . . Lugduni, Sumpt. Joan. Antonii Huguetan, & soc., 1679.
  [16], 606, [6] p.   plates.   26 cm.   [**3205**]
Added engraved title page.

—[The same.] . . . Ed. nova . . . Lugduni, Sumpt. Marci & Joan. Henrici Huguetan, 1683.
  [16], 606, [6] p.   plates.   26 cm.   [**3206**]
Added engraved title page.
Different setting of type.

—[English tr.] The anatomy of human bodies, comprehending the most modern discoveries and curiosities in that art. To which is added a particular Treatise of the small-pox and measles. Together with several practical observations and experienc'd cures. Written in Latin . . . Translated from the last and most correct and full edition . . . by William Salmon . . . London, Edward Brewster, MCDLXXXIX [i.e. 1689]
  [42], 616, [9], 237, [3] p.   illus.   33 cm.
                                          [**3207**]

—[The same.] . . . London, W. Whitwood, 1694.
  [42], 616, [9], 237, [3] p.   illus., port.   33 cm.
                                          [**3208**]
A reissue of the 1689 edition with portrait and new title page.

—[French tr.] L'anatomie du corps humain, composée en latin . . . établie sur les nouvelles découvertes des anatomistes modernes . . . Traduction nouvelle, par Mr. J. Prost . . . Tome premier [-second] Lyon, Anisson & Postuel, 1695.
  2 v.   plates.   25 cm.   [**3209**]

—De peste libri quatuor, truculentissimi morbi historiam ratione & experientia confirmatam exhibentes. Arenaci, Ex officina Joannis Jacobi, 1646.
  [12], 337, [9] p.   21 cm.   [**3210**]
With this is bound Sibyllenus, P. De peste liber absolutissimus. 1564.

—[The same.] Tractatus de peste, in quatuor libros distinctus; truculentissimi morbi historiam ratione & experientia confirmatam exhibens. Ab auctore emendatus, plurimisque in locis adauctus. Amstelaedami, Typis Joannis Blaeu, 1665.
  [16], 366, [8] p.   19 cm.   [**3211**]

—[Dutch tr.] Traktaat vande peste, in het welk deze zeer gevaarlikjke ziekte met reden en eigen ervinding bevestigd, en naaktelijk vertoont word . . . Uit de Latijnsche inde Nederduitsche taal getrouwelijk overgezet, door Jacob du Buisson . . . Middelburg, Pieter van Goetthem, 1672.
  [12], 35 p.; 38 p.; 42 p.; 162 [i.e. 164] p.   16 cm.
                                          [**3212**]

—Disputationum practicarum pars prima & secunda, de morbis capitis & thoracis. Ed. 2. priore locupletior & emendatior. Trajecti ad Rhenum, Apud Theodorum ab Ackersdyck, 1664.
  [8], 326 p.   14 cm.   [**3213**]
Pars secunda, p. [223]-326, has half title.
Bound with Pecquet, J. Experimenta nova anatomica. 1661.

—*praeses.* Disputationis medicae de chymia, pars prior . . . Trajecti ad Rhenum, Typis Gisberti à Zijll & Theodori ab Ackersdijck, 1657.
  [16] p.   20 cm.   [**3214**]
Diss. — Utrecht (J. B. van Lamsweerde, *respondent*)

—*See* PEST-BESCHRIJVING. 1664.

—*as subject. See* GRAEVIUS, J. G. Oratio funebris in exequiis viri . . . Isbrandi Diemerbroekii. 1675.

DIEMERBROECK, Tieman van [*fl.* 1668-1684] *respondent.* Disputatio medica inauguralis, de asthmate ... Trajecti ad Rhenum, Ex officina Frederici Strick, 1668.

[12] p.   20 cm.   [3215]

—, *ed. See* Diemerbroeck, I. van. Opera omnia. 1685, 1688.

DIENHEIM, Johann Wolfgang [*fl.* 1610] Medicina universalis; seu, De generali morborum omnium remedio liber, quo veritas facilitasque medicinae cujusdam catholicae, omnes omnino morbos curantis ostenditur, ad eandemque adipiscendam aditus aperitur ... Argentorati, Sumptibus Lazari Zetzneri, 1610.

[16], 78, [9] p.   15 cm.   [3216]

DIEPHOLD, Rudolph [*d. ca.* 1620] Cl^mo. viro, Dn. Gebhardo Hurlebusch ... medicinae doctori renunciato. Helmstadii, In Academia Julia, 1610.

[4] p.   20 cm.   [3217]
In verse.

DIEPHOUT, Reinier à [*fl.* 1668] *respondent.* Disputatio medica inauguralis de chylificatione laesa ... Lugduni Batavorum, Apud viduam & haeredes Joannis Elsevirii, 1668.

[11] p.   20 cm.   [3218]
Diss.—Leyden.

DIEPPE. Avis utile aux medecines, chirurgiens, & apotiquaires de la campagne. Paris, 1680.

2 p.   24 cm.   [3219]
Caption title.

DIETERICH, Helvicus. *See* Dietrich, Helwig [1601-1655]

DIETERICH, Johann Daniel [*fl.* 1636] *See* Horst, G. [1578-1636] Operum medicorum tomus primus [-tertius] 1660, 1661.

DIETERICH, Johann Konrad [1612-1669] Iatreum Hippocraticum: continens narthecium medicinae veteris et novae; ex nobilioribus medicis, tam veteribus, quam recentioribus, jucunda verborum serie, juxta ductum Aphorismorum Hippocratis ita compositum, ut & aliarum facultatum studiis queat inservire ... Ulmae Suevorum, Typis & impensis Balthasar. Kühnen, 1661.

[2], 1555 p.   21 cm.   [3220]

With this is bound (as issued) Hippocrates. Joh. Cunradi Dieterici ... Aphorismi Hippocratis illustrati. 1661.

—, *ed. See* Hippocrates. Joh. Cunradi Dieterici ... Aphorismi Hippocratis illustrati et Iatreo ejusdem praemissi. 1661.

DIETERICUS, Helvicus. *See* Dietrich, Helwig [1601-1655]

DIETERICUS, Jacobus Andreas [*fl.* 1696] *respondent. See* Sturm, J. C., *praeses.* Disquisitio physica de fulmine & cognatis tonitru ac fulgure. 1696.

DIETRICH, Balthasar [*fl.* 1684] *respondent.* Disputatio medica inauguralis de epilepsia ... Lugduni Batavorum, Apud Abrahamum Elzevier, 1684.

[22] p.   22 cm.   [3221]
Diss.—Leyden.

DIETRICH, Helwig [1601-1655] Novus orbis. In quo, quaecunque de nato et creato serio et joco sciri vel desiderari possunt, inusitata rerum varietate et mira elogiorum jucunditate omnia proponuntur ... Nunc primum ad multorum petitiones publici juris factus ... Argentorati, Typis Wilhelmi Christiani Glaseri, 1631.

[16], 272 (i.e. 264) p.   16 cm.   [3222]
Published in 1627 under title: Elogium planetarum coelestium et terrestrium macrocosmi et microcosmi.

—*respondent. See* Sennert, D., *praeses.* Positiones medicae de dysenteria. 1624.

DIETRICUS, Balthasar. *See* Dietrich, Balthasar [*fl.* 1684]

DIETZ, Johann Heinrich [*fl.* 1677-1680] *respondent.* Consultatio medica de epilepsia infantum. Quam disputationis loco proposuit Johannes Henricus Dietzius ... medicinae studiosus. anno MDCLXXVII ... Lugduni Batavorum, Apud Arnoldum Doude, 1678.

12 p.   22 cm.   [3223]
Diss.—Leyden.

—Μοσχοκαρυολογια; id est, Brevis ac succincta de nuce moschata dissertatio ... Giessae Hassorum, Apud viduam B. Friderici Kargeri, 1680.

[2], 46 p.   19 cm.   [3224]
Diss.—Giessen.

DIETZ, PHILIPP HEINRICH [*fl.* 1664-1667] *respondent. See* HEILAND, M., *praeses.* Disputatio medica de phantasia. 1664.

DIEU, LUDOVICUS DE [*fl.* 1693] *respondent.* Disputatio medica inauguralis de angina ... Trajecti ad Rhenum, Ex officina Francisci Halma, 1693.

    20 p.   24 cm.   **[3225]**

Diss. — Utrecht.

DIEUDONNÉ, CLAUDE. *See* DEODATUS, Claudius [*fl.* 1603-1628]

DIEUXIVOYE, BERTIN SIMON DE [*fl.* 1683-1717] *praeses.* Quaestio medica ... An functiones a fermentis? [Parisiis, 1694]

    [1], 8 p.   26 cm.   **[3226]**

Caption title.

Diss. — Paris (P. Hecquet, *respondent*)

DIGBY, *Sir* KENELM [1603-1665] Choice and experimented receipts in physick and chirurgery, as also cordial and distilled waters and spirits, perfumes, and other curiosities. Collected by ... Sir Kenelm Digby ... Translated out of several languages by G[eorge] H[artman] London, The author, 1668.

    [5], 308, [12] p.   front. (port.)   15 cm.

                               [3227]

With this is bound *his* The closet of ... Sir Kenelme Digbie K^t. opened. 1669.

—[The same.] ... The 2d ed. corr. & amended. London, Printed by Andrew Clark, for Henry Brome, 1675.

    [4], 146, [9] p.   15 cm.   **[3228]**

—[Dutch ed.] Nieuwe beproefde en wel ondersochte genees-middelen, ofte zeltsame verborgentheden: met verscheide aardige blanketsels, om de jufferlyke schoonheid te onderhouden ... Uit het Fransch vertaalt. Amsterdam, Jacob van Royen en Timotheus ten Hoorn, 1680.

    281, [6] p.   14 cm.   **[3229]**

—[The same.] *In* Theatrum sympateticum. 1697.

—[French ed.] Recueil des remedes et secrets tirez des memoires de Mr. ... Digby ... Avec plusieurs autres secrets & parfums, tous experimentez ... Par Jean Malbec de Trefel [sic] ... Paris, Chez l'auteur et Mille de Beaujeu, 1669.

    [12], 359, [3] p.   17 cm.   **[3230]**

"Table" bound before the text.

Compiled and translated by Jean Malbec de Tresfel partly from Digby's Choice and experimented receipts, and A choice collection.

—[The same.] Remedes souverains et secrets experimentez ... Avec plusieurs autres secrets & parfums curieux pour la conservation de la beauté des dames. Paris, Guillaume Cavelier, 1684.

    [4], 299 (i.e. 307), [27] p.   16 cm.   **[3231]**

—[The same.] ... Nouv. ed. Paris, Guillaume Cavelier, 1689.

    [4], 300, [28] p.   16 cm.   **[3232]**

—[The same.] Nouveaux secrets expérimentez, pour conserver la beauté des dames, et pour guérir plusieurs sortes de maladies ... Avec son Discours touchant la guérison des playes, par la poudre de sympathie. Tome I [-Tome II] 6. ed., rev., corr. & augm. ... La Haye, Etienne Foulque, 1700.

    2 v. in. 1.   fronts.   17 cm.   **[3233]**

—[German ed.] Medicina experimentalis Digbaeana, das ist: Ausserlesene und bewährte Artzney-Mittel, auss ... Herren ... Digby ... Manuscriptis, zusammen gebracht: welchen auch einige, so sonsten von vornehmen Personen herkommen, und gleichfals bewährt seynd, beygefügt worden. Samt etlichen andern angehänckten Experimenten und Secreten. Durch etliche Liebhaber der wahren natürlichen Wissenschafft übersetzt, und an Tag gegeben ... Franckfurt, In Verlegung Johann Peter Zubrodt, gedruckt bey Paul Hummen, 1670.

    [21], 216, [28] p.   18 cm.   **[3234]**

Compiled and translated partly from Digby's Choice and experimented receipts, and A choice collection.

—[The same.] ... Franckfurt, In Verlegung Johann Peter Zubrodts, gedruckt bey Paul Hummen sel. Wittib., 1672-1676.

    2 parts in 1 v.   illus.   18 cm.   **[3235]**

Part [2] has title: ... Zweyter Theil ... Sampt dreyen unterschiedlichen angehenckten Tractätlein, nahmentlich: Aurora chymica. Herrn Le Febre Erläuterung der vortrefflichen Hertzstärckung des Herrn Walther Ravleighs und W. T. Philo-Astro-Medici, Medulla chymischer Artzneyen ... Gedruckt bey Johann Andreae, 1676.

Compiled and translated partly from Digby's Choice and experimented receipts, and A choice collection.

—Another issue. Differs in that on p. [329] (part [2]) there are 3 additional lines printed: Aus dem

Englischen ins Deutsche versetzt durch Carolum-Aloysium Ramsay.   [3236]

—[The same.] . . . Franckfurt am Mäyn, In Verlegung Johann Melchior Bencards. Offenbach, Druckts Bonav. de Launoy, 1687.

     2 parts in 1 v.   front., illus.   18 cm.   [3237]

    The "Erläuterung" and the "Medulla" have special title pages with imprint: Offenbach am Mäyn, Druckts Bonaventura de Launoy, 1686.

    The Medulla was translated from English into German by Charles Aloysius Ramsay.

—[The same.] Ausserlesene, seltsame philosophische Geheimnüsse und chymische Experimente, wie auch sonderbahre und zuvor nie eröffnete Artzneyen, Menstrua und Alkaheste, sampt dem wahren Geheimnüss das Sal Tartari flüchtig zu machen: welche alle von dem . . . Herrn Kenelm Digby . . . zusammen gelesen . . . jetzo . . . ans Tages Liecht gebracht worden durch Georg Hartman. Aus der englischen in die deutsche Sprache . . . übersetzet von J[ohann] L[ange] M[edicinae] C[andidatum] . . . Hamburg, Auff Gottfried Schultzens Kosten, 1684.

     [8], 269, [11] p.   port., plates.   17 cm. [3238]

—Chymical secrets, and rare experiments in physick & philosophy . . . Containing many rare and unheard of medicines, menstruums, and alkahests . . . Published . . . by George Hartman . . . London, Will. Cooper, 1683.

     [16], 272 p.   17 cm.   [3239]

—The closet of . . . Sir Kenelme Digbie K^t. opened: whereby is discovered several ways for making of metheglin, sider, cherry-wine, &c. Together with excellent directions for cookery: as also for preserving, conserving, candying . . . London, Printed by E. C. for H. Brome, 1669.

     [4], 312, [11] p.   port.   15 cm.   [3240]

    Imperfect: p. 171-172 and portrait wanting.

    Bound with *his* Choice and experimented receipts in physick and chirurgery. 1668.

—Discours fait en une celebre assemblée . . . touchant la guerison des playes par la poudre de sympathie. Où sa composition est enseignée . . . Paris, Augustin Courbé et Pierre Moet, 1658.

     195, [2] p.   16 cm.   [3241]

—[The same.] Rouen & Paris, Augustin Courbé, 1660.

     195, [2] p.   17 cm.   [3242]

    A corrected reprint of the 1658 edition.

—[The same.] . . . Roüen, Antoine Maurry, 1673.

     248 (i.e. 246) p.   14 cm.   [3243]

    "Dissertation touchant la poudre de sympathie, traduite du latin du sieur Papin . . . Par le sieur Rault" (p. [153]-248) has half title.

—[The same.] . . . Paris, Charles Osmont, 1681.

     248 (i.e. 246), [2] p.   15 cm.   [3244]

    Different setting of type.

—[The same *as subject*] See Deusing, A. Sympathetici pulveris examen. 1662.

—[Latin tr.] Oratio de pulvere sympathetico . . . [&] Explicatio tituli aenei . . .

     1—192 p.   illus.   14 cm.   (*In* Theatrum sympatheticum. Norimbergae, 1660)   [3245]

    Half title and caption title.

—[The same.] *In* Theatrum sympatheticum. 1661, 1662.

—[Dutch tr.] D'eminente oratie . . . Ghedaen in een voortreffelijcke vergaderingh, over't ghenesen der wonden, door het poeder, toe-genaemt de sympathie, sonder de selve wonden te sien of aen te raecken . . . Uyt het Frans . . . ghetranslateert door J[ohannes] C[asteleyn] . . . Haerlem, Joannes Casteleyn, 1661.

     49, [3] p.   19 cm.   [3246]

    With this is bound Papin, N. Theatrum sympateticum. 1662.

—[The same.] *In* Theatrum sympateticum. 1681, 1697.

—[English tr.] A late discourse made in a solemne assembly of nobles and learned men at Montpellier . . . touching the cure of wounds by the powder of sympathy; with instructions how to make the said powders . . . Rendred faithfully out of French into English by R. White, gent. London, R. Lownes, and T. Davies, 1658.

     [10], 152, [1] p.   15 cm.   [3247]

    Imperfect: first preliminary and last leaf (blank?) wanting; p. 73-74 mutilated.

—[The same.] . . . The 2d ed. corr. and augm. . . . London, R. Lowndes and T. Davies, 1658.

     [10], 152, [5] p.   14 cm.   [3248]

    A reprint of the first edition published in the same year.

—[The same.] . . . 3d ed. corr. and augm. . . . London, R. Lowndes and T. Davies, 1660.

[10], 152, [6] p.   15 cm.   [3249]
Different setting of type.

—[German tr.] Eröffnung unterschiedlicher Heimlichkeiten der Natur, worbey viel . . . Reden von nützlichen Dingen . . . beygefüget, und vornemlich von einem wunderbaren Geheimnüss in Heilungen der Wunden, ohne Berührung, vermög dess Vitrioli, durch die Sympathiam, Discurssweise gehalten in einer hochansehnlichen Versamlung zu Montpelier . . . Ubersetzet von M. H. Hupka. Zum dritten Mahl gedruckt . . . Franckfurt, Balthasar Christoph Wust, 1664.

[1], 123, [7] p.; [1], 82, [6] p.   18 cm.   [3250]
"Petri Servii . . . Aussführliches Bedencken, von der insgemein so genannten Waffen-Salben; oder, Von den Wunderwercken der Natur und Kunst": p. [1]-82 (2nd group of paging) with half title; "Wie das Poudre de Sympathie vor allerhand Wunden und Seitenstechen zu machen": p. [4-6] at end.

—[The same.] . . . Zum fünfftenmal gedruckt . . . [Franckfurt] Verlegt von Balthasar Christoph Wusten, 1671.

[1], 132, [8] p.; 88, [8] p.   front.   18 cm.
                                              [3251]

—A discourse concerning the vegetation of plants . . . Spoken . . . at Gresham College, on the 23. of January, 1660. At a meeting of the Society for promoting philosophical knowledge by experiments. London, Printed by J. G. for John Dakin, 1661.

[1], 100, [1] p.   13 cm.   [3252]
Errata: p. [101]

—[Latin tr.] Dissertatio de plantarum vegetatione. Habita in Collegio Greshammensi . . . ad diem 23. Januarii 1660 . . . Ex Anglica in linguam Latinam versa. Amstelodami, Apud Jodocum Pluymert, 1663.

[8], 104 p.   14 cm.   [3253]
Translated by Olfert Dapper.

—Observations upon Religio medici . . . London, Printed by R. C. for Daniel Frere, 1643.

[1], 124 p.   15 cm.   [3254]
Keynes (B) 218.

—[The same.] . . . The 2d ed. corr. and amended. London, Printed by F. L. for Lawrence Chapman and Daniel Frere, 1644.

[1], 124 p.   15 cm.   [3255]
Keynes (B) 215.
Bound with Browne, Sir T. [Religio medici] 1645.

—[The same.] In Browne, Sir T. Pseudodoxia epidemica 1672 [and] Religio medici. 1659, 1678, 1682.

—Two treatises. In the one of which, the nature of bodies; in the other, the nature of mans soule; is looked into: in way of discovery, of the immortality of reasonable soules . . . Paris, Gilles Blaizot, 1644.

[44], 466 p.   illus.   36 cm.   [3256]

—[The same.] . . . London, John Williams, 1645.

[47], 429 p.; [10], 143, [1] p.   diagrs.   19 cm.
                                              [3257]
Part 2 has special title page: The second treatise: declaring, the nature and operations of mans soule.
With this is bound Ross, A. The philosophicall touchstone. 1645.

—[The same.] . . . London, John Williams, 1658.

[47], 429 p.; [10], 143 (i.e. 141), [1] p.   diagrs.
19 cm.   [3258]
Imperfect: sig. *2-3 wanting.
Part 2 has special title page dated 1657.
Different setting of type.

—[The same.] Of bodies, and of mans soul. To discover the immortality of reasonable souls. With two discourses Of the powder of sympathy, and Of the vegetation of plants . . . London, Printed by S. G. and B. G. for John Williams, 1669.

[55], 439 p.; [10], 231 p.   diagrs.   21 cm.
                                              [3259]
Part 2 has special title page: Second treatise: declaring the nature and operations of mans soul . . . The two discourses which follow the Second treatise have special title pages also.

—[Latin tr.] Demonstratio immortalitatis animae rationalis; sive, Tractatus duo philosophici, in quorum priori natura et operationes corporum, in posteriori vero, natura animae rationalis, ad evincendam illius immortalitatem, explicantur . . . Ex Anglico in Latinum versa opera & studio I[ohn] L[eyburn]. Praemittitur huic Latinae editioni praefatio metaphysica, authore Thoma Anglo [pseud. i.e. Thomas White] . . . Eidemque subnectuntur Institutionum peripeticarum libri quinque, cum Appendice theologica de origine mundi, ejusdem authoris. Francofurti, Secundum exemplar Parisiense, 1664.

[153], 610 p.; 246 p.   illus.   18 cm.   [3260]
Added engraved title page.
Tractatus secundus (p. [449]-585), Institutionum peripeticarum (p. [1]-158) and Appendix theologica de origine mundi (p. [159]-204) have half titles.

Includes also: "La poudre de sympathie . . . par Lazare Meysson-nier" p. [205]-228; "Laur. Straussii . . . Responsum ad examen pulveris sympathetici & secundinas Mussipontanas . . . Deusingii" p. [229]-246. Each item has half title.

—*See* BLANKAART, S. Theatrum chimicum. 1700.

—*as subject. See* HELVETIUS, J. F. Theatridium Herculis triumphantis. 1663; HIGHMORE, N. The history of generation. 1651; PAPIN, N. Theatrum sympateticum. 1662; ROSS, A. Medicus medicatus. 1645 [and] The philosophicall touch-stone. 1645; STRAUSS, L. Epistola ad . . . Dygbaeum. 1662.

DI GORDON, BERNARDO. *See* BERNARD DE GORDON [*fl. ca.* 1283–*ca.* 1308]

DIJK, CORNELIUS VAN. *See* DYK, Cornelis van [*fl.* 1665–1680]

DIJON. Collège des Médecins. *See* COLLÈGE DES MÉDECINS, Dijon.

DILECTUS, LUSITANUS [*fl.* 1642] Ocyrrhoes; seu, Praestantissimum morborum auxilium de venae sectione copiosa methodus . . . Venetiis, Apud Petrum Milochum, 1642.

[II], 223, [8] p.   24 cm.   [**3261**]

DILLENIUS, JUSTUS FRIEDRICH [1644–1720] *praeses.* Disputatio medica de pulsu . . . Gissae-Hassorum, Typis Henningi Mülleri, 1690.

24 p.   20 cm.   [**3262**]
Diss. — Giessen (J. W. Scheffer, *respondent*)

DILLY, ANTOINE. De l'ame des bêtes, ou apres avoir demontré la spiritualité de l'ame de l'homme, l'on explique par la seule machine, les actions les plus surprenantes des animaux. Par A[ntoine] D[illy] ***** Lyon, Anisson & Posuel, 1676.

[20], 359 p.   15 cm.   [**3263**]

—[The same.] Traitté de l'ame et de la connoissance des bétes, ou aprés avoir, demontré la spiritualité de l'ame de l'homme l'on explique par la seule machine, les actions les plus surprenantes des animaux, suivant les principles de Descartes. Par A[ntoine] D[illy] ***** Amsterdam, George Gallet, 1691.

[23], 276 p.   front.   14 cm.   [**3264**]

DIMEL, JOHANN WILHELM [*fl.* 1685] *respondent.* Disputatio medica inauguralis de morbis contagiosis

. . . Lugduni Batavorum, Apud Abrahamum Elzevier, 1685.

[24] p.   22 cm.   [**3265**]
Diss. — Leyden.

DINCKEL, DANIEL [*fl.* 1618] *respondent. See* SEBISCH, M. [1578–1674?] *praeses.* Disputatio de alimentorum facultatibus secunda. 1618.

DINCKEL, JOHANN RUDOLPH [*fl.* 1655] *respondent.* Disputatio . . . medica de chylificatione sive ventriculi coctione, ejusdemque concoctricis laesa actione . . . Argentorati, Ex typographeo Jacobi Thilonis, 1655.

[36] p.   18 cm.   [**3266**]
Imperfect: upper margins trimmed.
Diss. — Strasbourg.

DINCKEL, JOHANNES [1545–1601] *See* GOCLENIUS, R. [1547–1628] Physiologia crepitus ventris. 1607.

DINCKGREUE, JOHANNES [*fl.* 1675–1677] *respondent. See* WALDSCHMIDT, J. J., *praeses.* Disputatio medica de epilepsia. 1676.

DINET, JACQUES, *Father* [1580–1653] *See* DESCARTES, R. Meditationes de prima philosophia. 1650.

DINET, P. *See* REGIUS, H. Medicinae libri IV. 1657, 1668.

DINGHENS, LÉONARD FRANÇOIS [1648–1697] Fundamenta physico-medica . . . in sex libros divisa. Quibus accedit Tractatus de febribus. Lovanii, Typis Petri Sasseni, 1678.

[18], 396, [I] p.; 28, [4] p.   30 cm.   [**3267**]
The date of the imprint appears to have been M.DC.LXXVII. to which an I seems to have been subsequently added in print.
Imperfect: first page of Index capitum ([4] p. at end) printed on p. [15]

DIOCLES CARYSTIUS. Aurea ad Antigonum regem epistola, de morborum praesagiis, & eorumdem extemporaneis remediis. Ad haec, Arnaldi a Villa-Nova . . . Consilium ad regem Aragonum, de salubri hortensium usu. De syrmaismo, et ratione purgandi vomitum, ex Aegyptiorum inventi & formula. Jos. [sic] Langio autore. Antonii Mizaldi . . . cura & diligentia. Parisiis, Apud Claudium Morellum, 1607.

27, [I] ll.   18 cm. (Section [5] in Mizauld, Antoine. Opusculorum pars secunda. Parisiis, 1607)
                                                    [**3268**]

A reprint, with the omission of the translator's dedication, of the edition published in Paris in 1572.

—[The same.] Epistola de secunda valetudine tuenda. *In* Hygieia. 1628; Mizauld, A. Opusculorum pars prima [-secunda] 1607; Regimen sanitatis Salernitanum. Medicina Salernitana. 1605, 1611, 1612, 1622, 1624, 1628, 1638 [and] Schola Salernitana. 1649, 1657, 1667, 1683.

—[Latin and French tr.] *In* Regimen sanitatis Salernitanum. Le regime de santé de l'Eschole de Salerne. 1633, 1637, 1643, 1649, 1660.

—[German tr.] *In* Becher, J. J. Parnassus medicinalis illustratus. 1663.

DIOGENES, *of Sinope. See* DIOGENES, *the Cynic.*

DIOGENES, *the Cynic.* Letters. Greek and Latin. *In* Lubin, E., *ed.* and *tr.* Epistolae Hippocratis, Democriti, Heracliti. 1601.

DIOGENES LAERTIUS. Liber decimus de vita, moribus, placitisque Epicuri. Greek & Latin. *In* Gassendi, P. Opera omnia. 1658.

—*See* SEXTUS EMPIRICUS. Opera. 1621.

DIONIS, PIERRE [1643-1718] L'anatomie de l'homme, suivant la circulation du sang, & les dernieres découvertes. Démontrée au Jardin royal . . . 2. ed., corr. & augm. . . . Paris, Laurent d'Houry, 1694.
[36], 523, [35] p. plates, port. 19 cm.**[3269]**
Added engraved title page.

—[The same.] Nouvelle anatomie de l'homme . . . 3. ed., rev., corr. & augm. de deux tables tres-utiles. Paris, Laurent d'Houry, 1695.
[34], 523, [32] p. plates. 20 cm. **[3270]**
A reprint of the 1694 edition.

—Another issue with date altered from 1695 to 1696 and portrait added. **[3271]**

—[The same.] L'anatomie de l'homme . . . 3. éd., corr., & augm. d'une ample Dissertation sur la generation, & de plusieurs explications nouvelles. Paris, Laurent d'Houry, 1698.
[38], 671, [36] p. plates, port. 20 cm.**[3272]**
Added engraved title page.

—[Latin tr.] Anatomia corporis humani, juxta circulationem sanguinis & recentiores observationes: in Horto Regio Parisino ab ipso autore demonstrata . . . Amstelodami, Cramer & Perachon, 1696.
[22], 496, [23] p. front. (port.), plates. 20 cm. **[3273]**
Imperfect: portrait wanting.

—Another issue, with imprint: Genevae, Cramer & Perachon, 1696. **[3274]**

—Dissertation sur la generation de l'homme, ou l'on rapporte les diverses opinions des modernes sur ce sujet, avec des reflexions nouvelles, & plusieurs faits singuliers . . . Paris, Laurent d'Houry, 1698.
[2], 93 p. plates. 20 cm. **[3275]**
Also published as a part of the author's L'anatomie de l'homme. "Description d'une oreille du coeur extraordinairement dilatée": p. 85-93.

DIOSCORIDES, PEDANIUS, *of Anazarbos.* De materia medica. [Latin tr.] *In* Mattioli, P. A. Opera quae extant omnia. 1674.

—[French tr.] *In* Mattioli, P. A. Les commentaires. 1619, 1620, 1627, 1642, 1680.

—[German tr.] Kräuterbuch . . . von allerley wolriechenden Kräutern, Gewürtzen, köstlichen Oelen und Salben . . . und andern, so allein zur Artzney gehörig, Kräuterwein, Metalln, Steinen, allerley Erden, allem und jedem Gifft, viel und mancherley Thieren, und derselbigen heylsamen und nutzbaren Stück. In siben sonderbare Bücher underschieden. Erstlich durch Joannem Danzium von Ast . . . verteutscht, nun mehr aber von Petro Uffenbach . . . auffs newe ubersehen, verbessert, in ein richtige Form gebracht . . . mit dess . . . Hieronymi Braunschweig zweyen Büchern, als der Kunst zu destillieren, und dann dem heylsamen und vielfaltigen Gebrauch aller und jeden destillierten Wasser, vermehrt . . . Franckfurt am Mayn, Gedruckt durch Johann Bringern, in Verlegung Conrad Corthoys, 1610.
[11], 616, [33] p. illus., plate. 33 cm. **[3276]**
Pritzel 2322.

—[Italian tr.] *In* Mattioli, P. A. I discorsi. 1621, 1645.

—[Spanish tr.] Acerca de la materia medicinal, y de los venenos mortiferos. Traducidos de lengua griega, en la vulgar castellana, è ilustrado con claras, y sustanciales anotaciones, y con las figuras de in-umerables plantas exquisitas, y raras, por ... Andres de Laguna ... Va añadida una tabla para hallar remedio de todo genero de enfermedades, y otras cosas curiosas, nunca antes impress. Y aora en esta ultima impression corr., y enmendado de muchos er-rores que tenia conforme el catalogo nuevo del Santo Oficio ... Valencia, En la imprenta de Vicente Cabrera, a costa de Mateo Regil, 1677.

    [24], 617, [31] p. illus. 30 cm.   **[3277]**
    Added half title.

    —[The same.] ... Valencia, Por el heredero de Benito Mace, a expensas de Claudio Mace, 1695.

    [24], 617, [31] p. illus. 30 cm.   **[3278]**
    Imperfect: title page mutilated.
    Different setting of type.

    —[The same, *as subject*] *See* FALLOPPIO, G. Opera. 1606; VISCARDI, J. Explanationes aromatum. 1687.

    —*See* PONA, G. Monte Baldo descritto. 1617; ROLFINCK, W. Liber de purgantibus vegetabilibus. 1667; [STEPHANUS MAGNETES] Experiment Buch. 1623.

    —*as subject. See* CONTANT, J. Les oeuvres. 1628; FABER, Johannes. De nardo et epithymo adversus Josephum Scaligerum. 1607; FRANCKE, J. Veronica theézans. 1700; GOCKEL, E. Enchiridion medico-practicum de peste. 1669; HOFMANN, C. Variarum lectionum lib. VI. 1619; MAROGNA, N. Commentarius in tractatus Dioscoridis, et Plinii de amomo. 1608; PONA, G. Del vero balsamo de gli antichi commen-tario ... sopra l'Historia di Dioscoride. 1623.

DIOSKURIDES. *See* DIOSCORIDES, *Pedanius, of Anazarbos.*

DIRLEBER, BENEDICT [*fl.* 1649] *respondent.* Dodecas thesium inauguralium de passione colica flatulenta ... Lugduni Batavorum, Ex officina Fran-cisci Hackii, 1649.

    [12] p. 22 cm.   **[3279]**
    Diss.—Leyden.

DISCORSO d'astrologia e' fisonomia naturale, nel quale si discore della fisonomia, complessione, costumi, & infermità de gl' huomini, e delle donne, in qual si voglia mesi, e giorni dell'anno ... Venetia, et in Bassano, Per Gio. Antonio Remondini [1697?]

    36 p. illus. 16 cm.   **[3280]**

Giannantonio Remondini printed in Venice in 1697. Cf. Brown, p. 414.

DISCOURS chrétien sur l'établissement de l'Hôpital general de la ville d'Orleans ... Orleans, François Hotot, 1672.

    [4], 59 p. 25 cm.   **[3281]**
    Attributed to François Guerin.

DISCOURS de la methode pour bien conduire sa raison. 1637. *See* [DESCARTES, R.]

DISCOURS de l'origine, des moeurs, fraudes et impostures des ciarlatans. 1622. *See* [MERCURIO, G.]

DISCOURS des malades epidemiques. *See* POTEL, G. Traicté de la peste advenue en ceste ville de Paris. 1624.

DISCOURS prodigieux de deux filles, nées a Paris le 17. janvier 1605. Lesquelles s'entretenoient par le ventre inferieur, ayant deux testes, quatre yeux, quatre bras, quatre iambes & deux natures. Paris, Fleury Bourriquant, au mont S. Hilaire, pres le puits Certain, aux Fleurs Royalles [*ca.* 1606]

    11 p. 16 cm.   **[3282]**
    Fleury Bourriquant worked at this address from 1606. Cf. Renouard, p. 43.

DISCOURS sceptique sur le passage du chyle. 1648. *See* [SORBIÈRE, S.]

DISCOURS sur les hermaphrodits. 1614. *See* [RIOLAN, J., 1580-1657]

A DISCOURSE concerning the having many children. *See* [DUGARD, S.] Περὶ πολυπαιδίας. 1695.

A DISCOURSE concerning the period of humane life. 1677. *See* [ALLESTREE, R.]

A DISCOURSE of things above reason. *See* BOYLE, *Hon.* R.

A DISCOURSE, wherein the interest of the pa-tient ... is ... debated. 1669. *See* [COXE, T.]

DISCURSO serio-jocoso, sobre la nueva inven-cion del agua de la vida. 1682. *See* [GONZÁLEZ DE GODOY, P.]

DISCURSO, sobre el azucar rosado solutio. *See* RUIZ, F. Discurso sobre la composicion del azucar rosado solutivo. 1628.

DISCURSUS medicus de impotentia virili theoretico-practicus, antea in dissertatione quadam defensus: nunc vero ab eodem autore denuo revisus, et in lucem editus. Coloniae, Impensis Petri Martau, 1698.

48 p. 16 cm. [3283]

Possibly edited by Caspar Heinrich Schrey. Cf. DAL, 11893.

DISCURSUS medicus de mola ejus causis, signis, generatione et curandi modo. 1611. See KALT, A.

DISELIUS, JOHANN PETER [*fl.* 1692] *respondent. See* BEHRNAUER, G., *praeses.* Dissertationem inauguralem, de morbis archaelibus . . . exhibet. 1692.

The **DISPENSARY**; a poem. 1699, 1700. *See* [GARTH, *Sir* S.]

DISPENSATORIUM Brandenburgicum; seu, Norma, juxta quam in provinciis . . . Brandenburgici, medicamenta officinis familiaria dispensanda ac praeparanda sunt . . . a . . . Collegio medico . . . Berolini, Sumptibus Johannis Völckeri, imprim. Ulricus Liebpertus, 1698.

[32], 200 p.; 33 p. 31 cm. [3284]

"Tenor edicti medicinalis": p. [13–14]

Part [2] has special title page: Taxa; seu, Pretium omnium officinis marchiae usualium medicamentorum, jussu . . . electoralis Brandenburgicae statutum. Coloniae Brandenburgicae, Ulricus Liebpertus.

DISPENSATORIUM chymicum; hoc est, Nova et hactenus incognita rariora et praestantissima ad periculosissimos & mirabiles quosque morbos remedia conficiendi ratio, atque curandi methodus. Ex optimorum . . . auctorum praesertim Josephi Quercetani [i.e. Joseph Duchesne], Petri Baconis, Poterii, & aliorum . . . placitis digestum & in tres libros distributum; cui accessere Benedicti Faventini Medicationes empyricae. Item Camilli Tomaii curandorum morborum rationalis methodus, ac demum Nicolai Epiphanii succincta medicinalis practica, nec non aliquot medicamentorum compositiones praestantissimae. Accessit demum I. P. Lotichii M. D. De gummi (ut vocant) gotta sive laxativo Indico discursus theorico-practicus . . . Francofurti, Impensis Theobaldi Schönwetteri, typis Pauli Jacobi, 1626.

1 v. 18 cm. [3285]

Various pagings.

"J. P. Lotichii . . . De gummi (ut vocant) gotta laxativo Indico discursus theorico-practicus novus" has special title page.

DISPENSATORIUM pharmacorum omnium, tam Galenicorum, quam chymicorum, quae hodie in usu potiore sunt. Authore primo Valerio Cordo. Nunc vero opera & studio Collegii Medici inclytae Reipublicae Norimbergensis emendatius, ac . . . auctius redditum, & quarto publicatum. Norimbergae, Sumptibus Johannis Andreae Endteri, & Wolfgangi junioris haeredum, 1666.

[20], 286 p. front., tables. 30 cm. [3286]

Frontispiece has title: Dispensatorium Norimb.

DISPUTATIO inauguralis theoretica practica jus potandi breviter adumbrans. [German.] *See* MULTIBIBUS, B. Jus potandi; oder, Zech Recht. 1616.

DISPUTATIONES inaugurales de esculentis et poculentis. *See* WEIS-ET ROTHWEIN DE REBENSAFFT, J. Novae regulae sanitatis medico-physicae. 1657.

DISPUTATIONES medicae de natura atque facultatibus ligni sancti. 1602. *See* [CYNTHIUS, C.]

DISQUISITIO de mutuo. 1645. *See* SAUMAISE, C. de.

DISSALDEUS, FRANCISCUS. *See* DISSAUDEAU, François [*d.* 1623]

DISSAUDEAU, FRANÇOIS [*d.* 1623] Pharmaconetes, sive Pharmacitis biblos. *In* Cordus, V. Dispensatorium. 1627, 1651 [1652]

—, *ed.* and *tr. See* HIPPOCRATES. [De capitis vulneribus. French.] 1612, 1658.

DISSERTATIO de corporum naturalium παλιγγενεσια. [Jena? 1673?]

[8] p. 20 cm. [3287]

Caption title.

DISSERTATIO physico-medica, de febribus. In qua juxta normam philosophiae purioris & fundamenta Craanenia, clare & distincte utilia multa ad Oeconomiam animalem pertinentia, proponuntur. Auctore A. v. L. Med. Doct. Lugduni Batavorum, Apud Cornelium Boutesteyn, 1688.

[112] p. 14 cm. [3288]

DISSERTATION sur la generation des animaux. *See* La bibliotheque des acoucheurs et des sagesfemmes. 1693.

DISSERTATION sur la goutte. 1689. *See* [MAUDUIT, M. *Father*]

DISSERTATION sur les fievres pourprées. 1685. *See* COLLÈGE DES MÉDECINS, Dijon.

DISSERTATION sur les nouvelles reflexions de la nature de l'astme. Bordeaux, J. Mongiron-Millanges et Simon Boe, 1681.

95 p.   16 cm.   [3289]

DISSERTATION sur les ulceres des reins et de la vessie. Expliquées dans une lettre écrite à Mr. Rapin medecine de Dijon . . . Au sujet de la maladie de Monsieur l'abbé de Palleau. 2. ed. Dijon, J. Ressayre, 1685.

84 p.   15 cm.   [3290]

DISSERTATIONUM ludicrarum et amoenitatum, scriptores varii. Lugd. Batavor. Apud Franciscos Hegerum & Hackium, 1638.

7, [1], 567 p.   13 cm.   [3291]

Engraved title page.

In 1623 published under title: Argumentorum ludicrorum et amoenitatum scriptores varii.

Partial contents: Laus podagrae, Bilibaldi Pirckheimeri; Encomium febris quartanae, Guil. Menapii.

DISTEL, DANIEL CHRISTOPH [1666–1710] *respondent. See* SPERLING, P. G., *praeses.* Disputationem solennem medicam de incontinentia urinae . . . submittet M. C. D. D. 1697.

The **DISTILLER** of London. 1639, 1652. *See* MAYERNE, *Sir* T. T. de.

DITTRICH, JUSTINE. *See* SIEGEMUND, Justine Dittrich [1648–1705]

DIVERSI, PIETRO SALIO. *See* SALIUS DIVERSUS, Petrus [16th cent.]

DIVI LESCHI GENUS AMO. *See* SENDIVOGIUS, Michael [1566–1636]

DIVINI, Eustachio [*d.* 1695] Lettera . . . all'ill. sig. conte Carl'Antonio Manzini. Si ragguaglia di un nuovo lauoro, e componimento di lenti, che servono à occhialoni, ò semplici, ò composti. Roma, Giacomo Dragondelli, 1663.

[1], 5–62 p.   17 cm.   [3292]

DJĀBIR IBN ḤAYYĀN AL ṬARSOŪSĪ. *See* JĀBIR IBN ḤAIYĀN, al-Ṭarasūsī.

DOBRICIUS, JOANNES [*fl.* 1607] *respondent.* Determinatio tabis medica inauguralis . . . Basileae, Typis Excertierianis, 1607.

[16] p.   20 cm.   [3293]

Diss. — Basel.

[**DOBRZENSKY**, JACOBUS JOANNES WENCESLAUS. *fl.* 1659–1684] Praeservativum universale naturale. [Pragae, Typis Universitatis Carolo-Ferdinandeae, 1679]

[5], 5–31 p.   16 cm.   [3294]

—[The same.] . . . [Salisburgi, Typis Joan. Baptistae Mayr, 1680]

32 (i.e. 34), [1] p.   14 cm.   [3295]

—[German ed.] Allgemeines natürliches Praeservativ; oder, Verwahrungs-Mittel wider alle von gifftiger Lufft herrührende . . . Seuchen, kunstreich erwogen, und dem gemeinen Nutzen zum Besten eröffnet und mitgetheilet . . . Nürnberg, In Verlegung Johann Ziegers, 1680.

[32] p.   17 cm.   [3296]

—*praeses.* Hippocrates redivivus; sive, Theses medicae inaugurales primum quidem praeliminaria quaedam antiphysiologica, post ad usum quarundam partium appertinentia physiologica, demum securiorem medendi methodum & principia rerum Hippocratica continentes . . . [Pragae, Typis Georgii Czernoch, 1684]

[94] p.   15 cm.   [3297]

Diss. — Prague (J. I. F. Voita, *respondent*)

—, *ed. See* MARCI VON KRONLAND, J. M. Liturgia mentis. 1678.

DOBRZENTAEUS, Jacobus Joannes Wenceslaus. *See* DOBRZENSKY, Jacobus Joannes Wenceslaus [*fl.* 1659–1684]

The **DOCTORS** physician. *See* [FRÉMONT D'ABLANCOURT, N.]

DODEL, Philipp [*fl.* 1667] *respondent. See* ZWINGER, J., *praeses.* Disputatio theologica de circumcisione. 1667.

DODOENS, REMBERT [1517–1585] [Cruydeboeck. English] A new herbal; or, Historie of plants: wherein is contained the whole discourse and perfect description of all sorts of herbes and plants . . . and that not onely of those which are here growing in this our country of Engalnd [sic], but of all others also of forraine realmes commonly used in physicke. First set forth in the Dutch or Almaigne tongue . . . and now first translated out of French into English, by Henry Lyte ... Corr. and amend. London, Edward Griffin, 1619.

[24], 564 (i.e. 562), [30] p.   29 cm.   [3298]

Translation of the author's Cruydeboeck, written in Flemish. Nissen 512, 516.

—Medicinalium observationum exempla rara ... Hardervici, Apud viduam Thomae Henrici, impensis Henrici Laurentii, 1521 [i.e. 1621]

[16], 234, [6] p.   17 cm.   [3299]

"Antonii Benivenii ... De abditis nonnullis ac mirandis morborum ac sanationum causis liber, cum annotationibus Dodonaei": p. 94-204; "Medicinalium observationum exempla rara Valesci Tarantani, & Alexandri Benedicti": p. 205-217; "Historiae gestationis foetus mortui in utero, Matthiae Cornacis ... Egydii Hertogii ... Achillis Gassari": p. 218-234.

Bound with *his* Praxis medica. 1616.

—Praxis medica ... Amsterdami, Impensis Henrici Laurentii, 1616.

[8], 618, [8] p.   17 cm.   [3300]

The author's lectures on medicine, edited with annotations by Sebastian Egbertsz. de Vry.

With this is bound *his* Medicinalium observationum exempla rara. 1521 [i.e. 1621]

—[The same.] In D. Remberti Dodonaei Praxin artis medicae ... Sebastiani Egberti Cos. scholia, cum auctario annotationum Nicolai Fontani ... Amstelodami, Sumptibus Hendrici Laurentii, 1640.

[16], 565, [10] p.   17 cm.   [3301]

—Stirpium historiae pemptades sex, sive libri XXX. Varie ab auctore, paullo ante mortem, aucti & emendati. Antverpiae, Ex Officina Plantiniana, apud Balthasarem et Joannem Moretos, 1616.

[16], 872, [66] p.   illus.   38 cm.   [3302]

The author's last and most comprehensive herbal, including several of his previously published works. For contents cf. Bibl. Belg. 1.sér D117.

Nissen 517.

—[Dutch tr.] Cruydt-boeck ... volgens sijne laetste verbeteringe: met bijvoegsels achter elck capittel, vvt verscheyden cruydtbeschrijvers: item in 't laetste een Beschrijvinge vande Indiaensche gewassen, meest getrocken vvt de schriften van Carolus Clusius. Leyden, Inde Plantijnsche Druckerije van Françoys van Ravelingen, 1618.

[32], 1495, [56] p.   illus.   36 cm.   [3303]

Imperfect: first prelim. leaf (half-title) wanting.

Translation by Franciscus Raphelengien, edited by Justus Raphelengien.

Nissen 518.

—[The same.] ... Nu wederom van nieuws oversien ende verbetert. Antwerpen, Inde Plantijnsche Druckerije van Balthasar Moretus, 1644.

[36], 1492, [59] p.   illus.   41 cm.   [3304]

—[English tr.] *In* Gerard, J. The herball: or, Generall historie of plantes. 1633, 1636.

— *See* SCHOLTZ, L. Consiliorum medicinalium ... liber singularis. 1610.

DODONAEUS, REMBERTUS. *See* DODOENS, Rembert [1517-1585]

DÖBEL, JOHANN JAKOB [1640-1684] *praeses.* Disputatio medica inauguralis de morbo virgineo seu foedis virginum coloribus ... Rostochii, Typis Johannis Kilii, 1670.

[48] p.   20 cm.   [3305]

Diss. — Rostock (B. Barnstorff, *respondent*)

—, *ed. See* RIVÈRE, L. Opera medica universa. 1674, 1679, 1690, 1698.

DOEBEL, JOHANN JAKOB [1674-1743] *respondent. See* SCHAPER, J. E., *praeses.* Disputatione inaugurali valvularum vasorum lacteorum lymphaticorum, sanguiferorum dilucidationem ... submittit. 1694.

—*See* SCHAPER, J. E. Decanus Facultatis Medicae ... ad disputationem inauguralem de valvularum vasorum lacteorum, lympathicorum ac sanguiferorum dilucidatione a ... Johanne Jacobo Döbelio ... habendam ... invitat. 1694.

DÖBELN, JOHANN JACOB. *See* DOEBEL, Johann Jakob [1674-1743]

DÖHRING, CHRISTIAN [*fl.* 1663] *respondent. See* FRIDERICI, J. A., *praeses.* Exercitationem anatomicam de renibus ... subjicit ... 1663.

DÖRING, GEORG [*fl.* 1624] *respondent. See* INNICHENHÖFER, H., *praeses.* Ὑπολογια; sive, Tractatus jucundus physiologicus. 1624.

DÖRING, MICHAEL [*d.* 1644] Ἀκρόαμα medicophilosophicum, de opii usu, qualitate calefaciente, virtute narcotica, et ipsum corrigendi modo ... Jenae, Typis Johannis Beithmanni, impens. haered. Johannis Eyring & Johannis Perferti, 1620.

[16], 164, [9] p.   16 cm.   [3306]

[The same.] *In* Mutoni, N. Μιθριδατειοτεχνια. 1620.

—Bericht, wessen man sich in bevorstehender Infections-gefahr, nicht allein mit Praeserviren,

sondern auch mit Curiren verhalten solle. Auff . . .
der . . . Stadt Bresslaw, Verordnung . . . verfasset
. . . Bresslaw, Gedruckt durch Georgium Baumann,
1625.

[55] p.   18 cm.   [3307]

Signatures: [A]-F⁴, A⁴.

— De medicina et medicis adversus iatromastigas
et pseudiatros libri II. In quibus non solum generatim
medicinae origo, progressus, dignitas, & medici of-
ficium prolixe asseritur: sed etiam particulatim tam
Hippocraticae & Galenicae praestantia; quam empiricae, magicae, methodicae, & Paracelsicae usus
atque abusus excutitur . . . Giessae Hessorum, Typis
Nicolai Hampelii, 1611.

[8], 334 (i.e. 456) p.   16 cm.   [3308]

— Διατριβὴν de opobalsamo. *In* Mutoni, N.
Μιθριδατειοτεχνια. 1620.

— Epistola de nova, rara & admiranda herniae
uterinae, atque hanc justo tempore subsequentis partus caesarei historia, cum aliis nonnullis scitu utilibus
scripta ad Guilhelmum Fabricium Hildanum . . .
Witebergae, Ex officina Wolffgangi Meisneri, 1612.

[16] p.   19 cm.   [3309]

— Fasciculus quorundam tractatuum de peste; das
ist, Etliche unterschiedene Tractat von der Pest:
welche Theiles jetzo zum ersten Mahle herausser
gegeben: Theiles von newen ubersehen, und mit
nützlichen so wol Notis, als Marginalibus, verbessert:
Theiles aus dem Lateinischen in das Deutsche
ubergesetzet, unnd zu gemeines Wolstandes
Beförderung aus trewer Wolmeinung zum Drucke
verfertiget worden, durch Michaelem Döring . . .
Brieg, in Verlegung der Perfertischen Erben in
Bresslaw, 1631.

[125] p. 19 cm.   [3310]

Imperfect: upper margins trimmed with possible loss of
pagination.

— *respondent. See* SENNERT, D., *praees.* De febrium
malignarum differentiis & signis disputatio. 1607
[and] De febrium malignarum natura & causis
disputatio. 1607 [and] Quaestiones medicae controversae septem. 1607.

— *See* FABRICIUS VON HILDEN, W. Observationum
& curationum chirurgicarum centuriae. 1614, 1641;
[Dutch tr.] 1656 [and] Opera. 1646, 1682 [and] Wund-
Artzney, gantzes Werck. 1652; PLATTER, F. [1536-1614]

praees. De febrium malignarum curatione. 1607; SEN-
NERT, D. Operum in quinque tomos divisorum. 1666
[and] Operum in sex tomos divisorum tomus primus
[-sextus] 1676.

DÖRMER, AUGUST MICHAEL [*fl.* 1673] *respondent.*
See HELD, J. F., *praees.* Disputatio medico-chirurgica,
de partu Caesareo. 1673; WEDEL, G. W., *praees.*
Casum laborantis corysa . . . publice . . . proponit
A. M. D. 1673 [and] Disputationem inauguralem de
diarrhoea . . . exponit A. M. D. 1673.

DOGNON, R. Le bon cure; ou, Advis a messieurs
les curez touchant leurs charges. Avec les obligations,
expediens, precautions & industries considerables en
l'assistance deuë aux pestiferez . . . Rev., corr. &
augm. . . . Paris, Georges Josse, 1663.

[10], 331, [6] p.   15 cm.   [3311]

DOLÄUS, JOHANN [1651-1707] Opera omnia: exhibentia non modo encyclopaediam medicam
dogmaticam in qua affectus humani corporis interni,
et Encyclopaediam chirurgicam rationalem in qua
. . . Hippocratis, Galeni, Paracelsi, Helmontii,
Willisii, Sylvii, Cartesii, & aliorum sententiae de
morborum maxime causis & curatione perspiciantur
. . . superiora . . . in ultima hac editione longe auctiora & correctiora reddita, de novo offerentia I.
Tractatum de theriaca coelesti . . . II. Observationes
authoris rariores . . . III. Commercium ejus
epistolare cum . . . Johanne Jacobo Waldschmidio
. . . Venetiis, Sumptibus Joh. Jacobi Hertz, 1695.

2 v.   port.   34 cm.   [3312]

— Encyclopaedia chirurgica rationalis, in qua
omnes affectus externi corpus humanum unquam invasisse observati, tam veterum, quam recentiorum
in specie vero Galenicorum, Paracelsi, Helmontii,
Willisii, Sylvii, & Cartesianorum ex fundamentis,
quoad causas & curandi methodum solide pertractantur . . . Francofurti ad Moenum, Sumptibus
Friderici Knochii, 1689.

[35], 1602, [76] p.   front., port.   22 cm.
                                              [3313]

Added engraved title page.
Imperfect: portrait wanting.

— [The same.] Encyclopaedia chirurgica rationalis,
in duos tomos divisa. Tomus primus [-secundus]
[Venetiis, Apud Joannem Jacobum Hertz, 1690]

2 v. in 1.   port.   23 cm.   [3314]

Title from general half title.

—[The same.] Encyclopaedia chirurgica rationalis, in qua omnes affectus externi corpus humanum unquam invasisse observati ... Venetiis, Joh. Jacobi Hertz, 1695.

[4], 616, [30] p.; [1], 92 (i.e. 90) p. illus. 34 cm. [3315]

Part [2] has special title page: Johannis Dolaei ... Tractatus varii. Page [31] part [2] has half title: Joh. Jacobi Waldschmidt ... et Johannis Dolaei ... Dissertationes epistolicae de rebus medicis et philosophicis.

—Encyclopaedia, medicinae theoretico-practicae, qua tam veterum, quam recentiorum, Paracelsistarum nempe, Helmontianorum, Willisianorum, Sylvianorum, Cartesianorum, de causis & curationibus morborum sententiae exhibentur, addita simul authoris de his opinione ... Francofurti ad Moenum, Sumptibus Friderici Knochii, typis Johan-Georgii Drulmanni, 1684.

[23], 1038, [44] p. front. (port.) 21 cm. [3316]

—[The same.] ... Ed. nov. Amstelodami, Typis Andreae ab Hoogenhuysen, 1686.

[16], 739, [21] p. 20 cm. [3317]

—[The same.] ... Ed. 4. & ultima innumeris mendis expurgata. Amstelodami, Typis Andreae ab Hoogenhuysen, 1688.

[16], 739, [21] p. 21 cm. [3318]

Different setting of type.

—[The same.] ... Ed. nov. Venetiis, Apud Jo. Jacobum Hertz, 1690.

[16], 744, [32] p. 25 cm. [3319]

—[The same.] Encyclopaedia, medica dogmatica; in qua omnes affectus interni ... pertractantur, adeo ut in compendio quodam & uno intuitu tum veterum, tum recentiorum, Hippocratis, Galeni, Paracelsi, Helmontii, Willisii, Silvii, Cartesii, et aliorum sententiae de morborum internorum maxime causis & curatione perspiciantur: quibus ipsius authoris ad vera novaque artis medicae principia accommodatum judicium de sede affecta, diagnosi ... adjicitur ... Francofurti ad Moenum, Sumptibus Friderici Knochii, litteris Johannis Baueri, 1691.

[15], 774, 456, [47] p. port. 21 cm. [3320]

Added engraved title page.

—[English tr.] Systema medicinale, a compleat system of physick, theorical and practical. In six books ... Translated out of Latin into English, out of the most learned John Dolaeus being a summary of the ancient and modern way of practice, collected chiefly from Hippocrates, Galen, Paracelsus, Helmont, Willis, Sylvius, Cartesius, and others; wherein both the Galenick and chymick methods are ... brought into this portable volume ... Whereunto is annexed a prefatory discourse concerning the method of studying and practising physick ... Written by William Salmon ... London, Printed for T. Passinger, T. Sawbridge and T. Flesher, 1686.

[31], 516 p.; 360 p. front. (port.) 20 cm. [3321]

—See WALDSCHMIDT, J. J. Commercium literarium virorum. 1688 [and] Opera medico-practica. 1695 [and] Praxis medicinae rationalis succincta. 1690, 1691.

DOLÄUS, JOHANN DANIEL [*fl.* 1697] *respondent. See* HOFFMANN, F. [1660-1742] *praeses.* Dissertatio solennis medica de haemorrhagiarum genuina origine. 1697; STANGE, J. D., *praeses.* Diatriba de juvenis medici idea errante philosophico-medica. 1697.

DOLD, LEONHARD [1565-1611] *tr. See* LIBAVIUS, A. [*d.* 1616] Praxis alchymiae. 1604.

DOLDER, ZACHARIAS [*fl.* 1610] *respondent. See* STUPANUS, J. N., *praeses.* Σημειωτιcεs particularis cap. I. De affectibus. 1610.

DOLÉE, JEAN. *See* DOLÄUS, Johann [1651-1707]

DOLHOPFF, GEORG ANDREAS [*fl.* 1681] *comp.* Lapis animalis microcosmicus; oder, Die höchste Artzney, aus der kleinen Welt des menschlichen Leibs. Sampt einem Tractätlein vom Urin oder Harn des Menschen. Strassburg, In Verlegung Georg Andreas Dolhopffen, 1681.

[16], 80 p. 17 cm. [3322]

Sudhoff 412.

Contains excerpts from the works of Arnoldus de Villanova, Basilius Valentinus, Pierre Jean Fabre, Thomas Kessler, Konrad Khunrath, Paracelsus, George Ripley, Martin Schmuck, and others.

—Lapis vegetabilis; oder, Die höchste Artzney, auss dem Wein, auch andern Erden-Gewächsen. Sambt dem zehenden Buch der Archidoxen Philippi Theophrasti Paracelsi. Strassburg, In Verlegung Georg Andreas Dolhopff, 1681.

[4], 92 p. 16 cm. [3323]

Sudhoff 414.

Contains excerpts from the works of Basilius Valentinus, Joseph Duchesne, Konrad Khunrath, and others.

DOLLMANN, JOHANN CHRISTIAN [*fl.* 1700] *praeses.* Acquae supra-caelestes quas ex principio domestico demonstratas ... Vitembergae, Typis Christiani Kreusigii [1700]

[1], 13 p. 19 cm. [**3324**]

Diss. — Wittenberg (H. Voigt, *respondent*)

DOLPHINTON. *See* BROWN, Andrew [*fl.* 1687–1691]

DOMA, BERNHARDUS A. *See* BERNHARDUS, *a Doma.*

DOMERGUE [*fl.* 1687] Moyens faciles et asseurez pour conserver la santé, et se garantir & guerir de beaucoup de maladies sans prendre aucun remede, accompagnez d'un raisonnement sur L'oeconomie naturelle des esprits ... dans les corps animez ... Paris, Denys Thierry, 1687.

[4], 113, [2] p. 15 cm. [**3325**]

—[The same.] ... 2. ed. Paris, Nicolas le Gras, 1689.

[12], 108 p. 15 cm. [**3326**]

DOMPSELAER, GERARD [*fl.* 1671] *respondent.* Disputatio medica inauguralis, de universali atrophia ... Ultrajecti, Ex officina Cornelii à Vechten, 1671.

[28] p. 20 cm. [**3327**]

Diss. — Utrecht.

DOMUS anatomica Hafniensis brevissime descripta. *See* BARTHOLIN, T. Cista medica Hafniensis. 1662.

DONAT, CHRISTIAN [*fl.* 1665–1691] *praeses.* Dissertatio physica de somniis ... Wittebergae, Typis Johannis Borckardi [1671]

[24] p. 19 cm. [**3328**]

Diss. — Wittenberg (C. A. Vogel, *respondent*)

DONAT, JOHANN. Bericht wie sich die jenigen, bey welchen die bösen, gifftigen, pestilentischen Drüsen, Beulen, Apostemata, oder Carbunckel vormercket werden, oder schon aussgefahren sein, mit euserlichen Artzneyen, hierzu tauglichen vorsehen, und curiren sollen ... Durch Joan: Donatum ... Allen bekümmerten Inficirten dieser Stadt zu Trost und Nutze. Bresslaw, Inn Vorlegung David Müllers, gedruckt zur Neyss, durch Johannem Schubart, 1625.

[20] p. 19 cm. [**3329**]

DONATELLUS, JOANNES. *See* RUDIO, Eustachio [1551–1611]

DONATI, ANTONIO [1606–1659] De aëre Ravennati opusculum ... Ravennae, Typis Petri de Paulis, & Jo. Baptistę Joanelli, 1641.

8, 55 p. 21 cm. [**3330**]

—Trattato de semplici, pietre, et pesci marini, che nascono nel lito di Venetia, la maggior parte non conosciuti da Teofrasto, Dioscoride, Plinio, Galeno, & altri scrittori. Diviso in due libri ... Venetia, Pietro Maria Bertano, 1631.

[8], 120 p. illus. 23 cm. [**3331**]

DONATI, CHRISTIANUS. *See* DONAT, Christian [*fl.* 1665–1691]

DONATI, MARCELLO [1538?–1602] De historia medica mirabili libri sex. Jam primum in Germania editi, ab innumeris rerum & verborum erratis liberati, notis illustrati, & integro recentiorum observationum libro septimo completi, opera & studio Gregori Horsti ... Francofurti ad Moenum, Impensis Johan. Jacobi Porsii, typis Erasmi Kempfferi, 1613.

[24], 715, [17] p. 17 cm. [**3332**]

With this is bound: Scherb, P. Theses medicae. 1614.

DONATO D'EREMITA. *See* EREMITA, Donato d' [*fl.* 1624]

DONATO DI ROCCA. *See* EREMITA, Donato d' [*fl.* 1624]

DONATO, Antonio. *See* DONATI, Antonio [1606–1659]

DONATO, LEONARDO [1530?–1607] *See* CREMONINI, C. Oratio. 1606.

DONATUS, JOANNES. *See* DONAT, Johann.

DONCKERS, LAURENTIUS [1634–1700] Idea febris petechialis; sive, Tractatus de morbo punctuculari. Speciatim de eo, quo annis abhinc circiter tredecim Colonia ejusque vicinia afflictae fuere ... Lugd. Batavor., Apud Petrum vander Aa, 1686.

[62], 500, [34] p. 16 cm. [**3333**]

Added engraved title page.

DONDI DALL'OROLOGIO, JACOPO [*ca.* 1293–1359] *See* UFFENBACH, P. Thesaurus chirurgicae. 1610.

DONI, GIOVANNI BATTISTA [1593 *or* 4–1647] De restituenda salubritate agri Romani, opus posthumum . . . Florentiae, Ex Typographia sub signo Stellae, 1667.

[23], 192 p. illus., plates. 25 cm. [**3334**]

DONIA, Matteo [*fl. ca.* 1600] *ed. See* Ingrassia, G. F. In Galeni librum De ossibus. 1603.

DONINI, Girolamo [*fl.* 1631] *comp. See* Bologna. Laws, statutes, etc. Raccolta di tutti li bandi, ordini, e provisioni fatte per la città di Bologna. 1631.

DONNE, George. *See* Dunn, George [*fl.* 17th cent.]

DONNER-und Wetter-Gebet-Büchlein. *See* Geistreiches Donner und Wetter-Gebet-Büchlein. 1667.

DONNOLI, Francesco Alfonso [1636-1724] De iis, qui semel in die cibum capiunt. Liber, in quo demonstratur quibus corporibus, talis vivendi ratio possit esse idonea . . . Venetiis, Apud Benedictum Milochum, 1674.

[18], 340 p. 14 cm. [**3335**]
Imperfect: 1st prelim. leaf (blank?) wanting.

—Il medico pratico; cioè, Della vita attiva, con la qual può regolarsi ogni medico, che intende professar medicina pratica . . . Venetia, Francesco Valvasense, 1666.

[24], 300 p. front., port. 15 cm. [**3336**]

DONZELLI, Giuseppe [1596-1670] Additio apologetica ad suam de opobalsamo Orientali synopsim. Neapoli, Ex typographia Octavii Beltrani, 1640.

28 p. 22 cm. [**3337**]

—Lettera familiare . . . Sopra l'opobalsamo orientale adoperato in Roma dalli signore Antonio Manfredi, e Vincenzo Panuzzi in far le loro teriache. Al . . . signor Gio. Battista Paulucci . . . Padoa, Paolo Frambotti, 1643.

[24] p. 22 cm. [**3338**]

—Synopsis de opobalsamo orientali . . . Neapoli, Typis Francisci Sauii, 1640.

[18] p. 22 cm. [**3339**]

—Teatro farmaceutico dogmatico, e spagirico . . . Napoli, Giacinto Passaro, 1667.

[30], 660, [20] p. illus. 35 cm. [**3340**]
Added engraved title page.

—[The same.] . . . Con l'aggiunta in molti luoghi del dottor Tomaso Donzelli . . . et in questa 4. imp. corr., & accresciuto con un Catalogo dell'herbe native del suolo Romano del signor Gio. Giacomo Roggieri . . . Venetia, Paolo Baglioni, 1681.

[28], 811, [85] p. illus. 22 cm. [**3341**]
Imperfect: sig. 3f4-5 wanting.

—[The same.] . . . 5. imp. . . . Venetia, Paolo Baglioni, 1686.

[28], 811, [85] p. illus. 24 cm. [**3342**]
Imperfect: half title before title page and sig. 3-7 after title page wanting.
Different setting of type.

—[The same.] . . . 6. imp. . . . Venetia, Paolo Baglioni, 1696.

[24], 811, [85] p. illus. 23 cm. [**3343**]
Different setting of type.

—*See* Collegio degli speziali, Naples. Parere dell'almo Collegio de Spetiali di Napoli. 1640.

DONZELLI, Tommaso [1654-1702] *ed. See* Donzelli, G. Teatro farmaceutico dogmatico, e spagirico. 1681, 1686, 1696.

DONZELLINI, Girolamo [*d.* 1588] Remedium ferendarum injuriarum; sive, De compescenda ira . . . Lugduni Batavorum, Ex officina Joannis Maire, 1635.

[28], 257 p. 13 cm. [**3344**]

—, *ed. See* Giachini, L. In nonum librum Rasis . . . ad Almansorem . . . de partium morbis eruditissima commentaria. 1622.

—*See* Scholtz, L. Consiliorum medicinalium . . . liber singularis. 1610 [and] Epistolarum philosophicarum: medicinalium, ac chymicarum . . . volumen. 1610.

DOOLITTLE, Thomas [1632?-1707] אשיב ליהוה תגמלוהי ; or, A serious enquiry for a suitable return, for continued life, in and after a time of great mortality, by a wasting plague: (Anno 1665). Answered in XIII. directions. By Tho. Doolitel . . . London, Printed by R. I. for J. Johnson and sold by A. Brewster and R. Boulter, 1666.

[16], 291 p. 18 cm. [**3345**]

DOORISSELE, J. [*fl.* 1684-1685] *See* Ghent. Ordinances, local laws, etc. Ordonnantien ende statuten, gemaeckt by heer ende weth der stadt Gendt. 1685?

DOPPELMAYR, JOHANN GABRIEL [1671–1750] *respondent. See* STURM, J. C., *praeses.* Visionis sensum nobilissimum ex obscurae camerae tenebris luculenter-illustrans dissertatio optico-physica. 1699.

D'ORELL, HERMANN. *See* ORELL, Hermann d' [*fl.* 1669]

DORINGIUS, MICHAEL. *See* DÖRING, Michael [*d.* 1644]

DORLIX, PETR. *See* ARBERIUS. La physique d'uzage. 1664; NOUVEAU COURS DE MEDECINE. 1669, 1683.

DORN, Gerhard [16th cent.] [Clavis totius philosophiae chemisticae per quam potissima philosophorum dicta reserantur] [&] De artificio supernaturali [&] Tractatus de naturae luce physica ex genesi desumpta, juxta sapientiam Theophrasti Paracelsi [&] [Physica genesis; Phisica Hermetis Trismegisti; Physica Trithemii; Philosophia meditativa; Philosophia chemica] [&] Tractatus alter. De tenebris contra naturam, et vita brevi [&] De duello animi cum corpore [&] De lapidum preciosorum structura [&] Congeries Paracelsicae chemiae de transmutationibus metallorum [&] De genealogia mineralium ex Paracelso ...

192–591 p., vol. 1. illus. 20 cm. [*In* Zetzner, Lazarus, *ed.* Theatrum chemicum. Argentorati, 1659–61)   **[3346]**

Titles partly caption titles, partly supplied from table of contents.

— , *comp. See* PARACELSUS. Theophrastische Practica. 1618.

DORNAU, CASPAR [1577–1632] Casparis Dornavi Menenius Agrippa; hoc est, Corporis humani cum republica perpetua comparatio: observationibus historicis ... medicis illustrata. Hanoviae, Typis Wechelianis, apud haeredes Joannis Aubrii, 1615.

[12], 75 p. 19 cm.   **[3347]**

DORNAU, JOHANN GOTTFRIED [*fl.* 1651–1652] *respondent.* De apoplexia. *In* Rolfinck, W., *praeses.* Methodus cognoscendi & curandi adfectus capitis particulares. 1653.

— *See* ROLFINCK, W., *praeses.* Dissertatio de chylo et sanguine. 1652.

DORNAVIUS, CASPARUS. *See* DORNAU, Caspar [1577–1632]

DORNAVIUS, JOHANNES GOTTFRIED. *See* DORNAU, Johann Gottfried [*fl.* 1651–1652]

DORNCREILIUS, TOBIAS [1571–1605] Consilium von zweyen, ungewönlichen, newen unnd anklebischen Kranckheiten, die dieses 1602. Jahrs entstanden, und hin und wider heuffig grassiren. Gestellet durch D. Tobiam Dornkreyl ... Magdeburg, Bey Johan. Francken, 1602.

[24] p. 20 cm.   **[3348]**

—Dispensatorium novum ... continens descriptiones & usum praecipuorum medicamentorum ... pro ... Senatus Lunaeburgensis officina ordinatorum ... denuo ... auctius & emendatius editum: cui ... accessit ejusdem auctoris tractatus De purgatione utilissimus. Hamburgi, Ex Bibliopolio Frobeniano, 1604.

[24], 181 (i.e. 189) p. 13 cm.   **[3349]**

"De purgatione" (p. [97]–181 i.e. 189) has half title.

Imperfect: lower margins shaved, affecting imprint date on title page, supplied from a copy in the Wellcome Historical Medical Library.

—Kurtzer, doch gründtlicher ... Bericht von der angehenden, und hin und wieder bereit grassirenden Pestilentz dieses 1603. Jahrs ... Gestellet ... durch D. Tobiam Dornkreil ... Hamburg, Gedruckt [durch Paul Langen] in Verlegung M. Frobenii, 1604.

[6], 51 (i.e. 52), [1] p. 20 cm.   **[3350]**

—Medulla totius praxeos medicae aphoristica, quam ex medicorum excellentissimorum monumentis extractam in quatuor libros distribuit & maximam partem conscripsit Tobias Dorncreilius ab Eberhertz ... post hujus immaturam mortem auxit Joachimus Schelius ... post utriusque beatum obitum tandem explevit & absolvit Valentinus Andreas Möllenbroccius ... [Erfordiae] Sumptibus Christiani à Saher, typis excusa Arnstadio-Schmidianis, 1656.

[16], 624, [2] p. 20 cm.   **[3351]**

Errata: p. [625-6]

— , *ed. See* STOCKAR, J. Empirica. 1601.

DORNFELD, JOHANN [1643–1720] Humani corporis statura physice delineata ... Lipsiae, Typis Johannes Colerii [1674]

[20] p. 20 cm.   **[3352]**

Diss. pro loco—Leipzig.

DORNKREILIUS, Tobias. *See* Dorncreilius, Tobias [1571–1605]

DORPIUS, Martinus [1485–1525] *See* Erasmus, D. Μωρίας ἐγκώμιον. 1676.

DORSCH-VLEGEL; anders, Knuppel uit de sak, aan Doctor Jan Baptista van Lamsweerde toegeëigend. [Amsterdam?] "Goliath de Reus", 1677.
   12 p. 16 cm.   **[3353]**

DORSTEN, Johann Daniel [1643–1706] *praeses.* Disputatio medica de succi nutritii statu naturali & praeternaturali … Marpurgi Cattorum, Typis Johannis Jodoci Kürsneri, 1683.
   16 p. 18 cm.   **[3354]**
   Diss.—Marburg (J. W. O. Eggers, *respondent*)

—Exercitatio anatomica de monstro humano nupero … Marburgi Cattorum, Typis Joannis Henrici Stockenii [1684]
   48 p. plate. 21 cm.   **[3355]**
   Diss.—Marburg (K. P. Lombard, *respondent*)

—*See* Valentini, M. B. De monstrorum Hassiacorum ortu atque causis. 1684?

DORTMONT, Bonaventura van [*fl.* 1677] Aennemingh van de presentatie, van Mr. Andries Boekelman. Waer in aengewesen worden de quade practijken om sijn begaene misslagh, en sijn onwetenheyt te verschoonen, aengaende het afhalen van een doode vrucht. Amsterdam, Hieronymus Sweerts, 1677.
   32 p. 16 cm.   **[3356]**

—Antwoort, op het nootwendigh bericht, van Mr. Andries Boeckelman … Aengaende het af halen van een doode vrucht. Amsterdam, Hieronymus Sweerts, 1677.
   27 p. 16 cm.   **[3357]**

—Nootwendigh bericht, aen … Fredericus Ruysch, en … Andries Boeckelman … Amsterdam, Hieronymus Sweerts, 1677.
   [8] p. 16 cm.   **[3358]**

—Verklaring over de aen-neming van de presentatie van Mr. Andries Boekelman, over het verschil van het af-halen van een doode vrucht … Amsterdam, Alexander Lintman, 1677.
   31 p. 16 cm.   **[3359]**

—*See* Extraordinare Amsterdamsche Maendaegsche Courant. 1678; Koeckoecx naar sang. 1677; Sentiments d'un voyageur sur plusieurs libelles de ce temps. 1677.

—*as subject. See* Aanmerkingen. 1677; De amsteldamsche nyptang. 1678; De tweede onschult. 1678; Register der boeckjens. [1677–1678]; Schoppen is troef. 1678; Staetkundige bedencking, over het verschil tusschen den Heer Bonaventura Dortmond. 1677; Strijck op den bruy een sesjen. 1677.

D'ORVILLE, Petrus Fridericus. *See* Orville, Peter Friedrich d' [*fl.* 1684]

DOUGLAS, William [*b. ca.* 1665] *respondent.* Disputatio medica inauguralis de lue venerea … Lugduni Batavorum, Apud Abrahamum Elzevier, 1687.
   [16] p. 21 cm.   **[3360]**
   Diss.—Leyden.

DOUXCIEL, Ancelme Petit. *See* Petit Douxciel, Ancelme [*fl.* 1648]

DOUX DE CLAVES, Gaston. *See* Claves, Gaston Le Doux, *known as* Gaston de [*b. ca.* 1530]

DOYE, Jean Baptiste [*fl.* 1685–1716] *praeses.* Quaestio medica … An ischuriae emeticum? [Parisiis, Apud Franciscum Muguet, 1694]
   4 p. 24 cm.   **[3361]**
   Caption title.
   Diss.—Paris (J. Gelly, *respondent*)

DRACHSTEDT, Michael Friedrich [*fl.* 1685] *respondent. See* Fasch, A. H., *praeses.* Dissertatio medica inauguralis de febre quartana intermittente. 1685.

DRAGE, William [1637?–1669] A physical nosonomy; or, A new and true description of the law of God (called nature) in the body of man … Also in the second part of this book is a practice of physick … To which is added, a treatise of diseases from witchcraft … London, Printed by J. Dover, and sold by R. Tomlins and Geo. Calvert, 1665.
   [1], 415 p. 20 cm.   **[3362]**
   Errata inserted between sig. A1 and A2.
   The tract "A treatise of diseases from witchcraft" mentioned on the title page does not seem to have been included.

—[The same.] The practice of physick; or, The law of God (called nature) in the body of man ... Also in the second part of this book is a practice of physick ... To which is added, a treatise of diseases from witchcraft ... London, George Calvert, 1666.

415 p.   20 cm.   [3363]

A reissue of A physical nosonomy with new title page. Errata wanting.

DRAKE, JAMES [1667-1707] *tr. See* LE CLERC, D. The history of physick. 1699.

DRAKE, ROGER [1608-1669] Contra animadversiones Jac. Primrosii, in theses, quas ipse pro sanguinis motu circulari, sub paesidio Jo. Walaei, in ... Leidae Academia ... subjecerat, vindiciae.

167-240 p.   part [2].   20 cm. (*In* Recentiorum disceptationes de motu cordis. Lugduni Batavorum, 1647)   [3364]

Caption title.

—, *respondent. See* WALAEUS, J., *praeses.* Disputatio medica de circulatione naturali. 1640 [and] Theses de circulatione naturali. 1647.

[**DRAUD,** GEORG, 1573-1635] Bibliotheca exotica; sive, Catalogus officinalis librorum peregrinis linguis usualibus scriptorum ... La bibliotheque universail, contenant le catalogue de tous les livres, qui ont estè imprimes ce siecle passè, aux langues françoise, italiene, espaignole, & autres, qui sont aujourdhuy plus communes, depuis l'an 1500, jusques à l'an present 1610 ... Frankfourt, Pierre Kopf, 1610.

219 p.   21 cm.   [3365]

Imperfect: p. 217-19 mutilated affecting pagination.
Bound with *his* Bibliotheca librorum Germanicorum classica. 1611.

—Bibliotheca librorum Germanicorum classica. Das ist: Verzeichnuss aller und jeder Bücher, so fast bey dencklichen Jaren in teutscher Spraach von allerhand Materien hin und wider in Truck aussgangen, und noch den mehrertheil in Buchläden gefunden werden ... Franckfurt am Mayn, Getruckt durch Johann Saurn, in Verlegung Peter Kopffen, 1611.

[7], 563, [30] p.   21 cm.   [3366]

With this is bound *his* Bibliotheca exotica. 1610.

DRAWITZ, JOHANN [*fl.* 1642-1647] Bericht und Unterricht von der Kranckheit des schmertzmachenden Scharbocks woher derselbe entstehe und komme und wie solche Kranckheit zu curiren, zum andernmahl gedruckt ... corrigiret und mit einer

... Vorrede Hn. D. Johann Michaelis ... Leipzig, Verlegts Tobias Riese, Drucktens Henning Köhlers seel. Erben, 1658.

[66], 421 (i.e. 433), [31] p.   16 cm.   [3367]

Added engraved title page.

—[The same.] ... Zum drittenmahl gedruckt ... Leipzig, Verlegts Joh. Christoph. Tarnovius, gedruckt bey Johann Georgen, 1671.

[63], 421 (i.e. 433), [31] p.   17 cm.   [3368]

Added engraved title page.
Imperfect: Sig. Aviii—probably blank—wanting?
Different setting of type.

—, *respondent. See* ROLFINCK, W., *praeses.* De ichore ulcerum seroso. 1642.

DRECHSSLER, JOHANN GABRIEL [*d.* 1677] Disputatio I. De metallorum transmutatione, et imprimis de chrysopoeia oder Goldmachen ... Lipsiae, Vypis-Tiduae [sic] Joh. Wittigau [1673]

[16] p.   19 cm.   [3369]

Diss. pro loco—Leipzig.

—*praeses.* Discursus curiosus, at sobrius de nive prodigiosa, circa proxime praeteritum XX. Novembr. in Hungaria superiore coelo delapsa ... Lipsiae, Typis viduae Johannis Wittgau [1673]

19, [1] p.   illus.   20 cm.   [3370]

Diss.—Leipzig (D. Geisler, *respondent*)

—Disputatio II. de metallorum transmutatione, et imprimis de chrysopoeia oder Goldmachen ... Lipsiae, Typis viduae Joh. Wittigau [1673]

[16] p.   19 cm.   [3371]

Diss.—Leipzig (A. C. Platz, *respondent*)

— Dissertatio historico-physica de sermone brutorum ... Lipsiae, Typis viduae Joh. Wittigau [1673]

[24] p.   21 cm.   [3372]

Diss.—Leipzig (P. M. Rechtenbach, *respondent*)

DRELINCOURT, CHARLES [1633-1697] Opera varia. Lugd. Batav., Apud Cornelium Boutesteyn, 1693.

6 parts in 1 v.   14 cm.   [3373]

Contents: pt. [1] Clarissimum Monspeliensis Apollinis stadium, ed. 3.—pt. [2] De partu octimestri vivaci diatriba. Ed. 4.—pt. [3] La légende du Gascon; ou, La lettre de Charles Drelincourt, à Mr. Porrée, sur la méthode, prétendüe nouvelle, de trailler de la pierre; avec deus autres lettres à Mr. Le Prémier ... 3. éd., rev., & abrégée.—pt. [4] Praeludium anatomicum. Ed. 3.—pt. [5] Libitinae tropaea. Ed. alt.—pt. [6] Ἐυφημισμος Cardiaci contra viperinos calumniatorum morsus . . . — Each part (except part [6] which has half title) has special title page. Parts [1–2] and [4–5] are dated 1680. Parts [1–2] and [5] have imprint . . . Apud Felicem Lopez . . . ; part [3]: A Léïde, Chez Felix Lopez; and part [4]: . . . Apud Danielem à Gaesbeeck . . .

—Apologia medica, qua vetus illa depellitur calumnia, medicos sexcentis annis Roma exulasse. Lugduni Batavorum, Apud Cornelium Driehusium, 1671.

107, [1] p.   14 cm.   [3374]

—[The same.] Ed. alt. Lugduni Batavorum, Apud Felicem Lopez, 1672.

129 p.   31 cm.   [3375]

—De conceptione adversaria . . . Lugduni Batavorum, Apud Cornelium Boutesteyn, 1685.

[10], 58 p.   13 cm.   [3376]

Bound with *his* De foeminarum ovis. 1684.

—De foeminarum ovis, tam intra testiculos & uterum quam extra; ab anno 1666 ad retro secula . . . Lugd. Batav., Apud Danielem a Gaesbeeck, 1684.

[8], 98 p.   13 cm.   [3377]

With this are bound: *his* Experimenta anatomica. 1682.— *his* De conceptione adversaria. 1685.

—De foeminarum ovis historicae atque physicae lucubrationes . . . Ed. 2. physicis auctior. Lugd. Batav., Apud Danielem a Gaesbeeck, 1687.

[10], 190, [4] p.   14 cm.   [3378]

". . . De foeminarum ovis curae secundae . . ." (p. [III]–142) has special title page; ". . . Appendix de utero . . ." (p. [143]–185) has half title.

—De humani foetus membranis hypomnemata . . . Lugduni Batavorum, Apud Cornelium Boutesteyn, 1685.

134, [22] p.   15 cm.   [3379]

Published also as part [3] of *his* Opuscula de foetus humani conceptione.

—De partu octimestri vivaci diatriba. Ed. 3. . . . Parisiis, Apud Andream Cramoisy, 1668.

[8], 40 p.   21 cm.   [3380]

—[The same.] Quaestio medica de partu octimestri vivaci . . . Lugd. Batav., Ex officina Felicis Lopez de Haro, 1668.

48 p.   13 cm.   [3381]

—Experimenta anatomica, ex vivorum sectionibus petita. Edita per Ernestum Gottfried Heyseum . . .

Lugd. Batav., Apud Cornelium Boutesteyn, 1681.

[8], 70, [2] p.   14 cm.   [3382]

—[The same.] . . . Lugd. Batav., 1682.

70 p.   13 cm.   [3383]

Bound with *his* De foeminarum ovis. 1684.

—Experimenta anatomica, quibus adjecta sunt plurima curiosa super semine virili, foemineis ovis, utero, uterique tubis atque foetu. Lugd. Batav. Apud Cornelium Boutesteyn, 1684.

[10], 128 p.   14 cm.   [3384]

". . . Experimenta anatomica, ex vivorum sectionibus petita, edita per Ernestum Gottfried Heyseum . . . Ed. alt., ad fidem autographi Drelincurtiani revocata . . ." (p. [3]–75) has special title page.
—Copy 2.
With this is bound *his* Opuscula de foetus humani conceptione. 1685.

—Libitinae tropaea, pro concione, quum fasces academicos deponeret, computata; die . . . VIII. Feb. 1680. Ed. alt. Lugd. Batavor., Apud Felicem Lopez, 1680.

[12], 156 p.   13 cm.   [3385]

With this are bound: Ἐυφημισμος cardiaci contra viperinos calumniatorum morsus. [1680?]; — *his* Appendix ad Libitinae trophaea. 1680; —Alithophilus. Observationes extemporaneae. [1681?]

—Appendix ad Libitinae trophaea . . . [Lugduni Batavorum?] 1680.

12, [4], 13–84 p.   13 cm.   [3386]

Bound with *his* Libitinae tropaea. 1680.

—Opuscula de foetus humani conceptione, membranis, umbilico, nutritione atque partu . . . Lugduni Batavorum [Apud Cornelium Boutesteyn] 1685.

5 parts in 1 v.   14 cm.   [3387]

Contents: pt. [1] De conceptu conceptus, quibus mirabilia Dei super foetus humani formatione, nutritione atque partione, sacro velo hactenus tecta, systemate felici reteguntur. —pt. [2] De conceptione adversaria Ed. alt. —pt. [3] De humani foetus membranis hypomnemata. —pt. [4] De tunica foetus allantoide meletemata. —De foetuum pileolo sive galea emendationes. —pt. [5] Super humani foetus umbilico meditationes elencticae. —Each part has special title page. That of part [2] is dated 1686. The second treatise in part [4] has special title page also.
Bound with copy 2 of *his* Experimenta anatomica. 1684.

—Quaestiones quatuor cardinales . . . pro suprema Apollinari Daphne consequenda. Monspelii, Apud Danielem Pech, 1655.

20 p.   22 cm.   [3388]

—Super humani foetus umbilico meditationes elencticae . . . Lugduni Batavorum, Apud Cornelium Boutesteyn, 1685.

69, [1] p. 13 cm. [3389]

Published also as part [5] of *his* Opuscula de foetus humani conceptione.

—*praeses*. Disputatio medica de apoplexia . . . Lugduni Batavorum, Apud viduam & haeredes Johannis Elsevirii, 1671.

[16] p. 23 cm. [3390]

Diss. — Leyden (J. von Flammerdinge, *respondent*)

—Disputatio medica inauguralis, de suffocatione hypochondriaca in viro . . . Lugduni Batavorum, Apud Abrahamum Elzevier, 1688.

[32] p. 22 cm. [3391]

Diss. — Leyden (G. Walter, *respondent*)

—Dissertatio medica de nutritione foetus . . . Lugduni Batavorum, Apud Abrahamum Elzevier, 1682.

[16] p. 19 cm. [3392]

Diss. — Leyden (T. Kennedy, *respondent*)

—*respondent*. Disputatio anatomico-practica inauguralis de lienosis . . . Ed. alt. Lugduni Batavorum, Apud Cornelium Boutesteyn, 1693.

[64] p. 20 cm. [3393]

Diss. — Leyden.

—*See* ALITHOPHILUS, *pseud.* Alithophili Observationes extemporaneae. 1681?; ΕΥΦΗΜΙΣΜΟΣ cardiaci contra viperinos calumniatorum morsus. 1680? FELIX PUERPERA. 1684?

DRELINCURTIUS, CAROLUS. *See* DRELINCOURT, Charles [1633-1697]

DRESCHER, MATTHÄUS. *See* DRESSER, Matthäus [1536-1607]

DRESDEN. Rat. Ordinances, local laws, etc. Dess Raths zu Dressden Ordnung, wie bey ereignenden gefährlichen Seuchen, und anderen ansteckenden Kranckheiten die Inwohner, und Bürgerschafft hiesiger Churfl. Residenz-Stadt, sampt denen hierzu bestalten Bedienten auff einen und den andern Fall sich zu verhalten. Nebenst angefügten medicinischen Bedencken. Dressden, Gedruckt bey Christian Bergen, 1680.

[4], 23, [4] p.; [34] p. 21 cm. [3394]

Part [2] has special title page.
Imperfect? Sheet A of part [2] apparently skipped in signing.

DRESDENSIS, PETRUS. *See* PETRUS DRESDENSIS [d. 1440]

DRESLER, JOHANN LUDWIG [b. 1649] *See* WEDEL, G. W. Georgius Wolffgangus Wedelius . . . Facultatis Medicae decanus, lectori benevolo S. P. D. 1681.

DRESSER, MATTHÄUS [1536-1607] De partibus humani corporis & animae potentiis, libri duo, corr. & aucti denuo. Adjectae sunt ad finem morborum & medicamentorum communissimorum apellationes. Lipsiae, Impensis Jacobi Apelii [Imprimebat Michael Lantzenberger] 1607.

[10], 254, [22] p. 16 cm. [3395]

DRESSLER, JOHANN LUDWIG [*fl.* 1681] *respondent.* *See* CRAUSE, R. W., *praeses.* Dissertatio inauguralis medica de tabe. 1681.

DREXEL, JEREMIAS [1581-1638] Aloe amari sed salubris succi jejunium . . . Antverpiae, Typis vid. Joann. Cnobbari, 1638.

[18], 336, [2] p. 12 cm. [3396]

Engraved title page.

—Aurifodina artium & scientiarum omnium excerpendi solertia . . . monstrata . . . Cui annxea [sic] est Martini Kergeri M. D. Methodus excerpendi Drexeliana succinctior. Antverpiae, Apud viduam Joannis Cnobbari, 1658.

[21], 437, [13] p. 12 cm. [3397]

Added engraved title page.

—*See* GUARINONIUS, H. Hydroenogamia triumphpans. 1640.

DREY neue curieuse Tractätgen, von dem Trancke Cafe, sinesischen The, und der Chocolata. 1686, 1692. *See* [DUFOUR, P. S.]

DREY vortreffliche und noch nie im Druck gewesene chymische Bücher. Als I. Johannis Ticinensis . . . opusculum, genandt Processus de lapide philosophorum. II. Anthonii de Abbatia . . . aussgefärtigtes Send-Schreiben. III. . . . Edoardi Kellaei ausführlicher Tractat dem Käyser Rudolpho zugeschrieben . . . In teutscher Sprach übergesetzet . . . Hamburg, In Verlegung Johan Nauman, 1670.

160 p. 16 cm. [3398]

The second and the third treatises have half titles.

DREYER, Diricus [*fl.* 1677-1683] *respondent.* Disputatio medica inauguralis de menstruo fluxu sufflaminato ... Lugduni Batavorum, Apud Abrahamum Elzevier, 1683.

[12] p. 22 cm.   [**3399**]

Diss. — Leyden.

DREYSCHERFF, Joachim [*fl.* 1629] *respondent.* See Pfeiffer, J., *praes.* Disputatio physica. 1629.

DRIEL, Herman [*fl.* 1648-1655] *respondent.* Disputatio medica inauguralis de hepatis obstructione ... Lugduni Batavorum, Apud Franciscum Moyaert, 1648.

[8] p. 22 cm.   [**3400**]

Diss. — Leyden.

DRIVERE, Jérémie. *See* Dryvere, Jérémie de [1504-1554]

DROSSANDER, Andreas [1648-1696] *praeses.* De sale volatili disputatio chymico physica ... Upsalae, Henricus Keyser [1687]

[6], 37, [1] p. plate. 16 cm.   [**3401**]

Diss. — Uppsala (G. Browallius, *respondent*)

—Dissertatio physica de motu musculari ... Upsalae, Henricus Keyser [1692]

[6], 34 p. 15 cm.   [**3402**]

Diss. — Uppsala (J. Skovg, *respondent*)

—Tenuis & succincta contemplatio pororum ... Upsaliae, Henricus Keyser [1686]

[8], 85 p. 15 cm.   [**3403**]

Diss. — Uppsala (J. Zephyrinus, *respondent*)

DROÜIN, Vincent Denis [1660-1722] Description du cerveau, des principales distributions de ses dix paires de nerfs, & des organes des sens ... Par Mr Droüin ... Paris, Guillaume de Luyne, 1691.

[16], 125, [3] p. plates. 16 cm.   [**3404**]

DROYN, Gabriel [*fl.* 1584-1615?] Le royal syrop de pommes, antidote des passions melancoliques ... Paris, Jean Moreau, 1615.

[7], 152 p. 18 cm.   [**3405**]

DRUPWICH, Henricus a [*fl.* 1608] *respondent.* Disputatio medica de paralysi ... Marpurgi, Cattorum, Paulus Egenolphus, 1608.

[12] p. 21 cm.   [**3406**]

Diss. — Marburg.

DRYDEN, John [1631-1700] See Fracastoro, G. Syphilis. 1693.

DRYVERE, Jérémie de [1504-1554] *In* omnes Galeni de temperamentis libros epitome. *In* Hippocrates. Les Aphorismes. 1605, 1606, 162-?, 1627, 1628, 1646, 1660, 1671.

DUBÉ, Paul [17th cent.] Histoire de deux enfans monstreux nées en la paroisse de Septfonds au duché de S. Fergeau, le 20. juillet 1649 ... Paris, François Piot, 1650.

[2], 56, [2] p. 17 cm.   [**3407**]

—Le medecin et le chirurgien des pauvres. [Paris, Edme Couterot, 1671]

2 parts in 1 v. 15 cm.   [**3408**]

Title from half title.

Added engraved title page.

Each part has special title page. Part [1] has title: Le medecin des pauvres ... Rev. & augm. en cette 2. ed. de divers traitez, & particulierement du scorbut ... Par un docteur en medecine. Part [2] dated 1674 has title: Le chirurgien des pauvres.

—Another issue, part [1] in different setting of type. Imperfect: preliminary leaf (engraved title page?) wanting.   [**3409**]

—[The same.] 3. ed. 1676.   [**3410**]

—[The same.] Le medecin des pauvres ... 5. ed., rev., corr., & augm. de deux traitez. Paris, Edme Couterot, 1678.

2 parts in 1 v. 16 cm.   [**3411**]

Part [2] has special title page: Le chirurgien des pauvres.

—[The same.] Le medecin et le chirurgien des pauvres ... [Paris, Edme Couterot, 1680]

2 parts in 1 v. 14 cm.   [**3412**]

Added half title.

Each part has special title page: Nouv. ed. rev. & augm.

Author statement on title page of part [1]: Par un docteur en medecine de ce temps; part [2]: Par Mr. Dubé.

—[The same.] ... 1681.

2 parts in 1 v. 15 cm.   [**3413**]

Engraved title page and half title.

Each part has special title page. Pt. [2] has title: Le medecin [i.e. chirurgien] des pauvres ... Derniere ed. ... 1678.

—[The same.] Le medecin des pauvres ... Nouv. ed. rev. & augm. ... Agen, Antoine Bru, 1681.

2 parts in 1 v. 16 cm.   [**3414**]

Part [2] has special title page: Le chirurgien des pauvres ... Par un docteur en medecine, 3. ed.

—[The same.] ... Derniere ed., rev., corr., & augm. de deux traitez. Paris, Edme Coterot, 1686.

   2 parts in 1 v.   16 cm.   [**3415**]

—[The same.] Le medecin et chirurgien des pauvres ... 8. ed., rev., corr., & augm. de quelques traitez, & particulierement du quinquina. Paris, Edme Couterot, 1693.

   [89], 538 p.   front.   15 cm.   [**3416**]

—[The same.] Le medecin des pauvres ... Derniere ed., rev. & augm. Lyon, Laurens Bachelu fils, 1696.

   2 parts in 1 v.   16 cm.   [**3417**]

   Part [2] has title: Le chirurgien des pauvres ... with imprint: Lyon, François Sarrazin, 1693.

—[The same.] ... Derniere ed. Lyon, Jean Veyron, 1700.

   2 parts in 1 v.   16 cm.   [**3418**]

   Part [2] has special title page: Le chirurgien des pauvres ... Derniere ed., rev. & augm. Lyon, Pierre Thened, 1700.

—Medicinae theoreticae medulla; seu, Medicina animi et corporis ... Parisiis, Edmundum Couterot, 1671.

   [8], lix, [1], 351, [1] p.   16 cm.   [**3419**]

   Added engraved title page.

DUBOIS, Jacques [1478-1555] Jacobi Sylvii ... Opera medica, jam demum in sex partes digesta, castigata & indicibus necessariis instructa ... Opera et studio Renati Moraei ... Genevae, Apud Jacobum Chouët, 1634.

   [58], 204, 12, [205]-884, [31] p.   port.   33 cm.
                                               [**3420**]

   "Genevae" in imprint covered over with type ornaments and "Coloniae Allobrogum" printed above.

   Originally issued by Chouët in 1630.

   This copy contains both the cancel and the cancelland printing of the author's dedicatory epistle to Petrus Lysetus: the original (?) form, here cancelled by crossing through in ink, retained as p. [17-18] and the reprinted (?) form appearing as p. [57-58].

   Includes the Latin texts of Hippocrates' De natura hominis with the commentary of Galen, Galen's De ossibus ad tirones, and the younger Mesuë's De re medica libri tres (i.e. the principal pharmaceutical works attributed to Mesuë) edited with notes by Dubois.

—[The same.] Genevae, Apud Jacobum Chouët, 1635.

   [56], 204, 12, [205]-892 (i.e. 896), [31] p.   port.   33 cm.   [**3421**]

   Imperfect: p. [55-56] (half title and table of contents) wanting.

   An altered issue of Chouët's 1634 edition, with the addition of new "Consilia varia" (p. 885-892).

Contains (p. [17-18]) the author's epistle to Lysetus in the original (?) printing of the 1634 edition; the verso has been crossed out in ink; but the cancel (?) leaf has not been inserted.

—[De medicamentorum simplicium delectu. French.] La pharmacopee de M^e. Jacques Sylvius ... Qui est, la maniere de bien choisir, preparer les simples, & faire les compositions, despartie en trois livres. Faicte françoise par ... André Caille ... Derniere ed. ... Lyon, Jean Ant. Huguetan, 1604.

   [26], 686, [75] p.   12 cm.   [**3422**]

—*See* CORDUS, V. Dispensatorium. 1627, 1651, [1652]; [Dutch ed.] 1632, 1656; FONTEYN, N. Institutiones pharmaceuticae. 1633; GALENUS. De ossibus. 1665; MESUË [924 *or* 5-1015] Opera. 1602, 1623; SCHOLTZ, L. Consiliorum medicinalium ... liber singularis. 1610.

—*as subject. See* PARDOUX, B. Bartholomaei Perdulcis ... *In* Jac. Sylvii anatomen et in lib. Hippocratis De natura humana commentarii. 1643.

DUBOST, CLAUDIUS [*fl. ca.* 1620] *ed. See* VARANDA, J. de. Tractatus de morbis ventriculi. 1620.

DUBOURGDIEU, CAROLUS VALESIUS. Commentarii de peste, et exanthematibus ... Romae, Typis Ignatii de Lazaris, 1656.

   [8], 366, [1] p.   23 cm.   [**3423**]

   Errata: p. [367]

—, *ed. See* HIPPOCRATES. [Prognostica. Latin.] Aphorismi prognostici. 1659.

DU BOYS, JEAN. Methodus miscendi & conficiendi medicamenta, diligenter recognita, & a multis, quibus antea scatebat mendis, repurgata. Novae huic editioni accessit Hispalensium pharmacopoliorum recognitio, auctore D. Simone e Tovar ... Hagae-Comitis, Ex officina Theodori Maire, 1640.

   [6], 396, [22] p.; [6], 165, [2] p.   13 cm.
                                               [**3424**]

   Part [2] has special title page.

   First published in 1572 under title: In methodum miscendorum medicamentorum, quae in quotidiano sunt usu, observationes.

—Observationes in methodum miscendorum medicamentorum topicorum. *In* Bauderon, B. Pharmacopoea. 1639.

DU CANGE, CHARLES DU FRESNE, *sieur* [1610-1688] Caroli Du Fresne ... Glossarium ad scriptores mediae & infimae Latinitatis, in quo Latina vocabula novatae significationis, aut usus rarioris, barbara & exotica explicantur . . . Accedit Dissertatio de Imperatorum Constantinopolitanorum; seu, De inferioris aevi, vel imperii, uti vocant, numismatibus. Francofurti ad Moenum, Impensis Johannis Davidis Zunneri, typis Balthasaris Christophori Wustii, 1681.

> 3 v. in 2. illus., plates 36 cm.   **[3425]**
> Added engraved title page.
> Each volume has half title.

DU CASTEL, JEAN [*fl.* 1668] *respondent.* Disputatio medica inauguralis de lochiis . . . Lugduni Batavorum, Apud viduam & haeredes Joannis Elsevirii, 1668.

> [16] p. 24 cm.   **[3426]**
> Imperfect: sig. B2 wanting.
> Diss. — Leyden.

DU CHASTEAU, PIERRE VASC. *See* CASTELLO, Pedro Vasco [*fl.* 1616]

DU CHATEL, PIERRE. *See* CASTELLANUS, Petrus [1585–1632]

DUCHESNE, JOSEPH [*ca.* 1544–1609] Jos. Quercetani medici Opera medica: scilicet, Ad Jacobi Auberti Vindonis De ortu & causis metallorum contra chymicos explicationem, brevis responsio. De exquisita mineralium, animalium & vegetabilium medicamentorum spagyrica praeparatione & usu, perspicua tractatio. Sclopetrarius [sic] sive, De curandis vulneribus, quae sclopetorum & similium tormentorum ictibus acciderunt, liber. Antidotarium spagyricum adversus eosdem ictus. Lipsiae, Impensis Thomas Schüreri & Bartholomaei Voigt, 1614.

> 2 v. in 1. 16 cm.   **[3427]**
> "De mineralium, animalium, et vegetabilium spagyrica praeparatione, & usu" (v. [1], p. 63–152) has special title page, dated 1600.
> Vol. [2] has title: Josephi Quercetani medici Sclopetarius . . . Antidotarium spagyricum.

— Quercetanus redivivus; hoc est, Ars medica dogmatico hermetica, ex scriptis Josephi Quercetani . . . tomis tribus digesta: quorum I. Ars medica mediatrix, II. Ars medica auxiliatrix, III. Ars medica practica. Opera Joannis Schröderi . . . Francofurti, Apud Joannem Beyerum, 1648.

> 3 v. in 1. 21 cm.   **[3428]**
> Imperfect: Added engraved title page wanting.
> Errata leaf inserted at end of v. 3.

— [The same.] . . . Tribus tomis digesta, opera Joannis Schröderi . . . ante hac edita: hac autem secunda editione juxta exemplar Schröderianum revisa, variisque in locis correcta & aucta . . . Francofurti, Sumptibus haeredum Johannis Beyeri, 1679.

> 3 v. in 1. 21 cm.   **[3429]**
> Added engraved title page.

— [German ed.] Josephi Quercetani M. D. Drey medicinische Tractätlein. Das erste ein kurtze Antwort auff Jacobi Auberti Vindonis Ausslegung vom Ursprung und Ursachen der Metallen wider die Chymicos. Das andere von aussführlicher Bereitung der Mineralien, Thier, und Kräuter Artzneyen, wie dieselben spagyrisch . . . sollen zugerüstet und gebraucht werden. Das dritte ein Büchsen-Artzneybüchlein, darinnen aussführlichen berichtet wird, wie man die Wunden spagyrischer Weiss curiren . . . soll . . . auch von Zurüstung der Artzneyen, so man zu den geschossenen Wunden brauchen soll und muss. Von weyland dem edlen . . . Herren Josepho Quercetano . . . Lateinisch und Frantzösisch beschrieben, an jetzo aber . . . in die teutsche Sprache ubergesetzet. Durch M. Thomam Kesslern . . . Strassburg, In Verlegung Eberhardi Zetzners, 1631.

> [8], 96 (i.e. 94) p.; 117, [4] p. port. 20 cm.
>   **[3430]**

> Part [2] has special title page: Sclopetarius; das ist, Büchsen-Tractätlein . . . Und dann, Wie die Artzneyen . . . zubereiten seindt.
> Translation of Ad Jacobi Auberti . . . De ortu et causis metallorum contra chymicos explicationem . . . brevis responsio; De mineralium, animalium & vegetabilium medicamentorum spagyrica praeparatione & usu; Sclopetarius, and Antidotarium spagiricum. The same works had been published together in Latin in 1591 and later as the Opera medica.

— Ad Brevem Riolani excursum brevis incursio. *In his* Jos. Quercetani . . . Tetras gravissimorum totius capitis affectum 1617.

— [The same, *as subject.*] *See* RIOLAN, J. [1580–1657] Incursionum Quercetani depulsio. 1605.

— Ad Jacobi Auberti . . . De ortu et causis metallorum contra chemicos explicationem brevis responsio.

> 150–178 p., vol. 2. 20 cm. (*In* Zetzner, Lazarus, *ed.* Theatrum chemicum. Argentorati, 1659–61)
>   **[3431]**
> Caption title.

— [French tr.] *In his* Traicté familier. 1630, 1639, 1648.

—Jos. Quercetani ... Ad veritatem hermeticae medicinae ex Hippocratis veterumque decretis ac therapeusi; necnon vivae rerum anatomiae exegesi ipsiusque naturae luce stabiliendam, adversus cujusdam anonymi phantasmata responsio. Lutetiae Parisiorum, Apud Abrahamum Saugrain, 1604.

[16], 312 (i.e. 316), 68, [8] p.   17 cm.   **[3432]**

A reply to the Apologia pro Hippocratis et Galeni medicina adversus Quercetani Librum de priscorum philosophorum verae medicinae materia, generally attributed to the younger Jean Riolan.

—[The same.] ... Francofurti, Ex officina typographica Wolffgangi Richteri, impensa Conradi Nebenii, 1605.

[16], 300 p.   16 cm.   **[3433]**

With this is bound Servi, P. Ad librum de sero lactis Stephani Roderici Castrensis ... declamationes. 1634.

—[English tr.] The practise of chymicall and hermeticall physicke, for the preservation of health. Written in Latin by Josephus Quersitanus ... and translated into English by Thomas Timme ... London, Thomas Creede, 1605.

[206] p.   20 cm.   **[3434]**

Signatures: A⁴, *², B-2B⁴, 2C² (last leaf blank)
Imperfect: leaf [1] preceding title page, and "The fore-speech to the reader" (leaves signed *, *²) wanting.
STC 7276.
—Copy 2.   19 cm.
Imperfect: 1st and 2d prelim. leaves, including title page, wanting. "The fore-speech to the reader" present.

—Antidotarium spagiricum. *In his* Josephi Quercetani medici Sclopetarius; sive, De curandis vulneribus. 1614.

—[English tr.] *In* Paracelsus. One hundred and fourteen experiments and cures. 1652.

—[French tr.] *In his* Traicté de la cure ... des arcbusades. 1625.

—[German tr.] Spagirica, dess ... Herrn Josephi Quercetani ... Gründliche Beschreibung, der mineralischen, animalischen und vegetabilischen Artzneyen, derselben rechten Gebrauch und spagirische Bereitung ... Jetzo ... durch den ... Herrn Johannem Cupium ... ins Deutsch transferiret. Hall, Gedruckt durch Erasmum Hynitzsch, in Verlegung Joachimi Krüsicken, 1608.

[134] p.   16 cm.   **[3435]**

Bound with Thurneisser zum Thurn, Reise und Kriegs-Apotecken. 1602.

—[The same.] *In his* Josephi Quercetani medici sclopetarius. 1631.

—[De mineralium, animalium, et vegetabilium medicamentorum spagyrica preparatione et usu. English.] *In* Hester, J. The secrets of physick and philosophy. 1633.

—[French tr.] Traicté familier de l'exacte preparation spagyrique des medicamens, pris d'entre les mineraux, animaux & vegetaux. Avec une Breve response au livret de Jacques Aubert, touchant la generation & les causes des metaux ... Paris, Charles Morel, 1630.

152 (i.e. 160), [14] p.   18 cm.   (Part [2] in his La pharmacopee des dogmatiques reformee ... Avec un Traicté familier.)   **[3436]**

The two works were first published together in Latin in 1575 under title: Ad Jacobi Auberti De ortu et causis metallorum contra chymicos explicationem ... brevis responsio ... De exauisita mineralium, animalium, & vegetabilium medicamentorum spagyrica praeparatione & usu.

—[The same.] ... Rouen, Imprimerie de Louys Oursel, pour Corneille Pitresson, 1639.

152 (i.e. 160) p.   17 cm.   (Part [2] in his La pharmacopee des dogmatiques reformee ... Avec une Traicté familier.)   **[3437]**

Different setting of type.

—[The same.] ... Derniere ed. rev. & corr. de nouveau. Lyon, Hierosme de la Garde, 1648.

[1], 99, [11] p.   18 cm.   **[3438]**

Bound with (as issued?) *his* La pharmacopée des dogmatiques reformee. 1648.

—[Italian tr.] *In his* Le ricchezze della riformata farmacopea. 1646, 1655, 1665, 1684.

—Jos. Quercetani ... Liber de priscorum philosophorum verae medicinae materia, praeparationis modo, atque in curandis morbis, praestantia. Deque simplicium, & rerum signaturis tum externis, tum internis, seu specificis, a priscis & hermeticis philosophis ... comparatis atque introductis, duo tractatus. His accesserunt ejusdem Jos. Quercetani De dogmaticorum medicorum legitima & restituta medicamentorum praeparatione, libri duo. Itemque selecta quaedam consilia medica ... S. Gervasii, Apud haeredes Eustathii Vignon, 1603.

[24], 432 p.   17 cm.   **[3439]**

—[The same.] ... Aureliae Allobrogum, Apud Johannem Vignon, 1609.

[24], 432 p. 16 cm.   [3440]

Different setting of type.
With this is bound *his* Opera medica. Lugduni, 1600.

—[The same.] ... [Lipsiae] Impensis Thomae Schüreri & Barthol. Voigt, 1613.

[21], 480 p. 16 cm.   [3441]

Bound with Follinus, H. Amuletum Antonianum, 1618.

—[French tr.] Traicté de la matiere, preparation et excellente vertu de la medecine balsamique des anciens philosophes. Aquel sont adjoustez deux traictez, l'un des signatures externes des choses, l'autre des internes & specifiques, conformément à la doctrine & practique des hermetiques ... Paris, C. Morel, 1626.

[8], 215, [1] p. 17 cm.   [3442]

—[The same, *as subject*] See Riolan, J. [1580-1657] Apologia pro Hippocratis et Galeni medicina. 1603.

—Pestis alexicacus; sive, Luis pestiferae fuga, auxiliaribus selectorum utriusque medicinae remediorum copiis procurata. Authore Jos. Quercetano ... Parisiis, Apud Claudium Morellum, 1608.

[16], 527, [24] p. 18 cm.   [3443]

—[The same.] ... Nunc in Germania emendatius recusa. [Lipsiae] Impensis Thomae Schureri & Bartholomaei Voigt [Michael Lantzenberger excudebat] 1609.

[16], 461, [25] p. 16 cm.   [3444]

—[The same.] ... [Lipsiae] Impensis Thomae Schureri & Bartholomaei Voigt [Typis Tobiae Beyeri, excudebat Nicolaus Ball] 1615.

[16], 461, [25] p. 17 cm.   [3445]

Different setting of type.
Bound with *his* Tetras gravissimorum totius capitis affectuum. 1617.

—Pharmacopoea dogmaticorum restituta. Pretiosis selectisque hermeticorum floribus abunde illustrata. Auctore Jos. Quercetano ... 2. ed. ab eodem aucta & correcta. Parisiis, Apud Claudium Morellum, 1607.

[8], 919 (i.e. 621), [26] p. port. 17 cm.
                                        [3446]

Imperfect: added engraved title page and port. wanting.
Called "liber primus" in caption title. The projected 2d book, on external remedies (cf. pref.) was apparently never written.

—[The same.] ... Ed. 2. multis erratis repurgata ... [n. p.] David Anastasius, 1607.

[31], 510 p. 18 cm.   [3447]

—[The same.] ... Venetiis, Apud Joannem Antonium & Jacobum de Franciscis, 1608.

[24], 269 p. 23 cm.   [3448]

—[The same.] ... Ed. 3. Marburgi, Paulus Egenolphus, 1622.

[16], 448, [8] p. 18 cm.   [3449]

—[The same.] ... Ed. ult. multis erratis repurgata ... Genevae, Apud Petrum & Jacobum Chouët, 1628.

[32], 591 p. 17 cm.   [3450]

—[Excerpts.] *In* Renou, J. de. Dispensatorium medicum. 1615; Ziegler, A. Pharmacopoea spagyrica. 1628.

—[French tr.] La pharmacopee des dogmatiques reformee, et enrichie de plusieurs remedes excellents, choisis & tirez de l'art spagyrique. Avec un Traicté familier de l'exacte preparation spagyrique des medicaments pris d'entre les mineraux, animaux & vegetaux: et une Breve response au livret de Jacques Aubert, touchant la generation & les causes des metaux ... 2. éd., rev. & augm. de nouveau. Paris, Charles Morel, 1630.

[16], 509 (i.e. 549), [31] p.; 152 (i.e. 160), [14] p. port. 18 cm.
                                        [3451]

Added engraved title page dated 1629.
The first work is a translation of the Pharmacopoea dogmaticorum restituta. The second part of the book, containing the two other works, has special title page.

—[The same.] ... Derniere éd., rev. & augm. de nouveau. Rouen, De l'imprimerie de Ozee Seigneuré, pour Corneille Pitreson, 1639.

[12], 548, [44] p.; 152 (i.e. 160) p. port. 17 cm.
                                        [3452]

Part [2] has special title page with imprint: Rouen, De l'imprimerie de Louys Oursel, pour Corneille Pitresson, 1639.

—[The same.] ... Augm. en ceste derniere ed., de ce que l'autheur prevenu de mort n'y a peu adjouster pour la reformation des huiles, onguents, emplastres, & autres remedes externes, selon le mesme art des spagyriques, par L. Meysonnier ... Lyon, Hierosme de la Garde, 1648.

[16], 549, [31], 48 p. 18 cm.   [3453]

With this is bound (as issued?) *his* Traicté familier de l'exacte preparation spagyrique des medicamens. 1648.

—[Italian tr.] Le richezze della riformata farmacopea del sig. Giuseppe Quercetano ... Nuovamente de favella latina traportata in italiana dal sig. Giacomo Ferrari ... Venetia, Giovanni Guerigli, 1619.

[24], 256 p. 23 cm. [3454]

Added engraved title page: La farmacopea, overo, Antidotario riformato.

—[The same.] ... Venetia, Li Gueriglii, 1638.

[24], 256 p. 22 cm. [3455]

Half title: La farmacopea, overo, Antidotario riformato.
Different setting of type.

—[The same.] ... Et in quest'ultima impressione corretta, & aggionto La preparazione spagirica dei minerali, animali & vegetabili & loro uso; con un ristretto del medicamenti ch'appartengono alla chirurgia dell'istesso auttore. Tradotta nuovamente da Gio. Maria Ferro ... Venetia, Gli Guerigli, 1646.

[16], 264 p. 23 cm. [3456]

The Trattato della preparatione spagirica dei medicamenti ... & loro uso (p. 227-257, with special title page) is a translation of the De mineralium, animalium & vegetabilium medicamentorum spagyrica praeparatione et usu, to which has been added a translation of the list of spagyric medicaments used in surgery, with directions for their preparation, which was originally appended to the Antidotarium spagyricum.

—[The same.] ... Venetia, Li Guerigli, 1655.

[16], 264 p. 22 cm. [3457]

Imperfect: outer margins of p. 213-264 mutilated.
Different setting of type.

—[The same.] ... Venetia, I Guerigli, 1665.

[16], 264 p. 23 cm. [3458]

Different setting of type.

—[The same.] ... Venetia, Gio. Francesco Valvasense, 1684.

[16], 264 p. 23 cm. [3459]

Different setting of type.

—Le pourtraict de la santé. Où est au vif representée la regle universelle & particuliere, de bien sainement & longuement vivre. Enrichy de plusieurs preceptes, raisons, & beaux exemples, tirez des medecins, philosophes & historiens, tant grecs que latins, les plus celebres ... S. Omer, Charles Boscart, 1618.

[8], 598, [1] p. 15 cm. [3460]

Imperfect: p. 323-334 wanting.
Published originally in 1606 in both French and Latin. The author prepared the Latin version (Diaeteticon polyhistoricon) in somewhat abridged form.

—[Latin ed.] Jos. Quercetani ... Diaeteticon polyhistoricon ... Parisiis, Apud Claudium Morellum, 1606.

6 p., 171 (i.e. 170), 369-463 ll., [4] p. port. 17 cm. [3461]

Imperfect: 4 p. at end wanting.

—[The same.] ... Lipsiae, Impensis Thomae Schureri et Bartholomaei Voigtii [Michael Lantzenberger excudebat] 1607.

[8], 515, [1] p. 17 cm. [3462]

—Josephi Quercetani ... Tractatus duo: quorum prior inscribitur Diaeteticon polyhistoricum, alter vero Pharmacopoea dogmaticorum restituta ... Francoforti, Praelo Richteriano, impensis Johann. Theobaldi Schönwetteri, 1607.

[6], 134 p.; [6], 247, [9] p. port. 25 cm. [3463]

Part [2] has special title page.

—Jos. Quercetani ... Diaeteticon polyhistoricon ... Genevae, Apud Petrum Chouët, 1626.

418, [2] p. 17 cm. [3464]

—[German tr.] Josephi Quercetani M. D. Diaeteticon polyhistoricum; das ist, Natürliche Eechtmässigung dess gantzen menschlichen Lebens: wie nemlich es in jederley Anligen ... umb Vermeidung mancherley Seuchen könne und solle angestelt werden ... Lateinisch und Frantzösisch beschrieben ... nun aber von Johan Adolff Ringelstein ... in das Teutsche ubersetzet. Strassburg, In Verlegung Eberhardi Zetzners, 1625.

[8], 254, [14] p. port. 21 cm. [3465]

—Recueil des plus curieux et rares secrets touchant la medecine metallique & minerale, tirez des manuscripts, de feu Mre Joseph du Chesne ... Paris, Jean Brunet, 1641.

[8], 370, [12] p. port. 17 cm. [3466]

Imperfect: 3d and 4th prelim. leaves, containing privilege and portrait, and errata leaf wanting.

Added engraved title page, with date altered by hand from 1641 to 1648.

Contents. —Traicté de la medecine metallique. —Traicté de la medecine minerale. —Secrets particuliers.

—[The same.] ... Paris, Simeon Piget, 1648.
[8], 370, [13] p. port. 20 cm. **[3467]**

Errata: p. [13].
Added engraved title page dated 1641, altered by hand to 1648.
A reissue of the 1641 edition with new title page.

—Another issue, first signature has been reprinted with a change in the wording of the privilege on the 2d leaf. **[3468]**

Imperfect: first leaf (added engraved title page) wanting.

—Josephi Quercetani medici Sclopetarius; sive, De curandis vulneribus, quae sclopetorum et similium tormentorum ictibus acciderunt, liber. Ejusdem Antidotarium spagyricum adversus eosdem ictus. Lipsiae, Impensis Thomae Schüreri & Bartholomaei Voigt, 1614.
[8], 175, [16] p. 16 cm. (Vol. 2 of *his* Opera medica, Lipsiae, 1614) **[3469]**

—[French tr.] Traicté de la cure generale et particuliere des arcbusades. Avec l'Antidotaire spagirique, pour preparer & composer les medicamens ... Paris, Claude Morel, 1625.
[16], 248 p. 17 cm. **[3470]**

Bound with *his* Tetrade des plus grieves maladies de tout le cerveau. 1625.

—[German tr.] Josephi Quercetani medici Sclopetarius, das ist, Büchsen-Tractätlein, oder Buch von Heylung der Wunden ... Und dann Wie die Artzneyen wider gemelte Wunden und Schäden zubereiten seindt. Strassburg, In Verlegung Eberhardt Zetzners, 1631.
117, [4] p. 20 cm. (Part [2] in *his* Drey medicinische Tractätlein. Strassburg, 1631) **[3471]**

Translated by Thomas Kessler.
"Spagyrisches Artzney-Büchlein" (p. 88–117) is a translation of the Antidotarium spagiricum.

—Tetras gravissimorum totius capitis affectuum ... Adjectus est in eorundem morborum curatione, praeter vulgarem medendi methodum, ingens selectissimorum medicamentorum spagyricorum numerus ... Josepho Quercetano ... authore. Marpurgi, Typis Pauli Egenolphi, 1606.
[24], 488, [16] p. 16 cm. **[3472]**

—[The same.] ... 2. ed. Marpurgi, Typis Pauli Egenolphi, 1609.
[31], 488, [15] p. 17 cm. **[3473]**

—[The same.] ... Accessit hac tertia editione ejusdem Quercetani Ad Brevem Riolani excursum brevis incursio olim separatim edita. Marpurgi, Typis Pauli Egenolphi, 1617.
[24], 532, [17] p. 17 cm. **[3474]**

With this are bound *his* Pestis alexicacus. 1615; Scheunemann, H. Medicina reformata. 1617.

—[French tr.] Tetrade des plus grieves maladies de tout le cerveau ... Paris, Claude Morel, 1625.
[12], 499, [15] p. 17 cm. **[3475]**

With this is bound *his* Traicté de la cure generale et particuliere des arcbusades. 1625.

—[Excerpts] *In* Dolhopff, G. A., *comp.* Lapis vegetabilis. 1681.

—*See* BILLICH, A. G. Thessalus in chymicis redivivus. 1640; DISPENSATORIUM CHYMICUM. 1626; FIORAVANTI, L. Three exact pieces of Leonard Phioravant. 1652; HORST, J. D. Pharmacopoeia Galeno-chemica. 1651.

—*as subject. See* GOCKEL, E. Enchiridion medico-practicum de peste. 1669; [RIOLAN, J., 1580–1657] Brevis excursus in battologiam Quercetani. 1604; SALA, A. Processus ... de auro potabili. 1630.

DU CLOS. *See* COTTEREAU DU CLOS, Samuel [1598–1685]

DUCLOS, GASTON. *See* CLAVES, Gaston Le Doux, *known as* Gaston de [*b. ca.* 1530]

DU CLOS, SAMUEL COTTEREAU. *See* COTTEREAU DU CLOS, Samuel [1598–1685]

DUDITH, ANDRÁS, *Bp. of Pécs* [1533–1589] *See* SCHOLTZ, L. Epistolarum philosophicarum, medicinalium, ac chymicarum ... volumen. 1610.

DÜLCKEN, JOHANN HERMANN [*fl.* 1684] *respondent. See* FRANCK VON FRANCKENAU, G., *praeses.* Disputatio medica ordinaria et quidem prima de morbis acutis gravidarum. 1684.

DUEREN, JOHAN VAN [*fl.* 1687] De ontdekking der bedriegeryen vande gemeene pis-besienders, waar in naaktelijk vertoont werden hunne valsche waanen, doortrapte vonden, nietige uytvlugten, en hunne gevaarlijke genees oeffeningen; waar door zy de pis-brengers, en de zieken bedektelijk bedriegen, en schandelijk misleyden ... Amsterdam, Timotheus ten Hoorn, 1688.
[32], 426 (i.e. 424) p. 17 cm. **[3476]**

Added engraved title page.

DÜRER, ALBRECHT [1471–1528] [Vier Bücher von menschlichen Proportion. Dutch.] Beschryvinghe . . . van de menschelijcke proportion. Begrepen in vier . . . boecken . . . In't Latijn ende Hooghduytsch, tot Nurenbergh ghedruct . . . Ende nu in onse Nederlandtsche sprake over-gheset . . . Arnhem, Jan Jansz, 1622.

[1], 261, [5] p.   illus.   32 cm.   [**3477**]

"Elegia Bilibaldi Pirckeymheri in obitum Alberti Dureri": p. [4–5]

—[French tr.] Les quatre livres . . . de la proportion des parties & pourtraicts des corps humains. Traduicts par Loys Meigret . . . de langue latine . . . Arnhem, Jean Jeansz, 1613.

[2], 124 ll.   illus.   32 cm.   [**3478**]

—[The same.] . . . Rev. & cour. de nouveau. Arnhem, Jean Jeansz, 1614.

[2], 124. ll.   illus.   32 cm.   [**3479**]

A reissue of the 1613 edition with title page partly reset.

DU FAY, JAKOB FRIEDRICH [*b.* 1671] *respondent. See* HOFFMANN, F. [1660–1742] *praeses.* Disputatio inauguralis medica sistens malignitatis naturam et originem in morbis acutis. 1695.

—*See* HOFFMANN, F. [1660–1742] Propemticon inaugurale, de modo veterum balsamandi corpora. 1695.

[**DUFOUR**, PHILIPPE SYLVESTRE, 1622–1687?] De l'usage du caphé, du thé, et du chocolate. Lyon, Jean Girin & Barthelemy Riviere, 1671.

[24], 188 p.   illus.   15 cm.   [**3480**]

"Du chocolate discours curieux . . . par Antoine Colmenero de Ledesma . . . Traduit d'espagnol en françois . . . par René Moreau . . .": p. [73]–164; "Du chocolate dialogue entre un medecin, un indien, & un bourgeois. Composé par Barthelemy Marradon . . .": p. [165]–188. Items have half titles.

Attributed also to Jacob Spon. Cf. Mueller, p. 66.

—Traitez nouveaux & curieux du café, du thé et du chocolate. Ouvrage également necessaire aux medecins, & à tous ceux qui aiment leur santé. Par Philippe Sylvestre Dufour. Lyon, Jean Girin & B. Riviere, 1685.

[22], 445, [5] p.   illus., plates.   17 cm.

[**3481**]

Added engraved title page.

"Dialogue du chocolate. Entre un medecin, un indien & un bourgeois" (p. 423–445) is from the Spanish of Bartolomé Marradón.

—[The same.] . . . A quoy on a adjouté dans cette edition, la meilleure de toutes les methodes, qui manquoit à ce livre, pour composer l'excellent chocolate . . . La Haye, Adrian Moetjens, 1685.

[1], 403, [5] p.   plates.   13 cm.   [**3482**]

Added engraved title page.

"Dialogue du chocolate. Entre un medecin, un indien & un bourgeois" (p. 381–403) is from the Spanish of Bartolomé Marradón.

—[The same.] . . . 2. ed. Lyon, Jean Baptiste Deville, 1688.

[22], 444, [10] p.   illus., plates.   17 cm.

[**3483**]

Added engraved title page.

A reprint of the 1685 Lyons edition.

—[The same.] . . . 3. ed. La Haye, Adrian Moetjens, 1693.

[1], 404, [4] p.   plates.   14 cm.   [**3484**]

Added engraved title page.

A reprint of the 1685 The Hague edition.

—[Latin tr.] Tractatus novi de potu caphe, de Chinensium the, et de chocolata. Parisiis, Apud Petrum Muguet, 1685.

[9], 202, [4] p.   illus., plates.   15 cm.   [**3485**]

"Tractatus de chocolata" (p. 141–191) is mainly from the Spanish of Antonio Colmenero de Ledesma. "Dialogus de chocolata" (p. 192–202) is by Bartolomé Maradón.

Attributed to Jacob Spon. Cf. publisher's preface.

—[The same.] . . . a D. M. [i.e. J. J. Manget] notis illustrati. Genevae, Cramer & Perachon, 1699.

[6], 188 p.   front., plates.   16 cm.   [**3486**]

—[German tr.] Drey neue curieuse Tractätgen, von dem Trancke Cafe, sinesischen The, und der Chocolata, welche nach ihren Eigenschafften, Gewächs, Fortpflantzung, Praeparirung, Tugenden und herrlichen Nutzen sehr curieus beschrieben, und nunmehro in die hoch-teutsche Sprache übersetzet von dem, welcher sich jederzeit nennet Theae potum maxime colentem. Budissin, In Verlegung Friedrich Arnst, Druckts Joh. Wilhelm Krüger, 1686.

[8], 247 (i.e. 245), [3] p.   front., plates.   17 cm.

[**3487**]

"Geschpräche von der Chocolata, Unterredner sind, ein Medicus, Americaner, und gemeiner Bürger" (p. 235–247) is from the Spanish of Bartolomé Marradón.

Bound (as issued?) with Bontekoe, C. Kurtze Abhandlung von dem menschlichen Leben. 1686.

—[The same.] . . . Budissin, In Verlegung Friedrich Arnsts, 1692.

[6], 247 (i.e. 245), [3] p. front., plates. 16 cm.

[**3488**]

Different setting of type.

—[Excerpts. German] *See* [CHAMBERLAYNE, J.] *comp.* Schatzkammer rarer und neuer Curiositäten. 1689.

DU FOUR DE LA CRESPELIÈRE. Commentaire en vers françois, sur l'Ecole de Salerne, contenant les moyens de se passer de medecin, & de vivre long-temps en santé, avec une infinité de remedes contre toutes sortes de maladies, & un traitté des humeurs, & de la saignée, où sont adjoustez. La sanguification, circulation, et transfusion du sang, la poudre & l'onguent de sympathie, le thé, le caphé, le chocolate, et le grand secret de la pierre philosophale, ou la veritable maniere de faire de l'or, aussi en vers françois, et l'ouromantie, scatomantie, et hydromantie en prose. Par Monsieur D. F. C. . . . Paris, Gilles Alliot, 1671.

[60], 714 (i.e. 696) p. 15 cm. [**3489**]

Imperfect: added engraved title page wanting.
Includes Latin text of the Regimen sanitatis Salernitanum.
"Le serment d'Hippocrate en vers françois": p. 659–662.

—[The same.] . . . Paris, E. Langlois, & la veuve G. Alliot, 1674.

[60], 714 (i.e. 696) p. 15 cm. [**3490**]

A reissue of the 1671 edition with new title page.

—, *ed.* and *tr. See* HIPPOCRATES. Les Aphorismes. 1699.

—, *tr. See* DUPORT, F. La decade de medecine. 1694.

DU FRESNE, CHARLES, *seigneur du Cange. See* DU CANGE, Charles Du Fresne, *sieur* [1610–1688]

DUFRESNE, CLAUDE [*fl.* 1695–1712] *respondent. See* DAQUIN, P., *praeses.* Quaestio medica . . . An in apoplexia, praemissa venae sectione, feliciter purgatio? 1696.

DUGARD, SAMUEL [1645?–1697] The marriages of cousin Germans, vindicated from the censures of unlawfullnesse, and inexpediency. Being a letter written to his much honour'd T. D. . . . Oxford, Printed by Hen. Hall for Thomas Bowman, 1673.

[15], 116 p. 16 cm. [**3491**]

Wood ascribes the work to Dugard (cf. v. 4, col. 679), although it was said to be mostly taken from Jeremy Taylor's Ductor dubitantium.

—Περὶ πολυπαιδίας; or, A discourse concerning the having many children. In which the prejudices against a numerous offspring are removed. And the objections answered. In a letter to a friend . . . London, W. Rogers, 1695.

124, [4] p. 18 cm. [**3492**]

Ascribed to Samuel Dugard by Wood.

DUGARD, WILLIAM [1606–1662] *tr. See* PARACELSUS. Dispensatory and chirurgery. 1656.

DU GARDIN, LOUIS [*fl.* 1617–*ca.* 1631] Alexiloemos; sive, De pestis natura, causis, signis, prognosticis, praecautione, et curatione, epitome methodica per conclusiones distributa . . . Duaci, Typis Petri Auroii, 1617.

[16], 191, [1] p. illus. 16 cm. [**3493**]

With this is bound *his* La chasse-peste. 1617.

—[The same.] Ludovicus Gardinius Contra pestem; sive, De pestis natura, causis, signis, prognosticis, praecautione, et curatione . . . Accessit ejusdem Remedium erroris in ponderibus medicis. Duaci, Ex typographia Petri Auroi, 1631.

[12], 212, [1] p.; 47 (i.e. 45), [1] p. 15 cm.

[**3494**]

Part [2] has special title page, dated 1630.
With this is bound *his* Medicamenta purgantia. 1631.

—La chasse-peste; ou, Les remedes singuliers et familiers, dont chascun se pourra servir pour se preserver en temps pestiferé, et se guarir soy-mesme s'il est atteint de la peste . . . Douay, Pierre Auroy, 1617.

31, [1] p. 16 cm. [**3495**]

Bound with *his* Alexiloemos. 1617.

—De animatione foetus quaestio: in qua ostenditur, quod anima rationalis, ante organizationem non infundatur . . . Duaci, Typis Petri Auroy, 1623.

94, [1] p. 19 cm. [**3496**]

Imperfect: last leaf (errata and privilege) mutilated.
A reply to Thomas Feyens' De formatrice foetus.
Bound with Feyens, T. De formatrice foetus. 1620.

—Hortensii Manuductio, per omnes medicinae partes; seu, Institutiones medicinae . . . Duaci, Typis Petri Auroy, 1626.

[16], 408, [16] p.; [16], 304 p. illus. 18 cm.

[**3497**]

Part 2 has special title page.

—Ludovici Gardinii ... Medicamenta purgantia, simplicia & composita, selecta, usitata, & sufficientia. Accessit ejusdem Remedium erroris in ponderibus medicis. Duaci, Ex typographia Petri Auroy, 1631.

[12], 156 p.; 47 (i.e. 45), [1] p.   15 cm.   [3498]

Part [2] has special title page, dated 1630.
Bound with *his* Contra pestem. 1631.

—Remedes singuliers et familiers contre la peste, dont châcun se pourra servir pour se preserver en temps pestiferé, et se guerir soy-mesme s'il est atteint ... Bruxelles, François Foppens, 1668.

22, [1] p.   15 cm.   [3499]

DU HAMEL, Jean Baptiste [1624–1706] Operum philosophicorum tomus I [-tomus II] In quo continentur tractatus hi sequentes: I. Astronomia physica. II. De meteoris & fossilibus libri duo. III. De consensu veteris & novae philosophiae. Norimbergae, Sumptibus Johannis Ziegeri, literis Christophori Gerhardi, 1681.

2 v.   illus.   22 cm.   [3500]

Added engraved title page.
Contents of vol. 2: IV. De corporum affectionibus cum manifestis, tum occultis, libri duo. V. De mente humana libri quatuor. VI. De corpore animato libri quatuor.

—De corpore animato libri quatuor; seu, Promotae per experimenta philosophiae specimen alterum ... Parisiis, Apud Stephanum Michallet, 1673.

[23], 535, [12] p.   plates.   16 cm.   [3501]

—De corporum affectionibus cum manifestis, tum occultis, libri duo; seu, Promotae per experimenta philosophiae specimen, ubi non qualitates modo & vires corporum, sed & illustriora quae nostra hac aetate variis in locis facta sunt experimenta, breviter & aperte explicantur ... Parisiis, Apud Michaelem Le Petit & Stephanum Michallet, 1670.

[11], 556, [16] p.   plate.   16 cm.   [3502]

—De mente humana libri quatuor: in quibus functiones animi, vires, natura, immortalitas, simul & logica universa variis illustrata experimentis pertractantur ... Parisiis, Apud Michaelem Le Petit, 1672.

[22], 555, [9] p.   16 cm.   [3503]

DUIZING, Anton. *See* Deusing, Anton [1612–1666]

DU JON, François [1545–1602] *tr. See* De magorum daemonomania. 1603.

DU LAURENS, André [1558–1609] Andreae Laurentii ... Opera omnia. Partim jam antea excusa, partim nondum edita, nunc simul collecta, & ab infinitis mendis repurgata. Studio et opera Guidonis Patini ... Parisiis, Apud Joannem Foüet, 1628.

2 v. in 1.   port.   24 cm.   [3504]

—Operum Andreae Laurentii ... tomus alter. Continens Scripta therapeutica X. nimirum tractatum De crisibus, De mirabili strumas sanandi vi. De nobilitate visus, ejusque conservandi ratione. De melancholia, libris duobus absolutum. De senectute. De morbo articulari. De lepra. De lue venerea. Ejusdem Annotationes in artem parvam Galeni, & Consilia medica. Omnia nunc primum edita ... Francofurti, Impensis Gulielmi Fitzeri, 1628.

1. v.   32 cm.   [3505]

Various pagings.
Bound with *his* Historia anatomica. 1636.

—[French tr.] Toutes les oeuvres ... Recueillies et traduittes en francois, par ... Theophile Gelée ... Paris, P. Mettayer, 1613.

5 parts in 1 v.   illus., port.   36 cm.   [3506]

Engraved title page.
Parts [2–5] have half titles.

—[The same.] ... Paris, Pour Raphael du Petit Val a Rouen, 1621.

5 parts in 1 v.   illus., port.   36 cm.   [3507]

Engraved title page.
Parts [3–5] have half titles.
A reprint of the 1613 edition.

—[The same.] Rev., corr., et augm. en cette derniere ed. par G. Sauvageon ... Paris, Mathieu Guillemot, 1639.

[16], 597, [25] p.; 395 (i.e. 295) p.   illus.   37 cm.   [3508]

Part 2 has half title.

—[The same.] ... Paris, Michel Soly, 1646.

[16], 597, [19] p.;   [7], 395 (i.e. 295) p.   illus. 37 cm.   [3509]

Part [2] has half title.

—Another issue, with imprint: Paris, Augustin Courbe, 1646.

[3510]

Imperfect: half title wanting.

—[The same.] ... Rouen, La vefue de David du Petit Val, 1661.

[16], 572, [22] p.; [8], 488 (i.e. 286), [6] p. illus., port. 38 cm.   [**3511**]
Engraved title page.
Part [2] has half title.

—Andreae Laurentii ... De crisibus libri tres. Adjecta est Universalis quaedam methodus ad prognosin, & crises omnium morborum, sed praecipue acutorum morborum conferens ... Lugduni, Sumptibus Horatii Cardon, 1613.
[8], 137, [7] p. 18 cm.   [**3512**]
Bound with *his* Historia anatomica. 1605.

—[The same.] ... Francofurti, Ex officina typographica Nicolai Hoffmanni, sumptibus Jonae Rhodii, 1606.
[8], 160, [6] p. 19 cm.   [**3513**]

—Copy 2. 17 cm.
Last leaf (blank) wanting.
With this is bound Merindol, A. Selectae exercitationes VIII. 1617.

—De mirabili strumas sanandi vi solis Galliae regibus ... divinitus concessa liber unus. Et De strumarum natura, differentiis, causis, curatione quae fit arte & industria medica. Liber alter. Authore Andrea Laurentio ... Parisiis, Apud Marcum Orry, 1609.
[15], 293 (i.e. 307), [18] p. plate. 19 cm.   [**3514**]
Engraved title page.

—Discours de la conservation de la veue: des maladies melancholiques: des catarrhes: & de la vieillesse ... Rev. de nouveau & augm. de plusieurs chapitres. Paris, P. Mettayer, 1606.
[12], 274, [1] ll. 15 cm.   [**3515**]

—Another issue, with imprint: Paris, Marc Orry, 1606.   [**3516**]

—[The same.] ... Rouen, Claude Le Villain, 1615.
[8], 204 (i.e. 206) ll. 15 cm.   [**3517**]

—[The same.] ... Rouen, Claude Le Villain, 1620.
[8], 204 (i.e. 206) ll. 15 cm.   [**3518**]
Imperfect: leaves 25–34 wanting.
Different setting of type.

—[The same.] ... Rouen, Louys Loudet, 1630.
[8], 204 (i.e. 206) ll. 14 cm.   [**3519**]
Different setting of type.

—[Latin tr.] Discursus de visus nobilitate et conservandi modo. A Joanne Theodoro Schönlino ... ex clariss. Andreae Laurentii ... Gallico libello Latio adscriptus ... Monachii, Ex formis Bergianis apud viduam, 1618.
[12], 166 p. 13 cm.   [**3520**]
Engraved title page.

—[The same.] Discursus philosophicus et medicus de melancholia et catarrho, in quo de eorum differentiis, causis, signis et curandi ratione accurate disseritur, a Joanne Theodoro Schönlino ... ex clariss. Andreae Laurentii ... Gallico libello Latio adscriptus. Augustae [Apud Andream Aperger, sumptibus Sebastiani Mylii] 1620.
[22], 247 (i.e. 245), [1] p. 15 cm.   [**3521**]
Engraved title page.
Translation of the second and third treatises only.

—Copy 2. 14 cm.
With this is bound Camerarius, J. R. Sylloges memorabilium medicinae centuriae IV. 1624.

—[Italian tr.] Discorsi della conservatione della vista, delle malattie melanconiche, delli catarri, e della vecchiaia. Composti in lingua francese ... Tradotti ... e commentati da Fr. Gio. Germano ... Nap., Lazzaro Scorigio, 1626.
[8], 276, [4] p. 21 cm.   [**3522**]
Imperfect: title page mutilated.

—Andreae Laurentii ... Historia anatomica, humani corporis partes singulas uberrime enodans, novisque controversiis et observationibus illustrata ... Prodit e Francofurti Paltheniana, sumtibus Johnae Rhodii, 1602.
[16], 996, [43] p. illus. 21 cm.   [**3523**]

—[The same.] ... Lugduni, Apud Horatium Cardon, 1605.
[16], 893, [50] p. illus. 18 cm.   [**3524**]
With this is bound *his* De crisibus. 1613.

—[The same.] ... Venetiis, Apud Joan. Antonium & Jacobum de Franciscis, 1606.
[76], 918 (i.e. 908) p. illus. 17 cm.   [**3525**]

—[The same.] ... Francofurti, Excudebat Nicolaus Hoffmannus, sumptibus Jacobi Fischeri, 1615.
[16], 996, [43] p. illus. 19 cm.   [**3526**]

—[The same.] Historia anatomica humani corporis et singularum ejus partium multis controversiis & observationibus novis illustrata authore Andrea Laurentio ... Francofurti, Impensis Wilhelmi Fitzeri, 1636.

[16], 442, [21] p.   illus., port.   32 cm. [3527]

Enlarged and illustrated edition of the work published in Lyons in 1593 under title: Opera anatomica. A reprint of the edition published in Frankfurt in 1600.

With this is bound *his* Operum ... tomus alter. 1628.

—[French tr.] L'histoire anatomique, en laquelle toutes les parties du corps humain sont amplement declarees: enrichie de controverses & observations nouvelles ... De la traduction de Francois Sizé. Lyon, Simon Rigaud, 1631.

[38], 1451, [92] p.   port.   17 cm.   [3528]

Imperfect: port. and last leaf of index wanting; p. 699-706, 755-772, 1367, 1425 mutilated.

"Permissions" dated: 1620.

—[The same.] ... Lyon, Simon Rigaud [*ca.* 1631]

[38], 1451, [92] p.   port.   19 cm.   [3529]

Imperfect: title page wanting.

Title taken from the 1631 edition.

Different setting of type.

—[The same.] *as subject. See* LAUREMBERG, P. Procestria anatomica. 1619; RIOLAN, J. [1580-1657] Opera anatomica vetera. 1650 [and] Opuscula anatomica nova. 1649.

—*See* CROOKE, H. Μιχροχοσμογραφία A description of the body of man. 1615, 1618, 1631, 1651; VIGIER, J. [*fl.* 1608?] Tractatus absolutissimus et accuratissimus de catarrho. 1620.

—*as subject. See* ROSSELL, J. F. Ad sex libros Galeni De differentiis. 1627.

DULCO CLAVEUS, GASTON. *See* CLAVES, Gaston Le Doux, *known as* Gaston de [*b. ca.* 1530]

DULKEN, HEINRICH [*fl.* 1667] *respondent.* Disputatio medica inauguralis de nutritione ... Lugduni Batavorum, Apud viduam & haeredes Joannis Elsevirii, 1667.

[28] p.   20 cm.   [3530]

Diss.—Leyden.

—Another issue.

[28] p., [7] p.   23 cm.   [3531]

With Amicorum vota.

—Disputatio philosophica inauguralis, mentis humanae immortalitatem apodictice concludens ... Lugduni Batavorum, Apud viduam & haeredes Joannis Elsevirii, 1667.

[24] p.   23 cm.   [3532]

Diss.—Leyden.

DU MEZEREY, PIERRE. *See* POSTEL, N. Factum. 1685.

DUMMER, GEORG ADAM [*fl.* 1662-1665] *respondent. See* SCHENCK, J. T., *praeses.* De gravissimo et rarissimo capitis affectu caro disputatio inauguralis medica. 1665.

DU MOLIN, ANTOINE [*b. ca.* 1510] *See* INDAGINE, J. ab. La chiromance. 1638.

DU MONT, NICOLAUS [*fl.* 1690] *respondent.* Dissertationem inauguralem medicam de calculo renum et vesicae ... publice disputandum ... proponit ... Nicolaus du Mont ... Basileae, Typis Jacobi Bertschii [1690]

[20] p.   21 cm.   [3533]

Diss.—Basel.

—*See* HARDER, J. J., *praeses.* Exercitatio medica de chyli secretione et distributione. 1690.

DU MOULIN, ANTOINE [*b. ca.* 1510] *tr. See* INDAGINE, J. ab. Vraye et parfaicte chyromancie. [not before 1620]

DU MOULIN, PIERRE [1601-1684] *tr. See* PERRAULT, F. The devill of Mascon. 1658.

DUN, GEORGE. *See* DUNN, George [*fl.* 17th cent.]

DUN, PATRICK [*fl.* 17th cent.] *ed. See* LIDDEL, D. Artis conservandi sanitatem libri duo. 1651.

DUNCAN, DANIEL [1649-1735] La chymie naturelle; ou, L'explication chymique et mechanique de la nourriture de l'animal ... Imprimé à Montauban, & se vend a Paris, Laurent d'Houry, 1682.

[32], 339 p.   18 cm.   [3534]

Imperfect: part of preface bound between p. 338 and 339; p. 305-320 wanting.

—[The same.] ... Paris, Laurent d'Houry, 1683.

[28], 339 p.   18 cm.   [3535]

A reissue of the 1682 edition with new title page and without the author's Epistre.

—Seconde partie de La chymie naturelle; ou, L'explication chymique et mechanique de l'evacuation particuliere aux femmes ... Montauban, Samuel Dubois, 1686.

[36], 242, [2] p.   17 cm.   [3536]

—[The same.] Seconde et troisieme partie de La chymie naturelle; ou, L'explication chimique et mechanique de l'evacuation particuliere aux femmes, & de la generation ... Imprimées à Montauban, & se vendent a Paris, Laurent d'Houry & Daniel Horthemels, 1687.

[38], 242, [4] p.   18 cm.   [3537]

Contains part 2 only. A reissue of the 1686 Montauban edition with new title page and Table.

—Toisiéme partie de La chymie naturelle; ou, L'explication chymique et mechanique, de la formation et de la naissance de l'animal ... Montauban, Raymond Bro, 1686.

[44], 158 p.   18 cm.   [3538]

—Explication nouvelle et mechanique des actions animales. Où il est traité des fonctions de l'ame. Avec une methode facile pour démontrer exactement toutes les parties du cerveau ... Par M. Duncan ... Paris, Jean d'Houry, 1678.

[16], 447, [2] p.   16 cm.   [3539]

Errata: p. [449]

—Histoire de l'animal; ou, La connoissance du corps animé par la mechanique & par la chymie ... Paris, Laurent d'Houry & Daniel Horthemels, 1687.

[86], 255 p.   18 cm.   [3540]

DUNCAN, GUILLELMUS. Physiologia ... Tolosae, Apud Arnaldum Colomerium, 1651.

[18], 259 p.   22 cm.   [3541]

Imperfect: engraved title page wanting.

DUNN, GEORGE [*fl.* 17th cent.] The signes that doe declare a person to be infected with the pestilence ... London, Nathaniel Newbery [1636]

broadside. 32 x 20 cm.   [3542]

STC 7021.5

DUNSTAN, *Saint, Abp. of Canterbury* [909-988] *See* COLSON, L. Philosophia maturata. 1668.

DU PINET, ANTOINE, *sieur de Noroy* [1515?-1584?] *tr. See* MATTIOLI, P. A. Les commentaires. 1619, 1620, 1627, 1642, 1680.

DUPLEIX, SCIPION [1569-1661] Les causes de la veille et du sommeil, des songes, & de la vie & de la mort ... Lyon, Simon Rigaud, 1620.

[31], 208 p.   19 cm.   [3543]

Bound with (as issued?) *his* La curiosité naturelle. 1620.

—[The same.] ... Paris, Claude Sonnius, 1626.

[32], 240 p.   18 cm.   [3544]

Bound with (as issued?) *his* L'ethique. 1626.

—[The same.] ... Rouen, Adrian Ouyn, 1631.

[31], 208 p.   17 cm.   [3545]

—La curiosité naturelle redigee en questions selon l'ordre alphabetique ... Lyon, Simon Rigaud, 1620.

[23], 269 p.   19 cm.   [3546]

Imperfect: p. 7-10 wanting.

With this is bound (as issued?) *his* Les causes de la veille et du sommeil. 1620.

—[The same.] ... Rouen, Manassez de Preaulx, 1626.

[23], 269 p.   16 cm.   [3547]

Different setting of type.

—[The same.] ... Paris, Claude Sonnius, 1626.

[14], 296 p.   18 cm.   [3548]

Different setting of type.

Bound with (as issued?) *his* L'ethique. 1626.

—[English tr.] The resolver; or, Curiosities of nature. Written in French by Scipio Du Plesis ... London, N. & I. Okes, 1635.

[23], 408 p.   15 cm.   [3549]

Engraved title page.

STC 7362.

—L'ethique; ou, Philosophie morale ... Paris, Claude Sonnius, 1626.

[47], 413 p.   18 cm.   [3550]

With this are bound (as issued?): *his* La curiosité naturelle. 1626; *his* Les causes de la veille et du sommeil. 1626.

DU PLESSIS, CHARLES ARTHUR [*b. ca.* 1592] *ed. See* HIPPOCRATES. [Adaptations, etc. Latin.] Promptuarium Hippocratis in locos communes ordine alphabetico nec sine compendio digestum. 1683.

—*See* RIOLAN, J. [1580-1657] Encheiridium anatomicum et pathologicum. 1658, 1677.

DU PLESSIS, SCIPION. *See* DUPLEIX, Scipion [1569-1661]

DUPORT, François [1548-1624] Francisci Porti ... Medica decas, ejusdem authoris in singula librorum capita commentariis illustrata ... Lutetiae Parisiorum, Sumptibus Melchioris Mondiere [Excudebat Franciscus Jacquin] 1613.

[8], 462 (i.e. 460), [6] p.   24 cm.   [3551]

Books I-IV published in 1584 under title: De signis morborum libri quatuor.

—Another issue, with imprint: Lutetiae Parisiorum, Sumptibus Abrahami Saugrain, 1613.

[3552]

—[The same.] ... Nyorti, Ex typographia Joannis Moussat, 1624.

306 (i.e. 296), [11] p.   15 cm.   [3553]

Without the commentary.

—[French tr.] La decade de medecine; ou, Le medecin des riches & des pauvres ... Composé en vers latins ... nouvellement mis en vers françois par par [sic] Mr Du Four ... Paris, Laurent d'Houry, 1694.

[12], 493, [15] p.   17 cm.   [3554]

Added title page: Francisci Porti ... Medica decas ... In Latin and French.

DU PRADEL, Abraham. See Blegny, Nicolas de [1642?-1722]

DU PRAT, Abraham, tr. See Bartholin, C. [1585-1629] Institutions anatomiques. 1647.

DUPUIS, Guillaume [fl. 1536-1551] Guilielmi Puteani ... De occultis pharmacorum purgantium facultatib. deque veris ipsarum causis, libri duo. Quibus adjecta est appendicula, De purgatrice medicamentorum facultate. Auctore Jacobo Cusinoto, filio ... Lugduni, Sumpt. Michaelis Duhan, 1654.

[17], 206 p.   17 cm.   [3555]

Added engraved title page.

Published in 1552 under title: De medicamentorum quomodocunque purgantium facultatibus.

DURANTE, Castore [1529-1590] [De bonitate et vitio alimentorum centuria. English.] A treasure of health ... Wherein is shewn how to preserve health, and prolong life ... Translated out of Italian into English, by John Chamberlayne ... London, William Crook, 1686.

[6], 232 p.   15 cm.   [3556]

—[The same.] A family-herbal; or, The treasure of health; shewing how to preserve health and prolong life ... The 2d ed. ... London, W. Crooke, 1689.

[4], 12, 232 p.   15 cm.   [3557]

—[Italian tr.] Il tesoro della sanità ... Nel quale s'insegna il modo di conservar la sanità, & prolungar la vita. Et si tratta della natura de' cibi, de' rimedii, & de' nocumenti loro ... Venetia, Lucio Spineda, 1601.

[16], 270 p.   16 cm.   [3558]

—[The same.] ... Venetia, Domenico Farri, 1603.

[16], 324 p.   16 cm.   [3559]

Imperfect: p. 305-308 wanting.

—[The same.] ... Venetia, Gli heredi di Domenico Farri, 1606.

[16], 324 p.   15 cm.   [3560]

Different setting of type.

—[The same.] ... Venetia, Giacomo Sarzina, 1611.

[16], 324 p.   16 cm.   [3561]

Different setting of type.

—[The same.] ... Venetia, Domenico Imberti, 1611.

[16], 324 p.   15 cm.   [3562]

Different setting of type.

—[The same.] ... Torino [Gio. Domenico Tarino] 1612.

[32], 480 p.   13 cm.   [3563]

—[The same.] ... Di nuovo ristampato, & con somma diligenza corretto. Venetia, Lucio Spineda, 1614.

[16] 334 p.   15 cm.   [3564]

—[The same.] ... Di nuovo ristampato, & con somma diligenza corretto. Venetia, Marc' Antonio Zaltieri, 1616.

[16], 334 p.   15 cm.   [3565]

Different setting of type.

—[The same.] ... Venetia, Ghirardo & Iseppo Imberti, 1625.

[16], 334 p.   15 cm.   [3566]

A reissue of the 1616 Venice edition with new title page.

—[The same.] ... Venetia, Gio. Battista Cestaro, 1646.

[16], 320 p.   16 cm.   [3567]

—[The same.] . . . Venetia, Gio. Battista Brigna, 1663.

[6], 3-308 p. 17 cm. [**3568**]

—[The same.] . . . Venetia, Gio. Battista Cestari, 1668.

[6], 3-308 p. 14 cm. [**3569**]
Different setting of type.

—[The same.] . . . Venetia, Michiel'Angelo Barboni, 1675.

[6], 3-308 p. 17 cm. [**3570**]
Different setting of type.

—Herbario novo . . . Con figure, che rappresentano le vive piante, che nascono in tutta Europa, & nell'Indie orientali, & occidentali. Con versi latini, che comprendono le facoltà de i semplici medicamenti. Con discorsi, che dimostrano i nomi, le spetie, la forma, il loco, il tempo, le qualità, & le virtù mirabili dell' herbe . . . Venetia, Li Sessa, 1602.

[12], 492 (i.e. 480), [52] p. illus., ports. 32 cm. [**3571**]

Printer's error: p. 168 and 177 (i.e. 158 and 167) blank.

—[The same.] . . . Venetia, Appresso li Sessa, 1617.
[12], 492 (i.e. 480), [52] p. illus., ports. 30 cm. [**3572**]

Colophon: Trevigi, Angelo Reghettini Per li Sessa, 1617.

—[The same.] . . . Venetia, I Giunti, 1636.
[8], 515, [44] p. illus. 26 cm. [**3573**]
Imperfect: p. 103-106 wanting.

—[The same.] . . . Con aggionta in quest'ultima impressione de i discorsi à quelle figure, che erano nell'appendice, fatti da Gio. Maria Ferro . . . Venetia, Gio. Giacomo Hertz, 1667.

[12], 476, [27] p. illus. 33 cm. [**3574**]

—[German tr.] Hortulus sanitatis, das ist, Ein heylsam und nützliches Gährtlin der Gesundtheit. In welchem alle fürnehme Kräutter, die so wol in den beyderley Indien als an allen andern Orten der Welt zu finden, in einer wunderbaren Kürtze werden beschrieben. Erstlich von Castore Durante . . . in italienischer Sprach verfertigt, nunmehr aber in unsere hoch teutsche Sprach versetzt durch Petrum Uffenbachium . . . Franckfurt am Mayn, Getruckt durch Nicolaum Hoffmann, in Verlegung Jonae Rhodii, 1609.

[16], 1081, [50] p. illus. 25 cm. [**3575**]

DURASTANTE, GIANO MATTEO [16th cent.] De aceto scillino atque aloe. *In* Jessen, J. von. Adversus pestem consilium . . . disputatione. 1614 [1615]

Die DURCH seltsame Einbildung und Betriegery Schaden bringende Alchymisten-Gesselschafft, nach ihren gewöhnlichen Merckmahlen und Eigenschafften, welche sie von sich spühren lassen, nebst Anführung einiger Discurse, was von der Alchymie zu halten . . . worbey auch viele in Conversation gebräuchliche höffliche Reden . . . zubefinden, in einen nützlichen Lust-Spiele vorgestellet von J. D. K. Franckfurht [sic] und Leipzig, G. Heinrich Zickler, 1700.

[13], 227 (i.e. 223) p. plate. 14 cm. [**3576**]

DURELLE, JEAN, *Father* [*fl.* 1643] Onomatologie chirurgique; ou, Explication des mots grecs appartenans à chirurgie. Enrichie de recherches historiques, morales, & allegoriques tirées des SS. PP. & autres autheurs . . . Avec un petit Traicté de la correspondence des meteores du microcosme avec ceux du macrocosme . . . Lyon, Philippe Borde, 1644.

[48], 252, [23] p. 16 cm. [**3577**]
Errata: p. [23] at end.

DURET, CLAUDE [*d.* 1611] Histoire admirable des plantes et herbes esmerveillables & miraculeuses en nature: mesmes d'aucunes qui sont vrays zoophytes, ou plant-animales . . . avec leurs portraicts . . . selon les histoires, descriptions . . . des anciens & modernes Hebrieux, Chaldees . . . Allemans, & autres . . . Paris, Nicolas Buon, 1605.

[24], 341, [1] p. illus. 16 cm. [**3578**]

DURET, JEAN [1563-1629] Le general et souverain remede, contre la maladie pestilentieuse. Nouvellement mis en lumiere; par Mr. Duret . . . Paris, Jean de Bordeaux, 1623.

15 p. 17 cm. [**3579**]
Published by C. Morel in 1619 and 1623 under title: Advis sur la maladie. Cf. BNC, v. 45, col. 824.

—, *ed. See* HIPPOCRATES. Coacae praenotiones. 1621, 1658, 1665, 1668.

—, *tr. See* [MERCURIO, G.] Discours de l'origine, des moeurs, fraudes et impostures des ciarlatans. 1622.

DURET, LOUIS [1527-1586] In magni Hippocratis librum De humoribus purgandis, et in libros tres De diaeta acutorum Ludovici Dureti, Segusiani, commentarii interpretatione & enarratione insignes, a Petro Girardeto ... emendati, in ordinem distributi, ac primum in lucem prolati. Adjecta est sub finem accurata constitutionis primae libri 2. Epidemiⲱn ejusdem authoris interpretatio ... Parisiis, Apud Joannem Jost, 1631.

[16], 156, [4] p.; 130, [6] p.   18 cm.   **[3580]**

Includes Greek and Latin text of De humoribus and Latin texts of De diaeta acutorum (i.e. De victus ratione in morbis acutis) and Epidemiorum libri, book 2, section 1. The translations are by Duret.

—[The same.] ... Parisiis, Apud Joannem Jost, 1639.

[16], 156, [4] p.; 130, [6] p.   18 cm.   **[3581]**

A reissue of the 1631 edition with new title page.

—, *ed.* and *tr. See* HIPPOCRATES. Coacae praenotiones. 1621, 1658, 1665, 1668.

—, *ed. See* HOULLIER, J. Commentarius in Jacobi Hollerii ... librum De morbis internis. 1611 [and] De morbis internis liber. 1611 [and] De morbis internis libri II. 1603 [and] Omnia opera practica. 1623, 1635, 1664.

—*See* HOULLIER, J. *In* Aphorismos Hippocratis commentarii. 1613, 1620, 1632, 1646, 1675.

DURET, NOËL [1590–*ca.* 1650] *See* CULPEPER, N. Semeiotica Uranica. 1651, 1655, 1658.

DURETI, LODOVICO. *See* DURET, Louis [1527–1586]

DUREY, C. *See* DUREY, Claude [17th cent.]

DUREY, CLAUDE [17th cent.] De stupendo et lugendo infortunio. Ex lupo rabiente narratio verissima. Divione, Apud Joannem Grangier, 1661.

83, [1] p.   14 cm.   **[3582]**

Errata: p. [1]

DU RIVAGE. *See* LA MESNARDIÈRE, Hippolyte Jules Pilet de [1610–1663]

DUROY, HENRY. *See* REGIUS, Henricus [1598–1679]

DURRET, NATALIS. *See* DURET, Noël [1590–*ca.* 1650]

DURRIUS, JOHANN [*fl.* 1636–1640] *respondent. See* WENDLER, M. Disputationum physico-mathematicarum prima de maris nominibus. 1636.

DURSTON, W. [*fl.* 1682] *See* YONGE, J. Wounds of the brain proved curable. 1682.

DU RUEL, JEAN. *See* RUEL, Jean [1474?–1537]

DU SOUCY, FRANÇOIS, *Sieur de Gerzan. See* GERZAN, François Du Soucy, *sieur de* [*fl.* 17th cent.]

DUSSEN, PAULUS VAN DER [*fl.* 1699] *respondent.* Dissertatio medica inauguralis de ileo seu iliaca passione ... Lugduni Batavorum, Apud Abrahammum Elzevier, M DC XCXIX (i.e. 1699)

[20] p.   22 cm.   **[3583]**

Diss.—Leyden.

DUTAL, LOUIS FRANÇOIS [*fl.* 1700] *respondent. See* MAURIN, R., *praeses.* Quaestio medica. 1700.

DU TEIL, BERNARD [*fl.* 1636–*ca.* 1659] *tr. See* FERNEL, J. La chirurgie. 1667 [and] Les sept livres de la therapeutique universelle. 1648, 1650, 1668; GLAUBER, J. R. La consolation des navigants. 1659 [and] La description des nouveaux fourneaux philosophiques. 1659 [and] Le teinture de l'or. 1659 [and] Traitté de la medecine universelle. 1659.

DU TERTRE DE LA MARCHE, MARGUERITE. *See* LA MARCHE, Marguerite Du Tertre de [1638–1706]

DU VAIR, GUILLAUME [1556–1621] The morall philosophy of the Stoicks. Written originally in French by ... monsieur du Vaix ... Englished by Charles Cotton ... London, Henry Mortlock, 1664.

[6], 118 p.   15 cm.   **[3584]**

Imperfect: first preliminary leaf (blank?) wanting.

DU VAIX. *See* DU VAIR, Guillaume [1556–1621]

DU VAL, ANTOINE, *tr. See* [SENDIVOGIUS, M.] Lettre philosophique. 1671.

DU VAL, GUILLAUME [1572–1646] Historia monogramma; sive, Pictura linearis sanctorum medicorum et medicarum, in expeditum redacta breviarium. Adjecta est series nova, sive auctarium de sanctis praesertim Galliae, qui aegris opitulantur, certosque percurant morbos. Item Digressiuncula de plantis nomenclaturae sanctioris. Ipsa denique pietas Facultatis medicinae Parisiensis, nimirum ... oratio, ad sanctos medicos, & sanctas medicas. Preces pro rege, regina, et regia prole, singulis sabbathis post sacrum recitari solitae, in sacello Facultatis ... Accessit Praesentatio licentiandorum solenni oratione celebrata, die 29. Junii 1642 ... Parisiis, Apud viduam Hieronymi Blageart, 1643.

[14], 84 p.; [12], 3-23, [3] p. 23 cm. [**3585**]

Part [2] has special title page.

DUVAL, Jacques, *sieur d'Ectomare et Du Houvel* [*ca.* 1555–*ca.* 1615] Des hermaphrodits, accouchemens des femmes, et traitement qui est requis pour les relever en santé, & bien élever leurs enfans ... Rouen, David Geuffroy, 1612.

[16], 447, [11] p. illus. 17 cm. [**3586**]

—L'hudrotherapeutique [sic] des fontaines medicinales, nouvellement découvertes aux environs de Rouen ... Rouen, Jacques Besongne, 1603.

[12], 422 (i.e. 316), [6] p. 14 cm. [**3587**]

—Methode nouvelle de guarir les catarrhes et toutes maladies qui en despendent ... En ... laquelle se trouvent 71. paradoxes qui tous sont monstrez estre ortodoxes ... Rouen, David Geuffroy, 1611.

[26], 382, [5] p. illus. 17 cm. [**3588**]

DU VAL, Jan [*fl.* 1607] *tr. See* Wecker, J. J. Le grand dispensaire. 1609, 1610.

DUVAL, Jean [*fl.* 1615] Aristocratia humani corporis ... Parisiis, Apud Franciscum Jacquin, 1615.

[16], 169 (i.e. 173), [3] p. illus. 18 cm.

[**3589**]

DU VAUROÜY, Henry de Boyvin. *See* Boyvin du Vauroüy, Henry de [*b.* 1623]

DUVERDEN VAN VOORD, Johan van. *See* Bontekoe, C. Tractaat van het excellenste kruyd thee. 1685.

DUVERNEY, Guichard Joseph [1648–1730] Traité de l'organe de l'ouie, contenant la structure,

les usages & les maladies de toutes les parties de l'oreille ... Paris, Estienne Michallet, 1683.

[24], 210 p. plates. 17 cm. [**3590**]

—[Latin tr.] Tractatus de organo auditus, continens structuram, usum et morbos omnium auris partium ... E Gallico Latine versus. Norimbergae, Impensis Johannis Ziegeri, typis Joannis Michaelis Spörlini, 1684.

[12], 48 p. plates. 20 cm. [**3591**]

DU VIVIER, Daniel de. *See* Paracelsus. La petite chirurgie. 1623.

DUX, Aegidius. *See* Hertoghe, Gilles de [*fl.* 1549–1561]

DUYCK, Franco [*d.* 1628] Comparatio elegans venatoris et amatoris. Edita ex museo Joachimi Morsi ... Lugduni Batavorum, Excudebat Jacobus Marci, 1619.

[8] p. 21 cm. [**3592**]

DYGBAEUS, Kenelmus. *See* Digby, *Sir* Kenelm [1603–1665]

DYK, Cornelis van [*fl.* 1665–1680] Osteologia; of, Nauwkeurige geraamt beschryving van verscheyde dieren, nevens hare historien, uit de vermaartste, soo oude als nieuwe schrijvers, by een gebragt ... Amsterdam, Johannes ten Hoorn, 1680.

[12], 286, [2] p. plates. 17 cm. [**3593**]

Added engraved title page.
Imperfect: p. 21-22 wanting.

—*respondent.* Disputatio medica inauguralis de suffocatione hypochondriaca ... Lugduni Batavorum, Apud Wilhelmum ab Amstel, 1665.

[12] p. 19 cm. [**3594**]

Diss.—Leyden.

E

E. *See* Eizat, *Sir* Edward.

E., G., *ed. See* Vicary, T. The English mans treasure. 1613.

E., J. *See* Evelyn, John [1620–1706]

E., J. V. *See* Venette, Nicolas [*ca.* 1631–1698]

E., T. *chirurgo-medicus. See* Emes, Thomas [*d.* 1707]

E., T. H. R. B. *See* Boyle, *Hon.* Robert [1627–1691]

EBBLE, Johann Leonhard [*fl.* 1670] *praeses.* Principia entis naturalis intrinseca in fieri et facto esse ... dissertatione physica ... exponunt ...

Theodorus Viebegus . . . Lipsiae, Typis Joh. Wittigau [1670]

    [15] p. 19 cm.   **[3595]**

    Diss. — Leipzig (T. Viebeg, *respondent*)

EBELING, PETER [*fl.* 1682-1683] *respondent. See* WEDEL, G. W., *praeses.* Dissertatio medica de nutritione et atrophia. 1682.

EBELING, PETRUS SCHWENDUS. *See* SCHWENDI, Petrus [*fl.* 1685]

EBERHARD, JOHANN DAVID [*fl.* 1698] *respondent. See* WEDEL, G. W., *praeses.* Dissertatio inauguralis medica de tinctura bezoardica essentificata. 1698 [and] Dissertatio medica de ructu. 1698.

EBERHARD-KARLS-UNIVERSITÄT, Tübingen. Rector Academiae Tubingensis lect. ben. sal. Deerat nimirum & illud malis nostris & calamitatibus . . . [Tubingae] Typis Johann-Conradi Reisii [1695]
    broadside. 37 x 27 cm.   **[3596]**

    Eulogy of Elias Rudolph Camerarius.
    Bound with Metzger, G. B. Dissertatio . . . de acidulis. [1663]

EBERHART, HIERONYMUS [*fl.* 1645] *respondent. See* CONRING, H., *praeses.* Disputatio physiologica de vita et morte. 1645.

EBERLIN, GEORG [1585-1628] *respondent. See* CRÜGER, B., *praeses.* Disputatio medica tertia. 1610; SENNERT, D., *praeses.* Disputatio medica, de inflammatione. 1610.

    —*See* KNOBLOCH, T., *praeses.* Disputationes anatomicae. 1608, 1612.

EBERWEIN, HEINRICH. *See* CORDUS, Euricius [1484-1535]

EBHARDT, GOTTFRIED [*fl.* 1696] *respondent. See* SIMON, J. G., *praeses.* Faciem humanam ad similitudinem pulchritudinis coelestis figuratam occasione L. 17. si quis. C. de poenis . . . exponit G. E. 1696.

ECCHELLENSIS, ABRAHAM. *See* ABRAHAM ECCHELLENSIS [*d.* 1664]

ECCIUS, MELCHIOR [*fl.* 1611-1618] *respondent. See* SCHALLER, W., *praeses.* Positionum medicarum semicenturia de syncope. 1618.

ECHT, JOHANN [1515?-*ca.* 1568] *See* SENNERT, D. De scorbuto tractatus. 1624.

ECK, JOHANN WOLFFGANG SIGMUND [*b.* 1669] *respondent. See* SLEVOGT, J. A., *praeses.* Dissertatio medica inauguralis de cachexia. 1697.

    —*See* CRAUSE, R. W. Propemticum inaugurale de eo an, et quomodo aurora ut musis, ita quoque sanitati amica sit? 1697.

ECK, PAULUS, *de Sultzbach. See* ECK DE SULTZBACH, Paul [*fl.* 1489?]

ECK, PETER JOHANN [*fl.* 1655] *respondent. See* THAUVONIUS, A. G., *praeses.* Disputatio physica de sensibus. 1655.

ECK DE SULTZBACH, PAUL [*fl.* 1489?] Clavis philosophorum . . .
    1007-1014 p., vol. 4. 20 cm. (*In* Zetzner, Lazarus, *ed.* Theatrum chemicum. Argentorati, 1659-61)
    Caption title.   **[3597]**

ECKARDI, HIERONIMUS [*fl.* 1697] *respondent. See* WEDEL, G. W., *praeses.* Dissertatio medica de terrore. 1697.

ECKARDUS, FRIDERICUS. *See* ECKART, Friedrich [*fl.* 1607-1611]

ECKART, FRIEDRICH [*fl.* 1607-1611] *See* KNOBLOCH, T., *praeses.* Disputationes anatomicae. 1608, 1612.

ECKEBRECHT, PAUL [*fl.* 1679] *respondent. See* EISENHART, J., *praeses.* Exercitatio juridica de die critico vulnerum ac percussionum lethalium. 1679.

ECKELT, GEORG CHRISTOPHER [*fl.* 1678] *respondent. See* NEUMANN, C., *praeses.* Judicium discursu physico explicatum. 1678.

ECKHARD, JOHANN FRIEDRICH [*fl.* 1679-1680] *respondent. See* FRANCK VON FRANCKENAU, G., *praeses.* Dissertationem inauguralem de morbo virgineo . . . proponit J. F. E. 1680; WEDEL, G. W., *praeses.* Disputatio medica aegrum haemorrhoidibus dolentibus et immodicis laborantem exhibens. 1679.

ECKHARD, JOHANN WOLFFGANG [*fl.* 1687] *respondent. See* FASCH, A. H., *praeses.* Intemperies corporis humani morborum foecunda mater. 1687.

ECKARD, KONRAD [*fl.* 1662] *respondent. See* SCHENCK, J. T., *praeses.* Disputatio inauguralis medica de melancholiae διαγνωσει. 1662.

ECKHARD, VITUS [*fl.* 1655-1658] *respondent. See* SCHENCK, J. T., *praeses.* Disputatio inauguralis medica ... de tartaro microcosmico. 1658 [and] Guerneri Rolfincii ... Epitomes methodi cognoscendi & curandi affectus corporis humani particulares. 1655.

ECKHARDT, *Der getreue. See* ETTNER, Johann Christoph von [*b.* 1654]

ECKHARTH, *Der getreue. See* ETTNER, Johann Christoph von [*b.* 1654]

ECKOLT, DAVID [*fl.* 1662-1663] *respondent.* Disputatio inauguralis medica de diabete ... Argentorati, Typis Eberhardi Welperi, 1663.

    [20] p.   19 cm.   [3598]
Diss.—Strasbourg.

  —See SEBISCH, M. [1578-1674?] *praeses.* Disputatio medica de causis. 1662.

ÉCLUSE, CHARLES DE L'. *See* L'ÉCLUSE, Charles de [1526-1609]

EDELMANN, PETER [*fl.* 1681-1683] *respondent.* Disputatio medica inauguralis de causo ... Lugduni Batavorum, Apud Abrahamum Elzevier, 1683.

    [12] p.   22 cm.   [3599]
Diss.—Leyden.

  —See CRAUSE, R. W., *praeses.* Disputationem de hypercatharsi ... proponit. 1681.

EDELPHE. *See* PLANIS CAMPY, David de [*b.* 1589]

EDINBURGH. Royal College of Surgeons. *See* ROYAL COLLEGE OF SURGEONS OF EDINBURGH.

EDINGH, PAUL [*fl.* 1683] *See* VOTIVI APPLAUSUS AMICORUM IN HONOREM EXIMII ... DN. PAULI EDINGH. 1686.

EDIT du roy 1690?, 1692, 1697. *See* FRANCE. Sovereigns, etc. [1643-1715] (Louis XIV)

EDLER wolgeprobirter und bewehrter Haussartzt; das ist, Bewehrte und kräfftige Mittel für allerhand Gebrechen und Kranckheiten des menschlichen Leibes ... Hamburg, Gedruckt durch Arnold Lichtenstein, 1677.

    312, [9] p.   front.   14 cm.   [3600]

EDUARD, JOHANN [*fl.* 1631] *See* BURGERSDIJCK, F. P. Collegium physicum. 1642.

EDWARDS, *Doctor in physic and chirurgery. See* A RICH CLOSET OF PHYSICAL SECRETS. 1652.

EDWARDS, EDWARD [*fl.* 1637] The cure of all sorts of fevers ... with their definition, kindes, differences ... and manner of cure ... London, Printed by Thomas Harper, and sold by William Sheeres, 1638.

    [8], 53, [1] p.   19 cm.   [3601]
STC 7512.

EFFERARIUS. *See* FERRARIUS [*fl.* ca. 1200]

EFFEREN, LAURENTIUS [*fl.* 1660-1663] *respondent.* Dissertatiuncula de democriti heterodoxia in doctrina de nutritione foetus in utero. In Seger, G. Dissertatio anatomica de Hippocratis orthodoxia in doctrina de nutritione foetus humani in utero. 1660.

EGBERT, SEBASTIAN. *See* VRY, Sebastian Egbertszoon de [1563-1621]

EGENOLF, JOHANN AUGUSTIN [1632-1688] *praeses.* Disputatio physica de mistione ... [Lipsiae] Literis Quirini Bauchs [1654]

    [12] p.   19 cm.   [3602]
Diss.—Leipzig (F. Schmidt, *respondent*)

EGERLAND, JOHANN ERASMUS [*fl.* 1682-1685] *respondent. See* THILE, J., *praeses.* Dissertatio medica inauguralis de purpura epidemia scorbutica. 1685 [and] Dissertatio medico-chymica de minera martissolari. 1682.

EGGEBERT. SAMUEL [*fl.* 1651-1655] *respondent.* Disputatio medica inauguralis de angina ... Lugduni Batavorum, Ex officina Francisci Hackii, 1655.

    [12] p.   20 cm.   [3603]
Diss.—Leyden.

  —Disputatio medica inauguralis de epilepsia ... Lugduni Batavorum, Typis Wilhelmi Christiani Boxii, 1651.

    [15] p.   23 cm.   [3604]
Diss.—Leyden.

EGGEBRECHT, DANIEL [*fl.* 1627] *respondent.* Disputatio inauguralis de diarrhoea ... Basileae, Typis Joh. Jacobi Genathii [1627]

    [17] p.   19 cm.   [3605]
Diss.—Basel.

EGGERS, Johann Wilhelm Otto [*fl.* 1683–1685] *respondent.* Disputatio inauguralis medica de vulneribus in genere . . . Marburgi Cattorum, Typis Johannis Henrici Stockenii [1685]

    29 (i.e. 31) p.   20 cm.   **[3606]**

   Diss. — Marburg.

—*See* Dorsten, J. D., *praeses.* Disputatio medica de succi nutritii statu naturali. 1683.

EGGERT, Johann Andreas [*b.* 1666] *respondent. See* Crause, R. W., *praeses.* Disputatio inauguralis medica de febre hectica. 1695.

—*See* Slevogt, J. A. Decani Facultatis Medicae Jo. Hadriani Slevogtii . . . prolusio inauguralis de antichetico poterii. 1695.

EGIDIUS DE VADIS. *See* Aegidius de Vadis [*fl.* 1521?]

EGIDIUS ROMANUS. *See* Colonna, Egidio [1247?–1316]

EGLINGER, Nikolaus [1645–1711] *praeses.* Disputatio physiologico-medica de saliva . . . Basileae, Typis Jacobi Bertschii [1695]

    [16] p.   22 cm.   **[3607]**

   Diss. — Basel (S. Hoegger, *respondent*)

—Exercitatio chirurgico-medica de fracturis et luxationibus ossium . . . Basileae, Typis Joh. Rudolphi Genathii [1696]

    [23] p.   18 cm.   **[3608]**

   Diss. — Basel (J. K. Mosis, *respondent*)

—Positionum botanico anatomicarum centuria . . . [Basileae] Typis Jacobi Werenfelsii [1685]

    [16] p.   19 cm.   **[3609]**

   Diss. — Basel (J. K. Bauhin, *respondent*)

—*respondent.* Disputatio medica inauguralis de angina . . . Basileae, Typis Joh. Jacobi Deckeri [1661]

    [12] p.   22 cm.   **[3610]**

   Diss. — Basel.

—, *respondent. See* Stupanus, E. *praeses.* Disputatio medica in universam physiologiam. 1660.

EGLINGER, Samuel [1638–1673] *praeses.* [De] lienter[ico] et coeliac[o] affect[u] delineat[io] . . . Basileae, Typis Joh. Jacobi Deckeri [1667]

    [34] p.   18 cm.   **[3611]**

   Diss. — Basel (F. Platter, *respondent*)

—*respondent.* De nephritide theses disputat. inaugural. . . . Basileae, Typis Georgii Deckeri [1661]

    [20] p.   20 cm.   **[3612]**

   Diss. — Basel.

—, *respondent. See* Bauhin, J. K., *praeses.* Theses de humoribus. 1660.

[EGLINUS ICONIUS, Raphael, 1559–1622] Cheiragogia Heliana de auro philosophico necdum cognito [&] Disquisitio Heliana, de metallorum transformatione, &c. [&] Aphorismi Basiliani sive canones Hermetici . . . author Nicolaus Niger Hapelius [pseud.] de coelo terrestri, &c. Marpurgi Cattorum, Ex Officina Rudolphi Hutwelckeri, 1612.

    223 p.   16 cm.   **[3613]**

—[The same.] . . .

    265–287, 300–330 p., vol. 4.   20 cm.   (*In* Zetzner, Lazarus, *ed.* Theatrum chemicum. Argentorati, 1659–61)   **[3614]**

   Caption titles.

—Philochemicis Heliophilus a Percis Philochemicus [pseud.] S. Nova disquisitio de helia artista.

    214–246 p., vol. 4.   20 cm.   (*In* Zetzner, Lazarus, *ed.* Theatrum chemicum. Argentorati, 1659–61)   **[3615]**

   Running title.

EGLISHAM, George [*fl.* 1612–1642] *See* Barclay, W. Judicium. 1620.

EHINGER, Konrad Kaspar [*fl.* 1683] *respondent.* Disputatio medica inauguralis de odontalgia . . . Altdorffii, Literis Henrici Meyeri [1683]

    24 p.   20 cm.   **[3616]**

   Diss. — Altdorf.

EHRHARD, Johann David [*b.* 1676] *See* Slevogt, J. A. Decani Facultatis Medicae Jo. Hadriani Slevogtii . . . praelusio inauguralis de lapide bezoar. Jenae, Litteris Krebsianis [1698]

EHRHART, Balthasar [1639–1706] *respondent. See* Brotbeck, J. K. Commentarius medicus in historiam Galeni, de peste. 1661.

EHRLICH, Hieronymus Christian [*fl.* 1651] *respondent.* De vertigine. *In* Rolfinck, W., *praeses.* Methodus cognoscendi & curandi adfectus capitis particulares. 1653.

EHRLICH, JOHANN MARTIN [*fl.* 1684-1686] *respondent. See* CRAUSE, R. W., *praeses.* Disputatio inauguralis medica de ischuria. 1686; WEDEL, G. W., *praeses.* Disputatio medica, casum aegri hernia laborantis exhibens. 1684.

— *See* WEDEL, G. W. Propempticon inaugurale de fundamentis empiricorum. 1686.

EHRLICH, JOHANN THEODOR [*fl.* 1686-1688] *respondent. See* VESTI, J., *praeses.* Dissertatio medica de febri ardente maligna. 1686.

EHWALD, JOHANNES JACOBUS. *See* EWALD, Johann Jakob [*fl.* 1699]

EICHEL, JOHANN [*b.* 1666] *respondent. See* WEDEL, G. W., *praeses.* Disputatio inauguralis medica, de punctura nervorum. 1689.

— *See* WEDEL, G. W. Propempticon inaugurale de demonstratione Hippocratica. 1689.

EICHELBORN, GEORG [*fl.* 1654] *respondent. See* MOELLENBROCK, V. A., *praeses.* Disputatio medica de peste. 1654.

EICHHORN, JOHANN WILHELM [*fl.* 1674] *respondent. See* WEDEL. G. W., *praeses.* Disputationem inauguralem de febri petechiali . . . subjiciet J. G. E. 1674.

EICHLER, SALOMON [*fl.* 1667-1668] *respondent.* Disputationem physicam de putredine . . . submittit M. Salomon Eichler . . . Lipsiae, Typis Joh. Erici Hahnii [1667]

    [16] p. 20 cm.   **[3617]**
    Diss. — Leipzig.

— *See* AMMANN, P., *praeses.* Disputatio inauguralis medica de suffocatione uterina. 1668.

EICHOLTZ, JOHANN. *See* AICHHOLTZ, Johann [1520-1588]

EICHORN, JOHANN [*fl.* 1621-1623] *respondent. See* SCHENCK, E., *praeses.* Decas problematum medicorum. 1621.

EICHSTÄD, LAURENT [1596-1660] *praeses.* Disputatio generalis de osteologia humana ossium naturam, causas, numerum, partes, syntaxin usumque succincte exponens . . . Dantisci, Typis viduae Georgii Rhetii, 1648.

    [28] p. 20 cm.   **[3618]**
    Diss. — Danzig (J. Möller, *respondent*)

— Disputatio physiologica publica extraordinaria de peste . . . [Gedanum] David-Fridericus Rhetius [1657]

    [16] p. 19 cm.   **[3619]**
    Diss. — Danzig (J. Seidel, *respondent*)

EICKMEYER, JOHANNES ANTON [*fl.* 1698] *respondent.* Disputatio medica inauguralis de epilepsia uterina . . . Trajecti ad Rhenum, Ex officina Francisci Halma, 1698.

    [17], [3] p. 22 cm.   **[3620]**

EILERT, JOHANN CHRISTOPH [*fl.* 1661] *respondent. See* KIRCHMAYER, G. K., *praeses.* De montibus ignivomis. 1661.

EIMMARDUS, GEORGIUS CHRISTOPHORUS. *See* EIMMART, Georg Christoph [1638-1705]

EIMMART, GEORG CHRISTOPH [1638-1705] *respondent. See* VOGEL, C., *praeses.* Theorema geographicum de physica telluris rotunditate. 1658.

EINES ehrbarn Raths der Stadt Lübeck revidirte Pestordnung. 1639. *See* LÜBECK. Ordinances, local laws, etc.

EINES wol edlen . . . Rahts, der Stadt Nürnberg, Ordnung. 1679. *See* NUREMBERG. Ordinances, local laws, etc.

EINFELTIGER, kurtzer Bericht von der abscheulichen Seuch der Pestilentz, wie solche . . . nicht allein zu verhüten, sondern auch zu curirn seye: auss gnädigem Befelch dess . . . Herrn Philipps Ludwigen Pfaltzgraven bey Rhein, Hertzogen in Bayrn . . . Durch seiner . . . bestellte Medicos, für den gemeinen Mann in dero Fürstenthumb Neuburg . . . nutzlich zu gebrauchen . . . Laugingen, M. Jacob Winter [1606]

    28, [2] ll. illus. 19 cm.   **[3621]**

EIRENAEUS PHILOPONOS PHILALETHES. *See* STARKEY, George [1627-1665]

EISEN, KARL CHRISTOPH [1649-1690] *respondent.* De comate somnolento . . . Basileae, Typis Joh. Rodolphi Genathii [1674]

    [12] p. 19 cm.   **[3622]**
    Diss. — Basel.

—*See* GLASER, J. H., *praeses*. Casus medicus de mensium suppressione. 1673.

EISENHART, JOHANN [1643–1707] *praeses*. Exercitatio juridica de die critico vulnerum ac percussionum lethalium ... Helmestadi, Typis Henrici Davidis Mülleri, 1679.

[36] p. 20 cm. **[3623]**

Diss.—Helmstädt (P. Eckebrecht, *respondent*)

EISENHEIM, LUDWIG [*fl.* 1632] *respondent. See* SALTZMANN, J. R. [1573–1656] *praeses*. Disputatio medica de fame praeter-naturali et corrupta. 1632; SEBISCH, M. [1578–1674?] *praeses*. Exercitationes medicae. 1639 [and] Galeni Ars parva in disputationes triginta resoluta. 1633.

EISENMENGER, JOHANN CHRISTOPH [*fl.* 1613–*ca.* 1634] De foetu Mussipontano extra uterum in abdomine genito, ad Joh. Danielem Horstium. *In* Historia foetus Mussipontani. 1669; Sinibaldi, G. B. Geneanthropeiae. 1669.

—*See* STRAUSS, L. Resolutio casus Mussipontani foetus extra uterum in abdomine retenti. 1662.

—Kurtzer Bericht, wie die hitzige ansteckende Kopffkranckheit zu verhüten, und sampt ihren Zufällen zu curiren. Erstlich in Anno 1621. gestellt, jetzo aber ubersehen ... und in bessere Ordnung gebracht. Sampt aussführlichem Bericht von der gifftigen ansteckenden Rothen Ruhr, so Anno 1632, und 1633. regirt. Durch Joh. Christophorum Eysenmengern ... Heylbronn, Gedruckt bey Christoff Krausen, 1634.

[8], 157 (i.e. 153), [5] p. 13 cm. **[3624]**

—Nothwendiger Bericht, von dess ... Weinstein-Pulvers, rechtem Gebrauch, und wie dasselbige ... zu verfertigen. Auff Anlass Hern M. Ludovici Wolffharts ... in Truck aussgangener widerholter Schrifft, so er Experimentum cremoris tartari oder wahrhaffte Beschreibung dess Weinstein Saltz, was nemblich dessen Krafft und Würckung seye ec. genennet. Auss oberkeitlichem grossgünstigem Anbefehlen. Von dess ... Statt Heylbronn verordneten Physicis gestellt und jedermänniglich zur Nachrichtung gedruckt. Heylbronn, Gedruckt durch Christoff Krausen [1632?]

[1], 118 p. 14 cm. **[3625]**

Signed at end by Johann Christoph Eisenmenger and Ferdinand Herrscher.

Published also in the same year as part [2] of Ludwig Wolffhart's Experimentum cremoris tartari.

—*respondent. See* SCHLEGEL, P. M., *praeses*. Disputatio medica, de saluberrimo venarum. 1641.

EISENSCHMID, JOHANN CASPAR [1656–1712] *respondent*. Dissertatio inauguralis medica περι χοιραδιου; sive, De scrofulis ... Argentorati, Typis Johann-Jacobi Dolhopffi [1681]

[1], 25 p. 19 cm. **[3626]**

Diss.—Strasbourg.

EITERITZ, JOHANN CHRISTOPH ETTNER VON. *See* ETTNER, Johann Christoph von [*b.* 1654]

[**EIZAT**, Sir EDWARD] Apollo mathematicus; or, The art of curing diseases by the mathematicks, according to the principles of Dr. Pitcairn. A work ... never published in English before. To which is subjoined, A discourse of certainty, according to the principles of the same author ... [London] 1695.

142 p.; 26 p. 16 cm. **[3627]**

Imprint partly supplied from BMC, vol. 190, col. 661.

Part [2] has special title page with title: A discourse of certainty.

A satire on works by Archibald Pitcairne.

—*See* BROWN, A. The epilogue. 1699.

ELEMENS de botanique. 1694. *See* TOURNEFORT, J. P. de.

ELEONORA, *consort of* Ernest Joachim, *Prince of Anhalt. See* ELEONORA, *consort of* George I, *landgrave of Hesse-Darmstadt* [1551 or 2–1618]

ELEONORA, *consort of* George I, *landgrave of Hesse-Darmstadt* [1551 or 2–1618] *See* SECHS BÜCHER AUSERLESENER ARTZNEY UND KUNST-STÜCK. 1613, 1678.

ELEONORA, *duchess of Württemberg. See* ELEONORA, *consort of* George I, *landgrave of Hesse-Darmstadt* [1551 or 2–1618]

ELEONORA MARIA ROSALIA, *duchess of Troppau and Jägerndorf. See* TROPPAU UND JÄGERNDORF, Eleonora Maria Rosalia, *Herzogin zu* [1647–1704]

ELERS, JOHANNES [*fl.* 1678] *respondent. See* JOHRENIUS, C., *praeses*. Disputatio inauguralis medica de volatili & fixo. 1678.

ELICHMANN, JOHANN [*ca.* 1600–1639] *See* BEVERWIJCK. J. van. Epistolica quaestio de vitae termino, fatali, an mobili? 1636, 1651.

ELICI, Frediano [*d.* 1683] Arca novella di sanitá trattato fisico morale con alcune regole per conservarsi sano e vivere virtuosamente ... Lucca, Jacinto Paci, 1656.

[34], 296, [24] p. front. 16 cm.   [3628]

ELIOT, *Sir* Thomas. *See* Elyot, *Sir* Thomas [1490?-1546]

ELK besiet sig selven, of die schurft heeft, voelt waer 't jeut; soetelijk gediscoureerd over de twistsieke bytebaauvery van Lysjes kous: door Fokke Teekke, een flatige Fries, en Souwsje Douw, een Amsterdams kind ... [n. p., 1678]

16 p. 16 cm.   [3629]

ELLAIN, Nicolas [1534-1621] Advis sur la peste. Paris, David Douceur, 1606.

64 p. 17 cm.   [3630]

ELLENBERGER, Heinrich [1570-1624] *praeses.* Disputatio medica, de pleuritide ... Marpurgi Cattorum, Excudebat Paulus Egenolphus, 1603.

[39] p. 21 cm.   [3631]

Diss.—Marburg (T. Corbeius, *respondent*)

—Themata iatrochymica ... Marpurgi Cattorum, Ex chalcographia Rudolphi Hutwelckeri [1606]

[11] p. 20 cm.   [3632]

Diss.—Marburg (S. Gentersberger, *respondent*)

ELLIGER, Christian [*fl.* 1659] *respondent. See* Pichtel, B. J., *praeses.* Disputatio physica de speciebus sensibilibus. 1659.

ELLINGER, Adam [*fl.* 1659] *respondent. See* Kirchmayer, G. K., *praeses.* Ex physicis disputationem publicam, de aere ... sistet. 1659.

ELMENHORST, Heinrich [1632-1703] *respondent. See* Scheiner, P., *praeses.* Dissertatio physica de ignis elemento. 1653.

ELNBERGER, Adam Heinrich [*fl.* 1695] *respondent.* Dissertationem inaugural. medicam de passione hysterica, dem Aufsteigen der Mutter ... exponit Adamus Henricus Elnberger ... Duisburgi ad Rhenum, Apud Johannem Sas, 1695.

32 p. 20 cm.   [3633]

ELSEN, Aegidius van [*fl.* 1684] *respondent.* Disputatio medica inauguralis de partu difficili ... Lugduni Batavorum, Apud Abrahamum Elzevier, 1684.

[16] p. 22 cm.   [3634]

Diss.—Leyden.

ELSHOLTZ, Johann Sigismund [1623-1688] Anthropometria. Accessit doctrina naevorum ... Patavii, Typis Jo. Baptistae Pasquati, 1654.

[8], 99, [5] p. illus. 22 cm.   [3635]

—[The same.] Anthropometria; sive, De mutua membrorum corporis humani proportione, & naevorum harmonia libellus. Editio post Patavinam altera ... Francofurti ad Oderam, Praelo Andreae Becmani, apud Rupertum Völckern, 1663.

[12], 266 (i.e. 166), [1] p. plates. 17 cm.   [3636]

Imperfect: added engraved title page wanting.
Errata: p. [1] at end.
With this are bound: Höping, J. A. J. Institutiones chiromanticae. 1681.—Rehebold, Christian. Salomon & Marcolphus Justiniano-Gregoriani. 1678.

—[The same.] *In* Höchstfürtreflichtes chiromantisch- und physiognomisches Klee-Blat. 1695.

—Clysmatica nova; sive, Ratio, qua in venam sectam medicamenta immitti possint, ut eodem modo, ac si per os assumta fuissent, operentur: addita etiam omnibus seculis inaudita sanguinis transfusione. Ed. 2., variis experimentis ... illustrata. Coloniae Brandenburgicae, Ex officina Georgi Schultzii, impensis Danielis Reichelii, 1667.

[12], 68 p. plates. 15 cm.   [3637]

—[German tr.] Clysmatica nova; oder, Newe Clystier-Kunst, wie eine Arzney durch eröffnete Ader bey zu bringen, dass sie ihre Wirckung eben also verrichte, als wan sie durch den Mund genommen worden wäre ... Berlin, Bey Daniel Reicheln, 1665.

15 p. 15 cm.   [3638]

—De phosphoris observationes: quarum priores binae antea jam editae, tertia vero prima nunc vice prodit. Berolini, Literis Georgii Schultzii, 1681.

13, [2] p. plate. 18 cm.   [3639]

—Destillatoria curiosa; sive, Ratio ducendi liquores coloratos per alembicum, hactenus si non ignota, certe minus observata atque cognita. Accedunt Utis Udenii [pseud. i.e. Georg Wolffgang Wedel] & Guerneri Rolfincii Non-entia chymica. Berolini, Typis Rungianis, impensis Ruperti Volcheri, 1674.

[14], 176 p. front., illus. plate. 15 cm.   [3640]

—[English tr.] The curious distillatory; or, The art of distilling coloured liquors, spirits, oyls, &c. from vegitables, animals, minerals, and metals . . . Together with several experiments upon the blood (and its serum) of diseased persons . . . Written originally in Latin . . . put into English by T[homas] S[herley] . . . London, Printed by J. D. for Robert Boulter, 1677.

[15], III p.   front., illus.   16 cm.   [**3641**]

—*See* JASOLINO, G. Collegium anatomicum. 1668.

ELSNER, JOACHIM GEORG [1642-1676] *respondent.* *See* POSNER, C., *praeses.* Dissertatio physica de calido innato viventium. 1663.

ELVETIUS. *See* HELVÉTIUS, Jean Adrien [1661?-1727]

ELWERTH, JOHANN PHILIPP [*fl.* 1678] *respondent.* *See* WINCKLER, F. C., *praeses.* Casus curati phrenetici. 1678.

ELYOT, *Sir* THOMAS [1490?-1546] The castle of health, corrected, and in some places augmented by the first author . . . Now newlie perused, amended, and corrected, this present yeare, 1610. London, Company of Stationers, 1610.

[12], 140 p.   19 cm.   [**3642**]
Imperfect: p. 123-140 mutilated.
STC 7657.

EMERICUS, VALENTIN [*fl.* 1614-1616] *respondent.* Disputatio medica de hernia . . . Basileae, Typis Joh. Jacobi Genathii [1616]

[44] p.   19 cm.   [**3643**]
Diss. — Basel.

ÉMERY, *sieur d'.* Recueil de curiositez rares et nouvelles des plus admirables effets de la nature. Avec de beaux secrets gallans. Et la methode pour la disposition & preparation de ce qui est util & necessaire pour la vie des hommes . . . Recherchées par le sieur d'Emery. Paris, Louis Vendosme, 1674.

[12], 394 p.; [12], 203 p.   16 cm.   [**3644**]
Part 2 has special title page.
Attributed to Nicolas Lémery by NUC and BNC; to Antoine d'Emery by BMC.

—[The same.] . . . Recherchées par le sieur d'Hemery [sic] Paris, Louis Vendosme, 1676.

[12], 358, [1] p.; 136, [6] p.   15 cm.   [**3645**]

—[The same.] . . . Corr. . . . & augm. . . . Recherchées par le sieur d'Emery. Lausanne, David Gentil, 1681.

[8], 380 (i.e. 280), [31] p.; 173 (i.e. 137), [9] p.   15 cm.   [**3646**]

—[The same.] Recueil des curiositez rares & nouvelles des plus admirables effects de la nature & de l'art . . . Premiere [-Seconde] partie. Leide, suivant la copie de Paris, Pierre vander Aa, 1684.

[7], 344, [32] p.; 156, [12] p.   14 cm.   [**3647**]
Added engraved title page.
Part 2 has special title page.

—[The same.] . . . 1. partie [-2. partie] Derniére éd. . . . augm., rev., corr. . . . Paris, à Leide, Pierre Vander Aa, 1685.

[8], 648, [16] p.   plates.   14 cm.   [**3648**]
Added engraved title page.
Part 2 has special title page (p. [439]).

—[The same.] . . . Augmenté de plus de moitié, de merveilleux & beaux secrets gallands & autres, tres-utiles . . . de conserver leur santé . . . Composez par le Sr. d'Emery. 1. partie [-2. partie] Derniére ed. augm., rev., corr. . . . Suivant la copie de Paris. Leyde, Pierre van der Aa, 1688.

[10], 488, [32] p.; [1], 388, [26] p.   plates.   15 cm.   [**3649**]
Added engraved title page.
Part [2] has special title page.
Imperfect: p. 121-122 mutilated.

—[English tr.] Modern curiosities of art & nature. Extracted out of the cabinets of the most eminent personages of the French court . . . Made English from the original French. London, Matthew Gilliflower and James Partridge, 1685.

[45], 355, [5] p.   16 cm.   [**3650**]
Added engraved title page.

EMERY, ANTOINE d'. See ÉMERY, *sieur d'.* Recueil de curiositez rares. 1674, 1676, 1681, 1684, 1685, 1688; [English tr.] 1685.

EMES, THOMAS [*d.* 1707] A dialogue between alkali and acid: containing divers philosophical and medicinal considerations wherein a late . . . hypothesis, asserting alkali the cause, and acid the cure of all diseases; is proved groundless and dangerous. Being a specimen of the . . . mistakes and great ignorance of . . . John Colbatch. By T[homas]

E[mes] chirurgo-medicus . . . London, R. Cumberland and Thomas Speed, 1698.

[4], 108 p.   19 cm.   [**3651**]

—[The same.] . . . The 2d ed. London, Thomas Speed, 1699.

[6], 108 p.   18 cm.   [**3652**]

A reissue of the 1698 edition with new title page and with the addition of a list of books sold by Thomas Speed.

EMMENES, Jacob van [*fl.* 1650–1655] *respondent.* Disputatio medica inauguralis, de dysenteria . . . Ultrajecti, Ex officina Jacobi à Doeyenborgh, 1655.

[8] p.   20 cm.   [**3653**]

Diss. — Utrecht.

EMMEREZ, Guydo-Erasmus [*fl.* 1681–1695] *respondent. See* Delabre, J. C., *praeses.* Quaestio medica. 1681.

EMMERICH, Georg [1672–1727] *praeses.* Dissertatio academica sistens paradoxon physico-medicum de inspiratione . . . Regiomonti, Typis Friderici Reusneri [1698]

[12] p.   19 cm.   [**3654**]

Diss. — Königsberg (C. F. Hübner, *respondent*)

EMMERICH, Johann Christian [*fl.* 1695] *respondent. See* Ortlob, J. F., *praeses.* Disputatio medica inauguralis de ictero. 1695.

EMOHNE, Magdalena. *See* Eine rechte warhaffte Abcontrofactur eines wunderbarlichen Geschöpffs. 1616.

EMRICH, Johannes Christianus. *See* Emmerich, Johann Christian [*fl.* 1695]

ENCHIRIDION medicum. *See* [Valentinus, P. P.]

ENCHIRIDION physicae restitutae. *See* [Espagnet, J. d']

ENCHIRIDION practicum medico-chirurgicum; sive, De internorum externorumque morborum curatione . . . tractatus duo. I. Incerti, at magni authoris opus posthumum . . . II. Anthonii Chalmetei . . . Manuale chirurgicum . . . Genevae, Apud Petrum de le Roviere, 1621.

[15], 495 p.; [7], 351, [7] p.   18 cm.   [**3655**]

Part [2] has special title page: Enchiridion chirurgicum, externorum morborum remedia.

The first part was presumably outlined by Jean Fernel and completed by Julien Le Paulmier de Grentemesnil. [f. p. [3–4]]

—[The same.] . . . Genevae, Ex typographia Matthaei Berjon, 1627.

[16], 495 p.; [15], 351 p.   17 cm.   [**3656**]

Different setting of type.

—[The same.] . . . [Genevae?] Apud Petrum & Jacobum Chouët, 1644.

[16], 495 p.; [7], 351, [7] p.   17 cm.   [**3657**]

Different setting of type.

ENCKE, Friedrich [*fl.* 1687] *respondent. See* Limmer, C. P., *praeses.* Collegii Physici disputatorii disputatio quarta. 1687.

ENCKELMANN, Achatius Christophorus [*fl.* 1634–1636] respondent. *See* Sebisch, M. [1578–1674?] *praeses.* Collegii therapeutici disputatio I[–XIV] 1634 [i.e. 1635] [and] Examinis vulnerum partium dissimilarium pars I[–IV. & ultima] 1636 [i.e. 1637]

ENDTER, Johann Andreas. *See* Theatrum sympatheticum. 1660, 1661, 1662.

ENGELBRECHT, Georg [1638–1705] *praeses.* Discursum juridicum de peste et juribus circa tempus pestis, von dem was Recht ist zu Pest-Zeiten . . . Helmstadii, Typis Georg-Wolfgangi Hammii [1683]

[72] p.   18 cm.   [**3658**]

Diss. — Helmstedt (C. U. Blume, *respondent*)

ENGELBRECHT, Peter Christian [*fl.* 1691] *respondent. See* Schultz, C., *praeses.* Dissertatio academica, de chiromantiae vanitate. 1691.

ENGELEN, Engelbert [*fl. ca.* 1647] *respondent. See* Deusing, A., *praeses.* Synopsis medicinae universalis. 1649.

ENGELFREDUS, Annibal Dominicus Pimbiolus de. *See* Pimbiolo degli Engelfreddi, Annibale Domenico [*d.* 1731]

ENGELHARDT, Johann Lorenz [*fl.* 1669] *respondent. See* Sebisch, J. A., *praeses.* Dissertatio philologico-medica de Aesculapio inventore medicinae. 1669.

ENGELMANN, Gottfried [*fl.* 1662] *respondent.* Disputatio inauguralis medica de cholera . . . Basileae, Typis Joh. Jacobi Deckeri, 1662.

[8] p.   18 cm.   [**3659**]

Diss. — Basel.

ENGERING, GERHARD DANIEL [*fl.* 1689] *respondent.* Disputatio medica inauguralis de lithiasi renum et vesicae ... Trajecti ad Rhenum, Ex officina Francisci Halma, 1689.

18 p. 22 cm. [**3660**]

Diss.—Utrecht.

ENGLISH, PETER [*fl.* 1656] *tr. See* GALENUS [Methodus medendi. English.] Galen's method of physick. 1656.

The **ENGLISH** midwife enlarged, containing directions to midwifes ... Also instructions for women in their conceiving, bearing and nursing children. With two new treatises, one of the cure of diseases ... happening ... before and after childbirth. And another of the diseases, &c. of little children ... London, Rowland Reynolds, 1682.

[14], 320 p. front., illus., plates. 15 cm. [**3661**]

Plagiarized from Wolveridge's Speculum matricis. Cf. Spencer, p. 178.

The **ENGLISHMANS** doctor. *See* REGIMEN SANITATIS SALERNITANUM. The Englishmans doctor. 1608, 1609, 1624.

ENGRING, JOHANN CLEMENS [*fl.* 1685] *respondent.* Disputatio medica inauguralis de catarrho ... Lugduni Batavorum, Apud Abrahamum Elzevier, 1685.

[12] p. 22 cm. [**3662**]

Diss.—Leyden.

ENNICHMAN, ZACHARIAS [*fl.* 1659] *respondent.* Cleomenis omochilus ... Lugduni Batavorum, Apud Johannem Elsevirium, 1659.

[15] p. 19 cm. [**3663**]

Caption title reads: Cleomenis omochilus, Hippocrates v. Epid. li.

Diss.—Leyden.

—*See* SCHENCK, J. T., *praeses.* Historia plantarum generalis. 1656; VORSTIUS, A., *praeses.* Aphorismorum Hippocrateorum decades duae. 1659.

ENNIUS, QUINTUS. *See* FRANCK VON FRANCKENAU, G., praeses. De morbo Q. Enii poetae. 1694.

ENRIQUEZ, RODRIGO. *See* HARIZA, J. B. de. Instancias a un papel muy docto de ... Rodrigo Enriquez. 1670.

ENT, Sir GEORGE [1604-1689] Opera omnia medico-physica ... Nunc primum junctim edita, a plurimis mendis repurgata ... Lugduni Batavorum, Apud Petrum vander Aa, 1687.

[30], 629, [26] p. 17 cm. [**3664**]

Added engraved title page.

"Apolologia pro circuitione sanguinis. Qua respondetur Aemylio Parisano" (p. [13]-418) has half-title. "Ἀντιδιατριβη; sive, Animadversiones in Malachiae Trustoni, M. D. diatribam De respirationis usu primario" (p. [419]-629) has special title page.

—ʼΑντιδιατριβη; sive, Animadversiones in Malachiae Thrustoni, M. D. diatribam De respirationis usu primario ... Londini, Typis J. M. impensis autem Guil. Bromwich, 1679.

[3], 214 p. front. (port.) 18 cm. [**3665**]

—[The same.] Animadversiones in Malachiae Thrustoni, M. D. diatribam De respirationis usu primario ... Londini, Typis prostant vero venales at insigne Bibliorum in vico vulgo vocato Ludgatehill, 1685.

[8], 214 p. 18 cm. [**3666**]

A reissue of the 1679 edition with new title page.

—Apologia pro circuitione sanguinis. Qua respondetur Aemylio Parisano ... Ed. alt., auct. & accuratior. Londini, Typis M. F. impensis Gualteri Kettilby, 1685.

[20], 431 p. illus. 19 cm. [**3667**]

—*See* [PEACHIE, John] Some observations made upon the Barbado seeds. 1694; THRUSTON, M. De respirationis usu primario. 1670, 1671.

Der **ENTLARVTE** Marcktschreyer. *See* [ETTNER, J. C. von] Des getreuen Eckharts [pseud.] medicinischen Maul-Affens erster Theil. 1694.

EPHEMERIDORUM medico-physicarum Germanicarum. *See* MISCELLANEA CURIOSA.

The **EPHESIAN** and Cimmerian matrons. 1668. *See* [CHARLETON, W.]

EPICURUS. *See* CHARLETON, W. Physiologia Epicuro-Gassendo-Charltoniana. 1654.

EPIGRAMMATA regiorum medicinae professorum. *See* HIPPOCRATES. [Aphorismi. Greek and Latin.] Οι ʼΑφορισμοὶ πεξικοί τε καὶ ἔμμετροι. 1633.

EPIPHANIUS, *medicus. See* EPIPHANIUS, Nicolaus [*fl.* 1561]

EPIPHANIUS, Nicolaus [*fl.* 1561] Empyrica. *In* Dispensatorium chymicum. 1626; Renou, J. de. Dispensatorium medicum. 1615; Vittori, B. De curandis morbis ad tyrones practica magna. 1628.

EPIRIO, Fronimo. *See* Falconieri, Paolo [*d.* 1704]

EPISCOPUS, Andreas [*fl.* 1626] *respondent. See* Hoever, W., *praeses.* Methodus praecavendae curandaeque pestis. 1626.

EPPLIN, Johann Kaspar [*fl.* 1648-1649] *respondent. See* Sebisch, M. [1578-1674?] *praeses.* Galeni quinque priores libri. 1651.

ERASISTRATUS. *See* Aquenza y Mossa, P. De sanguinis missione. 1696; Porzio, L. A. Erasistratus; sive, De sanguinis missione. 1683.

ERASMUS, Desiderius [*d.* 1536] De sympathia et antipathia. *In* Mizauld, A. Harmonia superioris naturae mundi et inferioris. 1598.

—Μωρίας ἐγκώμιον. Stultitiae laus. Des. Erasmi Rot. declamatio, cum commentariis Ger. Listrii, & figuris Jo. Holbenii ... Accedunt ... Praefatio Caroli Patini. Vita Erasmi ... Vita Holbenii ... Epistola Erasmi ad Mart. Dorpium. Epistola Erasmi ad Th. Morum. Epistola Th. Mori ad Mart. Dorpium ... Basileae, Typis Genathianis, 1676.

    [80], 336, [11] p.   ports., illus.   20 cm.
                             [3668]
Added engraved title page by Holbein.
Edited by Charles Patin.

—, *tr. See* Sextus Empiricus. Opera. 1621.

—*See* Beverwijck, J. van. DD. virorum epistolae et responsa. 1665 [and] Epistolicae quaestiones, cum doctorum responsis. 1644.

ERASTUS, Thomas [1524-1583] De occultis medicamentorum proprietatibus. *In* Smet, H. Miscellanea ... medica. 1661.

—*See* Scholtz, L. Consiliorum medicinalium ... liber singularis. 1610 [and] Epistolarum philosophicarum: medicinalium, ac chymicarum ... volumen. 1610.

—*as subject. See* Claves, G. Le D., *known as* Gaston de. Apologia chrysopoeiae et argyropoeiae, adversus Thomam Erastum. 1602, 1659 [and] Claveus Germanicus. 1617 [and] Philosophia chymica. 1612; Hof-

mann, C. Animadversiones in Com. Montani ... De morbis. 1641.

ERAXISTRATUS. *See* Erasistratus.

ERB, Johann Christoph [*fl. ca.* 1686] Der treue und aufrichtige Medicus, kurtz abgebildet. Brieg, Druckts Johann Christoph Jacob, 1686.
    [11], 79 p.   14 cm.   **[3669]**

ERBEN VON BRANDAU, Matthias [*fl.* 17th cent.] Warhaffte Beschreibung von der Universal-Medicin, und Güldnen Tinctur Ursprung, Anfang, Mittel und Ende. Wie auch derselben Zubereitung nach der alten und neuen Philosoph. warhafften gründen, wobey auch noch viele andere curiöse Sachen zufinden. Aus des ... Autoris MSto zum Druck befördert und communiciret durch T. P. G. L. M. S. Leipzig, Zufinden in Lackischen Laden, 1689.
    [12], 148 p.   17 cm.   **[3670]**

ERBERFELDT, Heinrich [*fl.* 1674] *respondent. See* Meibom, H., *praeses.* Disputatio medica inauguralis de spiritibus ex vegetabilibus. 1674.

ERBINÄUS VON BRANDAU, Matthäus. *See* Erben von Brandau, Matthias [*fl.* 17th cent.]

ERDMANN, Adam. See Mirus, Adam Erdmann [1656-1727]

EREMITA, Donato d' [*fl.* 1624] Antidotario ... nel quale si discorre intorno all'osservanza, che deve tenere lo spetiale nell'elegere, preparare, componere, & conservare i medicamenti semplici, & composti. Diviso in libri tre: a quali si è agiunto il quarto libro intitulato L'arte distillatoria. Napoli, Secondino Roncagliolo, 1639.
    [6], 142 p.   illus.   33 cm.   **[3671]**
Engraved title page.
Only one book was published.

—Dell'elixir vitae ... libri quattro ... Napoli, Secondino Roncagliolo, 1624.
    [12], 182 p.   plates.   29 cm.   **[3672]**
Engraved title page.

ERESIUS, Theophrastus. *See* Theophrastus.

ERFURTH, Valer [*fl.* 1673] *respondent. See* Friderici, V., *praeses.* Διασκεψις historico-philologica de capillamentis vom Barücken. 1673.

ERHARDT, JOHANN GEORG [*fl. 1632*] *respondent.* *See* SEBISCH, M. [1578-1674?] *praeses.* Galeni Ars parva in disputationes triginta resoluta. 1633.

ERICH, FRANZ JOHANN [*b. 1665*] *respondent.* *See* WEDEL, G. W., *praeses.* Disputatio inauguralis medica de mensium fluxu immodico. 1688.

—*See* CRAUSE, R. W. Rudolfus Wilhelmus Crasius . . . Facult. Med. . . . decanus lectori benevolo salutem. 1688.

ERICI, NICOLAUS [*fl. 1688*] *respondent. See* BORCH, O., *praeses.* Disputatio medica inauguralis de phthisi. 1688.

ERITREO, JANO NICIO, *pseud. See* ROSSI, Gian Vittorio [1577-1647]

ERKELS, EBERHARDT [*fl. 1673*] *respondent.* Disputatio inauguralis medica de febre quartana intermittente . . . Basileae, Literis Jacobi Werenfelsii [1673]

[20] p. 19 cm. **[3673]**
Diss. — Basel.

ERKELS, FRIEDRICH GOTTFRIED SYLVESTER [*fl. 1686*] *respondent.* Disputatio inauguralis medica de inflammatione in genere . . . Basileae, Literis Jacobi Werenfelsii [1686]

[24] p. 19 cm. **[3674]**
Diss. — Basel.

ERLSFELD, JOHANN FRANZ LOEW VON. *See* LOEW VON ERLSFELD, Johann Franz, *Ritter,* [1648-1725]

ERMENGARD BLASII. *See* ARMENGANDUS BLASII [*fl. ca. 1280-1309*]

ERNDEL, CHRISTIAN HEINRICH. *See* ERNDL, Christian Heinrich [1676-1734]

ERNDL, CHRISTIAN HEINRICH [1676-1734] Dissertationem de usu historiae naturalis exoticogeographicae in medicina . . . publicae eruditorum censurae subjicit, Christianus Henricus Erndl . . . respondente Daniele Kiessling . . . Lipsiae, Typis Christiani Scholvini [1700]

[36] p. 19 cm. **[3675]**
Diss. — Leipzig (D. Kiessling, *respondent*)

—*respondent. See* RIVINUS, A. Q., *praeses.* Disputatio inauguralis de situ aegrorum commodo. 1700.

—*See* BOHN, J. Facultatis Medicae in Academia Lipsiensi p. t. procancellarius D. Johannes Bohn . . . L. S. D. 1700.

ERNESTI, JOHANN. *See* BURGGRAV, Johann Ernst [*fl. 1600-1629*]

ERNI, ANDREAS [*fl. 1675*] *respondent.* Disputatio medica de phthisi, Schwind- oder Lungensucht. 1675.

ERNON, LAURENTIUS [*fl. 1615*] *respondent. See* PAUW, P., *praeses.* Propositiones medicae-chirurgicae de capitis vulneribus. 1615.

ERNST, JOHANN PETER [*fl. 1679*] *respondent. See* VIRDUNG VON HARTUNG, H. K., *praeses.* Congressus inauguralis Herculeus quem cum Herculeo morbo id est epilepsia. 1679.

EROTIANUS. Vocum Hippocraticarum collectio. *In* Hippocrates. [Collected works. Greek and Latin] Τα ευρισκόμενα. 1657, 1662.

ERRARD, CHARLES [*d. 1689*] *illus. See* GENGA, B. Anatomia per uso et intelligenza del disegno. 1691.

ERRESALDE, PIERRE [*fl. 1652*] Nouveaux secrets rares et curieux. Donnés . . . par une personne de condition. Contenant divers remedes eprouvez . . . pour toutes sortes de maladies. Et divers secrets pour la conservation de la beauté des dames . . . Paris, Jean Baptiste Loyson, 1660.

[20], 280 p. 17 cm. **[3676]**

ERSFELD, NIKOLAUS WILHELM [*fl. 1682*] *respondent.* See FASCH, A. H., *praeses.* Dissertatio inauguralis medica de rhachitide. 1682.

ERYTHRAEUS, JANUS NICIUS, *pseud. See* ROSSI, Gian Vittorio [1577-1647]

ERYTHROPILUS, HEINRICH CHRISTOPH [*fl. 1675*] *respondent.* SEE MEIBOM, H., *praeses.* Exercitatio medica de phthisi. 1675.

ESAMINA da farsi da leprosi. *In* CROCE, G. A. della. Cirugia universale e perfetta. 1605, 1661.

ESBERG, JOHANN [1665-1735] *praeses.* Exercitium academicum mulieris philosophantes leviter adumbrans . . . Upsaliae, Recusum anno, 1700.

[26 +] p. 19 cm. **[3677]**
Imperfect: all after p. 26 wanting.
Diss. — Uppsala, 1699 (P. Hedengrahn, *respondent*)

ESCHENBACH, ANDREAS CHRISTIAN [1663–1722] *praeses.* De unctionibus gentilium ... Jenae, Literis Nisianis [1687]

112 p.   20 cm.   [3678]

Diss. – Jena (R. Verwey, *respondent*)

ESCHENBACH, JOHANN [*fl.* 1670–1672] *respondent. See* RIKEMANN, J., *praeses.* Satyriasin et priapismum publicae philiatrorum disquisitioni. 1670; ROLFINCK, W., *praeses.* Disputatio inauguralis medica de podagra. 1672.

ESCHENREUTTER, GALLUS. *See* ETSCHENREUT-TER, Gallus [*fl.* 1561–1571]

L'ESCHOLE DE SALERNE. 1650, 166–?, 1664. *See* MARTIN, L.

ESCRIVANO, JUAN, *tr. See* PORTA, G. B. della. I tre libri de' spiritali. 1606.

ESMARCH, HEINRICH CHRISTIAN [*fl.* 1681] *respondent. See* PECHLIN, J. N., *praeses.* Disputatio medica inauguralis de phrenitide. 1681.

[**ESPAGNET,** JEAN D', 17th cent.] Arcanum; or, The grand secret of Hermetick philosophy. *In* Dee, A. Fasciculus chemicus. 1650.

– Enchiridion physicae restitutae, in quo verus naturae concentus exponitur, plurimique antiquae philosophiae errores per canones & certas demonstra-tiones delucide aperiuntur. Tractatus alter inscrip-tus Arcanum Hermeticae philosophiae opus ... Utrumque opus ejusdem authoris anonymi Spes mea est in Agno [i.e. Jean d'Espagnet] Parisiis, Apud Nicolaum Buon, 1623.

[16], 196 p.; 96, [2] p.   18 cm.   [3679]

Errata: p. [1–2] at end.
Part [2] has special title page.

[–] [The same.] ... 4. ed. emend. & aucta. Rothomagi, 1647.

303 (i.e. 301) p.   illus.   12 cm.   [3680]

"Arcanum Hermeticae philosophiae opus" (p. [199]–300) has special title page.

– [The same, without part 2.] *In* Aubigné de la Fosse, N. Bibliotheca chemica. 1653.

[–] [English tr.] Enchyridion physicae restitutae; or, The summary of physicks recovered. Wherein the true harmony of nature is explained ... London, Printed by W. Bentley, and sold by W. Sheares and Robert Tutchein, 1651.

[20], 167 p.   13 cm.   [3681]

Imperfect: sig. A1 (blank except for signature) wanting.

[–] [French tr.] La philosophie naturelle restablie en sa pureté ... Avec le traicté de L'ouvrage secret de la philosophie d'Hermez, qui enseigne la matiere, & la façon de faire la pierre philosophale ... Paris, Edme Pepingué, 1651.

[32], 378, [6] p.   illus., plate.   17 cm. [3682]

Translated by Jean Bachou.

ESPICH, DANIEL [*fl.* 1647] *respondent. See* SEBISCH, M. [1578–1674?] *praeses.* Disputatio cheirurgica de ulceribus. 1647.

ESPICH, JOHANN JACOB [*fl.* 1685–1691] *respondent. See* MAPP, M., *praeses.* Quaestio medica physiologica de aquis. 1685.

ESSAIS d'anatomie. *See* BEDDEVOLE, D.

An **ESSAY** of the great effects of even languid and unheeded motion. *See* BOYLE, *Hon.* R.

An **ESSAY** touching the gravitation ... of fluid bodies. *See* [HALE, *Sir* M.]

An **ESSAY** towards a general history of whoring. From the creation of the world, to the reign of Augustulus ... and from thence down to the pres-ent year 1697 ... Vol. I. London, Richard Baldwin, 1697.

[24], 318 p.   18 cm.   [3683]

ESSAYES of anatomy. *See* BEDDEVOLE, D.

ESSEN, THEODOR VON [*fl.* 1681–1689] *respondent.* Dissertationem inauguralem theoretico-practicam de viribus et languore, quantenus se in omnes pene mor-bos diffundunt ... sistet Theodorus von Essen ... Duisburgi ad Rhenum, Apud Franconem Sas, 1681.

[1], 44 p.   20 cm.   [3684]

Diss. – Duisburg.

ESSENIUS, LEONARD [1676–1748] *respondent.* Dissertatio medica inauguralis de febre quartana ... Duisburgi ad Rhenum, Typis Johannis Sas, 1698.

32 p.   20 cm.   [3685]

Diss. – Duisburg.

ESTAT des maisons [de personnes] de la ville de Rouen. 1668–[1669] *See* ROUEN.

ESTATUTOS da veneravel Igreia, e hospital de Santo Antonio de Naçaõ Portuguesa de Roma. 1683.

See Igreja e Hospital de Santo António da Nação Portuguesa.

ESTEVAN DE VILLA, Fray. *See* Villa, Fray Esteban de [*d.* 1660]

ESTIENNE, Henri [1531-1598] Emendationes conjecturales [and] Henri Stephani nox IIII [-VII] et V [-VIII] atticis Auli Gellii vigiliis invigilatae. *In* Gellius, A. Noctes atticae. 1603.

—, *ed. See* Gellius, A. Noctes atticae. 1603.

—*See* Sextus Empiricus. Opera. 1621.

ETLICHE schöne und geistreiche Gebätte. *See* Martinus, J. Etliche Gewissens-Fragen von der Pestilentz. 1668.

ETMÜLLER, Michael. *See* Ettmüller, Michael [1644-1683]

ETNER, Johann Christoph von. *See* Ettner, Johann Christoph von [*b.* 1654]

ETSCHENREUTTER, Gallus [*fl.* 1561-1571] Von den aller heilsamsten und nutzlichsten Bädern, Saurbrunnen, und anderer Wasser, so in Teuschland bekandt und erfahren, auch ihrer Metallen un [sic] Mineralien Natur, Krafft, Tugend und Würkungen . . . Jetz wider von newem corrigiert, und mit etlichen Bädern gemehret. [n. p.] 1616.

[16], 151, [37] p. 16 cm. **[3686]**

With this is bound Ruland, M. III. Bücher, von Wasserbädern. 1613.

ETTEN, Hendrik van. *See* Leurechon, Jean [1591-1670]

ETTINGSHAUSEN, Heinrich [*fl.* 1695] *respondent.* Microcosmi lapidicinam in renibus & vesica . . . Erfordiae, Stanno Groschiano, 1695.

[24] p. 20 cm. **[3687]**

Diss.—Erfurt.

ETTMÜLLER, Ernst Michael. *See* Ettmüller, Michael Ernst [1673-1732]

ETTMÜLLER, Michael [1644-1683] Opera omnia theoretica et practica, in quibus universa praxis medica sive omnium totius humani corporis morborum dilucida descriptio . . . Secundum principia & experimenta chymica ac anatomica . . . Helmontii, Willisii, Sylvii [i.e. Frans de Le Boë] Tackenii, aliorumque neotericorum exhibetur. Accedit

chirurgia medica . . . Ut & methodus consultatoria . . . Lugduni, 1685.

[8], 427 p.; 436 p.; 112 (i.e. 212) p.; 362 p. 20 cm. **[3688]**

—Opera omnia: nempe, institutiones medicinae, cum notis; collegium practicum generale & speciale de morbis virorum, mulierum ac infantium. Collegium chirurgicum. Notae in Morelli Methodum de formulis medicamentorum praescribendis; in Ludovici dissertationes pharmaceuticas; & in Schroederi pharmacopoeam. Chymia rationalis; cum collegio casuali, et variis . . . dissertationibus aliis. Opus posthumum, post varias editiones mancas, nunc hinc inde suppletum . . . Cum praefatione D. Georgii Franci . . . Francofurti ad Moenum, Sumptibus Johannis Davidis Zunneri, Amstelodami prostat apud Henricum Wetstenium, 1688.

[12], 718, 628, 270, [52] p. 37 cm. **[3689]**

—Operum omnium medico-phisicorum ed. nov: caeteris omnibus tum correctior, tum auctior, tum vero facilior. Opera & studio Petri Chauvin . . . Tomus primus [-secundus] Lugduni, Sumptib. Thomae Amaulry, 1690.

2 v. 40 cm. **[3690]**

Partial contents of vol. 2: Schröderi dilucidati phytologia.—De compositione medicamentorum; sive, Commentarius in Schoderum & Morelli Methodum praescribendi formulas.—Danielis Ludovici . . . De pharmacia moderno seculo applicanda; dissertationes III. cum commentar Wolffgangi Wedelii, & Michaëlis Ettmulleri.

—Opera medica theoretico-practica; hoc est, Exercitationes et collegia omnia . . . in quibus universa doctrina & praxis medica, sive dilucida omnium totius humani corporis morborum descriptio . . . secundum ultimas b. autoris hypotheses harmonice connexa, ac prioribus editionibus duplo plus auctiora, correctioraque . . . Studio et cura Johannis Casp. Westphali . . . Francofurti ad Moenum, Impensis Johannis Davidis Zunneri, et Amstelodami, Apud Johannem Rips. 1696-1697.

2 v. in 3. 36 cm. **[3691]**

Partial contents of vol. 1: Collegium pharmaceuticum in Johannis Schroederi Pharmacopoeiam medico-chymicam.—Collegium pharmaceuticum, in Danielis Ludovici Pharmaciam moderno seculo applicandam.

—Opera omnia medico-physica, theoretica et practica. Editio postrema . . . ac prioribus editionibus duplo auctior . . . Tomus primus [-tertius] Venetiis, Apud Joannem Jacobum Hertz, 1700.

3 v.   37 cm.   [3692]

Imperfect: p. 1208 and p. 1033 of vol. 2 blank, lack text.

Partial contents of vol. 3: Collegium pharmaceuticum in Johannis Schroederi Pharmacopoeiam medico-chymicam. — Collegium pharmaceuticum in Danielis Ludovici Pharmaciam moderno seculo applicadam.

—[English tr.] Etmullerus abridg'd; or, A compleat system of the theory and practice of physic. Being a description of all diseases incident to men, women and children. With an account of their causes . . . and . . . methods of cure, both physical and chirurgical . . . Translated from the last ed. of the works of Michael Etmullerus . . . London, E. Harris, F. Hubbard and A. Bell, 1699.

[15], 677 (i.e. 659) p.   21 cm.   [3693]

Sig. M8 and sheet N(p. 175-192) apparently skipped in signing.

—[French tr.] Pratique generale de medicine de tout le corps humain . . . Trad. nouv. Tome premier [-second] Lyon, Thomas Amaulry, 1691.

2 v.   20 cm.   [3694]

—Opera pharmaceutico-chymica. Ejus scilicet I. Schröderus dilucidatus, seu Commentarius in Joh. Schröderi Pharmacopoeiam medico-chymicam. II. Commentarius in Danielis Ludovici dissert. De pharmacia moderno seculo applicanda. III. Pyrotechnia rationalis . . . Quibus . . . annexae sunt ejusdem Dissertationes selectae academicae . . . Lugduni, 1686.

5 parts in 1 v.   21 cm.   [3695]

Various pagings.

Parts [1], [3] & [5] have special half title pages.

—[Chirurgia medica. French.] Nouvelle chirurgie, medicale et raisonnée . . . avec une Dissertation sur l'infusion des liqueurs dans les vaisseaux . . . Nouv. trad. Lyon, Thomas Amaulry, 1690.

[24], 518, [29] p.   17 cm.   [3696]

Added engraved title page.

—[The same.] . . . Lyon, Thomas Amaulry, 1691.

[24], 518, [29] p.   16 cm.   [3697]

Added engraved title page.

Different setting of type.

—[The same.] Nouvelle pratique de chirurgie, medicale et raisonnée . . . avec divers remedes, et une Dissertation sur l'infusion des liqueurs dans les vaisseaux. Amsterdam, Jean Aubie, 1691.

[23], 464, [27] p.   15 cm.   [3698]

Added engraved title page.

—[De morbis virorum, mulierum et infantium. French.] Pratique de medecine speciale . . . sur les maladies propres des hommes, des femmes & des petits enfans, avec des Dissertations . . . sur l'epilepsie, l'yvresse, le mal hypochondriaque, la douleur hypochondriaque, la corpulence, & la morsure de la vipere. Trad. nouv. Lyon, Thomas Amaulry, 1691.

[12], 740, [15] p.   plate.   20 cm.   [3699]

—[The same.] 2. ed., . . . rev. corr. & augm. . . . Lyon, Thomas Amaulry, 1698.

[12], 740, [15] p.   20 cm.   [3700]

Imperfect: plate wanting.

—[De praescriptione formularum. French.] Methode de consulter et de prescrire les formules, de medecine . . . Oeuvre posthume. Lyon, Thomas Amaulry, 1698.

[14], 656, [68] p.   20 cm.   [3701]

—De virtute opii diaphoretica dissertatio . . . Lipsiae et Jenae, Sumptibus Joh. Bielkii, literis Krebsianis [ca. 1682]

48 p.   19 cm.   [3702]

First Jena edition published in 1682. Cf. Haller, vol. 3., p. 175.

—Medicus theoria et praxi generali instructus; hoc est, Fundamenta medicinae vera . . . Luci publicae nunc primum donata . . . Francofurti ac Lipsiae, Sumptibus Michaelis Güntheri, 1685.

[8], 168 p.; 173, [27] p.   plates.   21 cm.   [3703]

—[French tr.] Nouveaux instituts de medecine . . . Lyon, Thomas Amaulry, 1693.

[16], 620 (i.e. 624), [86] p.   19 cm.   [3704]

—Dissertationem medicam de chirurgia infusoria . . . p. p. Michael Ettmüller . . . respondente Georgio Friderico Stirio . . . Lipsiae, Apud Nicolaum Scipionem [1668]

[64] p.   21 cm.   [3705]

Diss. — pro loco—(G. F. Stirius, *respondent*)

Dissertations — Leipzig

—*praeses.* Abstrusum respirationis humanae negotium, exulante famosa vacui fuga, ex genuinis gravissimi hujus argumenti φαινομένων causis plenius erutum. Simul cum ardui istius Harveani, doctis omnibus 1. De gen. animal. exerc. de partu proposui, nec non bimembris hujus problematis solutione; cur animalia tam proper aeris inspirati cohibitique, praesentiam, quam in machina Boyliana pneumatica exhausta propter ejusdem aeris absentiam tam velociter quasi ex anima succumbant, brevique moriantur ... Lipsiae, Typis Jon. Georg, 1676.

[112] p. 21 cm.   [3706]

Z. Neukrantz, *respondent.*

—Another printing.   [3707]

—Cerebrum orcae vulgari supposititia spermatis ceti larva develatum ... Lipsiae, Apud Nicolaum Scipionem, 1678.

[24] p. 21 cm.   [3708]

Previously published in 1671. Cf. BMC.
Diss. — A. S. Scholtz, *respondent.*

—Disputatio inauguralis, de temulentia ... Lipsiae, Apud Nicolao Scipionem [1678]

[24] p. 21 cm.   [3709]

J. F. Ittig, *respondent.*

—Another printing, with imprint: Lipsiae, Stanno Coleriano [1678]   [3710]

—Disputatio medica de corpulentia nimia ... [Lipsiae] Typis Krügerianis [1681]

[52] p. 21 cm.   [3711]

G. M. Widemann, *respondent.*

—Disputatio medica de dolore hypochondriaco, vulgo sed falso putato splenetico ... Lipsiae, Apud Nicolaum Scipionem, 1683.

32 p. 21 cm.   [3712]

Diss. — 1671. E. Blum, *respondent.*

—Disputationem medicam de epilepsia ... submittit ... Godofredus Weinlig ... [Lipsiae] Typis Johannis Wilhelmi Krügeri [1676]

[24] p. 19 cm.   [3713]

G. Weinlig, *respondent.*

—[The same.] ... Lipsiae, Apud Nicolaum Scipionem, 1683.

24 p. 21 cm.   [3714]

Diss. — 1676. G. Weinlig, *respondent.*

—Dissertatio medica de malo hypochondriaco ... Proponet ... ad diem XIV. April. An. M.DC.LXXVI ... Lipsiae, Impensis Nicolai Scipionis, 1684.

15, [1] p. 20 cm.   [3715]

Diss. — 1676. J. C. Troppanniger, *respondent.*

—Dissertatio medica de medicis balneis artificialibus ... Lipsiae, Impensis Nicolai Scipionis [1672]

24 p. 21 cm.   [3716]

T. Müller, *respondent.*

—[The same.] Exercitium medicum de medicis balneis artificialibus quam ... subjiciet Theophilus Müller ... Lipsiae, Typis viduae Joh. Wittigau [1672]

[24] p. 19 cm.   [3717]

Different setting of type.
T. Müller, *respondent.*

—Dissertationes XIIX. medicae. Prodeunt adjecto indice locupletissimo. Francofurti & Lipsiae, Prostant apud Nicolaum Scipionem, 1685.

1 v. 21 cm.   [3718]

Various pagings.
Contains 18 Leipzig dissertations published or republished between 1663 and 1685; Ettmüller is either praeses or respondent.

—Exercitatio medica sistens ideam praescribendarum formularum ... Lipsiae, Typis viduae Galli Niemanni [1682]

[112] p. 21 cm.   [3719]

J. M. Merckell, *respondent.*

—Exercitationem therapeuticam de praecipitantium vero usu feroque abusu examini publico exponunt Michael Ettmüller ... et ... Jo. Wilhelmus Pauli ... Lipsiae, Literis Justini Brandii [1681]

92 p. 21 cm.   [3720]

J. W. Pauli, *respondent.*

—Exercitium medicum de dolore hypochondriaco, vulgo sed falso putato splenetico ... submittit ... Emanuel Blum ... Lipsiae, Typis Johannis Baueri [1671]

[32] p. 19 cm.   [3721]

E. Blum, *respondent.*

—Medicina Hippocratis chymica ... publico examini exponunt ... ad diem Octobr. A. 1670 ... Lipsiae, 1678.

[38] p. 20 cm.   [3722]

Diss. — 1670. H. Warnatius, *respondent.*
A reprint published in 1684 states date of examination as 1679.

—[The same.] Medicina Hippocratis chymica ... publico examine exponunt ... ad diem Octobr. Anno. 1679 ... Lipsiae, Impensis Nicolai Scipionis, 1684.

[32] p. 21 cm.   [3723]

Diss. — 1670. H. Warnatius, *respondent.*

—Parva magnorum morborum initia . . . Lipsiae, Typis Spörelianis [1676]

[35] p. 21 cm. [3724]

M. Preuss, *respondent.*

—Valetudinarum infantile . . . Lipsiae, Literis Johannis Georgi [1675]

[56] p. 21 cm. [3725]

G. Heintke, *respondent.*

—[The same.] . . . Lipsiae, Impensis Nicolai Scipionis, 1685.

[56] p. 21 cm. [3726]

Diss. — 1675. G. Heintke, *respondent.*

—Virtutem opii diaphoreticam . . . exponunt . . . Johannes Acoluth . . . Lipsiae, Stanno Brandiano [1679]

[46] p. 21 cm. [3727]

J. Acoluth, *respondent.*

—*respondent. See* FRIESS, M. F., *praes.* Examen coraliorum tincturae. 1665, 1679; SULTZBERGER, S. R., *praes.* Dissertationem inauguralem de morsu viperae . . . submittit M. M. E. 1666, 1679, 1685; WELSCH, G., *praes.* Dissertatio medica de singularibus. 1663.

—*See* PECHEY, J. A plain introduction to the art of physick. 1697; SCHRÖDER, J. La pharmacopée raisonée. 1698.

ETTMÜLLER, MICHAEL ERNST [1673-1732] Epistola anatomica, problematica, duodecima . . . ad . . . Fredericum Ruyschium . . . De cerebri corticali substantia, &c. Amstelaedami, Apud Joannem Wolters, 1699.

29, [3] p. plates. 22 cm. [3728]

"Frederici Ruyschii responsio . . .": p. [7]-29.

—*respondent. See* BOHN, J., *praes.* Dissertationem inauguralem de singultu . . . exponet. 1697.

—*See* Lectori benevolo Facultatis medicae in Academia Lipsiensi p. t. pro-cancellarius D. Johannes Bohn, P. P. salutem! 1697.

ETTNER, JOHANN CHRISTOPH VON [*b.* 1654] Manes Poteriani, i.e. Petri Poterii . . . Inventa chymica, anxie hactenus desiderata, secundum mentem autoris elaboranda ex autoris excellentissimi textu combinata, exhibente editione Francofurtensi Wilh. Richardi Stockii, anno M.DC.LXVI. adjunctis enchirisibus accuratissimis, producti a Joanne Christoph. Etner . . . Francofurti & Lipsiae, Apud haeredes Michael Rolachii [169-?]

[40] p. 20 cm. [3729]

An edition dated 1692 was published by Michael Rolach while the present edition was published by his heirs.

Based on portions of Pierre Potier's Opera omnia medica et chemica but apparently contains no exact quotations from it.

Includes (p. [36-40]) Ettner's Epistola de essentia salis armoniaci martialis (dated Nov. 12, 1689)

[—] [The same.] Arcana Petri Poterii . . . Inventa chymica anxie hactenus desiderata . . . Bononiae, Typis Julii Burzagii, 1700.

40 p. illus. 15 cm. (*In* Lémery, Nicolas. Corso di chimica. Bologna, 1700) [3730]

—Des getreuen Eckharts [pseud.] medicinischen Maul-Affens erster Theil; oder, Der entlarvte Marcktschreyer, in welchen vornehmlich der Marcktschreyer und Quacksalber Bossheit und Betrugereyen, wie dieselben zu erkennen und zu meiden; hernach bewertheste Artzney-Mittel in allerhand Kranckheiten . . . zu gebrauchen . . . vorgestellet worden. Franckfurt und Leipzig, Zu finden bey Michael Rorlachs sel. Erben. 1694.

[14], 540, [1] p. front. 17 cm. [3731]

Errata: p. [541]

—Dess getreuen Eckarths [pseud.] ungewissenhaffter Apotecker, in welchen wie ein rechtschaffener Apotecker beschaffen seyn, was er vor Tugenden an sich nehmen, und welcherley Laster er fliehen soll; hernach bewehrteste Artzeney-Mittel in allerhand Kranckheiten . . . zu gebrauchen . . . Augspurg und Leipzig, Bey Lorentz Kroniger und Gottlieb Göbels seel. Erben, 1700.

[12], 1288 p. front. 18 cm. [3732]

—Dess getreuen Eckharts [pseud.] unwürdiger Doctor, in welchem wie ein Medicus, der rechtschaffen handeln will, beschaffen seyn soll; hernach bewährteste Artzney-Mittel in allerhand Kranckheiten . . . zu gebrauchen . . . Augspurg und Leipzig, Bey Lorentz Kroniger und Gottlieb Göbels seel. Erben, 1697.

[10], 958 p.; 207 p. front., plates. 17 cm. [3733]

Part [2] has half title: Dess getreuen Eckarths Anhang, vorstellende einen rechtschaffenen und gewissenhafften Medicum.

—Dess getreuen Eckardts [pseud.] vertwegener Chirurgus, in welchem wie ein rechtschaffener

Chirurgus beschaffen seyn solle, was er für Tugenden an sich nehmen, und welcherley Laster er zu fliehen; hernach bewährteste Artzney-Mittel in allerhand Kranckheiten ... zugebrauchen ... Augspurg und Leipzig, Bey Lorentz Kroniger und Gottlieb Göbels seel. Erben, 1698.

[1], 2074 (i.e. 1074) p.   front.   17 cm.   [3734]

—*respondent. See* AMMANN, P., *praeses.* Disputatio chirurgica. 1674.

ETZLER, AUGUST [*fl.* 17th cent.] Isagoge physico-magico-medica. In qua signaturae non paucorum vegetabilium et animalium tam internae quam externae accurate depinguntur, ex quibus mundi superioris astralis, cum inferiori elementali mundo concordantia, & influentia, mirabilisque ... sympathia & antipathia rerum ... elucescunt ... Argentinae, Sumptibus Casspari Dietzelii, 1631.

[6], 176, [10] p.   18 cm.   [3735]

ETZLER, CHRISTIAN [*fl.* 1690] *respondent. See* BERGER, J. G. von, *praeses.* Exercitationem inauguralem de epilepsia ... p. p. C. E. 1690.

EUCLIDES. *See* CHALES, C. F. M. DE, *Father.* Cursus seu mundus mathematicus. 1690.

EUDOXUS PHILALETHES, *pseud. See* DONZELLINI, Girolamo [*d.* 1588]

EUFERARIUS. *See* FERRARIUS [*fl. ca.* 1200]

EUFRENIUS, ALBERTUS [1581-1626] Poëmata Alberti Eufreni Georgiadis ... poeseos et medicinae studiosi. Erotica. Basia. Coma, Sylva. Hieronimus ad Pammachium ... Lugduni Batavorum, Ex officina Christophori Guyotii, 1601.

[16], 160 p.   17 cm.   [3736]

"Alberti Eufreni ... Lima in praecendentia sua poëmata; et Appendix (p. 129-160) has special title page.

Albertus Eufrenius is sometimes considered to be a pseud. for Albert Jorisz Goedaert.

EUGALENUS, SEVERINUS [*b.* 1535] De scorbuto morbo liber ... Cui adjunctae quaedam observationes sunt, cum brevi & succincta cujusque curationis indicatione ... Nunc vero ordine meliore & triplici indice, in lucem productus a D. Josepho Stubendorfio ... Lipsiae, Michael Lantzenberger excudebat, impensis Bartholomaei Voigt, 1604.

[16], 321, [11] p.   16 cm.   [3737]

—[The same.] ... Anno 1624 ordine meliore & triplici indice in lucem productus a D. Josepho Stubendorfio ... Nunc denuo recognitus & editus. Jenae, Typis Johannis Beithmanni, Impensis Bartholomaei Voigt, 1623 [i.e. 1624?]

[16], 453, [56] p.   16 cm.   [3738]

Edited by Zacharias Brendel, *the elder.*

With this is bound Brucaeus, H. De scorbuto propositiones. 1589.

—[The same.] De morbo scorbuto liber cum observationibus quibusdam, brevique & succincta cujusque curationis indicatione ... Ed. ult. recognita & emendata. Hagae-Comitis, Typis Adriani Vlacq, 1658.

[16], 453, [51] p.   16 cm.   [3739]

Edited by Zacharias Brendel, the elder.

Different setting of type.

—Copy 2.

With this is bound (as issued?) Brunner, B. De scorbuto tractatus duo. 1658.

EUGENIUS φιλιατρός, *ed. See* WILLIS, T. The London practice of physick. 1685.

EUONYMUS PHILIATRUS, *pseud. See* GESNER, Konrad [1516-1565]

ΕΥΦΗΜΙΣΜΟΣ cardiaci contra viperinos calumniatorum morsus ... [Lugduni Batavorum? 1680?]

24 p.   13 cm.   [3740]

Contains letters concerning Drelincourt's Libitinae tropaea.

Bound with Drelincourt, C. Libitinae tropaea. 1680.

EURELIUS, ANDREAS [*fl.* 1687] *respondent. See* DAHLSTIERNA, G., *praeses.* Ηλεκτρον. 1687.

EURELIUS, GUNNO. *See* DAHLSTIERNA, Gunno [1661-1709]

EURETA MISOCOLO. *See* PONA, Francesco [1594-1652]

EUSTACHI, BARTOLOMEO [*d.* 1574] *See* GALENUS. De ossibus. 1665.

EUSTACHIO DA MATERA. *See* EUSTAZIO DA MATERA [13th cent.]

EUSTAZIO DA MATERA [13th cent.] De balneis Puteolanis. *In* Bartoli, S. Breve ragguaglio. 1667.

EUTH, JOANNES AEGIDIUS [*fl.* 1667-1700] Agonisma de hydrope curiosum. Ad recentiorum mentem delineatum. Hagae Comitis, Apud Nicolaum Wilt, 1700.

[24], 150, [2] p.   16 cm.   [3741]

—Anatome umbilici curiosa. Ad calcem Carmina in reges, principes, et alios sunt adjecta . . . Lugduni Batavorum, Apud Jord. Luchtmans, 1697.

176 p.   17 cm.   [3742]

—respondent. See ROLFINCK, W., praeses. Αγωνισμα iatrikon de hydrope. 1667.

EVAGRIUS SCHOLASTICUS [b. 536?] See MARCHINI, F. Belli divini; sive, Pestilentis temporis accurata. 1633.

EVELYN, JOHN [1620-1706] Fumifugium; or, The inconveniencie of the aer and smoak of London dissipated. Together with some remedies humbly proposed by J. E. . . . London, Printed by W. Godbid for Gabriel Bedel and Thomas Collins, 1661.

[12], 26 p.   19 cm.   [3743]

EVERAERTS, ANTHONY [d. 1679] Cosmopolitae [pseud.] Historia naturalis, comprehendens humani corporis atomiam [sic] & anatomicam delineationem, ab ipsis primis foetus rudimentis in utero, usque ad perfectum & adultum statum . . . Lugduni Batavorum, Apud Petrum van der Aa, 1686.

[6], 451, [21] p.   front.   14 cm.   [3744]

—Another issue, with imprint: Lugduni Batavorum, Typis Johannis Kellenaar, 1686.

[3745]

Imperfect: frontispiece bound after title page, and signature [*4] bound before *3.

—Novus et genuinus hominis brutique animalis exortus . . . Medioburgi, Ex officina Francisci Kroock, 1661.

[36], 288 p.   13 cm.   •   [3746]

—Verhandelinge van de pokken. In Blankaart, S. Venus belegert en ontset. 1688, 1696, [German tr.] 1689.

EVERAERTS, GILLES. See EVERARD, Giles.

EVERAERTS, MARTEN [fl. 1563-ca. 1613] tr. See PARACELSUS. De kleyne chirurgie. 1629.

—See RÜFF, J. 't Boeck vande vroet-wijfs. 1633, 1648, 1668, 1680.

EVERARD, GILES. De herba panacea, quam alii

tabacum, alii petum, aut nicotianam vocant, brevis commentariolus . . . Ultrajecti, Pro Davide ab Hoogenhuysen, 1644.

305 p.   14 cm.   [3747]

"Johannis Neandri . . . Tabacologia": p. [59]-146; "Epistolae et judicia clarissimorum aliquot medicorum de tabaco": p. [147]-197 (i.e. 195); "Misocapnus; sive, De abusu tobacci lusus regius [by James I of Great Britain]": p. [197]-223; "Hymnus tabaci, autore Raphaele Thorio": p. [225]-305. Items have special title pages.

—Panacea; or, The universal medicine, being a discovery of the wonderfull vertues of tobacco taken in a pipe, with its operation and use both in physic and chyrurgery . . . London, Simon Miller, 1659.

[16], 79, 55 p.   illus., port.   14 cm.   [3748]

Imperfect: front. (port.) wanting; title page mutilated, with loss of part of imprint.

Dedicatory letter signed: J. R.

Includes translations of Everard's De herba panacea, part of Neander's Tabacologia, and some passages from L'Écluse's edition of Monardes.

EVERARD, JOHN [1575?-1650?] tr. See HERMES TRISMEGISTUS. The divine pymander. 1650.

EVERART, MARTIN. See EVERAERTS, Marten [fl. 1563-ca. 1613]

EVERARTUS, AEGIDIUS. See EVERARD, Giles.

EVERDINGEN, JOHANNES VAN [fl. 1651] respondent. Disputatio medica inauguralis de spasmo . . . Trajecti ad Rhenum, Typis Gisberti à Zijll & Theodori ab Ackersdijk, 1651.

[12] p.   20 cm.   [3749]

Diss. —Utrecht.

EVERHARD, ANTON. See EVERAERTS, Anthony [d. 1679]

EVERHARDI, ANTHONIUS. See EVERAERTS, Anthony [d. 1679]

EVOLI, FLAMINIO. See FERRARI, G., ed. Idea theriacae. 1601.

EVONYMUS PHILIATRUS. See GESNER, Konrad [1516-1565]

EWALD, JOHANN JAKOB [fl. 1699] respondent. See STAHL, G. E., praeses. Disputatio medica inauguralis de hectica febre. 1699.

—See STAHL, G. E. Propempticon inaugurale de abstinentia et nausea carnium in morbis, praecipue acutis. 1699.

EWALDT, BENJAMIN [1674-1719] *respondent.* Dissertatio medica inauguralis de podagra ... Erfordiae, Typis Joh. Heinr. Groschii [1697]

47 p.   20 cm.   **[3750]**

Diss. — Erfurt.

Bound with Stahl, G. E., *praes.* Disputatio medica inauguralis de podagrae nova pathologia. [1698]

—*See* STAHL, G. E., *praes.* Dissertatio medica de impotentia virili. 1697.

EWALDT, JOHANN NIKOLAUS [*fl.* 1663-1665] *respondent. See* ROLFINCK, W., *praes.* Disputatio medica inauguralis, de χλωρωσευ. 1665.

EWICH, JOHANN VON [1525-1588] De officio fidelis et prudentis magistratus, tempore pestilentiae rempubl. a contagio praeservandi liberandique, libri duo ... Nunc recens iterum in lucem editi ... Bremae, Typis & impensis Arnoldi Wesseli, 1656.

[6], 152, [8] p.   17 cm.   **[3751]**

EXAMEN alchymisticum. 1676. *See* GASSMANN, F.

EXAMEN des esprits propres et naiz aux sciences. 1602, 1608, 1619. *See* HUARTE DE SAN JUAN, J.

EXAMEN leprosorum. *In* Croce, G. A. della. Cirugia universale e perfetta. 1605, 1661.

The **EXCELLENCIE** of physick and chirurgerie. 1652. *See* [HESTER, J.]

EXCELLENT directions for cookery. *See* HARTMAN, G. The true preserver and restorer of health. 1682, 1684, 1695.

EXERCITATIO medica de usu vini emetici in curatione febrium malignarum ad mentem Hippocratis. 1662. *See* RESTAURAND, R.

EXNER, KASPAR [*fl.* 1648] *respondent. See* WALTHER, J., *praes.* Disquisitio physica de pluvia. 1648.

EXNER, MELCHIOR [*fl.* 1620] *respondent. See* HARTRANFT, J., *praes.* Theoremata physica de sensibus internis. 1620.

The **EXPERIENCED** farrier; or, Farring compleated, in two books physical and chyrurgical, being pleasure to the gentlemen, and profit to the countrey-man ... By. E. R. Gent. London, Rich[ard] Northcott, 1678.

2 parts in 1 v.   front., illus.   20 cm.   **[3752]**

Part 2 has special title page.

Imperfect: last leaf (sig. 3c2) wanting; photocopy of the missing leaf, made from the original at the British Library, is bound in.

—[The same.] The experienc'd farrier; or, A compleat treatise of horsemanship, in two books physical and chyrurgical, fitted to the use, not only of gentlemen, but of all farriers, grooms, jockeys and breeders of horses ... The 2d ed. much enl. ... By E. R. Gent. London, W. Whitwood and A. Feltham, 1691/2.

[16], 418, [40] p.   front., illus.   22 cm. **[3753]**

"The second part of the Experienc'd farrier ... the 2d imp. much enl. and amended by A. O. London, Richard Northcott, 1680": p. [175]-418, [1-40].

EXPERIMENT Buch. 1623. *See* [STEPHANUS MAGNETES]

An **EXPERIMENTAL** discourse of some unheeded causes of the insalubrity and salubrity of the air. *See* BOYLE, *Hon.* R.

The **EXPERT** doctors dispensatory. 1657. *See* [MOREL, P.]

EXPLANATIONES aromatum. 1687. *See* VISCARDI, J.

EXTRACT uyt het register van de willekeuren der Stadt Amstelredam. 1655. *See* AMSTERDAM. Ordinances, local laws, etc.

EXTRAICT des registres de Parlement. 1664. *See* FRANCE. Parlement de Bretagne.

EXTRAORDINARE Amsterdamsche Maendaegsche Courant. Amsterdam, Gedrukt by Famianus de Bode, 1678.

47 p.   16 cm.   **[3754]**

Occasioned by the controversy between Andreas Boekelman and Bonaventura van Dortmont.

EYGEL, ANTONIUS [*fl.* 1672] Apologema pro urinis humanis; of, Verantwoordingh voor de menschelicke wateren. Tegen alle kleyn-achters der selver ... Ten tweeden: een beschrijvingh der selver wateren ... Ten derden: een weder-legging tegen de schriften der wateren van ... Forestus, en Stratenius ... Amsterdam, Voor den autheur, by Sierik Paulusz, 1672.

[32], 400, [5] p.   16 cm.   **[3755]**

Added engraved title page.

Errata: p. [405]

With this is bound *his* Nieuwe genees-konst. 1673.

—Nieuwe genees-konst; of, Mantissa medi-caminum, dat is, toegift van medicamenten, tegen de siecten, aengewesen zijnde door 't menschelick water in sijn drie voorgaende werken, dienende meerendeels voor menschen van 15, of 16 jaren tot 60, of 70. Amsterdam, Voor den autheur gedruckt by Sierik Paulusz, 1673.

107, [4] p. 16 cm. [3756]

Bound with *his* Apologema pro urinius humanis. 1672.

EYNATTEN, Maximilianus van [*d.* 1631] Manuale exorcismorum: continens instructiones, & exorcismos ad ejiciendos e corporibus obsessis spiritus malignos ... Antverpiae, Ex officina Platiniana apud Balthasarem Moretum, & viduam Joannis Moreti, & Jo. Meursium, 1626.

[16], 314, [2] p. 19 cm. [3757]

EYSDEN, Jan van [*fl.* 1676] *respondent. See* Craanen, T., *praeses.* Disputatio medica de hydrope. 1676.

EYSEL, Andreas. *See* Eyssel, Andreas [*fl.* 1693-1694]

EYSEL, Johann Philipp [1652-1717] Compendium physiologicum, modernorum dogmatibus accom-modatum, per quaestiones & responsiones distinc-tum, corporis humani fabricam, quoad omnes partes concinne describens ... Erfordiae, Impensis autoris, Stanno Groschiano [1698]

[12], 198, [10] p. 16 cm. [3758]

With this is bound Vesti, J. Oeconomia corporis humani [1688]

—Decanus Facultatis Medicae in Academia Er-furtensi Joannes Philippus Eyselius ... lectorem ... ad disputationem inauguralem ... invitat. Erfordiae, Charactere Kindlebiano [1696]

[8] p. 21 cm. [3759]

Program—Erfurt (with vita of G. S. Cronpusch)

Dissertations—Erfurt

—*praeses.* Disputatio inauguralis medica, de epilep-sia ... Erfordiae, Typis Groschianis [1698]

16 p. 20 cm. [3760]

D. Seyfart, *respondent.*

—Disputatio inauguralis medica, de febri petechiali ... Erfordiae, Literis Groschianis [1700]

19 p. 20 cm. [3761]

C. Hahn, *respondent.*

—Disputatio inauguralis medica, sistens aegrum haemoptyseos malignae ... Erfurti, Literis Kindle-bianis [1700]

24 p. 20 cm. [3762]

J. E. Vogler, *respondent.*

—Disputatio inauguralis medico chirurgica de her-niis ... Erfordiae, Praelo Groschiano [1697]

24 p. 20 cm. [3763]

J. G. Regemann, *respondent.*

—Disputatio medica inauguralis exhibens historiam de ruptura lienis ... Erfordiae, Prelo Mülleriano [1696]

[30] p. 20 cm. [3764]

M. Vanselow, *respondent.*

—Disputationem anatomico-medicam de glan-dularum natura et usu ... exponet Joh. Gottfried Nietner ... Erfurti, Stanno Kindlebiano [1694]

32 p. 18 cm. [3765]

J. G. Nietner, *respondent.*

—Dissertatio inauguralis medica, exhibens visionis statum naturalem at praeternaturalem ... Erfordiae, Stanno Groschiano [1696]

36 p. 18 cm. [3766]

T. Martius, *respondent.*

—Dissertationem inauguralem de chiragra, Zip-perle an Händen ... proponit Johannes Heinricus Lasius ... Erfordiae, Prelo Groschiano [1695]

24 p. 20 cm. [3767]

J. H. Lasius, *respondent.*

—Exercitatio medica de pleuritide ... Erfurti, Charactere Kindlebiano [1697]

25 (i.e. 24) p. 19 cm. [3768]

J. C. Wachtel, *respondent.*

—*respondent. See* Ruperti, C. H., *praeses.* Disser-tatio medica de syncope. 1675.

EYSENMENGER, Johann Christoph. *See* Eisenmenger, Johann Christoph [*fl.* 1613-ca. 1634]

EYSENSCHMIDIUS, Joannes Casparus. *See* Eisenschmid, Johann Caspar [1656-1712]

EYSSEL, Andreas [*fl.* 1693-1694] *praeses.* Chylum secundum & praeter naturam spectatum disputatione medica ... submittit ... Johannes Henricus Spiess ... Erfurti, Literis Kindlebii [1694]

24 p.   18 cm.   [3769]

Diss. — Erfurt (J. H. Spiess, *respondent*)

—*respondent*. Disputatio inauguralis medica, de febre infantum putrida, ex putredinali vermium seminario orta ... Erfurti, Literis Joh. Heinrici Groschii [1693]

20 p.   19 cm.   [3770]

Diss. — Erfurt.

EYSSEL, JOHANN PHILIPP. *See* EYSEL, Johann Philipp [1652–1717]

EYSSONIUS, HENRICUS [1620–1690] Dissertatio medica de foetu lapidefacto; in qua ejusdem in utero generatio, in abdomen irreptio, ultra viginti annos retentio, ac lapidescentia, aliaque huc spectantia, per circumstantias, & causas explicantur & confirmantur ... Groningae, Typis Joannis Draper, 1661.

[20], 243 p.   14 cm.   [3771]

Bound with Deusing. A. Foetus Mussipontani. 1662.

—Tractatus anatomicus & medicus, de ossibus infantis, cognoscendis, conservandis, & curandis. Accessit Volcheri Coiteri eorundem ossium historia. Groningae, Typis Johannis Cölleni, 1659.

[24], 216 p.   14 cm.   [3772]

"Volcheri Coiteri ... Tractatus anatomicus, de ossibus foetus abortivi, et infantis, dimidium annum nati: recensitus per Henricum Eyssonium ...": p. [169]–201.

—*See* HOBOKEN, N. Anatomia secundinae humanae repetita. 1675.

EYZAT, *Sir* EDWARD. *See* EIZAT, *Sir* Edward.

EZLER, AUGUSTUS. *See* ETZLER, August [*fl.* 17th cent.]

F

F. *See* LIAGNO, Teodoro Filippo di [*fl.* 17th cent.]

F., G., [*fl.* 1678] *ed. See* BURGGRAV, J. E. Lapadem vitae & mortis. 1678.

F., G. O. *See* APPROBIRTE LAND-UND FELD-APOTHECKEN. 1690.

F,. I. *See* FLETCHER, John [1556?–1613]

F., J. *See* FLENDER, Johann [*fl.* 17th cent.]; FRENCH, John [1616?–1657]; FRYER, John [*d.* 1733]

F., J., *tr. See* GLAUBER, J. R. A description of new philosophical furnaces. 1651.

F., L. de. *See* FONTENETTES, Louis de [1612–1661]

F., M. L. de. *See* FONTENETTES, Louis de [1612–1661]

F., P. *See* FELGENHAUER, Paul [*fl.* 1619–1659]; FLETCHER, Phineas [1582–1650]

F., R. *See* FITZGERALD, Robert [1638?–1698]

F., T., *tr. See* WILLIS, T. A plain and easie method. 1691.

F. A. M. D. *See* A., F., M. D.

F.P.P.R. *See* R., F. P. P. [*fl.* 1607]

FABER, ALBERT OTTO [*d.* 1686] De auro potabili medicinali ... Ex Anglico idiomate in Latinum translata ... Francofurti ad Moenum, Sumptibus Alberti Othonis Fabri, typis Joh. Theodorici Fridgenii, 1678.

32 p.   20 cm.   [3773]

—[German tr.] Von dem medicinalischen auro potabili ... Aus dem Englischen ins Hochteutsche übergesetzt ... Franckfurt, Amsterdam, und Dantzig, Bey Henrico Wilmsonio, & Bartelsonio, 1677.

23 p.   21 cm.   [3774]

FABER, ANTON [*fl.* 1615] *respondent*. Positiones medicae de ... quartana ... Basileae, Typis Joh. Jacobi Genathii, 1615.

[20], p.   19 cm.   [3775]

Diss. — Basel.

FABER, DAVID [*fl.* 1605] *respondent*. De gangraena et sphacelo determinatio ... Basileae, Typis Joannis Schroeteri, 1605.

[10] p.   18 cm.   [3776]

Diss. — Basel.

FABER, DAVID [*fl.* 1638] *respondent. See* SPERLING. J., *praeses*. De vita & morte. 1638.

FABER, GEORG [*fl.* 1619–*ca.* 1625] ed. *See* HAYNE, J. Drey unterschiedliche newe Tractätlein. 1620, 1663.

—, *tr. See* CATELAN, L. Ein newer historischer und medicinischer Tractat. 1627.

FABER, JOACHIM [*fl.* 1623] Speculatio singularis, circa dissidium medicum, de venae sectione in febre (dicta) Ungarica, seu petechiali. Das ist, Sonderbar embsige Nachsinn, und Betrachtung, dess under den Medicis endtstandenen Zwitrachts, oder Controvers, wegen dess gebrauchs der Aderläss in der ungarischen also genendten Kranckheit, innhaltend insonderheit wie, was Gestalt, und warumb die Aderläss . . . zugebrauchen seye . . . Newburg an der Thonaw, Getruckt durch Lorentz Danhauser, 1623.

[17], 88 p. 16 cm. [3777]

FABER, JOANNES REINHARDUS [*fl.* 1620–1623] *respondent. See* SEBISCH, M. [1578–1674?] *praeses.* Exercitationes medicae. 1639.

FABER, JOHANN [*fl.* 1621] Kurtzer und nothwendiger Underricht, wie sich ein jeder gering verständiger bey jetzt schwebenden gifftigen pestilentzischen Fiebern oder ungerischen Kranckheit, so woln zu derer Verhütung, als bedürfftiger Curation erzeigen und verhalten solle . . . Ingolstatt, Gedruckt bey Gregoris Hänlin, 1621.

[10], 75, [3] p. 14 cm. [3778]

—[The same.] *In* Kurtzer Underricht in Sterbensläuffen. 1662.

FABER, JOHANN JAKOB [*fl.* 1621–1623] *respondent. See* SEBISCH, M. 1578–1674?] *praeses.* Disputatio de purgatione septima. 1621 [and] Disputationes de recta ratione purgandi. 1621 [and] Exercitationes medicae. 1639.

FABER, JOHANN MATTHIAS [*d.* 1702] Strychnomania explicans strychni manici antiquorum, vel solani furiosi recentiorum, historiae monumentum, indolis nocumentum, antidoti documentum . . . Augustae, Vindelicorum, Sumptibus Theophili Goebelii, typis Joannis Schönigkii, 1677.

[10], 107, [21] p. front., plates. 20 cm. [3779]

—*respondent.* Nakir Arabum; seu, Flatus ambulativus . . . Argentorati, Typis Eberhardi Welperi, 1653.

[24] p. 19 cm. [3780]

—*respondent. See* SEBISCH, M. [1578–1674?] *praeses.* Galeni quinque priores libri. 1651.

FABER, JOHANN REINHARD [*fl.* 1620–1624] *respondent. See* SEBISCH, M. [1578–1674?] *praeses.* Disputationes de recta ratione purgandi. 1621.

FABER, JOHANNES [*ca.* 1570–*ca.* 1640] Aliorum Novae Hispaniae animalium Nardi Antonii Recchi imagines et nomina. *In* Hernández, F. Rerum medicarum Novae Hispaniae thesaurus. 1628, 1651.

—De nardo et epithymo adversus Josephum Scaligerum. Disputatio. Qua plantarum istarum vera descriptio continetur; Dioscoridis, Propertii & Ovidii loca declarantur, & a corruptela defenduntur: medicorum denique & pharmacopoeorum honos a Scaligeri calumniis vindicatur . . . Romae, Gullielmi Facciotti, 1607.

54, [1] p. 20 cm. [3781]

—In imagines illustrium ex Fulvii Ursini bibliotheca, Antverpiae a Theodoro Gallaeo expressas, commentarius . . . Antverpiae, Ex Officina Plantiniana, apud Joannem Moretum, 1606.

[8], 88, [11] p.; 151 (i.e. 168) p. plates. 22 cm. [3782]

Added engraved title page, inserted before plates, reads: Illustrium imagines, ex antiquis marmoribus, nomismatibus, et gemmis expressae: quae extant Romae, major pars apud Fulvium Ursinum. Ed. alt., aliquot imaginibus, et J. Fabri ad singulas commentario, auctior atque illustrior. Theodorus Gallaeus delineabat.

FABER, LUDWIG JOHANN [*fl.* 1696–1697] *respondent.* Dissertatio inauguralis medica de epilepsia . . . Marburgi Cattorum, Typis haered, Joh. Jodoci Kürsneri [1696]

20 p. 20 cm. [3783]

Date of presentation changed by hand from Die M DC XCVI to Die 7. Januarii M DC XCVII.
Diss. — Marburg.

FABER, MARTIN [*fl.* 1666] Dissertatio medica de asthmate . . . Giessae Hassorum, Typis Josephi Dieterici Hampelii [1666?]

40 p. 20 cm. [3784]

FABER, PETRUS JOANNES. *See* FABRE, Pierre Jean [*d. ca.* 1650]

FABER, TANAQUIL. *See* LE FÈVRE, Tanneguy [1615–1672]

FABIGER, JOHANN [*fl.* 1649] *respondent. See*

POMARIUS, S., *praeses*. De noctambulis disputatio prior. 1649, 1686.

FABRA, ALOYSIUS A. *See* FABRA, Luigi dalla [1655-1723]

FABRA, LUIGI DALLA [1655-1723] De Noceriana terra inter simplicia medicamenta absorbentia, ac dulcificantia pro medicinae usu. Ferrariae, Typis Antonii Carrarę, 1700.

    63, [1] p.   17 cm.   **[3785]**

FABRE, ANTOINE [*fl.* 1657?] Traitté des eaux minerales du Vivarez ... Avignon, I. Piot, 1657.

    [18], 124, [4] p.   21 cm.   **[3786]**

FABRE, JEAN [*fl.* 1697] Quaestiones medico-chymico-practicae duodecim ab ... Michaele Chicoyneau ... propositae ... pro regia chymiae professione vacante per obitum ... Arnaldi Fonsorbe ... Monspelii, Apud Honoratum Pech, 1697.

    [6], 22 p.   22 cm.   **[3787]**

    Thèse de concours—Montpellier.

FABRE, PIERRE JEAN [*d. ca.* 1650] Operum voluminibus duobus exhibitorum volumen prius. In quo I. Panchymicum; seu, Anatomia totius universi. II. Sapientia universalis; seu, Anatomia hominis & metallorum ... Francofurti, Sumptibus Joannis Beyeri, 1656.

    3 parts in 3 v. illus. 22 cm.   **[3788]**

    Part [2] has title: Sapientia universalis quatuor libris comprehensa. Videlicet 1. Quid sit sapientia, & de mediis ad eam perveniendi. 2. De cognitione hominis. 3. De medendis morbis hominum. 4. De meliorandis metallis.

    Part 3 (Opera reliqua) wanting.

—L'abregé des secrets chymiques. Ou l'on void la nature des animaux vegetaux & minereaux entierement découverte: avec ... un traitté de la medecine generale ... Paris, Pierre Billaine, 1636.

    [15], 392 p. 18 cm.   **[3789]**

—Another issue, with imprint: Paris, Anthoine de Sommaville, 1636.   **[3790]**

—Alchymista Christianus. In quo Deus rerum author omnium, & quamplurima fidei Christianae mysteria, per analogias chymicas & figuras explicantur ... Tolosae Tectosagum, Apud Petrum Bosc, 1632.

    [31], 236, [4] p. illus. 18 cm.   **[3791]**

—Chirurgia spagyrica ... In qua de morbis cutaneis omnibus spagyrice & methodice agitur ... Tolosae, Apud Petrum Bosc [En l'imprimerie de Jean Boude, par Nicolas d'Estey] 1626.

    176, [8] p. 17 cm.   **[3792]**

—Myrothecium spagyricum; sive, Pharmacopoea chymica, occultis naturae arcanis, ex Hermeticorum medicorum scriniis depromptis abunde illustrata ... Tolosae Tectosagum, Apud Petrum Bosc, 1628.

    448, [22] p. 18 cm.   **[3793]**

    "Insignes curationes variorum morborum, quos medicamentis chymicis jucundissima methodo curavit, Petrus Joannis Fabri ..." (p. [353]-448) has special title page.

—[The same.] ... Item: Insignes curationes variorum morborum, qui medicamentis chymicis ... curati fuere. Cum Chirurgia spagyrica, in qua de morbis cutaneis omnibus, spagyrice & methodice agitur ... Argentorati, Sumptibus heredum Lazari Zetzneri, 1632.

    [4], 380, [17] p.; 157 (i.e. 147), [4] p. 18 cm.   **[3794]**

    Imperfect: sig. 2B3-4 misbound after title page.

    "Insignes curationes variorum morborum ..." (p. [297]-380) and part [2] (Chirurgia spagyrica) have special title pages.

    With this is bound (as issued?) *his* Palladium spagyricum. 1632.

—[The same.] ... Tolosae Tectosagum, Apud Petrum Bosc, 1646.

    448, [22] p. 18 cm.   **[3795]**

    A reprint of the 1628 edition.

—Palladium spagyricum ... Tolosae, Apud Petrum Bosc, 1624.

    [14], 394, [17] p. 18 cm.   **[3796]**

    Engraved title page.

    Imperfect: engraved title page wanting; supplied in photocopy from British Museum.

—[The same.] ... Ed. 2. Argentorati, Sumptibus heredum Lazari Zetzneri, 1632.

    [10], 326, [14] p. 18 cm.   **[3797]**

    Bound with (as issued?) *his* Myrothecium spagyricum. 1632.

—Propugnaculum alchymiae. Adversus quosdam misochymicos ... qui ... dum chymiam stulte rident, nec tamen brutorum genia tenent. Ubi an sit lapis philosophorum, qui sit, & qua methodo, & via ipsum lapidem habuerunt antiqui, clarissime tractatur ... Tolosae, Apud Petrum Bosc, 1645.

    [4], 128, [4] p. 17 cm.   **[3798]**

—[Excerpts] *In* Dolhopff, G. A., *comp.* Lapis animalis microcosmicus. 1681.

—*See* HAUPTMANN, A. Epistola praeliminaris. 1650; LANGE, C. Opera omnia. 1688.

FABRI, HONORÉ [1606–1688] Pulvis Peruvianus vindicatus de ventilatore ejusdemque suscepta defensio ab Antimo Conygio [pseud.] hortatu Germani Poleconii. Romae, Typis heredum Corbelletti, 1655. 88 p. 16 cm.   [**3799**]

   "Pulvis febrifugus orbis Americani . . . ventilatus ratione, experientia, auctoritate a Joanne Jacobo Chifletio . . . 1653" (p. [45]-88) has special title page.

   "Antimus Conygius [pseud.] Peruviani pulveris febrifugi defensor repulsus a Melippo Protimo [pseud. i. e. Vopiscus Fortunatus Plemp] . . .": at end in manuscript.

—Tractatus duo: quorum prior est de plantis, et de generatione animalium: posterior de homine. Parisiis, Apud Franciscum Muguet, 1666.
   [12], 440, 142, [15] p.   25 cm.   [**3800**]
   Imperfect: plate wanting.

—[The same.] . . . Norimbergae, Sumtibus Wolfgangi Mauritii Endteri, & Johannis Endteri haeredum, 1677.
   [10], 582, [14] p.   plate.   24 cm.   [**3801**]

—Tractatus physicus de motu locali, in quo effectus omnes, qui ad impetum, motum naturalem, violentum, & mixtum pertinent, explicantur . . . Lugduni, Apud Joannem Champion, 1646.
   [32], 446, [3] p.   24 cm.   [**3802**]

—*See* BORELLI, G. A. Historia, et meteorologia incendii Aetnaei. 1670.

FABRI, JOHANN LORENZ [*fl.* 1666] *respondent. See* ROLFINCK, W., *praeses.* Ἰχνογράφημα theoreticopracticum de pyretologia. 1666.

FABRI DE HILDEN, GUILLAUME. *See* FABRICIUS VON HILDEN, Wilhelm [1560–1634]

FABRICE, GUILLAUME. *See* FABRICIUS VON HILDEN, Wilhelm [1560–1634]

FABRICIUS, GEORG [1516–1571] Methodus dignoscendarum syllabarum. *In* Smet, H. Prosodia. 1660.

FABRICIUS, HIERONYMUS, *ab Aquabendente* [*ca.* 1533–1619] Opera omnia anatomica & physiologica, hactenus variis locis ac formis edita; nunc vero certo ordine digesta, & in unum volumen redacta . . . Cum praefatione . . . Johannis Bohnii . . . Lipsiae, Sumptibus Johannis Friderici Gleditschii, excudebat Christianus Goezius, 1687.
   [12], 452, [24] p.   illus., plates.   36 cm.
                                 [**3803**]

—Opera anatomica. De formatu foetu. De formatione ovi, & pulli. De locutione, & ejus instrumentis. De brutorum loquela . . . Patavii, Sumptibus Antonii Meglietti, 1625.
   4 parts in 1 v.   illus., plates.   40 cm.   [**3804**]
   Parts [2-4] have special title pages dated 1621, 1603 and 1603 respectively.
   Imperfect: Title page, dedicatory epistle, and p. 151 of part [1] wanting.

—Operationes chirurgicae. In duas partes divisae. Quibus adjectum est pentateuchon antea editum, & alia quae in eo desiderari videbantur . . . Venetiis, Apud Paulum Meglietium, 1619.
   [20], 187 p.; [20], 178, [26] p.   33 cm. [**3805**]
   Imperfect: p. [25-26] mutilated affecting page.
   Part [2] has special title page.

—[The same.] Opera chirurgica . . . in duas partes divisa; quarum prior operationes chirurgicas per totum corpus humanum . . . comprehendit . . . Altera libros quinque chirurgiae jam ante in Germania impressos & sub nomine Pentateuchi chirurgici divulgatos complectitur. Francofurti, Excudebat Nicolaus Hoffmannus, impensis viduae & heredum Jonae Rosae, 1620.
   [16], 1096, [29] p.   19 cm.   [**3806**]
   ". . . Operum chirurgicorum pars posterior. Continens libros quinque chirurgiae, et jam ante haec per D. Joannem Hartmannum . . . sub nomine Pentateuchi divulgatos; nunc vero ab ipsomet authore denuo in lucem emissos . . . Francofurti, Typis Nicolai Hoffmanni, 1619" (p. [553]-1096) has special title page.

—[The same.] . . . Lugduni, Ex officina Joannis Pillehotte, sumpt. Joannis Caffin, & Francisci Plaignard, 1628.
   [24], 984 p.   17 cm.   [**3807**]
   ". . . Operum chirurgicorum pars posterior . . ." (p. [489]-984) has half title.

—[The same.] . . . Accesserunt huic postremae editioni icones instrumentorum, quae autor invenit. Patavii, Apud Franciscum Bolzettam, ex typographia Sebastiani Sardi, 1641.
   [26], 204 p.; [15], 187 p.   2 plates.   33 cm.
                                   [**3808**]

—[The same.] . . . Item, De abusu cucurbitularum in febribus putridis dissertatio: e museo
ejusdem. Patavii, Impensis Francisci Bolzettae, 1647.

[31], 204 p.; [4] p.; 187 p. 9 plates, ports.
32 cm.   [3809]

Imperfect: "Index operationum chirurgicarum" and "Index rerum
notabilium in operationibus chirurgicis" wanting.

"Hieronymi Fabricii ab Aquapendente vita. Ex elogiis . . . Jacobi
Philippi Tomasini . . .": p. [7-8]

—[The same.] . . . Ed. 25. . . . Patavii, Typis
Matthaei de Cadorinis, 1666.

[8], 364, 31 p. plates. 32 cm.   [3810]

—[Dutch tr.] De chirurgicale operatien . . . Inde
Nederduytsche tale over gheset door . . . Casparum
Nollens . . . s' Graven Haghe, Byde weduwe en
erfgenamen van wylen Hillebrant Jacobssz van
Wouw, 1630.

2 v. in 1. 21 cm.   [3811]

Engraved title page.

Vol. 2 has title: Het tweede deel vande chirurgicale werckinghen
. . . Vervattende vijf boecken, die wel eer door D. Joannem Har-
mannum . . . onder den naem van Pentateuche uyt-gegeven: doch
nu vanden autheur selfs verbetert zijn . . .

With this is bound (as issued?) Cabrol, B. Het anatomiicke A.
B. C. 1630.

—[French tr.] Oeuvres chirurgicales . . . Divisées
en deux parties. Dont l'une contient le pentateuque
chirurgical; l'autre, toutes les operations manuelles,
qui se practiquent sur le corps humain . . . Traduict
de latin en françois . . . Lyon, Pierre Ravaud, 1643.

[16], 584, [76] p.; [8], 470, [25] p. 19 cm.
                                                [3812]

Title page of part 1 is a cancel, and is mounted on cancelland
title page which differs only in reading "tient" for "contient" (line 9).

Part 2 has special title page.

—Another issue. Oeuvres chirurgicales . . .
Divisées en deux parties. Dont l'une tient le Pentateuque chirurgical . . . Lyon, Pierre Ravaud, 1643.

2 v. 17 cm.   [3813]

Imperfect: title page of vol. 1 mutilated with loss of date; vol.
1, p. 193-208, 225-226, 257-258, 271-272, last 2 leaves (blank) wanting; vol. 2, p. 143-144, 337-352, [493-495] wanting.

—[The same.] . . . Derniere ed., soigneusement
rev., & enrichie de diverses figures inventées par
l'autheur. Lyon, Pierre Ravaud, 1649.

[16], 936 (i.e. 930), [22] p. illus. 18 cm.
                                                [3814]

—[The same.] . . . Lyon, Jean Antoine Huguetan
& Marc Antoine Ravaud, 1658.

[16], 936 (i.e. 930), [22] p. illus. 17 cm.
                                                [3815]

Different setting of type.

—Another issue, with imprint: Lyon, Jean Antoine Hugueten.   [3816]

—[The same.] . . . Derniere ed., enrichie de
diverses figures. Lyon, Jean-Antoine Huguetan,
1666.

[16], 936 (i.e. 930), [22] p. illus. 18 cm.
                                                [3817]

—[The same.] . . . Dernire [sic] ed. Soigneusement rev., & enrichie de plusieurs figures inventées
par l'autheur. Lyon, Jean Antoine Huguetan &
Guillaume Barbier, 1670.

[16], 936 (i.e. 930), [22] p. illus. 19 cm.
                                                [3818]

Different setting of type.

—[The same.] . . . Lyon, Jean-Antoine Huguetan,
1674.

[16], 936 (i.e. 930), [22] p. illus. 18 cm.
                                                [3819]

Different setting of type.

—[German tr.] Wund-Artznei in II. Theile
abgetheilet. Der I. Theil erkläret in fünff
unterschiedlichen Büchern alle . . . Wunden . . . und
Verrenckungen. Der II. Theil eröffnet alle . . .
Handgriffe, der gantzen Wund-Artznei . . . Sambt
einen Anhang, vom Missbrauch des Schrepffens . . .
in die teutsche Sprach übersetzt, durch Johannem
Scultetum . . . Nürnberg, In Verlegung Johann
Daniel Taubers, Druckts Johann-Philipp Miltenberger, 1672.

2 v. in 1. front. (port.), plates. 22 cm.
                                                [3820]

Added engraved title page.

"Johannis Sculteti Noribergensis . . . Anhang. vom chirurgischen
Kurass . . .": 17 p. at end of vol. 2.

—Another issue, with date 1673.   [3821]

Imperfect: portrait, added engraved title page and signature a4
wanting.

—[The same.] . . . Zum andern Mal gedruckt,
und . . . verbässert. Nürnberg und Franckfurt,
Verlegts Johann Daniel Tauber, 1684.

2 v. in 1. front. (port.), plates. 21 cm.

[3822]

Added engraved title page.

"Hieronymi Fabricii ab Aquapendente, Rede von dem Missbrauch des Schrepffens . . .": p. 1–8; "Johannis Sculteti . . . Beschreibung . . . dess chirurgischen Kürasses . . .": p. 9–21 at end of vol. 2.

—[Italian tr.] L'opere chirugiche . . . divise in due parti. Nella prima si tratta de'tumori, delle ferite, ulcere, rotture, e slogature. Nella seconda dell'operationi principali di chirurgia; tradotte in lingua italiana . . . Bologna, Gioseffo Longhi, 1678.

[12], 359 p. plates. 34 cm. [3823]

—[The same.] . . . Et in questa seconda impressione aggiuntovi un Compendio della chirurgia di Marco Aurelio Severino . . . tradotto nell'italiano utilissimo a i professori di chirurgia . . . Padova, Giacomo Cadorino, 1684.

[8], 268, 265–288 p. plates. 35 cm. [3824]

—De brutorum loquela. Patavii, Ex typographia Laurentii Pasquati, 1603.

[6], 27 p. 42 cm. [3825]

Bound with Spiegel, A. van de. De humani corporis fabrica libri decem. 1627.

Published also as part [4] of *his* Opera anatomica. Patavii, 1625.

—De formatione ovi, et pulli tractatus accuratissimus . . . Patavii, Ex officina Aloysii Bencii, 1621.

[4], 68, [2] p. illus., plates. 42 cm. [3826]

Errata: [2] p. at end.

With this are bound: another issue of *his* De formatu foetu. 1600 [i.e. 1606?]; *his* De venarum ostiolis. 1603.

Published also as part [2] of *his* Opera anatomica. Patavii, 1625.

—De formatu foetu. Venetiis, Per Franciscum Bolzettam 1600 [i.e. 1606?]

[10], 151, [2] p. illus. 42 cm. [3827]

Engraved title page.

Colophon: Patavii, Ex typographia Laurentii Pasquati, 1604.

Dedicatory epistle dated 1606.

Imperfect: sig. a², b² wanting; Errata bound between p. 150–151.

Bound with Spiegel, A. van de. De humani corporis fabrica libri decem. 1627.

Published also as part [1] of *his* Opera anatomica. Patavii, 1625.

—Another issue. Bound with *his* De formatione ovi. 1621. [3828]

Imperfect: title page, p. 19–22, 63, 82 and 88 wanting, supplied in photocopy from copy 1 in National Library of Medicine: p. 94 and 100 printed in duplicate on p. 82 and 88 respectively; errata bound between p. 150–151.

—De gula, ventriculo, intestinis tractatus. Patavii, Typis Laurentii Pasquati, 1618.

[4], 184 (i.e. 174), [7] p. 20 cm. [3829]

Published also as part [2] of *his* Tractatus De respiratione & ejus instrumentis. 1625.

—De locutione et ejus instrumentis liber a Joanne Ursino editus M.DC.I. Patavii, Ex typographia Laurentii Pasquati, 1603.

[8], 27 p. illus. 42 cm. [3830]

Bound with Spiegel, A. van de. De humani corporis fabrica libri decem, 1627.

Published also as part [3] of *his* Opera anatomica. Patavii, 1625.

—De venarum ostiolis. Patavii, Ex typographia Laurentii Pasquati, 1603.

[2], 23 p. illus. 42 cm. [3831]

Bound with *his* De formatione ovi. 1621.

—Medicina practica. Necnon Aemilii Campilongi . . . tractatus De vermibus; De uteri affectibus; deque morbis cutaneis . . . Utrumque opus nunc primum prodit in lucem singulari studio atque opera Petri Bourdelotii . . . Parisiis, Apud Clodoueum Cottard, 1634.

[12], 799, [80] p. 24 cm. [3832]

Colophon: Parisiis, Ex officina typographia Natalis Charles, 1633.

—Pentateuchos cheirurgicum . . . publicis in Academia Patavina lectionibus ab auctore propositum: jam vero, contractiore paulo forma, capitibus distinctum, lucique datum, opera Johannis Hartmanni Beyeri . . . Francofurti, Typis Nicolai Hoffmanni, 1604.

[16], 586, [6] p. 18 cm. [3833]

—[German tr.] *In* Uffenbach, P. Ein newes Artzney Buch. 1605.

—[Spanish tr.] Crisol de la cirugia . . . Traducido en Castellano por don Pedro Gonzalez de Godoy . . . Madrid, Por Juan Garcia Infanzon, a costa de Gabriel de Leon [1676]

[8], 435 p. 30 cm. [3834]

Palau y Dulcet 14255.

—Tractatus anatomicus triplex quorum primus De oculo, visus; secundus De aure, auditus; tertius De laringe, vocis admirandam tradit historiam, actiones, utilitates . . . [Oppenheym?] Per Johann Theodorum de Bry, 1613.

[7], 163, [11] p. illus. 30 cm. [3835]

Engraved title page.

Imprint date may read M.DC.XIII or M.DC.XIV.

Johann Theodor de Bry worked in Oppenheim around 1613. Cf. Wellcome, vol. 1, p. 384.

With this is bound Morgagni, G. B. Adversaria anatomica prima. 1706.

— Tractatus De respiratione & ejus instrumentis. De ventriculo intestinis, & gula. De motu locali animalium, secundum totum. De musculi artificio, & De ossium dearticulationibus ... Patavii, Sumptibus Antonii Meglietti, 1625.

    1 v. illus. 21 cm.   **[3836]**

Various pagings.

Imperfect: Addenda to item [3], and duplicate of Errata to item 4 inserted after title page.

Contents. — [1] De respiratione, & ejus instrumentis liber primus. — [2] De gula, ventriculo, intestinis tractatus. — [3] De musculi fabrica. Pars prima [-tertia] — [4] De articulorum structura pars prima [-tertia]. Item [1] has colophon: Patavii, Typis Laurentii Pasquati, 1615. Item [2] has special title page with imprint: Patavii, Typis Laurentii Pasqati, 1618.

— Tractatus quatuor. Quorum I. De formato foetu. II. De locutione & ejus instrumentis. III. De loquela brutorum. IV. De venarum ostiolis, loquitur ... Francofurti, Impensis Jacobi de Zetter, typis Hartm. Palthenii, 1624.

    [12], 158, [9] p. plates. 32 cm.   **[3837]**

Errata: p. [9] at end.

Items 2-4 have special title pages.

— *See* PIGNORIA, L. De servis, et eorum apud veteres ministeriis, commentarius. 1613; THUILLE, J. Funus ... Hieronymi Fabricii ab Aquabendente ... celebratum a Joanne Thulio. 1619.

FABRICIUS, JAKOB [1577-1652] *praeses.* Theses medicae de ephialte sive incubone ... Rostochii, Joachimus Pedanus [1627]

    [12] p. 18 cm.   **[3838]**

Diss. — Rostock (W. Schmidt, *respondent*)

— *respondent. See.* SCHRÖTER, P. J., *praeses.* De incubone disputatio medica. 1602.

FABRICIUS, JAKOB [*fl.* 1699] *respondent.* Dissertatio inaug. medica de phthisi renali calculo vesicae complicata ... Gissae Hassorum, Typ. Johan. Reinhardi Vulpii [1699]

    20 p. 20 cm.   **[3839]**

Diss. — Giessen.

FABRICIUS, JÁNOS [*fl.* 1700] *respondent. See* HEUCHER, J. H., *praeses.* Ex historia naturali de vegetabilibus magicis generatim disserent M. Jo. Henr. Heucherus. 1700.

FABRICIUS, JOHANN PHILIPP [*fl.* [1664-1668] *respondent. See* STRAUSS, L., *praeses.* Conatus anatomici specimen quartum. 1664; WALDSCHMIDT, J. J., *praeses.* Astrologus medicus. 1681.

FABRICIUS, JOHANN WOLFFGANG [*fl.* 1626] *respondent. See* CHARSTADIUS, V., *praeses.* Disputationum medicarum prima de constitutione medicinae. 1626.

FABRICIUS, JOHANNES CHRISTOPH [*fl.* 1663] *respondent.* Disputatio medica inauguralis, de epilepsia ... Ultrajecti, Typis Meinardi à Dreuenen, 1663.

    [16] p. 20 cm.   **[3840]**

Diss. — Utrecht.

FABRICIUS HILDANUS, GUILHELMUS. *See* FABRICIUS VON HILDEN, Wilhelm [1560-1634]

FABRICIUS VON HILDEN, JOHANN [*fl.* 1637] *ed.* Lacrumae aeternae a singularibus amicis ... In obitum ... Guilhelmi Fabricii Hildani ... effusae, et a Johanne Fabricio Hild. fil. collectae. Arctopoli [1637]

    [83] p. 20 cm.   **[3841]**

The author's presentation copy to his mother.

FABRICIUS VON HILDEN, WILHELM [1560-1634] Opera quae extant omnia, partim antehac excusa, partim nunc recens in lucem edita ... Francofurti ad Moenum, Sumptibus Johannis Beyeri, 1646.

    [23], 1044, [19] p.; [16], 297, [14] p. illus. 34 cm.   **[3842]**

Part [2] has special title page.

Imperfect: added engraved title page of part [1] and part [2] wanting.

Partial contents. Part [1]: — Consilium, in quo de conservanda valetudine, item de thermis Valesianis, & acidulis Griesbachcensibus, earum facultatibus & usu, succincte agitur ... Accessit epistola ad ... Paulum Croquerum ... in qua de thermis ... Piperinis, & nonnullis aliis ... agitur. — Lithotomia vesicae ... ab ... Henrico Schobingero ... in Latinum translata. — Epistola, de nova ... herniae uterinae, atque ... partus caesarei historia ... Scripta ... a Michaele Döringio. — Tractatus sclopetariae curationis ... A ... Johan-Henrico Lavatero, Latina facta. — Part [2]: Marci Aurelii Severini ... De efficaci medicina libri III.

— Another issue, with new title page: ... Adjectis ob materiae Marci Aurelii Severini ... De efficaci medicinae libris tribus.

                                 [3843]

Added engraved title page.
Imperfect: part [2] wanting.

—[The same.] . . . Francofurti ad Moenum, Typis ac sumptibus Balth. Christophori Wustii, jun., 1682.

[36], 1044, [19] p.; [16], 272, [12] p. illus. 36 cm.   [3844]

Part [2] has special title page.
Imperfect: added engraved title page wanting.
A reprint of the 1646 edition.

—Another issue, with new title pages and sig. []:(5-6) of part [1] reset.

[3845]

Each part has added half title.
Part [2] has special title page with imprint: Francofurti, Sumptibus haeredum Joannis Beyeri, 1671.

—[German tr.] Wund-Artzney, gantzes Werck, und aller Bücher, so viel deren vorhanden . . . Alle von dem Authore auffs new übersehen . . . Aus dem Lateinischen . . . übersetzt, durch Friderich Greiffen . . . Hanaw, Getruckt bey Johann Aubry, Franckfurt am Mayn, In Verlegung Johann Beyers, 1652.

[28], 1338, [28] p. illus. 34 cm.   [3846]
Imperfect: p. 645-646 wanting.

—Another issue, variant state: p. 777, 785, 819 are numbered 781, 791, 820 consecutively.

[3847]

Imperfect: wormholes throughout.

—Anatomiae praestantia et utilitas; das ist, Kurtze Beschreibung der Fürtrefflichkeit, Nutz, und Nothwendigkeit der Anatomy oder kunstreichen Zerschneitung, und Zerlegung menschliches Leibs . . . Bern, Jacob Stuber, 1624.

234, [1] p. illus. 17 cm.   [3848]
Errata: p. [235]

—Consilium, in quo de conservanda valetudine, item de thermis Vallesianis, & acidulis Griesbachcensibus, earum facultatibus & usu succincte agitur . . . Accessit epistola ad . . . Paulum Croquerum . . . in qua de thermis Piperinis, & nonnullis aliis . . . agitur . . . Francofurti, Caelo & sumptibus Matthaei Meriani, 1629.

78 p. plate. 21 cm.   [3849]

—De combustionibus, quae oleo et aqua fervida, ferro candente, pulvere tormentario, fulmine, &

quavis alia materia ignita fiunt libellus; in quo differentiae, signa . . . et curatio, tum ipsarum combustionum tum omnium fere accidentium . . . describuntur. Cui accessit bustum, in quo accensi sunt odores suavissimi memoriae . . . viri D. Caroli Utenhovii, C. F. Basileae, Sumptibus Ludovici Regis, 1607.

[16], 107, [1] p. port., illus. 17 cm.   [3850]

—[Dutch tr.] In Baten, C. Hant-boeck. 1634, 1653; Wirsung. C. Medicyn-boeck. 1627.

—[English tr.] Experiments in chyrurgerie: concerning combustions or burnings, made with gun powder, iron shot, hot-water, lightning, or any other fiery matter whatsoever. In which is excellently described the differences, signs, prognostication and cures, of all accidents and burning themselves . . . Translated out of Latine by John Steer, chyrurgeon. London. Barnard Alsop, 1643.

[4], 66 (i.e. 60) p. illus. 19 cm.   [3851]

—De dysenteria, hoc est, cruento alvi fluore, liber unus. In quo hujus morbi causae, signa . . . curatio, & preservatio contientur . . . Item, quomodo symptomata . . . sint removanda . . . Oppenheimii, Ex typographia Hieronymi Galleri, aere Johan-Theodori de Bry, 1616.

22, [2], 157, [10] p. port. 17 cm.   [3852]

—[French tr.] Traitté de la dysenterie, c'est à dire, du flux de ventre sanguinolent, contenant ses causes, signes, prognostique, curation, & preservation . . . 2. ed. augm. . . . Oppenheim, Par Hierome Galler, aux despens de Jean-Theodore de Bry, 1617.

15, 102, [2] p. illus. 17 cm.   [3853]

—De gangraena et sphacelo, tractatus methodicus . . . Ed. 10. . . . In Oppenheimio, Ex Officina chalcographica Hieronymi Galleri, sumptibus & aere Johannis-Theodori de Bry, 1617.

241, [12] p. illus., port. 20 cm.   [3854]

—[The same.] In Fontanon, D. De morborum internorum curatione. 1607.

—[Dutch tr.] Nieuwe veldt-chirurgye, tracterende van kranckheden ende gebreken die in krijgh en oorlogh . . . den chirurgijns gemeenlijck voor- vallen. Item Een chirurgische reys-kiste; dat is, Beschrijvinge der medicamenten en instrumenten, daer mede een chirurgijn in der krijgh, soo ter zee als te lande sal voorsien zijn . . . In onse Nederduytsche tale . . .

overgeset door Ysbrandum Hieronymum Franck ...
Amsterdam, Jan Hendricksz. Boom, 1664.

[12], 188, [6], 142, [4] p.   illus.   20 cm.

[3855]

—[German tr.] Von dem heissen und kalten
Brandt, welcher Gangraena et Sphacelus, oder S.
Antonii und Martielis Fewr genannt wirdt, grund-
tlicher Bericht. Von solcher Schäden, Beschreibung
... und endlichen Heilung. Item: wie die verdorbene
Gliedmassen abzuschneiden ... und wie den
Zufälln, als Ohnmacht, Feber ... fürzukommen und
zu wehren ... Durch den Authorem selbst übersehen
... gemehret, und ins Teutsch ubergesetzt. Basel,
In Verlegung Ludwig Königs, 1603.

[22], 374 p.   illus., port.   16 cm.   [3856]

—[The same.] New Feldt Artzny Buch von Kranckheiten und Schäden, so in Kriegen den Wundart-
zen gemeinlich fürfallen. Als, heisser unnd kalter
Brandt, Braüne, unmässiges Bluten auss der Nasen,
rote Ruhr, geschossen Wunden, Gliedwasser, und
wie die erharte, und krumme Glieder zu erweichen
... sein. Item ein chirurgischer Reisskasten; das ist,
Beschreibung der Artzneyen und Instrumenten,
damit ein Wundartzet im Krieg soll versehen sein
... Jetzo durch den Authorn widerumb ubersehen
... und gebessert. Basel, In Verlegung Ludwig
Königs, 1615.

[38], 674 (i.e. 676), [8] p.   illus.   17 cm.

[3857]

—De vulnere quodam gravissimo & periculoso, ic-
tu sclopeti inflicto observatio et curatio singularis ...
In Oppenhemio, Typis Hieronymi Galleri, aere
Johan-Theodor de Bry, 1614.

77 p.   illus.   17 cm.   [3858]

—[Dutch tr.] *In* Wirsung, C. Medicyn-boeck. 1627.

—Lithotomia vesicae; that is, An accurate description of the stone in the bladder ... Wherein severall
wayes of operation are described, and the chirurgicall
instruments lively delineated. Written first in High
Dutch ... Afterward augmented by the author, and
first translated into Latin by Henricus Schobingerius
Sangalthensis; and now done into English by N. C.
... London, Printed by John Norton, and sold by
William Harris, 1640.

[16], 206 p.   illus., plates.   18 cm.   [3859]
STC 10658.

—Observationum & curationum chirurgicarum
centuriae. [Centuria I] In qua inclusae sunt viginti
& quinque, antea seorsim editae: reliqae nunc cum
nonnullis instrumentorum, ab autore inventorum
delineationibus ... in lucem prodeunt. Basileae,
Sumptibus Ludovici Regis, 1606.

[29], 298, [9] p.   illus., port.   17 cm.   [3860]

Bound with Holtzemius, P. Prognosis vitae et mortis. 1605.

—Observationum & curationum cheirurgicarum
centuria secunda. Epistolis nonnullis virorum ... nec
non instrumentis cheirurgicis, ab authore inuentis illustrata. Genevae, Apud Petrum & Jacobum Chouët,
1611.

[32], 432, [10] p.   illus., port.   17 cm.   [3861]

—Observationum & curationum cheirurgicarum
centuria tertia ... Accessit Epistola, de nova ... herniae uterinae, & partus caesarei historia, ad
authorem scripta a Michaele Doringio ... Item
authoris ad hunc responsio epistolica ... In Oppenhemio, Typis Hieronymi Galleri, aere Johan-
Theod. de Bry, 1614.

577, [1] p.   illus., port.   17 cm.   [3862]

—Observationum & curationum chirurgicarum
centuria V. Epistolis virorum doctorum, nec non instrumentis ab autore inventis illustrata. Francofurti, In Bibliopoleio Bryano, apud Matthaeum
Merianum, 1627.

[28], 331, [16] p.   illus.   21 cm.   [3863]

Errata: p. [16] at end.

With this is bound Marcquis, G. Decas pestifuga. 1627.

—Observationum & curationum chirurgicarum
centuriae [I–V] nunc primum simul in unum opus
congestae, ac in duo volumina distributae. Quorum
prius continet centurias I. II. & III. Lugduni, Sumptibus Joan. Antonii Huguetan, 1641.

2 v. in 1.   illus.   25 cm.   [3864]

"Epistola de nova ... hemiae uterinae atque ... partus caesarei
historia ... a Michaele Doringio ..." [&] "Guilhelmi Fabricii
Hildani ... responsio epistolica ...": p. [521]–568 at end of Centuria III.

Imperfect: port. wanting; Centuriae IV–V bound after title page
and preliminary matter of first volume, and Centuria I–III after
title page and preliminary material of Centuriae IV–V.

—[Dutch tr.] Aanmerkingen ... rakende de
genees ende heelkonst ... Nevens een brief van een
wonderlijk lijf-moeders-scheurzel, daar de vrucht
levendig uitgesneden is: beschreven door D. Michael
Doringius, en beantwoord door Fabricius Hildanus.

Uit de Latijnsche inde Nederduitsche taal overgezet, door Nicolaes van Assendelft ... Rotterdam, Arnout Leers, 1656.

[10], 358, 542, [32] p. illus., port. 24 cm. **[3865]**

—[French tr.] Observations chirurgiques ... Tirées de ses centuries, epitres, traités de la dysenterie, gangrene, brûlures, & autres oeuvres. Traduites ... & reduites en ordre par un D. Medecin ... Geneve, Pierre Chouët, 1669.

[19], 614, [19] p. plates. 22 cm. **[3866]**

Translated by Théophile Bonet. Cf. Barbier, 1875, vol. 3, col. 597.

Imperfect: plate 17 wanting; supplied in photocopy from vol. 2 of Bonet's Corps de medecine.

—[The same.] *In* Bonet, T., ed. Corps de medecine et de chirurgie. 1679.

—[Reisskasten. English.] Cista militaris; or, A military chest, furnished either for sea, or land, with convenient medicines, and necessary instruments. Amongst which is also a description of Dr. Lower's lancet, for the more safe bleeding. Written in Latin, by Gulielmus Fabritius Hildanus. Englished for publick benefit. London, Printed by W. Godbid, and sold by Moses Pitt, 1674.

[1], 30 p. illus. 17 cm. **[3867]**

Originally published under the title: Reisskasten, with his Von geschossenen Wunden, and in his Neues Feld-Artzneibuch. The later enlarged Latin version appeared in 1633 under title: Cista militaris. "A description of a lancet, for the more secure letting of blood, by Dr. Lower" (p. 1-6) is translated from his De corde, 3d ed., Amsterdam, 1671, p. 166-169.

—Another issue. 1674 [i.e. 1676] **[3868]**

Bound with Barbette, P. Thesaurus chirurgiae. 3d ed., London, 1676, with which it was issued as vol. [2]

—[The same.] *In* Barbette, P. Thesaurus chirurgiae. 1687.

—*See* ARNOUL, F, *Father.* Traictez curieux. 1673; PETRAEUS, H. Encheiridion cheirurgicum. 1625; SALMON, W. Iatricia. 1681, 1684, 1694; UFFENBACH, P. Thesaurus chirurgicae. 1610.

—*as subject. See* DÖRING, M. Epistola de nova ... herniae uterinae. 1612; FABRICIUS VON HILDEN, J., *ed.* Lacrumae aeternae a singularibus amicis ... In obitum ... Guilhelmi Fabricii Hidani ... effusae. 1637.

FABRIUS, ALBERTUS OTHO. *See* FABER, Albert Otto [*d.* 1686]

FABRIUS, JOACHIM. *See* FABER, Joachim [*fl.* 1623]

FABRIUS, PETRUS JOANNES. *See* FABRE, Pierre Jean [*d. ca.* 1650]

FABRIZIO, GIROLAMO. *See* FABRICIUS, Hieronymus, *ab Aquapendente* [*ca.* 1533-1619]

FABRIZIO D'ACQUAPENDENTE, GIROLAMO. *See* FABRICIUS, Hieronymus, *ab Aquapendente* [*ca.* 1533-1619]

FABROT, CHARLES ANNIBAL [1580-1659] Epistola ... de mutuo. Cum responsione Cl. Salmasii ad Aegidium Menagium. Lugduni Batavorum, Ex officina Joannis Maire, 1645.

32 p. 16 cm. **[3869]**

Misbound after p. 302 of Wissenbach's Confutatio, second work in this volume.

Bound with (as issued) Saumaise, C. Disquisitio de mutuo. 1645.

—Exercitationes duae. *In* Carranza, A. Tractatus novus ... de partu naturali et legitimo. 1629, 1630.

—, *ed. See* Raguseo, G. Epistolarum mathematicarum. 1623.

FABRUS, JOHANNES MATTHAEUS. *See* FABER, Johann Matthias [*d.* 1702]

FABRY VON HILDEN, JOHANN. *See* FABRICIUS VON HILDEN, Johann [*fl.* 1637]

FABRY VON HILDEN, WILHELM. *See* FABRICIUS VON HILDEN, Wilhelm [1560-1634]

FACIO, SILVESTRO [*fl.* 1550-1596] Paradoxes de la peste, ou il est monstré clairement comme on peut vivre & demeurer dans les villes infectées, sans crainte de la contagion, Traduicts en françois de l'italien ... par B. Barralis ... Paris, Fleury Bourriquant, 1620.

[8], 252, [1] p. 18 cm. **[3870]**

A dialogue between the author, Giuseppe Ratto, and Stefano Mari. Full names of the participants appeared in the Italian original, published in Genoa in 1584. This translation was also issued in 1620 without the author's name.

Privilege and errata on leaf at end.

FACTUM, pour les sieurs conseillers de la chambre de ville de Nancy appellans de deux sentences. 1647. *See* Lambert, N., defendant.

FACULTAS MEDICA PARISIENSIS. *See* UNIVERSITÉ DE PARIS. Faculté de médecine.

FACULTÉ DE MÉDECINE DE PARIS. *See* UNIVERSITÉ DE PARIS. Faculté de médecine.

FACULTÉ DE MÉDECINE DE TOULOUSE. *See* UNIVERSITÉ DE TOULOUSE. Faculté de médecine.

FACULTÉ DE MÉDECINE, Montpellier. *See* UNIVERSITÉ DE MONTPELLIER. Faculté de médecine.

FAGE, JOHN [*fl.* 1606] Speculum aegrotorum, the sicke-mens glasse; or, A plaine introduction wherby one may give a true, and infallible judgement, of the life or death or a sicke bodie, the originall cause of the griefe, how he is tormented and afflicted . . . and the day and houre in which he shall recover, or surrender his vitall breath. Whereunto is annexed a treatise of the foure humors . . . London, William Lugger, 1606.

    [72] p.   tables.   18 cm.   **[3871]**
<small>Imperfect: sig. E³ wanting; supplied in photocopy from Library of Congress.
STC 10665.</small>

FAGON, GUY CRESCENT [1638-1718] Quaestio medica . . . An ex tabaci usu frequenti vitae summa brevior? [Parisiis, Apud Franciscum Muguet, 1699]

    [8] p.   25 cm.   **[3872]**
<small>Diss. — Paris (C. Berger, *respondent*)</small>

    —*praeses. See* ANDRY DE BOISREGARD, N. De le génération des vers dans le corps de l'homme. 1700.

    —*See* VIEUSSENS, R. Réponse . . . a trois lettres . . . du sieur Chirac. 1698.

    —*as subject. See* PANTHOT, J. B. Lettre . . . écrite a . . . Gui Crescent Fagon . . . sur la maladie extraordinaire dont feu M. Jean De-Rhodes. 1695?

FAIRFAX, NATHANIEL [1637-1690] A treatise of the bulk and selvedge of the world. Wherein the greatness, littleness and lastingness of bodies are freely handled. With an answer to Tentamine de Deo, by S[amuel] P[arker] . . . London, Robert Boulter, 1674.

    [37], 201, [4] p.   illus.   17 cm.   **[3873]**

    —*respondent.* Disputatio medica inauguralis de lumbricis . . . Lugduni Batavorum, Apud viduam & haeredes Joannis Elsevirii, 1670.

    [8] p.   23 cm.   **[3874]**
<small>Diss. — Leyden.</small>

FAJARDO DE REQUESENS Y ZUÑIGA, LUIS [*fl.* 1599-1630] *See* VALENCIA. Laws, statutes, etc. Real crida y edicte. 1630.

FAHR, CHRISTOPH JOACHIM [*fl.* 1698] *respondent. See* BERGER, J. G. von, *praeses.* Dissertatio inauguralis de morbis oculorum. 1698.

FAHRNER, CHRISTOPH. *See* FARNER, Christoph [*fl.* 1655-1659]

FAIRCLOUGH, JOHN. *See* FEATLEY, John [1605?-1666]

FALAISE, NORMANDY. Religeuses hôpitalieres. Remedes des pauvres . . . Extrait de la lettre de la superieure desdites religeeuses du 30 Octobre 1679. [n. p., 1679?]

    p. 9-10   24 cm.   **[3875]**
<small>Signature C.
Caption title.</small>

FALCINELLI, BERNARDINO [*fl.* 1646-1649] Apologia di Bernardino Falcinelli . . . nella quale si difende . . . Francesco Carocci dalle censure fattegli dal sig. G. C. C. intorno all'aderenza della membrano col craneo. Firenze, Francesco Onofri, 1649.

    [8], 101. p.   15 cm.   **[3876]**

    —Instituzione alla cirugia . . . Firenze, Francesco Onofri, 1649.

    [16], 233+ p.   illus.   16 cm.   **[3877]**
<small>Imperfect: p. 231-232, and all after p. 233 wanting.</small>

    —[The same.] . . . Firenze, Gl'eredi dell'Onofri, 1688.

    [9], 206 p.   illus.   16 cm.   **[3878]**

    —Nuova dichiarazione, e comento ne' testi d'Ipocrate sopra le ferite del capo, con le sue figure, modo diconoscerle, e curarle . . . In questa 2. ed. ricorretto da moltissimi errori. Firenze, Francesco Onofri, 1657.

    [4], 256 p.   illus. 15 cm.   **[3879]**
<small>Includes Italian text of De capitis vulneribus.</small>

    —[The same.] . . . 3. ed. Firenze, Piero Matini, 1693.

    vi, 256 p.   illus.   16 cm.   **[3880]**
<small>Different setting of type.</small>

FALCINI, DOMENICO [*b. ca.* 1570] *illus. See* ASELLIO, G. De lactibus. 1627; 1640.

FALCK, Michael [1622–1676] Wohlerbauliche Buss-Predigten. Eines Theils über die Parabel vom verlohrnen Sohn, auss Luc. XV. in XXXV. gewöhnlichen Wochen-Predigten. Andern Theils über ... Buss-Texte Altes und Neues Testament, an sonderbahren offentlich angesetzten Buss-Bet-und Dank-Tagen in ... Dantzig ... Nebenst einem Anhange zweyer Krönungs-und Leichen-Predigten zum Druck heraus gegeben durch dessen aeltisten Sohn. Frankfurt am Mayn, In Verlegung Martin Hallervorden, gedruckt by Johann Andreae, 1681.

[14], 1074, [21] p.   front. (port.)   21 cm.
[3881]

FALCK, Nathanael [*fl.* 1685–1692] De discursu brutorum ex physicis ... Wittebergae, Praelo Matthaei Henckelii [1688]

[16] p.   19 cm.   [3882]

Diss. — Wittenberg (J. Decani, *respondent*)

FALCO, Jean. *See* Falcon, Jean [*fl.* 1491–1541?]

FALCON, Jean [*fl.* 1491–1541?] Remarques sur la Chirurgie de M. Guy de Chauliac ... Diligemment conferées avec toutes les impressions precedentes, & pour la plus part mises en langage plus intelligible; outre la traduction nouvelle de tous les textes latins de l'autheur ... Lyon, Jean Radisson, 1649.

[16], 1000, [54] p.   illus.   19 cm.   [3883]

Imperfect: p. 1-2 wanting; supplied in photocopy from the New York Academy of Medicine Library.

Published in 1559, with the quotations in Latin, under title: Notabilia supra Guidonem.

FALCONIERI, Paolo [*d.* 1704] *See* Redi, F. Lettera intorno all'invenzione degli occhiali. 1690 [and] Osservazioni intorno alle vipere. 1687.

FALLOPPIO, Gabriele [1523–1562] Opera genuina omnia, tam practica, quam theorica ... Quorum pars una, tota praesertim chirurgia, & tractatus de morbo gallico, methodusque consultandi ab auctore ad editionem concinnata ... nunc primum lucem adspicit; pars vero altera e volumine incondito Francofurti nuper editio desumpta, & repurgata ... Tomus primus [-tertius] ... Venetiis, Apud Jo. Antonium, & Jacobum de Franciscis, 1606.

3 v.   illus.   33 cm.   [3884]

Includes the author's De materia medicinali in lib. 1. Dioscoridis (vol. 1, p. 211-248), Commentarius in Hippocratis Coi librum de vulneribus capitis (vol. 2, p. 411-456) and his Expositio libri Galeni De ossibus (vol. 3, ll. 121-156).

— La chirurgia ... Tradotta dalla sua Latina nella lingua volgare, & novamente posta in luce per Gio. Pietro Maffei ... Nella quale ... si tratta de tutte le specie di tumori, di ulceri, e di ferite ... Venetia, Giacomo Anton. Somascho, 1603.

[18], 560 ll.   illus.   20 cm.   [3885]

— [The same.] ... Venetia, Appresso i Bertani, 1647.

[8], 430 ll.   illus.   25 cm.   [3886]

— [The same.] ... Venetia, Abondio Menafoglio, 1675.

[16], 669 p.   illus.   23 cm.   [3887]

— Secreti diversi, e miracolosi. Raccolti dal Faloppia, & approbati da altri medici di gran fama. Nuovamente ristampati, & à commun beneficio di ciascuno, distinti in tre libri ... Venetia, Gio. Battista Usso, 1618.

[31], 366 p.   15 cm.   [3888]

Edited by Borgaruccio Borgarucci.

— [The same.] ... Venetia, Appresso li Milochi, 1650.

[32], 366 p.   15 cm.   [3889]

Different setting of type.

— [The same.] ... Venetia, Giuseppe Tramontin, 1687.

[24], 358 p.   15 cm.   [3890]

Imperfect: upper margins trimmed.

— *See* Sánchez, F. Opera medica. 1636; Zunthus, H. De balneo thermali. 1615.

FALOPIA, Gabriello. *See* Falloppio, Gabriele [1523–1562]

A FAMILY-HERBAL; or, The treasure of health. 1689. *See* [Durante, C.]

FANIANUS, Joannes Chrysippus [16th cent.] De arte metallicae metamorphoseos ... [&] De jure artis alchemiae; hoc est, Variorum authorum & praesertim jurisconsultorum judicia & responsa ad quaestionem quotidianam: an alchimia sit ars legitima ...

33-63 p., vol. 1.   20 cm.   (*In* Zetzner, Lazarus, *ed.* Theatrum chemicum. Argentorati, 1659-61)
[3891]

Caption titles.

FANOISIUS, Guido [*fl.* 1668-1669] Dissertatio medica de morbo epidemio hactenus inaudito: praeterita aestate anni 1669. Lugduni-Batavorum, Apud Lothum de Haes, 1671.

[20], 52 p. 13 cm. [3892]

—*respondent.* Disputatio medica inauguralis de febribus intermittentibus ... Lugduni Batavorum, Apud viduam & haeredes Joannis Elsevirii, 1668.

[18] p. 23 cm. [3893]
Diss.—Leyden.

—, *tr. See.* Steno, N., Bp. Dissertatio de cerebri anatome 1671.

FARBIUS, Antimus. *See* Fabri, Honoré [1606-1688]

FARCY, Dominique de [*fl.* 1666-1700] *praeses.* Quaestio medica ... An asthmati humido nicotiana? [Parisiis, 1700]

4 p. 25 cm. [3894]
Caption title.
Diss.—Paris (R. J. Finot, *respondent*)

—Quaestio medica ... An paralysi sudorifica? [Lutetiae, 1674]

4 p. 24 cm. [3895]
Caption title.
Diss.—Paris (N. Pelletier, *respondent*)

FARFÁN, Augustin [*d.* 1604] Tratado breve de medicina y de todas las enfermedades ... Agora neuvamente añadido ... Mexico, En la Emprenta de Geronymo Balli, por Cornelio Adriano Cesar, 1610.

[4], 261, [5] ll. 22 cm. [3896]

FARINA, Tiberio. Informatione della podagra, e sua cura ... Roma, Filippo M. Mancini, 1672.

63, [1] p. 15 cm. [3897]

—Ortus, et occasus cujuslibet morbi epidemici seu maligni ... Romae, Ex typographia Mancini, 1672.

[8], 128 p. 16 cm. [3898]

FARINE, Jean. *See* Alithophilus. Alithophili Observationes extemporaneae, 1681?

La **FARMACOPEA** o'antidotario dell'eccellentissimo Collegio de'signori medici di Bergomo. 1680. *See* Collegio dei medici, Bergamo.

FARNECK, Johann Philipp [*fl.* 1686-1687] *respondent. See* Altwein, J. Disputatio inauguralis. 1687.

FARNER, Christoph [*fl.* 1655-1656] *See* Glauber, J. R. Apologia. 1655; [Latin tr.] 1655 [and] Glauberus ridivivus. 1656 [and] The works. 1689; Zipffell, J. Podagrischer Triumph. 1659.

FARNESIUS, Georg Theodor [*fl.* 17th cent.] Appendix bibliothecae medicophilosophico philologicae inclytae nationis Germanicae artistarum quae Patavii degit sub ... auspiciis ... bibliothecariis Georgio Theodoro Farnesio ... Christiano Barthio ... Patavii, Typis Petri Mariae Frambotti, 1680.

[8] p. 23 cm. [3899]
Bound with Stockhamer, F. Bibliotheca medico-philosophico-philologica. 1677.

FARQUHAR, Robertus [*fl.* 1699] *respondent.* Disputatio medico-anatomica inauguralis de organo olfactus ... Trajecti ad Rhenum, Ex officina Guilielmi vande Water, 1699.

20 p. 23 cm. [3900]
Diss.—Utrecht.

FARRA, Grassino. Trattato dell'ipocondria e suoi accidenti, con sua cura, & insignamento di rimedii ... Venetia, Per il Producimo, 1686.

[12], 126, [2] p. 14 cm. [3901]

—[The same.] ... Bologna, Longhi, 1699.

120 p. 14 cm. [3902]

FASCH, Augustin Heinrich [1639-1690]

Dissertation—Pro loco—Jena

—Dissertationem medico-chirurgicam de vesicatoriis ... publico examini exponet Augustinus Henricus Faschius ... Jenae, Stanno Bauhoferiano, 1673.

[28] p. 18 cm. [3903]

Programs—Jena

—Augustini Henrici Faschii ... Collegii Medici decani invitatio publica ad disputationem inauguralem de hectica. [Jenae, 1688]

8 p. 20 cm. [3904]
With vita of C. Krause.

—Augustinus Henricus Faschius ... Collegii Medici decanus ... S. P.D. lectori benevolo. [Jenae, 1687]

[8] p. 20 cm. [3905]
With vita of J. M. Heinsius.

—Augustinus Henricus Faschius ... Collegii Medici decanus S. P. D. lecturis! [Jenae, 1684]

[8] p.   21 cm.   [3906]

With vita of G. E. Stahl.

—Augustinus Henricus Faschius ... decanus salutem ... precatur lectori benevolo! [Jenae, 1681]

[8] p.   20 cm.   [3907]

With vita of G. F. Aeplinius.

—Augustinus Henricus Faschius ... Facultatis Medicae decanus, S. D. L. [Jena, 1687]

[8] p.   19 cm.   [3908]

With vita of J. Á. Hofsteter.

—Augustinus Henricus Faschius ... Facultatis Medicae X. decanus S. P. D. benevolo lectori! [Jenae, 1689]

[8] p.   20 cm.   [3909]

With vita of J. Glosemeyer.

—Augustinus Henricus Faschius ... Facultatis Medicae X. decanus S. P. D. benevolo lectori! [Jenae, 1689]

[8] p.   19 cm.   [3910]

With vita of K. J. Leicker.

—Augustinus Henricus Faschius ... Facultatis Medicae X. decanus S. P. D. benevolo lectori! [Jenae, 1689]

[8] p.   20 cm.   [3911]

With vita of J. Müller.

—Decanus Collegii Medici, Augustinus Henricus Faschius ... S. P. D. benigno lectori. [Jenae, 1681]

[8] p.   20 cm.   [3912]

With vita of J. A. Slevogt.

—Decanus Facultatis Medicae Augustinus Henricus Faschius ... ad ... de ictero disputationis solennitam ... invitat. [Jenae, 1685]

[8] p.   20 cm.   [3913]

With vita of J. M. Hoffmann.

—Decanus Facultatis Medicae Augustinus Henricus Faschius ... L. B. S. D. eumque ad hanc de lunbricis disputationem inauguralem officiose & amice invitat. [Jenae, 1685]

[8] p.   20 cm.   [3914]

With vita of J. G. Glytz.

Dissertations—Jena

—*praeses.* Ἄνθραξ pestilens dissertatione inaugurali explicatus ... Jenae, Typis Krebsianis [1681]

[2], 48 p.   19 cm.   [3915]

J. A. Slevogt, *respondent.*

—Castoreum publico ... examini committet ... Johannes Ernestus Krausoldt ... Jenae, Typis Johannis Nisii [1677]

[48] p.   20 cm.   [3916]

J. E. Krausoldt, *respondent.*

—Consultatio medica practica proponens aegrotum arthritico-nephriticum ... Jenae, Typis Samuelis Krebsii [1675]

[20] p.   20 cm.   [3917]

J. J. Bücking, *respondent.*

—De chylificatione laesa ... Jenae, Litteris Nisianis [1689]

[24] p.   20 cm.   [3918]

J. C. Schröter, *respondent.*

—Disputatio inauguralis medica, de aegra febre hectica laborante ... [Jenae] Literis Nisianis [1678]

24 p.   20 cm.   [3919]

E. Franz, *respondent.*

—Disputatio inauguralis medica de αυτοχειρια ... Jenae, Typis viduae Samuelis Krebsii [1681]

48 p.   20 cm.   [3920]

F. Hoffmann, *respondent.*

—Disputatio inauguralis medica de diarrhoea ... Jenae, Typis Nisianis [1682]

[24] p.   19 cm.   [3921]

D. Kanitz, *respondent.*

—Disputatio inauguralis medica de doloribus post partum ... Jenae, Literis Krebsianis [1683]

24 p.   20 cm.   [3922]

C. F. Gerber, *respondent.*

—Disputatio inauguralis medica de epilepsia ... Jenae, Typis Samuelis Krebsii [1686]

28 p.   19 cm.   [3923]

D. Boess, *respondent.*

—Disputatio inauguralis medica de praedictione mortis, vulgo vom Leben Absagen ... Jenae, Literis Krebsianis [1686]

[4], 26, [2] p.   19 cm.   [3924]

J. C. Schnetter, *respondent.*

—Disputatio inauguralis medica de suffocatione hysterica ... Jenae, Literis Krebsianis [1687]

36 p.   20 cm.   [3925]

Z. Waxmann, *respondent.*

—Disputatio inauguralis medica exhibens mulierem melancholia hypochondriaca laborantem ... Jenae, Literis Bauhoferianis [1674]

[32] p. 18 cm.   [3926]

J. C. Wachtel, *respondent.*

—Disputatio medica inauguralis de dysenteria ... Jenae, Literis Krebsianis [1684]

24 p. 21 cm.   [3927]

J. J. Hoffman, *respondent.*

—Disputatio medica inauguralis de dysenteria epidemica ... Jenae, Stanno Gollneriano [1678]

[24] p. 18 cm.   [3928]

J. B. Ziegler, *respondent.*

—Disputatio medica inauguralis de epilepsia ... Jenae, Exprimebat Joh. Nisius [1679]

[44] p. 19 cm.   [3929]

J. Fuhrmann, *respondent.*

—Disputatio medica inauguralis de suffocatione uterina ... Jenae, Prelo Krebsiano [1681]

[40] p. 19 cm.   [3930]

J. A. Schmid, *respondent.*

—Dissertatio anatomica de ovario mulierum ... Jenae, Literis Krebsianis [1681]

[1], 24, [2] p. 20 cm.   [3931]

J. M. Bertuch, *respondent.*

—Dissertatio inauguralis de asthmate ... Jenae, Literis Krebsianis [1684]

31, [1] p. 20 cm.   [3932]

M. Sprögel, *respondent.*

—Dissertatio inauguralis de circulatione lymphae, et catarrhis ... Jenae, Literis Nisianis [1682]

[1], 25, [1] p. 20 cm.   [3933]

J. G. Berger, *respondent.*

—Dissertatio inauguralis medica de arthritide vaga scorbutica ... Jenae, Exscripta literis Krebsianis [1683]

27, [1] p. 19 cm.   [3934]

B. Kruger, *respondent.*

—Dissertatio inauguralis medica de rhachitide ... Jenae, Typis viduae Samuelis Krebsii [1682]

28 p. 20 cm.   [3935]

N. W. Ersfeld, *respondent.*

—Dissertatio inauguralis medica purpuram puerperarum exponens ... Jenae, Stanno Bauhoferiano [1674]

34 p. 20 cm.   [3936]

S. Zeidler, *respondent.*

—Dissertatio medica de latice ... Jenae, Typis Bauhoferianis [1677]

16 p. 19 cm.   [3937]

A. Schemberger, *respondent.*

—Dissertatio medica de morbo dominorum & domino morborum ... [Jenae] Stanno Nisiano [1670]

[2], 62 p. 20 cm.   [3938]

P. H. Juch, *respondent.*

—Dissertatio medica inauguralis de febre quartana intermittente ... [Jenae] Litteris Krebsianis [1685]

16 p. 21 cm.   [3939]

M. F. Drachstedt, *respondent.*

—Dissertatio medica inauguralis de mola ... Jenae, Literis Krebsianis [1684]

24 p. 19 cm.   [3940]

N. L. Maas, *respondent.*

—Dissertatio medica inauguralis de morbo Hungarico ... Jenae, Literis Bauhoferianis [1682]

32 p. 19 cm.   [3941]

A. Löw, *respondent.*

—Dissertatio medica inauguralis de oedemate ... Jenae, Literis Krebsianis [1683]

23, [1] p. 20 cm.   [3942]

G. Grundel, *respondent.*

—Dissertatio medica inauguralis, spicilegium pestis exhibens ... [Jenae] Literis Krebsianis [1685]

[40] p. 20 cm.   [3943]

S. Rochliz, *respondent.*

—Dissertationem de myrrha ... submittet ... Simon Andreas Beckerus ... Jenae, Typis Samuelis Krebsii [1676]

[36] p. 20 cm.   [3944]

S. A. Becker, *respondent.*

—Dissertationem inauguralem de amore insano ... exponit Augustinus Severus Backhauss ... Jenae, Literis Krebsianis [1686]

21, [3] p. 20 cm.   [3945]

A. S. Backhauss, *respondent.*

—Dissertationem inauguralem de ανορεξια, seu fame abolita ... submittit Johannes Adamus Hofsteter ... Jenae, Typis Joh. Zach. Nisi [1687]

[23] p. 20 cm.   [3946]

J. Á. Hofsteter, *respondent.*

—Dissertationem inauguralem medicam de febre hectica . . . submittit . . . Christophorus Krause . . . Jenae, Excudebat Krebsius [1688]

24 p.   20 cm.   [**3947**]

C. Krause, *respondent.*

—Dissertationem medicam inauguralem de peste . . . subjicit Johannes Block . . . [Jena] Literis Nisianis [1681]

28, [8] p.   19 cm.   [**3948**]

J. Block, *respondent.*

—Dysenteriam . . . disquisitioni proponit David Valtherus . . . Jenae, Charactere Nisiano [1678]

[24] p.   20 cm.   [**3949**]

D. Valther, *respondent.*

—Historiam et curationem calculorum humanorum . . . examini sistii Johannes Carolus Heinlein . . . Jenae, Typis Johannis Nisii, 1676.

83, [1] p.   20 cm.   [**3950**]

J. K. Heinlein, *respondent.*

—Intemperies corporis humani morborum foecunda mater . . . Jenae, Literis Joch. Zach. Nisii [1687]

[8], 120, [8] p.   20 cm.   [**3951**]

J. W. Eckhard, *respondent.*

—Παρωτίδας physiologice & pathologice consideratas . . . Jenae, Literis Johannis Jacobi Bauhoferi [1683]

24 p.   20 cm.   [**3952**]

C. F. Gerber, *respondent.*

—Respirationis laesiones hypochondriaco-scorbuticas . . . publicae censurae exponit Georgius Fridericus Cellarius . . . Jenae, Typis Johannis Nisii [1677]

[32] p.   20 cm.   [**3953**]

G. F. Cellarius, *respondent.*

—Specimen inaugurale medicum de febre amatoria . . . Jenae, Literis Krebsianis [1689]

28 p.   19 cm.   [**3954**]

J. Müller, *respondent.*

—Specimen inaugurale medicum de morbillis . . . Jenae, Literis Krebsianis [1689]

24 p.   19 cm.   [**3955**]

B. Müller, *respondent.*

—Sterilitas . . . Jenae, Literis Krebsianis [1684]

[2], 46 p.   20 cm.   [**3956**]

J. M. Bertuch, *respondent.*

—*respondent. See* ROLFINCK, W., *praeses.* Θεα μισοπτωχος vulgo medicorum opprobrium podagra. 1663.

—*See* WEDEL, G. W., *praeses.* Dissertatio inauguralis medica, de apoplexia. 1680.

FASELT, CHRISTIAN [*ca.* 1638-1694] *praeses.* Exercitatio physica . . . de stillicidio sanguinis ex interemti hominis cadavere, praesente occisore . . . Wittebergae, Typis Johannis Haken, 1665.

[24] p.   19 cm.   [**3957**]

Diss. — Wittenberg (G. Voigt, *respondent*)

FASTERLING, MARTIN LUTHER [*d.* 1717] *respondent. See* SALTZMANN, J. P. De claudendis aedibus peste infectorum. 1681.

FAUCON, JEAN. *See* FALCON, Jean [*fl.* 1491-1541?]

FAUSIUS, JOHANN KASPAR [*d.* 1671] *praeses.* Disputatio inauguralis medica, de venenis, morbisque venenosis . . . Heidelbergae, Typis Aegidii Walteri, 1656.

24 p.   18 cm.   [**3958**]

Diss. — Heidelberg (J. Friderici, *respondent*)

FAUSIUS, JOHANN WILHELM [*fl.* 1675] *respondent.* Disputatio medica inauguralis de haemorrhoidibus . . . Lugduni Batavorum, Apud viduam & heredes Johannis Elsevirii, 1675.

[12] p.   21 cm.   [**3959**]

Diss. — Leyden.

FAUST, JOHANN [1632-1695] *praeses.* Exercitatio academica, nugis nonneminis opposita, qui temere dixit, & audacter confirmavit, logicam medico inutilem esse . . . Argentorati, Literis Johannis Pastorii [1677]

32 p.   19 cm.   [**3960**]

Diss. — Strasbourg (J. P. Sebisch, *respondent*)

—Quarta figura quam Galenus medicus et logicus doctissimus invenit, qui λόγον, adeoque logicam ineffabile bonum & donum omni animae indidit . . . Argentorati, Typis Josiae Staedelii, 1659.

[2], 19, [3] p.   19 cm.   [**3961**]

Diss. — Strasbourg (S. Taddel, *respondent*)

FAUST, JOHANN MICHAEL [1663-1707] *respondent.* Dissertatio inauguralis medica, σειπταρμου; sive, De sternutatione ... Argentorati, Literis Johannis Pastorii [1688]

40 p. 19 cm. [**3962**]

Diss. — Strasbourg.

—*See* Scheid, J. V., *praeses*. Quaestionum de visu dodecas. 1684.

FAUST, Johann Wilhelm [*fl.* 1666] *respondent*. *See* Rolfinck, W., *praeses*. Ordo et methodus cognoscendi & curandi maniam. 1666.

FAVENTINUS, Benedictus Victorius. *See* Vittori, Benedetto [*d.* 1561]

FAVINUS, Remius. *See* Flavianus, Remmius.

FAXARDO DE REQUESENS Y ZUÑIGA, Luis. *See* Fajardo de Requesens y Zuñiga, Luis [*fl.* 1599-1630]

FAY, Jacobus Fridericus du. *See* Du Fay, Jakob Friedrich [*b.* 1671]

FAZIO, Silvestro. *See* Facio, Silvestro [1550-1596]

FEAKE, John [*fl.* 1670] *respondent*. Disputatio medica inauguralis in Hippocratis Aphorismorum 51, sectionis 2 ... Lugduni Batavorum, Apud viduam & haeredes Joannis Elsevirii, 1670.

[16] p. 23 cm. [**3963**]

Dis. — Leyden.

FEATLEY, John [1605?-1666] Tranen eener barende-vrouwe, ofte eenige hertversterckende alleen spraken, seer profijtelyck ende troostelyck voor een vrouvwe als de ween om te baren beginnen te genaken ... Uyt Engels vertaelt door Abraham van Laren. Vlissinge, Abraham van Laren, 1665.

[23], 71 p. 14 cm. [**3964**]

Translation of A fountaine of teares.

With this is bound (as issued?) Goddelijcke vierschare. 1665.

FEBRIS china chinae expugnata. 1687. *See* [Nigrisoli, F. M.] *ed.*

FEBRIUM malignarum historia et curatio. 1660. *See* [Menjot, A.]

FECHT, Ernst Heinrich [*b.* 1678] *respondent*. *See* Schaper, J. E., *praeses*. Medicinae curiosae specimen quatuor quaestionum enodatione ostensum ... exponit. 1698.

FEDELE, Fortunato [1550-1630] Fortunati Fidelis ... Contemplationum medicarum libri

XXII. In quibus non pauca praeter communem multorum medicorum sententiam, notatu digna explicantur ... Panormi, Apud Joannem Baptistam Maringum, 1621.

[26], 311, [1] p. 21 cm. [**3965**]

—Fortunati Fidelis ... De relationibus medicorum libri quatuor. In quibus ea omnia, quae forensibus, ac publicis causis medici referre solent, plenissime traduntur ... Panormi, Apud Joannem Antonium de Franciscis, 1602.

[8], 352, [12] p. 21 cm. [**3966**]

Imperfect? Sheet 2z wanting?

—[The same.] ... Studio D. Pauli Ammanni ... Lipsiae, Impensis Joh. Christ. Tarnovii, literis Christiani Michaelis, 1674.

[30], 612, [43] p. 16 cm. [**3967**]

Added engraved title page.

—Copy 2. 17 cm.

Imperfect: sig. B⁸ (blank) wanting.

With this are bound: Maynwaring, E. Historia et mysterium luis venerae. 1675; Clarke, W. Naturalis historia nitri. 1675.

—[The same.] Schola jure-consultorum medica, relationum libris aliquot comprehensa, quibus principia medicinae in jus transsumta ex professo examinantur. Autore D. Thoma Reinesio ... Lipsiae, Impensis Johan. Christ. Tarnovii, literis Christiani Michaelis, 1679.

[14], 612, [43] p. 17 cm. [**3968**]

A reissue, with new title page and preliminary matter.

With this is bound Wandal, H. Vindicae libertatis Christianae. 1678.

—*See* Read, A. Chirurgorum comes. 1687.

FEDELISSIMI, Rainiero [*d.* 1614] Enchiridion pharmaceuticum medicamentorum omnium, que in Antidotario Florentino continentur, breviter facultates complectens ... Bononiae, Apud Bartholomaeum Cochium, 1617.

130, [1] p. 13 cm. [**3969**]

FEDERER, Johann Jacob. Brevis et compendiosa febris Ungaricae curandae, cognoscendae, et ab aliis febribus discernendae methodus. Partim a praestantissimis totius Italiae, Galliae, et Germaniae authoribus desumpta ... & lucem edita ... Friburgi Brisgoiae, Ex typographia Joannis Jacobi Böckleri, sumptibus Jo. Bernhardi Klumpii, 1624.

46 (i.e. 64), [8] p. 16 cm. [**3970**]

"Epigramma in . . . De febris Ungaricae cura . . . libellum . . . Per Joannem Petrum Haering . . .": [8] p. at end.

FEDRO VON RODACH, Georg [16th cent.] Opuscula iatro chemica quatuor. I. Praxis medico chemica. II. Halopyrgice, sive pestis medica-chemica curatio. III. Chirurgia minor. IV. Furnus chymicus . . . Partim nunquam antehac edita, partim nunc Latinitate donata . . . curante Joanne Andrea Schenckio . . . Francofurti, Typis Joannis Wolphii, sumptibus Antonii Hummii, 1611.

[7], 128, [7] p. 15 cm. [**3971**]

Imperfect: upper margins trimmed; p. [1-6] and 127-128 multilated.

—*See* Basilius Valentinus. Triumph-Wagen Antimonii . . . 1676.

FEHR, Heinrich [*fl.* 1610] *See* Stupanus, J. N. Gratiosi medicorum Basiliens. collegii decreto. 1610.

FEHR, Johann Michael [1610-1688] Anchora sacra; vel, Scorzonera, ad normam & formam Academiae naturae-curiosorum elaborata . . . Accessit Schediasma curiosorum de unicornu fossili Joh. Laurentii Bausch . . . Jenae, Typis Joh. Jacobi Bauhoferi, impensis Viti Jacobi Trescher [1666?]

[16], 204, [12] p. plates. 16 cm. [**3972**]

Added engraved title page inserted after index.

—Hiera picra; vel, De absinthio analecta, ad normam & formam Academiae Naturae Curiosorum selecta . . . Lipsiae, Impensis Viti Jacobi Trescheri, literis Johan-Erici Hahnii, 1667.

[16], 176, [4] p. 1 plate. 16 cm. [**3973**]

—[The same.] . . . Lipsiae, Impensis Viti Jacobi Trescheri, literis Johan-Erici Hahnii, 1668.

[16], 176, [4] p. 4 plates. 16 cm. [**3974**]

A reissue of the 1667 edition with new title page and additional plates.

—*See* Welsch, G. H. Epistolae mutuae Argonautae. 1677.

FEICKENS, Pierius [*fl.* 1652] *respondent.* Disputatio medica inauguralis historiam dysenterici proponens . . . Lugduni Batavorum, E typographeo Francisci Hackii, 1652.

[12] p. 23 cm. [**3975**]

Diss. — Leyden.

FEIERVARUS, Stephanus. *See* Fejérvári, István [*d.* 1688]

FEJÉRVÁRI, István [*d.* 1688] *respondent.* Disputatio medica inauguralis de scorbuto . . . Lugduni Batavorum, Apud Abrahamum Elzevier, 1684.

[12] p. 22 cm. [**3976**]

Diss. — Leyden.

FELDE, Joannes a. *See* Felden, Johann von [*d. ca.* 1668]

FELDEN, Johann von [*d. ca.* 1668] Tractatus de peste, divisus in partes duas, quarum prior continet speculationem physicam autore Johanne a Felde . . . posterior ea, quae artis medicae sunt propria, remedia nimirum contra pestem speculationi praemissae congruentia atque a multis seculis cum primis autem praecedenti anno comprobata. Autore Frid. Günt. Kircheim . . . Hall. Saxon. Sumpt. Simon Joh. Hübneri, 1681.

[24], 288 p. illus. 14 cm. [**3977**]

FELDNER, Caspar [*fl.* 1661] *respondent.* Theses medicae de suffocatione uteri . . . Altdorffii, E typographeo Johannis Göbelii [1661]

28 p. 20 cm. [**3978**]

Diss. — Altdorf.

FELGENHAUER, Paul [*fl.* 1619-1659] Anthora; das ist, Gifft-heil, oder Beschreibung des Giffts der Pestilenz, auch vieler andern gifftigen und gefährlichen Kranckheiten . . . Geschrieben durch P[aul] F[elgenhauer] . . . [Brehmen] 1677.

[56] p. 14 cm. [**3979**]

Later editions published as an addition to Elias Beynon's Barmhertziger Samariter.

—[The same.] . . . [n. p.] 1680.

[65] p. 14 cm. [**3980**]

Imperfect: upper margins trimmed with possible loss of pagination.

—[The same.] *In* Beynon, E. Barmhertziger Samariter. 1685, 1696, 1700.

FELICE, Antonio. *See* Marsigli, Antonio Felice [1649-1710]

FELICIANUS, Joannes Bernardus [*ca.* 1490-*ca.* 1552] *tr. See* Cremonini, C. De calido innato, et semine. 1634.

FELINI, Francesco. *See* Fellini, Francesco [1630-1711]

FELIPPO DI LIAGNO, Teodoro. *See* Liagno, Teodoro Filippo di [*fl.* 17th cent.]

FÉLIS, D. [*fl.* 1622-1645] Lavenicus criticus; seu, Antiqua judicationum morborum causa rediviva, et longissimis observationibus Avenione, huc usque factis, confirmata. Per N. E. D. E. D. F. M. D. . . . Avenione, Ex typographia Joannis Piot, 1645.

    [29], 354 (i.e. 254), [1] p. illus. 23 cm.

[3981]

Errata: p. [255]; p. [29] is another list of errata with different setting of type, marked by the printer to be discarded.

FELIX, Antonius, *Father* [*fl.* 1683] De ovis cochlearum epistola ad Marcellum Malpighium . . . cum Joh. Jacobi Harderi . . . epistolis aliquot, de partibus genitalibus cochlearum, generatione item insectorum ex ovo, ad praefatum abbatem, & D. Lucam Schröckium . . . Augustae Vindelicorum, Sumptibus Theophili Goebelii, literis Leonhardi Zachariae, 1684.

    [10], 58 p. plates. 17 cm.

[3982]

Bound with Gehema, J. A. De morbo vulgo dicto plica Polonica. 1683.

    —[The same.] *In* Malpighi, M. Opera omnia. 1687.

FELIX puerpera; seu, Observationes medicae, circa regimen puerperarum & infantium recens natorum ad . . . D. D. Drelincurtium, per M. M. M. Lugd. Batavor. Apud Petrum vander Aa [1684?]

    [8], 40 p. 13 cm.

[3983]

FELL, John, *Bp. of Oxford* [1625-1686] *ed. See* Nemesius, *Bp. of Emesa.* Περὶ φύσεως ἀνθρώπον βιβλίον ἐν.

FELLINI, Francesco [1630-1711] Apologemma jocosum in . . . Sebastianum Badum Venae sectionis apparentibus variolis defensorem . . . Auctore Francisco Felino . . . Genuae, Typis Petri Jo. Calenzani, 1664.

    216 p. 20 cm.

[3984]

Imperfect: p. 150-151 and 154-155 blank, lacking text.

FELTMANN, Gerhard [1637-1696] De dea podagra liber singularis. Bremae, Sumptibus Hermanni Braueri, 1693.

    214, [41] p. 16 cm.

[3985]

    —Tractatus de cadavere inspiciendo . . . Adjicitur disceptatio alterplex ad. L. per agrum. XI. C. de servit. & aqua. Quarum prior est De transitu exercitus

altera De vehiculis sibi obviis . . . Groningae, Typis Remberti Huysman, 1673.

    [8], 168 p.; 52, [12] p.

[3986]

With this is bound Garmann, C. F. De miraculis mortuorum. 1670.

    —[The same.] De cadavere inspiciendo liber unus . . . Adjiciuntur disceptationes binae ad L. per agrum. XI. C. de servit. & aqua. Quarum prima est De transitu exercitus. Altera, De vehiculis sibi obviis . . . Ed. alt. priore auctior & emendatior. Bremae, Typis & impensis Hermanni Braueri, 1692.

    [16], 320, [8] p. 21 cm.

[3987]

    —Tractatus de polygamia; das ist, Gewissenschafftes und schrifftmässiges Gespräch zwischen Weltmann und Sittmann, dem Gewissenlosen und Unschrifftmässigen, zwischen Monogamus und Polygamus, von der Vielweiberey gehaltenen Gespräch entgegen gesetzt. Leipzig, In Verlegung Matthäus Birckners, druckts Johann Köhler, 1677.

    [1], 217 p. 17 cm.

[3988]

FERARO, Battista. *See* Ferraro, Giovanni Battista [*d.* 1569?]

FERDINAND III, *Emperor of Germany* [1608-1657] Privilegium comitatus palat., & militiae auratae a Ferdinando III. Romanorum imperatore . . . concessum vener. nobilium Physicor. Collegio civitatis Mediolani. In Congressu electoral. Ratisbonae, 1653.

    [15] p. 22 cm.

[3989]

Bound with Collegio dei fisici, Milan. Decreta. 1645.

FERDINANDI, Epifanio [1569-1638] Aureus de peste libellus . . . Neapoli, Apud Dominicum Maccaranum, 1626.

    113, [11] p. 20 cm.

[3990]

    —Centum historiae; seu, Observationes, et casus medici, omnes fere medicinae partes . . . continentes . . . Nunc primum in lucem editae . . . Venetiis, Apud Thomam Baglionum, 1621.

    [28], 352 p. 33 cm.

[3991]

Preface by Cataldo Antonio Mannarino.

    —Theoremata medica et philosophica, mira doctrinae varietate . . . in tres libros digesta . . . Venetiis, Apud Thomam Ballionum, 1611.

    [32], 271 p. 36 cm.

[3992]

FERDINANDO I, *Grand Duke of Tuscany* [1549-1609] *See* Riforma dell ospedale detto di Mon'Agnesa. 16—?

FERDINANDO SICULO. *See* BALAMI, Ferdinando [*fl.* 1514–*ca.* 1552]

FERIET, JOHANN BENJAMIN. *See* FERIET DE MONDELANGE, Jean Benjamin [*fl.* 1700]

FERIET DE MONDELANGE, JEAN BENJAMIN [*fl.* 1700] *respondent.* De paralysi . . . Basileae, Typis Jacobi Bertschii [1700]

    [24] p.   19 cm.   **[3993]**
    Diss. — Basel.

FERMOSTHENES, JOHANN [*fl.* 17th cent.] Homicidium theriacale; das ist, Wie und durch was Betrug die Marckschreyer und Theriacks-Krämer unter dem Schein ihres wolbewehrten Theriacks approbirten Aesculapii, Electuari Regii, Secreti Balsami vitae, und dergleichen experimentirt-vermeyneten Medicamenten, die Einfältigen betriegen, und auffzuopffern pflegen. Kürtzlich entworffen von Johanne Fermosthene . . . [n. p.] 1672.

   .   [8] p.   20 cm.   **[3994]**

FERNÁNDEZ, ANDRÉS [*fl.* 1624] *ed. See* OBREGÓN, B. de. Instruccion de enfermeros. 1664.

FERNANDEZ, FRANCISCO. *See* HERNÁNDEZ, Francisco [*ca.* 1517–1587]

FERNÁNDEZ DE LA FUENTE, ANDRÉS [*fl.* 1640–1649] Avisos preservativos de peste. A la noble, y leal ciudad de Ecija . . . Ecija, Luis Estupiñan, 1649.

    52 ll.   22 cm.   **[3995]**
    Imperfect? ll. 11–12 wanting?

FERNEL, JEAN [1506 or 7–1558] Universa medicina: ab ipso quidem authore ante obitum diligenter recognita, & justis accessionibus locupletata. Postea autem studio et diligentia Guliel. Plantii . . . postremum elimata, et in librum Therapeutices septimum doctissimis scholiis illustrata. Ed. 7. Cui accessit ejusdem Fernelii Consiliorum liber, cum quibusdam clarorum medicorum Parisiensium responsis. Lugduni, Apud Joannem Veyrat et Thomam Soubron, 1602.

    4 v. in 1.   35 cm.   **[3996]**
    Sherrington 73. J 17.
    Contents. — [v. 1.] Physiologiae libri VII. Pathologiae libri VII. — [v. 2] Therapeutices universalis, seu Medendi rationis, libri septem. — Febrium curandarum methodus generalis. — De luis venereae curatione perfectissima, liber. — Consilium epileptico praescriptum. — [v. 3] De abditis rerum causis libri duo. — [v. 4] Consiliorum liber.

—[The same.] . . . Ed. 6. Qua nunc primum accedit Vita auctoris ab eodem Plantio luculenter exposita: & Consiliorum medicinalium libellus. Francofurti, Apud Claudium Marnium & heredes Joan. Aubrii, 1607.

    4 v. in 1.   ports.   18 cm.   **[3997]**
    Imprint varies: v. [2] and [4]: Hanoviae, Typis Wechelianis, apud Claudium Marnium & haeredes Joannis Aubrii.
    Vol. [4]: 4. ed.
    Sherrington 76. J 20.

—[The same.] . . . Ed. 6. . . . Hanoviae, Impensis Claudii Marnii heredum, Johannis & Andreae Marnii & consortum, 1610.

    4 v. in 1.   ports.   34 cm.   **[3998]**
    Vol. [4]: 5. ed.
    Sherrington 77. J 21.

—[The same.] . . . Ed. 8. . . . Lugduni, Apud Claudium Morillon, 1602–15 [v. 1, 1615]

    4 v. in 1.   35 cm.   **[3999]**
    Vol. [4] imperfect: p. 111–112 wanting.
    Vol. [2] has title page with imprint: Lugduni, Apud Joannem Veyrat, et Thomam Soubron, 1602; vols. [3]–[4] have half titles.
    A reissue of Veyrat's edition, with new title pages.
    Sherrington 78. J 22 (variant).

—[The same.] . . . Genevae, Apud Petrum & Jacobum Chouët, 1619.

    [16] 1172, [57] p.   24 cm.   **[4000]**
    Sherrington 79. J 23.

—[The same.] . . . Genevae, Petrus Aubertus, 1627.

    [16], 631 (i.e. 611), [53] p.; 484, 397, [63] p.   18 cm.   **[4001]**
    Sherrington 80. J 24.

—Another issue, bound in two volumes, without place of publication on title page.   **[4002]**

—[The same.] . . . Universa medicina. Ab ipso quidem autore ante obitum diligenter recognita, & justis accessionibus locupletata. Addita sunt ejus Fernelii Consilia: & Guliel. Plantii scholia in pharmacopoeam seu librum Therapeutices septimum. Editio postrema. Genevae, Typis Jacobi Stoer, 1637.

    [16], 1172, [57] p.   23 cm.   **[4003]**
    A reprint of the 1619 edition.
    Sherrington 81. J 25.

—[The same.] Universa medicina: a doctissimo et experientissimo medico diligenter recognita, & ab innumeris mendis & erroribus, quibus priores scatebant editiones repurgata, collatis invicemi vetustissimis & optimis exemplaribus. Ed. postrema. Addita sunt ejusdem Fernelii Consilia, & Guliel. Plantii scholia in pharmacopoeam seu librum Therapeutices septimum. Genevae, Apud Jacobum Crispinum, 1638.

[16], 647, [41] p.; 448, 397, [47] p.   18 cm.
                                                      [4004]

Sherrington 82. J 26 (variant)

—Another issue, with imprint: Genevae, Apud Jacobum Chouët, 1638.

[16], 647, [41] p.   17 cm.   [4005]
Contains Physiologia and Pathologia only.
Sherrington 82. J 26.

—[The same.] . . . Genevae, Apud Jacobum Chouët, 1644.

[16], 631 (i.e. 611), [53] p.; 484, 397, [63] p.   18 cm.   [4006]
A reprint of the 1627 edition.
Sherrington 84. J 28.

—[The same.] Universa medicina. Nova hac editione, quae obscura erant, illustrata, quae deficiebant, suppleta sunt. Lugduni Batavorum, Ex officina Francisci Hackii, 1645.

5 v. in 2.   19 cm.   [4007]
Engraved title page.
Vol. [2] has engraved title page: De morbis universalibus et particularibus.
Contents. — Vita Fernelii, auctore G. Plantio. — Physiologiae libri VII. — Pathologiae libri III. — Joannis Magiri Appendix de signis prognosticis. — Therapeutices universalis, seu Medendi rationis, libri VII. — Pathologiae liber IV. — Febrium curandarum methodus generalis. — Pathologie libri V, VI. — De luis venereae curatione perfectissima liber. — Pathologiae liber VII. — De abditarum rerum causis libri II. — Consiliorum medicinalium liber: ex ejus adversariis quadrigentarum consultationum selectus a Juliano Palmario.
Sherrington 85. J 29 (variant)

—[The same.] Universa medicina, primum quidem studio & diligentia Guilielmi Plantii . . . elimata, nunc autem notis, observationibus, & remediis secretis Joann. & Othonis Heurni . . . et aliorum praestantissimorum medicorum scholiis illustrata. Cui accedunt casus & observationes rariores, quas . . . Otho Heurnius . . . in diario practico annotavit . . . Trajecti ad Rhenum, Typis Gisberti à Zijll, & Theodori ab Ackersdijck, 1656.

2 v. in 1.   24 cm.   [4008]
Sherrington 86. J 30.

—[The same.] . . . Nunc demum opera Theophili Boneti . . . auctior adjectione Encheiridii medicopractici, incerti authoris, & Chirurgici Chalmetei, adeo ut singula illorum capita singulis Pathologiae Fernelii capitibus respondeant . . . Coloniae Allobrogum, Apud Samuelem de Tournes, 1679.

[32] 914 (i.e. 814), 17, [34] p.   port.   35 cm.
                                                      [4009]

Sherrington 87. J 31.

—Another issue, with imprint: Genevae, Apud Samuelem de Tournes, 1680.   [4010]

—La chirurgie . . . Avec les annotations de monsieur Simeon de Provanchieres . . . Tolose, Raymond Bosc, 1667.

[8], 278, [1] p.   17 cm.   [4011]
A commentary as much as a translation of the seventh book of the Pathologia. Cf. Sherrington 104. P 3.
"La methode de guerir par les medicamens exterieurs, entierement necessaires pour la guerison des maladies qui regardent la chirurgie. Tirée du sixième livre de la Therapeutique de messire Jean Fernel": p. [139]-278. This translation is extracted from the French version of the Therapeutices universalis libri VII done by B. Du Teil and published in Paris in 1648.

—Consiliorum liber, cui accesserunt responsa quaedam clarorum medicorum Parisiensium. Lugduni, Apud Bartholomaeum Vincentium, 1605.

174 p.   18 cm.   [4012]
Signatures: 3A-3L^8.
Printed on first page of many gatherings: "Tom. 2." This work apparently formed a part of vol. 2 of an edition of the author's Universa medicina.
Bound with *his* Therapeutices universalis . . . libri septem. 1605.

—De abditis rerum causis. *See* Riolan, J. [1538?-1605?] Praelectiones in libros physiologicos. 1601.

—[De naturali parte medicinae. French.] Les VII. livres de la physiologie . . . Traduits en françois par Charles de Saint-Germain . . . Paris, Jean Guignard le jeune, 1655.

[24], 384, [8], 385-773 (i.e. 775) p.   17 cm.
                                                      [4013]
Translation of the treatise on physiology from the author's Medicina (1554), originally published separately under title: De naturali parte medicinae. Cf. Sherrington. p. 190.
Sherrington 7. D 4.

—[The same.] *See* Riolan, J. [1538?-1605?] Praelectiones in libros physiologicos. 1601.

—De vacuandi ratione. *In* Hygieia. 1628.

—[Excerpts.] *In* Regimen sanitatis Salernitanum. Medicina Salernitana. 1605, 1611, 1612, 1622, 1624, 1628, 1638 [and] Schola Salernitana. 1649, 1657, 1667, 1683.

—[Febrium curandarum methodus generalis. French.] La methode generale de guerir les fievres ... Traduite en françois par Charles de Saint-Germain ... Paris, Chez Jean Guignard le jeune, 1655.

[14], 65 (i.e. 95) p.   19 cm.   [**4014**]
Sherrington 97. M 3.
Bound with *his* La therapeutique. 1668.

—[Pathologia. French.] La pathologie ... Mis en françois par A. D. M. ... Paris, La veuve de Jean Le Bouc, 1646.

[16], 580, [2] p.   18 cm.   [**4015**]
Not in Sherrington.

—[The same.] ... Paris, Jean Guignard, 1650.
[16], 580, [2] p.   18 cm.   [**4016**]
A reissue of the 1646 edition with new title page.
Sherrington 129. X 2.

—[The same.] ... 2. ed. Paris, En la boutique de Langelier, chez Jean Guignard le pere, 1660.

[16], 580 p.   19 cm.   [**4017**]
Different setting of type.
Sherrington 131. X 4.

—[Pathologia. Excerpts.] *In* Hartmann, J. Praxis chymiatrica. 1682.

—Pathologiae liber quartus De febribus. Aphorismorum de febribus loquentium explicatio, & praedicendi, curandique ratio singulis febribus adjecta, a Rutgero Loenio ... Amstelodami, Apud Aegidium Valkenier, CIƆ IƆ LXIV [i.e. 1664]

[16], 271, [1] p.   16 cm.   [**4018**]
Sherrington 135. Z

—Pharmacia Jo. Fernelii cum Guilel. Planti & Franc. Saguyerii scholiis ... nunc primum edita ... Hanoviae, Typis Wechelianis, apud Claud. Marnium & haeredes Jo. Aubrii, 1605.

[14], 3-348, [7] p.   15 cm.   [**4019**]
The unsigned Epistola is by Kaspar Bauhin, the editor.
Book 7 (On prescriptions) of the "Therapeutics" of the "Universal medicine", with notes by Saguyer in addition to those by Plancy. Cf. Sherrington 124. U.

—Therapeutices universalis; seu, Medendi rationis, libri septem, quam totius medicinae tertiam fecit partem, ad praxim perutilem & necessariam.

Lugduni, Apud Bartholomaeum Vincentium, 1605.
552 (i.e. 546), [30] p.   18 cm.   [**4020**]
Signatures: Aa-Zz, 2A-2N⁸.
Printed on first page of many gatherings: Tom. 2. This volume apparently formed a part of v. 2 of an edition of the author's Universa medicina.
With this is bound *his* Consiliorum liber. 1605.

—[The same.] *See* Horst, G. *praeses*. Theses medicae de verae sectione. 1622.

—[French tr.] Les sept livres de la therapeutique universelle ... Mis en françois par le sieur Du Teil. Paris, Chez la veufue Jean Le Bouc, 1648.

[14], 679, [9] p.   18 cm.   [**4021**]
Sherrington 91. K 4 (variant)

—[The same.] ... Paris, Jean Guignard, 1650.
[18], 679, [9] p.   18 cm.   [**4022**]
Imperfect: signatures of sheet a misbound.
A reissue of the 1648 edition with new title page and additional preliminary matter.
Not in Sherrington.

—[The same.] La therapeutique; ou, la methode ... de guerir les maladies. ... Traduction nouvelle & plus exacte que celle des editions precedentes. Paris, Chez Jean Guignard et René Guignard, 1668.

[16], 648 p.   19 cm.   [**4023**]
With this is bound *his* La methode generale de guerir les fievres. 1655.

—*See* BAYLEY, W. Two treatises concerning the preservation of eie-sight. 1616; ENCHIRIDION PRACTICUM MEDICO-CHIRURGICUM. 1621, 1627, 1644; GUY DE CHAULIAC. Le maistre en chirurgie. 1691, 1697; JONSTONUS, J. The idea of practical physick. 1657, 1661; RIVIÈRE, L. The practice of physick. 1658-61, 1672, 1678; VAUGHAN, W. Directions for health. 1626, 1633.

—*as subject. See* BAILLOU, G. de. Opuscula medica. 1643; BARTSCH, J. Exercitationum medicinalium ex Fernelio octava, nona et decima. 1624; HOFMANN, C. Rejectanea pathologica. 1639; LAGNEAU, D. Traicté pour la conservation de la santé. 1650; SALTZMANN, J. R. [1573-1656] *praeses*. Exercitationum medicinalium ex Fernelio tertia: De abdominis. 1622 [and] Exercitationum medicinalium ex Fernelio quinta: De capitis. 1623 [and] Exercitationum medicinalium ex Fernelio septima: De symptomatis. 1624; SEBISCH, M [1578-1674?] *praeses*. Exercitationum medicinalium ex Fernelio prima [-secunda] 1622 [and] Exercitationum medicinalium ex Fernelio sexta. 1623.

FERRAND, Antoine [*fl.* 16th cent.] *ed. See* FERRAND, Jean, *the younger.* De febribus libellus. 1602.

FERRAND, Jacques [*fl.* 17th cent.] De la maladie d'amour; ou, Melancholie erotique. Discours curieux qui enseigne à cognoistre l'essence, les causes, les signes, & les remedes de ce mal fantastique . . . Paris, Denis Moreau, 1623.

    [40], 270, [10] p.   17 cm.   **[4024]**
    Imperfect: p. 263–266 wanting.

    —[English tr.] Ἐρωτομανια; or, A treatise discoursing of the essence, causes, symptomes, prognosticks, and cure of love, or erotique melancholy . . . Oxford, Printed by L. Lichfield and sold by Edward Forrest, 1640.

    [39], 363 p.   15 cm.   **[4025]**
    STC 10829.
    Translated by Edmund Chilmead.

FERRAND, Jean, *the elder* [*fl.* 1570] De nephrisis et lithiasis, seu de renum, et vesicae calculi definitione, causis, signis, praedictione, praecautione & curatione. Ex Hippocrate, Dioscoride, Galeno, Avicenna, Aetio, & Paulo Aegineta, aliisque celeberrimis medicis, collectis . . . 2. ed. Parisiis, Apud Michaelem Sonnium, 1601.

    152 ll.   16 cm.   **[4026]**
    Bound with Ferrand, Jean, *the younger.* De febribus libellus. 1602.

FERRAND, Joannes Baptista [*fl.* 1647–1678]. *See* febribus libellus. Ex variis authoribus collectus . . . Parisiis, Apud Michaelem Sonnium, 1602.

    156 ll.   plate.   16 cm.   **[4027]**
    Edited by Antoine Ferrand.
    With this is bound Ferrand, Jean, *the elder.* De nephrisis et lithiasis. 1601.

FERRAND, Joannes Baptista [*fl.* 1647–1678].*See* TARDY, C. An biliosis purgatio ante cibum? 1661?

FERRANT, Louis, *ed. See* HIPPOCRATES. [Coacae praenotiones.] Coaca praesagia. 1657.

FERRANTE LONGOBARDI. *See* BARTOLI, Daniello, *Father* [1608–1685]

FERRANTE SICILIANO. *See* BALAMI, Ferdinando [*fl.* 1514–*ca.* 1552]

FERRARA, Camillo [*fl.* 1596] Nuova selva di cirugia, divisa in tre parti. Nella prima sono gli avvertimenti del manual, & artificioso modo di curare molte, e gravi infirmità del corpo humano. Nella

seconda sono molti medicamenti esquisiti, con le figure de' ferri, ò instrumenti necessarii per essercitar l'arte della cirugia. Nella terza parimente si contengono molti rari medicamenti per distillationi, con le figure in ultimo de' vasi, e fornelli appartenenti all'arte distillatoria. Del R. P. F. Gabriele Ferrara . . . Et in questa 3. impressione ampliato, & acresciuto di molti secreti dall'istesso autore . . . Venetia, Sebastian Combi, 1605[?]

    [32], 565 p.   illus.   15 cm.   **[4028]**
    Final figure of imprint date illegible.

    —[The same.] . . . Et aggiuntovi la quarte parte, che tratta delle qualità, & rimedii della peste . . . Venetia, Gio. Battista Combi, 1627.

    [32], 565, [16] p.; 86 p.   illus.   15 cm.   **[4029]**
    "Nuova selva di cirugia, per servire in tempo di peste. Libro quatro . . ." (86 p. at end) has special title page.

    —[Latin tr.] Sylva chirurgiae, in tres libros divisa: in quorum I. De observationibus chirurgicis, II. De medicamentis itidem ad chirurgiam pertinentibus, III. De medicamentis per destillationem acquisitis, & quam maxime etiam in chirurgia usurpandis agitur . . . Primo quidem a Gabriele Ferrara . . . Italico idiomate descripta & collecta: nunc vero per Petrum Uffenbachium . . . Latinitate donata, & in lucem emissa. Francofurti, Sumptibus Jacobi de Zetter, typis H. Palthenii, 1625.

    [16], 405, [33] p.   illus.   16 cm.   **[4030]**

FERRARA, Gabriele. *See* FERRARA, Camillo [*fl.* 1596]

FERRARI, Giacomo, *ed.* Idea theriacae, et mithridatii, ex . . . Antonii Berthioli pragmatia: ipsorumque interim ingredientium simplicium . . . discussio, & praesertim de viperis scitu dignissima . . . a Jacobo Ferrario . . . partim ex . . . Flamminii Evoli scriptis, partim ex propriis excerpta, & ad commune commodum edita. Venetiis, Apud Jo. Antonium & Jacobum de Franciscis, 1601.

    [8], 24 ll.   22 cm.   **[4031]**

    —, *tr. See* DUCHESNE, J. Le ricchezze della riformata farmacopea. 1619, 1638, 1646, 1655, 1665, 1684.

FERRARI, Giovanni Battista, *Cavalerizzo Napolitano. See* FERRARO, Giovanni Battista [*d.* 1569?]

FERRARI, Giovanni Battista, *Sanese. See* FERRARI, Giovanni Battista, *Father* [1584–1655]

FERRARI, Giovanni Battista, *Father* [1584-1655] Flora; overo, Cultura di fiori ... Distinta in quattro libri e trasportata dalla lingua latina nell'italiana da Lodovico Aureli Perugino. Roma, Pier'Ant. Facciotti, 1638.

[15], 520, [27] p. illus. 24 cm. [**4032**]
Engraved title page.
Errata: p. [27]

—In funere Marsilii Cagnati medici praestantissimi laudatio Joannis Baptistae Ferrarii ... Habita ... V. Kal. Augusti MDCXII. Romae, Apud Jacobum Mascardum, 1612.

[8] p. 22 cm. [**4033**]

FERRARI, Ognibene [16th cent.] De arte medica infantium libri IV. Ejusdem item de eadem Aphorismorum particulae tres: in Germania nunc primum edit. Lipsiae, Impensis Henningi Grossy, 1605.

[14], 278 (i.e. 294) p.; 26 p. 17 cm. [**4034**]
Part [2] has special title page: De arte medica infantium aphorismorum, particulae tres. Witebergae, Typis Wolffgangi Meisneri, 1604.

FERRARI, Pirro Antonio. *See* Ferraro, Pirro Antonio [16th-17th cent.]

FERRARIUS [*fl. ca.* 1200] De lapide philosophorum secundum verum modum formando ... [&] Thesaurus philosophiae.

143-165 p. vol. 3. 20 cm. (*In* Zetzner, Lazarus, *ed.* Theatrum chemicum. Argentorati, 1659-61) [**4035**]
Caption titles.

—Tractatus chemicus. *In* [Combach, L.] *ed.* and *tr.* Tractatus. 1647.

FERRARO, Giovanni Battista [d. 1569?] Trattato utile, e necessario ad ogni agricoltore. Per guarire cavalli, bovi, vacche, cani, asini, muli, & uccelli di gabbia; con il modo di castrar porci; & il rimedio di guarire le bestie bovine dal cancro volante. Et il modo di coltiva i giardini ... Bologna et in Bassano, Gio. Antonio Remondin [1673?]

96 p. illus. 16 cm. [**4036**]

—*See* Ferraro, P. A. Cavallo frenato ... Diviso in quattro libri. 1620.

FERRARO, Pirro Antonio [16th-17th cent.] Cavallo frenato ... Diviso in quattro libri. Et à questi quattro libri suoi, precede l'opera di Gio. Battista Fer-

raro suo padre, divisa in altri quattro libri ... dove si tratta il modo di conservar le razze, disciplinar cavalli, & il modo di curargli ... Venetia, Francesco Prati, 1620.

[4], 118, [2] p.; 256 p. illus. 34 cm. [**4037**]
Part [2] has special title page.

FERREIRA DA ROSA, Joao. *See* Rosa, João Ferreira da [*fl.* 1686-1695]

FERRER, Auger. *See* Ferrier, Auger [1513-1588]

FERRER DE VALDECEBRO, Andrés [1620-1680] Govierno general, moral, y politico, hallado en las fieras, y animales sylvestres, sacado de sus naturales propriedades ... con particular tabla para sermones varios tiempo, y de santos ... [Madrid, Diego Diaz de la Carrera, 1658]

[13], 205, [23] ll. illus. 20 cm. [**4038**]
Half title.
Added engraved title page.

—Govierno general, moral, y politico, hallado en las aves mas generosas, y nobles, sacado de sus naturales, virtudes, y propiedades ... Con quatro tablas diferentes, es la una para sermones varios de tiempo, y de santos ... Madrid, Melchor Alegre, 1670.

[20], 205, [15] ll. illus. 20 cm. [**4039**]

FERRERO, Charles Hyacinthe [1648-1730]. *See* Chales, C. F. M. de, *Father.* Cursus seu mundus mathematicus. 1690.

FERRI, Alfonso [1515-1595]. *See* Uffenbach, P. Thesaurus chirurgicae. 1610.

FERRIER, Auger [1513-1588] A generall diet. *In* Banister, J. A treatise of chirurgerie. 1633.

—Rimedi preservativi, e curativi in tempo di peste ... Tradotti dalla lingua francese nell'italiana ... Siena & Bologna, Presso Clemente Ferroni, ad instanza di Sebastiano Balestra, 1630.

29, [2] p. 20 cm. [**4040**]

FERRIOL, Petrus [*fl.* 17th cent.] *ed. See* Garcia Carrero, P. Disputationes medicae, et commentaria in fen. primam libri quarti Avicennae. 1628.

FERRIOLUS, Balthasar Andreas [17th cent.] Armamentarium physico-antipesticum; oder, Medicinalisch Zeug-Hauss, darinnen viele unterschiedliche Gegenwehr, und natürliche Mittel zu finden, welche wider den ... Pestilentz ...

gebraucht werden können . . . Franckfurt am Mäyn, Gedruckt und verlegt durch Johann Kuchenbeckern, 1666.

[8], 112 p.   17 cm.   **[4041]**

—Morbosi ventriculi infelix hactenus tentata cura; das ist, Warhaffte Arth und Natur der Däuung so im Magen geschiehet . . . Franckfurt am Mäyn, Bey Johann David Zunnern, 1668.

[16], 78 p.   16 cm.   **[4042]**
Bound with Charleton, W. Spiritus gorgonicus. 1650.

FERRO, GIOVANNI MARIA [*d.* 1682] *ed. See* DURANTE, C. Herbario novo. 1667.

—, *tr. See* DUCHESNE, J. Le ricchezze della riformata farmacopea. 1646, 1655, 1665, 1684.

—*See* IMPERATO, F. Historia naturale. 1672.

FERRO, SALADINO. *See* SALADINUS, Asculanus [*fl.* ca. 1430-1448]

FERRY, DAVID [*fl.* 1693] *respondent.* Disputatio medica inauguralis de ανορεξια . . . Lugduni Batavorum, Apud Abrahamum Elzevier, 1693.

[15] p.   22 cm.   **[4043]**
Diss. — Leyden.

FERVACQUIUS, ROBERTUS [*fl.* 1650] *ed. See* COLLEGIE DER MEDECYNE, Brussels. Statuta Collegii Medici Bruxellensis. 1650.

FESEL, WOLRAD ENGELHARD [*fl.* 1632-1633] *respondent. See* SEBISCH, M. [1578-1674?] *praeses.* Galeni Ars parva in disputationes triginta resoluta. 1633 [and] Prodromi examinis vulnerum singularum humani corporis partium. 1632.

FETTI, PIETRO [*fl.* 1613] *ed. See* MAGNI, P. P. Discorsi. 1613.

FEUERBERG, JOHANN [*fl.* 1556?] Fons sacer; das ist, Beschreibung des . . . heiligen Brunnen . . . in . . . Pyrmont . . . Vormahls beschrieben von Johanne Byrmontano, alias Feuerberg, und gedruckt zu Lemgo durch Conrad Grothen Erben, im Jahr 1597. Anitzo . . . auffs neue . . . verb. durch A. V. K. G. C. D. [i.e. Andreas von Keil genannt Cunaeus D.] [Lemgo? 1688?]

[10], 34 p.   17 cm.   **[4044]**
Dedication by Andreas von Keil dated 1688.
"Noch ein kleines Tractätlein vom Pyrmontischen Sauer-Brunnen und Bade, wie dieselben im Jahr 1560 sind gebrauchet

worden . . . Und . . . zum Druck befordert von Andrea von Keil" (p. 25-34) has special title page.

FEUEREISEN, JOHANN CHRISTIAN [*fl.* 1675] *respondent. See* HOFFKUNTZ, C., *praes.* Disputationem anthropologicam de unione . . . corporis humani . . . subjiciunt. 1675.

FEYENS, JEAN [*d.* 1585] Joannis Fieni . . . De flatibus humanum corpus molestantibus, commentarius novus ac singularis. In quo flatuum natura, causae & symptomata describunter, eorumque remedia facili & expedita methodo indicantur. Amstelodami, Apud Joannem Janssonium, 1643.

[16], 240, [3] p.   13 cm.   **[4045]**

—[The same.] Physographia, de flatibus morbisque flatuosis eorumque expedita curationis methodo, commentarius novus ac singularis olim a Joanne Fieno . . . nunc emendatior factus cum notis Henrici Laevini Fischeri . . . Hamburgi, Typis Henrici Werneri, 1644.

[3], 194, [4] p.   14 cm.   **[4046]**

—[English tr.] A new and needful treatise of spirits and wind offending mans body. Wherein are discovered their nature, causes and effects. By . . . Dr. Fienus. And englished by William Rowland . . . London, Printed by J. M. for Benjamin Billingsley and Obadiah Blagrave, 1668.

[14], 115, [5] p.   15 cm.   **[4047]**
Added title page (p. [7], sig A¹) reads: A new and excellent treatise of wind offending mans body . . . [Translated] By W. R. M. D. . . .

—[The same.] . . . Together with its speedy and easie remedy. [Translated] By W. R. M. D. . . . London, Benjamin Billingsley, 1676.

[12], 115 p.   15 cm.   **[4048]**

FEYENS, THOMAS [1567-1631] Thomae Fieni . . . De cauteriis libri quinque. In quibus vires, materia, modus, locus, numerus, tempus ponendorum cauteriorum, ex veterum Graecorum, Arabum, Latinorum, necnon neotericorum sententia quam dilucide explicantur. Lovanii, Apud Joan. Baptistam Zangrium, 1601.

[8], 258 ll.   plate.   15 cm.   **[4049]**

—De formatrice foetus liber in quo ostenditur animam rationalem infundi tertia die. Authore Thoma Fieno . . . Antverpiae, Apud Gulielmum a Tongris, 1620.

[16], 283, [2] p.   19 cm.   **[4050]**

With this is bound Du Gardin, L. De animatione foetus quaestio. 1623.

—[The same.] *See* DU GARDIN, L. De animatione foetus quaestio. 1623.

—De viribus imaginationis tractatus, authore Thoma Fieno ... Lovanii, In officina typographica Gerardi Rivii, 1608.

[16], 200 p. 18 cm. [4051]

—[The same.] ... Ed. postrema. Lugd. Batavorum, Ex Officina Elseviriana, 1635.

377, [7] p. 20 cm. [4052]

—[The same.] ... Ed. nova. Londini, Ex officina Rogeri Danielis, 1657.

334, [11] p. 12 cm. [4053]

Willems 1214. (Printed in Amsterdam by Louis and Daniel Elzevier.)

Device of the Elsevier press, Amsterdam, on title page.

—Another issue, with new title page and imprint: Amstelodami, Prostant apud Joannem Janssonium, 1658. [4054]

—Thomae Fieni ... Libri chirurgici XII. De praecipuis artis chirurgicae controversiis ... Opera posthuma, Hermanni Conringii cura nunc primum edita. Francofurti, Apud Thom. Matthiam Goezium, 1649.

[12], 108 (i.e. 110) p. 19 cm. [4055]

—[German tr.] D. Thomae Fieni ... Zwölff Bücher von der Wund-Arzney-Kunst, oder Chirurgia ... in lateinischer Sprach heraus gegeben von D. Hermanno Conringio, anjezo aber von einem Liebhaber der Kunst ins Deutsche übersetzet. Hiebey ist mit angefüget D. Johannis Friedrichs Schweizers Güldenes Kalb; J. R. H. Philosophischer Phönix &c. vom Stein der Weisen. Samt einer annehmlichen Zugabe der Chimiae, und ihren wahren Fundamenten. Nürnberg, Wolff Eberhard Felsecker, 1675.

[12], 200 p.; 66 p.; 28, [4], 35-44 p. 17 cm. [4056]

Added engraved title page.

Parts [2] and [3] have special title pages.

—Thomae Fieni Pro sua de animatione foetus tertia die opinione apologia adversus Ant. Ponce Sanctacruz ... Lovanii, Apud viduam Henrici Hasteni, 1629.

[16], 255, [1] p. 19 cm. [4057]

—Thomae Fieni ... Simiotice; sive, De signis medicis, tractatus ... Lugduni, Sumpt. Joannis Antonii Huguetan, & Marci Antonii Ravaud, 1664.

[12], 414, [10] p. 23 cm. [4058]

—Another issue, with new title page and imprint: Lugduni & vaeneunt Parisiis, Apud Gasparum Meturas patrem & filium, 1664. [4059]

—*See* FOLLINUS, H. Amuletum Antonianum; seu, Luis pestiferae fuga. 1618.

FEYERABEND, JOHANN BALTASAR [*fl.* 1681] *respondent.* Disputatio inauguralis medica de affectione coeliaca ... Argentorati, Typis Johannis Welperi [1681]

[28] p. 19 cm. [4060]

Diss.—Strasbourg.

FEYNES, FRANÇOIS [*d.* 1573] Medicina practica: in quatuor libros digesta ... Nunc primum e' bibliotheca ... Renati Moraei ... studiosorum usibus ... concessum. Lugduni, Sumpt. Joannis Antonii Huguetan, & Marci Anton. Ravaud, 1650.

[16], 740, [46] p. 24 cm. [4061]

FEYO, FRANCISCO SOARES. *See* SOARES FEYO, Francisco.

FICINO, MARSILIO [1433-1499] Libri III de vita. I. De studiosorum sanitate tuenda. II. De vita eorum producenda. III. De vita valida & longa coelitus comparanda. Omnibus literatis tam utiles quam necessarii. Moguntiae, Typis Nicolai Heyll, sumpt. Philippi Jacobi Fischeri, 1647.

[16], 196 p. 14 cm. [4062]

"Marsilii Ficini Apologia": p. [11-16]

With this is bound Bongars, J. Jacobi Bongarsii et Georgii Michaelis Lingelshemii epistolae. 1660.

—*See* VIGILANTIUS DE MONTE CUBITI, *pseud., ed.* and *tr.* Dreyfaches hermetisches Kleeblat. 1667.

FICK, JOHANN JAKOB [1663-1730] *praeses.* Dissertationem hanc de abortu epidemico ... publice ventilandam sistit ... H. T. Witte ... Jenae, Typis Gollnerianis [1697]

36 p. 21 cm. [4063]

Diss.—Jena (H. T. Witte, *respondent*)

—*respondent. See* BERGER, J. G. von, *praeses.* Disputationem de chylo ... submittit M. Johannes Jacobus Fickius ... 1686; CRAUSE, R. W., *praeses.* Disputatio inauguralis de morbis mammarum. 1689.

—*See* WEDEL, G. W. Propempticon inaugurale de anil, indico, glasto. 1689.

FIDELIS, FORTUNATUS. *See* FEDELE, Fortunato [1550–1630]

FIDENSA, EUSTACHIUS. *See* BONAVENTURA, *Saint, Cardinal* [1221–1274]

FIDENZA, GIOVANNI PIETRO. *See* BONAVENTURA, *Saint, Cardinal* [1221–1274]

FIDLER, ANDREAS [*fl.* 1666] *respondent. See* CLEMAS, M., *praeses.* Disputatio physica de putredine. 1666.

FIENUS, JOANNES. *See* FEYENS, Jean [*d.* 1585]

FIENUS, THOMAS. *See* FEYENS, Thomas [1567–1631]

FIERA, BATTISTA [1469–1538] Coena notis illustrata a Carolo Avantio ... Cui novissima hac editione accesserunt ... Marci Aurelii Severini ... epistolae duae: altera De lapide fungifero, altera De lapide fungimappa. Patavii, Typis Sebastiani Sardi, 1649.

[16], 208, [11] p. illus., port. 21 cm. **[4064]**
Dedication signed by Jacopo Avanzi.

FIERABRAS, HERVÉ [*fl.* 1550] Methode briefue et facile pour aisement parvenir a la vraye intelligence de la chirurgie: en laquelle est declaree l'admirable construction du corps humain ... Nouvellement rev. & corr. Paris, Claude Banqueteau, 1635.

[8], 344 p. illus., tables. 17 cm. **[4065]**

—[The same.] La vraye methode de la parfaicte chirurgie ... Divisée en trois livres ... Le tout rev. & corr. par M. Jean de Montigny ... Paris, Nicolas Bessin, 1648.

[20], 336 p. illus. 17 cm. **[4066]**

FIERAVANTI, LEONARDO. *See* FIORAVANTI, Leonardo [1517–1588].

FIGATELLI, GIOVANNI [17th cent.] Medico sacro che si piglia pensiero de gl'incurabili; e pratica rimedii preservativi, curativi, e confortativi; quando appunto l'huomo, dovendo far passaggio all'eternità dell'altra vita, ò per corso naturale, ò di morte violenta per mano della giustitia ... Opera ... distinta in quattro libri ... Venetia, Gio. Francesco Valvasense, 1677.

477 p. 15 cm. **[4067]**

FIGUEROA, CHRISTOVAL SUAREZ DE. *See* SUÁREZ DE FIGUEROA, Cristóbal [*ca.* 1571–1645]

FIGUEROA, FRANCISCO [*fl.* 1599–1631] Carte que ... escrivio a Francisco de Rioja, coronista de su Magestad; en que le dize, pierda el miedo a la peste causada de Unguentos, y polvos, que dizen ha corrido en Milan ... [Sevilla, 1631?]

19 ll. 29 cm. **[4068]**

FIGULUS, BENEDICTUS. *See* TOEPFER, Benedict [*fl.* 1607]

FIGULUS, GEORGIUS [*fl.* 1660] Novum & inauditum medicinae universalis speculum cabalistico-chymicum. Bruxellae, Typis Joannis Mommartii, 1660.

207, [33] p. 14 cm. **[4069]**

FIKKE, JOHANN JACOB. *See* FICK, Johann Jakob [1662 *or* 3–1730]

FILEATRO [*fl.* 1687] *See* TIXEDAS, C. Verdad defendida. 1688.

FILIPPO, TEODORO. *See* LIAGNO, Teodoro Filippo di [*fl.* 17th cent.]

FILIPPO NERI, *Saint* [1515–1595] *See* VITTORI, A. Medica disputatio. 1613 [and] Medicae consultationes. 1640.

FINCK, ISRAEL [*fl.* 1669] *respondent. See* KIRCHMAJER, T., *praeses.* Dissertatio physica de cruentatione cadaverum. 1669.

FINCK, JOHANN VINCENT [*fl.* 1615–1618] Encheiridion dogmatico-hermeticum morborum partium corporis humani praecipuorum curationes breves continens ... Lipsiae, Excudebat Laurentius Cober, impensis Eliae Rehefeldii & Johan. Grosii, 1618.

[16], 222, [2] p. 14 cm. **[4070]**

—[The same.] ... Lipsiae, Impensis Eliae Rehefeldii & Johan. Grosii [Typis Georgi Ligeri] 1626.

[16], 185, [3] p. 13 cm. **[4071]**

FINELLA, FILIPPO [*b. ca.* 1585] De metoposcopia astronomica de duodecim signis coelestibus. Antverpia, Ex Officina Plantiuiana [sic] apud Baldassarem Morenum [sic] 1650.

[8], 216 p. illus. 15 cm. **[4072]**
Presumably printed by Jacob Gaffarus of Naples. Cf. M. Sabbe. Falsche Moretusdrucke. Gutenberg Jahrbuch, 1929, p. 193–214.

—De metroposcopia; seu, Methoposcopia naturali. Liber primus [-tertius]. Antverpiae, Ex Officina
Plantiuiana [sic] apud Balthassarem [sic] Morenum
[sic] 1648.

    3 v. in 1.   illus.   17 cm.   [4073]

Imperfect: signatures of sheet + of vol. 3 wrongly imposed.
Vol. 2 has imprint: Antverpiae, Ex Officina Plantiniana, apud
Balthassarem [sic] Moretum, 1648.
    Printed by Jacob Gaffarus of Naples. Cf. M. Sabbe. Falsche
Moretusdrucke. Gutenberg Jahrbuch, 1929, p. 193-214.

—De quatuor signis, quae apparent in unguibus
manuum . . . Neap. Typis Jacobi Gaffari, 1649.

    68, [3] p. illus., port. 16 cm.   [4074]

With this are bound: *his* Primo libro de nevi. 1632; Indagine,
J. ab. Introductiones apotelesmaticę elegantes. Lugduni, 1556.

—Primo libro de nevi . . . Antverpie, 1632.
    [14], 102, [1] p.   illus. 16 cm.   [4075]

Bound with *his* De quatuor signis, quae apparent in unguibus
manuum. 1649.

—Soliloquium salium Philippi Finelli. Neap.,
Typis Jacobi Gaffari, 1649.

    [14], 130, [6] p.   front. (port.)   15 cm. [4076]

FINGER, Christian Gottfried [*fl.* 1694] *praeses.*
Dissertatio physica de quotidiano corporis humani
decremento . . . Lipsiae, Typis Christophori
Fleischeri [1694]

    [16] p.   20 cm.   [4077]

Diss.—Leipzig (G. S. Cronpusch, *respondent*)

—*respondent. See* Ortlob, J. F., *praeses.* Disputatio
inauguralis de dentitione puerorum difficili. 1694.

—*See* Bohn, J. Facultatis Medicae in Academia
Lipsiensi p. t. procancellarius, D. Johannes Bohn . . .
L. S. D. 1694.

FINOLDT, Melchior [*fl.* 1605] *ed.* and *tr. See*
Seitz, A. Manuale medicum. 1605.

FINOT, Raymond Jacques [*fl.* 1700-1746] *respondent. See* Farcy, D. de, *praeses.* Quaestio medica . . .
An asthmati humido nicotiana? 1700.

FINXIUS, David [*fl.* 1607] *respondent. See*
Siegfried, J., *praeses.* Disputatio de melancholia.
1607.

FIOCCHETTO, Giovanni Francesco
[1564-1642] Trattato della peste, et pestifero contagio
di Torino, &c . . . Torino, Gio. Guglielmo Tisma,
1631.

    [4], 315, [27] p.   17 cm.   [4078]

FIORAVANTI, Leonardo [1517-1588] Three exact pieces of Leonard Phioravant . . . viz. his Rationall secrets, and Chirurgery, reviewed, and revived. Together with a book of excellent experiments
and secrets, collected out of the practises of severall
expert men in both faculties [by John Hester]
Whereunto is annexed Paracelsus his One hundred
and fourteen experiments: with certain excellent
works of B. G. a Portu Aquitano [i.e. B. G. Penot]
Also Isaac Hollandus his secrets concerning his
vegetall and animall work. With Quercetanus [i.e.
J. Duchesne] his Spagyrick antidotary for gun-shot.
London, Printed by G. Dawson, and sold by Richard
Lownds and William Nealand, 1652.

    4 v. in 1.   19 cm.   [4079]

Sudhoff 370.
    Vols. [2-4] have imprint: London, Printed by G. D., 1652.
    "To the reader" signed: J. H. [and] W. J. [i.e. John Hester and
William Johnson]
    "Short animadversions upon the book lately published by one
who stiles himselfe Noah Biggs, Helmontii psittacum," signed W.
I., and a letter addressed to "Friend Culpeper," signed W. J., are
followed by "The epistle to the reader," signed W. I. M. B. From
this last epistle it appears that the collection was assembled by
William Johnson, chiefly from translations by John Hester.
    Vol. [1], a short discourse of the secrets . . . (180 p.) is composed
of selections from Fioravanti's Secreti rationali, Capricci medicinali,
and Fisica.

—La cirugia . . . Distinta in tre libri. Nel primo
de' quali; si discorrono molte utili cose nella materia
cirugicale. Nel secondo, si tratta della anatomia, &
sue parti, & si mostra quanto al cirugico sia
necessaria. Nel terzo, si scrivono molte ricette di
diversi autori. Con una gionta de secreti nuovi,
dell'istesso autore. Venetia, Lucio Spineda, 1610.

    23, 182 ll.   6 cm.   [4080]

Contents the same as those of the 16th century editions, except
that the author's dedicatory epistles are omitted.
    "Libri da noi posti in luce, & le materie che in essi si contengono.
Cap. 83": leaves 179-180.

—[The same.] . . . Venetia, Lucio Spineda, 1630.
    [16], 182 ll. 15 cm.   [4081]

Different setting of type.

—[English tr.] *In* [Hester, J.] The excellencie of
physick and chirurgerie. 1652.

—Del compendio de' secreti rationali . . . Libri
cinque . . . Venetia, Pietro Miloco, 1620.

    [24], 185 + ll. 15 cm.   [4082]

Imperfect: all after leaf 185 wanting.

—[The same.] . . . Aggiuntovi in questa nostra ultima impressione alcuni secreti cavati dal Regimento della peste dell'istesso autore . . . Venetia, Zaccaria Conzatti, 1660.

[32], 320 p. 16 cm. [4083]

Imperfect: p. 1-2, 307-308, and 317-318 wanting.

—[The same.] . . . Venetia, Li Prodotti, 1675.

[32], 295 p. 16 cm. [4084]

—[German tr.] Compendium oder Ausszug der Secreten, Gehaymnissen und verborgenen Künsten . . . Jetzund auss dem Italienischen . . . ins Teutsch versetzet. Darmbstadt, Gedruckt durch Johann Leinhosen, in Verlegung Johann Berners, 1624.

399 p. 16 cm. [4085]

Imperfect: p. 277-278, 283-284 wanting.
With this is bound *his* Corona; oder, Kron der Artzney. 1618.

—De' capricci medicinali . . . libri quattro . . . Di nuovo dall' istesso auttore in molti luoghi, di secreti importantissimi, ampliati . . . Con molta diligenza revisti, corretti, & ristampati. Venetia, Lucio Spineda, 1602.

[20], 267 ll. illus. 15 cm. [4086]

Published in 1561 under title: Capricci medicinali.

—[The same.] . . . Venetia, Comino Gallina, 1617.

[18], 230 ll. illus. 16 cm. [4087]

—[The same.] . . . Venetia, Il Cestaro, 1647.

[20], 267 ll. illus. 15 cm. [4088]

A reprint of the 1602 edition.

—[The same.] . . . Venetia, Valentino Mortali, 1670.

[32], 380 p. illus. 17 cm. [4089]

—[The same.] . . . Venetia, Giacomo Zattoni, 1680.

346 (i.e. 350), [17] p. illus. 15 cm. [4090]

—[German tr.] Corona; oder, Kron der Artzney . . . in vier sonderbare Bücher unterscheiden . . . Erstlich neuwlich in intaliänischer Spraach von dem Autore selbst in Truck verfärtiget. Nunmehr aber in unsere hochteutsche Spraach . . . versetzt. Franckfurt am Mayn, Gedruckt bey Nicolaus Hoffmann, in Verlegung Johann Berrner, 1604.

[7], 507, [13] p. illus. 16 cm. [4091]

—[The same.] . . . Franckfurt am Mayn, Gedruckt bey Anthoni Hummen, in Verlegung Johann Berrners, 1618.

[7], 512, [13] p. illus. 16 cm. [4092]

Bound with *his* Compendium oder Ausszug der Secreten. 1624.

—Della fisica . . . Divisa in libri quattro. Nelli quali si discorrono molte, & diverse materie molto importanti . . . Venetia, Giacomo Zattoni, 1678.

[32], 365, [1] p. 15 cm. [4093]

—[Excerpts. English] *In* [Hester, J.] The excellencie of physick and chirurgerie. 1652.

—Dello specchio di scientia universale . . . libri tre. Nel primo de' quali, si tratta di tutte l'arti liberali, & mecanice . . . Nel secondo si tratta di diverse scientie, & di molte belle contemplationi de filosofi antichi. Nel terzo si contengono alcune inventioni notabili . . . Nuovamente ristampato, & con molte cose aggionte . . . Venetia, Lucio Spineda, 1603.

[16], 347 ll. 15 cm. [4094]

Identical in contents with the edition published in Venice in 1572. Wants the "Additioni" at the end of the edition of 1583.

—[The same.] . . . Venetia, Ad instan. del Curti, 1679.

[30], 446 p. 16 cm. [4095]

Based on the edition published in Venice in 1572, but with most of the preliminary matter omitted.

—Discorsi sopra la chirurgia. *In* Rostinio, P. Compendio di tutta la cirugia. 1607, 1677.

—Il reggimento della peste . . . Nel quale si tratta che cosa sia la peste, & da che procede, & quello che doveriano fare i prencipi per conservar i suoi popoli da essa; & ultimamente, si mostrano mirabili secreti da curarla . . . Di nuovo ristampato, corretto, & ampliato di diversi bellissimi secreti, & di settantasette dottissimi afforismi . . . In questa ultima impressione aggiuntovi alcuni secreti dati in luce dall'autore avanti la sua morte, pertinenti alla materia del libro. Venetia, Lucio Spineda, 1626.

141, [6] ll. 15 cm. [4096]

—[The same.] . . . Venetia, Giacomo Zattoni, 1680.

189 ll. 15 cm. [4097]

—Il tesoro della vita humana . . . Diviso in libri quattro. Nel primo, si tratta delle qualità, & cause di diverse infermità . . . Nel secondo, si descrivono molti esperimenti [medici] . . . Nel terzo, vi sono diverse lettere . . . dove si discorre cosi in fisica, come in cirugia. Nel quarto . . . sono rivelati i secreti più importanti di esso autore. Di nuovo ristampato . . .

Venetia, Il Spineda, 1629.

[16], 327 ll. 15 cm. [4098]

—[The same.] ... Di nuovo ristampato, & con diligenza corretto. Venetia, Il Brigna, 1673.

[16], 592 p. 17 cm. [4099]

—A discourse upon chyrurgery: written by ... Leonardo Phioravanti ... With a declaration of many wonderfull matters necessary to be knowne; with most notable secrets found out by the said authour. Translated out of Italian by John Hester, and now newly published and augmensed ... by Richard Booth, gent. London, Edward Allde, 1626.

[4], 118 p. 18 cm. [4100]

Imperfect: p. 113-114 wanting.
STC 10882.
A new edition of the compilation published in London in 1580 under title: A short discours ... uppon chirurgerie, including translations of extracts from several different works of Fioravanti.

—, ed. See ROSTINIO, P. Compendio di tutta la cirugia. 1607, 1677.

—See VICARY, T. The English mans treasure. 1613, 1633, 1641 [and] The surgions directorie. 1651; VIGO, G.de. La prattica universale in cirugia. 1605, 1622, 1639, 1647, 1669, 1685.

FIORDIBELLO, ANTONIO, *Bp.* [1510-1574] Panegyricus Carolo V. Rom. imperatori dictus, ad superiorum temporum illustrationem, editus ex bibliotheca Joachimi Morsii. Lugduni Batavorum, Excudebat Jacobus Marci, 1619.

[4], 20 p. 21 cm. [4101]

FIRMIANUS, LUCIUS CAECILIUS LACTANTIUS. *See* LACTANTIUS, Lucius Caecilius Firmianus.

FIRNHABER, JOHANN JAKOB [*fl.* 1617] *respondent.* See RÖSSEL, P., *praeses.* Disputatio physica de unione animae rationalis cum corpore. 1617.

FISCHBECK, ANDREAS WILHELM [*fl.* 1682] *respondent. See* MEIBOM, H., *praeses.* Disputatio medica inauguralis de lue venerea. 1682.

FISCHER, CHRISTIAN FRIEDRICH [*fl.* 1689] *respondent. See* HAMBERGER, G. A., *praeses.* Dissertatio optica de coloribus. 1689.

FISCHER, CONRAD [*fl.* 1694] *respondent. See* VESTI, J., *praeses.* Disputatio inauguralis medica de atrophia. 1694.

FISCHER, EBERHARD [*fl.* 1610-1612] *respondent. See* CRÜGER, B., *praeses.* Disputatio medica sexta. 1610; SENNERT, D., *praeses.* Disputatio medica, de pleuritide. 1611.

FISCHER, ELIAS [*fl.* 1622] *respondent. See* TAMITIUS, A. Disputatio physica de anima. 1622.

FISCHER, HEINRICH LEVIN, *ed. See* FEYENS, J. Physographia. 1644.

FISCHER, JOHANN GEORG [*fl.* 1665] *respondent. See* HUNDESHAGEN, J. C., *praeses.* Disputatio physica de fulmine. 1665.

FISCHER, JOHANN HEINRICH [*fl.* 1681] *respondent. See* MIRUS, A. E., *praeses.* Disputatio physica de monstris. 1681.

FISCHER, JOHANN PETER [*fl.* 1684-1686] *respondent.* Disputatio medica inauguralis de gonorrhoea virulenta ... Lugduni Batavorum, Apud Abrahamum Elzevier, 1686.

[20] p. 18 cm. [4102]

Diss.—Leyden.

—See WEDEL, G. W., *praeses.* Dissertatio medica, de casu ab alto. 1684.

FISCHER, LEVIN [*fl.* 1620-ca. 1640] Corpus medicinae imperiale, facili idea per certa & apodictica neotericorum verae artis principia ac panacei remediorum methodicorum, chymiatricorum specificorum normam, digestum. Annexis examine candidatorum medicinae, hactenus consueto resolutione casuum & aphorismorum Hippocrat. genuina ... Hemipoli, Sumptibus Hynitzschianis, 1680.

[16], 796 (i.e. 776), [20] p. 17 cm. [4103]

—See MERCKLIN, G. A. Sylloge physico-medicinalium casuum incantationi vulgo adscribi solitorum. 1698.

FISCHER, ZACHARIAS [*fl.* 1673] *respondent. See* FRENZEL, S. F., *praeses.* De rerum futurarum praesensione naturali. 1673.

FISH, JOHN [*fl.* 1700] *respondent.* Dissertatio physico-anatomica inauguralis de variis praeparationibus & immutationibus quas subeunt in diversis corporis partibus assumpta ... Lugduni Batavorum, Apud Abrahamum Elzevier, 1700.

[2], 28 p. 21 cm. [4104]

Diss.—Leyden.

FISIONOMIA naturale. 1606. *See* INGEGNERI, G., *Bp. of Capo d'Istria.*

FISKE, NICHOLAS [*fl.* 17th cent.] *ed. See* HEYDON, *Sir* C. An astrological discourse. 1650.

FISONOMIA naturale di Gio: Battista dalla Porta, Giovanni Ingegnieri [e] Polemone; & Fisonomia celeste del medesimo Porta. [Padova, Pietro Paolo Tozzi, 1622]
4 parts in 1 v. illus., ports. 23 cm. **[4105]**
General half-title; each part has special title page; parts [2] and [3] dated 1623.
These four works were issued together in one volume by the same publisher again in 1627, but apparently without the general half-title.

FISSCHER, HEINRICH [*fl.* 1657] *respondent.* Disputatio medica inauguralis, de suffocatione uterina ... Trajecti ad Rhenum, Typis Theodori ab Ackersdijck & Gisberti à Zijll, 1657.
[16] p. 20 cm. **[4106]**
Diss. — Utrecht.

FITZGERALD, ROBERT [1638?-1698] Salt-water sweetned; or, A true account of the great advantages of this new invention both by sea and by land: together with a full and satisfactory answer to all apparent difficulties. Also the approbation of the Colledge of Physicians. Likewise a letter of ... Robert Boyle to a friend upon the same subject ... 3d ed. with additions. London, William Cadman, 1683.
[1], 11, [2] p. 19 cm. **[4107]**
Fulton (A) 236.

—[Latin ed.] Aqua salsa dulcorata; sive, Accurata novi hujus arteficii, quatenus tum maris, tum portuum incolis, utilis, descriptio. Accessit praeterea plena omnium alicujus momenti contra novum hoc adinventum objectionum solutio. Nec non approbatio Collegii medicorum Londinensis. Epistola denique ... Roberti Boylii hac super re ad amicum conscripta. Londini, Impensis Edvardi Brewster, 1683.
[32] p. 20 cm. **[4108]**
Fulton (A) 236.

FIVE wonders seene in England. Two at Barnstable, one at Kirkham, one in Cornwall, one in Little Britain in London. In all which places whereby Gods judgements are miraculously seene upon some ... The 2d impression with additions, and certificate from those who were eye witnesses thereof ... London, J. C., 1646.
[1], 6 p. 18 cm. **[4109]**

FLACCUS, AULUS PERSIUS. *See* PERSIUS FLACCUS, Aulus.

FLACH, NIKOLAUS ANTON [*fl.* 1681] *respondent.* Dissertatio medica inauguralis de callo ... Argentorati, Literis Staedelianis [1681]
32 p. 20 cm. **[4110]**
Diss. — Strasbourg.

FLACHS, ANDREAS [*fl.* 1660] *respondent. See* KIRCHMAYER, G. K., *praeses.* De aranea. 1660.

FLÄSCHER-BAADWASSER, das ist: seiner Situation, Ursprungs, Eigenschafft, Natur, Würkung, Gebrauchs ... kurtze Andeutung ... Bregentz, Getruckt bey Bartholome Schnell, 1669.
17, [1] p. 16 cm. **[4111]**

FLAMANT [*fl.* 1690] L'art de se conserver la santé; ou, Le medecin de soy-mesme. Avec un traité de quelques remedes ... pour la guerison de differentes maladies ... Paris, Estienne Michallet, 1692.
[24], 224, [12] p. 15 cm. **[4112]**

—[The same.] ... Amsterdam, Arnoux et Reniers Leers, 1692.
[24], 224, [12] p. 15 cm. **[4113]**
Imperfect: sig. ai and Kx wanting; sig. aii-aix mutilated. Different setting of type.

—[The same.] ... Paris, Estienne Michalet, 1693.
[16], 146, [6] p. 13 cm. **[4114]**

—Le veritable medecin; ou, Le moyen de se conserver la santé ... Avec plusieurs remedes simples ... Paris, Estienne Michalet, 1699.
[24], 379, [4] p. 16 cm. **[4115]**

FLAMEL, NICOLAS [*d.* 1418] Le sommaire philosophique. *In* La metallique transformation. 1618.

—Tractatus brevis; sive, Summarium philosophicum ...
172-179 p. 22 cm. (*In* Musaeum Hermeticum. Francofurti, 1678) **[4116]**
Caption title.

—*See* ARNAULD, P. Trois traitez de la philosophie naturelle. 1612; HOUPREGHT, J. F., *comp.* Aurifontina chymica. 1680; SALMON, W. Medicina practica. 1692; ZACAIRE, D. Opusculum philosophiae naturalis metallorum. 1659.

FLAMENT. *See* FLAMANT [*fl.* 1690]

FLAMINIUS, GULIELMUS [*fl.* 1693] *respondent.* Disputatio medica inauguralis de angina ... Lugduni Batavorum, Apud Abrahamum Elzevier, 1693.

[20] p. 22 cm. [4117]

Diss.—Leyden.

FLAMMERDINGE, JOHANN VON [*fl.* 1669-1671] *respondent.* Disputatio medica inauguralis de tumoribus lienis ... Lugduni Batavorum, Apud viduam & haeredes Joannis Elsevirii, 1671.

[42] p. plates. 22 cm. [4118]

Diss.—Leyden.

—*See* DRELINCOURT, C., *praeses.* Disputatio medica de apoplexia. 1671; LE BOË, F. de. Disputatio medica de ischuria. 1671; MATTHAEUS, P., *praeses.* Disputatio medica de passione iliaca. 1669.

FLAVIANUS, REMMIUS. Carmen de ponderibus et mensuris. *In* Celsus, A. C. De re medica libri octo. 1608, 1625; Serenus Sammonicus, Q. De medicina praecepta saluberrima. 1662.

FLAYDER [*fl.* 1669] *tr. See* LA FORGE, L. de. Tractatus de mente humana. 1669, 1673, 1688.

FLEMLØSE, PEDER JACOBSEN [*ca.* 1554-*ca.* 1598] En elementisch oc jordisch astrologia ... [Kiøbenhaffn, 1644]

[176] p. 16 cm. [4119]

Bound with Aalborg, N. M. Medicin eller laege-boog. 1640.

FLENDER, JOHANN [*fl.* 17th cent.] *ed. See* LA FORGE, L. de. Tractatus de mente humana. 1688.

FLETCHER, J., *M.D. of Cambridge. See* FLETCHER, John [1556?-1613]

FLETCHER, JOHN [1556?-1613]. The differences, causes, and judgements of urine: according to the best writers thereof ... London, John Legatt, 1641.

[15], 134, [16] p. illus. 15 cm. [4120]

FLETCHER, PHINEAS [1582-1650] The purple island; or, The isle of man. Together with Piscatorie eclogs and other poeticall miscellanies. By P[hineas] F[letcher] Cambridge, Printers to the Universitie, 1633.

[13], 181 p.; [1], 130 (i.e. 126), [2] p. 20 cm. [4121]

Printed by T. & J. Buck. Cf. Bowes. No. 49.
Part [2] and "Elisa, or, An elegie upon the unripe decease of

Sr. Antonie Irby ..." (p. [103]-130 at end) have special title pages. STC 11082.

FLETCHER, RICHARD [*fl.* 1676] A character of a true physician; or, A true chymist compared with a goose-quill pedant. With a short view of the frauds and abuses in physick, committed by the confederate prescribing doctoral methodists, with their combinators the apothecaries ... London, Printed for the author, 1676.

30, [1] p. 16 cm. [4122]

FLICCIUS, JOHANN HEINRICH [*fl.* 1685] *respondent. See* FRANCK VON FRANCKENAU, G., *praeses.* Disputatio inauguralis medica exhibens casum viri empyemate ex pleuritide laborantis. 1685.

FLÖSSERUS, JOANNES ERASMUS [*fl.* 1609] *See* SCHRÖTER, J. F., *praeses.* Αγωνισμα medicum. 1609.

FLOREBELLI, ANTONIO. *Bp. of Lavello. See* FIORDIBELLO, Antonio, *Bp.* [1510-1574]

FLOREBELLUS, ANTONIUS, Mutinensis. *See* FIORDIBELLO, Antonio, *Bp.* [1510-1574]

FLORENCE. Accademia Del Cimento. *See* ACCADEMIA DEL CIMENTO, Florence.

—**Arte de' Medici e Degli Speziali.** *See* ARTE DE' MEDICI E DEGLI SPEZIALI, Florence.

—**Collegio de' Medici.** *See* ARTE DE' MEDICI E DEGLI SPEZIALI, Florence.

—**(City) Magistrato di sanità.** Provisione de mol. mag. sig. uffitiali della sanita. Che li beccai mantenghino netti li scannatio, non si possa scannare ò suentrare bestie per le strade, che li minugìai votino le budella in Arno fuori delle porti ... Firenze, Heredi di Christofano Marescotti [1616]

[8] p. 21 cm. [4123]

—**(City) Ordinances, local laws, etc.** Instruzione del magistrato della sanità di Firenze, Per li rettori di giustizia di fuori ne casi di mali di contagio, che si scoprissero nelle loro jurisdizioni, in particolare per i contadi, e ville. Firenze, Zanobi Pignoni, 1630.

[8] p. 21 cm. [4124]

Signed by Niccolò Magnani.

—Ordini per la quarantena. Fiorenza, Per Zanobi Pignoni, 1630.

broadside. 47 x 30 cm. [4125]

Imperfect: mutilated with loss of text.
Signed by Niccolò Magnani.

—Proroga della quarantena . . . Fiorenza, Zanobi Pignoni, 1630.

    broadside.   42 x 30 cm.   **[4126]**

Signed by Niccolò Magnani.

FLORENTIUS, Henricus [*fl.* 1617–1637] *ed. See* Pauw, P. Tractatus de peste. 1637.

FLORES poetici quibus coronam doctoralem medicam . . . Jo. Jacobo Osvaldo . . . a . . . Jacobo Rot . . . collegii medic. . . . prodecano . . . impositam exornare dignati sunt gratulabundi . . . amici. Basileae, Literis Joh. Ludovici Koenig et Johan. Brandmylleri [1687]

    [8] p.   19 cm.   **[4127]**

Bound with Oschwald, J. J. Disputatio inauguralis medica. [1687]

FLORETUS A BETHABOR. Traum-Gesicht, welches Ben-Adam, zur Zeit der Regierung Rucharetz, des Königes von Adama, gehabt, und an Tag gegeben hat, Floretus à Bethabor. Mit noch einem andern Tractätlein von der Reise Friedrich Galli, nach der Einöde S. Michael. Hamburg, Johann Naumann, 1682.

    [15] p.   17 cm.   **[4128]**

FLORIBUS, Johann Martin [*b.* 1672] *respondent. See* Slevogt, J. A., *praeses.* Puellam variolis malignis laborantem . . . sistit J. M. F. 1699.

—*See* slevogt, J. A. Facultatis Medicae decani Jo. Hadriani Slevogtii . . . publica invitatio ad dissertationem inauguralem de puella. 1699.

FLORIDAN, *pseud. See* Birken, Sigmund von [1626–1681]

FLORIO, Michele [*fl.* 1656] Cladis epidemiae florentissimam Neapolitanam urbem devastantis lacrymabilis laconismus . . . Veronae, Apud Franciscum Rossi, 1661.

    [23], 114 p.   14 cm.   **[4129]**

FLORUS, Friedrich Christopher [*fl.* 1690] *respondent. See* Vesti, J., *praeses.* Dissertatio medica de colica. 1690.

FLOYER, *Sir* John [1649–1734] An enquiry into the right use and abuses of the hot, cold, and temperate baths in England . . . To this is added I. An extract of Dr. Jones's treaty on Buxton-bath . . . II. A letter from Dr. Clayton . . . concerning the use of St. Mungus-well. III. An abstract of some cures perform'd by the bath at Buxton . . . London, R.

Clavel, 1697.

    [70], 144 p.   16 cm.   **[4130]**

—Φαρμακο-βασανος; or, The touch-stone of medicines. Discovering the vertues of vegetables, minerals, & animals, by their tastes & smells. In two volumes . . . London, Printed for Michael Johnson, and sold at his shops, 1687.

    2 v. in 1.   20 cm.   **[4131]**

Imperfect: sig. A1 wanting.

Vol. 2 has half title.

". . . The sixth part . . ." (p. [249]–340) and "An appendix to the second part . . ." (p. [341]–416 at end of vol. 2) have special title pages dated 1690.

—Another issue, with imprint: London, Printed for Michael Johnson, and sold by Robert Clavel, 1687.

    Vol. 1 only.   **[4132]**

—The preternatural state of animal humours described, by their sensible qualities, which depend on the different degrees of their fermentation . . . To this treatise are added two appendixes. I. About the nature of fevers . . . II. Concerning . . . tumours, pains, and fluxes of humours . . . especially those in the gout and asthma . . . By the author of the Φαρμακο-βασανος. London, Printed by W. Downing for Michael Johnson and sold by Robert Clavel, Sam Smith and Benjamin Walford, 1696.

    [23], 264 p.   20 cm.   **[4133]**

—A treatise of the asthma. Divided into four parts . . . London, Richard Wilkin, 1698.

    [40], 247 p.   17 cm.   **[4134]**

—*See* Vallerius, N. Tentamina physico-chymica. 1699.

FLUCTIBUS, Robertus de. *See* Fludd, Robert [1574–1637]

FLUDD, Robert [1574–1637] Anatomie amphitheatrum effigie triplici, more et conditione varia, designatum . . . Francofurti [Typis Erasmi Kempferi] Sumptibus Johannis Theodori de Bry, 1623.

    [4], 331 p.   illus., port.   32 cm.   **[4135]**

Engraved title page.

Special title page (p. 1) reads: Sectionis primae portio tertia de anatomia triplici in partes tres divisa.

"Monochordum mundi symphoniacum; seu, Replicatio Roberti Flud . . . ad apologiam . . . Joannis Kepleri, adversus Demonstrationem suam analyticam, nuperrime editam . . ." (p. [287]–331) has special title page.

—Doctor Fludds answer unto M. Foster; or, The squesing of parson Fosters sponge, ordained by him for the wiping away of the weapon-salve ... London, Nathanael Butter, 1631.

[8], 144, 68 p. 19 cm.   [4136]

STC 11120.

—Responsum ad Hoplocrisma-spongum M. Fosteri ... ab ipso, ad unguenti amarii validitatem delendam ordinatum; hoc est, Spongiae M. Fosteri ... expressio seu elisio ... Goudae, Excudebat Petrus Rammazenius, 1638.

30, [1] ll. 33 cm.   [4137]

Errata: ll. [1]

—Discursus de unguento armario.

507-513 p. 21 cm. (*In* Theatrum sympatheticum auctum. Norimbergae, 1662)   [4138]

Caption title.

—Medicina catholica; seu, Mysticum artis medicandi sacrarium. In tomos divisum duos. In quibus metaphysica et physica tam sanitatis tuendae, quam morborum propulsandorum ratio pertractatur ... Francofurti, Typis Caspari Rötelii, impensis Wilhelmi Fitzeri, 1629-1631.

2 v. illus., plates, port. 32 cm., 33 cm.
                                            [4139]

Imperfect: folded plate entitled Medicamentosum Apollinis oraculum (at end of vol. 2) wanting.

Contents—Vol. 1 [pt. 1] Sanitatis mysterium ... Cui, in fine ... responsum ad Martini Mersenni calumnias annectitur, with half title.—[pt. 2] Sophiae cum moria certamen, in quo, lapis lydius a falso structore, Fr. Marino Mersenno ... reprobatus ... examinat, with caption title.—[pt. 3] Summum bonum ... insignis calumniatoris ... Marini Mersenni dedecus publicatum, with special title page.

Vol. 2 has title: Integrum morborum mysterium; sive, Medicinae catholicae tomi primi tractatus secundus, in sectiones distributus duas. Francofurti, Typis excusus Wolfgangi Hofmanni, prostat in officina Guilielmi Fitzeri, 1631. Includes: Καθολικον medicorum κατοπτρον: ... sive tomi primi, tractatus secundi, sectio secunda, de morborum signis ... 1631, with special title page.—Pulsus; seu, Nova et arcana pulsuum historia ... hoc est, portionis tertiae ars tertia, de pulsuum scientia, with half title.

—Philosophia moysaica. In qua sapientia & scientia creationis & creaturarum sacra vereque Christiana ... ad amussim & enucleate explicatur ... Goudae, Petrus Rammazenius, 1638.

[4], 152 (i.e. 144) ll. illus. 32 cm.   [4140]

—[English tr.] Mosaicall philosophy: grounded upon the essentiall truth or eternal sapience. Written first in Latin, and afterwards thus rendred into English ... London, Humphrey Moseley, 1659.

[6], 300 p. illus. 30 cm.   [4141]

"The second section ..." has special title page (p. [127]).

—Philosophia sacra & vere Christiana; seu, Meteorologia cosmica. Francofurti, Prostat in Officina Bryana, 1626.

[6], 303 p. illus., plate. 32 cm.   [4142]

Imperfect: sig.):(¹ (blank?) wanting.

Bound with vol. 2 of his Utriusque cosmi ... metaphisica ... historia. 1617-1621.

—Tractatus apologeticus integritatem Societatis de Rosea Cruce defendens. In qua probatur contra D. Libavii & aliorum ejusdem farinae calumnias, quod admirabilia nobis a Fraternitate R. C. oblata, sine improba magiae impostura, aut diaboli praestigiis & illusionibus praestari possint. Authore R. De Fluctibus ... Lugduni Batavorum, Apud Godefridum Basson, 1617.

196 p. illus. 16 cm.   [4143]

—Utriusque cosmi majoris scilicet et minoris metaphysica, physica atque technica historia in duo volumina secundum cosmi differentiam divisa. Tomus primus de macrocosmi historia in duos tractatus divisa ... Oppenhemii, Aere Johan-Theodori de Bry, typis Hieronymi Galleri, 1617-1621.

2 v. illus., plate. 32 cm.   [4144]

Engraved title page.

Vol. 1 part [2] has special engraved title page: Tractatus secundus de naturae simia; seu, Technica macrocosmi historia in partes undecim divisa ... 1618.

Vol. 2 has engraved title page: Tomus secundus de supernaturali, naturali, praeternaturali et contranaturali microcosmi historia, in tractatus tres distributa ... 1619.

"Tomi secundi tractatus primi, sectio secunda, de technica microcosmi historia, in portiones VII. divisa" has half title.

"Tomi secundi tractatus secundus, de praeternaturali utriusque mundi historia. In sectiones tres divisa ... Francofurti, Typis Erasmi Kempfferi, sumptibus Joan. Theodori de Bry, 1621" has special title page. This last item contains "Section prima" only. The other two sections were never completed.

With vol. 2 of this are bound *his* Veritatis proscenium. 1621; *his* Philosophia sacra. 1626.

—Veritatis proscenium, in quo aulaeum erroris tragicum dimovetur ... seu, Demonstratio quaedam analytica, in qua cuilibet comparationis particulae, in appendice quadam a Joanne Kepplero, nuper in fine Harmoniae suae mundanae edita; factae inter harmoniam suam mundanam, & illam Roberti Fludd, ipsissimis veritatis argumentis respondetur ... Francofurti, Typis Erasmi Kemfferi, sumptibus

Joan. Theodor. de Bry, 1621.

    54 p. illus. 32 cm. [**4145**]

Bound with vol. 2 of *his* Utriusque cosmi . . . metaphysica . . . historia. 1617-1621.

—*See* PRAETORIUS, J. Ludicrum chiromanticum Praetorii. 1661.

—*as subject. See* GASSENDI, P. Epistolica exercitatio, in qua principia philosophiae Roberti Fluddi medici reteguntur. 1630.

FOCHETTI, MADAMA. *See* FOUQUET, Marie (de Maupeou) *vicomtesse de Vaux* [1590-1681]

FÖGGLER, JÁNOS [*fl.* 1661] *respondent. See* SCHNEIDER, K. V., *praeses.* Disputatio inauguralis de phthisi. 1661.

FÖGGLERUS, JOHANNES BAPTISTA. *See* FÖGGLER, János [*fl.* 1661]

FÖRSTER, CHRISTIAN WILHELM [*b.* 1656] *respondent. See* DEHN ROTFELSER, J. F. Dissertationis [sic] inauguralis chymico-medica de experimentorum chymicorum. 1680; WEDEL, G. W., *praeses.* Dissertatio medica inauguralis de procidentia uteri. 1684.

—*See* WEDEL, G. W. Propempticon inaugurale de fundamentis methodicorum. 1684.

FÖRSTER, GOTTFRIED [*fl.* 1660-1663] *respondent. See* MÖBIUS, G., *praeses.* Dissertatio medica inauguralis de ardore ventriculi. 1660.

FÖRTER, DAVID [*fl.* 1602] *tr. See* BAUHIN, J. Ein new Badbuch. 1602.

FÖRTSCH, JOHANN PHILIPP [*fl.* 1681] *respondent. See* MAJOR, J. D., *praeses.* Disputatio medica inauguralis de petechiis. 1681.

FOES, ANUCE [1528-1595] Oeconomia Hippocratis alphabeti serie distincta. Opus . . . in quo dictionum apud Hippocratem omnium . . . usus explicatur, & velut ex amplissimo penu depromitur, ita ut lexici, & concordantiarum Hippocratearum vicem implere possit . . . Genevae, Typis & sumptibus Samuelis Chouët, 1662.

    [8], 418 p. 39 cm. [**4146**]

Edited by Étienne Le Clerc.

A separate issue of the last section of Chouet's two volume edition of Hippocrates' works, 1657-1662.

—, *ed.* and *tr. See* HIPPOCRATES. (Collected works. Greek and Latin] Τὰ εὑρισκόμενα. 1621, 1624 1657, 1662.

—, *tr. See* GALENUS. *In* Aphorismos Hippocratis commentaria. 1633; HIPPOCRATES. [Aphorismi. Greek and Latin. 1633] [and] [Aphorismi. English. 1665] [and] [Aphorismi. Adaptations, etc. Latin. 1647, 1669] [and] [Coacae praenotiones. 1660] [and] [Prognostica. Greek and Latin] 1645; MORALIS, G. Commentaria in magni Hippocratis Coi Aphorismos. 1648.

FOGEROLAEUS, FRANCISCUS. *See* FOUGEROLLES, François de [*ca.* 1560-1620]

FOGLIA, GIOVANNI ANTONIO [*fl.* 1620] De anginosa passione, crustosis malignisque tonsillarum, et faucium ulceribus. Per . . . Neapolis civitatem, multaque regni loca vagantibus . . . Neapoli, Ex typographia Tarquinii Longi, 1620.

    [8], 136 (i.e. 138), [1] p. 21 cm. [**4147**]

Errata: p. [139]

FOLIGNO, GENTILE DA. *See* GENTILE DA FOLIGNO [*d.* 1348]

FOLLI, CECILIO. *See* FOLLIO, Cecilio [1615-1660]

FOLLINUS, HERMANNUS [*fl.* 1612-1618] Amuletum Antonianum; seu, Luis pestiferae fuga. In duos libros distributa, multisque remediis usu & observatione cognitis expedita; cui accessit utilis libellus de cauteriis . . . Antverpiae, Apud Hieronymum Verdussium, 1618.

    [22], 310 (i.e. 312) p. port. 16 cm. [**4148**]

"De cauteriis" (p. 279-310, with special title page) is mainly extracted from the work of the same title by Thomas Feyens, to whom the work is dedicated.

With this are bound: Claves, Gaston Le Doux, known as Gaston de. Philosophia chymica. 1612. — Duchesne, J. Liber de priscorum philosophorum verae medicinae materia. 1613. — Billich, A. G. De tribus chymicorum principiis. 1621.

—Den Nederlandtsche sleutel van t' secreet der philosophie, in welck grondelijc bewesen wert, d' aert, so in 't generael, als in 't bysonder aller metallen . . . En die gheheele alchijmie, met haer verborgendtheden. Midtsgaders d' eerste materie der philosophen, dat is Quinta essentia des wijns met haren volcoinen ghebruyck, en verclaringhe aller duystere woorden des voorsz. constes, op dat Paracelsus claerijck in alles mach werden verstaen . . . Haerlem, Ghedruckt by Adriaen Rooman, door Daniel de Keyser, 1613.

    76 ll. illus. 15 cm. [**4149**]

With this are bound: Jacobs, H. Het schat der armen. 1609. — Paracelsus. Dat secreet der philosophien. 1612.

—Speculum naturae humanae; sive, Mores et temperamenta hominum usque ad intimos animorum sensus cognoscendi, olim ab Hermanno Follino ... Belgico idiomate concinnatum, & methodo Aristotelis illustratum, nunc vero studio et opera ejusdem filii Joannis Follini Latinitate donatum ... Coloniae Agrippinae, Apud Jodocum Kalcovium, 1649.

[20], 158 p. 14 cm.   [4150]

Bound with Follinus, J. Synopsis tuendae et conservandae bonae valetudinis. 1648.

—*See* FOLLINUS, J. Synopsis tuendae et conservandae bonae valetudinis. 1646.

FOLLINUS, JOANNES [*fl.* 1646–1649] Synopsis tuendae et conservandae bonae valetudinis. Ex probatissimis quibusque authoribus digesta ... Coloniae Agrippinae, Typis viduae Valentini Clementis, 1646.

[16], 231 (i.e. 221) p. 14 cm.   [4151]

Added engraved title page.

"Orationes duae, quarum prior est de natura febris peticularis ejusque curatione; posterior de studiis Hippocraticis conjungendis cum chymicis [habitae ab Hermanno Follino]" (p. [137]–231, i.e. 221) has special title page.

Bound with Regimen sanitatis Salernitanum. Schola Salernitana. 1649.

—[The same.] ... Ed. 2. auctior & correctior. Coloniae Agrippinae, Typis viduae Hartgeri Woringii, sumptibus Jodoci Kalcovii, 1648.

[24], 113 p. 14 cm.   [4152]

Added engraved title page.

With this are bound: *his* Tyrocinium medicinae practicae. 1648. — Follinus, H. Speculum naturae humanae. 1649. — Wier, J. Medicarum observationum rararum liber I. 1657.

—Tyrocinium medicinae practicae ex probatissimis authoribus digestum ... Coloniae Agrippinae, Typis viduae Hartgeri Woringii, sumptibus Jodoci Kalcovii, 1648.

[22], 194 p. 14 cm.   [4153]

Bound with *his* Synopsis tuendae et conservandae bonae valetudinis. 1648.

—, *tr. See* FOLLINUS, H. Speculum naturae humanae. 1649.

FOLLIO, CECILIO [1615–1660] *See* BERNARDI, F. L'ignoranza convinta. 1669.

FONES, THOMAS [*fl.* 1669] *respondent.* Disputatio medica inauguralis de opthalmia ... Lugduni Batavorum, Apud viduam & haeredes Joannis Elsevirii, 1669.

[8] p. 19 cm.   [4154]

Diss. — Leyden.

FONSECA, FERNANDO SOLIS DA [*fl.* 1584–1585] Regimento per a conservar a saude e vida. Em dous dialogos. O primeiro trata do regimento das seis cousas naõ naturais, o segundo, de qualidades do ar, de sitios, & mantimentos do termo da cidade de Lisboa ... Lisboa, Geraldo da Vinha, 1626.

[8], 76 ll. 14 cm.   [4155]

FONSECA, RODRIGO DE [*d.* 1622] Consultationes medicae singularibus remediis refertae ... Accessit de consultandi ratione breve compendium, & consultatio de plica Polonica ... Venetiis, Apud Joannem Guerilium, 1619–1622.

2 v. in 1. 32 cm.   [4156]

Vol. 2 has title: Consultationum medicinalium tomus secundus.

—[The same.] ... Francofurti ad Moenum, Typis Wechelianis, apud Danielem & Davidem Aubrios & Clementem Schleichium, 1625.

[32], 608 p. 16 cm.   [4157]

—[The same.] Consultationum medicinalium tomus primus [-secundus] In quo singularia remedia proponuntur ... Accessit de consultandi ratione breve compendium, & consultatio de plica Polonica ... Venetiis, Apud Joannem Guerilium, 1628.

2 v. in 1. 33 cm.   [4158]

Imperfect: p. 1–40 of vol. 1 wanting.
A reprint of the 1619–22 Venice edition.

—De tuenda valetudine, et producenda vita liber ... Florentiae, Apud Bartholomaeum Sermartellium juniorem, 1602.

[7], 124 p. 23 cm.   [4159]

Imperfect: p. 73–76 wanting.

—[The same.] ... Francofurti, Ex Officina Paltheniana, 1603.

[8], 292, [15] p. 17 cm.   [4160]

"De vera ratione curandi bubonis, atque carbunculi pestilentis, deque eorundem praecautione commentarius. Auctore Joan. Baptista Gemma ... 3. ed. prioribus emendatior, ac locupletior ..." (p. [189]–292) has special title page.

—[Italian tr.] Del conservare la sanita ... Tradotta dal latino in toscano da Poliziano Mancini da Montepulciano ... Firenze, Antonio Semartelli, 1603.

[8], 147, [9] p. 21 cm.   [4161]

—In septem Aphorismorum Hippocratis libros commentaria, eo ordine contexta, quo doctoratus puncta exponi consuevere. Quibus accessere ejusdem auctoris in singulas sententias adnotationes . . . Venetiis, Apud Joannem Antonium & Jacobum de Franciscis, 1608.

[4], 246 (i.e. 248) ll.   22 cm.   [4162]

—[The same.] . . . Accessit huic 3. ed. ejusdem auctoris Tractatus de remediis febrium acutarum, & pestilentium . . . Venetiis, Apud Joannem Guerilium, 1621.

[4], 248 ll.; [8], 112 p.   21 cm.   [4163]

Printer's error: sig. V3v, V4r, V5v, V6r blank, text supplied in manuscript.

Part [2] has special title page.

—[The same.] Commentaria in septem libros Aphorismorum Hippocratis . . . Accessit huic 4. ed. index aphorismorum . . . Venetiis, Apud Joannem Guerilium, 1628.

[8], 248 ll.   23 cm.   [4164]

A reprint of part [1] of the 1621 edition. The Tractatus de remediis febrium acutarum is not included.

—See GIACHINI, L. Methodus curandar. febrium. 1615.

FONT, CHARLES DE LA. See LA FONT, Charles de [d. 1707]

FONTAINE, GABRIEL [fl. 1655] D. Gabrielis Fontani . . . De veritate Hippocraticae medicinae firmissimis rationum & experimentorum momentis stabilita, & demonstrata; seu, Medicina antihermetica, in qua dogmata medica . . . contra Paracelsi, & Hermeticorum placita . . . promulgantur . . . Adjectus est . . . Apologeticon adversus Van-Helmont, ubi . . . demonstratur, quatuor humores Galenistarum non esse fictitios . . . Lugduni, Sumpt. Philip. Borde, Laur. Arnaud, & Cl. Rigaud, 1657.

[28], 464, [30] p.   [4165]

FONTAINE, JACQUES [d. 1621] Jacobi Fontani . . . Opera: in quibus universae artis medicae secundum Hippocratis & Galeni doctrinam, partes quatuor methodice explicantur. Praeponuntur libri duo De demonstratione medica ad artem medicinae comparandam penitus necessarii. Cum indicibus librorum, rerum item verborum. Parisiis, Apud Hadrianum Perier, 1612.

[4], 891 p.; 285 p.   25 cm.   [4166]

Imperfect: index "rerum" and "verborum" wanting.

"Alexandri Aphrodisei . . . De febribus liber": p. 271–285, at end.

—[The same.] . . . Accesserunt Commentaria in omnes Hippocratis Aphorismos absolutissima, & Crisium doctrina: nec non Consilia medica ejusdem autoris accuratissima. Cum indicibus librorum, rerum item & verborum. Coloniae Allobrogum, Apud Petrum Jacobum Chouet, 1613.

[4], 891 (i.e. 879) p.; 285 p.; 182 p.   25 cm.   [4167]

A reissue of the 1612 Paris editon. The first four leaves are reprinted, and the last three works (182 p. at end) added.

Imperfect: index "rerum" and "verborum" wanting.

"Commentaria in Hipp[ocratis] Aph[orismos] cum docta, brevi, fida, ac perspicua enarratione, novaque methodo" (p. [1]–95, part [3]) includes Latin text of the Aphorismi, in a subject arrangement.

—Jacobi Fontani . . . Commentaria in Hipp[ocratis] omnes Aph[orismos] cum docta, brevi, fida, ac perspicua enarratione, novaque methodo . . . Ejusdem tractatus absolutissimi, De crisiων & morborum causis, aliique nonnulli, in quo priori, Fracastorii sententia de cris. causis erudite defenditur . . . Parisiis, Apud Adrianum Beys, 1608.

[8], 215, [15] p.; 70 p.   15 cm.   [4168]

Includes Latin text of the Aphorismi, in a subject arrangement.

—De astrologia medica liber, in quo ex principiis naturalibus & corpori humano insitis probatur evidentissime vana esse ea omnia quae astrologi judiciarii de hominum moribus, institutis, morbis, crisibus & illorum morborum curationibus asserverunt. Authore Jacobo Fontano . . . Lugduni, Apud Thomam Soubron, 1620.

[5], 154 p.   15 cm.   [4169]

—Methodus generalis cognoscendi, praedicendi, et curandi morbos eorumque symptomata. Ad veterum, maximeque Hippocratis & Galeni normam exacta . . . Authore Jacobo Fontano . . . Avenione, Ex typog. Jacobi Bramerau, 1601.

[16], 324 p.   17 cm.   [4170]

With this is bound Rondelet, G. De ponderibus, sive de justa quantitate & proportione medicamentorum. Lugduni, 1563.

—[The same.] Methodus generalis et specialis cognoscendi & curandi morbos. Parisiis, Apud Hadrianum Beys, 1612.

7, [5], 184 p.   18 cm.   [4171]

Lacks the "Exercitationes tres" appended to the 1601 edition.

Bound with Brissot, P. Apologetica disceptatio. 1622.

—Jacobi Fontani . . . Practica curandorum morborum corporis humani, in quatuor libros distincta. Nunc primum in lucem edita. Parisiis, Apud

Adrianum Beys, M. XC. XI. [1611?]

[10], 572 p.   19 cm.   [4172]

—, *ed. See* ARISTOTELES. Phisiognomia. 1611.

—*See* CATELAN, L. Discours. 1614.

FONTAINE, JEHAN DE LA. *See* JEAN DE LA FONTAINE [*b.* 1381]

FONTANA, ALESSANDRO [*d.* 1554].*See* ROSTINIO, P. Trattato di mal francese. 1623.

FONTANON, DENYS [*d.* 1544?] De morborum internorum curatione libri quatuor ... Quibus accesserunt: Selectae observationes chirurgicae quinque & viginti, Gulielmi Fabricii Hildani ... Item ejusdem De gangraena & sphacelo tractatus methodicus & succinctus. Lugduni, Apud Antonium de Harcy, 1607.

[31], 839 p.   illus.   12 cm.   [4173]

"Gulielmi Fabricii Hildani De gangraena et sphacelo tractatus methodicus ..." (p. [707]-839) has special title page dated 1605.

FONTANUS, GABRIEL. *See* FONTAINE, Gabriel [*fl.* 1655]

FONTANUS, JACOBUS. *See* FONTAINE, Jacques [*d.* 1621]

FONTANUS, NICOLAUS. *See* FONTEYN, Nicolaas [*fl.* 1622-1644]

FONTE, LELIO DA. *See* BISCACCIANTI DA FONTE, Lelio [*d.* 1643]

FONTE EUGUBINO, LELIO A. *See* BISCACCIANTI DA FONTE, Lelio [*d.* 1643]

FONTECHA, JUAN ALONSO Y DE LOS RUYZES DE. *See* ALONSO Y DE LOS RUYZES DE FONTECHA, Juan [1560-1620]

FONTENETTES, LOUIS DE [1612-1661] *tr. See* HIPPOCRATES. [Aphorismi; Adaptations, etc. 1654]

FONTEYN, NICOLAAS [*fl.* 1622-1644] Nicolai Fontani Commentarius in Sebastianum Austrium ... De puerorum morbis. In frontispicia adjecti Aphorismi Hippocratis, noviter natorum adfectus enarrantes. Amstelodami, Apud Joannem Janssonium, 1642.

[16], 556 p.   plates.   13 cm.   [4174]

Includes the text of Austrius' work.

—Florilegium medicum, in quo flores universae medicinae, tam theoricae, quam practicae, per partes distinctas proponuntur, & raris, utilibus illustribusque quaestionibus exornantur ... Auctore Nicolao Fontano. Amstelredami, Apud Henricum Bernardi, 1637.

[40], 293 p.   13 cm.   [4175]

—Fons, seu origo febrium, earumque remedia ... Auctore Nicolao Fontano. Amsterdami, Apud Joannem Blaeu, 1644.

[32], 122 p.   14 cm.   [4176]

—Institutiones pharmaceuticae, ex Bauderonio & Du Boys in pharmacopoeorum gratiam potissimum concinnatae. Amstelodami, Ex typographia Jacobi Charpentier, 1633.

[12], 327, [20] p.   13 cm.   [4177]

—Nicolai Fontani Observationum rariorum analecta. Amstelodami, Sumptibus Henrici Laurentii, 1641.

[20], 126, [1] p.   illus.   20 cm.   [4178]

Errata: p. [127]

—Responsionum & curationum medicinalium liber unus. Auctore Nicolao Fontano ... Amstelodami, Typis Joannis Janssonii, 1639.

179, [21] p.   14 cm.   [4179]

—Syntagma medicum de morbis mulierum in libros IV. Distinctum a Nicolao Fontano ... Amstelodami, Apud Johannem Janssonium, 1644.

[16], 288 p.   13 cm.   [4180]

—, *ed. See* DODOENS, R. *In* D. Remberti Dodonaei Praxis artis medicae ... scholia. 1640; VESALIUS, A. Librorum ... de humani corporis fabrica epitome. 1642.

—*See* HIPPOCRATES. Aphorismi. Latin. 1633.

FONTRAILLES, JEAN [*fl.* 1696] Traité de physique et de chirurgie, ou l'on explique la sanguification, la circulation du sang ... les differentes causes des fiévres ... avec une explication succinte de l'anatomie ... Paris, La veuve de Claude Thiboust, et Pierre Esclassan, 1697.

[20], 376 p.   17 cm.   [4181]

FOOT, DANIEL [*fl.* 1651-1693]. *See* SIMPSON, W. Hydrological essayes. 1670.

FOPPENS, HADRIANUS [*fl.* 1661] *ed. See* SEIDEL, B. Liber, morborum incurabilium causas. 1662.

FOQUAUD, Jean. Nouvelle doctrine sur le suiet de la connoissance naturelle de l'animal. Ou il est traitté par occasion & d'une façon aussi nouvelle, des principes & causes ... Paris, Henry le Gras, 1658.

[8], 181 (i.e. 183) p.   19 cm.   **[4182]**

FORBERG, Georg. *See* Forberger, Georg [16th cent.]

FORBERGER, Georg [16th cent.] *tr. See* Locatelli, L. Theatro d'arcani ... nel quale si tratta dell'arte chimica. 1644, 1667.

FORD, Simon [1619?-1699] A discourse concerning God's judgments ... Preached ... at Old Swinford in Worcester-Shire and now publish'd to accompany the annexed narrative, concerning the man whose hands and legs lately rotted off in the neighbouring parish of Kings-Swinford, in Stafford-Shire; penned by another author [i.e. James Illingworth] ... London, Printed by A. C. for Henry Brome, 1678.

[8], 64 p.   18 cm.   **[4183]**

James Illingworth's narrative was issued separately under title: A just narrative, or, account of the man whose hands and legs rotted off.

FOREEST, Pieter van [1522-1597] Observationum et curationum medicinalium ac chirurgicarum, opera omnia ... Francofurti, Sumptibus haeredum D. Zachariae Palthenii, 1619.

1 v.   33 cm.   **[4184]**

Various pagings.

Contents. — [1-3] Observationum et curationum medicinalium; sive, Medicinae theoricae & practicae libri XXVIII [-liber XXIX & XXX-XXXII] — [4-5] Observationum et curationum chirurgicarum, libri quinque [-libri quatuor posteriores] Each item has special title page, dated respectively 1614, 1614, 1609, 1610, and 1611.

—[The same.] ... Francofurti, Typis Hartmanni Palthenii, sumptibus heredum D. Zachariae Palthenii, 1623.

2 v. in 3.   32 cm.   **[4185]**

A reissue of the 1619 edition with new general title page.

—[The same.] ... Francofurti, Prostant in Officina Paltheniana, Philippi Fieveti, 1634.

[34], 476, 166, 776, [29] p.   35 cm.   **[4186]**

Contains only *his* Observationum et curationum medicinalium; sive, Medicinae theoricae & practicae, libri XXVIII, with a special title page.

—[The same.] ... accesserunt ejusdem authoris Libri III. de incerto ac fallaci urinarum judicio adver-

sus uromantas & uroscopos ... Tomus primus [-quartus] Rothomagi, Sumpt. Joan. & Davidis Berthelin, 1653.

4 v. in 2.   36 cm.   **[4187]**

—[The same.] ... Francofurti, Prostant apud Johann. Andream & Wolffgangi Endteri jun. haeredes, 1660.

1 v.   33 cm.   **[4188]**

Various pagings.

Contents: — [1] Observationum et curationum medicinalium; sive, Medicinae theoricae & practicae, libri XXVIII. Item [1] has special title page with imprint: Francofurti, Prostant in Officina Paltheniana, Philippi Fieveti, 1634. — [2] Observationum et curationum chirurgicarum, libri quinque; — [3] ... Libri quatuor posteriores; [4] ... Observationum et curationum medicinalium; sive, Medicinae theoricae et practicae liber XXIX. Each item has special title page with imprint: Francofurti, Prostat apud Johannem Andream, & Wolfgangi Endteri junioris haeredes, 1661. — [5] Observationum et curationum medicinalium; sive, Medicinae theoricae et practicae libri XXX-XXXII. Item [5] has special title page with imprint: In Francoforto, Prodierunt e Collegio Musarum Paltheniano, 1631.

—De incerto ac fallaci urinarum judicio. (In *his* Observationum et curationum chirurgicarum, libri quinque ... Quibus accesserunt ... libri III. De incerto, ac fallaci urinarum judicio adversus uromantas & uroscopos ... 1610.)

—[English tr.] The arraignment of urines: wherein are set downe the manifold errors and abuses of ignorant urine-monging empirickes, cozening quacksalvers, women-physitians, and the like stuffe ... Collected ... and written first in the Latin tongue ... by Peter Forrest ... Newly epitomized, and translated ... by James Hart ... London, Printed by G. Eld for Robert Mylbourne, 1623.

[22], 122 (i.e. 120) p.   18 cm.   **[4189]**

Imperfect: sig. (*)1 (blank) wanting. Sheet A supplied in photocopy from Huntington Library.

STC 11180.

—[The same.] *In* Hart, J. The anatomie of urines. 1625.

—Observationum et curationum chirurgicarum libri quinque, de tumoribus praeter naturam, cum scholiis, in quibus eorum causa, signa, prognoses, ac curatio graphice depinguntur. [Lugduni Batavorum?] Ex Officina Plantiniana Raphelengii, 1610.

[8], 495, [15] p.   17 cm.   **[4190]**

With this is bound *his* Observationum et curationum chirurgicarum libri quatuor posteriores. 1610.

—[The same.] Observationum et curationum chirurgicarum, libri quinque ... De tumoribus praeter naturam sanguineis, biliosis, pituitosis, melancholicis, mixtis seu compositis ... Quibus accesserunt ejusdem libri III. De incerto, ac fallaci urinarum judicio adversus uromantas & uroscopos ... Francofurti, Apud Zachariam Palthenium, 1610.

247, [15] p. 32 cm. [4191]

With this is bound *his* Observationum et curationum chirurgicarum libri quatuor posteriores. 1611.

Issued also as item [4] of *his* Observationum et curationum medicinalium ac chirurgicarum, opera omnia. Francofurti, 1619.

—[The same.] ... Francofurti, Prostant in Officina Paltheniana Philippi Fieveti, 1634.

245, [15] p. 33 cm. [4192]

Bound with *his* Observationum et curationum medicinalium ... liber XXIX. 1631.

—Observationum et curationum chirurgicarum libri quatuor posteriores [i.e., Liber sextus -nonus] de vulneribus, ulceribus, fracturis, luxationibus. [Lugduni Batavorum?] Ex Officina Plantiniana Raphelengii, 1610.

[8], 479 p. 17 cm. [4193]

Bound with *his* Observationum et curationum chirurgicarum libri quinque. 1610.

—[The same.] Observationum et curationum chirurgicarum libri quatuor posteriores. Quorum I. De plagis, seu vulneribus cruentis. II. De ulceribus, III. De fracturis, IV. De luxationibus ... Francofurti, Apud Zachariam Palthenium, 1611.

174 p. 32 cm. [4194]

Bound with *his* Observationum et curationum chirurgicarum libri quinque. 1610.

Issued also as item [5] of *his* Observationum et curationum medicinalium ac chirurgicarum, opera omnia. 1619.

—[The same.] ... Francofurti, Prostant in Officina Paltheniana Philippi Fieveti, 1634.

170 p. 33 cm. [4195]

Bound with his Observationum et curationum medicinalium ... liber XXIX. 1631.

—Observationum et curationum medicinalium; sive, Medicinae theoricae & practicae, libri XXVIII [-Liber XXIX, -Libri XXX-XXXII] Francofurti, Prodeunt e Paltheniana Officina, 1602-1609.

2 v. in 3. illus. 31 cm. [4196]

Various pagings.

Liber XXIX (dated 1604) and Libri XXX-XXXII (dated 1609) have special title pages.

—Observationum et curationum medicinalium liber vigesimus-nonus, de arthritide & aliis affectibus partium externarum. [Lugduni Batavorum?] Ex Officina Plantiniana, Raphelengii, 1603.

[8], 240, [7] p. 17 cm. [4197]

—Observationum et curationum medicinalium; sive, Medicinae theoricae et practicae liber XXIX. De arthritide & aliis affectibus partium externarum ... In Francofurto, Prodiit e Collegio Musarum Paltheniano, 1631.

[4], 777-827 (i.e. 839) p. 33 cm. [4198]

With this are bound *his* Observationum et curationum medicinalium ... libri XXX-XXXII. 1631; *his* Observationum et curationum chirurgicarum libri quinque. 1634; *his* Observationum et curationum chirurgicarum libri quatuor posteriores. 1634.

—[German tr.] *In* Uffenbach, P., *ed.* and *tr.* Ein newes Artzney Buch. 1605.

—Observationum et curationum medicinalium liber XXX De venenis, & XXXI De fucis. [Lugduni Batavorum?] Ex Officina Plantiniana Raphelengii, 1606.

[8], 236, [12] p. 17 cm. [4199]

—Observationum et curationum medicinalium; sive, Medicinae theoricae et practicae libri XXX XXXI. et XXXII. De venenis, fucis & lue venerea ... In Francofurto, Prodierunt e Collegio Musarum Paltheniano, 1631.

[3], 169, [7] p. 33 cm. [4200]

Bound with *his* Observationum et curationum medicinalium ... liber XXIX. 1631.

—*See* BONET, T., *ed.* Corps de medecine et de chirurgie. 1679; EYGEL, A. Apologema pro urinis humanis. 1672; SALMON, W. Iatrica. 1681, 1684, 1694.

FORESTIER, JEAN [*fl.* 1646-1647] *praeses.* Quaestio medica ... An contumacibus morbis ex stibio purgatio? [Lutetiae, 1646]

6 p. 24 cm. [4201]

Diss. — Paris (L. Le Noir, *respondent*)

FORESTUS, NANNIUS [*fl.* 1631?] *respondent. See* BURGERSDIJCK, F. P., *praeses.* Collegium physicum. 1642.

FORESTUS, PETRUS. *See* FOREEST, Pieter van [1522-1597]

FORGE, LOUIS DE LA. *See* LA FORGE, Louis de [1632-1666]

A FORM of common prayer with thanksgiving to God. 1666. *See* CHURCH OF ENGLAND. Liturgy and ritual.

La FORME de la direction et oeconomie du Grand Hostel-Dieu. 1646, 1661. *See* HÔTEL-DIEU DE LYON.

A FORME of prayer, necessary to bee used in these dangerous times. 1626. *See* CHURCH OF ENGLAND. Liturgy and ritual.

FORMI, PIERRE [*d.* 1679] L'idée de la peste. Avec les remedes ... qu'on doit employer, tant en la preservation, qu'en la guerison de ce mal ... Montpelier, Chez P. du Buisson par P. Claverie, 1649.

    [23], 120 p.   12 cm.   [4202]

—Traité de l'adianton; ou, Cheveu de Venus contenant la description, les utilitez, & les diverses preparations galeniques & spagyriques de cette plante ... Montpelier, Pierre du Buisson, 1644.

    [16], 80 p.   illus.   17 cm.   [4203]

FORMY, SAMUEL [*fl.* 1590-1610] Traicté chirurgical des bandes, laqs, emplatres, compresses, astelles, et des bandages en particulier. Plus les observations des cures faictes, par les bandes, laqs & compresses emplatrées ... Montpelier, Pierre Dubuisson, M.CD.LI [i.e. 1651]

    [12], 240, [26] p.   tables.   18 cm.   [4204]
    Errata: p. [25-26]

FORORDNING om medicis oc apotecker. *See* COPENHAGEN. Ordinances, local laws, etc. Catalogus & valor medicamentorum simplicium & compositorum in officinis Hafniensibus prostantium. 1672.

FORREST, JAKOB [*fl.* 1690] *respondent. See* BOHN, J., *praeses.* Exercitatio academica. 1690.

FORREST, PETER. *See* FOREEST, Pieter van [1522-1597]

FORSTER, MARTIN. Tartarus hypochondriorum; das ist: Natur gemäss künstliche Beschreibung der Tartar Kranckheit, welche von dem Fabricatore morborum in cuciebitulis balnei hypochondriorum, von den Excrementis procreationum elementorum crescentium, &c. zusammen colligieret ... worden ... Gera, In Verlegung Jacob Apels, 1614.

    [18], 205, [1] p.   16 cm.   [4205]

"Antidotus loemo-polemica. Ist eine wahre ... Beschreibunge der Pest ..." (p. [121]-205) has special title page.

FORT, REMY [*fl.* 17th cent.] Le medicin d'armee; ou, Les entretiens de Polemaitre et de Leoceste, sur les maladies des soldats ... Paris, René Guignard, 1681.

    [12], 312 p.   16 cm.   [4206]

FORTI, RAYMUNDUS JOANNES. *See* FORTIS, Raimondo Giovanni [1603-1678]

FORTIS, RAIMONDO GIOVANNI [1603-1678] Consultationum et responsionum medicinalium centuriae quatuor ... Patavii, Typis Matthaei Bolzetta de Cadorinis, 1669-78.

    2 v.   ports.   32 cm.   34 cm.   [4207]
    Engraved title pages.
    Vol. 2 has imprint: Patavii, Sumptibus Petri Mariae Frambotti, 1678.

—[The same.] ... Accesserunt ejusdem consilia De febribus et de morbis mulierum ... Genevae, Sumptibus Leonardi Chouët, 1677-1681.

    2 v.   port.   35 cm.   [4208]
    Part [2] of vol. 1 has special title page.

—[The same.] ... Patavii, Sumptibus Jacobi de Cadorinis, 1700.

    [12], 475, [20] p.   port.   37 cm.   [4209]
    Contents as in the 1669-78 edition.
    Vol. 1 only.

—De febribus et morbis mulierum facile cognoscendis atque curandis ... Patavii, Typis heredum Pauli Frambotti, 1668.

    [20], 522 p.   23 cm.   [4210]

—[The same.] ... Patavii, Typis Petri Mariae Frambotti, 1694.

    [8], 146, [10] p.   36 cm.   [4211]

FORTIUS, JEAN. *See* FORTIS, Raimondo Giovanni [1603-1678]

FOSS, JOHANN [*fl.* 1617] *respondent.* Disputatio inauguralis de lethargo ... Lugduni Bathavorum, Ex officina Henrici Ludovici ab Haestens, 1617.

    [8] p.   21 cm.   [4212]
    Diss. — Leyden.

FOSTER, WILLIAM [1591-1643] Hoplocrismaspongus; or, A sponge to wipe away the weaponsalve. A treatise, wherein is proved, that the cure latetaken up amongst us, by applying the salve to the weapon, is magicall and unlawfull ... London, Printed by Thomas Cotes, for John Grove, 1631.

[16], 56 p. 18 cm. [4213]

Imperfect: upper margins shaved.
STC 11203.

—*as subject.* See FLUDD, R. Doctor Fludds answer unto M. Foster. 1631 [and] Responsum ad Hoplocrisma-spongum M. Fosteri. 1638.

FOUCAULT, TOUSSAIN [*fl.* 1646] See TARDY, C. Hippocratica purgandi methodus. 1646.

FOUCQUET, MARIE (de Maupeou) *vicomtesse de Vaux.* See FOUQUET, Marie (de Maupeou) *vicomtesse de Vaux.* [1590-1681]

FOUET, CLAUDE [*fl.* 1677] Le secret des bains et eaux minerales de Vichy en Bourbonnois ... dans lequel sont contenuës beaucoup de recherches & pensées curieuses utiles & necessaires pour les malades qui ont besoin des eaux minerales en general ... Paris, La veuve d'Olivier de Varennes, 1679.

[24], 148 p. 17 cm. [4214]

—[The same.] ... Paris, Laurent d'Houvry, 1686.

[24], 148 p. 17 cm. [4215]

A reissue of the 1679 edition with new title page.

—Nouveau sisteme des bains et eaux minerales de Vichy, fondé sur plusieurs belles experiences, & sur la doctrine de l'acide & de l'alcaly ... Paris, Robert Pepie, 1686.

[24], 306, [5] p. 16 cm. [4216]

FOUGEROLLES, FRANÇOIS DE [*ca.* 1560-1620] De senum affectibus praecavendis, nonnullisque curandis enarratio ... Lugduni, Sumptib. Joan. de Gabiano, & Laur. Durand, 1610.

128 p. 24 cm. [4217]

—Methodus in septem Aphorismorum libros ab Hippocrate observata omnibus tamen retro saeculis inaudita. Jam primum mirabili schematon artificio demonstrata ... Parisiis, Apud Adrianum Perier, 1612.

[16], 154 p. 23 cm. [4218]

Includes Latin text of the Aphorismi, generally following Niccolò Leoniceno's version.

—, *ed.* and *tr.* See *Porphyrius.* De non necandis ad epulandum animantibus libri IIII. 1620.

FOUQUET, MARIE (de Maupeou) *vicomtesse de Vaux* [1590-1681] Recueil de receptes où est expliquée

la maniere de guerir à peu de frais toute sorte de maux tant internes, qu'externes inveterez, & qui ont passé jusqu'à present pour incurables ... Lyon, Jean Certe, 1676.

[44], 342, [6] p. 15 cm. [4219]

Pref. signed by Delescure, the editor.
First ed. (1675) has title: Recueil de receptes choisies, experimentées et approuvées. Also published under titles: Les remèdes charitables; and Recueil de remèdes faciles et domestiques.

—[The same.] Les remedes charitables ... pour guerir a peu de frais toute sorte de maux tant internes, qu'externes, inveterez, & qui ont passé jusques à present pour incurables ... Augm. d'un tiers dans cette derniere ed. ... Lyon, Jean Certe, 1681.

[48], 456, [24] p. 16 cm. [4220]

—[The same.] ... Lyon, Jean Certe, 1682.

[48], 456, [24] p. 15 cm. [4221]

Imperfect: p. 407-408 wanting.
A reprint of the 1681 edition.

—Recueil de remedes faciles et domestiques; choisis, experimentez, & tres-approuvez pour toutes sortes de maladies internes & externes, inveterées, & difficiles à guerir. Recüeillis par les ordres charitables d'une illustre & pieuse dame pour soulager les pauvres malades. Augm. de plusieurs secrets, corr. & mis dans un meilleur ordre que les impressions precedentes ... Imprimé à Dijon, & se vend a Paris, Chez Estienne Michallet, 1683.

[24], 384, [24] p. 16 cm. [4222]

Part 2 (p. [193]-384) has special title page with imprint: Dijon, J. Ressayre, 1679.
Bound with Blegny, N. de. Le remede anglois pour la guerison des fievres. 1683.

—[The same.] ... Suivant l'imprimé à Paris ... Bruxelles, Eug. Henry Fricx, 1684.

[20], 330, [22] p. 14 cm. [4223]

—Les remedes charitables ... pour guerir a peu de frais toute sorte de maux tant internes, qu'externes, inveterez, & qui ont passé jusques à present pour incurables ... Augm. dans cette derniere ed. de la Methode que l'on pratique à l'Hôtel des Invalides pour guerir les soldats de la verole ... Lyon, Jean Certe, 1685.

[50], 476, [26] p. 16 cm. [4224]

A reprint of the 1682 Lyons edition.

—Recueil des remedes faciles et domestiques, choisis, experimentez, & tresapprouvez, pour toutes sortes de maladies, internes, & externes, inveterées,

& difficiles à guerir . . . 3. ed. Augmentée de quantité de secrets, corrigés & mise dans un meilleur ordre que les impressions precedentes . . . I. partie [-II. partie] Dijon, Jean Ressayre, 1686.

2 v. 16 cm. (Vol. 1: [24], 384, [24] p.; vol. 2: [40], 440 p.) [4225]

Vol. 1, part 2 (3. ed., 2. ptie.) has special title page (p. [193]) dated 1679.

Vol. 2 has title: Suite du Recueil des remedes faciles et domestiques, choisis, experimentez & approuvez pour toutes sortes de maladies internes & externes, inveterées & difficiles à guerir . . . Avec un regime de vie pour chaque complexion & pour chaque maladie; & un traité du lait: le tout par ordre alphabetique. Dijon, Jean Ressayre, 1687.

The "Approbation" signed by the regent of the Faculty of Medicine of Paris and the royal privilege (p. [40]) are both dated 1686.

Bound uniformly with the preceding Recueil, 1686, with which it was issued. In the "Avertissement" on p. [39] of the suite the Recueil is referred to as "le premier volume" and this as "ce second volume."

—Suite du Recueil des remedes faciles et domestiques, choisis, experimentez & approuvez pour toutes sortes de maladies internes & externes, inveterées & difficile à guerir, recuillis par les ordres charitables de . . . Madame Fouquet . . . Avec un regime de vie pour chaque complexion & pour chaque maladie; & un traité du lait: le tout par ordre alphabetique. Dijon, Jean Ressayre, 1689.

[40], 440 p. 16 cm. [4226]

Colophon (p. 408): A Dijon, par Jean Ressayre . . . 1687. Published also as vol. 2 of the Recueil.

—Les remedes charitables . . . pour guerir a peu de frais toute sorte de maux externes, invéterez, & qui ont passé jusques à present pour incurables. Augm. en cette ed. d'un grand nombre d'autres remédes faciles, & aussi experimentés, trouvé depuis peu dans les Mémoires de cette même pieuse dame . . . Lyon, Jean Certe, 1696.

2 v. 16 cm. [4227]

—[Italian tr.] I rimedii di madama Fochetti per sanare con pouchissima spesa tutta sorte d'infirmità interne, & esterne, invecchiate, e passate fino al presente per incurabili . . . Portati dal francese da Ludovico Castellini . . . Milano, Ambrogio Ramellati, 1683.

[24], 153 p.; [1], 132 p. 15 cm. [4228]

Pref. signed: De Lescure.
Part 2 has half title.

—[The same.] . . . Bologna, Gli HH. di Gio. Recal[dini] 1685.

[22], 178 p.; [1], 153, [1] p. 15 cm. [4229]

—[The same.] Rimedi caritativi . . . per guarire con poca spesa ogni sorte di mali, tanto interni, quanto esterni, inveterati, e che sin al presente sono passati per incurabili . . . Accresciuti d'un terzo in quest'ultima impressione. Divisi in due parti. Tradotii dalla lingua francese nell'italiana, da un sacerdote dell' ord. serafico de Min. Oss. Rif. della provincia di S. Tomaso Apostolo in Piemonte. Cuneo, Bartolomeo Strabella, 1685.

[24], 497, [27] p. 14 cm. [4230]

—[The same.] I rimedii di madama Fochetti per sanare con pochissima spesa tutta sorte d'infirmità interne, & esterne, invecchiate, e passate fino al presente per incurabili . . . Divisi in due parti, e portati dal francese da Lodovico Castellini . . . Bologna, Nella stamperia del Longhi (ca. 1688]

[24], 166 p.; [2], 168 p. 15 cm. [4231]

Part 2 has half title.

Probably reprinted from the edition printed by the heirs of Giovanni Recaldini in Bologna in 1685. It was examined by the same ecclesiastical officials as that edition; but the undated "Reimprimatur" statement which follows on p. [24] is here signed by "Fr. Petrus Martyr . . . S. Officii Bononiae provicarius," while the 1685 edition was approved by a different person as "vicarius." Petrus Martyr approved other works printed by Longhi in 1687 and 1688.

—[The same.] Secretii, overo rimedii di madama Fochetti. Per sanare con poca spesa ogni sorte d'infirmità interne, & esterne, invecchiate, e passate fino al presente per incurabili . . . Tradotti dal francese da Ludovico Castellini . . . Venetia, Stefano Curti, 1693.

312, [24] p. 16 cm. [4232]

Pref. signed: De Lescure.

—[The same.] . . . In questa nuova impressione aggiuntovi [sic] la terza parte che in essa opera si contiene . . . Venetia, Il Prodocimo, 1697.

336, 20, [24] p. 14 cm. [4233]

Part 3 has special title page: Aggiunta de' secreti di madama Fochetti. Del metodo, quale si tiene nell' Hospitale de gl'invalidi di Parigi per curare il mal francese. This is a translation of the "Methode que l'on pratique à l'Hôtel des invalides pour guerir les soldats de la verole" which was added to part 2 of the Recueil in the Lyons edition of 1685.

FOUR, DAVID DE [fl. 1675] respondent. See WEDEL, G. W., praeses. Disputatio medica de purgantibus rite adhibendis. 1675.

FOUR DE LA CRESPELIÈRE, Du. *See* Du Four de La Crespelière.

FOURE statutes, specially selected and commanded by His Majestie. 1609. *See* Gt. Brit. Laws, statutes, etc.

FOURESTIER, James, ed. See [Hester, J.] The excellencie of physick and chirurgerie. 1652.

FOURNEILLIS DES. *See* Cordemoy, Louis Géraud de [1626–1684]

FOURNIER, Denis [*d.* 1683] L'accoucheur methodique, qui enseigne la maniere d'operer dans tous les accouchements naturels et artificiels, tost, seurement & sans douleur . . . Paris, L'autheur et Sebastien Cramoisy, 1677.

[26], 522, [4] p. front. (port.), illus., plates. 15 cm.   [**4234**]

Imperfect: title page wanting; supplied in photocopy from College of Physicians of Philadelphia library.

One leaf inserted between p. 6 and 7; recto blank, verso numbered 6 has text.

—L'anatomie pacifique nouvelle et curieuse. Conforme à la doctrine d'Hippocrate & de Galien, qui donne les moyens d'accorder les recents avec les anciens, par des experiences nouvelles, principalement touchant les actions du coeur & des pulmons . . . Paris, L'autheur et Sebastien Cramoisy, 1678.

[16], 30, 64, [4], 65–104, 99–154 p. illus., plates., port. 23 cm.   [**4235**]

L'Alphabet chirurgical, lequel contient le compendium de l'osteologie par tables . . . l'abregé de la Myologie aussi par tables . . . 1672 has special title page inserted between p. 34 and p. 35.

—L'antiloimotechnie; ou, L'art qui chasse la peste et tous ses accidents, qui sont le pourpre, la petit verolle, la rougeolle pourprée, la dysenterie, les bubons . . . par une methode generalle de la medecine, & par un remede experimente . . . Paris, La veuve I. Rebuffé, 1669.

[36], 240 p. front., illus. 15 cm.   [**4236**]

—L'oeconomie chirurgicale, pour le r'habillement des os du corps humain, contenant l'osteologie, la nososteologie, et l'apocatastosteologie, ou la science et le discours des os, de leurs maladies, de leurs remedes . . . Et outre ce le traitté des bandages . . . suivant la methode d'Hippocrate, de Galien, d'Oribaze . . . Paris, François Clouzier, Robert de Ninville et Sebastien Cramoisy, 1671.

4 parts in 1 v.   illus., plates., port.   23 cm.   [**4237**]

Added engraved title page.

Part [2] has title: Explication des bandages . . . divisée en deux traitez . . . Paris, Pierre Josse, 1668. Part [3] has title: L'oeconomie chirurgicale pour le restablissement des parties molles du corps humain. Contenant les principes de chirurgie, & un traitté methodique de la garison de la peste . . . Paris, Chez François Clouzier et Sebastien Cramoisy, 1671. Part [3] has added engraved title page also. Part [4] has engraved title page: L'antiloimotechnie; ou, L'art qui chasse la peste.

FOX, Abraham Lenertzon [*fl.* 1632] *tr. See* Wirtz, F. An experimental treatise of surgerie. 1656.

FOY-VAILLANT, Jean. *See* Vaillant, Jean-Foi [1632–1706]

FRACANTIANUS, Antonius. *See* Fracanzano, Antonio [*d.* 1567]

FRACANZANO, Antonio [*ca.* 1567] *See* Scholtz, L. Consiliorum medicinalium . . . liber singularis. 1610.

FRACASSATI, Carlo [1630–1672] De cerebro et lingua. *In* Malpighi, M. Opera omnia. 1687.

—*See* Malpighi, M. Epistolae anatomicae. 1669.

—*as subject. See* Herfelt, H. G. Philosophicum hominis, de corporis humani machina. 1687.

FRACASTORIUS, Hieronymus. *See* Fracastoro, Girolamo [1483–1553]

FRACASTORO, Girolamo [1483–1553] Operum pars prior [-posterior]   [Genevae] Apud Samuelem Crispinum, 1621.

2 parts in 1 v.   illus.   17 cm.   [**4238**]
Baumgartner-Fulton 37.

—[The same.] Operum pars prior [-altera] [Genevae] Apud Petrum & Jacobum Chouët, 1622.

2 parts in 1 v.   17 cm.   [**4239**]
The Poemata is bound before Pars posterior.
Baumgartner-Fulton 38.

—Operum pars prior. Philosophica et medica continens, quorum elenchum pagina sequens indicat . . . [Genevae] Typis Jacobi Stoer, 1637.

[32], 657, [31] p. illus. 18 cm.   [**4240**]

Part [1] only.
Place of imprint blocked out.
Baumgartner-Fulton 41.

—De sympathia et antipathia rerum, liber unus.

[650]-704 p. 21 cm. (*In* Theatrum sympatheticum auctum. Norimbergae, 1662) **[4241]**
Caption title.

—Siphylis [sic], sive morbus Gallicus. *In* ΑΝΘΟΛΓΊΑ; seu, Selecta quaedam poemata Italorum. 1684.
Baumgartner-Fulton 16.

—[English tr.] Syphilis; or, A poetical history of the French disease. Written in Latin . . . Now attempted in English by N. Tate. London, Jacob Tonson, 1686.
[19], 84 p. 18 cm. **[4242]**
Baumgartner-Fulton 72.

—[The same.] Syphilis. Written (in Latin) . . . English'd by Mr. Tate. [London, Printed by R. E. for Jacob Tonson, 1693]
[16], 84 p. 19 cm. **[4243]**
Published as part [2] of John Dryden's Examen poeticum: being the third part of miscellany poems.
Baumgartner-Fulton 73.

—[Excerpts.] *See* LANCETTA, T. Raccolta medica. 1645.

—*See* FONTAINE, J. Jacobi Fontani . . . Commentaria in Hipp[ocratis] omnes Aph[orismos] 1608.

FRAGOSO, JUAN [*d.* 1597] Cirugia universal, aora nuevamente emendada, y añadida en esta 6. impression . . . Y mas otros quatro tratados. El primero es una suma de proposiciones contra ciertos avisos de cirugia. El segundo, de las declaraciones a cerca de diversas heridas, y muertes. El tercero, de los Aforismos de Hipocrates, tocantes a cirugia. El quarto, de la naturaleza, y calidades de los medicamentos simples. Alcala de Henares, En casa de Juan Gracian, 1621.
[4], 685, [38] p. 31 cm. **[4244]**
Imperfect: title page and p. 1-4 wanting, supplied in photocopy from Bibliothèque nationale, Paris.
"Tres tratados de cirugia" (p. [511]-616) has special title page.
The original version of the Cirugia universal appeared in Madrid in 1570 under title: Erotemas chirurgicos.
"Tratado tercero, de los aforismos de Hipocrates tocantes a la cirugia: con una breve exposicion sobre cada uno dellos" (p. 577-616) includes selections from the Aphorismi in Latin and Spanish.

—[Italian tr.] Della cirugia . . . parti due, nelle quali di tutte le cose, che alla cirugia appartengono, essattamente si ragiona. Tradotte dalla lingua spagnola nella italiana da Baldassar Grasso alias Grassia, con l'aggiunta di altre tre trattati utilissimi

alla cirugia del secondo Gio Fragoso. Palermo, Antonio Martarello, 1639.
[13], 424 (i.e. 240) p. 33 cm. **[4245]**
Although the three treatises at end are attributed here and in later editions of this Italian translation to a supposed Juan Fragoso II, they are apparently by Juan Fragoso, author of the first part of the work.
"Trattato terzo de gl'aforismi d'Hipp. pertinenti alla cirugia, con alcuna breve espositione sopra ciascheduno di quelli per il II. Giovanni Fragoso, &c." (p. 401-424 (i.e. 398-420)) includes selections from the Aphorismi in Latin and Italian.

—[The same.] . . . Venetia, Paolo Baglioni, 1662.
[16], 556 p. 23 cm. **[4246]**

—[The same.] . . . Venetia, Paola Baglioni, 1686.
[12], 519 p. 26 cm. **[4247]**

—Tratado de cirugia, sacado de la Cirugia universal, que escrivio el licenciado Juan Fragoso conforme se practica en el Hospital general de Madrid. Zaragoza, Por los herederos de Pedro Lanaja, 1692.
112 p. 15 cm. **[4248]**
An abridged version of the first part of Fragoso's Cirugia universal.
Edited by Gerónimo de Ayala.

—[Excerpts.] *In* Ayala, G. de. Principios de cirugia. [1683?], 1693.

—[Discursos de las cosas aromaticas, arboles y frutales, y de otras muchas medicinas simples que se traen de la India Oriental. Latin.] Aromatum, fructuum, et simplicium aliquot medicamentorum ex India utraque, et Orientali et Occidentali, in Europam delatorum, quorum jam est usus plurimus, historia brevis . . . Conscripta primum Hispanice . . . nunc Latine edita opera et ac studio Israelis Spachii . . . Argentinae, Excudebat Jodocus Martinus, 1601.
[8], 115, [1] ll. 16 cm. **[4249]**

FRAICHOT, CASIMIR. *See* FRESCHOT, Casimir [1640?-1700]

FRAIZER, *Sir* ALEXANDER [1610?-1681] *ed. See* HALL, J. Select observations on English bodies. 1679, 1683; MENZIES, J. A. sermon. 1681.

FRAMBESARIUS, NICOLAS ABRAHAM. *See* LA FRAMBOISIÈRE, Nicolas Abraham de.

FRAMBOISIÈRE, NICOLAS ABRAHAM DE LA. *See* LA FRAMBOISIÈRE, Nicolas Abraham de.

FRAMBOTTUS, PAULUS, *ed. See* CARDANO, G. *In*

Aphorismos Hippocratis commentaria luculentissima cum Graeco textu. 1653.

FRANC, Johann. *See* Francke, Johann [1648–1728]

FRANC, Louis, *tr. See* Beynon, E. Le samaritain charitable. 1673 [and] Suitte du Samaritain charitable. 1673.

FRANCE. Assemblée Générale du Clergé. *See* Assemblée charitable à Paris. Remedes. Pour les pauvres gens. [1677]; Remedes pour les pauvres gens de la campagne. 1672.

FRANCE. Conseil privé. Arrest, portant reglement des chirurgiens privilegiez. Extraict des registres du Conseil privé du roy. [n. p., 1668]

  15 p.   24 cm.   [4250]
  Caption title.

FRANCE. Laws, statutes, etc. Reglement de la cour, rendu sur les conclusions de … le procureur general du roy; faisant défenses à tous … personnes venants des costes de la Martinique & des Indes & autres lieux infectez de la peste … Du 10, avril 1699. Rennes, François Vatar, 1699.

  [4] p.   19 cm.   [4251]

FRANCE. Parlement. (Grenoble) *See* Notabel arrest van't Parlement 's Hoffs van Grenoble. 1637.

FRANCE. Parlement. (Paris) Arrest de la Cour de Parlement, sur l'enlevement des personnes frappees de contagion logees és chambres locantes, fermeture de leurs maisons, provision & nourriture de ceux qui resteront esdites maisons. Du septiesme aoust 1623. Paris, Fed. Morel, 1623.

  [6] p.   17 cm.   [4252]

—Arrest de nosseigneurs du Parlement, qui fait défenses à tous ceux qui ne sont point medecins de la Faculté de Paris, d'exercer la medecine dans la ville & fauxbourgs de Paris, á peine de cinq cens livres d'amende, & qui declare ladite amende encouruë. [Paris? 1698]

  [3] p.   20 cm.   [4253]
  Caption title.

—Ordonnances de la police generalle tenue en Parlement en la Chambre Sainct Louys, pour obvier à la contagion … Paris, Nicolas Alexandre, 1623.

  8 p.   18 cm.   [4254]

FRANCE. Parlement. (Rennes) *See* France. Parlement de Bretagne.

FRANCE. Parlement. (Toulouse) Arrest de la cour de Parlement de Toulouse. Portant defences a toutes personnes d'accoucher les femmes sans avoir presté serment devant les consuls des lieux. Donné le 18. mars 1681. Toulouse, J. Boude, 1681.

  4 p.   22 cm.   [4255]

FRANCE. Parlement de Bretagne. Extraict des registres de Parlement. Le procureur general du roy entré en la Cour, a remonté qu'il a en advis qu'en Hollande & ville d'Amsterdam, il est arrivé un mal contagieux … Fait en Parlement à Rennes le septiesme juin 1664. [Rennes?] 1664.

  [3] p.   19 cm.   [4256]
  Date changed by hand from 1644 to 1664.

FRANCE. Sovereigns, etc. [1643–1715] (Louis XIV) Declaration du roy, concernant la regie, gouvernement & administration des hôpitaux, maladeries, leproseries & autres lieux pieux. Avec l'arrest de registre du 30. decembre 1698. Toulouse, Claude-Gilles Le Camus, 1698.

  8 p.   23 cm.   [4257]
  Pagination altered by hand to ll. 92–95.

—Declaration du roy, donnée à Versailles au mois de decembre 1698. Portant reglement general pour la regie & administration des hôpitaux, léproseries, maladeries & autres lieux pieux, desunis de l'Ordre de Nostre-Dame de Mont-carmel & de S. Lazare, dans lesquels l'hospitalité a été établie … Grenoble, Alexandre Giroud, 1699.

  [1], 10 p.   24 cm.   [4258]

—Declaration du roy. Donnée par sa majesté à Versailles le 19. de Juillet 1696. Portant que nul ne pourra exercer la médecine dans aucune ville du royaume, sans avoir été reçû docteur dans quelqu'une des universitez … Publié en Parlement le 5. de Juillet 1700 … [Grenoble? 1700]

  [4] p.   24 cm.   [4259]
  At head of title: No. 329

—Declaration du roy, portant defences á ceux de la R[eligion] P[retenduë] R[eformée] de l'un & l'autre sexe, de se mesler dores-en-avant des accouchemens des femmes, tant de la Religion Catholique Apostolique, & Romaine, que de la R. P. R. Registrée à

Tolose en Parlement le vingt-deuxième mars 1680. Tolose, Jean Boude, 1680.

7 p.   22 cm.   [4260]

—Declaration du roy, portant qu'aucune personne ne pourra faire la fonction de medecin, ny pratiquer la medecine dans la ville & fauxbourgs de Paris, encore qu'ill ait obtenu des degrez dans les autres universitez du royaume, qu'il ne se soit presenté en ladite Faculté de Paris pour y prendre de nouveaux degrez . . . Donnée à Versailles le 29. mars 1696 . . . [Paris, François Muguet, 1696]

4 p.   20 cm.   [4261]
Caption title.

—Declaration du roy, portant que les demonstrateurs établis au jardin royal continuëront leurs leçons & exercices sur la vertu des plantes medecinales, & pharmacie tant ancienne que nouvelle; comme aussi qu'ils pourront faire audit jardin toutes operations chirurgicales, dissections, & démonstrations anatomiques, & qu'à cét effet le premier corps exécuté leur sera delivré par préference à tous autres. Donnée à S. Germain . . . le 20. janvier 1673 . . . Paris, Sebastien Mabre-Cramoisy, 1673.

7 p.   26 cm.   [4262]

—Declaration du roy, portant que les visites des blessez seront faites par les deux chirurgiens commis par le premier medecin, suivant l'ancien usage. Verifiée en Parlement le premier septembre 1671. Poitiers, Jean Fleuriau, 1672.

4 p.   24 cm.   [4263]

—Declaration du roy, registrée en Parlement, portant suppression de la Chambre royale des medecins des universitez provinciales à Paris. Avec l'arrest du Conseil d'éstat du 9, juin 1694. Et la réponse au libelle intitulé, Requeste importante pour les medecins de la Chambre royale contre les medecins de la Faculté de Paris . . . Paris, François Muguet, 1695.

61 p.   25 cm.   [4264]

—Edit du roy, donné à Fontainebleau au mois d'aoust 1661. Par lequel sa majesté défend à tous ses sujets, de donner à l'avenir aucuns deniers comptans, heritages au rentes aux communautez ecclesiastiques . . . (à l'exception de l'Hôtel-Dieu, du Grand hôpital de Paris, & de la Maison des incurables) à condition d'une rente leur vie durant . . . [Paris, Joseph Saugrain, 1690?]

8 p.   25 cm.   [4265]

Caption title.
Pagination altered by hand to 225–232.
"Edit du roy, donné à Versailles au mois de janvier 1690. Portant défenses à Hôpital general & autres, de prendre des rentes à fonds perdu plus bas que le denier vingt": p. 6–8.

—Edit du roy, donné à Versailles au mois de février 1692. Portant creation en titre d'offices formez & hereditaires de deux chirurgiens jurez dans chacune des grandes villes du royaume, terres & seugneuries de l'obéissance de sa majesté où il y a parlement, & autres cours, & d'un medecin juré ordinaire du roy en chacun ressort. Publié en audiance publique le 27, mars. 1692. Grenoble, Alexandre Giroud, 1697.

16 p.   25 cm.   [4266]

—Edit du roy, portant creation de deux chirurgiens jurez dans chacune des grandes villes, & un dans les autres du royaume . . . Donné à Versailles au mois de février 1692 . . . Paris, Guillaume Desprez, 1692.

15 p.   23 cm.   [4267]

—Reglemens que le roy veut estre executez dans l'Hôpital general de Paris, pour la correction des enfans de famille, & pour la punition des femmes débauchées, qui y seront renfermez . . . Paris, François Muguet, 1684.

8 p.   25 cm.   [4268]

FRANCESCO DI PIEDIMONTE [d. 1319] See Mesuë [924 or 5–1015] Opera. 1602, 1623.

FRANCESCO DI TERRANOVA. See Terranova, Francesco di, Father [fl. 1658]

FRANCINI, Horace de [16th–17th cent.] Hippiatrique . . . où est traicté des causes des maladies du cheval tant interieures qu'exterieures: le moyen de la guarir d'icelles; ensemble de la bonté & qualité d'iceluy . . . Paris, Marc Orry, 1607.

[15], 554 p.   22 cm.   [4269]
A free translation of the second part of Carlo Ruini's Dell'anatomia et dell'infermita del cavallo. Cf. Mennessier de la Lance.

FRANCISCI, Andrea Lischovino. See Lischovini, András Ferencz [fl. 1697–1703]

FRANCISCI, Martin [fl. 1694–1698] respondent. See Vater, C., praeses. Dissertationem inauguralem de vertigine . . . exponet M. F. 1698.

FRANCISCO, Joannes Franciscus de. Libellus

aureus de venae sectione contra empiricos. Francofurti & Lipsiae, Ex officina Hafniensi, Christiani Hauboldi & Johannis Liebe, typis Aubryanis, 1685.

[16], 78 p. 17 cm. [4270]

FRANCISCO DE LUQUE, CHRISTOBAL. *See* LUQUE, Cristóbal Francisco de [*fl.* 1682–1694]

FRANCISCUS DE FRANCISCO, JOANNES. *See* FRANCISCO, Joannes Franciscus de.

FRANCISCUS DE PEDEMONTIO. *See* FRANCESCO DI PIEDIMONTE [*d.* 1319]

FRANCK, BARTHOLOMAEUS [*fl.* 17th cent.] *See* ALITHOPHILUS, *pseud.* Alithophili Observationes extemporaneae. 1681?

FRANCK, BERNHARD MATTHIAS [1667–1701] *respondent.* Dissertatio medica inauguralis de catarrho . . . Altdorffii, Typis Henrici Meyeri [1690]

104 p. 20 cm. [4271]
Diss. — Altdorf.

—*See* HOFFMANN, J. M., *praeses.* Dissertatio anatomico-physiologica de gustu. 1689.

FRANCK, HIERONYMUS [*fl.* 1649] *respondent.* Disputatio medica inauguralis de lethargo . . . Trajecti ad Rhenum, Ex officina Johannis à Noortdyck, 1649.

[10] p. 20 cm. [4272]
Diss. — Utrecht.

FRANCK, ISBRANT JERONIMUSZ [1576–1643] *tr. See* FABRICIUS VON HILDEN, W. Nieuwe veldt-chirurgye. 1664.

FRANCK, JOHANN [*fl.* 1608–1609] *respondent. See* STUPANUS, J. N., *praeses.* Casus medicus theorico-practicus de anasarca. 1608.

FRANCK DE FRANCKENAU, GEORG FREDERIK. *See* FRANCK VON FRANCKENAU, Georg Friedrich [1669–1732]

FRANCK VON FRANCKENAU, GEORG [1643–1704] Bona nova anatomica; hoc est, noviter inventa per anatomicorum accuratam diligentiam dum in theatro anatomico cadaveris juvenis αυτοχειπος sollemnem sectionem celebrat . . . proposuit Georgius Francus . . . Heidelbergae, Literis Samuelis Ammonii [1680?]

32 p. 20 cm. [4273]

—De medicis philologis epistola ad . . .

Gothofredum Thomasium . . . Wittenbergae, Typis Matthaei Henckelii, 1691.

[28] p. 21 cm. [4274]

—De studiorum noxa, dissertatio in promotione trium medicinae doctorum solemniter habita VI. November M DC LXXIII. Ed. 2. Jenae, Apud Johann. Bielkium, 1695.

[48] p. 14 cm. [4275]
Bound with Wedel, G. W. Aphorismi aphorismorum. 1695.

—Georgii Franci . . . Institutionum medicarum synopsis . . . Annectitur methodus discendi medicinam . . . Heidelbergae, Sumbtibus Joh. Petri Zubrodt, excud. Wilhelm Walter, 1672.

68, [1] p. 13 cm. [4276]

—Lexicon vegetabilium usualium in quo plantarum, quarum usus usque innotuit, nomen cum synonymis Latinis, Graecis, Germanicis & interdum Arabicis, temperamentum, vires ac usus generalis & specialis atque praeparata . . . Argentorati, Sumtibus ac typis Josiae Staedelii, 1672.

[24], 142 p. 13 cm. [4277]
Added half title.

—Tractatus philologico-medicus de cornutis in quo varia curiosa delibantur ex theologorum, jctorum, medicorum . . . monumentis cum indice auctorum. Heidelbergae, Typis Samuelis Ammonii, 1676.

[2], 13 (i.e. 31), [3] p. 20 cm. [4278]

—In illustrissima Universitate Vitembergensi decani Facult. medicae Georgii Franci de Frankenau . . . propempticon inaugurale de ψαμμισμω. Vitembergae, Typis Christiani Schrödteri [1695]

[16] p. 19 cm. [4279]
Program — Wittenberg (with vita of J. J. Marchand)

Dissertations — Heidelberg
—*praeses.* Agonismata physico-medica sexta vice . . . Heidelbergae, Literis Samuelis Ammonii [1682]

4 p. 18 cm. [4280]
D. Nebel, *respondent.*

—Agonismata physico-medica nona vice . . . Heidelbergae, Literis Samuelis Ammonii [1683]

4 p. 19 cm. [4281]
J. W. Hansen, *respondent.*

—'Ατμογραφια microcosmica; hoc est, Disputatio inauguralis de halitu humano . . . Heidelbergae,

Typis Samuelis Ammonii [1681]

   32 p.   19 cm.   **[4282]**

D. Bscherer, *respondent.*

—Disputatio inauguralis de soldana . . . Heidelbergae, Typis Joh. Christiani Walteri [1674]

   12 p.   19 cm.   **[4283]**

J. H. Soldan, *respondent.*

—Disputatio inauguralis medica, de carbunculo . . . Heidelbergae, Literis Samuelis Ammonii [1682]

   20 p.   20 cm.   **[4284]**

A. Schachtler, *respondent.*

—Disputatio inauguralis medica de sterilitate muliebri . . . Heidelbergae, Typis Joh. Christiani Walteri [1673]

   20 p.   19 cm.   **[4285]**

J. V. Schade, *respondent.*

—Disputatio inauguralis medica exhibens casum viri colica laborantis . . . Heidelbergae, Typis Samuelis Ammonii [1681]

   20 p.   19 cm.   **[4286]**

A. Blommart, *respondent.*

—Disputatio inauguralis medica exhibens casum viri empyemate ex pleuritide laborantis . . . Heidelbergae, Excudebant heredes Walterian [1685]

   20 p.   19 cm.   **[4287]**

J. H. Fliccius, *respondent.*

—Disputatio medica de alapis sive colaphis . . . Heidelbergae, Typis Joh. Christiani Walteri [1674]

   [8] p.   20 cm.   **[4288]**

G. Wicken, *respondent.*

—Disputatio medica inauguralis de risu sardonio . . . Heidelbergae, Literis Samuelis Ammonii [1683]

   28 p.   19 cm.   **[4289]**

J. Richier, *respondent.*

—Disputatio medica inauguralis qua casum, dysuria ad stranguriam vergente laborantis, resolutum . . . exhibet Joh. Wilhelmus Christiani . . . Heidelbergae, Literis Samuelis Ammonii [1686]

   16 p.   21 cm.   **[4290]**

J. W. Christiani, *respondent.*

—Disputatio medica ordinaria, de lapicidina microcosmi in capite . . . Heidelbergae, Typis Joh. David. Bergmanni [1688]

   [4], 24 p.   20 cm.   **[4291]**

P. F. von Hasselt, *respondent.*

—Another issue, with title: Disputatio medica ordinaria, et quidem II. de lapicidina microcosmi in capite.   **[4292]**

—Disputatio medica ordinaria et quidem prima de morbis acutis gravidarum . . . Heidelbergae, Lit. Abr. Ludov. Walteri [1684]

   8 p.   19 cm.   **[4293]**

J. H. Dülcken, *respondent.*

—Disputatio medica qua lupanaria s. v. Huren-Häuser, ex principiis medicis qq. improbantur . . . Heidelbergae, Typis Joh. Christiani Walteri [1674]

   12 p.   18 cm.   **[4294]**

G. Wicken, *respondent.*

—Disputatio physico-medica de saliva et vasis salivalibus . . . Heidelbergae, Typis Joh. Christiani Walteri [1673]

   24 p.   20 cm.   **[4295]**

R. Lentilius, *respondent.*

—Disputationem inauguralem qua febris militum diaetetica, vulgo die bissher grassirende Hitzige Kranckheit . . . pertractatur examinandam propono . . . Petrus Appel . . . Heidelbergae, Typis Joh. Christiani Walteri, 1674.

   28 p.   19 cm.   **[4296]**

P. Appel, *respondent.*

—Disputationem medicam ordinariam de coryza . . . proponent Johannes Conradus Apffelstatt . . . Heidelbergae, Litt. Walterianis [1685]

   16 p.   20 cm.   **[4297]**

J. K. Apffelstatt, *respondent.*

—Dissertatio inauguralis medica de labiis leporinis, von Hasen-Scharten . . . [Heidelbergae] Imprimebat Joh. David Bergmann, Walterian. [1686]

   16 p.   20 cm.   **[4298]**

J. P. Hofmann, *respondent.*

—Dissertationem inauguralem de morbo virgineo . . . proponit Johannes Fridericus Eckhardus . . . Heidelbergae, Literis Samuelis Ammonii [1680]

   24 p.   20 cm.   **[4299]**

J. F. Eckhard, *respondent.*

—Satyrae medicae continuatio XV. de vitro et ὑαλοφαγοις von Glas-Frässern . . . Heidelbergae, Literis Samuelis Ammonii [1678]

   24 p.   18 cm.   **[4300]**

P. Kreps, *respondent.*

—Satyrae medicae, continuatio XVII. disputatione ordinaria disquirens quamdiu dormiendum . . . Heidelbergae, Literis Samuelis Ammonii [1682]

40 p.   20 cm.   [4301]

Date altered by hand from M DC LXXXI to M DC LXXXII.

J. K. Kissel, *respondent.*

—Satyrae medicae, continuatio XVIII. disputatione ordinaria disquirens de ovis paschalibus von Oster-Eyern . . . Heidelbergae, Literis Samuelis Ammonii [1682]

16 p.   19 cm.   [4302]

J. Richier, *respondent.*

—Specimen inaugurale quo medicus monstrosus . . . proponitur . . . examinandus a Jeremia Cotta . . . Heidelbergae, Typis Samuelis Ammonii [1677]

[4], 36 p.   20 cm.   [4303]

J. Cotta, *respondent.*

Dissertations — Wittenberg

—De morbo Q. Enii poetae; sive, Podagra ex vino . . . Wittenbergae, Prelo Goderitschiano [1694]

[4], 64 p.   19 cm.   [4304]

J. J. Chüden, *respondent.*

—Dissertatio inauguralis de hydrope ascite . . . Witteb., Typis Matthaei Henckelii [1690]

[28] p.   19 cm.   [4305]

J. D. Löser, *respondent.*

—Dissertatio inauguralis medica de theriaca coelesti . . . Wittenbergae, Typis Matthaei Henckelii [1691]

[40] p.   19 cm.   [4306]

J. D. Hoffstadt, *respondent.*

—Dissertationem inauguralem de hydrope . . . publice . . . examinandam sistit Heinricus Emanuel Rüel . . . Wittenbergae, Literis Kreusigianis [1693]

30, [2] p.   19 cm.   [4307]

H. E. Rüel, *respondent.*

—, ed. *See* MAXWELL, W. De medicina magnetica libri III. 1679; [German tr.] 1687; ZACCHIA, P. Quaestionum medico-legalium, tomi tres. 1688.

—*See* ETTMÜLLER, M. Opera omnia. 1688; FRANCK VON FRANCKENAU, G. F., ed. Georgii Franci . . . Catalogus variorum tractatuum. 1692; LANGE, C. Opera omnia. 1688.

FRANCK VON FRANCKENAU, GEORG FRIEDRICH [1669-1732] Georgii Friderici de Franckenau . . . Disquisitio epistolaris succi nutricii per nervos transitum ejusque effectus in corpore humano expendens . . . Lipsiae, Impensis Joh. Melchior Liebe. 1696.

96 p.   14 cm.   [4308]

—Ὀνυχολογια curiosa; sive, De unguibus tractatio physico-medica, non tantum eorum physiologiam ubi et de cornibus, sed et pathologiam ac therapiam tradens . . . Jenae, Sumtibus Johannis Bielkii, 1695.

[8], 52, [3] p.   19 cm.   [4309]

Preface by Georg Wolffgang Wedel.

—Another issue, dated 1696.   [4310]

—Georgius Fridericus Francus de Frankenau . . . philiatris S. P. D. eosdemque ad lectiones publicas . . . invitat . . . Wittenbergae, Prelo Goderitschiano [1693]

8 p.   20 cm.   [4311]

—ed. Georgii Franci . . . Catalogus variorum tractatuum, programmatum ac disputationum sub ejus praesidio habitarum, quae omnia olim in lucem prodierunt publicam, collectus atque editus ab auctoris filio Georgio Friderico Franco . . . Dresdae, Apud Johannem Riedelium, 1692.

24 p.   20 cm.   [4312]

—*respondent. See* BRUNNER, J. C., *praes.* Exercitatio anatomico-medica. 1688; HOFFMANN, J. M., *praes.* Exercitatio medica de pericardio. 1690; SCHELHAMMER, G. C., *praes.* Exercitationem inauguralem de epulide & parulide . . . p. p. G. F. F. 1692.

FRANCKE, JOHANN [1648-1728] Polycresta herba veronica ad botanices, philosophicae juxta et medicae cynosuram elaborata . . . Ulmae, Sumtibus & typis Gassenmayerianis, 1690.

272, [16] p.   14 cm.   [4313]

—Veronica theézans; id est, Collatio veronicae Europaeae cum theé chinitico. Accedit mantissae loco conjectura de alysso Dioscoridis . . . Ed. 2. auct. & corr. . . . Lipsiae & Coburgi, Apud Pfotenhauerum, literis Pentzoldi, 1700.

[14], 158, [10] p.   front., plates.   14 cm.
[4314]

—*respondent. See* METZGER, G. B., *praes.* Disputatio medica inauguralis de sterilitate muliebri. 1677.

—Marius, J. J. F. Castorologia explicans castoris animalis naturam & usum medico-chemicum. 1685.

FRANCKENAU, Georg Franck von. *See* Franck von Franckenau, Georg [1643-1704]

FRANCKENBERG, Abraham von. *See* Frankenberg, Abraham von [1593-1652]

FRANCKENSTEIN, Christian Friedrich [1621-1679] *praeses.* Academica de ephialte diatribe . . . Lipsiae, Literis Wittigavianis [1663]

[16] p.   18 cm.   [4315]

Diss. — Leipzig (J. Loss, *respondent*)

FRANCO, Gaspar dos Reis. *See* Reyes Franco, Gaspar de los [*fl.* 1658]

FRANCO, Miguel [*fl.* 1601] Discurso medicinal en el qual se declara la horden, que se a de tener para praeservarse de la peste y otras enfermedades . . . Cordova, Gabriel Ramos Bejarano, 1601.

[4], 9, [13] ll.   21 cm.   [4316]

FRANÇOIS, René. *See* Binet, Étienne, *Father* [1569-1639]

FRANCUS, Georgius. *See* Franck von Franckenau, Georg [1643-1704]

FRANCUS, Georgius Fridericus. *See* Franck von Franckenau, Georg Friedrich [1669-1732]

FRANCUS, Joannes. *See* Franck, Johann [*fl.* 1608-1609]

FRANCUS DE FRANCKENAU, Georgius Fridericus. *See* Franck von Franckenau, Georg Friedrich [1669-1732]

FRANEKER, Netherlands. **Universiteit.** *See* Academia Franekerana.

FRANEKER, Hoogeschool. *See* Academia Franekerana.

FRANK, Georg. *See* Franck von Franckenau, Georg [1643-1704]

FRANK, Jo. Nikolaus [*fl.* 1671] De corporum animorumque humanorum dissimilitudine discursus . . . Vinariae, Typis Schmidianis, 1671.

[7] p.   19 cm.   [4317]

FRANKE, Jean. *See* Francke, Johann [1648-1728]

FRANKENAU, Georg Frank von. *See* Franck von Franckenau, Georg [1643-1704]

FRANKENBERG, Abraham von [1593-1652] Raphael; oder Artzt-Engel . . . Auffgesetzt . . . im Jahr 1693 [i.e. 1639] . . . Amsterdam, Jacob von Felsen, 1676.

[4], 46, [1] p.   illus.   22 cm.   [4318]

Interleaved.

Added engraved half title.

A pirated German (?) reprint of Felsen's original edition published in the same year. Letters from J. Bruckner, Assistant Librarian, University College London, 8 & 28 October 1974.

—[The same.] Raphael; oder, Artzt-Engel . . . Auffgesetzt . . . im Jahr 1639 . . . Amsterdam, Franckfurt, und Leipzig, Druckts und verlegts Andreas Luppius gnädigst-priviliirter Buch-Händler zu Duissburg und Wesel [ca. 1687]

[4], 46, [1] p.   illus.   24 cm.   [4319]

Added engraved half title.

A reissue with new title page of Felsen's original edition of 1676. Letters from J. Bruckner, Assistant Librarian, University College London, 8 & 28 October 1974.

Privilege granted to Andreas Luppius in 1686. Cf. Benzing (A), p. 167.

FRANKENIUS, Johannes [1590-1661] *praeses.* De occultis medicamentorum simplicium qualitatibus in genere dissertatio medica . . . Upsaliae, Imprimebat Eschillus Matthiae, 1646.

[16] + p.   18 cm.   [4320]

Imperfect: all after p. [16] wanting.

Diss. — Uppsala (J. Simonis, *respondent*)

FRANKFURT AM MAIN. Ordinances, local laws, etc. Reformation; oder, Ernewerte Ordnung der Statt Franckfurt am Mayn, die Pflege der Gesundtheit betreffendt. Welche den Medicis, Apotheckern . . . zur Nachrichtung gegeben worden. Beneben dem Tax und Werth der Artzneyen, welche in den Apothecken allda zufinden. Jetzo abermals von newem getruckt. Franckfurt am Mayn, Durch Caspar Röteln, 1628.

28 p.; 57 p.   24 cm.   [4321]

Part [2] has special title page: Valor sive taxatio medicamentorum . . . quae in officinis Francofurtanis prostant.

—[The same.] . . . Franckfurt am Mayn, By Thomas Matthias Götzen, 1656.

III p.   19 cm.   [4322]

"Valor sive taxatio medicamentorum . . . quae in officinis Francofurtanis prostant . . ." (p. [25]-III) has special title page.

—[The same.] . . . Franckfurt am Mayn, Bey Johann David Zunnern, 1687.

184, [1] p.   20 cm.   [4323]

Errata: p. [185]

"Valor sive taxatio medicamentorum ... quae in officinis Francofurtanis prostant ..." (p. [25]–184) has special title page.

FRANKLIN, ROBERT [1630–1684] A murderer punished and pardoned; or, A true relation of the wicked life, and shameful-happy death of Thomas Savage ... executed at Ratcliff, for ... killing his fellow-servant ... To which is annexed a sermon preached at his funeral ... London, 1668.

48 p.   16 cm.   [4324]

Imperfect: margins trimmed.
Without the sermon.

FRANTZE, WOLFGANG. *See* FRANZ, Wolfgang [1564–1628]

FRANTZIUS, WOLFGANG. *See* FRANZ, Wolfgang [1564–1628]

FRANZ, ELIAS [*fl.* 1674–1678] *respondent. See* FASCH, A. H., *praeses.* Disputatio inauguralis medica, de aegra febre hectica laborante. 1678; WEDEL, G. W., *praeses.* Disputatio medica, exhibens aegrum laborantem colica. 1674.

FRANZ, WOLFGANG [1564–1628] Historia animalium sacra in qua plerorumque animalium praecipuae proprietates in gratiam studiosorum theologiae ... ad usum εικονολογιχον breviter accommodantur ... Witebergae, Sumtibus Zachariae Schureri & Johannis Gormanni, 1613.

[48], 888, [32] p.   17 cm.   [4325]

FRANZI, GIOVANNI BATTISTA [*b.* 1655] Pillola antivenerea; o sia, Mistura antiacida unico purificativo degl'umori ... Milano, Carlo Giuseppe Quinte, 1700.

[14], 166 p.   16 cm.   [4326]

FRANZIUS, THEODOSIUS CHRISTIANUS [*fl.* 1698] respondent. Dissertatio medica inauguralis de apoplexia ... Trajecti ad Rhenum, Ex officina Francisci Halma, 1698.

[16] p.   21 cm.   [4327]

Diss. — Utrecht.

FRANZOSI, GIROLAMO [*fl.* 1652] De motu cordis, et sanguinis in animalibus pro Aristotele, & Galeno adversus anatomicos neotericos libri duo ... Veronae, Typis Merulanis [1652?]

188, [2] p.   21 cm.   [4328]

Errata: p. [189]

—Tractatus apologeticus de semine pro Aristotele

adversus Galenum ... Veronae, Ex typographia Merulana, 1645.

95 p.   22 cm.   [4329]

FRASIER, Sir ALEXANDER. *See* FRAIZER, *Sir* Alexander [1610?–1681]

FRATTA E MONTALBANO, MARCANTONIO DELLA, *marchese* [1635–1695] Dell'acque minerali del regno d'Ungheria ... Venetia, Girolamo Albrizzi, 1687.

[8], 27 p.   illus.   23 cm.   [4330]

Imperfect: fold. map wanting; supplied in photocopy from the New York Academy of Medicine Library.

FRAUENDOERFFER, PHILIPP [*d.* 1702] Oniscographia curiosa; sive, Tractatus physico-medico-pharmaceuticus de asellis vulgo millepedibus, ad normam Imperialis Academiae Caesareo-Leopoldinae Naturae Curiosorum scriptus ... Brunae, Typis Francisci Ignatii Sinapi, 1700.

[14], 132, [8] p.   14 cm.   [4331]

Added engraved title page.

—Opusculum de morbis mulierum, ad mentem recentiorum constructum, & pluribus selectioribusque Hippocratis textibus munitum. Norimbergae, Impensis Johannis Ziegeri, 1696.

108 p.   14 cm.   [4332]

FRAUENDORFF, JOHANN CHRISTIAN [*fl. ca.* 1680] respondent. *See* RIEMER, J. praeses. Bella mulierum. 1680.

A FREE enquiry into the vulgarly receiv'd notion of nature. *See* BOYLE, *Hon.* R.

FREER, ADAM [*fl.* 1687] *respondent.* Disputatio medica inauguralis de partu difficili ... Lugduni Batavorum, Apud Abrahamum Elzevier, 1687.

[16] p.   21 cm.   [4333]

Diss. — Leyden.

FREGOSO, JUAN. *See* FRAGOSO, Juan [*d.* 1597]

FREHER, KARL JOECHIM [*fl.* 1677] *respondent.* De melancholia hypochondriaca positiones ... Basileae, Literis Jacobi Werenfelsii [1677]

[20] p.   20 cm.   [4334]

Diss. — Basel.

FREILAS, ALONSO DE [*fl.* 1605] Conocimiento, curacion, y preservacion de la peste ... Va añadido un tratado nuevo del arte de descontagiar las ropas de seda, telas de oro, y plata, tapicerias ... Con un discurso al fin, si los melancolicos pueden saber lo que està por venir: con la fuerça de su ingenio, ò soñando ... Jaen, Fernando Diaz de Montoya, 1606.

[20], 254, [10] ll. 20 cm. [4335]

Colophon: Jaen, Impresso en casa del autor, por Fernando Diaz de Montoya, 1605.

FREINSHEIM, JOHANN [1608-1660] Dissertatiuncula de calidae potu ... Argentorati, Sumptibus heredum Lazari Zetzneri, 1686.

56 p. 16 cm. [4336]

FREITAG, ARNOLD [ca. 1560-1614] tr. See PISANELLI, B. De esculentorum potulentorumque facultatibus. 1620, 1662.

—See BARICELLI, G. S. Hortulus genialis. 1620.

FREITAG, JOHANN [1581-1641] Aurora medicorum Galeno-chymicorum; seu, De recta purgandi methodo e priscae sapientiae decretis postliminio in lucem reducta, & medicamentis purgantibus simplicibus, compositisque tam veterum, quam neotericorum & chymiatrorum libri IV. ... Francofurti, Impensis Joannis Theobaldi Schönwetteri, 1630.

[16], 642, [30] p. 21 cm. [4337]

—De opii natura, et medicamentis opiatis ad omnes totius corporis affectus ... Groningae, Ex officina Joannis Sas, 1632.

[24], 241, [18] p.; [87] p. 16 cm. [4338]

"Casus aegritudinis a ... Jacobo Ottonis ... propositus ... ad Johannem Freitagium M. D.": p. [1-62]

—[... De unguento armario]

609-612 p. 21 cm. (*In* Theatrum sympatheticum auctum. Norimbergae, 1662) [4339]

Running title.

—Kurtzer Bericht von der Melancholia Hypochondriaca. Nebenst zwölff curiosen Fragen, und einer Analogia der grossen Welt mit der kleinen. Darbey dess Wundersteins der Weissheit und Reichthumbs nicht vergessen wird ... Franckfurt am Mayn, By Caspar Röteln, in Verlegung, Johann David Zunners, 1643.

[40], 513 p. 17 cm. [4340]

Added engraved title page, dated 1644.

—Noctes medicae; sive, De abusu medicinae tractatus ... Accessit dissertatio ... De sanitate & morbo novis verarum opinionum flosculis respersa, et Poematum juvenilium ejusdem auctoris manipulus

... Francofurti, Ex officina typographica Johannis Bringeri, sumptibus Joannis Berneri, 1616.

[32], 464 p. 20 cm. [4341]

Imperfect: lower part of title page mutilated.

"De sanitatis et morborum natura" and "Poematum juvenilium manipulus" have special title pages.

—*praes.* Disputatio medica calidi innati essentiam juxta veteris medicinę & philosophiae decreta explicans ... Groningae, Ex officina Johannis Sas, 1632.

[62] p. 16 cm. [4342]

Diss. — Groningen (K. Walther, *respondent*)

—Disputatio medica de morbis substantię, & cognatis quaestionibus contra hujus tempestatis novatores & paradoxologos ... Groningae, Ex Officina Sassiana, 1632.

56 p. 16 cm. [4343]

Diss. — Groningen (J. Martini, *respondent*)

—Disputatio medico philosophica de formarum origine ... Groningae, Typis Johannis Sas, 1633.

[72] p. 16 cm. [4344]

Imperfect: sig. C8 mutilated affecting text.

Diss. — Groningen (H. Welman, *respondent*)

—See SENNERT, D. Opera omnia in tres tomos distincta. 1641; WINCKLER, D. De opio tractatus. 1635.

FREITAG, JOHANN [1587-1654] *respondent. See* ARNISAEUS, H., *praes.* Observationes aliquot anatomicae. 1610.

—See SPERLING, J. Tractatus physico-medicus, de calido innato. 1634.

FREMERY, EMOND [*fl.* 1693] *respondent.* Disputatio medica inauguralis de facultatibus in genere et in specie de facultate naturali ... Lugduni Batavorum, Apud Abrahamum Elzevier, 1693.

[20] p. 22 cm. [4345]

Diss. — Leyden.

FRÉMONT D'ABLANCOURT, NICOLAS, [1625?-1693] Dialogues de la santé. De M^r de ***. Paris, Jacques Villery, 1683.

[10], 296, [1] p. 17 cm. [4346]

Errata: p. [297]

—Another issue, with imprint: Paris, Jean de la Caille, 1683. [4347]

—[The same.] ... Nouv. ed., rev. & corr.

Amsterdam, Henry Desbordes, 1684.

[6], 206 p.   14 cm.   **[4348]**

[−] [English tr.] The doctors physician; or, Dialogues concerning health. Translated out of the original French. London, Joseph Hindmarsh, 1685.

[8], 219 p.   15 cm.   **[4349]**

Later English editions have title: Health restor'd.

FRENCELIUS, SIMONUS FRIDERICUS. *See* FRENZEL, Simon Friedrich [*fl.* 1660–1679]

FRENCH, JOHN [1616?–1657] The art of distillation; or, A treatise of the choisest spagyricall preparations performed by way of distillation . . . together with the description of the chiefest furnaces and vessels used by ancient, and moderne chymists: also, a discourse of divers spagyrical experiments . . . and of the anatomy of gold and silver . . . All which are contained in six books . . . London, Printed by Richard Cotes and sold by Thomas Williams, 1651.

[24], 199, [16] p.   illus.   19 cm.   **[4350]**

Imperfect: p. 177–178 wanting; supplied in manuscript.

−[The same.] . . . The 2d ed. To which is added, The London-distiller . . . London, Printed by E. Cotes, for Thomas Williams, 1653.

[16], 191 p.; 64, [16] p.   illus.   20 cm.   **[4351]**

Part [2] has special title page dated 1652.

−[The same.] . . . To which is added in this 3d impr. Calcination and sublimation: in two books. As also The London-distiller . . . London, Printed by E. Cotes for T. Williams, 1664.

[16], 250, [22] p.; [1], 46, [3] p.   illus.   19 cm.   **[4352]**

Part [2] has special title page.

−[The same.] . . . 4th impr. . . . London, Printed by E. Cotes for T. Williams, 1667.

[16], 250, [22] p.; [1], 43, [3] p.   illus.   19 cm.   **[4353]**

Part [2] has special title page.
A reprint of the 1664 edition.

−The York-shire spaw; or, A treatise of four famous medicinal wells . . . near Knaresborow in York-shire . . . London, E. Dod, and N. Ekins, 1652.

[8], 124, [2] p.   15 cm.   **[4354]**

−[The same.] . . . London, Nath. Brook, 1654.

[8], 124, [2] p.   15 cm.   **[4355]**

A reissue of the 1652 edition with new title page.

−, *ed. See* HERMES TRISMEGISTUS. The divine pymander. 1650.

−, *tr. See* AGRIPPA VON NETTESHEIM, H. C. Three books. 1651; SENDIVOGIUS, M. A new light of alchymie. 1650, 1674.

FRENTZ, GERARDUS [*fl.* 1695–1696] Epistola anatomica, problematica quinta . . . ad . . . Fredericum Ruyschium . . . de vasis sanguiferis periostii tibiae, ut & viis, per quas vesicula fellea sarcinam acquirit. Amstelaedami, Apud Joannem Wolters, 1696.

10, [2] p.   plates.   22 cm.   **[4356]**

"Frederici Ruyschii responsio . . .": p. 5–10.

FRENTZELIUS, SIMONUS FRIDERICUS. *See* FRENZEL, Simon Friedrich [*fl.* 1660–1679]

FRENZEL, SIMON FRIEDRICH [*fl.* 1660–1679]

Dissertations — Wittenberg

−*praeses.* Causas corporum cruentorum, superioribus non modo annis, sed elapso cum maxime in Misnia, vicinisque oris conspicuorum . . . exponet . . . Gottfried Schultze . . . Wittebergae, Literis Matthaei Henckelii [1673]

[28] p.   18 cm.   **[4357]**

G. Schultze, *respondent.*

−De rerum futurarum praesensione naturali . . . Wittebergae, Literis Matthaei Henckelii [1673]

[32] p.   19 cm.   **[4358]**

Imperfect: upper margins trimmed.
Z. Fischer, *respondent.*

−Disputatio publica prima, de anima, maxime rationali, pro adstruenda ejusdem in homine unitate, contra pluralitatem animarum realiter et secundum substantiam in homine distinctarum . . . Wittebergae, Literis Johannis Borchardi [1663]

[16] p.   18 cm.   **[4359]**

J. Bugius, *respondent.*

−Disputatio publica secunda pro animae humanae unitate rationes producens contra pluralitatem animarum realiter et secundum substantiam in homine distinctarum . . . Wittebergae, Literis Johannis Borchardi [1663]

[16] p.   18 cm.   **[4360]**

K. Fritz, *respondent.*

−Disquisitionem naturalem de unicornu . . . publicae ventilatione sistit . . . Christianus Vater . . .

Wittebergae, Typis Johannis Wilckii, 1679.

    [24] p. 19 cm.   **[4361]**

   C. Vater, *respondent.*

—Monstrum humanum ventribus sine proportione et mutilis artubus, Wittebergae D. XXX Augusti, natum . . . Wittebergae, Typis Johannis Willkii [1674]

    [28] p. 19 cm.   **[4362]**

   T. Schepler, *respondent.*

—Serpentem . . . publicae eruditorum contemplationi sistit Arnoldus Berninck . . . Wittebergae, Ex officina Johannis Haken [1665]

    [68] p. 19 cm.   **[4363]**

   A. Berninck, *respondent.*

FRÈRE JACQUES. *See* BEAULIEU, Frère Jacques de [1651-1714]

FRERUS, JOANNES. *See* FRYER, John [*fl.* 1544-1571]

FRESBAUCH, HILARIUS. *See* WEIS- ET ROTHWEIN DE REBENSAFFT, J. Novae regulae sanitatis medico-physicae.

FRESCHOT, CASIMIR [1640?-1700] *ed. See* [GAYA, L. de] Cerimonie nuzziali di tutte le nationi del mondo. 1685.

FRESENIUS, JOHANN GEORG [*fl.* 1697] *respondent.* Disputatio inauguralis medica, de spasmo seu convulsione . . . Gissae-Hassorum, Imprimebat Henningus Müllerus [1697]

    20 p. 20 cm.   **[4364]**

   Diss. — Giessen.

FREUDENHAMMER, GEORG SIEGEFRID [*fl.* 1641-1646] Speculum theoriae-medicae, ex optimis, iisque diversissimis autoribus . . . concinnatum, & expolitum . . . [Amstelodami?] Typis Johannis Pauli, 1646.

    36, [1] p. 14 cm.   **[4365]**

   Errata: p. [37]

FREUND, JOHANN GEORG [*fl.* 1698] *respondent.* Disputatio inauguralis medica de semine masculino in statu s. & p. n. constituto . . . [Altdorffii] Literis Henrici Meyeri [1698]

    44 p. 21 cm.   **[4366]**

   Diss. — Altdorf.

FREY, JANUS CÄCILIUS [*d.* 1631] Opera quae reperiri potuerunt in unum corpus collecta. Parisiis, Apud Petrum David, 1645.

[7], 296, [8] p.; [8], 570 p. 17 cm.   **[4367]**

   Part [2] has special title page: Mens . . . centuriis II. axiomatum expressa. Ed. IV. auctior, & ordinatior.

   ". . . Admiranda Galliarum compendio indicatam" (p. [309]-507) and ". . . Scientiae et artes quotquot hactenus fuerunt aut supersunt omnes ordine & cum cura, distributae & descriptae . . ." (p. [509]-570) have special title pages.

—Opuscula varia nusquam edita, philosoph. medic. & curiosis omnibus utiliss. quorum haec est series. 1. Philosophia druidarum. 2. Cribrum philosophorum. 3. Propositiones de universo curiosiores. 4. Cosmographiae selectiora. 5. Dialectica veterum, praeceptis ad expeditam rerum notitiam utilissimis instructa. 6. Compendium medicinae . . . Parisiis, Apud Petrum David, 1646.

    [17], 523, [17] p. 17 cm.   **[4368]**

   Edited by Antoine Morand.

FREY, JOHANN [*fl.* 1645-1647] *respondent. See* SALTZMANN, J. R. [1573-1656] *praeses.* Disputatio medica de dysenteria. 1647; SEBISCH, M. [1578-1674?] *praeses.* Disputatio de naturalibus facultatibus prima [-octava & ultima] 1644 [i.e. 1645] [and] Galeni quinque priores libri. 1651.

FREY, JOHANN LUDWIG [*fl.* 1699] *respondent. See* ZWINGER, T., *praeses.* Dissertationem hanc philosophicam quae est de natura mentis humanae . . . tuebitur J. L. F. 1699.

FREY, LORENZ JOSEPH [*fl.* 1661] *respondent. See* KIRCHMAYER, G. K., *praeses.* De coralio. 1661.

FREYBURGER, JOHANN CLAUDIUS [*fl.* 1661] *respondent. See* SEBISCH, M. [1578-1674?] *praeses.* Problemata medica miscellanea. 1661.

FREYLAS, ALONSO DE. *See* FREILAS, Alonso de [*fl.* 1605]

FREYTAG, GOTTLIEB [*fl.* 1660] *respondent.* Disputatio medica inauguralis de lypothymia . . . Altdorffii, E typographeo Academico Hageniano [1660]

    [20] p. 19 cm.   **[4369]**

   Diss. — Altdorf.

—*See* HOFFMANN, M., *praeses.* Theses medicae de sanguine. 1660.

FREYTAG, JOHANN. *See* FREITAG, Johann [1587-1654]

FREYWALDT, DONAT [*fl.* 1608] *respondent. See* HORST, G. [1578-1636] *praeses.* Problematum medicorum θεραπευτικων decades priores quinque. 1608.

FREYWALDT, DONAT [*fl.* 1666-1667] *respondent. See* KORMART, G. Disputatio physica de elemento aquae Helmontii. 1667.

FREZZA, FABIO [*fl.* 1614-1623] Discorsi intorno a i rimedii d'alcuni mali, a i quali foggiace la citta, & il regno di Napoli ... Napoli, Per li heredi di Tarquinio Longo, 1623.

[8] 110, [1] p. 21 cm. **[4370]**

FRICCIUS, JOANNES. *See* FRICK, Johann [*fl.* 1607]

FRICCIUS, MELCHIOR. *See* FRICK, Melchior [1651-1703]

FRICK, JOHANN [*fl.* 1607] *See* KNOBLOCH, T., praeses. Disputationes anatomicae. 1608, 1612.

FRICK, MELCHIOR [1651-1703] Dissertatio medica de peste; seu, Nova methodus, cognoscendi & curandi pestem ... Ulmae, Typis haeredum Christiani Balthasaris Kühnen, 1684.

156 p. 14 cm. **[4371]**

—Historia et consultatio medica pro podagrico exhibita & examinata ... Ulmensi 1683.

[26] p. 19 cm. **[4372]**

—Icon podagrae; seu, Accurata delineatio repraesentans morbi podagrici historiam, causas, prognosin, et curationem ... Ulmae, Typis Gassenmejerianis, 1693.

[8], 230 p. 14 cm. **[4373]**
With this are bound: Sydenham, T. Tractatus de podagra et hydrope. 1686. — Sydenham, T. Additamenta nova ad ... Opera universa. 1689.

—Medicinischer Bericht von der sogenandten Colica scorbutica; oder scharbockischen Darmgicht, und der darauss entstehenden Paresi, dass ist: Lähmung, deren Ursprung, Ursachen, Kenn-und Vorsagungs-Zeichen, wie auch Curation beschrieben ... Ulm, Joh. Carl Gassenmeyer, [1676?]

[1], 67 p. 14 cm. **[4374]**
Imprint date worn, may read 1696; Latin edition published in 1696.

—Paradoxa medica, in quibus plurima curiosa & utilia contra communes medicorum opiniones pertractantur, & affectuum aliquot, ut apoplexiae, maniae, vulnerum venenatorum, hydrophobiae & aliorum theoria & praxis ostenditur. Ulmae, Sumptibus Georgii Wilhelmi Kühnen, 1699.

[12], 300 p. 15 cm. **[4375]**

—*respondent. See* CRAUSE, R. W., *praeses.* Disputatio inauguralis medica de alvi fluxu. 1674; SCHENCK, J. T., *praeses.* Dissertatio medica de poris corporis humani. 1670.

FRIDELIUS, JOHANNES. *See* FRIEDEL, János [*fl.* 1665-1668]

FRIDENRYCHIUS, SAMUEL [*fl.* 1652] *respondent. See* DEUSING, A., *praeses.* Disputationum anatomicarum octava. 1652.

FRIDERICH, ANTON GÜNTER [*fl.* 1652-1658] Disputatio physica de nutritiva facultate ... exhibet M. Anthonius Gunther Friederici ... respondente Johanne Töpffer ... Lipsiae, Excudebat Johannes Bauer, 1652.

[23] p. 19 cm. **[4376]**
Diss. — Leipzig (J. Töpffer, respondent)

—*respondent. See* LANGE, C., *praeses.* Disputatio inauguralis de malo literatis familiari. 1658.

FRIDERICI, DANIEL [*fl.* 1667] *respondent. See* AMMANN, P., *praeses.* Disputationem inauguralem de haemorrhagia ... subjicit ... D. F. 1667.

FRIDERICI, GOTTLIEB [*fl.* 1682] *respondent.* Disputatio medica inauguralis de gangraena et sphacelo ... Lugduni Batavorum, Apud Abrahamum Elzevier, 1682.

[16] p. 22 cm. **[4377]**
Imperfect: last leaf mutilated.
Diss. — Leyden.

FRIDERICI, JOHANN ARNOLD [1637-1672] Anatomen medicinae fundamentum in nobilioris sexus cadavere adornabit ... Jenae, Stanno Krebsiano [1665]

[15] p. 19 cm. **[4378]**

—Dissertationem, de sterilitate muliebri ... Johann-Arnoldus Friderici ... publicae artis cultorum censurae offert ... Jenae, Stanno Krebsiano [1664]

[40] p. 20 cm. **[4379]**
Diss. pro loco — Jena.

Dissertations — Jena

—*praeses.* Aloen publicae florae cultorum censurae exponit Gothofredus Beier ... Jenae, Typis Johannis Wertheri [1670]

    [28] p.   20 cm.   **[4380]**

G. Beier, *respondent.* ——

—Anatomia lienis ... Jenae, Aere Krebsiano [1669]

    [52] p.   19 cm.   **[4381]**

J. Ussleber, *respondent.*

—Consultatio medica de stupore manuum ... Jenae, Literis Wertherianis [1667]

    [23] p.   20 cm.   **[4382]**

P. M. Marci, *respondent.*

—De tentigine disputationem ... publico examini submittit ... Andreas Homberg ... Jenae, Typis Wertherianis, 1671.

    40 p.   21 cm.   **[4383]**

A. Homberg, *respondent.*

—Diatriba medica de spiritibus sylvestribus flatulentis ... Jenae, Expressit Johannes Gollner [1671]

    [28] p.   18 cm.   **[4384]**

J. J. Gotter, *respondent.*

—Disputatio inauguralis medica de imbecillitate ventriculi ... Jenae, Typis Wertherianis [1672]

    [32] p.   19 cm.   **[4385]**

S. P. Klettwich, *respondent.*

—Disputatio inauguralis medica de lienteria ... Jenae, Literis Wertherianis, 1670.

    [24] p.   19 cm.   **[4386]**

G. T. Wallich, *respondent.*

—Disputatio inauguralis medica de melancholia ... Jenae, Literis Wertherianis, 1671.

    [44] p.   19 cm.   **[4387]**

J. K. Fuchs, *respondent.*

—Disputatio medica de conceptione ... Jenae, Literis Müllerianis [1670]

    [62] p.   18 cm.   **[4388]**

B. Scharff, *respondent.*

—Disputatio medica de paeonia ... Jenae, Literis Johannis Wertheri [1670]

    [24] p.   20 cm.   **[4389]**

J. Geinitz, *respondent.*

—Disputatio medica de ventriculo ... Jenae, A calcographeo Samuelis Krebsii [1671]

    [24] p.   20 cm.   **[4390]**

C. E. Clauder, *respondent.*

—Disputatio medica inauguralis de morbo castrensi seu Hungarico ... Jenae, E calcographeo Krebsiano, 1666.

    [36] p.   19 cm.   **[4391]**

J. A. Zapff, *respondent.*

—Disputatio medica inauguralis, qua ... peripneumoniam ... publicae ... disquisitioni submittit Johannes Casparus Heim ... Jenae, Typis Johannis Nisii, 1666.

    [40] p.   19 cm.   **[4392]**

J. K. Heim, *respondent.*

—Disputationem inauguralem de cardialgia ... publicae ... censurae exponit Christianus Fridericus Richter ... Jenae, Literis Johannis Nisii [1671]

    [36] p.   19 cm.   **[4393]**

C. F. Richter, *respondent.*

—Disputationem medicam de corpulentia nimia publicae ... censurae ... submittit ...Joann Fridericus Held ... Jenae, Typis Nisianis [1670]

    [36] p.   20 cm.   **[4394]**

J. F. Held, *respondent.*

—Disputationem medicam de mania ex philtro ... publicae censurae submittit ... Georgius Tobias Wallich ... Jenae, Literis Wertherianis [1670]

    [48] p.   19 cm.   **[4395]**

G. T. Wallich, *respondent.*

—Dissertatio inauguralis medica, de δυστοκία naturali ... [Jenae] Literis Nisianis [1665]

    [24] p.   20 cm.   **[4396]**

A. W. Osann, *respondent.*

—Dissertatio inauguralis medica de mola ... Jenae, Typis Samuelis Adolphi Mülleri, 1670.

    [28] p.   20 cm.   **[4397]**

M. B. Burchardi, *respondent.*

—Dissertatio inauguralis medica de pica ... Jenae, Ex Molybdographia Krebsiana, 1668.

    [32] p.   19 cm.   **[4398]**

S. Ledel, *respondent.*

—Dissertatio medica de ῾υστερομανια ... Jenae, Literis Nisianis [1666]

    [28] p.   20 cm.   **[4399]**

Imperfect: title page and p. [9-14] mutilated.
J. K. Heim, *respondent.*

—Dissertatio medica de incubo . . . Jenae, Typis Joannis Nisii [1665]
[36] p. 20 cm.   **[4400]**
J. J. Ruttörffer, *respondent.*

—Dissertatio medica inauguralis de apoplexia . . . Jenae, Typis Johannis Wertheri, 1668.
[40] p. 19 cm.   **[4401]**
M. Merckel, *respondent.*

—Dissertatio medica inauguralis de stranguria . . . Jenae, Literis Krebsianis [1667]
[44] p. 20 cm.   **[4402]**
P. Wernic, *respondent.*

—Dissertatio medico-chirurgica de gangraena et sphacelo, per ἀφηεσιν και προφυγαξιυ chirurgico-pharmaceuticam tollendis & curandis . . . Jenae, Typis Nisianis, 1671.
[56] p. 20 cm.   **[4403]**
C. F. Pollmar, *respondent.*

—Dissertationem medicam de atrophia . . . examini sistit Samuel Chemnitius . . . Jenae, Literis Johannis Nisii [1672]
[52] p. 20 cm.   **[4404]**
S. Chemnitz, *respondent.*

—Dissertationem medicam de vertigine . . . publico . . . examini submittit Christophorus Richter . . . Jenae, Stanno Krebsiano, 1669.
[44] p. 20 cm.   **[4405]**
C. Richter, *respondent.*

—Exercitationem anatomicam de renibus . . . publicae . . . ventilationi subjicit Christianus Döhring . . . Jenae, Literis Samuelis Krebsii [1663]
[24] p. 19 cm.   **[4406]**
C. Döhring, *respondent.*

—Haemorrhagiae uteri menstruae praeternaturalis, θεωριαν και θεροπειαν ut specimen . . . exhibet . . . Johannes Otto Wurstschmidt . . . Jenae, E chalcographeo Nisiano, 1670.
[1], 32, [2] p. 19 cm.   **[4407]**
J. O. Wurstschmidt, *respondent.*

—Υοτερυδερίασις; sive, Uteri hydrops, disputatione inaugurali repraesentatus . . . Jenae, Typis Johannis Nisii, 1669.
[47] p. 19 cm.   **[4408]**
J. H. Laurentius, *respondent.*

—Ordo et methodus cognoscendi & curandi gravissimum intestini tenuioris affectum ileum . . . Jenae, Typis Samuelis Krebsii [1666]
[48] p. 18 cm.   **[4409]**
C. E. Stempel, *respondent.*

—Scrutinium hydrocephali, secundum διαγνωσιν προγνωσιν και θεραπειαν . . . Jenae, Typis Samuelis Adolphi Mülleri, 1669.
[36] p. 19 cm.   **[4410]**
J. P. Prükkel, *respondent.*

—Ταρακολόηια; sive, De tabaco dissertatio . . . Jenae, Literis Wertherianis [1667]
32 p. 20 cm.   **[4411]**
A. Hahn, *respondent.*

—*respondent. See* ROLFINCK, W., *praes.* Dissertatio inauguralis medica, qua . . . apoplexiam . . . offert disquisitioni M. J. A. F. 1661.

FRIDERICI, JOHANNES [*fl.* 1656] *respondent. See* FAUSIUS, J. K., *praeses.* Disputatio inauguralis medica, de venenis. 1656.

FRIDERICI, MICHAEL [*fl.* 1622] *respondent. See* SCHALLER, W., *praeses.* Centuria positionum medicarum de passione colica. 1622.

FRIDERICI, VALENTIN [1630-1702] *praes.* Διασκεψις historico-philologica de capillamentis vom Barücken . . . Lipsiae, Typis Joh. Erici Hahnii [1673]
16 p. 18 cm.   **[4412]**
Diss. — Leipzig (V. Erfurth, *respondent*)

—Disputatio physica de sapore . . . [Lipsiae] Typis Johannis Baueri [1654]
[16] p. 19 cm.   **[4413]**
Diss. — Leipzig (B. Seyler, *respondent*)

FRIDERICUS, KASPAR [*fl.* 1602] *respondent. See* ROOMEN, A. van, *praeses.* Disceptatio anatomica de partibus thoracis earumque convenienti administrandi ratione. 1602.

FRIEDEL, JÁNOS [*fl.* 1665-1668] *praeses.* Disputatio medica de pleuritide . . . Wittebergae, Typis Johannis Haken [1668]
[56] p. 20 cm.   **[4414]**
Diss. — Wittenberg (M. Kölsch, *respondent*)

—*respondent. See* SCHNEIDER, K. V., *praeses.* Disputatio inauguralis medica de angina. 1666.

FRIEDERICH, *Prince of Saxony. See* SAXONY. Laws, statutes, etc. Fürstliche sachs. bothaische medicinische Verordnung. 1680.

FRIEDERICH, ANTON GÜNTHER. *See* FRIDERICH, Anton Günter [*fl.* 1652–1658]

FRIEDERICH, PHILIPP ERNST [*fl.* 1685–1686] *respondent. See* ALBINUS, B. Dissertatio de fonte. 1685 [and] Dissertatio medica inauguralis, de missione sanguinis. 1686.

FRIEDERICI, ANTHONIUM GÜNTHER. *See* FRIDERICH, Anton Günter [*fl.* 1652–1658]

FRIEDLIBIUS, AMADEUS. *See* FRANKENBERG, Abraham von [1593–1652]

FRIES, HANS JAKOB [1586–1656] *respondent. See* LUCIUS, J. J., *praeses.* Disputatio medica de morborum natura et differentis. 1608.

FRIESE, ANDREAS WILHELM [*fl.* 1655–1656] *respondent. See* CONRING, H., *praeses.* Disputatio medica de epilepsia. 1656.

FRIESE, CHRISTOPH [*fl.* 1663] *respondent. See* PAULLI, J. H., *praeses.* Anatome anatomiae Bilsianae. 1663.

FRIESE, FRIEDRICH [1668–1721] *praeses.* Dissertationem physicam de curiosa et superstitiosa rusticorum physica ... submittit ... Johann Karl Ritter ... Lipsiae, Literis Christiani Scholvinii [1691]
[34] p. 18 cm.   [4415]
Diss. — Leipzig (J. K. Ritter, *respondent*)

FRIESE, HEINRICH [1630–1690] Disputatio medica qua defenditur, quod celebratissima illa per totam Europam hodie medicina thee arthritide conveniat ... Regiomonti, Praelo Reusneriano, 1684.
[8] p. 19 cm.   [4416]
Diss. pro loco — Königsberg (C. R. Hertz, *respondent*)

FRIESE, JOHANN JACOB [1586–1656] *See* FRIES, Hans Jakob [1586–1656]

FRIESE, JOHANN JACOB [*fl.* 1610–1612] *respondent. See* STUPANUS, J. N., *praeses.* Σημειοτιces particularis cap. I. De affectibus. 1610.

FRIESS, MARTIN FRIEDRICH [1632–1700]

Programs — Leipzig
Facultatis Medicae in Academia Lipsiensi h. t.

pro-cancellarius Martinus Fridericus Friess ... L. S. [Lipsiae, Literis Wittigavianis, 1689]
[8] p. 19 cm.   [4417]
With vita of J. C. Schamberg.

—Martinus Fridericus Friess ... pro-cancellarius, L. S. [Lipsiae, 1680]
[8] p. 20 cm.   [4418]
For diss. of J. D. Schmoller.

Dissertations — Leipzig
—*praeses.* De salivation ... Lipsiae, Typis Christiani Gözii [1684]
[28] p. 20 cm.   [4419]
J. F. Ortlob, *respondent.*

—Dentes eruditorum limae ultra perpoliendos ... subjicit ... Gabriele Malmo ... Lipsiae, Aere Coleriano [1654]
[20] p. 19 cm.   [4420]
G. Malmus, *respondent.*

—Examen coraliorum tincturae ... Lipsiae, Typis viduae Henningi Coleri [1665]
[27] p. 20 cm.   [4421]
M. Ettmüller, *respondent.*

—[The same.] Examen coraliorum tincturae ... P. P. ... ad diem XV. Septembr. M. DC. LXV ... Lipsiae, Denuo excudebat Nicolaus Scipio, 1679.
[27] p. 18 cm.   [4422]
M. Ettmüller, *respondent.*

—Inauguralis de podagra disputatio ... Lipsiae, Typis Johannis Erici Hahnii [1673]
[16] + p. 20 cm.   [4423]
Imperfect: all after p. [16] wanting.
J. S. Wider, *respondent.*

FRIESS, MARTIN FRIEDRICH [1632–1700] *respondent. See* MICHAELIS, J., *praeses.* De apoplexia disputationem inauguralem ... submittit M. F. F. 1657.

FRIESSEM, HERMAN VAN [*fl.* 1662] *respondent.* Disputatio medica inauguralis de temperamentis ... Lugduni Batavorum, Ex officina Salomonis Wagenaer, 1662.
[16] p. 21 cm.   [4424]
Diss. — Leyden.

FRIETZSCH, MATTHÄUS FRIEDRICH [*fl.* 1689] *respondent. See* HARDT, J. G., *praeses.* Dubium physicum quoad sonum in campana vulgo creditum extricatum. 1689.

FRIGGIO, Onofrio [*fl.* 17th cent.] Ricette galenistiche agionte al libro intitolato L'arte del spetiale di Fra Francesco Sirena date alla luce dal P. Onofrio Friggio ... Pavia, Gio. Ghidini, 1692.

24, 224 p.   22 cm.   [**4425**]

FRIGIMELICA, Francesco [1491-1559] De balneis metallicis artificio parandis, liber postumus novi argumenti e bibliotheca Joannis Rhodii. Patavii, Apud Sebastianum Elpidium, 1659.

[8], 45, [3] p.   16 cm.   [**4426**]

—[The same.] ... Norimbergae, Impensis Johannis Ziegeri, 1679.

44, [3] p.   17 cm.   [**4427**]

—See Hofmann, C. Pathologia parva. 1640.

FRIGIO, Jacopo Antonio [*fl.* 1608] In magni Hippocratis Prognostica Jacobi Antonii Phrygii ... explanatio. Apposita cuique fere loco ex Libris epidemiorum privata exempla ad confirmandas auctoris sententias, & ad praxim exercendam apprime utilia ... Ticini, Apud Marcum Grigium bibliopolam [Apud Petrum Bartolum] 1608.

[16], 453, [51] p.   15 cm.   [**4428**]
Errata; p. [46-51]
Includes Latin text of the Prognostica in Lorenzo Laurenziani's version.

FRIGIO, Pietro Francesco [1586 or 7-1659] Petri Francisci Phrygii ... Commentarii in historias epidemicas Hippocratis, in tres partes digesti ... Lugduni, Sumptibus Joan. Antonii Huguetan, 1644.

[16], 569, [34] p.   25 cm.   [**4429**]
Includes Greek and Latin text of the case histories from Epidemiorum libri 1 and 3.

FRIMEL, Johann [1632-1688] *praeses.* Disputationem physicam de aqua ... publice sistunt ... Johannes Frimel ... & ... Michael Desler ... Wittebergae, Literis Johannes Röhnerus [1657]

[16] p.   18 cm.   [**4430**]
Imperfect: upper margins trimmed.
Diss. — Wittenberg (M. Desler, *respondent*).

FRISCH, Gebhard [*fl.* 1694] Anatomia alchymiae, quae universalem viam et totius philosophiae Hermeticae doctrinam, ac divisiones exhibet ... Alkahest sermone emblematico ventilatur. Ipsummet lapidem et ejus compositionem docet disceptatio de lapide physico, in qua ... Geber, Comes Trevisanus, arcanum Hermeticum, Sendivogius, Philaletha, & Pantaleon explicantur, &

cujuslibet practica dispersa, ordinatim recollecta, & dilucidata traditur. Quae omnia ab authore D. Gebhardo Frischi ... composita Thomas Bergmiller ... typis imprimi curavit ... Parmae, Ex typographia Josephi Rosetti, 1695.

[16], 207, [1] p.   18 cm.   [**4431**]

FRISCHMUTH, Johann [1619-1687] Epistola gratulatoria ad ... Joh. Hadrianum Slevogtum ... qua simul de antrace, carbunculo, bubone & altauna, philologice disseritur. Jenae, Typis viduae Krebsianae, 1681.

[8] p.   20 cm.   [**4432**]

FRISE, Heinricus. *See* Friese, Heinrich [1630-1690]

FRISIMELICA, Franciscus. *See* Frigimelica, Francesco [1491-1559]

FRISIUS, Andreas., *ed. See* Mercuriale, G. De arte gymnastica. 1672.

FRISIUS, Christophorus. *See* Friese, Christoph [*fl.* 1663]

FRISIUS, Fridericus. *See* Friese, Friedrich [1668-1721]

FRISIUS, Joannes Jacobus. *See* Fries, Hans Jakob [1586-1656]

FRITSCH, Ahasverus [1629-1701] Diatribe juridica de jure ac privilegiis hospitalium ... Jenae, Sumptibus Johannis Bielcken, 1672.

[4], 44 p.   19 cm.   [**4433**]

—Medicus peccans; sive, Tractatus de peccatis medicorum. Norimbergae, Apud Wolfgangum Mauritium Endterum, 1684.

116 p.   14 cm.   [**4434**]

FRITSCH, Christian Ludwig [*fl.* 1697] *respondent. See* Thomasius, C., *praeses.* Dissertatio inauguralis de jure circa pharmacopolia civitatum. 1697.

FRITSCH, Gottfried [*fl.* 1665] *respondent. See* Sultzberger, S. R., *praeses.* De rore microcosmi. 1665.

FRITSCH, Johann [*fl.* 1626] *respondent. See* Ager, N. Disputatio physica ... de mente humana. 1626.

FRITSCH, Peter [*fl.* 1677-1691] *respondent. See* Posner, C., *praeses.* De manna. 1677.

FRITZ, KASPAR [*fl.* 1663] *respondent. See* FRENZEL, S. F., *praeses.* Disputatio publica secunda pro animae humanae unitate. 1663.

FRITZSCHE, BARTHOLOMÄUS [*fl.* 1608] *respondent.* Specimen inaugurale publicum thesium miscellarum politico-medicarum, physiologic. patholog. simiotic. diaetet. pharmaceut. chirurgic. & clinicarum ... Basileae, Ex officina Johannis Schroeteri, 1608.

    [20] p.   22 cm.   [**4435**]
    Diss. — Basel.

FRITZSCHEN, JOHANN [*fl.* 1673] *respondent. See* ARTOPÄUS, J. D., *praeses.* Dissertatio anti-Baroniana. 1673.

FRIZIMELICA, FRANCISCUS. *See* FRIGIMELICA. Francesco [1491–1559]

FRIZSCHIUS, BENJAMIN [*fl.* 1679] *respondent. See* ROHR, P., *praeses.* Dissertatio historico-philosophica de masticatione mortuorum. 1679.

FRÖLICH, GOTTFRIED [*fl.* 1688] *respondent. See* DEUBLINGER, D. O., *praeses.* Exercitatio philosophica. 1668.

FRÖLICH, JOHANN HEINRICH [*fl.* 1599–1613] *praeses.* Σημειωτιχὴ φοιβεία paradoxis & heterodoxis ... D. Felicis Plateri ... adornata ... Basileae, Typis Johan. Jacobi Genathii, 1612.

    [24] p.   19 cm.   [**4436**]
    Diss. — Basel (G. Obermeyer, *respondent*)

    —*respondent.* ῾Επτὰς δεκάδων ἰητρικῶν ἀμφιμιγέων ... Basileae, Typis Joan. Jacobi Genathii, 1611.

    [12] p.   illus.   22 cm.   [**4437**]
    Text in Latin.
    Diss. — Basel.

    —*respondent. See* PLATTER, F. [1536–1614] *praeses.* Theses miscellae. 1612.

FRÖLING, ANDREAS [*ca.* 1629–1683] *praeses.* De qualitatibus primis dissertatio physica ... Helmestadii, Typis Henningi Mulleri, 1658.

    [32] p.   18 cm.   [**4438**]
    Diss. — Helmstedt (J. Lechel, *respondent*)

FROHNE, JOHANN BERNHARD [*fl.* 1643] *respondent. See* GARPIUS, P., praeses. Disputatio physica de propagatione animae humanae. 1643.

FROIDMONT, LIBERT [1587–1653] Liberti Fromondi ... Meteorologicorum libri sex. Antver-piae, Ex Officina Plantiniana, apud Balthasarem Moretum & viduam Joannis Moreti, & Jo. Meursium, 1627.

    [12], 420, [18] p.   illus.   23 cm.   [**4439**]

FROMENT, PIERRE [*d.* 1715] Hypothese raisonnée, dans laquelle on fait voir que la cause interne de toutes les fievres, & generalement de toutes les autres maladies, vient des levains acides, acres ou salez qui se rencontrent dans les premieres voyes. Le tout expliqué sur les principes du celebre Monsieur Descartes ... Paris, Laurent d'Houry et l'auteur, 1694.

    [16], 322, [18] p.   16 cm.   [**4440**]

FROMHOLD, GUSTAV ENOCH [*fl.* 1682–1684] *respondent. See* LOSS, J., *praeses.* Disputatio inauguralis medica de cancro mammarum. 1684 [and] Exercitatio pathologica. 1682.

    —*See* LOSS, J. Jeremias Lossius ... anat. et botanices prof. publicus ... S.P.D. lecturis. 1683.

FROMMANN, JOHANN ANDREAS [1626–1690] Hypotyposis; sive, Summaria delineatio juris furiosorum singularis ... Argentinae, Ex officina Josiae Staedelii, 1656.

    83, [5] p.   19 cm.   [**4441**]

FROMMANN, JOHANN CHRISTIAN [*b. ca.* 1640] Discursus medicus de venae sectione in morbillorum declinatione oborta pleuritide administranda ... Lipsiae, Impensis Georgii Heinrici Frommanni, 1668.

    [8], 104, [4] p.   16 cm.   [**4442**]
    Imperfect: upper margins shaved.

    —Tractatus de fascinatione novus et singularis, in quo fascinatio vulgaris profligatur, naturalis confirmatur, & magica examinatur; hoc est, nec visu, nec voce fieri posse fascinationem probatur ... Norimbergae, Sumtibus Wolfgangi Mauritii Endteri, & Johannis Andreae Endteri haeredum, 1675.

    [79], 1067, [45] p.   21 cm.   [**4443**]
    Added engraved title page dated 1674.
    With this is bound Thumm, T. Tractatus theologicus. 1667.

    —Tractatus singularis de haemorrhoidibus problematum theoreticorum & practicorum centuria absoluta ... Norimbergae, Sumtibus Wolfgangi Mauritii Endteri, & Joh. Andreae Endteri haeredum, 1677.

    [40], 504, [52] p.   14 cm.   [**4444**]
    Added engraved title page.

—*praeses*. Exercitationem physico-medicam de consensu partium corporis humani ... publicae eruditiorum censurae sistunt ... Joh. Christianus Frommann ... ac ... Joh. Wolffgangus Schreiber ... [Coburgi] Typis Joh. Conradus Munch [1658]

[48] p. 18 cm.   [4445]

Diss.—Coburg (J. W. Schreiber, *respondent*)

—Exercitationis medicae prioris de haemorrhoidibus, problemata theoretica, ad circulationem sanguinis Harvejanam accommodata ... Coburgi, Johannes Conradus Monachus [1669]

[2], 44, [2] p. 18 cm.   [4446]

Diss.—Coburg (J. Röder, *respondent*)

—Problemata miscellanea tria ... Coburgi, Typis Ducalibus, imprimebantur per Johannem Conradum Monachum [1668]

[2], 24, [2] p. 20 cm.   [4447]

Diss.—Coburg (J. C. Walz, *respondent*)

—Quaestionis hujus physicae, an sanguis, quem Christus passionis suae initio sudavit, naturaliter promanarit ... Coburgi, Formis Ducalibus, imprimebat Johannes Conradus Mönch, 1665.

[24] p. 19 cm.   [4448]

Diss.—Coburg (H. Wernhöfer, *respondent*)

—*respondent*. See MÖBIUS, G., *praeses*. Disputatio inauguralis medica de dolore capitis. 1653.

FROMMER Christen Fast-Buss- and Bet-tägliche allerbeste Erquickstunden. *See* MÜHLMANN, J. Geistlicher Noth- und Todes-Schirm. 1680.

FROMONDUS, LIBERTUS. *See* FROIDMONT, Libert [1587-1653]

FRONTEAU, JEAN, *Father* [1614-1662] Dissertatio I. philologica ... de virginitate honorata, erudita, adorata, foecunda ... Lutetiae Parisiorum, Apud Sebastianum & Gabrielem Cramoisy, 1651.

[8], 45, [1] p. 21 cm.   [4449]

Imperfect: lower margin shaved, affecting text.
Bound with [Quillet, C.] Calvidii Leti [pseud.] Callipaedia. 1655.

FRONTO, JOANNES. *See* FRONTEAU, Jean, *Father* [1614-1662]

FROSTEN, ERNESTUS BOGISLAUS [*fl.* 1660] *respondent*. De tartaro. *In* Rolfinck, W., *praeses*. Dissertationes chimicae sex de tartaro. 1660, 1679.

FROWEIN, KASPAR [*fl.* 1686] *respondent*. Disputatio medica inauguralis de hydrope ascite ...

Lugduni Batavorum, Apud Abrahamum Elzevier, 1686.

[20] p. 22 cm.   [4450]

Diss.—Leyden.

FRÜEAUFF, NIKOLAUS DANIEL [*fl.* 1672] *respondent*. *See* RUMPEL, J. H., *praeses*. Dissertationem meteorologico-physicam de terrae motu ... censurae publice sistent D. N. F. 1672.

FRUNDECK, JOHANN LUDWIG VON [*fl.* 1660-1666] Tractatus de elixire arboris vitae; id est, Medicina mea universali ... Hagae-Comitis, Ex typographia Adriani Vlacq, 1660.

[4], 147, [1] p. 16 cm.   [4451]

FRYER, John [*fl.* 1544-1571] *See* HIPPOCRATES. [Aphorismi. Greek and Latin. 1633.]

FRYER, JOHN [*d.* 1733] A new account of East-India and Persia, in eight letters. Being nine years travels, begun 1672, and finished 1681. Containing observations made of the moral, natural, and artificial estate of those countries: namely, of their ... health, diseases ... London, Printed by R. R. for Ri. Chiswell, 1698.

[9], 427, [xxiv] p. illus., plates., port. 32 cm.
                                   [4452]

FUCHS, GILBERT. *See* FUSCH, Gilbert [*ca.* 1504-1567]

FUCHS, JOHANN [*fl.* 1607] *respondent*. Disputatio medica de cruenta expuitione ... Basileae, Typis Excertierianis, 1607.

[12] p. 20 cm.   [4453]

Diss.—Basel.

FUCHS, JOHANN KONRAD [*fl.* 1670-1671] *praeses*. *See* FRIDERICI, J. A., *praeses*. Disputatio inauguralis medica de melancholia. 1671.

—*respondent*. *See* SCHENCK, J. T., *praeses*. Exercitatio medica cura vexatorum ad veterum & recentiorum mentem exstructa. 1670.

FUCHS, JOHANN REINHARD [*fl.* 1686-1688] *respondent*. Thema ... de gutta rosacea ... Altdorffii, Stanno Schönnerstaedtiano [1688]

16 p. 20 cm.   [4454]

Diss.—Altdorf.

—*See* WEDEL, G. W., *praeses*. Dissertatio medica de clavo pedis. 1686.

FUCHS, Leonhart [1501-1566] Institutionum medicinae libri quinque: nunc denuo diligentissime recogniti, ab innumeris mendis repurgati, nonnullisque in locis auctiores redditi . . . Basileae, Typis Conradi Waldkirchii, 1605.

[15], 809, [77] p.   17 cm.   [4455]
Stübler 29E.

— [The same.] Institutionum medicinae; seu, Medendi methodi, ad Hippocrat. Galen. aliorumque veterum, et recentiorum medicorum celeberrimum scripta adytum . . . libri quinque . . . opera, & studio Emmanuelis Stupani . . . ab innumeris pene repurgati erroribus, plurimisque in locis auctiores redditi. Basileae, Sumptibus Ludovici Regis, 1618.

[12], 760, [58] p.   illus.   17 cm.   [4456]
Stübler 29F.

—, tr. See Hippocrates. [Aphorismi. Dutch. 1665] [and] [Aphorismi. Adaptations, etc. French. 1654]

— See Hippocrates [Aphorismi. English. 1655]

FUCHS, Petrus [fl. 1635] respondent. See Sebisch, M. [1578-1674?] praeses. Collegii therapeutici disputatio I[-XIV] 1634 [i.e. 1635]

FUCHS, Rémacle. See Fusch, Remaclus [ca. 1510-1587]

FUCHS, Samuel [1588-1630] Metoposcopia & ophthalmoscopia. Argentinae, Excudebat Theodosius Glaserus, sumptibus Pauli Ledertz, 1615.

[16], 140 p.   ports., illus.   16 cm.   [4457]

FUELDEZ, Antoine [fl. 1643] Observations curieuses, touchant la petite verole, vraye peste des petits enfans: et le bezahar son antidote. Contenant plusieurs rares secrets pour embellir le visage, & pour oster les difformitez que laisse aptes soy cette maladie . . . Lyon, Jean Antoine Huguetan, 1645.

[15], 157, [3] p.   17 cm.   [4458]

FUENTA LA PEÑA, Antonio de, Father [fl. 1676] El ente dilucidado. Discurso . . . que muestra ay en naturaleza animales irracionales invisibles, y quales sean . . . Madrid, Emprenta Real, acosta de Ju. Calatayud, 1677.

[22], 438, [18] p.   22 cm.   [4459]
Engraved title page.

FUENTE, Andrés Fernández de la. See Fernández de la Fuente, Andrés [fl. 1640-1649]

FÜRST, Johann Zacharias [fl. 1674-1692] Dialogus hygiasticus; id est, Colloquium physico medicum, inter Hygiophilum et Jatrophilum . . . Francofurti, Sumptibus authoris, typis Andreae Deutschmann, 1692.

[6], 3-150, [6] p.   13 cm.   [4460]

— respondent. See Leichner, E., praeses. Disputatio medica inauguralis de mania. 1674.

FÜRSTLICHE sachs. bothaische medicinische Verordnung. 1680. See Saxony. Laws, statutes, etc.

FUHRMANN, Josua [fl. 1676-1679] respondent. See Fasch, A. H., praeses. Disputatio medica inauguralis de epilepsia. 1679.

FULBERTI, Godefrido. See Buonanni, Filippo [1638-1725]

FULDA, Christoph [fl. 1603-1607] respondent. See Schröter, P. J., praeses. De diaeta aegrorum themata medica. 1607.

FULGINEO, Gentilis de. See Gentile da Foligno [d. 1348]

FULKE, William [1538-1589] A most pleasant prospect into the garden of naturall contemplation, to behold the naturall causes of all kinde of meteors: as well fierie and airie, as watrie and earthly . . . 2d ed. corr. and amend. London, Printed by John Haviland, and sold by James Boler, 1634.

[3], 71 ll.   15 cm.   [4461]
STC 11439.

A FULL relation concerning the wonderfull and wholsome fountain. At first discovered in Germany two miles from the city of Halberstadt . . . With a specification of those persons, which . . . were . . . cured by use of these waters. A list of the diseases . . . London, Printed by T. W. for Joshua Kirton, 1646.

[1], 21 p.   19 cm.   [4462]

FULLER, Thomas [1654-1734] See Bate, G. Pharmacopoeia Bateana. 1700.

FUNCCIUS, Carolus Ludovicus [fl. 1677] respondent. Disputatio medica inauguralis de haemorrhoidibus nimium conniventibus et coecis . . . Altdorffii, Typis Heinrici Meieri [1677]

40 p.   20 cm.   [4463]
Diss. — Altdorf.

—Another issue, includes laudatory poems.
44 p.   19 cm.   **[4464]**

FUNCCIUS, CHRISTIANUS. *See* FUNCK, Christian [1626–1695]

FUNCCIUS, CHRISTOPHORUS. *See* FUNK, Christoph [*fl.* 1608–1615]

FUNCK, CHRISTIAN [1626–1695] *respondent. See* MAUCKISCH, J., *praeses.* Aphorismi physici de pluvia. 1647.

FUNCK, DANIEL [*fl.* 1676–1678] *respondent. See* HOPFFER, B., *praeses.* Disputatio moralis de desperatione. 1678.

FUNCK, JOHANN BALTHASAR [17th cent.] *ed. See* BARNSTEIN, H. Tabacks Wunder Kunst. 1677.

FUNK, JOHANN MICHAEL [*fl.* 1694–1695] *respondent. See* BRUNO, J. P., *praeses.* Cholegraphia. 1694.

FUNCKE, CHRISTOPH [*fl.* 1653–1654] *respondent.* De paralysi. *In* Rolfinck, W., *praeses.* Methodus cognoscendi & curandi adfectus capitis particulares. 1653.

—*See* MÖBIUS, G., *praeses.* Discursus inauguralis de legitimo venaesectionis usu. 1654.

FUNDAMENTA vera chymiae. Paracelsus. Separate & ad maturitatem perducite. [n. p.] 1660.
15 p.   17 cm.   **[4465]**
With this is bound Index et manuductor chymicus. 1680.

FUNK, CHRISTOPH [*fl.* 1608–1615] *respondent.* Theses de sterilitate muliebri . . . Basileae, Typis Joh. Jacobi Genathii, 1615.
[16] p.   20 cm.   **[4466]**
Diss. — Basel.

FUNK, JOHANN MICHAEL [*fl.* 1694–1695] *respondent.* Cholegraphiae pars altera; h. e., Dissertatio therapeutica de bile vitiosa corrigenda . . . [Altdorffii] Excudebat Henricus Meyerus [1695]
30 p.   20 cm.   **[4467]**

FUOLI, CECILIO. *See* FOLLIO, Cecilio [1615–1660]

FURCK, SEBASTIAN [1589–1666] *engr. See* BOISSARD, J. J. Bibliotheca chalcographia. 1650–54.

FURICH, JOHANN NICOLAUS [*fl.* 1623] *respondent. See* SEBISCH, M. [1578–1674?] *praeses.* Exercitationes medicae. 1639.

FURLANUS, DANIEL [*d.* 1576] *tr. See* THEOPHRASTUS. Θεοφράστον . . . ἅπαντα. Theophrasti . . . Graece & Latine opera omnia. 1613.

FUSCH, GILBERT [*ca.* 1504–1567] *See* A BRIEFE DISCOURSE OF THE HYPOSTASIS. 1612?

FUSCH, REMACLUS [*ca.* 1510–1587] *See* BERNARD DE GORDON. Lilium medicinae. 1617.

FUSCONE, PIETRO PAOLO [*fl.* 1605] Trattato del bere caldo, e freddo . . . Dove si disputa, se conviene generalmente à tutti cosi sani, come amalati, & in particolare a' podagrosi il bevere del continovo l'acqua col vino, tanto calda quanto si può sufferire, overo molto fredda con neve, ò pure come ci vien data dalla natura. Aggiungendovisi in fine un capitolo, dove s'insegna il vero modo di conoscere le acque buone, e di correggere le triste. Genova, Giuseppe Pavoni, 1605.
[8], 388 (i.e. 390), [8] p.   22 cm.   **[4468]**

FUSCUS, REMACLUS. *See* FUSCH, Remaclus [*ca.* 1510–1587]

G

G., C. *See* GLASER, Christophe [*ca.* 1615–*ca.* 1673]

G., C. L. C. *See* LECLERC, Charles Gabriel [1644–1700?]

G., E. *See* GARDINER, Edmund.

G., E. *See* GRIMSTONE, Edward.

G., J. *See* GADBURY, John [1627–1704]

G., J. *See* GLAZEMAKER, Jan Hendrik [*d.* 1682]

G., J., *tr. See* PARÉ, A. The workes. 1649, 1665, 1678.

G., J. C. [*fl.* 1681] *ed. See* SPECULUM ASTROLOGICUM. 1693.

G., J. H. *See* GLAZEMAKER, Jan Hendrik [*d.* 1682]

G., R. *See* GOWER, Richard [*fl.* 17th cent.]

G., R., *M.D. See* GOCLENIUS, Rudolph [1572–1621]

G. T., M. B. *See* GUIDOTT, Thomas [1638–1706]

GABALIS. *See* VILLARS, N. P. H. *de Montefaucon.* Le Comte de Gabalis. 1675?

GABELKOVER, OSWALD [1539–1616] Artzneybuch, Darinnen ... fast für alle fess menschlichen Leibs Anligen und Gebrechen, ausserlesene und bewehrte Artzneyen, gemeinem Vatterland teutscher Nation zu gutem, auss vielen hohen und niders Stands Personen geschribnen Artzneybüchern zusamen getragen, und in den Truck verfertiget sind ... Und nun ... publiciert, an vielen Orten verbessert, und mit nutzlichen heilsamen Artzneyen gemehrt worden ... [Franckfurt] In Truck verfertiget durch Nicolaum Hoffmann, in Verlegung Johann Jacob Porschen, und Johann Berrners, 1610.
[12], 424 p.; [2], 434, [3] p. 21 cm. [**4469**]
Part [2] has special title page.
First published in 1589 under title: Nützlich Artzneybuch für alle des menschlichen Leibes Anliegen und Gebrechen.

—[The same.] ... [Franckfurt] In Verlegung Johann Jacob Porschen und Johann Berrners, 1618.
[12], 424 p.; [2], 434, [3], p. 21 cm. [**4470**]
Part 2 has special title page.
Different setting of type.

—[The same.] ... [Franckfurt] In Verlegung Johann Jacob Porschen s. Wittib und Johann Berrners s. Erben, 1641.
[12], 424 p.; [2], 434, [3] p. 21 cm. [**4471**]
Part 2 has special title page.
Different setting of type.

—[The same.] ... Von neuem von etlichen fürnehmen Medicis durchsehen, vermehret und verbessert. Franckfurt am Mayn, Johann Peter Zubrodt, 1680.
[6], 498, [14] p. port. 21 cm. [**4472**]

—Kurtzer Bericht: der fürstlichen Württembergischen Hoff Medicorum; wie sich mit Artzney ... zu dieser ... Zeit der Pestilentz, zuhalten ... Sampt hinzugethanem kurtzem Regiment, von ... der Artzney Doctorn, gestellt und zusamen getragen. Tübingen, Getruckt in der Gellischen Truckerey, 1608.
82 p. 16 cm. [**4473**]
"Wie sich vor der Pestilentz ... zuverhüten": p. 3–28; signed by Oswald Gäbelkover, Christoff Schwartz, and Ulrich Porta.

—[The same.] ... Stuttgardt, Getruckt bey Johann Weyrich Röszlin, 1626.
[1], 28 p. 18 cm. [**4474**]

Without the Regiment.
Signed at end by Oswald Gabelkover, Christoff Schwartz and Ulrich Porta.

GABELKOVER, WOLFGANG [*b. ca.* 1570] Curationum et observationum medicinalium. Centuria I [-VI] Tubingae, Typis Philippi Gruppenbachii, impensis Johannis Berneri, 1611–27.
6 v. in 1. 16 cm. [**4475**]
Imprint varies.
Imperfect: all leaves after sig. S8 of vol. 6 wanting.

—, *ed. & tr. See* BACCI, A. De gemmis et lapidibus pretiosis. 1603.

GABIANO, JOANNES FRANCISCUS DE [*fl.* 1558] *See* SOLENANDER, R. Consiliorum medicinalium ... sectiones quinque. 1609.

GABIR, ABU MUSA IBN ḤAIYĀN AL-AZDI [al-Safi] [*fl. ca.* 776] *See* JĀBIR IBN ḤAIYAN, al-Ṭarasūsī.

GĀBIR IBN ḤAYYĀN. *See* JĀBIR, IBN ḤAIYĀN, al-Ṭarasūsī.

GABLER, ANDREAS [*fl.* 1611] De conservanda valetudine; das ist, Nützlicher Bericht, wie menschliche Gesundheit zu erlangen, und bestendig zu erhalten sey. Dabey auch nicht allein ordentliche Mittel der Artzney angezeiget werden, wie man sich vor jtzt regierender Seuche (die Hauptkranckheit genant) ... verwahren soll, sondern auch wie man sich vor der ... Seuch der Pestilentz, welche ... im Monat September, und hernach in der edlen Provintz Schlesien ... grassiren wird ... auffhalten kan ... Pragaw, 1611.
[39] p. 18 cm. [**4476**]

[GABRIEL, SIONITA, 1577–1648] Arabia, seu Arabum vicinarumque gentium orientalium leges, ritus, sacri et profani mores, instituta et historia: accedunt praeterea varia per Arabiam itinera, in quibus multa notatu digna enarrantur. Amstelodami, Apud Joannem Janssonium, 1633.
297 (i.e. 287) p. illus. 11 cm. [**4477**]
Half title reads: De nonnullis orientalium urbibus, necnon indigenarum religione ac moribus, tractatus brevis. A Gabr. Sionita ... ac Joanne Hesronita.

GADALDINI, AGOSTINO [1515–1575] *ed. See* GALENUS. [Ars medica. Latin. 1606, 1663]; SCHOLA MEDICA. 1682–84.

GADBURY, JOHN [1627–1704] Collectio geniturarum; or, A collection of nativities, in CL genitures ... with ... observations ... historical and astrological ... London, James Cottrel, 1662.

    [15], 219 p. front. (port.), illus. 27 cm.
                                            [4478]

    In 3 parts, each with special title page.

—Philastrogus knavery epitomized, with a vindication of Mr. Culpeper, Mr. Lilly, and the rest of the students in that noble art, from all the false aspersions ... cast upon them, about the great eclipse of the sunne ... Written by J[ohn] G[adbury] ... London, 1652.

    15, [1] p. 19 cm.   [4479]

—Thesaurus astrologiae; or, An astrological treasury. Containing the choicest mysteries of that curious, but abstruse learning, relating to physick. Being the collections and experiments of a learned physitian and astrologer deceased, whose name is not known ... London, Thomas Passenger, 1674.

    [16], 272, [8] p. illus., plates. 17 cm. [4480]

GADEBUSCH, SAMUEL VALENTIN [*fl.* 1685] *respondent. See* HELLWIG, C. von, *praeses.* Disputatio medica inauguralis de affectione hypochondriaca. 1685.

GÄBELE, JOHANN. Dass Ihro käyserl. Majestät Leopoldus die Freyheit mitgetheilt, auch durch die Herren Doctores untersucht und abprobiert worden. ... Memmingen, Gedruckt bey Johann Valentin Mayer [not before 1658]

    [8], 382, [6] p. illus. 17 cm.   [4481]
    Caption title on p. 1: Des Wund-Artzney-Buches erster Theil.

GAEBELCHOVER, WOLFGANG. *See* GABELKOVER, Wolfgang [*b. ca.* 1570]

GÄBELKHOUER, OSSWALDT. *See* GABELKOVER, Oswald [1539–1616]

GAEN, JEAN [*fl.* 1661] *See* BLONDEL, F. Lettres ... au sieur Jaques Didier ... touchant les eaux minerales chaudes d'Aix & de Borcet. 1662.

GAESBEECK, LAURENS VAN [*fl.* 1663] *respondent. See* RAEI, J. de, *praeses.* Disputatio philosophica. 1663.

GAETKE, JOACHIM PETER [*fl.* 1698] *respondent. See* STAHL, G. E. *praeses.* Dissertatio medica inauguralis de vena portae porta malorum. 1698.

GAFFAREL, JACQUES [1601–1681] Curiositez inouyes; hoc est, Curiositates inauditae de figuris Per-

sarum talismannicis, horoscopo patriarcharum et characteribus coelestibus ... Latine, cum notis ... editae, opera M. Gregorii Michaelis ... Hamburgi, Apud Gothofredum Schultzen, prostant & Amsterdami, Apud Jansonio-Waesbergios, 1676.

    [62], 290, [1] p.; 498, [47] p. illus., plates. 16 cm.   [4482]

    Added engraved title page.
    Part [2] has special title page: M. Gregorii Michaelis ... Notae in Jacobi Gaffarelli Curiositates.

—, *ed. See* CAMPANELLA, T. Medicinalium, juxta propria principia, libri septem. 1635.

—*See* SOREL, C. Des talismans. 1636.

GAGLIARDI, DOMENICO [*fl.* 1689–*ca.* 1723] Anatomes ossium novis inventis illustratae ... Pars prima. Romae, Typis Joannis Jacobi Komarek, 1689.

    [16], 109, [3] p. plates. 19 cm.   [4483]
    No more published.
    Author's presentation copy, unsigned.

GAGLIARDI, GIOVANNI ANTONIO [*fl.* 17th cent.] *See* GAGLIARDI, U. De victus quantitate in febribus pestiferis. 1628.

GAGLIARDI, UBERTO. De victus quantitate in febribus pestiferis, malignis, et acutis ... Typis tradita per Jo. Antonium ejus filium ... Genuae, Apud Josephum Pavonem, 1628.

    50 p. 21 cm.   [4484]

GAGNON, F. A. D., *sieur de Saintigny* [*fl.* 1697] La recherche de la verité dans la medecine, où paroît l'homme sur un nouveau system qui fait voir comment il vit, le jeu de tous ses ressorts pour l'oeconomie naturelle de sa vie ... Paris, Jean de Nully, et l'auteur, 1698.

    [8], 442, [2] p. 18 cm.   [4485]

GAGO DE VADILLO, PEDRO [*fl.* 1630] Discursos de verdadera cirugia, y censura de ambas vias, y eleccion de la primera intencion curativa, y union de las heridas ... Madrid, Juan Gonçalez, 1632.

    [6], 171 ll. 21 cm.   [4486]
    Imperfect: last leaf (blank?) wanting.

—[The same.] Luz de la verdadera cirugia, y discursos de censura de ambas vias, y eleccion de la primera intencion curativa, y union de las heridas ... Corr., y enmendado en esta 3. imp. ...

Pamplona, Juan Nicol, 1692.

[4], 292, [2] p. illus. 21 cm.   [**4487**]

Imperfect: p. 253-4 mutilated.

GAIGNON, D. *See* GAGNON, F. A. D., *sieur de Sain-tigny* [*fl.* 1697]

GAILHARD, JEAN DE [*d.* 1707] Johannis Gailhardi Tolosatis De venae sectione disquisitio ubi quaestio an in apoplexia sit vena secanda … confirmatur. Hafniae & Lipsiae, Sumt. Samuelis Garmanni, 1699.

[4], 112 p. 14 cm.   [**4488**]

GAILLARD, JEAN [*fl.* 1685] *praeses.* Quaestiones medicae selectiores … Tolosae, Ex typographia Dominici Desclassan, 1685.

[4], 13 p. 22 cm.   [**4489**]

Diss. — Toulouse (S. Langlade, *respondent*)

GAIOTIUS, MARCUS ANTONIUS. *See* GAJOTIUS, Marcus Antonius [*fl.* 1646-1647]

GAIUS, BERNARDINUS. *See* CAIUS, Bernardinus [*fl.* 1596-1612]

GAJOTIUS, MARCUS ANTONIUS [*fl.* 1646-1647] *ed.* *See* HIPPOCRATES. [Aphorismi. Greek and Latin. 1647]

GALATHEAU, DE [*fl.* 1662-1674] Dissertation sur la digestion de l'estomach, touchant l'humeur acide … Paris, François Muguet, 1675.

116, [2] p. 17 cm.   [**4490**]

—*See* LAMY, G. Explication … des fonctions de l'ame sensitive. 1678, 1681, 1687.

GALE, THOMAS [1635?-1702] *ed.* Opuscula mythologica physica et ethica. Graece et Latine … Amstelaedami, Apud Henricum Wetstenium, 1688.

[30], 7-752, [8] p. 22 cm.   [**4491**]

Added engraved title page.

GALEANO, GIUSEPPE [1605-1675] *comp.* and *tr.* Del conservar la sanita libri sei de Galeno. Compendio, e traduzione del … Giuseppe Galeano … Palermo, Nicolò Bua, 1650.

[10], 115, [9] p. 15 cm.   [**4492**]

Il **GALENISTA** confuso; overo, L'arte convinta d'impostura nell'uso del salasso. 1697. *See* [CUSANI, R.]

GALENUS

Arrangement

I.   Collected works [Greek and Latin]

II.   Collected works [Latin]

III.   Selected works [Greek and Latin]

IV.   Selected works [Latin]

V.   Selected works [French]

VI.   Selected works [Spanish]

VII.   Selections, etc. [Greek and Latin]

VIII.   Selections, etc. [Latin]

IX.   Individual works (arranged alphabetically by standard Latin title)

X.   Recettario

XI.   References

I. Collected works [Greek and Latin]

1679. *In* Hippocrates. Collected works [Greek and Latin] 1679.

II. Collected works [Latin]

1609

—Opera ex octava Juntarum editione … Venetiis, Apud Juntas, 1609.

13 v. in 5. illus. 35 cm.   [**4493**]

Vol. [13] has title: Antonii Musae Brasavoli … Index refertissimus in omnes Galeni libros, qui ex octava Junctarum editione extant.

Edited by Fabius Paulinus.

J. A. Boni assisted A. M. Brasavola in the preparation of the index.

—Another printing, with same contents, but a different typesetting throughout, except the 4 preliminary leaves.

Vol. [13], the index, only.   [**4494**]

1625

—Opera ex nona Juntarum editione … Venetiis, Apud Juntas, 1625.

13 v. in 5. illus. 36 cm.   [**4495**]

A reprint.

III. Selected works [Greek and Latin]

1640

—Τῶν σωζομενων τινα … Opuscula varia … A … Theodoro Goulstono … Graeca recensita, mendisque … repurgata, & in linguam Latinam … traducta … Accessere ab eodem variae lectiones, & annotationes criticae. Londini, Typis Richardi Badger, sumptibus Ph. Stephani, & Ch. Meredith, 1640.

[24], 247, [27] p. 22 cm.   [**4496**]

Contents. — Exhortatio ad medicinam & artes. — Quod optimus medicus, idem & philosophus. — De optimo docendi genere. — De sectis. — De optima secta. — De animi perturbationibus. — De animi erratis. – De substantia naturalium facultatum. – Quod animi mores sequantur temperamentum corporis.

IV. Selected works [Latin]

1604. *In* Valleriola, F. Loci medicinae communes. 1604.

1624

—Αιτιολογικη και παθολογικη; sive, De morborum et symptomatum differentiis, et causis, libri sex Claudii Galeni ... una cum commentariis Jacobi Segarrae ... Opus nunc recens excusum, et ... correctum ... per Hieronymum Vincentium Salvador ... Valentiae, Michaelis Sorolla, 1624.

[8], 270, [17] ll. 21 cm.   [**4497**]

Translated by Gulielmus Copus.

1627. *In* Rossel, J. F. Ad sex libros Galeni De differentiis. 1627.

1645

—Francisci Vallesii ... Commentaria illustria, in Cl. Galeni Pergameni libros subsequentes, I. Artem medicinalem, II. De inaequali temperie libellum, III. Tertium de temperamentis librum, IIII. Quinque priores de simplicium medicamentorum facultate libros, V. Duos de differentia febrium, VI. Sex de locis patientibus libros. Tractatus medicinales. I. De urinis compendiaria tractatio, II. De pulsibus libellus, III. De febribus commentarius, IIII. Methodi medendi libri tres. Omnia recens prima hac editione publicata, opera & industria Joannis Petri Ayroldi Marcellini ... Francfurti, Apud Johannem Beyer, 1645.

[1] p., 1222 (i.e. 1184) columns, [10] p. 32 cm.
[**4498**]

A reissue with new title page of the 1594 edition.

Includes Latin versions of the Galenic texts. The Ars medica, De inaequali intemperie and De differentiis febrium were translated by the commentator; the third book of the De temperamentis by Thomas Linacre; the first five books of the De simplicium medicamentorum facultatibus by Theodoricus Gerardus; and the De locis affectis by Gulielmus Copus.

1680

—Praxis medica curiosa; hoc est, Galeni Methodi medendi libri XIV. Nova, eaque omnium accuratissima versione, & perpetuis plus vice simplici desideratis commentariis, et castigationibus ... illustrati a Casparo Hofmanno ... Adjectis nonnullis, in epidorpismatum vicem, cum primis De dictero illo, medice vivere esse pessime vivere, cum oratione

Joannis Georgii Volckameri ... Curante Sebastiano Scheffero, M. D. Francofurti, Impensis Joannis Justi Erythropili, typis Joannis Andreae, 1680.

3 parts in 1 v. 21 cm.   [**4499**]

Part [2] has special title page: Vita medica; hoc est Galeni Υγιεινων; sive, Methodi sanitatis tuendae libri VI.

Part [3] has caption title: Oratio prima [-quinta] De dictero illo, medice vivere esse pessime vivere [... Joannis Georgii Volckameri ... in laudem ... Caspari Hofmanni]

V. Selected works [French]

1605

—Les six principaux livres de la methode therapeutique de Claude Galien, avec le II. De l'art curatoire à Glaucon. Auquel est adiousté le livres Des tumeurs, contre nature ... Rev. & corr. ... Derniere ed. Lyon, Pierre Rigaud, 1605.

[8], 288 ll. 13 cm.   [**4500**]

A reprint of Tibault Payan's 1558 Lyon edition.

Includes versions of books 3–6 and 13–14 of Methodus medendi, all but book three translated by Jean Canappe. The version of the De tumoribus is that of Pierre Tolet.

Edited by Claude Martin.

1634 *In* Guidi G. [*ca.* 1500–1569] Les anciens et renommés autheurs de la medecine & chirurgie. 1634.

VI. Selected works [Spanish]

1624

—Therapeutica methodo de Galeno en lo que toca de cirugia. Recopilada de varios libros suyos, y adornada con ... paraphrases en muchos lugares obscuros: nuevamente troduzida en romance por Geronymo Murillo ... Añadido un tratado de Jacobo Holerio, y traduzidas las receptas de latin en romance ... Valencia, Miguel Sorolla, a costa de Juan Antonio Tavano, 1624.

[16], 440, [28] p.; 95, [5] ll. 16 cm. [**4501**]

Part [2] has special title page.

Contents. – Part [1] El tercero [-sexto] libros de la Therapeutica. – El libro De los tumores contra natura. – El decimotercio, y decimoquarto libros de la Therapeutica. – El segundo de la Arte curativa a Glaucon. – El De los tiempos de toda una enfermedad. Part [2] Tratado de la materia de cirugia. Compuesto por Jacobo Hollerio.

1651

—[The same.] ... Zaragoça, Juan de Ybar, 1651.

[16], 440, [28] p.; 95, [5] ll. 15 cm. [**4502**]

Part [2] has special title page with undated imprint: En Valencia, Por Miguel Sorrolla. A costa de Juan Antonio Tavano.

Different setting of type.

VII. Selections, etc. [Greek and Latin]

1655, 1675. *In* Rolfinck, W. Epitome methodi cognoscendi & curandi particulares corporis affectus. 1655, 1675.

VIII. Selections, etc. [Latin]

1604

—Epitome Galeni . . . operum, in quatuor partes digesta . . . per Dn. Andream Lacunam . . . collecta. Accesserunt ejusdem And. Lacunae Annotationes in Galeni interpretes . . . Item, De ponderibus & mensuris medicinalibus utilis commentarius . . . Editio postrema prioribus multo castigator atque correctior. Argentorati, Sumptibus Lazari Zetzneri, 1604.

[8] p., 1298 columns, [151] p.   illus.   33 cm.

[**4503**]

1616

—Ad artium liberalium studium capescendum oratio adhortaria [sic]. Item, quod optimus medicus, nisi etiam philosophus, non sit. Ex interpretatione nova Sixti Arcerii cum notis ejusdem . . . Franekarae, Apud viduam Romberti Doyema, 1616.

[4], 23, [15] p.   21 cm.   [**4504**]

1643

—Epitome Galeni operum, in quatuor partes digesta . . . Cum compendio ipsiusmet Galeni in Hippocratem, in calce hujus libri adjecto. Ed. nov. . . . expurgata. Auctore A. Lacuna. Lugduni, Sumpt. Joan. Caffin & Francisc. Plaignard, 1643.

[20], 636, [80] p.; 187 p.   illus.   37 cm.   [**4505**]

Part [2] has half title: Epitome commentariorum Galeni in Hippocratem ab. A. Lacuna. Includes: Enantiomata, sive, Contradictiones Galeni.

1672. *In* Clément, G. Sententiae principum medicorum. 1672.

1677, 1688. *In* Beckers, N. W. Florilegium Hippocraticum et Galenicum. 1677, 1688.

IX. Individual works.
Ars medica

Greek and Latin

1610. *In* Argenterio, G. Opera. 1610.

Latin

1606

—Ars medicinalis, Nicolao Leoniceno interprete.

Venetiis, Apud Franciscum Bolzettam, 1606.

159 p.   10 cm.   [**4506**]

"Ad Graecorum veterum exemplarium fidem ab Augustino Gadaldino, aliquibus in locis emendati [sic]" Cf. p. 5.

With this are bound: Hippocrates. Aphorismorum . . . sectiones septem. 1610 [i.e. 1611]; Hippocrates. Pronosticorum libri tres. 1611; Avicenna. Fen. I, lib. I. Canonis. 1611.

1607. *In* Oddi, O. degli. Expositio. 1607.

1612. *In* Santorio, S. Commentaria in Artem medicinalem Galeni. 1612.

1622

—[The same.] . . . Novissima hac editione argumentis & & [sic] divisionibus tum totius opusculi, tum singulorum capitum locupletata, a Joanne Thuilio . . . Patavii, Ex typographia Gasparis Crivellarii, 1622.

[10], 157 p.   11 cm.   [**4507**]

Imperfect: p. 103–106 wanting.

1631. *In* Santorio, S. Commentaria in Artem medicinalem Galeni. 1631.

1642

—[The same.] . . . Patavii, Typis Pauli Frambotti, 1642.

[11], 173 p.   14 cm.   [**4508**]

With this are bound: Avicenna. Fen. I. lib. I. Canonis. 1648; Hippocrates. Aphorismorum sectiones VII. 1649.

1660. *In* Santorio, S. Opera omnia. 1660.

1663

—[The same.] . . . Venetiis, Apud Turrinum, 1663.

116, [4] p.   11 cm.   (Part [2] in Schola medica in qua Hippocratis, Galeni, Avicennaeque . . . habentur fundamenta. Venetiis, 1663)   [**4509**]

"Ad Graecorum veterum exemplarium fidem ab Augustino Gadaldino, aliquibus in locis emendati [sic]." Cf. p. 5.

"Capita, sive puncta quae laureandis proponi solent in celeberrimis collegis": p. 113–116.

"Libri medici, chirurgici, chimici, & pharmacop. Latini": [4] p. at end.

1682. *In* Schola medica. 1682–1684.

English

1652

—Galens art of physick . . . Translated into English, and largely commented on . . . By Nich. Culpeper . . . London, Peter Cole, 1652.

[19], 120, [7] p.   front. (port.)   14 cm.   [**4510**]

—*as subject. See* RIOLAN, J. [1538?-1605?] In artem parvam Galeni commentarius. 1631; SEBISCH, M. [1578-1674?] Galeni Ars parva in disputationes triginta resoluta. 1633.

De alimentorum facultatibus
Latin
1633
—De alimentorum facultatibus libri III. Ex Martini Gregorii interpretatione; pluribus in locis, hac editione, emendata. Subjunctus est, alimentorum de quibus agit, index & nomenclator Graecus, Latinus, Gallicus, Belgicus. Lugduni Batavorum, Apud Asingam de Fries [Ex officina typographica Wilhelmi Christiani] 1633.
[4], 320, [43] p. 11 cm. [4511]

De antidotis. Selections.
Italian
1613
—L'antidotario di Claudio Galeno Pergameno interpretato da Michelangelo Angelico ... Nel quale si contengono di due libri de gli Antidoti, quello della Theriaca à Panfiliano, il Trattato dessa à Pisone, & il discorso de' sali theriacali ... Vicenza, Domenico Amadio, 1613.
[8], 131, [10] p. 21 cm. [4512]

De constitutione artis medicae
Latin
1626. *In* Valleriola, F. Artis medicae fundamina secundum Galenum. 1626.

De compositione medicamentorum secundum locos
Latin
—*as subject. See* HOULLIER, J. Ad libros Galeni De compositione medicamentorum. 1603.

De curandi ratione per venae sectionem. Selections, etc.
Latin
1649. *In* Guibert, P. Medici officiosi opera. 1649.
French
1633, 1636, 1639, 1640, 1641. *In* Guibert, P. Les oeuvres charitables.
1645. *In* Guibert, P. Le medecin charitable. 1645.

1647, 1649, 1653, 1656, 1657, 1660, 1670, 1674, 1678. *In* Guibert, P. Les oeuvres charitables.

—*as subject. See* SEBISCH, M. [1578-1674?] *praeses.* Problemata phlebotomica. 1631.

De decubitu infirmorum ex mathematica scientia.
—*See* IMBRASIUS, of Ephesus. Prognostica de decubitu.

De euchymia et cacochymia
—*as subject. See* SEBISCH, M. [1578-1674?] *praeses.* Disputatio medica de plethora et cacochymia. 1631.

De differentiis febrium
Latin
1626. *In* Vega, C. de. Opera omnia. 1626.
1651. *In* Navarro, J. B. Commentarii ad libros Galeni De differentiis febrium. 1651.

De methodo medendi ad Glauconem. Selections, etc.
Greek and Latin
1610. *In* Argenterio, G. Opera. 1610.
Latin
1606. *In* Argenterio, G. Opera. 1606.

De morbis et symptomatis libri sex
—*as subject. See* SEBISCH, M. [1578-1674?] *praeses.* Libri sex Galeni De morborum differentiis. 1632; ZAMORA Y CLAVERÍA, J. Pathologicae elucubrationes. 1659.

De naturalibus facultatibus
—*as subject. See* SEBISCH, M. [1578-1674?] Disputatio de naturalibus facultatibus prima [-octava & ultima] 1644 [i.e. 1645]

De optima doctrina
Greek and Latin
1621. *In* Sextus Empiricus. Opera. 1621.

De ossibus ad tirones
Greek and Latin
1603. *In* Ingrassia, G. F. In Galeni librum De ossibus. 1603.

1630

—Περὶ ὀστῶν τοῖς εἰαγομένοις [sic] . . . De ossibus ad tyrones liber. Ferdinando Balamio interprete, cum notis perpetuis Casp. Hofmanni . . . Francofurti ad Moenum, Typis Wechelianis, sumptibus Clementis Schleichii, & Petri de Zetter, 1630.

[4], 31 p.   35 cm.   [4513]

Greek and Latin in parallel columns.
Bound with Hippocrates. Liber prior de morbis mulierum, Parisiis, 1585.

— Copy 2.   34 cm.

Bound with Hofmann, Caspar. De thorace. 1627.

1665

—De ossibus Graece & Latine. Accedunt Vesalii, Sylvii, Heneri, Eustachii, ad Galeni doctrinam exercitationes. Ex bibliotheca Joannis van Horne. Lugduni Batavorum, Apud Danielem vander Boxe, 1665.

[12], 276 p.   14 cm.   [4514]

Special title page in Greek and Latin (p. [1] main group of paging): Γαληνοῦ περὶ ὀστῶν τοῖς εισαγομένοις . . . De ossibus ad tyrones.
The Latin text is slightly different from Ferdinando Balami's version.
"Andreae Vesalii et Jacobi Sylvii [i.e. Jacques Dubois] super libello Galeni De ossibus controversiae": p. 116-162; "Suscepit Renatus Henerus pro Vesalio Apologiam adversus has Sylvii Depulsiones, quem proinde sic animose satis adoritur": p. 163-196; "Sed nunc operae-pretium est audire, quomodo Bartholomaeus Eustachius, in examine ossium, Galeni partes, adversus recentiores anatomicos, praecipue vero Vesalium, acriter tueatur": p. 197-257; " ʹ Ἱπποκράτονς περι οστέων φυσιος" (Greek text and Latin translation, the latter with caption title "De ossium natura"): p. 258-265. (This is in five sections, of which the first four form the first chapter of the Mochlicus. The Latin translation is that of Janus Cornarius); "Aur. Cor. Celsus De positu & figura ossium totius humani corporis": p. 266-276.

Latin

1613. *In* Riolan, J. [1580-1657] Osteologia. 1614.

1634. *In* Dubois, J. Jacobi Sylvii . . . Opera medica. 1634.

1635. *In* Dubois, J. Jacobi Sylvii . . . Opera medica. 1635.

—*as subject. See* FALLOPPIO, G. Opera. 1606; RIOLAN, J. [1580-1657] Anthropographia. 1626; [French tr.] 1628-29 [and] Opera anatomica vetera. 1650.

De pulsibus ad tirones

Latin

1602. *In* Lavelli, J. De pulsibus ad tyrones. 1602.

1651. *In* Navarro, J. B. Commentarii ad libros Galeni De differentiis febrium. 1651.

De sanitate tuenda. Selections, etc.

Italian

1650. *See* GALEANO, G., *comp.* and *tr.* Del conservar la sanita libri sei de Galeno. 1650.

De semine

Latin

1634. *In* Cremonini, C. De calido innato, et semine. 1634.

De simplicium medicamentorum facultatibus

French

1610

—Deux livres des simples de Galien, c'est à sçavoir. Le cinquiesme, et le neufviesme. Traduits par . . . Jean Canape . . . Et de nouveau par luy revues & corrigez. Lyon, Pierre Rigaud, 1610.

184 (i.e. 186) p.   12 cm.   [4515]

Imperfect: sig. M6 (blank?) wanting.
A reprint of Benoist Rigaud's edition published in 1570.

—*as subject. See* SEBISCH, M. [1578-1674?] *praeses.* Galeni quinque priores libri. 1651.

De urinis

Latin

1651. *In* Navarro, J. B. Commentarii ad libros Galeni De differentiis febrium. 1651.

De usu partium

French

1608

—De l'usage des parties du corps humain, livres XVII. Escrits par Claude Galien, & traduicts fidelement du grec en françois. Paris, René Ruelle, 1608.

997, [10] p.   illus.   17 cm.   [4516]

A reprint of the 1566 Lyon edition translated by Claude Dalechamps. Cf. Barbier, vol. 4, p. 902.

1666

—[The same.] . . . Traduit du grec et latin. Et mis en bel ordre, par questions & responses . . . Par A. E. B. D. C. I. Paris, Jean d'Houry, 1666.

[16], 765, [15] p.   illus.   25 cm.   [4517]

—*as subject. See* HOFMANN, C. Commentarii in Galeni De usu partium corporis humani. 1625.

De venae sectione.
Selections, etc.

Latin

1661. *In* Brotbeck, J. K. Commentarius medicus in historiam Galeni, de peste. 1661.

In Hippocratis Aphorismos

Greek and Latin

1628. *In* Hippocrates. Aphorismi . . . Graece et Latine, una cum Galeni Commentariis. 1628.

1633

—In Aphorismos Hippocratis commentaria: ex interpretatione Anutii Foesii, & Gulielmi Plantii, cum annotationibus ejusdem. Editio novissima, a multis, quibus antea scatebat mendis, diligenter repurgata ab Adriano Toll . . . Lugduni Batavorum, Ex officina Joannis Maire, 1633.

[4], 800 (i.e. 798), [22] p.   14 cm.   **[4518]**

Includes Greek text of Hippocrates' Aphorismi, with the Latin translations by Foes and Plancy. Galen's commentaries are in Plancy's Latin translation.

1668. *In* Hippocrates. Aphorismi . . . Graece et Latine. 1668.

French

1605. (bk. 1 only) *In* Hippocrates. [Aphorismi.] 1605.

1606. *In* Hippocrates. [Aphorismi.] 1606.

162-?. *In* Hippocrates. [Aphorismi.] 162 ?

1622. *In* Hippocrates. Aphorismi. [Adaptations, etc. French.] 1622.

1627. *In* Hippocrates. [Aphorismi.] 1627.

1628. *In* Hippocrates. [Aphorismi.] 1628.

1646. *In* Hippocrates. [Aphorismi.] 1646.

1660. *In* Hippocrates. [Aphorismi.] 1660.

1671. *In* Hippocrates. [Aphorismi.] 1671.

Latin

1625. *In* Hippocrates. [Aphorismi.] 1625.

In Hippocratis De natura hominis librum

Latin

1634, 1635. *In* Dubois, J. Jacobi Sylvii . . . Opera medica. 1634.

In Hippocratis Prognostica

Latin

1626. *In* Vega, C. de. Opera omnia. 1626.

Linguarum Hippocratis explicatio

Greek

1657, 1662. *In* Hippocrates. Collected works [Greek and Latin] Τα ευρισκόμενα. 1657, 1662.

Methodus mendendi

English

1656

—Galen's method of physick: or, his great masterpeece, being the very marrow and quintessence of all his writings . . . Whereto is annexed a . . . commentary . . . by its translatour, Peter English . . . Edinburgh, Printed by A. A. for George Svintoun, and James Glen, 1656.

[4], 344 p.   13 cm.   **[4519]**

—*as subject. See* SEBISCH, M. [1578-1674?] Collegii therapeutici disputatio I[-XIV] 1634 [i.e. 1635] [and] Galeni Methodus medendi in quatuordecim disputationes resoluta. 1639.

Quod animi mores corporis temperamenta sequuntur

Greek and Latin

1617. *In* Hippocrates. [De medicamentis purgatoriis. Greek and Latin.] 1617.

Utrum medicinae sit an gymnastices hygieine

—*as subject. See* MINADOI, G. T. Medicarum disputationum liber primus. 1610.

X. Recettario

1611

—Recettario di Galeno, approvato, & molto utile alle infirmità, che sono sottoposti gli corpi humani. Con rimedii di conservare la sanità, e prolongar la vita, con altre nuove recette, che non erano ne gli altri prima restampate & altre da preservarsi contra il mal contagioso. Tradotto in lingua volgare, per . . . Giovanni Saracino . . . Venetia, Gio. Batt. Bonf., 1611.

79 ll.   illus.   15 cm.   **[4520]**

1645

—[The same.] . . . Venetia, Heredi dell'Imberti, 1645.

    79 ll. illus. 16 cm.   [**4521**]

Different setting of type.

1666

—[The same.] . . . Venetia, Giacomo Zattoni, 1666.

    152, [15] p. illus. 15 cm.   [**4522**]

1676

—[The same.] . . . Venetia, Benedetto Miloco, 1676.

    152, [14] p. illus. 14 cm.   [**4523**]

Imperfect: sig. G12 (blank?) wanting.

1683

—[The same.] . . . Venetia, Sebastian Menegatti, 1683.

    154, [14] p. illus. 14 cm.   [**4524**]

Imperfect: p. 107–108 mutilated.
Different setting of type.

1686

—[The same.] . . . Venetia, Giuseppe Tramontin, 1686.

    152, [15] p. illus. 14 cm.   [**4525**]

XI. References

—*See* ACAMPO, S. Commentaria in libros Galeni De differentiis febrium. 1642; AIGNAN, F. L'ancienne medecine. 1693; AMAT, J. C. Fructus medicinae. 1623; 1681; BAILLOU, G. de. Definitionum medicarum liber. 1639; BARIL, J. Physiologia humana. 1653; BERTOCCI, A. Methodus curativa. 1608; BRAVO DE SOBREMONTE RAMIREZ, G. Resolutionum, & consultationum medicarum. 1662; BRONZERIO, G. G. De innato calido et naturali spiritu disputatio. 1626; BROTBECK, J. K. Progymnasmatis medici pars prima. 1664; CAIMO, P. De febrium putridarum indicationibus juxta Galeni methodum colligendis. 1628; CALVO, J. Primera y segunda parte de la cirugia universal. 1647; CAMPOLONGO, O. Considerationi . . . intorno alla theriaca. 1614 [i.e. 1615]; CAPRILI, P. E. Libri duo. 1643; CARDANO, G. Contradicentium medicorum libri duo. 1607; CASERTA, F. A. Tractationes duae ad medicinae praxim pertinentes. 1623; CASTELLI, B. Castellus renovatus; hoc est, Lexicon medicum. 1682, 1688, 1700 [and] Lexicon medicum, Graeco Latinum. 1607, 1626, 1628, 1642, 1644, 1651, 1657, 1664, 1665, 1669, 1685; CASTELLI, P. De abusu circa dierum criticorum enumerationem. 1642; CASTELLO, P. V. Exercitationes medicinales. 1616; CASTILLO, J. de. Tractatus. 1683; CASTRO, R. de. De universa mulierum medicina. 1603, 1617, 1628, 1644, 1662, 1689; CNUTIUS, J. Compendium universae medicinae juxta doctrinam Hippocratis, & Galeni. 1608, 1679; CONRING, H., *praeses.* Commentariolum in Cl. Galeni lib. XIII. 1663; CONSTANTIN, A. Opus medicae prognoseos. 1613; CULPEPER, N. A physical directory. 1651 [and] Pharmacopoeia Londinensis. 1659; CUSAC, L. Reflexions sur la theorie et la pratique d'Hippocrate et de Galien. 1692, 1693; FONTAINE, G. D. Gabrielis Fontani . . . De veritate Hippocraticae medicinae firmissimis rationum & experimentorum momentis stabilita, & demonstrata. 1657; FRANZOSI, G. Tractatus apologeticus de semine pro Aristotele adversus Galenum. 1645; FREITAG, J. Aurora medicorum Galeno-chymicorum. 1630; GILLET, S. Galenus moralis ac mysticus. 1661; GORRIS, J. de [*fl.* 1572–1622] Opuscula quatuor. 1660; GREMBS, F. O. Arbor integra et ruinosa hominis. 1657, 1671; HELMONT, J. B. van. Opuscula medica inaudita. 1644, 1648; HOFMANN, C. Apologiae pro Galeno. 1668 [and] Pathologia parva. 1640 [and] Vita medica, hoc est Galeni ὑγιεινῶν. 1680; LANCETTA, T. Raccolta medica. 1645; MAGINET, P. La theriaque francoise. 1623; MAGINI, G. A. De astrologica ratione. 1607; MARINELLI, C. De morbis nobilioris animae facultates obsidentibus libri tres. 1615; MARIOTTI, C. De universarum febrium generibus tractatus ad Hippocratis, et Galeni mentem. 1654; NAVARRO, J. B. Commentarii ad libros Galeni De differentiis febrium. 1649, 1651; OBIZZI, I. Iatrastronomicon varios tractatus medicos. 1618; PÉREZ, A. Summa, y examem [sic] de cirugia, de lo mas necessario que en ella se contiene. 1634; PONCE DE SANTA CRUZ, A. [*d. ca.* 1650] Opuscula medica, et philosophica. 1624; PORZIO, L. A. Erasistratus; sive, De sanguinis missione. 1683; REYS TAVARES, M. dos. Controversias philosophicas, et medicas. 1667; ROMATET, C. Crisiologia medica. 1635; ROSS, A. Arcana microcosmi. 1651, 1652; RUDIO, E. Liber de anima. 1611; SALANDI, F. Tractatus de purgatione. 1607; SÁNCHEZ, F. Opera medica. 1636; SANTORIO, S. Methodi vitandorum errorum omnium. 1603, 1630; SASSONIA, E. De pulsibus libri tres. 1603; SCALIGER, J. J. Loci cujusdam Galeni difficillimi explicatio. 1619; SEBISCH, M. [1578–1674?] *praeses.* Liber Galeni de differentiis morborum in theses contractus. 1630; SELVATICO, G.

B. Galeni historiae medicinales a Jo. Baptista Silvatico ... enarratae. 1605; SENNERT, D. De chymicorum cum Aristotelicis et Galenicis consensu ac dissensu liber. 1629, 1655; SINAPI, M. A. Absurda vera. 1697; SØRENSEN, P. Idea medicinae philosophicae. 1660; STEFANI, G. Hippocratis Coi theologia. 1638; TRISSINO, A. Problematum medicinalium ex sententia Galeni libri sex posthumi. 1629; VALLES, F. De. Controversiarum medicarum et philosophicarum ... libri X. 1606, 1609, 1625; VOIGT, J. K. I. Tractatus medicus Galeno-chymicus. 1678.

GALEOTTI, Marzio. *See* MARZIO, Galeotto [15th cent.]

GALESI, BARTOLOMEO [*d.* 1635?] Epistola responsive ad ... Aloysium Card. Capponium ... super morbo hisce temporib. grassante cum suis antidotis ... [Bononiae] Apud Francisc. Cataneum, 1630.

[1], 101, [1] p.   21 cm.   [4526]

Engraved title page.

—Tractatus de podagra, 2. ed. auctus paralello terraemotus cum microcosmi motu: cui inferitur doctrina de genituris; de decubitibus aegrorum; de morbo Gallico; de physiognom. de insomniis; de veneficiis; de venenis. Agitur quaestio: an morbi per simplicem relationem curari possint. Afferuntur Aristot. auctoritates pro immateriali mentis humanae statu. Bononiae, Typis Francisci Catanii, 1633.

[38], 315 (i.e. 365), [9] p. illus. 21 cm.   [4527]

Has running title throughout: Liber primus.

Additional title page inserted after p. [143] reads: ... Varia physica & medica διδαγματα, complexa in tractatu de podagra ... Bononiae, Typis Clementis Ferronii [n. d.]

Imperfect: signatures of sheet + (index of books 4 and 5) wrongly imposed.

GALINA, FRANCESCO. *See* GALLINA, Francesco [1528-1608]

GALLAEUS, THEODORUS. *See* GALLE, Théodore [1571-1633]

GALLARATI, GIUSEPPE [*d.* 1694] Diatriba medico-sceptica de alcali, & acido ... Bolngna [sic] Giacomo Monti, 1688.

81 p. 15 cm.   [4528]

Bound with *his* Systema renovatum physiologiae medicae. 1684.

—Specimen medicum de febrifugis salinis per hypothesin mechanicam explicatis ... Bonnoiae

[sic], Typis Petri-Mariae de Montibus, 1694.

35 p. 15 cm.   [4529]

Bound with *his* Systema renovatum physiologiae medicae. 1684.

—Systema renovatum physiologiae medicae, juxta veterum philosophorum hypothesin, cui in hac 2. imp. accedit liber tertius De anima sensitiva ... Bononiae, Typis Jacobi Montii, 1684.

[24], 538 p. 15 cm.   [4530]

With this are bound: *his* Specimen medicum de febrifugis salinis. 1694; his Diatriba medico-sceptica de alcali. 1688.

GALLE, THÉODORE [1571-1633] *See* Faber Johannes. *In* imagines illustrium ex Fulvii Ursini bibliotheca ... commentarius. 1606.

GALLEGO, BENITO MATAMOROS VÁZQUEZ. *See* MATAMOROS VÁZQUEZ GALLEGO, Benito [*fl.* 1622]

GALLEGO, SEBASTIAN DE [*fl.* 17th cent.] *ed. See* MONTEMAYOR, C. Medicina y cirugia de vulneribus capitis. 1664.

GALLEGO BENÍTEZ DE LA SERNA, JUAN. *See* GALLEGO DE LA SERNA, Juan [*fl.* 1621-1640]

GALLEGO DE LA SERNA, JUAN [*fl.* 1621-1640] Opera physica, medica, ethica, quinque tractatibus comprehensa: quorum I. Agit de principiis generationis omnium viventium. II. De conservatione infantis in utero, de bono & malo pariendi modo ... III. De puerorum alendi ratione, & sanitate tuenda ... IV. De communi puerorum educandi ratione, inscriptus; Ethica puerorum. V. De optimi regis educandi ratione. Lugduni, Sumptibus Jacobi & Petri Prost, 1634.

[12], 324, [18] p.; [4], 136, [11] p. 37 cm. [4531]

Part [2] has special title page: Tractatus duo posteriores.

—Recte ac dogmatice medendi vera methodus ... In sex tractatus distributum ... Parisiis, Sumptibus Antonii Bertier, 1639.

[16], 495, [37] p. 37 cm.   [4532]

—*See* CHIFFLET, J. J. De morte ... D. Francisci de Paz. 1640.

GALLERATI, GIUSEPPE. *See* GALLARATI, Giuseppe [*d.* 1694]

GALLI, FRIEDRICH. *See* GALLUS, Friedrich.

GALLINA, FRANCESCO [1528-1608] *ed. See* BENZI, U. Regole della sanità. 1620; PISANELLI, B. Trattato de' cibi. 1612.

GALLO, ANDREA [16th cent.] Fascis aureus de peste, ac febre pestilentiali, qua ejus venenum atrocissimum per praecautionem ac curationem partim eradicatur, partim demetitur ... Francofurti, Ex officina typographica Joannis Saurii, 1606.

[16], 622, [9] p.   17 cm.   [**4533**]

Published in 1565 under title: Fascis de peste.
Edited by Peter Uffenbach.
"Epicedium ... D. Andreae de Gallis ... scriptum ... a Doct. Laurentio Span a Spanouu": p. 616–622.

— [The same.] Homo afflictus & jacens; in quem astra, elementa, meteora ... conspirant, mugiunt, saeviunt, funestamque important pestem ... sublevatur ... curatur ... variaque ejus symptomata resecantur ... Francofurti, Impensis Egenolphi Emmelii, 1608.

[16], 622, [9] p.   17 cm.   [**4534**]

A reissue of Fascis aureus de peste ... 1606, with new title page and preliminary matter reset.

— *See* SCHOLTZ, L. Consiliorum medicinalium ... liber singularis. 1610.

GALLUS, FRIEDRICH. *See* FLORETUS A BETHABOR. Traum-Gesicht. 1682.

GALLUS, PANCRATIUS [*fl.* 1607] *respondent. See* VARUS, A., *praeses.* Themata medica περι της φρενιτιδος. 1607.

GALTERIUS, MARCUS ANTONIUS. Consultatio, et oratio habitae in foelici urbe Panormi. Panormi, Apud Joannem Antonium de Franciscis, 1626.

95, [9] p.   23 cm.   [**4535**]

GALTIER, LOUIS DE. Enchiridion therapeutique et prophilactique pourpre; ou, Manuel contenant ... maniere de traitter & guarir la maladie epidemique ... appellée ... le pourpre ou le tacq, avec le moyen de s'en preserver ... Paris, Theodore Pepingue, 1645.

[8], 78 p.   17 cm.   [**4536**]

GALVANI, DOMENICO [*d.* 1649] Delle fontanele trattato ... diviso in duo libri. L'uno pertinente alla teorica, nel qual si discorre intorno all'essenza, e l'utile delle fontanele, sedagni, inanellationi, ustioni, & vessicatorii, l'altro alla prattica ... [Padova, Gasparo Crivellari, 1620]

[8], 80, [4] ll.   illus   21 cm.   [**4537**]

GAMBS, JOHANN FRIEDRICH [*fl.* 1694] *respondent.* Disputatio inauguralis medica de phrenitide ...

Basileae, Typis Jacobi Bertschii [1694]

[16] p.   19 cm.   [**4538**]

Diss. — Basel.

GANDOLF, MAXIMILIAN, *count, Cardinal, Prince-Archbishop of Salzburg* [*d.* 1687] *See* SALZBURG, Austria. (Diocese) Archbishop, 1668–1686 (Maximilian Gandolf) Instructio practica, de officio parochorum aliorumque curatorum pro tempore pestis expositorum. 1680.

GANIVET, JEAN [*fl.* 1431–1434] Amicus medicorum, continens differentias, I. De numero coelestium orbium, &c. II. De distinctione zodiaci, &c. III. De inquisitione epidemiorum & mortis. IV. De modis conservandi sanitatem & obviandi aegritudinibus. Cui acceserunt opusculum, Coeli enarrant; liber Abrahami Avenezrae De diebus criticis; directorium de figura coeli in Amicum medicorum; et Astronomia Hippocratis. Omnia primum a Gondisalvo Toledo ... in lucem emissa. Nunc vero denuo revisa et utillissimis annotatiunculis in margine locupletata. Francoforti, Typis Nicolae Hoffmanni, sumptibus Jacobi Fischeri, 1614.

617, [18] p.   diagrs., tables.   14 cm.   [**4539**]

Reprinted mainly from the 1550 Lyons edition. Both "Coeli enarrant" and "De diebus criticis" of Abraham Ibn Ezra are probably also the work of Ganivet. Cf. Thorndike v. 4 (1934) p. 139.
Gondisalvus Toledo's "Epistola astrol. defensiva": p. 3–19.

GANS, JOHANN LUDWIG [*fl.* 1620–1630] Corallorum historia, qua mirabilis eorum ortus, locus natalis, varia genera, praeparationes chymicae quamplurimae, viresque eximiae proponuntur. Francofurti, Sumptibus Lucae Jennisii, 1630.

[16], 174 p.   illus.   17 cm.   [**4540**]

Last leaf (blank) wanting.

— [The same.] ... Ed. nova ex variis auctoribus aucta. Francofurti, Apud Hermannum à Sande, 1669.

[24], 248 p.   illus.   14 cm.   [**4541**]

With this is bound Pierer, G. P. De natta dissertatiuncula medica. 1669.

— *respondent. See* SEBISCH, M. [1578–1674?] *praeses.* Disputatio de purgatione quinta. 1621 [and] Disputationes de recta ratione purgandi. 1621.

GANTZLAND, ANDREAS [*fl.* 1628–1636] *respondent. See* MICHAELIS, J., *praeses.* Themata miscellanea. 1636.

GARBERS, JAKOB [*fl.* 1693] *respondent.* Disputatio medica inauguralis de diureticis ... Lugduni

Batavorum, Apud Abrahamum Elzevier, 1693.

[16] p. 22 cm.   [4542]

Diss. — Leyden.

GARCES Y RIBERA, FRANCISCO SALADO. *See* SALADO GARCÉS Y RIBERA, Francisco [*fl.* 1644-1654]

GARCÍA, BALDASSAR. *See* GRASSO, Baldassar.

GARCÍA, PEDRO. [*fl.* 1681-1685] *See* GARCÍA CONDE, Pedro [*fl.* 1681-1685]

GARCIA CARRERO, PEDRO [16th-17th cent.] Disputationes medicae, et commentaria in fen. primam libri quarti Avicennae: in quibus non solum quae pertinent ad theoricam; sed etiam ad praxim, locupletissime reperiuntur ... Opera et industria ... Petri Ferriol ... Burdigalae, Apud Guillelmum Millangium, 1628.

8, 1122, [14] p.   35 cm.   [4543]

—Disputationes medicae super fen primam libri primi Avicenae, etiam philosophis valde utiles ... Compluti, Ex officina Joannis Gratiani, apud viduam, 1611.

[8], 1398, [31] p.   30 cm.   [4544]

—*See* REYS TAVARES, M. dos. Controversias philosophicas, et medicas. 1667.

GARCÍA CONDE, PEDRO [*fl.* 1681-1685] Verdadera albeyteria ... Dividido en quatro libros ... Lleva diferentes estampas, donde vàn delineadas las enfermedades ... Madrid, Impresso a costa del autor. Por Antonia Gonzalez de Reyes, 168[5]

[23], 636, [6] p. illus., port. 28 cm. [4545]

Imperfect: outer margin of title page mutilated.

GARCIA D'ORTA. *See* ORTA, Garcia d' [1501 *or* 2?-1568]

GARCIA SALAT, VICENTE [*d.* 1614] Utilissima disputatio de dignotione et curatione febrium ... Valentiae, Ex typographia Fuster, expensis Joannis Laurentii Cabrera, 1652.

[8], 191, [1] p.   21 cm.   [4546]

GARDIN, LOUIS DU. *See* DU GARDIN, Louis [*fl.* 1617-*ca.* 1631]

GARDINER, EDMUND. The triall of tabacco. Wherein his worth is most worthily expressed ... as also the complexions, dispositions, and constitutions of such bodies, & persons as are fittest ... to take it. By E[dmund] G[ardiner] ... London, By H.

L. for Mathew Lownes, 1610.

[6], 58 ll. 19 cm.   [4547]

Imperfect: title page mutilated, affecting text. STC 11564.

GARENCIÈRES, THÉOPHILE DE [*ca.* 1610 — *ca.* 1680] The admirable virtues, and wonderful effects of the true and genuine tincture of coral, in physick ... London, Printed by W. R. for Samuel Sprint, 1676.

[11], 83 p.   15 cm.   [4548]

—Angliae flagellum; seu, Tabes Anglica. Numeris omnibus instructa ubi omnia quae ad ejus tum cognitionem cum curationem pertinent ... aperiuntur ... [London] Excudit T. W. pro Richardo Whitaker, 1647.

[7], 185, [13] p.   12 cm.   [4549]

Imprint partly supplied from Wing G254.

—A mite cast into the treasury of the ... city of London; being a brief and methodical discourse of the nature, causes, symptoms, remedies and preservation from the plague, in ... 1665. Digested into aphorismes ... London, Thomas Ratcliffe, 1665.

[4], 11 p. 19 cm.   [4550]

Bound with Bradwell, S. A watch-man for the pest. 1625.

GARMANN, CHRISTIAN FRIEDRICH [1640-1708] De miraculis mortuorum. Lipsiae, Impensis Christiani Kirchneri, Chemnitii, Typis Joh. Gabr. Güttneri, 1670.

[16], 112, [8] p.   20 cm.   [4551]

Bound with Feltmann, G. Tractatus de cadavere inspiciendo. 1673.

—Homo ex ovo; sive, De ovo humano dissertatio. Chemnitii, Sumptibus authoris, typis Johannis Gabrielis Gütneri, 1672.

[4], 28 p.   20 cm.   [4552]

—[The same.] ... Chemnitii, Sumptibus authoris, typis Johannis Gabrielis Gütneri, 1682.

[4], 28 p.   19 cm.   [4553]

Different setting of type.

—Oologia curiosa duabus partibus absoluta, ortum corporum naturalium ex ovo demonstrans. Cygneae, Literis Christiani Bittorffii; sumptibus Johannis Christoph. Weidneri [1691]

[8], 240 p.   21 cm.   [4554]

—*respondent. See* WELSCH, G., *praeses.* Discursus physico-medicus de gemellis et partu numerosiore. 1667.

GARMERS, JOHANN [1628-1700] *respondent. See* CONRING, H., *praeses.* Disquisitionem de venae sectione . . . publice examinandam proponent . . . C. G. 1651.

—, *ed. See* ROSSI, F. Nocturnae exercitationes in medicas historias. 1660.

—*See* BECKE, D. von der. Dissertatio anatomico-practica de procidentia uteri. 1683.

GARNERUS, GEORGIUS. *See* GARNIER, Georges [1550-1614]

GARNIER, GEORGES [1550-1614] Ἐπιτομή; seu, Βραχυλογία λοιμώδης. Desumpta ex magno libro Georgii Garneri . . . de peste, quae grassata est Venetiis anno Domini 1576, & Bruntruti, anno Domini 1582 . . . revisa atque multis . . . remediis locupletata . . . Bruntruti, Apud Christophorum Krakau, 1610.

[13], 201, [21] p. 16 cm. [**4555**]

GARNIER, PIERRE [*d.* 1710?] Novelles formules de medecine, latines et francoises, pour le grand Hôtel-Dieu de Lyon . . . Augmentées par l'auteur d'un Traité de la verole. 2. ed. Lyon, La veuve de Jean-Baptiste Guillimin, 1699.

[48], 423 (i.e. 234) p.; [1], 116, [3] p. 17 cm. [**4556**]

Part [2] has half title.

GARNIERE, JACQUES DE. Esbauchement de l'accord des controverses de ceux qui font estat de la cognoissance des simples medicamens: et principalement des plantes . . . Lyon, Thomas Soubron, 1618.

27 p. 15 cm. [**4557**]

GARON, LOUIS [*ca.* 1580–*ca.* 1636] Exilium melancholiae; das ist, Unlust Vertreiber; oder zwey tausend lehrreiche . . . Sprüche . . . auss Ludovici Caron [sic] frantzösischem Tractat, La chasse ennuy . . . intitulirt, und andern guten Authorn colligirt, und . . . übergesetzet . . . Strassburg, Gedruckt und Verlegt durch Josias Städel, 1669.

[8], 563, [37] p. 18 cm. [**4558**]

Imperfect: several pages mutilated.

GARPIUS, PETER [*fl.* 1642-1643] *praeses.* Disputatio physica de anima, potiori parte hominis . . .

Regiomonti, Typis Reusnerianis, 1642.

[8] p. 19 cm. [**4559**]

Diss. — Königsberg (J. Oldenburg, *respondent*)

—Disputatio physica de propagatione animae humanae . . . Regiomonti, Typis Reusnerianis, 1643.

[20] p. 19 cm. [**4560**]

Diss. — Königsberg (J. B. Frohne, *respondent*)

[**GARTH,** *Sir* SAMUEL, 1661-1719] The dispensary; a poem. London, John Nutt, 1699.

[3], 84 p. 22 cm. [**4561**]

First appeared in 1699 in "broadside paper form." Cf. Harvey Cushing, "Dr. Garth: the Kit-Cat poet." *In* Johns Hopkins Hospital bulletin, v. 17 (1906) p. 5.

A satire on the opponents of the dispensary organized by the Royal College of Physicians.

—[The same.] . . . In six canto's . . . The 2d ed., corrected by the author. London, John Nutt, 1699.

[25], 94 p. fronts., plates, port. 20 cm.
[**4562**]

Manuscript notes in the text explaining fictitious or abbreviated names.

—[The same.] . . . The 3d ed., corrected by the author. London, John Nutt, 1699.

[23], 94 p. front. 20 cm. [**4563**]

—[The same.] . . . The 4th ed., with additions. London, John Nutt, 1700.

[23], 96 p. front. 20 cm. [**4564**]

—Oratio laudatoria, in aedibus Collegii Regalis Med. Lond. 17mo· die Septembris . . . Londini, Impensis Abelis Roper, 1697.

[3], 16 p. 21 cm. [Harveian oration, 1697]
[**4565**]

GARTNER, ANDREAS [*fl.* 1603-1605] *respondent. See* SENNERT, D., *praeses.* De symptomatum caussis disputatio prima. 1605.

GARTZ, GILIAN [*fl.* 1642] *respondent. See* SCHLEGEL, P. M., *praeses.* Disputatio medica de epilepsia. 1642.

GARUFI, NICCOLO ANDREA [*fl.* 17th cent.] *See* AVELLINO, F. Oratio in exornandis philosophiae. 1660.

GARZONI, MARINO [*fl.* 1688-1692] L'arte di ben conoscere, e distinguere le qualità de' cavalli, d'introdurre, e conservare una razza nobile, e di risanare il cavallo da' mali, à quali soggiace . . . 2. impr. Venetia, Andrea Poletti, 1700.

[14], 328 p. plates. 23 cm. [**4566**]

GARZONI, Ottaviano. *See* Garzoni, Tommaso [1549?-1589]

GARZONI, Tommaso [1549?-1589] L'hospidale de' pazzi incurabili ... Nuovamente ristampato, & corretto ... Serravalle di Venetia, Ad instanza di Roberto Meglietti [Per Marco Claseri] 1605.

119, [1] p.   21 cm.   **[4567]**

"Capitolo di Theodoro Angelucci á Tomaso Garzoni sopra la Pazzia": p. 100-107; "Capitolo del Sig. Guido Casoni in lode della pazzia": p. 108-112; "Capitolo dell'auttore all'Angelucci in lode della pazzia": p. 113-119.

—[The same.] Nuovamente ristampato, & con somma diligenza ricoretto ... Venetia, Giorgio Valentini, & Antonio Giuliani, 1617.

[8], 90 (i.e. 94) p.   24 cm.   **[4568]**

—[French tr.] L'hospital des fols incurables ... Tirée de l'italien ... par François de Clarier, sieur de Long-val ... Paris, François Julliot, 1620.

[4], 267, [1] p.   18 cm.   **[4569]**

—La piazza universale di tutte le professioni del mondo. [Excerpts.] *In* Suárez de Figueroa, C. Plaza universal de todas ciencias. 1629.

—Il serragli de gli stupori del mondo ... Diviso in diece appartamenti, secondo i vari, & ammirabili oggetti. Cioè di mostri, prodigii, prestigii, sorti, oracoli ... curiositá astrologica ... Arricchita di varie annotationi dal ... Bartolomeo Garzoni ... Venetia, Appresso Ambrosio et Bartolomeo Dei, fratelli, 1613.

[60], 787, [1] p.   23 cm.   **[4570]**

GASPARI. *See* Gasparis, Stefano de [*fl. ca.* 1640]

GASPARIS, Stefano de [*fl. ca.* 1640] Liquoris artificialis pro opobalsamo Orientali in conficienda theriaca Romae adhibiti physica oppugnatio ... Romae, Ex tipographia Antonii Landini, 1640.

[22], 287, [28] p.   15 cm.   **[4571]**

Engraved title page.

—*See* Campi, B. Baldassari, e Michel Campi al sig. Antonio Manfredi ... In dilucidotione, e confermatione maggiore di alcune cose state da noi dette nella risposta al sig. Gaspari medico. 1641; Nemi, N. Imbiancatura di Nicolò Nemi da Novi. 1640.

GASSARUS, Achilles Pirminius. *See* Gasser, Achilles Pirminius [1505-1577]

GASSENDI, Pierre [1592-1655] Opera omnia in sex tomos divisa ... Hactenus edita auctor ante obitum recensuit ... Posthuma vero totius naturae explicationem complectentia, in lucem nunc primum prodeunt, ex bibliotheca ... Henrici Ludovici Haberti Mon-Morii ... Lugduni, Sumptibus Laurentii Anisson, & Joan. Bapt. Devenet, 1658.

6 v. in 3.   front. (port.), illus.   37 cm.   **[4572]**

Edited in collaboration with François Henry.

"...Samuelis Sorberii praefatio, in qua de vita, et moribus Petri Gassendi disseritur" (p. [1-30], vol. 1). "... Diogenis Laertii Liber decimus de vita, moribus, placitisque Epicuri, cum nova interpretatione, et notis" (p. 1-236, vol. 5) with text in Greek and Latin, includes extracts from Epicurus.

—Abregé de la philosophie de Gassendi ... Par F[rançois] Bernier ... Lyon, Anisson & Posuel, 1678.

8 v.   illus.   17 cm.   **[4573]**

—Epistolica exercitatio, in qua principia philosophiae Robert Fluddi medici reteguntur; et ad recentes illius libros, adversus R. P. F. Marinum Mersennum ... scriptos, respondetur. Cum appendice aliquot Observationum coelestium. Parisiis, Apud Sebastianum Cramoisy, 1630.

[43], 360, [2] p.   18 cm.   **[4574]**

"Ad ... Marinum Mersennum, Francisci Lanovii judicium de Roberto Fluddo": p.[23-29]

—Viri illustris Nicolai Claudii Fabricii de Peiresc, senatoris Aquisextiensis vita ... Ed. 3. auctior, correctior, & distinctior. Hagae-Comitum, Ex typographia Adriani Vlacq, 1655.

[8], 300, [16] p.   port.   21 cm.   **[4575]**

"Peireskii laudatio habita in concione funebri Academicorum Romanorum. Die Decemb. 21. an. 1637. Jo. Jacobo Buccardo ... perorante": p. 257-275; "Gabrielis Naudaei ad Petrum Gassendum, de Peireskii obitu epistola": p. 276-279; "Ad vitam ... Pereskii auctarium ... [by] Petrus Borellus ...": p. 281-289.

—*See* Pineau, S. De integritatis & corruptionis virginum notis. 1639, 1640, 1641, 1650, 1663, 1690.

—*as subject. See* Charleton, W. Physiologia Epicuro-Gassendo-Charltoniana. 1654; Quillet, C. Callipaedia. 1655.

GASSER, Achilles Pirminius [1505-1577] Curationes et observationes medicae, e bibliotheca Georgii Hieronymi Velschii, cum ejusdem notis.

46, [10] p.   20 cm.   (Part [3] *in* Welsch, Georg Hieronymus. Sylloge curationum. Aug. Vindel., 1667)   **[4576]**

—Another issue, with new title page dated 1668.

                                                         [4577]

—*See* Dodoens, R. Medicinalium observationum exempla rara. 1621.

GASSMANN, Franz. Bifolium metallicum; seu, Medicina duplex, pro metallis & hominibus infirmis, a proceribus artis hermeticae, sub titulo lapidis philosophici inventa, elaborata & posteritati transmissa ... denuo recognita a Pantaleone [pseud., i.e. Franz Gassmann] hermeticae sophiae perito. Noribergae, Apud Pauli Fürstii, 1676

55 p. 16 cm. [4578]

—Examen alchymisticum, quo, ceu Lydio lapide, adeptus a sophista & verus philosophus ab impostore dignoscuntur, institutum in gratiam magnatum & eorum, qui, ex defectu multae lectionis & vulcanicae experientiae, punctum chymicum plenarie non intelligunt ... Authore Pantaleone [pseud., i.e. Franz Gassmann] ... Noribergae, Apud Pauli Fürstii viduam & haeredes, 1676.

43 (i.e. 44) p. 16 cm. [4579]
Imperfect: p. 45-48 (blank?) wanting?

—*See* Deux traitez nouveaux sur la philosophie naturelle. 1689.

GASTALDI, Geronimo [d. 1685] Tractatus de avertenda et profliganda peste politico-legalis eo lucubratus tempore, quo ipse loemocomiorum primo, mox sanitatis commissarius generalis fuit, peste Urbem invadente anno MDCLVI & LVII ... Bononiae, Ex Camerali typographia Manolessiana, 1684.

[69], 792, [116] p. illus. 40 cm. [4580]
Imperfect: sig. a1 mutilated; groups of pages misbound throughout.

GASTO, Flaminius [*fl.* 1659] Tractatus de peste ... Gorlicensis, Typis Christophori Zipperi, 1660.

[159] p. 14 cm. [4581]
Signatures: A-F12, G8.
Dedicatory letter dated from Glogau, 28 October 1659. The present Latin treatise may be wholly or in part based on the elder Flaminius' Discurs vom rechten Nutz etlicher gebräuchlicher Artzneyen, bey wehrenden Sterbensleufften. Cf. Adam, p. 197, and Jöcher, p. 878.

GATENARIA, Mauo. *See* Gatinaria, Marco [d. 1496]

GATFORD, Lionel [d. 1665] Λογος Ἀλεξιφαϱμακος; or, Hyperphysicall directions in time of plague. Collected out of the sole authentick dispensatory of the chief physitian both of soule and body, and disposed more particularly ... according to the method of those physicall directions printed by command of the lords of the councell at Oxford 1644 ... Oxford, H. Hall, 1644.

[1], 35 p. 19 cm. [4582]

GATHMANN, Reinhard. *See* Solenander, Reiner [1524-1601]

GATINARIA, Marco [d. 1496] De medendis humani corporis malis practica uberrima ... Jam ante etiam edita, nunc vero denuo revisa, et omni, qua fieri potuit ... emaculata ... Accesserunt Blasii Astarii, & Caesaris Landulphi opuscula De febribus, ac insuper Sebastini Aquilae Quaestio de febribus & tractatus De morbo Gallico ... Francofurti, Typis Nicolai Hoffmanni, impensis Joannis Berneri, 1604.

[14], 473, [7] p. 17 cm. [4583]
With this are bound: Stockar, J. Praxis morborum. 1609.— Stockar, J. Empirica. 1601.—Hollings, E. Medicamentorum oeconomia nova. 1615.

GATTA, Geronimo [*fl.* 1657] Di una gravissima peste, che nella passata primavera, & estate dell'anno 1656. depopulò la città di Napoli ... Napoli, Luc'Antonio di Fusco, 1659.

[36], 248, [40] p. 22 cm. [4584]

GAUB, Johann [*fl.* 1695-*ca.* 1720] Epistola problematica prima [-tertia] ad Fredericum Ruyschium ... de pilis, pinguedine, septoque scroti; nec non de papillis pyramidalibus; ut & de corpore reticulari, sub cuticula sito, &c. Amstelaedami, Apud Johannem Wolters, 1696.

31 (i.e. 32) p. plates. 24 cm. [4585]
Signatures: A-D4.
Each Epistola is followed by the answer of Frederik Ruysch. Problemata secunda [-tertia] have half titles.

—[Another printing] ... Amstelaedami, Apud Joannem Wolters, 1696.

13 p., 16 p., 16 p. illus. 22 cm. [4586]
Signatures: A-B4; A-B4; A-B4.

—*respondent.* Disputatio medica inauguralis, de pituita ... Harderovici, Apud Albertum Sas, 1698.

[28] p. 23 cm. [4587]
Diss. — Harderwijk.

GAUDAEUS, Samuel. *See* Gaudé, Samuel.

GAUDANUS, Theodoricus. *See* Gerardus, Theodoricus.

GAUDÉ, SAMUEL, *ed. See* VALLES, F. de. Commentaria in Prognosticum Hippocratis. 1655 [and] Commentaria in quatuor Hippocratis libros De ratione victus in morbis acutis. 1655 [and] Commentaria, in septum libros Hippocrat. De morbis popularibus. 1654 [i.e. 1655]

GAULTIER, JEAN. Traité de la maladie venerienne, ou grosse verole. Contenant la vraye cognoissance du mal, & sa vraye curation . . . Tolose, Raymond Colomiez, 1617.

    [1], 12, [10], 127 p.   14 cm.   **[4588]**

GAURICO, POMPONIO [*ca.* 1482-1530] *See* INDAGINE, J. ab. Introductiones apotelesmaticae. 1603, 1622, 1630, 1663, 1672.

GAUTERON, ANTOINE [1660-1737] Quaestiones medico-chymico-practicae duodecim ab Michaele Chicoyneau [et al.] . . . propositae pro regia chymiae professione vacante per obitum . . . Arnaldi Fonsorbe . . . Monspelii, Apud Honoratum Pech, 1697.

    [6], 20, [2] p.   22 cm.   **[4589]**
Thèse de concours — Montpellier.

GAVALDÁ, FRANCISCO, *Father* [1618-1668] Memoria de los sucessos particulares de Valencia, y su reino en los años 1647 y 48, tiempo de peste . . . Valencia, Silvestre Esparsa, 1651.

    [188] p.   20 cm.   **[4590]**
Signatures: a¹², A-D⁴, E⁶, F-T⁴, V³.

GAVET, JACQUES [*b.* 1674] Nova febris idea; seu, Novae conjecturae physicae, circa febris naturam. Quibus praemittitur . . . explicatio motus fermentationis, generationis animantium, materiae & motus sanguinis, motus cordis & arteriarum, tandemque secretionis humorum. Genevae, Sumptibus Societatis, 1700.

    [12], 264 p.   illus.   15 cm.   **[4591]**

GAVET DE RUMILLY, JACQUES. *See* GAVET, Jacques [*b.* 1674]

GAVINELLUS, FAUSTINUS [*fl.* 17th cent.] *ed. See* MALPIGHI, M. Opera posthuma. 1698.

GAY, BRICE, *tr. See* COURTIN, G. Les oeuvres anatomiques et chirurgicales. 1656.

[**GAYA**, LOUIS DE] Cerimonie nuzziali di tutte le nationi del mondo . . . Venetia, Steffano Curti, 1685.

    [12], 161, [7] p.   15 cm.   **[4592]**
Translation by Casimir Freschot of Cérémonies nuptiales de

toutes les nations.
    Edited by Giovanni Domenico Rossi.

GAYANT, LOUIS [*d.* 1673] *See* JASOLINO, G. Collegium anatomicum. 1668.

GAYLARD, JOSEPH [*b. ca.* 1657] *respondent.* Disputatio medico-physica inauguralis de convulsione, seu motibus convulsivis ubi ex conjunctione animae cum corpore eorum natura clarius explicatur . . . Lugduni Batavorum, Apud Abrahamum Elzevier, 1688.

    [12] p.   21 cm.   **[4593]**
Diss. — Leyden.

GAYTON, EDMUND [1608-1666] Hymnus de febribus . . . Londini, Imprimatur a Thoma Warreno [1655]

    [15], 54 p.   19 cm.   **[4594]**
Imprint partly supplied from Wing G413.

GAZA, THEODORUS [1398-1478] *tr. See* THEOPHRASTUS. De historia plantarum libri decem, Graece & Latine. 1644 [and] Θεοφράστον . . . ἅπαντα. Theophrasti . . . Graece & Latine opera omnia. 1613.

—*See* GUASTAVINO, G. Commentarii in priores decem Aristotelis Problematum sectiones. 1608.

GAZOLA, GIUSEPPE [1661-1715] *See* ZAPATA, D. M. Verdadera apologia en defensa de la medicina racional philosophica. 1691.

GEBAUER, MELCHIOR [1656-1726] *respondent. See* SCHMID, J. A., *praeses.* Dissertatio academica de sectis physicorum in genere. 1676.

GEBER, ABOU MOUSSAH DJAFAR AL SALI. *See* JĀBIR IBN ḤAIYĀN, al-Ṭarasūsī.

GEBLER, JOHANN WILHELM [*fl.* 1650] *respondent. See* HOFFMANN, M., *praeses.* Theses medicae de generatione et usu partium. 1650.

GEELMANN, GEORG. *See* GELMAN, Georg [*fl.* 1640-1652]

GEERDINXIUS, JOSAPHATUS [*fl.* 1623] *respondent.* Disputatio medica inauguralis de apoplexia . . . Lugduni Batavorum, Ex officina Isaaci Elseverii, 1623.

    [12] p.   21 cm.   **[4595]**
Diss. — Leyden.

GEHEMA, JANUS ABRAHAMUS A [1645-1700] De morbo vulgo dicto plica Polonica. Literulae ad . . .

D. Corn. Bontekoe ... Hagae-Comitis, Apud Petrum Hagium, 1683.

27 p. 16 cm. [4596]

With this is bound Felix, A., *Father*. De ovis cochlearum epistola. 1684.

—Diaetetica vera sanae rationi ac experientiae certae innixa in gratiam vitam & sanitatem longam exoptantium conscripta ... Sedini, Impensis Johann. Adami Pleneri, 1690.

[6], 72 p. 14 cm. [4597]

—Eroberte Gicht, durch die chinesche Waffen der Moxa. Worin aus genugsamer Erfahrung angewiesen wird, dass die beste ... Genesung, so bisshero noch erfunden worden, bestehe, in dem alhier angeführten Methodo oder Curirungs-Kunst ... Hamburg, Auff Godfried Schultzens Kosten, 1683.

108 p. 14 cm. [4598]

With this is bound *his* Der reformirte Apotheker. 1688.

—Grausame medicinische Mord-Mittel, Aderlasse, Schröpffen, Purgiren, Clistiren, Juleppen, und Ohnmacht-machende Hertzstärckungen, wodurch unbedachtsame Geness-und Heilmeister so viel tausend ... Menschen jämmerlich vom Leben zum Tode helffen ... Brehmen, 1688.

[16], 102 p. 16 cm. [4599]

—Der krancke Soldat bittende dass er hinführo besser möge conserviret, mitleidiger tractiret, und vorsichtiger curiret werden ... Sampt einer woleingerichteten Feld-Apotecke vorgestellet ... [Stettin] Verlegts Johann Adam Plener, 1690.

[166] p. 14 cm. [4600]

Imprint partly supplied from Kośmiński.
Bound with *his* Der qualificirte Leib-Medicus. 1690.

—Der qualificirte Leib-Medicus ... [Stettin] Verlegts Johann Adam Plener, 1690.

[46] p. 14 cm. [4601]

Imprint partly supplied from Kośmiński.
With this is bound *his* Der krancke Soldat. 1690.

—Der reformirte Apotheker, fürstellende ein ohnmaassgebliches Project, wie und welcher Gestalt die heutige Apotheken billich zu reformiren ... weren ... Bremen, In Verlegung Hermann Brauers, 1688.

67 p. 14 cm. [4602]

Bound with *his* Eroberte Gicht. 1683.

—Von den heutigen Arcanis antipodagricis; oder ... Geheimbten Mitteln wieder das Podagra ...

[n. p.] In Verlegung des Autoris, 1685.

[23] p. 20 cm. [4603]

—Der wohlversuchte Feld-Medicus, anweisende die Missbräuche, welche bisshero bey Anstellung der Feld-Medicorum ... eingeschlichen. Sambt einem ohnmaassgeblichen Project, wie und auff was Weise alles könne remediret ... werden ... Rostock, Gedruckt bey Jacob Richeln, 1689.

[26], 68 p. 14 cm. [4604]

Bound with copy 2 of Lanzoni, G. Tractatus de balsamatione cadaverum. 1696.

—*See* GEUDER, M. F. Heilsame medicinische Lebens Mittel. 1689; HORLACHER, C. Die höchstschädliche Würckung des Aderlassens. 1691.

GEHLER, MICHAEL [*fl.* 1607-1611] *respondent.* Theses de plica ... Basileae, Apud Excertierianos, 1607.

[16] p. 20 cm. [4605]

Diss.—Basel.

GEHMA, JANUS ABRAHAMUS A. *See* GEHEMA, Janus Abrahamus a [1645-1700]

GEHRIG, CHRISTOPH [*fl.* 1692] *respondent. See* PETRI VON HARTENFELS, G. C. *praes.* Dissertatio medica inauguralis de anorexia seu apositia. 1692.

GEIDELIN, SAMUEL [*fl.* 1662-1663] *respondent.* Disputatio inauguralis medica de suppressione mensium ... Argentorati, Typis Eberhardi Welperi, 1663.

[32] p. 20 cm. [4606]

Diss.—Strasbourg.

—*See* SEBISCH, M. [1578-1674?] *praeses.* Disputatio ... medica de ophthalmia. 1662.

GEIER, JOHANN DANIEL [1660-ca. 1735] Schediasma, de montibus conchiferis ac glossopetris alzeiensibus ... Francofurti et Lipsiae, Prostat apud Georg. Heinr. Oehrlingium, excudit Joh. Zach. Nisius, 1687.

22, [2] p. plate. 20 cm. [4607]

—Tractatus physico-medicus de cantharidibus ... Lipsiae et Francofurti, Prostat apud Georg. Heinr. Oehrlingium, excudit Joh. Zach. Nisius, 1687.

[16], 75, [4] p. 21 cm. [4608]

GEIGER, DANIEL [1595-1664] Responsum medicum defensivum ad Johannis Helwigii ... de morbo ac morte ... Cardinalis Wartenbergici & c. cui condigna talionis opera, in calce accedit Instrumentum publicum retorsionis legitime factae . . . Augustae Vindelicorum, Typis Johannis Praetorii, 1662.

[36] p.   19 cm.   [4609]

"Instrumentum retorsionis legitime" has German text.

GEIGER, MALACHIAS [1606–1671] Fontigraphia; oder, Brunnen Beschreibung dess miraculosen Heilbronnens bey Benedictbeuren . . . [München?] 1636.

[23], 137 p.   16 cm.   [4610]

Engraved title page.

—Kelegraphia; sive, Descriptio herniarum cum earundem curationibus tam medicis quam chirurgicis . . . Monachii [Apud Nicolaum Henricum] 1631

[40], 288, [15] p.   front. (port.) illus.   17 cm.
                                        [4611]

Engraved title page.
Imperfect: portrait and p. 115–116 wanting.

—Kurzer Underricht und Guetachten wie mann sich bey jetzigen Sterbens Lauffe praeservieren unnd da jemand inficiert wurde curieren solle . . . Müchen, 1649.

[1], 29 p.   plates.   20 cm.   [4612]

Engraved title page.

—Margaritologia; sive, Dissertatio de margaritis, in qua post varia ad margaritas pertitientia, demonstratur, margaritas Bavaricas in usu medicinali, viribus et effectibus aequivalere Orientalibus et Occidentalibus elaborata . . . [Monachii, Formis Cornelii Leysserii] 1637.

[12], 79, [1] p.   plates.   17 cm.   [4613]

Engraved title page.

—Microcosmus hypochondriacus; sive, De melancholia hypochodriaca tractatus . . . Curatio hujus affectus, in quantum sanabilis et curabilis est, ex triplici curationis fonte, diaetetico, chirurgico, & pharmaceutico desumpta . . . Quibus emblemata varia, tam Galenica quam Hermetica . . . cum explicationibus suis addita sunt . . . Monachii, Apud Lucam Straub, 1652.

[38], 524, [11] p.   plates.   20 cm.   [4614]

Added engraved title page, dated 1651.

GEILFUS, BERNHARD WILHELM [*fl.* 1674–1676] *respondent.* Disputatio inauguralis de moxa . . . Marpurgi Cattorum, Typis Salomonis Schadewitzii, 1676.

[2], 30 p.   20 cm.   [4615]

Diss.—Marburg.

—*See* WALDSCHMIDT, J. J., *praeses.* Disputatio

medica de chylificatione. 1674.

GEILFUS, JOHANN CHRISTOPH. Trutz Podagram; das ist, Kurtzes Bedencken wider das Podagram . . . Augspurg, Johann Schultes, 1658.

[46] p.   16 cm.   [4616]

Signatures: A–B⁸, C⁶.

GEILFUS, JOHANN GOTTFRIED [*fl.* 17th. cent.] Unterricht vom Sauer- und Brodel Brunnen zu Langen-Schwalbach. [n. p.] 1662.

48 p.   17 cm.   [4617]

Bound with Horst, J. D. Kurtze Beschreibung. 1659.

—[The same.] . . . Zum dritten Mahl auffgelegt. Franckfurt, In Verlegung Johan David Zunnern, 1682.

32 p.   16 cm.   [4618]

GEINITZ, JOHANN [*fl.* 1670–1677] *respondent. See* FRIDERICI, J. A. *praeses.* Disputatio medica de paeonia. 1670.

GEISELBRUNNER, ELIAS [*fl.* 1614–1620] *respondent. See* SEBISCH, M. [1578–1674?] *praeses.* Disputationes de recta ratione purgandi. 1621.

GEISENDÖRFFER, BALTHASAR. *See* GYSENDÖRFFER, Balthasar [*fl.* 1660]

GEISLER, DAVID [*fl.* 1673] *respondent. See* DRECHSSLER, J. G., *praeses.* Discursus curiosus, at sobrius de nive prodigiosa. 1673.

GEISSLER, AUGUSTIN [*fl.* 1685?] *respondent. See* BOHN, J., *praeses.* Dissertationes chymico-physicae. 1685.

GEISSLER, ELIAS [*fl.* 1674–1676] Disputatio historico-physica de amphibiis . . . Lipsiae, Typis Johann-Erici Hahnii [1676]

[16] p.   23 cm.   [4619]

Diss. pro loco—Leipzig.

GEISSLER, FRIEDRICH [*fl.* 17th. cent.] Excellens nostri viridis panacea Leonis cabalistice desumta, ex illo spaientum antiquorum, aenigmate: visitabis interiora terrae, rectificando, invenies occultum lapidem verae . . . medicinae . . . Norimbergae, Sumptibus viduae & haeredum B. Pauli Fürstii, typis Christophori Gerhardi, 1678.

47 p.   plates.   15 cm.   [4620]

Text in German.

GEIST-REICHES Donner und Wetter-Gebet-Büchlein; das ist, Christlicher Unterricht, wie sich ein jeder vor, inn- und nach schwerem Donner- und Hagel-Wetter, Christlich erzeigen und verhalten soll . . . Nürnberg, Joh. Philipp Miltenberger, 1667.

[24], 144 p. front. 14 cm. **[4621]**

With this are bound: Geistliches Feigenblat. 1666; Lutz, C. Geistliche Apotecke. 1666.

GEISTLICHE Artzney in Zeit der Pest, ansteckenden Kranckheiten, und betrübten Zeiten, andächtig zu betten. Gezogen aus dem Psalter St. Bonaventura, von unser lieben Frauen Mutter Gottes Maria, bestehend in 5. Psalm, jeden von 12. Versen: nebst des trostreichen Gebett, O edler Himmels-Stern etc. [n. p., 16--?]

[16] p. 14 cm. **[4622]**

GEISTLICHES Feigenblat; d. i., Unterschiedliche Gebete, Fürbitte und Danksagunge, auf etzliche gewisse Fälle wider . . . der gifftigen Pestilentz . . . [n. p.] 1666.

141 p. 14 cm. **[4623]**

Bound with Geist-reiches Donner und Wetter-Gebet-Büchlein. 1667.

GEITZINGER, FRIEDRICH [*fl.* 1672-1673] *respondent. See* PURPIUS, A., *praeses.* Humanae nutritionis rationem. 1672.

GELÉE, THÉOPHILE [*ca.* 1566-1650] L'anatomie francoise en forme d'abbregé recueillie des meilleurs autheurs qui ont escrit de cette science . . . Dieppe, Nicolas Acher, 1623.

[18], 485 (i.e. 486), [10] p. 17 cm. **[4624]**

—[The same.] . . . A Dieppe [Chez Nicolas Acher] et se vend a Paris chez Augustin Courbé, 1629.

[15], 485 (i.e. 486), [10] p. 17 cm. **[4625]**

Different setting of type.

—[The same.] . . . Rouen, Jean Bouley, 1630.

[8], 479, [9] p. 18 cm. **[4626]**

Bound with Pigray, P. Epitome des preceptes de medecine et chirurgie. 1625.

—[The same.] . . . Rev., corr., & de beaucoup augm. en ceste derniere ed., par l'autheur. Paris, Charles Sevestre, 1632.

[8], 479, [9] p. 17 cm. **[4627]**

Different setting of type.

—[The same.] . . . Paris, André Soubron, 1635.

[8], 479, [9] p. 17 cm. **[4628]**

Different setting of type.

—[The same.] . . . Rouen, Jean Berthelin, 1642.

[8], 479, [9] p. 17 cm. **[4629]**

Different setting of type.

—[The same.] . . . Rev., corr., & de nouveau augm. en cette derniere ed., d'un petit Traité anatomique des valvules [par. G. Sauvageon] Rouen, Robert Daré, 1654.

[8], 470, [10] p. 18 cm. **[4630]**

—[The same.] . . . Rev., & corr. dans tout le cours du livre, & outre le Traité des valvules, d'un autre Des veines lactées [par G. Sauvageon] Augm. d'un Discours des veritez anatomiques & chirurgicales. Par Gabriel Bertrand . . . Paris, Jean Doury, 1656.

[14], 531, 5-128 p. 18 cm. **[4631]**

—[The same.] . . . Rev., corr. & augm. dans tout le cours du livre, & outre le Traicté des valvules, d'un autre, Des veines lactées. Par . . . Guillaume Sauvageon . . . Paris, Jean Bessin, 1658.

[4], 582, [10] p. 17 cm. **[4632]**

—[The same.] . . . Rev., corr. & de beaucomp augm. en cette derniere ed. par l'autheur. Lyon, Horace Huguetan, 1665.

[8], 479, [9] p. 17 cm. **[4633]**

—[The same.] . . . Rev. & augm. dans tout le cours du livre, & outre le Traité des valvules, d'un autre Des veines lactées. Par G. Sauvageon . . . Avec un Discours des veritez anatomiques & chirurgicales. Par Gabriel Bertrand . . . Paris, Jean Doury, 1668.

[14], 531 p.; [2], [5]-128 p. 18 cm. **[4634]**

Part [2] has special title page dated 1661.

—[The same.] . . . Rev., corr., & de nouveau augm. en cette derniere ed., d'un petit Traitté anatomique des valvules [par G. Sauvageon] Roüen, Jacques Besongne, 1668.

[8], 470 (i.e. 490) p. 17 cm. **[4635]**

Imperfect: "Table des livres et chapitres" ([10] ? p. at end) wanting.

—[The same.] . . . Rev. & augm. dans tout le cours du livre, & outre le Traité des valvules, d'un autre Des veines lactées. Par G. Sauvageon . . . Avec un Discours des veritez anatomiques & chirurgicales. Par Gabriel Bertrand . . . Derniere ed. Paris, Jean d'Houry, 1671.

[16], 624 p. 18 cm. **[4636]**

—[The same.] . . . Rev., corr. & de beaucoup

augm. en cette derniere ed. par l'autheur. Lyon, Estienne Baritel, 1673.

[8], 479, [9] p.   17 cm.   [4637]

—[The same.] ... Rev., corr., & de nouveau augm. en cette derniere ed., d'un petit Traitté anatomique des valvules [by G. Sauvageon], Rouen, Julien Courant, 1679.

[8], 470 (i.e. 490), [10] p.   17 cm.   [4638]

GELÉE, THÉOPHILE [ca. 1566-1650] tr. See DU LAURENS, A. Toutes les oeuvres. 1613, 1621, 1639, 1646, 1661.

GELEN, SIGISMUND [1497-1554] See PLINIUS SECUNDUS, C. Naturalis historiae, tomus primus [-tertius]. 1668-1669.

GELI, CLAUDIO. See GELLI, Claudio.

GELIDUS, THEOPHILUS. See GELÉE, Théophile [ca. 1566-1650]

GELLI, CLAUDIO. Risposta ... ad un certo libro contra medici rationali ... Milano, Gio. Battista Bidelli, 1617.

84 p.   15 cm.   [4639]
Bound with Bovio, Z. T. Il fulmine contro de' medici putatitii rationali. 1617.

—[The same.] ... Padova, Pietro Paolo Tozzi, 1626.

81 p.   15 cm.   [4640]
Bound with Bovio, Z. T. Flagello de' medici rationali. 1626.

—Another issue.

81 p.   15 cm.   [4641]
(Part [3] in Bovio, Z. T. Opere contra medici putaticii rationali. Padova, 1626)

—[The same.] In Bovio, Z. T. Opere. 1676.

—as subject. See BOVIO, Z. T. Melampigo. 1617, 1626.

GELLI, GIOVANNI BATTISTA [1498-1563] De naturae humanae fabrica: dialogi decem. In quibus Ulysses, cum aliis quibusdam Graecis, qui in varias belluarum formas transmutati erant, de hominis animantiumque reliquorum praestantia ac miseria disputat ... Opusculum ... nunc multis in locis restitutum & in Latinum conversum: auctore Johann Wolfio ... Ambergae, Typis Michaëlis Forsteri, 1609.

353, [2] p.   14 cm.   [4642]
Translation of Gelli's La Circe.

GELLIUS, AULUS. Noctes atticae; seu, Vigiliae atticae, quas nunc primum a magno mendorum numero magnus veterum exemplarium numerus repurgavit. Henrici Stephani noctes aliquot Parisinae atticis A. Gellii noctibus, seu vigiliis invigilatae. Cui adjectae sunt ejusdem Stephani in Gellium, conjecturae & emendationes posteriores ... Francofurti, Ex Officina Zavhario-Paltheniana, 1603.

[15], 494, [126] p.; [4], 182 p.   17 cm.
       [4643]

With this is bound Strobelberger, J. Systematica universae medicinae adumbratio. 1627.

GELLY, JEAN [fl. 1694-1714] respondent. See DOYE, J. B., praeses. Quaestio medica. 1694.

GELMAN, GEORG [fl. 1640-1652] Tripartita; das ist, Dreyfache chyrurgische Blumen, in welchen zu finden, erstlich die anatomische Beschreibung dess Haupts ... der Brust ... der eussern Glieder ... Franckfurt am Mäyn, Gedruckt bey Johann Kempffern, in Verlegung Thomae Matthiae Götzens, 1652.

[8], 447, [36] p. plates. 20 cm.   [4644]
Added engraved title page.
Last section is interleaved.
Imperfect: plates of first eleven figures of the head wanting.

—[The same.] Chirurgiae tripartita flora; das ist, Dreyfache chyrurgische Blumen, in welchen zu finden, erstlich die anatomische Beschreibung und Figuren des Haupts ... der Brust ... der eussern Glieder ... Franckfurth und Jehna, In Verlag Johann Meyers, 1680.

[8], 488, [52] p. front. (port.), plates. 21 cm.
       [4645]

Imperfect: all pages after sig. c^4 and all plates after the 3d figure of the arm, at end, wanting.

GELSTHORP, PETER [d. 1719] respondent. Disputatio medica inauguralis, de variolis ... Trajecti ad Rhenum, Ex officina Francisci Halma, 1687.

24 p.   22 cm.   [4646]
Diss.—Utrecht.

GEMIGNANI, CAMMILLO. Thesoro di sanita nel quale si contiene alcuni particolari secreti ... Perugia & Firenze, 1612.

[8] p.   16 cm.   [4647]

GEMMA, GIOVANNI BATTISTA [ca. 1545-1608] See FONSECA, R. de. De tuenda valetudine, & producenda vita liber. 1603.

GENASPE, RUDOLPH [*b.* 1670] *respondent. See* CRAUSE, R. W., *praeses.* Dissertatio medica inauguralis de abortu. 1697; WEDEL, G. W., *praeses.* Dissertatio medica de foetore praeternaturali. 1696.

—*See* SLEVOGT, J. A. Decani Facultatis Medicae Jo. Hadriani Slevogtii ... prolusio inauguralis qua argumenta potiora aequivocam generationem asserentium proponuntur. 1697.

GENATH, JOHANN JACOB [1582-1654] *comp.* Decas I. [-Decas VI.] disputationum medicarum select. ... nunc de novo recusarum ... Basileae [Sumptibus Johan. Jacobi Genathii] 1618.

[1061] p. illus. 20 cm. **[4648]**

Each decas has special title page, that of Decas I, II, III, IV, V, and VI dated 1618, 1619, 1620, 1620, 1621 and 1622 respectively.
Includes 60 mostly Basel theses, dated from 1601-1621.

GENDRE, ANTONIUS [*fl.* 17th cent.] De febre epidemica in Montis-Albani obsidione grassata, medica dissertatio ... Nunc primum in lucem prodit ... Lugduni, Sumpt. Antonii Chard, 1626.

[16], 532 (i.e. 472), [15] p. 18 cm. **[4649]**

GENDRON, CLAUDE DESHAIES-. *See* DESHAIES-GENDRON, Claude [*ca.* 1663-1750]

A GENERAL collection of discourses of the virtuosi of France. 1664. *See* [RENAUDOT, E.]

La GENERATION de l'homme. 1676. *See* HOUPPEVILLE, G. de.

GENGA, BERNARDINO [1636?-1734?] Anatomia chirurgica; cioè, Istoria anatomica dell'ossa, e muscoli del corpo humano con la descrittione de vasi più riguardevoli che scorrono per le parti esterne, & un breve trattato del moto, che chiamano circolatione del sangue ... Roma, Nicolò Angelo Tinassi, 1672.

[25], 455, [1] p. 16 cm. **[4650]**

Added engraved title page.
Imperfect: title page wanting; supplied in photocopy.

—[The same.] ... In questa seconda impressione riformata, & accresciuta di molte riflessioni pathologiche chirurgiche ... Roma, Dom. Ant. Ercole, 1686.

[33], 332, [16] p. 16 cm. **[4651]**

Added engraved title page.

—[The same.] ... in questa nuova impressione riformata, & accresciuta di molte riflessioni pathologiche chirurgiche ... Bologna, Il Longhi [1686?]

[32], 332, [16] p. 16 cm. **[4652]**

Different setting of type.

—[The same.] ... Bologna, Il Longhi, 1687.

[32], 332, [16] p. 16 cm. **[4653]**

Different setting of type.

—[The same.] ... Roma et Firenze, Gl'eredi dell'Onofri, 1687.

[24], 446, [16] p. 16 cm. **[4654]**

—Anatomia per uso et intelligenza del disegno ricercata non solo su gl'ossi, e muscoli del corpo humano; ma dimostrata ancora su le statue antiche più insigni di Roma. Delineata in più tavole con tutte le figure in varie faccie, e vedute. Per istudio della Regia Academia di Francia pittura e scultura sotto la direzzione di Carlo Errard gia direttore di essa in Roma. Preparata su'i cadaveri dal dottor Bernardino Genga ... Con le spiegazioni et indice del sig^r. canonico Gio. Maria Lancisi ... Roma, Domenico de Rossi, herede di Gio. Jacomo de Rossi, 1691.

59 ll. incl. 43 plates. 48 cm. **[4655]**

Variant copies have "libro primo" on the title page, although no more was published. Also issued with only 40 plates.
Plates 40-41 signed: F. Andriot. The others are unsigned.

—In Hoppocratis Aphorismos ad chirurgiam spectantes. Commentaria ... Latino, ac Italico idiomate ad communiorem intelligentiam exarata. Romae, Typis Rev. Cam. Apost., 1694.

[34], 494 p. port. 16 cm. **[4656]**

Added engraved title page.
Includes selected Aphorismi in Latin (in Niccolò Leoniceno's version) and in Italian.

—[The same.] ... Bononiae, Typis Longi, M.DC. CXVII [i.e. MDCXCVII]

[32], 494 p. 16 cm. **[4657]**

Different setting of type.

GENGE, JOHANN MELCHIOR [*fl.* 1684-1687] *respondent. See* ALBINUS, B. Dissertatio de thee. 1684 [and] Dissertatio solennis medica, de hydrophobia. 1687.

GENIATES A CORDO. *See* SIMON GENUENSIS.

GENIUS, MICHAEL [*fl.* 1669] *respondent.* Disputatio medica inauguralis de melancholia hypochondriaca ... Lugduni Batavorum, Apud viduam & haeredes Joannis Elsevirii, 1669.

[42] p. 19 cm. **[4658]**

Diss. — Groningen.

GENIUS παντουλιδαμας ad diam scholam apud Parisios empirico-methodicam in cauto nuper igne raptam in lyra . . . Parisiis, 1654.

[1], 133 p.   22 cm.   [4659]

Concerns controversy with Charles Guillemeau.

GENNIP, PHILIPP A [*fl.* 1616] *respondent. See* VORSTIUS, A. E., *praeses.* Theses medicae de convulsione quarum patrocinium volente. 1616.

GENOA. Laws, statutes, etc. Sucinto fatto per informatione al trono sereniss.^{mo} nella causa dell'arte della speciaria. Genoua, Per Gio. Battista Celle e Benedetto Semino [*ca.* 1694]

3 p.   23 cm.   [4660]

GENSEL, JÁNOS ÁDÁM. [*b.* 1677] *respondent. See* WEDEL, G. W., *praeses.* Dissertatio medica, aegrum ischuria laborantem exhibens. 1699.

GENTERSBERGER, SAMUEL [*fl.* 1606] *respondent. See* ELLENBERGER, H., *praeses.* Themata iatrochymica. 1606.

GENTILE DA FOLIGNO [*d.* 1348] *See* MESUË [924 *or* 5-1015] Opera. 1602, 1623.

GENTILIBUS, GENTILIS DE, *de Fulgineo. See* GENTILE DA FOLIGNO [*d.* 1348]

GENTMAN, ADRIAAN [*fl.* 1667-1669] *respondent.* Disputatio medica inauguralis de vermibus . . . Ultrajecti, Ex officina Antonii Smytegelt, 1669.

[28] p.   23 cm.   [4661]

Diss. — Leyden.

— Disputatio philosophica inauguralis de visione . . . Lugduni Batavorum, Apud viduam & haeredes Joannis Elsevirii, 1669.

[16] p.   23 cm.   [4662]

Diss. — Leyden.

GENUENSIS, SIMON. *See* SIMON GENUENSIS.

GENUESER Eytelkeit und Trauer-Kleid. Kurtze Beschreibung der Ankunfft, statlichen Gebäu, fürstlichen Palläst, Pracht und Herrligkeit, der . . . Stadt Genua. Wie . . . Gott . . . in grossem Wollust leben lassen, unlangst mit einer erschröcklichen Pestilentz heimgesuchet . . . [n. p.] 1657.

[48] p.   19 cm.   [4663]

GEOFFRETUS, ALEXANDER [*fl.* 1663] Quaestio medica pyretologica & Consultationes medicinales.

Liburni, Apud Jo. Vincentinm [sic] Bonfilium, 1664.

96 p.   16 cm.   [4664]

GEOPHILUS, JOSEPH [*fl.* 1625-1666] Iatromathematicus liber de febribus malignis, et pestiferis generali, & particulari febrium Messapiae, methodo diserte disceptis, in quo aliqua scitu digna continentur, tam in astrologia, quam in medicina . . . Venetiis, Ex typographia Marci Philippi, 1666.

[8], 168, [8] p.   illus.   23 cm.   [4665]

GEORG WILHELM, *Herzog von Braunschweig-Lüneburg* [1624-1705] *See* BRUNSWICK (DUCHY) Laws, Statutes, etc.

GEORG WILHELMS, *Hertzogen zu Braunschweig und Lüneburg, etc.* . . . Verordnunge. 1680. *See* BRUNSWICK (DUCHY) Laws, Statutes, etc.

GEORGE, LORD BISHOP OF CHESTER. SEE HALL, George, *Bp. of Chester* [1612?-1668]

GEORGI, ANDREAS CASPAR [*fl.* 1682-1687] *respondent. See* LOSS, J., *praeses.* Disputationem de nuce vomica . . . proponit Andreas Caspar Georgi. 1683; VATER, C., *praeses.* De dyspnoea. 1684; VESTI, J., *praeses.* Disquisitio inauguralis medica de febre Hungarica. 1687.

GEORGIUS RAGUSAEUS. *See* RAGUSEO, Giorgio [*ca.* 1579-1622]

GEORGIUS, MATTHAEUS. *See* GIORGI, Matteo.

GEQUIER, PIETER [*fl.* 1669] *respondent.* Disputatio medica inauguralis de usu venae-sectionis in medicina . . . Lugduni Batavorum, Apud viduam & haeredes Joannis Elsevirii, 1669.

[36] p.   23 cm.   [4666]

Diss. — Leyden.

GÉRARD DE CRÉMONE LE JEUNE, *dit. See* GERARDUS, Cremonensis, *of Sabbioneta* [*fl. ca.* 1255-1259]

GERARD, JOHN [1545-1612] The herball; or, Generall historie of plantes. Gathered by John Gerarde . . . very much enlarged and amended by Thomas Johnson . . . London, Adam Islip, Joice Norton and Richard Whitakers, 1633.

[37], 1630, [48] p.   illus.   35 cm.   [4667]

1 v. in 2.

Engraved title page.

Imperfect: first and last leaves (blank) wanting.

"A catalogue of the Brittish [i.e. Welsh] names of plants, sent me by Master Robert Davyes of Guissaney in Flint-Shire": p. [31-32] at end.

STC 11751. Hunt 223.

—[The same.] ... 1636.

[37], 1630, [49] p. illus. 36 cm.   **[4668]**

Engraved title page.

Imperfect: first and last leaves (blank) wanting.

Different setting of type.

STC 11752. Hunt 230.

GERARDI, JOANNES [*fl.* 1665] *respondent.* Disputatio medica inauguralis de tristitia ... Lugduni Batavorum, Ex officina Salomonis Wagenaer, 1665.

[12] p. 22 cm.   **[4669]**

Diss.—Leyden.

GERARDUS CREMONENSIS [1113 *or* 14-1187] *tr. See* AVICENNA. Avicennae Arabum medicorum principis. 1608 [and] Fen. I. lib. I. Canonis. 1648; SANTORIO, S. Commentaria in primam fen primi libri Canonis Avicennae. 1646 [and] Opera omnia. 1660; WELSCH, G. H. Exercitatio de vena medinensi. 1674.

GERARDUS, CREMONENSIS, *of Sabbioneta* [*fl. ca.* 1255-1259] Geomancie astronomique de Gerard de Cremone, pour savoir les choses passées, les presentes, & les futures. Avec des observations necessaires pour les medecins, les chirurgiens ... Traduite par le sieur de Salerne. Et augm. en cette dern. imp. de plusieurs questions, & d'autres curiositez. Paris, L'auteur, 1669.

[12], 258, [6] p. illus. 15 cm.   **[4670]**

Imperfect: Sig. [â 7-8] wanting?

GERARDUS, JOANNES GULIELMUS [*fl.* 1650] *ed. See* MORONE, M. Directorium medico-practicum, 1650.

GERARDUS, SABLONETANUS. *See* GERARDUS, Cremonensis, *of Sabbioneta* [*fl. ca.* 1255-1259]

GERARDUS, THEODORICUS, *tr. See* Galenus, Francisci Vallesii ... Commentaria illustria, in Cl. Galeni Pergameni libros. 1645.

GERBER, CHRISTIAN FRIEDRICH [*fl.* 1682-1683] *respondent. See* FASCH, A. H., *praeses.* Disputatio inauguralis medica de doloribus post partum. 1683 [and] Παρωτίδας physiologice & pathologice consideratas. 1683; WEDEL, G. W., *praeses.* Disputatio medica sistens aegrum laborantem vertigine. 1682.

GERBER, FRIEDRICH [*fl.* 1652-1655] *respondent.* De incubo. *In* Rolfinck, W., *praeses.* Methodus

cognoscendi & curandi adfectus capitis particulares. 1653.

—*See* MÖBIUS, G., *praeses.* Disputatio inauguralis medica de scirrho lienis. 1655.

GERBER, GEORG SALOMON [*fl.* 1685] *praeses.* Driff Helmontii ... disputatione inaugurali ... publice examinandum proponit praeses M. Georgius Salomon Gerberus ... respondente Johanne Melchior. Thilo ... Erfordiae, Stanno Groschiano [1685]

28 p. 20 cm.   **[4671]**

Diss. — Erfurt (J. M. Thilo, *respondent*)

GERBEZIUS, MARCUS [*ca.* 1658-1718] Intricatum extricatum medicum; seu, Tractatus de morbis complicatis ... Labaci, Typis Josephi Thaddaei Mayr, 1692.

[26], 459, [20] p. 16 cm.   **[4672]**

Added engraved title page.

Errata: p. [20] at end.

GERDES, JOHANN [*ca.* 1656-1700] Programma, quo ... ad dissertationem inauguralem ... Henrici Anhalt ... d. 21, Aug. ... ventilandam ... invitat Johannes Gerdes ... decanus. Rostochii, Typis Joh. Wepplingii [1690]

[8] p. 20 cm.   **[4673]**

Imperfect: p. [7-8] mutilated.

Program — Rostock (with vita of H. Anhalt)

—*praeses.* Disputatio inauguralis medica de hydrophobia ... Gryphiswaldiae, Literis Danielis Benjaminis Starckii [1697]

[27] p. 20 cm.   **[4674]**

Diss. — Greifswald (P. J. Hielm, *respondent*)

—Ideam errantem ac furibundam, in hydrophobia conspicuam ... publicae eruditorum censurae ventilandam, exhibebit ... Henricus Anhalt ... Rostochii, Typis Johannis Wepplingii [1689]

[6], 48 p. 20 cm.   **[4675]**

Diss. — Rostock (H. Anhalt, *respondent*)

—Ideam errantem in ecstasi s. enthusiasmo conspicuam ... sistit ... M. Joh. Jac. Stolterfoht ... Gryphiswaldiae, Literis Danielis Benjaminis Starckii [1692]

[52] p. 19 cm.   **[4676]**

Diss. — Greifswald (J. J. Stolterfoht, *respondent*)

—[The same.] Ideam errantum in ecstasi seu enthusiasmo conspicuam ... sistit ... M. Joh. Jac.

Stolterfoht . . . D. 28 April A. O. R. M.DC.XCII
. . . Gryphiswaldiae, Litteris Starckianis, 1693.

[40] p.   19 cm.   [4677]

—*respondent.* See Loss, J., *praes.* Dissertatione inaugurali morborum ab imaginatione ortorum. 1681;
Schneider, K. V., *praes.* Disputatio medica de
peste. 1680.

GERENZANO, Carlo Giuseppe. *See* Gerenzano
Portigliotto, Carlo Giuseppe [1644–1722]

GERENZANO PORTIGLIOTTO, Carlo
Giuseppe [1644–1722] L'armeria d'Esculapio munita
d'arcani di salute, registrati, e ristretti nello scrigno
di vita, sotto le chiavi di tre indici principali; per
ritrovare, e pratticare . . . li migliori rimedii Galenici,
e spagirici, ad espugnare, provisionalmente, morbi
subitanci, e cronici . . . Milano, Agnelli, 1694.

252 p.   14 cm.   [4678]
Imperfect: p. 3–4 wanting.

—Il morbifugo universale; o sia, La polve viperina
espugnatrice di tutte le infermita . . . Sal volatile
viperino, con le prodigiose cure fatte con questo . . .
Milano, Agnelli, 1693.

[24], 300 p.   16 cm.   [4679]
Imperfect: p. [13–14] mutilated.

—La vipera rediviva; o siano, L'impareggiabili
prerogative del sal volatile viperino, nuovamente fab-
bricato . . . Milano, Ambrogio Ramellati [1688]

48 p.   16 cm.   [4680]

GERET, Andreas [*fl.* 1673–1674] *praes.* Infans
monstrosus Wittebergae D. 30 Augusti, anno
M.DC.LXXIV natus . . . Wittebergae, Typis
Johannis Borcardi [1674]

[16] p.   19 cm.   [4681]
Diss. — Wittenberg (P. Hüttlinger, *respondent*)

GERHARDI, Friedrich Wilhelm [*fl.* 1697]
respondent. See Hoffman, F. [1660–1742] *praes.* Dissertatio inauguralis sistens fermentorum morbificorum
ejectionem e medicina. 1697.

GERICIUS, Fridericus [*fl.* 1606] *respondent.*
Theses de pleuritide exquisita . . . Basileae
Rauracorum, Typis Johannis Schroeteri, 1606.

[10] p.   20 cm.   [4682]
Diss. — Basel.

GERLACH, Johann Gottfried [*fl.* 1667] *respondent.* See Rolfinck, W., *praes.* Dissertatio medica de
dysenteria. 1667.

GERLACH, Nathaniel [1667?–1715] *respondent. See*
Albinus, B. Disputatio medica inauguralis, de
elephantiasi. 1694.

GERLING, Gerhard [*b.* 1651] *respondent.*
Disputatio medica inauguralis de febribus . . .
Lugduni Batavorum, Apud viduam & heredes
Johannis Elsevirii, 1677.

[40] p.   21 cm.   [4683]
Diss. — Leyden.

GERMAIN, Charles de Saint. *See* Saint Germain, Charles de [*fl.* 1650–1655]

GERMAIN, Claude [*fl.* 1650–1672] Orthodoxe;
ou, De l'abus de l'antimoine, dialogue . . . pour
detromper ceux qui donnent ou prennent le vin &
pouldre emetique . . . Paris, Chez Thomas Blaise [De
l'imprimerie de Sebastien Martin] 1652.

[40], 442, [16] p.   illus.   26 cm.   [4684]

GERMAIN, Jean, *Father* [*fl.* 1625–1637] La parfaite quint-essence de la chirurgie reduite in cinq parties. Avec un Antidotaire ou description de plusieurs
excellents remedes pour la guerison de diverses
maladies . . . Paris, Pierre Billaine, 1638.

[15], 270 (i.e. 370), [16] p.   17 cm.   [4685]
Imperfect: sig. a1–3 mutilated.

—, *ed.* and *tr.* See Du Laurens, A. Discorsi della
conservatione della vista. 1626.

GERMANO, Giovanni. *See* Germain, Jean, *Father*
[*fl.* 1625–1637]

GERMANUS, Johannes [*fl.* 1675] *See* Porz, J. D.
Demonstratio brevis medico chyrurgica de
tumoribus. 1679.

GERMBERG, Hermann [*fl.* 1580–1599] *ed.* See
Junius, H. Nomenclator octilinguis. 1602.

GERNER, Adam [*fl.* 1634] *respondent. See* Sebisch,
M. [1578–1674?] *praes.* Collegii therapeutici
disputatio I[-XIV] 1634 [i.e. 1635]

GERNER, Andreas [*fl.* 1633–1638] *respondent.*
Disputatio medica inauguralis, de angina exquisita
. . . Argentorati, Typis Mauritii Caroli, 1638.

[15] p.   18 cm.   [4686]
Diss. — Strasbourg.

—See Sebisch, M. [1578–1674?] *praes.* Galeni Ars
parva in disputationes triginta resoluta. 1633.

GERNER, JOHANN [*fl.* 1622] *respondent.* Disputatio medica inauguralis de pica et malacia . . . Basileae, Typis Joh. Jacobi Genathii [1622]

[12] p.   19 cm.   **[4687]**

Diss. — Basel.

GERRESHEIM, ADOLPH FRIEDRICH [*fl.* 1680-1682] *respondent. See* VEHR, I., *praeses.* Delirium ex ventriculo . . . disputatione inaugurali . . . sistitur ab A. F. G. 1682.

GERRESHEIM, JOHANN WILHELM [*fl.* 1679] *praeses.* Diatribe academica de nexu principiorum physicorum in homine . . . Francofurti ad Oderam, Typis haeredum Johannis Ernesti [1679]

[44] p.   19 cm.   **[4688]**

Diss. — Frankfurt an der Oder (G. G. Knobeloch, *respondent*)

GERSDORFF, HANS VON [*d.* 1529] Chirurgia; ofte, Velt-boeck van den . . . M. Scheel-Hans . . . Overgheset uyt den Hoochduytsche in onse Nederlantsche tale, door Jan Pauwelszoon . . . Amsterdam, Cornelis Claess, 1605.

[12], 175 (i.e. 187) p.   illus.   21 cm.   **[4689]**

Imperfect: p. [5-8] wanting; p. 169-170 in duplicate.

GERSDORFF, JOHANN VON. *See* GERSDORFF, Hans von [*d.* 1529]

GERSTMANN, FLORIAN [*fl.* 1620-1622] *respondent. See* SCHALLER, W., *praeses.* Centuria positionum medicarum de passione colica. 1622.

GERSTMANN, FLORIAN [*fl.* 1651-1656] *respondent.* De mania. *In* Rolfinck, W., *praeses.* Methodus cognoscendi & curandi adfectus capitis particulares. 1653.

—*See* MICHAELIS, J., *praeses.* Diatriben medicam de asthmate . . . submittit . . . F. G. 1656.

GERTRUX, VALENTINE. *See* GREATRAKES, Valentine [1629-1683]

GERVASI, DOMENICO [*d.* 1711] Delle dilogationi trattato chirurgico . . . Lucca, Salvatore Marescandoli, e fratelii, 1673.

[12], 377, [12] p.   21 cm.   **[4690]**

[GERZAN, FRANÇOIS DU SOUCY, *sieur de, fl.* 17th cent.] Sommaire de la medecine chymique . . . Avec un recuel de divers secrets de medecine. Paris, Pierre Billaine, 1632.

[16], 433 p.   17 cm.   **[4691]**

—Le vray tresor de la vie humaine, où l'on void, comme il est possible de chasser les maladies sans incommoder les malades, par un remede qui guerit sans nous nuire; et nettoye nos corps sans les user . . . Premiere partie. Paris, L'autheur, 1653.

[7], 252 p.   16 cm.   **[4692]**

GESNER, DANIEL [*fl.* 1625] *respondent. See* SCHALLER, W., *praeses.* Sesquicenturia positionum medicarum de arthritide. 1625.

GESNER, JEREMIAS [*fl.* 1614] *See* MONARDES, N. Ein nützlich und lustig Gespräche. 1615.

GESNER, JEREMIAS [*fl.* 1616] *respondent.* De epilepsia theses . . . Basileae, Typis Joh. Jacobi Genathii [1616]

[15] p.   19 cm.   **[4693]**

Diss. — Basel.

GESNER, KONRAD [1516-1565] De raris & admirandis herbis, quae, sive quod noctu luceant, sive alias ob causas, lunariae nominantur, & obiter de aliis etiam rebus, quae in tenebris lucent, commentariolus. Ed. 2. emendatior. Cum iconibus quibusdam herbarum novis. Hafniae, Typis Matthiae Godicchenii, Impensis Petri Hauboldi, 1669.

82, [22] p.   illus.   16 cm.   (Part [2] *in* Bartholin, Thomas. De luce hominum & brutorum libri III. Hafniae, 1669)   **[4694]**

—Historiae animalium liber primus [-liber V] . . . Ed. 2 novis iconibus nec non observationibus non paucis auctior, atque etiam multis in locis emendatior . . . Francofurti, In bibliopolio Henrici Laurentii [Ex officina typographica Egenolphi Emmelii], 1617-1621 [v. 1, 1620]

5 v. in 3   illus.   39 cm.   **[4695]**

Contents. — Liber primus, de quadrupedibus viviparis. — Liber II. de quadrupedibus oviparis. — Liber III, de avium natura. — Liber IV, de piscium & aquatilium animantium natura. Continentur in hoc volumine Guilielmi Rondeleti . . . & Petri Bellonii . . . de aquatilium singulis scripta. — Liber V. de serpentium natura. Ex variis schedis et collectaneis ejusdem compositus per Jacobum Carronum . . . Adjecta est ad calcem, scorpionis insecta historia a D. Casparo Wolphio . . . conscripta. Last item has special title page.

—[Selections. English] *In* Topsell, E. The history of four-footed beasts. 1658.

—Thesaurus Euonymi Philiatri [pseud.] de remediis secretis. *In* Vege, P. de. Pax methodicorum. 1620.

—[French tr.] Quatre livres des secrets de medecine, et de la philosophie chimique. Faicts francois par M. Jean Liebaut ... Rouen, Jean Baptiste Behourt, 1628.

[7], 297, [14] ll. illus. 17 cm. [4696]

Translation of the second part of Thesaurus Euonymi Philiatri [pseud.] de remediis secretis, published in 1569 under title: Euonymus. De remediis secretis, liber secundus.

—[The same.] Secrets de medecine et de la philosophie chimique. Par M. Jean Liebaut ... Rouen, Nicolas L'Oyselet, 1643.

[7], 297, [14] ll. illus. 18 cm. [4697]

Different setting of type.

—[German tr.] Köstlicher Artzneyschatz dess wolerfarnen unnd weytberümpten Euonymi Philiatri [pseud.]: darinnen behalten sind viel heimlicher bewärter Artzneystucken, fürnemlich aber die Art unnd Eigenschafft der gebranten Wasseren und Oelen: sampt grundtlicher Beschreibung, wie man die selbigen ... heilsamlich gebrauchen sölle: dessgleyhen von Bereitung allerhand Weinen ... Erstlich ... in Latein beschrieben: hernach von Johann Rudolph Landenberger ... ins Teutsch ubersetzt, unnd ... vermehret ... Zürych, 1608.

2 parts in 1 v. illus. 19 cm. [4698]

"Ander Theil" has special title page and was translated by Hans Jakob Nüscheler.

—, tr. See AELIANUS, C. Περί ζώων ὶδιότητος βιβλία ιζ ... De animalium natura libri XVII. 1611.

—See MOFFETT, T. Insectorum, sive minimorum animalium theatrum. 1634.

GESSELIN, JEAN [fl. 1634] ed. See GUIDI, G. [ca. 1500-1569] Les anciens et renommés autheurs de la medecine & chirurgie. 1634.

GESSNER, CONRAD. See GESNER, Konrad [1516-1565]

GESTRIN, MARTIN ERICI [1594-1648] praeses. Disputatio physica de intellectu humano ... Ubsaliae, Impressa ab Eschillo Matthiae [1646]

[12] p. 18 cm. [4699]

Diss. — Uppsala (N. Zenius, respondent)

Des GETREUEN Eckharts [pseud.] medicinischen Maul-Affens erster Theil. 1694. See [ETTNER, J. C. von]

Dess GETREUEN Eckarths [pseud.] ungewissenhaffter Apotecker. 1700. See [ETTNER, J. C. von]

Dess GETREUEN Eckarts [pseud.] unwürdiger Doctor. 1697. See [ETTNER, J. C. von]

Dess GETREUEN Eckardts [pseud.] vertwegener Chirurgus. 1698. See [ETTNER, J. C. von]

GEUDER, MELCHIOR FRIEDRICH [fl. 1684-1692] Diatriba de fermentis variarum corporis animalis partium specificis & particularibus ... Cui subjicitur Dissertatio de ortu animalium. Amstelaedami, Apud Joannem Wolters [Campis, Typis Caspari Cotii] 1689.

[7], 341, [1] p. 16 cm. [4700]

—Heilsame medicinische Lebens Mittel, denen grausamen medicinischen Mord-Mitteln, Herrn D. Jan. Abrah. à Gehema entgegen gesetzt ... Ulm, Georg Wilhelm Kühn, 1689.

[20], 114 p. 16 cm. [4701]

—respondent. See CAMERARIUS, E. R., praeses. Disputatio inauguralis medica de vomitu aquae ex gula. 1686.

—, ed. and tr. See HAVERS, C. Osteologia nova. 1692.

—, tr. See TAUVRY, D. Nova anatomia ratiociniis illustrata. 1693, 1694.

—See ALETHOPHILUS, J. M. Unvorgreiffliches Bedencken. 1691; HORLACHER, C. Die höchstschädliche Würckung des Aderlassens. 1691.

GEULINCX, ARNOLD [1624-1669] Annotata praecurrentia ad Renati Cartesii Principia, operis oeconomiam succincta analysi evolventia, & philosophiae Renatae dogmata singulari verborum compendio insigni cum perspicuitate comprehendentia. Quae olim in privatis suis collegiis discipulis ad calamum dictavit ... Dordraci, Ex officina Theodori Goris, 1690.

[4], 107 p. illus. 20 cm. [4702]

GEUS, JAN DE. See ANTWOORD op seker boekjen, rakende de genesinge van een hooft-wonde. 1687

GEUSIUS, JACOBUS [d. 1671] ed. and tr. See ARCEO, F. Kortbondige, ende rechte middel, en kunst. 1667.

GEUSS, WOLFF [fl. 1576-1608] Methodus curandorum morborum mathematica; qua morborum depellendorum ex astrorum ... influxu ratio ... ostenditur. Cui & locorum hylegialium, & thematum coelestium structura adjecta. Nunc primum publici juris facta ... Francofurti, Excudebat Wolffgangus Richterus, impensis Antonii Hummii, 1613.

[8], 54 p. illus., table. 21 cm. [4703]

Imperfect: table mutilated.

With this is bound (as issued?) Tabulae chiromanticae. 1613.

GEYER, JOHANN DANIEL. *See* GEIER, Johann Daniel [1660–*ca.* 1735]

GEYGER, DANIEL. *See* GEIGER, Daniel [1595–1664]

GHEBODEN ende uyt-gheroepen by mijne heeren, den onderschouteth ... ende raedt der stadt van Antwerpen. 1646? *See* Antwerp. Ordinances, local laws, etc.

GHEERAERDS, THEODORICUS. *See* GERARDUS, Theodoricus.

GHELEN, SIGMUND. *See* GELEN, Sigismund [1497–1554]

GHENT. Ordinances, local laws, etc. Ordonnantien ende statuten, gemaeckt by heer ende weth der stadt Gendt, ende geapprobeert by Syne Majesteyt, op't faict van de medicyne, raekende de doctoren, apotecarissen, ende chirurgyns. Gendt, Jan Meyer [1685?]

46, [12] p. 22 cm. [4704]

Includes reprints of ordinances of the city of Ghent dated 1663 and 1664; an ordinance by Philip IV of Spain in 1665; and two ordinances signed by J. Doorissele in 1684 and 1685 respectively.

GHERARDO DA SABBIONETA. *See* GERARDUS, Cremonensis, *of Sabbioneta* [*fl. ca.* 1255–1259]

GHEZZI, MARIANO. De i bagni di San Casciano, libri due ... Opera ... ne la quale si spiegano esattamente la natura, l'efficacia, e gl'effetti segnalati di quei fonti febei ... A cui s'aggiunge nel fine un Discorso, sopra il fumaiolo della città di Castro, e de i maravigliosi suoi effetti. Ronciglione, Gli heredi di Domenico Dominici, 1617.

[16], 98 (i.e. 95), 8 p. 20 cm. [4705]

Imperfect: Discorso sopra il fumaiolo della città di Castro (8 pages at end) wanting.

GHIRARDELLI, CORNELIO. Cefalogia fisonomica divisa in dieci deche, dove conforme à documenti d'Aristotile, e d'altri filosofi naturali, con brevi discorsi ... si esaminano le fisonomie di cento teste humane che intagliate si vedono in quest'opera ... Aggiontivi altretanti sonetti di diversi ... poeti ... Et additioni a ciascun discorso sell'Inquieto Academico Vespertino. Bologna, Presso gli heredi

di Evangelista Dozza e compagni, 1630.

[20], 628, [19] p. illus., port. 24 cm. [4706]

Colophon: Bologna, Presso Clemente Ferroni ad instanza de gli heredi di Evangelista Dozza, e compagni, 1630.

Engraved title page.

Illus. on p. 181 covered by slip cancel.

Inquieto Academico Vespertino is possibly a pseudonym for Ovidio Montalbani. Cf. BMC.

—Another issue; date on engraved title page could be read 1670.

[4707]

—[The same.] ... Bologna, Gio. Recaldini, 1674.

[15], 661, [1] p. illus. 16 cm. [4708]

GHIRARDELLI, LORENZO [1600–1641] Il memorando contagio sequito in Bergamo l'anno 1630 historia ... Bergamo, Per li fratelli Rossi, 1681.

[8], 361 p. 24 cm. [4709]

GHIRINZANA, LAZZARO [17th cent.] In septem libros Aphorismorum magni Hyppocratis ... animadversiones Hyppocraticae, ad veram atque exactam eorum intelligentiam comparandam, in quibus multa Hyppocratis loca contradicentia concilliantur & difficilia dilucidantur brevi compendio ... Genuae, Ex officina typographica Joannis Marię Farroni [1649]

441 (i.e. 459), [12] p. 23 cm. [4710]

Signatures: A–3M, +4.

Imprint partly supplied from Pescetto, v. 1, p. 271.

Includes Latin text of the Aphorismi, generally following Niccolò Leoniceno's version.

GIACHINI, LIONARDO [*fl.* 1527–1546] In nonum librum Rasis ... ad Almansorem ... de partium morbis eruditissima commentaria: sive praxis in omnes corporis praeter naturam affectus. Opera ac diligentia Hieronymi Donzellini ... emendata ac perpolita ... Lugduni, Sumptibus Antonii Pillehotte, 1622.

[20], 508, [58] p. 23 cm. [4711]

Imperfect: p. 507 mutilated.

" ... Praecognoscendi methodus. De rationali curandi arte. De acutorum morborum curatione. Quaestiones naturales" (p. [395]–508) has half title.

—Methodus curarandar. febrium, per Rodericum Fonsecam ... in lucem edita. Cui accescere ejusdem Fonsecae, quę ad operis absolutionem febres desiderabantur ... Pisis, Apud Jo. Fontanum, 1615.

[39], 288 p. 21 cm. [4712]

GIACOBINI, Giovanni Domenico. *See* Giacobini, N. Virtù mirabili della triaca. 1667.

GIACOBINI, Nicolao. Virtù mirabili della triaca ... che con ogni essattezza hanno fabricata, e con tutta fede dispensano ... i fratelli Nicolao, e Gio Domenico Giacobini ... Torino, Gio. Sinibaldo, 1667.

8 p.   21 cm.   [4713]

GIANNELLI, Basilio [1662-1716] Varii componimenti per la ricuperata salute del rè ... Napoli, Giacomo Raillard, 1696.

[4], 31, [1] p.   21 cm.   [4714]
Text partly in Spanish.

GIAPPI, Marco Antonio. *See* Ciappi, Marco Antonio [*fl.* 1577-1601]

GIAQUINTO, Trivulso [*fl. ca.* 1640] Ragguaglio primo venuto di Parnaso l'anno M.DC.XXXX. sopra il balsamo d'Arabia, con il quale li spetiali Antonio Manfredi, e Vincenzo Panutio hanno composto in Roma la lor theriaca l'anno. 1639 ... Trento, Santo Zanetti, 1640.

[8] p.   22 cm.   [4715]

—Ragguaglio secondo venuto di Parnaso l'anno M.DC.XXXX. sopra il balsamo d'Arabia, con il quale li spetiali Antonio Manfredi, e Vincenzo Panutio hanno composto in Roma la lor theriaca l'anno 1639 ... Venetia, Guidabuono Domasciocchi, 1640.

[12] p.   22 cm.   [4716]

[GIBSON, Thomas, 1647-1722] The anatomy of humane bodies epitomized ... By a Fellow of the College of Physicians, London. London, Printed by M. Flesher for T. Flesher, 1682.

[7], 510 p.   plates.   19 cm.   [4717]
Imperfect: p. 401-416 wanting; p. 343-344 in duplicate.

—[The same.] ... The 2d. ed., corr. and inl. ... London, Printed by J. Heptinstall, for Tho. Flesher, 1684.

[15], 590 (i.e. 592) p.   plates.   20 cm. [4718]

—[The same.] ... The 3d. ed. ... London, Awnsham Churchil, 1688.

[15], 585 (i.e. 587), [18] p.   plates.   20 cm.
                                           [4719]

—[The same.] ... The 4th ed. corr. and inl. ... London, Printed by T. W. for Awnsham and John Churchill, 1694.

[15], vi, 626 p.   plates.   21 cm.   [4720]

—[The same.] ... The 5th ed., corr. and inl. ... London, Printed by T. W. for Awnsham and John Churchill, and sold by Timothy Childe, 1697.

[14], vi, 626 p.   plates.   20 cm.   [4721]
Imperfect: title page mutilated affecting text; sig. A 1 wanting? Different setting of type.

—*See* Cooke, J. Mellificium chirurgiae. 1693.

GICHTL, Michael [*fl.* 1608-1609] *respondent.* Theses medicae de morbo Ungarico ... Basileae, Per Joan. Jacob. Genathium 1609.

[23] p.   20 cm.   [4722]
Diss. — Basel.

GIENDDER, Johann. Der geistliche Seelen-Artzt, versehen mit General-Artzney, wider alle erdenckliche Melancholey, aus den jetzigen Welt-Stand gerichtet; auss dem Grund göttlicher H. Schrifft ... ausserlesenen Sprichwörtern ... medicinalischen Haupt-Regeln ... durch nützliche Recipe vorgeschrieben ... Regenspurg zu Statt am Hoff, In Verlegung Quirini Heyl, 1696.

[62], 288, [8] p.   front.   21 cm.   [4723]
With this is bound Greef, V. Tuba D. Vincentii, 1692.

GIESELER, Johann Friedrich [*fl.* 1672-1674] *respondent.* Disputatio medica inauguralis de calculo vesicae ... Lugduni Batavorum, Apud viduam & heredes Johannis Elsevirii, 1674.

[23] p.   22 cm.   [4724]
Diss. — Leyden.

—*See* Posner, C., *praeses.* Disputatio physica de principiis generationis. 1672.

GIESELER, Laurentius. *See* Giesler, Lorenz [*d.* 1685]

GIESLER, Lorenz [*d.* 1685] Observationes medicae de peste Brunsvicensi anni M DC LVII. Brunsvigae, Sumptibus Christoph-Friderici Zilligeri, 1663.

[135] p.   21 cm.   [4725]
Upper margins trimmed.

—*respondent. See* Conring, H., *praeses.* Disputatio medica inauguralis de scorbuto. 1644.

GIESWEIN, Johann Philipp [*fl.* 1665-*ca.* 1676] Hodegus medicus; sive, Systema universae materiae medicae, Galeno-chemicum, medicamenta tum universalia ... tum affectuum humani corporis fere omnium particularia ... & specifica ... continens ... Francofurti ad Moenum, Sumptibus haeredum Johannis Beyeri, 1676.

[72], 1670, [25] p. 18 cm.   [4726]

Errata: p. [23-25] at end.

—*respondent.* Disputatio inauguralis medica de febre maligna ... Giessae Hassorum, Typis Friederici Kargeri, 1665.

48, [6] p. 20 cm.   [4727]

Diss.—Giessen.

—*See* STRAUSS, L., *praes.* Disputatio medica, de suffocatione uterina. 1665.

GIFANIUS, OBERTUS. *See* GIFFEN, Hubert van [1533?-1604]

GIFFEN, HUBERT VAN [1533?-1604] *See* LUCRETIUS CARUS, Titus. De rerum natura libri sex. 1686.

GIGANTE, CASPARUS. *See* GIGAS, Caspar [*fl.* 1660-1662]

GIGAS, CASPAR [*fl.* 1660-1662] *respondent.* De antimonio. *See* ROLFINCK, W., *praes.* Dissertationes chimicae sex de tartaro. 1660; SCHENCK, J. T., *praes.* Disputatio inauguralis medica de palpitatione cordis. 1662.

GIGAS, GOTTFRIED [*fl.* 1664-1668] *respondent.* Disputatio medica inauguralis de lipothymia ... Lugduni Batavorum, Apud viduam & haeredes Joannis Elsevirii, 1668.

[16] p. 23 cm.   [4728]

Diss.—Leyden.

—*See* SCHENCK, J. T., *praes.* Dissertatio methodum cognoscendi & curandi obstructiones continens. 1665.

GIGLIO, FRANCESCO MARIA. *See* NIGRISOLI, Francesco Maria [1648-1727 or 8]

GIL DE MURO, MATIAS DE LERA. *See* LERA GIL DE MURO, Matías de [*fl.* 1657]

GILBAU, FELIX JULIANUS RODRIGUEZ Y DE. *See* RODRÍGUEZ, Félix Julían [*d.* 1693]

GILBERT, PHILIBERTUS. *See* GUIBERT, Philbert [1579?-1633]

GILBERT, WILLIAM [1540-1603] *See* CABEI, N. Philosophia magnetica. 1629.

GILBERTUS LYMBURGENSIS. *See* FUSCH, Gilbert [*ca.* 1504-1567]

GILDEBRIEF, by die vande gerechte der stadt Leyden gemaect. 1637. *See* LEYDEN. Ordinances, local laws, etc.

GILES OF ROME. *See* COLONNA, Egidio [1247?-1316]

GILG, GEORG WOLFFGANG [*fl.* 1685-1691] *respondent.* Dissertatio medica inauguralis de memoriae laesione ex nimio veneris usu oriunda ... [Altdorffii] Literis Henrici Meyeri [1691]

16 p. 20 cm.   [4729]

Imperfect: title page mutilated.

Diss.—Altdorf.

GILG, JOHANN GEORG [*fl.* 1653] *respondent.* Disputatio medica inauguralis de epilepsia ... Basileae, Typis Georgii Deckeri [1653]

[8] p. 20 cm.   [4730]

Diss.—Basel.

GILIO, FRANCISCUS MARIA. *See* NIGRISOLI, Francesco Maria [1648-1727 or 8]

GILLENIUS, JOHANN WERNER [*fl.* 1680] *respondent.* Disputatio medica inauguralis de variolis ... Marburgi Cattorum, Typis Joh. Henrici Stockenii, 1680.

30 p. 19 cm.   [4731]

Diss. — Marburg.

GILLES, PIERRE [1489-1555] *tr. See* AELIANUS, C. Περί ζώων ἰδιότητος βιβλία ιζ' ... De animalium natura libri XVII. 1611.

GILLET, SERVAIS [1599-*ca.* 1662] Galenus moralis ac mysticus, praescribens alexipharmaca, et amuleta, ad utriusque hominis sanitatem praeservandam, conservandam, restaurandam praesentanea ... Ed. 2. ... correctior & auctior. Lovanii, Typis Georgii Lipsii, 1661.

[32], 120 (i.e. 320), [2] p. 16 cm.   [4732]

GILPIN, RICHARD [1625-1700] The comforts of divine love. Preach'd upon the occasion of the much lamented death of the Reverend Mr. Timothy Manlove. With his character, done by another hand. London, Tho. Parkhurst and Sarah Button, 1700.

[10], 46 p. port. 16 cm.   [4733]

"A short character of Mr. Timothy Manlove" (p. [3-6]) signed: J. T.

GINTRIO, Burchardus Sallius. *See* Balde, J. *Father*. Solatium podagricorum libri duo. 1661.

GIORGI, Matteo. Phlebotomia liberata; sive, Apologia pro sanguinis missione in febribus, aliisque morbis magnis, qua respondetur Dominico La Scala ... Accedit de febribus dissertationis prodromus in epistola ad Paulum Franciscum Bruni ... Genuae, Antonii Casamarae, 1697.

[16], 224 p. 21 cm. [**4734**]

GIPHANIUS, Obertus. *See* Giffen, Hubert van [1533?-1604]

GIRALDI, Giovanni Battista [1662-1732] Rupes insuperabilis in pelago medico ... Bononiae, Ex Camer. Typographia, 1693.

105, [1] p. 15 cm. [**4735**]

"Morborum exitialium tyrannica saevitia syntomia in medicam historiam redacta ..." (p. [89]-105) has special title page.

—*See* Malpighi, M. Opera posthuma. 1697.

GIRALDINI, Pier Francesco [*fl.* 1626] Discorso sopra la pietra belzuar minerale ... Firenze, Zanobi Pignoni [1626]

106, [8] p. 22 cm. [**4736**]

Engraved title page.
Imperfect: p. [9-10] (blank?) wanting.

GIRARD, François [*fl.* 1675-1678] *praeses*. Quaestio medica ... An inveteratae & contumaci dysenteriae lactis potio? [Parisiis, Apud Franciscum Muguet, 1678]

4 p. 25 cm. [**4737**]

Diss. — Paris (C. Hugot, *respondent*)

—*respondent. See* Pelletier, N., *praeses*. Quaestio medica ... An magnis lienibus ferrum. 1675.

GIRARD, Jacques [*fl.* 1549-1583] *See* Bacon, R. De l'admirable pouvoir et puissance de l'art & de nature. 1629.

GIRARD, Jacques, *de Tournus. See* Girard, Jacques [*fl.* 1549-1583]

GIRARD DE TOURNUS, Jacques. *See* Girard, Jacques [*fl.* 1549-1583]

GIRARD DES BERGERIES, Jean-Jacob [1614-1681] L'apothiquaire charitable, contenant la nature, l'usage & les proprietés des mineraux, plantes, & animaux, qui servent à la medecine ... Avec un grand nombre de compositions & receptes bien choisies contre la plus part des maladies ...

Geneve, Jean Herman Widerhold, 1673.

[7], 207 p. 18 cm. (Part [2] *In* La medecine domestique. Geneve, 1673) [**4738**]

—Le gouvernement de la santé, où sont contenus non seulement les preceptes les plus seurs pour s'y conserver, châcun selon son âge, son temperament & sa constitution, mais encore plusieurs conseils & remedes, pour prevenir les maux & les incommodités les plus communes de la vie. Avec un traitté de la nature, proprietés, & droit usage de tout ce qui sert de viande, & breuvage en ces quartiers de l'Europe ... Geneve, Jean Herman Widerhold, 1673.

[16], 174 p. 18 cm. (Part [1] *In* La medecine domestique. Geneve, 1673) [**4739**]

GIRARDELLI, Lorenzo. *See.* Ghirardelli, Lorenzo [1600-1641]

GIRARDET, Pierre [17th cent.] *ed. See* Duret, L. *In* Magni Hippocratis librum De humoribus. 1631, 1639.

GIRAUD, Jacques [*fl.* 1549-1583] *See* La metallique transformation. 1618.

GIRAULT, Jean [*fl.* 1610?] *See* Dalechamps, J. Chirurgie françoise. 1610.

GIRINZANA, Lazarus. *See* Ghirinzana, Lazzaro [17th cent.]

GIRNT, Jeremias [*fl.* 1627-1628] *respondent. See* Sennert, D., *praeses*. De pleuritide disputatio. 1627.

GIROLAMI, Ansano Francesco [*fl.* 1698] Il trionfo della china china ... Firenze nel Garbo, Giuseppe Manni, 1699.

viii, 52, [5] p. 15 cm. [**4740**]

Errata: p. [57]
Bound (as issued) with Helvétius, J. A. Trattato delle perdite del sangue. 1699.

GISELER, Laurentius. *See* Giesler, Lorenz [d. 1685]

GIVRIUS, Petrus. *See* Le Givre, Pierre [1618-1684]

GKISLEY, Gabriel. *See* Grisley, Gabriel [*fl.* 1655-ca. 1661]

GLACAN, Nellanus. *See* O'Glacan, Nial [*fl.* 1629-1655]

GLADBACH, JOHANN BERNHARD [*d.* 1728] Kurtze Abhandelung von dem Schwalbacher Sauerbrunnen, wie derselbe zu Erhaltung der Gesundheit und Abwendung vieler sonst unheilbahren Kranckheiten eines jeden Constitution nach entweder kalt oder warm gemacht, könne gebraucht werden . . . Franckfurt am Mäyn, Verlegts Johann Friderich Knoch, gedruckt bey Johann Bauern, 1699.

40 p.   20 cm.   [**4741**]

—Praxeos medicae idea novissima in qua secundum solidiora verae physicae & sanioris medicinae fundamenta, omnium morborum origo ex quatuor cardinalibus concatenata serie deducitur, eorumque succincta ac perspicua medendi methodus explanatur . . . Herbornae, Typis & sumptibus Jo. Nicolai Andreae, 1694.

[24], 499, [29], p.   18 cm.   [**4742**]
With this is bound: Jüngken, J. H. Modernae praxeos medicae vade mecum. 1694.

—*respondent.* Dissertatio medica inauguralis demonstrans omnium febrium unam eandemque esse causam . . . Lugduni Batavorum, Apud Abrahamum Elzevier, 1692.

[24] p.   20 cm.   [**4743**]
Diss.—Leyden.

GLADBACH, JOHANN PETER [*fl.* 1669] *respondent.* Disputatio medica inauguralis de ictero flavo . . . Lugduni Batavorum, Apud viduam & haeredes Joannis Elsevirii [1669]

[12] p.   23 cm.   [**4744**]
Diss.—Leyden.

GLADO, JOHANN BENJAMIN [*fl.* 1696–1697] *respondent. See* PAULI, J. W., *praeses.* Diatriben inauguralem medicam de anorexia . . . submittit. 1696.

GLANDORP, MATTHIAS [1595 *or* 6–1636] Methodus medendae paronychiae. Cui accessit Decas observationum. Bremae, Typis Villerianis [Impensis M. Johannis Willii & Georgii Hoismanni] 1623.

[14], 206, [1] p.   16 cm.   [**4745**]
Engraved title page.

—Speculum chirurgorum, in quo quid in unoquoque vulnere faciendum, quidve omittendum, praemissa partis affectae anatomica explicatione, observationibusque . . . adjunctis . . . pertractatur . . . Bremae, Typis Thomae Villeriani [Impensis M. Johannis Willii & Johannis Benthemii] 1619.

[15], 257, [15] p.   illus.   17 cm.   [**4746**]

—Matthiae Ludovici Glandorp . . . Tractatus de polypo narium affectu gravissimo observationibus illustratus. Bremae, Typis Wesselianis [Sumtibus authoris] 1628.

[8], 60, [4] p.   port.   23 cm.   [**4747**]
Engraved title page.

GLANDORP, MATTHIAS LUDWIG. *See* GLANDORP, Matthias [1595 *or* 6–1636]

GLANVIL, ECEBOLIUS. *See* GLANVILL, Joseph [1636–1680]

GLANVILL, JOSEPH [1636–1680] Essays on several important subjects in philosophy and religion . . . London, Printed by J. D. for John Baker and Henry Mortlock, 1676.

1 v.   21 cm.   [**4748**]
Various pagings.
Contains 7 essays, each with half title.

—Lux Orientalis; or, An enquiry into the opinion of the Eastern sages, concerning the praeexistence of souls. Being a key to unlock the grand mysteries of providence, in relation to mans sin and misery. London, 1662.

[40], 192 p.   16 cm.   [**4749**]
Bound with *his* The vanity of dogmatizing. 1661.

—Plus ultra; or, The progress and advancement of knowledge since the days of Aristotle. In an account of some . . . late improvements of practical . . . learning . . . London, James Collins, 1668.

[34], 149, [6], p.   17 cm.   [**4750**]

—Saducismus triumphatus; or, Full and plain evidence concerning witches and apparitions. In two parts. The first treating of their possibility, the second of their real existence . . . With a letter of Dr. Henry More on the same subject. And an authentick, but wonderful story of certain Swedish witches; done into English by Anth. Horneck . . . London, J. Collins, and S. Lowndes, 1681.

[9], 58, [16], 3–180 p.; [16] 328 (i.e. 338) p.   front., illus., plate.   20 cm.   [**4751**]
Both parts and An appendice to the first part have special title pages.
"An account of what happened in the Kingdom of Sweden . . . in relation to the persons that were accused for witches . . . by Anthony Horneck": p. [311]–338.

—[The same.] . . . The 3d. ed with additions . . . London, Printed for A. L. and sold by Roger Tuckyr, 1700.

8 parts in 1 v. front., illus., plate. 20 cm.
[**4752**]

Each part has special title page.

—The vanity of dogmatizing; or, Confidence in opinions. Manifested in a discourse of the shortness and uncertainty of our knowledge, and its causes; with some reflexions on peripateticism; and an apology for philosophy ... London, Printed by E. C. for Henry Eversden, 1661.

[32], 250, [6] p. 16 cm.   [**4753**]

With this is bound *his* Lux Orientalis. 1662.

—[The same.] Scepsis scientifica; or, Confest ignorance, the way to science; in an essay of the vanity of dogmatizing, and confident opinion. With a reply to the exceptions of the learned Thomas Albius [pseud. i.e. Thomas White] ... London, E. Cotes, for Henry Eversden, 1665.

[35], 184 p.; [16], 92 p. 21 cm.   [**4754**]

Part [2] has special title page: Scir$\frac{e}{1}$tuum nihil est; or, The authors defence of the vanity of dogmatizing, against the exceptions of ... Tho. Albius. ...

—*See* STUBBS, H. A censure upon certain passages contained in the history of the Royall Society. 1671 [and] The Lord Bacons relation of the sweating-sickness examined. 1671 [and] The plus ultra reduced to a non plus. 1670.

GLANVILLA, BARTHOLOMAEUS DE. *See* BARTHOLOMAEUS ANGLICUS [13th cent.]

GLANVILLE, BARTHOLOMEW DE. *See* BARTHOLOMAEUS ANGLICUS [13th cent.]

GLAREANO, SCIPIO, *pseud. See* APROSIO, Angelico [1607–1681]

GLASER, CHRISTOPHE [*ca.* 1615–*ca.* 1673] Traite de la chymie, enseignant par une brieve et facile methode toutes ses plus necessaires preparations ... Paris, L'autheur, 1663.

[16], 378, [3] p. plate. 17 cm.   [**4755**]

Engraved title page.

—[The same.] ... 3. ed. Rev. & augm. ... Lyon, Jean Thioly, 1670.

[20], 394, [3] p. plates. 18 cm.   [**4756**]

—[The same.] ... Nouv. ed. Rev. & augm. ... Paris, Jean d'Houry, 1674.

[12], 439, [11] p. plates. 16 cm.   [**4757**]

Added engraved title page.

—[The same.] ... 4. ed. Rev. & augm. par l'autheur. Bruxelles, Gille t'Serstevens, 1676.

[12], 364 (i.e. 394), [10] p. 15 cm.   [**4758**]

—[English tr.] The compleat chymist; or, A new treatise of chymistry ... Written in French ... Now ... Englished by a fellow of the Royal Society ... London, John Starkey, 1677.

[16], 285, [2], p. 19 cm.   [**4759**]

—[German tr.] Novum laboratorium medico-chymicum; das ist, Neu-eröffnete chymische Artzney- und Werk-Schul, in drey Bücher abgetheilet ... aus den besten ... Authoribus zusammen gelesen, und also erstesmals in frantzösischer Sprache verabfasset worden durch C[hristophe] G[laser] Anjetzo aber ... in das Hoch-Teutsche übersetzet von Johann Marschalck ... Deme beygefügt ein Anhang, handlend von dem Grund und Erkanntniss der Natur ... Nürnberg, In Verlegung Michael und Johann Friderich Endtern, 1677.

[56], 666, [13] p. front., plates. 17 cm.
[**4760**]

Errata: p. [13] at end.
Frontispiece has title: Chymische Artzney-und Werck-Schul.

—[The same.] Chimischer Wegweiser; das ist, Sichere Anweisung zur chimischen Kunst, darinnen durch einen kurtzen Weg ... gewiesen wird, wie man allerley Artzneyen durch die Chimie bereiten kan ... Übersetzet von einem Philochimico. Jena, Verlegts Joh. Jac. Bauhofer, 1684.

[12], 446, [13] p. front., plates. 14 cm.
[**4761**]

Translated by Jean Menudier.

GLASER, JOHANN ADAM [*fl.* 1688] *respondent. See* RINGMACHER, D. Dissertationem de variis philosophorum circa principia corporum naturalium, praessertim viventium, placitis ... p. p. ... M. D. R. 1688.

GLASER, JOHANN HEINRICH [1629–1675] Tractatus posthumus de cerebro ... Nunc primum luci publicae expositus opera Joh. Jacobi Staehelini ... Basiliae, Typis Jacobi Bertschii, 1680.

[16], 231, [9] p. 17 cm.   [**4762**]

Added engraved title page.

—*praes*. Casus medicus de mensium suppressione, eorumque per aures excretione, ut et febre tertiana notha . . . Basileae, Typis Jacobi Werenfelsii [1673]

    [27] p. 20 cm.   **[4763]**

    Diss.—Basel (K. C. Eisen, *respondent*)

—Disputatio chirurgico-medica de herniis in genere, singulisque earum differentiis in specie . . . Basileae, Typis Jacobi Bertschii [1673]

    [32] p. 19 cm.   **[4764]**

    Diss.—Basel (J. Hoegger, *respondent*)

—[Dissertatio casualis de caro apoplexia terminato] . . . Basileae, Typis Jacobi Bertschii [1672]

    [20] p. 19 cm.   **[4765]**

    Diss.—Basel (H. Martini, *respondent*)

—Dissertatio historiae medicae de scrofulis . . . Basileae, Typis Jacobi Bertschii [1672]

    [20] p. 19 cm.   **[4766]**

    Diss.—Basel (M. Harder, *respondent*)

—Dissertatio medica de ictero nigro . . . Basileae, Typis Jacobi Bertschii [1673]

    [18] p. 20 cm.   **[4767]**

    Diss.—Basel (J. J. Harder, *respondent*)

—*respondent. See* STRASBURG, J. G., *praes*. De dolore colico positiones medicas. 1650; STUPANUS, E., *praes*. Signorum medicorum doctrina. 1649.

GLASER, JOHANN KONRAD [*fl.* 1677–1682] *respondent. See* RIVINUS, A. Q., *praes*. Dissertatio de spiritu hominis vitali. 1681.

GLAUBER, JOHANN RUDOLPH [1604?–1670] Opera chymica, Bücher und Schrifften, so viel deren von ihme bisshero an Tag gegeben worden. Jetzo von neuem . . . übersehen, auch . . . vermehret . . . Franckfurt am Mayn, In Verlegung Thomae Matthiae Götzens, 1658–59.

    2 v. in 1. plates. 21 cm.   **[4768]**

    Vorrede of vol. 2 signed by J. M. D.

—[English tr.] The works . . . containing great variety of choice secrets in medicine and alchymy in the working of metallick mines, and the separation of metals . . . Translated . . . and published . . . by . . . Christopher Packe . . . London, Printed by Thomas Milbourn for the author, and sold by D. Newman and W. Cooper, 1689.

    3 parts in 1 v. illus., plates. 40 cm. **[4769]**

    Part 2 has special title page; part 3 caption title.

    There are 11 plates, including a duplicate of the one preceding p. 189.

    Includes his controversy with Christoph Farner, and Paracelsus' The book touching the tincture of natural things.

—Apologia; oder, Verthaidigung, gegen Christoff Farners Lügen und Ehr-abschneidung. [Amsterdam?] 1655.

    88 p. 17 cm.   **[4770]**

—[Latin tr.] Apologia contra mendaces Christophori Farnneri calumnias, ex Germanico in Latinum idioma trans-fusa. Amstelodami, 1655.

    [94 p. 17 cm.   **[4771]**

—De auri tinctura; sive, Auro potabili vero was solche sey, und wie dieselbe von einem falschen und sophistischen Auro potabili zu unterscheiden und zu erkennen . . . Und wo zu solche in Medicina könne gebraucht werden . . . Amsterdam, Gedruckt bey Johann Fabeln, 1646.

    39, [1] p. 15 cm.   **[4772]**

    Imperfect: upper margin of title page mutilated.

—[The same.] . . . Amsterdam, Johan Jansson, 1662.

    32 p. 16 cm.   **[4773]**

—[Latin ed.] De auri tinctura; sive, Auro potabili vero. Quid sit & quommodo differat ab auro potabili falso & sophistico quomodo spagyrice praeparandum & quomodo in medicina usurpandum . . . Amsterodami, Prostant apud Joannem Janssonium, 1651.

    22 p. 17 cm.   **[4774]**

    Bound (as issued?) with *his* Furni novi philosophici. 1651.

—[French tr.] La teinture de l'or; ou, Le veritable or potable; sa nature . . . sa preparation spagirique, & son usage dans la medecine . . . Mise en françois par le S^r Du Teil. Paris, Thomas Jolly, 1659.

    22 p. 19 cm.   **[4775]**

    With this is bound *his* Traitté de la medecine universelle. 1659.

—De Elia Artista; oder, Wass Elias Artista für einer sey, und wass er in der Welt reformiren . . . werde, wann er kombt? Nemblich: die wahre spagirische Medicin, der alten aegyptischen Philosophen, welche . . . er wiederumb herfürziehen, solche renoviren, und durch newe Inventiones . . . illustriren . . . wirdt . . . Amsterdam, Bey Johan Waesberge, und der Witwe Elizaei Weyerstraet, 1668.

    71 p. 16 cm.   **[4776]**

—De igne secreto philosophorum; oder, Geheimen Fewr der Weisen. Dadurch die Philosophi nicht allein ihre universal Medicin gegen natürliche Kranckheiten des Menschen aussgezeitiget, sondern auch particulariter alle geringe Metallen . . . figirt und Cupellen beständig gemacht haben . . . Amsterdam, Bey Johan Jansson a Waesberge, und Wittwe von Elisaeo Weierstraet, 1669.

54, [1] p.   16 cm.   [4777]

Errata: p. [55]

—De lapide animali, oder von dieser animalischen Materi, oder subjecto . . . Was es eigentlich für ein Materi sey, unnd wie eine wahre universal Medicin darauss bereiret werden könne . . . Amsterdam, Bey Johan Jansson a Waesberge, und Wittwe Elizei Weierstraet, 1669.

60 p.   16 cm.   [4778]

Evidently intended as the sixth Centuria following on the Reicher Schatz- und Sammelkasten, 1660-1668. Cf. Duveen, p. 257.

—De purgatorio philosophorum; oder, Von dem Fegfewer der Weysen . . . Welches Fegfewer von den alten Philosophis Ysopaica genant worden: welches so viel, als Ars lavandi per Ignem . . . zu sagen ist. Neben beygefügtem Unterricht, wie auss allen Metallen . . . durch hülffe dass Salis Mundi ein lebendiger Mercurius in Copia zu bereiten sey . . . Amsterdam, Bey Johan Waesberge, und der Witwe Elizaei Weyerstraet, 1668.

70 p.   16 cm.   [4779]

—De tribus lapidibus ignium secretorum; oder, Von den drey alleredelsten Gesteinen, so durch drey secrete Fewer gebohren werden: und erstlich von dem Lapide Philosophorum . . . Zum andern, von dem obern- und untern Donnerstein . . . Und zum dridten, wie des Basilii Stein Ignis auss dem Antimonio durch Kunst zu bereiten sey . . . Amsterdam, Bey Johan Waesberge, und der Witwe Elizaei Weyerstraet, 1667.

94 p.   16 cm.   [4780]

Includes letter by Johannes Pontanus (p. 27-31)

—[Explicatio oder Ausführliche Erklärung. Latin.] Explicatio tractatuli, qui miraculum mundi inscribitur, nuper a Joh. Rud. Glaubero editi, tam plana quam solida, in rei veritatis testimonium, & artes amore prosequentium utilitatem . . . Francofurti, Impensis Thomae Matthiae Götzens, 1656.

62 p.   17 cm.   [4781]

Ferguson (A) p. 325.

—Explicatio; oder, Ausslegung über die Wohrten Salomonis: In herbis, verbis, & lapidibus, magna est virtus. Sampt beygefügtem tractätlein De quinta essentia metallorum . . . Amsterdam, Johan Jansson, 1663.

101 p.   plate.   16 cm.   [4782]

—[Latin tr.] Explicatio verborum Salomonis: in herbis, verbis & lapidibus magna est virtus. Una cum adjuncta tractatiuncula De quinta essentia metallorum . . . Amsterdami, Prostant apud Joannem Janssonium, 1664.

88 p.   17 cm.   [4783]

—[Furni novi philosophici; oder, Beschreibung einer new-erfundenen Distillir-Kunst. Latin.] Furni novi philosophici; sive, Descriptio artis destillatoriae novae; nec non spirituum, oleorum, florum, aliorumque medicamentorum illius beneficio, facilima quadam & peculiari vie e vegetabilibus, animalibus & mineralibus, conficiendorum & quidem magno cum lucro . . . Amsterodami, Prostant apud Joannem Janssonium, 1651.

6 parts in 1 v.   illus., plates.   17 cm.   [4784]

Parts 1-5 and Annotationes in appendicem quintae partis have special title pages.

With this is bound (as issued?) *his* De auri tinctura. 1651.

—[English tr.] A description of new philosophical furnaces; or, A new art of distilling, divided into five parts. Whereunto is added a description of the tincture of gold, or the true aurum potabile; also, the first part of the mineral work . . . Set forth in English, by J. F. D. M. London, Richard Coats, for Thos. Williams, 1651.

[16], 452, [12] p.   illus.   19 cm.   [4785]

Each chapter has special title page dated 1652.

—[French tr.] La description des nouveaux fourneaux philosophiques; ou, Art distillatoire, par le moyen duquel sont tirez les esprits, huiles, fleurs, & autres medicaments: par une voye aisée & avec grand profit, des vegetaux, animaux, & mineraux . . . Traduit . . . par le sieur Du Teil. Paris, Thomas Jolly, 1659.

6 parts in 1 v.   plates.   19 cm.   [4786]

Parts 1-5 and Annotations sur l'appendix de la cinquiesme partie (bound between part 2 and 3) have special title pages.

[—] Glauberus concentratus; oder, Laboratorium Glauberianum; darinn die Specification, und Taxation dehren medicinalischen, und chymischen Arcanitäten, welche in ermeldtem Laboratorio, von viel

Jahren zu Jahren nach einander bereitet . . . Sambt aller dehren . . . Instrumenten, welche im Laboratorio gebrauchet . . . Amsterdam, Bey Johan Waesberge, und der Witwe Elizaei Weyerstraet, 1668.

75 p.; 15 p.   16 cm.   [**4787**]

"Catalogus librorum . . .": 15 p. at end.

[—] Glauberus ridivivus [sic]; dass ist, Der von falschen und gifftigen Zungen ermorte . . . nun aber . . . wieder auffgestandene Glauber. Oder klarer Beweiss dass Farners . . . falschgenante Apologia nichts anders als lauter . . . Lügen sein . . . Amsterdam, Johan Jansson, 1656.

109 p.   17 cm.   [**4788**]

—Gründliche und warhafftige Beschreibung, wie man auss der Weinhefen einen guten Weinstein in grosser Menge extrahiren sol . . . Amsterdam, 1654.

32 p.   17 cm.   [**4789**]

—[Latin tr.] Vera ac perfecta descriptio, qua ratione ex vini fecibus bonum plurimumque tartarum sit extrahendum . . . Amstelodami, Prostant Apud Joannem Janssonium, 1655.

28 p.   17 cm.   [**4790**]

—Kurtze Erklährung, über die höllische Göttin Proserpinam Plutonis Haussfrawen, was die philosophische Poëten, als Ovidius, Virgilius, und andere darduch [sic] verstanden haben; und wie durch Hülff dieser Proserpinae die Seelen der abgestorbenen metallischen Leibern auss der chimischen Höllen, in den philosophischen Himmel geführet werden . . . Ambsterdam, Bey Johan Jansson von Waesberge, und der Witwe Elizaei Weyerstraet, 1667.

56 p.   16 cm.   [**4791**]

—Libellus dialogorum; oder, Gespräch-Buchlein, zwisschen einigen Lieb-habern der hermetischen Medicin, Tincturam universalem betreffend . . . Amsterdam, Johan Jansson, 1663.

91 p.   plate.   16 cm.   [**4792**]

—[Latin tr.] Libellus dialogorum; sive, Colloquia, nonnullorum Hermeticae medicinae, ac tincturae universalis studiosorum, in gratiam eorum, qui Hermeticam philosophiam amplectuntur . . . Amstelodami, Apud Joannem Janssonium, 1663.

91 p.   plates.   17 cm.   [**4793**]

—Libellus ignium; oder, Feur Büchlein darinnen

von unterschiedlichen frembden und biss Dato noch gantz unbekandten Feuren gehandelt . . . Amsterdam, Johan Jansson, 1663.

61, [1] p.   16 cm.   [**4794**]

—Miraculum mundi; oder, Aussführliche Beschreibung der wunderbaren Natur, Art, und Eigenschafft des grossmächtigen Subjecti, von den alten Menstruum universale oder Mercurius Philosophorum genandt . . . Amsterdam, 1653.

3 parts in 1 v.   17 cm.   [**4795**]

Part [2] (bound after part [3]) has special title page: Miraculi mundi continuatio . . . Amsterdam, Johan Jansson, 1657.

Part [3] has special title page: Miraculi mundi ander Theil. Oder dessen vorlängst geprophezeiten Eliae Artistae triumphirlicher Einritt . . . Amsterdam, Johan Jansson, 1660.

"Ph. Theophrasti Bombast, ab Hohenheim . . . De tinctura physicorum . . .": p. 50–96, part [2], with text in German.

With this is bound *his* Explicatio. 1656.

—Annotationes in nuper editam Continuationem Miraculi mundi, secreta ibidem contenta, aurumque potabile verum, cujus simul mentio ibidem facta est, explicantes & defendentes . . . Amstelodami, Apud Joannem Janssonium, 1659.

37 p.   16 cm.   [**4796**]

—Explicatio; oder, Uber dass unlängst, von Joh. Rud. Glaubern aussgebenes (Miraculum mundi, intitulirtes) Tractätlein aussfuhrliche Erklährung . . . Amsterdam, Johan Jansson, 1656.

110 p.   17 cm.   [**4797**]

Bound with *his* Miraculum mundi. 1653.

—Novum lumen chimicum; oder, Eines newerfundenen und der Weldt noch niemahlen bekandgemachten hohen Secreti Offenbahrung: dardurch . . . gezeiget wird, dass in der gantzen Welt, so wohl in den Kalten, als hitzigen Landen allenthalben guth zu finden, und mit nutzen herauss zu ziehen . . . Ambsterdam, Bey Johan Jansson vom Waesberge und Elizee Weyerstraet, 1664.

43, [2] p.   16 cm.   [**4798**]

—[Latin tr.] Novum lumen chymicum; hoc est, Cujusdam recens inventi & mundo nondum unquam patefacti secreti ardui revelatio, qua mundo caeco clarum atque inexstinguibile lumen ante oculos collocatur . . . quod per universum terrarum orbem aeque in frigidis ac in calidis regionibus passim aurum probum inveniri atque utiliter elici possit . . . Amstelodami, Apud Joannem Janssonium a Waesberge, & Elisaeum Weyerstraet, 1664.

45 p.   17 cm.   [**4799**]

—[English tr.] *In* Cooper, W. The philosophical epitaph. 1673–75.

—Operis mineralis; oder, Vieler künstlichen . . . metallischen Arbeitten Beschreibung erster Theil [-dritter Theil] . . . Amsterdam, 1651.

   3 parts in 1 v.   17 cm.   **[4800]**

Part [2] has special title page dated 1652.

Part 3 has special title page: Operis mineralis dritter Theil: darinnen unter der Explication über dess Paracelsi Büchlein, Coelum philosophorum oder Liber vexationum genandt, der Metallen transmutationes in genere gelehret . . . 1652.

—[Latin tr.] Operis mineralis. Pars prima [-pars tertia] . . . Amsterodami, Prostant apud Joannem Janssonium, 1651.

   3 parts in 1 v.   17 cm.   **[4801]**

Part 2 has special title page dated 1652.

Part 3 has special title page: Operis mineralis pars tertia, in qua titulo commentarii in libellum Paracelsi Coelum philosophorum sive Liber vexationum dictum, metallorum transmutationes in genere docentur . . . In Latinum idioma ex Germanico conversa . . . 1652.

—Pharmacopaeae spagyricae; oder, Gründlicher Beschreibung, wie man aus den Vegetabilien, Animalien und Mineralien, auff eine besondere und leichtere Weise, gute . . . Artzneyen zurichten und bereiten soll. Erster Theil [-Siebender Theil] . . . Amsterdam, Bey Johan a Waesberge, und der Witwe Elizee Weyetstraet [sic] 1668.

   10 parts in 1 v.   plate.   17 cm.   **[4802]**

In addition to the seven parts there are three appendices supplementing part 7.

Each part has special title page dated 1668, 1656, 1657, 1661, 1663, 1664, 1667, 1667, 1668, 1668 respectively; parts 2–5 were printed by Johan Jansson.

—Another issue.   **[4803]**

Part 7 only. Pages 8–9 paged 2–3.

—[Latin tr.] Pharmacopoea spagyrica; sive, Exacta descriptio, qua ratione ex vegetabilibus, animalibus & mineralibus . . . medicamenta fieri praepararique possint. Pars prima [-quinta pars] . . . Amsterodami, Apud Joannem Janssonium, 1654.

   5 parts in 1 v.   plate.   17 cm.   **[4804]**

Each part has special title page dated 1654, 1656, 1661, 1661, 1663, respectively.

—Reicher Schatz- und Sammelkasten; oder, Appendix generalis, über alle dessen heraussgegebene Bücher . . . In decem Centuriis . . . beschrieben, und an Tag geben. Amsterdam, Johan Jansson, 1660.

   198 p.; 158, [1] p.; [5], 87 p.   illus.   16 cm.   **[4805]**

Contains five Centurias.

"... Zweite Centuria ..." and "... Die dritte, vierdte und fünffte Centuria ... Amsterdam, Bey Johan Waesberg und der Witwe Elisaei Weyerstraet, 1668" have special title pages.

At the end of the fifth centuria (p. 87) the publication of a sixth centuria is promised, and this appeared in 1669 under title: De lapide animali.

—[Latin tr.] Arca thesauris opulentia; sive, Appendix generalis omnium librorum hactenus editorum . . . In decem centurias distributum. Amstelaedami, Apud Johannem Janssonium, 1660.

   189 p.; 149, [1] p.   illus.   17 cm.   **[4806]**

Part 2 has special title page: Opulenti thesauri, et arcae thesaurariae; sive, Appendicis generalis, centuria secunda . . . 1661.

The text of part 2 is followed by a duplicate of its title page, but with slightly different text.

—[Teutschlands Wohlfart.] Des Teutschlandts Wohlfart erster Theil [-sechster und letzter Theil] Darinnen von des Weins, Korns und Holtzes concentrirung, sambt deroselben nutzlichern . . . Gebrauch, gehandelt wirdt . . . Amsterdam, Johan Jansson, 1656.

   7 parts in 1 v.   plates.   17 cm.   **[4807]**

Parts 1–6 and Appendix uber des Teutschlandes Wohlfahrt, fünfften Theil (bound between parts 5 and 6) dated 1656, 1657, 1659, 1659, 1660, 1660, 1661 respectively, have special title pages.

—Tractatus de medicina universali; sive, Auro potabili vero. Oder aussführliche Beschreibung einer wahren Universal Medicin . . . Amsterdam, Johan Jansson, 1657.

   80 p.   16 cm.   **[4808]**

—[Latin tr.] Tractatus de medicina universali; sive, Auro potabili vero, hoc est, accurata descriptio verae medicinae universalis . . . Amstelodami, Apud Joannem Janssonium, 1658.

   75, [2] p.   18 cm.   **[4809]**

—[French tr.] Traitté de la medecine universelle; ou, Le vray or potable . . . Mis en françois par le Sʳ Du Teil. Paris, Thomas Jolly, 1659.

   61, [1] p.   19 cm.   **[4810]**

Bound with *his* La teinture de l'or. 1659.

—Tractatus de natura salium; sive, Dilucida descriptio, perfecta explanatione declarans naturam, proprietates, & usus salium vulgo notorum . . . cum demonstratione . . . quod sal (post Deum & solem,) unicum sit principium . . . Item tractatulus . . . de salium, metallorum, & planetarum signatura . . . Amsterodami, Apud Joannem Janssonium, 1659.

[16], 96 p.　17 cm.　　　　　　　　**[4811]**

Translated from the German.

—Tractatus de signatura salium, metallorum, et planetarum; sive, Fundamentalis institutio . . . monstrans, quo pacto . . . non solum salium, metallorum, atque planetarum, sed etiam appellationum, & nominum ipsis impositorum vires, significatio, natura, & proprietates, non ex libris, aut scriptis, sed nuda ipsorum signatura, circuli & quadrati ope, cognosci, addisci, & supputari queant . . . Amstelodami, Apud Joannem Janssonium, 1659.

44 p.　illus.　17 cm.　　　　　　**[4812]**

Translated from the German.

—Trost der Seefahrenten: darinnen gelehret . . . wirt, wie sich die Seefahrende vor Hunger und Durst, wie auch solchen Kranckheiten so ihnen auff langwiriger Reise begegnen möchten, versorgen und bewahran können . . . Amsterdam, Johan Jansson, 1657.

102, [5] p.　18 cm.　　　　　　　**[4813]**

Errata: p. [107]

—[Latin tr.] Consolatio navigantium: in qua docetur, & deducitur, quomodo per maria peregrinantes a fame ac siti immo etiam morbis . . . sibi providere ac suppetiari liceat . . . Amstelodami, Apud Joannem Janssonium, 1657.

96 p.　16 cm.　　　　　　　　　**[4814]**

—[French tr.] La consolation des navigants. Dans laquelle est enseigné à ceux qui voyagent sur mer un moyen de se garantir de la faim & de la soif, voire mesme des maladies qui leur pourroient survenir durant un long voyage . . . Traduite . . . par le sieur Du Teil. Paris, Thomas Jolly, 1659.

64 p.　19 cm.　　　　　　　　　**[4815]**

—[Von den dreyen Anfängen der Metallen. Latin.] Tractatus de tribus principiis metallorum, videlicet sulphure, mercurio & sale philosophorum, quemadmodum illa in medicina, alchymia aliisque artibus associatis utiliter adhiberi valeant . . . Amstelodami, Apud Joannem Janssonium à Waesberge, & viduam Elizaei Weyerstraet, 1667.

109 p.　17 cm.　　　　　　　　　**[4816]**

—See HARPRECHT, J. Sudum philosophicum, pro secretis chymicis perspiciendis. 1660.

GLAUBERUS concentratus. 1668. *See* [GLAUBER, J. R.]

GLAUBERUS ridivivus. 1656. *See* [GLAUBER, J. R.]

GLAZEMAKER, JAN HENDRIK [*d.* 1682] *tr. See* REGIMEN SANITATIS SALERNITANUM. Schoola Salernitana. [Dutch tr.]: 1658.

—*See* LESSIUS, L. De schat der soberheit. 1681.

GL'INDIRIZZI dell'arte dello spetiale medicinalista. 1658? *See* UNIVERSITÀ DI BOLOGNA. Collegio de medicina.

GLISSON, FRANCIS [1597–1677] Opera medico-anatomica, in unum corpus collecta, & tribus voluminibus comprehensa . . . Lugd. Batavor., Apud Petrum vander Aa, 1691–1711 [v. 1, 1711]

3 v. in 1.　front. (port.), illus., plates.　14 cm.

　　　　　　　　　　　　　　　　　[4817]

Title pages of vol. 1 and 3 are dated 1691. Each vol. has also special title page dated 1711, 1711 and 1691 respectively.

Contents: v. 1. Tractatus de rachitide. v. 2. Anatomia hepatis. v. 3. Tractatus de ventriculo & intestinis.

—Anatomia hepatis. Cui praemittuntur quaedam ad rem anatomicam universe spectantia. Et ad calcem operis subjiciuntur nonnulla de lymphaeductibus nuper repertis . . . Londini, Typis Du-Gardianis, impensis Octaviani Pullein, 1654.

[48], 458, [13] p.　illus., plates.　17 cm.

　　　　　　　　　　　　　　　　　[4818]

—[The same.] . . . Amstelaedami, Sumptibus Joannis Ravesteinii, 1659.

[48], 552, [12] p.　illus., plates.　14 cm.

　　　　　　　　　　　　　　　　　[4819]

Added engraved title page.

—[The same.] . . . Ed. nova. caeteris emendatior. Amstelodami, Apud Joannem Janssonium et Elizaeum Weyerstraten, 1665.

[48], 423, [18] p.　illus., plates.　14 cm.

　　　　　　　　　　　　　　　　　[4820]

Added engraved title page.

—[The same.] . . . Ed. nov., prioribus emendatior. Hagae-Comitum, Apud Arnoldum Leers, 1681.

[48], 552, [12] p.　illus., plates.　14 cm.

　　　　　　　　　　　　　　　　　[4821]

Added engraved title page.

—De rachitide; sive, Morbo puerili, qui vulgo the rickets dicitur, tractatus ... adscitis in operis societatem Georgio Bate, & Adhasuero Regemortero ... Londini, Typis Guil. Du-gardi, impensis Laurentii Sadler & Roberti Beaumont, 1650.

[30], 416 (i.e. 414) p.   illus.   17 cm.   [4822]
Imperfect: sig. A1 (blank?) wanting.

—[The same.] ... Ed. 2. priori adcuratior longe, & emendatior. Londini, Typis Th. Roycroft, impensis Laurentii Sadler, 1660.

[22], 378 (i.e. 380) p.   illus.   15 cm.
[4823]

—[The same.] ... Ed. 3. ... Lugduni Batavorum, Ex officina Cornelii Driehuysen, & Felicis Lopez, 1671.

[20], 427, [1] p.   illus.   16 cm.   [4824]
Added engraved title page.

—[The same.] ... Ed. postrema. Hagae-Comitis, Apud Arnoldum Leers, 1682.

[18], 412 p.   illus.   14 cm.   [4825]

—[English tr.] A treatise of the rickets: being a disease common to children ... Published in Latine, by Francis Glisson, George Bate, and Adhasuerus Regemorter ... Translated by Phil Armin. Enl. corr., and ... amended ... By Nich. Culpeper ... London, Printed by John Streater, and sold by George Sawbridge, 1668.

[4], 373 (i.e. 363), [4] p.   illus.   15 cm.
[4826]
Signatures: A^2, C–Z^8, Aa–Bb^8.
Imperfect: p. [2–4] at end mounted and mutilated.

—Tractatus de natura substantiae energetica; seu, De vita naturae, ejusque tribus primis facultatibus, I. perceptiva, II. appetitiva, & III. motiva, naturalibus, &c. ... Londini, Typis E. Flesher, prostat venalis apud H. Brome, & N. Hooke, 1672.

[53], 534, [1] p.   front., port.   20 cm. [4827]
Errata: p. [535]

—Tractatus de ventriculo et intestinis. Cui praemittitur alius, De partibus continentibus in genere; & in specie, de iis abdominis ... Londini, Typis E. F., prostat venalis apud Henricum Brome, 1677.

[8], 509, [27] p.   illus., plates, port.   21 cm.
[4828]
Imperfect: port. wanting.

—[The same.] ... Amstelodami, Apud Jacobum

Juniorem, 1677.

[32], 591 p.   illus., plates, port.   15 cm.
[4829]
With this are bound Riolan, J. [1580–1657] Incursionum Quercetani depulsio. 1605; Riolan, J. [1580–1657] Censura demonstrationum Harveti pro veritate alchymiae. 1606.

—*See* BARTHOLIN, T. Opuscula nova anatomica. 1670.

GLOBICZ, JOANNES DANIEL, *ed. See* HIPPOCRATES. Aphorismi. Latin. 1681.

GLOCK, JOHANN GEORG [*fl.* 1690] *respondent. See* CAMERARIUS, E. R., *praeses.* Theses medicae de catalepsi epileptica. 1690.

GLOCKEN, JOHANN GEORG [*fl.* 1691] *respondent. See* CAMERARIUS, E. R., *praeses.* Dissertatio medica inauguralis. In qua obex curationis morborum ... monstratur. 1691.

GLOCKIUS, JOHANN GEORGIUS à. *See* GLOCKEN, Johann Georg [*fl.* 1691]

GLOGAU (FÜRSTENTUM) **Ordinances, local laws, etc.** Kurtzer Bericht; oder, Extract, wie sich in dem Königl. Erb-Fürstenthumb Glogau bey jetzo aller Orten gefährlichen Zeiten sowohlen vor- als in- und nach der Pest zuverhalten. [Grossglogau] 1680.

[32] p.   19 cm.   [4830]
Signed by Graf Johann Bernhardt von Herberstein.

GLOGER, JOHANN [*fl.* 1622] *respondent. See* MÜLLER, J. [1598–1672] *praeses.* Στοιχειολογὶα disputatio III de aqua. 1622.

GLOSEMEYER, JOHANN [*b.* 1664] *respondent. See* CRAUSE, R. W., *praeses.* Disputatio inauguralis medica de apoplexia. 1689; VATER, C., *praeses.* Existentiam & motum spirituum animalium in nervis ... defendet J. G. 1687.

—*See* FASCH, A. H. Augustinus Henricus Faschius ... Facultatis Medicae X. decanus S. P. D. benevolo lectori! 1689.

GLOSSOGRAPHIA. 1674. *See* BLOUNT, T.

GLOXIN, PAUL BENJAMIN [*fl.* 1649] *respondent.* Theses de hydrope ... Argentorati, Excudebat Johannes Pickel, 1649.

[27] p.   19 cm.   [4831]
Diss.—Strasbourg.

GLUD, SØREN PEDER [*fl.* 1686] Quinque sensus

exteriores eorumque organa vera . . . proponit Severinus Petri Glud philos. baccal., respondente Erico Munch. Hafniae, Literis Christiani Weringii, 1686.

[2], 16 p.   19 cm.   [4832]

GLÜCK, Friedrich Gottfried [*fl.*1685] *respondent. See* Berger, J. G. von. Dissertationem medicam de mania . . . sistit . . . F. G. G. 1685.

GLÜCKRADT, Christopher, *pseud. See* Hartmann, Johann [1568–1631]

GLYTZ, Johann Georg [*b.* 1658] *respondent. See* Crause, R. W., *praeses.* Disputatio medica inauguralis de lumbricis. 1685; Hoffmann, F. [1626–1675] *praeses.* Morbum convulsivum a viso spectro . . . exponit . . . J. G. G. 1682.

—*See* Fasch, A. H. Decanus Facultatis Medicae Augustinus Henricus Faschius . . . L. B. S. D. eumque ad hanc de lunbricis disputationem inauguralem officiose & amice invitat. 1685.

GMELIN, Georg Friedrich [*fl.* 1699–1700] *respondent. See* Camerarius, R. J., *praeses.* De convenientia plantarum in fructificatione et viribus. 1699; Zeller, J. G., *praeses.* Disputatio inauguralis medica de gonorrhoea virulenta utroque in sexu. 1700.

GNOSIUS, Dominicus [*fl.* 1608] *ed. See* Hermes Trismegistus. Tractatus vere aureus. 1610.

GOBBO DI SANCASCIANO, Il, *pseud. See* Bertini, Anton Francesco [1658–1726]

GOCKEL, Christoph Erasmus [*fl.* 1694–1695] Disputatio inauguralis medica de herpete . . . [Altdorffii] Excudebat Henricus Meyer [1695]

[4], 16 p.   20 cm.   [4833]

—*respondent. See* Hoffmann, J. M., *praeses.* Exercitatio medica de aere morbifico. 1694.

GOCKEL, Eberhard [1636–1703] Consiliorum et observationum medicinalium decades sex . . . Augustae Vindelicorum, Impensis Theophili Göbelii, typis Joh. Jacobi Schönigkii, 1683.

[14], 550, [56] p.   front. (port.)   18 cm.
                                                 [4834]

—Discursus politico-historico-medicus de ira; oder, Politische, historische, und medicinische Betrachtung dess Zorns, und deren darauss entspringenden Unfällen . . . und . . . Kranckheiten: . .

auch wie demselben zu begegnen . . . seye . . . Nördlingen, Friderich Schultes, 1667.

132 p.   15 cm.   [4835]

—Enchiridion medico-practicum de peste. Atque ejus origine, causis & signis prognosticis, quin etiam praeservationis ac curationis modo & antidotis; partim ex probatissimorum medicorum (utpote Jos. Quercetani [i.e. J. Duchesne], Gregor Horstii, Raym. Mündereri, Ath. Kircheri, aliorumque) scriptis . . . concinnatum; cui annexus est Libellus de venenis . . . Augustae Vindelicorum, Impensis Gottlieb Goebelii, typis Joannis Schönigkii, 1669.

[10], 125, [14] p.; 119 , [5] p.   front. (port.) 17 cm.   [4836]

Part [2] has special title page: Libellus alter de venenis. Eorum causis & antidotis. Ex optimis & probatissimis hinc inde notatis auctoribus, in primis Theo. Paracelso, Petro Aponensi, Henrico a Bra, Dioscoride, Jo. Bauhino, Jo. Praevotio, &c. congestus.

—Gallicinium medico-practicum; sive, Consiliorum, observationum et curationum medicinalium novarum centuriae duae, cum dimidia . . . Ulmae, Impensis Georgii Wilhelmi Künnen, 1700.

[24], 749, [47] p.   front. (port.), plates.   22 cm.
                                                 [4837]

Errata: p. [46–47]
"Appendix, que in se continet Observationum medicinalium decades V. Quibus accessit Additamentum, videlicet modus inspiciendi vulnera lethalia . . .": p. [621]–749.

GOCLENIUS, Rudolph [1547–1628] Physiologia crepitus ventris, et risus, recognita . . . et iterato edita . . . Cum ritu depositionis scholasticae. Francofurti, Prostat in Officina Paltheniana, 1607.

[7], 173, [1] p.   16 cm.   [4838]

"Friderici Widebrandi, typus depositionis scholasticae heroico carmine descriptus": p. 74–90; —"De origine, caussis, typo, et ceremoniis illius ritus, qui vulgo in scholis depositio appellatur, oratio M. Johannis Dinckelii": p. 93–123; —"Judicium Dn. Doctoris Martini Lutheri, de depositione in academiis usitata. Witebergae": p. 125–128; —"Theses de risu, fletu, et locutione respondente Johanne Kuhl . . .": p. 169–173.

Attributed also to Rudolph Goclenius the younger. Cf. BMC and Wellcome.

—, *ed. See* Seidel, B. Physica. 1656.

GOCLENIUS, Rudolph [1572–1621] Acroteleution astrologicum, triplex hominum genus circa divinationem ex astris in scenam producens, falsamque astrologiam a vera . . . distinguens . . . Annexus . . . est tractatus integer correctior . . . Cypriani Leovitii . . . De conjunctionibus magnis, eclipsibus solaribus

& cometis, cum eorundem effectuum historica expositione ... Marpurgi, Apud Paulum Egenolphum, 1618.

78 p.; 84 p.   21 cm.   [4839]

Part [2] has special title page: De conjunctionibus magnis insignioribus superiorum planetarum ... auctore Cypriano Leovitio.

—De vita proroganda; hoc est, Animi corporisque vigore conservando, salubriterque producendo tractatus ... Moguntiae, Typis Joannis Albini, impensis Conradi Meulli, 1608.

[16], 628, [26] p.   17 cm.   [4840]

Imperfect: p. [15-16] at beginning, p. 7-10, 627-628, and p. [24-26] wanting.

—Loimographia, in qua graves quaedam arduaeque quaestiones, medicorum quorumdam ignorantiam & errorem in curanda peste detengentes explicantur ... Quid in specie in peste Marpurgensi hoc anno 1611. evenerit ... lector passim insertum reperiet ... Francofurti, Impensis Petri Musculi & Ruperti Pistorii, 1613.

[16], 247 p.   17 cm.   [4841]

Bound with copy 2 of *his* Tractatus novus de magnetica vulnerum curatione. 1613.

—Another issue. Part of preliminary matter reset.

[12], 247 p.   16 cm.   [4842]

Imperfect: recto of sig. (:)4 and recto of sig. (:)2 interchanged; sig. (:)(:)3-4 wanting?

—Mirabilium naturae liber, concordias et repugnantias rerum in plantis, animalibus, animaliumque morbis & partibus, manifestans, nunc primo in lucem datus ... Adjecta est in fine brevis & nova defensio magneticae curationis vulnerum ex solidis principiis. Francofurti, Typis Egenolphi Emmelii, impensis Joan. Carol. Unckelii, 1625.

[15], 303 p.   16 cm.   [4843]

Imperfect: wormholes on p. 152-161.

—Copy 2. 17 cm.

With this are bound: Minaeus, F., *Father*. Justa Ludovici Justi. 1622; Sossius, G. De vita Henrici Magni. 1522 (i.e. 1622); Université de Paris. Decretum. 1626.

—Oratio qua defenditur vulnus non applicato etiam remedio, citra ullum dolorem curari naturaliter posse, si instrumentum tantum vel telum quod sauciavit, seu quo vulnus est inflictum, peculiari unguento inunctum, obligetur. Inserta sunt notatu digna de memoria acuenda ... Marpurgi Cattorum,

Ex officina Rodolphi Hutwelckeri, 1608.

70, [1] p.   16 cm.   [4844]

Errata: p. [71]

—Physiognomica et chiromantica specialia, hactenus tanquam secretissima suppressa, nunc vero primum ... in lucem emissa ... Accesserunt in fine Memorabilia experimenta & observationes chiromanticae cum speciali judicio, hactenus a nemine visae. Francofurti, Apud Joannem Carolum Unckelium, 1625.

170 (i.e. 190) p.   illus.   16 cm.   [4845]

—[The same.] ... Hallis Saxonum, Typis Johannis Rappoldti, impensis Johannis Naumanni, 1652.

157 p.; 31, [1] p.   illus.   16 cm.   [4846]

Errata: p. [1] at end.

Part [2] has special title page, with imprint: Hamburgi, Sumptibus Johanni Naumanni, 1651.

—[The same.] Physignomica [sic] et chiromantica specialia ante annos aliquot in lucem emissa ... nunc denuo recognita ... aucta, & restituta, ut sic fere absolutam, atque integram physiognomiam humanam ... exhibeant ... Hamburgi, Apud Johannem Naumannum, 1661.

280 p.   illus.   17 cm.   [4847]

Imperfect: p. 272-280 wanting.

"Memorabilia experimenta, et observationes chiromanticae ..." (p. [235]-278 (?)) has special title page.

—Synarthrosis magnetica, opposita infaustae anatomiae Joh. Roberti ... pro defensione Tractatus de magnetica vulnerum curatione ... Marpurgi, Apud Jonam Saurium, impensis Petri Musculi, 1617.

227, [1] p.   16 cm.   [4848]

—Tractatus de magnetica curatione vulneris, citra ullam & superstitionem & dolorem, & remedii applicationem. Ed. 3. ... corr. & locupletior ... Marpurgi, Ex Officina Hutwelckeriana, 1610.

276 p.   14 cm.   [4849]

Bound with Puteanus, E. Ovi encomium. 1617.

—[The same.] Tractatus novus de magnetica vulnerum curatione, citra ullum et dolorem, et remedii applicationem ... Huic annexus est alter, de luxuriosis ac portentosis nostri seculi conviviis ... Francofurti, Impensis Petri Musculi, & Ruperti Pistorii, 1613.

[6], 174 p.   17 cm.   [4850]

—Copy 2.

With this is bound *his* Loimographia. 1613.

—[The same.] Tractatus de manetica [sic] vulnerum curatione, citra ullam superstitionem, dolorem, & remedii etiam applicationem ... [&] ... Synarthrosis magnetica, opposita infaustae anatomiae Joh. Roberti ... pro defensione Tractatus de magnetica vulnerum curatione ...

[177]–225 and [237]–308 p. 21 cm. (In Theatrum sympatheticum auctum. Norimbergae, 1662)   [4851]

Half titles.

—[The same.] *In* Longinus, C., *ed.* Trinum magicum. 1616, 1673.

—Tractatus de portentosis luxuriosis ac monstrosis nostri seculi conviviis, eorumque artificibus, auctoribus, origine & asseclis, denuo recognitus, & auctus ... Accessit etiam in fine questio: an symposia homini Christiano sint fugienda, liceatque huic cum impiis convivari. Marpurgi, Typis Rodolphi Hutwelckeri, 1609.

114 (i.e. 141), [1] p. 14 cm.   [4852]

—Uranoscopiae, chiroscopiae, metoposcopiae, et ophthalmoscopiae, contemplatio, qua probatur, divinationem ex astris, lineisque manuum, fronte, facie & oculis nec impiam esse nec superstitiosam. Ed. nova.: cui accessit totius Physiognomię ... demonstratio. Francofurti, Impensis Joh. Theob. Schönwett., 1608.

290 p. illus. 13 cm.   [4853]

With this is bound Aesopus. Fabularum selectarum partes duae. 1608.

—Uraniae divinatricis, quoad Astrologiae generalia, libri II. *In* Nifo, A. De auguriis libri II. 1614.

—Weiss und Weg, sich for der schweren Seuche der Pestilentz ... zubewahren. Auch wie denen, so damit beladen, durch darzu dienende Artzneyen zu helffen seye. Sampt Anzeigung vieler nothwendigen Dingen, als nemblich, Essen, Trincken, und Lufft betreffendt ... Auss alten und newen lateinischen Scribenten und Artzten zusammen gezogen und ins Teutsch gesetzt ... Marpurg, Rudolff Hutwelcker, 1607.

[II], 138 (i.e. 139) p. 15 cm.   [4854]

Imperfect: Title page mutilated.

—, *ed.* and *tr. See* [STEPHANUS MAGNETES] Experiment Buch. 1623.

—*See* GOCLENIUS, R. [1547–1628] Physiologia

crepitus ventris. 1607.

—*as subject. See* ROBERTI, J., *Father.* Goclenius heautontimorumenos. 1618; Tractatus novi de magnetica vulnerum curatione. 1662.

GODALL, CHARLES. *See* GOODALL, Charles [1642–1712]

GODARTIUS, JOHANNES. *See* GOEDAERT, Johannes [1617 or 20–1668]

GODDARD, JONATHAN [1617?–1675] Arcana Goddardiana. *In* Bate, G. Pharmacopoeia Bateana. 1691, 1700.

—A discourse setting forth the unhappy condition of the practice of physick in London, and offering some means to put it into a better ... London, John Martyn and James Allestry, 1670.

62 p. 20 cm.   [4855]

First page blank.

GODDELIJCKE vierschare, op-gheright, in 't haedt-huys, van 's menschen herte. Voor gestelt in een 't samen-spraeck; tusschen de Heere Jesus, Godts gherechtigheyt, ende den gevangenen sondaer. Uyt het Enghels vertaelt door Abraham van Laren. Vlissinghe, Ghedruckt by Abraham van Laren, 1665.

11, [1] p. 14 cm.   [4856]

Bound with (as issued?) Featley, J. Tranen eener barendevrouwe. 1665.

GODELMANN, JOHANN GEORG [1559–1611] Tractatus de magis, veneficis et lamiis, deque his recte cognoscendis et puniendis ... Publice in Academia Rostochiana olim praelectus, & in tres libros distributus ... Francofurti, Ex officina typographica Joannis Saurii, impensis Nicolai Bassaei, 1601.

3 v. in 1. 22 cm.   [4857]

Vol. 2 has title: Liber secundus de lamiis. Vol. 3 has title: Liber tertius, quomodo contra magos, veneficas, et lamias procedatur. A reprint of the 1591 edition.

With this is bound copy 3 of Riva di San Nazzaro, G. F. Illustris de peste tractatus juridicus. Lipsiae, 1598.

GODFREY, ROBERT. Various injuries & abuses in chymical and Galenical physick. Committed both by physicians & apothecaries, detected ... London, Printed by John Darby, for Richard Jones, 1674.

[14], 208 p. 15 cm.   [4858]

First blank leaf present.

GODI, GIOVANNI CESARE [d. 1710] Lucubratiunculae ... a Michaele Angelo Molinetto ... Venetiis,

Ex Antonii Bosii typis, 1686.

[6], 28 p. 28 cm. [4859]

GODIN, NICOLAS [b. 1509] tr. See VIGO, G. de. La pratique et chirurgie. 1610.

GODOY, PEDRO DE. See GONZÁLEZ DE GODOY, Pedro [fl. 1673-1682]

GODOY, Pedro Gonzalez De. See GONZÁLEZ DE GODOY, Pedro [fl. 1673-1682]

GODSCHED, JOHANNES. See GOTTSCHED, Johann [1668-1704]

GÖBEL, CHRISTOPH [fl. 1628] respondent. See RASPE, G. Disputatio decima-nona, de visu et auditu. 1628.

GÖBEL, JOHANN MELCHIOR [fl. 1684] respondent. Disputatio medica inauguralis de lacte ejusque vitiis ... Lugduni Batavorum, Apud Abrahamum Elzevier, 1684.

[24] p. 22 cm. [4860]
Diss. — Leyden.

GOEBEL, MARTIN [fl. 1682] respondent. See CYPRIAN, J., praeses. Dissertatio physica de hominis definitione. 1682.

GÖBEL, SEVERIN [1530-1612] Kurtze Erinnerung von Verhütung und Abschaffunge der pestilentzische Seuchen zum Memorial in Reim gefasset ... Königsberg, Gedruckt bey Georg Osterbergers Widwen, 1602.

[12] p. 19 cm. [4861]

GÖCKEL, CHRISTIAN LUDWIG [1662-1738] respondent. See WEDEL, G. W., praeses. Disputatio inauguralis medica de hydrope. 1685 [and] Dissertatio medica de convulsione. 1683.

GÖCKEL, RUDOLPH. See GOCLENIUS, Rudolph [1572-1621]

GOEDAARD, JOHANNES. See GOEDAERT, Johannes [1617 or 20-1668]

GOEDAERT, ALBERT JORISZ. See EUFRENIUS, Albertus [1581-1626]

GOEDAERT, JOHANNES [1617 or 20-1668] [Metamorphosis naturalis. Latin] Johannes Goedartius De insectis, in methodum redactus, cum notularum additione. Opera M. Lister ... Item Appendicis ad historiam animalium Angliae, ejusdem

M. Lister, alt. ed. hic quoque exhibetur ... Londini, Excudebat R. E., sumptibus S. Smith, 1685.

[7], 356 p.; [4], 45 p. plates. 21 cm. [4862]
The Appendix has special title page.

—Metamorphosis et historia naturalis insectorum ... Cum commentariis D. Joannis de Mey ... Medioburgi, Apud Jacobum Fierensium [1700] [& Johannem Martinum, 1667]

3 v. illus., plates. 16 cm. [4863]
Each vol. has added engraved title page. Vols. 1 and 3 are without the translator's name. Date of Dedicatio of vol. 1: 1700; that of vol. 2: 1667; vol. 3 is not dated.

Vol. 2 has title: Metamorphoseos ... pars secunda, de insectis ... Latinitate donata, commentariis et notis ... illustrata ... a Paulo Veezaerdt.

—[English ed.] Of insects. Done into English, and methodized, with the addition of notes. The figures etched upon copper, by Mr. F[rancis] Pl[ace]. York, Printed by John White, for M. L., 1682.

[6], 140 p. plates. 21 cm. [4864]
Edited and translated by Martin Lister.

—[French tr.] Metamorphoses naturelles; ou, Histoire des insectes observée tres-exactement suivant leur nature & leurs proprietez ... Amsterdam, George Gallet, 1700.

3 v. plates, port. 16 cm. [4865]
Each vol. has added engraved title page.
Imperfect: in vol. 1 lower margin of the title page trimmed.
Includes the commentaries of Johannes de Mey.

GOEDDAEUS, HERMANN [fl. 1612-1615] respondent. See PETRAEUS, H., praeses. Disputatio medica de natura. 1615.

GÖDELMANN, JOHANN GEORG. See GODELMANN, Johann Georg [1559-1611]

GÖLICKE, ANDREAS OTTOMAR [1670?-1744?] Epistola anatomica, problematica nona ... Ad ... Fredericum Ruyschium ... De cursu arteriarum per piam matrem cerebrum involventem, de tertia cerebri meninge, de arteriis membranarum cavitates ossis frontis supra narium radices ... Amstelaedami, Apud Joannem Wolters, 1679 (i.e. 1697).

13, [2] p. illus. 22 cm. [4866]
"Frederici Ruyschii responsio...": p. [7]-13.

—respondent. See HOFFMANN, F. [1660-1742] praeses. Dissertatio inauguralis medica de purgantibus specificis. 1696.

GÖSGEN, DAVID [*fl.* 1689–1690] *praeses.* Dissertatio physica de monstris ... Lipsiae, Literis Christophori Guntheri [1690]

[16] p.   19 cm.   [**4867**]

Diss. — Leipzig (M. G. Schuster, *respondent*)

GÖTSCHL, THEOPHIL, *Father* [*fl.* 1682] *respondent.* See BANHOLZER, J., *Father, praeses.* Oculus per quaestiones acroamaticas et exotericas explicatus. 1682.

GÖTZ, MATTHIAS [*fl.* 1607] *respondent.* De paralysi et anima intellectiva ὑπομνηματισμοί ... Basileae, Typis Joan. Schroeteri, 1607.

[15] p.   19 cm.   [**4868**]

Diss. — Basel.

GOETZE, GEORG HEINRICH [1667–1728] De theologis pseudo-medicis; seu, Num theologo artem medicam exercere liceat? Disquisitio. Lipsiae, Typis Heinrici Richteri, 1700.

[28] p.   20 cm.   [**4869**]

GOGLER, CARL VON [17th cent.] Hauss- und Feld-Apothec, darinnen befindlich wie nicht allein der Mensch bey gesunden Tagen, seinen Leib ... bestes verwahren solle ... so auch der Mensch ... allbereit mit Kranckheit angegriffen wäre ... zu erhalten. Und seynd diese Recept meistens allbereit ... probirt gut befunden ... aber ... niemals an Tag kommen ... Franckfurt am Mayn, Martin Hallervorden, 1667.

[4], 113, [5] p.   33 cm.   [**4870**]

—Erneuerte Hauss- und Feld-Apotheck; oder, Stadt- und Land Artzney-Buch, darinnen zu finden wie sich der Mensch beydes vor allerhand Zufällen, als auch in denenselben verhalten solle ... Nunmehr ... in Vielen verbessert ... Franckfurt am Mäyn. In Verlegung Martin Hallervorden in Königsberg. Getruckt bey Johann Andreae, 1678.

[13], 394, [6] p.   18 cm.   [**4871**]

Added engraved title page.

GOHL, DANIEL. See GOHL, Johann Daniel [1674–1731]

GOHL, JOHANN DANIEL [1674–1731] *respondent. See* STAHL, G. E., *praeses.* Dissertatio inauguralis medica de haemorrhoidum internarum motu. 1698.

—See STAHL, G. E. Propempticon inaugurale de στοχάσμω medico. 1698.

GOLDAMMERUS, CASPARUS GOTHOFREDUS [*b.* 1673] *respondent. See* SLEVOGT, J. A., *praeses.* Dissertatio medico-chirurgica inauguralis de ambustione ejusque remediis. 1698.

—See WEDEL, G. W. Propempticon inaugurale de Mose chimico. 1698.

GOLDAST, MELCHIOR [1578–1635] Paradoxon de honore medicorum ad v. cl. Hermannum Conerdingium ... in quo praeceptum Jesu Sirachi apodictice explicatur ... Francofurti ad Moenum, Sumptibus Rulandiorum, typis haeredum Joannis Bringeri, 1620.

26 p.   23 cm.   [**4872**]

A GOLDEN practice of physick. 1662. *See* PLATTER, F. [1536–1614]

GOLDSCHMIDT, ANDREAS [1512–1559] Succini historia. *In* Crato von Krafftheim, J. Consiliorum & epistolarum medicinalium ... liber. 1620, 1671.

GOLIUS, JACOBUS [1596–1667] Lexicon Arabico-Latinum, contextum ex probatioribus Orientis lexicographiis. Accedit index Latinus ... Lugduni Batavorum, Typis Bonaventurae & Abrahami Elseviorum, prostant Amstelodami apud Johannem Ravesteynium, 1653.

[12], 16 p., 17–2922 col., [40] p.   37 cm.

                                                   [**4873**]

Imperfect: title page mutilated affecting imprint. Imprint supplied from NUC.

GOLLES, ADRIAN [*fl.* 1668] Abregé de l'oeconomie du grand et petit monde, divisé en trois parties. La premiere traite de la diverse nature & difference des estres ... La seconde, l'histoire anatomique des principales parties du corps. La troisiéme, l'histoire des facultez de l'ame & du corps, avec un discours de la sanguification & de la circulation du sang ... Rouen, François Vaultier le jeune, 1670.

[23], 413, [16] p.   15 cm.   [**4874**]

GOLLETI, ANTOINE. Les oeuvres medicinales de l'herboriste d'Attigna ... Tome premier [-troisieme] Lyon, Jean Thioly & Antoine Boudet, 1695.

3 v.   in 1.   16 cm.   [**4875**]

GOMES, MANOEL [*b. ca.* 1580] Tractaet vande peste inhoudende d'oorsaecken, teeckenen, remedien soo verhoedende als ghenesende ... Hantwerpen, Joachim Trognesius, 1603.

56 p.   17 cm.   [**4876**]

Published the same year in Latin under title: De pestilentiae curatione methodica tractatio.

GOMESIUS MIEDES, Bernardinus. *See* Gómez Miedes, Bernardino [1521-1589]

GOMEZ, Imanuel. *See* Gomes, Manoel [*b. ca.* 1580]

GÓMEZ DE HUERTA, Jerónimo [1573-1643] *ed.* and *tr. See* Plinius Secundus, C. Historia natural. 1624-29.

GÓMEZ DE LA PARRA Y ARÉVALO, Alfonso [*fl.* 1621] Polyanthea medicis speciosa, chirurgis mirifica, myrepsicis valde utilis & necessaria. In quinque partes divisa . . . Matriti, Ex Officina Joannis Gonçalez, 1625.

 [6], 180, [8] ll. 22 cm.   **[4877]**

GÓMEZ MIEDES, Bernardino [1521-1589] Αλογραφια; sive, Diascepseon de sale libri quatuor . . . Nunc vero denuo revisi . . . per Petrum Uffenbachium . . . Ursellis, Ex officina typographica Cornelii Sutorii, sumptibus Joan. Berneri, 1605.

 [39], 679, [17] p. 17 cm.   **[4878]**

GOMMESIUS, Emanuel. *See* Gomes, Manoel [*b. ca.* 1580]

GONÇALEZ, Gregorio. *See* González, Gregorio [*fl.* 1621-22]

GONÇALVES, Antonio. Tratado de gonorrea pello. *In* Cruz, A. de. Recopilaçam de cirurgia. 669 [i.e. 1669]

GONSALVE DE TOLEDO. *See* Toledo, Gondisalvus [*fl.* 1496-1508]

GONTIER, Pierre [*fl.* 1668] Exercitationes hygiasticae; sive, De sanitate tuenda et vita producenda, libri XVIII . . . Lugduni, Sumptibus Antonii Jullieron, 1668.

 [20], 560, [44] p. 24 cm.   **[4879]**
Errata: p. [43-44]

GONZÁLEZ, Gregorio [*fl.* 1621-22] *ed. See* Oviedo, L. de. Methodo de la coleccion y reposicion de las medicinas simples. 1622, 1692.

[GONZÁLEZ DE GODOY, Pedro, *fl.* 1673-1682] Discurso serio-jocoso, sobre la nueva invencion del agua de la vida, y sus apologias. En que entre burlas, y veras, se dizen veras, y burlas; aora nuevamente sacado à luz por un quidan, que queriendo tener fama, no tiene nombre. Mantua Carpentana, Impresso por un vezino de ella, 1682.

 [4], 26 p. 20 cm.   **[4880]**
Palau 103101 (variant state.)

[—] Segundo discurso serio-jocoso sobre la nueva invencion de la agua de la vida en que respondiendo a una apologia, entre veras, y burlas, se hazen las burlas veras . . . [Zaragonza?] 1682.

 24 p. 21 cm.   **[4881]**
Imperfect: wormhole on p. 23-24.
Palau 103102.

— , *tr. See* Fabricius, H., *ab Aquapendente.* Crisol de la cirugia. 1676.

GOODALL, Charles [1642-1712] The Colledge of Physicians vindicated, and the true state of physick in this nation faithfully represented: in answer to a scandalous pamphlet, entituled, The corner stone . . . London, Printed by R. N. for Walter Kettilby, 1676.

 [12], 191, [6] p. 18 cm.   **[4882]**

—The Royal College of Physicians of London founded and established by law; as appears by letters patents, acts of Parliament, adjudged cases, &c. And An historical account of the college's proceedings against empiricks and unlicensed practisers . . . London, Printed by M. Flesher, for Walter Kettilby, 1684.

 [11], 288, [52], 305-472, [11] p. 21 cm. **[4883]**
"An historical account": [52], 305-472 p., with special title page.

—*respondent.* Disputatio medica inauguralis de haemorrhagiis scorbuticis . . . Lugduni Batavorum, Apud viduam & haeredes Joannis Elsevirii, 1670.

 [8] p. 23 cm.   **[4884]**
Diss. — Leyden.

GOODSCHALK, Diederik [*fl.* 1689] Prodromus de ossium tum generatione, tum corruptione interna . . . Lugd. Batavorum, Apud Petrum de Graaf, 1691.

 60, [1] p. 16 cm.   **[4885]**
With this are bound: Chrouet, W. Dissertatio medico-physica de trium oculi humorum aliarumque ejus partium origine. 1688. — Nuck, A. Defensio ductuum aquosorum. 1691. — Toornburg, K. Kort vertoog van de anatomia. 1691.

—*respondent.* Disputatio medica inauguralis de transpiratione . . . Lugduni Batavorum, Apud Abrahamum Elzevier, 1689.

 [32] p. 23 cm.   **[4886]**
Diss. — Leyden.

GOODWIN, PHILIP [*d.* 1699] The mystery of dreames, historically discoursed; or a treatise, wherein is clearly discovered, the secret yet certain good or evil ... truth or falsity ... of mens differing dreames ... London, Printed by A. M. for Francis Tyton, 1658.

[61], 361, [28] + p.   17 cm.   [**4887**]

Imperfect: last leaf (blank?) wanting.

GORDONIUS, BERNARDUS. *See* BERNARD DE GORDON [*fl. ca.* 1283-1308]

GORGES, *Sir* ARTHUR [*d.* 1625] *tr. See* BACON, F., viscount St. Albans. The essays. 1668.

GORIO, CAMILLO [*fl.* 17th cent.] Brevis discursus de fractura brachii et an in ipsa conveniant ferulae ... Romae, Ex typographia Jacobi Mascardi, 1617.

28 p.   23 cm.   [**4888**]

—Disceptatio unica de chalcantho, ejusque oleo, an ullum habeat locum in febribus putridis. Romae, Ex typographia Jacobi Mascardi, 1616.

31 p.   23 cm.   [**4889**]

GORIS, GERARD [*fl.* 1685-1715] Medicina contempta, propter λογομαχιαν vel ignorantiam medicorum. Discursus ... in quo de integerrimae artis vitiis, ob artificum indolem & mores, vulgique errores ... tractatur. Accedit Appendicula observationum & curationum aliquot medicarum. Lugduni Batavorum, Apud Abrahamum de Swart, 1700.

[20], 336, [12] p.   21 cm.   [**4890**]

—*respondent.* Disputatio medica inauguralis de diarrhoea ... Lugduni Batavorum, Apud Abrahamum Elzevier, 1685.

[16] p.   22 cm.   [**4891**]

Diss.—Leyden.

GORMANN, JOHANN ANDREAS [*fl.* 1695] *respondent. See* VATER, C., *praeses.* Dissertationem inauguralem de morbo laterali acuto ... subjicit J. A. G. 1695.

GORMELEN, ESTIENNE. *See* GOURMELEN, Étienne [1538-1593]

GORRAEUS. *See* GORRIS.

GORRIS, JEAN DE [1505-1577] Opera. Definitionum medicarum libri XXIIII. A Joanne Gorraeo filio ... locupletati & accessione magna adaucti ... Nicandri Theriaca et Alexipharmaca cum interpretatione & scholiis ejusdem J. Gorraei ... Hippocratis libelli De genitura, De natura pueri, Jusjurandum, De arte, De prisca medicina, De medico, eodem J. Gorraeo interprete cum annotationibus & adjectis unicuique libello brevibus scholiis. Formulae remediorum quibus vulgo medici utuntur authore Petro Gorraeo ... Parisiis, Apud Societatem Minimam, 1622.

[II], 722, [I] p.; [4], 166, [I] p.   illus., 2 tables.   36 cm.   [**4892**]

Imperfect: 1 table wanting; dedicatory epistle for Nicander's Theriaca bound between p. 12 and 13 in part [2].

Colophon: Parisiis, Apud Josephum Cottereau, Sebastianum Chappelet, Abrahamum Pacard, Jacobum Quesnel, Dionisium Moreau et Samuelem Thiboust.

Each work by Hippocrates and Nicander in Greek and Latin, with special title pages.

—Definitionum medicarum libri XXIIII, literis Graecis distincti. Ab authore ante obitum recogniti, magnaque accessione aduacti, & nunc denuo ... editi. Adjectus in calce Latinograecus index ... Francofurti, Typis Wechelianis apud Claudium Marnium, & heredes Joannis Aubrii, 1601.

[8], 543, [I] p.   illus., port., table.   35 cm.   [**4893**]

A page for page reprint of the 1578 edition.
Edited by Jean de Gorris, the younger.
Contains corrections by Friedrich Sylbert (p. 539-543)

—, *ed. See* MORESCOTTUS, A. Compendium medicinae totius. 1604.

—*See* CHIAVENNA, G. A. Clavis Clavennae aperiens naturae thesaurum. 1648; GORRIS, J. de [*fl.* 1572-1622] Opuscula quatuor. 1660.

GORRIS, JEAN DE [*fl.* 1572-1622] Opuscula quatuor. Quaestiones duae cardinalitiae matutinis disputationibus ad discutiendum propositae in scholis medicorum Parisiensium. I. An medicorum Parisiensium frequentes phlebotomiae jure vel injuria accusantur? II. An methodus medendi medicorum Parisiensium omnium saluberrima? Quaestionis utriusque assertiones singulae confirmantur ex enarratis Hippocratis & Galeni locis. Item De usu venaesectionis ad curandos morbos δεύτεραιφροντίδες: secundae cogitationes. Nec non Brevis animadversio in libellum Joannis Lanaei ... quo Aphorismos Hippocratis in novum ordinem digessit. Parisii, Apud Gasparum Meturas, 1660.

[8], 105, [3], 105-206 p.   24 cm.   [**4894**]

The Brevis animadversio has special title page dated 1659.
Attributed also to Jean de Gorris, the elder. Cf. BNC.

—, *ed. See* GORRIS, J. de [1505–1577] Opera. Definitionum medicarum libri XXIIII. 1622.

—, *tr. See* [MERCURIO. G.] Discours de l'origine, des moeurs, fraudes et impostures des ciarlatans. 1622.

—*See* GORRIS, J. de [1505–1577] Definitionum medicarum libri XXIIII. 1601.

GORRIS, PIERRE DE [*fl.* 1511] Formulae remediorum. [Greek and Latin.] *In* Gorris, J. de [1505–1577] Opera. Definitionum medicarum libri XXIIII. 1622.

—[Latin tr.] . . . Coloniae Allobrogum, Apud Petrum & Jacobum Chouët, 1612.

158, [2] p.   13 cm.   **[4895]**

"Doctrinae et praecepta quaedam ex probatissimis quibusque medicis desumpta": p. 127–144; —"Loci aliquot Philippi Melanth. in libro De anima, de moderatione cibi & potus, item somni & vigiliarum": p. 145–150; —"Polybius De salubri victus ratione privatorum, Guinterio Joanne Andernaco interprete": p. 150–158.

—*See* MORESCOTTUS, A. Compendium medicinae totius. 1604.

GORUS, CAMILLUS. *See* GORIO, Camillo [*fl.* 17th cent.]

GOSKY, ANTON UDALRICH [1636–1696] *respondent.* Disputatio solennis de marasmo, sive marcore: macilentia item & gracilitate sanorum; macilentia & gracilitate aegrotantium; crassitie & corpulentia sanorum naturali; crassitie & magnitudine corporis morbosa aegrorum . . . Argentinae, Typis Eberhardi Welperi, 1658.

[59] p.   19 cm.   **[4896]**

Diss. — Strasbourg.

GOSKY, LEOPOLD DIETRICH [1670–1700] *respondent. See* ALBINUS, B. Dissertatio inauguralis medico chirurgica de catarrhacta. 1695.

GOSKY, MARTIN [*fl.* 1610 – *ca.* 1666] *respondent. See* ARNISAEUS, H., *praeses.* Disputatio medica de apoplexia, 1610 [and] Disputatio medica de lue venerea. [1610]

GOTHA (FÜRSTENTUM). Nothwendig-und nützlicher Unterricht, so wol vor Jedermänniglichen, als sonderlich vor die bestellten Wehemütter oder Heb-ammen im Fürstenthumb Gotha. Wornach sich dieselbige vor-in-und nach ereigneten Geburts-Fällen bey denen schwangern . . . und der Geburt allbereit entladenen Weibes-Personen . . . richten und achten sollen. Auff sonderbahre fürstliche Anordnung . . . zusammen getragen und gestellet von denen vorordneten Medicis zu Gotha. Gotha, Gedruckt durch Johan Michael Schalln, 1658.

[24] p.   19 cm.   **[4897]**

Imperfect: upper margins trimmed affecting text (and pagination?)

GOTTER, JOHANN JAKOB [*fl.* 1671–1672] *respondent. See* FRIDERICI, J. A., *praeses.* Diatriba medica de spiritibus sylvestribus flatulentis. 1671; PETRI VON HARTENFELS, G. C., *praeses.* Diatribe inauguralis medica de suffocatione uterina. 1672.

GOTTFRIED, JOHANN WILHELM [*fl.* 1698] *respondent. See* VESTI, J., *praeses.* Dissertationem inauguralem de variolis . . . subjicit . . . J. W. G. 1698.

GOTTLOB. *See* FRITSCH, Ahasverus [1629–1701]

GOTTLOB B., A. [*fl.* 1678] *ed. See* MONTESNYDER, J. de. Tractatus de medicina universali. 1678.

GOTTSCHED, JOHANN [1668–1704] *praeses.* Dissertatio physiologica de motu musculorum, ex fundamentis physico-mechanicis demonstrata . . . Regiomonti, Praelo Reusneriano [1694]

[44] p.   20 cm.   **[4898]**

Diss. — Königsberg (R. Wagner, *respondent*)

—Exercitatio practica, sistens medicum castrensem exercitui Moscovitarum praefectum . . . Regiomonti, Typis Friderici Reusneri haeredum [1700]

[4], 40 p.   20 cm.   **[4899]**

Diss. — Königsberg (J. D. Blumentrost, *respondent*)

—*respondent.* Disputatio medico-practica de anathrepsi, seu renutritione eorum, qui ob diuturnam famen et inediam, in terrae sterilitatibus, bellis, obsidionibus, peregrinationibus &c. emaciati sunt . . . Regiomontii, Typis Reusnerianis [1694]

[40] p.   18 cm.   **[4900]**

Diss. — Königsberg.

GOTTSCHICH, MELCHIOR [*fl.* 1638] *respondent. See* HOEVER, W., *praeses.* Disputatio medica de arthritide. 1638.

GOTTSMANN, JOHANN GOTTFRIED [*fl.* 1668] *respondent. See* JOHNIUS, A. G., *praeses.* Disputatio physica de terrae motu. 1668.

GOTTWALD, JOHANN CHRISTOPH [*fl.* 1695] *respondent. See* SCHAPER, J. E. Dissertatio inauguralis de viscido. 1695.

—*See* SCHAPER, J. E. Facultatis Medicae ... decanus ... ad disputationem inauguralem de viscido, sanitatis offendiculo ... candidati Dn. Johannis Christophori Gottwalds ... habendam ... invitat. 1695.

GOTTWALDT, CHRISTOPH [1636-1700] *respondent. See* LE BOË, F. de, *praeses.* Disputatio medica de vasis lymphaticis ... Lugduni Batavorum, Apud Johannem Elsevirium, 1661.

GOULSTON, THEODORE [1572-1632] *ed.* and *tr. See* GALENUS. [Selected works. Greek and Latin. 1640]

GOUPIL, JACQUES. *See* GOUPYL, Jacques [*ca.* 1525-1564]

GOUPYL, ANDRÉ. *See* GOUPYL, Jacques [*ca.* 1525-1564]

GOUPYL, JACQUES [*ca.* 1525-1564] *ed. See* JOANNES ACTUARIUS. De differentiis urinarum. 1688 [and] De urinis libri VII. 1670.

GOURMELEN, ÉTIENNE [1538-1593] Les oeuvres chirurgicales ... [Paris, Gaspar Meturas, 1647]

4 parts in 1 v. table. 19 cm. [4901]
General half title. Each part has special title page.
The author of "Réplique à une apologie" is Gourmelen himself speaking in the person of one of his pupils, B. Compérat.
Contents. — [pt. 1] Le guide des chirurgiens. Fait en latin, depuis translaté de latin en françois, par Germain Courtin. Ensemble Le sommaire de toute la chirurgie. Derniere ed., rev., corr., & de beaucoup augm. de la main de l'autheur. — [pt. 2] Le sommaire de toute la chirurgie, composez en latin par Gourmelen et traduits en françois par André Malesieu. — [pt. 3] Replique a une apologie publiée sous le nom de Ambroise Parè contre Estienne Gourmelen, par B. Comperat. — [pt. 4] Advertissement et conseil a messieurs de Paris, tant pour se preserver de la peste, comme aussi pour nettoyer la ville & les maisons qui y ont esté infectées (p. [59]-80 at end).

—Le guide des chirurgiens. Fait en latin, & redigé en trois livres selon l'ordre d'Hippoc. & autres anciens medecins ... Depuis translaté de latin en françois, par M. Germain Courtin ... & enrichy d'argument sur chacun livre ... Dern. ed., rev., corr., & ... augm. de la main de l'autheur ... Paris, Olivier de Varennes, 1619.

[23], 282, [2] p. plate. 18 cm. [4902]
With this is bound *his* Le sommaire de toute la chirurgie. 1607.

—Le sommaire de toute la chirurgie, contenant six livres. Composez en latin ... et traduits en françois par M. Andre Malesieu ... Paris, Olivier de Varennes, 1607.

[8], 72 p. 18 cm. [4903]
Bound with *his* Le guide des chirurgiens.

—*See* PARDOUX, B. Bartholomaei Perdulcis ... Universa medicina. 1630, 1640, 1649, 1650.

GOUTHIÈRE, JACQUES [1568-1638] Tiresias seu caecitatis encomium. *In* Admiranda rerum admirabilium encomia. 1666, 1677.

GOWER, RICHARD [*fl.* 17th cent.] *tr. See* LE BOË, F. de. A new idea of the practice of physic. 1675 [and] Of childrens diseases. 1682.

GOYKENS, ELBERT [*fl.* 1649] *respondent.* Disputatio medica inauguralis de ileo ... Trajecti ad Rhenum, Ex officina Johannis à Noortdyck, 1649.

[8] p. 20 cm. [4904]
Diss. — Utrecht.

GRAAF, REINIER DE [1641-1673] Opera omnia. Lugd. Batav., Ex Officina Hackiana, 1677.

[32], 717, [2] p. illus., plates. port. 19 cm. [4905]
Engraved title page.

—Opera omnia. Lugd., Sumpt. Jo. Ant. Huguetan & soc., 1678.

xx, [1], 390 p. front. (port.), illus., plates. 20 cm. [4906]
Engraved title page.

—[Dutch tr.] Alle de wercken, so in de ontleedkunde, als andere deelen der medicyne ... Amsterdam, Abraham Abrahamse, 1686.

[32], 671 p. illus., plates, port. 19 cm. [4907]
Added engraved title page.
Imperfect: printer's error, p. [207] lacks illustration.

—De mulierum organis generationi inservientibus tractatus novus. Demonstrans tam homines & animalia caetera omnia, quae vivipara dicuntur, haud minus quam ovipara ab ovo originem ducere ... Lugduni Batav., Ex Officina Hackiana, 1672.

[24], 334, [16], p. front. (port.), illus., plates. 16 cm. [4908]
Added engraved title page.
With this is bound *his* Partium genitalium defensio. 1673.

—De virorum organis generationi inservientibus,

de cliisteribus et de usu siphonis in anatomia. Lugd. Batav. et Roterod., Ex Officina Hackiana, 1668.

[32], 234, [14] p.   front. (port.), plates.   17 cm.   [4909]

Engraved title page.

With this is bound *his* Tractatus anatomico-medicus de succi pancreatici natura. 1671.

—[French tr.] Histoire anatomique des parties genitales, de l'homme et de la femme, qui servent a la generation: avec un Traité du suc pancreatique, des clisteres et de l'usage du syphon . . . Traduit . . . par Monsieur N. P. D. M. . . . Bale, Emanuel Jean George König. Et se vend à Lyon chez Hilaire Baritel, M.DC.LXCIX. (i.e. 1699?)

3 parts in 1 v.   plates.   19 cm.   [4910]

Part [2] has half title, part [3] caption title.

—Partium genitalium defensio . . . Lugd. Batav., Ex Officina Hackiana, 1673.

[7], 83 p.   16 cm.   [4911]

Includes letter to V. F. Plemp.

Bound with *his* De mulierum organis generationi inservientibus. 1672.

—Tractatus anatomico-medicus de succi pancreatici natura & usu . . . Lugd. Batavorum, Ex Officina Hackiana, 1671.

[22], 216, [14] p.   plates.   17 cm.   [4912]

Added engraved title page.

". . .Epistola ad . . . D. Lucam Schacht . . . de partibus genitalibus mulierum": p. 209-216.

Bound with *his* De virorum organis generationi inservientibus. 1668.

—[English tr.] De succo pancreatico; or, A physical and anatomical treatise of the nature and office of the pancreatick juice . . . Translated by Christopher Pack . . . London, N. Brook, 1676.

[24], 151, [17] p.   plates.   17 cm.   [4913]

—[French tr.] Traitté de la nature et de l'usage du suc pancreatique, ou plusieurs maladies sont expliquées, principalement les fievres intermittentes . . . Paris, Olivier de Varennes, 1666.

[20], 156, [12] p.   plates.   15 cm.   [4914]

Imperfect: p. 5-8 and plate 1 wanting.

—*respondent. See* LE BOË, F. de, *praeses.* Disputatio medica de natura & usu succi pancreatici. 1664.

—*See* PECHLIN, J. N. Jani Leoniceni Veronensis [pseud.] Metamorphosis. 1672, 1673; VESLING, J. Syntagma anatomicum. 1666, 1677, 1696.

GRABA, JOHANN ANDREAS [1625-1669] Ελαφ-ογϱαφια; sive, Cervi descriptio physico-medico-chymica, in qua tam cervi in genere, quam in specie ipsius partium consideratio theorico-practica instituitur, ad multifarium usum praesertim medicum, omnibus fere corporis humani affectibus ceu panacea apprime conveniens: secundum leges ac methodum Academiae Naturae Curiosorum elaborata, multisque medicinae secretis instructa . . . Jenae, Impensis Viti Jacobi Trescher, typis Johannis Nisii, 1667.

312, [37] p.   16 cm.   [4915]

—Another issue, dated 1668.

[4916]

—*respondent.* Disputatio medica inauguralis, exhibens casum laborantis affectu hypochondriaco cum symptomatibus scorbuticis . . . Giessae Cattorum, Typis Josephi Dieterici Hampelii, 1658.

31 p.   18 cm.   [4917]

Date altered by hand from M.DC.VIII to M.DC.LVIII.

Diss.—Giessen.

GRABE, MARTIN SILVESTER [1674-1727] *praeses.* Theses medicae de phthisi . . . Regiomonti, Typis Friderici Reusneri haeredum [1700]

[12] p.   18 cm.   [4918]

Diss.—Königsberg (M. P. Hartmann, *respondent*)

—*respondent.* Dissertatio medica inauguralis de renum calculo . . . Lugduni Batavorum, Apud Abrahamum Elzevier, 1700.

22, [2] p.   22 cm.   [4919]

Diss.—Leyden.

GRACCHUS, SEMPRONIUS MASSILIENSIS. *See* MANITIUS, Samuel Gotthelf [d. 1698]

GRACHT, JACOB VAN DER [1593-1652] Anatomie der wtterlicke deelen van het menschelick lichaem. Dienende om te verstaen, ende volkomentlick wt te beelden alle beoerlicheit des selven lichaems . . . s'Graven Hagae, Door den auteur, 1634.

[65] p.   illus.   41 cm.   [4920]

Engraved title page.

GRÄBER, KASPAR [*fl.* 1668] *respondent. See* THILO, G., *praeses.* Exercitatio e philosophia naturali de succino. 1668.

GRAEBNER, DAVID. *See* GREBNER, David von [1655-1737]

GRAEF, REGNIER DE. *See* GRAAF, Reinier de [1641-1673]

GRAEF, THEODOR VAN DE [*fl.* 1676] *respondent.* Disputatio medica inauguralis de catalepsi ... Lugduni Batavorum, Apud viduam & haeredes Johannis Elsevirii, 1676.

[12] p.   22 cm.   **[4921]**

Diss. — Leyden.

GRAETZ, JOHANN HEINRICH [*fl.* 1691-1697] Epistola anatomica, problematica sexta ... ad ... Fredericum Ruyschium ... de arteria & vena bronchiali, nec non de polypis bronchiorum ejectis, venae & arteriae pulmonalis ramos mentientibus. Amstelaedami, Apud Joannem Wolters, 1696.

12, [3] p.   illus.   22 cm.   **[4922]**

"Frederici Ruyschii responsio ...": p. 10-12.

— Another printing.

11, [2] p.   illus.   24 cm.   **[4923]**

"Frederici Ruyschii responsio ...": p. 9-11.

— Epistola anatomica, problematica septima ... Ad ... Fredericum Ruyschium ... De pia matre, ejusque processibus. Amstelaedami, Apud Joannem Wolters, 1696.

14 p.   illus.   22 cm.   **[4924]**

"Frederici Ruyschii responsio ...": p. [7]-10.

— Epistola anatomica, problematica octava ... Ad ... Fredericum Ruyschium ... De structura nasi cartilaginea, vasis sanguiferis arteriosis mebranae & cavitatis tympani & ossiculorum auditus eorumque periostio. Amstelaedami, Apud Joannem Wolters, 1697.

13, [2] p.   illus.   22 cm.   **[4925]**

"Frederico Ruyschii responsio ...": p. 9-13.

— *respondent. See* HOFFMANN, F. [1660-1742] *praeses.* Disputatio solennis medica de hydrope pericardii rarissimo. 1697; LIMMER, C. P., *praeses.* Disputatio physico-medica de monstroso abortu Dessaviensi. 1694.

GRAEVIUS, JOANNES GEORGIUS [1632-1703] Oratio funebris in exequiis viri ... Isbrandi Diemerbroekii ... Habita A. D. XVII Novembris anni M DC LXXIV. Ultrajecti, Ex officina Meinardi a Dreunen, 1675.

24 p.   24 cm.   **[4926]**

GRAFENBERG, JOHANNES SCHENCK VON. *See* SCHENCK VON GRAFENBERG, Johannes [1530-1598]

GRAFFENRIED, FRANZ LUDWIG VON [*fl.* 1651] *ed. See* BAUHIN, J. Historia plantarum universalis. 1650-1651.

[GRAINDORGE, ANDRÉ, 1616-1676] In fictilem figuli exercitationem de principiis foetus: animadversiones seu dissertatio ad mentem Aristotelis de principio materiali generationis foetus. Narbonae, Typis Guillelmi Besse, 1658.

[6], 176 p.   18 cm.   **[4927]**

Concerns Raymond Restaurand's Figulus.

GRAMAN, GEORG [*fl.* 1618-1630] Ein sonderliche chymische Reise und Hauss Apoteca, sampt aussführlichem Bericht, was für Unterscheid zwischen der Galenischen und Paracelsischen Medicin sey, und wie mit denen auss Edelsteinen, Mineralien ... und Saltzen ... die Gesundheit ein lange Zeit erhalten, und dann auch allerhand gefährliche Kranckheiten ... mit kleiner Dosi ... gantz sicher ... selbst curirt ... [Erfurt, Gedruckt bey Joachim Mechlers Erben, in Verlegung Johan. Birckners, 1618]

[40], 160, [7] p.   16 cm.   **[4928]**

Place of imprint supplied from J. Benzing p. 106.

— [The same.] New zugerichte, sehr nützliche chymische Reise und Hauss Apotheca ... zum ander Mal verbessert ... Schleusingen, Gedrucket in der Steinmannischen Druckerey [durch Peter Schmieden, in Verlegung Johan Victor Mohrs] 1630.

[64], 176, [8] p.   17 cm.   **[4929]**

GRAMANN, JOHANN [16th-17th cent.] *See* LIBAVIUS, A. [*d.* 1616] Appendix necessaria Syntagmatis arcanorum chymicorum. 1615.

GRAMANN, MELCHIOR [*fl.* 1616] *respondent.* Hunc de apoplexia discursum ... proponit M. Melchior Gramannus ... Marpurgi Cattorum, Ex Officina Rodolphi Hutwelckeri, 1616.

[15] p.   18 cm.   **[4930]**

Diss. — Marburg.

GRAMM, CAESO [1640-1673] *praeses.* Quaestiones physicae metamorphosin, qua uxor Lothi in statuam salinam est conversa ... [Kilonii] Joach. Reimannus, 1669.

[24] p.   19 cm.   **[4931]**

Diss. — Kiel (K. Jansen, respondent)

— *respondent.* Dissertatiuncula de cotyledonibus seu acetabulis uteri. *See* SEGER, G. Dissertatio anatomica de Hippocratis orthodoxia in doctrina de nutritione foetus humani in utero. 1660.

GRAMMANN, GEORGE. *See* GRAMAN, Georg [*fl.* 1618–1630]

IL GRAN VILLANO. *See* CARLO, *called* Il gran villano.

GRANA angelica; or, The rare and singular vertues and uses of those angelical and innocent pils, discovered and left to posterity, by Doctor Patrick Anderson ... [London?] 1679.

broadside. 42 x 32 cm. port. [4932]

GRANADO, ALONSO. Dudas a la aniquilacion, y defensa de las sangrias del tovillo ... Sevilla, Juan Lorenço Machado, 1653.

48 p. 20 cm. [4933]

GRAND Hôstel-Dieu de Nostre-Dame de Pitié. *See* HÔTEL-DIEU DE LYON.

Le GRAND mareschal françois; ou il est traité de la connoissance des chevaux, de leurs maladies, & de leur guerison ... Recueilly et divisé en trois traitez, par trois divers autheurs ... Paris, Jean Promé, 1653.

[6], 226 p.; 119 p.; 137 p.; [21] p. 17 cm. [4934]

—[The same.] Le grand maréchal expert, et françois ... Derniere ed., rev. & corr. de nouveau ... Lyon, Antoine Tomaz, 1682.

[8], 328, [19] p. illus., plate. 15 cm. [4935]

GRANDES materias ingenia parva non sustinent, & in ipso conatu ultra vires ausa, succumbunt. 1685. *See* BORROMEO, A.

GRANDI, DOMENICO [*fl.* 1636] *See* REGGIO EMILIA (CITY) Ordinances, local laws, etc. Sospensione per occasione di peste. 1636.

GRANDI, JACOBO [1646–1691] De laudibus Sanctorii oratio ... [Venetiis] Apud Joannem Franciscum Valvasensem [1671?]

18 p. 21 cm. [4936]

—*See* RIVIÈRE, L. Opera medica universa. 1686, 1687, 1700.

GRANDI, LAZZARO [*fl.* 1666] Alfabeto di secreti medicinali, et altri curiosi, e dilette-voli d'ogni materia con l'arte facile d'uccellare, e pescare ...

Milano, Francesco Vigone, 1666.

[8], 256 p. 17 cm. [4937]

—[The same.] ... Et in questa 2. impr. aggiontovi dallo stesso auttore numerosi altri di consideratione. Milano, Francesco Vigone, 1670.

[8], 243 p. 15 cm. [4938]

—[The same.] ... Et in questa 3. impr. aggiontovi dallo stesso auttore numerosi altri secreti di consideratione. Milano, Francesco Vigone, 1681.

[8], 267 p. 15 cm. [4939]

—[The same.] ... Bologna, Il Longhi [1694?]

217, 22 p. 16 cm. [4940]

GRANDI, PIETRO [*fl.* 1641] Illustriss. Gabellae syndicorum nomenclatura pro parte ... Collegii Medicae Facultatis ab anno Domini 1508. usque ad annum 1641 inclusive ... Bononiae, Typis Nicolai Tebaldini, 1641.

[16] p. 23 cm. [4941]

The list of names is continued in manuscript to 1653.

GRANDI DI GAIATO, JACOBO. *See* GRANDI, Jacobo [1646–1691]

GRANDIER, URBAIN [1590–1634] *See* [AUBIN, N.] Histoire des diables de Loudun. 1694.

GRANDIS, PETRUS DE. *See* GRANDI, Pietro [*fl.* 1641]

GRANDORGAEUS, ANDREAS. *See* GRAINDORGE, André [1616–1676]

GRANGIER, BALTAZAR, *Bp.* [*d.* 1679] *See* TRÉGUIER, France (Diocese) [1646–*ca.* 1679] (Baltazar Grangier) Remedes pour les pauvres gens. 1678.

The GRANTS and acts of Parliament, in favours of the College and Corporation of Surgeons of Edinburgh. 1696. *See* ROYAL COLLEGE OF SURGEONS OF EDINBURGH.

GRAPHEUS, BENVENUTUS. *See* GRASSUS, Benevenutus [*fl.* 12th cent.]

GRAS, HENRI [*d.* 1665] *ed. See* RANCHIN, F. Opuscula medica. 1627; SAPORTA, A. De tumoribus praeter naturam. 1624; VARANDA, J. de. Opera omnia. 1658.

GRASECCIUS, GEORGIUS [*fl.* 1605] Examen του μικροκοσμικου θεατρου in quo ceu viva imagine fabrica humani corporis masculum repraesentantis ejusque praecipuae partes affabre τη αὐτοψια demonstrantur . . . Argentinae, Sumptibus authoris, 1605.

[16], 722, [31] p.   16 cm.   [**4942**]

Engraved title page.

GRASECK, GEORG. *See* GRASECCIUS, GEORGIUS [*fl.* 1605]

GRASS, SAMUEL [1653-1730] *respondent. See* WEDEL, G. W., *praeses.* Disputation medica inauguralis de paralysi 1677.

GRASS, SIGMUND [*fl.* 1648-1649] *praeses.* Exercitatio medica de pleuritide . . . [Wittenbergae] Excudebat Johannes Röhnerus [1649]

[24] p.   19 cm.   [**4943**]

Diss.—Wittenberg (J. Tarnov, *respondent*)

—*respondent. See* SCHNEIDER, K. V., *praeses.* Disputatio de vera natura & recta ratione curandae phthisews conscripta. 1648.

GRASSEK, GEORG. *See* GRASECCIUS, Georgius [*fl.* 1605]

GRASSETTI, GIOVANNI BATTISTA [*fl.* 1609-1684] La vera, e falsa astrologia, con l'aggiunta della vera, e della falsa chiromanzia. Opera di Gio. Battista Tasgresti . . . Roma, Giuseppe Corvo, 1683.

[24], 308 p.   illus.   17 cm.   [**4944**]

GRASSEUS, JOANNES. *See* GRASSHOFF, Johann [*d.* 1623]

GRASSHOFF, JOHANN [*d.* 1623] Arca arcani artificiosissimi de summis naturae mysteriis . . . Constructa ex rustico ejus majore & minore, & physica naturali rotunda per visionem cabalisticam chemicam descripta . . .

294-323 p., vol. 6.   illus.   20 cm. (*In* Zetzner, Lazarus, *ed.* Theatrum chemicum. Argentorati, 1659-61)   [**4945**]

Caption title.

—Aureus tractatus de philosophorum lapide. Ab adhuc vivente, sed anonymo philosopho Germanice in lucem emissus, nunc autem Latinitate donatus. Francofurti, Apud Hermannum a Sande, 1677.

52 p.   22 cm. (*In* Musaeum Hermeticum. Francofurti, 1678)   [**4946**]

Translation of Ein güldener Tractat vom philosophischen Stein, originally published in Hermannus Condeesyanus' (pseud. of Johann Grasshoff) Dyas chymica tripartita. Another translation

of the original German text appeared in Johann Rhenanus' Opera chymiatrica. Cf. Ferguson, vol. 2, p. 264, 462.

—Mysterium occultae naturae. Anonymi discipuli Johannis Grassei dicti . . . De duobus floribus astralibus agricolae minoris, in ejus arca arcani artificiosissimi contentis . . .

523-542 p., vol. 6   20 cm. (*In* Zetzner, Lazarus, *ed.* Theatrum chemicum. Argentorati, 1659-61)   [**4947**]

Caption title.

—Ein philosophischer und chemischer Tractat. Genannt: Der kleine Baur: von der Materia und Erkantnuss dess . . . Subjecti Universalis Magni & illius praeparatione. Sampt beygefügtem Commentariis Johannis Walchii [i.e. Johann Grasshoff] . . . Und in dieser andern Edition ist das Supplementum von grünen Underzug beygedruckt . . . Strassburg, In Verlegung Eberhard Zetzners, 1658.

[16], 368, [13] p.   16 cm.   [**4948**]

"Elucidatio testamenti Raymundi Lullii": p. 363-368.

GRASSI, BENVENUTO. *See* GRASSUS, Benevenutus [*fl.* 12th cent.]

GRASSI, GIUNIO PAOLO [*d.* 1574] *tr. See* ARETAEUS. Ιατρικά. Aetiologica . . . morborum acutorum & diuturnorum. 1603 [and] Libri septem. 1700.

GRASSI, PAOLO [1562-1622] Mortis repentinae examen. Una cum brevi methodo praesagiendi, & praecavendi omnes, qui subeunt illius periculum. Per Paulum Crassum . . . nunc primum editum . . . Mutinae, Apud Julianum Cassianum, 1612.

98, [12] p.   15 cm.   [**4949**]

—Ragionamenti domestici intorno alla natura de' sogni . . . Bologna, Bartolomeo Cochi, 1613.

86, [1] p.   20 cm.   [**4950**]

GRASSIA, BALDASSAR. *See* GRASSO, Baldassar.

GRASSIUS, SIGISMUNDUS. *See* GRASS, Sigmund [*fl.* 1648-1649]

GRASSO, BALDASSAR, *tr. See* FRAGOSO, J. Cirugia universal. [Italian tr.] 1639, 1662, 1686.

GRASSUS, BENEVENUTUS [*fl.* 12th cent.] De oculis eorumque egritudinibus et curis. English. In Hippocrates. [Aphorismi. English. 1610]

GRATAROLI, GUGLIELMO [1516-1568] Monita; seu, Praecepta tuendae sanitatis. *In* Hygieia. 1628.

—, *tr. See* Bracesco, G. De alchemia. 1673.

—*See* Indagine, J. ab. Introductiones apotelesmaticae. 1603, 1622, 1630, 1663, 1672; Rantzau, H. De conservanda valetudine liber. 1604, 1617; Turba philosophorum. 1610.

GRATII, Salustio [*fl.* 1600] *tr. See* Huarte de San Juan, J. Essamina de gl'ingegni de gli huomini acconci. 1603.

GRATRICK, Valentine. *See* Greatrakes, Valentine [1629–1683]

GRAUEL, Johann Philipp [*fl.* 1675] *respondent. See* Wedel, G. W., *praeses.* Aegrum hypochondriacum ... publice examinandum proponit ... J. P. G. 1675.

GRAUNT, John [1620–1674] Natural and political observations mentioned in a following index, and made upon the bills of mortality ... London, Printed by Tho. Roycroft, for John Martin, James Allestry, and Tho. Dicas, 1662.

[16], 85, [1] p. tables. 18 cm. **[4951]**

Imperfect: upper margins of title page, p. [15–16] and lower margin of p. 77–78 trimmed; table placed after p. 76 in facsimile. Attributed also to Sir William Petty. Cf. Hull.

—[The same.] ... The 2d ed. London, Printed by Tho. Roycroft, for John Martin, James Allestry, and Tho. Dicas, 1662.

[16], 79 p. table. 19 cm. **[4952]**

Imperfect: p. 67–70 wanting, supplied in photocopy from Harvard University library.

—[The same.] ... The 3d ed. much enl. London, Printed by John Martyn, and James Allestry, 1665.

[29], 205 p. tables. 18 cm. **[4953]**

—[The same.] ... The 4th impression. Oxford, Printed by William Hall, for John Martyn, and James Allestry, 1665.

[29], 205 p. plates. 17 cm. **[4954]**

Different setting of type.

—[The same.] ... The 5th ed., much enl. London, Printed by John Martyn, 1676.

[38], 150 p. plate. 18 cm. **[4955]**

GRAVEROL, François [1636–1694] *See* Sorbière, S. Sorberiana. 1694.

GRAVESANDE, Isaac 's [*fl.* 1691] *respondent.* Disputatio medica inauguralis de angina vera & spuria ... Lugduni Batavorum, Apud Abrahamum

Elzevier, 1691.

[12] p. 22 cm. **[4956]**

Diss.—Leyden.

GRAVIUS, Cornelius [*fl.* 1685] *respondent.* Dissertatio medica inauguralis de apoplexia ... Lugduni Batavorum, Apud Abrahamum Elzevier, 1685.

[20] p. 22 cm. **[4957]**

Diss.—Leyden.

GT. BRIT. Admiralty. Commission for Sick and Wounded. *See* [Baston, S.] Baston's case vindicated. 1695.

GT. BRIT. Court of wards and liveries. *See* Gt. Brit. Sovereign [1603–1625] (James I) A commission with instructions and directions, granted by his Maiestie. 1618.

GT. BRIT. Laws, statutes, etc. Certain orders thought meet to be put in execution against the infection of the plague ... London, Robert Barker and by the assignes of John Bill, 1641.

broadside. 34 × 24 cm. **[4958]**

Imperfect: upper margin shaved.

—Certaine statutes especially selected, and commanded by His Majestie ... Also certaine orders thought meete by His Majestie and his Privie Counsell, to bee put in execution, together with ... medicines against ... the plague, set downe by the Colledge of the Physicians ... also a decree of the Starre-Chamber, concerning buildings and in-mates. London, Robert Barker and John Bill, 1630.

[15], 68, [32], [83]–95, 107–117 p. 20 cm. **[4959]**

Colophon: London, Robert Barker, 1609.
STC 9342.

—Foure statutes, specially selected and commanded by His Majestie to be carefully put in execution by all justices and other officers of the peace throughout the realme. Together with a proclamation, a decree of the Starre-Chamber, and certaine orders depending upon the former lawes, more particularly concerning the citie of London, and counties adjoyning. London, Robert Barker, 1609.

[6], 117 p. 18 cm. **[4960]**

Imperfect: sig. A1 wanting.
STC 9341.

GT. BRIT. Parliament. Six severall orders of the Lords and Commons assembled in Parliament ... An order for provision of beds, and other necessaires for maymed and sicke souldiers, within the counties of Berks, Buckingham, Middlesex, and Surrey, or other places, where the said souldiers shall reside . . . [London?] E. P. for T. S., 1643.

[1], 6 p.   19 cm.   [4961]

GT. BRIT. Privy Council. At the Court at Whitehall the ninth of January 1683 . . . Whereas by the grace and blessing of God, the kings and queens of this realm . . . have had the happiness by their sacred touch . . . to cure those who are afflicted with the disease called the kings-evil . . . London, Assigns of John Bill deceas'd and Henry Hills and Thomas Newcomb, 1683.

broadside.   35 x 29 cm.   [4962]

—Orders thought meet by His Maiestie, and his Privie Councell, to be executed throughout the counties of this realme, in such . . . places, as are, or may be hereafter infected with the plague, for the stay of further increase of the same. Also an advice set downe by the best learned in physicke within this realme, containing sundrie good rules and easie medicines . . . London, John Bill, 1625.

[24] p.   19 cm.   [4963]
STC 9245.2
Bound with Bradwell, S. Physick for the sicknesse, commonly called the plague. 1636.

—[The same.] . . . London, Robert Barker and John Bill, 1629.

[26] p.   19 cm.   [4964]
Signatures: A⁵, B–C⁴ (A1 and 2 apparently cancel an original A1)
STC 9245.6

—*See* GT. BRIT. LAWS, STATUTES, ETC. Certaine statutes especially selected, and commanded by His Majestie. 1630.

GT. BRIT. Sovereign [1603–1625] (James I) A commission with instructions and directions, granted by his Maiestie to the Master and counsaile of the Court of wards and liveries, for compounding for wards, ideots, and lunaticks. And given . . . the eleventh day of December 1618. London, Bonham Norton and John Bill, 1618.

[4], 30 p.   21 cm.   [4965]
STC 9239.

GT. BRIT. Sovereign [1625–1649] (Charles I) A proclamation declaring His Majesties pleasure touching orders to be observed for prevention of dispersing the plague . . . Given . . . the two and

twentieth day of April, in the twelfth yeere of our reigne . . . London, Robert Barker and the assignes of John Bill, 1636.

broadside.   41 x 30 cm.   [4966]
STC 9063.

—A proclamation for restraint of unnecessarie resorts to the court. For that the infection of the plague weekely increaseth . . . Given . . . the sixe and twentieth day of June . . . London, Bonham Norton and John Bill, 1625.

broadside.   38 x 30 cm.   [4967]
STC 8786.

—A proclamation for the adjournement of part of Trinitie terme. For as much as the infection of the plague is at this present greatly increased . . . Given . . . the eighteenth day of June . . . London, Bonham Norton and John Bill, 1625.

broadside (in 2 leaves).   37 x 29 cm.   [4968]
STC 8785.

—A proclamation prohibiting the keeping of Bartholomew faire, and our Ladie faire in Southwarke . . . Given the six and twentieth day of July, in the yeere of our Lord God, 1636. . . . London, Robert Barker, and by the assignes of John Bill, 1636.

broadside.   38 x 30 cm.   [4969]
STC 9070.

—A proclamation to prohibit the keeping of this next Sturbridge faire . . . Given . . . the twentieth day of August, in the twelfth yeere of our reigne, 1636 . . . London, Robert Barker, and by the assignes of John Bill, 1636.

broadside.   38 x 30 cm.   [4970]
STC 9071.

GT. BRIT. Sovereign [1660–1685] (Charles II) A proclamation for the better ordering of those who repair to the court for their cure of the disease called the kings-evil . . . Given . . . the fourth day of July, 1662 . . . London, John Bill and Christopher Barker, 1662.

broadside (in 2 leaves).   29 x 27 cm.   [4971]

GT. BRIT. Sovereign [1685–1688] (James II) At the council-chamber in Whitehall, Monday the 22th. of October, 1688. [London, Charles Bill, H. Hills and Th. Newcomb, 1688]

[4] p.   36 cm.   [4972]
An account, with the evidence of doctors, surgeons and midwives, of the birth of the Prince of Wales.

—At the council-chamber in Whitehall, Monday the 22. of October, 1688. [London, Charles Bill, Henry Hills and Thomas Newcomb, 1688]

40 p. 30 cm.   [4973]

Caption title.

An account, with the evidence of doctors, surgeons and midwives, of the birth of the Prince of Wales.

The GREAT preservative of mankinde. *See* [BARKER, Sir R.]

GREATARICK, VALENTINE. *See* GREATRAKES, Valentine [1629-1683]

GREATRAKES, VALENTINE [1629-1683] A brief account of Mr. Valentine Greatraks, and divers of the strange cures by him lately performed. Written by himself in a letter addressed to the Honourable Robert Boyle Esq. Whereunto are annexed the testimonials of several . . . persons of the chief matters of fact therein related. London, J. Starkey, 1666.

[1], 96 p. front. (port.) 20 cm.   [4974]

Imperfect: lower part of front. mutilated.

—*See* [LLOYD, D.] Wonders no miracles. 1666; STUBBS, H. The miraculous conformist. 1666.

[GREAVES, *Sir* EDWARD, 1608-1680] Morbus epidemius anni 1643; or, The new disease with the signes, causes, remedies, &c. . . . Oxford, Leonard Lichfield, 1643.

[1], 25 p. 19 cm.   [4975]

GREAVES, JOHN [1602-1652] *See* RAUWOLFF, L. A collection of curious travels & voyages. 1693.

GREBNER, DAVID VON [1655-1737] Medicina vetus restituta; sive, Paragraphe Hippocratico-Galenica in Theodori Craanen, Tractatum physico-medicum de homine . . . Lipsiae, Apud Davidem Fleischerum, literis Johannis Georgii [1695]

[26], 706, [70] p. front. (port.) 21 cm.   [4976]

Added engraved title page.

—Copy 2.

2d and 3d preliminary sheets interchanged.

With this are bound *his*: Tractatus philologico-physico-medici septem. [Vratislaviae? 1712?]; Mantissa operum. Javoriae, 1708.

GREEF, VINCENTIUS [*fl.* 1674] *ed.* and. *tr.* Tuba D. Vincentii; das ist, Erschallende Possaun dess H. Vincentii Ferreii . . . Anfangs Lateinisch beschrieben ab A. R. P. Vincent, Greef . . . jetzt aber . . . nit nur verteutscht, sondern auch in 30. formierten

Predigen . . . abgetheilt . . . Beschriben und formiert durch R. P. F. Fridericum Behm . . . Kempten, Caspar Roll, 1692.

[24], 418, [5] p. 21 cm.   [4977]

Bound with Giendder, J. Der geistliche Seelen-Artzt. 1696.

GREENFIELD, JOHN. *See* GROENVELDT, Jan [1647-1710]

GRÉGOIRE, MARTIN [*d.* 1552] *tr. See* GALENUS. De alimentorum facultatibus libri III. 1633.

GREGORIUS A SANCTO VINCENTIO. *See* SAINT-VINCENT, Grégoire de, *Father* [1584-1667]

GREGORIUS NAZIANZENUS, *Saint, Patriarch of Constantinople. tr. See* NEMESIUS, *Bp. of Emesa.* Περὶ φύσεως ἀνθρώπον βιβλίον ἕν.

GREGORIUS Papa XIII ad perpetuam rei memoriam. 1675. *See* CATHOLIC CHURCH. *Pope,* 1572-1585 (Gregorius XIII)

GREGORIUS, MARTINUS. *See* GRÉGOIRE, Martin [*d.* 1552]

GREGORY, *of Nazianzus, Saint, Patriarch of Constantinople. See* GREGORIUS NAZIANZENUS, *Saint, Patriarch of Constantinople.*

GREIFF, FRIEDRICH [1601-1668] *tr. See* FABRICIUS VON HILDEN. W. Wund-Artzney, gantzes Werck. 1652.

GREIFF, SEBASTIAN. Wundartzeney, vor dessen aus Phil. Theophrast. Paracelsi Schrifften colligiret, und aus . . . selbst eigener Erfahrung . . . beschrieben und hinterlassen . . . Jetzo aber auff begeren revidiret . . . durch Johann Mercker . . . Schleusingen, Typis Schmuccianis, gedruckt durch Thomam Marckart, in Verlegung Salomon Grunners, 1622.

[10], 101 p. 16 cm.   [4978]

"Kurtzer Discurs von dem Zipperlein, aus H. D. Lippen . . . und andere Medicorum Schrifften zusammen getragen . . .": p. 95-101.

GREIFFENFELD, PETRUS. *See* GRIFFENFELD, Peder Schumacher, *greve af* [1635-1699]

GREISEL, JOHANN GEORG [*d.* 1684] Tractatus medicus de cura lactis in arthritide, in quo . . . diaeta lactea optima arthritidem curandi methodus proponitur . . . Viennae Austriae, Typis Joannis Jacobi Kürner, 1670.

[45], 253, [39] p. 14 cm.   [4979]

—[The same.] ... Budissinae, Impensis Joh. Wilischii, typis Andreae Richteri, 1681.

[41], 240, [26] p. 13 cm. [4980]

With this is bound: Gufer, J. Tabulae medicae. 1690.

GREMBS, FRANZ OSWALD [*fl.* 1657–*ca.* 1682] Arbor integra et ruinosa hominis; id est, Tractatus medicus theorico practicus in tres libros divisus; in quo sana et morbosa hominis natura ... demonstratur ac simul de rerum principiis ... de usu & defectibus partium humani corporis, de anima, de febribus, peste, venenis, vita longa, & brevi, & tandem de remediis Paracelsicis, juxta consensum et dissensum Hippocratis, Galeni et Helmontii ... disseritur ... Francofurti, Typis Johannis Georgii Spörlin, sumptibus Wilhelmi Serlini, 1657.

[22], 240 (i.e. 340), 385–112 (i.e. 512), [32] p. 20 cm. [4981]

Added engraved title page.

—[The same.] ... Ed. 2. Francofurti, Sumptibus Wilhelmi Richardi Stockii, 1671.

[6], 240 (i.e. 340), 385–512, [32] p. 20 cm. [4982]

Imperfect: first preliminary leaf wanting.
Preliminary matter contains Proemium ad lectorem and Index only.

GRENTEMESNIL, JULIEN LE PAULMIER DE. *See* LE PAULMIER DE GRENTEMESNIL, Julien [1520–1588]

GRETRAKES, VALENTINE. *See* GREATRAKES, Valentine [1629–1683]

GREULICH, JOHANN GEORG [*fl.* 17th cent.] Χοληλογια; sive, Themata paradoxa de bile sana & aegra: illa sanitatis, hac morborum causa: rationi, Hippocratis authoritati, atque observationibus medicis congruentia ... Francofurti, Apud Hermannum a Sande, literis Balthas. Christoph. Wustii, Jun., 1682.

129 (i.e. 128) p. 17 cm. [4983]

Bound with *his* Curandi hydropis vera methodus. 1681.

—Curandi hydropis vera methodus, quam ex causis sibi noviter observatis deduxit, perque experientiam confirmavit; ac modo una cum Dissertatione de bile ... Francofurti, Apud Hermannum a Sande, 1681.

[8], 62 p. 17 cm. [4984]

With this is bound *his* Χοληλογια; sive, Themata paradoxa de bile. 1682.

GREULINCK, JOHANN HEINRICH [*fl.* 1693–1697] *praeses.* De multiplicatione hominis, secundum utramque essentiae partem, disputationem physicam primam ... publice defendet Petrus Berger ... Halae Magdeburgicae, Literis Chr. Henckelii [1697]

[1], 30 p. 20 cm. [4985]

Diss.—Halle (P. Berger, *respondent*)

—*respondent. See* HOFFMANN, F. [1660–1742] *praeses.* Dissertatio physico-chymica experimentalis de generatione salium. 1693.

GREULING, JOHANN HEINRICH. *See* GRUELINCK, Johann Heinrich [*fl.* 1693–1697]

GREVENBROICH, WILHELM VON. *See* INSULANUS MENAPIUS, Gulielmus [*d.* 1556]

GREVERUS, JODOCUS. *See* GREWER, Jodocus [16th cent.]

GRÉVIN, JACQUES [1538–1570] *See* VALVERDE, J. de. A. Vesalii en Valverda Anatomie. 1647.

GREW, NEHEMIAH [1641–1712] The anatomy of plants. With an idea of a philosophical history of plants, and several other lectures, read before the Royal Society ... [London] Printed by W. Rawlins, for the author, 1682.

[21], 24, [10], 304 (i.e. 300), [19] p. plates. 32 cm. [4986]

Contents:—An idea of a philosophical history of plants. 2d. ed.—The anatomy of plants, begun. 1st book: General account of vegetation. 2d ed. 2d book: The anatomy of roots, 2d ed. 3d. book: The anatomy of trunks, 2d ed. 4th book: The anatomy of leaves, flowers, fruits and seeds. In four parts.—Several lectures read before the Royal Society. Items have special title pages.

—The anatomy of vegetables begun. With a general account of vegetation founded thereon ... London, Spencer Hickman, 1672.

[31], 198 (i.e. 186), [17] p. plates. 17 cm. [4987]

—[French tr.] Anatomie des plantes qui contient une description exacte de leurs parties & de leurs usages, & qui fait voir comment elles se forment, & comment elles croissent ... Paris, Lambert Roulland, 1675.

[26], 215, [13] p. front., illus., plates. 15 cm. [4988]

Translated by Louis Le Vasseur.

—[The same.] . . . 2. ed. Paris, Antoine Dezallier, 1679.

[26], 215, [12] p. front., illus., plates. 15 cm.
[**4989**]
A reissue of the 1675 edition with new title page and without the colophon.

—[The same.] . . . Et L'ame des plantes par M^r. Dedu . . . Avec un Receuil d'experiences & observations curieuses faites par M^{rs}. Grew & Boyle . . . Leide, Pierre van der Aa, 1685.

[12], 310 p.; [1], 106 p. 15 cm.   [**4990**]
Added engraved title page.
Fulton(A) 131.
"De l'ame des plantes, de leur naissance, de leur nourriture & de leurs progrez. Essay de physique par M. Dedu" (p. [247]-310) has special title page.
Part [2] has special title page: Recueil d'experiences et observations curieuses sur le combat, qui procede du mélange des corps. Sur les saveurs, et sur les odeurs. Par . . . Nehem. Grew, & Rob. Boyle.

—The comparative anatomy of stomachs and guts. In Royal Society of London. Museum Regalis Societatis. 1681, 1694.

—[Experiments in consort of the luctation arising from the affusion of several menstruums upon all sorts of bodies. French.] Recueil d'experiences et observations sur le combat, qui procede du mélange des corps, sur les saveurs, sur les odeurs, sur le sang, sur le lait . . . Paris, Estienne Michallet, 1679.

[17], 262, [2] p. front., plate. 17 cm. [**4991**]
Imperfect: front. and plate wanting.
Fulton(A) 130.
The Experiences sur les saveurs et sur les odeurs, is by Hon. Robert Boyle, and the Observations sur le sang et sur le lait, by Anthony van Leeuwenhoek.
Translated by Louis Le Vasseur.

—Tractatus de salis cathartici amari in aquis Ebeshamensibus, et hujusmodi aliis contenti natura & usu . . . Londini, S. Smith & B. Walford, 1695.

[11], 96 p. 16 cm.   [**4992**]

—[English ed.] A treatise of the nature and use of the bitter purging salt contain'd in Epsom, and such other waters . . . London, 1697.

64 p. 17 cm.   [**4993**]

—*respondent.* Disputatio medica-physica inauguralis de liquore nervoso . . . Lugduni Batavorum, Apud viduam & haeredes Joannis Elsevirii, 1671.

[8] p. 23 cm.   [**4994**]
Diss. — Leyden.

—, *comp. See* ROYAL SOCIETY OF LONDON. Museum Regalis Societatis. 1681, 1694.

GREWER, JODOCUS [16th cent.] Secretum . . .
699-721 p., vol. 3. 20 cm. (In Zetzner, Lazarus, ed. Theatrum chemicum. Argentorati, 1659-61)   [**4995**]
Caption title.

GREY, THOMAS DE LA. *See* DE LA GREY, Thomas.

GRIDA sopra il sepelire le bestie morte. 1634. *See* MODENA. Ordinances, local laws, etc.

GRIDA sopra la custodia delle porte della città di Modana. 1657. *See* MODENA. Ordinances, local laws, etc.

GRIDA sopra l'espurgatione della città per conservatione della sanità. 1629. *See* MODENA. Ordinances, local laws, etc.

GRIENDEL, JOHANN FRANZ [*fl.* 1676-1687] Micrographia nova; sive, Nova & curiosa variorum minutorum corporum singularis cujusdam & noviter ab autore inventi microscopii . . . descriptio . . . Norimbergae, Sumptibus Johannis Ziegeri, 1687.

[8], 64 p. plates. 22 cm.   [**4996**]

—[German tr.] Micrographia nova; oder, Neu-curieuse Beschreibung verschiedener kleiner Körper, welche vermittelst eines absonderlichen von dem Authore neuerfundenen Vergrösser-Glases verwunderlich gross vorgestellet werden . . . Nürnberg, In Verlegung Johann Ziegers, 1687.

[8], 64 p. plates. 20 cm.   [**4997**]

GRIENDELIUS VON ACH, JOHANNES FRANCISCUS. *See* GRIENDEL, Johann Franz [*fl.* 1676-1687]

GRIFFENFELD, PEDER SCHUMACHER, *greve af* [1635-1699] *See* BARTHOLIN, T. Quaestiones nuptiales. 1670.

GRIFFITH, JOHN [*fl.* 17th cent.] *See* [PEACHIE, John] Some observations made upon the Brasillian root. 1682.

GRIFFITH, RICHARD [1635?-1691] A-la-mode phlebotomy no good fashion; or, The copy of a letter to Dr. Hungerford, complaining of . . . the phantastick behaviour and unfair dealing of some London physitians when they come to be consulted withal about sick persons living . . . in the country. Whereupon a fit occasion is taken to discourse of the profuse way of blood-letting . . . London, Printed by T[homas] B[raddyll] for Joseph Hindmash, 1681.

[30], 209, [3] p. 18 cm. [4998]

GRILLOT, JEAN, *Father* [1588-1647] Lugdunum lue affectum, et refectum; sive, Narratio rerum memoria dignarum Lugduni gestarum ab Augusto mense anni 1628. ad Octobrem anni 1629 . . . Lugduni, Sumptibus Francisci de la Bottiere, 1629.

117, [2] p. 17 cm. [4999]

—[French ed.] Lyon affligé de contagion; ou, Narré de ce qui s'est passé de plus memorable en ceste ville, depuis le mois d'aoust de l'an 1628. jusques au mois d'octobre de l'an 1629 . . . Lyon, François de la Bottiere, 1629.

142, [2] p. 17 cm. [5000]

GRIM, HERMANNUS NICOLAUS. *See* GRIMM, Hermann Nicolaus [1641-1711]

GRIMALDI, FRANCESCO MARIA, *Father* [1613-1663] Physico-mathesis de lumine, coloribus, et iride, aliisque adnexis libri duo . . . Opus posthumum. Bononiae, Ex typographia haeredis Victorii Benatii, impensis Hieronymi Berniae, 1665.

[21], 535, [16] p. illus. 27 cm. [5001]
Added title page.
Edited by Jeronimo Bernia.

GRIMBERG, NICOLAUS [1649-1746] Kurtze Beschreibung des Nieren und Blasen Steins; das ist, Gründtliches Bedencken von beyder Natur und Eigenschafften, deroselben Nahmen, Ursachen, de materiali & efficiente tam diagnosticis, quam pathognomicis, nicht minder auch von dem Utero Dulech. und der Cura prophylactica & therapeutica . . . Hafniae, Sumptibus authoris, literis Justini Hög [1695?]

[8], 52 p. 15 cm. [5002]
Imperfect: outer and lower margins trimmed.

—Observationes medicae . . . Amstelodami, Apud Janssonio Waesbergios, 1689.

[12], 72, [8] p. 14 cm. [5003]

GRIMESTONE, EDWARD. *See* GRIMSTONE, Edward.

GRIMM, HERMANN NICOLAUS [1641-1711] Compendium medico-chimicum; seu, Accurata medendi methodus, quae excellentissimis medicamentis, tam Europae, quam Indiae Orientali proficuis, repleta, rariores praeterea observationes, & curiosam op-

timorum medicamentorum, in libelli hujus formulis contentorum, praeparationem exhibet. Bataviae, Ex officina Abrahami van den Eede, 1679.

[16], 307, [1] p. 15 cm. [5004]

—[The same.] . . . Auctior & emendatior. Augustae Vindelicorum, Impensis Theophili Göbelii, typis Johan. Jacob. Schönigii, 1684.

[12], 475, [11] p. 17 cm. [5005]

GRIMM, JOHANN CASPAR [1662-1728] Kurtze historische, physicalische und medicinische Relation einiger Mirabilium Naturae . . . in specie von einem Monstrobicorporeo, oder von einer Wunder-Geburth, so in diesem 1700sten Jahr . . . von einer Frau in Pombsen . . . an das Tage-Licht gekommen . . . [Leipzig] In Verlegung des Autoris, gedruckt bey Justus Reinholdens seel. Witben, 1700.

[28] p. plate. 20 cm. [5006]

—*respondent. See* BOHN, J., *praeses.* Dissertationem inauguralem de torminibus colicis . . . publice ventilandam . . . sistit, J. C. G. 1689.

—*See* AMMANN, P. Pro-cancellarius . . . Paulus Ammann lecturis S. 1689.

GRIMSTONE, EDWARD, *tr. See* ACOSTA, J. de. The naturall and morall historie. 1604.

GRINAU, P., [*fl.* 1687] *tr. See* AVERROËS. Averroeana: being a transcript of several letters from Averroes. 1695.

GRINDL, JOHANN FRANCISCUS. *See* GRIENDEL, Johann Franz [*fl.* 1676-1687]

GRISLEUS, GABRIEL. *See* GRISLEY, Gabriel [*fl.* 1655-*ca.* 1661]

GRISLEY, GABRIEL [*fl.* 1655-*ca.* 1661] Desenganos para a medicina, ou, botica para todo pay de familias. Consiste na declaracão das qualidades, & virtudes de 260 ervas, com o uso dellas, tamben de 60. agoas estiladas, com as regras de arte da estilação . . . Lisboa, Henrique Valente de Oliveira, 1656.

[10], 182 ll. 16 cm. [5007]

—*See* RAY, J. Stirpium Europaearum extra Britannias nascentium sylloge. 1694.

GRISONE, FEDERICO [16th cent.] Ordini de cavalcare, et modi di conoscere le nature de' cavalli, di emendare i lor vitii . . . Di nuovo migliorati, & accresciuti di postille, & di tavola. Aggiungevisi una

Scielta di notabili avvertimenti, per far eccellenti razze & per rimediare alle infermita de' cavalli . . . Venetia, Andrea Muschio, 1610.

[12], 163, [1] p.; 70, [11] p.　illus., plates.　23 cm.

[5008]

Part [2] has special title page.

—[The same.] . . . Venetia, Andrea Muschio, 1620.

[12], 163, [1] p.; 70, [11] p.　illus.　23 cm.

[5009]

Different setting of type.

GROB, HANS ULRICH [1571–1621] *respondent. See* PETRAEUS, H., *praeses.* Disquisitio hermetica de origine formarum e seminio virtute plastica instructo. 1612.

GROBIUS, GEORG ANDREAS [*fl.* 1666] *respondent. See* BOHN, J. Disputatio medica, de cholera. 1666.

GROBIUS, JOHANNES ULRICUS. *See* GROB, Hans Ulrich [1571–1621]

GROELLMANN, JOHANNES DANIEL [*fl.* 1683] *respondent.* Disputatio medica . . . inauguralis, de philtris, quorum historiam, naturam, ac effectuum malorum curam . . . publicae disquisitioni subjicit . . . Ultrajecti, Typis Appelarianis, 1683.

[51] p.　19 cm.

[5010]

Diss.—Utrecht.

GROEN, JAN VAN DER [*fl.* 17th cent.] Den Nederlandtsen hovenier. *In* 't Vermakelijck landt-leven. 1686.

—[French ed.] Le jardinier du Pays-Bas, ou sont déscrites toutes sortes de belles maisons de plaisance & de campagne, & comment on les peut planter, semer, & embellir de plusieurs herbes, fleurs, & arbres rares . . . Bruxelles, Chez la vefue Vleugart, 1681.

[30], 180, [2] p.　illus.　21 cm.　**[5011]**

"24 nouveaux . . . modelles de parterres a la françoise": p. [75]–82; "Deux cens modelles, pour ceux qui se plaisent au jardinage . . .": p. [83]–137; "Boutiques a remedes enseignant, de quelle maniere il faut preparer les medicines pour guerir les maladies des animaux": p. [139]–156; "Traité des abeilles ou mouches a miel . . .": p. [157]–180. Items have special title pages.

GROENENDAAL, CONRAD VAN [*fl.* 1698] *respondent.* Disputatio medica inauguralis de haemoptysi . . . Trajecti ad Rhenum, Ex officina Francisci Halma, 1698.

13, [2] p.　21 cm.　**[5012]**

Diss.—Utrecht.

GROENENDYCK, CORNELIS À [*fl.* 1668] *respondent.* Disputatio medica inauguralis de sterilitate in utroque sexu . . . Lugduni Batavorum, Apud viduam & haeredes Joannis Elsevirii, 1668.

[10] p.　24 cm.　**[5013]**

Diss.—Leyden.

GROENEVELD, JOANNES. *See* GROENVELDT, Jan [1647–1710]

GROENEWEGEN, ALBERT VAN [*fl.* 1653] *respondent.* Disputatio medica inauguralis de nephritide . . . Lugduni Batavorum, Ex officina Francisci Hackii, 1653.

[8] p.　23 cm.　**[5014]**

Diss.—Leyden.

GROENE-WOLT, JOANNES, *respondent. See* DEUSING, A., *praeses.* Synopsis medicinae universalis. 1649.

GROENVELDT, JAN [1647–1710] De tuto cantharidum in medicina usu interno . . . Londini, Typis J. H. prostant venales apud Johannem Taylor, 1698.

[3], xvi, 135, [1] p.　15 cm.　**[5015]**

—Dissertatio lithologica variis observationibus & figuris illustrata . . . Ed. 2, priori multo auctior & emendatior. Londini, Typis M. Flesher, impensis Abeli Swalle, 1687.

[29], 70 p.　plates.　20 cm.　**[5016]**

Imperfect: first preliminary leaf (blank?) wanting.

—[English tr.] Λιθολογια. A Treatise of the stone & gravel their causes, signs, & symptoms, with methods for their prevention and cure. And some account also of the manner of the collotian section. Written in Latin . . . and rendred into English . . . London, Printed by H. C. for J. T. and sold by Rob. Clavel, 1677.

[7], 69 p.　16 cm.　**[5017]**

—*See* READ, A. Chirurgorum comes. 1687.

GROIEAN, NICOLAUS. *See* GROSJEAN, Nicolas [*fl.* 1665–1670]

GROMMEE, ABRAHAM [*fl.* 1679–1684] *respondent.* Disputatio medica inauguralis continens praxin morborum soporosorum . . . Lugduni Batavorum, Apud Abrahamum Elzevier, 1684.

[19] p.　22 cm.　**[5018]**

Diss.—Leyden.

GRONOVIUS, JOANNES FREDERICUS [1611–1671] *praeses*. Disputatio medico-chirurgic inauguralis de hydrocephalo ... Lugduni Batavorum, Ex typographia Severini Matthaei, 1661.

[12], p. 21 cm.				**[5019]**

Diss.—Leyden (A. A. Huxholtz, respondent)

—*See* PLINIUS SECUNDUS, C. Naturalis historiae, tomus primus [-tertius] 1668–1669.

GROOT, HUGO DE [1583–1645] H. Grotii et aliorum dissertationes de studiis instituendis. Amsterodami, Apud Ludovicum Elzevirium, 1645.

[12], 687 p. 14 cm.				**[5020]**

Engraved title page.

A collection of 24 essays by 21 authors of which 2 are of medical interest.

—*See* REGIMEN SANITATIS SALERNITANUM. Schola Salernitana. 1649, 1657, 1667, 1683.

GROOT, THEODOOR DE [*fl.* 1671] *respondent*. Disputatio medica inauguralis de arthritide ... Lugduni Batavorum, Apud viduam & haeredes Joannis Elsevirii, 1671.

[16] p. 23 cm.				**[5021]**

Diss.—Leyden.

GROS, SIMON. *See* GROSS, Simon [*fl.* 1679–1680]

GROS, WILHELM [*fl.* 1606] *respondent*. *See* BARTHOLIN, C. Astrologia. 1616.

GROSCESIUS, JOANNES. *See* CHROŚCIEJOWSKI, Jan Hieronim [*fl.* 1583–1612]

GROSGEBAUER, PHILIPP. *See* GROSSGEBAUER, Philipp [1653–1711]

GROSJEAN, NICOLAS [*fl.* 1665–1670] *respondent*. De θρομβωσει; h. e., Lactis in mammis coagulatione ... Basileae, Ex typographia Deckeriana [1670]

[28] p. 19 cm.				**[5022]**

Diss.—Basel.

GROSS, HENNING. *See* GROSSE, Henning [d. 1649]

GROSS, SIMON [*fl.* 1679–1680] *respondent*. *See* NÜSSLER, W., *praeses*. Dissertatio physica de anima brutorum. 1680.

GROSSAEUS, JOANNES. *See* GRASSHOFF, Johann [d. 1623]

GROSSE, HENNING [d. 1649] *See* SENNERT, D. Operum in quinque tomos divisorum. 1666.

Das **GROSSE** Planeten-Buch, welches aus dem Platone, Ptolomeo, Hali, Albumasar, Barlaam, und Johann Konigsperger, aufs fleissigste zusammen gezogen. Benebst der Geomantie, Physiognomie und Chiromantie, wie auch der alten Weiber Philosophie und kleinen Cosmographie. Darinnen nicht nur was dem Menschen für Glück, Unglück, Reichthum, gute und böse Zeit begegnen kann; ingleichen wie einem jeden alle Jahre seine Revolution zu setzen, und ein Mensch durch alle Monate des Jahrs sich verhalten soll, kürzlich und deutlich berichtet, sondern auch alle Länder und Wasser beschrieben werden ... [n.p., not before 1694]

[22], 412 p. front., illus., plates. 19 cm.				**[5023]**

Imperfect: title page trimmed and mounted with loss of the imprint. Vorrede partly misbound after p. 402 and p. 406.

Vorrede signed: M. Sebastianus Brenner [i.e. S. Prenner]

Engraved frontispiece with title Groses Planeten Buch is signed "Brühl sc. Lips." [i.e. possibly Nikolaus Brühl, Cf. Thieme-Becker, vol. 5, 105]

Similar titles are listed by Sabattini, nos. 270–273, under the name of Wolffgang Hildebrand, with a cross reference from Sebastian Brenner to Hildebrand. The authorship, however, cannot as yet be ascertained.

GROSSER, GABRIEL [*fl.* 1694] *respondent*. *See* LANGE, C. J., *praeses*. Hominem aerometrum ... in dissertatione publica considerandum ... sistet ... G. G. 1694.

GROSSGEBAUER, PHILIPP [1653–1711] Αυτοσχεδιασμα de loquela brutorum von der Sprache der Thiere quo ad declamationes oratorio-dialogisticas cras, Deo dante, ipsis Calend. Sept. audita hora nona in auditorio Lycei nostri consueto quadruplici idiomate a frugi bonaeque indolis discipulis memoriter recitandas patronos ac fautores artium liberalium decenter humiliterque invitat Philippus Brossgebaur [sic] rector. [Vinariae? 1698]

19 p. 19 cm.				**[5024]**

GROSSI, TOMMASO. *See* GROSSO, Tommaso [*fl.* 17th cent.]

GROSSMANN, THOMAS [*fl.* 1651] *respondent*. *See* SEBISCH, M. [1578–1674?] *praeses*. Galeni quinque priores libri. 1651.

GROSSO, TOMMASO [*fl.* 17th cent.] Lectiones de febribus, in quibus praeter hanc exactissimam febrium doctrinam: infinita problemata, plures etiam Hypocratis, Galeni, Avicennae, & aliorum auctorum controversiae explicantur, concilianturve. Accessit quaestio de vino exhibendo in febribus a principio ... Venetiis, Apud Joannem Guerilium, 1627.

[48] 294 p. 23 cm. [5025]

—Quaestio unica. An morbi, qui in Italia, & praesertim in Gallia Cysalpina, hoc anno evagantur, sub nomine pestis, an vero inter febres pestilentiales connumerari debeant ...Venetiis, Apud Marcum Antonium Broiollum, 1631.

[20], 95, [1] p. 23 cm. [5026]

—Tractatus in sex propositiones divisus. De natura, differentiis, & usu, sex rerum non naturalium, corpora nostra alterantium, quae sunt aer, cibus & potus, motus & quies, somnus & vigilia, repletio, & exinanitio, & animi affectiones ... Venetiis, Apud Joannem Guerilium, 1617.

[16], 329, [32] p. 21 cm. [5027]

GROSSUS, Thomas. *See* Grosso, Tommaso [*fl.* 17th cent.]

Das GROSZE Planeten-Buch. *See* Das Grosse Planeten-Buch.

GROTIUS, Hugo. *See* Groot, Hugo de [1583–1645]

GROTIUS À DESWIG. Daniel Meno Matthias [*fl.* 1687] *respondent. See* Bartholin, C. [1655–1738], *praeses*. Disputatio inauguralis medico anatomica de formatione et nutritione foetus in utero. 1687.

GROVE, Robert [1634–1696] Carmen de sanguinis circuitu, a Gulielmo Harvaeo ... primum invento. Adjecta sunt, miscellanea quaedam. Londoni, Typis R. E., impensis Qualteri Kettilby, 1685.

[4], 40 p. 21 cm. [5028]

GRUBE, Hermann [1637–1698] Analysis mali citrei compendiosa ... Hafniae, Apud Danielem Paulii, literis Henrici Gödiani, 1668.

[8], 72 p. 17 cm. [5029]
—Copy 2. 16 cm.
With this is bound Huenerwolf, J. A. Anatomia paeoniae. 1680.

—Commentarius de modo simplicium medicamentorum facultates cognoscendi, ad praxin medicam directus ... Cui praefixa Thomae Bartholini Epistola de simplicibus medicamentis inquilinis cognoscendis. Hafniae & Francofurti, Ex bibliopolio Danielis Paulli, 1669.

[16], xxix, 173 (i.e. 171), 18 p. illus. 17 cm. [5030]

—De arcanis medicorum non arcanis commentatio ex inventis recentiorum Harveianis, Bartholianis, Sylvianis, Willisianis & ceteris in gratiam tyronum breviter concinnata ... Cui praefixa Thomae Bartholini De transplantatione morborum epistola. Hafniae, Ex bibliopolio Danielis Paulli, 1673.

[22], 80, 272 p. 16 cm. [5031]
"Th. Bartholini De transplantatione morborum dissertatio epistolica": 80 p., with special title page.
With this is bound *his* De transplantatione morborum. 1674.

—De ictu tarantulae, & vi musices in ejus curatione, conjecturae physico-medicae. Francofurti, Ex bibliopolio Hafniensi, Danielis Paulli, 1679.

[14], 76, [10] p. illus. 17 cm. [5032]

—De transplantatione morborum. Analysis nova. Hamburgi, Apud Gothofredum Schultze & Amsterodami, Apud Joannem Janssonium a Waesberge, 1674.

[6], 87 (i.e. 89), [9] p. 16 cm. [5033]
Bound with *his* De arcanis medicorum. 1673.

—*praeses.* Conflictus academicus de temperamento ... Jenae, Literis Johannis Wertheri, 1666.

20 p. 19 cm. [5034]
Diss.—Jena (S. Ledel, *respondent*)

—*respondent. See* Schuyl, F., *praeses.* Disputatio medica inauguralis, de gonorrhoea. 1666.

GRUBEL, Johann Georg. *See* Grübel, Johann Georg [*fl.* 1672–1674]

GRUBER, Christoph Friedrich [1650–1694] *respondent.* Dissertationem de stranguria inauguralem ... proponit Georgii Andreae Dilhopffii [1674]

20 p. 20 cm. [5035]
Diss.—Strasbourg.

GRUE, Johann Joachim la [*fl.* 1682] *respondent.* Disputatio medica inauguralis de ascite ... Lugduni Batavorum, Apud Abrahamum Elzevier, 1682.

[16] p. 22 cm. [5036]
Diss.—Leyden.

GRUE, Philippe La. *See* La Grue, Philippe [17th cent.]

GRUE, Thomas. *See* La Grue, Thomas [*fl.* 1661]

GRÜBEL, Christian [1642–1715] *praeses.* De salutatione ... [Jenae] Literis Joh. Jacobi Bauhoferi [1675]

[64] p. 20 cm. [5037]
Diss.—Jena (S. Besser, *respondent*)

GRÜBEL, JOHANN GEORG [*fl.* 1672–1674] *praeses.* Dissertatio anatomica de ductu chylifero Pecquetiano . . . Jenae, Typis Bauhoferianis [1674]

[2], 22 p. 19 cm.   **[5038]**

Diss.—Jena (J. A. Slevogt, *respondent*)

—*respondent. See* ROLFINCK, W., *praeses.* Disputatio medica de strangulatione uteri. 1672.

GRÜBELING, FRANZ HEINRICH [*fl.* 1699–1701] *respondent. See* MEIBOM, H., *praeses.* Exercitatio medico chirurgica de catheterismo. 1699.

GRUEBER, JOHANN [1623–1665] *See* KIRCHER, A. La Chine. 1670.

GRÜGENER, MICHAEL. *See* CRÜGENER, Michael [*fl.* 1648–1679]

GRÜLING, JOHANN GERHARD [*fl.* 1681–1686] *respondent. See* HOFFMANN, F. [1660–1742] *praeses.* De cinnabari antimonii exercitatio medico-chymica. 1681.

GRÜLING, PHILIPP [1593–1667] Curationum dogmatico-hermeticarum, in certis locis, & notis personis optime expertarum & rite probatarum centuria prima . . . Lipsiae, Typis & sumptibus heredum Gothofredi Grossii, 1638.

[12], 284 p. 16 cm.   **[5039]**

Included, with revisions, in his Observationum et curationum medicinalium dogmatico-hermeticarum . . . centuriae VII, published 1662–66.

—De triplici in medicina universalis evacuationis genere et in specie: 1. De venaesectione . . . 2. De medicamentis purgantibus . . . 3. De sudoriferis, diureticis . . . Novum ac posthumum opus multiplici experientia ac fida ratione elaboratum et chymicis potissimum observationibus illustratum . . . Francofurti & Lipsiae, Sumptibus Georgi Heinrici Frommanni, 1671.

3 parts in 1 v. 21 cm.   **[5040]**

Added engraved title page.
Parts 2–3 have special title pages dated 1670.
Edited by Philipp Gerhard Grüling.

—Deutsches Artzney-Buch, darinnen nicht allein zu finden, wie man allerley Früchte, Wurtzeln, Beeren, Schalen und anders einmachen, die Oehle, Saltze, Essentien, Spiritus, und Conserven nach der Apotheker Kunst praepariren, sondern auch alle Kranckheiten . . . mit offt experimentirten Artzney-Mitteln curiren und abwenden soll. Wobey mit angefüget dess sel. Autoris beyde Tractat Von der Pest und Kinder-Kranckheiten . . . Franckfurt und Leipzig, Georg Heinrich Fromman, 1676.

[14], 539, [5] p. front. (port.), illus. 21 cm.   **[5041]**

Imperfect: p. 65–72 and 161–168 wanting.
Edited by Philipp Gerhard Grüling.

—Florilegium chymicum, hoc est, libellus insignis de quorundam medicamentorum chymicorum, ut-pote: essentiarum, magisteriorum, extractorum, salium, tincturarum, florum, crocorum, oleorum, spirituum, faecularum, balsamorum, aquarum, pulverum, &c., vera praeparatione, recto usu & certa dosi, multis exemplis, observationibusque illustratus . . . Lipsiae, Impensis Gothofredi Grosii [Johannes-Albertus Minzelius excudebat] 1631.

[24], 476, [27] p. 14 cm.   **[5042]**

With this are bound: Blochwitz, M. Anatomia sambuci. 1631.— Santorio, S. Ars Sanctorii Sanctorii de statica medicina. [1624]

—Florilegium Hippocrateo-Galeno chymicum novum longe pluris priore auctum & quasi pro-dromus practici operis propediem insecuturi, in quo praescribitur plurimorum medicamentorum . . . con-ficiendorum certa ratio: una cum ipsorum virtute, usu, dosi, notis, observationibus et exemplis quamplurimis. Lipsiae, Sumptibus haeredum Godofredi Grosii, excudebat Timotheus Ritzsch, 1644.

[24], 479 p. 21 cm.   **[5043]**

Interleaved.

—[The same.] Florilegii Hippocrateo-Galeno-chymici novi et quasi prodromi Medicinae practicae proxime insequentis ed. 3. variis & infinitis locis, longeque pluris priore altera aucta . . . Lipsiae, Sumptibus Georgii Henrici Frommanni, 1665.

[20], 578 (i.e. 568), [12] p. 21 cm.   **[5044]**

—Medicinae practicae libri quinque, in quibus non modo omnes fere corporis humani morbi describuntur, verum etiam eorum causae, signa, prognoses et curationes prolixius depinguntur . . . Lipsiae, Sumptibus Georgii Heinrici Frommanni, 1668.

[22], 601, [5] p. front. (port.) 21 cm.

      [5045]

With this is bound *his* Observationum et cura-tionum medicinalium . . . centuriae VIII. 1668.

—[The same.] . . . Jam editione hac plane nova, post obitum authoris, diligenter recensiti, & prope infinitis iisque optimis experimentis ac observationibus locupletati. Lipsiae, Sumptibus Georg. Heinr. Frommanni, literis Johannis Coleri, 1673.

[22], 923, [4] p. front. (port.) 20 cm.
[5046]

Added engraved title page.
"Editio secunda."

—Observationum et curationum medicinalium dogmatico-hermeticarum, in certis locis & notis personis optime expertarum & probatarum, centuriae VII. Cum appendice quorundam medicamentorum secretiorum in lucem edita. Lipsiae, Sumpt. Georgii Heinrici Frommani, 1662–1666.

7 parts in 1 v. front. (port.) 20 cm. [5047]

Each part has special title page or half title.
Imprint varies: centuriae 2-7, Northusae, Johann Erasmus Hynitzsch.
Centuriae 5-7 have also additional special title page: Triga centuriarum curationum medicinalium dogmatico-hermeticarum ... opera et studio Philippi Gerhardi Grülingii ... denuo revisa ...

—[The same.] ... Lipsiae, Sumptibus Georgii Heinrici Frommanni, 1668.

8 parts in 1 v. 21 cm. [5048]

Each part has special title page.
Part [8] has title: Tractatus novus de calculo et suppressione urinae.
Bound with *his* Medicinae practicae libri quinque. 1668.

—Tractat von Kinder Kranckheiten und allerhand beschwerlichen Zufällen, woher sie kommen, was daraus zu urtheilen und wie solche curiret werden können ... Nordthausen, Johann-Erasmus Hynitzsch, 1660.

[8], 104 p. 19 cm. [5049]

GRÜLING, PHILIPP GERHARD [*fl.* 1671-1721] Tractatus novus von Weiber-Kranckheiten und allerhand beschwerlichen Symptomatibus, woher sie kommen und wie solche curirt werden können ... Franckfurt, Georg Heinrich Fromman, 1675.

[8], 5-64, [4] p. 20 cm. [5050]

—[The same.] ... Franckfurt und Leipzig, Georg Heinrich Fromman, 1680.

62, [2] p. 21 cm. [5051]

—, ed. See GRÜLING, P. De triplici in medicina universalis evacuationis genere et in specie. 1671 [and] Deutsches Artzney-Buch. 1676 [and] Observationum et curationum medicinalium dogmatico-hermeticarum. 1662-1666.

GRÜNDLICHER Bericht von dem Nativitaetstellen. *See* TREW, A. Nucleus astrologiae correctae. 1651.

GRÜNDTLICHE Unterrichtungen, wornach man sich zur Zeit eingeschlichener böser Seuche, der abschewlichen Pestilentz, so wol zu deren Abwendung, als auch wie man sich zuverhalten, wann dieselbe jemands ergriffen, und darvon verlangt befreyet zuwerden ... Costantz, Bey David Hautt dem jüngern, 1667.

96 p. 13 cm. [5052]

GRÜZMANN, DANIEL [*fl.* 1667] *praeses.* Dissertatio academica in qua aves paradisiacas & primario harum regem ... sistit Nicolaus Bonenberg ... Jenae, Literis Bauhoferianis [1667]

[23] p. illus. 20 cm. [5053]

Diss.—Jena (N. Bonenberg, *respondent*)

GRUMMET, CHRISTOPH [*fl. ca.* 1677] Das Blut der Natur ... Dressden, In Verlegung des Autoris, gedruckt durch Melchior Bergens seel. nachgelassene Wittbe und Erben, 1677.

[23] p. 19 cm. [5054]

GRUNDEL, GYÖRGY [*b.* 1659] *respondent. See* FASCH, A. H., *praeses.* Dissertatio medica inauguralis de oedemate. 1638; WEDEL, G. W., *praeses.* Dissertatio medica sistens aegrum laborantem syncope. 1682.

—*See* WEDEL. G. W. Georgius Wolffgangus Wedelius ... Facultatis Medicae decanus, lectori benevolo S. P. D. 1683.

GRUNDMANN, AUGUST DAVID [*fl.* 1693] *respondent.* Dissertatio medica inauguralis de medicamentis uterinis ... Lugduni Batavorum, Apud Abrahamum Elzevier, 1693.

[20] p. 20 cm. [5055]

Diss.—Leyden.

GRUNDMANN, VALENTIN [*fl.* 1623] *respondent. See* INNICHENHÖFER, H., *praeses.* Ὑπνολογια; sive, Tractatus jucundus physiologicus. 1624.

GRUNINGK, ADAM [*fl.* 1630] *respondent. See* MÜLMANN, P., *praeses.* Disputatio physica de insomnii. 1630.

GRUVE, JOHANN FRIEDRICH [*fl.* 1685-1692] *respondent. See* KÖRBER, J. L., *praeses.* Exercitium medicum de ecclipsi microcosmica ... exponet J. F. G. 1685.

GRUVE, MATTHIAS [*ca.* 1623-1683] *praeses.* Disputatio physica de origine animae humanae ... Erffurti, Literis Dedekindianis [1673]

[34] p. 19 cm. [5056]

Diss.—Erfurt (J. G. Berckhoff, *respondent*)

GRUVIUS *See* GRUVE.

GSELL, JOHANN HEINRICH [*fl.* 1692] *respondent. See* CAMERARIUS, E. R., *praeses.* Dissertatio inauguralis medica de febre intermittente anomala. 1692 [and] Dissertatio medica de febribus in genere. 1692.

GUACCIUS, FRANCISCUS MARIA. *See* GUAZZO, Francesco Maria [*d. ca.* 1640]

GUALDO, PAOLO [1553-1621] Vita Joannis Vincentii Pinelli patricii Genuensis ... Augustae Vindelicorum [Christophorus Mangus] 1607.

[16], 140, [8] p. port. 21 cm. [5057]

"Joannis Boteri ad Joannem Vincentium Pinellum sylva, cui titulus, Otium honoratum": p. 129-140.

GUALTHER, LUDWIG FRIEDRICH [*fl.* 1698-1715] *respondent. See* STAHL, G. E., *praeses.* Disputatio medica inauguralis de inflammationis vera pathologia. 1698.

—*See* STAHL, G. E. Propempticon inaugurale de aestimatione partium & laesionum. 1698.

GUARGUANTI, ORAZIO [1554-1611] De theriacae virtutibus paraphrasis [Italian]. *In* Melich, G. Avertimenti nelle compositioni de' medicamenti per uso della spetiaria. 1605, 1648, 1678.

—Responsa varia, ad varias aegritudines. Et in primis tres tractatus, unus de dysenteria, alter de morbo gallico, & tertius de febre pestilentiali, & de peste ... Huc accedit exactissima cognitio sedandi, & curandi fluxus. R. P. E. Cypriani Mantegarrii ... summo studio, summoque labore collecta, serie digesta, & ... in lucem edita ... Venetiis, Apud Ambrosium & Batholomeum Dei, 1613.

[14], 295, [24] p. port. 22 cm. [5058]

Colophon: Venetiis, Excudebat Ambrosius Dei, 1603.

GUARINONI, CRISTOFORO [*d.* 1601 or 2] Consilia medicinalia in quibus universa praxis medica exacte pertractatur ... Venetiis, Apud Thomam Baglionum, 1610.

[12], 738 (i.e. 742) p. 34 cm. [5059]

—De natura humana sermones quatuor, Veronae in consessu literatorum habiti ... Francoforti, Im-

primebat Joannes Saurius, sumptibus Nicolai Steinii, 1601.

164 p. illus. 21 cm. [5060]

With this are bound: *his* Sententiarum Aristotelis ... interpretatio. Francoforti, 1601.—Denaisius, P. Apologia meri imperii. 1601.

—Sententiarum Aristotelis de anima seu mente humana interpretatio ... Francoforti, Imprimebat Joannes Saurius sumptibus Nicolai Steinii, 1601.

94 p. 21 cm. [5061]

Includes portions of the text of Aristoteles' De anima.
Bound with *his* De natura humana sermones quatuor. 1601.

GUARINONIUS, HIPPOLYTUS [1571-1654] Die Grewel der Verwüstung menschlichen Geschlechts. In sieben ... Bücher ... abgetheilt ... Ingolstatt, Andreas Angermayr, 1610.

[72], 1330, [2] p. port. 33 cm. [5062]

Errata: p. [2] at end.

—Hydroenogamia triumphpans [sic]; seu, Aquae vinique connubium vetustum, sanctum salutare, necessarium pro ... patre Hieremia Drexelio ... Oenohydromachiae triumphatae, oppositum. Heillig und heilsamber Wasser, und Wein Heürath ... Oeniponti, Apud Michaelem Wagner, 1640.

[16], 428, [36] p. 16 cm. [5063]

Engraved title page.

—Pestilentz Guardien, für allerley Stands Personen, mit Säuberung der inficierten Haüser, Beth-Leingewandt, Kleider, &c. ... Ingolstadt, Getruckt durch Andream Angermayr, 1612.

203 [i.e. 265], [1] p. 16 cm. [5064]

GUASTAVINO, GIULIO [*d. ca.* 1633] Commentarii in priores decem Aristotelis Problematum sectiones ... Lugdoni, Sumptibus Horatii Cardon, 1608.

[8], 395, [12] p. 37 cm. [5065]

Includes the first ten books of Problemata in Greek and in Theodorus Gaza's Latin version.

—Locorum de medicina selectorum liber [-Liber alter] ... Nunc primum in lucem emissus ... Lugduni, Sumptibus Horatii Cardon, 1616-25.

2 v. 24 cm., 22 cm. [5066]

Vol. 2 has imprint: Florentiae, Ex typographia Sermartelliana, 1625.

GUAZZO, FRANCESCO MARIA [*d. ca.* 1640] Compendium maleficarum, ex quo nefandissima in genus humanum opera venefica, ac ad illa vitanda remedia conspiciuntur ... In hac ... secunda aeditione ...

remediis locupletatum. His additus est exorcismus potentissimus ad solvendum omne opus diabolicum; nec non modus curandi febricitantes . . . Mediolani, Ex Collegii Ambrosiani typographia, 1626.

[16], 391 p.　illus.　21 cm.　　　　[5067]
Engraved title page.

GUCKELIN, LUDWIG CHRISTOPH [*fl.* 1695-1699] *respondent. See* CRAUSE, R. W., *praeses.* Dissertatio inauguralis medico-chirurgica de sclopetorum vulneribus. 1695.

— *See* LENTILIUS, R. Ad . . . Ludovicum Christophorum Guckelinum . . . de hydrophobiae caussa et cura dissertatio. 1700.

GUDENUS, URBAN FERDINAND VON [*fl.* 1662] *respondent. See* SEBISCH, M. [1578-1674?] *praeses.* Problemata medica varia. 1662.

GUEINZ, CHRISTIAN [1592-1650] *praeses.* Disputatio de sale . . . In Salinis Salanis [Halae] Typis Christophori Salfeldii, 1639.

[12] p.　19 cm.　　　　　　[5068]
Diss. — Halle (Gymnasium) (P. Zesen, *respondent*)

Ein **GÜLDENER** Tractat vom philosophischen Stein. *See* [GRASSHOFF, J.] Aureus tractatus de philosophorum lapide. 1677.

GUELFAGLIONE, GIULIO CESARE BENEDETTI. *See* BENEDETTI, Giulio Cesare [*d.* 1656]

GUENELLON, PIETER [*fl.* 1667-1689] Epistolica dissertatio, de genuina medicinam instituendi ratione: ad Johannem Munnicks . . . Amstelodami, Apud Adrianum a Gaasbeek, 1680.

80 p.　13 cm.　　　　　　[5069]

—, *tr. See* PORTAL, P. De Practyk der vroed' meesters, en vroed' vrouwen. 1690.

GÜNTER, JOHANN [*fl.* 1625] *praeses.* Disputatio medica de peste . . . Lipsiae, Typis excribebat Georgius Liger [1625]

[23] p.　19 cm.　　　　　　[5070]
Diss. — Leipzig (V. Hertel, *respondent*)

GÜNTHER, CHRISTIAN [*fl.* 1683] *respondent. See* BOHN, J., *praeses.* Dissertationum chymico-physicarum sexta de menstruis. 1683.

GÜNTHER, GEORG [*fl.* 1691] *respondent. See* LIMMER, C. P., *praeses.* Dissertatio anatomica de cute. 1691.

GÜNTHER, JACOB [*fl.* 1625] Consilium de praecavendo & curando morbo epidemico. Kurtze Raths-Erteilung und Unterricht von der gemeinen pestilentialischen Haupt-Kranckheit und Epidemial-Feber: wie sich ein jeder darvor hütten und vorwahren . . . oder . . . curiren sol . . . Brieg, Gedruckt druch [sic] Augustinum Gründer, 1625.

[56] p.　18 cm.　　　　　　[5071]
Imperfect: upper margins trimmed with possible loss of pagination.

GUENTHER, JOHANN, *von Andernach. See* GUINTERIUS, Joannes, *Andernacus* [1505-1574]

GÜNTHER, SIMON [*fl.* 1608] Hortulus sanitatis amoenissimus; hoc est, De tuenda et conservanda bona valetudine . . . Spira, Typis Augustini Scheideri, impensis authoris, & Heliae Kembachii, 1608.

155, [11] p.　13 cm.　　　　[5072]

GÜNZ, GOTTFRIED [*fl.* 1691] *respondent. See* WÄCHTLER, C. J., *respondent.* Verisimilia de stellis novis . . . ostendunt ac defendunt M. Christophorus Jacobus Wächtler. 1691.

GÜNZEL, JOHANN GEORG [*fl.* 1690] *respondent.* Dissertatio inauguralis medica . . . de somno atque insomniis brevibus complexa . . . Trajecti ad Rhenum, Ex officina Francisci Halma, 1690.

[23] p.　20 cm.　　　　　　[5073]
Diss. — Utrecht.

GUERICKE, OTTO VON [1602-1686] Experimenta nova (ut vocantur) Magdeburgica de vacuo spatio primum a R. P. Gaspare Schotto . . . nunc vero ab ipso auctore perfectius edita, variisque aliis experimentis aucta . . . Amstelodami, Apud Joannem Janssonium à Waesberge, 1672.

[16], 244, [4] p.　illus., plates.　32 cm.
　　　　　　　　　　　　　　　[5074]

Added engraved title page.
With this are bound: Borelli, G. A. Philosophia de motu animalium. 1704; Aynscom, F. X., Father. Expositio ac deductio geometrica. 1656.

GUÉRIN, FRANÇOIS. *See* DISCOURS CHRÉTIEN SUR L'ÉTABLISSEMENT DE L'HÔPITAL GENERAL DE LA VILLE D'ORLEANS. 1672.

GUÉRIN, JACQUES A. [*fl.* 1651-*ca.* 1656] Le chirurgien charitable . . . Tirée des plus celebres autheurs

... 3. ed. augm. par l'autheur ... Bordeaux, Pierre du Coq, 1663.

[15], 216 p.   17 cm.   [5075]

—[The same.] Le parfait chirurgien charitable; ou, Le veritable moyen de bien connoistre & guarir les maladies, externes du corps humain. 8. ed., rev., corr., & enrichie de plusieurs ... traitez de medecine ... Et augm. en cette derniere ed. ... Et de l'emplastre de manus Dei. Rouen, François Vaultier [not before 1667]

[21], 314 p.; [1], [5]-16 p.   15 cm.   [5076]

Part [2] has special title page: Methode particuliere pour bien faire le merveilleux emplatre appellé manus Dei ... 1663.

La GUERISON du cancer au sein. 1693. *See* HOUPPEVILLE, G. de.

GUERRERO, DIDACUS RODERICUS. *See* RODRÍGUEZ GUERRERO, Diego.

GÜTH, JAKOB ERNST [*fl.* 1688] *respondent. See* WOLF, Jakob, *praeses.* Dissertatio medica de urinae incontinentia. 1688.

GÜTNER, JOHANN DAVID [*fl.* 1685] *respondent. See* THILE, J., *praeses.* Theses inaugurales de tussi 1685.

GÜTTNER, JOHANN DAVID [*fl.* 1678] *respondent. See* RECHENBERG, A., *praeses.* De mundi anima. 1678.

GUFER, JOHANN [*fl.* 1667] Tabulae medicae; seu, Medicina domestica ... Das ist Kleine Hauss-Apothek, darinnen allerhand schöne Experimenta oder Artzneyen ... beschriben ... Augspurg, In Verlegung Gottlieb Göbels, gedruckt bey Jacob Koppmayer, 1679.

[47], 306, [27] p.   14 cm.   [5077]

Added engraved title page.
With this is bound Schorer, C. Reglen der Gesundheit. 1668.

—[The same.] ... Augspurg, In Verlegung Lorentz Kronigers und Gottlieb Göbels seel. Erben, 1690.

[35], 306, [27] p.   13 cm.   [5078]

Added engraved title page.
Bound with Greisel, J. G. Tractatus medicus. 1681.

GUGGER, JOHANN JAKOB [*fl.* 1607-1611] *respondent.* Theses medicae miscellae ex partibus medicinae quinque ... Basileae, Per Joan. Jacob. Genathium, 1609.

[12], p.   22 cm.   [5079]

Diss. — Basel.

GUIBELET, JOURDAIN [*fl.* 1603-1631] Examen de l'Examen des esprits ... Paris, La veufve Jean de Heuqueville, et Louys de Heuqueville, 1631.

[24], 813, [54] p.   18 cm.   [5080]

A criticism of Juan Huarte de San Juan's Examen de ingenios. Issued also in the same year under the imprint of Michel Soly, to whom the royal privilege (p. [49] at end) was originally granted May 16, 1631.
"Correction des fautes": p. [52-54] at end.

—Trois discours philosophiques. Le I. De la comparaison de l'homme avec le monde. Le II. Du principe de la generation de l'homme. Le III. De l'humeur melancholique. Mis de nouveau en lumiere par Jourdain Guibelet, Evreux, Antoine Le Marié, 1603.

[11], 286 (i.e. 300), [8] ll.   plates.   17 cm.
                                        [5081]

Engraved title page.
First leaf of the first gathering (blank?) cancelled.

GUIBERT, NICOLAS [*ca.* 1547-*ca.* 1620] *See* LIBAVIUS, A. [*d.* 1616] Appendix necessaria Syntagmatis arcanorum chymicorum. 1615.

GUIBERT, PHILBERT [1579?-1633] Les oeuvres charitables ... Sçavoir, Le medecin charitable. Le prix et valeur des medicamens. L'apotiquaire charitable. La maniere d'embaumer les corps morts. Paris, Denys Langlois, 1627.

4 v. in. 1.   front. (port.)   15 cm.   [5082]

Vol. [1]: 13. ed., 1626; vol. [2]: 4. ed. rev. & corr.; vol. [3]: 3. ed. rev. & augm. par l'autheur; vol. [4]: 1. ed.

—Premiere partie des oeuvres charitables ... [Scavoir, Le medecin charitable. Le prix & valeur de medicamens. L'apotiquaire charitable. La maniere d'embaumer les corps morts. Les tromperies du bezoard descouvertes. Le choix des medicamens. Le traité du sené. La maniere de faire gelées. La maniere de faire confitures. Et Le traité de la conservation de santé] ... Rev. & augm. de nouveau ... Paris, Jean Jost, 1632.

[12], 602 (i.e. 646), [14] p.   port.   15 cm.
                                        [5083]

Added engraved title page dated 1631 reads: Les oeuvres du medecin charitable.
Some treatises have special title pages.
Le Traite de la conservation de la santé wanting.
Le traite du sené is by Antoine Mizauld.

—Toutes les oeuvres charitables ... Sçavoir, Le medecin charitable. Le prix & valeur des medicamens. L'apothicaire charitable. La maniere d'embaumer les corps morts. Les tromperies du bezoard descouvertes. Le choix des medicamens. Le traité du sené. La maniere de faire toutes sortes de gelées. La maniere de faire diverses confitures. Le discours de la peste. Le traité de la saignée. Et la Methode agreable & facile pour se purger doucement, & sans aucun dégoust. Rev. corr. & augm. en ceste derniere ed. par l'autheur. Paris, Jean Jost, 1633.

[11], 1046 (i.e. 1063), [22] p.   18 cm.   **[5084]**

Added engraved title page.

Imperfect: title page wanting; supplied in photocopy from Wellcome. Wormholes on p. 717-742 and 801-816.

Items have special title pages.

Includes also Petit traité de la conservation de santé, with special title page.

Le traité de la saignée includes considerable portions of the Galenic text.

—[The same.] . . . Paris, Jean Jost, 1636.

346 (i.e. 874), [33] p.   15 cm.   **[5085]**

Added engraved title page dated 1633.

With the addition of La conservation de santé and without Les tromperies du bezoard descouvertes.

—[The same.] . . . Paris, Jean Jost, 1639.

[14], 880, [30] p.   port.   18 cm.   **[5086]**

Added engraved title page.

—[The same.] . . . Lyon La vefve de C. Rigaud, & Philippe Borde, 1640.

[9], 766 p.   18 cm.   **[5087]**

Added title page reads: Le medecin charitable . . . 18. edition.

Some treatises have special title pages with various imprints.

A reprint of the 1633 edition.

—Another issue, with imprint: Lyon, Nicolas Gay, 1640.

[5088]

Bound with Vaussard, G. L'operateur des pauvres. 1642.

—[The same.] . . . Rouen, De l'imprimerie de Ozee Seigneure pour Corneille Piiresson, 1641.

[10], 880, [27] p.   18 cm.   **[5089]**

Imperfect: sig. a6 (blank) wanting.

Contents as in the 1636 Paris edition.

—[The same.] . . . Rouen, David Ferrand, 1645.

[10], 880, [29] p.   17 cm.   **[5090]**

—[The same.] . . . Paris, Julian Jacquin, 1647.

[10], 880, [29] p.   port.   17 cm.   **[5091]**

Imperfect: [29] p. (Index) wanting.

Different setting of type.

—[The same.] . . . [Lyon, Jean Huguetan, 1649]

[10], 766 p.   18 cm.   **[5092]**

Le prix et valeur des medicamens; L'apothiquaire charitable; and Seconde partie des oeuvres du medecin charitable, have special title pages with imprint: Lyon, Guillaume Chaunod, 1648.

Contents as in the 1640 Lyon edition.

Imprint supplied from added title page: Le medecin charitable.

—[The same.] . . . Paris, Julian Jacquin, 1653.

[10], 880, [29] p.   port.   18 cm.   **[5093]**

Contents as in the 1636 Paris edition.

—[The same.] . . . Rouen, Jean Viret, 1656.

[31], 672 p.   18 cm.   **[5094]**

—[The same.] . . . Paris, Jean Jost, 1657.

[8], 660, [20] p.   19 cm.   **[5095]**

—[The same.] . . . Paris, Chez Estienne Loyson [De l'imprimerie de Sebastien Martin] 1660.

[8], 600, [14] p.   19 cm   **[5096]**

—[The same.] . . . Paris, Chez Pierre Le Mercier [De l'imprimerie de Sebastien Martin] 1670.

[8], 580, [20] p.   19 cm.   **[5097]**

—[The same.] . . . [Lyon, Jean Baptiste de Ville, 1674]

[10], 766 p.   18 cm.   **[5098]**

Imprint supplied from added title page: Le medecin charitable . . . 24. edition.

Contents as in the 1640 Lyon edition.

Some treatises have special title pages with various imprints.

—[The same.] . . . Rouen, Louis Coste, 1678.

[8], 672, [24] p.   16 cm.   **[5099]**

Contents as in the 1636 Paris edition.

—[Latin tr.] Medici officiosi opera . . . centies antehac Gallice edita, nunc primum Latine reddita. Parisiis, Typis viduae Theod. Pepingué, & Steph. Maucroy, 1649.

[16], 760 p.   port.   18 cm.   **[5100]**

Added engraved title page.

Translation by Guillaume Sauvageon.

—[English tr.] The charitable physitian with The charitable apothecary. Written in French . . . and now . . . translated into English . . . by I. W. London, Printed by Thomas Harper, and sold by Lawrence Chapman, 1639.

[7], 173, [8] p.   19 cm.   **[5101]**

STC 12457.

Contains The charitable physitian, shewing the manner to make . . . remedies, The charitable apothecaire, and The charitable physitian shewing the manner to embalme a dead corps, each with special title page.

—Another issue, with imprint: London, Printed by Thomas Harper, and sold by William Sheeres, 1639.

[5102]

Title page a cancel.
STC 12457.5.

—L'apothiquairie du medecin charitable. Enseignant à faire en la maison les medicamens composez avec grande facilité, peu de frais, & peu de temps ... Paris, Denys Langlois, 1625.

[16], 70 (i.e. 170), [1] p.   15 cm.   [5103]
Bound with *his* Le medecin charitable. Paris, 1626.

—[The same.] Traicté de l'apothicairie du medecin charitable ... Lyon, Claude Armand, dit Alphonse, 1626.

[20], 168 + p.   15 cm.   [5104]
Imperfect: all after p. 168 wanting.
Bound with *his* Le medecin charitable. Lyon, 1626.

—[The same.] ... Derniere ed., rev. & augm. par l'autheur. Paris, Denys Langlois, 1628.

[22], 163, [2] p.   14 cm.   [5105]

—[L'apothiquaire charitable. ca. 1640]
7-208 p.   17 cm.   [5106]
Imperfect: all pages before p. 7 wanting.
Contains: L'apothiquaire charitable; Traité de la conservation de santé; Traité du sené, by Antoine Mizauld.
Bound with Vaussard, G. L'operateur des pauvres. 1642.

—L'apotiquaire charitable ... Augmenté de trois nouveaux traités, scavoir, La maniere de faire diverses confitures. La conservation de santé, par un bon & legitime usage des choses requises pour bien & sainement vivre. Et La maniere de faire gelées de chair, de poisson & cordiales ... Augmenté de L'operateur des pauvres ... Ensemble le secret du baulme policreston ... Troyes, Nicolas Oudot, 1646.

192 p.; [1], 78 p.; 46 p.   17 cm.   [5107]
Imperfect: p. 79-80 mutilated.
Part [2] has special title page: Methode agreable et facile, pour avoir des fruicts és jardins.—Part [3] has special title page: L'operateur des pauvres; ou, La fleur d'operation necessaire aux pauvres ... Ensemble le secret du baulme policreston, sa vertu, & autres secrets admirables. Par M. G. Vaussard ... Rev., & corr. par l'autheur.
Bound with *his* Le medecin charitable. 1645.

—Le medecin charitable & profitable au public. Enseignant la maniere de faire, & preparer en la maison, avec facilité & peu de frais les remedes propres à toutes maladies ... Avec un preservatif asseuré contre la peste ... preparé par la Faculté de Medecine de Paris ... A costé de chacun remede est cotté combien il peut couster ... Paris, Jean de Bordeaux, 1623.

47 (i.e. 49) p.   17 cm.   [5108]
Imperfect: p. 7-24 wanting; upper margins trimmed; wormholes throughout.
With this are bound: Le medecin reformé. 1623;—Response au Medecin reformé. 1623.

—Le medecin charitable. Enseignant la maniere de faire & preparer en la maison avec facilité & peu de fraiz les remedes propres à toutes maladies, selon l'advis du medecin ordinaire. Augmenté de nouveau de plusieurs remedes ... Paris, Denys Langlois, 1624.

89, [5] p.   15 cm.   [5109]
Bound with Heurtault, P. Le preservatif contre la peste. 1621.

—[The same.] ... Avec un preservatif asseuré contre la peste, composé & preparé par la Faculté de Medecine de Paris, assemblée pour cet effect. A costé de chaque remede est cotté combien il peut couster ... Lyon, Claude Armand, dit Alphonse, 1626.

[6], 63, [3] p.   15 cm.   [5110]
With this are bound: *his* Traicté de l'apothicairie du medecin charitable. 1626; Marque, J. de. Methodique introduction a la chirurgie. 1628.

—Le medecin charitable ... 12. ed. Paris, Denys Langlois, 1626.

101, [6] p.   15 cm.   [5111]
Contents as in the 1624 ed.
With this are bound *his*: Le prix et valeur des medicamens. 1625; L'apothiquairie du medecin charitable. 1625.

—[The same.] ... Augmenté d'un Discours du sené touchant ses vertus & proprietez, en suite un Advis salutaire de Galien sur la saignée. Ensemble La maniere d'embaumer les corps morts, avec un amble traicté de la peste ... Troyes, Nicolas Oudot, 1645.

[4], 268 p.   17 cm.   [5112]
Imperfect: p. 4 mutilated; upper margins of p. 235 trimmed.
The Traité du sené is by Antoine Mizauld, and Advis salutaire sur la saignée includes considerable portions of the Galenic text.
With this is bound *his* L'apotiquaire charitable. 1646.

—[The same, as subject.] *See* LAGNEAU, D. Traicté pour la conservation de la santé. 1650.

—Le prix et valeur des medicamens tant simples

que composés, desquels on se sert à la medecine . . . Paris, Denys Langlois, 1625.

71, [1] p. 15 cm. [5113]

Bound with *his* Le medecin charitable. Paris, 1626.

GUIDARELLUS, DOMINICUS [*fl.* 1641-1647] *See* COLLEGIO DEI MEDICI, Rome. Ordini. 1641; VATICAN. Protomedico generale. Tavola de prezzi delle robbe di spetiaria per tutto lo Stato Ecclesiastico. 1648.

GUIDE, PHILIPPE [*d.* 1718] Observations anatomiques, faites sur plusieurs animaux au sortir de la machine pneumatique . . . Paris, Thomas Moette, 1674.

[12], 45, [3] p. plate. 15 cm. [5114]

GUIDI, GUIDO [*ca.* 1500-1569] Vidi Vidii . . . Opera omnia; sive, Ars medicinalis, in qua cuncta quae ad humani corporis valetudinem praesentem tuendam, & absentem revocandam pertinent, methodo exactissima explicantur. Quae per Vidum Vidium juniorem diligentissime recognita, ac multis . . . partibus aucta, diuque expetita, nunc primum in Germania tota simul luci data . . . Francofurti ad Moenum, Typis & sumptibus Wechelianorum, apud Danielem & Davidem Aubrios & Clementem Schleichium, 1626.

3 v. in 2. illus. 37 cm. [5115]

—Les anciens et renommés autheurs de la medecine & chirurgie. Hippocrate: Des ulceres, Des fistules, Des playes de la teste, avec les commentaires de Guy Vide sur chacun livre. Hippocrate: Des fractures, Des articles, De l'officine du chirurgien, avec les commentaires de Galien. Galien: Des bandes. Oribase: Des lacqs, Des machines & engins. Le tout traduit fidelement du grec & du latin en françois par un docteur en medecine . . . Paris, Pierre Menard, 1634.

[4], 1148, [41] p. illus. 19 cm. [5116]

Translation of the collection edited by Guido Guidi and first published in 1544 under title: Chirurgia è Graeco in Latinum conversa.

Oribasius' Des lacqs and Des machines et engins are translations of books 43 and 45 of his Συναγωγαὶ ἰατριχαί.

Dedicatory epistle signed by Eustache d'Aubin and Jean Gesselin, the editors.

—Another issue, with imprint: Paris, Jean Gesselin, 1634.

[5117]

—Vidi Vidii . . . De anatome corporis humani

libri VII. Nunc primum in lucem editi . . . Venetiis, Apud Juntas, 1611.

[14], 342, [8] p.; 124 (i.e. 122) p. illus. 33 cm. [5118]

Part [2] has caption title: Vivi Vidii De chirurgia liber primus [-quartus]

GUIDI, GUIDO [16th-17th cent.] *ed. See* GUIDI, G. [*ca.* 1500-1569] Vidi Vidii . . . Opera omnia. 1626.

GUIDO DE CAULIACO. *See* GUY DE CHAULIAC, [*ca.* 1300-1368]

GUIDO, JEAN [*fl.* 1540] De mineralibus tractatus in genere . . . libri quatuor . . . Venetiis, Apud Thomam Ballionum, 1625.

[8], 208 (i.e. 198), [40] p. 23 cm. [5119]

GUIDON. *See* GUY DE CHAULIAC [*ca.* 1300-1368]

GUIDOTT, THOMAS [1638-1706] De thermis Britannicis tractatus. Accesserunt observationes hydrostaticae, chromaticae, & miscellaneae, uniuscujusque balnei apud Bathoniam naturam . . . exhibentes . . . Londini, Excudebat Franciscus Leach, sumptibus authoris, veneunt apud S. Smith, 1691.

[29], 412 p.; [1], 28, [16] p. front., illus., plates. 21 cm. [5120]

Part [2] has special title page: Observationum centuria, pleniorem in thermarum Bathoniensium naturam inquisitionem complectens.

—A discourse of Bathe, and the hot waters there. Also, some enquiries into the nature of the water of St. Vincent's rock, near Bristol: and that of Castle-Cary. To which is added, A century of observations, more fully declaring the nature . . . of the baths. With an account of The lives, and character, of the physicians of Bathe . . . London, Henry Brome, 1676.

[31], 200 p. illus., plates. 19 cm. [5121]

Added engraved title page.

A century of observations, and The lives . . . of the physicians of Bathe, have special title pages, the last one dated 1677.

—Gideon's fleece; or, The sieur de Frisk. An heroick poem. Written on the cursory perusal of a late book, call'd The conclave of physicians. By a friend of the muses . . . London, Sam. Smith, 1684.

[8], 30, [1] p. 19 cm. [5122]

Preface signed by Philo-Musus, pseud.

Concerns Gideon Harvey's The conclave of physicians.

—A quaere concerning drinking Bath-water, at

Bathe, resolved. By Eugenius Philander [pseud.] London, George Sawbridge, 1673.

[1], 26 p.   17 cm.   [5123]

—See JORDEN, E. A discourse of natural bathes. 1669, 1673.

GUIDUCCI, MARIO [1584-1646] *See* RONDINELLI, F. Relazione del contagio stato in Firenze l'anno. 1630. e 1633. 1634.

GUIGO DE CHAULHACO. *See* GUY DE CHAULIAC [*ca.* 1300-1368]

GUILANDINUS, MELCHIOR [1519 *or* 20-1589] De medicina Indorum. *In* Alpini, P. De medicina Aegyptiorum. 1645.

—Hortus Patavinus. Cui accessere . . . conjectanea synonimica plantarum eruditissima . . . Publicante Joan. Georg. Schenckio . . . Francofurti, Excudebat Mathaeus Becker, impensis Jo. Theo. & Jo. Israel de Brii, 1600. [Impensis vidua Johannis Theodori de Bry, 1608]

[10], 93 p.   plate.   17 cm.   [5124]

—See ALPINI, P. De plantis Aegypti. 1638-40.

GUILHEMET, TANNEQUIN. *See* GUILLAUMET, Tannequin [*fl.* 1575-1622]

GUILHELMUS TECENENSIS. *See* TECENENSIS, Guilhelmus [*fl.* 16th-17th cent.]

GUILLAUMET, TANNEQUIN [*fl.* 1575-1622] Livre xenodocal; c'est à dire, Hospitalier, ou lieu de pauvre sejour . . . Lyon, Pierre Rigaud, 1611.

[14], 146 p.   15 cm.   [5125]

Bound with copy 2 of *his* Traicté de maladie nouvellement appelee cristaline. 1611.

—Traicté de maladie nouvellement appelee cristaline, diligemment disputee suivant la doctrine nouvelle & ancienne . . . Lyon, Pierre Rigaud, 1611.

[24], 104 (i.e. 106), [14] p.   15 cm.   [5126]

—Copy 2.

With this are bound *his*: Livre xenodocal. 1611; Traicté des ouvertures. 1611.

—Traicté second de la maladie appellee cristaline. Autrement maladie Indiene, ou rongne Espagnole . . . Nismes, Jean Vaguenar, 1614.

[37], 174, [26] p.   15 cm.   [5127]

—Traicté des ouvertures, trous et ulceres spontanees, selon la doctrine nouvelle & ancienne . . .

Lyon, Pierre Rigaud, 1611.

96 p.   15 cm.   [5128]

Bound with copy 2 of *his* Traicté de maladie nouvellement appelee cristaline. 1611.

GUILLEMEAU, CHARLES [1588-1656] Cani miuro; sive, Curto fustis; hoc est, Caroli Guillemei . . . responsio pro se ipso ad alteram alogiam . . . Curti, Mompel. canis cellarii [i.e. Simeon Curtaudus] Lutetiae Parisiorum, 1654.

[4], 38 p.   23 cm.   [5129]

Concerns the Seconde apologie de l'université en medecine de Montpellier, in fact written by Isaac Cattier.

—Defensio altera, adversus impias, impuras . . . anonymi copreae calumnias ac contumelias. [Paris? 1648?]

49 p.   23 cm.   [5130]

Caption title.

Imprint supplied from BMC.

[—]Traicté des abus qui se commettent sur les procedures de l'impuissance des hommes & des femmes. Paris, Abraham Pacard, 1620.

42, [7] p.   17 cm.   [5131]

—[The same.] *In* Guillemeau, J. De la grossesse et accouchement des femmes. 1620, 1643.

—*praeses*. Question cardinale a disputer aux escholes de medecine . . . La methode d'Hippocrate est-elle la plus certaine, la plus seure, & la plus excellente de toutes, à guarir les maladies? . . . Paris, Nicolas Boisset, 1648.

[16], 94, 15 p.   23 cm.   [5132]

Text of dissertation in French and Latin.

Diss.—Paris (J. P. Moreau, *respondent*)

—, *ed.* and *tr. See* HIPPOCRATES. Aphorismi. Adaptations, etc. French. 1622.

—*See* GENIUS παντουλιδαμασ AD DIAM SCHOLAM APUD PARISIOS EMPIRICO-METHODICAM. 1654; LENONIS GUILLEMEI SCHOLAE PARISIENSIS EMPIRICO-METHODICAE DOCTORIS. 1654.

GUILLEMEAU, JACQUES [1550-1613] De la grossesse et accouchement des femmes; du gouvernement de'celles et moyen de survenir aux accidents qui leur arrivent, ensemble de la nourriture des enfans . . . Rev. et augm. . . . Avec un traitté de l'impuissance, par Charles Guillemeau . . . Paris, Abraham Pacard, 1620.

[20], 1049 p.; 42, [67] p.   illus.   18 cm.   [5133]

Engraved title page.

Imperfect: p. 41-42 of part [2] supplied in photocopy.

Part [2] has special title page: Traicté des abus qui se commettent sur les procedures de l'impuissance des hommes & des femmes.

— De la grossesse et accouchement des femmes, du gouvernement d'icelles; & moyen de survenir aux accidens qui leur arrivent: ensemble de la nourriture des enfans . . . Rev. & augm. . . . Avec un traité de l'impuissance, & un autre de la generation. Par M. Charles Guillemeau . . . Paris, Jean Jost, 1643.

[52], 803, [68] p. illus. 19 cm. [5134]

Added engraved title page dated 1642.

"Traité sur les abus qui se commettent sur les procedures de l'impuissance des hommes & des femmes": p. 775-803.

— [English tr.] Child-birth; or, The happy deliverie of women . . . Together with the diseases, which happen to women . . . and the meanes to helpe them. To which is added, a treatise of the diseases of infants . . . with the cure of them . . . London, A. Hatfield, 1612.

[16], 246 p.; [14], 118 p. illus. 20 cm. [5135]

Part 2 has special title page: The nursing of children . . . Together: with the meanes to helpe and free them, from all such diseases as may happen unto them.

STC 12496.

Bound with [Roeslin, Eucharius] The byrth of mankinde. [1613]

— [The same.] . . . London, Printed by Anne Griffin, for Joyce Norton, 1635.

[15], 247 p.; [14], 118 p. illus. 19 cm. [5136]

STC 12497.

— Les oeuvres de chirurgie . . . Augmentees et mises en un et enrichies de plusieurs traitez, pris des leçons de M^e. Germain Courtin . . . Paris, Nicolas Buon, 1612.

[50], 863, [32] p. illus. 36 cm. [5137]

— [The same.] . . . Rouen, Chez Jean Viret, François Vaultier, Clement Malassis et Jacques Besongne [De l'imprimerie de Pierre Maille] 1649.

[50], 863, [32] p. illus. 36 cm. [5138]

Different setting of type.

— Traité des maladies de l'oeil, qui sont en nombre de cent treize, ausquelles il est sujet . . . Lyon, Pierre Rigaud, 1610.

[30], 243, [3] p. 13 cm. [5139]

— [Dutch tr.] Hondert en dertien gebreken en genesinge der oogen . . . Vermeerdert door Mr.

Johannes Verbrigge . . . Nebens een kleyne beschrijvinge der tanden. Amsterdam, Jan Claesz. ten Hoorn, 1678.

[24], 232 p. front. 15 cm. [5140]

— [English tr.] A treatise of one hundred and thirteene diseases of the eyes, and eye liddes. The second time published, with some profitable additions . . . by Richard Banister . . . London, Imprinted by Felix Kyngston, for Thomas Man, 1622.

2 parts in 1 v. 15 cm. [5141]

Signatures: a–e^{12}, A–O^{12}, P.5.

Part [2] has special title page: A worthy treatise of the eyes. (Signature: e^9)

A reprint of A worthy treatise of the eyes, published in London, 1587-88, preceded by Banister's Breviary of the eyes.

Translated from the French by Anthony Hunton. Cf. Wellcome. STC 12499.5.

—, tr. See PARÉ, A. Wundt Artzney. 1601, 1635.

GUINTERIUS, JOANNES, *Andernacus* [1505-1574] Gynaeciorum commentarius, de gravidarum parturientium, puerperarum & infantium, cura. Nunc primum e Schenkiana bibliotheca in lucem emissus. Accessit elenchus auctorum in re medica cluentium, qui gynaecia scriptis clararunt & illustrarunt. Opera et studio Joan. Georgii Schenkii . . . Argentorati, Impensis Lazari Zetzneri, 1606.

56 p. 16 cm. [5142]

"Πίναξ auctorum in re medica . . . qui gynaecia, sive muliebria pleno argumento sive ex instituto scriptis excoluerunt & illustrarunt; e magno opere Pandectarum, et partitionum medicinalium propediem publicando . . . succinctius exscriptus": p. [37]-56, with special title page.

—, ed. See ORIBASIUS. *In* Aphorismos Hippocratis commentaria hactenus non visa. 1658.

—, tr. See GORRIS, P. de [*fl.* 1511] Formulae remediorum, quibus vulgo medici utuntur. 1612; REGIMEN SANITATIS SALERNITANUM. De conservanda bona valetudine. 1607, 1619 [and] Schola Salernitana. [Dutch tr.] 1658; VALLERIOLA, F. Artis medicae fundamina secundum Galenum. 1626.

— *See* SENNERT, D. De febribus libri IV. 1628, 1633, 1641, 1653.

GUIOTIUS, JOANNES. *See* GUYOT, Jean [*fl.* 1579]

GUIOTUS DE GARAMBERIO, JOANNES. *See* GUYOT, Jean [*fl.* 1579]

GUISSON, PIERRE [*fl.* 1665] Epistolica dissertatio de anonymo libello . . . ubi potissimum eventilatur principiorum chymicorum hypothesis. *In* Potier, P. Opera omnia medica, et chemica. 1666, 1698.

GUITIUS, JOANNES. *See* GUYOT, Jean [*fl.* 1579]

GULDINER APFFEL. 1635. *See* [TILEMANN, J.]

GULER VON WEINECK, JOHANN [1562-1637] Fiderisser Sawrbrunn: das ist, seiner Situation, Ursprungs, Natur, Würckung, Gebrauchs, und was darvon zu wüssen nutz und nothwendig, kurtze Andeütung ... Durch ... Johann Gulern von Weineck ... vermehret, und ... an Tag gegeben durch Andresen seinen Sohn ... [n. p.] 1642.

15 p.   21 cm.   [**5143**]

Imperfect: p. 3-4 wanting.

—, *ed. See* GULER VON WEINECK, J. Fiderisser Sawrbrunn. 1642.

GULIDEOLUS MORDICUS. *See* MORIDCUS, Gulideolus.

GULLMANN, BENEDIKT [*fl.* 1693-1697] *respondent.* *See* ORTLOB, J. F., *praeses.* Dissertatio medica de hydrae in hypochondriis nidulantis origine. 1696.

GULLMANN, BENEDIKT [*fl.* 1693-1697] *See* RIVINUS, A. Q. L. S. D. ... procancellarius Augustus Quirinus Rivinus. 1697.

GULSTON, THEODORE. *See* GOULSTON, Theodore [1572-1632]

GUMMERT, JOHANN [*fl.* 1681] *respondent.* [De peste] ... Argentorati, Typis Joh. Jacobi Folhopffii [1681]

[16] p.   20 cm.   [**5144**]

Diss. — Strasbourg.

GUMPERTZ, SALOMON [*fl.* 1684] *respondent.* Disputatio medica inauguralis de cephalalgia ... Lugduni Batavorum, Apud Abrahamum Elzevier, 1684.

[22] p.   22 cm.   [**5145**]

Diss. — Leyden.

GUNTER, JASPER. Catalogus librorum medicorum, juridicorum, mathematicorum, philologicorum ex bibliothecis Gasp. Gunteri Med. Doct. ... Una cum nonnullis libris Gallicis, Italicis, Hispanicis, &c. ... Quorum auctio habebitur Londini ... vicesimo die Martii, 168¾. Per Edvardum Millingtonum, bibliopolam. [London] 1684.

28 p.   23 cm.   [**5146**]

GUNTHER, ANTON. *See* BILLICH, Anton Günther [1598-1640]

GUNTHER, JOHANN [*fl.* 1608] *respondent.* Theses de methodo medendi ... Basileae, Per. Joan. Jacob. Genathium, 1608.

[8] p.   22 cm.   [**5147**]

Diss. — Basel.

GUSTEL, JOHANN GEORG [*fl.* 1618] *respondent.* Disputatio medica de hydrope ... Basileae, Joh. Jacobus Genathius [1618]

[23] p.   19 cm.   [**5148**]

Diss. — Basel.

GUTHERIUS, JACOBUS. *See* GOUTHIÈRE, Jacques [1568-1638]

GUTHIERRES, JACQUES. *See* GOUTHIÈRE, Jacques [1568-1638]

GUTIÉRREZ, LÁZARO JUAN. *See* LÁZARO GUTIÉRREZ, Juan [*fl.* 17th cent.]

GUTISCHOVIUS, GERARDUS. *See* GUTSCHOVEN, Gérard van [1615-1668]

GUTSCHOVEN, GÉRARD VAN [1615-1668] Description de cinq corps embaûmez et anatomisez, par le Sr Louis de Bils ... Bruxelles, G. Scheybels [1662?]

8 p.   19 cm.   [**5149**]

—*See* PLEMP, V. F. Ophthalmographia. 1659.

GUTTA podagrica: a treatise of the gout ... What diet is good for such as are troubled therewith. And some approved medicines and remedies for the same. Perused by P[hilemon] H[olland] Dr. in physick. London, Thomas Harper, 1633.

[5], 49 p.   19 cm.   [**5150**]

Editor's preface signed: H[enry] H[olland]
Attributed also to William Holland, son of Philemon and brother of Henry. Cf. Silvette, p. x, and p. 23.
STC 12539.

GUTTMANN, GOTTFRIED [*fl.* 1695] *respondent.* *See* HÄSSLER, J. J., *praeses.* De foeminis fortitudine sagata claris. 1695.

GUTZMER, JOHANN ALBERT [*fl.* 1700] *respondent.* *See* WILDVOGEL, C., *praeses.* Disputatio inauguralis de jure manus dextrae vom Rechte der Rechten Hand. 1700.

GUY DE CHAULIAC [*ca.* 1300–1368] [Chirurgia magna. Dutch.] De chirurgije van Guido de Cauliaco, seer profijtelijck voor alle chirurgijns. Uyt de Latijnsche in de Nederduytsche tale overgeset. Nu van nieuws oversien ende merckelijck verbetert door P. Nieustadt ... Amsterdam, Theunis Jacobsz, 1646.

[8], 430, [10] p. illus. 21 cm.   **[5151]**

A revision, by Pieter Nieustadt, of the Flemish translation by Josse van Sterthem of the Chirurgia magna; the translation was first published in Ghent ca. 1553. Cf. the editor's Voor-reden (p. [6]) and Nicaise, p. cxxxiv (no. 26–27)

—[French tr.] La grande chirurgie ... composée l'an de grace 1363. Resituée par M. Laurens Joubert ... Rouen, De l'imprimerie de Raphael du Petit Val, Chez David du Petit Val, 1615.

[32], 711, [24] p. port. 18 cm.   **[5152]**

With this is bound (as issued?) Joubert, L. Annotations ... sur toute la chirurgie de M. Guy de Chauliac. 1615.

—[The same.] ... Tournon, Claude Michel, 1619.
[28], 694, [14] p. 17 cm.   **[5153]**

—[The same.] ... Rouen, David du Petit Val, 1641.
[32], 711, [24] p. port. 17 cm.   **[5154]**
A reprint.

With this is bound (as issued?) Joubert, L. Annotations ... sur toute la chirurgie de M. Guy de Chauliac. 1641.

—[The same.] ... En ceste derniere ed., on a corrigé plusieurs fautes & manquements ... Lyon, Simon Rigaud, 1642.
[24], 605 (i.e. 601), [21] p. port. 18 cm.   **[5155]**

With this is bound (as issued?) Joubert, L. Annotations ... sur toute la chirurgie de M. Guy de Chauliac. Lyon, 1642.

—[The same.] ... Rouen, David du Petit Val. 1649.
[32], 711, [24] p. port. 18 cm.   **[5156]**
A reprint.

With this is bound (as issued?) Joubert, L. Annotations ... sur toute la chirurgie de M. Guy de Chauliac. 1649.

—[The same.] ... Lyon, Jacques Ollier, 1659.
[32], 711, [24] p. port. 18 cm.   **[5157]**
A reprint.

With this is bound (as issued?) Joubert, L. Annotations ... sur toute la chirurgie de ... Guy de Chauliac. 1659.

—[The same.] ... Traduite nouvellement en françois, & enrichie de plusieurs remarques, tant de theorie que de prattique, en forme de commentaire. Par Maistre Simon Mingelousaulx ... 1. ed.

Bourdeaux, Jacq. Mongiron Millanges, Pierre Du Cocq, Simon Boé, 1672.

[40], 460 (i.e. 462) p.; 760 p.; 175 p. 19 cm.   **[5158]**

Also issued in two volumes in the same year. Cf. Nicaise, p. cli, no. 57.

—[The same.] ... Tome premier [-second] ... Bourdeaux, & se vend a Paris, Chez Laurent d'Houry, 1683.

2 v. 19 cm.   **[5159]**

A reissue of the sheets of the Bordeaux edition of 1672, with new title pages, some slight typographical changes, and differences in arrangement.

—[The same. French excerpts.] *In* Courtin, G. Leçons anatomiques et chirurgicales. 1612, 1656.

—[The same, *as subject.*] *See* FALCON, J. Remarques sur la Chirurgie de M. Guy de Chauliac. 1649.

—Les fleurs du grand Guidon, c'est à dire, les sentences principales de certains chapitres ... Par M. Racul [sic] ... Paris, Jacques de La Carrieres [n. d.]

128 p. illus. 11 cm.   **[5160]**

An abridgment by Jean Raoul of the Chirurgia magna.

—[The same.] ... Par Maistre Jean Raoul chirurgien ... Rouen, Daniel Loudet, 1646.
142 p. 14 cm.   **[5161]**

Imperfect: Sig. f12 (blank?) wanting.
Bound with Hippocrates. Les aphorismes. 1646.

—[The same.] ... Rouen, Jacques Besongne, 1660.
142 p. 14 cm.   **[5162]**

Different setting of type.
Issued also as part [2] of Hippocrates. Les Aphorismes ... Derniere ed. ... augm. des Fleurs du grand Guidon. Rouen, 1660.

—[The same.] ... Corr. & augm. De la pratique de chirurgie, avec plusieurs experiences & secrets. Et de la methode de consulter pour les jeunes chirurgiens. Extraicte des leçons de ... L. Meysonnier ... Lyon, Simon Potin, 1673.
[8], 216, [12] p. 15 cm.   **[5163]**

—[The same.] ... Pau, Jerôme Du Poux, 1693.
[4], 108 p. 15 cm.   **[5164]**

Imperfect: contains Les Fleurs only.

—Le maistre en chirurgie; ou, L'abregé de la Chirurgie de Guy de Chauliac ... Dressé en faveur des jeunes aspirans. Par Mr Verduc, maître chirurgien juré de Paris. Paris, Laurent d'Houry, 1691.

[24], 286, [1] p.   15 cm.   **[5165]**

Errata: p. [1] at end.

Described in the publisher's epistle in the 3d edition (1704) as chiefly the work of Laurent Verduc, the younger, though the first two editions were commonly attributed to the elder Laurent Verduc.

In his epistle, Verduc acknowledges that he took the "Traité des choses naturelles, non naturelles, & contre nature" (p. 51-101) from the works of Jean Fernel.

—[The same.] . . . 2. éd., revuë & augmentée d'un Manuel instructif sur l'osteologie. Mar. M. Verduc . . . Paris, Laurent d'Houry, 1697.

[16], 366, [2] p.   17 cm.   **[5166]**

Contents as in the 1691 ed. except for the "Avis du libraire" which is omitted.

"Manuel instructif sur l'osteologie" (by the younger Laurent Verduc): p. 193-248.

—[Italian tr.] Il maestro in chirurgia; o, Compendio della Chirurgia di Guido da Chauliaco . . . Tradotto dalla francese nella nostra lingua toscana da Giulio Cesare Arizzarra . . . e in questa traduzione ampliato di moltissime materie, con aggiunta in principio delle condizioni del buon chirurgo, ed in fine d'un trattatto de' tumori, e fistole dell'ano . . . Coll'aggiunta Dell' operazioni chirurgiche fondate sopra la struttura della parte, segni, sintomi, e loro esplicazioni, e un'idea generale delle ferite, di Giuseppe della Charriere. Firenze, Piero Matini, 1697.

468 p.   front.   15 cm.   **[5167]**

The treatise by La Charrière is a translation of Traité des opérations de chirurgie . . . et une idée générale des playes.

—*See* Abeille, S. L'anatomie de la teste. 1689 [and] Le parfait chirurgien. 1696; Joubert, L. Annotations . . . sur toute la chirurgie de M. Guy de Chauliac. 1615, 1619, 1641, 1642, 1649, 1659; Lambert, A. Les commentaires. 1662, 1671, 1677; Ranchin, F. Questions en chirurgie. 1604, 1627, 1628; [Dutch tr.] 1662.

GUYBERT, Philbert. *See* Guibert, Philbert [1579?-1633]

GUYON, Louis, *sieur de la Nauche* [*d. ca.* 1630] Les diverses leçons . . . Divisees en cinq livres. Contenans plusieurs histoires . . . recueillis des autheurs grecs, latins, françois . . . Rev., corr., & augm. par l'autheur en ceste 2. ed. . . . Lyon, Claude Morillon [1610]

[24], 913, [21] p.   16 cm.   **[5168]**

Imprint partly supplied from colophon.

Imperfect: vol. 1 only, title page mutilated affecting imprint; upper margins trimmed.

Vol. 2 was published in 1613. Cf. BNC.

—Le miroir de la beauté, et santé corporelle. Contenant toutes les difformitez & maladies, tant internes qu'externes, qui peuvent survenir au corps humain. Avec leurs definitions, causes, signes & remedes usitez de toute ancienneté, modernes & spagirics; ensemble les prognostics . . . Derniere ed., rev., & corr. d'une infinité de fautes: et augm. d'un Traicté des maladies extraordinaires, & nouvelles. Par M. L. Meyssonnier . . . Lyon, Claude Prost, 1643.

1 v.   18 cm.   **[5169]**

Imperfect: vol. 1 only; added engraved title page wanting.

—[The same.] . . . Le cours de medecine en francois, contenant Le miroir de beauté et santé corporelle, par M. Louys Guyon Dolois, sieur de la Nauche . . . et la Theorie avec un accomplissement de practique selon les principes tant dogmatiques, que chymiques, adjoustées à cette 4. ed. . . . par M. Lazare Meyssonnier . . . Lyon, Claude Prost, 1664.

2 v. in 1.   illus., plates.   23 cm.   **[5170]**

Imperfect: 3d-4th prelim. leaves (sig. ẽ2-3) in v. 2 wanting; fold. plate in Theorie de la medecine wanting.

Le miroir de la beauté et santé corporelle, first published in 1615, was reprinted with additions by Lazare Meyssonnier, and beginning in 1664 appeared under title: Le cours de medecine.

The Theorie de la medecine by Lazare Meyssonnier has special title page and separate pagination.

—[The same.] . . . 5. et derniere ed. . . . augm. d'un discours des maladies veneneuses qui manquoient à la precedente, & d'une methode pour apprendre en bref la medecine par l'usage de la doctrine de l'auteur mise à la fin. Lyon, J. Ant. Huguetan, & Guill. Barbier, 1671.

2 v. in 1.   illus., plates.   24 cm.   **[5171]**

Contents as in the 1664 ed.

—[The same.] . . . 6. et derniere ed. . . . Lyon, Daniel Gayet, & Jaques Faeton, 1673.

2 v. in 1.   plates.   24 cm.   **[5172]**

Imperfect: plate in Theorie de la medecine wanting.

—[The same.] . . . 7. et derniere ed. . . . Lyon, Guillaume Barbier, 1678.

2 v. in 1.   plates.   24 cm.   **[5173]**

GUYOT, Jean [*fl.* 1579] Divinae naturae, artisque sacrae triumphus. Hoc est, enarratio . . . insignis, rari . . . at naturalis, non miraculosi affectus

... Basileae, Typis Georgii Deckeri, 1653.
70, [1] p.   16 cm.   [5174]

GWINNE, Matthew [1558?–1627] Aurum non aurum; sive, In assertorem chymicae sed verae medicinae desertorem Fra. Antonium adversaria ... Antverpiae, Prostant apud Hieronymum Verdussen, 1613.

[12], 251 [1] p.   21 cm.   [5175]
Imperfect: p. [1–8] mutilated.

GWYNN, Matthaeus. *See* Gwinne, Matthew [1558?–1627]

GWYNTHER VON ANDERNACH, Johann. *See* Guinterius, Joannes, Andernacus [1505–1574]

GYRALDUS, Johannes Baptista. *See* Giraldi, Giovanni Battista [1662–1732]

GYSENDÖRFFER, Balthasar [*fl.* 1660] *respondent*. *See* Stupanus, E., *praeses*. Disputatio physico-medica de humanae mentis facultatibus. 1660.

H

H., A. *See* Hay, Alexander [*fl.* 1689–1697]

H., A. *See* Hunton, Anthony [*ca.* 1560–1624]

H., D. D. D. V. *See* Valverde de Horozco, Diego de [17th cent.]

H., F. *See* Herring, Francis [*d.* 1628]

H., H. *See* Holland, Henry [1583–1650?]

H., H., *tr. See* Bontekoe, C. Fragmenta. German.

H., I. [*fl.* 1616] *ed. See* Scheunemann, H. Medicina reformata. 1617.

H., J., *Esquire. See* Halfpenny, John.

H., J., *D. M. L. See* Portatile medicum. 1680.

H., J., *M. A. See* Harris, John [1641?–1682]

H., J., *Oxon. See* Harding, John.

H., J. R. *See* Rist, Johannes [1607–1667]

H., P., *Dr. in physick. See* Holland, Philemon [1552–1637]

H., R. J., *tr. See* Bontekoe, C. Kurtze Abhandlung von dem menschlichen Leben. 1686.

H., S. *See* Regimen Sanitatis Salernitanum. The Englishmans doctor. 1624.

H., S. *See* Stubbs, Henry [1632–1676]

H., S. *See* [Valentinus, P. P.] Enchiridion medicum. 1612.

H., S., *tr. See* Hippocrates. [Aphorismi. English.] 1610, 1655.

H., S., *student in physic. See* Haworth, Samuel [*b.* 1660?]

H., S., *student in physicke. See* Hobbes, Stephen [*fl.* 1596–1610]

H. D. M. *See* Desmarets, Henri.

H. S. P. *See* P., H. S. [*fl.* 1682]

HAACK, Johann Friedrich [*fl.* 1678] *respondent*. *See* Amling, J. Dissertatio inauguralis. 1678.

HAARLEM. Collegium Medicum. *See* Collegium Medicum, Haarlem.

HAARLEM. Ordinances, local laws, etc. Alsoo mijn heeren van den gherechte deser stadt Haerlem ... die ghepleeght ende ghehouden werd int begraven van de persoonen die van de heete sieckte der peste zijn gestorven ... Haerlem, Adriaen Roman, 1636.
broadside.   50 x 41 cm.   [5176]

HAARLEM. Senate. *See* Pharmacopoea Harlemensis senatus auctoritate munita. 1693.

HABDARRAHMAN ASIUTENSIS. *See* al-Suyūtī [1445–1505]

HABERKORN, Adam [*fl.* 1638–1641] *praeses. See* Rolfinck, W., *praeses*. Disputatio medica, de febris malignae natura et curatione. 1638.

HABERLAND, János Godofréd [*fl.* 1689] *respondent*. *See* Vesti, J., *praeses*. Disputatio medica inauguralis de medico felici et infelici. 1689.

HABERMAN, Kaspar [*fl.* 1663] *praeses*. Discursus physicus de habitibus naturalibus intellectus et voluntatis et influxu eorum ... Lipsiae, Typis Johannis Wittigau [1663]

[16] p. 20 cm. [5177]

Diss.—Leipzig (F. Christiani, *respondent*)

HABERMASS, GEORG CHRISTOPH [*fl.* 1687–1690] *respondent. See* ORTLOB, J. F. De rhachitide. 1687; VESTI, J., *praeses*. Disputatio inauguralis medica de abortu. 1690.

HABERSACK, JOHANN KARL [*fl. ca.* 1673–1679] Relation, in welcher beygebracht wird, was gestalten die Wiennerische Neustatt mit der Pest angesteckt worden, sie man sich ... verhalten, was für Praeservativ-Mittel gebraucht ... worden ... Wienn, Leopold Voigt, 1681.

[6], 138, [14] p. 15 cm. [5178]

Imperfect: title page mutilated.

HABERT DE MONTMOR, HENRI LOUIS [*d.* 1679] *ed. See* GASSENDI, P. Opera omnia. 1658.

HABICOT, NICOLAS [1550–1624] Antigigantologie; ou, Contrediscours de la grandeur des geans ... Paris, Jean Corrozet, 1618.

[8], 182, [1] p. 19 cm. [5179]

—Gygantosteologie; ou, Discours des os d'un geant ... Paris, Jean Houzé, 1613.

[12], 60 (i.e. 61) p. table. 18 cm. [5180]

—Paradoxe myologiste, par lequel est demonstré contre l'opinion vulgaire ... que le diaphragme, n'est un seul muscle ... Paris, Jean Houzé, 1610.

[8], 61 p. 18 cm. [5181]

—Problemes sur la nature, preservation, et cure de la maladie pestilentielle ... Paris, Jean Houzé, 1607.

[14], 200, [8] p. 16 cm. [5182]

—Problesmes medecinaux et chirurgicaux ... Paris, Jean Corrozet, 1617.

110 p. 18 cm. [5183]

—Semaine, ou, practique anatomique. Par laquelle est enseigné par leçons le moyen de desassembler les parties du corps humain les unes d'avec les autres, sans les interesser ... Paris, Martin Colet, 1631.

321 (i.e. 320), [4] p. tables. 17 cm. [5184]

—[The same.] ...Nouv. ed., rev., & corr. ...

Paris, Michel Robin, 1660.

320, [4] p. tables. 19 cm. [5185]

Different setting of type.

HABRECHT, ISAAC [*d.* 1633] *ed. See* ZETZNER, L., *ed.* Theatrum chemicum. 1659–61.

HABRISCH, ELIAS [*fl.* 1630] *respondent. See* SEBISCH, M. [1578–1674?] *praeses*. Exercitationes medicae. 1639.

HADDEN, JAAKOB VAN [*fl.* 1656] Pleuris; ofte, Zyde-wees genesing sonder aderlaten ... Amsterdam, Jacob Lescaille, 1657.

29 p. 14 cm. [5186]

Imperfect: lower margins trimmed.

—Pleuris; ofte, Zyde-wees genesinge zonder aderlaten tegen Joan Baptist van Lamzweerdes ... nadenkinge vaster gesteld ... Amsterdam, Voor Gebrant Schagen [Gedrukt by Kornelis de Bruyn] 1660.

[8], 87, [1] p. 16 cm. [5187]

HAEBERLIN, BALTHASAR [*fl.* 1623] *respondent. See* SEBISCH, M. [1578–1674?] *praeses*. Exercitationes medicae. 1639.

Ein HÄITERER philosophischer Tag. *See* HARPRECHT, J. Sudum philosophicum, pro secretis chymicis perspiciendis. 1660.

HÄNDEL, CHRISTOPH CHRISTIAN [*d.* 1734] *respondent. See* OMEIS, M. D., *praeses*. Dissertatio de eruditis Germaniae mulieribus. 1688.

HAERING, JOHANN PETER. *See* FEDERER, J. J. Brevis et compendiosa febris Ungaricae curandae ... methodus. 1624.

HÄRLIN, JOHANN KASPAR [*fl.* 1675–1677] *respondent. See* METZGER, G. B., *praeses*. Dissertatio inauguralis medica de haemorrhoidum statu s. et p. n. 1677.

HAESBAERT, JAN WILLEM [*fl.* 1668] *respondent*. Disputatio medica inauguralis de fame laesa ... Lugduni Batavorum, Apud viduam & haeredes Joannis Elsevirii, 1668.

[12] p. 21 cm. [5188]

Diss.—Leyden.

HAESBERT, MARTIN JOHANN [*fl.* 1679] *respondent*. Dissertationem inauguralem de hydrope, von der Wassersucht ... exponit Martinus Johannes

Haesbaert . . . Marpurgi Cattorum, Typis Caspari & Josephi-Dieterici Göringiorum [1679]

[1], 30 p.   20 cm.   [5189]

Diss. — Marburg.

HÄSSLER, JOHANN JAKOB [*fl.* 1695] *praeses.* De foeminis fortitudine sagata claris . . . Lipsiae, Literis Johannis Coleri [1695]

[40] p.   19 cm.   [5190]

Diss. — Leipzig (G. Guttmann, *respondent*)

HÄYNER, CHRISTIAN [*fl.* 1671] *respondent. See* MADEWEIS, F., *praeses.* De filamentis d. Virginis. 1671.

HAFACKER, GILLES [*fl.* 1678] Leer om leer, voor Petrus van den Bosch . . . nevens een geluckwensching aen sijn vader, Mr. Gerard van den Bosch, over het horribel mirakel, aen sijne soon geschiet dat hy van stom sprekende is geworden . . . Utrecht, Johannes Borculo, 1678.

32 p.   16 cm.   [5191]

HAFENREFFER, JAKOB [*fl.* 1676-1677] *respondent. See* BROTBECK, J. K., *praeses.* Disputatio medica de hydrope ascite. 1676; METZGER, G. B., *praeses.* Urocriterium brevibus thesibus exhibitum. 1677.

HAFENREFFER, SAMUEL [1587-1660] Monochordon symbolico-biomanticum. Abstrusissimam pulsuum doctrinam, ex harmoniis musicis dilucide, figurisque oculariter demonstrans . . . Ulmae, Typis & impensis Balthasari Kühnen, 1640.

[14], 146 p.   illus., plates.   16 cm.   [5192]

Imperfect: Last preliminary leaf wanting? Preliminary leaves and p. 1-4 mutilated.

—Nosodochium, in quo cutis, eique adhaerentium partium, affectus omnes, singulari methodo, et cognoscendi et curandi . . . traduntur; quod etiam variis medicamentis Galencis, chymicis, cosmeticis . . . est illustratum . . . sub calcem adjecti tibicines, lectorem, Arabica, Graeca, Latina & Germanica contenta, indagare succincte informant. Renovatum & plurimis in locis auctum . . . Ulmae, Typis & expensis Balthasar. Kühnen, 1660.

554, [25] p.   illus., plates.   17 cm.   [5193]

Added engraved title page.
Errata: p. [23-25]

—Officina iatrica, continens pharmaca selecta Hippocratico-Galenica, & Hermetico-Paracelsica, juxta morborum seriem, causarumque indicem disposita & condita . . . Ulmae, Apud Balthasar

Kühnen, 1653.

[16], 204, [3] p.   17 cm.   [5194]

Added engraved title page.
Errata: p. [3] at end.

—πανδοχεῖον αἰλόδερμον in quo cutis eique adhaerentium partium, affectus omnes, singulari methodo, et cognoscendi & curandi . . . traduntur . . . Tubingae, Typis & expensis Joh. Contr. Geysleri, 1630.

[14], 582, [25] p.   17 cm.   [5195]

Errata: p. [25]
Bound with Cornacchini, M. Methodus. 1628.

—Raphael artem medicam feliciter cum inchoandi, tum continuandi, absolvendi, tractandique fideliter informans. Nec non rationes peregrinandi, et pharmacopolia visitandi aphoristice docens. Revelatus per Samuelem Hafenrefferum . . . Tubingae, Theodoricus Werlin, 1622.

[1], 101 p.   13 cm.   [5196]

"Caroli Paschalii oratio" (physician's prayer, from Paschal's Christianae preces): p. 67-73.

—[The same.] Raphael artem medicam explanans, cum Velo temporis, & Anchora precum hac II. editione auctior: productus per Samuelem Hafenrefferum . . . Francofurti, Impensis Joan. Berneri, 1629.

144 p.   illus., plate.   15 cm.   [5197]

"De velo temporis commonefactio" (p. 96-121) contains calendar tables. "In anchoram precum" (p. 122-144) contains miscellaneous prayers, including Charles Paschal's "Precatio pro felicitate praxeos."

—Copy 2. 16 cm.

With this are bound: Strobelberger, J. S. Brevissima manuductio ad curandos pueriles affectus. 1625; Münster, J. Discussio eorum quae ab Abrahamo Schopffio . . . scripta sunt. 1603.

—[The same.] Raphael ὅδιος de arte medica, velo temporis, litationibus, tertium locupletior ingrediens, ad ἀκροατήιον Apollineum divertere persuasus; a Samuele Hafenreffero . . . Ulmae, Typis & impensis Balthasari Kühnen, 1642.

[3], 355, [17] p.   illus., plates, tables.   16 cm.
                                                 [5198]

Added engraved title page: Raphael artem medicam pandens Veloque temporis Anchoram precum affigens Thessalos III salutans . . .

"De velo temporis commonefactio" (p. 195-245) contains calendar tables.

"In anchoram precum" (246-283) contains miscellaneous prayers, including Charles Paschal's "Precatio pro felicitate praxeos."

"Aphorismorum Hippocratis sectio I[-VII]: p. 284-328; "Hippocratis Coi Praesagiorum. Liber I[-III]": p. 328-355.

HAGA, David de Haga, *Baron von de. See* Spina, David de [1662-1710]

HAGEDORN, Christoph [*b.* 1663] *respondent. See* Schelhammer, G. C., *praeses.* Dissertationem inauguralem medicam de febrifugorum natura agendi et applicandi modo ... publicae ... disquisitioni sistit ... C. H. 1694.

—*See* Crause, R. W. Decanus ... Collegii Medici Rudolfus Guilielmus Crausius ... lectori benevolo S. P. D. 1694.

HAGELSHEIM, Gottfried Held von. *See* Held von Hagelsheim, Gottfried [1670-1724]

HAGEN, Friedrich Kaspar [17th-18th cent.] *See* Stübner, A. G., *praeses.* De lunae viribus in haec inferiora et inprimis oceanum. 1700.

HAGEN, Johann Heinrich [1669-1708] *respondent. See* Hoffmann, F. [1660-1742] *praeses.* Disputatio solennis medico-practica tradens historiam variolarum epidemice Halae grassantium. 1699.

HAGEN, Johann von. *See* Indagine, Joannes ab [*ca.* 1467-1537]

HAGENBUT, Johann. *See* Cornarius, Janus [1500-1558]

HAGENDORN, Ehrenfried [1640-1692] Cynosbatologia ad normam Academiae Naturae-Curiosorum adornata. Jenae, Impensis Johannis Bielckii, 1681.

[28], 191, [14] p.   plates.   17 cm.   [5199]
Engraved title page.
Bound with Nenter, Georg Philipp. Theoriae hominis aegroti. Argentorati, 1716.

—Observationum et historiarum medico-practicarum rariorum centuriae tres, quibus annexa Analecta quaedam ad historias nonnullas illustrandas. Francofurti & Lipsiae, Sumptibus Johannis Wilischii, literis Johannis Coleri, 1698.

[12], 423, [46] p.   illus., plates.   17 cm.
                                          [5200]
Added engraved title page.
Errata: p. [43-46]

—Tractatus physico-medicus, de catechu; sive, Terra Japonica, in vulgus sic dicta, ad norman Academiae Naturae-Curiosorum. Jenae, Impensis Johannis Bielkii, typis Samuelis Krebsii, 1679.

[23], 81, [1] p.   front.   17 cm.   [5201]

—*respondent. See* Schenck, J. T., *praeses.* Disputationem inauguralem de macie puerorum ex fascino ... submittit ... E. H. 1667.

HAGENS, Johann. *See* Haghens, Jan [*fl.* 1574-1604]

HAGENS, Matthijs. *See* Haghens, Matthijs [*fl.* 1616]

HAGER, Abraham Achatius [*fl.* 17th cent.] Aloe chorae salitiana ... Alteburgi, Typis Joh. Bernh. Bauerfinccii [1663]

[12] p.   19 cm.   [5202]

HAGER, Achatius [*fl.* 1661] *respondent.* Disputatio medica inauguralis de febribus in genere ... Lugduni Batavorum, Ex officina Petri Didier, 1661.

[20] p.   19 cm.   [5203]
Diss. — Leyden.

HAGER, Johann Joachim [*fl.* 1666-1670] Judicium et consilium medicum, uber die zu dieser Zeit grassirende Durchfälle, wie man sich dabey verhalten, praeserviren und ... curiren solle ... Weissenfels, Johann Brühl, 1676.

[32] p.   20 cm.   [5204]

—*respondent. See* Rolfinck, W., *praeses.* Disputatio medica inauguralis de salivatione. 1670.

HAGER, Lorenz [*fl.* 1594] *See* Nutzlicher unnd kurtzer Bericht, Regiment und Ordnung. 1611.

HAGHENS, Jan [*fl.* 1574-1604] Den lust-hof der medecijnen: inhoudende den gront van alle cranckheden ende ghebreken ... Beschreven ende nagelaten by ... Joannes Hagius, ende nu eerst int licht ghebracht door ... Matthijs Haghens ... Dordrecht, Isaack Jansz. Canin, 1616.

[12], 617, [36] p.   port.   31 cm.   [5205]

—*See* Vigo, G. de. Medecyn boec, ende chyrurgie. 1614.

HAGHENS, Matthijs [*fl.* 1616] *ed. See* Haghens, J. Den lust-hof der medecijnen. 1616.

HAGIUS, Christoph [*fl.* 1650] *respondent. See* Seelmann, C., *praeses.* Mors homini inevitabilis. 1650.

HAGIUS, Joannes. *See* Haghens, Jan [*fl.* 1574-1604]

HAGUE. Collegium Medicum. *See* Collegium Medicum, Hague.

HAHN, Adam [*fl.* 1667–1668] *respondent. See* Friderici, J. A., *praeses.* Ταραχολόγια; sive, De tabaco dissertatio. 1667.

HAHN, Christian [*fl.* 1700] *respondent. See* Eysel, J. P., *praeses.* Disputatio inauguralis medica, de febri petechiali. 1700.

HAHN, Sigmund [1664–1742] *respondent. See* Rivinus, A. Q., *praeses.* Dissertatio physiologica de visu. 1686.

HAIM. *See* Haimo, *Bp. of Halberstadt* [*d.* 853]

HAIMO, *Bp. of Halberstadt* [*d.* 853] Epistola . . . de quatuor lapidibus philosophicis materiam suam ex minori mundo desumentibus.

    497–501 p., vol. 6. 20 cm. (*In* Zetzner, Lazarus, *ed.* Theatrum chemicum. Argentorati, 1659–61)   [**5206**]
    Caption title.

HAINLIN, Sebastian [1594–1663 *respondent. See* Hofmann, C., *praeses.* Disputatio de venarum origine secundum Aristotelem. 1615.

HAINTZEL, Tobias Jakob [*fl.* 1662–1663] *respondent.* Disputatio inauguralis de catarrho . . . Argentorati, Typis Eberhardi Welperi, 1663.
    16 p.   19 cm.   [**5207**]
    Diss. — Strasbourg.

    —*respondent. See* Sebisch, J. A., *praeses.* Disputatio exhibens problemata quaedam anatomica. 1662.

HAIO, Gerbrandus [*fl.* 1618] *respondent.* Disputatio inauguralis de apoplexia . . . Lugduni Batavorum, Henricus ab Hastens, 1618.
    [11] p.   21 cm.   [**5208**]
    Diss. — Leyden.

HAIUS, Alexandrus. *See* Hay, Alexander [*fl.* 1689–1697]

HAKE, Robert [*fl.* 1688] *respondent. See* Schrader, F., *praeses.* Exercitatio medica de doloribus. 1688.

HAKEWILL, George [1578–1649] The vanitie of the eye . . . The 3d. ed. by the author . . . Oxford, Joseph Barnes, 1615.
    [6], 170, [18] p.   13 cm.   [**5209**]
    STC 12622.

HALBACH, Christian [*fl.* 1657] *respondent.*

Disputatio inauguralis medica de dolore capitis . . . [Altdorffii] Charactere Georgi Hagen [1657]
    [28] p.   22 cm.   [**5210**]
    Diss. — Altdorf.

HALBERSTADT. Ordinances, local laws, etc. Rahts zu Halberstadt abgefassete Apotheken-Ordnung und revidirte Taxa. Halberstadt, Zu finden in Christian Genschen Buchhandlung, 1697.
    [23], 74, [18] p.   22 cm.   [**5211**]
    Added engraved half title.

HALBERSTÄDTISCHES Pest-Bedencken, beides zur Praeservation und Curation, auff obrigkeitlichen Befehl, von denen Medicis daselbst gestellet und ausgefertiget. [n. p.] 1680.
    24 p.   14 cm.   [**5212**]
    A reprint of Kurtzer und einfältiger Bericht, wie man in Zeit der jetzo regierenden Pestilentz . . . verhalten soll, published in Halberstadt in 1597.

HALBMAYER, Johann Georg [*fl.* 1624–1626] *respondent. See* Ager, N. Disputatio physica de nutritione. 1624; Charstadius, V., *praeses.* Disputationum medicarum secunda de sanitate ejusque subjecto. 1626; Sebisch, M. [1578–1674?] *praeses.* Exercitationes medicae. 1639.

[**HALE**, Sir Matthew, 1609–1676] An essay touching the gravitation, or non-gravitation of fluid bodies, and the reasons thereof. The 2d ed. with Some occasional additions. London, Printed by W. Godbid for William Shrowsbury, 1675.
    [6], 88, 23 p.   illus.   16 cm.   [**5213**]

    —The primitive origination of mankind, considered and examined according to the light of nature . . . London, Printed by William Godbid, for William Shrowsbery, 1677
    [11], 380 p.   front. (port.), illus.   33 cm.   [**5214**]

HALFPENNY, John. The gentleman's jockey, and approved farrier: instructing in the natures, causes, and cures of all diseases incident to horses . . . With divers other curiosities collected by the long practice . . . of J[ohn] H[alfpenny] Esquire [and others]. The 4th ed. . . . London, Hen. Twyford and Nath. Brook, 1676.
    [16], 300, [4] p.   illus.   18 cm.   [**5215**]
    Imperfect: sig. A2 mutilated.
    Mainly extracted from Gervase Markham's works. Cf. Smith, vol. 1, p. 323.

HALL, Francis, *Father* [1595-1675] *See* Boyle, *Hon.* R. New experiments physico-mechanical, touching the air. 1662, 1682 [and] Nova experimenta physico-mechanica de vi aëris elastica. 1669.

HALL, George, *Bp. of Chester* [1612?-1668] A fast-sermon, preached to the lords in the high-court of Parliament assembled, on the day of solemn humiliation for the continuing pestilence, Octob. 3. 1666 . . . London, Timothy Garthwait, 1666.

    [1], xxx p. 20 cm.   **[5216]**

HALL, John [1575-1635] Select observations on English bodies: or, Cures both empericall and historicall, performed upon . . . persons in desperate diseases. First, written in Latine . . . Now put into English . . . by James Cooke . . . London, John Sherley, 1657.

    [24], 316 p. 15 cm.   **[5217]**
    Imperfect: first preliminary leaf (longitudinal label) wanting.

  —[The same.] . . . To which is now added, An hundred like counsels and advices, for several honourable persons, by the same author. In the close is added, Directions for drinking of the bath-water, and Ars cosmetica, or Beautifying art, by H. Stubbs . . . London, Printed by J. D. for Benjamin Shirley, 1679.

    [30], 350 p. port. (front.) 18 cm.   **[5218]**
    Imperfect: Directions for such as drink the bath-water, and Ars cosmetica (p. 337-350) wanting.
    "Directions for such as drink the bath-water" are "revised and approved by Sir Alexander Frasier."

  —[The same.] . . . London, William Marshall, 1683.

    [30], 350 p. port. 18 cm.   **[5219]**
    Imperfect: port. wanting.
    A reissue of the 1679 edition, with new title page.

HALL, Joseph, *Bp. of Norwich* [1574-1656] *See* Butler, J. Ἁγιαστρολογία. 1680.

HALLING, Pieter [*fl.* 1678] Bekentmakinge aen Doctor van Yperen. [Amsterdam, 1678]

    [2] p. 16 cm.   **[5220]**
    Written in answer to allegations by Jan Baptist van Lamsweerde.

HALLYWELL, Henry [1640?-1703] Melampronoea; or, A discourse of the polity and kingdom of darkness . . . With a solution of the . . . objections brought against the being of witches . . . London, Walter Kettilby, 1681.

    [16], 118 p. 16 cm.   **[5221]**

HALMAAL, Jacob van [*fl.* 1689] Ontleding over d'Amsterdamsche apotheek; ofte, Nodige opmerkingen over de handelingen der compositien en praeparatien van de selve . . . Amsterdam, Jan ten Hoorn, 1689.

    [16], 246, [10] p. plates. 16 cm.   **[5222]**
    Added engraved title page.

HAMAND, Henry. Ourography: or, Speculations on the excrements of urine . . . Also, a philosophicall discourse of the colours of urine, with the art of mixing them, according to quantity, number, and weight . . . London, Francis Eglesfield, 1655.

    [16], 83, [29] p. col. illus. 15 cm.   **[5223]**
    Imperfect: preliminary leaves (p. [1-4]) and p. [24, 25, 29] mutilated; p. 65-80 wanting.

  —[The same.] . . . London, Printed by R. D. for Francis Eglesfield and sold by William Ballard, 1656.

    [16], 83, [29] p. illus. 15 cm.   **[5224]**
    Imperfect: title page mutilated.
    A reissue of the 1655 edition with new title page.

HAMBERGER, Georg Albrecht [1662-1716] *praeses.* Dissertatio optica de coloribus . . . Jenae, Litteris Krebsianis [1689]

    40 p. 20 cm.   **[5225]**
    Diss.—Jena (C. F. Fischer, *respondent*)

  —Dissertatio physica de elatere . . . Jenae, Literis Christophori Krebsii [1699]

    35, [1] p. plate. 20 cm.   **[5226]**
    Diss.—Jena (C. Wedel, *respondent*)

HAMBUT, Johann. *See* Cornarius, Janus [1500-1558]

HAMEL, Joachim Friedrich [*fl.* 1691] *respondent.* *See* Albinus, B. Dissertatio solennis medica de cardialgia. 1691.

HAMEL, Marin [*fl.* 1657] Discours sommaire et methodique de la cure & preservation de la peste . . . Rouen, 1658.

    [8], 75 p. 15 cm.   **[5227]**

HAMER, Johann Hermann [*fl.* 1692] *respondent.* Dissertatio inauguralis medica, sistens medicinam renunciatoriam . . . Erfordiae, Typis Joh. Henr. Groschi [1692]

    32 p. 20 cm.   **[5228]**
    Diss.—Erfurt.

HAMEY, BALDWIN [1600-1676] Dissertatio epistolaris de juramento medicorum, qui Ὅρκος Ἱπποκράτους dicitur: in qua ... Balduinus Hamey, M. D., veterem vulgarem versionem improbans, aliam substituit novam; exploratis aliquot virorum doctorum judiciis ... Editore Adamo Littleton ... Londini, Prostat apud Guilielmum Birch, 1693.

[3], 3, [7], 32 p. 20 cm. [5229]

Greek and Latin texts of Hippocrates' Jusjurandum: 3 p., preceding preface.

"Versio vulgaris primi & secundi articuli in Ὅρκω Hippocratico recognita per B. H." (p. 1-7) is dated 1674.

HAMMEN, LUDOVICUS VON [1652?-1689] De herniis dissertatio academica. Accedunt de crocodilo ac vesicae mendaci calculo epistolae et responsiones ... Ed. 3. Lugduni Batavorum, Apud Cornelium Boutesteyn, 1681.

[6], 135 p. 14 cm. [5230]

Includes correspondence by J. N. Pechlin.

HAMMER, MARTIN [*fl.* 1602-1605] [Die erste Predigt, darinnen von Blattern gehandelt wird ... Die andere Leichpredigt, bey der christlichen Leichsbestattung Annae Gundermans ... welches den 20. Octobris des 1605. Jahrs, an den Blattern ... gestorben ... Leipzig, Gedruckt durch Valentin Am Ende, typis haeredum Beyeri, 1606]

[95] p. 19 cm. [5231]

Imperfect: title page wanting.
Title from caption titles, imprint from colophon.

HAMMERER, JOHANN KARL [*fl.* 1665-1669] *respondent. See* SEBISCH, J. A., *praeses.* Disputatio exhibens problemata quaedam anatomica. 1665.

HAMMERICUS, FRIEDRICH [*fl.* 1660-1666] *respondent.* Disputationem medicam inauguralem de carbunculo pestilentiali ... examini submittit Fridericus Hammericus ... Lugduni Batavorum, Apud viduam & haeredes Johannis Elsevirii, 1666.

[24] p. 21 cm. [5232]

Diss.—Leyden.

—*See* BARTHOLIN, T., *praeses.* Spicilegium secundum ex vasis lymphaticis. 1660.

HAMPAANEAH hammeguelleh. *See* HEYDON, J.

HAMPE, JOHANNES HARDOVICUS [*fl.* 1676-1678] *respondent.* Dissertationem inauguralem medicam de rhagadibus ... submittit Johannes Hardovicus Hampe ... [Argentorati] Literis Georgii Andreae

Dolhopffii, imprimebat Johannes Schütz [1678]

[4], 40 p. 18 cm. [5233]

Imperfect: upper margins trimmed.
Diss.—Strasbourg.

—*respondent. See* WEDEL, G. W., *praeses.* Dissertationem medicam de suffimentis ... submittet ... J. H. H. 1676.

—, *ed. See* PAULLI, S. Παρεκβασις. 1678.

HAMUSCO, JUAN VALVERDE DE. *See* VALVERDE, Juan de.

HAN, BALTHASAR [*fl.* 1613-1635] *respondent. See* WOLF, M., *praeses.* Ἑπτας problematum physicorum ... proponit: B. H. ... 1613.

—*See* SENNERT, D. Practicae medicinae. 1636-54.

HANBUT, JOHANN. *See* CORNARIUS, Janus [1500-1558]

HANDEL, GOTTFRIED [*fl.* 1671] *respondent. See* ROLFINCK, W., *praeses.* Dissertatio medica inauguralis de pleuritide. 1671.

HANDRIOT, FRANÇOIS. *See* ANDRIOT, François [*d.* 1704]

HANDSCH, GEORG [1529-1578] *tr. See* MATTIOLI, P. A. Kreutterbuch. 1611, 1626, 1678, 1696.

HANEMANN, JOHANN LUDWIG. *See* HANNEMANN, Johann Ludwig [1640-1724]

HANHARD, JOHANN ULRICH [*fl.* 1685] *respondent.* Disputatio inauguralis medica de salibus in genere ... Basileae, Typis Emanuelis König & Ludovici heredum [1685]

[24] p. 19 cm. [5234]

Diss.—Basel.

HANNAEUS, GEORGIUS [1647-1699] Facultati Medicae & ... Regia Academia Hafniensis, medicinae doctoribus ... meum hunc foetum Apollineum submisse consecro ... [Hafniae, 1684]

[4], 49, [5] p. 20 cm. [5235]

Caption and running title reads: Aphonologia.
Imperfect? Title page wanting?

—*See* BARTHOLIN, R. Erasmius Bartholinus ... Facultatis Medicae decanus, L. S. 1684.

HANNASCH, CASPAR [*fl.* 1657] *respondent.* Disputatio medica inauguralis de miscellaneis

medicis ... Basileae, Typis Georgii Deckeri [1657]
[16] p. 20 cm. [5236]
Diss. — Basel.

HANNEKEN, BALTHASAR MENO [*fl.* 1700–1704]
respondent. See VATER, C., *praeses.* Exercitationem
medicam de hemiplegia ... exhibebit ... B. M. H.
1700.

HANNEMANN, JOHANN LUDWIG [1640–1724]
Ovum Hermetico-Paracelsico-Trismegistum; i.e.,
Commentarius-philosophico-chemico-medicus, in
quandam epistolam Mezahab dictam de auro, et
historia philosophico-chemico-medica de eodem
metallo nativo & artificiali. In quo et 108 quaestiones
chemicae ab ... D. D. Morhofio propositae ...
solvuntur ... Una cum Fasciculo epistolarum ad
quosdam nostri seculi medicos celeberrimos, & Appendice apologetico. Francofurti, Impensis Friderici
Knochii, 1694.
[68], 440, 28, [14] p. 18 cm. [5237]

HANNEMANN, TOBIAS THOMAS MICHAEL JOEL
DIETRICH [*fl.* 1697] *respondent. See* WALDSCHMIDT, W.
U., *praeses.* Dissertatio inauguralis exhibens
pathologiae animatae specimen. 1697.

HANSEN, JOHANN WILHELM [*fl.* 1683] *respondent.
See* FRANCK VON FRANCKENAU, G., *praeses.* Agonismata
physico-medica nona vice. 1683.

HANT, SYBRAND [*fl.* 1687] *respondent.* Progym-
nasma medicum inaugurale de duelech sive de λιθιασι
... Lugduni Batavorum, Apud Abrahamum
Elzevier, 1687.
[20] p. 21 cm. [5238]
Diss. — Leyden.

HAPELIUS, NICOLAUS NIGER. *See* EGLINUS
ICONIUS, Raphael [1559–1622]

HARANGUE de la goutte a messieurs ses hostes
ou elle mesme fait son apologie, son panegyrique,
& montre enfin les moyens dont on se peut servir
pour la rendre plus traittable. Geneve, Jean Herman
Widerhold, 1673.
[2], 61 p. 18 cm. [5239]
Published also as part [5] of La medecine domestique. Geneve,
1673.

HARBECH, THOMAS [*fl.* 1669] *respondent.*
Disputatio medica inauguralis de rheumatismo ...
Lugduni Batavorum, Apud viduam & haeredes

Joannis Elsevirii, 1669.
[8] p. 23 cm. [5240]
Diss. — Leyden.

HARDER, CHRISTOPH [1625–1689] *respondent. See*
SEBISCH, M. [1578–1674?] *praeses.* Disputatio de
naturalibus facultatibus prima [-octava & ultima] 1644
[i.e. 1645] [and] Disputatio medica de calculo renum.
1647.

HARDER, JOHANN JAKOB [1656–1711] Apiarium
observationibus medicis centum ac physicis experimentis plurimis refertum ... cum responsione
ad invectivam Joh. Baptist. de Lampsweerde cap.
XXIV. Hist. nat. molar. uteri ... Basileae, Impensis
Johann. Philippi Richteri, typis Jacobi Bertschii,
1687.
[12], 376, 12 p. plates. 21 cm. [5241]
Imperfect: lower margin of title page trimmed with loss of date.
With this is bound Bohn, J., *praeses.* Dissertationes chimico-
physicae. 1685.

—Dissertatio anatomico-practica; viscerum
praecipuorum structuram et usum adumbrans.
Basileae, Typis Jacobi Bertschii, 1686.
[32] p. 20 cm. [5242]

—Paeonis [pseud.] et Pythagorae [pseud., i.e. J.
C. Peyer] Exercitationes anatomicae et medicae
familiares bis L. Hecatombe, non Hecatae, sed illustri Academiae Naturae Curiosorum sacra.
Basileae, Prostat apud Emanuel König & fil., typis
Jacobi Bertschii, 1682.
[16], 280 p. 18 cm. [5243]

—Another issue, with different title vignette.
[5244]

—Prodromus physiologicus naturam explicans
humorum nutritioni et generat. dicatorum ...
Basileae, Literis Jacobi Bertschii, 1679.
[16], 192 p. 17 cm. [5245]
Includes correspondence by J. K. Peyer.

—Alexander Pfisterus ... Franc. Sebas. Vorster
... Paulus Ancillon ... Johannes Hoferus ... digni
habiti sunt quibus summi doctoratus medici ...
privilegia conferrentur, voce manuque Joh. Jacobi
Harderi ... Ad que ... d. XIV. Maji ann. M. D.
C. LXXXIX. solenniter peragenda invitantur ...
Basileae, Typis Jacobi Bertschii [1689]
broadside. 34 x 25 cm. [5246]
Program — Basel.
Bound with Vorster, F. S., *respondent.* Experimenta. [1689]

—*praeses.* Dissertatio anatomico-practica viscerum praecipuorum structuram et usum adumbrans ... Basileae, Typis Jacobi Bertschii [1685]

[32] p.   20 cm.   [**5247**]

Diss.—Basel (J. Burgauer, *respondent*)

—Dissertatio medica de νοσταλγία oder Heimwehe ... Basileae, Typis Jacobi Bertschii [1688]

[16] p.   20 cm.   [**5248**]

Diss.—Basel (J. Hofer, *respondent*)

—Exercitatio medica de chyli secretione et distributione ... Basileae, Typis Jacobi Bertschii [1690]

[12] p.   19 cm.   [**5249**]

Diss.—Basel (N. Du Mont, *respondent*)

—Exercitatio medica de chylificatione ... Basileae, Typis Jacobi Bertschii [1688]

[18] p.   20 cm.   [**5250**]

Diss.—Basel (P. Ancillon, *respondent*)

—Exercitatio medica de sanguinis motu vitali ... Basileae, Typis Jacobi Bertschii [1694]

[16] p.   17 cm.   [**5251**]

Diss.—Basel (J. J. Weiss, *respondent*)

—Exercitatio medica naturalem atque praeternaturalem sanguificationis in humano corpore historiam exponens ... Basileae, Typis Jacobi Bertschii, 1690.

[16] p.   23 cm.   [**5252**]

Diss.—Basel (A. Hertzog, *respondent*)

—*respondent.* Disputatio medica inauguralis, de asthmate ... Basileae, Literis Jacobi Bertschii [1676]

[32] p.   19 cm.   [**5253**]

Diss. — Basel.

—Dissertatio medico chirurgica de empyemate ... [Basileae] Typis Jacobi Bertschii [1675]

[20] p.   19 cm.   [**5254**]

Diss. — Basel.

—*respondent. See* GLASER, J. H., *praeses.* Dissertatio medica de ictero nigro. 1673.

—*See* FELIX, A. *Father.* De ovis cochlearum epistola. 1684; MARSIGLI, A. F. De ovis cochlearum epistola. 1684; PEYER, J. K. Parerga anatomica et medica septem. 1681.

HARDER, MATTHAEUS [*fl.* 1672–1675] *respondent.* Disputatio inauguralis medica, de cataracta, seu suffusione ... Basileae, Typis Jacobi Bertschii [1675]

[20] p.   20 cm.   [**5255**]

Diss. — Basel.

—*See* GLASER, J. H., *praeses.* Dissertatio historiae medicae de scrofulis. 1672.

HARDERUS, JOHANNES [*fl.* 1663] *respondent.* Disputatio medica inauguralis de partu septimestri, tam ictorum responsis, quam medicorum placitis insigni ... Lugduni Batavorum, Ex officina Jacobi Voorn, 1663.

[16] p.   24 cm.   [**5256**]

Diss. — Leyden.

HARDING, JOHN, *tr. See* BASILIUS VALENTINUS. The triumphant chariot of antimony. 1660, 1661; PARACELSUS. Archidoxis. 1660.

HARDOUIN DE SAINT JACQUES, PHILIPPUS. *See* HARDUIN DE SAINT JACQUES, P.

HARDT, FRIEDRICH CHRISTOPH [*fl.* 1693] *praeses.* Porositatis omnibus in corporibus adsertio ... Lipsiae, Typis Goezianis [1693]

[24] p.   21 cm.   [**5257**]

Diss. — Leipzig (C. R. Preiss, *respondent*)

HARDT, JOHANN GOTTLIEB [*d.* 1713] *praeses.* Dubium physicum quoad ignis receptum calorem extricatum ... Lipsiae, Literis Christiani Gözii [1686]

[24] p.   20 cm.   [**5258**]

Diss. — Leipzig (M. Schrader, *respondent*)

—Dubium physicum quoad sonum in campana vulgo creditum extricatum ... publicae ventilationi sistet ... Matthaeus Fridericus Frietzsch ... Lipsiae, Typis Christiani Goezii [1689]

[24] p.   19 cm.   [**5259**]

Diss. — Leipzig (M. F. Frietzsch, *respondent*)

HARDUIN DE SAINT JACQUES, PHILIPPUS, *ed. See* UNIVERSITÉ DE PARIS. Faculté de médecine. Codex medicamentarius. 1638, 1639, 1645.

HARDY, SÉBASTIEN [*fl.* 17th. cent.] *tr. See* LESSIUS, L. Deux traittez. 1623 [and] Le vray regime de vivre. 1646.

HARINGTON, *Sir* JOHN [1561–1612] *tr. See* REGIMEN SANITATIS SALERNITANUM. The Englishmans doctor. 1608, 1609, 1624.

HARIZA, JUAN BALTHAZAR DE. Instancias a un papel muy docto de ... Rodrigo Enriquez, medico que fue en la ciudad de Ezija, y aora lo es de la de Sevilla, sobre averiguar la causa de unos accidentes que entonces padecia una señora religiosa . . . Granada, Francisco Sanchez, 1670.

[8], 76 ll.; 23 ll.   22 cm.   [5260]

"Parecer del Doctor don Rodrigo Enriquez . . .": 23 ll. at end.

HARMENS, PETER [*fl.* 1687] *respondent. See* HELWIG, C. Disputatio medica inauguralis de suffocatione uterina. 1687.

HARMES, HEINRICH [1636-1670] *praeses.* Disputatio medica de peste . . . Bremae, Typis Hermanni Braueri [1668]

28 p.   19 cm.   [5261]

Diss. — Bremen. Gymnasium (J. Keuchler, *respondent*)

HARMES, MARTIN [*fl.* 1681-1685] *respondent.* Diatriba inauguralis de acidularum usu earundemque vero operandi modo . . . Marburgi Cattorum, Typis Johannes Henrici Stockenii, 1685.

64 p.   20 cm.   [5262]

Diss. — Marburg.

—*See* WALDSCHMIDT, J. J., *praeses.* Disputatio medica de ventriculi et intestinorum morbis. 1684.

HARMONIA et disharmonia taxarum; das ist, Vergleichung der oesterreichischen, rheinländischen ober-und-nieder-sächsischen Apothecker Taxe. Mit kurtzen Anmerckungen, warum etliche Misshelligkeiten eingeschlichen . . . Hannover und Wolffenbüttel, Verlegts Gottfried Freytag, druckts Joh. Peter Grimmen, 1700.

[1], 109 (i.e. 107), [15] p.   22 cm.   [5263]

HARO, DAVID DE [*fl.* 1631?] *respondent. See* BURGERSDIJCK, F. P., *praeses.* Collegium physicum. 1642.

HARPOCRAS. *See* HARPOCRATION, Valerius.

HARPOCRATE. *See* HARPOCRATION, Valerius.

HARPOCRATION, VALERIUS. Λεξικὸν τῶν δέκα ῥητόρων . . . Lexicon decem oratorum. Nicolaus Blancardus . . . emendavit, disposuit, Latine vertit, ac elenchum veterum scriptorum adjecit. Subjiciuntur Philippi Jacobi Maussaci notae, & Dissertatio critica . . . Accesserunt Henrici Valesii Notae & animadversiones in Harpocrationem, & Maussaci notas. Lugduni Batavorum, J. a Gelder incepit, J.

A. de la Font perfecit, 1683.

[24], 432 p.; 141, [11] p.   25 cm.   [5264]

Text in Greek and Latin.

—*See* KIRANUS, *King of Persia.* Moderante auxilio redemptoris supremi, Kirani Kiranides. 1638, 1681; [English tr.] 1685.

HARPRECHT, JOHANN [*b.* 1610?] Lucerna salis philosophorum; hoc est, Delineatio nuda desiderati illius principii tertii mineralium Sendivogiani, sive salis pontici, quod est subjectum omnis mirabilitatis . . . nec non clavis artis Gebricae . . . Communicata a filio Sendivogii [pseud., i.e. Johann Harprecht] . . . Amstelodami, Apud Henricum Betkium, 1658.

167, [1] p.   16 cm.   [5265]

—Sudum philosophicum, pro secretis chymicis perspiciendis; sive, Duo libelli concernentes famosum illum modernum scriptorem chymicum per anagramma vocatnm [sic] Vah! Longus verbo, sed nil supra! [i.e. Johann Rudolf Glauber] Quorum prior exhibet seriem praecipuorum ejus secretorum . . . Posterior autem ostendit ejusdem hallucinationem circa mercurium philosophorum, aurum potabile, ac metallorum transmutationem . . . Zu Teutsch, Ein häiterer philosophischer Tag, umb die chymische Geheimnüsse zu erkennen; oder, Zwei Büchlein anlangend den itzig beschrienen chymischen Scribenten welches Nahmen dieses Anagramma begreiffet: So so! Er will pur Geld naus habn. Deren das Erste eine verzeuchnüss seiner . . . Geheimnüssen verfasset . . . Das Andere aber zeiget seine Irrsahlen, betreffent den Mercurium philosophorum, Aurum potabile, und metallische Transmutation: von welchen aber hierin . . . gehandelt wird durch den Sohn Sendivogii . . . [n. p.] 1660.

294 p.   16 cm.   [5266]

In Latin and German.

—*See* JOHANNES ISAACI, H. Opus vegetabile. 1695.

HARRIS, JOHN [1641?-1682] The divine physician: prescribing rules for the prevention, and cure of most diseases, as well of the body, as the soul . . . In two parts. By J[ohn] H[arris] M. A. . . . London, Printed by H[enry] B[ridges] for Will. Whitwood, and sold by George Rose, 1676.

[14], 201, [6] p.   15 cm.   [5267]

Imperfect: first preliminary leaf (blank?) wanting.

HARRIS, WALTER [1647-1732] De morbis acutis infantum ... Londini, Impensis Samuelis Smith, 1689.

[13], 146, [2] p.   17 cm.   [**5268**]

—[The same.] Tractatus de morbis acutis infantum variis observationibus illustratus. Genevae, Sumptibus Cramer & Perachon, 1696.

[8], 44 p.   22 cm.   [**5269**]

—[The same.] De morbis acutis infantum ... Amstelodami, Apud Georgium Gallet, 1698.

[8], 51, [4] p.   20 cm.   [**5270**]
Bound with Lister, M. Octo exercitationes medicinales. 1698.

—[The same.] *In* Morton, R. Opera medica. 1696, 1697, 1699.

—[English tr.] An exact enquiry into, and cure of the acute diseases of infants ... Englished by W[illiam] C[ockburn] M. S. With a preface in vindication of the work. London, Sam. Clement, 1693.

[28], 139 p.   14 cm.   [**5271**]
Imperfect: p. [21-22] mutilated; p. 28 wrongly printed.

—[German tr.] Gründlicher Bericht von den schnellen und gefährlichsten Kranckheiten junger Kinder. Nebenst angehengten Observationen ... zusammen getragen und ... in lateinischer Sprach herausgegeben anjetzo aber in das Hochteutsche übersetzt, und mit einem fernern Anhang von andern Zuständen junger Kinder und beygefügtem ... Anmerckungen vermehrt. Franckfurt und Leipzig, Zu finden bey Georg Wilhelm Kühnen, 1691.

[15], 212 p.; 279 p.   14 cm.   [**5272**]
Part [2] has half title.

—A description of the king's royal palace and gardens at Loo. Together with a short account of Holland. In which there are some observations relating to their diseases ... London, Printed by K. Roberts, and sold by T. Nutt, 1699.

[4], 41 (i.e. 43) p.   plate.   22 cm.   [**5273**]

—Pharmacologia anti-empirica; or, A rational discourse of remedies both chymical and Galenical ... Together with some remarks on the causes and cure of the gout ... London, Richard Chiswell, 1683.

[31], 332, [12] p.   18 cm.   [**5274**]

—, *tr. See* BLEGNY, N. de. New and curious observations on the art of curing the venereal disease. 1676;

LÉMERY, N. An appendix to A course of chymistry. 1680 [and] A course of chymistry. 1686, 1698.

HARRISON, HENRY [*d.* 1692] The last words of a dying penitent: being an exact account of the passages ... on which was grounded the first suspicion of his being concerned in the ... murder of Dr. Clinch ... Written with his own hand after condemnation ... London, Randal Taylor, 1692.

[1], 31 p.   21 cm.   [**5275**]

HARSCHER, MATTHIAS [1596-1651] *respondent. See* BRUNN, J. J. von, *praeses.* De morborum causis. [1617]

HARSCHER, MATHIAS [*fl.* 1665-1668] *respondent.* Dissertatio inauguralis de lethargo ... Basileae, Excudebat Jacobus Werenfelsius [1668]

[8] p.   19 cm.   [**5276**]
Diss. — Basel.

HARSCHLEBEN, JOHANN ALBERT. *See* HARSSLEBEN, Johann Albert [*fl.* 1666-1668]

HARSSLEBEN, JOHANN ALBERT [*fl.* 1666-1668] *respondent. See* ROLFINCK, W., *praeses.* Dissertatio medica de partu difficili. 1666; SCHENCK, J. T., *praeses.* Disputatio inauguralis medica de ... pestilentia. 1668.

HART, JAMES [*fl.* 1607-1633] The anatomie of urines. Containing the conviction and condemnation of them. Or, the second part of our discourse of urines. Detecting ... the manifold falshoods ... in the judgement of diseases by the urines onely ... Collected, as well out of the ancient Greeke, Latine, and Arabian authors, as out of our late famous physitians of severall nations ... translated out of the originall tongues, together with ... the authors owne observations ... Never heretofore published. London, Printed by Richard Field for Robert Mylbourne, 1625.

[18], 127, [1] p.   19 cm.   [**5277**]
STC 12887ª.
The first part of the discourse, entitled The arraignment of urines ... London, 1623, is an epitomized translation by James Hart of a work by Pieter van Foreest.

—Κλινική; or, The diet of the diseased. Divided into three bookes. Wherein is set downe at length the whole matter and nature of diet for those in health, but especially for the sicke ... Collected as well out of the writings of ancient philosophers ... and ...

moderne writers . . . London, Printed by John Beale, for Robert Allot, 1633.

[14], 28, 411, [16] p.   29 cm.   [5278]

STC 12888.

—*respondent.* Positiones de pleuritide . . . Basileae, Ex officina Johannis Schroeteri, 1609.

[11] p.   20 cm.   [5279]

Diss. — Basel.

—, *tr. See* FOREEST, P. van. The arraignment of urines. 1623.

HARTENFELS, GEORG CHRISTOPH VON. *See* PETRI VON HARTENFELS, Georg Christoph [1633-1718]

HARTIG, AMAND [*fl.* 1630] *respondent. See* SEBISCH, M. [1578-1674?] *praeses.* Libri sex Galeni De morborum differentiis. 1632.

HARTIG, CHRISTIANUS [*fl.* 1623] *respondent. See* SEBISCH, M. [1578-1674?] *praeses.* Exercitationes medicae. 1639.

HARTIG, JOHANN JAKOB [*fl.* 1623] *respondent. See* SEBISCH, M. [1578-1674?] *praeses.* Exercitationes medicae. 1639.

HARTLIB, SAMUEL [*d.* 1662] *See* CHYMICAL, MEDICINAL, AND CHYRURGICAL ADDRESSES. 1655.

HARTMAN, GEORGE [*fl.* 1668-*ca.* 1682] The family physitian; or, A collection of choice . . . remedies, for the cure of almost all diseases . . . Containing some hundreds of . . . receipts . . . Together with the true English wineceller . . . with a collection of the choicest . . . cosmetick remedies . . . London, Richard Wellington, 1696.

[15], 528 p.   plates.   18 cm.   [5280]

—The true preserver and restorer of health: being a choice collection of . . . remedies for all distempers . . . Selected from, and experienced by the most famous physicians . . . of Europe. Together with Excellent directions for cookery . . . London, Printed by T[homas] B[raddyll] for the author, 1682.

[20], 351, [1] p.; 80, 32 p.   illus., plates.   17 cm.
                                                    [5281]

Imperfect: plate and p. 3-10 of first group of second part wanting; supplied in photocopy from Library of Congress.

The second part has special title page: Excellent directions for cookery . . . with A collection of . . . receipts for making of metheglin.

—[The same.] . . . The 2d ed. with additions . . . London, Printed by T[homas] B[raddyll] and are to be sold by Randol Taylor, 1684.

[15], 352 p.; 80, 32 p.   illus.   16 cm.   [5282]

The special title page of the second part is dated 1682.

—[The same.] . . . The 2d ed. with additions . . . London, Printed for A. and J. Churchill [1695]

[15], 352 p.; 80, 32, [12] p.   illus., plate.   16 cm.
                                                    [5283]

Imperfect: imprint date partly erased, may read 1695.
The special title page of the second part is dated 1682.

—, *ed.* and *tr. See* DIGBY, *Sir* K. Choice and experimented receipts in physick. 1668, 1675.

—, *ed. See* DIGBY, *Sir* K. Ausserlesene . . . chymische Experimente. 1684 [and] Chymical secrets. 1683.

HARTMAN, HARTMANN [*fl.* 1653] *respondent.* Theses inaugurales de carbunculo . . . Lugduni Batavorum, Ex officina Francisci Moyardi, 1653.

[8] p.   23 cm.   [5284]

Diss. — Leyden.

HARTMANN, CHRISTIANUS [*fl.* 1630] *respondent. See* SEBISCH, M. [1578-1674?] *praeses.* Exercitationes medicae. 1639.

HARTMANN, GEORG EVERHART [*fl.* 1633-1659] *ed. See* CROLL, O. Basilica chymica. 1635, 1643, 1658, 1670.

—*See* HARTMANN, J. Praxis chymiatrica. 1633, 1634, 1639, 1682.

HARTMANN, HIERONYMUS ERHARD [*b.* 1677] *respondent. See* WEDEL, C., *praeses.* Centuria thesium de theriaca. 1700.

HARTMANN, JOHANN [1568-1631] Opera omnia medico-chymica, in quibus praxis ejus chymiatrica, notae in Basilicam Crollii & Beguinii Tyrocynium, Disputationes chymico medicae, Tractatus de opio, Miscellanea medico chymica & Introductio in vitalem philosophiam continentur. Partim antehac seorsim impressa, partim vero jam ex authoris MSS. non dum antea editis collecta, & in unum volumen congesta atque pluribus aucta a Conrado Johrenio . . . Francofurti ad Moenum, Impensis viduae

Seylerianae, typis Balthas. Christophori Wustii, junioris, 1684.

7 parts in 1 v.   illus., plate.   36 cm.   [5285]

Each part has half title.
The Tractatus de opio was edited by J. G. Pelshofer.

—[The same.] . . . Francofurti ad Moenum, Apud Wolffgangum Röderum, Typis Bonaventurae de Launoy, 1694.

7 parts in 1 v.   illus., plate.   36 cm.   [5286]

Imperfect: sig.) : ( ) : (wanting.
A reissue of the 1684 edition with new title page and sig.) : (2 reset.
The Tractatus de opio was edited by J. G. Pelshofer.

—Anthropologia physico-medico-anatomica . . . in qua totius humani corporis mechanica structura describitur, partiumque usus, atque operandi modus examinatur . . . Venetiis, Typis Joannis Baptistae Tramontini, 1696.

[14], 350, [2] p.   port.   23 cm.   [5287]

Errata: [2] p.

—Disputationes chymico-medicae; pleraque . . . ab aliquot medicinae candidatis . . . censurae publicae expositae, & hac 2. ed. auctiores editae. Accessit Philosophus, sive naturaeconsultus medicus, initio professionis chymiatricae ab ipso propositus. Marpurgi, Typis Pauli Egenolphi, 1614.

[8], 36, 387 p.   21 cm.   [5288]

—Officina sanitatis; sive, Praxis chymiatrica plane aurea. Antehac a Johanne Hartmanno . . . conscripta . . . Nunc . . . locupletata a Johanne Hiskia Cardilucio . . . Noribergae, Sumptibus Wolfgangi Mauritii Endteri, & Johannis Andreae Endteri haeredum, 1677.

[16], 1231, [41] p.   front.   22 cm.   [5289]

"Zodiacus medicus; sive, Libellus de concordantia rerum medicarum cum zodiaco coelesti . . . Authore Johanne Hiskia Cardilucio . . ." (p. [1083]-1231) has half title.

—Praxis chymiatrica . . . edita a Johanne Michaelis . . . et Georgio Everharto Hartmanno . . . Lipsiae, Sumptibus Gotofredi Grossii, [Exprimebat Joannes Albertus Minzelius] 1633.

[15], 238 (i.e. 246), [31] p.   21 cm.   [5290]

—[The same.] . . . Huic editioni adjectus est, propter affinitatem materiae, tractatus novus, De oleis variis chimice destillatis. Francofurti, Apud Casparum Rötelium, 1634.

[8], 652, [52] p.   17 cm.   [5291]

"Tractatus, Joannis Ernesti . . . De oleis variis arte chymica destillatis": p. 434-652.

—[The same.] . . . Huic postremae editioni adjecti sunt propter affinitatem materiae, tres tractatus novi. I. De oleis variis chymice distilatis. II. Basilica antimonii Hameri Poppii . . . III. Marci Cornachini D. M. Methodus, qua omnes humani corporis affectiones ab humoribus copia, vel qualitate peccantibus . . . curantur. Genevae, Sumptibus Petri Chouët, 1639.

631, [33] p.; 112, [13] p.   plates.   16 cm.
[5292]

Part [2] has half title.
"Tractatus Joannis Ernesti . . . De oleis variis arte chymica destillatis": p. 397-594.

—Praxis chymiatrica, recognita & emendata prae omnibus hactenus editionibus. Lugd. Batavorum, Apud Jacobum Voorn, 1663.

[6], 366, [34] p.   14 cm.   [5293]

Interleaved.
Edited by J. A. van der Linden.

—[The same.] . . . Addita Pathologia J. Fernelii, cujus singula capita singulis illius praxis capitibus praefixa sunt. Cura Theop. Boneti . . . Accedunt tractatus tres. I. [Joannis Ernesti] De oleis chymice distillatis &c. II. Basilica antimonii Humeri Poppii . . . III. M. Cornachini Methodus in pulverem. Genevae, Sumptibus Leonardi Chouet, & socii, 1682.

[12], 494, 33 p.; 329, 29 p.   plates.   18 cm.
[5294]

Part [2] has half title.

—[English tr.] Praxis chymiatricae; or, The practise of chymistry. In Croll, O. Bazilica chymica. 1670.

—Tractatus physico-medicus, de opio . . . publice praelectus Marpurgi anno 1615. Nunc vero primum in lucem editus a Johanne-Georgio Pelshofero . . . Wittenbergae, Apud haeredes Clementis Bergeri, typis Johannis Rohneri, 1635.

[6], 173, [29] p.   16 cm.   [5295]

—, ed. See CROLL, O. Basilica chymica. 1635, 1643, 1658, 1670.

—See BÉGUIN, J. Tyrocinium chymicum. 1643, 1650, 1659, 1669. CROLL, O. Königlicher chymischer und artzneyischer Palast. 1684. LIBAVIUS, A. [d. 1616] Appendix necessaria Syntagmatis arcanorum chymicorum. 1615.

HARTMANN, Johann [*fl.* 1697] *respondent. See* Waldschmidt, W. H., *praeses.* Dissertatio chymico-medica de salis volatilis cornu cervi crystallisatione volatili essentiali. 1697.

HARTMANN, Konrad Georg [*fl.* 1686] *respondent. See* Wedel, G. W., *praeses.* Disputatio medica inauguralis de Somno praeternaturali. 1686.

HARTMANN, Martin [*fl.* 1666–1670] *praeses.* Magni Hippocratis Coi Aphorismi VI sectionis VI, in quo vitiorum renum & vesicae in senioribus prognosis traditur, resolutio ... Jenae, Literis Wertherianis [1670]

    [1], 21, [1] p.   18 cm.   **[5296]**

Without a dedication on the verso of the title page.
Diss.—Jena (J. S. Dicelius, *respondent*)

HARTMANN, Melchior Philipp [1685?–1765] *respondent. See* Grabe, M. S., *praeses.* Theses medicae de phthisi. 1700.

HARTMANN, Philipp Jakob [1648–1707] Succini Prussici physica & civilis historia cum demonstratione ex autopsia & intimiori rerum experientia deducta ... Francofurti, Impensis Martini Hallervordi, typis Johannis Andrea, 1677.

    [1], 291 p.   plate.   17 cm.   **[5297]**

Added engraved title page.

Dissertations—Königsberg

—*praeses.* Disquisitio de phoca sive vitulo marino ... Regiomonti, Typis Friderici Reusneri [1683]
    [2], 30 p.   20 cm.   **[5298]**

Imperfect: p. 29–30 bound before p. 1.
M. F. Thormann, *respondent.*

—Exercitationum anatomicarum ... de originibus anatomicae prima [-quarta] ... Regiomonti, Typis Friderici Reusneri haeredum, 1683.
    66 (i.e. 74) p.   20 cm.   **[5299]**

Each Exercitatio has special title page.
Imperfect: t. p. of the 3d exercise supplied in manuscript.
A. Harweck, F. W. Latter, T. F. Stadlander and C. Woschki, *respondents.*

—Exercitationum anatomicarum in publicas lectiones de iis, quae contra peritiam veterum anatomicam afferuntur in genere, prima ... Regiomonti, Typis Friderici Reusneri haeredum [1684]
    [4], 40, [4] p.   19 cm.   **[5300]**

J. S. Lange, *respondent.*

—Exercitationum anatomicarum in publicas lectiones de iis, quae contra peritiam veterum anatomicam afferuntur in genere, secunda ... Regiomonti, Typis Friderici Reusneri haeredum [1687]
    [4], 66, [2] p.   19 cm.   **[5301]**

J. H. Panring, *respondent.*

—Exercitationum anatomicarum in publicas lectiones de iis quae contra peritiam veterum anatomicam afferuntur in specie, secunda ... Regiomonti, Typis Friderici Reusneri haeredum [1693]
    [2], 31–70 p.   21 cm.   **[5302]**

J. Schmidt, *respondent.*

—Theses de causis pestis in aëre ... Regiomonti, Ex Typographia Reichiana, 1687.
    [11] p.   illus.   20 cm.   **[5303]**

A. Hartwich, *respondent.*

HARTRANFT, Johann [*fl.* 1620] *praeses.* Theoremata physica de sensibus internis, de potentia appetitiva et locomotiva, nec non de somno, vigilia & somniis ... Lipsiae, Excudebatur typis Friderici Lanckisii [1620]
    [15] p.   19 cm.   **[5304]**

Diss.—Leipzig (M. Exner, *respondent*)

HARTSOEKER, Nicolaas [1656–1725] Essay de dioptrique ... Paris, Jean Anisson, 1694.
    [24], 233, [1] p.   illus., plate.   24 cm.
                                       [5305]

—Principes de physique ... Paris, Jean Anisson, 1696.
    [20], 236 p.   illus.   26 cm.   **[5306]**

—*See* Andry de Boisregard, N. De la génération des vers dans le corps de l'homme. 1700.

HARTSTEIN, Heinrich [*fl.* 1655] *respondent. See* Heiland, M., *praeses.* Dissertationem physiologicam de principiis generationis humani corporis materialibus ... examini sistit ... H. H. 1655.

HARTUNG, Hieronymus Conradus Virdungi ab. *See* Virdung von Hartung, Hieronymus Konrad [*fl.* 1679]

HARTWICH, Abraham [*fl.* 1687–1688] *respondent. See* Hartmann, P. J., *praeses.* Theses de causis pestis in aëre. 1687.

HARTWIG, CHRISTIAN [*fl.* 1604-1609] *respondent.*
Disputatio medica de hydrope ... Basileae, Typis
Johannis Schroeteri, 1609.

[8] p.   20 cm.   [5307]

Diss. — Basel.

—*See* SENNERT, D., *praeses.* De methodo medendi
disputatio IX, de purgationis quantitate. 1604.

HARTWIG, JOHANN [*fl.* 1659-1660] *respondent. See*
KIRCHMAYER, G. K., *praeses.* Ex physicis disputationem publicam, de calido innato ... sistet. 1659,
1660.

HARVET, ISRAEL [*fl. ca.* 1597-1605] Animadversiones in Joannis Antarveti [pseud., i.e. Jean Riolan
the younger] ... Apologiam pro judicio scholae Parisiensis, de alchymia. Francoforti, Impensis Claudii
Marnii, & hered. Joannis Aubrii, 1604.

172 p.   16 cm.   [5308]

"Animadversiones pro G. Baucyneto, in Joannis Antarveti ...
Apologiam pro judicio scholae Parisiensis, de alchymia ad Harveti
& Baucyneti recoctam cramben": p. [3]-96; "Animadversiones pro
J. Harveto, in Joannis Antarveti ... Apologiam pro judicio scholae
Parisiensis, de alchymia ad Harveti & Baucyneti recoctam
cramben": p. 97-172.

Attributed to Gulielmus Baucynetus by BNC.

—Demonstratio veritatis doctrinae chymicae,
adversus Joan. Riolani Comparationem veteris
medicinae cum nova, Hippocraticae cum Hermetica,
dogmaticae cum Spagyrica ... Hanoviae, Typis
Wechelianis, apud Claudium Marnium & haeredes
Joan. Aubrii, 1605.

123, [5] p.   17 cm.   [5309]

—[The same, as subject] *See* RIOLAN, J. [1580-1657]
Censura demonstrationum Harveti pro veritate
alchymiae. 1606.

HARVEY, GIDEON [1640?-1700?] Archelogia
philosophica nova; or, New principles of philosophy.
Containing philosophy ... Metaphysicks ...
Dynamilogy ... Religio philosophi ... Physicks ...
London, Printed by J. H. for Samuel Thomson, 1663.

[14], 103 p.; [1], 441, [1] p.   illus.   20 cm.
                                                   [5310]

Part 2 has special title page.

—The art of curing diseases by expectation: with
remarks on a supposed great case of apoplectick fits.

Also ... observations on coughs, consumptions ...
London, James Partridge, 1689.

[4], 224 p.   15 cm.   [5311]

—[Latin ed.] Ars curandi morbos expectatione;
item De vanitatibus, dolis, & mendaciis medicorum.
Accedunt his praecipue supposita, & phaenomena,
quibus veterum recentiorumque dogmata de
febribus, tussi, phthiae, asthmate, apoplexia, calculo
renum & vesicae, ischuria & passione hysterica convelluntur; aliaque verisimiliora traduntur ... Juxta
exemplar Londinense. Amstelodami, 1695.

[6], 302, p.   17 cm.   [5312]

With this are bound: [Venette, N.] Traité du scorbut. 1671;
Menon, D. L'ecole de Salerne. 1695.

—Casus medico-chirurgicus; or, A most
memorable case of a noble-man, deceased. Wherein
is shewed, his lordship's wound, the various diseases
survening, how his physicians and surgeons treated
him ... London, M. Rooks, 1678.

[6], 160 p.   16 cm.   [5313]

—Copy 2.

Author's portrait pasted on page facing title page.

—[The same.] ... The 2d ed. ... London, James
Partridge, 1685.

[6], 160 p.   17 cm.   [5314]

Imperfect: sheet A wrongly imposed.
A reissue of the 1678 edition with new title page.

—The conclave of physicians, detecting their intrigues, frauds, and plots, against their patients. Also
a peculiar discourse of the Jesuits bark ... London,
James Partridge, 1683.

[17], 228 p.   15 cm.   [5315]

—[The same.] ... In two parts ... London,
James Partridge, 1686.

[24], 138 p.; [1], 124 p.   15 cm.   [5316]

Each part has special title page. That to part 2 has date: 1685.

—[The same, as subject.] *See* A DIALOGUE BETWEEN
PHILIATER AND MOMUS. 1686; GUIDOTT, T. Gideon's
fleece; or The sieur de Frisk. 1684.

—De febribus tractatus theoreticus, et practicus
praecipue, quo praxin curandarum febrium continuarum modernam esse lethiferam & barbaram,
abunde patefit ... Londini, Impensis Gulielmi
Thackerey, 1672.

[6], 75, [2] p.   18 cm.   [5317]

—The disease of London; or, A new discovery of the scorvey . . . Together with anatomical observations, and discourses on convulsions, palsies . . . and small pox, with their . . . remedies . . . London, Printed by T. James, for W. Thackery, 1675.

[13], 296 p.   17 cm.   [5318]

—The family physician, and the house apothecary . . . London, T. R., 1676.

[24], 165 (i.e. 167) p.   15 cm.   [5319]

—[The same.] . . . The 2d ed. rev. by the author. London, M. R., 1678.

[24], 165 p.   15 cm.   [5320]

—Great Venus unmasked; or, A more exact discovery of the venereal evil, or French disease . . . Together with . . . cures of . . . gonorrhoea . . . With discourses of the scurvy, manginess, and plague. The 2d ed. . . . London, Printed by B. G. for Nath. Brook, 1672.

[8], 161 (i.e. 163), [4] p.   port.   17 cm.   [5321]

Imperfect: sheet M wrongly imposed.

—Morbus Anglicus; or, The anatomy of consumptions . . . To which are added, some brief discourses of melancholy, madness, and distraction occasioned by love. Together with certain new remarques touching the scurvy and ulcers of the lungs . . . Never before published . . . London, Nathaniel Brook, 1666.

[8], 250, [5] p.   14 cm.   [5322]

—[The same.] . . . The 2d. ed. . . . London, Printed by Thomas Johnson, for Nathanael Brook, 1672.

[4], 154 p.   front. (port.)   17 cm.   [5323]

Date altered by hand from 1672 to 1674.

"A discourse of the plague . . . The 2d ed. . . . 1673" (p. [129]-154) has special title page.

—[The same.] Morbus Anglicus; or, A theoretick and practical discourse of consumptions, and hypochondriack melancholy . . . Likewise a discourse of spitting of blood . . . [London] William Thackeray [1672?]

[9], 252 p.   13 cm.   [5324]

Imprint partly supplied from Wing H 1071.

—A new discourse of the smallpox, and malignant fevers, with an exact discovery of the scorvey . . . Together with anatomical observations . . . on convulsions, palsies, apoplexies, rheumatisms, and gouts . . . London, Printed by H. Hodgskin for James Partridge, 1685.

[4], 200 p.   16 cm.   [5325]

—The vanities of philosophy & physick: together with directions and medicines easily prepared by any of the least skill . . . Comprizing moreover hypotheses different from those of the schools throughout almost the whole art of physick, and particularly relating to indigestion . . . fevers, consumption, stone, gravel . . . London, A. Roper, R. Basset, W. Turner, 1699.

[8], 184 p.   19 cm.   [5326]

—[The same.] . . . The 2d. ed., much enl. London, W. Turner, 1700.

[8], 143 p.   18 cm.   [5327]

—See [MERRET, C.] The accomplisht physician. 1670.

HARVEY, JOHN [1563?-1592] tr. See HERMES TRISMEGISTUS. The learned work. 1657?

HARVEY, WILLIAM [1578-1657]

De motu cordis

—Exercitatio anatomica de motu cordis et sanguinis in animalibus . . . Francofurti, Sumptibus Guilielmi Fitzeri, 1628.

72 p.   illus.   19 cm.   [5328]

Keynes (D) 1. (Without errata leaf.)

—De motu cordis & sanguinis in animalibus, anatomica exercitatio. Cum refutationibus Aemylii Parisani . . . et Jacobi Primirosii . . . Lugduni Batavorum, Ex officina Joannis Maire, 1639.

[8], 267, 84 p.   plates.   20 cm.   [5329]

Keynes (D) 3.

—[The same.] . . . Cui postrema hac editione accesserunt Cl. V. Johannis Walaei . . . Epistolae duae, quibus Harveii doctrina roboratur. Patavii, Apud Sebastianum Sardum, sumptibus Dominici Ricciardi, 1643.

[11], 227 p.   illus.   15 cm.   [5330]

Imperfect: p. 95-96 wanting.

Keynes (D) 4.

—[The same.] . . . De motu cordis & sanguinis in animalibus anatomica exercitatio. Cum refutationibus Aemylii Parisani . . . et Jacobi Primrosii . . .

[4], 267 p.; 84, [4] p.   plates.   20 cm.   (In

Recentiorum disceptationes de motu cordis. Lugduni Batavorum. 1647)   [5331]

Half title.

Keynes (D) 6.

Part [2] has half title: Jacobi Primrosii ... Exercitationes, & animadversiones in librum Guilielmi Harveii ... De motu cordis et circulatione sanguinis.

— Exercitatio anatomica de motu cordis & sanguinis. Cum praefatione Zachariae Sylvii ... Accessit Dissertatio de corde Doct. Jacobi de Back ... Roterodami, Ex officina Arnoldi Leers, 1648.

[40], 216 p.; [2], 219, [8] p.   illus.   14 cm.
                    [5332]

Added engraved title page.

Errata: p. [8] at end.

Keynes (D) 7.

Part [2] has special title page.

— [The same.] Exercitationes anatomicae, de motu cordis & sanguinis circulatione ... Accessit Dissertatio de corde Doct. Jacobi de Back ... Roterodami, Ex officina Arnoldi Leers, 1654.

[32], 285, [19], p.; 252, [24] p.   illus.   14 cm.
                    [5333]

Added engraved title page wanting.

Keynes (D) 8.

Part [2] has special title page: Jacobi de Back ... Dissertatio de corde ... Ed. altera.

— [The same.] ... Roterodami, Ex officina Arnoldi Leers, 1660.

[32], 285, [19] p.; 252, [24] p.   illus.   14 cm.
                    [5334]

Added engraved title page dated 1661.

Keynes (D) 9.

"Exercitationes anatomicae duae de circulatione sanguinis, ad J. Riolanum, J. filium": p. 173-285.

Part [2] has special title page: Jacobi de Back ... Dissertatio de corde. Ed. 3.

— [The same.] ... Quibus accesserunt Jo. Walaei, De motu chyli & sanguinis, epistolae duae ... Londini, Ex officina R. Danielis, 1660.

[40], 464, [23] p.   plates.   13 cm.   [5335]

Without the engraved title page dated 1661 present in most copies.

Imperfect: p. 5-20 wanting; supplied in photocopy; pages 88-89 are blank (not 87-88 as in Keynes)

Keynes (D) 10.

"Jacobi de Back ... Dissertatio de corde ... Editio altera" (p. [283]-464, [1]-[23]) has special title page.

— Exercitationes anatomicae, de motu cordis & sanguinis circulatione ... Accessit Dissertatio de corde ... Jacobi de Back ... Roterodami, Ex officina Arnoldi Leers, 1671.

[32], 285, [19] p.; 252, [24] p.   illus.   14 cm.
                    [5336]

Keynes (D) 11.

Added engraved title page dated 1661.

The two parts are from different copies and are bound separately.

Part [2] has special title page: Jacobi de Back ... Dissertatio de corde ... editio quarta.

With part [2] of this is bound: Collectanea de diuturna graviditate. 1662.

— [Dutch tr.] Vande beweging van't hert, ende bloet. Vit het Latijn vertaalt door N. van Assendelft ... Amstelodam, Cornelis Last, 1650.

[26], 97, [3] p.   16 cm.   [5337]

Imperfect: added engraved title page wanting.

Keynes (D) 18.

With this are bound: Walaeus, J. Twee brieven van de beweginge des chyls ende des bloeds. 1650; Tulp, N. De drie boecken der medicijnsche aenmerkingen. 1650.

— [English tr.] The anatomical exercises ... concerning the motion of the heart and blood. With the preface of Zachariah Wood ... To which is added Dr. James de Back his Discourse of the heart ... London, Printed by Francis Leach, for Richard Lowndes, 1653.

[38], 111 p.; [20], 123 p.; [2], 86 p.   17 cm.
                    [5338]

Keynes (D) 19. (With p. 5 correctly numbered, but with 6 additional errors in paging not recorded by Keynes.)

The title page is a cancel, without the lines to Harvey (by Z. Wood, i.e. Z. Sylvius) on the verso.

Back's work and the Two anatomical exercises have special title pages.

The first work is a translation of Exercitatio anatomica de motu cordis et sanguinis in animalibus.

"Two anatomical exercitations concerning the circulation of the blood, to John Riolan the son ... The author, William Harvey": [2], 86 p. at end.

— [The same.] ... London, Richard Lowndes and Math. Gilliflower, 1673.

[24], 107 p.; [20], 172 (i.e., 176) p.   front., (port.)
17 cm.   [5339]

Keynes (D) 20. (Portrait and error in paging not mentioned)

Part [2] has special title page with imprint: London, Printed by T. R., 1673.

"Two anatomical exercitations concerning the circulation of the blood. To John Riolan the son ... The author, William Harvey" (p. [105]-172) has special title page.

—[The same.] *In* Parisano, E. Nobilium exercitationum libri duodecim de subtilitate. 1623–43; Spiegel, A. van de. Opera quae extant, omnia. 1645.

—[The same, *as subject*.] *See* RIOLAN, J. [1580–1657] Opera anatomica vetera. 1650 [and] Opuscula anatomica nova. 1649.

De circulatione sanguinis

—Exercitationes duae anatomicae de circulatione sanguinis. Ad Joannem Riolanum filium … Roterodami, Ex officina Arnoldi Leers, 1649.

[2], 140, [1] p. 15 cm.   [5340]
Keynes (D) 32.

—[The same.] Exercitatio anatomica, de circulatione sanguinis. Ad Joannem Riolanum filium … Parisiis, Apud Gaspardum Meturas, 1650.

81, [1] p. 14 cm.   [5341]
Errata: p. [82]
Keynes (D) 33.
Bound with copy 2 of Riolan, Jean (1580–1657). Encheiridium anatomicum. 1648.

De generatione animalium

—Exercitationes de generatione animalium. Quibus accedunt quaedam De partu; De membranis ac humoribus uteri; & De conceptione … Londini, Typis Du-Gardianis: impensis Octaviani Pulleyn, 1651.

[28], 301, [1] p. 23 cm.   [5342]
First prelim. leaf and final leaf, both blank, wanting.
Added engraved title page.
Keynes (D) 34.

—[The same.] … Amstelodami, Apud Ludovicum Elzevirium, 1651.

568, [5] p. 14 cm.   [5343]
Added engraved title page with imprint: Londini, Apud Octavianum Pulleyn, 1651.
Keynes (D) 35.

—[Another issue.] … Amstelodami, Apud Ludovicum Elzevirium, 1651.

568, [5], p. 13 cm.   [5344]
Title page and added engraved title page closely trimmed and mounted.
Keynes (D) 36 (The issue with the imprint on the added engraved title page the same as that on the title page)

—[The same.] … Amstelodami, Apud Joannem Janssonium, 1651.

[34], 415, [4] p. 14 cm.   [5345]
Added engraved title page.
Keynes (D) 37.

—[The same.] … Ed. novissima a mendis repurgata. Amstelaedami, Apud Joannem Ravesteynium, 1651.

[28], 388, [3] p. 14 cm.   [5346]
Engraved title page.
Keynes (D) 38.

—[The same.] … Ed. novissima a mendis repurgata. Amstelaedami, Apud Joannem Ravesteynium, 1662.

[28], 388, [3] p. 14 cm.   [5347]
Engraved title page.
Keynes (D) 39.

—[The same.] … Patavii, Typis heredum Pauli Frambotti, 1666.

[35], 604, [5] p. 15 cm.   [5348]
Engraved title page.
Keynes (D) 40.

—Observationes et historiae omnes & singulae e Guilielmi Harvei libello De generatione animalium excerptae, & in accuratissimum ordinem redactae. Item Wilhelmi Langly De generatione animalium observationes quaedam. Accedunt Ovi faecundi singulis ab incubatione diebus factae inspectiones; ut et Observationum anatomico-med. decades quatuor; denique Cadavera balsamo condiendi modus. Studio Justi Schraderi, M. D. Amstelodami, Typis Abrahami Wolfgang, 1674.

[34], 240 p. plates. 13 cm.   [5349]
Keynes (D) 41.

—Exercitationes de generatione animalium. Quibus accedunt quaedam De partu; De membranis ac humoribus uteri; & De conceptione … Ed. novissima a mendis repurgata. Hagae Comitis, Apud Arnoldum Leers, 1680.

[36], 582, [4] p. 14 cm.   [5350]
Engraved title page.
Keynes (D) 42.

—[English tr.] Anatomical exercitations, concerning the generation of living creatures: to which are added particular dicourses, of births, and of conceptions, &c. … London, Printed by James Young, for Octavian Pulleyn, 1653.

[46], 566 (i.e. 556), [1] p. front. (port.) 17 cm.   [5351]
Keynes (D) 43.

—[The same, *as subject*.] *See* VORST, J. De generatione animantium conjectura. 1667.

—*See* Betts, J. De ortu et natura sanguinis. 1669.

—*as subject. See* Bartholin, T. Defensio vasorum lacteorum et lymphaticorum adversus Joannem Riolanum. 1655 [and] Opuscula nova anatomica. 1670; Ettmüller, M., praeses. Abstrusum respirationis humanae negotium. 1676; Garth, Sir S. Oratio laudatoria. 1697; Grove, R. Carmen de sanguinis circuitu. 1685; Grube, H. De arcanis medicorum non arcanis commentatio. 1673; Herfelt, H. G. Philosophicum hominis, de corporis humani machina. 1687; Jasolino, G. Collegium Anatomicum. 1668; Leichner, E. De motu sanguinis exercitatio anti-Harveiana. 1645; Primrose, J. Exercitationes. 1630; Rall, G. F. De generatione animalium. 1669; Rogers, G. Oratio anniversaria. 1682; Rolfinck, W. Ordo et methodus cognoscendi & curandi febres generalis. 1658; Ross, A. Arcana microcosmi. 1652; Walaeus, J., praeses. Disputatio medica de circulatione naturali. 1640 [and] Theses de circulatione naturali. 1647.

HARVIEU. *See* Hervieu, Julien Placide [1671-1746]

HARWARD, Simon [*fl.* 1572-1614] Phlebotomy; or, A treatise of letting of blood, fitly serving, as well for an advertisement ... to ... chirurgians, as also to give a caveat ... to all men to beware of the ... dangers, which may ensue upon rash ... letting of bloud. Comprehended in two bookes ... London, Imprinted by F. Kingston for Simon Waterson, 1601.

[15], 130, [6] p. 17 cm. **[5352]**
STC 12922.

HARWECK, Adam [1661-1703] *praeses.* Dissertatio medica, de affectu hypochondriaco ... Regiomonti, Typis Reusnerianis [1696]

[16] p. 19 cm. **[5353]**
Diss.—Königsberg (J. T. Strasburg, *respondent*)

—*respondent. See* Hartmann, P. J., *praeses.* Exercitationum anatomicarum ... de originibus anatomicae prima [-quarta] 1683.

HASCARD, Pierre. *See* Haschaert, Pierre [16th cent.]

HASCHAERT, Pierre [16th cent.] *See* Baten, C. Hant-boeck der chirurgyen. 1634, 1653.

HASCHARDUS, Petrus. *See* Haschaert, Pierre [16th cent.]

HASE, Simon [*fl.* 1607-1614] *See* Knobloch, T., praeses. Disputationes anatomicae. 1608, 1612.

HASEN. *See* Avicenna [980?-1037]

HASEVEN, Gerbrand [*fl.* 1699] *respondent.* Dissertatio physico-medica inauguralis de corporis humani perspirabilitate ... Lugduni Batavorum, Apud Abrahamum Elzevier, 1699.

[22] p. 22 cm. **[5354]**
Diss.—Leyden.

HASOLLE, James, *pseud. See* Ashmole, Elias [1617-1692]

HASSARDUS, Petrus. *See* Haschaert, Pierre [16th cent.]

HASSELT, Johann Heinrich [*fl.* 1659] *respondent. See* Conring, H. *praeses.* Disputatio medica inauguralis de podagra. 1659, 1678.

HASSELT, Philipp Friedrich von [*fl.* 1688] *respondent. See* Franck von Franckenau, G., *praeses.* Disputatio medica ordinaria, de lapicidina microcosmi in capite. 1688 [and] Disputatio medica ordinaria, et quidem II. de lapicidina microcosmi in capite. 1688.

HAST, Johann Georg [*fl.* 1691] *respondent. See* Schelhammer, G. C., *praeses.* Disputationem inauguralem de suffusione vulgo vom Staar ... examini subjiciet ... J. G. H. 1691.

HASTEVILLE, de. La parfaicte et entiere curation de la sterilite. Mise en lumiere en faveur des jeunes dames, tardiues à engendrer, les premieres années de leur mariage. Par le Chevalier de Hasteville ... Leyde, Gaspar de Launay, 1655.

[1], 486 (i.e. 488) p. 17 cm. **[5355]**
Imperfect: p. 61-90 and 235-236 wanting.

HATTENBACH, Johann [*fl.* 1609] *respondent. See* Libavius, A. [*d.* 1616] *praeses.* De linguis originalibus Sacrae Scripturae. 1609.

HAUCK, Ferdinand Anton [*fl.* 17th cent.] *tr. See* Schuss frey in dem Krieg Gottes. 1692.

HAUCKE, Friedrich [*fl.* 1681] *respondent.* Dissertatio medica inauguralis de vi medicinali ...

Basileae, Literis Johannis Ludovici König & Johannis Brandmylleri [1681]

[16] p.　19 cm.　　　　　　　　　[5356]

Diss. – Basel.

HAUENREUTER, Johann Ludwig. *See* Hawenreuter, Johann Ludwig [1548–1618]

HAUPTMANN, August [1607–1674] Epistola praeliminaris, tractatui de viva mortis imagine mox edendo sacrata, et D. D. Petro Joanni Fabro . . . officiosa menta consecrata. Francofurti, Apud Thomam Matthiam Götzen, typis Joannis Kempfferi, 1650.

23 p.　17 cm.　　　　　　　　　[5357]

—Sedula gratiosorum fontium, qui Hornhusii, pervestigatio; Das ist, Hornhausischer Gnaden Brünnen eigentliche Erforschung . . . Leipzig, In Verlegung Henning Schürers, Gedruckt bey Timoth. Hönen, 1647.

[8], 166 p.　16 cm.　　　　　　　[5358]

—Uhralter wolckensteinischer warmer Badt- und Wasser-Schatz, zu unser lieben Frawen auf dem Sande genand, welcher durch wahre chymische Kunst . . . wieder gefasset und aufgeführet. Auch was er eigentlich in sich halte, und worzu er . . . als Heylung gekränckter Gesundheit nützlich. Nebenst vielen andern . . . Anmerckungen . . . Leipzig, In Verlegung Andreen Löfflers, gedruckt bey Johann Bauern, 1657.

[20], 252, [42] p.　illus.　16 cm.　　　[5359]

Includes letter by Athanasius Kircher.
With this is bound: Schrey, C. H. Neugefasster . . . wolckensteinischer . . . Wasser-Schatz. 1696.

—*respondent.* Bilem ejusque usum, cumprimis juxta neotericorum quorundam mentem, vel ulterioris indaginis causa, levi calamo adumbratum . . . exhibet . . . [Lipsiae] Typis Bauchianis [1653]

[26] p.　19 cm.　　　　　　　　[5360]

Diss. – Leipzig.

—*See* Lange, C., *praeses.* Curationem calculi humani . . . p. p. A. H. 1652 [and] De genuino acidulas egranas salubriter usurpandi modo. 1651 [and] Generationem calculi humani . . . p. p. A. H. 1650; Schrey, C. H. Neugefaster . . . wolckensteinischer Warmer-Bahd- und Wasser-Schatz. 1696.

HAUPTVOGEL, Johann Friedrich [*fl.* 1693] *respondent. See* Crell, L. C., *praeses.* Disputationem historico-physicam de locustis . . . publice habebunt . . . J. F. H. 1693.

HAUSDORFF, Salomon Gottlob [*b.* 1677] *respondent. See* Wedel, G. W., *praeses.* Dissertatio inauguralis medica de aegro cachectico. 1700.

—*See* Slevogt, J. A. Facultatis Medicae decani Jo. Hadriani Slevogtii . . . prolusio inauguralis de natura morborum per morbos curatrice. 1700.

HAUSER, Johann Jakob [*fl.* 1690–1711] *respondent.* Disputatio medica inauguralis de ischuria integra urinae suppressione . . . Basileae, Typis Jacobi Bertschii [1690]

[16] p.　19 cm.　　　　　　　　[5361]

Diss. – Basel.

HAUSMANN, Salomon Gerhard [*fl.* 1655] *respondent. See* Schenck, J. T., *praeses.* De sero sanguinis. 1655.

HAUSS Apoteck; oder, Ein gemein nützliches Haussartzney Büchlein, darinnen allerhand Artzneyen für den gemeinen Mann, der in der Eil die Apotecken nicht haben kan oder sonsten dieselbigen zu ersuchen vermögens nicht were, und also hiemit ihm selbsten mit geringem Unkosten zu Hülffe kommen kan . . . Wittenberg, Lorentz Seuberlich, 1613.

[2], 172, [10] p.　20 cm.　　　　[5362]

Running title: Von gemeiner Hauss Artzney.
Published in Colmar in 1684 under title: Ein nutzliches Hand Büchlein.
Bound with Sechs Bücher auserlesener Arzney und Kunst-Stück. 1613.

HAUSTED, Peter [*d.* 1645] *tr. See* Thorius, R. Hymnus tabaci. 1651.

HAUTIN, Jean [*d.* 1615] *ed. See* Houllier, J. Omnia opera practica. 1664.

HAUTNORTHON, Josephat Friedrich, *pseud? See* Harprecht, Johann [*b.* 1610?]

HAUWENREUTER, Johann Ludwig. *See* Hawenreuter, Johann Ludwig [1548–1618]

HAVENREUTER, Johann Ludwig. *See* Hawenreuter, Johann Ludwig [1548–1618]

HAVERS, Clopton [1660?–1702] Osteologia nova; or, Some new observations of the bones . . . with the manner of their accretion, and nutrition, communicated to the Royal Society in several discourses. I. Of the membrane ... and internal structure of the bones. II. Of accretion ... and of venereal nodes. III. Of the medulla ... IV. Of the mucilaginous glands ... To which is added a fifth discourse Of the cartilages ... London, Samuel Smith, 1691.

[15], 294, [2] p. plates. 18 cm. [5363]

—[Latin tr.] Osteologia nova; sive, Novae quaedam observationes de ossibus, et partibus ad illa pertinentibus; quarum occasione ossium accretio & nutritio ... exponuntur. Quinque discursibus ... Regiae Societati Londinensi per intervalla communicate ... idiomate Anglico Londini editae ... Nunc ... in Latinum idioma conversae & editae ... Cura Melchioris Friderici Geuderi ... Francofurti & Lipsiae, Apud Georgium Wilhelmum Kühnium, 1692.

[16], 343, [39] p. plates. 18 cm. [5364]

—respondent. Disputatio medica inauguralis de respiratione ... Trajecti ad Rhenum, Ex officina Francisci Halma, 1685.

23 p. 22 cm. [5365]
Diss.—Utrecht.

HAVERS, George [fl. 1663] tr. See [RENAUDOT, E.] A general collection of discourses of the virtuosi of France. 1664 [and] Another collection of philosophical conferences of the French virtuosi. 1665.

HAWENREUTER, Johann Ludwig [1548-1618] praeses. Disputatio physica de natura terrae ... Argentorati, Excudebat Marcus ab Heyden, 1616.

[8] p. 18 cm. [5366]
Diss.—Strasbourg (L. Hüenerer, respondent)

—Disputatio physica de primis corporum naturalium principiis ... Argentorati, Typis Conradi Scher, 1616.

[12] p. 18 cm. [5367]
Diss.—Strasbourg (J. Simon, respondent)

—, ed. See THURNEISSER ZUM THURN, L. Zehen Bücher von kalten ... Wassern. 1612.

—See ARISTOTELES. Commentarii ... In libros Metaphysicorum Aristotelis. 1604.

[HAWES, Richard] The poore-mans plaster-box. Furnished with diverse excellent remedies for sudden mischances, and usuall infirmities ... Where-

unto is added certaine directions, whereby a man may know by what meanes a person (being found dead) came by his death ... London, Printed by Tho. Cotes, for Francis Grove, 1634.

[1], 44 p. 18 cm. [5368]
STC 12942.

HAWORTH, Samuel [b. 1660?] Ἀνθρωπωλογία; or, A philosophic discourse concerning man. Being the anatomy both of his soul and body ... By S[amuel] H[aworth] student in physic ... London, Stephen Foster, 1680.

[36], 211, [5] p. 16 cm. [5369]

—A description of the Duke's Bagnio, and of the mineral bath and new spaw thereunto belonging. With an account of the ... medicinal vertues of the spaw ... London, Sam. Smith, 1683.

[8], 117, [3] p. front. (port.) 16 cm. [5370]

—The true method of curing consumptions, wherein 1. the vulgar method is discovered to be useless ... 2. A new method ... is describ'd. 3. The ... cause of this distemper, explain'd. And 4. several remarkable observations on persons cured ... related ... London, Samuel Smith, 1683.

[26], 134 (i.e. 146), [8] p. front. 15 cm. [5371]

Imperfect: frontispiece wanting.

HAY, Alexander [fl. 1689-1697] Tyrocinium pharmaceuticum; sive, Collectanea Galeno-Spagyrica, Scoto-Britannica, medicamentorum simplicium & compositorum ... in praxi authoris ... observata ... Edinburgi. Excudebant haeredes & successores Andreae Anderson, prostant venales in officina Jacobi Wardlaw, 1697.

[8], 180, [4] p. 15 cm. [5372]
Imperfect: lower margin of title page trimmed.

—See SAINT GERMAIN, C. de. The royal physician. 1689.

HAYE, François de la. See LA HAYE, François de [fl. 1689-1693]

HAYMO, See HAIMO, Bp. of Halberstadt [d. 853]

HAYN, Jean de. See INDAGINE, Joannes ab [ca. 1467-1537]

HAYNE, Johann. Drey unterschiedliche newe Tractätlein, deren Erstes von astralischen Kranckheiten ... Das Andere, von tartarischen Kranckheiten ... Das Dritte, begreifft in sich das Fundament ... wie man die Urinen ... erkennen möge ... Nun ... in Truck verfertiget, durch Georg Fabrum ... Franckfurt am Mayn, Getruckt bey Paul Jacob, in Verlegung Johan Dreutels, 1620.

[24], 348, [32] p. illus., plates. 16 cm.   [**5373**]

Imperfect: p. [197]–202 wanting.

—[The same.] ... Vormahls durch Georg Fabrum ... nunmehr ... benebenst einer Vorrede Hrn. D. Johannis Schröderi auff dass neue Truck verfertiget. Franckfurt am Mayn, In Verlegung Thomae Matthiae Götzens, 1663.

[44], 348, [32] p. illus., plates. 17 cm.   [**5374**]

HAYNPOL, Johann. See Cornarius, Janus [1500–1558]

HAZARD, Pierre. See Haschaert, Pierre [16th cent.]

HEADRICH, John [*fl.* 17th cent.] *ed.* Arcana philosophica; or, Chymical secrets, containing the ... medicines of Dr. Wil and Rich. Russel chymists, viz. I. Species vitae ... II. Tinctura regalis ... III. Species coroborativa ... IV. Species proprietatis. V. Species minor. VI. A pestilential cordial ... As also several ... chymical processes and spagerick preparations ... Likewise four ... treatises, viz. The I. of fevers, the II. of the jaundies, the III. of madness, and the IV. of diarrhaeas ... by ... Paracelsus ... London, Printed by Henry Hills, and sold by Eben. Tracy, 1697.

[17], 128, [7] p. 17 cm.   [**5375**]
Sudhoff 424.

HEBENSTREIT, Georg [*fl.* 1605–1607] Πεμπτας una quaestionum miscellarum, politico-medicarum ... Tubingae, Typis Philiperti Brunnii, 1627.

[2], 77 p. 14 cm.   [**5376**]

—*respondent.* See Platter, F. [1536–1614] *praeses.* Disputatio medica de mola matricis. 1607; Sennert, D., *praeses.* De differentiis symptomatum disputatio. 1605.

HEBENSTREIT, Johann Baptista [*d.* 1638] *See* Horst, G. [1578–1636] Operum medicorum tomus primus [-tertius] 1660, 1661.

HEBENSTREIT, Johann Paul [1664–1718] *praeses.* De locustis, immenso agmine aerem nostrum implentibus, et quid portendere putentur ... Jenae, Impensis Salomonis Schmidii, literis Krebsianis [1693]

65 (i.e. 53) p. plate. 19 cm.   [**5377**]
Diss.—Jena (C. Prange, *respondent*)

—De remediis adversus locustas, imprimis pontificiorum quorundam methodo expellendi eas per excommunicationem aquam lustralem, & exorcismum ... Jenae, Literis Wertherianis [1693]

[38] p. 19 cm.   [**5378**]
Diss.—Jena (J. G. Lippoldt, *respondent*)

HEBICH, Lorenz [*fl.* 1628] *respondent.* See Hoever, W., *praeses.* Disputatio medica de corporis humani singularumque partium doloribus. 1628.

HEBIUS, Tarraeus. See Barth, Kaspar von [1587–1658]

HECHLER, Johann Wilhelm [*fl.* 1665] *praeses.* Disquisitio physica de noctambulis ... subjicit ... die 29 Julii 1665. Gissae Cattorum, Recusa literis Kargerianis, 1682.

28 p. 20 cm.   [**5379**]
Diss.—Giessen, 1665 (J. H. Lotichius, *respondent*)

HECHSTETTER, Philipp. See Hoechstetter, Philipp [*ca.* 1579–1635]

HECHT, Joachim Sigismund [*fl.* 1673] *respondent.* See Meibom, H., *praeses.* Exercitatio medica de cancro mammarum. 1673.

HECHTEL, Johann Leonhard [*b.* 1666] *respondent.* See Crause, R. W., *praeses.* Dissertatio inauguralis medica de abscessu. 1690; Wedel, G. W., *praeses.* Dissertatio medica de naevis maternis. 1688.

—See Wedel, G. W. Propempticon inaugurale de animalitate hominis. 1690.

HECKHELER, Johann [*fl.* 1691] *respondent.* See Mapp, M., *praeses.* Dissertatio medica de potu thee. 1691.

HECQUET, Joannes. See Hecquet, Philippe [1661–1737]

HECQUET, PHILIPPE [1661-1737] *respondent. See* DIEUXIVOYE, B. S. de, *praeses.* Quaestio medica. 1694; PUYLON, C. [*fl.* 1660-1696] *praeses.* Quaestio medica ... An chronicorum morborum medicina, in alimento? 1695.

HÉDELIN, FRANÇOIS, *abbé d'Aubignac. See* AUBIGNAC, François Hédelin d', *Father* [1604-1676]

HEDEN, NIKOLAUS CHRISTOPH [*fl.* 1678-1681] *respondent. See* CRAUSE, R. W., *praeses.* Disputatio inauguralis medica de odontalgia. 1681.

HEDEN, NIKOLAUS LEONHARD [*fl.* 1669-1676] *respondent. See* WEDEL, G. W., *praeses.* Disputatio inauguralis medica de epilepsia hysterica. 1676.

HEDENGRAHN, PEHR [*fl.* 1699] *respondent. See* ESBERG, J., *praeses.* Exercitium academicum mulieris philosophantes leviter adumbrans. 1700.

HÉDOUVILLE, *sieur de, pseud. See* SALLO, Jean Denis de [1626-1669]

HEER, HENRI DE [1570-1636] Observationes medicae oppido rarae, in Spa & Leodii animadversae, cum medicamentis aliquot selectis, & ut volunt secretis ... Leodii, Apud Arnoldum a Corsuvaremia, 1630.
[216] p. 16 cm. [5380]
Signatures: A-N ^{8}, O^4.

—[The same.] ... Accessit ejusdem autoris Spadacrene, ed. 2. ... in publicum emissa ... a Joanne Michaelis ... Lipsiae, Apud Andream Kühnen, typis Timothei Hönii, 1645.
2 parts in 2 v. (348 p.; 144 p.), 14. 12 cm. [5381]
Imperfect: title page of part [1] mutilated.
Part [2] has special title page: Spadacrene; hoc est, Fons Spadanus; ejus singularia, bibendi modus ... Ed. alt. auct. & corr.

—Spadacrene; hoc est, Fons Spadanus, accuratissime descriptus ... Et Observationum medicarum oppido raratum liber unicus ... Ed. corr. ... Lugduni Batavorum, Apud Franciscum Moiardum & Adrianum Wyngaerden, 1645.
[22], 159, [17] p.; [8], 254, [21] p. 13 cm. [5382]
Part [2] has half title.
Imperfect: first preliminary leaf (blank?) wanting.

—[The same.] ... Ut et Observationes medicae oppido rarrae in Spa & Leodii animadversae ... Ed.

nov. ... Lugd. Batav., Apud Petrum vander Aa, 1685.
[22], 159, [17] p.; [6], 254, [19] p. 16 cm. [5383]
Part [2] has special title page.
Imperfect: first preliminary leaf (blank?) wanting.
Different setting of type.

HEER, MARTIN [1643-1707] Kurtzer Bericht, wie sich nicht alleine Haus-Vatër, Haus-Mütter, Jung und Alt ja jedwede Menschen in diesem gefährlichen Seuchen der Pest-Zeit hierinnen verhalten und mit Haus-Artzneyen versorgen sollen ... Nebst einem Anhange vieler nützlichen ... Pest-Mittel, so zuvor niemals im Druck kommen ... Leipzig, Gedruckt bey Eliä Fiebigs seel. Wittwe [1680]
[8] p. 18 cm. [5384]

—[The same.] Kurtzer Bericht, wie sich Hauss-Väter und Mütter, auch jedermänniglich in dieser gefährlichen Pest-Zeit verhalten und mit Artzneyen versorgen soll ... Nebenst einem Anhange vieler nützlichen ... Pest-Mittel, wie auch drey ... Remedia wieder die Pestilentz ... zu gebrauchen. Görlitz, 1680.
[16] p. 20 cm. [5385]

—*respondent. See* ALBERTI, V. Disputatio physica. 1661; WELSCH, G., *praeses.* Disputationem inauguralem de morbis haereditariis in genere ... subjicit M. H. 1665.

HEER, NATHANAEL [*fl.* 1700] *respondent. See* BERGER, J. G. von, *praeses.* Dissertationem solennem de difficultate respirandi ... p. p. 1700.

HEEREBORT, ADRIANUS. *See* HEREBOORT, Adrianus [*fl.* 1631]

HEERFORDT, CHRISTOPHER [1609-1679] *See* BARTHOLIN, T. Dissertatio prima [-secunda] de theriaca. 1671.

HEERS, HENRI DE. *See* HEER, Henri de [1570-1636]

HEGNER, HANS HEINRICH [*fl.* 1678-1694] Waarhafte und eigentliche Beschreibung des heilsamen ... Lörli-Bads, in der Statt Winterthur gelegen ... Zürich, Heinrich Müller, 1678.
8 p. 18 cm. [5386]

HEGNER, JOHANN HEINRICH [*fl.* 1666] *respondent. See* BAUHIN, H. *praeses.* Disputatio medica de tertiana intermittente exquisita. 1666.

HEGNER, JOHANN HEINRICH [*fl.* 1700] *respondent.* Theses medicae de paronychia ... Basileae, Typis Jacobi Bertschii [1700]

[20] p. 19 cm. [**5387**]
Diss. — Basel.

HEIDANUS, ANTONIUS. *See* HEIDE, Antonius de [1646–*ca.* 1693]

HEIDANUS, CASPARUS [*fl.* 1668] *respondent. See* MATTHAEUS, P., *praeses.* Disputatio medica de scorbuto. 1668.

HEIDE, ANTONIUS DE [*ca.* 1646–1693] Anatome mytuli, Belgice mossel ... Subjecta est Centuria observationum medicarum ... Amstelodami, Apud Janssonio-Waesbergios, 1684.

[15], 199, [1] p. plates. 16 cm. [**5388**]
Centuria observationum medicarum (p. 51–199) has half title. With this is bound Peyer, J. J. Observationes quaedam anatomicae. Lugduni Batavorum, 1719.

— [Dutch tr.] Ontleedinge des mossels, en Ontleedgenees- en heelkundige waarnemingen ... uit het Latyn vertaalt door Theod. Jansson. van Almeloveen ... Nog des selfs Nieu ligt der apothekers, of noodige aanmerkinge omtrent de misslagen in't bereiden der artzenye ... Amsteldam, Joannes en Gillis Janssonius van Waasberge, 1684.

[8], 288 (i.e. 248), [4] p.; [8], 82, [2] p. illus., plates. 16 cm. [**5389**]

— Experimenta circa sanguinis missionem, fibras motrices, urtica [sic] marinam &c. Accedunt ... Observationes medicae; nec non, Anatome mytuli. Ed. nova. Amstelodami, Apud Janssonio-Waesbergios, 1686.

[7], 206, [2] p.; 48 p. plates. 16 cm. [**5390**]

Imperfect: title page mutilated.
Contents: [1] ... Experimenta (p. 1–48). — [2] Centuria observationum medicarum (p. 51–199) with half title. — [3] Anatome mytuli (p. 1–48). Items 2–3 are in the same setting of type as in the 1684 edition of Anatome mytuli.

— Nieu ligt der apotekers, aanwijsende de onkennis ontrent de kragt der genees-middelen ... Beneffens eenige ontleedgenees en heel-kundige waarnemingen ... Amsterdam, By d'erfgenamen van Joannes Janssonius van Waasberge, 1682.

[12], 201, [3] p. 16 cm. [**5391**]

—, *ed. See* VOORDE, C. van de. Nieuw lichtende fakkel der chirurgie. 1680.

— *See* NEUES LIECHT VOR DIE APOTHECKER. 1690, 1700.

HEIDER, CHRISTIAN [*fl.* 1660] *respondent. See* SIEGFRIED, C. E. [*fl.* 1655–1681] *praes.* Disputatio physica de terra. 1660.

HEIDER, MARTIN [*fl.* 1623] *respondent. See* SENNERT, D., *praeses.* De scorbuto disputatio. 1623.

HEIGEL, AMBROSIUS [*fl.* 1681] *respondent.* Disputatio medica inauguralis opium, qua naturam & usum ejus exhibens ... Altdorffii, Litteris Henrici Meyeri [1681]

43 p. 23 cm. [**5392**]
Diss. — Altdorf.

HEIGL, ANDREAS [*fl.* 1637] *respondent. See* HOEVER, W., *praeses.* Disputatio medica de apoplexia. 1637.

HEILAND, JOHANN DANIEL [*fl.* 1675–1680] *respondent.* Disputatio medica inauguralis de apoplexia ... Lugduni Batavorum, Apud viduam & haeredes Joannis Elzevirii, 1680.

[10] p. 21 cm. [**5393**]
Diss. — Leyden.

HEILAND, MICHAEL [*fl.* 1646–1676] Monstri Hassiaci disquisitio medica ... Gissae Hassorum, Excudebat Fridericus Kargerus [1664]

48 p. 21 cm. [**5394**]
Date of imprint supplied from BMC.
Imperfect: engraving wanting.

— [The same.] Historia infantis monstrosi. *In* Blasius, G. Observationes medicae rariores. 1667.

— *praeses.* Disputatio medica de phantasia ... Giessae Hassorum, Typis Josephi Dieterici Hampelii, 1664.

12 p. 20 cm. [**5395**]
Diss. — Giessen (P. H. Dietz, *respondent*)

— Dissertationem physiologicam de principiis generationis humani corporis materialibus ... examini sistit publico Heinricus Hartstein ... Lipsiae, Typis Johannis Baueri, 1655.

[24] p. 19 cm. [**5396**]
Diss. — Leipzig (H. Hartstein, *respondent*)

—Theses inaugurales medicas de lue venerea
. . . Lipsiae, Prelo Johannis Baueri [1663]

[44] p.   19 cm.   [*5397*]

Diss.—Leipzig (G. Cretzschmar, *respondent*)

—*respondent.* De fistula dissertatio medica . . . Lipsiae, Excudebat Quirinus Bauch, 1653.

[30] p.   18 cm.   [*5398*]

—De signaturis disputationem phytologicam pp. M. Michael Heiland, et Antonius Marquard . . . Lipsiae, Typis Timothei Hönii [1646]

[20] p.   21 cm.   [*5399*]

Diss.—Leipzig (A. Marquart, *respondent*)

—*See* HOPP, J., *praeses.* De purpura dissertatio medica. 1652.

HEILBRONNER, JACOB [1548-1618] *See* PISTORIUS, J. Daemonomania Pistoriana. 1601.

HEILMANN, JOHANN JACOB [*fl.* 1613-1661] *ed.* and *tr. See* ZETZNER, L., *ed.* Theatrum chemicum. 1659-61.

—, *tr. See* VIGENÈRE, B. de. Tractatus de igne et sale. 1661.

HEIM, F. [*fl.* 17th cent.] *engr. See* BOISSARD, J. J. Bibliotheca chalcographica. 1650-54.

HEIM, JOHANN KASPAR [*fl.* 1666] *respondent. See* FRIDERICI, J. A., *praeses.* Disputatio medica inauguralis, qua . . . peripneumoniam . . . publicae . . . disquisitioni submittit J. C. H. 1666 [and] Dissertatio medica de ὑστερομανια. 1666.

HEIMBACH, JOHANN VON [*fl.* 1610] *respondent.* Specimen inaugurale . . . de morbi sacri διαγνώσει & θεραπεία . . . Basileae, Typis Joan. Jacobi Genathii, 1610.

[16] p.   plate.   20 cm.   [*5400*]

Diss.—Basel.
Bound with Stupanus, J. N. Positiones iatricae de phrenitide. 1607.

—*See* PLATTER, F. [1536-1614] Felix Platerus . . . decreto. 1610.

HEIMBURGER, J. E. [*fl.* 1679] *respondent. See* RIVINUS, A. Q., *praeses.* Dissertatio physiologica de bile. 1679, 1688.

HEIMREICH, JOHANN [1676-1730] *praeses.* Dissertatio physica de chylificatione . . . Jenae, Typis Pauli Ehrichii [1698]

22 p.   20 cm.   [*5401*]

Diss.—Jena (J. A. Arens, *respondent*)

—*respondent. See* CRAUSE, R. W., *praeses.* Theses medicae inaugurales, quas . . . examini exponit. 1700.

—*See* WEDEL, G. W. Propempticon inaugurale de cirsio Dioscoridis. 1700.

HEINE, NIKOLAUS [*fl.* 1609-1610] *respondent.* Theses medicae de phrenitidis theoria et therapia . . . Basileae, Typis Johannis Schroeteri, 1609.

[31] p.   20 cm.   [*5402*]

Diss.—Basel.

—*See* PLATTER, F. [1536-1614] Felix Platerus . . . decreto. 1610.

HEINECCIUS, ABRAHAMUS. *See* HEINICK, Abraham [*fl.* 1613-1627]

HEINICK, ABRAHAM [*fl.* 1613-1627] *praeses.* Exercitium physicum de oscitatione . . . Wittebergae, Excusum typis Johannis Haken, 1627.

[24] p.   19 cm.   [*5403*]

Diss.—Wittenberg (J. B. Crüger, *respondent*)

HEINIUS, JOHANN GEORG [*fl.* 1676] *respondent. See* MAY, H. *praeses.* Disquisitio physica de animae rationalis ortu. 1676.

HEINLEIN, JOHANN KARL [*fl.* 1676-1677] *respondent. See* CRAUSE, R. W., *praeses.* Disputatio medica inauguralis de spasmo cynico. 1677; FASCH, A. H., *praeses.* Historiam et curationem calculorum humanorum . . . examini sistit . . . J. K. H. 1676.

HEINLIN, SEBASTIANUS. *See* HAINLIN, Sebastian [1594-1663]

HEINRICH, HEINRICH. *See* HENRICI, Heinrich [*fl.* 1697-1713]

HEINRICI, HEINRICUS. *See* HENRICI, Heinrich [*fl.* 1697-1713]

HEINS, JOHANN [1585-1666] Joh. Henisii . . . Kurtzer, gründlicher und vollkommener Bericht von der Pestilentz, was derselbigen Natur, Ursprung und Eygenschafft, auch wie man sich darvor . . . verwahren, und da jemandt damit behafft, wiederumb darvon entledigen solle. Erstlich in lateinischer

Sprach beschrieben, volgendts aber ... in das Teutsch gebracht ... Aupspurg [sic], Gedruckt durch Andream Aperger, in Verlegung Sebastian Müllers, 1621.

[16], 60 p.   17 cm.   [5404]

— *respondent.* De peste discursum medicum ... proponit ... M. Johannes Henisius ... Basileae, Typis Joh. Jacobi Genathii, [1611]

[23] p.   19 cm.   [5405]

Diss. — Basel.

HEINS, Nicolaas. *See* Heinsius, Nicolaas [1656?–1718]

HEINS, Tobias [*fl.* 1656–1680?] Kurtzer und wohl-gemeinter Unterricht, wie doch bey itzt hin und wieder grassirender und ansteckenden Seuche, oder höchstgefährlichen Pest-Fiebern sich männiglich ... curiren könne ... Berlin, Rupert Völcker [1680?]

48 p.   14 cm.   [5406]

Rupert Völcker bought his Berlin shop in 1660 and owned it until he died in 1697. Cf. Benzing (B).

— *respondent.* Τοῦ μικροκοσμικοῦ κατακδύσματος 'εξέτασις; s., De ascite dissertatio ... Basileae, Typis Georgii Deckeri [1656]

[20] p.   20 cm.   [5407]

Diss. — Basel.

HEINSIUS, Daniel [1580–1655] *ed. See* THEOPHRASTUS. Θεοφράστον ... 'άπαντα. Theophrasti ... Graece & Latine opera omnia. 1613.

HEINSIUS, Ernst [*fl.* 1687] Lapis offensionis in febrium curatione purgatio, sive discursus medicus, de purgantium validiorum abusu in febribus ... Lipsiae, Apud Mauritii Georgii Weidmanni, 1693.

47 p.   20 cm.   [5408]

— *respondent. See* Albinus, B. Disputatio inauguralis medico-chirurgica de paracentesi thoracis. 1687 [and] Dissertationem medicam de cantharidibus ... submittet ... E. H. 1687.

HEINSIUS, Johann Michael [*b.* 1658] *respondent. See* Crause, R. W., *praeses.* Dissertatio inauguralis medica de strumis. 1687.

— *See* Fasch, A. H. Augustinus Henricus Faschius ... Collegii Medici decanus ... S. P. D. lectori benevolo. 1687.

HEINSIUS, Nicolaas [1620–1681] Nicolai Heinssii Dan. F. Elegia ad fontem medicatum Driburgicum agri Paderani. [n. p., n. d.]

[4] p.   19 cm.   [5409]

Paged in handwriting: 5046–5049.
Bound with Hörnyk, M. De acidularum. [1615?]

HEINSIUS, Nicolaas [1656?–1718] De kwynende Venus; ofte, Een korte doch naukeurige verhandeling van de pokken ... als ook de schadelykheid van 't kwylen, onmatig sweeten en veelvoudig purgeren in dese siekte ... Beneffens een Aanhang van verscheyde aanmerkingen, omtrent het genesen deser kwaal door gemelde genees-middelen ... Amsterdam, Nathanael Holbeex en Johannes Broers, 1697.

[14], 286 p.   17 cm.   [5410]

— [German tr.] Schmachtende Venus; oder, Curieuser Tractat von spanischen Pocken und so genanten Frantzosen, darinnen die bissher im Brauch gewesene Salivations- und Schwitz-Cur gäntzlich verworffen, und eine gantz neue ... Methode ... gewiesen wird. Nebst einem Anhang etlicher auf die neue Manier curirten Patienten. Aus dem Holländischen übersetzet von Heinr. Elias Hundertmarck ... Franckfurt und Leipzig, Verlegts Christoph Hülsse, 1700.

[21], 15–186, [2] p.; 118, [4] p.   front.   17 cm.
                                                        [5411]

Part [2] has half title.
With this is bound Boerhaave, Herman. Verhandlung der Venus-Seuche. Bremen, 1737.

— Naukeurige verhandeling van het podagra, en d'algemeene jigt, vervattende der selver eerste oorsprong, en begintzelen in het bloed, als ook den aard en ware eygenschap van des selfs pynelijk ferment. Beneffens verscheide ... recepten ... Amsterdam, Jan ten Hoorn, 1698.

[24], 276, [6] p.   17 cm.   [5412]

Added engraved title page.

HEINSIUS, Ulrich [*fl.* 1681–1684] *praeses.* Dissertatio historico-zoologica de alce ... Jenae, Joh. Jacob. Bauhofer [1681]

[64] p.   illus.   20 cm.   [5413]

Diss. — Jena (P. Lentner, *respondent*)

HEINTKE, Georg [*fl.* 1673–1675] *respondent. See* Bohn, J., *praeses.* Exercitationum physiologicarum prima ... [-decima tertia] 1674; Ettmüller, M., *praeses.* Valetudinarum infantile. 1675, 1685.

HEINTZ, JOHANN [*fl.* 1621] *respondent.* Disputatio de epilepsia ... Lipsiae, Excudebat Fridericus Lanckisch, 1621.

    [30] p.   19 cm.   [5414]
    Diss.—Leipzig.

HEINZ, JOHANN LEONHARD [*fl.* 1678?] *respondent.* Tractatus medicus de affectibus soporosis ... Argentorati, Apud Josiam Staedelium, 1678.

    40 p.   21 cm.   [5415]
    Diss.—Strasbourg.

HEINZELMANN, JOHANN [1629-1678] *respondent. See* SPERLING, J., *praeses.* Aphorismi physici de igne. 1646.

HEISEN, JAKOB [*fl.* 1684] *respondent.* Disputatio medica inauguralis de fluxu mulierum menstruo ejusque suppressione ... Lugduni Batavorum, Apud Abrahamum Elzevier, 1684.

    [20] p.   22 cm.   [5416]
    Diss.—Leyden.

HEISIUS, DANIEL GERHARD [*fl.* 1695] *respondent. See* STROLTERFOHT, J. J., *praeses.* Disputatio medicophysica de idea errante in monstrorum generatione. 1695.

HEISTERMAN, THEODOR [*fl.* 1680] Disputatio medica inauguralis de suppressione mensium ... Lugduni Batavorum, Apud viduam & haeredes Joannis Elzevirii, 1680.

    [12] p.   21 cm.   [5417]
    Diss.—Leyden.

HELBACH, FRIEDRICH [*fl.* 1604] Oenographia, Weinkeller oder Kunstbuch vom Wein, das ist: Aussführliche und eigentliche Beschreibung ... dess Weins, seiner Natur, Eygenschafft und Tugendt ... darinnen auch angezeigt wirdt alles was vom Weinstock, Wein und desselbigen Artzney Mag gesagt werden. Sampt nützlichem ... Bericht aller Kräuterwein ... welche, zu notturfftigen Artzneyen können praefpariert werden ... Darneben auch von Kräuter Essig und Bier gehandelt wirdt. Franckfort am Mayn, Bey Matthias Beckern, In Verlegung Peter Kopffen, 1604.

    [18], 328, [16] p.   20 cm.   [5418]
    Imperfect: all pages after p. 321 mutilated.

HELBIG, JOHANN OTTO. *See* HELLWIG, Johann Otto von, baron [1654-1698]

HELBIGK, CHRISTOPH [*fl.* 1685-1688] *respondent. See* WEDEKIND, J. K. Dissertatio inauguralis medica de alkahest. 1685.

HELBLING, FERDINAND [*fl.* 17th cent.] *ed. See* HELBLING, J. C. Elixir vitae. 1663.

HELBLING, JOHANN CASPAR [*fl.* 1614-1617] Elixir vitae; das ist, Eine hertzstärckende, und diaphoretische, oder schweisstreibende Artzney ... Von ... Ferdinando Helbling ... in offentlichen Truck gegeben. Bregentz am Bodensee, Getruckt bey Bartholome Schnell, 1663.

    38 p.   17 cm.   [5419]

HELCHER, HANSS HEINRICH [1671 or 2-1729] *respondent. See* ORTLOB, J. F., *praeses.* Disputatio inauguralis medica de rheumatismo. 1696.

    —*See* BOHN, J. Lectori benevolo Facultatis Medicae in Academia Lipsiensi p. t. procancellarius, D. Johannes Bohn ... S. D. 1696.

HELCHER, JOH. HEINRICH. *See* HELCHER, Hanss Heinrich [1671 or 2-1729]

HELD, GOTTFRIED [*b.* 1670] *See* WEDEL, G. W. Propemticum inaugurale de minio lunari. 1695.

HELD, JOHANN FRIEDRICH [*fl.* 1670-1673] *praeses.* Disputatio medico-chirurgica, de partu Caesareo ... Erfordiae, Literis Joh. Georgii Hertzii, 1673.

    [20] p.   19 cm.   [5420]
    Diss. — Erfurt (A. M. Dörmer, *respondent*)

    —*respondent. See* FRIDERICI, J. A., *praeses.* Disputationem medicam de corpulentia nimia publicae ... censurae ... submittit ... J. F. H. 1670; ROLFINCK, W., *praeses.* Disputatio inauguralis medica de phrenitide. 1672.

HELD VON HAGELSHEIM, GOTTFRIED [1670-1724] *respondent. See* WEDEL, G. W., *praeses.* Dissertatio inauguralis medica de thermis. 1695.

HELLBERG, ANDREAS HERMANN [*fl.* 1678] *respondent. See* MEIBOM, H., *praeses.* Disputatio medica inauguralis de vomitu. 1678.

HELLENIUS, WILHELMUS [*fl.* 1668] *respondent.* Disputatio medica inauguralis de asthmate ... Lugduni Batavorum, Apud viduam & haeredes Joannis Elsevierii, 1668.

    [12] p.   24 cm.   [5421]
    Diss.—Leyden.

HELLOT, MARC ANTOIN [*fl.* 1672–1676] *praeses.* Quaestio medica . . . An demorsis a cane rabido colocynthis? [Parisiis, Apud Franciscum Muguet, 1676]

4 p.   25 cm.   **[5422]**

Diss.—Paris (J. Thomasseau, *respondent*)

HELLWAG, JOHANN FRIEDRICH [*fl.* 1677] *respondent. See* METZGER, G. B., *praeses.* Dissertationem inauguralem medicam de passione hysterica . . . submittit . . . J. F. H. 1677.

HELLWIG, CHRISTOPH VON [1642–1690] *See* HELWIG, Christoph [1642–1690]

HELLWIG, CHRISTOPH VON [1663–1721] *respondent. See* PETRI VON HARTENFELS, G. C., *praeses.* Disputatio medica inauguralis virginem chlorosi. 1693.

HELLWIG, JAKOB [*fl.* 1669] *respondent. See* SCHWIMMER, J. M., *praeses.* Disputatio physica de antipathia. 1669.

HELLWIG, JOHANN [1609–1674] Ἀλφάβητον ἰατρικόν; hoc est, Brevis totius medicinae Hippocraticae in paucas tabellas redactae delineatio . . . Noribergae, Typis & sumptibus Wolffgangi Endteri, 1631.

[2], 38 ll.   37 cm.   **[5423]**

—Observationes physico-medicae, posthumae, in lucem editae, scholiisque adauctae a Luca Schröckio . . . Augustae Vindelicorum, Apud Theophilum Goebelium, literis Koppmayerianis, 1680.

[11], 422, [14] p.   plates.   21 cm.   **[5424]**

Added engraved title page.

—*See* GEIGER, D. Responsum medicum defensivum ad Johannis Helwigii. 1662.

HELLWIG, JOHANN OTTO VON, *baron* [1654–1698] Introitus in veram atque inauditam physicam epistola ex India Orientali in Europam ad . . . Academiam Naturae Curiosorum transmissa apertus . . . Hamburgi, Apud Gothofredum Schultze, 1680.

32 p.   16 cm.   **[5425]**

HELMICH, JOHANN MICHAEL [*fl.* 1676] *respondent. See* VATER, C., *praeses.* De chymicorum principio. 1676.

HELMONT, FRANCISCUS MERCURIUS VAN, *baron* [1618–1699] Alphabeti vere naturalis Hebraici . . . delineatio. Quae simul methodum suppeditat, juxta quam qui surdi nati sunt sic informari possunt, ut

non alios saltem loquentes intelligant, sed & ipsi ad sermonis usam perveniant . . . Sulzbaci, Typis Abrahami Lichtenthaleri, 1667.

[35], 107, [1] p.   front., plates.   14 cm.   **[5426]**

—[Dutch ed.] Een zeer korte afbeelding van het ware natuurlyke Hebreuwse A. B. C. welke te gelyk de wyse vertoont, volgens welke die doof geboren syn, sodanig konnen onderwesen werden, dat sy niet alleenig andere die spreken konnen, verstaan, maar selfs tot het gebruik van spreken komen . . . Door Franciscus Mercurius van Helmont . . . Als mede een verhandeling om de doof-geboorene te leeren spreken. Door Joh. Conrad. Amman . . . Amsterdam, Pieter Rotterdam, 1697.

[48], 200, [4] p.   plates.   14 cm.   **[5427]**

Added engraved title page.

Imperfect: p. 83–86 wanting; supplied in photocopy from Western Reserve University Library.

Amman's Surdus loquens has special title page (p. [145]).

—[German ed.] Kurtzer Entwurff des eigentlichen Natur-Alphabets der heiligen Sprache: nach dessen Anleitung man auch Taubgeborne verstehend und redend machen kan . . . Sultzbach, Abraham Lichtenthaler, 1667.

[45], 167 p.   front., plates.   14 cm.   **[5428]**

Imperfect: upper margins trimmed.

—The paradoxal discourses of F. M. van Helmont, concerning the macrocosm and microcosm, or the greater and lesser world, and their union. Set down in writing by J. B. and now published. London, Printed by J. C. and Freeman Collins, for Robert Kettlewel, 1685.

[16], 127 p.; 215, [1] p.   plates.   19 cm.   **[5429]**

Includes F. M. van Helmont's Imperial patent of nobility in Latin (p. 206–215).

—The spirit of diseases; or, Diseases from the spirit: laid open in some observations concerning man, and his diseases. Wherein is shewed how much the mind influenceth the body in causing and curing of diseases . . . The first part. London, Sarah Howkins, 1694.

[14], 215, [1] p.   17 cm.   **[5430]**

Translation of Aanmerkingen . . . over den mensch en desselfs ziektens, Amsterdam, 1692. NUC, vol. 239, p. 605.

—, *ed. See* HELMONT, J. B. van. Opuscula medica inaudita. 1648 [and] Oriatrike; or, Physick refined.

1662 [and] Ortus medicinae. 1648, 1651, 1652, 1655, 1667, 1682.

HELMONT, JEAN BAPTISTE VAN [1577-1644]

Works and Collections

Ortus medicinae; id est, Initia physicae inaudita. Progressus medicinae novus, in morborum ultionem ad vitam longam ... Edente ... Francisco Mercurio van Helmont ... Nostra autem haec ed. emend. ... Venetiis, Apud Juntas, & Joan. Jacobum Hertz, 1651.

[52], 700 p.   illus.   33 cm.   [5431]

"Doctrina inaudita, de causis ... & resolutione lithiasis ..." (p. [506]-700) has special title page and includes his treatises titled De febribus, Scholarum humoristarum passiva deceptio (i.e. De humoribus Galeni), and De peste.

—[The same.] ... Edente ... Francisco Mercurio van Helmont, cum ejus praefatione ex Belgico translata. Ed. nova ... multam partem adauctior reddita & exornatior. Amsterodami, Apud Ludovicum Elzevirium, 1652.

[35], 894 (i.e. 884), [48] p.   front. (port.), illus.   20 cm.   [5432]

"... Opuscula medica inaudita. I. De lithiasi. II. De febribus. III. De humoribus Galeni. IV. De peste. Ed. 3. multo emendatior ..." (p. [637]-894 (i.e. 884)) has special title page.

—[The same.] ... Ed. 4, in qua ... quaedam auth. fragmenta adjecti fuerunt ... Tractatum De lithiasi, Febr., Humoribus, & Peste qui in aliis desiderabantur. Lugduni, Sumptibus Joannis Baptistae Devenet, 1655.

[22], 487 p.; 192, [58] p.   illus.   36 cm.   [5433]

Engraved title page.
Imperfect: engraved title page mutilated, general t. p. wanting.
Part [2] has special title page: Opuscula medica inaudita ... Ed. 5 multo emendatior.

—[The same.] ... Lugduni, Sumptibus Joan. Ant. Huguetan, & Guillielmi Barbier, 1667.

[24], 487 p.; 192, [58] p.   illus.   37 cm.   [5434]

Engraved title page.
General title page: Opera.
Part 2 has special title page: Opuscula medica inaudita ... Ed. 6 multo emendatior.
Different setting of type.

—Another issue. Text partly reset.

[5435]

—[The same.] Opera omnia. Additis his de novo tractatibus aliquot posthumis ejusdem authoris, maxime curiosis pariter ac perutilissimis, antehac non in lucem editis ... Francofurti, Sumptibus Johannis Justi Erythropili, typis Johannis Philippi Andreae, 1682.

[39], 765, [73] p.; [16], 275, [43] p.   illus.   22 cm.   [5436]

Added engraved title page.
Part [2] has special title page: Opuscula medica inaudita.
Contents as in the previous editions of Ortus medicinae with the addition of Tractatus novus posthumus ... de virtute magna verborum ac rerum (p. 753-765).
Edited by Franciscus Mercurius van Helmont.

—[Dutch tr. Extracts.] Dageraad; ofte, Nieuwe opkomst der geneeskonst, in verborgen grondregulen der nature ... Not in't licht gesien, en van den autheur zelve in't Nederduits beschreven, 1660. Rotterdam, Joannes Naeranus, 1660.

[18], 404 p.   21 cm.   [5437]

—[English tr.] Oriatrike; or, Physick refined ... Being a new rise and progress of phylosophy and medicine, for the ... prolongation of life ... Now ... rendered into English ... by J[ohn] C[handler] ... London, Lodowick Loyd, 1662.

[44], 1161 (i.e. 1167), [22] p.   front. (port.), illus.   31 cm.   [5438]

"Opuscula medica inaudita; that is , Unheard of little works of medicine. Being treatises 1. Of the disease of the stone. 2. Of fevers. 3. Of the humors of Galen. 4. Of the pest or plague" (p. 815-1161) has special title page.
Edited by Franciscus Mercurius van Helmont.

—[French tr.] Les oeuvres ... traittant des principes de medecine et physique, pour la guerison assurée des maladies: de la traduction de M. Jean Le Conte ... Lyon, Jean Antoine Huguetan & Guillaume Barbier, 1670.

[8], 396 p.   23 cm.   [5439]

—Another issue.

[5440]

New title page dated 1671.

—Opuscula medica inaudita. I. De lithiasi. II. De febribus. III. De humoribus Galeni. IV. De peste. Coloniae Agrippinae, Apud Jodocum Kalcoven, 1644.

3 parts in 1 v.   16 cm.   [5441]

Items I, II, and IV have special title pages.

—[The same.] ... Ed. 2. multo emendatior. Amsterodami, Apud Ludovicum Elzevirium, 1648.

3 parts in 1 v.   22 cm.   [5442]

"Scholarum humoristarum passiva deceptio atque ignorantia ..." (p. 68-115 of part [2]) has caption title.

Edited by F. M. van Helmont.

Bound with (as issued) *his* Ortus medicinae. 1648.

Single Works

—De mag[netica] vulnerum curatione. Disputatio, contra D. Joan. Roberti ...

[457]-507 p. 21 cm. (*In* Theatrum sympatheticum auctum. Norimbergae, 1662)   **[5443]**

Half title.

—Deliramenta catarrhi; or, The incongruities, impossibilities, and absurdities couched under the vulgar opinion of defluxions ... The translator and paraphrast Dr. Charleton ... London, Printed by E. G. for William Lee, 1650.

[12], 75 p. 19 cm.   **[5444]**

Imperfect: p. 65-75 mutilated.

Translation of Catarrhi deliramenta.

—Febrium doctrina inaudita ... Antverpiae, Apud viduam Joan. Cnobbari, 1642.

200, [20] p. 12 cm.   **[5445]**

Errata: p. [19-20]

—Fundamenta medicinae recens jacta, sub unum conceptum & intuitum breviter contracta, de causis ac principiis morborum constitutivis, jam a temporibus Hippocratis medici, XII. seculorum oblivione sepultis ... ultimis vero his nostris diebus ... manifestatis ... ac evulgatis per ... Joannem Baptistam Helmontium. Ulmae, Sumptibus Georgii Wilhelmi Kühn, 1680.

100 p.; 273, [22] p. 14 cm.   **[5446]**

Part [2] has half-title: Pro supplemento introductorii sequuntur adnotata ex relectione operis Johann. Baptistae van Helmont.

—Ortus medicinae; id est, Initia physicae inaudita. Progressus medicinae novus, in morborum ultionem, ad vitam longam ... Edente ... Francisco Mercurio Van Helmont, cum ejus praefatione ex Belgico translata. Amsterodami, Apud Ludovicum Elzevirium, 1648.

[36], 800 (i.e. 808) p. illus., port. 22 cm.

                              [5447]

With this is bound (as issued) *his* Opuscula medica inaudita. 1648.

—[Pharmacopolium ac dispensatorium modernum. French] *In* Massard, J. Traité des panacées. 1681; [Dutch tr.] 1687.

—Praecipiolum; or, The immature-mineral-electrum. *In* Collectanea chymica. 1684.

—Propositiones notatu dignae, depromptae ex ejus disputatione de mag: vulnerum curatione. Parisiis, edita. Additae sunt censurae ... theologorum, & medicorum ex autographis optima fide descriptae. Leodii, Typis Joannis Tournay, 1634.

[20] p. 20 cm.   **[5448]**

Bound with Plemp, V. F. Animadversio. 1642.

—A ternary of paradoxes. The magnetick cure of wounds. The nativity of tartar in wine. The image of God in man ... Translated, illustrated, and ampliated by Walter Charleton ... London, Printed by James Flesher for William Lee, 1650.

[52], 144 p. front. 19 cm.   **[5449]**

—[The same.] ... London, Printed by James Flesher for William Lee, 1650.

[43], 147 p. front. (port.) 18 cm. **[5450]**

Imperfect: lower part of margins trimmed.

Added engraved title page reads: ... The second impression, more reformed, and enlarged with some marginal additions.

—Tumulus pestis ... Coloniae Agrippinae, Apud Jodocum Kalcoven, 1644.

180, [3] p. 17 cm.   **[5451]**

Errata: p. [3]

—[German tr.] Tumulus pestis; das ist, Gründlicher Ursprung der Pest ... Nebenst Beyfügung der wahren Ursach und Grund allerhand Fieber ... Aus dem Niederländischen übersetzt durch Johannem Henricum Seyfrid. Sulzbach, Druckts Abraham Liechtenthaler, 1681.

[8], 375 p. 14 cm.   **[5452]**

—*See* DIDIER, J. Refutation de la doctrine nouvelle du sieur Helmont touchant les fievres. 1653; MERCKLIN, G. A. Sylloge physico-medicinalium casuum incantationi vulgo adscribi solitorum. 1698; PORZIO, L. A. Erasistratus; sive, De sanguinis missione. 1683.

—*as subject. See* CONRING, H., *praeses.* Disputatio medica inauguralis de pleuritide. 1654; DOLÄUS, J. Encyclopaedia chirurgica rationalis. 1689, 1690, 1695 [and] Encyclopaedia, medicinae theoretico-practicae. 1684, 1686, 1688, 1690, 1691 [and] Opera omnia. 1695 [and] Systema medicinale, a compleat system of physick. 1686; ETTMÜLLER, M. Opera omnia theoretica et practica. 1685; FONTAINE, G. D. Gabrielis Fontani ... De veritate Hippocraticae medicinae firmissimis rationum & experimentorum momentis stabilita, & demonstrata. 1657; GREMBS, F. O. Arbor integra et ruinosa hominis. 1657, 1671; LA SCALA, D. Phlebotomia damnata. 1696; NITSCHKE, E., respondent. Disputatio medica inauguralis de custode errante Helmontii. 1670; PISONI, O. Cruentum periculum. 1695; POLEMANN, J. Novum lumen medicum. 1659, 1660, 1699; ROLFINCK, W. Ordo et methodus cognoscendi & curandi febres generalis. 1658; [STARKEY, G.] Liquor alchahest. 1675 [and] Natures explication and Helmont's vindication. 1657.

HELMSTADT. Universität. *See* JULIUS UNIVERSITÄT, Helmstedt.

HELMSTEDT. Academia Julia. *See* JULIUS UNIVERSITÄT, Helmstedt.

HELMSTEDT. Universität. *See* JULIUS UNIVERSITÄT, Helmstedt.

HELVETIUS, ADRIAAN. *See* HELVÉTIUS, Jean Adrien [1661?-1727]

HELVETIUS, CHRISTIAN LEBRECHT [*fl.* 1683] *respondent. See* BOHN, J., *praeses.* Dissertationes chymico-physicae. 1685.

HELVÉTIUS, JEAN ADRIEN [1661?-1727] Lettre . . . sur la nature et la guerison du cancer. Paris, Jean Cusson, 1691.

18 p. illus. 25 cm.   [*5453*]

Imperfect: p. 9-12 wanting.

—Methode pour guerir toute sorte de fievres, sans rien faire prendre par la bouche . . . Paris, La veuve de Nicolas Oudot, 1694.

62 p. 13 cm.   [*5454*]

—[The same.] . . . 2. ed. rev. & augm. Paris, Laurent d'Houry, 1697.

[18], 100 p. 16 cm.   [*5455*]

—[Italian tr.] *In* [Les admirables qualitez du kinkina] Italian. 1694.

—Traité des pertes de sang de quelque espece qu'elles soient, avec leur remede specifique, nouvellement découvert . . . Accompagné de sa Lettre sur la nature & la guerison du cancer. Paris, Laurent d'Houry, 1697.

[14], 168 p. plate. 17 cm.   [*5456*]

—[Italian tr.] Trattato delle perdite del sangue con il loro rimedio specifico nuovamente scoperto . . . e

tradotto in italiano . . . Firenze nel Garbo, Giuseppe Manni, 1699.

[1], xii, 82, [2] p. 15 cm.   [*5457*]

General title page reads: Specifico contro le perdite del sangue [&] Il trionfo della china china.

With this is bound (as issued) Girolami, A. F. Il trionfo della china china. 1699.

HELVETIUS, JOHANN FRIEDRICH [1629 *or* 30-1709] Amphitheatrum physiognomiae medicum. Runder Schauplatz, der artzeneyschen Gesicht-Kunst. Ist eine Verhandelung, der edelen Gesicht-Kunst, durch eusserliches Anschauen der Zeichen, nicht allein die innerlichen Gemüths-bewegungen dess Menschen, sondern auch . . . seines Liebesgebrechen und Kranckheiten . . . zuerkennen: noch zum überfluss auch dessen eignen Natur übereinkommende Geness-Mittel . . . Heydelberg, Samuel Broun, 1660.

[44], 130 p. 16 cm.   [*5458*]

—[Latin ed.] Microscopium physiognomiae medicum; id est, Tractatus de physiognomia, cujus ope non solum animi motus simul ac corporis defectus interni, sed & congrua iis remedia noscuntur . . . Amstelodami, Apud Janssonio-Waesbergios, 1676.

[102], 244, [4] p. ports., plate. 17 cm.   [*5459*]

—[Dutch ed.] Amphitheatrum physiognomiae medicum; dat is, Schouw-plaets der medicinale gesicht-konst. Sijnde een verhandelinge van de edele gesichtkonst, door't uyterlijcke aenschouwen van de tekenen, omme niet alleen de innerlijcke bewegingen des menschen gemoets, maer oock . . . sijn lichemelijcke gebreecken ende kronckheden . . . te erkennen; ende ten overvloet noch der selver eygen natuyr overeen-komende genoes-middel uyt . . . 's Graven-Hage, Levijn van Dyck, 1664.

[48], 311 p. 16 cm.   [*5460*]

—Den ontwapenden pest-doodt in den theriakelpot. Waer in aenghewesen werdt, hoe hem een yder in de besmettelijcke sieckte dienen kan . . . s'Graven-Hage, Christoffel Doll, 1664.

41 (i.e. 61) p. 16 cm.   [*5461*]

—Diribitorium medicum, de omnium morborum accidentiumque in & externorum definitionibus ac curationibus, ex saporibus, odoribus foetoribusque, provenientibus a fermentorum, effervescentiarum aut putrefactionum salibus, sulphuribus vel mercuriis, quae male inveniuntur in succis alibilibus bene constitutis omnium ventriculorum, glandularum vasorumque lymphaticorum totius corporis. Amstelodami, Apud Joannem Janssonium a Waesberge, 1670.

[16], 176 p.   16 cm.   [5462]

— Mors morborum; das ist, Der Kranckheiten Todt. Darin kürtzlich verhandelt wird, wie man ohne grosse umbschweiffige Reden, ein gewisses Urtheil von allerley Gebrechen fellen soll, zwischen der Nothwendigkeit und der Nothdürftigkeit einen festen Bundt aufzurichten ... Heydelberg, Samuel Broun, 1661.

[7], 31 p.   18 cm.   [5463]

— Theatridium Herculis triumphantis; ofte, Kleyn schouw-tooneel, van den triumpherenden Hercules. Met volkomen kennisse der natuyrlijcke dingen, bestaende in sympathia, ende antipathia, magice ende magnetice. Midtsgaders, grondighe weder-legginghe der schrifften van Sijn Excell. Digby, aengaende poudre sympathie ... s'Graven-Hage, Johannes Tongerloo, 1663.

[16], 199, [1] p.   port.   17 cm.   [5464]

— Vitulus aureus, quem mundus adorat & orat, in quo tractatur de rarissimo naturae miraculo transmutandi metalla, nempe quomodo tota plumbi substantia vel intra momentum ex quavis minima lapidis veri philosophici particula in aurum obryzum commutata fuerit ...

[815]-863 p.   22 cm.   (*In* Musaeum Hermeticum. Francofurti, 1678)   [5465]

— [English tr.] The golden calf, which the world adores, and desires: in which is handled the most rare and incomparable wonder of nature, in transmuting metals ... Written in Latin ... and faithfully Englished. London, John Starkey, 1670.

129 p.   15 cm.   [5466]
Translated by William Cooper. Cf. Ferguson (A).

— [The same.] *In* Cooper, W. The philosophical epitaph of W[illiam] C[ooper] 1673-75.

— [German tr.] *In* Feyens, T. Zwölff Bücher von der Wund-Arzney-Kunst. 1675.

HELVIGIUS, CHRISTOPHORUS. *See* HELWIG, Christoph [1642-1690]

HELWICH, CHRISTIAN [1666-1740 *or* 44] *praeses.* Exercitatio academica, exponens sententiam peripateticorum de calido et frigido ... Regiomonti, Typis Reusnerianis [1695]

[20] p.   19 cm.   [5467]
Diss. — Königsberg (D. Vogel, *respondent*)

— *respondent.* De apoplexia ... Altdorffii, Henricus Meyer [1695]

16 p.   20 cm.   [5468]
Diss. — Altdorf.

HELWICH, CHRISTOPH. *See* HELWIG, Christoph [1642-1690]

HELWICH, JAKOB FRIEDERICH [*fl.* 1700] *respondent. See* VATER, C., *praeses.* Dissertatio inauguralis medica de venenis eorundemque antidotis. 1700 [and] Machinae humanae organa animalia in specie dicta. 1700.

HELWIG, CHRISTIAN [1666-1770] *See* HELWICH, Christian [1666-1740 *or* 44]

HELWIG, CHRISTOPH [1642-1690] De studii botanici nobilitate oratio ... Lipsiae, Literis Christiani Michaelis [1666]

[19] p.   20 cm.   [5469]

— Facultatis Medicae decanus Christophorus Helvigius ... ad inauguralem de sanguine disputationem quam ... habebit ... Nicolaus Schultze ... invitat. Gryphiswaldiae, Typis Danielis Benjaminis Starckii [1683]

[8] p.   20 cm.   [5470]
Program — Greifswald (with vita of N. Schultze)

— Programma quo ad inauguralem de vulneribus disputationem, quam ... Matthaeus Clemasius ... habebit ... invitat ... rector Medicaeque Facultatis decanus Christophorus Helvigius. Gryphiswaldiae, Typis Matthaei Doischeri [1674]

[8] p.   20 cm.   [5471]
Program — Greifswald (with vita of M. Clemas)

— Programma, quo decanus Facultatis Medicae Christophorus Helvigius ... ad inauguralem de peste disputationem, quam ... Christianus Lemcke ... habebit ... invitat. Gryphiswaldiae, E typothesia B. Doischeri, 1682.

[8] p.   20 cm.   [5472]
Program — Greifswald (with vita of C. Lemcke)

—Programma, quo decanus Facultatis Medicae Christophorus Helvigius . . . ad inauguralem disputationem, quam de pleuritide . . .subjiciet . . . Philippus Ösler . . . invitat. Gryphiswaldiae, Literis Danielis Benjaminis Starckii [1686]

[8] p.   20 cm.   [5473]

Program — Greifswald (with vita of P. Ösler)

Dissertations — Greifswald

—*praeses.* Delineatio medica apoplexiae . . . Gryphiswaldiae, Literis Danielis Benjaminis Starckii [1686]

[44] p.   20 cm.   [5474]

F. Schütte, *respondent.*

—Disputatio inauguralis medica de pleuritide . . . Gryphiswaldiae, Literis Danielis Benjaminis Starckii [1686]

[32] p.   20 cm.   [5475]

P. Ösler, *respondent.*

—Disputatio medica inauguralis de affectione hypochondriaca . . . Gryphiswaldiae, Literis Danielis Benjaminis Starckii, 1685.

[32] p.   20 cm.   [5476]

S. V. Gadebusch, *respondent.*

—Disputatio medica inauguralis de peste . . . Gryphiswaldiae, E typothesia Beati Matthaei Doischeri, 1682.

[32] p.   20 cm.   [5477]

C. Lemcke, *respondent.*

—Disputatio medica inauguralis de suffocatione uterina . . . Gryphiswaldiae, Literis Danielis Benjaminis Starckii [1687]

47, [1] p.   19 cm.   [5478]

P. Harmens, *respondent.*

—Dissertationem chirurgicam de vulneribus cum fracturis & luxationibus sive conjunctis eorum praecipuis & symptomatibus . . . submittit M. Matthaeus Clemasius . . . Gryphiswaldiae, Excudebat Matthaeus Doischer, 1674.

[64] p.   20 cm.   [5479]

M. Clemas, *respondent.*

—Dissertationem inauguralem medicam de sanguine . . . submittit Nicolaus Schultz . . . Gryphiswaldiae, Typis Danielis Benjaminis Starckii [1683]

40 p.   20 cm.   [5480]

Day, month and year of the presentation written on title page by contemporary hand.

N. Schultz, *respondent.*

—*respondent.* Exercitationem medicam ad text. XXII. sect. II. lib. II. Epid. Hippocr. de fluore muliebri . . . publico eruditorum examini sistit . . . Christophorus Helvigius . . . Basil., Typis Joh. Jacobi Deckleri [1666]

[35] p.   22 cm.   [5481]

Diss. — Basel.

HELWIG, Jakob Friedrich. *See* Helwich, Jakob Friederich [*fl.* 1700]

HELWIG, Johannes. *See* Hellwig, Johann [1609–1674]

HEMEL, Florian [*fl.* 1627] *respondent.* Disputatio inauguralis medica de sterilitate mulierum . . . Basileae, Typis Joh. Jacobi Genathii [1627]

[10 +] p.   20 cm.   [5482]

Imperfect: all after p. [10] wanting.

Diss. — Basel.

HEMMER, Ambrosius [*fl.* 1624] *respondent. See* Innichenhöfer, H., *praeses.* Υπνολογια; sive, Tractatus jucundus physiologicus. 1624.

HEMMER, Christoph [*fl.* 1695] *respondent. See* Bartholin, C. [1655–1738], *praeses.* Dissertatio medica inauguralis de spina ventosa. 1695.

HEMMING, J. [*fl.* 1666–1690] *ed. See* Willis, T. A plain and easie method. 1691.

HEMPEL, Christian [*fl.* 1685] *praeses.* Ex ungue hominem publicae eruditorum disquisitioni . . . Christianus Hempelius . . . & . . . Johannes Spiesmacher . . . sistunt. Lipsiae, Literis Brandianis [1685]

[16] p.   plate.   19 cm.   [5483]

Diss. — Leipzig (J. Spiesmacher, *respondent*)

HEMPEL, Johann [*fl.* 1611–1614] *See* Horst, G. [1578–1636] Dissertatio de natura thermarum. 1618.

HEMSING, Rotgerus [1604–1643] Non semel ilios vexata est; oder, Ablehnung etzlicher ungeräumbter Dinge, so in dem newlich aussgegebenen . . . Georgii Lothi Messer-tractat zufinden, nebest einer . . . verbesserten Relation von dem 29. May newen Calenders 1635. verschluckten, und den 9 Julii alhie zue Königssberg aussgeschnittene Messer ... Elbing, Gedruckt bey Wendel Bodenhausen, 1635.

[52] p. illus. 20 cm. [5484]

HEMSTERHUIS, SIBOUT [*b. ca.* 1629] Historia et analysis arthritidis vagae ... Leovardiae, Typis Schelteni Joachimi, 1666.

[10], 178, [2] p. 14 cm. [5485]

Errata: [2] p.

—Messis aurea triennalis, exhibens; anatomica: novissima et utilissima experimenta ... Lugduni Batavorum, Ex officina Adriani Wyngaerden, 1654.

[16], 347, [10] p. plates. 14 cm. [5486]

Imperfect: plate facing p. 190 wanting.

Includes also Jean Pecquet's Experimenta nova anatomica; Thomas Bartholin's De lacteis thoracicis historia anatomica, De lacteis thoracicis dubia anatomica, Vasorum lymphaticorum historia nova; Olof Rudbeck's Nova exercitatio anatomica, exhibens ductus hepaticos aquosos et vasa glandularum serosa, Variae anatomicae observationes.

—[The same.] Messis aurea exhibens; anatomica: novissima et utilissima experimenta ... Huic editioni accesserunt De vasis lymphaticis tabulae Rudbeckianae ... Heidelbergae, Typis Adriani Wyngaerden, 1659.

[14], 370, [39] p. illus., plates. 17 cm. [5487]

Title page pasted on verso of engraved title page.

Contents as in the 1654 Leyden edition, with the addition of 13 plates accompanied by text.

HEMSTERHUYS, SIBOLDUS TIBERIUS. *See* HEMSTERHUIS, Sibout [*b. ca.* 1629]

HENAULT, GUILLAUME DE. *See* HÉNAUT, Guillaume de [*fl.* 1655-1663]

HÉNAUT, GUILLAUME DE [*fl.* 1655-1663] Clypeus, quo tela in Pecqueti cor, a ... Carolo le Noble ... conjecta, infriguntur [sic] & eluduntur ... Rothomagi, Apud Jullianum Courant, 1655.

71 p. 16 cm. [5488]

—Le thrône de la medecine ... Avec les statuts & ordonnances concernants la pharmacie. Rouen, Jacques Besogne, 1663.

[12], 108 p. 18 cm. [5489]

HENCKEL, ELIAS HEINRICH [*fl.* 1654-1688] De philtris, eorumque efficacia ac remediis. Francofurti, Impensis Nicolai Försteri, 1690.

[8], 95 p. illus. 16 cm. [5490]

—Ordo et methodus cognoscendi & curandi energumenos seu a Stygio Cacodaemone obsessos ... Francofurti & Lipsiae, Sumptibus Nicolai Försteri, 1689.

[14], 240, [16] p. 16 cm. [5491]

Imperfect: outer margin of title page trimmed.

HENDEL, ANDREAS [*fl.* 1610] *respondent. See* STUPANUS, J. N., *praeses.* Σημειωτιces particularis cap. I. De affectibus. 1610.

HENERUS, RENATUS [*fl.* 1554] *See* GALENUS. De ossibus. 1665.

HENISCH, GEORG [1549-1618] *ed. See* ARETAEUS. Ιατρικά. Aetiologica ... morborum acutorum & diuturnorum. 1603.

—, *tr. See* MIZAULD, A. Artztgarten. 1616.

HENISIUS, Joannes. *See* HEINS, Johann [1585-1666]

HENNICKE, GOTTFRIED [*fl.* 1686-1700] De panaceis tractatio medico-chymica. Curiosis experimentis ac ratiociniis illustrata. Francofurti ad Moenum, Sumptibus Christiani Genschii, 1689

39 p. 17 cm. [5492]

—*respondent. See* BRUNNER, J. C., *praeses.* Festo seculari Heidelbergensis Academiae tertio ... panaceas ... examini apponet Gottfried Hennicke. 1686.

—, *tr. See* THOMSON, G. Chymiatrorum acus magnetica. 1686.

HENNIG, GOTTOFREDUS. *See* HENNICKE, Gottfried [*fl.* 1686-1700]

HENNIN, HEINRICH CHRISTIAN [*ca.* 1655-1703] *tr. See* SWAMMERDAM, J. Historia insectorum generalis. 1693.

HENNING, HEINRICH CHRISTIAN. *See* HENNIN, Heinrich Christian [*ca.* 1655-1703]

HENNINGER, JOHANN SIGISMUND [1667-1719] *respondent.* Disputatio inauguralis medica de cephalalgiae curatione ... Argentorati, Typis Johannis Pastorii [1692]

[52] p. 20 cm. [5493]

Diss. — Strasbourg.

HENNINIUS, HEINRICH CHRISTIAN. *See* HENNIN, Heinrich Christian [*ca.* 1655-1703]

HENRI IV, *King of France* [1553–1610] *See* Sossius, G. De vita Henrici Magni libri IV. 1522 (i.e. 1622)

HENRI DE MONDEVILLE. *See* Mondeville, Henri de [14th cent.]

HENRICI, Heinrich [*fl.* 1697–1713] *respondent. See* Hoffmann, F. [1660–1742] *praeses.* Disputatio medica inauguralis de inedia magnorum morborum.

HENRICUS DE SAXONIA [13th cent.] *See* Albertus Magnus. Tractatus Henrich de Saxonia. 1615.

HENRION, Denis [*d. ca.* 1640] Nottes [sic] sur les recreations mathematiques. In Mydorge, C. Examen du livre des Recreations mathematiques et de ses problemes en geometrie. 1638.

HENRION, Didier. *See* Henrion, Denis [*d. ca.* 1640]

HENRIQUES, Semuel Baruh [*fl.* 1674] *respondent.* Disputatio medica inauguralis, de epilepsia … Ultrajecti, Ex officina Meinardi à Dreunen, 1674.
　　8 p.　20 cm.　　　　　　　　**[5494]**
Diss. — Utrecht.

HENRY, François [1615–1686] *ed. See* Gassendi, P. Opera omnia. 1658.

HENSHAW, Nathaniel [1627?–1673] Aerochalinos; or, A register for the air; in five chapters. 1. Of fermentation. 2. Of chylification. 3. Of respiration. 4. Of sanguification. 5. That often changing the air, is a friend to health … Dublin, Samuel Dancer, 1664.
　　[12], 98 p.　17 cm.　　　　　**[5495]**

—[The same.] … The 2d. ed. … London, Benj. Tooke, 1677.
　　[23], 166, [2] p.　14 cm.　　　**[5496]**

HENTSCHEL, Samuel [*fl.* 1659–1662] *praeses.* Disquisitionem naturalem de asteria gemma … proponunt … Samuel Hentschel … & … Joh. Heinricus Laurentius … Witteb[ergae], Typis Johannis Borckardi [1662]
　　[20] p.　19 cm.　　　　　　　**[5497]**
Diss. — Wittenberg (J. H. Laurentius, *respondent*)

HENTZSCHEL, Michael [*fl.* 1658] *respondent. See* Sperling, J., *praeses.* Disputatio physica de meteoris aqueis. 1658.

HEPBURNE, George [*fl.* 1693] *respondent. See* Pitcairne, A., *praeses.* Dissertatio de motu sanguinis per vasa minima. 1693.

HEPNER, Paul [*fl.* 1608–1610] *respondent. See* Sennert, D., *praeses.* Disputatio medica de ophthalmia. 1608; Platter, F. [1536–1614] Felix Platerus … decreto. 1610.

HEPPIUS, Johannes Casparus [*b.* 1600 *respondent. See* Sebisch, M. [1578–1674?] *praeses.* Exercitationes medicae. 1639.

HERACLITUS, *of Ephesus.* [Letters. Greek and Latin] *In* Lubin, E., *ed.* and *tr.* Epistolae Hippocratis Democriti, Heracliti. 1601.

HERAEUS, Christian [*fl.* 1679] *respondent.* Disputatio medica inauguralis de phthisi … Lugduni Batavorum, Apud viduam & heredes Johannis Elsevirii, 1679.
　　[10] p.　21 cm.　　　　　　　**[5498]**
Diss. — Leyden.

HERBERT, George [1593–1633] *tr. See* Lessius, L. Hygiasticon. 1634 [and] The temperate man. 1678.

HERBST, Johann Jeremias, *respondent.* Dissertatio inauguralis medica de renum et vesicae calculo … Marburgi Cattorum, Typis Philippi Casimiri Mülleri [not before 1673]
　　[4], 20 p.　19 cm.　　　　　**[5499]**
Diss. — Marburg.

HERCKLITZ, Valentin Gottfried [*fl.* 1700] *respondent. See* Jenichen, G. A., *praeses.* De cultu heroinarum sago vel toga illustrium. 1700.

HEREBOORT, Adrianus [*fl.* 1631] *respondent. See* Burgersdijck, F. P., *praeses.* Collegium physicum. 1642.

HEREDIA, Pedro Miguel de [*d. ca.* 1661] Opera medica; in quatuor tomos divisa … [Lugduni, Sumptib. Philippi Borde, Laurentii Arnaud, Petri Borde, et Guill. Barbier, 1665]
　　4 v. in 2.　port.　36 cm.　　**[5500]**
Title from general half title.
Posthumous edition by Pedro Barea de Astorga.
Vol. 2 includes Latin text of 38 case histories from books 1 and 3 of Hippocrates' De morbis popularibus (i.e. Epidemiorum libri).
Contents.—v. 1. De febribus syntagma universale.—v. 2. Historiae epidemicae; seu, Commentaria in Hippocratem De morbis popularibus.—v. 3. De morbis acutis totius corporis humani.

De somno & vigilia. De natura delirii et ejus causis. — v. 4. Affectuum particularium tractatus aliquot. De morbis mulierum & utero-gerentium.

—[The same.] . . . [Lugduni, Sumptibus Laurentii Arnaud, & Petri Borde, 1673]

4 v. in 2.   port.   37 cm.   [5501]

Each volume has title page with statement: Ed. altera perquam accurate recognita, ac emendata cura & diligentia D. Petri Barea de Astorga . . .

"Quaest[io] posthuma, de febribus eradicatu difficilibus" (v. 1, p. 546–555) and "Tractatus . . . de expurgatione minorativa" (v. 4, p. 143–160) are added to the contents of the first edition.

—[The same.] . . . [Lugduni, Sumptib. Petri Borde, Joan. & Petri Arnaud, 1688–90 [v. 1, 1690]

4 v. in 2.   36 cm.   [5502]

A page for page reprint of the 1673 edition.

HERFELD, Henricus Gerhardus. *See* Herfelt, Heinrich Gerritsen [*fl.* 1678–1685]

HERFELT, Heinrich Gerritsen [*fl.* 1678–1685] Philosophicum hominis, de corporis humani machina, deque centro nobili, sede, seu vinculo mentis, tractans; confirmatum observationibus anatomicis . . . D. D. Willisii, Bartholini, Malpighii, Fracassati, Harvei, aliorumque: methodo . . . D. Cartesii concinnatum. Lugd. Batavor., Apud Jordanum Luchtmans, 1687.

[60], 462, [22] p.   illus.   17 cm.   [5503]

Added engraved title page.

—*respondent.* Disputatio inauguralis medica de affectione hypochondriaca . . . Duisburgi ad Rhenum, Apud Franconem Sas, 1678.

12 p.   20 cm.   [5504]

Diss. — Duisburg.

HERFORD, Marcus [*fl.* 1678] *respondent. See* Crause, R. W., *praeses.* Dissertatio medica inauguralis de tussi. 1678.

HÉRIGONE, Pierre. *See* Henrion, Denis [*d. ca.* 1640]

HERING, Honorius [*fl.* 1637–1639] Microcosmus melancholicus; seu, Tractatus singularis de melancholia in genere, et affectione hypochondriaca in specie, una cum appendice variorum exemplorum & medicamentorum . . . ex optimis autoribus collectorum . . . Bremae, Typis Wesselianis, ac sumptibus Georgii Hoismanni haeredum, 1683.

212 p.   13 cm.   [5505]

—Σχεδιασμα ιατρικον; seu, Consilium medicinale extemporaneum febrium erraticarum per oras hasce septentrionales . . . disseminatarum . . . theorian & therapian per aphorismos breviter delineatam exhibens . . . Bremae, Typis Wesselianis & sumptibus Georgii Hoismanni haeredum, 1638.

70 p.   13 cm.   [5506]

—Syntagma medicam theorico-practicum tripartitum de arthritide in genere, & podagra in specie, una cum appendice variorum medicamentorum antipodagricorum probatissimorum ex optimis autoribus collectorum . . . Bremae, Apud haeredes Hoismannianos, typis Wesselianis, 1639.

142 p.   14 cm.   [5507]

—Tractatus de pestilentia singularis, cui accessit fasciculus medicamentorum antipestilentialium insigniorum . . . Bremae, Typis Wesselianis, ac sumptibus Georgii Hoismanni haeredum, 1638.

801 p.   14 cm.   [5508]

HERING, Johann Ernst [*fl.* 1659–1669] *praeses.* Disputatio physica de hydromantia, quoad sagas probandas per aquam frigidam . . . [Wittenberg] In Officina Finceliana exscribebat Michael Meyer [1667]

[20] p.   19 cm.   [5509]

Diss. — Wittenberg (G. Kartner, *respondent*)

—Ex physicis de ortu avis Britannicae . . . publicam sententiarum collationem instituet Johannes Junghans . . . Wittebergae, Literis Michaelis Wendt, 1665.

[16] p.   19 cm.   [5510]

Diss. — Wittenberg (J. Junghans, *respondent*)

—*respondent. See* Simon, J., *praeses.* Ex physicis de generatione aequivoca. 1659.

HERING, Johann Jakob [*d.* 1723] *respondent. See* Bohn, J., *praeses.* Dissertatio medica inauguralis de haemorrhoidibus caecis. 1694.

HERLICIUS, David. *See* Herlitz, David [1557–1636]

HERLIN, Johann Heinrich [*fl. ca.* 1685] Biga remediorum generosorum, sive de remediis sudoriferis, cum praemissis de sudore, ac analepticis, discursus phisiologico-therapeuticus . . . Lipsiae, Sumptibus Joh. Christian. Wohlfart, 1693.

38 p.   20 cm.   [5511]

HERLINUS, Bernhardus [*fl.* 1670-1681] Consilium sanitatis; oder, Wohlmeynender Rath und Bericht, woraus des Menschen Gesundheit und Kranckheit entspringe, auch wie vollkommene Gesundheit zu erkennen und zu erhalten . . . Sampt einem Anhang, vom Missbrauch der wahren Physiognomiae, entgegen-gesetzt dem . . . Bericht von der Physiognomia Herrn Philippi Mayens anno 1681. in Dressden gedruckt. Coburg, Johann-Conrad Mönch, 1682.

384 p. 16 cm. [5512]

— *respondent. See* Petri von Hartenfels, G. C., *praeses.* Ignem microcosmicum . . . submittit . . . B. H. 1670.

HERLITZ, David [1557-1636] Consilium politico-physicum, gründliches Bedencken, und getrewer Rath, was eine Stadt, in welcher, den vorgangenen Herbst, die Pest ein wenig angefangen, künfftigen Frühling . . . fürnehmen solle, und insonderheit wie man die Lufft rectificiren . . . möge. Alles gantz new . . . zum Theil aus den . . . berümbtesten Medicis, arabischer, griechischer, lateinischer, und deutscher Sprachen . . . zusammen getragen . . . Franckfurt an der Oder, Bey Friedrich Hartman gedruckt, in Vorlegung Martini Gucks, 1621.

[8], 144 p. 19 cm. [5513]

— [The same.] . . . Nürnberg, *In* Verlegung Georg Endters dess Eltern, 1623.

[8], 144 p. 19 cm. [5514]

Different setting of type.

— De cura gravidarum, puerperarum & infantum. Newe Frawen Zimmer; oder, Gründtliche Unterrichtung, von den Schwangern unnd Kindelbetterinnen, was ihnen vor, in, und nach der Geburt zu wissen von Nöthen sey . . . Jetzo zum viertdenmahl wider ubersehen, und . . . vermehret . . . Alten Stettin, Gedruckt durch Joachim Rheten, 1609.

[16], 234, [1] p. port. 20 cm. [5515]

— [The same.] . . . Jetzo zum 4. Mahl wider ubersehen, und . . . vermehret . . . Magdeburgk, Gedruckt bey Johann Francken, 1613.

[188] p. 21 cm. [5516]

Bound with Sechs Bücher auserlesener Artzney und Kunst-Stück, 1613.

— [The same.] . . . Jetzo auffs newe . . . ubersehen, und . . . verbessert . . . Alten Stettin,

Gedruckt durch Johann Christoff Landtrachtingern, 1618.

[26], 426 p. 16 cm. [5517]

— [The same.] . . . Jetzo . . . zum vierdten Mahl . . . ubersehen, und . . . verbessert . . . Alten Stettin, By David Rheten, 1628.

[30], 484 p. 17 cm. [5518]

Imperfect: sig. A8 (blank?) wanting.

With this is bound Huxholtz, W. Unterricht der Hebammen. 1652.

— De variolis vel papulis. Notwendige und kurtze Erinnerung, von den jtzt [sic] grassierenden Bocken oder Blattern . . . Lübeck, Bey Nathan Amsedern, 1609.

[24] p. 19 cm. [5519]

Imperfect: upper margins trimmed possibly affecting pagination.

HERLS, Cornelis [*d.* 1625] Examen der chyrurgie . . . Seer nut ende dienstelijck alle jonge chyrurgyns, ende insonderheyt die haer begheven na Oost ofte West-Indien . . . 2. druck, van vele fauten gesuyvert. Middelburgh, By de weduwe ende erfgenamen van Symon Moulert [n. d.]

378, [5] p. 15 cm. [5520]

Voor-reden signed by G. M., the editor.

— [German tr.] Examen chirurgiae; oder, Der Wund-Artzney, in Frag und Antwort zusammen getragen . . . Anfangs in niederländischer Sprache beschrieben, nunmehro aber das erstemal ins Hochteutsche übersetzt, an vielen Orten verbessert . . . Nürnberg, In Verlegung Johann Hoffmanns, 1676.

[18], 666, [30] p. 14 cm. [5521]

HERMAN, Paul. *See* Hermann, Paul [1640?-1695]

HERMANN, Christian [*fl.* 1670] *respondent. See* Posner, C., *praeses.* Dissertatio academica de somniis vigilantium. 1670.

HERMANN, Daniel [1543?-1601] De rana et lacerta succino Prussiaco insitis. *In* Crato von Krafftheim, J. Consiliorum & epistolarum medicinalium . . . liber. 1620, 1671.

HERMANN, David. Manuale anatomicum; das ist: Kurtze Beschreibung und Erzehlung aller unnd jeglicher Glieder unnd Theil dess gantzen menschlichen Cörpers, auss den Authoribus auffskürtzest . . . ausgezogen, und in dieses kleine

Tractätlein gebracht . . . Nürnberg, In Verlegung Wolffgang Endters, 1630.

272, [12] p.   13 cm.   [5522]

Bound with Contarini, G., *Cardinal.* De elementis eorumque mixtionibus. 1633.

HERMANN, JOHANN AUGUST [*fl.* 1668–1670] *respondent. See* BOHN, J., *praeses.* Exercitationum physiologicarum prima . . . [-decima tertia] 1674?; LEICHNER, E., *praeses.* Disputatio inauguralis medica, de cholera humida. 1670.

HERMANN, MARTIN [*fl.* 1655] *respondent. See* ITTIG, J., *praeses.* Disputatio meteorologica. 1655.

HERMANN, PAUL [1640?–1695] Horti Academici Lugduno-Batavi catalogus exhibens plantarum omnium nomina, quibus anno MDCLXXXI ad annum MDCLXXXVI hortus fuit instructus ut & plurimarum in eodem cultarum & a nemine hucusque editarum descriptiones & icones . . . Lugduni Batavorum, Apud Cornelium Boutesteyn, 1687.

[20], 699 (i.e. 703) p.   illus.   20 cm.   [5523]

Added engraved title page.

—*praeses.* Disputatio medica de hydrope . . . Lugduni Batavorum, Apud Abrahamum Elzevier, 1693.

[16] p.   18 cm.   [5524]

Diss. — Leyden (H. von Schiffart, *respondent*)

—Paradisi Batavi prodromus. *In* Tournefort, J. P. de. Schola botanica. 1689.

—*See* BIDLOO, G. Oratio, in funere . . . Pauli Hermanni. 1695.

HERMANN, PÉTER [*fl.* 1700] *respondent. See* ROESCHEL, J. B., *praeses.* Disputationem physicam primam de fontium origine . . . submittit . . . P. H. 1700.

HERMANNI, PHILIPPUS [16th cent.] Een constich distillier-boeck, inhoudende die rechte ende waerachtige conste, om alderhande wateren, cruyden, bloemen, wortelen ende alle andere dingen te leeren distillieren, opt alderconstichste beschreven . . . Van nieus oversien, gecorrigeert ende verbetert. Amsterdam, Broer Jansz [1622]

[144] p.   illus.   15 cm.   [5525]

Date of imprint supplied from Forbes, p. 159, 379.
Includes a section (p. [118–125]) on the distillation of wine.

—*See* HESTER, J. The secrets of physick and philosophy. 1633; PARACELSUS. Dat secreet der philosophien. 1612.

Les HERMAPHRODITES. *See* [ARTUS, T., *sieur d'Embry*]

HERMES TRISMEGISTUS. De decubitu infirmorum. *In* Culpeper, N. Astrologicall judgment of diseases. 1655, 1658.

—The divine pymander . . . in XVII. books. Translated formerly out of the Arabick into Greek, and thence into Latine, and Dutch, and now out of the original into English; by . . . Doctor Everard. London, Printed by Robert White, for Tho. Brewster, and Greg. Moule, 1650.

[16], 215 p.   15 cm.   [5526]

Preface signed by the editor: J[ohn] F[rench]
— Copy 2.
With this is bound *his* The learned work. [1657?]

—The learned work . . . intituled iatromathematica. That is . . . physical mathematiques . . . directed unto Ammon . . . Lately Englished by John Harvey . . . [London? 1657?]

[2], 31 p.   15 cm.   [5527]

Signatures: M⁷⁻⁸, N–O⁸.
Published in 1657 as part [2] of Ralph Williams' Physicall rarities. Cf. BMC.
Bound with copy 2 of *his* The divine pymander. 1650.

—Sesthien boecken . . . uyt het Griecx ghebracht in ons Neder-duytsch: en, in versen af-gedeelt, nevens veel annotatien . . . Met eene . . . voor-rede uyt het Latijn, van Franciscus Patricius. Amstelredam, Pieter la Burgh [1652]

[8], 423 (i.e. 325) p.   14 cm.   [5528]

—Tabula smaragdina. *In* Tabula smaragdina. 1659.

—Tractatus vere aureus, de lapidis philosophici secreto, in capitula septem divisus: nunc vero a quodam anonymo, scholiis . . . illustratus . . . Tandem opera & studio Dominici Gnosii . . . in lucem editus . . . Lipsiae, Sumptibus Thomae Schureri [Valentinus am Ende imprimebat] 1610.

[16], 276, [2] p.   illus.   17 cm.   [5529]

—[The same.] Tractatus aureus de lapidis physici secreto, in capitula septem divisus, nunc vero a quodam anonymo scholiis illustratus . . .

592–705 p., vol. 4   illus.   20 cm.   (*In* Zetzner, Lazarus, *ed.* Theatrum chemicum. Argentorati, 1659–61)   **[5530]**

Caption title.

—*See* CONRING, H. De Hermetica . . . medicina liber unus. 1648 [and] De Hermetica . . . medicina libri duo. 1669; DORN, G. [Clavis totius philosophiae chemisticae. 1659]. SALMON, W. Medicina practica. 1692.

A HERMETICALL banquet, drest by a spagiricall cook: for the better preservation of the microcosme. London, Andrew Crooke, 1652.

[35], 161 p.   15 cm.   **[5531]**

Imperfect: sig. A1 (blank?) wanting.

Attributed sometimes to Thomas Vaughan or to James Howell. Cf. Halkett-Laing, vol. 9, p. 131.

HERMONDAVILLE, HENRI DE. *See* MONDEVILLE, Henri de [14th cent.]

HERNÁNDEZ, FRANCISCO [*ca.* 1517–1587] Rerum medicarum Novae Hispaniae thesaurus; seu, Plantarum animalium mineralium Mexicanorum historia ex Francisci Hernandi . . . relationibus . . . a Nardo Antonio Reccho . . . collecta ac in ordinem digesta a Joanne Terrentio . . . notis illustrata. Nunc primum . . . studio et impensis Lynceorum publici juris facta . . . Romae, Ex typographeio Jacobi Mascardi, 1628.

[1], 950, [34] p.; 90, [6] p.   illus., table.   34 cm.   **[5532]**

Engraved title page.

"Aliorum Novae Hispaniae animalium Nardi Antonii Recchi imagines et nomina. Joannis Fabri . . . expositione": p. [457]–840; - "Fabii Columnae . . . in Nardi Antonii Recchi rerum medicarum Novae Hispaniae volumen. Annotationes . . .": p. [841]–899; - "Phylosophicarum tabularum ex frontispiciis naturalis theatri principis Federici Caesii . . . desumpta prima pars . . .": p. [901]–950; - "Historiae animalium et mineralium Novae Hispaniae liber unicus . . . Francisco Fernandez authore . . .": 90 p. Except the last one, items have half titles.

—[The same.] . . . Romae, Ex typographeio Vitalis Mascardi, 1651.

[16], 950 (i.e. 958), [22] p.; 90, [6] p.   illus., table.   34 cm.   **[5533]**

Engraved title page.

A reissue of the 1628 edition with new title page, preliminary matter added, and some dedicatory epistles replaced with new ones. 8 new pages inserted after p. [456]

12 pages of Index medicamentorum Novae Hispaniae not present. Appendix to p. 917 inserted after p. 950.

Hunt 247.

HERODICUS, *pseud. See* FRAUENDOERFFER, Philipp [*d.* 1702]

HEROLD, HIERONYMUS [*d.* 1566] *See* SCHOLTZ, L. Epistolarum philosophicarum: medicinalium, ac chymicarum . . . volumen. 1610.

HÉRON, GILES [*fl.* 1600–1604] *See* RIOLAN, J. [1580–1657] Incursionum Quercetani depulsio. 1605.

HERRICHEN, JOHANN GOTTFRIED [1629–1705] De thea herba doricum melydrion. [Amstelodami, 1688]

[8] p.   18 cm.   **[5534]**

Text in Greek.

Place and date supplied in manuscript on title page. Imprint in BMC: [Leipzig? 1670?]

HERRING, FRANCIS [*d.* 1628] Certaine rules, directions, or advertisments for this time of pestentiall contagion; with a caveat to those that weare about their neckes impoisoned amulets as a preservative from the plague. First published for . . . the city of London, in . . . 1603. And now reprinted for the said citie . . . Whereunto is added certaine directions, for the poorer sort of people . . . London, William Jones, 1625.

[22] p.   19 cm.   **[5535]**

STC 13240.

—[The same.] Preservatives against the plague; or, Directions and advertisements for this time of pestilentiall contagion . . . Also a caveat to those that weare about their necks impoisoned amulets as a preservative . . . First published . . . in . . . 1603 and 1625 . . . London, Jasper Emerie, 1641.

[22] p.   19 cm.   **[5536]**

Imperfect: sig. C4 (blank?) wanting.

—A discovery of certaine strategems. *In* Oberndörfer, J. The anatomyes of the true physition. 1602, 1605.

—A modest defence of the caveat given to the wearers of impoisoned amulets, as preservatives from the plague . . . Likewise that unlearned . . . opinion, that the plague is not infectious . . . is . . . glansed at, and refuted by way of preface . . . London, Printed by Arnold Hatfield for William Jones, 1604.

[13], 37 p.   19 cm.   **[5537]**

STC 13248.

—, *tr. See* OBERNDÖRFER, J. The anatomyes of the true physition. 1602, 1605.

HERRSCHER, FERDINAND [*fl.* 1632] *See* EISENMENGER, J. C. Nothwendiger Bericht. 1632?

HERSTELLE, DANIEL ANDREAS [*fl.* 1699-1701] *respondent. See* SCHRADER, F., *praeses.* De signis medicis exercitatio prima [-tertia] 1699-1700.

—*See* SCHRADER, F. Programma quo exercitationes medicas publice habendas significat ad easque . . . invitat F. S. 1699.

HERT, JOHANN CHRISTOPH [1649-1731] *respondent.* Dissertatio inauguralis medica, de catarrho suffocativo . . . Giessae, Typis Friderici Kargeri [1673]
     32 p.   20 cm.   [**5538**]
     Diss. — Giessen.

HERTEBRODT, JOHANN MICHAEL [*fl.* 1667] *respondent.* Dissertatio inauguralis medica de peste . . . Argentorati, Literis Johannis Welperi, 1667.
     16 p.   20 cm.   [**5539**]
     Diss. — Strasbourg.

HERTEL, JOHANN MICHAEL [*d.* 1711] *praeses.* Medicinae theoricae, generalis, ac compendiariae veteris, et novae conjunctio. Seu utriusque qua dissonae, ac controversae conciliatio . . . Ingolstadii, Typis Thomae Grass [1700]
     [32], 313, [6] p.   front. (port.)   16 cm.   [**5540**]
     Diss. — Ingolstadt (J. P. Zimmer, *respondent*)

HERTEL, VALENTIN [*fl.* 1620-1625] *respondent. See* GÜNTER, J., *praeses.* Disputatio medica de peste. 1625.

—*See* STROBELBERGER, J. S. Epistolaris concertatio super variis . . . quaestionibus. 1625

HERTELIUS, MICHAEL. *See* HERTEL, Johann Michael [*d.* 1711]

HERTELIUS, VALENTIN. *See* HERTEL, Valentin [*fl.* 1620-1625]

HERTODT, JOHANN FERDINAND [1647-1714] Crocologia; seu, Curiosa croci regis vegetabilium enucleatio continens illius etymologiam, differentias . . . usum mechanicum, pharmaceuticum, chymico-medicum, omnibus pene humani corporis partibus destinatum . . . Ad normam et formam S. R. I. Academiae Naturae Curiosorum congesta . . . Jenae, Sumptibus Viti Jacobi Trescheri, typis Johannis Nisii, 1671.
     [19], 283, [5] p.   fronts., plate.   16 cm.   [**5541**]

—Opus mirificum sextae diei; id est, Homo physice, anatomice, & moraliter in potiores suas partes dissectus . . . Jenae, Sumtibus viti Jacobi Trescheri, typis Johannis Nisii, 1671.
     [4], 78 p.   front.   17 cm.   [**5542**]

—Tartaro-mastix Moraviae per quem rariora & admiranda a natura in faecundo hujus regionis gremio effusa, comprimis tartarus, illiusque effectus morbosi . . . examinantur, & cura tam therapeutica quam prophylactica proponitur . . . Viennae Austriae, Typis Susannae Rickesin viduae, 1669.
     [18], 263, 11 p.   16 cm.   [**5543**]
     Added engraved title page.

HERTOGHE, GILLES DE [*fl.* 1549-1561] *See* DODOENS, R. Medicinalium observationum exempla rara. 1621.

HERTZ, CONRAD RUDOLPH [*fl.* 1678-1687] *respondent. See* FRIESE, H. Disputatio medica qua defenditur, quod celebratissima illa per totam Europam hodie medicina thee arthritide conveniat. 1684; KALCKHOFF, J. C. Dissertatio inauguralis. 1678; RAST, G. *praeses.* Ebrietas medice considerata. 1682; WEDEL, G. W., *praeses.* Disputationem inauguralem de scorbuto . . . proponit C. R. H. 1687.

HERTZOG, ANASTASIUS [*fl.* 1695] *respondent.* Disputatio inauguralis medica de gangraena et sphacelo . . . Basileae, Typis Jacobi Bertschii [1695]
     [16] p.   19 cm.   [**5544**]
     Diss. — Basel.

—*See* HARDER, J. J., *praeses.* Exercitatio medica . . . sanguificationis in humano corpore historiam exponens. 1690.

HERTZOGIUS, RUDOLPHUS. *See* HERZOG, Rudolf [*fl.* 1645]

HERVÉ-FIERABRAS. *See* FIERABRAS, Hervé [*fl.* 1550]

HERVELT, JACOB VAN [*fl.* 1693] Geneeskundige aanmerkingen in sijn dagelijkse practyk voorgevallen; zaamgesteld na de oprechte wysbegeerte en nieuwe geneeskunde. Als mede een regte manier om de Venus-qualen, met haren aanhang, grondig en op een seer korte wyse te geneesen . . . Amsterdam, Jan teen Hoorn, 1693.
     [8], 295, [42] p.   illus.   16 cm.   [**5545**]
     Added engraved title page.

HERVET, Gentian [1499–1584] *See* Sextus Empiricus. Opera. 1621.

HERVIEU, Julien Placide [1671–1746] *See* Les secrets de la medecine des chinois. 1671.

HERWIG, Henning Michael. The art of curing sympathetically or magnetically . . . With a discourse concerning the cure of madness, and an Appendix to prove the reality of sympathy . . . Written originally in Latin . . . London, Tho. Newborough, R. Parker, and P. Buck, 1700.

[15], 151 p.   15 cm.   [5546]

HERWIG, Johann Friedrich [*fl.* 1688] *respondent. See* Wedel, G. W., *praeses.* Disputatio medica, sistens aegrum quartana laborantem. 1688.

HÉRY, Thierry de [*ca.* 1500–*ca.* 1560] La methode curatoire de la maladie venerienne; vulgairement appellee grosse vairolle, & de la diversité de ses symptomes . . . Plus est adjousté un traitté de la maniere de faire le baume de François Arcaeus. Et l'emplastre de Paracelse, telle qu'il l'a donnee en son livre de la guarison des playes. Paris, Eustache d'Aubin, 1634.

[18], 208 (i.e. 210), [1] p.   17 cm.   [5547]

Imperfect: sig. A1 wanting.

—[The same.] . . . Paris, Jean Dehoury, 1660.
[12], 208 (i.e. 212) p.   18 cm.   [5548]

—[The same.] . . . Paris, Jean d'Houry, 1674.
[12], 208 (i.e. 212) p.   18 cm.   [5549]

A reissue of the 1660 edition, with original imprint covered by lower portion of another title page, as above.

HERZBERG, Godofredus Sigismundus Schlegel. *See* Schlegel, Gottfried Sigmund [*fl.* 1691]

HERZOG, Johann Friedrich [*fl.* 1678] *respondent. See* Lyncker, N. C. von, *praeses.* Disputatio inauguralis juridica de fatalibus. 1678.

HERZOG, Rudolf [*fl.* 1645] *respondent. See* Horne, J. van. Miscellanea . . . anatomica et chirurgica. 1645.

HERZOG, Samuel [*fl.* 1697–1698] *respondent. See* Camerarius, E., *praeses.* Quaestionem casuistarum medico-legalem, an liceat medico pro salute matris abortum procurare? 1697; Camerarius, R. J., *praeses.* De colica paretico-epileptica. 1698.

HESPORN, Franz [*fl.* 1679] *respondent. See* Major, J. D., *praeses.* Positiones medicae variae earumque praecipuae de podagra. 1679.

HESSE, Adam [*fl.* 1699] *respondent. See* Hoffmann, F. [1660–1742] *praeses.* Dissertatio medicina inauguralis, de praecipuo studiosorum morbo. 1699.

HESSE, Johann Christian [*fl.* 1684] *respondent. See* Schmid, C. [*fl.* 1684] *praeses.* Dissertatio physica de prodigiis sanguineis vulgo creditis. 1684. .

HESSE-DARMSTADT, Eleonora, *Landgräfin von. See* Eleonora, *consort of George I, landgrave of Hesse-Darmstadt* [1551 or 2–1618]

HESTEAU, Clovis, *sieur de Nuisement* [*fl.* 1578–1594] Poeme philosophic de la verité de la phisique mineralle, ou sont refutees les obiections que peuvent faire les incredules & ennemis de cet art. Auquel est naïfvement & veritablement depeinte la vraye matiere des philosophes. Par le sieur de Nuisement . . . Paris, Jeremie Perier & Abdias Buisard, 1620.

80 p.   17 cm.   [5550]

Bound with *his* Traittez de l'harmonie . . . du vray sel. 1621.

—Traittez de l'harmonie et constitution generalle du vray sel, secret des philosophes, & de l'esprit universelle du monde, suivant le troisiesme principe du cosmopolite . . . Recueilly par le sieur de Nuisement . . . Paris, Jeremie Perier et Abdias Buisard, 1621.

[28], 332 (i.e. 312) p.   illus.   17 cm.   [5551]

With this is bound *his* Poeme philosophic. 1620.

—[Latin tr.] Tractatus de vero sale secreto philosophorum, & de universali mundi spiritu, Gallice primo scriptus . . . nunc simplicissimo stylo Latine versus a Ludovico Combachio . . . Lugduni Batavorum. Apud Arnoldum Doude, 1671.

[16], 224 p.   14 cm.   [5552]

Bound with copy 2 of Rhijne, Willem ten. Meditationes in magni Hippocratis textum xxiv De veteri medicina. 1672.

[—][English tr.] Sal, lumen, & spiritus mundi philosophici; or, The dawning of the day, discovered by the beams of light: shewing, the true salt and secret of the philosophers. The first and universal spirit of the world. Written originally in French afterwards turned into Latin by . . . Lodovicus Combachius . . . And now transplanted into Albyons garden, By R[obert] T[urner] . . . [London] Printed by J. C. and sold by Nath. Ekins, 1657.

[30], 220, [2] p.   14 cm.   [5553]

—*See* Vigilantius de Monte Cubiti, *ed.* and *tr.* Dreyfaches hermetisches Kleeblat. 1667.

[HESTER, JOHN, d. 1593] The excellencie of physick and chirurgerie, collected out of approved practises, and learned observations of many expert men in both faculties. London, G. D[awson] 1652.

[10], 92 (i.e. 72) p. 19 cm. (Vol. [3] in Fioravanti, Leonardo. Three exact pieces ... Together with a book of excellent experiments and secrets, collected [by John Hester] ... London, 1652)   [5554]

Reprinted (with omission of the dedication and the latter part of the note to the reader, both by the editor, James Fourestier) from the edition published in London in 1594 under title: The pearle of practise.

"A supplement or addition ... This appendix ... containeth both philosophicall discourses, of the causes and cures of ... sundry diseases: as also many pithie discourses, of the vertues and use of many vegetables, animals, &c. culled ... out of the Physicks and Chirurgery of Sir Leonardo Phioravante ...": p. 45-92.

— The secrets of physick and philosophy, divided into two bookes: in the first is shewed the true and perfect order to distill, or draw forth the oyles of all manner of gummes, spices, seedes ... In the second is shewed the true and perfect order to prepare ... all manner of minerals ... First written in the German tongue by ... Theophrastus Paraselsus [sic], and now published in the English tongue, by John Hester ... London, Printed by A. M. for William Lugger, 1633.

[24], 196, [15] p. 14 cm.   [5555]

Imperfect: preliminary leaf (half title?) wanting.
STC 19182.
Sudhoff 356, 184.
Earlier London editions (1575, 1580, 1596) were published under title: The key of philosophie. Also published anonymously in London in 1633 under title: A storehouse of physicall and philosophicall secrets.
Part 1 is "a loose paraphrase, not a translation" of Duchesne's De exquisita mineralium, animalium, & vegetabilium medicamentorum spagyrica praeparatione & usu, perspicua tractatio. Part 2 probably is derived from Paracelsus. Cf. P. H. Kocher, John Hester, Paracelsan in Joseph Quincy Adams memorial studies, 1948, p. 629-630.

[—The same.] A storehouse of physicall and philosophicall secrets. Teaching to distill all manner of oyles from gummes, spices, seedes ... London, Thomas Harper, 1633.

[4], 57, [1] p. 18 cm.   [5556]
Imperfect: sig. D⁸ (last blank leaf) wanting.
STC 19182.5.
Issued also as vol. [3] of Banister, John. The workes. London, 1633. 19 cm.

—, ed. See FIORAVANTI, L. Three exact pieces of Leonard Phioravant. 1652; PARACELSUS. One hundred and fourteen experiments and cures. 1652.

—, tr. See FIORAVANTI, L. A discourse upon chyrurgery. 1626; VICARY, T. The English mans treasure. 1613, 1633, 1641 [and] The surgions directorie. 1651.

HESTERBERG, ERICH [fl. 1691] respondent. See VESTI, J., praeses. Exercitium medicum inaugurale, proponens chlorosin ... exponet E. H. 1691.

HETEROPOLITANUS, PROBUS, pseud. See LE BON, Jean [d. 1583?]

HETTENBACH, ERNESTUS, respondent. See SENNERT, D. De scorbuto tractatus. 1624.

HETTMAYER, GEORG IGNAZ [fl. 1676-1688] Uhrsprung, Gelegenheit, alter Beschreibung, Würckung, Nutzen und Gebrauch des uhralten Joannis-Bad, im Königreich Böhaimb, am Riesen-Geburg ... gelegen, beschrieben ... im Jahr 1676 ... Glatz, Gedruckt bey Mathaeo Erich, 1680.

79 p. 15 cm.   [5557]

—[The same.] ... Beschrieben ... im Jahr 1676. und zum erstenmahl in Druck ausgeben im Jahr 1680. Jetzo aber, nebst einem vermehrten Anhang ... zum andernmahl in Druck befördert ... Glatz, Andreas Franc. Pega, 1688.

95 p. 15 cm.   [5558]

HETZER, CHRISTOPH LUDWIG [fl. 1649] respondent. See SEBISCH, M. [1578-1674?] praeses. Galeni quinque priores libri. 1651.

HEUCHER, JOHANN HEINRICH [1677-1747] praeses. Ex historia naturali de vegetabilibus magicis generatim disserent M. Jo. Henr. Heucherus ... & Joannes Fabricius ... Wittebergae, Typis Johannis Hakii, 1700.

[18] p. 19 cm.   [5559]
Diss.—Wittenberg (J. Fabricius, respondent)

HEUNISCH, AUGUST FRIEDRICH [fl. 1699] respondent. See SPERLING, P. G., praeses. Dissertatio inauguralis medica de fame canina. 1699.

HEURNE, JOHAN VAN [1543-1601] Opera omnia. Edidit ... Ottho Heurnius ... [Lugduni

Batavorum] Ex Officina Plantiniana Raphelengii, 1609 [i.e. 1611]

 3 v. illus., port., tables. 23 cm. **[5560]**

General title page in vol. [1] only; vol. [2-3] have special title pages. The separately paged works have special title pages dated 1603-11.

Contents. — [v. 1] Vita auctoris. — [pt. 1] Institutiones medicinae, ed. alt. 1609. — [pt. 2] Praxis medicinae nova ratio, editio postrema. 1609. — [v. 2] Praxis medicinae particularis. 1609 [i.e. 1611] — [v.3] In praecipuos libros Hippocratis Coi commentaria. 1609.

—Opera omnia. Edidit . . . Ottho Heurnius . . . [Lugduni Batavorum] Ex Officina Plantiniana Raphelengii, 1611 [i.e. 1615]

 1 v. in 8 parts. illus., fold. tables. 21 cm.

[5561]

The separately paged works have special title pages dated 1602-15.

Contents. — Vita auctoris. — [pt. 1] Institutiones medicinae; ed. alt. 1611. — [pt. 2] Praxis medicinae nova ratio; ed. postrema. 1609. — [pt. 3] De morbis qui in singulis partibus humani capitis insidere consueverunt. 1608. — [pt. 4] De morbis oculorum, aurium, nasi, dentium et oris liber. 1602. — [pt. 5] De morbis pectoris liber. 1602. — [pt. 6] De febribus liber. 1610. — [pt. 7] De peste liber. 1615. — [pt. 8] De gravissimis morbis mulierum liber; item De morbis ventriculi, aliique. 1610.

—Opera omnia: tam ad theoriam, quam ad praxin medicam spectantia . . . Juxta Otthonis Heurnii . . . recensionem ac oeconomiam fideliter expressa, ac duos in tomos tributa. Postrema editio: prioribus, non tantum augustiore forma, sed & typorum nitore, & mendarum raritate, infinities tum luculentior, tum accuratior. Lugduni, Sumptibus Joannis Antonii Huguetan & Marci Antonii Ravaud, 1658.

 2 v. illus., port., tables. 38 cm. **[5562]**

Half title: Opera omnia in duos tomos divisos. Vol. 2 has title: Operum omnium . . . tomus secundus.

The author's commentaries on Hippocrates (v. 2, p. 137-478) include the Hippocratic texts in Greek and Latin.

—De febribus liber. [Lugduni Batavorum] Ex Officina Plantiniana Raphelengii, 1610.

 [8], 124 p. 22 cm. **[5563]**

A reprint of the 1598 Leyden edition.

With this are bound *his:* De peste liber. 1615; De morbis qui in singulis partibus humani capitis insidere consueverunt. [Lugduni Batavorum] 1594.

—De gravissimis morbis mulierum liber, De humana felicitate liber, & De morbis novis et mirandis epistola. Edidit . . . Ottho Heurnius . . . [Lugduni Batavorum] Ex Officina Plantiniana Raphelengii, 1607.

 [12], 101, [3] p. 22 cm. **[5564]**

—De gravissimis morbis mulierum liber; item De morbis ventriculi, aliique . . . Edidit . . . Ottho Heurnius . . . [Lugduni Batavorum] Ex Officina Plantiniana Raphelengii, 1610.

 61, [3] p.; 32, [3] p. 21 cm. **[5565]**

Part [2] has half title: . . . De morbis ventriculi liber; Responsum ad . . . Joannem Banchemium . . . nullum esse aquae innationem lamiarum indicium; Oratio de medicinae origine.

Bound with *his* De morbis qui in singulis partibus humani capitis insidere consueverunt. 1608.

—De humana felicitate. *In his* De gravissimis morbis mulierum liber. 1607.

—De morbis novis et mirandis epistola. *In his* De gravissimis morbis mulierum liber. 1607.

—De morbis oculorum, aurium, nasi, dentium et oris, liber; editus . . . ab . . . Othone Heurnio. [Lugduni Batavorum] Ex Officina Plantiniana Raphelengii, 1602.

 [16], 95, [4] p. table. 21 cm. **[5566]**

Bound with (as issued) *his* De morbis pectoris liber. 1602.

—Another issue.

 [8], 95, [4] p. 21 cm. (Vol. 1, part 4 *in his* Opera omnia. [Lugduni Batavorum] 1611 [i.e. 1615])

[5567]

Without the folded table and without p. [9-16] (commendatory verses) of the original issue.

—[The same.] . . . 1608.

 [8], 96 (i.e. 66), [6] p. (incl. table) 21 cm.

[5568]

A reprint, omitting some commendatory verses, of the 1602 Leyden edition.

Bound with *his* De morbis qui in singulis partibus humani capitis insidere consueverunt. 1608.

—De morbis pectoris liber, editus . . . ab . . . Othone Heurnio. [Lugduni Batavorum] Ex Officina Plantiniana Raphelengii, 1602.

 [16], 181, [3] p. 21 cm. **[5569]**

Caption title: De partium spirabilium morbis.

With this is bound (as issued) *his* De morbis oculorum, aurium, nasi, dentium et oris, liber. 1602.

—Another issue.

 [8], 181, [3] p. 21 cm. (Vol. 1, part 5 *in his* Opera omnia. [Lugduni Batavorum] 1611 [i.e. 1615])

[5570]

Without p. [9-16] (commendatory verses) of the original issue.

—[The same.] . . . 1608.

 [4], 127, [5] p. 21 cm. **[5571]**

A reprint, omitting some commendatory verses, of the 1602 Leyden edition.

Bound with *his* De morbis qui in singulis partibus humani capitis insidere consueverunt. 1608.

—De morbis qui in singulis partibus humani capitis insidere consueverunt. Hic ... morborum ideae, causae, & cujusque causae morbificae, partisque aegrae signa, prognoses, & curatio rationalis & empirica graphice depinguntur ... [Lugduni Batavorum] Ex Officina Plantiniana Raphelengii, 1608.

[8], 245, [11] p.   21 cm.   [5572]

With this are bound *his*: De morbis oculorum, aurium, nasi, dentium et oris liber. 1608; De morbis pectoris liber. 1608; De gravissimis morbis mulierum liber; item De morbis ventriculi. 1610; De peste. 1611.

—De morbis ventriculi liber: Responsum ad ... Joannem Banchemium ... nullum esse aquae innatationem lamiarum indicium: Oratio de medicinae origine, Aesculapidum, ac Hippocratis stirpe & scriptis. Edidit ... Ottho Heurnius ... [Lugduni Batavorum] Ex Officina Plantiniana Raphelengii, 1608.

[8], 62, [2] p.   20 cm.   [5573]

—[The same.] *In his* De gravissimis morbis mulierum liber. 1610.

—De peste liber. [Lugduni Batavorum] Ex Officina Plantiniana Raphelengii, 1611.

37, [3] p.   21 cm.   [5574]

Bound with *his* De morbis qui in singulis partibus humani capitis insidere consueverunt. 1608.

—[The same.] ... 1615.

37, [3] p.   22 cm.   [5575]

Different setting of type.

Bound with *his* De febribus liber. 1610.

—De studio medicinae bene instituendo dissertatio. *In* Groot, H. de. H. Grotii et aliorum dissertationes de studiis instituendis. 1645.

—In Hippocratis Coi De hominis natura libros duos, commentarius. Edidit ... Ottho Heurnius ... [Lugduni Batavorum] Ex Officina Plantiniana Raphelengii, 1609.

[8], 52, [2] p.   21 cm.   [5576]

Includes Greek text of De natura hominis, with Heurne's Latin translation.

With this are bound: Hippocrates. Prolegomena et Prognosticorum libri tres. Lugduni Batavorum, 1597; his In Hippocrates

Coi De victus ratione in morbis acutis librum primum [-quartum] ... commentarius. 1609. —copy 2 of Hippocrates. Aphorismi. 1609. —Copy 2.

Bound with Hippocrates. Prolegomena et Prognosticorum libri tres. Lugduni Batavorum, 1597.

—[The same.] ... 1611.

32 p.   23 cm.   (Part 1 *in his* In praecipuos libros Hippocratis Coi commentaria. [Lugduni Batavorum] 1609 [i.e. 1611] Opera omnia [v. 3]   [5577]

A reprint, omitting the commendatory verses and index, of the 1609 Leyden edition.

—In Hippocratis Coi De victus ratione in morbis acutis librum primum [-quartum] ... commentarius. Edidit ... Ottho Heurnius ... [Lugduni Batavorum] Ex Officina Plantiniana Raphelengii, 1609.

2 v.   21 cm.   [5578]

Includes Greek text of De victus ratione in morbis acutis, with Heurne's Latin translation.

Bound with *his* In Hippocratis Coi De hominis natura libros duos, commentarius. 1609.

—Copy 2.

Bound with Hippocrates. Prolegomena et Prognosticorum libri tres. Lugduni Batavorum, 1597.

—[The same.] ... 1611.

125, [3] p.   23 cm.   (Part 3 *in his* In praecipuos libros Hippocratis Coi commentaria. [Lugduni Batavorum] 1609 [i.e. 1611] Opera omnia [v. 3])   [5579]

Half title.

A reprint of the 1609 Leyden edition. Books 3–4 have special half title.

—In praecipuos libros Hippocratis Coi commentaria ... Edidit ... Ottho Heurnius ... [Lugduni Batavorum] Ex Officina Plantiniana Raphelengii, 1609.

4 parts.   23 cm.   (Vol. 3 *in his* Opera omnia. [Lugduni Batavorum] 1609[-11])   [5580]

Parts have special title pages dated 1603-11.

Includes Hippocratic texts in Greek and Latin.

Contents. — [pt. 1] In Hippocratis Coi De hominis natura libros duos commentarius. 1611. — [pt. 2] Hippocratis Coi prolegomena, et Prognosticorum libri tres; cum paraphrastica versione & brevibus commentariis. 1603. — [pt. 3] In Hippocratis Coi De victus ratione in morbis acutis libros quatuor commentarius. [dedication 1609] — [pt. 4] Hippocratis Coi Aphorismi ... brevi enarratione, fidaque interpretatione ... illustrati. 1609.

—Institutiones medicinae. Ed. alt., priore emendatior, opera ... Othonis Heurnii. [Lugduni

Batavorum] Ex officina Plantiniana Raphelengii, 1609.

    [23], 588 p. 14 cm.   [**5581**]

Preface by the original editor, Pieter Pauw.

Contains also his Modus ratioque studendi eorum, qui medicinae operam suam dicarunt.

—[The same.] . . . 1609.
    [8], 176, [8] p. 23 cm. [Vol. 1, part 1 *in his* Opera omnia. [Lugduni Batavorum] 1609[-11]
                                  [**5582**]

Another edition issued by the same press in the same year. Without the commendatory verses.

—[The same.] . . . 1611 [i.e. 1615]
    [8], 176, [7] p. 21 cm. [Vol. 1, part 1 *in his* Opera omnia. [Lugduni Batavorum] 1611 [i.e. 1615]
                                    [**5583**]

A reprint of the 1609 Leyden edition. Index shortened by one page.

—[The same.] . . . Lugduni Batavorum, Ex officina Joannis Maire, 1627.
    [16], 583 p. 13 cm.   [**5584**]

—[The same.] . . . 1638.
    [24], 612, [11] p. 13 cm.   [**5585**]

Errata: p. [11]

—Oratio de medicinae origine. *In his* De morbis ventriculi liber. 1608.

—Praxis medicinae nova ratio: qua, libris tribus methodi ad praxin medicam, aditus facilimus aperitur ad omnes morbos curandos. Ed. postrema, emendatior, opera . . . Otthonis Heurnii . . . [Lugduni Batavorum] Ex Officina Plantiniana Raphelengii, 1609.
    [8], 376, [12] p. illus., tables. 21 cm. [**5586**]

"Tabulae ponderum & mensurarum antiquae & recentioris medicinae": 3 folded leaves inserted at end.

—[The same.] . . . Ex accurata recensione Zachariae Sylvii . . . Roterodami, Ex officina Arnoldi Leers, 1650.
    [36], 721, [21] p. illus. 20 cm.   [**5587**]

Added engraved title page with title: Methodus ad praxin medicam.

Imperfect: p. 23-24 mutilated.
Interleaved.

—Praxis medicinae particularis . . . Edidit . . . Ottho Heurnius . . . [Lugduni Batavorum] Ex Officina Plantiniana Raphelengii, 1609 [i.e. 1611]

6 parts. 23 cm. [Vol. 2 *in his* Opera omnia. [Lugduni Batavorum] 1609 [i.e. 1611]   [**5588**]

Parts have special title pages dated 1608-11.

Contents. — [pt. 1] De morbis qui in singulis partibus humani capitis insidere consueverunt. 1608. — [pt. 2] De morbis oculorum, aurium, nasi, dentium et oris liber. 1608. — [pt. 3] De morbis pectoris liber. 1608. — [pt. 4] De gravissimis morbis mulierum liber; item De morbis ventriculi, aliique. 1610. — [pt. 5] De febribus liber. 1610. — [pt. 6] De peste liber. 1611.

—, ed. and *tr. See* HIPPOCRATES. [Aphorismi. Greek and Latin] 1601, 1609, 1611, 1615, 1617, 1623, 1633, 1638, 1664, 1688, 1690.

—, ed. *See* HIPPOCRATES. [Selected works. Greek and Latin] 1611.

—, *tr. See* HIPPOCRATES. [Selected works. Greek and Latin] Aphorismi Graece, & Latine. 1607, 1627 [and] [Aphorismi. Latin.] 1623, 1631, 1646, 1663; SCHÖNFELD, P. J. Synopsis medica super Pharmacopoeiam Augustanam pro praecipuis humani corporis affectibus. 1677.

—*See* BROEKHUIZEN, D. van. Secreta alchimiae magnalia D. Thomae Aquinatis. 1602; FERNEL, J. Universa medicina. 1656, 1679; HIPPOCRATES. [Aphorismi. English] 1655; [Collected works. Greek and Latin] 1657, 1662.

HEURNE, OTTO VAN [1577-1652] *praeses.* Disputatio medica de hydrope . . . Lugduni Batavorum, Ex officina Zachariae Smetii, 1621.
    [7] p. 20 cm.   [**5589**]

Diss. — Leyden (J. Le Piper, *respondent*)

—, ed. *See* HEURNE, J. van. De gravissimis morbis mulierum liber. 1607, 1610 [and] De morbis oculorum, aurium, nasi, dentium et oris, liber. 1602, 1608 [and] De morbis pectoris liber. 1602, 1608, 1611 [i.e. 1615] [and] De morbis ventriculi liber. 1608 [and] *In* Hippocratis Coi De hominis natura libros duos. 1609, 1611 [and] *In* Hippocratis Coi De victus ratione. 1609, 1611 [and] *In* praecipuos libros Hippocratis Coi commentaria. 1609 [and] Institutiones medicinae. 1609, 1611, 1627, 1638 [and] Opera omnia. 1609 [i.e. 1611], 1611 [i.e. 1615], 1658 [and] Praxis medicinae particularis. 1609 [i.e. 1611]

—*See* FERNEL, J. Universa medicina. 1656, 1679.

HEURNIUS. *See* HEURNE.

HEURTAULT, PIERRE. Le preservatif contre la peste. Avec le moyen de garir ceux qui en sont affligez ... Caen, Jean de Bally, 1621.

59 p. 15 cm. [5590]

With this is bound Guibert, P. Le medecin charitable. 1624.

— Traicté de la phlebotomie. Où selon la doctrine des anciens & modernes approuvez, est contenuë la maniere de bien & artificiellement saigner ... Caen, Jean de Basly, 1622.

[10], 66 ll. 16 cm. [5591]

HEYDE, ANTONIUS DE. *See* HEIDE, Antonius de [1646–*ca*. 1693]

HEYDE, HERMANN VAN DER. *See* HEYDEN, Hermann van der [1572–*ca*. 1650]

HEYDE, LAZARUS AB. *See* HEYDEN, Lazarus von [*fl*. 1625–1631]

HEYDEN, HERMANN VAN DER [1572–*ca*. 1650] Discours et advis sur les flus de ventre douloureux, soit qu'il y ayt du sang ou point. Sur le troussegallant: dict cholera morbus: la peste: les effects signalés & incroyables de l'eau: la vraye generation & asseureé curatio de la goutte: les fievres tierces & quartes, causées de l'infection des poldres & terres avoisinées de la mer & d'autres marascageuses. Avec addition d'un appendice de la goutte, & de la sciatique en particulier: & des nouveaux discours sur l'hydropisie, colique, toux ordinaire & phtisique, gravelle, & la jaunisse (pour estre accidens aux susdictes fievres survenans & suyvans) & sur la morsure des chiens enragés ... Gand, Servais Manilius, 1643, et l'addition, 1645.

[10], 182, [2] p. 19 cm. [5592]

Imperfect: printer's mark excised from title page, with damage to the privilege on the verso.

A leaf (sig. b1) with a complimentary poem addressed to the author is inserted before p. 1 of the text.

The original French edition of 1643 ended at p. 120. Reissued with a cancel title page and the addition (p. 121–174) in 1645. Includes the author's "Advertissement & responce sur quelques objections" (p. 175–182).

Errata at end.

— Another issue. 20 cm. [5593]

Imperfect: all pages after p. 120 wanting.
Contains an insert of one unsigned leaf between p. 70–71.

— [Latin tr.] Synopsis discursuum ... idiomate Gallico editorum ... Latinitati donata ... In qua ... compendiose deducuntur ... utilia, dictis discursibus contenta. Et praecipue, seri lactis in fluxu torminali, & maxime dysenterico - acquae frigidae ... effectus, podagrae dolores vel sistentis, vel ... demulcentis ... et aceti vini, in praeservatione a peste ... facultates ... commendantur. Multis additis observationibus novis ... Gandavi, Ex officina Servatii Manilii, 1649.

[24], 202, [3] p. 15 cm. [5594]

Errata: p [3] at end.
Imperfect: sheets E and F transposed.

— [English tr.] Speedy help for rich and poor; or, Certain physicall discourses touching the vertue of whey ... Of cold water ... Of wine-vinegar ... Written in Latine ... London, Printed by James Young, for O. P. and sold by John Saywell, 1653.

[34], 211, [2] p. 15 cm. [5595]

Imperfect: first preliminary leaf and last leaf (blank?) wanting.

HEYDEN, LAZARUS VON [*fl*. 1625–1631] *respondent*. *See* SEBISCH, M. [1578–1674?] *praeses*. Disputatio de crisibus posterior. 1627 [and] Exercitationes medicae. 1639.

—, *tr. See* CASTELLANI, G. M. Ausführliche und nothwendige Verzeichniss. 1665.

HEYDENREICH, GOTTFRIED [*fl*. 1677] *respondent*. *See* LOSS, J., *praeses*. Disputatio medica de salivae natura. 1677.

HEYDENREICH, JUSTUS RUDOLF [*fl*. 1675–1677] *respondent*. *See* WEDEL, G. W., *praeses*. Dissertatio medica proponens juvenem melancholia laborantem. 1675.

HEYDER, SIGMUND ADAM [*fl*. 1699] *respondent*. *See* SPERLING, P. G., *praeses*. Dissertatio inauguralis medica exhibens choleram. 1699.

HEYDON, *Sir* CHRISTOPHER [*d*. 1623] An astrological discourse, manifestly proving the powerful influence of planets and fixed stars upon elementary bodies, in justification of the verity of astrology. Together with an astrological judgment upon the great conjunction of Saturn and Jupiter 1603 ... London, Printed by John Macock, for Nathaniel Brooks, 1650.

[14], 111 p. illus. 14 cm. [5596]

To the reader signed by the editor: Nicholas Fisk.

HEYDON, JOHN [*b.* 1629] Hammeguleh hampaaneah; or, The Rosie Crucian crown set with seven angels, 7 planets ... and their occult powers, upon the 7 mettalls and miraculous vertues in medicines ... Whereunto is added Elhavareuna Presoria, Regio lucis, and Psonthon ... London, Printed by P. L. for Samuel Speed, 1665.

[26], 54 p.; [4], 44 p. 17 cm. **[5597]**

Part [1] contains the first and second book, part [2] the third book of The Rosie Crucian crown. The latter has special title page: Hampaaneah hammegulleh; or, The Rosie crucian crown ... Whereunto is added, a perfect full discovery of the pantarva, and elixirs of metals. By Eugenius Theodidactus [pseud.] London, Printed for the author, 1664.

HEYE, FRIEDRICH [*fl.* 1662] *respondent. See* TAPPE, J., *praeses. Disputatio medica de febri ephemera.* 1662.

HEYLAND, MICHAEL. *See* HEILAND, Michael [*fl.* 1646-1676]

HEYNSIUS, PIETER [*fl.* 1669] *respondent.* Disputatio medica inauguralis continens casum de pleuritide vera ... Lugduni Batavorum, Apud viduam & haeredes Joannis Elsevirii, 1669.

[12] p. 23 cm. **[5598]**

Diss.—Leyden.

HEYSE, ERNST GOTTFRIED [1655 or 6-1692] *respondent. See* BOHN, J., *praeses.* Dissertationes chymico-physicae. 1685.

—, *ed. See* DRELINCOURT, C. Experimenta anatomica. 1681, 1682, 1684.

HEZMANSEDER, GEORG [*fl.* 1607] *See* KNOBLOCH, T., *praeses.* Disputationes anatomicae. 1608, 1612.

HIAERNE, URBAIN. *See* HJÄRNE, Urben [1641-1724]

HIBNER, ISRAEL. *See* HIEBNER, Israel [*fl.* 1648]

HIDDINGH, GERARDUS [*fl.* 1661] *respondent.* Disputatio medica inauguralis, de asthmate ... Lugduni Batavorum, Ex officina Francisci Moyaert, 1661.

[8] p. 21 cm. **[5599]**

Diss.—Leyden.

HIEBNER, ISRAEL [*fl.* 1648] Mysterium sigillorum, herbarum & lapidum; oder, Vollkommene Cur und Heilung aller Kranckheiten Schäden

und Leibes- auch Gemüths-Beschwerungen durch underschiedliche Mittel ohne Einnehmung der Artzney. In 4. Classen ... abgetheilet ... [Erffurdt] In Verlegung Johann Birckners, 1651.

[2], 166, [39] p. illus. 20 cm. **[5600]**

Errata: p. [37-39]

—[The same.] ... [Erffurdt] In Verlegung Johann Caspar Birckners, 1696.

[1], 166, [31] p. illus. 21 cm. **[5601]**

A page for page uncorrected reprint of the 1651 edition omitting some commendatory verses and the errata.

HIEBNER VON SCHNEEBERGK, ISRAEL. *See* HIEBNER, Israel [*fl.* 1648]

HIELM, PETER J. [*fl.* 1697] *respondent. See* GERDES, J., *praeses.* Disputatio inauguralis medica de hydrophobia. 1697.

HIENLIN, WOLFFGANG FRIEDRICH [*fl.* 1699-1700] *respondent. See* HOFFMANN, F. [1660-1742] *praeses.* Dissertatio inauguralis medico-practica de diarrhoea. 1700 [and] Dissertatio physico-medica de causis caloris naturalis. 1699.

HIERNE, URBANUS. *See* HJÄRNE, Urban [1641-1724]

HIERONYMI, JOANNES GEORGIUS [*fl.* 1672-1683] *respondent. See* MEIBOM, H., *praeses.* Disputatio medica inauguralis de sanguinis eductione. 1674 [and] Dissertatio medica de atrophia. 1672.

—*See* REISKE, J. De glossopetris Lüneburgensibus ad ... Joh. Georg. Hieronymi ... epistolica commentatio. 1684.

HIERONYMUS, PRESBITER. *See* JEROME, *Saint.*

HIERONYMUS, *Saint. See* JEROME, *Saint.*

HIERONYMUS MERCURIALIS. *See* MERCURIALE, Girolamo [1530-1606]

HIESELER, LAURENTIUS. *See* GIESLER, Lorenz [*d.* 1685]

HIFIPETO, *pseud. See* BRONZERIO, Giovanni Girolamo [1577-1630]

HIGHMORE, NATHANIEL [1613-1685] Corporis humani disquisitio anatomica; in qua sanguinis circulationem in quavis corporis particula plurimis typis novis, ac aenygmatum medicorum succincta dilucidatione ornatam prosequutus est ... Hagae-Comitis, Ex officina Samuelis Broun, 1651.

[14], 262, [8] p.   illus., plate.   30 cm.   [5602]

Added engraved title page.

—De hysterica & hypochondriaca passione, responsio epistolaris ad Doctorem Willis ... Londini, Sumptibus Roberti Clavel, 1670.

[1], 30 p.   20 cm.   [5603]

—Exercitationes duae. Quarum prior De passione hysterica: altera De affectione hypochondriaca ... Oxon., Excudebat A. Lichfield, impensis R. Davis, 1660.

[9], 184 p.   14 cm.   [5604]

—[The same.] ... Ed. 2. Oxon., Excudebat A. Lichfield, impensis R. Davis, 1660.

[8], 184 p.   14 cm.   [5605]

Different setting of type.

—[The same.] ... Ed. 2. priori emendatior. Amstelodami, Apud Casparum Commelinum, 1660.

[8], 136 p.   14 cm.   [5606]

—[The same.] ... Ed. 3. priori emendatior. Jenae, Typis Gollnerianis, 1677.

[10], 248 p.   13 cm.   [5607]

—The history of generation. Examining the several opinions of divers authors, especially that of Sir Kenelm Digby, in his Discourse of bodies ... To wich is joyned A discourse of the cure of wounds by sympathy ... especially by that powder, known chiefly by the name of Sir Gilbert Talbots powder ... London, Printed by R. N. for John Martin, 1651.

[14], 141 p.   plates.   18 cm.   [5608]

Imperfect: first preliminary leaf and last leaf (blank?) wanting.

—See VESLING, J. Syntagma anatomicum. 1666, 1677, 1696; WILLIS, T. Affectionum quae dicuntur hystericae et hypochondriacae pathologia spasmodica vindicata. 1671.

HILAIRE, S. See SAINT HILAIRE, sieur de [fl. 1665–1698]

HILARIUS A SANCTO ANASTASIO [fl. 1637] Thaumaturgus eucharisticus Augustanis Vindelicis divino munere concessus; sive, De prodigiose mirabili sacramento, ad S. Crucem Augustae, annis amplius quadringentis, rubea carnis specie

visendo, historia ... Augustae Vindelicorum, Typis Andreae Apergeri, 1637.

[2], 366, [20] p.   16 cm.   [5609]

Errata: p. [17–20]

HILARIUS, JUSTUS. Hortulus medicus. In Lavinheta, B. de. Opera omnia. 1612.

HILBRAND, JOHANN PHILIPP [fl. 1664–1668] praeses. Dissertatio medica de κεφαλαλγια ... Jenae, Typis Johannis Jacobi Bauhoferi [1668]

[24] p.   19 cm.   [5610]

Diss.—Jena (J. P. Hoechstetter, respondent)

HILCHEN, JOHANN PHILIPP [fl. 1693] respondent. Disputatio inauguralis medica aegrum pleuritide laborantem exhibens ... Altdorffii, Literis Henrici Meyeri [1693]

[20] p.   20 cm.   [5611]

Diss. — Altdorf.

HILDANUS, GUILHELMUS FABRICIUS. See FABRICIUS VON HILDEN, Wilhelm [1560–1634]

HILDANUS, JOHANNES FABRICIUS. See FABRICIUS VON HILDEN, Johann [fl. 1637]

HILDEBRAND, ANDREAS. See HILTEBRAND, Andreas [d. 1637]

HILDEBRAND, WOLFFGANG. Neu vermehrt, vortrefflich, ausserlesen curieuses Kunst und Wunderbuch, darinnen begriffen, wunderbahre Geheimnüsse und Kunststücke, wie man nemlich mit dem gantzen menschlichen Cörper, zahmen und wilden Thieren, Vogeln, Fischen ... Pflantzungen ... verrichten ... mit ... Beschreibung des Paradiss Lustgarten und ausserlesenen Planetenbuche. Darinne eine ... Beschreibung der Physiognomiae, Chiromantiae und Distillir-Kunst ... Franckfurt am Mayn, In Henning Grossens Buchladen, 1690.

[2], 990 (i.e. 986) p.   illus., plates, tables.   18 cm.   [5612]

Running titles: Das erste [-vierdte] Buch Magiae Naturalis (p. 20–486); Kunst und Wunder-Buchs anderer [-dritter] Theil (p. 468–990).

The second section of Dritter Theil has half title: Ander Theil des Planeten Buchs. Tabula vel Canon nach des Mondes Lauff durch die 12. himmlische Zeichen, was darinnen fürzunehmen und zu lassen. Durch Martinum Albertum (p. 865).

The "Anhang" is not present.

—See DAS GROSSE PLANETEN-BUCH. [not before 1694]

HILDEN, WILHELM FABRICIUS VON. *See* FABRICIUS VON HILDEN, Wilhelm [1560-1634]

HILDESHEIM, FRANZ [1551-1614] De cerebri et capitis morbis internis spicilegia. In quibus primo morbi cujusque catholica proponuntur: inde consilia & curationes variae attexuntur; denique empyrica morborum remedia ipiusque auctoris experimenta historica adferuntur ... Francofurti, Excudebat Erasmus Athleta, sumptibus Egenolphi Emmelil, 1612.

[16], 784, [48] p.   18 cm.   [5613]

HILKEN, JAN [*fl.* 1689] *respondent.* Disputatio medica inauguralis de sterilitate ... Lugduni Batavorum, Apud Abrahamum Elzevier, 1689.

[51] p.   21 cm.   [5614]
Diss.—Leyden.

HILLE, PETRUS [*fl.* 1684] *respondent. See* CRAUSE, R. W., *praeses.* Disputatio medica inauguralis de palpitatione cordis. 1684; RIVINUS, A. Q., *praeses.* Dissertatio medica de febribus malignis. 1684.

HILLEL BEN SAMUEL [*ca.* 1220-*ca.* 1295] *tr. See* HIPPOCRATES. Sententiae definitivae Graece, Latine, Hebriace. 1647.

HILLER, JOHANN HEINRICH [*fl.* 1677-1678] *respondent. See* METZGER, G. B., *praeses.* Disputatio medico anatomica de humoribus uteri. 1677 [and] Dissertationem medicam inauguralem de medicamentis sternutatoriis ... subjicit J. H. H. 1678.

HILLER, SILVESTER [*fl.* 1697] *respondent. See* HOFFMANN, F. [1660-1742] *praeses.* Dissertatio medico-chirurgica inauguralis, de synovia. 1697.

HILLING, GREGOR [1619-1680] *respondent. See* SEBISCH, M. [1578-1674?] *praeses.* Collegii therapeutici disputatio I[-XIV] 1634 [i.e. 1635]

HILTEBRAND, ANDREAS [*d.* 1637] *tr. See* QUATTRAMI, E. Tractatus brevis de praeservatione & curatione pestis. 1618.

HILTMANN, PHILIPP [*fl.* 1626] *respondent. See* CHARSTADIUS, V., *praeses.* Disputationum medicarum decima de methodo medendi in genere. 1626; SEBISCH, M. [1578-1674?] *praeses.* Exercitationes medicae. 1639.

HILTPRAND, JOHANN [*fl.* 1583] Nutzliche Underweisung zur die Hebammen und schwangeren Frawen: darauss nit allein die Hebammen, wie sie in Antrettung ihres ... schweren Standts geschaffen seyn ... sondern auch die Frawen, wie sie sich vor, in, und nach der Geburt verhalten sollen, zu lernen ... Mit einem kurtzen Bericht ... etlicher bey den schwangeren Frawen, Kindtbetterin unnd Kindern fürfallenden Kranckheiten, wie auch denselben durch heylsame ertzneyische Mittel zuhelffen sey ... Auffs new uberlesen ... unnd ... zum andernmal in Truck verfertigt ... Ingolstadt, Getruckt in der Ederischen Truckery durch Andream Angermayr, 1601.

[8], 227, [4] p.   illus.   21 cm.   [5615]

—Ein sehr nutzliche Ordnung und Regiment, wie man sich zu disen jetzigen gefährlichen Zeiten vor der Pestilentz, welche in Oesterreich diss Jar ... eingerissen, hüten soll, unnd wie dieselbige zuvertreiben und zucuriern sey. Jetzt zum andernmal gemehret und gebessert in Truck geben. Mit ... Bericht, was die jetzt regierende pestilentzische, faule, hitzige Fieber (welche man in gemeyn die ungarische Kranckheit nennet) seynd ... [Ingolstadt,] Getruckt durch Andream Angermayer, 1607.

[16], 336 p.   plates.   17 cm.   [5616]
Published in 1584 in Nuremberg under title: Regiment.

HIMSELIUS, GEORGIUS [*fl.* 1676] *respondent. See* SCHNEIDER, K. V., *praeses.* Disputationem medicam ... contra ineptam opinionem Nicolai Chesneau, de spasmorum subjecto ... habebit G. H. 1676.

HINCHLOÜS, HENRY [*fl.* 1617] *respondent.* Theses inaugurales de sanguinis missione ... Lugduni Batavorum, Typis Isaaci Elzevirii, 1617.

[7] p.   20 cm.   [5617]
Diss.—Leyden.

HIPPIUS, JOHANN CHRISTIAN [*fl.* 1666-1668] Disputatio medica inauguralis de hectica ... Lipsiae, Literis Wittigavianis [1668]

[22] p.   19 cm.   [5618]
Diss. pro loco—Leipzig.

—*respondent. See* MACASIUS, J. C., *praeses.* Disputatio medica de calculo renum. 1666.

HIPPOCRATES

Arrangement

I. Collected works [Greek and Latin]

1621

—Τὰ εὑρισκόμενα . . .Opera omnia quae extant in VIII. sectiones ex Erotiani mente distributa. Nunc denuo Latina interpretatione & annotationibus illustrata, Anutio Foesio . . . authore: adjecta sunt ad VI. sectionem Palladii scholia Graeca in librum Περὶ ἀγμῶν, & sua Latinitate donata [a Jacobo Santalbino] His praeterea accessere variae in omnes Hippocr. libb. lectiones Braecae, ex reconditissimis manuscriptis exemplaribus . . . collectae, antea quidem partim Frobeniano codici, partim verbosissimis Galeni commentariis: nunc autem ipsissimis textus paginis ac lineis . . . applicatae: necnon etiam quorundam doctiss. virorum in aliquot Hippocr. libros observationes. Omnia nunc ab innumeris, quibus prior scatebat editio, vitiis repurgata . . . Francofurti, In officina Danielis ac Davidis Aubriorum & Clementis Schleichii, 1621.

[12], 1344, [48] p.   40 cm.   [**5619**]

A reissue of the edition published by the same press in 1620. Conjectural emendations by Aemilius Portus: p. [1345-1350]

1624

—Another issue. 1624.

[**5620**]

Only the date line is altered.

1657

—[The same.] . . . Huic novissimae omniumque emendatissimae editioni accesserunt Hippocratis libri De medicamentis purgantibus cum commentariis Joannis Heurnii & De structura hominis [Nicolao Petreio Corcyraeo interprete] Item Erotiani & dictionum Herodoti lexica cum Galeni Glossarum Hippocratis explicatione: & denique gemino indice eorum qui in Hippocratis scripta commentati sunt, vel eum quavis alia ratione illustrarunt . . . Genevae, Typis & sumptibus Samuelis Chouët, 1657.

[48], 1344, [53] p.   40 cm.   [**5621**]

The main text is reprinted page for page from the Foes edition printed in Frankfurt in 1620 and reissued in 1621 and 1624. The present publication, the editorship of which some authorities ascribe to Étienne Le Clerc, is clearly edited by Chouet. Cf. "Typographus lectori."

Erotian's Vocum Hippocraticarum collectio, Galen's Linguarum Hippocratis explicatio, and selections from the Lexicon Herodoteum and from the De dialectis, by Gregorius, archbishop of Corinth p. [14-38] are in Greek only.

Conjectural emendations by Aemilius Portus: p. [1345-1350]

1662

—[The same.] . . . Genevae, Typis & sumptibus Samuelis Chouët, 1657-62 [i.e. 1662]

2 v.   front. (port.)   40 cm.   [**5622**]

Vol. 2 has special title page: . . . Operum omnium tomus secundus, sectionem septimam, et octavam . . . ac denique Foesii Oeconomiam complectens.

Chouet's edition of Hippocrates' works was previously issued in one volume in 1657. Foes' Oeconomia Hippocratis (with special title page and independent paging) was also issued separately in 1662.

"Finis tomi primi" added at end of p. 933; blank leaf mounted over original p. 934; p. 935-936 cancelled. Fold with special title page and cancel p. 934-936 at beginning of vol. 2.

1665

—Opera omnia. Graece & Latine edita, et ad omnes alias editiones accommodata. Industria & diligentia Joan. Antonidae vander Linden . . . Lugduni Batavorum, Apud Danielem, Abrahamum & Adrianum à Gaasbeeck, 1665.

2 v. in 1.   port.   20 cm.   [**5623**]

Added engraved title page.

Latin translation by Janus Cornarius.

Van der Linden was prevented by death from preparing also "suas observationes singulari tomo." Cf. printer's pref. Listed in Krieg 1954, p. 323.

Willems no. 897; ". . . Edition incontestablement imprimé par la veuve de Jean [Elzevier] pour la compte de Gaasbeek."

Dedication signed by the editor's son, Henricus Antonides van der Linden.

1679

—Hippocratis Coi, et Claudii Galeni . . . Opera. Renatus Charterius . . . plurima interpretatus, universa emendavit, instauravit, notavit, auxit, secundum distinctas medicinae partes in tredecim tomos digessit, & conjunctim Graece & Latine primus edidit. Lutetiae Parisiorum, Apud Andream Pralard, 1679.

13 v. in 9.   10 plates (v. 12)   43 cm.   [5624]

Engraved portraits of Hippocrates and Galen on title pages of v. 1, 7, and 11.

Vols. 9, 10, and 12 were edited after Chartier's death by François Blondel and Antoine Le Moine. The other volumes are reissues, with imprint dates on the title pages altered to 1679 by means of cancel slips; vols. 1–6, 8, and 13 were originally published in 1639; vol. 7 and 11 in 1649. Vol. 9 incorrectly dated 1689.

The index volume promised in Chartier's preface was never published.

Includes miscellaneous selections from other ancient Greek medical authors.

Contents.—v. 1. Quae ad vitam, ac genus tum Hippocratis, tum Galeni spectant.—v. 2. Quae in artem medicam introducunt, opuscula.—v. 3. Elementa, temperamenta, humores.—v. 4. Dissectiones, aut partes.—v. 5. Quae ad animam spectant facultates, functiones, spiritus.—v. 6. Ad sanitatem tuendam spectantia.—v. 7. Quae ad morbos, morborum causas, & symptomata spectant.—v. 8. Τα σεμειωτικά.—v. 9. Permixta opera.—v. 10. Quae ad morborum curationem spectant.—v. 11. Ad aegrotantium victus rationem spectantia.—v. 12. Ad chirurgium spectantia.—v. 13. Quae ad pharmaciam & medicamenta spectant.

—Additamenta in Hippocratem. [n. p., 17–]

[85] p.   43 cm.   [5624.1]

Binder's title.

A collection of title pages and prefatory material from vols. 1, 2, and 6 of the original issue, together with manuscript copies of J. F. de Villiers' Lettre ... sur l'edition ... des oeuvres d'Hippocrate & de Galien, publiés par Rene Chartier (from Jean Goulin's Mémoires littéraires ... et bibliographiques, Paris, v. 2, 1776, p. 211–227) and of Eduard Sandifort's De Charteriana editione operum Hippocratis & Galeni (from his Exercitationes academicae, Leyden, v. 1, 1783, p. 113–127)

II. Collected works [Latin]
1610

—Opera, quibus addidimus commentaria Joann. Marinelli ... Nova, & argumenta in singulos libros per Joan. Culman. Geppingen. sunt addita. Vincentiae, Sumptibus Francisi Lenii & Orlandi Jadrae [Apud Jo. Petrum Joanninium] 1610.

2 v. in 1.   33 cm.   [5625]

Vol. [1] is based on Johann Culmann's edition of Cornarius' translation, with "Liber de hominis structura" translated by Nicolas Petreius.

Vol. [2] has special title page: Commentaria Joan. Marinelli in lib. Hippocratis.

A page for page reprint (except for a different dedication in v. [1]) of the 1575 Venice edition.

1619

—[The same.] ... Venetiis, Apud Hieronymum & Alexandrum Polum, 1619.

2 v. in 1.   34 cm.   [5626]

A page for page reprint of the 1610 Vicenza edition.

1679

—[The same.] ... Venetiis, Typis Abbundii Menfolii, 1679.

2 v. in 1.   33 cm.   [5627]

A reprint (except for different dedication in v. [1]) of the 1610 Vicenza edition.

III. Collected works [French]
1667

—Les oeuvres du grand Hippocrate ... ou toutes les causes de la vie, de la naissance & de la conservation de la santé; les signes & les symptomes de toutes les maladies sont nettement expliquées, avec leur guerison, par les lumieres du mouvement circulaire, et autres nouvelles experiences. Par ... Claude Tardy ... Paris, Chez l'auteur, Jean du Bray, Claude Barbin, 1667.

2 v.   23 cm.   [5628]

Vol. 1 only.

1697

—Les oeuvres ... Traduites en françois, avec des remarques. Et conferées sur les manuscripts de la Bibliotheque du roy. Paris, Claude Barbin, 1697.

2 v.   17 cm.   [5629]

Colophon (v. 1): A Paris, De l'imprimerie d'Antoine Lambin, 1696.

General title page. Special title page for each volume has imprint: La Compagnie des libraires, 1697.

Edited and translated by André Dacier.

"La vie d'Hippocrate, a Monseigneur le chancelier": v. 1, p. [97–157]; "A Monsieur D ..." (letter from Eusèbe Renaudot, on Syriac and Arabic translations): v. 1, p. [158–171]

Errata: v. 2, p. [544–546]

Contents.—v. 1. De l'art de la medecine. De l'ancienne medecine. La loy. Le serment. Du medecin. De la decence. Les preceptes. De la nature humaine. Des chairs, ou Des principes. Des vents. De l'usage des choses humides.—v. 2. Le premier [-troisième] livre de la diete. De la diete salubre. De l'air, de l'eau & des lieux.

IV. Selected works [Greek and Latin]
1607

—Aphorismi Graece, & Latine, una cum Prognosticis, Prorrheticis, Coacis, & aliis decem ejusdem opusculis: pleraque ex interpretatione Johannis

Heurnii ... [Lugduni Batavorum] Ex Officina Plantiniana Raphelengii, 1607.

[4], 715 p.   10 cm.   [5630]

Contents.—Aphorismi.—Prognostica.—Prorrhetica, seu Praedictiones, ex editione Johannis Opsopoei.—Praeceptiones.— De carnibus, sive De principiis.—De purgatoriis remediis.—De veteri medicina.—De medico.—De arte.—De elegantia.— Jusjurandum.—Lex.—Aphorismi interjecti, seu Sectio octava Aphorismorum ex editione Ant. Musae Brasavolae.—Coacae praenotiones, ex editione Johannis Opsopoei.

1611

—Prolegomena, et Prognosticorum libri tres: cum paraphrastica versione & brevibus commentariis Johannis Heurnii ... Lugduni Batavorum, Ex Officina Plantiniana, apud Franciscum Raphelengium, 1603 [i.e. 1611]

184, [7] p.   23 cm.   (Part 2 in Heurne, Johan van. In praecipuos libros Hippocratis Coi commentaria. [Lugduni Batavorum] 1609 [i.e. 1611] Opera omnia [v. 3])   [5631]

1619

—Chirurgia, nunc primum Graece restituta Latinitate donata, & commentariis illustrata. A Steph. Manialdo ... Parisiis, Apud Joann. Libert, 1619.

23, [1], 397 (i.e. 429) p.   17 cm.   [5632]

Contents.—De medico sive chirurgi institutione.—De vulneribus.—De haemorrhoidibus.—De fistulis.—De vulneribus capitis.

1622. *In* Gorris J. de. [1505-1577] Opera. Definitionum medicarum libri XXIIII. 1622.

1627

—Aphorismi Graece, & Latine, una cum Prognosticis, Prorrheticis, Coacis, & aliis decem ejusdem opusculis, aphoristica brevitate conscriptis. Pleraque ex interpretatione Johannis Heurnii ... Iterata editio, commodior. Lugduni Batavorum, Ex officina Johannis Maire, 1627.

[4], 637 p.   13 cm.   [5633]

Contents as in the 1607 Leyden edition.

1631

—Aphorismi Graeco-Latini e regione. Ex optima versione cum indice novo ... Adjecta sunt ejusdem Hippocratis Prognostica, & insigniores Cornelis Celsi sententiae. Parisiis, Apud Savinianum Pigoreav, 1631.

2 parts in 1 v.   11 cm.   [5634]

Added engraved title page.

Part [2] has special title page.
Dedicatory epistle signed by Guy Patin.

1658. *In* Heurne, J. van. Opera omnia. 1658; Varanda, J. de. Opera omnia. 1658.

V. Selected works [Latin]

1609. *In* Heurne, J. van. In praecipuos libros Hippocratis Coi commentaria. 1609.

1663. *In* Cardano, G. Opera omnia. 1663.

VI. Selected works [French]

1634. *In* Guidi, G. [*ca.* 1500-1569] Les anciens et renommés autheurs de la medecine & chirurgie. 1634.

Selected works

Adaptations, etc.

Latin

1683

—Promptuarium Hippocratis in locos communes ordine alphabetico, nec sine compendio digestum ... Labore & industria ... Caroli Arturi Plessei ... Opus posthummum. Rotomagi, Sumptibus viduae Jacobi Lucas, 1683.

[14], 607, [1] p.   front. (port.)   24 cm.   [5635]

1685

—Hippocrates contractus, in quo magni Hippocratis ... opera omnia, in brevem epitomen, summa diligentia redacta habentur. Studio & opera Thomae Burnet ... Edinburgi, Excudebat J. Reid, sumptibus Georgii Mosman, 1685.

[8], 219 (i.e. 217), [18] p.   16 cm.   [5636]

"Additamentum": p. [218-219]; "Errata perpauca": p. [235]

1686

—[The same.] ... Londini, Johan. Malthus, 1686.

[8], 219 (i.e. 217), [18] p.   16 cm.   [5637]

A reissue of the 1685 Edinburgh edition with new title page.

VII. Selections, etc. [Greek and Latin]

1655. *In* Rolfinck, W. Epitome methodi cognoscendi & curandi particulares corporis affectus.

1656. *In* Linden, J. A. van der. Selecta medica. 1656.

1665. *In* Peyssonel, J. de. De temporibus humani partus. 1665.

1666. *In* Peyssonel, J. de. De temporibus humani partus. 1666.

1675. *In* Rolfinck, W. Epitome methodi cognoscendi & curandi particulares corporis affectus. 1675.

1677. *In* Cortnumm, J. De morbo attonito liber unus. 1677 [and] Nova, utilis ac curiosa apoplexiam. 1677.

1684.

—Ἀφορισμοὶ νεώτεροι. Aphorismi novi, ex Hippocratis operibus nunc primum collecti, & in suas quinque classes digesti, notisque illustrati. Studio Jacobi Sponii . . . Lugduni, Apud Anissonios, Joan. Posuel & Cl. Rigaud, 1684.

[22], 406, [14] p.   16 cm.   [**5638**]

1685. *In* Cortnumm, J. De morbo attonito liber unus. 1685.

VIII. Selections, etc. [Latin]

1604. *In* Valleriola, F. Loci medicinae communes. 1604.

1626. *In* Riolan, J. [1580-1657] Anthropographia. 1626.

1637

—Manuale medicorum, seu, Σύναξ ις Aphorismorum Hypocratis, Praenotionum, Coacarum, & Praedictionum, secundum propriam morborum omnium nomenclaturam, alphabetico digesta ordine. Labore & industria . . . Honorati Bicaissii . . . Parisiis, Apud Andream Soubron, 1637.

[16], 356 p.   12 cm.   [**5639**]

1650. *In* Riolan, J. [1580-1657] Opera anatomica vetera. 1650.

1659

—[The same.] . . . Londini, Typis Tho. Roycroft, impensis Jo. Martin, Ja. Allestry, & Tho. Dicas, 1659.

[8], 356 p.   12 cm.   [**5640**]

Apparently reprinted from the 1637 Paris edition.

1660

—[The same.] . . . Genevae, Sumptibus Petri Chouët, 1660.

[6], 225 p.   14 cm.   [**5641**]

1666. *In* Barra, P. De veris terminis partus humani libri tres ex Hippocrate. 1666.

1672. *In* Clément, G. Sententiae principum medicorum. 1672.

1677. *In* Becker, N. W. Florilegium Hippocraticum et Galenicum. 1677.

1682. *In* Restaurand, R. Hippocrates de natura lactis. 1682.

1685. *In* Cortnumm, J. Nova, utilis ac curiosa apoplexiam. 1685.

1688. *In* Becker, N. W. Florilegium Hippocraticum et Galenicum. 1688.

1696. *In* Frauendoerffer, P. Opusculum de morbis mulierum. 1696.

IX. Selections, etc. [French]

1628. *In* Riolan, J. [1580-1657] Anthropographia. French. 1628.

X. Selections, etc. [German]

1663. *In* Becher, J. J. Parnassus medicinalis illustratus. 1663.

XI. Individual works
Aphorismi
Greek

1633. *In* Galenus. In Aphorismos Hippocratis commentaria. 1633.

1655. (bk. 2 only) *In* Cureau de la Chambre, M. Novae methodi pro explanandis Hippocrate & Aristotele specimen. 1655.

1657. *In his* Aphorismi. [Adaptations, etc. Latin.] 1657.

1664. *In* Rogers, J. Analecta inauguralia. 1664.

Greek and Latin

1601

—Aphorismi Graece, & Latine. Brevi enarratione, fidaque interpretatione ita illustrati, ut ab omnibus facile intelligi possint. Cum historiis, observationibus, cautionibus, & remediis selectis A. J. Heurnio . . . [Lugduni Batavorum] Ex Officina Plantiniana, apud Christophorum Raphelengium, 1601.

[16], 512, [16] p.   14 cm.   [5642]

1606. *In* Offredi, D. In librum Aphorismorum Hippocratis commentaria aphoristica. 1606.

1607. *In his* [Selected works. Greek and Latin] 1607.

1609

—[The same.] . . . Ed. alt., multo emendatior. [Lugduni Batavorum] Ex Officina Plantiniana Raphelengii, 1609.

[10], 512, [14] p.   12 cm.   [5643]

Imperfect: upper margins trimmed.

Apparently a reprint of the 1601 Leyden edition. Three poems are omitted from the preliminaries.

1609

—[The same.] . . . [Lugduni Batavorum] Ex Officina Plantiniana Raphelengii, 1609.

161, [5] p.   21 cm.   [5644]

A corrected reprint of the second edition, which was published in Leyden in the same year. The commendatory verse is omitted.

Bound with *his* Prolegomena et Prognosticorum libri tres. Lugduni Batavorum, 1597.

—Copy 2.

Bound with Heurne, Johan van. In Hippocratis Coi De hominis natura libros duos commentarius.

1610. (bks. 1, 2, 4 only) *In* Argenterio, G. Opera. 1610.

1611

—[The same.] . . . [Lugduni Batavorum] Ex officina Plantiniana Raphelengii, 1611.

161, [5] p.   21 cm.   [5645]

Different setting of type.

1612. (bk. 1 only) *In* Cachet, C. Controversiae theoricae . . . in primam Aphorismorum Hippocratis sectionem. 1612.

1613. *In* Houllier, J. In Aphorismorum Hippocratis commentarii. 1613.

1615

—[The same.] . . . Edictio [sic] postrema, accuratior & emendatior. Lugduni, Sumptibus viduae Antonii de Harsy, 1615.

[8], 494 (i.e. 497), [15] p.   15 cm.   [5646]

Imperfect: sig. Y 12 (blank?) wanting.

1617

—[The same.] . . . Ed. postrema, accuratior & emendatior. Lugduni, Sumptibus viduae Antonii de Harsy, 1617.

[8], 494 (i.e. 497), [15] p.   15 cm.   [5647]

A reissue of the 1615 Lyons edition with new title page.

1620. *In* Houllier, J. In Aphorismos Hippocratis commentarii. 1620.

1623

—[The same.] . . . Lugduni Batavorum, Apud Joannem Maire, 1623.

[12], 512, [15] p.   14 cm.   [5648]

1625

—Aphorismi et Prognostica, Joanne Butino interprete & commentatore. Adjectus est novus index in quo aphorismi per locos communes dispositi, & in certa classes distributi ex tempore oculis repraesentantur . . . Genevae, Apud Petrum & Jacobum Chouët, 1625.

[102], 394, [12] p.   13 cm.   [5649]

The main texts, in Greek and Latin, are from Jean Butin's edition of the Aphorismi and Prognostica published in Lyons in 1580. The Aphorismi are here changed from Butin's subject arrangement into traditional order and an index of subjects (based on several authorities) is prefixed to them.

"Hippocratis Coï Jusjurandum," "Hippocratis Lex," and "Hippocratis genus et vita ex Sorano": p. [8–27] "Insigniores aliquot sententiae selectae ex libris Aurelii Cornelii Celsi": p. 377–394.

1625

—Another issue, with imprint: Aureliopoli, Apud Petrum & Jacobum Chouët, 1625.

Imperfect: p. [17–32] (1st group) and [12] p. at end wanting.   [5650]

1627. *In his* [Selected works. Greek and Latin] 1627.

1628

—Ἀθορισμοί. Aphorismi . . . Ex recognitione A. Vorstii M. P. Lugd. Batavorum, Ex Officina Elzeviriana, 1628.

[4], 231 p.   port.   10 cm.   [5651]

Engraved title page.

The earlier of two variant issues of 1628.

Willems 297.

Copinger 2284.

"Aphorismi interjecti, sue sectio octava": p. 210–221.

"Lex": p. 222–231.

1628

—Aphorismi . . . Graece et Latine in novum ordinem digesti, et in sectiones septem distributi, cum argumentis in eosdem. Authore Joanne Lanaeo . . . Parisiis, Apud Ludovicum Julianum, 1628.

[32], 185, [11] p.   19 cm.   [5652]

The Latin version of the Aphorismi is by Niccolò Leoniceno. "De officio medici. Carmen Joannis Lanay": p. [4–11], at end, following errata.

1628

—Aphorismi . . . Graece et Latine, una cum Galeni Commentariis: Nicolao Leoniceno . . . interprete. Quibus accesserunt adnotamenta marginalia . . . Ed. postrema prioribus multo castigatior. Genevae, Ex typographia Petri Chouët, 1628.

620, [18] p.   12 cm.   [5653]

Apparently reprinted from the 1549 Lyons edition.

1631

—Aphorismorum . . . liber primus. Heurnio interprete. Singulis aphorismis subjungitur nunc primum carmen alternum Graecum . . . Cantabrigiae, 1631.

[4], 14 p.   19 cm.   [5654]

Imperfect: last leaf (blank?) wanting.

Greek text, with Latin translation by Johan van Heurne and Greek metrical version by Ralph Winterton.

STC 13519.

1631. *In his* [Selected works. Greek and Latin] 1631.

1632. *In* Houllier, J. In Aphorismos Hippocratis commentarii. 1632.

1633

—Οἱ Ἀφορισμοὶ πεξικοί τε καὶ ἐμμετροι . . . Aphorismi, soluti & metrici. Interprete Joanne Heurnio . . . Metaphrastis, Joanne Frero . . . et Radulpho Wintertono . . . Cantabrigiae, Thomas Buck & Rogerus Daniel, 1633.

[14], 292 p.; [2], 45 p.   15 cm.   [5655]

STC 13518.

Leaves signed ¶ 2–3, perhaps inserted, contain Ralph Winterton's dedicatory epistle to William Laud as Bishop of London and Chancellor of Oxford.

"Censurae" of six Cambridge professors, dated April 10th–16th, 1633: p. [7–10]

The Greek text of book 1, with corresponding Latin translation by Johan van Heurne and Greek metrical version by Ralph Winterton, was published at Cambridge in 1631 under title: Aphorismorum Hippocratis liber primus.

John Fryer's Latin metrical version was published in London in 1567 under title: Hippocratis . . . Aphorismi versibus scripti. Winterton rendered into Latin verse book 7, aphorisms 60–75, which were omitted by Fryer. Cf. p. [13]

"Epigrammata regiorum medicinae professorum Cantabrigiensis atque Oxoniensis . . . in Radulphi Wintertoni metaphrasin nuper editam . . . Quibus accedunt epigrammata therapeutica ejusdem": [2], 45 p. at end, with special title page.

—Another issue, without the dedicatory epistle to William Laud and without the "Epigrammata" at end.

[5656]

—Another issue, without the dedicatory epistle to William Laud. Statements on p. [7] and [10] are undated.

[5657]

1633

—Aphorismorum sectiones octo; ex interpretatione Anutii Foesii. Quibus accedit methodus, qua Aphorismi, in certum ordinem digesti, & accurate dispositi, exhibentur a Joanne Ernesto Scheffler . . . Lugduni Batavorum, Ex officina Joannis Maire, 1633.

[8], 280 p.   10 cm.   [5658]

Imperfect: title page mutilated.

"Perutilis & luculenta methodus qua omnes in universum Hipp. Aphorismi . . . accuratè digesti ac dispositi sunt, opera . . . Joanne Ernesto Scheffler (p. [223]–280) has special title page.

1634

—Aphorismorum Hippocratis textus, Latino versu redditus, & commentario brevi illustratus. Per Guiliel. Odry . . . Parissis [sic] Apud Joannem Jost, 1634.

[8], 207 p.   15 cm.   [5659]

1638

—Aphorismi Graece & Latine; brevi enarratione; fidaque interpretatione ita illustrati, ut ab omnibus facile intelligi possint. Cum historiis, observationibus, cautionibus, & remediis selectis. A. J. Heurnio . . . Ed. altera, multa [sic] emendatior. Lugduni Batavorum, Ex officina Joannis Maire, 1638.

522 (i.e. 512), [16] p.   14 cm.   [5660]

1641

—Aphorismi, Graeco et Latine sermone expressi, breviter & nervose secundum rationis & experientiae ductum enodati & eo digesti ordine, ut non solum quilibet morbus suos adjunctos habeat Aphorismos, verum etiam, praeter succinctas annotationes, appositis ubique splendeat regulis practicis, & allegatis probatissimorum authorum, tam priscorum, quam neotericorum ... In usum primum privatum conscripti opera, industria, & jusdicio magni olim illius Tobiae Knoblochii ... Publico bono dati nunc ab haeredibus ... Noribergae, Literis & impensis Wolfgangi Endteri, 1641.

[23], 533, [27] p.   front.   16 cm.   [5661]
Added engraved title page.

1646. *In* Houllier, J. In Aphorismos Hippocratis commentarii. 1646.

1647

—Sententiae definitivae Graece, Latine, Hebriace: Marci Antonii Gajotii ... studio. Opus novum, nec hactenus elaboratum ... Romae, Sumptibus Simonis Pellopei [Ex typographia Ludovici Grignani, excudebat Joannes Andreas Lotus] 1647.

[16], 242, [6] p.   17 cm.   [5662]
Engraved title page.
Greek, Latin and Hebrew in parallel columns. The Latin translation is a new recension by Gajotius; the Hebrew he edited from two manuscript copies. Cf. "Ad lectorem" p. [13-14] According to Steinschneider (p. 660) this Hebrew translation was made from the Latin version of Constantinus Africanus, very probably by Hillel ben Samuel in Italy toward the end of the 13th century.

1653. *In* Cardano, G. In Aphorismos Hippocratis commentaria luculentissima cum Graeco textu. 1653.

1655. (bk. 2 only) *In* Cureau de la Chambre, M. Novae methodi pro explanandis Hippocrate ... specimen. 1655.

1657. (bk. 1 only) *In* Naldi, M. Aphorismorum Hippocratis explanatio. 1657.

1661

—Joh. Cunradi Dieterici ... Aphorismi Hippocratis illustrati et Iatreo ejusdem praemissi. Ulmae, Apud Balthasar Kühnen, 1661.

[4], 160 p.   21 cm.   [5663]
Bound with (as issued) Dieterich, J. K. Iatreum Hippocraticum, 1661.

1661

—Αθορισμοί. Aphorismi ... Ex recognitione A. Vorstii. Lugduni,Sumptib. Antonii Cellier, 1661.

[4], 231, [1] p.   port.   10 cm.   [5664]
Engraved title page.

A reprint, nearly page for page like the 1628 Elsevier edition. "Lex": p. 222-231.

1662. (bk. 2 only) *In* Cureau de la Chambre, M. Novae methodi pro explanandis Hippocrate ... specimen. 1662.

1664

—Aphorismi Graece & Latine; brevi enarratione; fidaque interpretatione ita illustrati, ut ab omnibus facile intelligi possint.Cum historiis, observationibus, cautionibus, & remediis selectis. A. J. Heurnio ... Ed. 3, multo emendatior. Hagae Comitis, Ex typographia Adriani Vlacq, 1664.

512, [16] p.   14 cm.   [5665]
Corresponds page for page with the 1638 Leyden edition.

1668

—Aphorismi ... Graece et Latine; una cum Galeni commentariis: Nicolao Leoniceno ... interprete. Necnon Joan. Signoreti ... Excerpta aphoristica, cum symbola. Accesserunt adnotamenta marginalia ... Editio postrema prioribus multo castigatior. Lugduni, Sumpt. Laurentii Anisson, 1668.

620, [18] p.; 191 p.   13 cm.   [5666]
Contents and paging of the first part (620, [18] p.) the same as those of the 1628 Geneva edition. The Aphorismi are differently numbered after p. 600.
The "excerpta" in Signoretus' work are based on Galen's commentaries on the Aphorismi. Only the first three of the seven sections of the work are here printed.

1671. (bk. 5 only) *In* Metzger, G. B. Disputatio inauguralis medica. 1671.

1675?

—'Αθορισμοί. Aphorismi ... Hos edi accuravit, interpretationem novam adjecit, loca parallela plurima ex ipso Hippocrate collegit, et indicem locupletissimum subjunxit Lucas Verhoofd ... Lugd. Batav., Apud Danielem à Gaesbeeck [1675?]

[20], 279, [78] p.   port.   10 cm.   [5667]
Added engraved title page.
Dedication is dated Dec. 1675.
Errata: p. [76-78]
Verhoofd's Latin translation is evidently based mainly on that of Janus Cornarius. Includes the spurious "Aphorismi interjecti. Sectio octava" (p. 267-279).

1675. *In* Houllier, J. In Aphorismos Hippocratis commentarii. 1675.

1685

—'Αθορισμοί . . . Aphorismi. Variorum auctorum maxime Hippocratis & Celsi. Locis parallelis illustrati. Subjiciuntur Celsi sententiae.Studio & cura Theodori Janssonii ab Almeloveen . . . Amstelaedami, Apud Henricum Wetstenium, 1685.

[16], 181, [37], 30 p. port. 13 cm.   [5668]

Added title page.

Latin translation by Lucas Verhoofd. Includes also Verhoofd's index to the Aphorismi.

"Aphorismi interjecti. Sectio octava": p. 173-181.

1688

—Aphorismi Graece & Latine; brevi enarratione; fidaque interpretatione ita illustrati, ut ab omnibus facile intelligi posint. Cum historiis, observationibus, cautionibus, & remediis selectis. A J. Heurnio . . . Ed 4. multo emendatior. Amstelodami, Ex officina Gerbrandi Schagen, 1688.

512, [16] p. 14 cm.   [5669]

A reissue, with pages [1]-24 reprinted, of the third edition, The Hague, 1664.

1690

—[The same.] . . . Juxta exemplar Lugduni Batavor. Jenae, Apud Henrich. Christoph. Crökerum, 1690.

[11], 512, [15] p. front. (port.) 14 cm.   [5670]

Text mainly page for page like the 1601 Leyden edition but with the errata corrected.

Latin

1601. (bk 1 only) *In* Capivaccio, G. Tractatus. 1601.

1603. (bk 1 only) *In* Capivaccio, G. Opera omnia. 1603.

1605. *In his* [Aphorismi. French] 1605.

1606. *In his* [Aphorismi. French] 1606.

1606. (bks. 1, 2, 4 only) *In* Argenterio, G. Opera. 1606.

1608. *In* Fontaine, J. Jacobi Fontani . . . Commentaria in Hipp[ocratis] omnes Aph[orismos] 1608.

1610 [i.e. 1611]

—Aphorismorum . . . sectiones septem: quibus ex Antonii Muse commentariis adjecta fecit [sic] & octava. Et ad imminuendum studiosorum laborem singuli aphorismi selecti fuere, tam ad febres, quam ad morbos singulos attinentes: ut facile unusquisque uno intuitu quaecunque in aphorismis continentur cernere possit. P. Francisco Oclerio . . . authore. Vicentiae, Apud Franciscum Lenium, 1610 [i.e. 1611]

[48], 96 p. 10 cm.   [5671]

Translated by Niccolò Leoniceno. Section 8 is a collection of spurious aphorisms translated by Antonio Musa Brasavola.

Following the present work is the author's Pronosticorum, libri tres. Vicentiae, 1611, which was issued with it.

Bound with Galenus. Ars medicinalis. 1606.

1612. (bk 1 only) *In* Cachet, C. Controversiae theoricae . . . in primam Aphorismorum Hippocratis sectionem. 1612.

1612. *In* Fougerolles, F. de. Methodus in septem Aphorismorum libros ab Hippocrate observata. 1612.

1613. *In* Fontaine, J. Jacobi Fontani . . . Opera. 1613.

1613. *In* Le Maistre, R. Doctrina Hippocratis. 1613.

1617. (bk 1 only) *In* Capivaccio, G. Opera omnia. 1617.

1617. *In* Canonieri, P. A. In septem aphorismorum Hippocratis . . . interpretationes. 1617-18.

1618. (bk 1 only) *In* Celi, A. Antonini Caelii . . . Introductio universalis ad medicam facultatem. 1618.

1619. *In his* [Adaptations, etc. Latin] 1619.

1619. *In* Mercuriale, G. In omnes Hippocratis Aphoriamorum libros. 1619.

162?. *In his* [Aphorismi. French] 162?.

1620. *In his* [Aphorismi. French] 1620.

1621. (Selections) *In* Fragoso, J. Cirugia universal. 1621.

1621. *In* Mercuriale, G. In omnes Hippocratis Aphorismorum libros. 1621.

1622

—Aphorismorum . . . in septem sectiones sive libellos divisio. Cui adjectus est index duplex copiosissimus . . . Accesserunt itidem ejusdem authoris Prognosticorum, sive De praesagiis morborum libri tres. Herbipoli, Ex typis & officina Joannis Volmari, 1622.

94, [39], 54 (i.e. 44) p. 11 cm.   [5672]

"... Prognosticorum libri tres ... [Guilielmo Coppo ... interprete]" (44 p. at end) has special title page.

Latin translations of the Aphorismi by Niccolò Leoniceno, with the spurious section 8 (p. 90–94) translated by Antonio Musa Brasavola. The indexes prepared by Pietro Francesco Occlerio.

1623

—Aphorismi Nicolao Leoniceno ... interprete. Una cum annotationibus quibusdam, & circa textum praecipus Joannis Manelphi ... Romae, Sumptibus Joannis Manelphi, apud haeredem Bartholomaei Zannetti, 1623.

126, [1] p.   12 cm.   [**5673**]

Errata: p. [1]

"Liber octavus" (spurious) translated by Antonio Musa Brasavola: p. 119–123.

"Jusjurandum" in Johan van Heurne's version: p. 124–126.

1626. *In* Vega, C. de. Opera omnia. 1626.

1627. *In his* [Aphorismi. French] 1627.

1628. *In his* [Aphorismi. French] 1628.

1629. (bk I only) *In* Santorio, S. Commentaria in primam sectionem Aphorismorum Hippocratis. 1629.

1629. (bk I only) *In* Zecchi, G. In primam D. Hipp. Aphorismorum sectionem ... lectiones. 1629.

1631. *In* Aristoteles. Aristotelis, aliorumque philosophorum, ac medicorum problemata. 1631.

1631. *In* Mercuriale, G. In omnes Hippocratis Aphorismorum libros. 1631.

1633

—Aphorismi ... methodice dispositi. Quibus accedit Tractatus de extractione foetus mortui per uncum, auctore Nicolao Fontano ... Amsteldami, Typis Jacobi Carpentier, 1633.

[12], 125, [1] p.   13 cm.   [**5674**]

Hippocratic text translated by Niccolò Leoniceno.

"Lex" and "Jusjurandum" (p. 4–8) in the versions by Janus Cornarius.

1633. *In* Galenus. [In Hippocratis Aphorismos. Greek and Latin]

1639

—Thesaurus Hippocraticus; sive, Aphorismi ... in classes & certos titulos ordine dispositi atque succinctis rationibus illustrati a Bernhardo Langwedelio ... Hamburgi, Typis Jacobi Rebenlini, impensis Zachariae Hertelii, 1639.

[24], 324, [9] p.   13 cm.   [**5675**]

Added engraved title page.

Errata: p. [9] at end.

The Latin text of the Aphorismi is from Adolph Vorstius' edition, Leyden, 1628.

With this is bound *his* Aphorismi, seu, Axiomata. Bruxellae, 1647.

1639. (Selections) *In* Fragoso, J. Della cirugia. 1639.

1642. *In* Fonteyn, N. Nicolai Fontani Commentarius in Sebastianum Austrium ... De puerorum morbis. 1642.

1642. *In* Hafenreffer, S. Raphael ὅδιος de arte medica. 1642.

1644. (bks. 1, 2, 4 only) *In* Locatelli, L. Theatro d'arcani ... nel quale si tratta dell'arte chimica. 1644.

1645. *In his* [Aphorismi. French] 1645.

1646

—Aphorismi Nicolao Leoniceno ... interprete. Una cum annotationibus quibusdam, & circa textum praecipue Joannis Manelphi ... a quo in hac secunda editione plurimae aliae annotationes adjectae fuerunt ... Romae, Apud Manelphum Manelphium, sumptibus Jo. Baptistae Subissati, 1646.

6, [2], 152, [16] p.   12 cm.   [**5676**]

Contents as in the 1623 Rome edition.

With this is bound: Manelfi, G. Prognostica in febribus. Romae, 1646.

1646. *In his* [Aphorismi. French] 1646.

1647. *In his* [Adaptations, etc. Latin.] 1647.

1647. *In* Lorenz, G. F. Georgii-Friderici Laurentii Exercitationum in non nullos minus absolute veros Hippocratis Aphorismos. 1647.

1648. (bks. 1–2 only) *In* Moralis, G. Commentaria in magni Hippocratis Coi Aphorismos. 1648.

1649

—Aphorismorum sectiones VII. Nicolao Leoniceno ... interprete. Accessit octava ex Ant. Musae Brasavoli commentariis. Cum gemino Aphorismorum, ac rerum indice Francisci Oglerii. Item Prognosticorum lib. III. Guilielmo Copo interprete. Patavii, Typis Pauli Frambotti, 1649.

[36], III p.   14 cm.   [**5677**]

Bound with Galenus. Ars medicinalis. 1642.

1649. *In* Albanese, G. A. Aphorismorum Hippocratis expositio peripatetica. 1649.

1649. *In* Ghirinzana, L. In septem libros Aphorismorum magni Hyppocratis . . . animadversiones Hyppocraticae. 1649.

1650. *In* Tilemann, J. Aphorismi Hippocratis. 1650.

1653

—Ars parva; sive, Aphorismorum sectiones VII. quibus, ordine resolutivo tradi universam medicinam, ab ipso Hippocrate, demonstratur; summa a brevitate . . . aphorismus per aphorismum, vel explicatur, vel limitatur, vel roboratur. Auctore Georgio Morali . . . Venetiis, Apud Juntas, 1653.

[64], 353, [59] p.   11 cm.   **[5678]**

1653. *In* Cardano, G. In Aphorismos Hippocratis commentaria luculentissima cum Graeco textu. 1653.

1653. (bks. 1–2 only) *In* Cigalini, P. In Aphor. Hippocratis lib. primum et secundum lectiones. 1653.

1654. *In his* [Aphorismi. Adaptations, etc. French] 1654.

1655. *In* Moralis, G. Enchiridium medicum. 1455 (i.e. 1655)

1658. *In* Oribasius. In Aphorismos Hippocratis commentaria hactenus non visa. 1658.

1660. *In his* [Aphorismi. French] 1660.

1660. (bk. 1 only) *In* Santorio, S. Opera omnia. 1660.

1660. *In* Tilemann, J. Aphorismi Hippocratis. 1660.

1662. (Selections) *In* Fragoso, J. La cirugia. 1662.

1663

—Aphorismi, Nicolao Leoniceno . . . interprete. Una cum annotationibus quibusdam, & circa textum praecipue Joannis Manelphi . . . Accessere & Prognostica itemque Aphorismi selecti ad singulos morbos. Quibus accedunt quaedam medica apophthegmata scitu in primis necessaria non antea typis tradita. Venetiis, Apud Turrinum, 1663.

16, 3–194 p.   11 cm.   (Part 1 in Schola medica in qua Hippocratis, Galeni, Avicennaeque . . . habentur fundamenta. Venetiis, 1663)   **[5679]**

Manelfi's annotations are from his edition of the Aphorismi as printed in Rome in 1623. "Liber octavus" (spurious) translated by Antonio Musa Brasavola: p. 106–109.

"Aphorismi selecti ad singulos morbos" (p. 7–14, 1st group) is P. F. Occlerio's classed index to the Aphorismi.

The Prognostica (p. 113–114) is translated by Gulielmus Copus.

The "medica apophthegmata" (p. 155–194, with caption title, Collectiones medicinae, de medici atque aegroti officio) here anonymous and stated not to have been printed before, are by Alessandro Benedetti; they were printed several times in the 15th and 16th centuries.

". . . Jusjurandum" (Johan van Heurne's version): p. 110–112.

1665. (bk. 1 only) *In* Cabotin, A. Commentaire en vers sur les Aphorismes d'Hypocrate. 1665.

1665. *In his* [Aphorismi. Dutch] 1665.

1666. *In his* (Aphorismi. French] 1666.

1667. *In* Latioso, A. In Hippocratis Aphorismos . . . commentarii. 1667.

1667. (bks. 1, 2, 4) *In* Locatelli, L. Theatro d'arcani . . . nel quale si tratta dell'arte chimica. 1667.

1669. *In his* [Adaptations, etc. Latin] 1669.

1671. *In his* [Aphorismi. French] 1671.

1673. *In* Cardilucius, J. H., *ed.* and *tr.* Neuaufgerichtete Stadt- und Land-Apotheke. 1673–80.

1674

—Aphorismorum . . . sectiones septem. Quibus ex Antonii Musae commentariis adjecta fuit, & octava. Et ad imminuendum studiosorum laborem singuli aphorismi selecti fuere, tam ad febres, quam ad morbos singulos attinentes: ut facile unusquisque uno intuitu quaecunque in aphorismis continentur cernere possit. P. Francisco Occlerio . . . authore. Venetiis, Apud Nicolaum Pezzana, 1674.

[48], 96 p.   12 cm.   **[5680]**

Apparently a reprint of the 1611 Vicenza edition.

With this is bound (as issued) *his* Prognostica. Latin. 1674.

1680. *In* Sorbait, P. de. Commentaria & controversiae in omnes libros Aphorismorum Hippocratis. 1680.

1681

—Tripus medicinae, oracula Hippocratica divulgans; seu, Hippocratis Aphorismorum omnium in III. sectiones nova digestio, ad mentem ipsius in Aphorismo primo insinuatam. At sic sectiones positae sunt, ut in prima Aphorismi curativi, in secunda curativi & prognostici, in tertia curativi, prognostici & reliqui contineantur. Singulae vero sectiones in certas subsectiones divisae, & rursus Aphorismi singuli secundum connexionem, quam invicem habent . . . dispositi sunt . . . Aphorismi denique ex Tilemanno juxta recognitionem Vorstii, interpositis adnotationibus Visceri, & subnexa vel saltem citata versione Celsi (quae deinde sequitur) describuntur . . . Authore Joanne Daniele Globicz . . . Noribergae, Sumtibus Johannis Ziegeri, typis Andreae Knorzii, 1681.

    [4], 216, [54] p.   14 cm.   **[5681]**

Adolph Vorstius' Latin text of the Aphorismi (p. 79-184) was printed with Johannes Tilemann's Synopsis Aphorismorum Hippocratis, Marburg, 1643, reprinted in 1650 and 1660 under title: Aphorismi Hippocratis facile methodo digesti. Johann Vischer's annotations are from his Enarratio brevis Aphorismorum Hippocratis, Tübingen, 1591.

"Ex libris De re medica quaedam": p. 185-215, are selections, mainly from the Aphorismi.

1682. (bks. 1-2 only) *In* Barisano, F. D. Magnus Hippocrates medico-morlis. 1682.

1684

—Aphorismorum . . . sectiones septem; quibus Antomii [sic] Musae commentariis adjecta fuit, & octava. Et ad imminuendum studiosorum laborem singuli Aphorismi selecti fuere, tam ad febres, quam ad morbos singulos attinentes, ut facile unusquisque uno intuitu quaecunque in Aphorismis continentur cernere possit; P. Francisco Occlerio . . . authore. Patavii, Apud Cadorinum, 1684.

    [48], 83 p. 43 p.   12 cm.   (Part [3] *in* Schola medica in qua Hippocratis, Galeni, Avicennaeque . . . habentur fundamenta. Patavii, 1682-84)

                                  [5682]

"Hippocratis . . . Prognosticorum, libri tres" (43 p. at end) has special title page, with imprint: Patavii, Typis Jacobi de Cadorinis, 1684.

Books 1-7 of the Aphorismi translated by Niccolò Leoniceno; book 8 (spurious) translated by Antonio Musa Brasavola. The Prognostica translated by Gulielmus Copus.

1685. *In his* [Aphorismi. French] 1685.

1685. *In* Osorio y Peralta, D. Principia medicinae. 1685.

1686. (Selections) *In* Fragoso, J. La cirugia. 1686.

1693. (bks. 1-4) *In* Tozzi, L. In Hippocratis Aphorismos commentaria. 1693.

1694. *In* Genga, B. In Hippocratis Aphorismos. 1694.

1697. *In* Genga, B. In Hippocratis Aphorismos. 1697.

1697. (bks. 1-4) *In* Sinapi, M. A. Absurda vera. 1697.

1699. *In his* [Aphorismi. French] 1699.

1699. *In his* [Adaptations, etc. Latin] 1699.

Dutch

1606. *In* Baten, C. Handboek der cirurgijen. 1606.

1634. *In* Baten, C. Handboek der cirurgijen. 1634.

1640. *In* Chaumette, A. Handt-boeck der chirurgie. 1640.

1653. *In* Baten, C. Handboek der cirurgijen. 1653.

1658

—Aphorismi Hippocratis; Dat is, Afgesonderde, kort-bondige spreucken vanden out wijs-ervarensten arts Hippocrates . . . Uyt het Griecks . . . vertaelt . . . door Michael Tatinghof . . . Amsterdam, Voor Abraham de Wees [gedruckt by Christoffel Cunradus] 1658.

    [20], 264, [2] p.   10 cm.   **[5683]**

Imperfect: p. 147-148 and 185-186 mutilated.

1665

—Aphorismi. Dat zijn: kort en bondige leeringen, of regulen; aanwijzende de oorzaken en eigenschappen der ziekten; en de maniere van genesinge der zelve. Uit geleid en verciert met Nederduitsche aanteikeningen . . . Door Ernestum Ras . . . Midwlburg, Sibrand Jordens, 1665.

    [10], 385, [37] p.   port.   17 cm.   **[5684]**

Added engraved title page.

Includes the Latin translation by Leonhart Fuchs.

English

1610

—The whole aphorismes of great Hippocrates . . . Translated into English . . . of the Greek and Latin tongs. Whereunto is annexed A short discourse of the nature and substance of the eye, with many excellent and approved remedies for the cure of most the diseases thereof . . . With an exact table shewing the substance of every aphorism. London, Printed by H. L. for Richard Redmer, 1610.

[21], 198, [4] p. 13 cm. [5685]

Dedicatory epistle signed by S. H., the editor, probable translator of the Aphorisms. According to E. Arber's *A transcript of the registers of the Company of Stationers of London, 1554–1640* [New York, P. Smith, 1950] vol. 3, p. 200, the book was "...translated into Englishe, devided into 8 books by FF: B. Doctor of phisique."

"The life of Hippocrates": [4] p. at end.

"A briefe discourse upon the nature & substance of the ey," is an abridged translation of "De oculis eorumque egritudinibus et curis" by Benevenutus Grassus.

STC 13521.

1655

—The aphorisms ... With an exact table shewing the substance of every aphorism, and a short comment on each one, taken out of those larger notes of Galen, Heurnius, Fuchsius, &c. London, Humphrey Moseley, 1655.

[22], 179 p. front. (port.) 13 cm. [5686]

"Hippocrates his life out of Soranus": p. [3–10]

"Hippocrates his oath": p. [11–13]

The translation is similar to the 1610 London edition, translated by S. H.

1662. *In* Cooke, J. Mellificium chirurgiae. 1662.

1665

—The eight sections of Hippocrates Aphorismes review'd and rendred into English: according to the translation of Anutius Foesius. Digested into an exact and methodical form and divided into several chapters, wherein every aphorisme is reduced to its proper subject ... Wherein also many aphorisms are significantly interpreted which were neglected in the former translation ... London, Printed by W. G. for Rob. Crofts, 1665.

[4], 167, [1] p. port. 16 cm. [5687]

1676. *In* Cooke, J. Mellificium chirurgiae. 1676.

1685. *In* Cooke, J. Mellificium chirurgiae. 1685.

1693. *In* Cooke, J. Mellificium chirurgiae. 1693.

French

1605

—Les Aphorismes ... avec le commentaire de Galien sur le premier livre. Traduicts de grec en françois par M. J. Breche. Avec annotations sur ledict premier livre: ensemble certaines paraphrases servans de brief commentaire, dupis le second livre

jusques à la fin du septiesme, par ledict Breche. Plus, les Aphorismes de J. Damascene [i.e. the elder Mesuë] ... ensemble un Epitome sur les trois livres des temperamens de Galien [par Jérémie de Dryvere] Le tout nouvellement reveu & corrigé. Lyon, Jean Ant. Huguetan, 1605.

[2], 254 ll. 12 cm. [5688]

Includes Niccolò Leoniceno's Latin version of Hippocrates' Aphorismi.

A page for page reprint of the edition published in 1600.

1606

—[The same.] ... Rouen, Romain de Beauvais, 1606.

[2], 254 ll. 12 cm. [5689]

1620

—Les Aphorismes ... ausquelles sont contenues toutes les loix, decrets, & arrests de la vraye medecine dogmatique. Traduittes de nouveau en françois, enrichies de tresbelles & riches notes, & doctes commentaires sur chasque sentence; rengées & disposées par lieux communs, & selon la disposition des parties du corps humain. Par M. Jean Vigier ... Lyon, Jean Ant. Huguetan, 1620.

[16], 602, [1] p. 12 cm. [5690]

Includes Latin text of the Aphorismi, generally following Niccolò Leoniceno's version.

162–?

—[The same.] Les Aphorismes ... avec le commentaire de Galien sur le premier livre. Traduits de grec en françois par M. J. Breche. Avec annotations sur ledit premier livre: ensemble certaines paraphrases servans de brief commentaire, depuis le second livre jusques à la fin du septiéme, par ledit Breche. Plus les Aphorismes de J. de Damascene [i.e. the elder Mesuë] ... Ensemble une Epitome sur les trois livres des temperamens de Galien [par Jérémie de Dryvere] Paris, Antoine Bourriquant [162–?]

430 p. 14 cm. [5691]

Typography resembles that of the Paris edition dated 1627 published by P. Gaultier.

Includes Niccolò Leoniceno's Latin version of Hippocrates' Aphorismi.

1627

—[The same.] ... Paris, Philippes Gaultier, 1627.

367 p. 13 cm. [5692]

Typography resembles that of the undated Paris edition published by A. Bourriguant, from which it probably was reprinted.

1628

—[The same.] ... Lyon, Claude Chastellard, 1628.

479 p. 12 cm. [**5693**]

Includes Latin text of Hippocrates' Aphorismi.

1642. *In his* [Aphorismi. Adaptations, etc. French] 1642.

1645

—Les sept livres d'Aphorismes ... en latin et en françois, enrichis de tres-beaux et tres-doctes discours en forme de paraphrases, et d'explications tres-judicieuses prises des anciens & nouveaux autheurs ... Par Me Michel Le Long ... Paris, Nicolas & Jean de la Coste, 1645.

[8], 954, [37] p. 24 cm. [**5694**]

The Latin version is that of Guillaume Plancy.

1646

—Les Aphorismes ... avec le commentaire de Galien sur le I. livre. Traduits de grec en françois par M. J. Breche. Avec annotations sur ledit premier livre: ensemble certaines paraphrases servans de brief commentaire, depuis le second livre jusques à la fin du septiéme, par ledit Breche. Où a esté adjousté de nouveau les Aphorismes de J. de Damascen [i.e. the elder Mesuë] ... ensemble un Epitome sur les trois livres des temperamens de Galien [par Jérémie de Dryvere] Rouen, Daniel Loudet, 1646.

515 (i.e. 551) p. 14 cm. [**5695**]

Imperfect: p. 319–330, 477–478 wanting.
The title page is a cancel.
Includes Niccolò Leoniceno's Latin version of the Aphorismi.
With this is bound: Guy de Chauliac. Les fleurs du grand Guidon. 1646.

1654. *In his* [Aphorismi. Adaptations, etc. French] 1654.

1660

—[The same.] ... Derniere ed. rev. & corr. & augm. des Fleurs du grand Guidon. Rouen, Jacques Besongne, 1660.

[4], 571 (i.e. 531) p.; 142 p. 14 cm. [**5696**]

Imperfect: title page (a cancel) mutilated.
"Les fleurs du grand Guidon ... par Maistre Jean Raoul" has special title page.

1666

—Les Aphorismes ... traduits par Me J. Vigier ... Rev. & augm. de notes & commentaires sur châque sentence, rangées methodiquement par lieux communs, & selon la disposition des parties du corps humain. Avec ... la Vie, le Serment, & les Prognostiques d'Hippocrate ... Paris, Jean d'Houry, 1666.

[84], 684, [92] p. 16 cm. [**5697**]

Imperfect: p. 467–470 wanting.
The main work, with Vigier's commentaries and including the Latin text, generally following Niccolò Leoniceno's version, was previously published in Lyons in 1620. The present editor, who translated the accompanying works, has signed the dedicatory epistle: I. L. D.

1668

—Les aphorismes ... traduits nouvellement en françois suivant la verité du texte grec [par Lazare Meyssonnier] avec un meslange de paraphrases, d'eclaircissement és lieux plus obscurs, et la clef de cette doctrine par le moyen de la circulation du sang, & d'autres nouvelles découvertes de ce siecle en anatomie & chymie ... Lyon, Chez Pierre Compagnon [De l'imprimerie de Marcelin Gautherin] 1668.

[36], 290 (i.e. 288) p. 16 cm. [**5698**]

Dedicatory epistle and "advis au lecteur" signed by L. Meyssonnier, the translator.
With this is bound (as issued) Meyssonnier, L. Le medecin charitable abbregé. [1668]

1671

—Les Aphorismes ... Dern. ed., rev. & corr. Rouen, Chez Clement Malassis [De l'imprimerie de L. Cabut] 1671.

[4], 571 (i.e. 531) p. 15 cm. [**5699**]

A reprint of the 1660 Rouen edition with the same error in paging. It does not include Les fleurs du grand Guidon, which Louis Cabut printed separately in 1671. Cf. Lepreux, v. 3, p. 93–94.

1684

—Les aphorismes ... Lyon, Piere Compagnon & Robert Taillandier, 1684.

[36], 313 (i.e. 321), [3] p. 15 cm. [**5700**]

A reprint of the 1668 Lyons edition including Lazare Meyssonnier's Le medecin charitable abbregé (p. [273–306]) which was issued with that edition.
Error in paging: numbers 89–96 duplicated. Pages [25–32] are misbound with conjugate leaves paged 305–312.
"Sommaire des sentimens de M. L. Meyssonnier, extrait de ses oeuvres sur les cometes de 1664 & 1665": p. 307–312.

1685

—Aphorismes . . . traduits en francois. Avec des explications physiques, & des annotations curieuses . . . Paris, Estienne Michallet, 1685.

    2 v. in 1.   17 cm.   **[5701]**

Includes Latin text.

1699

—Les Aphorismes . . . rangez selon l'ordre des parties du corps humain. Avec des nouvelles explications, divers remedes & plusieurs observations de pratique sur les maladies, par M. Du Four . . . Paris Laurent d'Houry, 1699.

    [14], 616, [20] p.   17 cm.   **[5702]**

Imperfect: leaf paged 595-596 wanting. Cancel for leaf paged 593-594 inserted after the original leaf.

Includes the Latin text.

German

1673. *In* Cardilucius, J. H., *ed.* and *tr.* Neuaufgerichtete Stadt- und Land-Apotheke. 1673-80.

Hebrew

1647. *In his* [Aphorismi. Greek and Latin.] 1647.

Italian

1621. *In* Rosaccio, G. Il medico del dottore in . . . medicina . . . Giuseppe Rosaccio libri tre. 1621.

1639. (Selections) *In* Fragoso, J. Della cirugia. 1639.

1662. (Selections) *In* Fragoso, J. La cirugia. 1662.

1667. *In* Latioso, A. In Hippocratis Aphorismos . . . commentarii. 1667.

1686. (Selections) *In* Fragoso, J. La cirugia. 1686.

1694. *In* Genga, B. In Hippocratis Aphorismos. 1694.

1697. *In* Genga, B. In Hippocratis Aphorismos. 1697.

Spanish

1621. (Selections) *In* Fragoso, J. Cirugia universal. 1621.

1634. *In* Pérez, A. Summa, y examem [sic] de cirugia, de lo mas necessario que en ella se contiene. 1634.

Aphorismi

Adaptations, etc.

Greek and Latin

1633. *In his* [Aphorismi. Greek and Latin] Οι ’Αφορισμοὶ πεξικοί τε καὶ ἐμμετροι. 1633.

1634

—Aphorismi versibus Graecis et Latinis expositi. Per M. Gerardum Denisotum . . . Cujus selectiora aliquot epigrammata addita sunt huic operi, studio & sumptibus Jacobi Denisot nepotis in lucem editi. Parisiis, Apud Fiacrium Dehors, 1634.

    [16], 166, [1] p.   port.   19 cm.   **[5703]**

Errata: p. [167]

Latin

1619

—Aphorismi paraphrasi poetica olim illustrati a Reginaldo Sturmio, nunc denuo de novo parvo hoc opusculo seorsim comprehensi, ac Asclepiadeis hominibus exhibiti a Johanne Junckern . . . [Erfurt] Impensis Johannis Birckneri, 1619.

    [1], 45 ll.   13 cm.   **[5704]**

Originally published in Lyons in 1583 under title: In septem libros Aphorismorum Hippocratis paraphrasis poetica. Omits as spurious all after aphorism 79, book 7.

1622. *In his* [Adaptations, etc. French] 1622.

1634. *In his* [Aphorismi. Latin] 1634.

1634. *In his* Aphorismi. [Adaptations, etc. Greek and Latin] 1634.

1647

—Aphorismi; seu, Axiomata . . . septem libris comprehensa, versu heroïco explicata a Joan. Bapt. de Conde . . . Bruxellae, Ex typographia Joannis Mommarti, 1647.

    91, [17] p.   13 cm.   **[5705]**

Includes prose text "ex interpretatione Anutii Foesii & Gulielmi Plantii."

Bound with *his* Thesaurus Hippocraticus, sive Aphorismi. 1639.

1657

—Aphorismi metrica paraphrasi translati ab H. v. Poort M. D. Trajecti ad Rhenum, Typis Gisberti a Zyll, & Theodori ab Ackersdijck, 1657.

    167, [1] p.   12 cm.   **[5706]**

Includes Greek text of the Aphorismi.

1669

—Aphorismi aurei, septem libris comprehensi, versu heroico explicati ... [n. p.] 1669.

99, [20] p. 13 cm. [5707]

Previously printed in Brussels in 1647 with the author of the poetic version, Joannes Baptista de Conde, named on the title page, and with the accompanying prose translation identified as "ex interpretatione Anuti Foesii & Gulielmi Plantii."

1696. *In his* [Prognostica. Adaptations, etc. Latin] 1696.

1699

—Aphorismi poeticis salibus aspersi, authore Antonio Palmerio ... Neap., Typis Felecis Mosca. 1699.

[10], 156 p. front. 15 cm. [5708]

Includes Niccolò Leoniceno's Latin version.

French

1622

—Aphorismes de chirurgie tirez d'Hippocrate avec les commentaires. Nouvellement mis en lumiere, par Charles Guillemeau ... Paris, Abraham Pacard, 1622.

[8], 462 (i.e. 492), [14] p. 14 cm. [5709]

Includes French and Latin text of selections from Hippocrates' Aphorismi and French text of selections from Galen's In Hippocratis Aphorismos.

1642

—Les Aphorismes d'Hypocrate mis en vers françois ... Par le sieur de Launay, chirurgien. Rouen, Jean Viret, 1642.

[16], 152 (i.e. 142) p. 16 cm. [5710]

1654

—Hippocrate dépaïsé: ou la version paraphrasee de ses Aphorismes; en vers françois. Par M. L. de F. Paris, Edme Pepingué, 1654.

[24], 174, [2] p. 24 cm. [5711]

Dedicatory epistle signed: Louis de Fontenettes.

Latin text of the Aphorismi translated by Leonhart Fuchs printed in the margins.

Italian

1667. *In* Latioso, A. In Hippocratis Aphorismos ... commentarii. 1667.

—*as subject. See* BEVERWIJCK, J. van. Exercitatio in Hippocratis aphorismum de calculo. 1641.

See CLETI, E. Dilucidatio in Aphor. 22. primae sect. pro defensione interpretationis Marsilii Cagnati.

1621; FEAKE, J., *respondent*. Disputatio medica inauguralis. 1670; FONSECA, R. de. In septem Aphorismorum Hippocratis libros commentaria. 1608, 1621, 1628; GORRIS, J. de [*fl.* 1572–1622] Opuscula quatuor. 1660; MANELFI, G. Responsio brevis ad annotationes Prosperi Martiani. 1621; MARZIANI, P. In Hippocratis aphorismum XXII sectionis primae expositio. 1617; MORALIS, G. Manuductio ad universam Aphorismorum doctrinam. 1653; PARACELSUS. Erster [-zehender] Theil der Bücher und Schrifften. 1603; (bk. 7 only) PARDO, J. Tratado del vino aguado. 1661; SAUMAISE, C. de. Interpretatio Hippocratei aphorismi LXIX. sectione IV. de calculo. 1640; WEDEL, G. W. Aphorismi aphorismorum. 1695;

Coacae praenotiones

Greek and Latin

1621

—Coacae praenotiones ... Interprete & enarratore Ludovico Dureto ... Editio recens illustrata. Lutetiae Parisiorum, Sumptibus Petri Billaine, 1621.

[12], 578, [54] p. 35 cm. [5712]

Edited by Jean Duret.

Corresponds page for page with the 1588 Paris edition. Omits the errata note, but the errors are not all corrected in the text.

1621

—Another issue, with imprint: Lutetiae Parisiorum. Sumptibus viduae Joannis Meiat, 1621. [5713]

1657

—Coaca praesagia, brevi enarratione illustrata, decerpta a Galeno, Hollerio, Dureto, Foësio, Jacotio, & aliis non inferioris natae viris. In formam encheiridii ad usum faciliorem composita. Authore D. Lud. Ferrant ... Discrepantes reconciliante, variantes explicante, dubios denique obfirmante. Lutetiae Parisiorum, Apud Joannem Pocquet, 1657.

3, [9], 679, [61] p. 15 cm. [5714]

Privilege and errata: p. [60–61]

1658

—Coacae praenotiones ... Interprete & enarratore Ludovioco Dureto ... Lutetiae Parisiorum, Sumptibus Gaspari Meturas, 1658.

[12], 578, [54] p. 37 cm. [5715]

Different setting of type.

1660

—Coacae praenotiones, Graece & Latine ... Cum versione D. Anutii Foesii ... et notis Joh. Jonstoni ... Amstelaedami, Ex Officina Elzeviriana, 1660.

[12], 577, [107] p.   13 cm.   **[5716]**

1665

—Coacae praenotiones ... Interprete & enarratore Ludovico Dureto ... Genevae, Apud Stephanum Gamonet, 1665.

[12], 578, [54] p.   38 cm.   **[5717]**
Different setting of type.

1668

—[The same.] ... Lutetiae Parisiorum, Apud Casparum Meturas, 1668.

[12], 578, [54] p.   37 cm.   **[5718]**
A reissue, with cancel title page, of the 1665 Geneva edition.

Greek

1629. *In* Horst, G. [1578-1636] Ἐξετάσεων παθολογικῶν. 1629.

1622. *In* Horst, G. [1578-1636] Prognosis febrium. 1622.

Latin

1654. *In* Millo, G. Naturae morbos decernentis arcanum opus. 1654.

De aere, aquis, et locis
Greek and Latin

1646, 1655. *In* Martin, J. Praelectiones in librum Hippocratis ... De aere, aquis, et locis. 1646, 1655.

—*as subject. See* BALDI, B. Disquisitio iatro-physica. 1637.

De alimento
Latin

1635-1639. *In* Castro, E. R. de. Commentarius in Hippocratis Coi, libellum De alimento. 1635-39.

De capitis vulneribus
Greek and Latin

1616. *In* Pauw, P. Succenturiatus anatomicus. 1616.

1632. *In* Cortesi, G. B. Tractatus de vulneribus capitis. 1632.

Latin

1608. *In* Parma, I. Praxis chirurgica. 1608.

1639. *In* Aranzi, G. C. In librum Hippocratis De vulneribus capitis commentarius. 1639.

Dutch

1634, 1653. *In* Baten, C. Hant-boeck der chirurgyen. 1634, 1653.

French

1612

—Le livre ... des plaies de teste. Thresor de chirurgie. Traduict du grec, corrige et commente, par M. Francois Dissaudeau ... Saumur, Thomas Portau, 1612.

[14], 416, [21] p.   16 cm.   **[5719]**
Errata: p. [417]

1658

—[The same.] ... Rouen, Louys Du Mesnil, 1658.

[24], 416, [16] p.   16 cm.   **[5720]**

Italian

1657. *In* Falcinelli, B. Nuova dichiarazione. 1657.

1693. *In* Falcinelli, B. Nuova dichiarazione. 1693.

—*as subject. See* FALLOPPIO, G. Opera. 1606.

De corde
Latin

1657. *In* Restaurand, R. Monarchia microcosmi. 1657.

De corde
Adaptations, etc.
French

1683. *In* Barra, P. Hippocrate, de la circulation du sang et des humeurs. 1683.

—*as subject. See* SEGER, G. Dissertatio de Hippocratis libri περι καρδιης ortu legitimo. 1661.

De diebus judicatoriis

Adaptations, etc.

Latin

1696. *In his* [Prognostica. Adaptations, etc.] 1696.

De fracturis

Dutch

1691. *See* VERDUC, L. Het parische verband-huis. 1691.

De humoribus

Greek and Latin

1631. *In* Duret, L. In magni Hippocratis librum De humoribus. 1631.

1639. *In* Duret, L. In magni Hippocratis librum De humoribus. 1639.

De insomniis

Latin

1628. *In* Colle, G. De cognitu difficilibus in praxi ex libello Hippocratis De insomniis. 1628.

1659. *In* Scaliger, J. C. In librum De insomniis Hippocratis commentarius auctus nunc & recognitus. 1659.

—*as subject. See* LINDEN, J. A. van der, *praes.* Hippocrates de circuitu sanguinis, exercitatio I, III, IV. 1659 [and] Exercitatio V–XIII. 1660; TARDY, C. Traitté du mouvement circulaire du sang et des esprits. 1654.

De internis affectionibus

Greek and Latin

1637. *In* Martin, J. Praelectiones in librum Hippocratis ... De morbis internis. 1637.

De locis in homine

Latin

1638

—Liber de locis in homine. Commentariis illustratus a Francisco Perla ... Romae, Apud Bernardinum Tanum, 1638.

[16], 424, [36] p.   21 cm.   [5721]

The Latin translation is that of Janus Cornarius.

De medicamentis purgatoriis

Greek and Latin

1617

—Περὶ τῶν φαρμάκων καθαιρόντων ... De pharmacis purgantib. libellus. Ex Cujaciano cod. a R. P. S. J. exscriptus: hactenus in plerisque Hippocratis editionibus desideratus. Fed. Morellus ... Lat. vertit & notis illustravit. Accessit Galeni corollarium hactenus ineditum e Bibliotheca Reg. eodem interprete. Lutetiae, Apud Federicum Morellum, 1617.

60 p.   15 cm.   [5722]

"Epilogus seu corollarium lib. Galeni, Quod animi mores corporis temperamenta sequantur": p. 37–59.

"Fed. Morelli curae novae ad lib. Theophili De urinis": p. 59–60. Morel's edition of this work was published in Paris in 1608.

De morbis

Greek and Latin

1630. (Selections) *In* Bartsch, J. Inaugurales theses Hippocraticae. 1630.

Latin

1602. *In* Salius Diversus, P. Commentaria in Hippocratis libros quatuor De morbis. 1602.

1612. *In* Salius Diversus, P. Commentaria ... in Hippocratis ... De quaesitis universalibus ad medicinam spectantibus. 1612.

1646. *In* Salius Diversus, P. Commentaria in Hippocratis libros quatuor De morbis. 1646.

De morbo sacro

Latin

1631. *In* Ponce de Santa Cruz, A. [*d. ca.* 1650] Praelectiones Vallisoletanae, in librum magni Hipp. Coi De morbo sacro. 1631.

De natura hominis

Greek and Latin

1609. *In* Heurne, J. van. In Hippocratis Coi De hominis natura libros duos. 1609.

1611. *In* Heurne, J. van. In Hippocratis Coi De hominis natura libros duos. 1611.

Latin

1634. *In* Dubois, J. Jacobi Sylvii ... Opera medica. 1634.

1635. *In* Dubois, J. Jacobi Sylvii ... Opera medica. 1635.

—*as subject. See* PARDOUX, B. Bartholomaei Perdulcis ... In Jac. Sylvii anatomen et in lib. Hippocratis De natura humana commentarii. 1643; De natura hominis. *See* SALDO, G. F. Artis medicae liber primus. 1628.

De ossium natura

Greek and Latin

1665. *In* Galenus. De ossibus. 1665.

De prisca medicina

Latin

1681. *In* Porzio, L. A. In Hippocratis librum De veteri medicina ... paraphrasis. 1681.

Dutch

1687. *In* Massard, J. Verscheide verhandelingen raakende de panacéen. 1687.

French

1681. *In* Massard, J. Traité des panacées. 1681.

—*as subject. See* RHIJNE, W. ten. Meditationes in magni Hippocratis textum xxiv De veteri medicina. 1672.

De salubri victus ratione

Latin

1605. *In* Regimen sanitatis Salernitanum. Medicina Salernitana. 1605.

1607. *In* Regimen sanitatis Salernitanum. De conservanda bona valetudine. 1607.

1611. *In* Regimen sanitatis Salernitanum. Medicine Salernitana. 1611.

1612. *In* Regimen sanitatis Salernitanum. Medicine Salernitana. 1612.

1619. *In* Regimen sanitatis Salernitanum. De conservanda bona valetudine. 1619.

1622. *In* Regimen sanitatis Salernitanum. Medicine Salernitana. 1622.

1624. *In* Regimen sanitatis Salernitanum. Medicine Salernitana. 1624

1628. *In* Hygieia. 1628.

1628. *In* Regimen sanitatis Salernitanum. Medicine Salernitana. 1628.

1638. *In* Regimen sanitatis Salernitanum. Medicine Salernitana. 1638.

1649. *In* Regimen sanitatis Salernitanum. Schola Salernitana. 1649.

1657. *In* Regimen sanitatis Salernitanum. Schola Salernitana. 1657.

1667. *In* Regimen sanitatis Salernitanum. Schola Salernitana. 1667.

1683. *In* Regimen sanitatis Salernitanum. Schola Salernitana. 1683.

Dutch

1658. *In* Regimen sanitatis Salernitanum. Schoola Salernitana. 1658.

De septimestri partu

Greek and Latin

1665. *In* Peyssonel, J. de. De temporibus humani partus. 1665.

1666. *In* Barra, P. De veris terminis partus humani libri tres ex Hippocrate. 1666.

1666. *In* Peyssonel, J. de. De temporibus humani partus. 1666.

—*See* TARDY, C. In libellos Hippocratis De septimestri et octimestri partu. 1651.

De ulceribus

Italian

1690

—Libro ... dell'ulcere. Con le note pratiche chirurgiche di Giuseppe Cignozzi. Firenze, Nella stamperia di Pier Matini, ad istanza di Niccolò Taglini, 1690.

379, [1] p.   19 cm.   [5723]

Errata: p. [380]

De victus ratione

Latin

1624. (bk. 1 only) *In* Ponce de Santa Cruz, A. [*d. ca.* 1650] Opuscula medica, et philosophica. 1624.

1657. (Selections, bk. 1 only) *In* Restaurand, R. Monarchia microcosmi. 1657.

De victus ratione in morbis acutis

Greek and Latin

1609. *In* Heurne, J. van. In Hippocratis Coi De victus ratione. 1609.

1611. *In* Heurne, J. van. In Hippocratis Coi De victus ratione. 1611.

Latin

1631. *In* Duret, L. In magni Hippocratis librum De humoribus. 1631.

1639. *In* Duret, L. In magni Hippocratis librum De humoribus. 1639.

1655. *In* Valles, F. de. Commentaria in quatuor Hippocratis libros De ratione victus in morbis acutis. 1655.

—*See* TARDY, C. Traitté du mouvement circulair du sang et des esprits. 1654.

De virginum morbis

Latin

1635. *In* Stefani, G. In Hippocratis Coi libellum De virginum morbis commentarius. 1635.

Adaptations, etc.

Latin

1648. *In* Tardy, C. In libellum Hippocratis De virginum morbis commentatio paraphrastica. 1648.

French

1645. *In his* [Prognostica. French] 1645.

Epidemiorum libri

Greek

1644. (bks. 1–2 only) *In* Frigio, P. F. Petri Francisci Phyrigii . . . Commentarii in historias epidemicas Hippocratis. 1644.

Greek and Latin

1623. (bk. 2 only) *In* Mercuriale, G. In secundum lib. Epid. Hipp. 1626.

Latin

1602. (bks. 1, 3 only) *In* Mercuriale, G. Commentarii eruditissimi, in Hippocratis Coï Prognostica. 1602.

1621. (bks. 1–7) *In* In Valles, F. de. In Hippocratis libros De morbis popularibus commentaria. 1621.

1631. (bk. 2 only) *In* Duret L. In magni Hippocratis librum De humoribus. 1631.

1639. (bk. 2 only) *In* Duret, L. In magni Hippocratis librum De humoribus. 1639.

1644. (bks. 1, 3 only) *In* Frigio, P. F. Petri Francisci Phrygii . . . Commentarii in historias epidemicas Hippocratis. 1644.

1653. (bks. 1–7) *In* Valles, F. de. In Hippocratis libros De morbis popularibus commentaria. 1652 [i.e. 1653]

1655. (bks. 1–7 only) *In* Valles, F. de. Commentaria, in septem libros Hippocrat. De morbis popularibus. 1654 [i.e. 1655]

1656. (bk. 1 only) *In* Castro, E. R. de. Expositiones in aliquos Hippocratis aegrotos. 1656.

1665. (bks. 1, 3 only) *In* Heredia, P. M. de. Opera medica. 1665.

1673. (bks. 1, 3 only) *In* Heredia, P. M. de. Opera medica. 1673.

1690. (bks. 1, 3 only) *In* Heredia, P. M. de. Opera medica. 1690.

Adaptations, etc.

Latin

1661. *In* Valles, F. De. Imber aureus. 1661.

Epistolae

Greek and Latin

1601. *In* Lubin, E., *ed.* and *tr.* Epistolae Hippocratis, Democriti, Heracliti. 1601.

French

1632

—La conference et entreveuë d'Hippocrate et de Democrite. Tiree du grec, et commentee par Marcellin Bompart . . . Paris, La vefue Philippe Gaultier, 1632.

[24], 96, 88 (i.e. 68), [2] p. 17 cm. **[5724]**

A selection from the Epistolae.

Contents.—Le senat et peuple abderitain a Hippocrate.—Hippocrate au senat et peuple des Abderites.—Hippocrate a Philopemene.—Hippocrate a Denis.—Hippocrate a Damaget.—Hippocrate a Philopemene.—Hippocrate a Crateva.—La conference d'Hippocrate enoncee en céte lettre. Hippocrate salut et liesse a Damaget.

Epistolae. Ad Ptolemaeum regem de hominis fabrica

Latin

1633. *In* Stefani, G. In Hippocratis Coi libellum De hominis structura commentarius. 1633.

Jusjurandum

Greek and Latin

1627. *In* Ranchin, F. Opuscula medica. 1627.

1643

—ʿΟρκος; sive, Jusjurandum. Recensitum, & libro commentario illustratum, a Joanne Henrico Meibomio. Lugduni Batavorum, Ex officina Jacobi Lauwiickii [Typis Wilhelmi Christiani] 1643.

    [16], 232 p.   20 cm.   [5725]

Greek and Latin texts of the Jusjurandum: p. [9–11] "Idem Jusjurandum Latinis expressum, a Scaevola Sammarthano, Silvarum lib. I": p. [12–14]

1693. *In* Hamey, B. Dissertatio epistolaris de juramento medicorum. 1693.

Latin

1623. *In his* [Aphorismi. Latin] 1623.

1633. *In his* [Aphorismi. Latin] 1633.

1646. *In his* [Aphorismi. Latin] 1646.

1663. *In his* [Aphorismi. Latin] 1663.

1677. *In* Schönfeld, P. J. Synopsis medica super Pharmacopoeiam Augustanam pro praecipuis humani corporis affectibus. 1677.

English

1611. [i.e. 1612] *In his* [Prognostica. English] 1611 [i.e. 1612]

1634. *In his* [Prognostica. English] 1634.

1655. *In his* [Aphorismi. English] 1655.

1655. *In his* [Prognostica. English] 1655.

French

1639. *In* Bertrand, G. Les veritez anatomiques et chirurgicales. 1639.

1666. *In his* [Aphorismi. French] 1666.

Adaptations, etc.

Latin

1643. In his [Jusjurandum. Greek and Latin] 1643

French

1633. *In* Regimen sanitatis Salernitanum. Le regime de santé de l'Eschole de Salerne. 1633.

1637. *In* Regimen sanitatis Salernitanum. Le regime de santé de l'Eschole de Salerne. 1637.

1639. *In* Marque, J. de. Methodique introduction à la chirurgie. 1639.

1643. *In* Regimen sanitatis Salernitanum. Le regime de santé de l'Eschole de Salerne. 1643.

1647. *In* Marque J. de. Methodique introduction à la chirurgie. 1647.

1649. *In* Regimen sanitatis Salernitanum. Le regime de santé de l'Eschole de Salerne. 1649.

1652. *In* Marque, J. de. Methodique introduction à la chirurgie. 1652.

1660. *In* Regimen sanitatis Salernitanum. L'Escole des medecins de Salerne. 1660.

1671. *In* Du Four de La Crespelière. Commentaire en vers françois, sur l'Ecole de Salerne. 1671.

1680. *In* Marque, J. de. Methodique introduction a la chirurgie. 1680.

Lex.

Greek and Latin

1628. *In* [Aphorismi. Greek and Latin] 1628.

1661. *In his* [Aphorismi. Greek and Latin] 1661.

Latin

1637. *In* Stefani, G. In Hippocratis Coi Legem commentarius. 1637.

1633. *In his* [Aphorismi. Latin] 1633.

French

1645. *In his* [Prognostica. French] 1645.

Mochlicus

Greek and Latin

1665. *In* Galenus. De ossibus. 1665.

Prognostica
Greek and Latin

1625. *In* [Aphorismi. Greek and Latin] 1625.

1631. *In* [Selected works. Greek and Latin] 1631.

1645

—Vates medicus Hippocraticus; seu ... Prognosticorum liber, commentariis et notis illustratus. In lucem emissus a Bartholomaeo Horn ... Stralesundii, Literis Michaelis Mederi, & impensis Otthonis Ruymanni, 1645.

[4], 313, [15] p. 15 cm. [5726]

Includes Anuce Foe's Latin translation with commentary by Horn.

Latin

1602. (bk. 1 only) *In* Lavelli, J. De pulsibus ad tyrones. 1602.

1608. *In* Frigio, J. A. In magni Hippocratis Prognostica Jacobi Antonii Phrygii ... explanatio. 1608.

1611

—Pronosticorum, libri tres ... Vicentiae, Apud Franciscum Lenium, 1611.

48 p. 10 cm. [5727]

Translated by Gulielmus Copus.

Bound with Galenus. Ars medicinalis. 1606; and with Hippocrates. [Aphorismi. Latin] Aphorismorum ... sectiones septem: quibus ... adjecta fecit [sic] & octava. 1610 [i.e. 1611] with which it was issued. The title page is conjugate with the last page of the Aphorismi.

1622. *In his* [Aphorismi. Latin] 1622.

1626. *In* Vega, C. de. Opera omnia. 1626.

1642. *In* Hafenreffer, S. Raphael ὅδιος de arte medica. 1642.

1649. *In his* [Aphorismi. Latin] 1649.

1655. *In* Valles, F. de. Commentaria in Prognosticum Hippocratis. 1655.

1659

—Aphorismi prognostici ... in febribus acutis commentariis illustrati ... auctore Carolo Valesio Dubourgdieu ... a quo habitae sunt extremo anno M.DC.LVIII. excurrenteque M.DC.LIX. subjectae praelectiones ... Romae, Sumptibus Nicolai Angeli Tinassii, 1659.

[8] p., [1], 939 (i.e. 941) columns, [32] p. 33 cm. [5728]

1663. *In his* [Aphorismi. Latin] 1663.

1674

—Pronosticorum, libri tres ... 1674.

46 p. 12 cm. [5729]

Translated by Gulielmus Copus.

Bound (as issued) with *his* [Aphorismi. Latin] 1674.

168-? *In* Cardilucius, J. H., *ed.* and *tr.* Neuaufgerichtete Stadt- und Land-Apotheke. 1673–80.

1684. *In his* [Aphorismi. Latin] 1684.

English
1611 [i.e. 1612]

—The presages of divine Hippocrates: divided into three parts. With the protestation or oath which Hippocrates caused his schollers to make at their entrie with him to their studies. The whole collected and translated by Peter Lowe ... London, Thomas Purfoot, 1611 [i.e. 1612]

[31] p. 20 cm. (Part [2] *in* Lowe, Peter. A discourse of the whole art of chyrurgerie ... With The presages of divine Hippocrates. The 2d ed. London, 1612) [5730]

Translated from the French version by Pierre Verney.

Published in 1597 under title: The books of the presages of devyne Hyppocrates. Cf. Finlayson, p. 31.

1634

—[The same.] ... London, Thomas Purfoot, 1634.

[31] p. 20 cm. (Part [2] *in* Lowe, Peter. A discourse of the whole art of chyrurgerie ... With The presages of divine Hippocrates. The 3d ed. London, 1634) [5731]

1651. *In* Culpeper, N. Semeiotica Uranica. 1651.

1655

—The presages ... London, R. Hodgkinsonne, 1655.

457–487 p. 19 cm. (*In* Lowe, Peter. A discourse of the whole art of chyrurgery ... With The presages of divine Hippocrates. The 4th ed. London, 1654 [i.e. 1655]) [5732]

1655. *In* Culpeper, N. Semeiotica Uranica. 1655.

1655. *In* Lowe, P. A discourse of the whole art of chyrurgerie. 1654 [i.e. 1655]

1658. *In* Culpeper, N. Semeiotica Uranica. 1658.

French

1645

—Les prognostics d'Hippocrate, avec son Serment, et son traicté Des maladies des vierges. Mis en françois par le Sieur de Mirabeau . . . Paris, Antoine de Sommaville, 1645.

[31], 96, [46] p.   15 cm.   **[5733]**

"La loy d'Hippocrate": p. [25-31] The "Serment" is not present.

1666. *In* Hippocrates. Les aphorismes. 1666.

German

1663. *In* Becher, J. J. Parnassus medicinalis illustratus. 1663.

168-? *In* Cardilucius, J. H., *ed.* and *tr.* Neuaufgerichtete Stadt- und Land-Apotheke. 1673-80.

Adaptations, etc.

Latin

1661

—Caroli Sponii . . . Sibylla medica; Hippocratis libellum Prognosticon, heroico carmine Latine exprimens . . . Lugduni, Sumptib. Joan. Antonii Huguetan, & Marci Antonii Ravaud, 1661.

34 p.   23 cm.   **[5734]**

1696

—Prognosticorum et Aphorismorum Hyppocratis faelix recordatio a Paulo Hieronymo Bimio . . . relata in memoriae beneficium pro ingenuis medicinae tyronibus. Mediolani, Typis haeredum de Ghisulphis, 1696.

[12], 104 p.   24 cm.   **[5735]**

Contains Latin verse translations of Prognostica, Aphorismi, and De diebus judicatoriis.

XII. References

—Astrologia; Astronomia; De esse aegrorum secundum lunam; De medicorum astrologia; De significatione mortis et vitae secundum cursum lunae et aspectus planetarum. *See* IMBRASIUS, *of Ephesus.* Prognostica de decubitu.

—*as subject. See* AIGNAN, F. L'ancienne medecine. 1693; AMMANN, P. Irenicum Numae Pompilii, cum Hippocrate. 1689; ANDREAE, T. Sacrosancta triade annuente trias exercitationum de mente et corpore. 1679; BAILLOU, G. de. Definitionum medicarum liber.

1639; BARIL, J. Physiologia humana. 1653; BARRA, P. De veris terminis partus humani libri tres ex Hippocrate. 1666 [and] Hippocrate, de la circulation du sang et des humeurs. 1683; BENEDETTI, G. C. Epistolarum medicinalium libri decem. 1649 [and] Tutelaris columna. 1644; BERTOCCI, A. Methodus curativa. 1608; CAPRILI, P. E. Libri duo. 1643; CASERTA, F. A. Tractationes duae ad medicinae praxim pertinentes. 1623; CASTELLI, B. Castellus renovatus; hoc est, Lexicon medicum. 1682, 1688, 1700 [and] Lexicon medicum, Graeco Latinum. 1607, 1626, 1628, 1642, 1644, 1651, 1657, 1664, 1665, 1669, 1685; CASTELLI, P. De abusu circa dierum criticorum enumerationem. 1642; CASTELLO, P. V. Exercitationes medicinales. 1616; CASTRO, R. de. De universa mulierum medicina. 1603, 1617, 1628, 1644, 1662, 1689; CNUTIUS, J. Compendium universae medicinae juxta doctrinam Hippocrates, & Galeni. 1608, 1679; CONSTANTIN, A. Opus medicae prognoseos. 1613; CRUSIUS, D. Theatrum morborum Hermetico-Hippocraticum. 1615-16; CUSAC, L. Reflexions sur la theorie et la pratique d'Hippocrate et de Galien. 1692, 1693; DALECHAMPS, J. Chirurgie françoise. 1610; DIETERICH, J. K. Iatreum Hippocraticum. 1661; ETTMÜLLER, M. Medicina Hippocratis chymica. 1678, 1684; FOES, A. Oeconomia Hippocratis alphabeti serie distincta. 1662; FONTAINE, G. D. Gabrielis Fontani . . . De veritate Hippocraticae medicinae firmissimis rationum & experimentorum momentis stabilita, & demonstrata. 1657; GREMBS, F.O. Arbor integra et ruinosa hominis. 1657, 1671; GUILLEMEAU, C., *praeses.* Question cardinale a disputer aux escholes de medecine. 1648; HARTMANN, M., *praeses.* Magni Hippocratis Coi Aphorismi VI sectionis VI. 1670; HELLWIG, J. Ἀλφάβητον ἰατρικόν. 1631; HELWIG, C., *respondent.* Exercitationem medicam ad text. XXII. sect. II. lib. II. Epid. Hippocr. de fluore muliebri . . . publico eruditorum examini sistit . . . Christophorus Helvigius. 1666; LANCETTA, T. Raccolta medica. 1645; LANGWEDEL, B. Colloquium Romano-Hippocraticum. 1648; LIBAVIUS, A. [*d.* 1616] Appendix necessaria Syntagmatic arcanorum chymicorum. 1615; LINDEN, J. A. van der. Meletemata medicinae Hippocraticae. 1668; MANELFI, G. Prognostica in febribus in communi, et ad mentem Hippocratis. 1623, 1646; MARINELLI, G. Commentaria . . . in lib. Hippocratis. 1610, 1619, 1679; MARIOTTI, C. De universarum febrium generibus tractatus ad Hippocratis, et Galeni mentem. 1654; MARZIANI, P. Apologeticus liber. 1617 [and] Magnus Hippocrates . . . notationibus explicatus. 1626, 1652; MERCURIALE, G. Commentarii eruditissimi, in Hippocratis Coï Prognostica. 1602; MICHAULT, J. Le barbier medecin. 1672; MONIGLIA, G. A. Celer excursus in librum . . . Hippocratis de decenti ornatu. 1700; [NIGRISOLI, F. M.] *ed.* Febris china chinae expugnata. 1687, 1700; OBIZZI, I. De multiplici in medicina abusu. 1618; PEYSSONEL, J. de. De temporibus humani partus. 1665, 1666; RESTAURAND, R. Exercitatio medica de usu vini emetici in curatione febrium malignarum ad mentem Hippocratis. 1662 [and] Hippocrate de l'usage du boire a la glace. 1670, 1677 [and] Hippocrate de l'usage du china-china. 1681; [Italian tr.] 1695 [and] Hippocrates de inustionibus. 1681; RIOLAN, J. [1580–1657] Osteologia. 1614; ROLFINCK, W. Ordo et methodus cognoscendi & curandi febres generalis. 1658 [and] *praeses.* Commentarius in Hippocratis primum libri Aphorismum. 1662; ROMATET, C. Crisiologia medica. 1635; SÁNCHEZ, F. Opera medica. 1636; SAVOT, L. Nova, seu verius nova-antiqua de causis colorum sententia. 1609; SCHNEIDER, K. V. Liber de catarrhis. 1664; SCHUYL, F. Pro veteri medicina. 1670; SEBISCH, M. [1578–1674?] Dissertatio περι θειου. 1643; SEGER, G. Dissertatio anatomica de Hippocratis orthodoxia in doctrina de nutritione foetus humani in utero. 1660; SENNERT, D. De scorbuto tractatus. 1624; SINIBALDI, G. B. Hippocratis . . . antiphωνων libri quinque. 1650; SØRENSEN, P. Idea medicinae philosophicae. 1660; STEFANI, G. Hippocratis Coi theologia. 1638; TACHENIUS, O. Antiquissimae Hippocraticae medicinae clavis manuali experientia in fontibus elaborata. 1669, 1671, 1672, 1673, 1697 [and] Hippocrates chimicus. 1666, 1668, 1669, 1671, 1673 [and] Otto Tachenius his Hippocrates chymicus. 1677, 1690; TARDY, C. Hippocratica purgandi methodus. 1646; TINELLI, Z. Medicarum consultationum juxta Magni Hyppocratis doctrinam. 1605; VOIGT, J. K. I. Tractatus medicus Galeno-chymicus. 1678.

HIPPODAMUS, JOHANNES. *See* LANGE, Johann [*fl.* 1596–1604]

HIPPOLYTUS redivivus; id est, Remedium contemnendi sexum muliebrum. Autore S. I. E. D. V. M. W. A. S. [Netherlands] 1644.
 108 p. 14 cm.   **[5736]**
 "Poematia aliquot ejusdem argumenti": p. 91–108.

HIRNHAIM, HIERONYMUS, *Father* [1637–1679] De typho generis humani; sive, Scientiarum humanarum, inani ac ventoso tumore, difficultate, labilitate . . . praesumptione, incommodis, et periculis, tractatus . . . Pragae, Typis Georgii Czernoch, 1676.
 [8], 448, [6] p. 20 cm.   **[5737]**
 Imperfect: p. [3–4] following title page mutilated.

HIRSCHVOGEL, MICHAEL [*fl.* 1617] *respondent. See* SALTZMANN, J. R. [1573–1656] *praeses.* Disputatio medica de calculo renum et vesicae. 1617.

HISTOIRE des diables de Loudun. *See* [AUBIN, N.]

HISTOIRE des plantes de l'Europe, et des plus usitées qui viennent d'Asie, d'Afrique, & d'Amerique . . . Avec un abregé de leurs qualitez, & de leurs vertus specifiques. Divisées en deux tomes, & rangée suivant l'ordre du pinax de Gaspard Bauhin . . . Lyon, Jean-Bapt. De Ville, 1680.
 2 v. ([48], 866, [80] p.) illus. 17 cm. **[5738]**

 Dedication signed: Jean Baptiste De Ville.
 Attributed to Nicolas Deville. Cf. Sargent, p. 200.

—[The same.] . . . Tome premier [tome II] Lyon, Jean-Bapt. De Ville, 1689.
 [48], 866, [80] p. illus. 17 cm. **[5739]**
 Tome II has special title page (p. [443]).
 Different setting of type.

HISTOIRE des ouvrages des sçavans. *See* BASNAGE, H., *sieur de Beauval.*

HISTOIRE merveilleuse et espouventable, d'un monstre engendré dans le corps d'un homme, nommé Ferdinand de la Febue, au Marquisat de Cenete en Espagne. Imprimé premierement à Madric [sic] . . . Paris, Thibault du Val, 1622.
 12 (i.e. 14) p. 16 cm.   **[5740]**

HISTORIA flagellantium de recto et perverso flagrorum usu apud Christianos. *See* [BOILEAU, J.]

HISTORIA foetus Mussipontani extra uterum in abdomine reperti et lapidescentis cum adjectis variorum excellentissimorum virorum commentis. Francofurti, Sumptibus Joannis Petri Zubrodt, 1669.
 [1], 158 (i.e. 174), [1] p.; 70 p.; 69, [1] p.; 72 p. 21 cm.   **[5741]**
 "Antonii Deusingii . . . Consideratio physico anatomica foetus Mussipontani, extra uterum, in abdomine detenti, tandemque lapidescentis . . .": p. 11–55; "Antonii Deusingii . . . Foetus

Mussipontani, extra uterum in abdomine geniti, secundinae detectae: quibus multa naturae admiranda & abstrusa in lucem eruuntur ...": p. 81-118; "Historiae inauditae rationes et mechanica ... Honoratus Maria Lautier ..." [&] "Responsio adversus medicum Massiliensem anonimum super Muscipontano prodigo ... Honoratus Maria Lautier": p. 1-70; "Antonio Deusingii ... Vindiciae foetus extra uterum geniti. Contra tenebrionem Bernhardum a Doma ...": p. [1]-69; "Judicia varia celeberriorum virorum de foetus Mussipontani explicatione a Laurentio Straussio instituta": p. [1]-51; "Johann Christoph Eisenmengerus de foetu Mussipontano extra uterum in abdomine genito ...": p. [53]-72. Items have half titles.

HJÄRNE, URBAN [1641-1724] Een uthförlig berättelse om the nyys opfundne suurbrunnar widh Medewij uthi Östergöthland, huru the bäst skole brukas, och på hwad sätt i medlertijdh diaeten anställes; och huru man åthskillig tillfällen som brunngästerna undertijden wederfaras, kan bäst förekomma; Therjämpte några nödwändige frågor och ytterst några förledne åhrs curer opteknade ... Stockholm, Joh. Georg Eberdt, 1680.

[8], 197, [3] p. 15 cm. [**5742**]

Imperfect: title page and p. 137-138 mutilated.

HOBBES, STEPHEN [1596-1610] Margarita chyrurgica: containing a compendious practise of chyrurgerie. Selected, and translated, out of the works of the most famous physitions, and chyrurgians of this age. With a supplie of manie excellent emplasters, unguents, baulmes, waters, and wounddrinkes, used in chyrurgerie ... By S[tephen] H[obbes] student in physicke ... London, T.C. for Richard Bonian, and Henry Walley, 1610.

[8], 262 (i.e. 260), 142 p. 16 cm. [**5743**]

STC 13538.

HOBBES, THOMAS [1588-1679] Problemata de vacuo. *See* BOYLE, *Hon.* R. Tractatus. In quibus continentur, I. Suspiciones de latentibus quibusdam qualitatibus aeris. 1676, 1679.

—Vita. *In* Thomae Hobbes Angli Malmesburiensis philosophi vita. 1682.

—*tr. See* SPRAT, T., *Bp. of Rochester.* The plague of Athens. 1683.

—*See* BOYLE, *Hon.* R. New experiments and observations touching cold. 1665, 1683 [and] New experiments physico-mechanical, touching the air. 1662, 1682.

HOBBES, THOMAS [*fl.* 1678-1684?] *See* HOBBS, Thomas [*fl.* 1678-1684?]

HOBBS, STEPHEN. *See* HOBBES, Stephen [*fl.* 1596-1610]

HOBBS, THOMAS [*fl.* 1678-1684?] *See* YONGE, J. Currus triumphalis. 1679.

HOBERWESCHEL, ANDREAS [*fl.* 1609] *respondent.* Theoremata de uroscopia in genere ... Basileae, Typis Joan. Jacobi Genathii, 1609.

[20] p. 19 cm. [**5744**]

Diss. — Basel.

HOBOKEN, NICOLAAS [1632-1678?] Anatomia secundinae humanae, quindecim figuris ... illustrata ... Cum annexo s. Spicilegio epistolarum, rem potissimum generatoriam referentium. Trajecti ad Rhenum, Apud Johannem Ribbium, 1669.

221 (i.e. 219), [11] p. front. (port.), plates. 16 cm. [**5745**]

Added engraved title page.

—Anatomia secundinae humanae repetita ... et quadraginta quatuor figuris ... illustrata ... Praemittuntur literae ... Henr. Eyssonii ... cum autoris responsionibus ... Ultrajecti, Apud Johannem Ribbium, 1675.

[32], 548, [12] p. plates. 16 cm. [**5746**]

Added engraved title page.

—Anatomia secundinae vitulinae, triginta octo figuris ... illustrata ... Praemittuntur literae ... Thom. Bartholini, cum autoris ad eundem responsionibus ... Ultrajecti, Apud Johannem Ribbium, 1675.

[22], 288, [12] p. plates. 17 cm. [**5747**]

Added engraved title page: Secundiae vitulinae anatomia ... 1672.

—Cognito physiologica medica, accuratissima ... methodo tradita. Qua humani corporis sanitas, & quae eam significant imprimis, ac probant, hominis actiones, omni numero absolutae ... explicantur. Praeter praefixam autoris Orationem, de medicorum nobilitate, Steinfurti habitam ... Ultrajecti, Ex officina Henrici Versteegh, 1670.

[32], 352 p. 21 cm. [**5748**]

HOBS, THOMAS. *See* HOBBS, Thomas [*fl.* 1678-1684?]

Der HOCH- und löblichen Herren Fürsten . . . neue Infections-Ordnung. See Silesia. Laws, statutes, etc. Der hoch- und löblichen Herren Fürsten und Stände im Hertzogthum Ober- und Nieder Schlesien neue Infections-Ordnung. 1680, 1681.

HOCHREUTINER, JACOB [*fl.* 1682–1728] *respondent.* Dissertatio inauguralis medica exhibens generalem scirrhi descriptionem . . . Basileae, Typis Jacobi Bertschii [1682]

[26] p.	21 cm.	**[5749]**

Diss. — Basel.

HOCHSTATT, JOHANN WILHELM [*fl.* 1637–1638] *respondent.* See SALTZMANN, J. R. [1573–1656] *praeses.* Disputatio medica de urinarum causis in genere. 1638; SEBISCH, M. [1578–1674?] *praeses.* Examinis vulnerum partium dissimilarium pars I[–IV. & ultima] 1636 [i.e. 1637]

HOCHSTETTER, JOHANN PHILIPP. *See* HOECHSTETTER, Johann Philipp [*fl.* 1668–1674]

HOCHSTETTER, PHILIPP. *See* HOECHSTETTER, Philipp [*ca.* 1579–1635]

HODENCQ, MICHAEL DE [*fl.* 1681–1695] *praeses.* Quaestio medica . . . An cujuslibet causa morbi una e sex rebus non naturalibus? [Parisiis, Apud Franciscum Muguet, 1690]

4 p.	26 cm.	**[5750]**

Caption title.

Diss. — Paris (P. Caron, *respondent*)

HODGES, NATHANIEL [1629–1688] Λοιμολογία; sive, Pestis nuperae apud populum Londinensem grassantis narratio historica . . . Londini, Typis Gul. Godbid, sumptibus Josephi Nevill, 1672.

[14], 246, [6] p.	table.	17 cm.	**[5751]**

Imperfect: first preliminary leaf (blank?) wanting.

Table inserted before p. 1 has title: Parochiarum in . . . civitate Londinensi synopsis, funerum anno Dom. 1665. exhibens rationem.

Carem elegiacum ([6] p. at end) written by Adam Littleton.

—Vindiciae medicinae & medicorum; or, An apology for the profession and professors of physick. In answer to the several pleas of illegal practitioners . . . As also an account of the present pest . . . London, Printed by J. F. for Henry Broom, 1666.

[15], 225 p.	18 cm.	**[5752]**

—*See* THOMSON, G. Λοιμοτομια; or, The pest anatomized. 1666.

HÖCHER, JOHANN ADAM [*fl.* 1698] *respondent. See* MÖLLER, G. C., *praeses.* Disputatio physico-medica de saccharo. 1698.

HOECHSTETTER, JOHANN PHILIPP [*fl.* 1668–1674] *respondent. See* HILBRAND, J. P., *praeses.* Dissertatio medica de καφαλαλγια. 1668; SCHENCK, J. T., *praeses.* Dissertatio medica de cinnamomo. 1670.

—, *ed. See* HOECHSTETTER, P. Observationum medicinalium decades sex. 1674.

HOECHSTETTER, PHILIPP [*ca.* 1579–1635] Observationum medicinalium decades sex antehac editae; quibus nunc accessere quatuor decades aliae, nunquam hactenus visae: continentes historias, quaesita, observata, variaque monita medica . . . Francofurti & Lipsiae, Impensis Laurentii Sigism. Cörneri, 1674.

[92], 754, [16] p.; 456, [8] p.	16 cm.	**[5753]**

Part [2] has special title page: Rararum observationum medicinalium pars posthuma.

Dedicatio by Johann Philipp Hoechstetter, the editor.

The first 3 decades were published in 1624 under title: Rararum observationum medicinalium decades tres.

—Rararum observationum medicinalium decades tres. Continentes, historias medicas, theorica & practica varia [Pars secunda, continens decades tres sequentes, nimirum, quartam, quintam & sextam . . .] Augustae Vindelicorum, Typis Andreae Apergeri [Joannis Praetorii] sumptibus Sebastiani Mylii, 1624–1627.

2 v.	plate.	16 cm.	**[5754]**

—*respondent. See* BAUHIN, K., *praeses.* Praeludia anatomica. 1601.

HÖCHSTFÜRTREFLICHTES chiromantisch- und physiognomisches Klee-Blat, bestehend aus drey . . . Tractaten . . . erstlich des . . . Ronphyle Hand-Wahrsagung; zum Andern; Niclas Spadons Schauplatz der Curiositäten . . . drittens D. D. Johann Sigmund Eltzholtzens Anthropometrie oder Mess-Kunst des menschlichen Cörpers, welchen wegen Gleichheit der Materie Dominici de Rubeis Physiognomische Tafeln, Cardani Metoposcopie und Melampus von den Mählern des menschlichen Cörpers miteingeruckt etc. Alles aus dem Frantzösischen, Italiänischen, Lateinischen und Griechischen . . .

übersetzt ... durch I. G. D. T. Nürnberg, In Verlegung Johann Ziegers, 1695.

[30], 112 p.; 208 p.; 550 p. front., illus., plates. 17 cm. [**5755**]

General title page.
Each part has special title page. Part [1] originally translated by Rampalle. Part [3] translated by S. T. D. N.
With this are bound: Ingeber, Johann. Chiromantia. Franckfurt am Mayn, 1692; - Speculum astrologicum. 1693.

HÖFER, WOLFGANG [1614–1661] Hercules medicus; sive, Locorum communium medicorum tomus primus in quo plerorumque humani corporis affectuum curationes attinguntur, & quidquid in iisdem vel theorico vel practico consideratione praecipua dignum est, compendiose & utiliter pertractatur, cum subjectis, ubi quadrant, Aphorismis Hippocratis ... Viennae Austriae, Apud Joannem Jacobum Kürner, 1657.

[24], 383, [15] p. illus. 20 cm. [**5756**]

Added engraved title page.
Imperfect: wormholes on p. 331–346.
No additional volume appears to have been published.

—[The same.] Hercules medicus; sive, Locorum communium medicorum tomus unicus. In quo plerorumque humani corporis affectuum curationes compendiose pertractantur, cum subjectis, ubi quadrant, Hippocr. aphorismis, nec non Helmontianis de causis morborum, opinionibus ... [Noribergae] Impensis Mich. & Joh. Frider. Endterorum, 1665.

[1], 432, [22] p. illus. 14 cm. [**5757**]

[The same.] Hercules medicus; sive, Locorum communium liber ... ex probatissimis autoribus laborioso studio collectus, propriisque observationibus & experientia confirmatus & illustratus ... Nunc denuo ex autoris autographo recognitus, locisque innumeris auctus, nec non consiliis aliquot, ac sub finem annexa etiam ipsi olim Medicationum familiarium farragine locupletatus ... Noribergae, Sumtibus Michaël & Johan. Friderici Endterorum, 1675.

2 v. in 1. illus. 21 cm. [**5758**]

Added engraved title page.

—Another issue.
2 v. Title page reset. [**5759**]

HÖFFER, HENRIK ADOLF [*fl.* 1652] *respondent. See* SEBISCH, M. [1578–1674?] *praeses.* Disputatio de dolore. 1652.

HÖGER, CONRAD [1660–1738] *respondent. See* STURM, J. C., *praeses.* Dissertationem inauguralem de ignibus tantum-lucentibus ... sistet C. H. 1698.

HOEGGER, JACOB [*fl.* 1673] *respondent. See* GLASER, J. H., *praeses.* Disputatio chirurgico-medica de herniis in genere. 1673.

HOEGGER, SEBASTIAN [1660–1731] *respondent.* Dissertationem inauguralem de salivae statu morboso ... defendet Sebastianus Hoeggerus ... Basileae, Typis Jacobi Bertschii [1696]

[54] p. 19 cm. [**5760**]

Diss. — Basel.

—*See* EGLINGER, N., *praeses.* Disputatio physiologico-medica de saliva. 1695.

HÖHL, PAUL [*fl.* 1608] *respondent.* Διάσκεψις περὶ τῆς γαγγραίνας καὶ τοῦ σφακέλου ... [De gangraena et sphacelo]. [Basileae] Typis Johannis Schroeteri, 1608.

[16] p. 20 cm. [**5761**]

Diss. — Basel.

HÖLDERLIN, WILHELM FRIEDRICH [*fl.* 1690–1691] *respondent. See* CAMERARIUS, E. R., *praeses.* Dissertatio medica posterior, de cichorio. 1691.

HOELTERHOFF, ENGELBERTUS. *See* HOLTERHOFF, Engelbert [*fl.* 1665–1676]

HOELTICH, FRANZ HEINRICH [*d.* 1697] Quaest. foemina non est homo, videbunt publice Franciscus Henricus Hoeltich ... & Johannes Casparus Waltz ... a d. XIV. Decembris, anno 1672. Wittebergae, Typis Christiani Schrödteri [1672?]

[24] p. 19 cm. [**5762**]

Christian Schrödter printed in Wittenberg from 1674 till 1723. Cf. Benzing (A), p. 475.

—[The same.] Qu. foemina non est homo, vulgo ob die Weiber Menschen seyn oder nicht? Videbunt publice Francisc. Henr. Hoeltich... & Johannes Casparus Waltz ... a d. XIV. Decembris, anno 1688. Wittebergae, Typis Christiani Schrödteri [1688?]

[24] p. 19 cm. [**5763**]

Different setting of type.

HÖNIG, JOHANN HEINRICH [*fl.* 1654–1658] *See* SALTZMANN, J. R. [1573–1656] Dissertatio de mixtione. 1654.

HÖNN, JOHANN CORNELIUS [1656–1684] *respondent.* Disputationem inauguralem de trepanatione ... publice ... submittit Johannes Cornelius Hönn ... Altdorfii, Literis Henrici Meyeri [1678]

  19 p. 20 cm.   **[5764]**

 Diss. — Altdorf.

HÖPING, JOHANN ABRAHAM JAKOB [*fl.* 1673] Institutiones chiromanticae; oder, Kurtze Unterweisung, wie man aus denen Linien, Bergen, und Nägeln derer Hände, und denn aus der Proportion des Gesichts ... auch das Jahr ... in welchen einem was Glück-oder Unglückliches bevorstehet, muthmasslich judiciren kan. Sampt einer gantz neuen ... Harmoniâ, oder Ubereinstimmung aller Linien ... mit Fleiss verfertiget ... Zum dritten Mahl jetzt gedruckt, und ... vermehret ... Jena, In Verlegung Matthaei Birckners, Gedruckt bey Samuel Krebsens seel, nachgel. Wittwen, 1681.

  2 v. in 1. illus. 17 cm.   **[5765]**

 Vol. [2] has title: Chiromantia harmonica; das ist, Ubereinstimmung der Chiromantiae oder Linien in denen Händen ...
 Bound with Elsholtz, J. S. Anthropometria. 1663.

HÖRNICAEUS, LUDOVICUS. *See* HÖRNIGK, Ludwig von [1600–1667]

HOERNICK, MATTHAEUS. *See* HÖRNYK, Matthias [*fl.* 1614]

HÖRNIGK, LUDWIG VON [1600–1667] Gründliche Antwort auff die Frag: ob die Composition und Praeparation der Artzneyen den Materialisten und Trochisten zu gestatten sey? ... [n. p.] 1645.

  27 p. 20 cm.   **[5766]**

—Langen-Schwalbacher Saurbrunnen und Bäder, sampt deren Eygenschafft und rechtem Gebrauch, jetzo zum andern Mahl aussfürlich für alle und jede in 100 Fragen beschrieben und vermehrt ... Franckfurt am Mayn, Bey Anthoni Hummen, 1640.

  [16], 260, [26] p. 18 cm. **[5767]**

 Added engraved title page.

—Medicaster apella; oder, Juden Artzt. Strassburg, Gedruckt und verlegt durch Mary von der Heiden, 1631.

  [16], 383, [23] p. 17 cm. **[5768]**

 Engraved title page.

—Nützliche und curiöse Fragen die Apothecker und Materialisten betreffend, samt dero gründlichen und richtigen Beantwortung ... Franckfurt am Mayn, Zu finden in Henning Grossens Buchhandlung, 1697.

  52 p. 22 cm.   **[5769]**

—Politia medica; oder, Beschreibung dessen was die Medici ... Apothecker, Materialisten, Wundtärzt, Barbierer ... Patienten oder Krancke selbst zu thun, und was, auch wie sie in Obacht zu nehmen ... Franckfurt am Mayn, Bey Clemens Schleichen, und Mitverwandten, 1638.

  [8], 222 (i.e. 202), [13] p. 20 cm. **[5770]**

 Errata pasted on blank p. [13]

—*respondent. See* HORST, G. [1578–1636] Ἐξετάσεων παθολογικῶν. 1629 [and] Prognosis febrium. 1622.

HÖRNYK, MATTHIAS [*fl.* 1614] De acidularum, quae ad Egram sunt, viribus ... epistola ad Jessenium. Pragae, Typis Pauli Sessii [1615?]

  [8] p. 19 cm.   **[5771]**

 With this is bound Heinsius, N. [1620–1681] Elegia ad fontem medicatum Driburgicum. [n. p., n. d.]

HÖRSCHER, FERDINANDUS [*fl.* 1623–1624] *respondent. See* SEBISCH, M. [1578–1674?] *praeses.* Exercitationes medicae. 1639.

HOESCHEL, DAVID [1556–1617] *See* VALERIANO BOLZANI, G. P. Hieroglyphica. 1631. 1678.

HOEST, DANIEL DE [*fl.* 1670] *respondent.* Disputatio medica inauguralis de vomitu ... Lugduni Batavorum, Apud viduam & haeredes Joannis Elsevirii, 1670.

  [16] p. 23 cm.   **[5772]**

 Diss. — Leyden.

HOEST, NICOLAAS DE [*fl.* 1689] *respondent.* Disputatio medica inauguralis de sputo sanguinis ... Lugduni Batavorum, Apud Abrahamum Elzevier, 1689.

  [36] p. 18 cm.   **[5773]**

 Diss. — Leyden.

HÖVELL, GEORG [*fl.* 1639] *respondent. See* MASIUS, J., *praeses.* Decas positionum exhibens fabricam & usum oculi humani quam ... examini subjiciunt. 1639.

HOEVEN, CONRAD VAN [*fl.* 1659–1663] *respondent.* Disputatio medica inauguralis de pleuritide . . . Ultrajecti, Ex officina Meinardi à Dreunen, 1663.
[24] p.   19 cm.   [5774]
Diss. — Utrecht.

HOEVER, WOLFGANG [*fl.* 1599–1638]

Dissertations — Ingolstadt

—*praeses.* Disputatio medica de angina . . . Ingolstadii, Typis Gregorii Haenlini [1638]
[4], 8, [2] p.   19 cm.   [5775]
M. R. Schmuz, *respondent.*

—Disputatio medica de apoplexia . . . Ingolstadii, Gregorii Haenlini typis edita [1637]
[2], 16, [2] p.   19 cm.   [5776]
A. Heigl, *respondent.*

—Disputatio medica de arthritide . . . Ingolstadii, Typis Wilhelmi Ederi [1638]
[4], 7, [1] p.   19 cm.   [5777]
M. Gottschich, *respondent.*

—Disputatio medica de corporis humani singularumque partium doloribus . . . Ingolstadii, Gregori Haenlini typis edita [1628]
[4], 26, [2] p.   19 cm.   [5778]
L. Hebich, *respondent.*

—Methodus praecavendae curandaeque pestis . . . Ingolstadii, Typis Gregorii Haenlini, 1626.
[4], 21, [2] p.   19 cm.   [5779]
A. Episcopus, *respondent.*

HOFER, JOHANN [1669–1752] *respondent.* Disputatio medica inauguralis de hydrope uteri . . . Basileae, Typis Jacobi Bertschii [1689]
[16] p.   20 cm.   [5780]
Diss. — Basel.

—*See* HARDER, J. J., *praeses.* Dissertatio medica de νοσταλγία oder Heimwehe. 1688.

—*as subject. See* HARDER, J. J. Alexander Pfisterus. 1689.

HOFFKUNTZ, CHRISTIAN [1651–1711] *praeses.* Disputationem anthropologicam de unione et communione mentis et corporis humani . . . Christianus Hoffkuntz . . . & . . . Johann-Christian Feuereisen

. . . subjiciunt . . . Lipsiae, Typis viduae Johannis Wittigau [1675]
[36] p.   20 cm.   [5781]
Diss. — Leipzig (J. C. Feuereisen, *respondent*)

HOFFMAN, JOHANN [*fl.* 1627] Sehlen Artzney wider die Sucht der Pestilentz und alle ihre Zufälle auss der Apotecken des H. Geistes von den kräfftigsten Würtzeln Kreutern und Blumen dess Paradeises göttliches Wortes zusammen gezogen und in Reÿmen verfasset . . . [Augspurg, Gedruckt bey Johann Ulrich Schonigk, 1627]
[24], 352, [7] p.   13 cm.   [5782]
Engraved title page.

HOFFMANN, ABRAHAM [*fl.* 1696–1698] *respondent. See* ORTLOB, J. F., *praeses.* Scrutinium recidivarum. 1696; RIVINUS, A. Q., *praeses.* Dissertationem medicam inauguralem de cholera . . . exponet. 1698.

HOFFMANN, ANDREAS [*fl.* 1693] *respondent. See* KELLER, J. C., *praeses.* Dissertationem physicam de visu . . . submittet . . . A. H. 1693.

HOFFMANN, CHRISTIAN [*fl.* 1668–1671] Problema physicum an ex homine & bruto generari possit homo? . . . [Jenae] Typis Joh. Jacobi Bauhoferi [1671]
[40] p.   20 cm.   [5783]
Diss. pro loco — Jena (J. Melchin, *respondent*)

HOFFMANN, CHRISTOPH MORITZ [*fl.* 1690] *respondent.* De enteroscheocele, sive hernia intestino-scrotali, dissertationem inauguralem . . . publico submittit . . . Christoph. Mauricius Hoffmann . . . [Altdorffii] Typis Henrici Meyeri [1690]
28 p.   20 cm.   [5784]
Diss. — Altdorf.

HOFFMANN, FRIEDRICH [1626–1675] Appendix de modo insultum apoplecticum curandi lethifero . . . Lipsiae, Sumptibus Christiani Kirchneri, literis Christiani Michaelis, 1668.
[14] p.   19 cm.   [5785]
Bound with *his* Opus de methodo medendi. 1668.

—Cardianastrophe admiranda; seu, Cordis inversio . . . observata a collegio medico civitatis Hallensis in anatomia cadaveris sexus foeminei . . . Lipsiae, Impensis Christiani Kirchneri, typis Johannis Erici Hahnii, 1671.
[18], 28, [8] p.   plates.   20 cm.   [5786]

—Clavis pharmaceutica Schröderiana; seu, Animadversiones cum annotationibus in Pharmacopoeiam Schröderianam Baconianis, Cartesianis, & Helmontianis principiis illustratae & Dn. D. Johannis Michaelis ... & aliorum celeberrimorum medicorum arcanis concinnatae ... cum Thesauro pharmaceutico quorundam medicorum nostri seculi. Halae Saxonum, Sumptibus Christophori Mylii, 1675.

[50],706, [34] p.; [7], 117, [11] p.   front. (port.), plate.   21 cm.   [**5787**]

Part [2] has special title page.
Imperfect: lower part of title page, including imprint, trimmed.

—[The same.] ... Ed. 2. multis in locis correctior, nec non ex manuscripto B. auctoris necessariis additionibus auctior ... Halae Saxonum, Apud viduam et haeredes Mylianos, 1681.

[46], 706, [36] p.; [7], 117, [11] p.   front. (port.), plate.   21 cm.   [**5788**]

Different setting of type.

—Opus de methodo medendi, juxta seriem Wallaeianam, annexis fundamentis astrologicis, ex veterum ac recentiorum scriptis concinnatum, dogmaticis, Paracelsicis, Helmontianis, Harveianis principiis & propriis observationibus illustratum ... cum praefatione ... D. Johannis Michaelis. Lipsiae, Impensis Christiani Kirchneri, literis Christiani Michaelis, 1668.

[28], 448 p.   19 cm.   [**5789**]

Imperfect? Index wanting? Cf. BNC.
Includes considerable portions of J. B. van Helmont's works.
With this is bound *his* Appendix de modo insultum apoplecticum curandi lethifero. 1668.

—*praeses.* Morbum convulsivum a viso spectro ... publicae disquisitioni exponit Johann George Glytz ... Jenae, Typis Nisianis [1682]

24 p.   19 cm.   [**5790**]

Diss. — Jena (J. G. Glytz, *respondent*)

—*respondent. See* POMARIUS, S., *praeses.* De modo visionis disputatio quarta. 1650; ROLFINCK, W., *praeses.* Disputatio medica inauguralis de dysenteria. 1651.

—*See* SCHRÖDER, J. Pharmacopoea Schrödero-Hoffmanniana illustrata et aucta. 1687 [and] Trefflich-versehene medicin-chymische Apotheke. 1685 [and] Vollständige und nutzreiche Apotheke. 1693 [and] SCHULTZ, G. Scrutinium cinnabarinum. 1679?

HOFFMANN, FRIEDRICH [1660-1742] De affectu cataleptico rarissimo dissertatio epistolaris ad ... Georgium Wolffgangum Wedelium ... Francofurti ad Moenum, Ex Officina Grossiana, 1692.

32 p.   19 cm.   [**5791**]

—De studiis per regulas diaeteticas facilitandis, et prolonganda litteratorum vita ... dissertatio ... Halae Magdeburgicae, Apud Joh. Gothofredum Renger, 1697.

70 p.   17 cm.   [**5792**]

—Demonstrationes physicae curiosae, experimentis et observationibus mechanicis ac chymicis illustratae. Halae Magdëburgicae, Apud Christoph. Andream Zeitlerum, 1700.

56 p.   21 cm.   [**5793**]

—Exercitatio acroamatica de acidi et viscidi pro stabiliendis omnium morborum causis, & alcali fluidi, pro iisdem debellandis, insufficientia ... Francofurti ad Moenum, Sumptibus Christiani Genschii, 1689.

[8], 72 p.   17 cm.   [**5794**]

—Exercitatio medico-chymica de cinnabari antimonii ejusque eximiis viribus, usuque in morbis secretiori, quo ipso via ex illa veram panaceam conficiendi aperitur. Adjecta sunt experimenta ac ratiocinia varia curiosa. Lugduni Batavorum, Apud Petrum vander Aa, 1685.

157, [7] p.   15 cm.   [**5795**]

Added engraved title page.

—[The same.] ... Ed. 2. Francofurti ad Moenum, Sumptibus Christiani Genschii, 1689.

106, [2] p.   18 cm.   [**5796**]

—Fundamenta medicinae ex principiis naturae mechanicis in usum philiatrorum succincte proposita ... Halae Magdeburgicae, Impens. Simon Johan. Hübneri, literis viduae Salfeldianae, 1695.

[16], 238 p.   16 cm.   [**5797**]

Programs — Halle

—Propemticon inaugurale, de animae ac corporis commercio. Halae, Magdeburgicae, Typis Christoph. Andr. Zeitleri [1695]

8 p.   20 cm.   [**5798**]

—Another printing: Halae, Typis Christoph. Salfeld [1695]

8 p.   19 cm.   [**5799**]

—Another printing, without imprint.
[26]-44 (i.e. 33) p. 18 cm. **[5800]**
With vita of J. K. Hofsteter.

—Propemticon inaugurale de chinae chinae modo operandi, usu et abusu. Halae, Viduae literis Salfeldianae [1694]
[8] p. 19 cm. **[5801]**
With vita of J. B. Schondorff.

—Propempticon inaugurale de febrium novahypothesi. Halae, Literis Salfeldii [1694]
[8] p. 20 cm. **[5802]**
With vita of C. W. Sattler.

—Propempticon inaugurale de mechanica febrium doctrina Hippocratica ... [Halae, 1696]
[8] p. 20 cm. **[5803]**
With vita of S. Alischer.

—Propemticon inaugurale de medicamentorum prudenti applicatione. Halae, Typis Christoph. Andr. Zeitleri [1694]
[8] p. 19 cm. **[5804]**
With vita of J. C. Klimm.

—Another printing, with imprint: Halae, Literis Salfeldianis [1694]

[5805]

—Propemticon inaugurale, de modo veterum balsamandi corpora. Halae Magdeburgicae, Literis Christiani Henckelii [1695]
[8] p. 19 cm. **[5806]**
With vita of J. F. Du Fay.

—Propempticon inaugurale de pane grossiori Westphalorum, vulgo Bonpournickel. [Halae Magdeb., 1695]
[12] p. 19 cm. **[5807]**
With vita of I. Huszti.

—Propemticon inaugurale, de vapore carbonum fossilium innoxio. Halae Magdeburgicae, Typis Christiani Henckelii [1695]
[8] p. 20 cm. **[5808]**
With vita of H. J. Siemens.

Dissertation — Jena

—*praeses.* De cinnabari antimonii exercitatio medico-chymica ... Jenae, Literis Krebsianis [1681]
51, [1] p. 21 cm. **[5809]**
J. G. Grüling, *respondent.*

Dissertations — Halle

—*praeses.* Analysin chymico-medicam reguli antimonii medicinalis ... publicae disquisitioni exponet ... Joannes Samuel Carl ... Halae Magdeburgicae, Praelo excudebat Chr. Henckelius, 1698.
[1], 38 p. 20 cm. **[5810]**
J. S. Carl, *respondent.*

—Disputatio inauguralis medica de amputatione membrorum sphacelatorum, eorumque secura medela ... Halae. Magdeb., Literis Christiani Henckelii [1696]
[40] p. 20 cm. **[5811]**
Includes Hoffmann's Epistola gratulatoria to Barnstorff (p. [33-40])
E. Barnstorff, *respondent.*

—Disputatio inauguralis medica de apepsia ... Halae, Magdeb., Aere Henckeliano [1696]
[20] p. 20 cm. **[5812]**
J. G. Schultz, *respondent.*

—Disputatio inauguralis medica de chinae chinae modo operandi, usu et abusu ... Halae, Literis viduae Salfeldinae [1694]
[20] p. 20 cm. **[5813]**
J. B. Schondorff, *respondent.*

—Disputatio inauguralis medica, de saliva et ejus morbis ... Halae Magdeburgicae Typis Christoph. Salfeld. [1694]
32 p. 19 cm. **[5814]**
J. G. Hoyer, *respondent.*

—Disputatio inauguralis medica, de terebinthina ... Halae Magdeburgicae, Typis Christiani Henckelii [1699]
[1], 22 p. 20 cm. **[5815]**
J. Wilhelmi, *respondent.*

—Disputatio inauguralis medica sistens febris quartanae tutam ac felicem curationem ... Halae Magdeb., Aere Henckeliano [1696]
[20] p. 20 cm. **[5816]**
S. Alischer, *respondent.*

—Disputatio inauguralis medica sistens malignitatis naturam et originem in morbis acutis ... Halae Magdeburgicae, Literis Christiani Henckelii [1695]
[40] p. 20 cm. **[5817]**
J. F. Du Fay, *respondent.*

—Disputatio inauguralis medica sistens novam febrium intermittentium hypothesin, ex ipsis principiis mechanicis deductam ... Halae, Literis Salfeldii [1694]

20 p. 20 cm.					[5818]

C. W. Sattler, *respondent.*

—Disputatio inauguralis medico-chymica de nitro, ejus natura et usu in medicina ... Halae, Literis Salfeldii [1694]

[20] p. 20 cm.					[5819]

C. G. Schmalkalden, *respondent.*

—Another printing, with imprint: Halae, Chrstoph [sic] Andreae Zeitler [1694]

[5820]

Page [2] is blank.

—Disputatio medica inauguralis de inedia magnorum morborum remedio ... Halae Magdeb., Literis Chr. Henckelii [1698]

[1], 22 p. 20 cm.				[5821]

H. Henrici, *respondent.*

—Disputatio medica inauguralis de medicamentis specificis, eorumque agendi modo ... [Halae] Typis Christoph. Andr. Zeitleri [1694]

24 p. 20 cm.					[5822]

J. C. Klimm, *respondent.*

—Disputatio medica inauguralis, de salubritate fluxus haemorrhoidalis ... Halae Magdeb., Literis Christiani Henckelii [1697]

[2], 24, [2] p. 19 cm.				[5823]

G. A. Agricola, *respondent.*

—Disputatio solennis medica de hydrope pericardii rarissimo ... [Halae Magdeburgicae] Typis Christoph. Andreae Zeitleri [1697]

32 p. plate. 20 cm.				[5824]

J. H. Graetz, *respondent.*

—Disputatio solennis medica, de somnabulatione ... Halae, Typis Christophori Salfeldii [1695]

[32] p. 19 cm.					[5825]

J. K. Hofsteter, *respondent.*

"Friderici Hoffmanni ... decani, propemticon inaugurale, de animae ac corporis commercio ...": p. [25–32], an invitation to the dissertation of J. K. Hofsteter, has half title.

—Another printing, with imprint: Halae Magdeburgicae, Typis Christoph Andr. Zeitleri [1695]

24 p. 20 cm.					[5826]

—Disputatio solennis medico-practica tradens historiam variolarum epidemice Halae grassantium ... Halae Magdeburgicae, Literis Chr. Henckelii [1699]

40 p. 20 cm.					[5827]

J. H. Hagen, *respondent.*

—Another issue. Page 2 is blank.

[5828]

—Dissertatio inauguralis chirurgico-medica de membris fractis ... Halae Magdeb., Literis Chr. Henckelii [1700]

43, [1] p. 19 cm.				[5829]

G. F. Otto, *respondent.*

—Dissertatio inauguralis chymico-medica de mirabili sulphuris antimoniati fixati efficacia in medicina ... [Halae] Typis Christoph. Andreae Zeitleri [1699]

23, [1] p. 19 cm.				[5830]

J. Schockwitz, *respondent.*

—Dissertatio inauguralis medica de anthelminthicis ... Hallae, Typis Christoph. Andreae Zeitleri [1698]

27 p. 19 cm.					[5831]

G. Sikardus, *respondent.*

—Dissertatio inauguralis medica, de genuino et simplicissimo doloris podagrici remedio ... Halae Magdeb., Literis Christiani Henckelii [1697]

[1], 30 p. 22 cm.				[5832]

I. Király, *respondent.*

—Dissertatio inauguralis medica de mechanica operandi ratione medicamentorum sic dictorum alterantium ... Halae, Typis Christoph. Andreae Zeitleri [1698]

24 p. 18 cm.					[5833]

G. W. Müller, *respondent.*

—Dissertatio inauguralis medica de opiatorum nova eaque mechanica operandi ratione ... Halae Magdeb., Literis Chr. Henckelii [1700]

24 p. 19 cm.					[5834]

J. Descazals, *respondent.*

—Dissertatio inauguralis medica de purgantibus specificis ... Halae, Typis Christophori Andreae Zeitleri [1696]

20 p. 20 cm.					[5835]

A. O. Gölicke, *respondent.*

—Dissertatio inauguralis medica de remediorum evacuantium mechanica operandi ratione . . . Halae, Typis Christoph. Andreae Zeitleri [1698]

24 p. 19 cm. [5836]

M. Segnitz, *respondent.*

—Dissertatio inauguralis medico-chirurgica, de fistularum nova, tuta ac compendiosa sanatione . . . Halae Magdeburgicae, Literis Christiani Henckelii [1697]

[40] p. 20 cm. [5837]

J. N. Röper, *respondent.*

—Dissertatio inauguralis medico-practica de diarrhoea in febribus malignis, aliisque acutis morbis salutari . . . [Halae] Typis Christoph. Andreae Zeitleri [1700]

32 p. 19 cm. [5838]

W. F. Hienlin, *respondent.*

—Dissertatio inauguralis medico-practica, de pleuritide et peripneumonia, qua diversae de his autorum sententiae expenduntur . . . Halae Magdeb., Literis Chr. Henckelii [1699]

[24] p. 19 cm. [5839]

J. C. Pezold, *respondent.*

—Dissertatio inauguralis medico-practica de podagra retrocedente in corpus . . . Halae Magdeburg., Typis Johannis Jacobi Krebsii [1700]

20 p. 18 cm. [5840]

J. V. Vogel, *respondent.*

—Dissertatio inauguralis physico-medica de natura morborum medicatrice mechanica . . . Halae Magdeburgicae, Typis Christiani Henckelii [1699]

[40] p. 18 cm. [5841]

S. Cellarius, *respondent.*

—Dissertatio inauguralis physico-medica de potentia ventorum in corpus humanum, ubi simul agitur de ascensu & descensu argenti vivi in barometro . . . [Halae] Typis Christoph. Andreae Zeitleri [1700]

32 p. 20 cm. [5842]

C. Ockel, *respondent.*

—Dissertatio inauguralis sistens fermentorum morbificorum ejectionem e medicina . . . [Halae] Typis Christoph. Andreae Zeitleri [1697]

29, [3] p. 21 cm. [5843]

F. W. Gerhardi, *respondent.*

—Dissertatio medica de imaginatione, morborum causa . . . Halae, Literis Salfeldianis [1694]

[4], 28 p. 20 cm. [5844]

J. N. Röper, *respondent.*

—Dissertatio medica de necessaria salivae inspectione ad conservandam et restaurandam sanitatem . . . Halae, Typis Christoph. Andreae Zeitleri [1698]

28 (i.e. 20) p. 19 cm. [5845]

J. J. Baier, *respondent.*

—Dissertatio medica de pulverum sternutatoriorum vero usu et abusu . . . Halae Magdeburgicae, Typis Chr. Henckelii [1700]

32 p. 20 cm. [5846]

F. Camel, *respondent.*

—Dissertatio medica inauguralis, exhibens salis volatilis genesin, usum, & abusum in medicina . . . Halae Magdeb., Typis Christoph. Salfeldii [1696]

[28] p. 20 cm. [5847]

G. E. Berner, *respondent.*

—Dissertatio medicina inauguralis, de praecipuo studiosorum morbo, ejusque genuiuis [sic] causis . . . Halae, Typis Christoph. Andreae Zeitler [1699]

27, [1] p. 20 cm. [5848]

A. Hesse, *respondent.*

—Dissertatio medico-chirurgica inauguralis, de ἰσχαίμος; seu, Sanguinem sistentibus . . . Halae Magdeb., Literis Chr. Henckelii [1698]

[32] p. 19 cm. [5849]

G. Hoffmann, *respondent.*

—Dissertatio medico-chirurgica inauguralis, de synovia, ejusque origine . . . Halae Magdeb., Literis Chr. Henckelii [1697]

[32] p. 20 cm. [5850]

S. Hiller, *respondent.*

—Dissertatio medico-practica inauguralis sistens historiam febris malignae epidemicae petechizantis hactenus Halae grassantis . . . [Halae] Typis Christoph. Andreae Zeitleri [1699]

30 p. 20 cm. [5851]

P. Sanfftleben, *respondent.*

—Dissertatio physico-chymica experimentalis de generatione salium . . . Halae Magdeburgicae, Litteris Salfeldii [1693]

[32] p. 20 cm. [5852]

J. H. Greulinck, *respondent.*

—Dissertatio physico-medica de causis caloris naturalis et praeternaturalis in corpore nostro . . . [Halae] Typis Christoph. Andreae Zeitleri [1699]

26, [2] p.   20 cm.   [5853]

W. F. Hienline, *respondent.*

—Dissertatio solennis de prudenti medicamentorum applicatione in tempore . . . [Halae] Typis Christophori Salfeldii [1695]

[24] p.   20 cm.   [5854]

Imperfect: lower margin of title page trimmed affecting imprint.
I. Huszti, *respondent.*

—Dissertatio solennis medica de haemorrhagiarum genuina origine atque curatione ex principiis mechanicis . . . Halae Magdeb., Literis Chr. Henckelii [1697]

[32] p.   20 cm.   [5855]

J. D. Doläus, *respondent.*

—Dissertatione physico-medica inaugurali affectus hereditarios, illorumque originem . . . eruditorum placidae disquisitioni proponet Antonius Philippus Bornemann . . . Halae Magdeburgicae, Typis Christiani Henckelii [1699]

32, [2] p.   19 cm.   [5856]

Imperfect: lower margin of title page trimmed.
A. P. Bornemann, *respondent.*

—Exercitatio physico-medica, de infusi veronicae efficacia praeferenda herbae thee . . . Halae Magdeburgicae, Typis Christoph. Andreae Zeitleri [1694]

24 p.   20 cm.   [5857]

C. W. Sattler, *respondent.*

—Exercitatio physico-medica de mentis morbis, ex morbosa sanguinis circulatione ortis . . . Halae Magdeburgicae, Literis Chr. Henckelii [1700]

[4], 34, [2] p.   20 cm.   [5858]

J. J. Stange, *respondent.*

—Philosophiae experimentalis axiomaticae dissertatio prima de corporibus, illorumque principiis et affectionibus . . . Hallae Magdeburgicae, Typis Christoph. Andr. Zeitleri, 1695.

[16] p.   19 cm.   [5859]

I. Huszti, *respondent.*

—Specimen medicum solenne de mercurio et medicamentis mercurialibus selectis, ad expugnandos, sine salivatione morbos corporis humani rebelles

. . . Halae Magdeburgicae, Literis Chr. Henckelii [1700]

44, [3] p.   20 cm.   [5860]

J. van den Velde, *respondent.*

—*respondent. See* FASCH, A. H., *praeses.* Disputatio inauguralis medica de αυτοχειρια. 1681.

—, *ed. See* POTIER, P. Opera omnia practica & chymica. 1698.

HOFFMANN, FRIEDRICH [*fl.* 1687] *praeses.* Disputatio physica, de imaginationis natura ejusque viribus . . . Jenae, Literis Krebsianis [1687]

[30] p.   21 cm.   [5861]

Diss. — Jena (M. P. Oldekop, *respondent*)

HOFFMANN, GODFRYD [*fl.* 1698] *respondent. See* HOFFMANN, F. [1660–1742] *praeses.* Dissertatio medico-chirurgica inauguralis, de ισχαίμος. 1698.

HOFFMANN, JOHANN JUSTUS [*fl.* 1684] *respondent. See* FASCH, A. H., *praeses.* Disputatio medica inauguralis de dysenteria. 1684.

—*See* WEDEL, G. W. Propempticon inaugurale de bile. 1684.

HOFFMANN, JOHANN MARTIN [*b.* 1658] *respondent. See* WEDEL, G. W., *praeses.* Exercitatio medica aegrum paralysi laborantem sistens. 1682.

—*See* FASCH, A. H. Decanus Facultatis Medicae Augustinus Henricus Faschius . . . ad . . . de ictero disputationis solennitam . . . invitat. 1685.

HOFFMANN, JOHANN MORITZ [1653–1727] Anatomen corporis foemini, in theatro anatomico exhibiturus, quotquot sacra isthaec amant & aestimant, primumque viventium hospitium pia curiositate nosse cupiunt . . . [Altdorfii] Typis Henrici Meyeri [1682?]

[8] p.   19 cm.   [5862]

—Dissertationes anatomico-physiologicae, ad . . . D. Johannis van Horne . . . Microcosmum; seu, Brevem manuductionem ad historiam corporis humani annotatae, & experimentis atque observationibus recentioribus illustratae, annexa . . . Epistola de genitalibus Dn. D. van Horne, cum notis Joh. Swammerdamii . . . Altdorffii Noricorum, Typis Henrici Meyeri, 1685.

[8], 328, [11] p.   tables.   20 cm.   [5863]

Dissertations — Altdorf

—*praeses.* De glandulis renalibus exercitationem anatomico-medicam ... subjicit ... Fridericus Jacobus Bruno ... [Altdorffii] Literis Henrici Meyeri [1683]

23 p. 20 cm. [5864]

F. J. Bruno, *respondent.*

—De odoramentis et suffimentis dissertatio medica publica ... [Altdorffii] Literis Henrici Meyeri [1686]

[4], 36 p. 19 cm. [5865]

J. J. Cnopff, *respondent.*

—Disputatio medica aegrum asthmate laborantem exhibens ... Altdorffii, Literis Henrici Meyeri [1681]

[6], 26 p. 19 cm. [5866]

J. B. Cramer, *respondent.*

—Disputatio medica publica de carie ossium ... Altdorfii, Literis Henrici Meyeri [1681]

31 p. 20 cm. [5867]

M. Masson, *respondent.*

—Disputatio medica publica de dolore in genere ... Altdorffii, Literis Schönnerstaedtianis [1682]

19, [1] p. 20 cm. [5868]

D. Zollikofer, *respondent.*

—Disputatio medica publica de medicamentis martialibus ... [Altdorffii] Literis Henrici Meyeri [1685]

56 p. 19 cm. [5869]

J. G. Beuttel, *respondent.*

—Disputatio medica publica de omento ... [Altdorffii] Excudit Henricus Meyer [1695]

24 p. 19 cm. [5870]

J. Vierzigmann, *respondent.*

—Disputatio medica publica de ὑδροκεφάλῳ ... Altdorffii, Aere Heinrici Meyeri [1695]

40 (i.e. 39) p. 20 cm. [5871]

M. C. Cramer, *respondent.*

—Dissertatio anatomico-physiologica de gustu, atque experimentis & observationibus novissimis circa illum habitis ... Altdorfii, Literis Henrici Meyeri [1689]

44 p. 19 cm. [5872]

B. M. Franck, *respondent.*

—Dissertatio medica de anorexia ... Altdorffii, Literis Schönnerstaedtianis [1685]

20 p. 20 cm. [5873]

J. J. Kornmann, *respondent.*

—Dissertatio medica publica de vena portae ... Altdorfii, Literis Schönnerstaedtianis [1687]

[6], 33 p. 20 cm. [5874]

J. G. Ayrer, *respondent.*

—Dissertatio physiologico-pathologica de cuticula & cute ... [Altdorffii] Literis Henrici Meyeri [1685]

52 p. 18 cm. [5875]

K. D. Metzger, *respondent.*

—Dissertationem medicam de aepothpia sive microcosmi aeolia ... submittit Matthias Henricus Winter ... Altdorffii, Literis Henrici Meyeri [1680]

[4], 28 p. 20 cm. [5876]

M. H. Winter, *respondent.*

—Exercitatio anatomico-physiologica de fluidorum catholicorum foetus motu ... [Altdorffii] Literis Henrici Meyeri [1695]

20 p. 20 cm. [5877]

K. Rayger, *respondent.*

—Another issue. [5878]

Page 2 is blank.

—Exercitatio medica de aere morbifico ... [Altdorffii] Excudit Henricus Meyer [1694]

[6], 20 p. 20 cm. [5879]

C. E. Gockel, *respondent.*

—Exercitatio medica de pericardio ... Altdorfii, Literis Henrici Meyeri [1690]

[8], 32 p. 20 cm. [5880]

G. F. Franck von Franckenau, *respondent.*

—Exercitatio medica de salivatione mercuriali ... [Altdorffii] Typis Henrici Meyeri [1692]

27 p. 20 cm. [5881]

A. Untzelmann, *respondent.*

—Exercitatio physiologico-medica de suturis cranii humani earumque usu ... [Altdorffii] Literis Henrici Meyeri [1691]

26 (i.e. 28) p. 20 cm. [5882]

D. H. Meibom, *respondent.*

—Θεωρήματα ἰατρικά de differentiis alimentorum et medicamentorum ... Altdorffii, Typis Heinrici Meyeri [1677]

24 p. 19 cm. [5883]

J. C. Ayrer, *respondent.*

—*respondent. See* STURM, J. C., *praeses.* Magnorum mundi corporum magnetismus. 1671.

HOFFMANN, MORITZ [1622–1698] Botanotheca Laurembergiana; hoc est, Methodus conficiendi herbarium vivum ad usum societatis medicae in universitate Altdorffina Norimbergensium accommodata ... Altdorffii, Typis Georgii Hagen, 1662

[28] p. 19 cm. [5884]

—Florae Altdorffinae deliciae hortenses; sive, Catalogus plantarum horti medici quibus auctior erat A. C. cIɔIɔc Lx. ... Altdorffii, Typis Georgii Hagen [1660?]

[58] p. 20 cm. [5885]

—Historia vituli monstrosi. *In* Blasius, G. Observationes medicae rariores. 1677.

—Kurtzer ... Bericht, von denen ... grassirenden ... gifftigen Pest-Fiebern, wie dieselbe zeitlich zu tractiren seynd, damit sie nicht tödtlich werden mögen: auf ... Befehl eines ... Magistrats dess Heil. Röm. Reichs Stadt Nürnberg ... erkläret ... Nürnberg, Gedruckt bey Michael Endter, 1680.

[38] p. 21 cm. [5886]

—Prudentiae medicae ex sanguine pro salute mortalium agendorum rationes exponentis fundamenta in incluta Norimbergensium Universitate Altdorffina publ. disputata ... A. C. cIɔIɔc LXV. [Altdorffii] Typis Georgii Hagen [1665]

[64] p. front. 16 cm. [5887]

Frontispiece dated 1650.

—[The same.] Prudentiae medicae ex sanguine pro salute mortalium agendorum rationes exponentis fundamenta in incluta Norimbergensium Universitate Altdorffina A. C. cIɔIɔcLXII. & seqq. publice disputata ... [Altdorffii] Typis Henrici Meyeri, 1672.

[8], 56 p. 17 cm. [5888]

—[The same.] ... Ed. 3. [Altdorffii] Typis Henrici Meyeri, 1690.

[8], 56 p. 17 cm. [5889]

Different setting of type.

—Sciagraphia morborum contagiosorum ex natura sanguinis praecavendor. & curandorum in Universitate Altdorffina ... per dispp. XL. familiares exhibita A. C. cIɔIɔcLXVI. & seqq. Altdorffii, Typis Henrici Meyeri, 1672.

[8], 80 p. 17 cm. [5890]

—Synopsis institt. medicinae ex sanguinis natura vitam longiorem artem breviorem promittentis methodo nova perfacilique in Universitate Altdorffina Norimbergensium disputata ... Altdorffii, Typis Georgii Hagen, 1663.

[64] p. 17 cm. [5891]

— Copy 2.

With this is bound Whitaker, T. Tractatus de sanguine uvae. 1655.

Dissertations — Altdorf

—*praeses.* Ασκημα ἰατρικόν de alimentorum coctione prima, s. fermentatione chylosi dicta salva et laesa ... Altdorffii, Literis Johannis Göbelii [1662]

32 p. 19 cm. [5892]

J. D. Ulstätt, *respondent.*

—Disputatio medica de tumoribus praeter naturam in genere ... Altdorphii, Typis Georgii Hagen [1649]

[20] p. 20 cm. [5893]

J. P. Bruno, *respondent.*

—Θεώρημα ἰατρικόν de appetitu depravato pica dicto ... Altdorffii, Stanno Göbeliano [1662]

[4], 32 p. 18 cm. [5894]

J. F. Hubrigk, *respondent.*

Theses medicae de generatione et usu partium eidem inservientium contra vulgarem de quibusdam opinionem ... Altdorphii, Typis Georgii Hagen [1650]

[24] p. 21 cm. [5895]

J. W. Gebler, *respondent.*

—Theses medicae de sanguine, ejusque observatione quas contra vulgarem de quibusdam opinionem ... publice defendere conabitur ... Altdorphii, E typographeo Academico Hageniano [1660]

[40] p. 18 cm. [5896]

Imperfect: sig. E1 wanting.

G. Freytag, *respondent.*

—Theses medicae de venaesectionis necessitate ... [Altdorffii] E Typothesia Academica Hageniana, 1661.

[40] p. 20 cm. [5897]

B. Zorn, *respondent.*

—Theses summariae medicae de procidentia uteri ... Altdorfii, Literis Henrici Meyeri [1695]

12 p. 20 cm. [5898]

E. H. Wedel, *respondent.*

—*See* RAY, J. Stirpium Europaearum extra Britannias nascentium sylloge. 1694.

HOFFMANN, SAMUEL [*fl.* 1620] *praeses.* Disputatio medica de lumbricorum in humano corpore generatione, causis et curatione ... Helmaestadii, Typis heredum Jacobi Lucii, 1620.

[12] p. 19 cm. [5899]

Diss. — Helmstedt (W. E. Scheffer, *respondent*)

HOFFMANNUS, CASPARUS. *See* HOFMANN, Caspar [*d.* 1584]

HOFFSTADT, JOHANN DIETRICH [*fl.* 1680-1692] Panacea coelestis Hoffstadiana; oder, Kurze Beschreibung dess himmlischen Theriacks ... mit seinen kostbahren Ingredientien ... und nutzbarem Gebrauch ... Hanau, Gedruckt mit Joh. Adolph Aubrys Schrifften, 1693.

168, [8] p. 16 cm. [5900]

—*respondent. See* FRANCK VON FRANCKENAU, G., *praeses.* Dissertatio inauguralis medica de theriaca coelesti. 1691.

HOFFVENIAS, PER. *See* HOFFWENIUS, Petrus [1630-1682]

HOFFWENIUS, PETRUS [1630-1682] *praeses.* Disputatio medica de phlebotomia ... Upsaliae, Henricus Curio [1671]

[18] p. 20 cm. [5901]

Diss. — Uppsala (E. N. Holmdorphius, *respondent*)

—*respondent. See* LINDEN, J. A. van der, *praeses.* Hippocrates de circuitu sanguinis, exercitatio IV. 1659.

HOFLANDT, JUSTUS [*fl.* 1667] *respondent.* Disputatio medica inauguralis de pleuritide ...

Lugduni Batavorum, Apud viduam & haeredes Joannis Elsevirii, 1667.

[8] p. 24 cm. [5902]

Diss. — Leyden.

HOFMAN, JOHANN. *See* HOFFMAN, Johann [*fl.* 1627]

HOFMAN, LAURENTIUS. *See* HOFMANN, Lorenz [1582-1630]

HOFMANN, CASPAR [*d.* 1584] *See* SCHOLTZ, L. Consiliorum medicinalium ... liber singularis. 1610 [and] Epistolarum philosophicarum: medicinalium, ac chymicarum ... volumen. 1610.

HOFMANN, CASPAR [1572-1648] Animadversiones in Com. Montani libros quinque De morbis, et Thomae Erasti anatomen eorundem, nec non ant-Erastica ejusdem Montani. Cum auctario de causa continente. Amstelrodami, Apud Joannem Janssonium, 1641.

[23], 315, [20] p. 14 cm. [5903]

—Apologiae pro Galeno; sive, Χρηστοματείων libri tres. Tomus prior [-posterior] ... Ex bibliotheca Guidonis Patini ... Lugduni, Sumptibus Laurentii Anisson, 1668.

[8], 355, [20] p.; [1], 556, [39] p. illus. 24 cm. [5904]

Part [2] has special title page.
Edited by Guy Patin.

—Commentarii in Galeni De usu partium corporis humani lib. XVII. cum variis lectionibus in utrumque codicem, Graecum & Latinum ... Francofurti ad Moenum, Typis Wechelianis, Apud Danielem & Davidem Aubrios, & Clementem Schleichium, 1625.

[16], 364, [48] p. 33 cm. [5905]

Imperfect: p. [47-48] mutilated.

—De calido innato et spiritibus, syntagma in duos libros tributum, cum praefatio de sectis philosophorum. Francofurti ad Moenum, Apud Thomam Matthiam Götzium, 1667.

[3], 116 p. 20 cm. [5906]

Imperfect: upper margins of p. 115-116 trimmed.

—De generatione hominis libri quatuor. Contra Mundinum Mundinium. Adjecimus sententiam ejusdem De formarum origine secundum Aristotelem ... Francofurti ad Moenum, Typis Wechelianis, sumptibus Clementis Schleichii, & Petri de Zetter, 1629.

[10], 145 p.   31 cm.   [5907]

Bound with copy 2 of *his* De thorace. 1627.

—De ichoribus, et in quibus illi apparent, affectibus, collectanea . . . Lipsiae, Typis Nerlichianis, excudebat Justus Jansonius, impensis Eliae Rehefeldii, & Johannis Grosii [1617]

[53] p.   17 cm.   [5908]

—De locis affectis libri tres. His praemisimus septenarium controversiarum huc facientium . . . Noribergae, Typis Wolfgangi Endteri, 42 [i.e. 1642]

[8], 213, [1] p.   port.   13 cm.   [5909]

Added engraved title page, dedication, and colophon dated 1642.

—De medicamentis officinalibus . . . libri duo. Accesserunt quasi Paralipomena, quae vel ex animalibus, vel ex mineralibus petuntur . . . Parisiis, Apud Casparum Meturas, 1647.

[24], 707 p.   24 cm.   [5910]

—[The same] . . . Quibus accesserunt, quasi Paralipomena, remedia medicinalia, quae vel ex animalibus, vel ex mineralibus petuntur. Nec non . . . syntagma De calido innato et spiritibus . . . cui . . . adjunctus . . . liber De partibus similaribus . . . Jenae, Sumptibus Tobiae Oehrlingii, 1686.

[24], 563 p.; 116 p.; 136 p.   port.   22 cm.

[5911]

—De thorace, ejusque partibus commentarius tripartitus. In quo discutiuntur praecipue ea, quae inter Aristotelem & Galenum controversa sunt. Francofurti, Typis & sumptibus Wechelianorum, apud Danielum & Davidem Aubrios & Clementem Schleichium, 1627.

[8], 101, [1] p.   34 cm.   [5912]

With this is bound copy 2 of Galenus. Περὶ ὀστῶν τοῖς ε'ιαγομενοις. De ossibus ad tyrones. 1630.

— Copy 2. 31 cm.

With this is bound *his* De generatione hominis. 1629.

—De usu lienis, cerebri et de ichoribus. Lugd. Batavorum, Apud Franciscos Hegerum et Hackium, 1639.

[16], 168, [14], 169-294 (i.e. 298), [24] p.   13 cm.   [5913]

Engraved title page.

". . . De usu cerebri, secundum Aristotelem diatribe": p. [1-14], 169-240.

—De usu lienis secundum Aristotelem, liber singularis. [Lipsiae] Excudebant haeredes Valent. am Ende, impensis Johannis Börneri sen. & Eliae Rehefeldii, 1615.

[15], 149, [1] p.   16 cm.   [5914]

—Institutionum medicarum libri sex . . . Lugduni, Sumptib. Joan. Antonii Huguetan, 1645.

[32], 779, [90] p.   23 cm.   [5915]

Added engraved title page.

Epistola dedicatoria by Charles Spon.

—[The same, as subject] *See* RIOLAN, J [1580-1657] Opera anatomica vetera. 1650 [and] Opuscula anatomica nova. 1649.

—Institutionum suarum medicarum epitome, in sez libros digesta. Ex ipsius auctoris autographo edita. Heidelbergae, Sumptibus Johannis Petri Zubrodt, 1672.

[12], 511, [1] p.   14 cm.   [5916]

—Pathologia parva, in qua methodus Galeni practica explicatur, quam olim Fr. Frisimelica promiserat . . . Jenae, Typis Ernesti Steinmanni, impensis Joh. Reiffenbergeri, 1640.

143, p.   16 cm.   [5917]

—Rejectanea pathologica, qua de morbis formae et materiae, a Fernelio, Argenterioque per somnum visis . . . Helmaestadii, Typis heredum Jacobi Lucii, impensis Jeremiae Rixneri, 1639.

[63] p.   16 cm.   [5918]

—Relatio historica judicii acti in Campis Elysiis coram Rhadamanto contra Gelenum, cum approbatione Apollonis in Parnasso, communicata per Mercurium . . . Norimbergae, Typis Wolffgangi Endteri, 1642.

[1], 65, [4] p.   13 cm.   [5919]

Imperfect: p. [1]-2 bound after p. 18.

—Tractatus tres Du usu lienis secundum Arist. Cerebri secundum eunde et De ichoribus aucti et correcti. Francofurti, Apud Thomam Matthiam Götzium [1664?]

[26], 174, [14], 175-302, [24] p.   14 cm.

[5920]

Engraved title page.

Edited by Sebastian Scheffer.

Bound with copy 2 of Regimen sanitatis Salernitanum. Schola Salernitana. 1667.

—[The same.] Tractatus de usu lienis cerebri, et de ichoribus; adnexo insimul Francisci de Le Boe . . . experientia medica undequaque refertissimo, omnia & singula auctius, correctius, limatius edita. Lipsiae, Apud Tobiam Oehrlingium, typis Joannis Philippi Andreae, 1682.

[23], 174, [14], 175-302, [24] p.; [10], 113 p. 14 cm. [5921]

Added engraved title page.
Part [2] has special title page: Francisci de Le Boe Sylvii . . . Collegium medico-practicum dictatum 1660. Francofurti, Apud Thomam Matthiam Götzium, 1664.
With this is bound: Swalve, B. Pancreas pancrene. 1678.

—Variarum lectionum lib. VI. In quibus loca multi Dioscoridis, Athenaei, Plinii, Hippocratis, Aristotelis, Galeni, aliorum, qua illustrantur, qua explicantur . . . Lipsiae, [Laurentius Kober excudebat] impensis Eliae Rehefeldii & Johan. Grosii, 1619.

[22], 332, [14] p. 16 cm. [5922]

—Vita medica, hoc est Galeni ὑγιεινῶν; sive, Methodi sanitatis tuendae libri VI. Nova, eaque omnium accuratissima versione, & perpetuis commentariis et castigationibus . . . illustrati a Casparo Hofmanno . . . curante Sebastiano Scheffero, D. M. Francofurti, Impensis Joannis Justi Erythropili, typis Joannis Andreae, 1680.

[8], 56 p. 19 cm. [5923]

"Oratio quinta . . . Joannis Georgii Volckameri . . . in laudem . . . Caspari Hofmanni, anno MDC IL. scripta": p. 28-56.

—praeses. Disputatio de venarum origine secundum Aristotelem . . . Altorfii, Apud Cunradum Agricolam [1615]

[20] p. 19 cm. [5924]

Diss.—Altdorf (S. Hainlin, respondent)

—Disputatio medica de natura pulsuum . . . Altdorphii, Typis descripsit Balthasar Scherffius [1628]

[16] p. 18 cm. [5925]

Diss.—Altdorf (C. Kern, respondent)

—Theses de hepate, ejusque usu secundum Aristotelem . . . Altorphii, Apud Balthasarum Scherffium [1621]

[20] p. 19 cm. [5926]

Diss.—Altdorf (D. Bucretius, respondent)

—Theses de pulmone, ejusque usu secundum Aristotelem . . . Altorfii, Typis Scherffianis [1622]

[12] p. 19 cm. [5927]

Diss.—Altdorf (P. Weissensehe, respondent)

—, ed. and tr. See GALENUS. Praxis medica curiosa. 1680.

—, ed. See GALENUS. Περὶ ᾽οστῶν τοῖς εἰαγομένοις . . . De ossibus ad tyrones liber. 1630.

—See BARTHOLIN, T. Anatomicae vindiciae Cl. v. Casparo Hofmanno . . . aliisque oppositae. 1648; REINESIUS, T. Ad viros clariss. D. Casp. Hoffmannum. Christ. Ad. Rupertum . . . epistolae. 1660.

HOFMANN, CHRISTIAN. See HOFFMANN, Christian [fl. 1668-1671]

HOFMANN, FRIEDRICH. See HOFFMANN, Friedrich [fl. 1626-1675]

HOFMANN, GEORG BERNHARD [fl. 1700] respondent. Dissertationem de scorbuto inauguralem . . . examini submittit M. Georgius Bernhardus Hofmann . . . Argentorati, Literis Johannis Welperi [1700]

15 p. 22 cm. [5928]

Diss.—Strasbourg.

—See MAPP, M., praeses. Theses medicae de erysipelate. 1700.

HOFMANN, JOHANN GEORG [fl. 1665] respondent. See SCHURTZFLEISCH, K. S., praeses. De nive. 1665.

HOFMANN, JOHANN MORITZ. See HOFFMANN, Johann Moritz [1653-1727]

HOFMANN, JOHANN PHILIPP [fl. 1686] respondent. See FRANCK VON FRANCKENAU, G., praeses. Dissertatio inauguralis medica de labiis leporinis. 1686.

HOFMANN, LORENZ [1582-1630] De vero usu & fero abusu medicamentorum chymicorum commentatio . . . Halae Saxonum, 1611.

[31], 139, [16] p. 20 cm. [5929]

Date altered by hand from M.DC.XI. to M.DC.XIX.

—, ed. See BRUNNER, B. Consilia medica. 1617.

HOFMANN, MORITZ. See HOFFMANN, Moritz [1622-1698]

HOFMANN, PAUL [*fl.* 1689–1693] *respondent. See* BERGER, J. G. von, *praeses.* Exercitationem inauguralem de morbis senum ... p. p. 1693.

—*See* BERGER, J. G. von. Ordinis medici ... decanus ... lectori ... S. P. D. 1693.

HOFMANNUS, JOHANNES MARTINUS. *See* HOFFMANN, Johann Martin [*b.* 1658]

HOFSTADT, JOHANN DIETRICH. *See* HOFFSTADT, Johann Dietrich [*fl.* 1680–1692]

HOFSTETER, JÁNOS ÁDÁM [1660–1716?] *respondent. See* FASCH, A. H. *praeses.* Dissertationem inauguralem de ανοϱεξια, seu fame abolita. 1687.

—*See* FASCH, A. H. Augustinus Henricus Faschius ... Facultatis Medicae decanus, S. D. L. 1687.

HOFSTETER, JÁNOS KRISTÓF [*fl.* 1689–1695] *respondent. See* HOFFMANN, F. [1660–1742] *praeses.* Disputatio solennis medica, de somnabulatione. 1695.

—*See* HOFFMANN, F. [1660–1742] Propemticon inaugurale, de animae ac corporis commercio. 1695.

HOFSTETTER, JOHANN ADAM. *See* HOFSTETER, JÁNOS ÁDÁM [1660–1716?]

HOGELANDE, CORNELIUS AB. *See* HOGHELANDE, Cornelis van [*b.* 1590]

HOGELANDE, THEOBALD DE. *See* HOGHELANDE, Theobaldus van [*ca.* 1560–1608?]

HOGEMADE, JACOB VAN [*fl.* 1666] *respondent.* Disputatio medica inauguralis de epilepsia ... Lugduni Batavorum, Ex officina Petri & Cornelii Hackii, 1666.

    [20] p. 23 cm.   **[5930]**
Diss.—Leyden.

HOGHELANDE, CORNELIS VAN [*b.* 1590] Cogitationes, quibus Dei existentia; item animae spiritalitas, et possibilis cum corpore unio, demonstrantur: nec non, brevis Historia oeconomiae corporis animalis, proponitur, atque mechanice explicatur. Amstelodami, Apud Ludovicum Elzevirium, 1646.

    [28], 296, [22] p. 14 cm.   **[5931]**

—[The same.] ... His accedit tractatus De praedestinatione. Lugduni Batavorum, Apud Johannem a Gelder, 1676.

    [30], 159, [6], 163–269 p. 15 cm.   **[5932]**

"Exercitationes philosophicae miscellaneae de natura hominis, et speciatim de conjunctione mentis cum corpore" (p. [6], 163–269) has special title page with imprint: Amstelodami, Apud Petrum Parrival, 1676.

    Bound with Charleton, W. Exercitationes physico-anatomicae, de oeconomia animali. 1678.

—*See* NOUVEAU COURS DE MEDECINE. 1669, 1683.

HOGHELANDE, THEOBALDUS VAN [*ca.* 1560–1608?] De alchimiae difficultatibus liber. In quo docetur, quid scire quidque vitare debeat verae chemiae studiosus ad perfectionem aspirans ...

    109–191 p., vol. 1. 20 cm. (*In* Zetzner, Lazarus, *ed.* Theatrum chemicum. Argentorati, 1659–61)   **[5933]**
Caption title.

—De historia transmutationis metallorum. *In* Resch, J. U. Osiandrische Experiment von Sole. 1659.

HOHBERG, MARTIN [*fl.* 1681] *respondent. See* WEDEL, G. W., *praeses.* Dissertatio medica, sistens aegrum laborantem dolore ischiadico. 1681.

HOHELANDE, EWALD VON. *See* HOGHELANDE, Theobaldus van [*ca.* 1560–1608?]

HOHENLOHE (GRAFSCHAFT) Kurtzer Unterricht von Allerhandtmitteln, und Artzney, deren man sich in jetziger Zeit ... regierender Nfection [sic] und Seuch der Pestilentz ... so wol zur Praeservation als Curation, nützlichen zu gebrauchen. Also zusammen getragen ... durch der Graveschafft Hoenloe etc. bestelte Hoff Medicos. Nürnberg, Abraham Wagenmann, 1608.

    [67] p. 21 cm.   **[5934]**

HOJER, CHRISTIAN FRIEDRICH [*b.* 1662] *respondent. See* WEDEL, G. W., *praeses.* Disputatio inauguralis medica de cardialgia. 1688.

—*See* WEDEL, G. W. Propempticon inaugurale de tetragono Hippocratis. 1688.

HOLBEIN, HANS, *the younger* [1497–1543] *See* ERASMUS, D. Μοϱίας 'εγκώμιον. 1676.

HOLDER, WILLIAM [1616–1698] Elements of speech: an essay of inquiry into the natural production of letters: with an Appendix concerning persons deaf & dumb ... London, Printed by T. N. for J. Martyn, 1669.

    [7], 168 p. 17 cm.   **[5935]**

[–]Supplement to the Philosophical transactions of July, 1670. With some reflexions on Dr. John Wallis, his letter there inserted. London, Henry Brome, 1678.

[1], 14 p. 22 cm. [**5936**]

—*See* WALLIS, J. A defence of the Royal Society. 1678; WEPFER, J. J. Observationes anatomicae. 1675, 1681.

HOLDERHOFF, ENGELBERTUS. *See* HOLTERHOFF, Engelbert [*fl.* 1665–1676]

HOLL, JOHANN SEBALD [*b.* 1670] *respondent. See* STAHL, G. E., *praeses.* Dissertatio medica inauguralis de requisitis bonae nutricis. 1698 [and] Propempticon inaugurale de pathologia salsa. 1698.

HOLLAND, ADAM [*fl.* 1687] *respondent.* Disputatio medica inauguralis de hysterica passione … Lugduni Batavorum, Apud Abrahamum Elzevier, 1687.

[16] p. 21 cm. [**5937**]
Diss. — Leyden.

HOLLAND, HENRY [1583–1650?] *ed. See* BAUDERON, B. Pharmacopoea. 1639; GUTTA PODAGRICA: A TREATISE OF THE GOUT. 1633.

HOLLAND, PHILEMON [1552–1637] *tr. See* BAUDERON, B. Pharmacopoea. 1639; PLINIUS SECUNDUS, C. The historie of the world. 1601, 1634; REGIMEN SANITATIS SALERNITANUM. Regimen sanitatis Salernitanum. Regimen sanitatis Salerni. 1617, 1634, 1649.

—*See* GUTTA PODAGRICA: A TREATISE OF THE GOUT. 1633.

HOLLAND, WILLIAM [*d.* 1632] *See* GUTTA PODAGRICA: A TREATISE OF THE GOUT. 1633.

HOLLAND (PROVINCE) **Laws, statutes, etc.** Resolutie vande Ed. Groot Mog. heeren staten van Hollandt ende West-Vrieslandt. Behelfende middelen ende praecautien tegens het voorstetten vande pest. 's Graven-Hage, By de erfgenamen van wylen Hillebrandt Jacobssz van Wouw, 1664.

[14] p. 19 cm. [**5938**]

HOLLANDUS, JOANNES ISAACUS. *See* JOHANNES ISAACI, Hollandus [15th cent.]

HOLLERIUS, JACOBUS. *See* HOULLIER, Jacques [*d.* 1562]

HOLLIER, JACQUES. *See* HOULLIER, Jacques [*d.* 1562]

HOLLINGS, EDMUND [1556?–1612] De salubri studiosorum victu; hoc est, De literatorum omnium valetudine conservanda, vitaque diutissime producenda, libellus … Ingolstadii, Typis Ederianis, per Andream Angermarium, 1602.

[14], 145 p. 16 cm. [**5939**]

—Medicamentorum oeconomia nova; seu … Nova medicamentorum, in classes, sedes, atque familias, distribuendorum ratio … Ingolstadii, Typis Ederianis, per Andraeam Angermarium, 1610.

303 p. 16 cm. [**5940**]

—[The same.] … Ingolstadii, Typis Ederianis, per Elisabetham Angermariam, viduam, 1615.

303 p. 17 cm. [**5941**]
A reissue of the 1610 edition with new title page and preliminary matter reset.
Bound with Gatinaria, M. De medendis humani corporis malis practica uberrima. 1604.

HOLLYNGUS, EDMUNDUS. *See* HOLLINGS, Edmund [1556?–1612]

HOLMDORPHIUS, ERICUS N. [*fl.* 1671] *respondent. See* HOFFWENIUS, P., *praeses.* Disputatio medica de phlebotomia. 1671.

HOLMES, NATHANIEL. *See* HOMES, Nathaniel [1599–1678]

HOLSATUS, JOHANNES RIST. *See* RIST, Johannes [1607–1667]

HOLST, JACOB [*d. ca.* 1680] *See* BARTHOLIN, T. De flammula cordis epistola. 1667.

HOLSTEN, GABRIEL [*fl.* 1699] *respondent. See* ROBERG, L. Dissertatio medica varios effluviorum effectus breviter ostendens. 1699.

HOLSTEIN, JOHANN [*fl.* 1608] *respondent.* Themata medica de scirrho … Basileae, Per Joan. Jacob. Genathium [1608]

[8] p. 20 cm. [**5942**]
Diss. — Basel.

HOLTERHOFF, ENGELBERT [*fl.* 1665–1676] Discursus medicus ostendens errores medicorum in curationibus aliquorum praecipuorum et frequentius occurentium morborum ... Coloniae Agrippinae, Typis Joh. Henrici Kopp, 1676.

[4], 40 p.   20 cm.   **[5943]**

Title page and Epistola dedicatoria in duplicate.

— *respondent.* Disputatio medica inauguralis de bile ... Lugduni Batavorum, Ex officina Danielis, Abrahami & Adriani a Gaesbeeck, 1665.

[16] p.   21 cm.   **[5944]**

Diss. — Leyden.

HOLTZAPFEL, JAKOB [*fl.* 1661-1665] Medicina ab opprobriis vindicata et medicus indigne vapulans, oratio. Recitavit publice in Academia Lipsiensi ... Lipsiae, Typis Johannis Wittigau, 1661.

[16] p.   32 cm.   **[5945]**

Bound with Universität Leipzig. Decanus communitatis. [1661]

—*respondent. See* ISRAEL, J., *praeses.* Disputatio medica inauguralis de febribus. 1665.

—*See* UNIVERSITÄT LEIPZIG.

HOLTZEIM, PETRUS. *See* HOLTZEMIUS, Petrus [1570-1651]

HOLTZEM, PIETER. *See* HOLTZEMIUS, Petrus [1570-1651]

HOLTZEMIUS, PETRUS [1570-1651] Descriptio fontis medicati S. Antonii, vulgo Tilleborn dicti, prope Andernacum. Coloniae Agrippinae, In Officina Birckmannica sumptibus Hermanni Mylii, 1620.

[51] p.   16 cm.   **[5946]**

— Essentia hellebori extracta, in gratiam novorum hujus patriae & saeculi medicorum ... Coloniae Agrippinae, In Officina Birckmannica, sumptibus Hermanni Mylii, 1616.

[1], 46 p.   16 cm.   **[5947]**

— Essentia hellebori rediviva, secundo extracta, sive rectificata, & aucta, in gratiam novorum hujus patriae, & saeculi medicorum ... Coloniae Agrippinae, In Officina Birckmannica, sumptibus Hermanni Mylii, 1623.

68 p.   18 cm.   **[5948]**

— Prognosis vitae et mortis, longitudinis et brevitatis, resolutionis & permutationis morbi, duobus libris distincta ... Coloniae, Apud Gerardum Grevenbruch, 1605.

[12], 304, [34] p.   17 cm.   **[5949]**

With this is bound Fabricus von Hilden, W. Observationum & curationum chirurgicarum centuriae. 1606.

—, *ed. See* PHARMACOPOEA, SIVE DISPENSATORIUM COLONIENSE. 1628.

HOLTZMANN, WILHELM. *See* XYLANDER, Gulielmus [1532-1576]

HOLTZMEYER, PETER. *See* HOLZMEYER, Peter [*fl.* 1578]

HOLZMEYER, PETER [*fl.* 1578] *See* PANCKOW, T. Herbarium. 1673.

HOMATI, STANISLAO. *See* OMATI, Stanislao [*fl.* 1674-75]

HOMBERG, ANDREAS [*fl.* 1671-1673] *respondent. See* FRIDERICI, J. A., *praeses.* De tentigine disputationem ... publico examini submittit. 1671; MEIBOM, H., *praeses.* Exercitatio medica de cephalagia. 1672; SCHNEIDER, K. V., *praeses.* Disputatio inauguralis de fracturis cranii. 1673.

HOMERUS. *See* BRENDEL, A., *praeses.* De Homero medico. 1700; LASENA, P. Homeri nepenthes; seu, De abolendo luctu liber. 1624; PETIT, P. Homeri nepenthes. 1689.

HOMES, NATHANIEL [1599-1678] Daemonologie and theologie. The first, the malady, demonstrating the diabolicall arts, and devillish hearts of men. The second, the remedy: demonstrating, God a rich supply of all good ... London, Printed by Tho. Roycroft, and sold by Jo. Martin, and Jo. Ridley, 1650.

[12], 208 p.; 31 p.   15 cm.   **[5950]**

Part [2] has special title page.

HOMEYER, MARTIN [*fl.* 1676] *respondent. See* CONRING, H., *praeses.* Disputatio medica inauguralis de haemoptysi. 1676; MEIBOM, H., *praeses.* Disputatio medica de variolis et morbillis. 1676.

HOMMA, LAURENTIUS [*d.* 1681] *See* HOOGHT, E. van der. Omstandig beright. 1693.

HOMMART, JACOB. *See* L'HOMMART, Jacob [*b.* 1666]

HOMMEL, SEBASTIAN [*fl.* 1679] *respondent. See* MÜLLER, J. [*fl.* 1672-1679] *praeses.* Disputatio physica da lapide fulminari. 1679.

HONAIN IBN ISHĀQ. *See* HUNAIN IBN ISHĀK, al-'Ibādī [809?-873]

HONCAMP, MATTHIAS [*fl.* 1690] *tr. See* SCARLATTINI, O. Homo et ejus partes figuratus. 1695.

HONEIN IBN ISHĀK. *See* HUNAIN IBN ISHĀK, al-'Ibādī [809?-873]

HONESTIS, CHRISTOPHORUS DE [*d.* 1392] *See* MESUË [924 *or* 5-1015] Opera. 1602, 1623.

HONOLD, MATTHIAS [*fl.* 1687-1721] *praeses.* Dissertatio physica de visu ... Ulmae, Typis Christiani Balthasaris Kühnii haered. [1694]

    [26] p.   plate.   19 cm.   **[5951]**
Diss.—Ulm. Gymnasium (U. Juni, *respondent*)

HONORIBUS doctoralibus meritissimis ... Dn. Thomae Cademani Angli, inclytae nationis Anglicae in alma Universitate Patavina consiliarii dignissimi ... Patavii, Ex typographia Joannis Baptistae de Martinis, 1620.

    broadside.   36 x 25 cm.   **[5952]**
Collection of six poems published on the occasion when Cademan received his M.D. degree.

HONUPHRIIS, FRANCISCUS DE [*fl.* 1691] Abortus bicorporeus monoceps Romae anno MDCXCI. editus in Academia Physico-Mathematica examinatus ... Dissertatio epistolaris ad ... Franciscum Redi ... Romae, Typis Rev. Camerae Apostolicae, 1691.

    15 p.   plate.   23 cm.   **[5953]**

HOOGEVEEN, GERARD VAN [*fl.* 1616] *respondent.* Disputatio medica de tabe ... Lugduni Batavorum, Ex officina Johannis Boudewini, 1616.

    [8] p.   20 cm.   **[5954]**
Diss.—Leyden.

HOOGHLANT, CORNELIS SCHAGEN [*fl.* 1655] *respondent.* Disputatio medica inauguralis de hepatitide ... Lugduni Batavorum, Ex officina Adriani Wyngaerden, 1655.

    [11] p.   22 cm.   **[5955]**
Diss.—Leyden.

HOOGSTRATEN, DAVID VAN [1658-1724] *tr. See* MUYS, J. Redelyke heelkonstoeffening. 1684.

HOOGHT, EVERARD VAN DER [1642-1716] Omstandig beright, van Balthasar Bekker ... van sijne particuliere onderhandelinge met D. Laurentius Homma, sal. ged. in sijn leven mede predicant aldaar. Benessens d' ontdekte lagen van Everhardus van der Hooght, en Jakob Lansman tegen denselven. Amsterdam, Daniel vanden Dalen, 1693.

    [1], 22 p.   21 cm.   **[5956]**
Linde 117.

HOOGT, EVERT. *See* HOOGHT, Everard van der [1642-1716]

HOOKE, ROBERT [1635-1703] Lectures and collections made by Robert Hooke ... Cometa, containing observations of the Comet in April, 1677 ... Mr. Boyle's observation made on two new phosphori ... Microscopium, containing Mr. Leeuwenhoeck's two letters ... The author's discourse and description of microscopes, improved for discerning the nature and texture of bodies. P. Cherubine's accusations answered. Mr. Young's letter containing several anatomical observations. London, John Martyn, 1678.

    [8], 112 p.   plates.   24 cm.   **[5957]**
Keynes (A) 22.

—Micrographia; or, Some physiological descriptions of minute bodies made by magnifying glasses. With observations and inquiries thereupon ... London, Jo. Martin and Ja. Allestry, 1665.

    [35], 246, [10] p.   plates.   31 cm.   **[5958]**
Keynes (A) 6.

—[The same.] ... London, Printed for James Allestry 1667.

    [35], 246, [10] p.   plates.   30 cm.   **[5959]**
Keynes (A) 7a

HOOLA, THEODORUS [*fl.* 1699] *respondent.* Disputatio medica inauguralis de nephritide ... Lugduni Batavorum, Apud Abrahamum Elzevier, 1699.

    [20] p.   20 cm.   **[5960]**
Diss.—Leyden.

HOOLWERF, JACOB AB [*fl.* 1698] *respondent.* Dissertatio medica inauguralis de haemoptoe ... Lugduni Batavorum, Apud Abrahamum Elzevier, 1698.

    [27] p.   19 cm.   **[5961]**
Diss.—Leyden.

HOOPFER, BENEDICTUS. *See* HOPFFER, Benedikt [1643-1684]

HOORN, JOHAN VON [1662-1724] Den swenska wäl-öfwade jord-gumman hwilken grundeligen underwijser huru med en hafwande handlas, en wåndande hielpas, en barna-qwinna handteras, och det nyfödda barnet skiötas skal ... Stockholm, Nathanael Goldenaus, 1697.

[22], 20, [4], 328, [20] p.   plates, port.   17 cm.
[**5962**]

Added engraved title page.
Imperfect: signature **5-8 wanting?

HOORN, WILLEM VAN [*fl.* 1697] *respondent.* Exercitium philosophico-medicum inaugurale continens positiones quasdam theoreticas de multorum causis ... Lugduni Batavorum, Apud Abrahamum Elzevier, 1697.

[19] p.   22 cm.   [**5963**]
Diss.—Leyden.

HOORN, WILLEM VAN DEN [*fl.* 1660] *respondent.* Disputatio medica inauguralis, de pleuritide ... Trajecti ad Rhenum, Typis Theodori ab Ackersdijck & Gisberti à Zijll, 1660.

[8] p.   20 cm.   [**5964**]
Diss.—Utrecht.

—*See* LINDEN, J. A. VAN DER, *praeses.* Hippocrates de circuitu sanguinis, exercitatio IX. 1660.

HOORNBEEK, JOHANNES [1617-1666] *See* VARIORUM TRACTATUS THEOLOGICI DE PESTE. 1655.

HOORNE, JEAN VAN. *See* HORNE, Johannes van [1621-1670]

HOORNE, JOHAN VAN. *See* HOORN, Johan von [1662-1724]

HOPE, SIR WILLIAM, *bart.* [*fl.* 1687-1725] *See* SOLLEYSEL, J. de. The compleat horseman. 1696.

HOPFER, BENEDICTUS. *See* HOPFFER, Benedikt [1643-1684]

HOPFFER, BENEDIKT [1643-1684] *praeses.* Disputatio moralis de desperatione ... Tubingae, Typis Johann-Henrici Reisii, 1678.

20 p.   19 cm.   [**5965**]
Diss.—Tübingen (D. Funck, *respondent*)

HOPFNER, JOHANN WILIBALD [*fl.* 1640] *respondent. See* SCHLEGEL, P. M., praeses. Disputatio medica de erysipelate. 1640 [and] Disputatio solemnis et inauguralis medica, de haemorrhagia in genere. 1640.

HÔPITAL DE LA CHARITÉ, LYONS. *See* LYONS. Aumône générale. Institution de l'aumosne generale de Lyon. 1647, 1662.

HÔPITAL DE SAINT ROCH, ROUEN. *See* ROUEN. Recit de ce qui s'est passé en l'establissement des Hospitaux de Saint Louis & de S. Roch de la ville de Roüen. 1654.

HÔPITAL GÉNÉRAL, ORLEANS. *See* DISCOURS CHRÉTIEN SUR L'ÉTABLISSEMENT DE L'HÔPITAL GENERAL DE LA VILLE D'ORLEANS. 1672.

HÔPITAL GÉNÉRAL, PARIS. L'Hospital general de Paris. Paris, François Muguet, 1676.

[1], 123 p.; 7, 4, 3, 3 p.   23 cm.   [**5966**]
In addition to a Histoire de l'Hospital general de Paris, contains 4 Declarations du Roy, dated 23 Mars 1680, pertaining to the administration of the hospital.

—*See* FRANCE. Sovereigns, etc. [1643-1715] (Louis XIV) Edit du roy. 1690? [and] Reglemens que le roy veut estre executez dans l'Hôpital general de Paris. 1684.

HOPP, JOHANN [1616-1654] Disputatio chirurgico-medica de gangraena et sphacelo ... Lipsiae, Imprimebant haeredes Friderici Lanckisch [1646?]

[35] p.   19 cm.   [**5967**]
Date supplied from Jöcher, vol. 2, col. 1701.

—*praeses.* Catarrhus suffocativus disputationis thesibus resolutus ... Lipsiae, Typis Johannis Baueri, 1651.

[24] p.   19 cm.   [**5968**]
Diss.—Leipzig (J. W. Buch, *respondent*)

—De purpura dissertatio medica ... Lipsiae, Excudebat Quirinus Bauch [1652]

[28] p.   19 cm.   [**5969**]
Diss.—Leipzig (M. Heiland, *respondent*)

—Διάσκεψις φυσιολογικη και παθυλογικη ventriculi humani in theses redacta ... Lipsiae, Typis haeredum Timothei Hönii [1649]

[28] p.   19 cm.   [**5970**]
Diss.—Leipzig (B. Kreckler, *respondent*)

—Diatribe medica de phthisi ... Lipsiae, Typis haeredum Timothei Hönii [1648]

[28] p.   19 cm.   [**5971**]
Diss.—Leipzig (P. J. Sachs von Lewenhaimb, *respondent*)

HOPPIUS, CHRISTIAN [*fl.* 1652] *praeses.* Disputatio physica de principiis corporum naturalium ... Lipsiae, Literis Quirini Bauch, 1652.

[15] p. 19 cm. [**5972**]

Diss.—Leipzig (G. Lehne, *respondent*)

HOPPIUS, JOHANN. *See* HOPP, Johann [1616–1654]

HORARUM fallax mors incertissima rerum attamen horarum cur tibi cura datur. [1601?] *See* LIAGNO, T. F.

HORCH, HEINRICH [1652–1729] *respondent. See* WALDSCHMIDT, J. J., *praeses.* Disputatio medica de veneni pestilentialis. 1675.

HORING, MICHAEL [*fl.* 1618] *tr. See* PARACELSUS. Theophrastische Practica. 1618.

HORLACHER, CHRISTOPH MICHAEL [*b.* 1672] *See* VESTI, J. Facultatis Medicae ... decanus, Justus Vesti ... benevolo lectori S. P. D. 1689.

HORLACHER, CONRAD [*fl.* 1684–1691] Allgemeine Schatz-Kammer neu- und offt bewehrter ... Artzneÿen; oder, Gründliche Erklärung ... der vornehmsten ... und besten Artzneyen, dess ... D. Johann Michaelis seel. die in seinen ... Operibus medico-chirurgicis ... enthalten. Anbey vorstellend, was in unterschiedlichen theils anderer ... Medicorum, theils auch selbst eigener Erfahrung bewehrt befunden worden ... verfertiget durch Conrad Horlacher ... Ulm, In Verlag Georg Wilhelm Kühnen, 1694.

[15], 208 p. 17 cm. [**5973**]

—Christ-mitleidige ... Entdeck- Beschreib- und Eröffnung der bisshero den mehrern Theil verborgnen ... Stein-Cur, und an Statt dessen mit grossem Schaden und Schmertzen der Patienten, gemeinen Gebrauch nach, üblichen Stein-Schneidens: eines in Wahrheit sehr grausamen Artzney-Mittels ... Ulm, George Willhelm Kühn, 1694.

30 p. 17 cm. [**5974**]

—Die höchstschädliche Würckung des Aderlassens und Purgierens, mit zehen Beweissgründen, und Beantwortung der vornehmsten Einwendungen, auch kürtzlicher Betrachtung der von D. Geudern dem D. Gehemae entgegen gesetzten Apologi (in welcher die Purgir-Mittel, un das Aderlassen

vergebens geretter) ... Franckfurt und Leipzig, In Verlag Georg Wilhelm Kühn, 1691.

[3], 32 (i.e. 39) p. 16 cm. [**5975**]

Bound with Neu-vermehrtes ... Aderlass-Büchlein. [*ca.* 1670]

—Methodus urinoscopiae perfacilis ac perspicua, singularibus theorematibus inclusa, & semi-centuria circiter observationum propriae praxeos confirmata: additis quoque aliorum experimentis ... Ulmae, Apud Georg. Wilhelmum Kühn, 1691.

60 p. 13 cm. [**5976**]

Imperfect: upper and outer margins on p. 16, 20–21 and 37 trimmed.

—Theatrum arcanorum divinae sapientiae; oder, Gnadenreicher Schauplatz der göttlichen Weissheit ... welche erhellet in und auss denen vielfachen Wunder-Geheimnüssen der wahren Medicin, als nemlich ... Eröffnung der sichern ... Wassersuchts, podagrischer Kranckheit, ob Zipperleins, der Fieber, Pest, Ruhr und Hals Bräune, wie auch der Krätze, und Luis Venere oder so genannten Frantzosen-Cur und Heilungs-Art ... Franckfurt am Mayn, In Velegung Johann David Zunners, 1699.

[14], 520 p. front. 17 cm. [**5977**]

Frontispiece has title: Theatrum clementiae divinae, e vera medicina conspicuae.

Imperfect: outer margin of title page trimmed.

—Ungemeine Erörter- und ... Eröffnung, der ohnschmertzlich- und nicht gefährlichen Cur, oder Art und Weiss die öffters in Praxi vorkommende Brüch ... der Gedärm ... sicher zu heilen ... Ulm, In Verlag Georg Wilhelm Kühnen, 1695.

[2], 73 p. 17 cm. [**5978**]

—Vestgegründeter Beweiss, dass die eingeführten Meinungen von denen Catarrhis oder so genannten Haupt- und Steckflüssen, etc. nicht bessern Grund als alte Weiber-Mährlein haben. Samt angefügter Erläuterung ... wie sie zu curiren seyn. Nürnberg, In Verlegung dess Authoris, zu finden bey Wolffgang Moritz Endter, 1691.

[7], 110 p. 17 cm. [**5979**]

Imperfect: p. 110 mutilated.

—*respondent. See* METZGER, G. B., *praeses.* Σκιαγραφια suturarum cranii humani earumque veri usus. 1684.

—*See* ALETHOPHILUS, J. M. Unvorgreiffliches Bedencken. 1691.

HORN, Bartholomaeus [1614–1694] *ed. See* Hippocrates. [Prognostica Greek and Latin] 1645.

HORN, Caspar [1583–1653] Kurtzer und nothwendiger Bericht von der fremden, vorhin bey uns unbekannten, jetzt aber allhier eingreiffenden Kranckheit, dem Schorbock . . .

[1]–118 p. 14 cm. (*In* Viel-vergröster und hellerpolirter Schorbocks-Spiegel. Nürnberg, 1659.

Half title.   [5980]

—, *ed. See* Jābir ibn Ḥaiyān, al-Ṭarasūsī. Gebri Arabis Chimai. 1668.

—*See* Rötenbeck, J. Speculum scorbuticum. 1633.

HORN, Christopher. De auro medico philosophorum; id est, De illo occulto salutari, solari omnium mineralium, vegetalium, et animalium corporum, spiritu, seu balsamo vivifico, & maxume alexiterio, bezoartico, theriacali . . . dialogus scholasticus . . . Francofurti, Typis Wolffgangi Richteri, impensis Antonii Hummii, 1615.

[12], 88 p. 16 cm.   [5981]

Imperfect: first signature wrongly imposed.

—[The same.]
869–912 p., vol. 5. 20 cm. (*In* Zetzner, Lazarus, *ed.* Theatrum chemicum. Argentorati, 1659–61)
                                                           [5982]

Caption title.

—Hortulus medicus: Hippocraticus, spagyricus, Hermeticus, poeticus: studiosae philosophiae physicae juventuti adornatus . . . Cassellis, Ex Officina Typographica Mauritiana, opera Wilhelmi Wesselii, 1610.

[50] p.   20 cm.   [5983]

HORN, Georg [1620–1670] Arca Mosis; sive, Historia mundi. Quae complectitur primordia rerum naturalium omniumque artium ac scientiarum. Lugd. Bat. & Roterod., Ex Officina Hackiana, 1668.

[33], 220, [20] p.   14 cm.   [5984]

Added engraved title page dated 1669.
Imperfect: wormholes on p. 55–70.

—[The same.] . . . Lipsiae, Impensis fratrum Johann. & Frieder. Lüderwald, literis Johann-Erici Hahnii, 1675.

[35], 220, [23] p.   14 cm.   [5985]

Added engraved title page dated 1669.
Different setting of type.

—Historiae naturalis et civilis, ad nostra usque tempora, libri septem. Lugduni Batavorum, Apud Lothum de Haes, 1670.

[1], 19, 374 p.   14 cm.   [5986]

Added engraved title page.

—, *ed. See* Jābir ibn Ḥaiyān, al-Ṭarasūsī. Gebri Arabis Chimai. 1668; Schmitz, J. A. Medicinae practicae compendium. 1653, 1659.

HORN, Georg Konrad de [*fl.* 1689] *respondent. See* Albinus, B. Dissertatio medica inauguralis de salivatione mercuriali. 1689.

HORN, Henry [*fl.* 17 cent.] The perfect and compleat bel-man; or, The bel-man's diurnal. Being, above an hundred stanza's, for festival, and other common days. With good exhortations to well-minded people of all sorts, for their instruction. London, William Holeman, 1666.

[63] p.   14 cm.   [5987]

Imperfect: lower margin of p. [55] trimmed.

HORN, Joannes van. *See* Horne, Johannes van [1621–1670]

HORN, Johan von. *See* Hoorn, Johan von [1662–1724]

HORN, Johann Kaspar [*fl.* 1629] *respondent. See* Rolfinck, W., *praes.* Disputatio medica de melancholia. 1629.

HORNANUS, Adrianus Junius. *See* Junius, Hadrianus [1511–1575]

HORNE, Barthold [*fl.* 1664] *respondent. See* Tappe, J. *praes.* Disputatio inauguralis medica de ileo. 1664.

HORNE, Johannes van [1621–1670] Epistola de genitalibus. *In* Hoffmann, J. M. Dissertationes anatomico-physiologicae. 1685.

—Introduction methodique a la chirurgie. *In* Bonet, T., ed. Corps de medecine et de chirurgie. 1679.

—Μικροκοσμος; seu, Brevis manuductio ad historiam corporis humani . . . Lugduni Batavorum, Ex officina Jacobi Chouët, 1660.

[12], 126, [6] p.   13 cm.   [5988]

Added engraved title page.

—[The same.] ... Secundum edita. Lugduni Batavorum, Apud Jacobum Chouët [Typis Daniel Wilhelmi vander Boxe] 1662.

 [8], 142, [16] p. 13 cm. **[5989]**

Added engraved title page.

—[The same.] ... Tertium edita. Lugduni Batavorum, Apud Jacobum Voorn, 1665

 [10], 160, [16] p. table. 14 cm. **[5990]**

—[The same.] ... Quartum edita. Accessit huic editioni Epistola ad ... Guernerum Rolfincium ... perscripta, observationum in sexus utriusque partibus genitalibus specimen exhibens ... Lugduni Batavorum, 1675.

 [11], 156 p. 14 cm. **[5991]**

Added engraved title page.
Bound with Wedel, G. W. Theoremata medica. 1677

—[The same.] *In* Hoffmann, J. M. Dissertationes anatomico-physiologicae. 1685.

—Μιχϱοτεχνη; seu, Methodica ad chirurgiam introductio. Ed. alt. Lugd. Batav., Apud Gaasbekios, 1668.

 [16], 264, [12] p. 14 cm. **[5992]**

Added engraved title page.

—[Dutch tr.] Kort-begrijp der ontleed- en heelkonst ... Vertaald door Quiryn van Vissendiep. Leyden, Petrus vander Meersche, 1669.

 [16], 253, [1] p. table. 17 cm. **[5993]**

Added engraved title page.
Translation of Μιχϱοϰοσμος and Μιχϱοτεχνη.

—Novus ductus chyliferus. Nunc primum ... descriptus & eruditorum examini expositus ... Lugduni Batavorum, E typographeo Francisci Hackii, 1652.

 [38] p. illus. 19 cm. **[5994]**

—Waerschouwinge, aen alle lieff-hebbers der anatomie. Teegens de gepretendeerde weetenschap der selver, van ... Louijs de Bils ... onlangs uytgegeeven. Leyden, By Daniel ende Abraham van Gaasbeeck [ghedruckt by Daniel Willemsz. vander Boxe, incompagny met de weduwe van Willem Christiaans vander Boxe] 1660.

 [32] p. 20 cm. **[5995]**

Contains Lodewijk de Bils' Aan alle ware lief hebbers der anatomie.

—Miscellanea ... anatomica et chirurgica ... Basileae, Typis Georgii Deckeri, 1645.

 [8] p. 22 cm. **[5996]**

Diss. pro loco—Basel (R. Herzog, *respondent*)

—*praeses.* Dissertationis anatomicae de ductu chylifero, pars prior ... Lugduni Batavorum, Apud Johannem Elsevirium, 1660.

 [12] p. 21 cm. **[5997]**

Diss.—Leyden (A. Stephanides, *respondent*)

—, *ed. See* BOTALLO, L. Opera omnia. 1660; GALENUS. De ossibus. 1665.

—*See* BILS, L. de. Kort bericht over de waarschouwinge. 1660 [and] Responsio. 1661; DEUSING, A. Appendix ad Dissertationem de hepatis officio. 1661; SEVERINO, M. A. De la medecine efficace. 1668; STENO, N., *Bp.* Observationes anatomicae. 1662, 1680; SWAMMERDAM, J. Miraculum naturae. 1672, 1679, 1680.

—*See* also HEURNE, Johan van [1543–1601]

HORNE, OTTO VAN. *See* HEURNE, Otto van [1577–1652]

HORNECK, ANTHONY [1641–1697] *tr. See* GLANVILL, J. Saducismus triumphatus. 1681, 1700.

HORNICK, LUDWIG VON. *See* HÖRNIGK, Ludwig von [1600–1667]

HORNIUS, CHRISTIANUS. *See* HORN, Christopher.

HORNIUS, CHRISTOPHORUS. *See* HORN, Christopher.

HORNUNG, HENNING [*fl.* 1637] *respondent. See* KIEPER, A., *praeses.* Disputatio ... de fulmine. 1637.

HORNUNG, JOHANN MICHAEL [*fl.* 1662–1664] *respondent. See* SEBISCH, M. [1578–1674?] *praeses.* Problemata medica miscellanea. 1662.

HORNUNG, JOHANNES [*fl.* 1611–1625] De uroscopia fraudulenta discursus. Kurtzer Bericht von dem unvollkommenen und betrüglichen Urtheil des menschlichen Borns oder Harns ... Herborn [Christoph Corvinus] 1611.

 41, [2] p. 18 cm. **[5998]**

Printer's name supplied from Benzing (A), p. 191.

—Notwendiger chirurgischer Unterricht, wie man allerley Brandtschäden, von Fewer, glüenden Eisen, Höltzern, heissen Oelen, und Wassern. Item von

Büchsenpulvern, Donnerstraalen und ander vergleichen Verletzungen verursacht, unnd dem menschlichen Leib zugefügt, gründtlich erkennen, und ... curiren soll ... Nürnberg, Gedruckt bey Simon Halbamayern, 1622.

144 p. illus. 16 cm. [5999]

With this are bound: Horst, Gregor. Kurtzer Bericht von den rothen Ruhr. 1622. — Schöpf, J. Ulmischer Paradiss Garten. 1622.

—ed. Cista medica, qua in epistolae clarissimorum Germaniae medicorum, familiares, & in re medica, tam quoad Hermetica & chymica, quam etiam Galenica principia, lectu jucundae & utiles, cum diu reconditis experimentis asservantur. Potissimum ex posthuma ... Sigismundi Schnitzeri ... bibliotheca ... elaboratae ... Noribergae, Sumptibus Simonis Halbmayri [1626?]

[24], 516 p. illus. 19 cm. [6000]

Preface by Gregor Horst.

HOROSCO, DIEGO DE VALVERDE. *See* VALVERDE DE HOROZCO, Diego de [17th cent.]

HORREL in de wacht; ofte, Samen-spraeck tusschen een Professor van Leyden, en een Doctor van Amsterdam. Leyden, Jan de Koussenaer, 1677.

22 p. 16 cm. [6001]

HORSCHT, JACOBUS. *See* HORST, Jakob [1537-1600]

HORST, GEORG [*fl.* 1663-1666] *respondent.* Dissertatio inauguralis de siriasi ... Basileae, Typis Joh. Jacobi Deckeri [1665]

[8] p. 20 cm. [6002]

Diss. — Basel.

HORST, GREGOR [1578-1636] Operum medicorum tomus primus [-tertius] ... cura Gregorii Horstii, Junioris ... Norimbergae, Sumptibus Johann. Andreae & Wolffgangi Jun. haeredum Endterorum, 1660.

3 v. in 1. port. 36 cm. [6003]

Added engraved title page.

Imperfect: first 6 prelim. leaves (including title page, half title, and added engraved title page) of vol. 1, and 7th prelim. leaf and p. 215-216 and 431-432 of vol. 2 wanting; supplied in photocopy from the University of Michigan Library. Lower corners of leaves torn away in latter part of vol. 3 affecting the text from p. 229 to end.

Partial contents. — vol. 1. Institutiones medicae. Dissertationes medicae quatuor. — vol. 2. Observationes et epistolae medicinales tertia hac editione in ordinem redactae et auctae cura Jo. Danielis

Horstii. — vol. 3. Centuria problematus Θεραπευτικῶν. Exercitationes de febribus quatuor. Prognosis febrium. De tuenda sanitate studiosorum liber 2. Consilium dysentericum. Angeli Salae Tractatus de peste, ex Gallico sermone ab authore Latinitate donatus. Herbarium Horstianum. Institutiones physicae. Opusculum de vite vinifera ... conscriptum ... a Jacobo Horstio. Oratio funebris, qua authori parentavit J. D. Dieterich. J. B. Hebenstreitti Horstias, seu, Familiae Horstianae descriptio.

—[The same.] Operum medicorum tomus ... Goudae, Sumptibus Gulielmi vander Hoeve, 1661.

3 v. port. 25 cm. [6004]

Vol. 3 has imprint: Amstelodami, Sumptibus Pieter La Burgh, 1661.

Added engraved title page.

—Bericht von der hitzigen Kranckheit, sonsten auch die ungarische Fiebersucht, Fleckenfieber, oder Haupt-Schwachheit genand. Mit angehencktem Rath wider die Urschlechten oder Rinds-Blattern und Röteln ... an Tag gegeben von D. Joh. Daniele Horstio ... Franckfurt, Drucks und Verlags Balthasar Christoph Wusts, 1663.

[18], 150 p. 15 cm. [6005]

—Büchlein von dem Schorbock ... Mit angehencktem Rath in Pest Zeiten. Giessae, Typis Nicolai Hampelii, 1611.

[12], 148 p. 15 cm. [6006]

Imperfect: lower margin of title page mutilated.

—[The same.] ... Auffs newe durchsehen und vermehret. Giessen, Gedruckt durch Nicolaum Hampelium, 1615.

[12], 196 p. 16 cm. [6007]

"Tractälein von dem Schurbauch, beschrieben von ... Johann Weyern ...": p. 163-196.

—Büchlein von dem Schorbock ...

[255]-445 p. 14 cm. (*In* Viel-vergröster und hellerpolirter Schorbocks-Spiegel. Nürnberg, 1659) [6008]

Half title.

—Centuria problematum medicorum Θεραπευτικων, in qua gravissimorum affectuum cognitio & curatio juxta principia Hippocratica, Galenica & spagyrica pulchre deducitur ... Partim in illustri Witeberga anno MDCVIII partim in inclyta Giessa anno subsequenti publice disputandi causa proposita ... Witebergae, Sumptibus Clementis Bergeri, typis vero Johann. Schmidt, 1610.

[16], 404, [24] p. 16 cm. [6009]

—[The same.] ... Ed. nova, ab ipso autore ... aucta. Accessit Consultationum et epistolarum medicinalium de re medica varia liber tertius ... Noribergae, Prostat apud Wolfgang. Endter, typis Ulmanis, 1636.

[24], 240 (i.e. 530), [14] p.   21 cm.   **[6010]**

Imperfect: p. 197-198 (i.e. p. 297-298) mutilated.

Bound with *his* Observationum medicinalium ... libri IV. priores. Ulmae, 1628.

—De natura humana libri duo, quorum prior de corporis structura, posterior de anima tractat, ultimo elaborati, commentariis aucti ... Cum praefatione de anatomia vitali & mortua ... Francof. ad Moenum, Typis Erasmi Kempferi, sumptibus Clem. Bergeri, 1612.

[16], 510, [14] p.   illus., plates, port.   21 cm.

[6011]

With this is bound *his* Ἐξετασεων παθολογικων De morbis ... liber. 1612.

—De tuenda sanitate studiosorum et literatorum libri duo ... Giessae, Typis & sumptibus Casparis Chemlini, 1615.

[24], 235, [2] p.   14 cm.   **[6012]**

—[The same.] ... Ed. 2. corr. Giessae, Typis & sumptibus Casparis Chemlini, 1617.

[24], 377 p.   14 cm.   **[6013]**

—[The same.] ... Ed. nova, multis additionibus, inprimisque remediis selectis ... aucta. Marpurgi Cattorum, Typis ac sumptibus Casparis Chemlini, 1628.

[12], 292, [1] p.   15 cm.   **[6014]**

Errata: p. [1] at end.

—Disputationum medicarum viginti, continentes universae medicinae delineationem locis Hippocraticis & Galenicis ut plurimum illustratam ... Accesserunt ... Jacobi Horstii ... disputationes theoreticae & practicae. Wittebergae, Excudebat Joann. Schmidt, sumptibus Clementis Bergeri, 1609.

565, [19] p.   17 cm.   **[6015]**

Contains 20 Wittenberg and 21 Helmstädt theses.

—[The same.] Medicarum institutionum compendium, disputationibus universae medicinae delineationem, locis Hipp. & Galenicis ut plurimum illustratam, continens: olim in Academia Wittebergensi studiosae juventuti propositum. Accesserunt ... Jacobi Horstii ... disputationes theoreticae &

practicae. Ed nova, cui adjecta est Methodus medendi Ferneliana enucleata, & controversiis illustrata ... Wittebergae, Sumptibus Bergerianis, typis haeredum Christiani Tham, 1630.

[14], 565, [19] p.   16 cm.   **[6016]**

Imperfect: The Methodus medendi wanting.

—Gregor. Horstii D. Dissertatio de causis similitudinis et dissimilitudinis in foetu, respectu parentum, publice ... dicta, cum Johanni Huldaricho Streittero ... laurea doctoralis ... ab eodem IIX Decembr. anno M DC XVII imponeretur, cui annexa est resolutio quaestionis de diverso partus tempore ... Giessae, Ex officina typographica Casparis Chemlini, 1618.

[4], 59 p.   20 cm.   **[6017]**

—Dissertationes medicae tres De natura amoris, De natura thermarum, De causis similitudinis et dissimilitudinis in foetu, respectu parentum, antehac in Academia Gissensi propositae et discussae, quibus annexae sunt resolutiones illustrium quarundam quaestionum medicarum. Marpurgi, Ex officina typographica Casparis Chemlini, 1627.

[56] p.; [63] p.; [4], 59 p.   20 cm.   **[6018]**

Parts [2] and [3] have special title pages with imprint: Giessae, Ex officina typographica Casparis Chemlini, 1618.

With this is bound Müller, Jakob. Disquisitio medica. 1627.

—[The same.] ... Ed. nov. Marpurgi, Casparus Chemlinus, 1642.

[179] p.   21 cm.   **[6019]**

"Dissertatio de natura thermarum" has special title page.

— Ἐξετάσεων παθολογικῶν, De morbis, eorumque causis ac symptomatibus liber, cum declaratione quaestionum controversarum. Accesserunt ejusdem De febribus cognoscendi et curandis exercitationes. Olim in academia ... proposita, jam autem ab autore vicissim revisae. Marpurgi Cattorum, Typis ac sumptibus Casparis Chemlini, 1629.

[24], 471 p.   16 cm.   **[6020]**

Contains 11 Giessen and Wittenberg theses.

"Appendix continens Prognosin febrium potissimum continuarum & malignarum earumque accidentium. Juxta textum Hippocraticum declaratam, & tribus exercitationibus propositam" (p. 373-471) is a reprint of the Prognosis febrium published separately in 1622, containing 3 Giessen theses by Ludwig von Hörnigk, Franciscus Monhemius, and Johann Nicolaus Baumann and including the Greek text of Coacae praenotiones nos. 1-160, with commentary by Horst.

— Ἐξετάσεων παθολογικῶν, De morbis, eorumque causis liber, cum declaratione controversiarum, in gratiam studiosae juventutis in Academia Giessena, per semestre vernale anno M. DCXII. propositus. Giessae, Apud Casparem Chemlinum, 1612.

    [16], 158 p.   21 cm.   [6021]
    Contains six Giessen theses.
    Bound with *his* De natura humana libri duo. 1612.

— Kurtze nohtwendige [sic] Bericht, erstlich, von den Urschlechten oder Kinds-Blattern, wie auch Masern, Röteln, Rotesucht oder Kindsflecken, Zum andern von den roten Ruhr. Zum dritten von der in Anno 622 ... miteinreissenden newen Hauptschwachheit. Zum vierdten, wie man sich in einreissenden Pestzeiten zu verhalten habe ... Giessen, Caspar Chemlin, 1624.

    [8], 137, [12] p.   16 cm.   [6022]

— Kurtzer Bericht von den Urschlechten oder Kindsblattern, wie auch Masern, Röteln oder Kindsflecken ... Giessen, Caspar Chemlin, 1621.

    56 p.   17 cm.   [6023]

— Kurtzer Bericht von der rothen Ruhr, erstlichen dem gemeinen Mann zur Nachrichtung vor etlichen Jahren zu Giessen Deutsch beschrieben ... Jetzo aber ... vermehret ... Ulm, Gedruckt durch Johann Medern, 1622.

    [2], 44, [1] p.   16 cm.   [6024]
    Bound with Hornung, J. Notwendiger chirurgischer Unterricht. 1622.

— [The same.] ... Ulm, Gedruckt durch Johann-Sebastian Medern, 1634.

    37 p.   16 cm.   [6025]

— Observationum medicinalium singularium libri quatuor I. De febribus. II. De morbis capitis. III. De morbis pectoris. IV. De morbis viscerum concoctionis. Singulari et ad praxin accommodata methodo hactenus in Academia Giessena suis auditoribus propositi, jam ... revisi, casibus novis additis plurimum aucti, & ad praelum ab autore ... elaborati. His accessit epistolarum et consultationum medicarum, a clariss. Germaniae medicis potissimum, & aliis etiam cum autore communicatarum ... Ulmae Suevorum, Ex officina typographica Jonae Saurii, 1625.

    [16], 584 p.   illus., port.   21 cm.   [6026]
— Copy 2.

With this is bound *his* Observationum medicinalium ... libri quatuor posteriores. Ulmae Suevorum, 1628.

— [The same.] ... Ed. nova: cui auctuarium Pharmaceuticar. exercitationum, Galenicum, & spagyricum, recens additum ... Ulmae, Typis Saurianis, 1628.

    [16], 584 p.   illus., port.   21 cm.   [6027]
    Part [1] is a reissue of the 1625 edition with new, engraved title page.
    Part [2] (Pharmaceuticarum exercitationum decas) with special title page, bound as fourth item in this volume.
    With this are bound *his*: Observationum medicinalium singularium libri quatuor posteriores. 1637; Centuria problematum medicorum. 1636; Prognosis febrium. 1622.

— Observationum medicinalium singularium libri quatuor posteriores. I. De morbis mulierum. II. De morbis contagiosis & malignis. III. De doloribus partium externarum. IV. De chirurgicis quibusdam casibus. His accessit epistolarum & consultationum medicinalium, a cl. Germaniae medicis potissimum, & aliis cum autore communicatarum liber secundus ... Ulmae Suevorum, Typis Saurianis, 1628.

    [32], 643, [3] p.   21 cm.   [6028]
    Engraved title page.
    Bound with copy 2 of *his* Observationum medicinalium ... libri quatuor. 1625.

— [The same.] ... Ed. nova completa ... Heilbrunnae, Typis Christoph. Kraus, 1631.

    [24], 652 p.   21 cm.   [6029]
    "Complementum ad librum secundum epistolarum et consultationum medicinalium, continens novem superstites sectiones, in prima editione omissas ..." (p. [513]–642) has special title page.

— [The same.] ... Liber secundus. Ed. nova completa ... Norimbergae, Typis Wolffgangi Endteri, 1637.

    [24], 652 p.   21 cm.   [6030]
    A reissue of the 1631 edition with title pages and dedicatory epistles reset.
    Bound with *his* Observationum medicinalium ... libri IV. priores. 1628.

— Prognosis febrium potissimum continuarum et malignarum, juxta textum Hippocraticum in principio Coacarum praenotionum ... Gissae Hessorum, Typis Nicolai Hampelii, 1622.

    [8], 52 p.   20 cm.   [6031]
    Contains 3 Giessen theses by L. von Hörnigk, F. Monhemius and J. N. Baumann.
    Includes the Greek text of Coacae praenotiones nos. 1–160, with commentary by Horst.

—[The same.] . . . Ed. II. corr. Gissae Hessorum, Typis Nicolai Hampelii, 1622.

[8], 52 p.   21 cm.   [6032]

Mainly page for page like the first edition but with slight typographical differences and textual alterations. The Corrigenda are omitted on p. [8], but are not corrected in the text.

Bound with *his* Observationum medicinalium . . . libri IV. priores. Ulmae, Typis Saurianis, 1628.

—Σκεψις. Physica medica de casu quodam . . . singulari, ex quo subsequentia problemata deducuntur. I. An corpus humanum post mortem aliquot septimanis colore . . . floridum . . . absque . . . putredine incipiente naturaliter . . . durare possit? II. An fluxus sanguinis cadaveris humani occisi tam in principio coedis, quam post aliquot septimanas praesentiam interfectoris indicet? Accessit brevis responsio ad eundem casum a facultate medica Viennensis Academiae conscripta. Witebergae, Typis Meisnerianis, impensis Clement. Bergeri, 1606.

[8], 125, [1] p.   15 cm.   [6033]

" . . . De mixtis in genere . . . respondente Francisco Omichio . . . anno M.D.CIII . . .": p. 77-104; " . . . De animae facultatibus . . . Publice . . . an. M.D.CIII . . . proposita, respondente Paulo Claus . . .": p. 105-125.

—[The same.] Σκέψις de naturali conservatione et cruentatione cadaverum, ubi ex casu quodam admirando . . . duo problemata . . . deducuntur. Accessit brevis responsio ad eundem casum Facultatis medica Viennensis Academiae conscripta. Ed. nova . . . Exercitatione de somno et somniis aucta. Witebergae, Typis M. Georgii Mulleri, sumptibus Clement. Bergeri, 1608.

[16], III p.   17 cm.   [6034]

" . . . De mixtis in genere . . . respondente Francisco Omichio . . . anno M.DC.III . . .": p. 58-78; " . . . De animae facultatibus . . . Publice . . . M.DC.III . . . proposita, respondente Paulo Claus . . .": p. 78-94; " . . . Exercitatio de somno et somniis. Publice . . . anno M.DC.VI . . . proposita, respondente Daniele Langio . . .": p. 94-III.

Bound with Martini, G. Commentatiuncula. 1621.

—Dissertatio de natura amoris, in . . . Academiae Giessenae . . . proposita, cum tres . . . viri juvenes artis medicae laurea doctorali . . . IV. Non. April. anno M D C X I . . . coronarentur. Additis resolutionibus quaestionum Dnn. candidatorum, de cura furoris amatorii, de philtris, atque de pulsu amantium. Giessae, Excudebat Casparus Chemlinus, 1611.

[64] p.   19 cm.   [6035]

Program—Giessen (with the responses of C. Bilitzer, L. Jungermann and M. Schönwalder)

—Dissertatio de natura thermarum, in . . . Academiae Giessenae . . . proposita, cum . . . Johanni Hempelio . . . xv Cal. Sept. An. M. D C. XIV imponeretur. Cui annexa est resolutio quaestionis, de modo, quo mineralium virtutes aquis subterraneis communicantur. Giessae, Ex officina typographica Casparis Chemlini, 1618.

[63] p.   19 cm.   [6036]

Program—Giessen, 1614 (with the response of J. Hempel)

—*praeses.* De natura motus animalis et voluntarii exercitatio singularis, ex principiis physicis, medicis, geometricis & architectonicis deducta . . . Giessae, Ex typographia Casparis Chemlini, 1617.

[26] p.   illus.   19 cm.   [6037]

Diss.—Giessen (J. Müller, *respondent*)

—Disputatio de morbis puerorum juxta Hippocratem . . . Giessae, Ex officina libraria Casparis Chemlini, 1618.

[11] p.   19 cm.   [6038]

Diss.—Giessen (J. G. Obele, *respondent*)

—Problematum medicorum θεραπευτιχων decades priores quinque . . . Wittebergae, Typis Cratonianis, per Joan Gorman, 1608.

[112] p.   21 cm.   [6039]

Contains 5 dissertations each with special title page.

Diss.—Wittenberg (*Respondents*: J. J. Anomeous, D. Freywaldt, J. Köppe, W. Schaller and M. Walther)

—Theses medicae de venae sectione, ex lib. 2. De meth. med. Joh. Fernelii deductae, et controversis quaestionibus de eadem materia illustratae . . . Ulma, Typis Johannis Mederi, 1622.

[2], 30 p.   18 cm.   [6040]

Diss.—Ulm, Gymnasium (M. Merk, *respondent*)

—Tractatus de scorbuto; seu, De magnis Hippocratis lienibus, Pliniique stomacace scelotyrbe . . . Giessae Hassorum, Excudebat Nicolaus Hampelius, 1609.

[8], 69, [3] p.   21 cm.   [6041]

Contains 2 dissertations each with special title page.

Diss.—Giessen (*Respondents*: J. Degenhardus and Ph. Weber)

—*See* ABANO, P. D'. Conciliator enucleatus. 1615, 1621; GOCKEL, E. Enchiridion medico-practicum de peste. 1669; HORNUNG, J., *ed.* Cista medica. 1626?

—, *ed. See* DONATI, M. De historia medica mirabili libri sex. 1613; HORST, J. Herbarium Horstianum. 1630.

—, *tr. See* SALA, A. Tractatus, de praeservatione . . . pestis. 1641.

HORST, GREGOR [1626–1661] *ed. See* HORST, G. [1578–1636] Operum medicorum tomus primus [-tertius] 1660, 1661.

HORST, GREGOR [*fl.* 1677] *respondent.* Dissertationem hanc inauguralem de mania . . . submittit Gregorius Horstius . . . Gissae, Typis viduae Friderici Kargeri, 1677.

    20 p.   19 cm.   **[6042]**

Diss.—Giessen.

HORST, JAKOB [1537–1600] Disputationes catholicae de rebus secundum & praeter naturam. *See* HORST, G. [1578–1636] Disputationum medicarum viginti. 1609 [and] Medicarum institutionum compendium. 1630.

—Herbarium Horstianum; seu, De selectis plantis et radicibus libri duo, olim medicinae candidatis in Academia Julia anno M.D.LXXXVII a . . . Jacobo Horstio . . . propositi, in compendium redacti . . . pluribusque simplicibus . . . aucti . . . per Gregor. Horstium . . . Accessit praedicti Dn. D. Jacobi Horstii Opusculum de vite vinifera . . . Marpurgi, Typis & impensis Casparis Chemlini, 1630.

    [8], 414 p.   17 cm.   **[6043]**

The Opusculum de vite vinifera has special title page.

—*See* HORST, G. [1578–1636] Operum medicorum tomus primus [-tertius] 1660, 1661; LIDDEL, D. Ars medica. 1628.

HORST, JOHANN DANIEL [1616–1685] Epistolarum medicinalium decas . . . Francofurti, Apud Wilhelmum Serlinum & Georgium Fickwirthum, 1656.

    86 p.   20 cm.   **[6044]**

—Judicium de chirurgia infusoria Jo. Danielis Majoris . . . [Frankfurt am Main] Apud Georg Fickwirt, 1665.

    118 p.   15 cm.   **[6045]**

Imprint partly supplied from BMC.
"D. Joh. Danielis Majoris . . . Prodromus inventae a se chirurgiae infusoriae . . .": p. 17–63; —"Epistola . . . Jo. Tackii . . .": p. 95–108.

—Kurtze Beschreibung der Sauer-Brunnen zu Langen-Schwalbach und Dönningstein; wie auch dess Embser- Verstädter- Brodel- und Wissbades.

Franckfurt, In Verlegung Georg Fickwirths, 1659.

    [21], 190 p.   17 cm.   **[6046]**

With this are bound: Geilfus, J. G. Unterricht vom Sauer- und Brodel Brunnen. 1662; Mayer, M. Kurtze Beschreibung [1666?]

—Kurtzer Bericht vom Saur- und Brodel-Bronnen [sic] zu Langen-Schwalbach . . . Franckfurt am Mayn, 1680.

    16 p.   16 cm.   **[6047]**

Imperfect: outer margins of p. 4–6 trimmed.

—Manuductio ad medicinam, in Academia Marpurgensi studiosae juventuti ante annos vicenos primum praelecta . . . Ed. 4. . . . Ulmae, Typ. & impens. Balth. Kühnen, 1660.

    [12], 242, [29] p.   front., (port.).   14 cm.

                                  [6048]

Added engraved title page.

—Observationum anatomicarum decas. Additae sunt epistolae, quibus singularia scitu digna, lactearum nempe thoracicarum, & vasorum lymphaticorum natura, embryonisque per os nutritio . . . exponuntur. Francofurti, Apud Wilhelmum Serlinum & Georgium Fickwirthum, 1656.

    34 p.   20 cm.   **[6049]**

The Epistolae is not present.

—Pharmacopoeia Galeno-chemica, catholica post Renodaeum, Quercetanum, aliosque . . . adornata selectissimisque medicamentorum compositionibus, experimentis, & observationibus . . . adaucta. Accesserunt Institutiones pharmaceuticae . . . Francofurti ad Moenum, Impensis Joannis Godofredi Schönwetteri, 1651.

    2 v. in 1.   front.   35 cm.   **[6050]**

Imperfect: frontispiece wanting.

—,*ed. See* HORST, G. [1578–1636] Bericht von der hitzigen Kranckheit, 1663 [and] Operum medicorum tomus primus [-tertius] 1660, 1661; RIVIÈRE, L. Opera medica universa. 1669, 1674, 1679, 1686, 1687; SCHRÖDER, J. Pharmacopoeia medico-chymica. 1677, 1681; ZACCHIA, P. Quaestionum medico-legalium tomi tres. 1666, 1673–74, 1688.

—*See* KOLHANS, T. L. Litterae . . . de spiritu animali. 1658; SINIBALDI, G. B. Geneanthropeiae. 1669; STRAUSS, L. Resolutio casus Mussipontani foetus extra uterum in abdomine retenti. 1662.

HORTA, GARCIA DA. *See* ORTA, Garcia d' [1501 or 2?–1568]

HORTENSIUS, Ludovicus. *See* Du Gardin, Louis [*fl.* 1617–*ca.* 1631]

HORTI Beaumontiani exoticarum plantarum catalogus. 1690. *See* [Kiggelaer, F.]

HORTULANUS. Practica vera alkimica . . . Parisiis probata & excerpta, sub anno Domini 1358 . . .

912–934 p., vol. 4. 20 cm. (*In* Zetzner, Lazarus, *ed.* Theatrum chemicum. Argentorati, 1659–61) [6051]
Caption title.

HOSPICE DE LA CHARITÉ, Lyons. *See* Hôpital de la charité, Lyons.

HOSPITAL GENERAL DE MADRID. *See* Obregón, B. de. Instruccion de enfermeros. 1664.

HOSPITAL MAGGIORE DI COMO. Insruttione [sic], et ordini per il buon governo dell' Hospital Maggiore di Como, Et memoria delli carichi, a quali e tenuto lo stesso hospitale . . . Como, Nicolo Caprani [1650?]
[1], 82, [39] p. 21 cm. [6052]

HOSPITAL ZUM HEILIGEN GEIST, Nuremberg. *See* Pfann, J. Biblische Emblemata und Figuren. 1626.

HOSPITALE MAGGIORE DI MILANO. *See* Ospedale maggiore di Milano.

HOSPITAUX GENERAUX . . . Pour l'examen des pauvres . . . Reglemens des directeurs de l'hospital general . . . Paris, 1680.
8 p. 24 cm. [6053]
Caption title.

HÔTEL-DIEU DE LYON. Au bureau de l'Hôtel-Dieu . . . de Lyon, tenu le . . . septiéme jour du mois de May 1690 . . . [Lyons, 1690?]
[10] p. 23 cm. [6054]

—Au bureau du Grand Hôtel-Dieu . . . de Lion . . . le . . . 15. jour du mois de Janvier 1696 . . . [Lyons, 1696?]
[2] p. 23 cm. [6055]

—La forme de la direction et oeconomie du Grand Hostel-Dieu de Nostre Dame de Pitié du pont du Rhosne de la ville de Lyon. Lyon, Jean Jullieron, 1646.
[20], 116, 4, 18, 2, 24 p. plate. 23 cm. [6056]

—[The same.] . . . Lyon, 1661.
[12], 116, 4, 10, 2 p. illus. 23 cm. [6057]

—Reglement pour la pharmacie. Arrété au bureau de l'Hôtel-Dieu . . . de Lyon . . . le dix-neufviéme Mars 1690 . . . [Lyons, 1690?]
[4] p. 23 cm. [6058]

HÔTEL-DIEU DE NOSTRE-DAME DE PITIÉ. *See* Hôtel-Dieu de Lyon.

[**HOTMAN,** Antoine, 1525?–1596] Traicté de la dissolution du mariage par l'impuissance & froideur de l'homme, ou de la femme. 2. ed., rev. & augm. Paris, Robert Estienne, 1610.
52 ll. 17 cm. [6059]
Imperfect: ll. 29–32 wanting, supplied in photocopy from McGill Univ., Osler Library.

HOTTINGER, Johann Heinrich [1680–1756] Dissertatio de crystallis . . . Tiguri, Ex typographeo Bodmeriano, 1698.
[1], 44 p. plate. 19 cm. [6060]

—*respondent.* Dissertatio inauguralis medica de fastidio medicamentorum . . . Basileae, Literis Jacobi Bertschii [1698]
[25] p. 20 cm. [6061]
Diss. — Basel.

HOTTINGER, Salomon [1649–1713] *praeses.* Αϱτολογια; seu, Disputationum de pane hujus natura usu legitimo, et noxio abusu, prima . . . Tiguri, Typis Bodmerianis [1696]
[24] p. 19 cm. [6062]
Diss. — Zürich (H. Steiner, *respondent*)

HOULLIER, Jacques [*d.* 1562] Jacobi Hollerii . . . De morbis internis libri II: illustrati doctissimis ejusdem auctoris scholiis & observationibus non antea excusis: deinde Ludovici Dureti . . . in eundem adversariis: & Ant. Valetii . . . exercitationibus luculentis. Ejusdem Hollerii De febribus, De peste, De remediis κατὰ τόπους in Galeni libros, De materia chirurgica. His recens accessit Therapia puerperarum, auctore Joan. Le Bon . . . Omnia multo correctius, quam antea unquam edita. Francofurdi, Apud Nicolaum Hoffmannum, sumptib. Jonae Rhodii, 1603.
2 v. 13 cm. [6063]

Vol. [2] contains 3 works, the first two of which have special title pages with imprint: Francofurdi, Apud Nicolaum Hoffmannum, impensis haeredum Petri Fischeri, 1603.

Contents. — [v. 1] De morbis internis liber I. De morbis internis, febrium historiam & curationem continens, liber II. De peste libellus — [v. 2] Ad libros Galeni De compositione medicamentorum χατὰ τόπους, periochae VIII. Nunc denuo multo quam antea unquam castigatiores editae. De materia chirurgica libri III. Nunc multo correctius, quam antea umquam in lucem editi. Therapia puerperarum, auctore Joanne Le Bon (p. 477-518)

—Jacobi Hollerii ... Omnia opera practica. Doctissimis ejusdem scholiis & observationibus illustrata: deinde Lud. Dureti ... in eundem enarrationibus, annotationibus, & Antonii Valetii ... exercitationibuc lucuplentis. Accessit etiam ... Therapia puerperarum J. Le Bon ... Genevae, Jacobus Stoer, 1623.

[16], 584, 315 (i.e. 317), [18] p. 24 cm. [6064]

Combines Houllier's text and scholia, as edited by Valet and published in Paris in 1577 under title "De morbis internis libri II," with Duret's fuller commentary on De morbis internis alone, which was edited by R. Chartier and published in Paris in 1611.

—[The same.] ... Genevae, Apud Petrum & Jacobum Chouët, 1635.

[24], 584, 315 (i.e. 317), [18] p. 24 cm. [6065]

Different setting of type.

Contents as in the 1623 Geneva edition, except that a note to the reader and 4 p. of errata have been added.

—[The same.] ... Cum ... observationibus D. Joannis Hautin ... Accessit etiam ... Therapeia puerperarum Joan. Le Bon ... Parisiis, Apud Jacobum Dallin, 1664.

[12], 693 (i.e. 657), [12] p. 37 cm. [6066]

—Jacobi Hollerii ... Ad libros Galeni De compositione medicamentorum χατὰ τόπους periochae VIII. Nunc denuo multo quam antea unquam castigatiores editae. Francofurdi, Apud Nicolaum Hoffmannum, impensis haeredum Petri Fischeri, 1603.

[1]-161 p., vol. 2. 13 cm. (In his De morbis internis ... De remedii χατὰ τόπους in Galeni libros ... Francofurdi, 1603) [6067]

—Ludovici Dureti ... Commentarius in Jacobi Hollerii ... librum De morbis internis auctoris scholiis illustratum. Nunc primum publicavit & recensuit Renatus Charterius ... Parisiis, Ex Officina Plantiniana, apud Adrianum Perier, 1611.

[12], 716 (i.e. 654), [2] p. 23 cm. [6068]

"Theoremata Lud. Dureti": p. 689-703.

"Singulares aliquot Hollerii observationes, quae ad consilia curandi pertinent": p. 703-[717]

—[The same.] Jacobi Hollerii ... De morbis internis liber, auctoris scholiis illustratus, et Ludovici Dureti ... scholia [sic] amplissimis nunc primum prodeuntibus auctus. Has Renatus Charterius ... recensuit, publicavit. Cum indice rerum ... Parisiis, Ex Officina Plantiniana, apud Adrianum Perier, 1611.

[12], 716 (i.e. 654), [14] p. 22 cm. [6069]

Another issue with new title page and the addition of an index rerum.

—[De materia chirurgica. French.] In Tagault, J. La chirurgie. 1629, 1645.

—[Italian tr.] In Croce, G. A. della. Cirugia universale e perfetta. 1605, 1661; Tagault, J. Institutione di cirugia ... distinta in libri cinque. 1607.

—[Spanish tr.] Tratado de la materia de cirurgia. Compuesto por Jacobo Hollerio ... interpretado por Geronymo Murillo ... Y aora nuevamente en esta ultima impression traduzidas las recatas [sic] de latin en romance por ... Antonio Pablo Serrano ... Valencia, Miguel Sorolla, a costa Juan Antonio Tavano [1624]

95, [5] ll. 15 cm. (Part [2] in Galenus. Therapeutica methodo ... en lo que toca cirugia ... Añadido un tratado de Jacobo Holerio. Valencia, 1624) [6070]

—[The same.] ... Valencia, Miguel Sorrolla, a costa de Juan Antonio Tavano [n. d.] [i.e. Zaragoça, Juan de Ybar, 1651]

95, [5] ll. 15 cm. (Part [2] in Galenus. Therapeutica, methodo ... en lo que toca a cirurgia ... Añadido un tratado de Jacobo Hollerio. Zaragoça, 1651) [6071]

Different setting of type.

—Jacobi Hollerii ... In Aphorismos Hippocratis commentarii septem. Recens per Joan. Liebautium ... in lucem editi: ejusdemque scholiis doctissimis illustrati ... [Genevae] Apud Petrum & Jacobum Chouët, 1613.

[8], 472, [14] ll. 18 cm. [6072]

Contains the text of the Aphorismi in Greek and in the Latin translation by G. Plancy.

The commentary is edited from a manuscript of Houllier's lectures which was given to Liébault by Alexis Gaudinus, a student of Houllier. Liébault's scholia are drawn in part from the lectures of Louis Duret. Cf. Liébault's dedication, leaves [5-6]

"Spuriorum aphorismorum Hippocratis liber unus, ceu . . . liber octavus Aphorismorum": leaves 463-472.

Reprinted nearly page for page (with the errata corrected) from the 1582 Paris edition.

—[The same.] . . . Genevae, Apud Petrum & Jacobum Chouët, 1620.

[8], 472, [14] ll.   18   cm.   [6073]

Different setting of type.

—[The same.] . . . Genevae, Apud Petrum & Jacobum Chouët, 1632.

[8], 472, [14] ll.   18   cm.   [6074]

Different setting of type.

—[The same.] . . . Genevae, Ex typographia Petri Chouët senioris, 1646.

[8], 472, [14] ll.   17   cm.   [6075]

Different setting of type.

—[The same.] . . . Ed. novissima. Genevae, Sumptibus Leonardi Chouët, 1675.

[8], 472, [14] ll.   18   cm.   [6076]

Different setting of type.

—See UFFENBACH, P. Thesaurus chirurgicae. 1610.

HOUPPEVILLE, GUILLAUME DE [d. 1726] La generation de l'homme par le moyen des oeufs, & la production des tumeurs impures par l'action des sels, défendues par Eudoxe & Philotime, contre Antigene . . . Rouen, Jacques Lucas, 1676.

[20], 205, [2] p.   16   cm.   [6077]

—La guerison du cancer au sein. Rouen, La veuve de Loüis Behourt & Guillaume Behourt fils, 1693.

[16], 256, [10] p.   15   cm.   [6078]

—Another issue, with date changed from M.DC.XCIII. to M.DC.XCIII.I.   [6079]

HOUPREGHT, JOHN FREDERICK [fl. 17th cent.] comp. Aurifontina chymica; or, A collection of fourteen small treatises concerning the first matter of philosophers, for the discovery of their (hitherto so much concealed) mercury . . . London, William Cooper, 1680.

[22], 272, [4] p.   12   cm.   [6080]

Imperfect: sig. A1 (blank?) wanting.

Probably compiled and edited by William Cooper, the publisher. Cf. Ferguson (A), Vol. I, p. 58.

Includes treatises by Bernardus Trevirensis, N. Flamel, R. Lull, G. Ripley.

HOUTEN, FREDERIK VAN [fl. 1686] respondent. Disputatio medica inauguralis, de angina . . . Ultrajecti, Ex officina Francisci Halma, 1686.

II, [1] p.   22   cm.   [6081]

Diss.—Utrecht.

HOVIUS, BERNARD [fl. 1700] respondent. Disputatio medica inauguralis de hydrope in genere . . . Lugduni Batavorum, Apud Abrahamum Elzevier, 1700.

[16] p.   21   cm.   [6082]

Diss.—Leyden.

HOW, GEORGIUS. See HOWE, George.

HOW, WILLIAM [1620-1656] ed. See L'OBEL, M. de. Stirpium illustrationes. 1655.

HOWE, GEORGE [b. 1654 or 5-1710] respondent. Disputatio medica inauguralis de circulatione sanguinis in foetu humano, ejusque nutritione, & meconio . . . Lugduni Batavorum, Apud viduam & heredes Johannis Elsevirii, 1679.

[12] p.   23   cm.   [6083]

Diss.—Leyden.

HOWELL, JAMES [1594?-1666] See A HERMETICALL BANQUET. 1652; RUMSEY, W. Organon salutis. 1657, 1659, 1664.

HOYER, JOHANN GEORG [1663-1738] respondent. See HOFFMANN, F. [1660-1742] praeses. Disputatio inauguralis medica, de saliva. 1694.

HRABANUS MAGNENTIUS. See HRABANUS MAURUS, Abp. of Mainz [784?-856]

HRABANUS MAURUS, Abp. of Mainz [784?-856] See MERBITZ, J. V. De varietate faciei humanae. 1676.

HUARTE DE SAN JUAN, JUAN [1529?-1588] Examen de ingenios para las sciencias, donde se muestra la diferencia de habilidades, que ay enlos hombres; y el genero de letras, que a cada uno responde en particular . . . [Amberes] La Oficina Plantiniana, 1603.

[16], 464 p.   14   cm.   [6084]

Place of publication supplied from Palau.

This reprint of the text of the original edition (Baeza, 1575) was first issued by the Plantin press in 1593; in it the original dedication to Philip II of Spain has been altered to a notice "Al lector," all references to the King being omitted.

—[The same.] ... Tercera edicion de muchos querida. Leyde, Juan Maire, 1652.

[16], 464 p. 15 cm. [6085]

Different setting of type.

—[The same.] Examen de ingenios para las ciencias en el qual el lector hallara la manera de su ingenio, para escoger la ciencia en que mas ha de aprovechar: y la diferencia de habilidades que ay enlos hombres, y el genero de letras, y artes que a cada uno responde en particular ... Agora nuevamente emendado por el mismo autor, y añadidas muchas cosas curiosas, y provechosas ... Madrid, Por Melchor Sanchez, a costa de Gabriel de Leon, 1668.

[8], 346, [1] p. 22 cm. [6086]

Reprint of the enlarged edition which was first published in Baeza in 1594.

—[Latin tr.] Scrutinium ingeniorum pro iis, qui excellere cupiunt; perpetua linguae Castelanae translatione Latinitate donatum: interprete Aeschacio Majore Dobreborano [pseud. i.e. Joachimus Caesar] ... Ed. 2. [Jenae?] Sumptibus Johannis Victorini Mohr, bibliopolae, 1637.

[40], 743, [45] p. 17 cm. [6087]

Place of publication supplied from Benzing (A) p. 447, and Benzing (B) p. 482.

Chapters 18–23 are contained in a separate section (p. [561]–743) with special title page (Aeschacii Majoris Scrutinii ingenior [sic] e lingua Hispana in Latiarem translati reliquarium qui generari fierique ingeniosi ac sapientes possint liberi ...) and a new note by the translator.

Translation (with the addition of much other material) of the enlarged edition which was first published in Baeza in 1594.

—[English tr.] Examen de ingenios. The examination of mens wits. In which, by discovering the varietie of natures, is shewed for what profession each one is apt, and how far he shall profit therein ... Translated out of the Spanish ... by M. Camillo Camilli. Englished out of his Italian by R[ichard] C[arew] Esquire. London, Adam Islip, 1604.

[16], 333, [2] p. 19 cm. [6088]

A reprint of the first edition of this translation, published in London in 1594.

STC 13894.

—[The same.] ... London, Printed by Adam Islip for Thomas Adams, 1616.

[16], 333, [2] p. 18 cm. [6089]

Different setting of type.

Margins closely cropped, affecting dedication and headlines.

STC 13895.

—[The same.] Examen de ingenios; or, The tryal of wits. Discovering the great difference of wits among men, and what sort of learning suits best with each genius. Published originally in Spanish ... And made English from the most correct edition by Mr. Bellamy ... London, Richard Sare, 1698.

[40], 502, [2] p. 19 cm. [6090]

Translation of the enlarged edition which was first published in Baeza in 1594.

—[French tr.] Examen des esprits propres et naiz aux sciences. Où par merveilleux & utiles secrets ... est demonstree la difference des graces & habilitez qui se trouvent aux hommes, & à quel genre de lettres est convenable l'esprit de chacun ... Traduit d'espagnol en françoys, par Gabriel Chappuis. Derniere ed. Rouen, Theodore Reinsart, 1602.

[14], 208 ll. 14 cm. [6091]

Chappuys' translation first published in 1580 under title: Anacrise, ou parfait jugement et examen des esprits propres et naiz aux sciences.

—[The same.] Anacrise; ou, Parfait jugement et examen des esprits propres & nez aux sciences ... Composé en espagnol ... & mis en françois ... par Gabriel Chappuis ... De nouv. rev. & corr. Lyon, Jean Didier, 1608.

[15], 320 (i.e. 319) ll. 14 cm. [6092]

—[The same.] Examen des esprits propres et naiz aux sciences. Où par merveilleux & utiles secrets ... est demonstrée la difference des graces & habilitez qui se trouvent aux hommes, & à quel genre de lettres est convenable l'esprit de chacun ... Traduit d'espagnol en françois, par Gabriel Chappuis. Derniere ed. Rouen, Matthieu Gorgeu, 1619.

[8], 208 ll. 15 cm. [6093]

Different setting of type.

—[The same.] L'examen des esprits pour les sciences. Ou se montrent les differences d'esprits qui se trouvent parmy les hommes, & à quel genre de science chacun est propre en particulier ... Nouvellement traduit suivant l'ancien original. Et augm. suivant la derniere impression d'Espagne. Paris, Jean Guignard le fils, 1661.

[56], 650 (i.e. 653), [22] p. 15 cm. [6094]

Translated by Charles Vion Dalibray.

—Another issue, with imprint: Paris, Charles de Sercy, 1661. [6095]

—[The same.] ... Rev., corr., & mis en meilleur ordre, en cette derniere ed. ... Lyon, Gabriel Blanc, 1668.

[36], 126 (i.e. 428), [18] p. 15 cm.   **[6096]**
Imperfect: printer's privilege (one leaf at end) wanting.

—[The same.] ... Augm. de plusieurs additions nouvelles par l'auteur selon la derniere impression d'Espagne. Le tout traduit de l'espagnol par François Savinien d'Alquie. Amsterdam, Jean de Ravestein, 1672.

[64], 629 p. 14 cm.   **[6097]**
Added engraved title page.

—[Italian tr.] Essamina de gl'ingegni de gli huomini acconci ad apparare qual si voglia scienza ... Nella quale discorrendosi della diversità delle nature loro si viene à scoprire à qual'essercitio ciascuno piu atto sia, e qual giovamento ne possa trarre. Di lingua castigliana in pura italiana da Salustio Gratii recata ... Di nuovo diligentemente riveduta, e ricorretta, e di molti errori purgata ... Venetia, Mattheo Valentini, 1603.

[48], 470 p. 16 cm.   **[6098]**

—*as subject. See* GUIBELET, J. Examen de l'Examen des esprits. 1631.

HUARTE NAVARRO, JUAN DE DIOS. *See* HUARTE DE SAN JUAN, Juan [1529?-1588]

HUBER, ERHARD [*fl.* 1696] *respondent.* Disputatio medica inauguralis de nephritide ... Trajecti ad Rhenum, Ex officina Francisci Halma, 1696.

14, [2] p. 19 cm.   **[6099]**
Diss.—Utrecht.

HUBNER, BARTHOLOMAEUS [*fl.* 1578-1593] *praeses. In* Lipsius, D. Tractatus de hydropsis. 1624, 1678.

HUBRECHT, JAN [*fl.* 1678] *respondent.* Disputatio medica inauguralis de calculo renum ... Lugduni Batavorum, Apud viduam & heredes Joannis Elsevirii, 1678.

[19] p. 21 cm.   **[6100]**
Diss.—Leyden.

HUBRIGK, JOHANN FRIEDRICH [*fl.* 1660-1662] *respondent. See* HOFFMAN, M., *praeses.* Θεώρημα ἰατρικόν. 1662.

HUCHER, JEAN [*d.* 1603] De febrium differentiis, causis, signisque & curatione libri quatuor ... Lugduni, Apud Antonium de Harsy, 1601.

[64], 429, [23] p. 18 cm.   **[6101]**

—De prognosi medica libri duo ... Lugduni, Apud Antonium de Harsy, 1602.

[32], 161, [14] p. 18 cm.   **[6102]**

—De sterilitate utriusque sexus, opus in quatuor libros distributum: cui annexus est liber De diaeta et therapeia puerorum. Genevae, Apud Gabrielem Cartier, 1609.

[30], 910 p. 18 cm.   **[6103]**

—[The same.] ... Nunc primum in lucem editum ... Aureliae Allobrogum, Apud Samuelem Crispinum, 1610.

[30], 910 p. 18 cm.   **[6104]**
A reissue of the 1609 edition with new title page.

HÜBLER, CHRISTOPHORUS. *See* HÜBLER, Johann Christoph [*fl.* 1695]

HÜBLER, JOHANN CHRISTOPH [*fl.* 1695] Dissertatio historico-physica, de pluviis prodigiosis ... Erfurti, Literis Kindlebianis [1695]

20 p. 17 cm.   **[6105]**
Diss. pro loco — Erfurt (H. P. Juch, *respondent*)

HÜBNER, CHRISTOPH FRIEDRICH [*fl.* 1698] *respondent. See* EMMERICH, G., *praeses.* Dissertatio academica sistens paradoxon physico-medicum de inspiratione. 1698.

HÜBNER, JOHANN CHRISTOPH [*fl.* 1666-1667] *respondent. See* SCHENCK, J. T., *praeses.* Disputatio inauguralis medica de singultu. 1667.

HÜBNER, JOHANN HEINRICH [*fl.* 1688] *respondent. See* VEHR, I., *praeses.* Disput. inauguralis medica, de febre virginum amatoria. 1688.

HÜBNER, JOHANN VALENTIN [*fl.* 1674] *respondent.* Dissertatio inauguralis de tarantismo ... Argentorati, Typis Johannis Wilhelmi Tidemanni [1674]

[20] p. 20 cm.   **[6106]**

HÜENERER, LORENZ [*fl.* 1616] *respondent. See* HAWENREUTER, J. L., *praeses.* Disputatio physica de natura terrae. 1616.

HÜLLINGER, WENCESLAUS [*fl.* 1636] Hydriatria Carolina; das ist, Kurtze Besreibung [sic] was das weit-berühmte, Käyser - Carlsbad vor köstliche Mineralien mit sich führet, zu was Krankheit es dienstlich, und wie man solches recht brauchen soll. Anno. M.DC.XXXVIII ... zum ersten Mal heraus gegeben; anjetzo ... auff das newe an das Liecht gebracht. Prag, Gedruckt durch Johann Michael Störitz in Verlegung Andreas Bechers in Carls-Bad, 1692.

[4], 84 p.   16 cm.   [6107]

With this is bound (as issued?) Strobelberger, J. S. Kurtze Unterweisung. 1692.

HUENERWOLF, Jakob Augustin [1644-1685] Anatomia paeoniae, in qua natales et qualitates paeoniae, itemque praeparationes et medicamenta ex ea varia cum virtutibus et usu ad plurimos humani corporis affectus exhibentur ... Arnsteti, Typis Henrici Meureri, 1680.

[2], 110, [8] p.   16 cm.   [6108]

Bound with copy 2 of Grube, H. Analysis mali citrei compendiosa. 1668.

HÜNERWOLFF, Johann Friedrich [*fl.* 1695] *respondent. See* Wedel, G. W., *praeses.* Dissertatio inauguralis medica de aegilope. 1695.

HUERTA, Geronimo de. *See* Gómez de Huerta, Jerónimo [1573-1643]

HUERTE, Garcia de. *See* Orta, Garcia d' [1501 *or* 2?-1568]

HÜTTLINGER, Peter [*fl.* 1674] *respondent. See* Geret, A., *praeses.* Infans monstrosus Wittebergae D. 30 Augusti, anno M.DC.LXXIV natus. 1674.

HUGHES, William [*fl.* 1652-1683] The American physitian; or, A treatise of the roots, plants ... herbs, &c. growing in the English plantations in America. Describing the place ... temperature, vertues and uses of them, either for diet, physick, &c. Whereunto is added a discourse of the cacao-nut-tree, and the use of its fruit ... London, Printed by J. C. for William Crook, 1672.

[21], 159, [5] p.   14 cm.   [6109]

HUGO SENENSIS. *See* Benzi, Ugo [1376-1439]

HUGO, Johann Georg [*fl.* 1698-1699] *respondent. See* Vater, C., *praeses.* Disputatio inauguralis medica. 1699; Wedel, G. W., *praeses.* Dissertatio medica de austerorum et acerborum natura. 1698.

HUGOT, Claude [*fl.* 1677-1678] *respondent. See* Girard, F., *praeses.* Quaestio medica ... An inveteratae & contumaci dysenteriae lactic potio? 1678.

HUHN, Georg [*fl.* 1643-1644] *respondent. See* Conring, H., *praeses.* Disputatio medica de palpitatione cordis. 1643 [and] Disputatio medica inauguralis de peripneumonia. 1644; Tappe, J., *praeses.* Disputatio medica de mania. 1644.

HULSE, Edward [1631-1711] *respondent.* Disputatio medica inauguralis de hydrope ... Lugduni Batavorum, Apud viduam & haeredes Joannis Elsevirii, 1668.

[11] p.   24 cm.   [6110]

Diss. — Leyden.

HULSIUS, Eduard. *See* Hulse, Edward [1631-1711]

HUMMEL, Johann Christian [*fl.* 1688-1689] *respondent. See* Camerarius, E. R., *praeses.* Dissertatio medica prior de coryza sicca. 1688.

HUMMELSTEIN, Michael Friedrich Lochner von. *See* Lochner von Hummelstein, Michael Friedrich [1662-1720]

HUNAIN IBN ISHĀK, al-'Ibādī [809?-873] *See* Avicenna. Avicennae Arabum medicorum principis. 1608.

HUNAULD, Pierre [1664-1728] Discours physique, sur les proprietez de la sauge. *In* Bontekoe, C. nouveaux elemens de medecine. 1698.

HUNAYN IBN-ISHĀQ. See Hunain ibn Ishāk, al-'Ibādī [809?-873]

HUNDERTMARCK, Heinrich Elias [1664-1739] *respondent.* Disputatio medica inauguralis, delineationem medici genuini exhibens ... Trajecti ad Rhenum, Ex officina Francisci Halma, 1695.

[4], 20 p.   20 cm.   [6111]

Diss. — Utrecht.

—, *tr. See* Heinsius, N. [1656?-1718] Schmachtende Venus. 1700.

HUNDESHAGEN, Johann Christoph [1635-1681] Discursus physicus de stillicidio sanguinis in hominis violenter occisi, cadavere conspicui, an sit sufficiens praesentis homicidae indicium? ... Jenae, Sumptibus Christoph. Enoch Buchta, 1679.

[86] p.   19 cm.   [6112]

—Tractatus singularis de pluralitate animarum in homine realiter distinctarum ... Quarta vice auctius & emendatius editus. Jenae, Typis Gollnerianis, cIɔ cIɔ LXXV [i.e. 1675]

[64] p. 19 cm. [6113]

—*praeses.* Disputatio academica de imaginatione ejusque viribus ... Jenae, Litteris Joh. Jacobi Bauhoferi, 1665.

[32] p. 18 cm. [6114]

Diss. — Jena (J. Kisner, *respondent*)

—Disputatio academica de sanguinis stillicidio ex cadavere hominis occisi ad praesentiam homicidae ... Jenae, Typis Samuelis Adolphi Mülleri, 1669.

[40] p. 19 cm. [6115]

Diss. — Jena (A. F. Kraussold, *respondent*)

—Disputatio physica de fulmine ... Jenae, Characteribus Johannis Nisii, 1665.

[28] p. 20 cm. [6116]

Diss. — Jena (J. G. Fischer, *respondent*)

—Disputationem meteorologicam de ventis ... examini subjiciet Johann-Fridericus Peuschelius ... Jenae, Typis Georgii Sengenwaldi, 1667.

[26] p. illus. 20 cm. [6117]

Diss. — Jena (J. F. Peuschel, *respondent*)

HUNGERFORD, FRANCIS [*fl.* 1681] *See* GRIFFITH, R. A-la-mode phlebotomy no good fashion. 1681.

HUNTINGDON, ROBERT. *See* HUNTINGTON, Robert, *Bishop of Raphoe* [1637–1701]

HUNTINGTON, ROBERT, *Bishop of Raphoe* [1637–1701] *See* RAUWOLFF, L. A collection of curious travels & voyages. 1693.

HUNTON, ANTHONY [*ca.* 1560–1624] *See* GUILLEMEAU, J. A treatise of one hundred and thirteene diseases of the eyes. 1622.

HUPKA, M. H. [*fl.* 17th cent.] *tr. See* DIGBY, Sir K. Eröffnung unterschiedlicher Heimlichkeiten der Natur. 1664, 1671.

HURLEBUSCH, GEBHARD [*fl.* 1610] *respondent. See* PARCOV, F., *praeses.* De angina. 1610.

—*See* DIEPHOLD, R. Cl^mo. viro, Dn. Gebhardo Hurlebusch ... medicinae doctori renunciato. 1610.

HURTER, EMMANUEL [*fl.* 1649] *respondent. See* STUPANUS, E., *praeses.* Signorum medicorum doctrina. 1649.

HURTER, MELCHIOR [*fl.* 1679] *respondent.* Disputatio inauguralis medica de empyemate ... Argentorati, Literis Jo. Friderici Spoor [1679]

23 p. 19 cm. [6118]

Diss. — Strasbourg.

al-HUSAIN IBN 'ABD ALLĀH, ABŪ 'ALĪ. *See* AVICENNA, 980?–1037.

HUSANUS JOHANNES [*fl.* 1608] *respondent. See* LUCHTEN, A., *praeses.* De melancholia. 1608.

HUSER, JOHANN [*fl.* 1589] *ed. See* PARACELSUS. Chirurgische Bücher und Schrifften. 1605, 1618 [and] Erster [-zehender] Theil der Bücher und Schrifften. 1603 [and] Opera Bücher und Schrifften. 1603, 1616.

HUSWEDEL, JOHANN ALBERT [*ca.* 1618–1674] *respondent. See* KIJPER, A., *praeses.* Disputatio physica de anima rationali. 1640.

HUSZTI, ISTVÁN [*b.* 1671] *respondent. See* HOFFMANN, F. [1660–1742] *praeses.* Dissertatio solennis de prudenti medicamentorum applicatione in tempore. 1695 [and] Philosophiae experimentalis axiomaticae dissertatio. 1695.

—*See* HOFFMANN, F. [1660–1742] Propempticon inaugurale de pane grossiori Westphalorum, vulgo Bonpournickel. 1695.

HUSZTI, STEPHANUS. *See* HUSZTI, István [*b.* 1671]

HUTH, JOHANN CHRISTOPH [*fl.* 1695] *respondent. See* MAPP, M., *praeses.* Dissertatio medica de potu chocolatae. 1695.

HUTH, JOHANN PHILIPP [*fl.* 1661–1663] *respondent. See* SEBISCH, M. [1578–1674?] *praeses.* Disputatio medica de affectione hypochondriaca. 1661.

HUTH, JOHANN PHILIPP [*fl.* 1685]. *respondent.* Disputatio medica inauguralis de hernia vera ... Lugduni Batavorum, Apud Abrahamum Elzevier, 1685.

[16] p. 22 cm. [6119]

Diss. — Leyden.

HUTYER, PIERRE [*fl.* 1700–1707] Discours anatomique du corps humain avec un abrégé de la pratique de medecine suivant l'acide et l'amer ...

Moulins, La veve [sic] de Claude Vernoy, M VII. C. (i.e. 1700?)

[1], viii, [6], 35, 142, [10] p. 15 cm. **[6120]**

Approbations dated 1699 and 1700.

HUXHOLTZ, ADAM ANDREAS [*fl.* 1659–1661] *See* GRONOVIUS, J. F., *praeses.* Disputatio medico-chirurgic [sic] inauguralis de hydrocephalo. 1661.

HUXHOLTZ, JOHANN LUDWIG [*d.* 1718] *respondent.* Disputatio medico-chirurgica inauguralis de fontanellis … Marburgi Cattorum, Typis Salomonis Schadewitzii, 1673.

[1], 22 p. 19 cm. **[6121]**

Diss. - Marburg.

HUXHOLTZ, WOLRAD [1619?–1671] Unterricht der Hebammen. Darinnen gehandelt wird im ersten Theil, wie sich eine Hebamme in allen … Begebenheiten bey … gebährenden Weibern … zu verhalten habe … Im andern Theil, wie eine Hebamme, in denen Gebrechen, die von schwären Geburthen herrühren, und dem Augenschein unterworffen seyn, sich bey den Weibesbildern verhalten solle … Cassel, Gedruckt bey Salomom Schadewitz, in Verlegung Johann Schützens, 1652.

[14], 83, [3] p.; [4], 50, [3] p. 17 cm. **[6122]**

Part 2 has half title.
Bound with Herlitz, D. De curationibus gravidarum. 1628.

HUYBERTS, ADRIAN [*fl.* 1675] A corner-stone laid towards the building of a new colledge (that is to say, a new body of physicians) in London. Upon occasion of the … proceedings acted in the name of the society called the Colledge of Physicians … It being an apology for the better education of physicians … London, Printed for the author, 1675.

[1], 38 p. 20 cm. **[6123]**

—*as subject. See* GOODALL, C. The Colledge of Physicians vindicated. 1676.

HUYGENS, CHRISTIAAN [1629–1695] Traité de la lumiere. Où sont expliquées les causes de ce qui luy arrive dans la reflexion, & dans la refraction du cristal d'Islande. Par C[hristian] H[uygens] D. Z. Avec un Discours de la cause de la pesanteur. Leide, Pierre vander Aa, 1690.

[8], 180 p. illus. 23 cm. **[6124]**

HYGEA AUGUSTANA. 1682. *See* SCHROECK, L.

HYGIAE et panaceae parente … Casparus Bauhinus. 1610. *See* BAUHIN, K.

HYGIEIA; id. est, Bonae valetudinis conservandae thesaurus locupletissimus: in quo quicquid ad eam rem pertinet, ex probatissimis quibusque auctoribus traditur, docetur & explicatur … Luxemburgi, Excudebat Hubertus Reuland, 1628.

[16], 120, 440 p. 14 cm. **[6125]**

Contents. — [1] Medicus domesticus; seu, Medicina charitativa (p. [1]-120) — [2] De conservanda bona valetudine, liber scholae Salernitanae, with same contents as in the 1605 Frankfurt edition of Regimen sanitatis Salernitanum (p. 1-415) — [3] Hyppomnemata; seu, Praecepta sanitatis. Ex aureo Henrici Ranzovii De conservanda valetudine libello (p. [416]-433) — [4] Monita; seu, Praecepta tuendae sanitatis, ex Guilielmi Grataroli libello (p. 443-440)

—Another issue, with imprint: Coloniae Agrippinae, Typis Petri à Brachel, 1628.

[6126]

HYPHANTES, JOHANNES. *See* WEBSTER, John [1610-1682]

HYPSICLES. *See* CHALES, C. F. M. de, *Father.* Cursus seu mundus mathematicus. 1690.

I

I., A.E.B.D.C., *ed.* and *tr. See* GALENUS. De l'usage des parties du corps humain. 1666.

I., H. *See* JACOBS, Heyman.

I., H. I., *ed. See* BECHER, J. J. Medicinische Schatz-Kammer. 1700.

I., M. C., *ed. See* LE CHEMIN FRAYÉ ET INFAILLIBLE AUX ACCOUCHEMENS. 1689.

I., S. *See* JANSONIUS, Samuel.

I., W. *See* RECORDE, R. The urinal of physick. 1651.

I., W., *gent. See* JAR, W.

I.A.P.G.S.P.D. *See* PAËPP, Johann [*d.* 1613]

I. M., M. M. [*fl.* 1684] *See* FELIX PUERPERA. 1684?

I.M.D.V.C.A.P. *See* MICHAULT, Jean [1632-1694]

I. W. *See* W., I.

IÄGERSCHMIDT, Johann Victor. *See* Jägerschmidt, Johann Victor [*fl.* 1683–1684]

IANIKE, Joachim. *See* Janike, Joachim [*fl.* 1607]

IASOLINI, Giulio. *See* Jasolino, Giulio [1538–1622]

al-'IBĀDĪ, Hunain Ibn Ishāk. *See* Hunain Ibn Ishāk, al-'Ibādī [809?–873]

IBN al-WĀFID. *See* 'Abd al-Rahmān ibn Muhammad, *called* Ibn Wāfid [999–1068]

IBN EZRA, Abraham ben Meïr [1092–1167] De luminaribus et diebus criticis. *In* Ganivet, J. Amicus medicorum. 1614.

—*See* Culpeper, N. Semeiotica Uranica. 1651, 1655, 1658.

IBN ISHĀK, Hunain, al-'Ibādī. *See* Hunain ibn Ishāk, al-'Ibādī [809?–873]

IBN MĀSAWAYH, Abū Zakariyyā' Yūhanna *See* Mesuë [*d.* 857]

IBN MĀSAWAYH, Yūhannā *See* Mesuë [*d.* 857]

IBN RUSHD. *See* Averroës [1126–1198]

IBN RUSHD, Abū al-Walīd Muhammad ibn Ahmad, *called*. *See* Averroës [1126–1198]

IBN SĪNĀ. *See* Avicenna, 980?–1037.

IBN ZAKARĪYĀ. *See* Muhammad ibn Zakarīyā, Abū Bakr, al-Rāzī [865–925]

IBN ZUHR, 'Abd al-Malik. *See* Avenzoar [*d. ca.* 1162]

ICONIUS, Raphael Eglinus. *See* Eglinus Iconius, Raphael [1559–1622]

IENTSCHIUS, Joachimus. *See* Jentsch, Johann [*fl.* 1607]

IGNOTA febris. 1691? *See* Maynwaring, E.

IGREJA E HOSPITAL DE SANTO ANTÓNIO DA NAÇÃO PORTUGUESA. Estatutos da veneravel Igreia, e hospital de Santo Antonio de Naçaõ Portuguesa de Roma. Roma, Impressa na Rev. Cam. Apost., 1683.

153 p. 22 cm. [6127]

IKEN, Heinrich [*fl.* 1682–1685] *respondent.* Disputatio medica inauguralis, de furore uterino . . . Lugduni Batavorum, Apud Abrahamum Elzevier, 1685.

[24] p. 22 cm. [6128]
Diss. — Leyden.

ILLINGWORTH, James [1625–1693] A just narrative, or, account of the man whose hands and legs rotted off: in the parish of Kings-Swinford, in Stafford-Shire . . . London, Printed by A. C. for Henry Brome, 1678.

[4], 12, [8] p. 18 cm. [6129]
Issued also as part [2] of Simon Ford's A discourse concerning God's judgments.

ILLMER, Friedrich Ferdinand [*fl.* 1698] *praeses.* Disputatio medica de pulsu et respiratione . . . Viennae Austriae, Typis Leopoldi Voigt [1698]

[16] p. 19 cm. [6130]
Diss. — Vienna (J. J. Zebriacher, *respondent*)

ILLUSTRISSIMI signori. Perche . . . havendo io N. de N. sperimentato la virtù . . . di un oglio, che in poche hore sana la pleuritide, ò sia maldi punta, ò come dicono altri, mal di costa; havendo guarito da molti anni . . . tutte quelle persone, che l'hanno usato . . . hò stimato cosa honorifica, anzi ufficio di grande carità verso il prossimo far imprimere il detto secreto, cioè il modo di fare, e di usare l'oglio sudetto, & inviarlo alli signori presidenti degli hospitali di tutte le città d'Italia, anzi dell'Europa; accio à tutti giovar possa . . . [Ferrara, Alfonso, e Gio. Battista Maresti, 1669]

[2] p. 31 cm. [6131]

ILLUSTRIUM Hollandiae & Westfrisiae ordinum alma Academia Leidensis. 1614. *See* [Meurs, J. van, 1579–1639]

ILMER, Georg [*fl.* 1669] *praeses.* Dissertatio physico-philologica de tilia . . . Lipsiae, Stanno Christiani Michaelis [1669]

[16] p. 20 cm. [6132]
Diss. — Leipzig (D. Lindner, *respondent*)

IMBRASIUS, *of Ephesus.* Prognostica de decubitu. *In* Bovio, Z. T. Melampigo. 1617, 1626; Ganivet, J. Amicus medicorum. 1614; Pleier, C. Medicus-criticus-astrologus. 1627.

—[French tr.] *In* Lagneau, D. Traicté pour la conservation de la santé. 1650.

IMMENS, DAVID [*fl.* 1685] *respondent.* Disputatio medica inauguralis de mammarum cancro . . . Trajecti ad Rhenum, Ex officina Francisci Halma, 1685.

8 p.   22 cm.   [6133]

Diss.—Utrecht.

IMPERATO, FERRANTE [*ca.* 1550–*ca.* 1631] Historia naturale . . . nella quale . . . si tratta della diversa condition de minere, pietre pretiose, & altre curiosità. Con varie historie di piante & animali, sin' hora non date in luce. In questa 2. imp. aggiontovi da Gio. Maria Ferro . . . alcune annotationi alle piante nel libro vigesimo ottavo . . . Venetia, Combi, & La Noù, 1672.

[8], 696, [8] p.   illus., plate.   36 cm.   [6134]

IMPERIALE, GIOVANNI. *See* IMPERIALI, Giovanni [1596?–1670]

IMPERIALI, GIOVANNI [1596?–1670] Musaeum historicum et physicum . . . In primo illustrium literis virorum imagines ad vivum expressę continentur, additis elogiis . . . In secundo animorum imagines, sive ingeniorum naturę, differentię, causę, ac signa physice perpenduntur . . . Venetiis, Apud Juntas, 1640.

[16], 122 (i.e. 212) p.; [8], 219, [22] p.   ports.   23 cm.   [6135]

Engraved title page.

Printing error: p. 47, (part [1]) lacks portrait.

Part [2] has half title: Musaeum physicum; sive, De humano ingenio. Colophon on p. 219 dated 1639.

Errata: p. [21–22]

—Le notti beriche; overo, De' quesiti, e discorsi fisici, medici, politici, historici, e sacri libri cinque . . . Venetia, Paolo Baglioni, 1663.

[12], 390, [20] p.   25 cm.   [6136]

—Pestis anni MDCXXX, historico-medica . . . Vincentiae, Apud haeredem Francisci Grossi, 1631.

[8], 71 p.   22 cm.   [6137]

IMPERIALIS, JOANNES. *See* IMPERIALI, Giovanni [1596?–1670]

IN fictilem figuli exercitationem de principiis foetus. 1658. *See* [GRAINDORGE, A.]

IN libros Ethicorum Aristotelis ad Nicomachum . . . disputationes. 1616. *See* UNIVERSIDADE DE COIMBRA. Collegium Conimbricense Societatis Jesu.

IN speculo teipsum contemplare Dr. Black. A looking-glass for the Black-band of doctors. Wherein may be seen the ignorance and malice of these physicians, who have clubbed under the name of Dr. Black, for suppressing by their scriblings, and other calumnies, so great a benefite to the world, as the new cure of fevers. Contained in a 2d Letter written by Philander [pseud.] to his friend in the countrey Philomathes [pseud.] In defence of Dr. Broun. Edinburgh, Heir of Andrew Anderson, 1692.

47, [1] p.   18 cm.   [6138]

Concerns controversy over Sydenham's new methods of treatment.

With this are bound: Capon, John. The new booke of Mr. John Capons wits. [n. p., 17--?]—An essay for reforming the modern way of practising medicine. Edinburgh, 1727.

INCORPORATION OF CHIRURGIONS IN EDINBURGH. *See* ROYAL COLLEGE OF SURGEONS OF EDINBURGH.

INDAGINE, JOANNES AB [*ca.* 1467–1537] Introductiones apotelesmaticae in physiognomiam, astrologiam naturalem, complexiones hominum, naturas planetarum. Cum periaxiomatibus de faciebus signorum . . . Quibus . . . accessit Gulielmi Grataroli . . . opuscula De memoria reparanda, augenda, conservanda; De praedictione morum naturarumque hominum; De mutatione temporum . . . et Pomponii Guarici . . . tractatus De symmetriis, lineamentis & physiognomia, ejusque speciebus, etc. Urseliis, Apud Cornelium Sutorium, impensis Lazari Zetzneri, 1603.

387 p.   illus.   16 cm.   [6139]

—[The same.] . . . Argentorati, Sumptibus haeredum Lazari Zetzneri, 1622.

384 p.   illus.   19 cm.   [6140]

—[The same.] . . . Argentorati, Sumptibus haeredum Lazari Zetzneri, 1630.

384 p.   illus.   19 cm.   [6141]

Different setting of type.

Imperfect: all pages between title page and p. 97 and p. 115–118 wanting.

—[The same.] . . . Augustae Trebocorum, Sumptibus Simonis Paulii, 1663

384 p.   illus.   17 cm.   [6142]

Different setting of type.

—[The same.] . . . Augustae Trebocorum, Sumptibus Simonis Paulli, 1672.

384 p.   illus.   16 cm.   [6143]

A reissue of the 1663 edition with new title page.

The Prognostica de decubitu is known both as the pseudo-Hippocratic De esse aegrorum secundum lunam (Astronomia, De medicorum astrologia, etc.) and as the pseudo-Galenic De decubitu infirmorum ex mathematica scientia. It has also appeared under the name of Hermes Trismegistus with the title De decubitu infirmorum. Under the title De diebus decretoriis it has been ascribed to Pietro d'Abano as author; his name is associated with the text as translator.

It is attributed to Imbrasius of Ephesus in a Bodleian manuscript and was compiled in Egypt probably during the Ptolemaic period. Cf. S. Weinstock, in the Classical quarterly, v. 42, 1948, p. [41]-43.

—[French tr.] Vraye et parfaicte chyromancie et phisionomie, part le regard, des membres de l'homme. La diffinition des faces des signes. Reigles astronomiques du judgement des maladies. Plus, l'astrologie naturelle. La cognoissance de la complexion des hommes selon la domination des planettes. Traduction nouvelle. Paris, Jacques Villery [not before 1620]

[10], 380 (i.e. 381) p. illus. 16 cm.   [6144]
The two Jacques Villerys printed between 1620 and 1683. Cf. Goldsmith.
Translated by Antoine Du Moulin.

[The same.] . . . La chiromance et phisiognomie par le regard des membres de l'homme . . . Le tout mis en françois par Antoine du Moulin . . . Rouen, Jacques Cailloüé, 1638.

[8], 337 p. illus., port. 14 cm.   [6145]

INDEX et manuductor chymicus, in quo possibilitas transmutationis metallorum clare ostenditur, & simul via ad inveniendum lapidem philosophorum aperitur. [n. p.] 1680.

[40] p. 17 cm.   [6146]
Bound with Fundamenta vera chymiae. 1660.

INDIANO, Domenico. Varii secreti di medicina, et altri . . . Nuovamente posti in luce. Venetia, Bologna et Siena, Salvestro Marchetti, 1616.

[8] p. 16 cm.   [6147]

INFERIGNO, *accademico della Crusca, See* Rossi, Bastiano de [*fl.* 1585-1605]

INGEBER, Johann. Chiromantia; metoposcopia & physiognomia curioso-practica; oder, Kurtze Anweisung, wie man aus den vier Haupt-Linien in der Hand . . . von dess Menschen Gesundheit und Kranckheit . . . urtheilen kan . . . Sambt einer . . . noch nie in Druck gegebenen Abmessung der Linie

Honoris . . . Franckfurt am Mayn, Verlegts Georg Heinrich Ehrling, 1692.

[7], 180, [4] p. front., plates. 17 cm.
    [6148]
Added engraved title page.
Bound with Höchstfürtreflichtes chiromantischund physiognomisches Klee-Blat. 1695.

INGEGNERI, Angelo [1550-*ca.* 1613] *ed. See* Ingegneri, G., *Bp. of Capo d'Istria.* Fisionomia naturale. 1606.

INGEGNERI, Giovanni, *Bp. of Capo d'Istria* [*fl.* 1595] Fisionomia naturale nella quale con ragioni tolte dalla filosofia, dalla medicina, e dall'anatomia . . . si dimostra, come dalle parti del corpo humano, per la sua naturale complessione, si possa ageuolmente conietturare, quali sieno l'inclinationi, e gli affetti dell'animo altrui . . . Napoli, Gio. Jacomo Carlino, 1606.

[8], 166 p. 21 cm.   [6149]
Dedicatory epistle signed by Angelo Ingegneri, the editor.

—[The same.] . . . Vicenza, Pietro Paolo Tozzi, 1615.

60, [4] p. (Part [2] *in* Porta, G. B. della. Della fisonomia dell' huomo. 1615)   [6150]

—[The same.] . . . Padova, Pietro Paolo Tozzi, 1623.

64 p. (Part [2] *in* Fisonomia naturale di Gio: Battista dalla Porta, Giovanni Ingegnieri[e] Polemone. 1622)   [6151]
Reprint of the edition issued by the same publisher in Vicenza in 1615.

—[The same.] . . . Padova, Pietro Paolo Tozzi, 1626.

64 p. 21 cm. (Part [2] *in* Porta, G. B. della. Della fisonomia dell'huomo. 1627)   [6152]

—[The same.] *In* Porta, G. B. della. Della fisionomia dell'huomo. 1644, 1668.

INGRASSIA, Giovanni Filippo [1510-1580] In Galeni librum De ossibus . . . commentaria, nunc primum sedulo in lucem edita, & apte naturam imitantibus iconibus insignita, quibus appositus est Graecus Galeni contextus, una cum nova & fideli ejusdem Ingrassiae in Latinum versione . . . Panormi, Ex typographia Jo. Baptistae Maringhi, 1603.

[6], 276, [10] p. illus., port. 30 cm. [6153]

A note to the reader, by Matteo Donia, supplies biographical and bibliographical data on the author.

—, ed. *See* SICILY, Protomedico. Constitutiones. 1657.

INGRASSIA, PHILIPPUS. *See* INGRASSIA, Giovanni Filippo [1510–1580]

INNICHENHÖFER, HEINRICH [*b.* 1602] *praeses.* Υπνολογια; sive, Tractatus jucundus physiologicus, in disputationes [-prima -octava] aliquot redactus . . . in quo de somnii natura et essentia in genere . . . per quaestiones exacte pertractatur . . . Wittebergae, Ex officina typographica Christiani Tham, 1624.

[132] p. 20 cm. **[6154]**

Each dissertation has special title page dated 1623–1624.

DISS. — WITTENBERG (*Respondents:* G. Döring, V. Grundmann, A. Hemmer, I. Mylius, F. Richter, E. Schochius, J. Strössenreuter, J. Wolfrom)

INNOCENS, GUILLAUME DES. *See* DES INNOCENS, Guillaume [*d. ca.* 1610]

INQUIETO ACADEMICO VESPERTINO, *pseud. See* GHIRADELLI, C. Cefalogia fisonomica. 1630, 1670, 1674.

INSA, ANTONIO JUAN. Officina medicamentorum, et methodus recte eadem componendi, cum variis scholiis et aliis . . . ex sententia Valentinorum pharmacopolarum. Auctore . . . Antonio Johanne Insa, et Johanne Baptista Catarroja; tum, & . . . Gulielmo Salvador Borras, & Francisco Johanne Molina . . . Rocho Linyerola. Valentiae, Apud Johannem Chrysostomum Garriz, 1601.

[12], 412, [12] p. 29 cm. **[6155]**

—[The same.] . . . Segundo tomo: La farmaceutica de Francisco Velez de Arciniega. Tercero tomo: Examen de boticarios, por . . . Fr. Estevan de Villa. 2 impr. Vàn añadidas las tarifas del Reyno de Aragon, y ciudad de Zaragoça . . . Çaragoça, Por Gaspar Tomas Martinez, a costa de Matias de Lezaun, 1698.

3 v. in 1. 30 cm. **[6156]**

Vol. [2] has title: Theoria pharmaceutica. Sectiones septem, Regularum universalium a Joanne Mesue Damasceno scriptarum aliquot, simpliciumque medicaminum electiones, Hispanicam in linguam translatas, Latinis in ipsas annotationibus continens. Francisco Velez ab Arciniega . . . authore.

INSRUTTIONE [sic], et ordini per il buon governo dell' Hospital Maggiore di Como. 1650? *See* HOSPITAL MAGGIORE DI COMO.

INSTITUTIONES rei herbariae. 1700–1703. *See* TOURNEFORT, J. P. de.

INSTRUCTION pour elever, nourrir, dresser, instruire & penser toutes sortes de petits oyseaux de voliere, que l'on tient en cage pour entendre chanter. Avec un petit Traité pour les maladies des chiens. Paris, Charles de Sercy, 1674.

[12], 84 p. 15 cm. **[6157]**

INSTRUMENTA curationis morborum deprompta ex pharmacia Galenica & chymica. 1686. *See* TENQUE, J.

INSTRUMENTUM instrumentorum. 1604. *See* LEEMANN, B.

INSTRUTTIONE generale per purgare ogni sorte di robba. 1630. *See* TRIBUNALE DELLA SANITÀ DI MILANO.

INSTRUZIONE DEL MAGISTRATO DELLA SANITÀ DI FIRENZE. 1630. *See* FLORENCE (CITY) ORDINANCES, LOCAL LAWS, ETC.

INSULAE Ceyloniae thesaurus medicus; vel, Laboratorium Ceylonicum. A Bartholomeo Pielat . . . Latinitate donatum. Amstelodami, Apud Henricum & Theodorum Boom, 1679.

[24], 167 p. 15 cm. **[6158]**

INSULANUS MENAPIUS, GULIELMUS [*d.* 1556]. Encomium febris quartanae. *In* Admiranda rerum admirabilium encomia. 1666, 1677 [and] Dissertationum ludicrarum et amoenitatum, scriptores varii. 1638.

INTRODUCTIO anatomica. *See* LAUREMBERG, P. 'Ανωνυμου εισαγωγη ἀνατομιχε, cum interpretatione. 1618.

INTROITUS apertus. *See* CARDILUCIUS, J. H., ed. Magnalia medico-chymica. 1676; [PHILALETHES, E.] Der vortreffliche Tractat. 1676.

IRENICUM Numae Pompilii, cum Hippocrate. 1689. *See* AMMANN, P.

IRETON, JOHN, *tr. See* REMMELIN, J. A survey of the microcosme. 1675.

IRVINE, CHRISTOPHER [*d*. 1693] Medicina magnetica; or, The rare and wonderful art of curing by sympathy, laid open in aphorismes, proved in conclusions, and digested into an easy method ... By C. de Iryngio ... [London] 1656.

[14], 110 p.   17 cm.   **[6159]**

Imprint partly supplied from Wing I 1053.
"The weapon-salve, according to the description of ... Oswald Crollius": p. 102-110.

—, *ed. See* WALAEUS, J. Medica omnia. 1660.

—, *tr. See* BLOCHWITZ, M. Anatomia sambuci. 1655, 1670, 1677.

IRYNGIO, CHRISTOPHORUS DE. *See* IRVINE, Christopher [*d*. 1693]

ISAAC BEN SOLOMON ISRAELI. *See* ISRAELI, Isaac [ca. 832–ca. 932]

ISAAC HOLLANDUS. *See* JOHANNES ISAACI, *Hollandus* [15th cent.]

ISAAC ISRAELI, *the elder. See* ISRAELI, Isaac [ca. 832–ca. 932]

ISAAC, *Judaeus. See* ISRAELI, Isaac [*ca. 832–ca. 932*]

ISAACI, JOHANNES. *See* JOHANNES ISAACI, *Hollandus* [15th cent.]

ISAAK, *called the Hollander. See* JOHANNES ISAACI, Hollandus [15th cent.]

ISERMANN, CHRISTOPH [*fl*. 1699] *respondent. See* VESTI, J., *praeses.* Dissertatio inauguralis physico-medica. 1699.

ISHAK IBN SULAIMĀN, AL-ISRA'ILI. *See* ISRAELI, Isaac [*ca. 832–ca. 932*]

ISIDORE OF SEVILLE. *See* ISIDORUS, *Saint, Bp. of Seville* [*d*. 636]

ISIDORUS HISPALENSIS. *See* ISIDORUS, *Saint, Bp. of Seville* [*d*. 636]

ISIDORUS, *Saint, Bp. of Seville* [*d*. 636] Etymologiarum libri. *In* Mesuë [924 or 5-1015] Opera. 1602, 1623.

ISING, GEORG EBERHARD [*fl*. 1688] *respondent. See* POSNER, C., *praeses.* Dissertatio physica de animae adcessu in generatione hominis. 1688.

ISRAEL, JAKOB [*b*. 1621] *praeses.* Disputatio medica inauguralis de febribus in genere ... Heidelbergae, Ex officina Joh. Christiani Walteri, 1665.

[27] p.   18 cm.   **[6160]**

Diss.—Heidelberg (J. Holtzapfel, *respondent*)

—Disquisitio inauguralis medica de appetitu ejusque varie affecti speciebus ... Heidelbergae, Typis Adriani Wyngaerden, 1662.

16 p.   19 cm.   **[6161]**

Diss.—Heidelberg (J. K. Stetter, *respondent*)

—Dissertatio inauguralis medica de ligatione vulgo von Nestel Knöpffen ... Heidelbergae, Typis Joh. Christiani Walteri [1672]

24 p.   19 cm.   **[6162]**

Diss.—Heidelberg (J. G. Rosa, *respondent*)

ISRAELI, ISAAC [*ca. 832–ca. 932*] Thesaurus sanitatis de victus salubris ratione alimentorum facultatibus ciborumq. varietate ac delectu; sive, De dietis universalibus & particularibus libri II. Ab Isaaco Judaeo ... conscripti, & nunc primum Latinitate donati, opera Jo. Posthii ... Antverpiae, Sumptibus Gasparis Belleri, 1607.

[7], 605 p.   17 cm.   **[6163]**

ITTIG, JOHANN [1607-1676] *praeses.* Disputatio meteorologica de igne fatuo ... [Lipsiae] Literis Wittigianis [1655]

[20] p.   19 cm.   **[6164]**

Diss.—Leipzig (M. Hermann, *respondent*)

—Disputatio physica de anima humana ... [Lipsiae] Prelo Wittigaviano [1655]

[23] p.   18 cm.   **[6165]**

Diss.—Leipzig (J. Schultz, *respondent*)

ITTIG, JOHANN FRIEDRICH [*fl*. 1670-1678] *respondent.* Dissertatio de fontibus quam consensu inclutae Facult. philosophicae pub. proponunt M. Johannes Fridericus Ittigius ... & Jacobus Smalcius ... Lipsiae, Typis viduae John. Wittigau [1672]

[12] p.   19 cm.   **[6166]**

Diss.—Leipzig (J. Schmaltz, *respondent*)

—*See* ETTMÜLLER, M., *praeses.* Disputatio inauguralis, de temulentia. 1678; ITTIG, T. De lacrymis dissertatio physica. 1670.

ITTIG, Thomas [1643-1710] De lacrymis dissertatio physica ... Lipsiae, Typis Joh. Wittigau [1670] [24] p.   19 cm.   [6167]

Diss.—Leipzig (J. F. Ittig, *respondent*)

ITZSTEIN, Heinrich [*fl.* 1621] *respondent. See* Ager, N. Disputatio physica de auditu. 1621.

IVIE, *Sir* Thomas [*fl.* 1650-1653] Alimony arrign'd; or, The remonstrance and humble appeal of Thomas Ivié esq. from the High Court of Chancery, to His Highness the Lord Protector ... Wherein are set forth the unheard-of practices and villanies of lewd and defamed women, in order to separate man and wife. London, 1654.

[2], 52 p.   22 cm.   [6168]

J

J., J. H. See Sonderbahre nutzliche auch nöthige Anmerkungen eine sorgfältige Aufferziehung der jungen Kinder. 1688.

J., W. *See* Jar, W.

J. B. B. D. *See* Butler, John, B. D.

J. C. M. D. *See* Crull, Jodocus [*d.* 1713?]

J. D. *See* Davies, John [1625-1693]

J. G. *See* G., J.

J. G. *See* Glazemaker, Jan Hendrik [*d.* 1682]

J. G. R. M. C. *See* C., J. G. R. M.

J. H. D. M. L. *See* H., J., D. M. L.

J. L. M. C. *See* Lange, Johann [*fl.* 1667-1696]

J. P. W. D. *See* Wurfbain, Johann Paul [1655-1711]

J. R. *See* Rogers, John [1627-1665?]

J. R. H. *See* Rist, Johannes [1607-1667]

J. V. B. *See* Verbrugge, Johannes.

J. W. *See* W., I.

JĀBIR IBN ḤAIYĀN, al-Ṭarasūsī. Gebri Arabis Chimai; sive, Traditio summae perfectionis et investigatio magisterii innumeris locis emendta, a Caspare Hornio ... Accessit ejusdem Medulla alchimiae Gebricae. Omnia edita a Georgio Hornio. [Lugduni Batavorum, Apud Arnoldo Doude, 1668]

[19], 179 (i.e. 279) p.   14 cm.   [6169]

Added engraved title page: Gebri Arabis. Chimicae cum correctione, et Medulla G. Horni, has imprint.

—Gebri ... Summa perfectionis magisterii in sua natura, ex Bibliothecae Vaticanae exemplari undecunque emendatissimo edita, cum ... delineatione vasorum & fornacum. Denique libri investigationis magisterii & testamenti ejusdem Gebri, ac Aurei trium verborum libelli [Kallid Rachaidibi] & Avicennae ... Mineralium additione castigatissima. Gedani, Apud Brunonem Laurentium Tancken, 1682.

[23], 278 (i.e. 272) p.   plates.   16 cm.   [6170]

Added engraved title page: Gebri regis Arabum Chymia. Dantisci, Apud Brunonem Laurentium Tancken, 1682.

Includes Expositio epistolae Alexandri regis (p. 254-260); Authoris ignoti Philosophici lapidis secreta (p. 261-264); Merlini Allegoria (p. 265-269); and Rachaidibi, Veradiani, Rhodiani, et Kanidis ... De Materia philosophici lapidis acutissime colloquentium fragmentum (p. 270-277)

—*See* Bracesco, G. De alchemia. 1673; Harprecht, J. Lucerna salis philosophorum. 1658; Philalethes, E. Enarratio methodica trium Gebri medicinarum. 1678; Salmon, W. Medicina practica. 1692; Vogel, E. Liber de lapidis physici conditionibus. 1659.

JĀBIR, Musa ibn Ḥaiyān. *See* Jābir ibn Ḥaiyān, al-Ṭarasūsī.

JACCHAEUS, Gilbert [*ca.* 1585-1628] Institutiones medicae. Lugduni Batavorum, Apud Joannem Maire, 1624.

[14], 311 p.   14 cm.   [6171]

—[The same.] ... Ed. 3., prout autor eam ante mortem recognovit emendata. Lugduni Batavorum, Ex officina Joannis Maire, 1653.

428 p.   illus.   14 cm.   [6172]

JACCHEY, Gilbert. *See* Jacchaeus, Gilbert [*ca.* 1585-1628]

JACCHINUS, Leonardus. *See* Giachini, Lionardo [*fl.* 1527-1546]

JACHMAN, Georg [*fl.* 1674-1675] *respondent. See* Loss, J., *praeses.* Exercitatio anatomica. 1674, 1675.

JACKSON, Henry [*fl.* 1644-1660] *tr. See* Berengario, J. Μιϰϱοϰοσμογϱαφία; or, A description of the body of man. 1664.

JACKSON, Joseph. Enchiridion medicum theoretico-practicum; sive, Tractatus, de morborum theoria & praxi. (Cui subnectitur Appendix de lue venerea) . . . Juxta exemplar Londinense. Amstelodami, Apud Georgium Gallet, 1697.

[22], 192 p.   front.   14 cm.   [**6173**]

—Another issue, dated 1698.

[**6174**]

JACOB Da[niel vo]n Pisspen, auss dem Land Lünenburg, sein Spanne di[e Z]oll und er ist 96. Zoll lang, und kan in die höhe reichen 126. [Zoll. Sei]nes Alters drithalben und zwanzig Jahr, im [Jahr] 1613. [n. p., n. d.]

broadside.   illus.   28 x 35 cm.   [**6175**]
Imperfect: part of text worn through.

JACOBAEER, Andreas [*fl.* 1685] *respondent. See* Veter, C., *praeses.* Dissertatio physico-medica de febrium natura. 1685.

JACOBAEUS, Holger [1650-1701] De compendium institutionum medicarum in gratiam tyronum medicinae . . . Hafniae, Prostat apud J. M. Liebe, 1694.

[7], 118 p.   16 cm.   [**6176**]
Imperfect: sig. H8 (blank?) wanting.

—De ranis observationes. Accessit Caspari Bartholini Th. F. De nervorum usu in motu musculorum epistola. Parisiis, Apud Ludovicum Billaine, 1676.

[16], 108, [4] p.   plates.   17 cm.   [**6177**]
Imperfect: Tabula prima-quinta wanting.

—[The same.] . . . Parisiis, Apud Renatum Guignard, 1682.

[16], 108, [4] p.   plates.   18 cm.   [**6178**]
Imperfect: Tabula tertia wanting.
A reissue of the 1676 edition with new title page.
Bound with Bartholin, C. [1655-1738] Diaphragmatis. Parisiis, 1682.

—De ranis et lacertis observationes. Hafniae, Impensis Johannis M. Lieben, 1686.

[16], 134 p.   16 cm.   [**6179**]
Imperfect: plates wanting; outer margins trimmed.

—Oratio in obitum . . . Thomae Bartholini. Accessit operum Th. Bartholini editorum catalogus. Hafniae, Typis viduae Cornificii Luft, 1681.

[1], 36 (i.e. 38) p.   23 cm.   [**6180**]
Bound with copy 2 of Worm, W. Oratio in excessum . . . Thomae Bartholini. 1681.

—*praeses.* Dissertatio de natura & usu salium volatilium . . . Hafniae, Literis Johannis Philippi Bockenhoffer [1693]

16 p.   19 cm.   [**6181**]
Diss.—Copenhagen (C. Kempe, *respondent*)

—Dissertatio de vermibus et insectis . . . Hafniae, Literis Johan. Philip. Bockenhoffer [1696]

23 p.   20 cm.   [**6182**]
Diss.—Copenhagen (J. B. Winslow, *respondent*)

—Dissertatio medica inauguralis de febri lipyria . . . Hafniae, Joh. Jac. Bornheinrich [1695]

[40] p.   20 cm.   [**6183**]
Diss.—Copenhagen (P. Deichmann, *respondent*)

—, *ed. See* Ariosto, F. De oleo montis Zibinii. 1698.

JACOBI, Heyman. *See* Jacobs, Heyman.

JACOBI, Johann Ernest [*fl.* 1687-1689] *respondent. See* Behrens, G. H., *praeses.* Dissertatio inauguralis medica de lue Pannonica. 1687; Vesti, J., *praeses.* Dissertatio medica inauguralis de lue venerea. 1689.

JACOBI, Johannes [*fl.* 1661-1665] Problemata miscellanea circa fundamenta medicinae physiologicae occurrentia olim in Athenaeo Salano ventilata, jam vero denuo edita . . . Jenae, Sumtibus, Joh. Ludw. Neuenhahnii, 1662.

[1], 86 p.   19 cm.   [**6184**]

JACOBI, Ludwig Friedrich [*d.* 1715] *praeses.* Disputatio medica de anima, causa morborum proxima . . . Erfordiae, Typis Groschianis [1691]

28 p.   20 cm.   [**6185**]
Diss.—Erfurt (G. A. Logan, *respondent*)

—, *respondent. See* Cramer, C., *praeses.* Archeus faber febrium intermittentium. 1679.

JACOBI, Ludwig Konrad [*fl.* 1675] *respondent.* Disputatio inauguralis exhibens medicationem aegri, febri maligna graviter decumbentis ... Marburgi Cattorum, Typis Salomonis Schadewitzii, 1675.

[2], 46 p. 20 cm. **[6186]**

Diss.—Marburg

—*See* Waldschmidt, J. J., *praeses.* Exercitatio medica de cura lactis podagricorum solatio et certo podagrae remedio. 1675.

JACOBI, Michael [*fl.* 1664] *respondent. See* Schenck, J. T., *praeses.* Disputatio medica de causo. 1664.

JACOBS, Friedrich Heinrich [*fl.* 1699] *respondent. See* Tribbechov, J., *praeses.* De lectione fontium ut vulgo appellatur cursoria. 1699.

JACOBS, Heyman. Den cleynen herbarius; ofte, Kruydt-boexken, inhoudende die kracht ende operatie van ghemeene kruyden ende bekende vruchten ... waer deur men ... zijn gesonthz mach onder houden, en allerhande siekten can ghenesen. Van nieus oversien ende verm. per H[eyman] J[acobs] ... Amstelredam [1602?]

[191] p. 14 cm. **[6187]**

Imperfect: margins trimmed with possible loss of pagination and part of the imprint.

Bound with *his* Het schat der armen. Emrick, 1603.

—[The same.] ... Dordrecht, Abraham Andriesz, [Isaac Andriessz] 1637.

192 p. 15 cm. **[6188]**

—Copy 2.

With this is bound *his* [Van den schat der armen. Antwerpen? 1661?]

—[The same.] ... Dordrecht, Jan Barentsz Smient, 1660.

192 p. 15 cm. **[6189]**

Imperfect: title page mutilated.
Different setting of type.

—[The same.] ... Amsterdam, Gijsbert de Groodt [Enchuysen, Ghedruckt by Jan Broersz] 1683.

192 p. 15 cm. **[6190]**

Different setting of type.

—Het schat der armen; oft, Een medecijn boecx-ken, dienstelijck voor alle menschen, inhoudende

hoemen sijn gesontheyt onderhouden sal ... Emrick, Christoffel van Hartochvelt, 1603.

[182] p. 14 cm. **[6191]**

With this are bound: *his* Den cleynen herbarius. Amstelredam [1602?]; Simons, Guilliame. Den troost der aermen. Gendt [17--]

—[The same.] ... Amstelredam, Hendrick Barentssz, 1609.

[4], 184 (i.e. 185), [2] p. 15 cm. **[6192]**

Bound with Follinus, H. Den Nederlandtsche sleutel. 1613.

—[The same.] ... Haerlem, Abraham Casteleyn, 1661.

160+ p. illus. 15 cm. **[6193]**

Imperfect: all pages after p. 160 wanting; title page mutilated.

—[The same.] [Van den schat der armen, oft, Een medecijn-boeckxken, dienstelijck voor alle menschen, inhoudende hoemen zijne gesontheyt onderhouden sal ... Op een nieuv oversien ... en verm. ... Antwerpen? 1661?]

[1], 177, [1+] p. 15 cm. **[6194]**

Imperfect: title page, and all pages after p. [178] wanting.
Title and imprint supplied from BMC. That edition has 181 pages.
Running title: Het eerste [-tweede] deel van't schat der armen.
Bound with copy 2 of *his* Den Cleynen herbarius. 1637.

JACOBSEN, Holger. *See* Jacobaeus, Holger [1650-1701]

JACOBUS DE DONDIS. *See* Dondi dall' Orologio, Jacopo [*ca.* 1293-1359]

JACOPO DE' DONDI. *See* Dondi dall' Orologio, Jacopo [*ca.* 1293-1359]

JACOZ, Siméon [*fl.* 1656] *ed. See* Rivière, L. Institutiones, Observationes, et Praxis medicae. 1664, 1674 [and] Opera medica universa. 1663, 1672 [and] Observationum medicarum. 1659, 1662.

JACQUELOT, P. *See* Jaquelot, Pierre [*fl.* 1630]

JACQUES, Frere. *See* Beaulieu, Frère Jacques de [1651-1714]

JACQUES, Jacques [*fl.* 1657-1673] Le fautmourir, et les excuses inutiles qu'on apporte a cette necessité. Rev. corr. & augm. de nouveau des excuses d'un partisan & d'un savetier à la mort. Le tout en vers burlesques ... Lyon, Jean-Baptiste Deville, 1669.

[14], 470 p. 15 cm. **[6195]**

Added engraved title page.

—Le medecin liberal, qui donne, gratis, des remedes salutaires contre les frayeurs de la mort. 3. partie, & suite du Faut-mourir . . . Lyon, Charles Matheuet, 1666.

[13], 215 p.   15 cm.   **[6196]**
Added engraved title page.

JAEGER, JOHANN GEORG [*fl.* 1692] *respondent. See* VIRDUNG VON HARTUNG, P. W., *praeses.* Disputatio medica deictero flavo. 1692.

JÄGER, JOHANN GERHART [*fl.* 1631] *respondent. See* SEBISCH, M. [1578–1674?] *praeses.* Libri sex Galeni De morborum differentiis. 1632.

JÄGER, PHILIPP FRIEDRICH [*fl.* 1683–1684] *respondent. See* CAMERARIUS, E. R., *praeses.* Disquisitio medica inauguralis de phlogosibus vagis cum scorbuto. 1684 [and] Modus subitaneae refectionis enucleatus. 1683.

JÄGERNDORF, ELEONORA MARIA ROSALIA, *Herzogin zu Troppau und. See* TROPPAU UND JÄGERNDORF, Eleonora Maria Rosalia, *Herzogin zu* [1647–1704]

JÄGERSCHMIDT, JOHANN VICTOR [*fl.* 1683–1684] *respondent.* Infantem epilepticum cognoscendum curandumque . . . examini exponit Johann-Victor Jägerschmidt . . . [Altdorffii] Literis Henrici Meyeri [1684]

[16] p.   20 cm.   **[6197]**
Diss.—Altdorf.

—*See* SEERUP, G. N., *praeses.* Triumphus lithargyriatorum. 1700.

JÄSCHKE, GEORG FRIEDRICH [*fl.* 1700–1702] *respondent. See* BOHN, J., *praeses.* De medici officio dissertatio quinta. 1700.

JAHN, FRIEDRICH AUGUST [1646–1716] *respondent. See* ALBERTI, V. Dissertationem historico-physicam de pluvia prodigiosa . . . submittit F. A. J. 1667, 1674.

JAHN, JAKOB EUGEN [*fl.* 1672] *respondent. See* BOHN, J., *praeses.* Dissertatio medica de polypo narium 1672.

JAHN, JOHANN GOTTFRIED [*fl.* 1671] *respondent. See* MERBITZ, J. V., *praeses.* Schediasma physicum de infantibus supposititiis. 1671.

JAHN, PETER [*fl.* 1673] *praeses.* De lupo disputatio physica . . . [Witebergae] Apud Danielis Schmatzii [1673]

[16] p.   18 cm.   **[6198]**

Diss.—Wittenberg (J. Wolf, *respondent*)

JALĀL al-DĪN, AL-SUYŪTĪ. *See* AL-SUYŪTĪ [1445–1505]

JAMES I, *King of Great Britain* [1566–1625] Misocapnus; sive, De tobacci lusus regius. *In* Everard, G. De herba panacea. 1644.

[JAMET, NOËL PHILIBERT, *fl.* 17th cent.] Traité de la circulation des esprits animaux. Divisé en quatre parties. Par un religieux de la Congregation de Saint Maur. Paris, Chez la veuve de Louis Billaine, 1682.

[40], 248 p.   16 cm.   **[6199]**
Attributed also to Jean Bonet.

JANFORTI, RAIMONDO GIOVANNI. *See* FORTIS, Raimondo Giovanni [1603–1678]

JANI, JOHANNES FRIEDRICH [*fl.* 1682] *respondent.* Disputatio medica inauguralis, de martialium operandi modo & usu . . . Ultrajecti, Apud Gulielmum Clerck, 1682.

[12] p.   22 cm.   **[6200]**
Diss.—Utrecht.

JANICH, PETER [*fl.* 1606–*ca.* 1617] *respondent. See* KECKERMANN, B., *praeses.* De fulmine disputatio. 1606.

—, *ed. See* Varanda, J. de. Formulae remediorum internorum et externorum. 1617 [and] Physiologia et Pathologia. 1619 [and] Tractatus de affectibus renum et vesicae. 1617.

JANIKE, JOACHIM [*fl.* 1607] *See* KNOBLOCK, T., *praeses.* Disputationes anatomicae. 1608, 1612.

JANS, LYSBET. *See* JANSZ, Lijsbeth.

JANSEN, KORNEL [*fl.* 1669] *respondent. See* GRAMM, C., *praeses.* Quaestiones physicae metamorphosin. 1669.

JANSONIUS, SAMUEL. Korte en bondige verhandeling, van de voortteeling en t' kinderbaren met den aankleve van dien . . . Gedaan door S[amuel] J[ansonius] . . . 4. druck . . . verb. . . . Amsterdam, Timotheus ten Hoorn, 1695.

[16], 167 p.   plates.   16 cm.   **[6201]**
Added engraved title page.
Imperfect: plates 1–5 and 7 wanting.

—[The same.] . . . 5. druck . . . verb. . . . Amsterdam, Timotheus ten Hoorn, 1699.

[16], 167 p. plates. 17 cm. [6202]

Added engraved title page.

JANSSON, THEODOOR, *van Almeloveen. See* ALMELOVEEN, Theodoor Jansson van [1657-1712]

JANSZ, LIJSBETH. *See* BOEKELMAN, A. De onschult of zamenspraak tusschen de geesten van imandt en niemandt. 1678.

JANUENSIS, SIMON. *See* SIMON GENUENSIS.

JANUS, FRIDRICH AUGUST. *See* JAHN, Friedrich August [1646-1716]

JANUS, JACOBUS-EUGENIUS. *See* JAHN, Jakob Eugen [*fl.* 1672]

JANUS, JAKOB [*fl.* 1624-1627] *praeses.* Dissertatio medica de morbis haereditariis, centum thesibus inclusa . . . Witebergae, Typis Augusti Boreck [1627]

[36] p. 19 cm. [6203]

Diss.—Wittenberg (B. Cörner, *respondent*)

—*respondent. See* SCHALLER, W., *praeses.* Disputatio medica qua hypotyposis universae medendi methodi breviter proponitur. 1625 [and] Sesquicenturia positionum medicarum de arthritide. 1625.

JAPYN, ARNOLD [*fl.* 1669] *respondent.* Disputatio medica inauguralis de respirationis laesione . . . Lugduni Batavorum, Apud viduam & haeredes Joannis Elsevirii, 1669.

[11] p. 23 cm. [6204]

Diss.—Leyden.

JAQUELOT, PIERRE [*fl.* 1630] L'art de vivre longuement, sous le nom de Medee, laquelle enseigne les facultez des choses qui sont continuellement en nostre usage, & d'où naissent les maladies. Ensemble la methode de se comporter en icelles, & le moyen de pourvoir à leurs offences . . . Lyon, Louis Teste-Fort, 1630.

[16], 241 p. 18 cm. [6205]

—[The same.] . . . Lyon, et se vendent a Paris chez Jean Jost, 1632.

[16], 241 p. 18 cm. [6206]

A reissue of the 1630 edition with new title page.

JAR, W., *ed. See* KENT, E. (Talbot) G., *countess of.* A choice manuall. 1653, 1654.

JASOLINO, GIULIO [1538-1622] Collegium anatomicum clarissimorum trium virorum Julii Jasolini . . . Marci Aurelii Severini . . . Bartholomaei Cabrolii . . . per quos singulos collatae operae posteriore paginae facie patescent. Francofurti, Apud Hermannum a Sande, 1668.

[2], 20 (i.e. 68) p.; 54, [2] p.; [20], 192, [23], 28 p. plates, illus. 21 cm. [6207]

Part [2] has special title page: Marci Aurelii Severini quaestiones anatomicae quatuor. Prima, de aqua pericardia. Secunda, de cordis adipetertia. Tertia, de poris cholidochis. Quarta, osteologia pro Galeno adversus argutatores epidochae in totidem alias Julii Jasolini. Part [3] has special title page: Celeberrimorum anatomicorum Severini, Castrensis, Jasolini et Cabrolii varia opuscula anatomica. Praemissae sunt observationes chirurgiae infusoriae hominibus adhibitae; Dissertatio de generatione animalium Theodori Aldes [pseud. i.e. Matthew Slade] . . . contra Harveium, & nova ductus thoracici cum emulgente communio. M. Gayani . . . ex Gallico sermone in Latinum versa.

Concerns the works of Johann Sigismund Elsholtz, William Harvey, Johann Daniel Major, Adriaan van de Spiegel, Giovanni Trullio, Johann Vesling, and others.

Bound with copy 2 of Sinibaldi, G. B. Geneanthropeiae. 1669.

—*See* SEVERINO, M. A. Zootomia democritaea. 1645; VOLCKAMER, J. G. [1616-1693] Collegium anatomicum. 1654.

JAXHEIM, FRIEDRICH LUDWIG VON [*fl.* 1699] *respondent. See* KIRCHMAJER, S., *praeses.* Dissertatio de variis gentium moribus et indole. 1699.

JEAN DE HAYN, *chartreux. See* INDAGINE, Joannes ab [*ca.* 1467-1537]

JEAN DE LA FONTAINE [*b.* 1381] La fontaine des amoureux de science. *In* La metallique transformation. 1618.

JEAN DE MEUN [*d.* 1305?] Demonstratio naturae, quam errantibus chymicis facit, dum de sophista & stolido spiratore carbonario conqueritur . . . Francofurti, Apud Hermannum a Sande, 1677.

[145]-171 p. 22 cm. (*In* Musaeum Hermeticum. Francofurti, 1678) [6208]

Imprint on p. [145]

—Les remonstrances de natur à l'alchymiste errant. *In* La metallique transformation. 1618.

JEAN DE SAINT-AMAND. *See* SAINT-AMAND, Jean de [13th cent.]

JEHRING, JOHANN CHRISTIAN [*fl.* 1663] *respondent.* See ROLFINCK, W., *praeses.* Exercitatio medica de genuina calculorum in humano corpore. 1644.

JELTSCH, DAVID KASPAR [*fl.* 1684] *respondent.* See BOHN, J. *praeses.* Dissertationes chymico-physicae. 1685.

JENICHEN, GEORG [1641-1718] *praeses.* Disputatio physica, de fulmine ... Lipsiae, Literis Hahnianis [1663]

[16] p. 20 cm. [6209]

Diss.—Leipzig (F. C. Berens, *respondent*)

JENICHEN, GOTTLIEB AUGUST [*fl.* 1699-1700] *praeses.* De cultu heroinarum sago vel toga illustrium ... Lipsiae, Literis Joh. Andreae Zschauens [1700]

[24] p. 19 cm. [6210]

Diss.—Leipzig (V. G. Hercklitz, *respondent*)

—*respondent.* See MÜLLER, G. E. Dissertatio physica de saltu naturae. 1699.

JENICHEN, GOTTLOB FRIEDRICH [1680-1735] *praeses.* Disputatio physica de genesimantia ... Lipsiae, Literis Johan. Andreae Zschauens [1699]

[24] p. 21 cm. [6211]

Diss.—Leipzig (Z. Dezius, *respondent*)

JENTSCH, JOHANN [*fl.* 1607] See KNOBLOCH, T., *praeses.* Disputationes anatomicae. 1608, 1612.

JEROME, *Saint.* See SCHMID, J. A., *praeses.* Dux foemina facti haereseos vel autor vel fautor. 1697.

JERSIN, DIONYSIUS [*fl.* 1656] *respondent.* See OSTENFELD, C., *praeses.* Exercitationum de medicinae fundamentis prodromus. 1656.

JESSEN, JOHANN VON [1566-1621] Adversus pestem consilium, cum ejusdem de mithridatio, & theriaca disputatione. His annexi Jani Matthaei Durastantis De aceto scillino atque aloe medicamentis valetudini tuendae, vitae proprogandae singularibus, tractatus duo. Nec non Nicolai Curtii ... libellus ... anno 1575. Patavii propositus De medicamentis lenientibus, praeparantibus & purgantibus. Giessae, Typis Casparis Chemlini, 1614 [i.e., 1615]

341, [1] p. 14 cm. [6212]

Curtius' treatise has special title page dated 1615.

—Anatomiae, Pragae, anno M.D.C. abs se solenniter administratae historia. Accessit ejusdem De ossibus tractatus. Wittebergae, Excudebat Laurentius Seuberlich, impensis Samuelis Selfisch, 1601.

[15], 160 p.; 35, [4] ll. 17 cm. [6213]

Part [2] has special title page.

—De cavenda tollendaque peste ad patronos et amicos consilium. Pragae, Typis Schumanianis, 1606.

[32] p. 19 cm. [6214]

—De ossibus tractatus. Wittebergae, Excudebat Laurentius Seuberlich, impensis Samuelis Selfisch, 1601.

35, [4] ll. table. 18 cm. [6215]

—De sanguine, vena secta, dimisso judicium notis & castigationibus ad hodierna & vera artis medicae principia accommodatum a Jacobo Pancratio Brunone ... Norimbergae, Sumtibus Michaelis & Joh. Friderici Endterorum, 1668.

[24], 264, [24] p. 14 cm. [6216]

—Institutiones chirurgicae, quibus universa manu medendi ratio ostenditur. Witebergae, Excudebat Laurentius Seuberlich, impensis Samuelis Selfisch, 1601.

[8], 106, [6] ll. port. 17 cm. [6217]

—, *ed.* See CAMPOLONGO, E. Σημειωτιϰη. 1601; HÖRNYK, M. De acidularum. 1615? See RIOLAN, J. [1538?-1605?] Chirurgia. 1601, 1618, 1638.

—See LIDDEL, D. Ars medica. 1628.

JESSENIUS A JESSEN, JOANNES. See JESSEN, Johann von [1566-1621]

JESSINSKÝ, JAN. See JESSEN, Johann von [1566-1621]

JIMÉNEZ SAVARIEGO, JUAN [*b.* 1568] Tratado de peste, donde se contienen las causas, preservacion, y cura, con algunas questiones curiosas al proposito ... Antequera, Claudio Bolan, 1602.

4, CLXXII (i.e. CLXXX), [12] ll. 20 cm. [6218]

JOANNES XXI, *Pope.* See JOHANNES XXI, *Pope* [*d.* 1277]

JOANNES ACTUARIUS [13th cent.] De urinis libri VII ... Trajecti ad Rhenum, Ex officina Gisberti a Zyll, 1670.

[14], 320, 461 (i.e. 459), [5] p. 17 cm. [6219]

Ambrogio Leone's translation of Περὶ οὔρων, edited by Jacques Goupyl.

"Jodoci Willichii De probationibus urinarum, cum scholis medicis Hyeronimi Reusneri . . . & Remedia plurima ex urina desumpta": p. 309-320, 1-300 (2d and 3d groups of paging); "Thomae Willis Dissertatio de urinis": p. 301-378; "Guielmi [sic] Strateni . . . Disputationes medicae tres de erroribus popularibus, de fallaci urinarum judicio": p. [379]-408; "Aristotelis . . . De coloribus liber, Coelio Calcagnino interprete . . . Cui subjicitur Antonii Thylesii . . . De coloribus libellus": p. [409]-461.

—De differentiis urinarum lib. I . . . [&] De judiciis urinarum lib. I-II . . . [&] De causis urinarum lib. I-II . . . [&] De praevidentiis ex urinis. lib. I-II . . . Ambrosio Leone Nolano interprete, summa cura & diligentia a Jacobo Goupylo recogniti.

308 p. 16 cm. (*In* Willich, Jodocus. Exercitationes . . . de urinis libri IV. Amstelodami, 1688)   **[6220]**

Caption title.

JOANNES ANTARVETUS, *pseud.* *See* RIOLAN, Jean [1580-1657]

JOANNES DAMASCENUS [*d.* 857] *See* MESÜE [*d.* 857]

JOANNES DE LASNIORO. *See* LAAZ, Johann von [*fl.* 15th cent.]

JOANNES DE RUPESCISSA [*fl.* 1328-1365] De consideratione quintae essentiae. *In* Lull, R. Tractatus. 1616.

—Liber . . . de confectione veri lapidis philosophorum . . .

189-197 p., vol. 3. 20 cm. (*In* Zetzner, Lazarus, *ed.* Theatrum chemicum. Argentorati, 1659-61)   **[6221]**

Caption title.

—Liber lucis . . .

284-295 p., vol. 3. illus. 20 cm. (*In* Zetzner, Lazarus, *ed.* Theatrum chemicum. Argentorati, 1659-61)   **[6222]**

Caption title.

—[The same.] *In* Broekhuizen, D. van. Secreta alchimiae magnalia D. Thomae Aquinatis. 1602.

—*See* CARDILUCIUS, J. H., *ed.* Magnalia medicochymica. 1676; LAVINHETA, B. de. Opera omnia. 1612.

JOANNES, HESRONITA [*fl.* 17th cent.] *See* [GABRIEL, S.] Arabia. 1633.

JOANNES TICINENSIS. *See* JOHANN VON TETZEN.

JOANNINI, GIOVANNI BATTISTA. *See* JUANINI, Juan Bautista [1636-1691]

JOANNITIUS. *See* ḤUNAIN IBN ISḤĀḲ, al-'Ibādī [809?-873]

JOBELOT, CLAUDIO FRANCESCO [*fl.* 1695] *tr.* *See* LÉMERY, N. Corso chimico. 1695.

JOEHRENIUS, CONRAD. *See* JOHRENIUS, Conrad [1653-1716]

JOEL, FRANCISCUS [1510-1579] Operum medicorum . . . tomus primus [-sextus] in quo universae medicinae compendium succinctis quaestionibus & tabulis comprehensum, & in Academia Gryphiswaldensi ante complures annos publice traditum . . . In lucem editus a Matthaeo Bachmeistero . . . Hamburgi, Typis Henr. Carstens, 1616-1631.

6 v. in 2. plates. 20 cm.   **[6223]**

Imprint varies: Lunaeburgi, Excudebat Andreas Michaelis, 1622 (vol. 4); Rostochii, Typis Mauritii Saxonis, impensis Johan. Hallervord, 1629, 1631 (vol. 5-6).

Vols. 5-6 edited by Franciscus Joel, the author's grandson.

—[The same.] . . . Rostochii, Joachimi Wildii, 1622-1652 [v. 1, 1652]

6 v. in 2. plates. 21 cm.   **[6224]**

Imprint varies: Rostochii, Literis Nicolai Kilii, sumptibus Joachimi Wilden, 1648 (vol. 2); Rostochii, Apud Joachimum Wilden, 1650 (vol. 3); Lunaeburgi, Excudebat Andreas Michaelis, 1622 (vol. 4); Rostochii, Typis Mauritii Saxonis, impensis Johan. Hallervord, 1629, 1631 (vol. 5-6).

—Opera medica, ante complures annos utilitatis publicae causa in lucem edita, nunc rev., emend. . . . Amstelraedami, Apud Joannem Ravesteinium, 1663.

[8], 571, [13] p.; 295, [15] p. plates. 21 cm.   **[6225]**

Added engraved title page.
Edited by the publisher.

—De generali methodo medendi, & remediis usitatioribus liber. *In* Cordus, V. Dispensatorium. 1651.

JOEL, FRANCISCUS [1595-1631] *ed.* *See* JOEL, F. [1510-1579] Operum medicorum . . . tomus primus [-sextus] 1616-1631; 1622-1652 [v. 1, 1652]

JOEPSER, JAKOB JOSEPH [1627-1695] Isagoge; seu, Manuductio ad vitam longiorem: variis, de tuenda . . . valetudine, dissertationibus illustrata, & selectis, tum veterum, tum recentiorum medicorum scitis placitisque stabilita ... Noribergae, Sumtibus Michaelis & Johan. Friderici Endterorum, 1680.

[32], 688, [25] p. front. 21 cm.   **[6226]**

Errata: p. [25] at end.

JOHANN ERNST, *Prince of Saxony* [1658–1729] *See* SAXONY. Laws, statutes, etc. Des ... Herrn Johann Ernstens, Hertzogs zu Sachsen ... Anordnung. 1680.

JOHANN GEORG III, *Elector of Saxony* [1647–1691] *See* LEIPZIG. Ordinances, local laws, etc. Raths der Stadt Leipzig ... Ordnung und Taxa. 1689.

JOHANN GEORG DER ANDER, *Hertzog zu Sachsen. See* JOHANN GEORG III. *Elector of Saxony* [1647–1691]

JOHANN VON TETZEN. Processus de lapide philosophorum. In Drey vortreffliche und noch nie im Druck gewesene chymische Bücher. 1670.

[**JOHANNES XXI,** *Pope, d.* 1277] Libro de medicina llamado Thesoro de pobres. Con un Regimiento de sanidad. Agora nuevamente corregido y emendado, por Arnaldo de Villanova. Barcelona, Francisco Dotil, 1611.

73, [3] ll. 15 cm.   **[6227]**

JOHANNES DE SANCTO AMANDO. *See* SAINT-AMAND, Jean de [13th cent.]

JOHANNES ISAACI, *Hollandus* [15th cent.] Fragmentum de lapide philosophorum.

126–129 p., vol. 2 20 cm. (*In* Zetzner, Lazarus, *ed.* Theatrum chemicum. Argentorati, 1659–61)   **[6228]**

Caption title.

—Operum mineralium Joannis Isaaci Hollandi; sive, De lapide philosophico.

304–515 p., vol. 3. illus. 20 cm. (*In* Zetzner, Lazarus, *ed.* Theatrum chemicum. Argentorati, 1659–61)   **[6229]**

Caption title.

—Opus vegetabile. Worin er den treuhertzigen Filiis doctrinae, getreu warhaffter Massen umbständlichen Unterricht gibt, und den ... Weg anzeigt ... aus den Vegetabilien ... die wahre philosophische Quinta Essentia zu ziehen, und ein ... wunder-würckenden Medicinal-Stein zu perficiren ... Aus niederländischen Manuscriptis ... verhochdeutschet, und zu ... Druck ... hergegeben

vom Sohn Sendivogii genannt J.F.H.S. [i.e. Josephat Friedrich Hautnorthon, pseud. (?) of Johann Harprecht] Amsterdam, Bey Johann Caspar Meyern, 1695.

144 p. illus. 16 cm.   **[6230]**

—Tractatus de urina quomodo per spiritum ejus omnes tincturae sint extrahendae.

566–568 p., vol. 6. 20 cm. (*In* Zetzner, Lazarus, *ed.* Theatrum chemicum. Argentorati, 1659–61)   **[6231]**

Caption title.

—Tractatus duo chemici. *In* [Combach, L.] *ed.* and *tr.* Tractatus. 1647.

—*See* BASILIUS VALENTINUS. Triumph-Wagen Antimonii. 1676; FIORAVANTI, L. Three exact pieces of Leonard Phioravant. 1652. PARACELSUS. One hundred and fourteen experiments and cures. 1652. PENOT, B. G. De denario medico. 1608.

JOHANNES PAUPERUM. Abbrevatio de secretis secretorum ...

131–139 p., vol. 3. 17 cm. (*In* Artis auriferae. Basileae, 1610)   **[6232]**

Caption title.

JOHANNES TICINENSIS. *See* JOHANN VON TETZEN.

JOHANNITIUS. *See* ḤUNAIN IBN ISḤĀḲ, al-'Ibādī [809?–873]

JOHGTIJS, DANIEL. *See* JONCTYS, Daniel [1600–1654]

JOHN XXI, *Pope. See* JOHANNES XXI, *Pope* [*d.* 1277]

JOHN, SCHWEICKHARD, *Abp. and Elector of Mentz. See* SCHWEIKARD VON KRONENBERG, Johann, *Abp. of Mainz* [*d.* 1626]

JOHNIUS, ALEXANDER GOTTFRIED [*fl.* 1665–1668] *praeses.* Disputatio physica de terrae motu ... Lipsiae, Typis Johannis Coleri [1668]

[24] p. 19 cm.   **[6233]**

Diss.—Leipzig (J. G. Gottsmann, *respondent*)

—*respondent. See* WEISSE, J. S., *praeses.* Disputatio physico-philologica de sale. 1665.

JOHNSON, ROBERT [*b.* 1640?] Enchiridion medicum; or, A manual of physick. Being a compendium of the whole art, in three parts. Viz. I. Of diseases of the head. II. Of diseases of the breast. III. Of diseases of the belly ... The 2d. ed., with additions ... London, Printed by J. Heptinstall, for Brabazon Aylmer, 1684.

[16], 317, [7] p. port. 19 cm.   **[6234]**

Imperfect: port. wanting.

[**JOHNSON**, THOMAS, *d.* 1644] Mercurius botanicus; sive, Plantarum gratia suscepti itineris, anno M.DC.XXXIV. descriptio ... Huic accessit de Thermis Bathonicis tractatus. Londini, Thom. Cotes, 1634.

2 parts in 1 v. plate. 15 cm.   **[6235]**

Imperfect: upper and lower margins trimmed, with possible loss of pagination.

Part [2] has special title page.

—, *ed. See* BAUDERON, B. Pharmacopoea. 1639; GERARD, J. The herball: or, Generall historie of plantes. 1633, 1636.

—, *tr. See* PARÉ, A. The workes. 1634, 1649, 1665, 1678.

JOHNSON, WILLIAM [*d.* 1665] Lexicon chymicum. Cum obscuriorum verborum, et rerum Hermeticarum, tum phrasium Paracelsicarum, in scriptis ejus, et aliorum chymicorum, passim occurrentium, planam explicationem continens ... Londini, Excudebat G. D. impensis Gulielmi Nealand, 1652.

[18], 250 p. 15 cm.   **[6236]**

Lacks part [2] published in 1653.

—[The same.] ... Londini, Excudebat G. D. impensis Gulielmi Nealand, 1657.

[12], 228 p. 17 cm.   **[6237]**

Possibly lacks part [2].

—[The same.] ... Londini, Excudebat G. D. impensis Gulielmi Nealand, 1660.

[12], 259 p.; [24], 72, [11] p. 17 cm. **[6238]**

Part 2, including Vita Paracelsi, has special title page: Lexicon chymicum ... Lib. secundus. Londini, Excudebat G. D. et prostant venales apud L. Sadler, 1660.

—[The same.] ... Francof. & Lipsiae, Apud Joh. Henr. Ellingerum, 1678.

[12], 272 p.; [13], 72 p. 17 cm.   **[6239]**

"Vita Paracelsi": p. [7-13] in part 2.

Bound with Blankaart, S. Lexicon medicum Graeco-Latinum. 1683.

—, *ed. See* FIORAVANTI, L. Three exact pieces of Leonard Phioravant. 1652.

JOHNSTON, JAMES [*fl.* 1693] *respondent. See* PITCAIRNE, A., *praeses*. Dissertatio de caussis diversae molis. 1693.

JOHNSTON, JOHN. *See* JONSTONUS, Joannes [1603-1675]

JOHRENIUS, CONRAD [1653-1716] *praeses.* De affectione hypochondriaca diatribe ... Rinthelii, G. C. Wächter, 1678.

[10], 72 p. 19 cm.   **[6240]**

Diss.—Rinteln (N. C. Mohr, *respondent*)

—Disputatio inauguralis de pleuritide ... Rintelii, Typis Wächteri, 1678.

16 p. 20 cm.   **[6241]**

Diss.—Rinteln (F. O. Maas, *respondent*)

—Disputatio inauguralis medica de volatili & fixo, sanitatis humanae conservativo, destructivo & restaurativo ... Rinthelii, Excudebat G. C. Wächter [1678]

44 p. 20 cm.   **[6242]**

Diss.—Rinteln (J. Elers, *respondent*)

—Dissertatio solennis de epilepsia ... Francofurti ad Viadrum, Literis Christophori Zeitleri [1700]

31, [1] p. 21 cm.   **[6243]**

Diss.—Frankfurt an der Oder (J. W. Monschein, *respondent*)

—, *ed. See* HARTMANN, J. Opera omnia medicochymica. 1684, 1694.

JOHRENIUS, JOHANN MARTIN [*fl.* 1673] *praeses.* Disputatio philosophica de sede animae rationalis ... Marburgi Cattorum, Typis Salomonis Schadewitzii, 1673.

[1], 18 p. 19 cm.   **[6244]**

Diss.—Marburg (N. Wittich, *respondent*)

JOHRON, CONRAD. *See* JOHRENIUS, Conrad [1653-1716]

JOLY, HENRY. Discours d'une estrange ... maladie hypochondriaque venteuse, qui à duré onze ans, accompagnee de l'hysterique passion, avec leurs noms ... & leurs remedes ... Paris, Catherine Niverd, vefue de Claude de Monstr'oeil, 1609.

[8], 72 p. 17 cm.   **[6245]**

Imperfect? p. 57-64 wanting?

JON, FRANÇOIS DU. *See* DU JON, François [1545–1602]

JONAS PHILOLOGUS, *pseud. See* GUINTERIUS, Joannes, Andernacus [1505–1574]

JONCQUET, DENIS [*d.* 1671] Hortus; sive, Index onomasticus plantarum, quas excolebat Parisiis annis 1658. & 1659. Accessit ... Stirpium aliquot paulo obscurius denominatarum officinis, Arabibus, aliis, per Casparum Bauhinum explicatio. Parisiis, Apud Franciscum Clousier, 1659.

     [18], 140 p.; 47 p.   port.   24 cm.   **[6246]**
    Added engraved title page.
    Imperfect: portrait wanting.
    Part [2] has half title.

JONCTYS, DANIEL [1600–1654] *tr. See* SENNERT, D. Verhandelingh der toover-sieckten. 1638, 1646.

JONDOT, PHILIBERT. Traité des causes et necessitez de la saignée, et des maladies principales, où il s'en faut servir ... Paris, Jean Henault, 1662.

     [16], 236, [3] p.   16 cm.   **[6247]**

JONES, JOHN [*fl.* 1562–1579] *See* FLOYER, Sir J. An enquiry into the right use and abuses of the hot, cold, and temperate baths in England. 1697.

JONES, JOHN [1645–1709] The mysteries of opium reveald ... London, Richard Smith, 1700.

     [9], 371 p.   illus., plate.   22 cm.   **[6248]**

— Novarum dissertationum de morbis abstrusioribus tractatus primus. De febribus intermittentibus, in quo obiter febris continuae natura explicatur ... Londini, Typis H. H., impensis Gualteri Kettilby, 1683.

     [24], 279, [1] p.   19 cm.   **[6249]**

— [The same.] ... Hagae-Comitum, Apud Arnoldum Leers, 1684.

     [12], 236 p.   16 cm.   **[6250]**

— *See* PIENS, F. H. Tractatus de febribus in genere. 1689.

JONES, ZACHARY. *See* LE LOYER, P., *sieur de La Brosse.* A treatise of specters. 1605.

JONG, PIETER DE [*fl.* 1693] *respondent.* Disputatio medica inauguralis de specificiis ... Lugduni Batavorum, Apud Abrahamum Elsevier, 1693.

     [16] p.   22 cm.   **[6251]**
    Diss. — Leyden.

JONGE, CORNELIS DE [*fl.* 1684] *respondent.* Disputatio medica inauguralis, de phthisi sive tabe vera ... Harderovici, Apud Albertum Sas, 1684.

     [12] p.   22 cm.   **[6252]**
    Diss. — Harderwijk.

JONGH, JOHANNES DE [*fl.* 1694] *respondent.* Disputatio medica inauguralis de uteri suffocatione ... Trajecti ad Rhenum, Ex officina Francisci Halma, 1694.

     12 p.   18 cm.   **[6253]**
    Diss. — Utrecht.

JONGH, LAURENS DE [*fl.* 1685] *respondent.* Disputatio medica inauguralis de peste ... Lugduni Batavorum, Apud Abrahamum Elzevier, 1685.

     [28] p.   22 cm.   **[6254]**
    Diss. — Leyden.

JONGHE, ADRIAAN DE. *See* JUNIUS, Hadrianus [1511–1575]

JONSIUS, FRIDERICUS [*fl.* 1696–1698] *respondent. See* SCHELHAMMER, G. C., *praeses.* Dissertatio inauguralis de spina ventosa. 1698.

JONSTONUS, JOANNES [1603–1675] Enchiridion ethicum, ex sententiosissimis dictis concinnatum et in libros tres distinctum. Bregae Silesiorum, Sumptibus Casparis Mülleri, typis Tschornianis, 1658.

     [4], 220 p.   13 cm.   **[6255]**

— Historiae naturalis de quadrupedibus libri ... Amstelodami, Apud Joannem Jacobi fil. Schipper, 1657.

     6 parts in 4 v.   plates.   38 cm.   **[6256]**
    Engraved title page.
    Parts 2–6 have special title pages; those to parts 3, 4 and 5 are engraved.
    Contents: [1] De quadrupedibus. — [2] De exanguibus aquatis. — [3] De piscibus et cetis. — [4] De avibus. — [5] De insectis. — [6] De serpentibus.

— Idea hygieines recensita. Libri II. Johannes Jonstonus ... cum cura revidit. Jenae, Sumptibus Viti Jacobi Trescheri, typis Johannis Nisii, 1661.

     [20], 396 p.   14 cm.   **[6257]**
    With this is bound: Tilemann, J. Guldiner Apffel. 1635.

— Idea universae medicinae practicae libris VIII absoluta ... Amsterodami, Apud Ludovicum Elzevirium, 1644.

     [12], 759 p.   14 cm.   **[6258]**
    Engraved title page.

—[The same.] . . . Venetiis, Sub signo Minervae, 1647.

[8], 580 (i.e. 590), [15] p.   16 cm.   **[6259]**

—[The same.] Idea universae medicinae practicae libris XII absoluta, ed. hac quatuor accessere . . . Amstelodami, Apud Ludovicum Elzevirium, 1648.

[30], 756 p.   17 cm.   **[6260]**

Engraved title page.

—[The same.] . . . Ed. praeter Venetam 3., multo auct. & emend. Amstelodami, Apud Ludovicum Elzevirium, 1652.

[32], 752 p.   16 cm.   **[6261]**

Imperfect: p. 449-452 wanting.

—[The same.] . . . Ed. nov., prioribus auct. & emend. Lugduni, Apud Hieronymum de la Garde & Joannem Girin, 1655.

[24], 752 p.   19 cm.   **[6262]**

—[English tr.] The idea of practical physick in twelve books . . . They contain the marrow of all the works of Daniel Sennertus, and Fernelius, and twenty five physitians more . . . Written in Latin by John Johnston . . . And Englished by Nich. Culpeper . . . London, Peter Cole, 1657.

1 v.   27 cm.   **[6263]**

Various pagings.
Imperfect: sig. O4 and Ee4 mutilated.
Contents at end.

—[The same.] . . . There is now added . . . divers physical treatises. And many hundred famous and rare cures, partly collected out of other authors, and partly experiments dayly practiced. By Abdiah Cole . . . The 2d ed. London, Peter and Edward Cole, 1661.

1 v.   28 cm.   **[6264]**

Various pagings.
Imperfect: sig. O4 mutilated.
A reissue of the 1657 edition with new title page and preliminary matter partly reset. Contents bound after the Preface.

—Naturae constantia; seu, Diatribe in qua . . . mundum, nec ratione sui totius, nec ratione partium . . . perpetuo in pejus ruere, ostenditur. Amstelodami, Apud Guilielmum Blaeu, 1632.

[6], 182 (i.e. 164) p.   12 cm.   **[6265]**

Imperfect? First preliminary leaf wanting?

—Syntagma universae medicinae practicae libri XIV . . . Jenae, Ex officina Johannis Nisii, sumptibus Viti Jacobi Trescheri, 1674 [1673]

[42], IIII, [1] p.   front. (port.)   18 cm.   **[6266]**

Added engraved title page.

—Another issue. 19 cm. Added engraved title page lacks privilege; date erased to read MDCLXXIII. Title page and front. (port.) wanting.

[6267]

—[The same.] *In* Bonet, T. Polyalthes. 1691-1693.

—Thaumatographia naturalis, in decem classes distincta, in quibus admiranda I. Coeli. II. Elementorum. III. Meteororum. IV. Fossilium. V. Plantarum. VI. Avium. VII. Quadrupedum. VIII. Exanguium. IX. Piscium. X. Hominis. Amsterdami, Apud Guilielmum Blaeu, 1632.

[12], 501 p.   14 cm.   **[6268]**

—[The same.] Amstelodami, Apud Joannem Jansonium, 1633.

[6], 578 (i.e. 576), [2] p.   13 cm.   **[6269]**

—[The same.] Amstelodami, Apud Joannem Janssonium, 1661.

[11], 498, [3] p.   14 cm.   **[6270]**

—[The same.] . . . Amstelodami, Apud Joannem Janssonium et Elizeum Weyerstraet, 1665.

495, [3] p.   15 cm.   **[6271]**

Added engraved title page.

—[English tr.] An history of the wonderful things of nature, set forth in ten severall classes. Wherein are contained I. The wonders of the heavens. II. Of the elements. III. Of meteors. IV. Of minerals. V. Of plants. VI. Of birds. VII. Of four-footed beasts. VIII. Of insects . . . IX. Of fishes. X. Of man . . . Rendred into English, by a person of quality. London, John Streater, 1657.

[14], 354 p.   29 cm.   **[6272]**

—, *ed. See* HIPPOCRATES. Coacae praenotiones. 1660.

—*See* AD THERIACAE ANDROMACHI. 1642; MICHAELIS, J. Opera. 1688, 1698.

JOÓ, FERENC. *See* JOEL, Franciscus [1510-1579]

JOOSTENS, PÂQUIER [d. 1590?] De alea libri duo. Amsterodami, Apud Ludovic. Elzevirium, 1642.

[59], 213, [43] p.   11 cm.   **[6273]**

Engraved title page.
Dedicatory epistle by M. Z. Boxhorn, the editor.
Copinger 2571.
First published in 1561 under title: Alea; sive De curanda ludendi in pecuniam cupiditate, libry II.

JORDAAN, LAURENS. *See* JORDAEN, Laurens [*fl.* 1655–1658]

JORDAEN, LAURENS [*fl.* 1655–1658] *See* BILS, L. de. Specimina anatomica. 1661 [and] Waarachtig gebruik der tot noch toe gemeende gijlbuis. 1658; PARENT, A. Anatomisch vertoon van het ghehoor by ... Louys de Bils. 1655.

JORDAN, ELIAS [*fl.* 1627–1628] *respondent. See* MÜLLER, Jakob, *praeses.* Disquisitio medica φυσιολογικὴ calidi innati et influentis. 1627.

JORDAN, HIERONYMUS [*fl.* 1639–1650] De eo quod divinum aut supernaturale est in morbis humani corporis, ejusque curatione, liber. 1. Accessit Consilium pro nobili foemina, rarissimo cordis affectu laborante. 2. Morbi D. Joachimi Läger ... veneficio illati, historia. 3. Discursus D. Hermanni Conringii De angelis. 4. Disputatio inauguralis de paralysi, sub eodem Conringio habita ab H[ieronymus] I[ordano] ... Francofurti ad Moenum, Impensis Joan. Godofredi Schönwetteri, 1651.
[86], 269, [47] p. 20 cm. [6274]
Engraved title page.

—, *respondent See* CONRING, H., *praeses.* Disputatio de sale. 1639 [and] Disputatio medica de paralysi. 1644.

JORDÁN, THOMÁS, [1539–1586] *See* SCHOLTZ, L. Consiliorum medicinalium ... liber singularis. 1610.

JORDEN, EDWARD [1569–1632] A briefe discourse of a disease called the suffocation of the mother. Written uppon occasion which hath been of late taken thereby, to suspect possession of an evill spirit, or some such like supernaturall power. Wherein is declared that divers strange actions and passions of the body of man, which ... are imputed to the divell, have their true naturall causes, and do accompanie this disease ... London, John Windet, 1603.
[4], 25 ll. 19 cm. [6275]
STC 14790.

—A discourse of naturall bathes, and minerall waters. Wherein first the originall of fountaines in generall, is declared ... And lastly, of the nature and uses of bathes, but especially of four bathes at Bathe in Sommerset-shire. The 2d ed. ... enl. ... London, Thomas Harper, 1632.
[12], 142 p. 19 cm. [6276]
STC 14792.

—[The same.] ... The 3d ed. rev. and enl. with some particulars of the authors life. To which is added, An appendix concerning Bathe ... and the virtues of the hot waters there. By Thomas Guidott, M. B. London, Thomas Salmon, 1669.
[24], 167 p.; [9], 60 p. table. 17 cm. [6277]
Part [2] has special title page with imprint: London, Printed by J. Streater for Geo. Sawbridge, 1669.

—[The same.] ... And in this 4th ed., A quaere concerning drinking bath-water at Bathe, is resolved. To which is added, An appendix concerning Bathe ... and the virtues of the hot waters there. By Thomas Guidot, M. B. London, George Sawbridge; Thomas Salmon in Bathe, 1673.
[24], 167 p.; [9], 60 p.; [1], 26 p. 17 cm. [6278]
Part [2] has special title page with imprint: London, Printed by J. Streater for Geo. Sawbridge, 1669. Part [3] has special title page: A quare concerning drinking bath-water, at Bathe resolved. By Eugenius Philander [pseud., i.e. Thomas Guidott] London, George Sawbridge, 1673.

JORDIS, JOHANNES PHILIPP [*fl.* 1680] *respondent.* Disputatio medica inauguralis, de incubo ... Ultrajecti, Typis Appelarianis, 1680.
[22] p. 20 cm. [6279]
Diss. — Utrecht.

JORMANN, JOHANN ANDREAS [*fl.* 1693] *respondent. See* VATER, C., *praeses.* Judicium e sanguine per venae sectionem emisso. 1693.

JOSEPHUS, FLAVIUS. The famous and memorable workes of Josephus ... Translated out of the Latin, and French, by Tho. Lodge ... London, Printed by J. L. for Andrew Hebb, 1632.
[10], 812 (i.e. 816), [26+] p. 34 cm. [6280]
Imperfect: all pages after p. [26] wanting; title page mutilated.
"The lamentable ... history of the wars ... of the Jewes ... London, Printed by I. L. for Simon Waterson, 1632" (p. [555–763]) has special title page.

JOSSELYN, JOHN [*fl.* 1630–1675] New Englands rarities discovered: in birds, beasts, fishes, serpents, and plants of that country. Together with the physical and chyrurgical remedies wherewith the natives constantly use to cure their distempers, wounds and sores ... London, G. Widdowes, 1672.

[5], 114, [2] p. illus., plate. 15 cm. **[6281]**

JOSSIO, Nicandro [16th cent.] Tractatus novus ... De voluptate et dolore, de risu et fletu, somno et vigilia, deque fame & siti ... Cui accesserunt Antonii Laurentii ... De risu, ejusque causis et effectis, dilucide ac philosophice tractatis, libri duo ... Francofurti, Typis Wolffgangi Richteri, sumptibus Joannis Theobaldi Schönwetteri, 1603.

446 p. 16 cm. **[6282]**

JOUBERT, Isaac, *tr. See* Joubert, L. La premiere et seconde partie des Erreurs populaires. 1601.

—*See* Joubert, L. Annotations ... sur toute la chirurgie de M. Guy de Chauliac. 1615, 1619, 1641, 1642, 1649, 1659.

JOUBERT, Laurent [1529-1583] Annotations ... sur toute la chirurgie de M. Guy de Chauliac. Avec L'interpretation des langues dudit Guy: (c'est à dire, l'explication de ses termes plus obscurs) ... Rouen, De l'imprimerie de Raphael du Petit Val. Chez David du Petit Val, 1615.

32, 403, [11] p. illus., ports. 18 cm. **[6283]**

Interpretation des langues is by Issac Joubert.
Bound with (as issued?) Guy de Chauliac. La grande chirurgie. 1615.

—[The same.] ... Tournon, Claude Michel, 1619.

8, 403 (i.e. 401), [6] p. illus. 17 cm. **[6284]**

Imperfect: last leaf (index) mutilated.

—[The same.] ... Rouen, David du Petit Val, 1641.

[32], 403, [12] p. illus., port. 17 cm. **[6285]**

Bound with (as issued?) Guy de Chauliac, La grande chirurgie. 1641.

—[The same.] ... En ceste derniere ed., on a corrigé plusieurs fautes & manquements ... Lyon, Simon Rigaud, 1642.

[16], 355, [5] p. illus., ports. 18 cm. **[6286]**

Bound with (as issued?) Guy de Chauliac. La grande chirurgie. 1642.

—[The same.] ... Rouen, David du Petit Val, 1649.

32, 403, [11] p. ports. 18 cm. **[6287]**

Imperfect: p. 369-384 bound in wrong order.
Bound with (as issued?) Guy de Chauliac. La grande chirurgie. 1649.

—[The same.] ... Lyon, Jacques Olier, 1659.

32, 405, [8] p. illus., ports. 18 cm. **[6288]**

Bound with (as issued?) Guy de Chauliac. La grande chirurgie. 1659.

—La premiere et seconde partie des Erreurs populaires, touchant la medecine & le regime de santé ... Avec plusieurs autres petits traitez ... Rouen, Raphael du Petit Val, 1601.

2 parts in 1 v. 17 cm. **[6289]**

Part [2] has special title page dated 1600.
"Deux paradoxes de luy mesme, traduits par Isaac son fils": part [2], p. 180-211; "Question vulgaire, quel langage parleroit un enfant qui n'auroit jamais ouy parler": part [2], p. 212-227.

—, *ed.* and *tr. See* Guy de Chauliac. La grande chirurgie. 1615, 1619, 1641, 1642, 1649, 1659.

—*See* Bachot, G. Erreurs populaires touchant la medecine et regime de santé. 1626 [and] Troisiesme des erreurs populaires. 1626; Citois, F. Abstinens confolentanea, cui obiter annexa est pro Juberto apologia. 1602.

JOURNAL DE MEDECINE; ou, observations des plus fameux medecins, chirurgiens & anatomistes de l'Europe ... Avril [-Octobre] 1686. Paris, Daniel Horthemels, 1686.

60 p.; 46, [1] p.; 59 p.; 285, [19] p. plates. 17 cm. **[6290]**

Each group of paging has special title page.
Fourth group of paging has caption title: IV. Journal de medecine aust-octobre ... Nouvelles conjectures sur les organes des sens, où l'on, propose un nouveau sistème d'optique.

—Supplement. *See* Brunet, C. Supplement du volume des Journaux de Médecine de l'année M. DC. LXXXVI. 1687.

Le **JOURNAL DES SÇAVANS,** de l'an M. DC. LXV [-M. DC. LXVI] Par le sieur de Hedouville [pseud., i.e. Jean Denis de Sallo] Amsterdam, Pierre le Grand, 1684.

750, [16] p. illus. 14 cm. **[6291]**

Imperfect: p. 571-598 wanting.

JOURNU. Dissertation generale sur le sang ... Toulouse, J. Boude, 1694.

[12], 50, [4] p. 16 cm. **[6292]**

JOUVANCI, Nicolas de [*fl.* 1674-1675] *praeses.* Quaestio medica ... An nitidus faciei color bene moratorum viscerum index? [Parisiis, Apud Franciscum Muguet, 1675]

4 p.   25 cm.   [6293]

Diss. — Paris (J. Thomasseau, *respondent*)

—*See* BACHOT, E. Vesperiae et pileus doctoralis. 1675.

JOUYSE, DAVID [*fl.* 1622] Examen du livre de Lamperiere sur le sujet de la peste. Avec un Bref . . . discours de la preservation et cure de la maladie, suivy d'un advertissement adressé à Lamperiere . . . Rouen, David Geuffroy, 1622

[16], 325, [2] p.   18 cm.   [6294]

—*See* LAMPÉRIÈRE, J. de. L'ombre de necrophore vivant chartier de l'Hostel Dieu. 1622.

JUANINI, JUAN BAUTISTA [1636-1691] Cartas escritas a los . . . doctores . . . Francisco Redi . . . y . . . Juan Mathias de Lucas . . . en las quales se dize, que el sal azido, y alcali, es la materia que construye los espiritus animales, el oficina de los quales, es en los anteriores ventriculos del celebro . . . Madrid, Imprenta Real, Andres Blanco, 1691.

[20], 96 p.   22 cm.   [6295]

—Dissertation physique, ou l'on montre les mouvemens de la fermentation, les effets des matieres nitreuses dans les corps sublunaires, & les causes qui alterent la pureté de l'air de Madrid . . . Traduit d'espagnol en françois par Jean-Joseph Courtial . . . Toulouse, D. Desclassan, 1685.

[6], 102, [1] p.   15 cm.   [6296]

JUBILIUM votivum, in honorem . . . D. Samuelis Bouvier, postquam praemissa publica disputatione summis cum encomiis in . . . Batavorum Academia Lugdunensi Med. Doct. crearetur, ab amicis acclamatum . . . Lugduni Batavorum, Apud viduam & haeredes Johannis Elsevirii, 1670.

[8] p.   23 cm.   [6297]

JUCH, GUSTAV PROSPER [*b.* 1660] respondent. *See* VATER, C., *praeses.* Historiam et curam bubonis inguinalis cum perforatione intestini & eruptione lumbricorum . . . submittit G. P. J. 1693.

—*See* VATER, C. Collegii Medici decanus Christianus Vater . . . benevolo lectori S. P. D. 1693.

JUCH, HERMANN PAUL [1676-1756] respondent. *See* HÜBLER, J. C. Dissertatio historico-physica, de

pluviis prodigiosis. 1695; STAHL, G. E., *praeses.* Disputatio medica medico-pathologica. 1697 [and] Dissertatio inauguralis de motu sanguinis haemorrhoidali. 1698; WERCKMEISTER, F. H., *praeses.* Dissertatio medica, de genio. 1697.

—*See* STAHL, G. E. Propempticon inaugurale de morbis contumacibus. 1698.

JUCH, PAUL HEINRICH [1649-1733] *respondent. See* FASCH, A. H., *praeses.* Dissertatio medica de morbo dominorum. 1670.

JUDEL, ELIAS KASPAR [*b.* 1659] *See* WEDEL, G. W. Propempticon inaugurale de radice amara Homeri. 1692.

JUDICIA e multis quaedam virorum reverendorum . . . de laboribus Dn. Petri Kirstenii . . . Lipsiae, Excudebat Laurentius Cober, typis Tobiae Beyeri, 1611.

[11] p.   30 cm.   [6298]

Imperfect: wormholes throughout.
Edited by Moritz Schröter.

The JUDICIALL of urine. *See* RECORDE, R. The urinal of physick. 1651, 1665.

JÜNGKEN, JOHANN HELFRICH [1648-1726] Chirurgia manualis; oder, Kurtzer . . . Begriff, derer zu der Chirurgie in Specie gehörigen Operationen oder Hand-Arbeiten . . . Denen bey dieser 2. Ed. beygefüget einige Kurtze anatomische Fragen über diejenigen Theile des menschlichen Cörpers, welche der Chirurgus absonderlich wol fassen und wissen muss. Nürnberg, Verlegts Joh. Zieger und Georg Lehmann, druckts Abraham von Werth, 1700.

[15], 516, [24] p.; 154 p.   front., illus., plates.   18 cm.   [6299]

Part [2] has special title page.

—Chymia experimentalis curiosa, ex principiis mathematicis demonstrata; in qua ex triplici regno, remedia generosiora a neotericis et aliis hactenus inventa, fideliter exhibentur: adjunctis singulariorum remediorum formulis . . . Francofurti, Apud Hermannum à Sande, typis Joannis Andreae, 1681.

[22], 898 p.   illus.   18 cm.   [6300]

Imperfect: added engraved title page.
Errata: p. 897-898.

—[The same.] . . . Medicus praesenti seculo accommodandus, per veram philosophiam spagiricam, rerum naturalium veris fundamentis exornandus, & faciliori omnis generis morbos curandi methodo illustrandus ... Francofurti, Sumptibus authoris, typo Joannis Dieterici Friedgenii, 1682.

[22], 841, [7] p.   port.   17 cm.   [6301]

—[The same.] Chymia experimentalis curiosa, sive, Medicus praesenti seculo accommodandus ... Ed. postrema cum indicibus & priori auctior. Francofurti, Apud Hermannum à Sande, typis Balt. Christophori Wustii, jun., 1684.

[20], 840, [4] p.   18 cm.   [6302]

—[The same.] ... Francofurti ad Moenum, Sumtibus Alberti Ottonis Fabri, typis Joh. Dieterici Friedgenii, 1689.

[16], 841, [6], 119 p.   front. (port.)   17 cm.
           [6303]

A reprint (except that the dedications are omitted and the errata are corrected) of the 1682 edition. A new part (119 p. at end) has been added, with half title: Medici praesenti seculo accommodandi pars tertia ... The first two parts had been published in 1681 under the title: Chymia experimentalis curiosa.

—Fundamenta medicinae modernae eclectica, ubi physices compendio praemisso ad Cartesii potissimum mentem conscripto, ex celeberrimis neotericis scriptoribus medicis talis per omnes medicinae partes traditur selectus ... Francofurti, Impensis Johannis Ziegeri, typis Joh. Philippi Andrae, 1693.

[16], 864 (i.e. 862), [50] p.   18 cm.   [6304]

—Lexicon chimico-pharmaceuticum in duas partes divisum, quarum prior continet processus selectos chimicos ... Altera pars composita pharmaceutica tam usualia, quam alia his subordinata, & rationi consentanea exhibet ... Norimbergae, Impensis Johannis Ziegeri & Georgii Lehmanni, typis Melch. Gottfr. Heinii, typis Melch. Gottfr. Heinii, 1699.

1 v. ([32], 265, [13] p.; 423, [36] p.)   19 cm.
           [6305]

Part [2] has half title.

—Manuale pharmaceuticum; sive Lexici pharmaceutici continuatio, composita pharmaceutica tum usualia, tum minus usualia notissimarum pharmacopoearum, aliorumque celeberrimorum authorum hinc inde multum celebrata & usu recepta, tum alia juxta eorum mentem & censuras adornata, continens

... Francofurti ad Moenum, Sumptibus Friderici Knochii, 1698.

[16], 910 p.   18 cm.   [6306]

—Modernae praxeos medicae vade mecum, pro memoria sublevanda conscriptum ... Norimbergae, Sumptibus Johannis Ziegeri, 1694.

464 p.   18 cm.   [6307]

"Brevis Thomae Sydenhammi morbos curandi methodus ex ejus operibus excerpta": p. [375]-464.

Bound with Gladbach, J. B. Praxeos medicae idea novissima. 1694.

—Praxis medica; sive, Corporis medicina, morborum internorum corporeae machinae fere omnium, et fiendi et curandi methodum, juxta modernorum practicorum saniora principia, nudis exhibens terminis. Francofurti, Impensis Joannis Ziegeri, typis Joann. Phil. Andreae, 1689.

[15], 1020, [4] p.   18 cm.   [6308]

Added engraved title page.

—[The same.] ... Ed. alt. Francofurti, Impensis Joannis Ziegeri, et Georgii Lehmanni, typis Joann. Philippi Andreae, 1698.

[15], 1020, [2] p.   18 cm.   [6309]

Different setting of type.

Added engraved title page.

—Vernünftiger und erfarner Leib-Artzt, welcher lehret, wie ein Mensch, so von der Medicin keine Profession machet, so wohl seinen eigenen Cörper erkennen, sich vor allerhad Zufällen bewaren, als auch in Kranckheiten geschwinde raten möge. Leipzig, Thomas Fritsch, 1699.

[1], 742, 24 p.   plates.   17 cm.   [6310]

—, ed. See AGRICOLA, J. Deutlich- und wolgegründeter Anmerckungen über die chymische Artzneyen. 1686.

—See SPINA, D. de. Manuale sive lexicon pharmaceutico-chymicum. 1700; TILING, M. Opiologia nova. 1697.

JÜRGENS, JOACHIMUS [*fl.* 1676] *respondent.* See BORCH, O., *praeses.* Dissertatio medica de alimentorum cursu. 1676.

JULIAN, *maestro.* See JOHANNES XXI, *Pope* [d. 1277]

JULIÁN, PEDRO. See JOHANNES XXI, *Pope* [d. 1277]

JULIANO, *pseud.* See JOHANNES XXI, *Pope* [d. 1277]

JULIUS Papa III. Meritis devotionis vestrae. 1674. *See* Catholic Church. *Pope,* 1550-1555 (Julius III).

JULIUS UNIVERSITÄT, Helmstedt. Medizinische Fakultät. Kurtze, nohtwendige Ordnung und Raht, auch Verzeichnus und Taxa der Artzneyen, welche wider die jetzo gifftige und geschwinde grassirende Pestilentz in den Apoteken allhiero, der studierenden Jugend in der löblichen Julius Universitet, und der gemeinen Burgerschafft zu Helmstadt zum besten gestellet, durch die Professores Facultatis Medicae daselbsten. Helmstadt, Gedruckt durch Jacobum Lucium, 1609.
[15] p. 19 cm. [6311]

JUNCKEN, Johann Helfrich. *See* Jüngken, Johann Helfrich [1648-1726]

JUNCKER, Christian [1668-1714] Schediasma historicum, de ephemeridibus; sive, Diariis eruditorum, in nobilioribus Europae partibus hactenus publicatis. In appendice exhibetur Centuria foeminarum eruditione et scriptis illustrium ... Lipsiae, Sumtibus Joh. Fried. Gleditsch, 1692.
[18], 306, [12] p.; [6], 138 p. 14 cm. [6312]
The appendix has half title.

JUNCKER, Johann [*fl.* 1618-1624] Compendiosa methodus therapeutica: qua morborum fere incurabilium medicationes docentur per solam diaetam, et ligni guaiaci diversi-mode praeparati administrationem ... [Schleusinga] Typis Hieronymi Steinmanni, 1624.
[144] p. 20 cm. [6313]
Hieronymus Steinmann printed in Schleusingen from 1622 to 1629. Cf. Benzing (A), p. 382.

—, *ed. See* Hippocrates. Aphorismi. [Adaptations, etc. Greek and Latin]. 1619

JUNGERMANN, Ludwig [1572-1653] *See* Horst, G. [1578-1636] Dissertatio de natura amoris. 1611.

JUNGHANS, Johann [*fl.* 1665] *respondent. See* Hering, J. E., *praeses.* Ex physicis de ortu avis Britannicae ... publicam sententiarum collationem instituet J. J. 1665.

JUNI, Ulrich [*fl.* 1694-1697] *respondent. See* Honold, M., *praeses.* Dissertatio physica de visu. 1694.

JUNGKEN, Johann Helfrich. *See* Jüngken, Johann Helfrich [1648-1726]

JUNIUS, Franciscus. *See* Du Jon, François [1545-1602]

JUNIUS, Hadrianus [1511-1575] Epistolae, quibus accedit ejusdem vita & oratio De artium liberalium dignitate. Nunquam antea edita ... Dordrechti, Apud Vincentium Caimax, MDLII [i.e. MDCLII?]
[24], 648 p. 13 cm. [6314]
Edited by his son Petrus Hadrianus.
The same publisher issued Hadrianus' Batavia in 1652. Cf. NUC.

— Nomenclator octilinguis omnium rerum propria nomina continens ... Nunc vero renovatus, auctus & in capita LXXVII. sic distinctus ... Accessit huic postremae ed. alter Nomenclator ... Hermanni Germbergii opera & studio ... [Genevae], Excudebat Jacobus Stoer, 1602.
[16], 634, [73] p. 18 cm. [6315]
Imprint partly supplied from BNC.

JUNIUS, Petrus [*d.* 1594] *ed. See* Junius, H. Epistolae. MDLII [i.e. MDCLII?]

JUNKER, Johann. *See* Juncker, Johann [*fl.* 1618-1624]

JURGENS, Joachimus. *See* Jürgens, Joachimus [*fl.* 1676]

La JUSTE refutation des injustes louanges qu'impudemment a osé donner un medecin du roy, à Jules Mazarin, le plus scelerat de tous les hommes, & qui est en execration à Dieu, aux anges, & à toute la nature. Paris, François Noel, 1649.
8 p. 23 cm. [6316]

JUSTEL, Henri [1620-1693] *See* Vossius, I. Observationum ad Pomp. Melam appendix. 1686.

JUSTUS, Pascasius. *See* Joostens, Pâquier [*d.* 1590?]

JUVALTA, Fortunat von [*fl.* 1660-1662] *respondent. See* Burckhardt, J. R., *praeses.* Exercitatio medica de dysenteria. 1660.

K

K., I. C., *tr. See* PARACELSUS. Zween underschiedene Tractat. 1608.

K., J. D. [*fl.* 1699] *See* DIE DURCH SELTSAME EINBILDUNG UND BETRIEGERY SCHADEN BRINGENDE ALCHYMISTEN-GESELSCHAFFT. 1700.

K., T. *See* THE KITCHIN-PHYSICIAN. 1680.

KÄSEBERG, FRIEDRICH [*b.* 1658] *respondent. See* WEDEL, G. W., *praeses.* Disputato medica inauguralis de morbis a fascino. 1682 [and] Dissertatio medica de gibbere. 1681.

—*See* CRAUSE, R. W. Rudolfus Wilhelmus Krauss . . . Facult. Medic. . . . decanus, lectori benevolo S. P. D. 1682.

KAHLE, ADAM [*b.* 1665] *respondent. See* BARTHOLIN, C., *praeses.* Dissertatio inauguralis de diaeta jejunantium. 1693.

—*See* RØMER, O. C., *praeses.* Rector Regiae Universitatis Hafniensis Dn. Olaus Rømer L. S. 1693.

KAHLER, JOHANN [1649-1729] *praeses.* Dissertatio catoptrica, de reflexione luminis, ejusque effectu . . . Rinthelii, Typis Wichteri, 1682.
    [1], 18 p. plate. 19 cm.   **[6317]**
    Diss. — Rinteln (J. L. a Baumbach, *respondent*)

—Dissertatio hydrographica de oceano ejusque proprietatibus & vario motu . . . Rinthelii, Typis Godofredi Casperi Wächters [1679]
    [1], 46 p. illus. 19 cm.   **[6318]**
    Diss. — Rinteln (J. H. Steuber, *respondent*)

KALCKHOFF, JOHANN CHRISTIAN [*fl.* 1674-1678] Dissertatio inauguralis physico-chymico-medica de fontibus soteriis, Gesund-Brunnen, quam . . . pro licentia . . . in arte medica . . . doctoralia rite capessendi Joh. Christianus Kalchoff . . . Respondente Conr. Rudolpho Hertz . . . submittit . . . Erfurti, Literis Hertzianis [1678]
    [32] p. 20 cm.   **[6319]**
    Diss. — Erfurt.

—*respondent. See* CRAMER, C., *praeses.* Dissertationem de transmutatione metallorum . . . submittet. 1675.

KALCKHOVEN, JOST [*d.* 1669] *ed. See* KIRCHER, A. Magnes. 1643.

KALCOVEN, JODOCUS. *See* KALCKHOVEN, Jost [*d.* 1669]

KALINKA, JÁNOS [*fl.* 1657] *respondent. See* SPERLING, J., *praeses.* Disputatio physica de monstris. 1657.

KALINKIUS, JOHANNES. *See* KALINKA, János [*fl.* 1657]

KALKAR, JAN. *See* CALCAR, Jan Stephan von [1499–*ca.* 1546]

KALLEN, BERNARDUS à [*fl.* 1653-1655] Apologia prima . . . pro solutione, vel extractione auri sine corrosivo, contra invidiam & ignorantiam. Francofurti ad Moenum, Apud Joannem Gottofredum Schönwetterum, 1653.
    [8] p. 19 cm.   **[6320]**

—Apologia prima juncto appendice ad Parisienses. Pro solutione vel extractione auri sine corrosivo contra invidiam & ignorantiam. Item corvus deplumatus ab eodem authore in gratiam veritatus editus loco apologiae secundae. Francofurti, Apud Joann. Gottofr. Schönwetterum, 1656.
    [14] p. 19 cm.   **[6321]**

KALLHARDT, ELIAS [*fl.* 1660] *respondent. See* KIRCHMAYER, G. K., *praeses.* Ex physicis de risu. 1660.

KALLID RACHAIDIBI. *See* KHĀLID IBN YAZĪD, al-Umawi.

KALT, ANDREAS. Discursus medicus de mola ejus causis, signis, generatione et curandi modo. Constantiae, Ex typographaeo Nicolai Kalt, 1611.
    [24] p. 17 cm.   **[6322]**
    Written in collaboration with Hieronymus Sandholzer.

KALTSCHMIED, FRIEDRICH [*fl.* 1665-1668] *respondent. See* SCHENCK, J. T., *praeses.* Dissertationem inauguralem de paralysi . . . submittit . . . F. K. 1668 [and] Μαϱαθϱολογια; sive, De foeniculo dissertatio. 1665.

KAMMERMEISTER, JOACHIM. *See* CAMERARIUS, Joachim.

KAMPER, FLORENTIJN [*fl.* 1669] *respondent.* Disputatio medica inauguralis de empyemate . . . Lugduni Batavorum, Apud viduam & haeredes Joannis Elsevirii, 1669.

[12] p.   23 cm.   **[6323]**

Diss. — Leyden.

KAMPER, JOHANN LEOPOLD [*b.* 1671] *respondent. See* CRAUSE, R. W., *praeses.* Dissertatio inauguralis medico-chirurgica de hirudinibus. 1695.

— *See* WEDEL, G. W. Propemticum inaugurale de valvulis conniventibus. 1695.

KANID. *See* KANIS.

KANIS. *See* JĀBIR IBN ḤAIYĀN, al-Ṭarasūsi. Gebri . . . Summa perfectionis magisterii in sua natura. 1682.

KANITZ, DAVID [*b.* 1651] *respondent. See* FASCH, A. H., *praeses.* Disputatio inauguralis medica de diarrhoea. 1682.

— *See* CRAUSE, R. W. Rudolffus Wilhelmus Kraus . . . Facult. Med. . . . decanus. L. B. S. 1682.

KAPPEN, NIKOLAUS VAN DER [*fl.* 1682] *respondent. See* RYCKE, T., *praeses.* Disputatio medica inauguralis de sanguificatione. 1682.

KARDILUK, JOHANN HISKIAS. *See* CARDILUCIUS, Johannes Hiskias [17th cent.]

KARTNER, GABRIEL [*fl.* 1667] *respondent. See* HERING, J. E., *praeses.* Disputatio physica de hydromantia. 1667.

KAST, JOHANN JOACHIM [*fl.* 1683-1688] *respondent.* Dissertatio inauguralis medico-chirurgica de gangraena et sphacelo . . . Argentorati, Literis Joh. Friderici Spoor [1688]

[2], 46 p.   20 cm.   **[6324]**

Diss. — Strasbourg.

— *See* MAPP, M., *praeses.* Dissertatio medica qua primarium catameniorum vitium, h. e. suppressionem . . . submittit . . . 1686; SCHEID, J. V., *praeses.* Quaestionum decades duae de magnete. 1683.

KATSCH, JOHANN [*fl.* 1689] *respondent. See* BERGER, J. G. von, *praeses.* Dissertationem inauguralem de metallorum solutione . . . p. p. 1689.

KATZSCHIUS, JOHANNES [*fl.* 1549-1556] De gubernanda sanitate. In BECHER, J. J. Parnassus medicinalis illustratus. 1663.

— *See* HYGIEIA. 1628; REGIMEN SANITATIS SALERNITANUM. Medicina Salernitana. 1605, 1611, 1612, 1622, 1624, 1628, 1638 [and] Schola Salernitana. 1649, 1657, 1667, 1683.

KAUDERBACH, CHRISTOPH HEINRICH [*fl.* 1661] *respondent. See* MULLER C., *praeses.* Exercitatio anthropologica de cute. 1661.

KAULIZ, MICHAEL [*fl.* 1690-1694] *respondent. See* CRAUSE, R. W., *praeses.* Dissertatio inauguralis medica de febre quartana intermittente. 1694; WEDEL, G. W., *praeses.* Dissertatio medica de oblivione. 1690.

KAZUNGIUS, AEGIDIUS [*fl.* 1680-1682] *respondent. See* CRAMER, C., *praeses.* Dissertatio inauguralis medica de inundatione microcosmi. 1682.

KECK, THOMAS [*fl. ca.* 1644] *See* BROWNE, *Sir* T. Religio medici. 1656, 1659, 1678, 1682.

KECKERMANN, BARTHOLOMAEUS [*ca.* 1571-1608 or 9] *praeses.* Cursus philosophici disputatio XIX. De homine. Instituenda publice in Gymnasio Dantiscano . . . Respondente Georgio Paulo . . . Dantisci, Typis Martini Rhodi, 1605.

[35] p.   19 cm.   **[6325]**

Diss. — Danzig. Gymnasium (G. Paulus, *respondent*)

— De fulmine disputatio physica extraordinaria . . . Dantisci, Typis Guilhelmi Guilmothani, 1606.

[36] p.   19 cm.   **[6326]**

Diss. — Danzig. Gymnasium (P. Janich, *respondent*)

KEEREN, JAN VAN [*fl.* 1658] *respondent.* Disputatio medica inauguralis de cholera . . . Lugduni Batavorum, Ex officina Jacobi à Mylendonck, 1658.

[8] p.   24 cm.   **[6327]**

Diss. — Leyden.

KEERWOLFF, BARTHOLOMAEUS [*fl.* 1693-1697] Epistola anatomica, problematica decima . . . ad . . . Fredericum Ruyschium . . . De auricularum cordis, earumque fibrarum motricium structura. Amsteledami, Apud Joannem Wolters, 1697.

10, [1] p.   illus.   22 cm.   **[6328]**

"Frederici Ruyschii responsio . . .": p. 5-7.

KEESSEL, GODFRIED VAN DER [*fl.* 1684] *respondent.* Disputatio medica inauguralis de phrenitide ... Lugduni Batavorum, Apud Abrahamum Elzevier, 1684.

[16] p.   22 cm.   [6329]
Diss.—Leyden.

KEGEL, MARTIN [*fl.* 1670] *respondent. See* ROMANUS, P. F., *praes.* [Diatribes juridicae de medico] 1670.

KEGELER, CASPAR [*fl.* 1518-1529] Ein heilsam, nutzbar und hülffreichs Regiment. Wieder die Pestilentz und das gifftige Pestilentz Fieber (die Schweissucht genant) und sonsten mancherley gifftige und tödtliche Kranckheiten, anfengklich durch Herrn Caspar Keglern ... weiland Professoren und Physicen zu Leipzigh, mit vielen gewissen Experimenten zusammen gebracht, und darnacher zum ersten und andern Mal, Aō 1518. und 1529. bey seinem Leben selbsten, auch ferners nach Absterben, durch seinen Sohn Melchior Keglern ... Aō 1566. zum dritten, itzo aber, von dem Nepote, Doctor Caspar Keglern ... aus erwenten seines Grossvatern seligen eigenem Manuscripto und alten Exemplarien ... revidiret und das vierdte Mahl, wolmeinende gedruckt worden ... Dressden, Christian Bergen, 1607.

[21], 46, [2] p.   20 cm.   [6330]

The large red "A" on the title page designates this as the authorized edition, which alone is reliable for the special remedies and their dosages.
Previously published under title: Ein nützliches und tröstlichs Regiment wider die Pestilentz.

KEGELER, CASPAR [*fl.* 1607] *ed. See* KEGELER, C. [*fl.* 1518-1529] Ein heilsam, nutzbar und hülffreichs Regiment. 1607.

KEGELER, MELCHIOR [16th cent.] *See* KEGELER, C. [*fl.* 1518-1529] Ein heilsam, nutzbar und hülffreichs Regiment. 1607.

KEGLER, CASPAR. *See* KEGELER, Caspar [*fl.* 1518-1529]

KEIL, ANDREAS VON [*fl.* 1665-1688] Andreae Cunaei ... Beschreibung des Pyrmontischen Sauer-Brunnen ... Anjetzo auffs neue übersehen und von vielen Druckfehlern gesaubert, auch ... vermehret. Lemgo [Heinrich Wilhelm Meyer] 1697.

[25], 75 p.   17 cm.   [6331]

H. W. Meyer printed in Lemgo from 1690 to 1722. Cf. Benzing (A), p. 276.
Imperfect: title page mutilated.

—Diversorum morborum descriptio; das ist, Beschreibung aller hitzigen ... Fieber, Bräunen, Brust-und Hauptkranckheit ... Ruhr ... und ... der Pestilentz samt dero An-und Zufällen, woraus dieselben entstehen, ob und wie solche aus denen Himmelszeichen, Constellationen der Gestirn, Gewitter, Esmeten und derogleichen zu verkündigen ... und zu curiren sey ... Anno 1683 ausgefertiget ... Anitzo zum andernmahle von dem Autore durchsehen und heraus gegeben ... Zelle, Hieronymus Fridrich Hoffmann, 1688.

[15], 152 p.   17 cm.   [6332]

—, *ed. See* FEUERBERG, J. Fons sacer. 1688?

KEIL, JACOBUS. *See* KEILL, James [1673-1719]

KEILL, JAMES [1673-1719] The anatomy of the humane body abridged; or, A short and full view of all the parts of the body. Together with their several uses drawn from their compositions and structures ... London, William Keblewhite, 1698.

[24], 328, [8] p.   16 cm.   [6333]

— *See* LÉMERY, N. A course of chymistry. 1698.

KEILL, JOHN [1671-1721] *See* BURTHOGGE, R. Of the soul of the world. 1699.

KEITWERDT, HEINRICH WILHELM [*fl.* 1680] *respondent.* Disputatio inauguralis medica de sanguificatione ... Duisburgi ad Rhenum, Apud Franconem Sas, 1680.

24 p.   20 cm.   [6334]
Diss.—Duisburg.

KELCK, JAN [*fl.* 1695] *respondent.* Dissertatio medica inauguralis de fluxu menstruo ... Lugduni Batavorum, Apud Abrahamum Elzevier, 1695.

[27] p.   18 cm.   [6335]
Diss.—Leyden.

KELLAEUS, EDUARDUS. *See* KELLEY, Edward [1555-1595]

KELLER, JOHANN CHRISTIAN [*fl.* 1693] *praeses.* Dissertationem physicam de visu ... publicae ... censurae submittet ... Andrea Hoffmann ... Lipsiae, Typis Andrae Zeidleri [1693]

[36] p.   19 cm.   [6336]
Diss. — Leipzig (A. Hoffmann, *respondent*).

KELLER, SAMUEL [*fl.* 1586] *tr.* *See* MELICH, G. Dispensatorium medicum. 1601.

KELLEY, EDWARD [1555-1595] Ein schöner tractat . . . an den Römischen Kayser Rudolpho Secundo. *In* Drey vortreffliche und noch nie im Druck gewesene chymische Bücher. 1670.

—Excerpta . . . ex epistolis. *In* [Combach, L.] *ed.* and *tr.* Tractatus. 1647.

KELLNER, DAVID [*fl.* 1668-1690] Kurtze Anleitung, wie man sich wegen hin und wieder heftig grassirenden und gar nahe ruckenden Pest-Seuche . . . durch . . . heilsame Artzney-Mittel, so wol . . . bewahren, als . . . dieselbe heilen und vertreiben könne . . . Aus denen bewährtesten Pest-Schrifften zusammen getragen . . . Schleusingen, Sebast. Göbel [1680?]

96 p.   14 cm.   [**6337**]

—*respondent. See* MEIBOM, H., *praeses.* Disputatio medica inauguralis de oleorum stillatitiorum natura et usu in genere. 1670 [and] Exercitatio medica de ossium constitutione naturali et praeternaturali. 1668.

KELLNER, DAVID HEINRICH [*fl.* 1683] *respondent. See* RIVINUS, A. Q., *praeses.* Exercitatio medica de febribus intermittentibus. 1683.

KELLY, EDWARD. *See* KELLEY, Edward [1555-1595]

KELNER, DAVID. *See* KELLNER, David [*fl.* 1668-1690]

KEMP, WILLIAM [*fl.* 1665] A brief treatise of the nature, causes, signes, preservation from, and cure of the pestilence . . . London, D. Kemp, 1665.

[5], 94 (i.e. 92), [2] p.   18 cm.   [**6338**]

KEMPE, CHRISTIAN [*fl.* 1693] *respondent. See* JACOBAEUS, H., *praeses.* Dissertatio de natura & usu salium volatilium. 1693.

KEMPER, THEODULUS [*fl.* 1677-1683] *praeses.* Dissertatio anatomico-medica de valvularum in corporibus hominis et brutorum natura, fabrica et usu mechanico . . . Jenae, Literis Bauhoferianis [1683]

[1], 38 p.   20 cm.   [**6339**]

Diss. — Jena (J. E. Richelmann, *respondent*)

—*respondent. See* SCHELHAMMER, G. C., *praeses.* Exercitatio medica de capitis dolore. 1678; WEDEL, G.

W., *praeses.* Dissertatio medica inauguralis de syncope. 1680.

KENNEDUS, THOMAS. *See* KENNEDY, Thomas [*fl.* 1682]

KENNEDY, THOMAS [*fl.* 1682] *respondent. See* DRELINCOURT, C., *praeses.* Dissertatio medica de nutritione foetus. 1682.

KENT, ELIZABETH (TALBOT) GREY, *countess of* [1581-1651] A choice manuall; or, Rare and select secrets in physick and chyrurgery . . . Whereto are added several experiments of the virtues of Gascon pouder, and lapis contra-yarvam, by a professor of physick. As also most exquisite waies of preserving, conserving, candying, &c. The 2d ed. London, Printed by G. D. and sold by William Shears, 1653.

[15], 206 p.; [18], 140 p.   front. (port.)   12 cm.

[**6340**]

Imperfect: three leaves after title page mutilated.
Part [2] has special title page: A true gentlewomans delight . . . Published by W. I[ar] gent.

—[The same.] . . . The 4th ed. London, Printed by G. D. and sold by William Shaers, 1654.

[15], 206 p.; [18], 140 p.   front. (port.)   12 cm.

[**6341**]

Different setting of type.
Part [2] has special title page: A true gentlewomans delight . . . Published by W. J[ar] gent.

KENTMANN, JOHANNES [1518-1574] *See* SENNERT, D. De febribus libri IV. 1628, 1633, 1641, 1653.

KEPHALE, RICHARD [*fl.* 17th cent.] Medela pestilentiae: wherein is contained several theological queries concerning the plague, with approved antidotes, signes, and symptoms; also an exact method for curing that epidemical distemper . . . London, Printed by J. C. for Samuel Speed, 1665.

[7], 87, [1] p.   20 cm.   [**6342**]

KEPLER, JOHANN [1571-1630] Ad vitellionem paralipomena, quibus astronomiae pars optica traditur; potissimum de artificiosa observatione et aestimatione diametrorum deliquiorumque solis & lunae. Cum exemplis insignium eclipsium . . . de modo visionis, & humorum oculi usu, contra opticos & anatomicos . . . Francofurti, Apud Claudium Marnium & haeredes Joannis Aubrii, 1604.

[16], 449, [18] p.   illus., plates.   22 cm.

[**6343**]

—*See* FLUDD, R. Anatomiae amphitheatrum effigie triplici, more et conditione varia, designatum. 1623 [and] Veritatis proscenium. 1621.

KEPLER, LUDWIG [1607–1663] *respondent. See* SEBISCH, M. [1578–1674?] *praeses.* Libri sex Galeni De morborum differentiis. 1632.

KEPPLERUS, LUDOVICUS. *See* KEPLER, Ludwig [1607–1663]

KER, JOHANES [*fl.* 1697] *respondent.* Disputatio physico-medica inauguralis de secretionis animalis efficiente & ordine … Lugduni Batavorum, Apud Abrahamum Elzevier, 1697.

     [24] p.   22 cm.   **[6344]**
Diss. — Leyden.

KERCKRING, THEODOR [1640–1693] Anthropogeniae ichnographia; sive, Conformatio foetus ab ovo usque ad ossificationis principia, in supplementum Osteogeniae foetuum. Amstelodami, Sumptibus Andreae Frisii, 1671.

     [8], 14 p.   illus.   24 cm.   **[6345]**
Bound with his Spicilegium anatomicum. 1670.

—Spicilegium anatomicum, continens observationum anatomicarum rariorum centuriam unam; nec non Osteogeniam foetuum … Amstelodami, Sumptibus Andreae Frisii, 1670.

     [24], 280 p.   illus., plates.   24 cm.   **[6346]**
Added engraved title page.
The Osteogenia foetuum has special title page.
With this is bound his Anthropogeniae ichnographia. 1671.

—*See* BASILIUS VALENTINUS. Commentarius in Currum triumphalem antimonii Basilii Valentini. 1671, 1685 [and] Triumphant chariot of antimony. 1678; [VERDUC, J. B.] Nouvelle osteologie. 1689.

KERCKWYCK, CHRISTOFFEL COCK VAN. *See* COCK VAN KERCKWIJK, Christophorus [*d.* 1678]

KERFBYL, JOHANNES [*fl.* 1659–1660] *respondent.* Disputatio medica inauguralis, de dysenteria … Lugduni Batavorum, Ex officina Francisci Moiardi, 1560 [i.e. 1660]

     [8] p.   19 cm.   **[6347]**
Diss. — Leyden.

KERGER, MARTIN [*fl.* 1657–1663] De fermentatione liber phisico-medicus. Cui de inseparabilitate formarum materialium & vita singularia sunt innexa

… Wittebergae, Sumtibus haered. D. Tobiae Moevii, & Elerdi Schumacheri, typis Johannis Borckardi, 1663.

     [8], 254, [14] p.   21 cm.   **[6348]**
Bound with Möbius, G. Epitome institutionum medicarum. 1663.

—*See* DREXEL, J. Aurifodina artium & scientiarum omnium excerpendi solertia … monstrata. 1658.

KERN, CHRISTOPH [1592–1656] *respondent. See* HOFMANN, C., *praeses.* Disputatio medica de natura pulsuum. 1628.

KERN, JOHANN [*fl.* 1671] *praeses.* De Witteberga dissertationem historicam … submittit Bertholdus Magnus Brüning … Wittebergae, Literis Wendianis, excudebat Daniel Schmatz, 1671.

     [16] p.   20 cm.   **[6349]**
Diss. — Wittenberg (B. M. Brüning, *respondent*)

KERNER, ARNOLD [*fl.* 1608–1626] Λοιμολογία; das ist, Kurtzer, doch gründlicher Discurs, von der gifftpeyenden Seuche der Pestilentz, was nemlich derselben Natur … und wie die Gesunde zu praeserviren, und die damit befallene … zu curiren … Leipzig, Gedruckt bey Gregorio Ritzschen, in Vorlegung Bartholomaei Voigts, 1626.

     [8], 152 p.   19 cm.   **[6350]**

—Tetras chymiatrica, proponens praestantiam et in medicina efficaciam, auri, mercurii, antimonii, & vitrioli, & medicamentorum ex illis pacatorum [sic]: opposita misochymis eadem sat frivole calumniantibus … Erphordiae, Ex typographeo Johannis Röhbock, impensis Johannis Birckneri, 1618.

     [283] p.   16 cm.   **[6351]**
Bound with Brendel, Z. Chimia in artis formam redacta. 1641.

—*respondent.* Mensium suppressionis ratio et curatio … Basileae, Ex officina Johannis Schroeteri, 1608.

     [18] p.   20 cm.   **[6352]**
Diss. — Basel.

KERNER, TOBIAS [*fl.* 1686] *respondent.* Disputatio medica inauguralis, continens miscellanea medico-practica … Ultrajecti, Ex officina Francisci Halma, 1686.

     16 p.   22 cm.   **[6353]**
Diss. — Utrecht.

KESLER, Thomas. *See* Kessler, Thomas [*fl.* 1616-1630]

KESMANN, Johann [*fl.* 1613] *respondent. See* Labavius, A. [*d.* 1616] *praeses.* De theriaca Andromachi senioris. 1613.

KESSLER, Franz Thomas. *See* Kessler, Thomas [*fl.* 1616-1630]

KESSLER, Johann Elias [*fl.* 1668-1671] *respondent.* Exercitationem academicam de immoderata adbibendi consuetudine. Vom übermässigen Zutrincken ... submittit Johannes Elias Kessler ... Jenae, Literis Johannis Wertheri [1668]

[48] p. 20 cm.   [*6354*]
Diss. − Jena.

KESSLER, Johann Friedrich [*fl.* 1660] *respondent. See* Klein, N., *praeses.* Disquisitio philologico-physica de magnete. 1660.

KESSLER, Thomas [*fl.* 1616-1630] Zweyhundert ausserlesene chymische Process, und Stücklein, theils zur innerlichen, theils zur Wund, und aüsserlichen Artzney dienstlich, biss anhero in Geheim verhalten; anjetzo aber mit vielen guten ... Handgriffen verbessert ... Strassburg, Gedruckt bey Johanne Keppen, in Verlegung Johannis Philippi Sartorii, 1628.

[14], 204, [1] p. 16 cm.   [*6355*]

−Keslerus, redivivus; das ist, Fünff hundert ausserlesene chymische Process und Artzneyen, theils zu innerlichen und eusserlichen Leibskranckheiten, theils auch zu Verbesserung der mindern Metallen hochnutzlich. Deren erstlich vier hundert durch M. Thomam Keslerum ... an Tag gegeben und zum vierdten Mal auffgelegt, an jetzo aber von einem vornehmen Chymico auffs new ubersehen, und mit hinzusetzung dess fünfften hunderten in formliche Ordnung ... gesetzet ... Franckfurt am Mayn, In Verlegung Johann Behers, 1641.

[14], 536, [13] p. 17 cm.   [*6356*]
Imperfect: wormholes on p. 189-240.

−[The same.] Fünffhundert ausserlesene chymische Process und Stücklein, theils zur innerlichen, theils zur Wund-und eusserlichen Artzney, theils aber auch zur Versetzung und Verbesserung der mindern Metall dienstlich; anjetzo mit vielen ...

Handgriffen verbessert ... Nürnberg, In Verlegung Wolffgang Endters, 1645.

4 parts in 1 v. illus. 17 cm.   [*6357*]
Parts 2-4 have special title pages dated 1641, 1641, 1645 respectively. Imperfect: p. 11-22 and 27-38 of part [1] wanting.
With this are bound: Schmuck, M. Secretorum naturalium ... thesauriolus. 1649. - [Schmuck, M.] De occulta ... curatione ... tractatus. 1649.

−[Excerpts] *In* Dolhopff, G. A., *comp.* Lapis animalis microcosmicus. 1681.

−, *tr. See* Duchesne, J. Josephi Quercetani medici Sclopetarius; das ist, Büchsen-Tractätlein, oder Buch von Heylung der Wunden. 1631 [and] Josephi Quercetani M. D. Drey medicinische Tractätlein. 1631.

KEST, Franz [*fl.* 1614-1621] *praeses.* Themata disputationis ordinariae de vertigine ... Lipsiae, Johann Glück [1621]

[22] p. 19 cm.   [*6358*]
Diss. − Leipzig (F. Meurer, *respondent*)

−*respondent. See* Schilling, S., *praeses.* Themata disputationis ordinariae de gonorrhoea. 1614.

KESTLER, Johann Stephan [*fl.* 1675] *comp. See* Kircher, A. Physiologia Kircheriana experimentalis. 1680.

KESTNER, Heinrich Andreas [*fl.* 1686] *respondent. See* Wedel, G. W., *praeses.* Dissertationem medicam inauguralem de transplantatione morborum ... submittit M. H. A. K. 1686.

−*See* Wedel, G. W. Propempticon inaugurale de amello Virgilii. 1686.

KETELAAR, Vincent [1627-1679] Commentarius medicus de aphthis nostratibus, seu Belgarum Sprouw ... Lugd. Batavorum, Typis Adriani Severini, 1672.

58 p. 14 cm.   [*6359*]
Imperfect: p. 58 mutilated.

−*praeses.* Disputatio medica inauguralis de scorbuto ... Lugduni Batavorum, Apud Franciscum Moyaert, 1650.

[12] p. 23 cm.   [*6360*]
Diss. − Leyden.

KETTENES, Cornelis [*fl.* 1668] *respondent.* Exercitatio medica inauguralis de aphthis ... Lugduni

Batavorum, Apud viduam & haeredes Joannis Elsevirii, 1668.

[12] p.   23 cm.   [6361]
Diss. — Leyden.

KETTNER, FRIEDRICH GOTTLIEB [*d.* 1739] *praeses.* Dissertatio historica de mumiis Aegyptiacis . . . Lipsiae, Literis Christiani Scholvinii [1694]

[24] p.   19 cm.   [6362]
Diss. — Leipzig (J. S. Suschky, *respondent*)

KEUCHEN, JOHANN [*fl.* 1614] *respondent.* Theses medicae de tertiana . . . Basileae, Typis Joh. Jacobi Genathii [1614]

[8] p.   22 cm.   [6363]
Diss. — Basel.

KEUCHENIUS, ROBERTUS [1636–1673] Notae ad Samonicum. In Serenus Sammonicus, Q. De medicina praecepta saluberrima. 1662.

KEUCHLER, JOHANN [*fl.* 1668] *respondent. See* HARMES, H., *praeses.* Disputatio medica de peste. 1668.

KEURE en ordonnantie. 1696. *See* AMSTERDAM. Ordinances, local laws, etc.

KEYL, ANDREAS VON. *See* KEIL, Andreas von [*fl.* 1665–1688]

KEYSER, JOHANN GEORG [*fl.* 1665–1668] *respondent.* Rarissimum nec non gravissimum humani corporis affectum tetanum . . . publice . . . submittit Joh. Georgius Keyser . . . [Altorfii] Praelo Schönnerstaedtiano, 1668.

36 p.   19 cm.   [6364]
Diss. — Altdorf.

KHALAF IBN 'ABBĀS, ABŪ AL-QĀSIM. *See* ABULCASIS [936?–1013?]

KHĀLID IBN YAZĪD, AL-UMAWĪ. Rachaidibi [pseud., i.e. Khālid ibn Yazīd] . . . De materia philosophici lapidis . . .

255–259 p., vol. 1   17 cm.   (*In* Artis auriferae. Basileae, 1610)   [6365]
Caption title.

—[German tr.] [Rachaidibi Schreiben von der Materia Lapidis]

344–360 (i.e. 350) p., part 1.   19 cm.   (*In* Morgenstern, Philipp, *ed.* and *tr.* Turba philosophorum. Basel, 1613)   [6366]
Title from table of contents.

—Liber secretorum alchemiae compositus per Calid filium Jazichi, translatus ex Hebraeo in Arabicum, & ex Arabico in Latinum, incerto interprete [&] Liber trium verborum Kallid autissimi [sic]

208–231 p., vol. 1   17 cm.   (*In* Artis auriferae. Basileae, 1610)   [6367]
Caption titles.

—Liber trium verborum Kalid regis acutissimi . . .

186–190 p., vol. 5.   20 cm.   (*In* Zetzner, Lazarus, *ed.* Theatrum chemicum. Argentorati, 1659–61)   [6368]
Caption title.

—[German tr.] Das Buch der Geheimnussen der Alchimiae, gemacht durch den Calid, Iazichi Sohn, aus dem Hebraischen in Arabisch bracht, unnd auss dem Arabischen in Latein . . . jetzt aber verteutscht . . . [&] Das Buch der dreyer Wörter, dess vermischten Kallidts . . .

274–309 p., part 1   19 cm.   (*In* Morgenstern, Philipp, *ed.* and *tr.* Turba philosophorum. Basel, 1613)   [6369]
Caption titles.

—*See* JĀBIR IBN ḤAIYĀN, al-Ṭarasūsī. Gebri . . . Summa perfectionis magisterii in sua natura. 1682; SALMON, W. Medicina practica. 1692.

KHONIUS, ALPHONSUS. *See* KHONN, Alphons [*fl.* 1662–1671]

KHONN, ALPHONS [*fl.* 1662–1671] *respondent.* Disputatio medica inauguralis de catalepsi . . . Argentorati, Typis excudit Joh. Pastorius, 1662.

32 p.   19 cm.   [6370]
Diss. — Strasbourg.

—*respondent. See* SEBISCH, J. A., *praeses.* Dissertatio solennis de instrumento olfactus. 1662.

—, *tr. See* ZACCHIA, P. De affectionibus hypochondriacis libri tres. 1671.

KHUENBURG, MAXIMILIANUS GANDOLPHUS, *Graf von. See* GANDOLF, Maximilian, *count, Cardinal, Prince-Archbishop of Salzburg* [*d.* 1687]

KHUNRATH, HEINRICH [1560–1605] Amphitheatrum sapientiae aeternae solius verae, Christiano-kabalisticum, divino-magicum, nec non

physico-chymicum tetriunum, catholicon ...
[Hanoviae, Guilielmus Antonius, 1609]

[1], 60, 222, [1] p. plates, port. 31 cm.
[6371]

Engraved title page.
Edited by Erasmus Wolfart.

—De igne magorum philosophorumque secreto externo & visibili; das ist, Philosophische Erklährung, von, und uber dem ... Gludt und Flammenfewer der uhralten Magorum oder Weysen ... Beneben andern zweyen Tractätlein: deren das erste ein ... Judicium ... eines erfahrnen Cabalisten und Philosophen uber die 4. Figuren dess grossen Amphitheatri D. Henrici Khunradi. Das ander, von der Tinctur Antimonii und Oleo Stibii von Theophrasto beschrieben, aber bissher felschlich undter dem Namen Rogerii Baconis aussgesprengt, jetzt nun mehr restituirt, ergäntzt, und ... an Tag geben. Strassburg, In Verlegung Lazari Zetzners, 1608.

[8], 157 p. 15 cm.   [6372]

Imperfect: outer margins trimmed.
Sudhoff 286.
The works by Paracelsus, Von der Tinctur Antimonii, and Oleo Stibii, were edited by Benedict Toepfer.

—Quaestiones tres, per-utiles ... cum curationem, tum praecautionem absolutam ... arenae, sabuli, calculi, podagrae, gonagrae, chiragrae, aliorumque morborum tartareorum microcosmi seu mundi minoriis, hominis puta, concernentes; das ist, Hochnützliche ... drei Fragen, die gründliche ... Curation ... so wol auch Praecaution, oder verhutung Sandes, grieses Steins, Zipperleins und anderer mehr tartarischer Kranckheiten Microcosmi ... Leipzig, Thomas Schürer [Eissleben, Gedruckt durch Barthel Hörnigk] 1607.

[53] p. 16 cm.   [6373]

In Latin and German.

—Warhafftiger Bericht vom philosophischen Athanore ... Ed. 3., & auct. ... [Magdeburg] In Verlegung des Autoris, 1615.

[1], 60, [1] p. illus. 16 cm.   [6374]

KHUNRATH, Konrad [*fl.* 1594-1604] Medulla destillatoria et medica tertium aucta & renovata; das ist, Gründliches und vielbewehrtes Destillier und Artzney Buch, darinnen begriffen, wie der Spiritus Vini ... auch allerley köstliche Oliteten, Spiritus, Salia, &c. auss mancherley Animalibus, Mineralibus und Vegetabilibus, künstlich können destillirt, und in quintam Essentiam zur höchsten Exaltation gebracht: auch vermittelst solcher Extractionum, Aurum potabile, allerly herliche Medicamenta ... praeparirt, und in allerhand vorfallenden ... Kranckheiten heylsamlich gebraucht werden ... Und jetzt von einem Hochgelährten ... der Artzney und Chymiae ... in Druck befördert ... Hamburg, Ex Bibliopolio Frobeniano, 1605.

[15], 628 (i.e. 640), [35] p. 23 cm.   [6375]

—[The same.] ... Hamburg, Ex Bibliopoliò Frobeniano, 1621-1623 [v. 1, 1623]

2 v. ([10], 628 (i.e. 640), [35] p.; [8], 360 (i.e. 630), [24] p.) 20 cm.   [6376]

Imperfect: title page, and sig. b. 2 and 4 of vol. 1 wanting; last two leaves of Register mutilated.

—[The same.] ... Hamburg, Ex Bibliopolio Frobeniano, 1638.

[14], 384, [26] p.; [8], 365, [27] p. 23 cm.
[6377]

Added engraved title page.
Part [2] has special title page.

—[Excerpt.] Traité des vertus de l'esprit de sel philosophique. Dont fait mention le fameux medecin Conrad Kunraths, dans son livre intitulé Medulla distillatoria, partie premiere page 59, imprimé à Hambourg l'an 1638. Traduit de latin en françois. Par ... Antoine le Maire ... 2. ed. Paris, L'autheur, 1686.

12 p. 21 cm.   [6378]

In Latin and French.

—[Excerpts.] *In* Dolhopff, G. A., *comp.* Lapis animalis microcosmicus. 1681 [and] Lapis vegetabilis. 1681.

KIEPER, Albert [*fl.* 1636-1637] *praeses.* Disputatio II corollariorum duorum posteriorum disputationi de fulmine, quod Regiomonti turrim nitrariam percussit, suffixorum uberiorem declarationem & probationem continens ... Regiomonti, Typis Laurentii Segebadii, 1637.

[8] p. 19 cm.   [6379]

Diss. — Königsberg (H. Hornung, *respondent*)

KIESEWETTER, Johann Augustin [*fl.* 1684-1694] *respondent.* See Bohn, J., *praeses.* Dissertationes chymico-physicae. 1685; Musculus, B. J. Specimen inaugurale de pleuritidis natura et cura. 1685.

KIESSLING, DANIEL [*fl.* 1700] *respondent. See* ERNDL, C. H. Dissertationem de usu historiae naturalis exotico-geographicae in medicina ... subjicit ... D. K. 1700.

KIESSLING, JOHANN JACOB. *See* KISLING, Johann Jakob [*b.* 1644]

KIESSLING, JOHANN SIEGFRIED [*fl.* 1678–1682] *respondent. See* RIVINUS, A. Q., *praeses.* Dissertatio medica de ischuria. 1682 [and] Dissertatio physiologica de nutritione. 1678.

KIEVIT, BALTHAZAR [*fl.* 1686] *respondent.* Disputatio medica inauguralis de inflammatione ... Lugduni Batavorum, Apud Abrahamum Elzevier, 1686.

    [16] p. 22 cm. **[6380]**
Diss. — Leyden.

[KIGGELAER, FRANCISCUS, *fl.* 1690] Horti Beaumontiani exoticarum plantarum catalogus, exhibens plantarum minus cognitarum & rariorum nomina, quibus idem hortus anno domini M DC LXXXX instructus fuit. Hagae-Comitis, 1690.

    [4], 42 p. 18 cm. **[6381]**

— , *ed. See* COMMELIN, J. Horti medici Amstelodamensis. 1697–1701.

KIGGETARIUS, FRANCISCUS. *See* KIGGELAER, Franciscus [*fl.* 1690]

KIJPER, ALBERT [1605?–1655] Anthropologia corporis humani contentorum, et animae naturam et virtutes secundum circularem sanguinis motum explicans. Lugduni Batavorum, Ex officina Adriani Wijngaerden [1650?]

    [12], 123 (i.e. 665), [28] p. 21 cm. **[6382]**
Engraved title page.
Imperfect: printed title page wanting?

— [The same.] ... Cui accedit ejusdem responsio ad pseud-apologema V. F. Plempii. Lugduni Batavorum, Apud Johannem Elsevirium, 1660.

    [8], 26, 123 (i.e. 665), [30] p. 22 cm. **[6383]**
Different setting of type.

— Collegium medicum, viginti sex disputationibus ... complectens, quae ad institutiones pertinent. Accedent ejusdem Disputationes physico-medicae miscellaneae, atque politicae de origine & jure magistratus, de jure belli, & de foederibus. Lugduni Batavorum, Apud Johannem Meyer, 1655.

    [296] p. 17 cm. **[6384]**

— Institutiones medicae, ad hypothesin de circulari sanguinis motu compositae. Subjunguntur ejusdem Transsumpta medica, quibus continentur medicinae fundamenta. Amstelodami, Apud Joannem Janssonium, 1654.

    [16], 346 p.; [8], 161, [2] p. 20 cm. **[6385]**
Part [2] has special title page.

— Institutiones physicae. Adjecta est Confutatio pseud-apologematis Plempiani. Tomus posterior ... Lugduni Batavorum, Ex officina Adriani Wyngaerden, 1647.

    [1], 724, [2] p. 13 cm. **[6386]**
Vol. 2 only.

— *praeses.* Disputatio physica de anima rationali ... Lugduni Batavorum, Ex officina Joannis Maire, 1640.

    [12] p. 18 cm. **[6387]**
Diss. — Leyden (J. A. Huswedel, *respondent*)

— *See* PLEMP, V. F. Fundamenta medicinae ad scholae acribologiam aptata. 1644, 1654.

KILIAN, LUCAS [1579–1637] *illus. See* [REMMELIN, J.] Visio prima [-tertia] 1613.

KILLMAN, DANIEL [*fl.* 1623] *respondent. See* AGER, N. Disputatio physica de somno, insomniis et vigilia. 1623.

KIMBERLEY, SAMUEL [*fl.* 1688] *See* COLE, W. A physico-medical essay concerning the late frequency of apoplexies. 1689.

La KINAKINA. *See* LES ADMIRABLES QUALITEZ DU KINKINA. Ital. 1694.

al-KINDI. *See* YAʿKUB IBN ISḤĀK IBN ṢUBBĀḤ, Abū Yúsuf, al-Kindī [*d. ca.* 873]

KINNER, DANIEL [*fl.* 1685–1686] *respondent. See* BOHN, J., *praeses.* Dissertationes chymico-physicae. 1685 [and] Dissertationum chymico-physicarum decima quarta de solutione. 1685; RIVINUS, A.Q., *praeses.* Dissertatio medica de thoracis empyemate. 1686.

KINNER, GEORG FRIEDRICH [*fl.* 1682–1683] *respondent. See* WEDEL, G. W., *praeses.* Disputatio medica aegrum erysipelate laborantem exhibens. 1682 [and] Disputatio medica inauguraiis de raucedine. 1683.

KIPPING, HEINRICH [*ca.* 1623-1678] Responsum novum; sive, Naenia apologetica. Ad quam vivus vidensque lectulo componitur J. S. K. olim in Bohemica militia veterinarius Cacula, nunc in ludo Cerdoniano jorristico quintae classis subpraeceptor donatisticus, quartae classis expectans beanus, geisteranae sectae praedicans heri, hodie vespillo, et ad tumulum producitur. Hardiowisci [i.e. Bremae] Excudebat Smolcius Caminipurgator Nadolicensis, 1667.

[136] p. 13 cm. [6388]

Place of printing supplied from Weller, vol. 1, 272.

—*See* SCHILLING, L. Anti-corollarium Kippingianum. 1673.

KIRÁLY, ISTVÁN [*d.* 1726] *respondent. See* HOFFMANN, F. [1660-1742] *praeses.* Dissertatio inauguralis medica, de genuino et simplicissimo doloris podagrici remedio. 1697.

KIRANI KIRANIDES. *See* KIRANUS, *King of Persia.*

KIRANIDES. *See* KIRANUS, *King of Persia.*

KIRANUS, *King of Persia.* Moderante auxilio redemptoris supremi, Kirani Kiranides, et ad eas Rhyakini [pseud., i.e. Andreas Rivinus] Koronides. Quorum ille in quaternario tam librorum, quam elementari, e totidem linguis, primo de gemmis XXIV, herbis XXIV, avibus XXIV, ac piscibus XXIV ... ad tetrapharmacum constituendum agit; inde libro II de animalibus XL, lib. III de avibus XLIV sigillatim, et lib. IV de LXXIV piscibus iterum, eorumque viribus medicamentosis: hic vero ... MS. post semi-millenarium annorum ex inemendatissimo primum edidit, 2. notis ... illustravit, 3. praefatione isagogica ornavit ...[Leipzig, Aera C., 1638]

[18], 159, [23] p. 17 cm. [6389]

Place of imprint supplied from Kestner.

Special title page (p. [17]) reads: Liber physico-medicus Kiranidum Kirani, i.e. Regis Persarum ... post D. fere annos nunc primum e membranis Latine editus cum notis. Qui multis adhuc seculis ante Syriace, Arabice & Graece scriptus & versus extitit. Cum autem reliquae translationes interciderint, haec semibarbara non omnino sepelienda, nec ita totum opusculum

obliterandum fuit. De quo quid sentiendum sit, requiratur in C. Barthii Advers. & Lexico Harpocrationis ...

[—] [The same.] Mysteria physico-medica, ob augustissimos suos natales, uberrimamque rerum haud quotidianarum, quibus referta sunt segetem, curioso obtutu quam-maxime veneranda. Multis abhinc seculis Syriace, Arabice, & Graece conscripta; iterata nunc vice e membranis Latinis publicae luci exposita. Francofurti, Impensis Joannis Justi Erythropili, 1681.

201, [13] p. 14 cm. [6390]

—[English tr.] The magick of Kirani ... and of Harpocration; containing the magical and medicinal vertues of stones, herbs, fishes, beasts, birds ... Now published and translated into English from a copy found in a private hand. [n. p.] 1685.

[24], 156, [13] p. 17 cm. [6391]

KIRBY, RICHARD [*fl.* 1681-1683] Vates astrologicus; or, England's astrological prophet, fortelling what is likely to befall Great-Britain and Ireland ... as also France, Holland, Spain ... To which is added a treatise of the pestilence, both for the prevention and cure thereof ... London, Thomas Malthus, 1683.

[12], 48 p. illus. 22 cm. [6392]

Imperfect: upper margins of p. 33-36 and lower margin of p. 43 trim.ned.

With this is bound Clarke, Richard. A warning to the world. London, 1759.

KIRCH, JOHANN ADAM [*fl.* 1696] *respondent. See* RIVINUS. A. Q., *praeses.* Disputationem inauguralem medicam de frigoris damno ... submittit ... J. A. K. 1696.

—*See* BOHN, J. Lectori salutem Facultatis Medicae in Academia Lipiensi p. t. procancellarius, D. Johannes Bohn. 1696.

KIRCHBERGER, JOHANN HEINRICH. Aphorismi; seu, Canones medicinales de peste. Das ist: Kurtze Erinnerungspuncten von der Pest, wie man es mit einem und andern ... zur Pestzeit halten soll ... Nürmberg, Gedruckt durch Balthasar Scherffen, 1625.

[68] p. illus., plates 20 cm. [6393]

KIRCHEIM, FRIEDRICH GÜNTHER [*fl.* 1675-*ca.* 1681] *respondent.* Disputatio medica inauguralis de procidentia uteri ... Basileae, Typis Jacobi Bertschii [1675]

    [20] p. illus. 19 cm.   **[6394]**
Diss. — Basel.

  —*See* FELDEN, J. von. Tractatus de peste. 1681.

KIRCHENN, GEORG LUDWIG [*fl.* 1635-1636] *respondent.* Ἀμφισβήτημα ἰατρικον περὶ τῶ λοιμῶ; id est, Disceptatio de pestis natura, praeservatione & curatione ... Marpurgi Cattorum, Typis exscribebat Casparus Chemlinus, 1635.

    [32] p. 19 cm.   **[6395]**
Diss. — Marburg.

KIRCHENN, PHILIPP LUDWIG [*fl.* 1687-1694] *respondent. See* VIRDUNG VON HARTUNG, P. W., *praeses.* Disputatio inauguralis medica de colica. 1694.

KIRCHER, ATHANASIUS [1602-1680] Ars magna lucis et umbrae in decem libros digesta ... Romae, Sumptibus Hermanni Scheus, ex typographia Ludovici Grignani, 1646.

    [38], 935, [15] p. illus., plates. 32 cm.
                                [6396]
Imperfect: added engraved title page wanting.

  —La Chine ... illustrée de plusieurs monuments ... et de quantité de recherchés de la nature ... A quoy on à adjousté de nouveau les questions ... que le ... grand duc de Toscane a fait ... au P. Jean Grubere touchant ce grand empire. Avec un dictionaire chinois & françois ... qui n'a pas encores paru au jour. Traduit par F. S. Dalquié. Amsterdam, Jean Jansson à Waesberge, & les heritiers d'Elizée Weyerstraet, 1670.

    [16], 367, [12] p. illus., plates. 38 cm.
                                  [6397]
Added engraved title page dated 1667.

  —Magnes; sive, De arte magnetica opus tripartitum ... Romae, Ex typographia Ludovici Grignani, sumptibus Hermanni Scheus, 1641.

    [48], 916, [16] p. illus., plates. 26 cm.
                                  [6398]
Added engraved title page.
Errata: p. [15-16] at end.
Liber tertius has special title page.

  —[The same.] ... Ed. 2. post Romanam multi corr. Coloniae Agrippinae, Apud Jodocum Kalcoven, 1643.

    [28], 797, [39] p. illus., plates. 20 cm.
                                  [6399]

Imperfect: added engraved title page wanting.
"Literae P. Martini Martini ... in quibus plures observationes magneticae, aliaque scitu digna adnotantur": p. [35-39]
Edited by Jost Kalckhoven.

  —[The same.] ... Ed. 3. ab ipso authore recognita, emendataque, ac multis novorum experimentorum problematis aucta. Romae, Sumptibus Blasii Deversin, & Zanobii Masotti, typis Vitalis Mascardi, 1654.

    [32], 618, [28] p. illus. 34 cm.   **[6400]**
Added engraved title page.

  —[Excerpts. Dutch] *In* Theatrum sympateticum. Dutch. 1681, 1697.

  —Magneticum naturae regnum; sive, Disceptatio physiologica de triplici in natura rerum magnete, juxta triplicem ejusdem naturae gradum digesto: inanimato, animato, sensitivo ... Romae, Typis Ignatii de Lazaris, 1667.

    [1], 5-136 p. 24 cm.   **[6401]**

  —Musurgia universalis; sive, Ars magna consoni et dissoni in X. libros digesta ... Romae, Ex typographia haeredum Francisci Corbelletti, 1650.

    2 v. in 1. illus., plates. 34 cm.   **[6402]**
Added engraved title pages.
Vol. 2 has imprint: Romae, Typis Ludovici Grignani, 1650.
Edited by Jacobus Viva.

  —Phonurgia nova, sive conjugium mechanico-physicum artis & naturae paranympha phonosophia concinnatum ... Campidonae, Per Rudolphum Dreherr, 1673.

    [45], 229, [16] p. port., plate, illus. 34 cm.
                                  [6403]

Added half-title, and added engraved title page.

  —Physiologia Kircheriana experimentalis, qua ... naturalium rerum scientia per experimenta physica, mathematica, medica ... comprobatur ... Quam ex vastis operibus ... P. Athanasii Kircheri extraxit, & in hunc ordinem per classes redegit ... Joannes Stephanus Kestlerus ... Amstelodami, Ex officina Janssonio-Waesbergiana, 1680.

    [8], 248, [8] p. illus. 40 cm.   **[6404]**
Added engraved title page.

  —Scrutinium physico-medicum contagiosae luis, quae pestis dicitur ... Romae, Typis Mascardi, 1658.

    [16], 252, [15] p. 22 cm.   **[6405]**

—[The same.] . . . Cum praefatione D. Christiani Langii . . . Lipsiae, Apud haered. Schüreri & Götzii, Typis Bauerianis, 1659.

[47], 427, [53] p. 14 cm. [6406]

—[The same.] . . . Annexoque tractatu ejusdem de thermis Carolinis . . . Lipsiae, Sumptibus haered. Schurerianor & Joh. Fritzschii, Typis Johannis Baueri, 1671.

[16], 148, [26] p. 20 cm. [6407]
Appendix wanting.

—[German tr.] Natürliche und medicinalische Durchgründung der laidigen ansteckenden Sucht, und so genanten Pestilentz . . . Erstlich . . . in lateinischer Sprach beschriben . . . Anjetzo aber . . . in die teutsche Sprach übersetzet, im Jahr 1680 . . . Augspurg, Verlegt bey Johann Caspar Brandan, gedruckt bey Jacob Koppmayer [1680?]

[8], 302, [17] p. 17 cm. [6408]

—Sententia de unguento armario, ex libro III. ejusdem De arte magneta desumpta.

567-573 p. 21 cm. (In Theatrum sympatheticum auctum. Norimbergae, 1662) [6409]
Caption title.

—See GOCKEL, E. Enchiridion medico-practicum de peste. 1669; HAUPTMANN, A. Uhralter wolckensteinischer warmer Badt-und Wasser-Schatz. 1657; PETRUCCI, G. Prodomo apologetico alli studi chircheriani. 1677; REDI, F. Esperienze intorno a diverse cose naturali. 1671, 1686, 1687.

KIRCHHEIM, FRIEDRICH GARTH. See KIRCHEIM, Friedrich Günther [fl. 1675-ca. 1681]

KIRCHHOFF, GOTTFRIED. See KIRCHOFF, Gottfried [fl. 1692-1713]

KIRCHHOFF, JOHANN ADAM [fl. 1687] respondent. See BOHN, J., praeses. Exercitatio physiologica. 1687.

KIRCHMAIER. See KIRCHMAJER; KIRCHMAYER.

KIRCHMAJER, KARL CHRISTIAN [fl. 1687] respondent. See ROESER, J. G., praeses. Dissertatio physica. 1687; THILE, J., praeses. Theelogia medica. 1690.

KIRCHMAJER, SEBASTIAN [1641-1700] praeses. Disputatio physica de salsedine aquae marinae . . . Wittebergae, Typis Johannis Haken, 1666.

[16] p. 18 cm. [6410]
Diss.—Wittenberg (T. Kirchmajer, respondent)

—Dissertatio de variis gentium moribus et indole . . . Rotenburgi, Literis Noachi de Millenau, 1699.

28 p. 21 cm. [6411]
Diss.—Rothenburg ob der Tauber? Gymnasium? (F. L. von Jaxheim, respondent)

—Dissertatio physica de corpore humano . . . Ratisponae, Typis Augusti Hanckwitz, 1680.

[24] p. 20 cm. [6412]
Diss.—Regensburg (J. J. Knopff, respondent)

—Exercitationem physicam de indiciis in inquisitione venarum metallicarum observandis . . . submittit . . . Immanuel Lehmannus . . . Wittebergae, Typis Johannis Haken, 1666.

[16] p. 19 cm. [6413]
Diss.—Wittenberg (I. Lehmann, respondent)

KIRCHMAJER, THEODOR [1645-1715] Dissertatio physica de virgula divinatrice . . . Wittebergae, Typis Danielis Schmatz [1669]

[24] p. 19 cm. [6414]
Diss. pro loco—Wittenberg (J. H. Martius, respondent)

Dissertations — Wittenberg

—praeses. De locustis ex zoologia physica . . . [Wittenbergae] Typis Hakianis [1669?]

[16] p. 19 cm. [6415]
G. H. Ursin, respondent.

—Διασκεψις physica, qua vanitas pulveris sympathetici, ut vulgo vocant, ostenditur, & vis ejus curandi vulnera naturalis rejicitur . . . disputatio prima, publicae physicorum censurae exponenda, a . . . Johanne Büngero . . . Wittebergae, Literis Wendianis excud. Daniel Schmatz [1672]

[24] p. 20 cm. [6416]
J. Bünger, respondent.

—Dissertatio physica de cruentatione cadaverum, fallaci illo praesentis homicidae indicio . . . Wittebergae, Excudebat Matthaeus Henckelius [1669]

[16] p. 20 cm. [6417]
I. Finck, respondent.

—Elegantissimum ex phisicis thema de hominibus apparenter mortuis . . . publicae ventilationi sistent M. Theodorus Kirchmajer . . . & Christophorus Nottnagel . . . Wittebergae, Typis Matthaei Henckelii [1669]

[16] p. 19 cm. [6418]
C. Nottnagel, respondent.

—[The same.] . . . Wittenbergae, Typis Matthaei Henckelii, 1670.

[16] p.   20 cm.   [6419]

A reprint of the 1669 edition; the date of the defense of the thesis is "d. 15 Maji, A. 1670" instead of "d. 15 Maji, A. 1669."

C. Nottnagel, *respondent.*

—Schediasma physicum de viribus mirandis toniconsoni . . . Wittenbergae, Literis Wendianis excud. Daniel Schmatz, 1672.

[28] p.   19 cm.   [6420]

G. A. Beer, *respondent.*

—*respondent.* See KIRCHMAJER, S., *praeses.* Disputatio physica de salsedine aquae marinae. 1666.

KIRCHMANN, JOHANN. [1575-1643] De funeribus Romanorum libri quatuor cum appendice . . . Accessit et [sic] Funus parasiticum Nicolai Rigaltii. Lugd. Batav., Apud Hackios, 1672.

[48], 641 (i.e. 649), [45] p.; 24 p.   plates.   15 cm.   [6421]

Added engraved title page.
Part [2] has special title page.
With this is bound (as issued?) *his* In funere . . . Pauli . . . Merulae . . . oratio. 1672.

—In funere . . . Pauli . . . Merulae . . . oratio, in qua de vita scriptisque ejus disseritur. Lugd. Batav., Ex Officina Hackiana, 1672.

[8], 64 p.   15 cm.   [6422]

Bound (as issued?) with *his* De funeribus Romanorum libri quatuor. 1672.

KIRCHMAYER, GEORG KASPAR [1635-1700] De passionum animi & corporis morborum traduce, dissertatio epistolica . . . Wittenbergae, Imprimebat Johannes Wilkius, 1684.

[4], 36 p.   19 cm.   [6423]

—Noctiluca constans & per vices fulgurans, diutissime quaesita, nunc reperta; dissertatione brevi praevia de luce, igne, ac perennibus lucernis . . . Wittebergae, Typis Matthaei Henckelii, 1676.

[24] p.   19 cm.   [6424]

Dissertations — Wittenberg

—*praeses.* Ad Plin. Secund. Hist. nat. II, 105 & 107 de ignium miraculis, locisque semper-ardentibus, singulatim de carbone fossili . . . disseret Christianus

Scheibner . . . Wittenbergae, Typis Christiani Schrödteri [1693]

[24] p.   20 cm.   [6425]

C. Scheibner, *respondent.*

—De aranea, inprimis vero de tarantulis . . . Wittebergae, Typis Johannis Borckardi [1660]

[16] p.   19 cm.   [6426]

A. Flachs, *respondent.*

—De coralio, balsamo et saccharo . . . [Wittenbergae] Exprimebat Matthaeus Henckelius, 1661.

[22] p.   19 cm.   [6427]

L. J. Frey, *respondent.*

—De montibus ignivomis . . . [Wittenbergae] Typis Johanis Borckardi [1661]

[22] p.   18 cm.   [6428]

J. C. Eilert, *respondent.*

—De vitae humanae unitate, animae, in, cum, et sub semine, propagatione . . . Wittebergae, Typis Johannis Röhneri [1661]

[20] p.   18 cm.   [6429]

Imperfect: upper margins trimmed.
M. Schwertner, *respondent.*

—Ex physicis de risu . . . Wittebergae, Typis Johannis Haken [1660]

[16] p.   19 cm.   [6430]

Imperfect: upper margins trimmed with possible loss of pagination.
E. Kallhardt, *respondent.*

—Ex physicis disputationem publicam, de aere . . . sistet . . . Adamus Ellingerus . . . [Hala Magdeburgicae] Literis haered. Melchioris Oelschlegelii [1659]

[16] p.   18 cm.   [6431]

A. Ellinger, *respondent.*

—Ex physicis disputationem publicam, de calido innato, corporis animaeque vinculo . . . sistet . . . Johannes Hartwig . . . ad d. Octob. A.O.R. M.DC.LIX horis locoque solitis. [Hala Magdeburgicae] Literis haered. Melchioris Oelschlegelii [1659]

[16] p.   18 cm.   [6432]

J. Hartwig, *respondent.*

—[The same.] . . . ad d. 29 Octobr. A.O.R. M.DC. LX horis locoque solitis. Wittebergae, Literis Henckelianis [1660]

[16] p.   20 cm.   [6433]

—Ex physicis disputationem publicam de sale . . . sistet respondens Conradus Wilhelmus Brazius . . . [Wittenbergae] Literis Henckelianis [1659]

[16] p. 19 cm. [6434]

C. W. Brazius, *respondent*.

—Ferax metallor. atque mineralium Dübensis saltus, prope Schmidebergam, in Saxoniae electorali circulo . . . Wittebergae, Typis Christiani Schrödteri [1692]

[16] p. 19 cm. [6435]

J. Schockwitz, *respondent*.

—Metallo-metamorphosis, principiis ac experimentis curiosis metallurgicis asserta . . . Wittenbergae, Typis Christiani Schrödteri [1693]

[1], 24 p. 19 cm. [6436]

Imperfect: p. 1-2 mutilated.

L. K. Mayer, *respondent*.

—Τετϱας quaestionum ilustrium anthropologico-physicarum . . . Wittebergae, Typis Michaelis Wendt [1659]

[16] p. 18 cm. [6437]

S. Virna, *respondent*.

KIRCHOF, ALBERT [*fl.* 1614-1623] *See* BACMEISTER, J. [1563-1631], *praeses*. Disputatio inauguralis de peste. 1623.

KIRCHOFF, GOTTFRIED [*fl.* 1692-1713] *respondent*. Disputatio medica inauguralis de natura morborum medica . . . Lugduni Batavorum, Apud Abrahamum Elzevier, 1692.

[24] p. 19 cm. [6438]

Diss.—Leyden.

KIRCHOVIUS, ALBERTUS. *See* KIRCHOF, Albert [*fl.* 1614-1623]

KIRKRINGIUS, THEODORUS. *See* KERCKRING, Theodor [1640-1693]

KIRSTEN, GEORG [1613-1660] *respondent*. *See* SEBISCH, M. [1578-1674?] *praeses*. Exercitationes medicae. 1639.

KIRSTEN, MICHAEL [1620-1678] Epigrammata. *In* Casserio, G. Julii Casserii Placentini Anatomische Tafeln. 1656, 1683.

KIRSTEN, PETER [1577-1640] Liber de vero usu et abusu medicinae. Una cum praefatione inclytae

Facultatis medicae in Academia Lipsiensi. Breslae, Sumptibus authoris [1610]

[1], 14, 122, [21] p. 16 cm. [6439]

With this is bound *his* Trewe Warnung. Bresslaw, 1610.

—[German tr.] Trewe Warnung von rechtem Gebrauch und Missbrauch der Artzney . . . Darnach ins Deutsche vorseget . . . Darzu auch kommen ist, eine Vorrede der löblichen Facultet der Medicorum in Leipzig, 1610.

[1], 14, 127, [33] p. 16 cm. [6440]

Bound with *his* Liber de vero usu et abusu medicinae. [1610]

—, *ed.* and *tr. See* AVICENNA. القانون لا بن سبنا

من با ب شوا بو تد ; id est, Liber secundus De canone canonis. 1609.

—*See* JUDICIA E MULTIS QUAEDAM VIRORUM REVERENDORUM . . . DE LABORIBUS DN. Petri Kirstenii. 1611.

KISLING, ANTON [*fl.* 1629-1631] *respondent. See* SEBISCH, M. [1578-1674?] *praeses*. Problemata phlebotomica. 1631.

KISLING, JOHANN [*fl.* 1620] *respondent. See* SEBISCH, M. [1578-1674?] *praeses*. Disputatio de arteriotomia. 1620.

KISLING, JOHANN CHRISTIAN [*fl.* 1652-1656] *respondent*. De singultu disputationem inauguralem . . . examini submittit Johannes Christianus Kislingius . . . Argentorati, Typis Eberhardi Welperi, 1656.

[23] p. 19 cm. [6441]

Diss.—Strasbourg.

—*See* SEBISCH, M. [1578-1674?] praeses. Disputatio solennis de fame et siti. 1655; ZEISOLD, J., *praeses*. Disputatio physica de humoribus corporis humani. 1652.

KISLING, JOHANN JAKOB [*b.* 1644] *respondent. See* MAJOR, J. D., *praeses*. Disputatio medica inauguralis de tactis fulmine. 1673. *See* MARCH, K. Programma. 1673.

KISNER, JOHANN [*fl.* 1665-1670] *respondent*. Disputatio medica inauguralis de suffocatione hypochondriaca . . . Lugduni Batavorum, Apud viduam & haeredes Joannis Elseviri, 1670.

[24] p. 23 cm. [6442]

Diss.—Leyden.

—Dissertatio medico chirurgica inauguralis de laesione tendinum ... Lugduni Batavorum, Apud Abrahamum Elzevier, 1699.

[68] p. plate. 21 cm.   **[6443]**

Diss.—Leyden.

—*See* HUNDESHAGEN, J. C., *praeses.* Disputatio academica de imaginatione. 1665.

—*as subject. See* VOTA AMICORUM. 1670.

KISNER, JOHANN ERASMUS [*b.* 1662] *respondent. See* WEDEL, G. W., *praeses.* Disputatio inauguralis medica de empyemate. 1686.

—*as subject. See* WEDEL, G. W. Propempticon inaugurale de morbis senum Salomonaeis. 1686.

KISSEL, JOHANN HEINRICH [*fl.* 1688] *respondent.* Disputatio medica inauguralis de asthmate ... Trajecti ad Rhenum, Ex officina Francisci Halma, 1688.

II, [1] p. 22 cm.   **[6444]**

Diss.—Utrecht.

KISSEL, JOHANN KONRAD [*fl.* 1681–1684] *respondent. See* FRANCK VON FRANCKENAU, G., *praeses.* Satyrae medicae, continuatio XVII. 1682; WINCKLER, F. C., *praeses.* Disputatio inauguralis medica de siriasi. 1684.

The KITCHIN-PHYSICIAN; or, A guide for good-housewives in maintaining their families in health. Wherein are described the natures, causes, and symptoms of all diseases ... Prescribing ... proper medicines both in physick and chirurgery ... Published ... by T. K. doctor in physick. London, Samuel Lee, 1680.

[10], 134 p. plate. 15 cm.   **[6445]**

KITCHEN-PHYSICK. *See* COCKE, T.

KITTEL, JOHANN [*fl.* 1611–1616] *respondent.* Disputatio medica de variolis et morbillis ... Basileae, Typis Joan Jacobi Genathii, 1616.

[16] p. 19 cm.   **[6446]**

Diss.—Basel.

KLAUNIG, ANDREAS [*fl.* 1668] *respondent. See* BOHN, J., *praeses.* Exercitationum physiologicarum prima ... [-decima tertia] 1674?

KLAUNIG, GOTTFRIED [1676–1731] *respondent.* Dissertatio medica inauguralis de spasmo ...

Lugduni Batavorum, Apud Abrahamum Elzevier, 1699.

24 p. 22 cm.   **[6447]**

Diss.—Leyden.

—*See* RIVINUS, A. Q., *praeses.* Medicum superstitiosum ... examini sistit ... G. K. 1698.

KLAUSING, HEINRICH [1675–1745] *praeses.* Prima de motu corporum naturalium disputatio ... Witenbergae, Typis Christiani Schrödteri [1700]

[16] p. 19 cm.   **[6448]**

Diss.—Wittenberg (H. Labin, *respondent*)

KLEIN, CONRADUS [*fl.* 1624] *respondent. See* SEBISCH, M. [1578–1674?] *praeses.* Exercitationes medicae. 1639.

KLEIN, FRANZ [*fl.* 1680–1688] Convivium lacteum pro podagricis animo desolatis, tortura enervatis, cura desperatis, mundo ingratis, coelo destinatis ... Paratum a ... Francisco Kleinio ... dum ... Joannem Adamum Bautz ... medicinae doctorem ... inauguravit ... Herbipoli, Typis haeredum Zinck, per Martinum Richter [1688]

40 p. 20 cm.   **[6449]**

—*praeses.* Stephanus Brion ... dissertationem inauguralem de catarrho ... subibit [sic] ... Herbipoli, Typis Eliae Michaelis Zinck [1682]

[7], 24 (i.e. 25) p. 20 cm.   **[6450]**

Diss.—Würzburg (S. Brion, *respondent*)

KLEIN, JAKOB [*fl.* 1658?] *respondent. See* SPERLING, J., *praeses.* An virgula mercurialis agat ex occulta qualitate disquisitio philosophica. 1666.

KLEIN, NIKOLAUS [*fl.* 1660] *praeses.* Disquisitio philologico-physica de magnete ... Lipsiae, Typis Johannis Baueri [1660]

[28] p. 19 cm.   **[6451]**

Diss.—Leipzig (J. F. Kessler, *respondent*)

KLEINKNECHT, JOHANN JAKOB [*fl.* 1677] *respondent. See* METZGER, G. B., *praeses.* Disputatio medica inauguralis de ictero albo virginum. 1677.

KLERCQ, PIETER DE [*fl.* 1670] *respondent.* Disputatio-medico-chirurgica inauguralis de fracturis cranii ... Lugduni Batavorum, Apud viduam & haeredes Joannis Elsevirii, 1670.

[15] p. 23 cm.   **[6452]**

KLETT, Georg Benedikt [*fl.* 1700] *respondent. See* Stübner, A. G., *praeses.* Novem ex philosophia naturali paradoxa. 1700.

KLETTWICH, Simon Philipp [*fl.* 1672] *respondent. See* Friderici, J. A., *praeses.* Disputatio inauguralis medica de imbecillitate ventriculi. 1672.

KLETWICH, Johann Christoph [*fl.* 1688–1689] *respondent. See* Albinus, B. Dissertatio de phosphoro. 1688; Vehr, I., *praeses.* Disputatio inauguralis de suspirio et suspirioso. 1689 [and] Dissertationem physico medicam de oxyregmia ... exponit ... J. C. K. 1689.

Het KLEYN vroetwijfs-boek. *See* Roeslin, E.

KLIMM, Johann Christoph [*fl.* 1694–1724] *respondent. See* Hoffmann, F. [1660–1742] *praeses.* Disputatio medica inauguralis de medicamentis specificis, eorumque agendi modo. 1694.

—*See* Hoffmann, F. [1660–1742] Propemticon inaugurale de medicamentorum prudenti applicatione. 1694.

KLINCKHAAMER, Laurens [*fl.* 1650] *respondent.* Disputatio medica inauguralis de nephritide ... Lugduni Batavorum, Apud Davidem Lopez de Haro, 1650.
[11] p. 22 cm. **[6453]**
Diss.—Leyden.

KLIPPER, Johann Peter [*fl.* 1657–1659] *respondent.* Respirationem ... disputabunt M. Johannes Petrus Klipperus ... et Isaacus Thilo ... Lipsiae, Typis haered. Koleri, 1659.
[12] p. 18 cm. **[6454]**
Diss.—Leipzig.

—See Ammann, P., *praeses.* Theses physicae de nutritione. 1657.

KLOBIUS, Justus Fidus [*fl.* 1649–1666] Ambrae historiam ... exhibet Justus Fidus Klobius ... Wittenbergae, Sumptibus haered. D. Tobiae Mevii & Elerdi Schumacheri, typis Matthaei Henckelii, 1666.
[8], 76 p. plates. 20 cm. **[6455]**
Imperfect: one of two folded maps wanting.

KLOSE, Friedrich Wilhelm [*fl.* 1693–1702] *respondent. See* Bohn, J., *praeses.* Dissertationem inauguralem de angina ... examini exponit ...

F. W. K. 1696; Ortlob, J. F. *praeses.* Ἀντίπραξιν partium oeconomiae animalis legibus minus conformen. 1693.

KLUG, Daniel Gottfried [*fl.* 1675] *respondent.* De fluxu chyli in fluore muliebri gonorrhoea coeliaca urinis lacteis et lactis abundantia thematis novi summaria et theses ... Altdorfii, Typis Henrici Meyeri [1675]
[16] p. 18 cm. **[6456]**
Diss.—Altdorf.

KLUG, Georg Philipp [*fl.* 1647] *respondent. See* Möbius, G., *praeses.* Disputatio medica dogmaticorum. 1647.

KLUGE, Johann [*fl.* 1611–1613] *respondent.* Disputatio medica de cholera ... Basileae, Typis Joannis Schroeteri, 1613.
[8] p. 19 cm. **[6457]**
Diss.—Basel.

—*See* Sennert, D., *praeses.* Disputatio medica de dysenteria. 1611.

KLUGIUS, Johannes. *See* Kluge, Johann [*fl.* 1611–1613]

KNAUT, Christian [1654–1716] *respondent. See* Crause, R. W., *praeses.* Disputatio inauguralis de fermentatione in sanguine non existente. 1682.

KNAUTH, Christopher [1638–1694] *respondent. See* Rolfinck, W., *praeses.* De phthisi disputationem inauguralem ... submittit ... C. K. 1664.

KNEUSSEL, Christoph Friedrich [*fl.* 1695–1698] *respondent.* Dissertatio inauguralis medica de haemorrhagia uterina matronae abortientis, vulgo von dem angegangenen Hertz-Geblüt, ex praxi clinica desumpta ... Gissae-Hassorum, Typis Henningi Mülleri [1698]
24 p. 18 cm. **[6458]**
Diss.—Giessen.

—*See* Valentini, M. B., *praeses.* Disputatio medica, de ipecuanha. 1698.

KNIPHOF, Johann Melchior [*b.* 1660] *respondent. See* Schröder, C. P., *praeses.* Dissertatio inauguralis medica de requisitis veri medici. 1692; Vesti, J., *praeses.* Disputatio inauguralis medica qua aegrum artuum tremore correptum. 1694.

—*as subject. See* VESTI, J. Facultatis Medicae . . . decanus Justus Vesti . . . benevolo lecotri S. P. D. 1694.

KNIPS-MACOPPE. ALESSANDRO [1662-1744] De aortae polypo epistola medica . . . Carolo Patino . . . qua ejusdem abditissimum morbum a polypo arteriam magnam insidente dependere demonstratur, ac de ejus natura, dignotione, & curatione disseritur. Cum ejusdem cadaveris historia anatomica eventum comprobante . . . Lugduni, Sumptibus Cadorini, 1693.

    [8], 31, [1] p.   plate.   22 cm.   **[6459]**

KNISEL, JOHANN SAMUEL [*fl.* 1687-1690] *respondent. See* CAMERARIUS, E. R., *praeses.* Historiam pleuritidis et abscessus pectoris cum succedente colica spasmodica et gutta serena, & in eam commentarium . . . submittit . . . S. J. K. 1690; ZELLER, J. G., *praeses.* Dissertatio anatomica de vasorum lymphaticorum administratione. 1687.

KNOBELOCH, GEORG GOTTLIEB [*fl.* 1679-1684] *respondent. See* ALBINUS, B. Disputatio medica inauguralis de atrophia. 1684; GERRESHEIM, J. W., *praeses.* Diatribe academica de nexu principiorum physicorum in homine. 1679.

KNOBLADCH, HIERONYMUS. *See* Knoblauch, Hieronymus [*fl.* 1648-1649]

KNOBLAUCH, HIERONYMUS [*fl.* 1648-1649] *respondent. See* RIVINUS, A., *praeses.* Δεντέραι φροντίδες φιλοσοφικώτσραι. 1649.

KNOBLOCH, JOHANN [*fl.* 1607] *See* KNOBLOCH, T., *praeses.* Disputationes anatomicae. 1608, 1612.

KNOBLOCH, TOBIAS [*fl.* 1601-1607] *praeses.* Disputationes anatomicae explicantes mirificam corporis humani fabricam & usum . . . Witebergae, Typis Cratonianis, per Johannem Gorman, impensis Pauli Helwigii, 1608.

    [457] p.   illus.   20 cm.   **[6460]**

Contains 20 Wittenberg theses, each with special title page dated 1607. (Respondents: J. Wilkofer, no. 1; J. Janike, no. 2 & 22; G. Hezmanseder, no. 3; J. Frick, no. 4; C. Bilitzer, no. 5; G. Eberlin, no. 6; L. Baudiss, no. 7 & 21; S. Hase, no. 8 & 11; T. Bohemus, no. 9 & 16; F. Eckart, no. 10; J. Knobloch, no. 12; S. Stangius, no. 13 & 14; A. Bogner, no. 15; J. Widholtz, no. 17; J. Stotmeister, no. 18; N. Olschlegel, no. 19; J. Jentsch, no. 20)

—[The same.] Disputationes anatomicae et psychologicae, recens editae, & plurimis in locis

locupletatae . . . additis humani corporis affectibus praecipuis . . . [Lipsiae] Prelo Meisneriano, Sumptibus Pauli Helwigii, 1612.

    [16], 713, [29] p.   illus.   16 cm.   **[6461]**
Imprint partly supplied from Linden.
Without the special title pages.

—Kurtzer Bericht von dem Podagra, und andern Gliedsüchten . . . Wittemberg, Gedruckt bey Wolffgang Meissnern, in Vorlegung Paul Helwigens, 1606.

    [8], 110 p.   16 cm.   **[6462]**

—, *ed. See* HIPPOCRATES. Aphorismi. 1641.

KNOEFFEL, ANDRZEJ. *See* CNÖFFEL, Andreas [*d.* 1658]

KNÖRING, FRANTZ XAVER VON. Viaticum balneantium; das ist, Neue erholde Bad-Ordnung, in welcher aller denckwürdig in Pusterthall sich befindenden mineralischen Bad-Wässern . . . beschriben wird . . . Brixen, Joseph Schueshegger, 1700.

    [14], 157, [1] p.   15 cm.   **[6463]**

KNOGLER, JÁNOS KRISTÓF [*fl.* 1653] *respondent. See* SEBISCH, J. A., *praeses.* Theoremata anatomica miscellanea de variis humani corporis partibus. 1653.

KNOPFF, JOHANN JAKOB [*fl.* 1680] *respondent. See* KIRCHMAJER, S., *praeses.* Dissertatio physica de corpore humano. 1680.

KNORR VON ROSENROTH, CHRISTIAN [1636-1689] *ed. See* PORTA, G. B. della. Magia naturalis. 1680.

—, *tr. See* BROWNE, *Sir* T. Pseudodoxia epidemica [German.] 1680.

KOBER, DANIEL [*fl.* 1626] *respondent. See* AGER, N. Disputatio physica de luna. 1626.

KOBER, TOBIAS [*ca.* 1570-*ca.* 1612] Observationum Castrensium et Ungaricarum, decas prima, Austriaca [-decas secunda, Silesiaca; - decas tertia, Suevica] . . . Francofurti, E Collegio Paltheniano, 1606.

    120 p.; 112 p.; 1-32, 401-466 p.   18 cm.
                                      [6464]
Parts 2-3 have special title pages.

—Observationum medicarum Castrensium Hungaricarum decades tres. In usum publicum hoc tempore recusae . . . Cum indice & praefatione

Henrici Meibomii. Helmstad. & Gardelegensis, Sumptibus Friderici Lüderwaldi, 1685.

[12], 61 p.; 56 p.; 50, [10] p. 21 cm. **[6465]**

Parts 2–3 have half titles.

KOCH, CHRISTIAN GOTTLIEB [*b.* 1676] *respondent.* See SLEVOGT, J. A., *praeses.* Dissertatio inauguralis medica exhibens foeminam mola laborantem. 1700.

—See SLEVOGT, J. A. Facultatis Medicae decani Jo. Hadriani Slevogtii . . . prolusio inauguralis, de partu thamaris difficili et perinaeo inde rupto. 1700.

KOCH, JOHANN DANIEL [*fl.* 1644] *respondent.* See SCHMITNER, A., *praeses.* Disputatio medica de paresi ex colica. 1644.

KOCH, JOHANN WILHELM [*fl.* 1697] *respondent.* See ALBINUS, B. Dissertatio medica inauguralis, de partu naturali. 1697.

KØBENHAVNS UNIVERSITET. MEDICINSK FACULTET. *See* UNIVERSITAS REGIA HAFNIENSIS. Facultas medica.

KÖCKERT, JOHANN [*fl.* 1664–1665] *respondent.* Dissertatio inauguralis medica de renum et vesicae calculo . . . Basileae, Typis Johan. Jacobi Deckeri [1665]

[19] p. 22 cm. **[6466]**

Diss. — Basel.

—See SCHNEIDER, K. V., *praeses.* Dissertatio de morbo comitiali medica. 1664.

KOECKOECX naar sang . . . Amsterdam, Lijsbeth Jansz, 1677.

[8] p. 16 cm. **[6467]**

Poem concerning Andreas Boekelman and Bonaventura van Dortmont.

De KOECKOECX-ZANGH van de nachtuylen van het collegie Nil volentibus arduum, huylende met eenen naare geest: Dr. Ruysch en Boeckelman zijn de beest. Of een blyeyndende zamenspraak tusschen een doctor, proponent, en poeet. Zwol, Autheur [1677]

33, [2] p. 16 cm. **[6468]**

KÖFFERLIN, KASPAR FRANZ XAVER [*fl.* 1694] *respondent.* Dissertationem inauguralem de vitiis spirituum et humorum . . . publice examinandam offert . . . Casp. Francisc. Xaver Köfferlin . . . Basileae, Typis Joh. Jacobi Battierii [1694]

[32] p. 21 cm. **[6469]**

Diss. — Basel.

KOEHLER, ADAM GOTTLIEB [*b.* 1667] *respondent.* See CRAUSE, R. W., *praeses.* Disputatio inauguralis medica de fulmine tactis. 1694.

—See SCHELHAMMER, G. C. Programma conscriptum occasione inauguralis . . . Adami Gottlieb Koehleri, disputationis de fulmine tactis. 1694.

KÖHLER DE MOHRENFELD, GEORG GOTTLIEB [*b.* 1675] *respondent. See* STAHL, G. E., *praeses.* Dissertatio inauguralis medica tradens novam pathologiam calculi renum. 1698.

—*as subject. See* STAHL, G. E. Prolusio inauguralis de certitudine artis medicae. 1698.

KÖHN, HUBERT [*fl.* 1663] *respondent. See* POSNER, C., *praeses.* Disputatio physica de principatu partium. 1663.

KÖLICHEN, CASPAR [*fl.* 1664] *respondent. See* BARTHOLIN, T., *praeses.* Disputatio medica inauguralis de gutta seu morbo articulari. 1664.

KÖLSCH, MÁRTON [*fl.* 1668] *respondent. See* FRIEDEL, J., *praeses.* Disputatio medica de pleuritide. 1668.

KÖNIG, CHRISTOPHER [*fl.* 1630] *respondent. See* ZEIDLER, J., *praeses.* De mania themata medica. 1630.

KÖNIG, EMANUEL [1658–1731] Regnum vegetabile, physice, medice, anatomice . . . enucleatum . . . Accessit Selectus remediorum e triplici regno juxta norman & ductum pharmacie Ludovicianae cum Appendice compositionis artificiosae eorundem secundum celeberr. D. Georg. Wolfg. Wedelium. Basileae Rauracorum, Prostat apud Emanuelem & Joh. Georgium König, 1688.

[16], 186, [2] p.; 166, [14] p. 21 cm. **[6470]**

Part [2] has half title: Ludovicus enucleatus dilucidatus et auctus. With this is bound his Regni vegetabilis pars altera. Basileae, 1696.

—Regni vegetabilis pars altera plantarum descriptionem, classes et differentias, figuram . . . virtutes et usus proponens . . . methodo Bauhiniana enumeratio plantarum indigenarum seu in Helvetia

& circa Basileam sponte nascentium cum earundem synonymis & nova dispositione ex florum & seminum configuratione juxta Rob. Morison, & Joh. Rajum ... Basileae, Ex officina typographica Emanuelis & Joh. Georgii Regum, 1696.

[16], 271, [9] p.   21 cm.   **[6471]**
Bound with his Regnum vegetabile. 1688.

—*respondent.* Dissertationem inauguralem physico-medicam eviscerantem, enumerantem et emedullantem regnum animale ... proponit M. Emanuel König ... Basileae, Typis Emanuelis König & filiorum [1682]

[12], 174, [2] p.   20 cm.   **[6472]**

—*See* ROTH, J., *praeses.* Disputationem physico-medicam generalia regni vegetabilis enucleantem ... submittit E. K. 1680.

—*See* MURALT, J. von. Chirurgische Schrifften. 1691.

KÖNIG, JAKOB JOSEPH [*fl.* 1699] *respondent. See* VICARIUS, J. J. F., *praeses.* Disceptatio medica ... de malo hypochondriaco. 1699.

KÖNIGSBERG. ACADEMIA ALBERTINA. *See* ALBERTUS UNIVERSITÄT.

KÖNIGSBERG. ALBERTUS UNIVERSITÄT. *See* ALBERTUS UNIVERSITÄT.

KÖNIGSBERG. UNIVERSITÄT. *See* ALBERTUS UNIVERSITÄT.

KÖPPE, JOACHIM [*fl.* 1604-1609] *respondent. See* HORST, G. [1578-1636] *praeses.* Problematum medicorum θεραπευτιϰων decades priores quinque. 1608; SENNERT, D., *praeses.* De methodo medendi disputatio III, de indicantium consensu ac dissensu. 1604 [and] Quaestiones medicae controversae quinque, pro disputatione prima propositae. 1607.

KÖPPING, GABRIEL [*fl.* 1612] De euthanasia. Gründlicher und warer Bericht, von der rechten Sterbekunst, in welcher verfasset ist, der ... Schatz christlich und wol sterben, auff dass wir der ewigen Verdamnuss, ritterlich entfliehen mögen ... [Hoff, Gedruckt durch Matthaeum Pfeilschmiedt] 1612.

[48] p.   19 cm.   **[6473]**
In verse.

KÖRBER, HERMANN FRIEDRICH [*fl.* 1674-1677] *respondent. See* SCHENCK, J. T., *praeses.* Disputationem

inauguralem de cholera ... subjicit ... 1653; WEDEL, G. W., *praeses.* Exercitatio chimica de menstruis. 1674.

KÖRBER, JOACHIM LUDWIG [*fl.* 1682-1685] *praeses.* Exercitium medicum de ecclipsi microcosmica ... publicae exponet M. Joan. Frederich Gruvius ... Erffurti, Typis Joh. Henrici Groschii [1685]

24 p.   20 cm.   **[6474]**
Diss.—Erfurt (J. F. Gruve, *respondent*)

KÖSTER, DANIEL KONRAD [*fl.* 1690] *respondent. See* PETERMANN, A., *praeses.* Disputatio medica de pleuritide. 1690.

Ein **KÖSTLICH** Kinder-Pulver. *See* BECHER, J. J. Medicinische Schatz-Kammer. 1700.

KOHLER, MATERNUS [*fl.* 1619] *respondent. See* SEBISCH, M. [1578-1674?] *praeses.* Disputatio de alimentorum facultatibus tertia. 1619.

KOHLREUTER, SIGISMUND [1534-1599] *See* SENNERT, D. De febribus libri IV. 1628, 1633, 1641, 1653.

KOKUYT, ISAAC [*fl.* 1685] *respondent.* Disputatio medica inauguralis de melancholia ... Lugduni Batavorum, Apud Abrahamum Elzevier, 1685.

[20] p.   22 cm.   **[6475]**
Diss.—Leyden.

KOLB, JOACHIM JOHANN [*fl.* 1682] *respondent.* Dissertatio inauguralis medica aegrum syncope laborantem exhibens ... Erfurti, Literis Kirschianis [1682]

[24] p.   19 cm.   **[6476]**
Diss.—Erfurt.

KOLHANS, TOBIAS LUDOVICUS. Litterae ... de spiritu animali, ad ... J. D. Horstium ... [n. p.] 1658.

29 p.   17 cm.   **[6477]**
Bound with Castro, E. R. de. Variae exercitationes medicae. 1656.

—, *ed. & tr. See* ROCHAS, H. DE. Notabilia excerpta. 1663.

KOLLEGIUM DER AERZTE, NUREMBERG. *See* Dispensatorium pharmacorum omnium. 1666; KOLLEGIUM DER AERZTE, REGENSBURG. Kurtzer, sehr nothwendig-und treuhertziger Bericht. 1680; NUREMBERG. Ordinances, local laws, etc. Verneuerte

Gesetz, Ordnung und Tax . . . dess . . . Reichs Statt Nürmberg. 1624, 1700.

KOLLEGIUM DER AERZTE. REGENSBURG. Kurtzer, sehr nothwendig- und treuhertziger Bericht, wie sich jedermänniglich für jetzt besorglichen, geschwinden, und gefährlichen, anderwerts starck eingerissenen Seuche der Pestilentz . . . zeitlichen bewahren und vorsehen soll. Auff . . . Befehl gestellet durch die Medicos Ordinarios der Statt Regenspurg. Regenspurg, Gedruckt bey Augusto Hanckwitzen, 1679.

 [15] p. 19 cm.   **[6478]**

—[The same.] . . . Auff . . . Befehl gestellet durch die Medicos Ordinarios der Stadt Regenspurg und Nürnberg. [Regensburg?] 1680.

 67 p. 14 cm.   **[6479]**
 "Amuleta contra pestem": p. 25-31, signed Michael Wez.
 "Consilium Noribergense": p. 32-50.

KOLWECK, JOHANN [*fl.* 1621-1631] Tractat von dess . . . heylsamen . . . unser lieben Frawen Pfefers Bad, inn Ober Schweitz gelegen, wunderthätiger Natur . . . Krafft und Würckungen . . . Dilingen, Erhardt Lochner, 1631.

 [8], 302, [2] p. illus. 16 cm. **[6480]**

KONGL. May:tz i nader uthgifne sidste medicinal-ordningar. 1699. *See* SWEDEN. Laws, statutes, etc.

KOPFF, ARPOLD PHILIPP [*fl.* 1686-1691] *respondent. See* WEDEL, G. W., *praeses.* Exercitatio medica, de cephalalgia in genere. 1686.

KOPP, WILHELM. *See* COPUS, Gulielmus [*ca.* 1460-1532]

KOPPE, JOACHIM. *See* KÖPPE, Joachim [*fl.* 1604-1609]

KOPPEN, JOHANN DANIEL [*fl.* 1680] *respondent.* Dissertatio inauguralis medica de imbecillitate ventriculi . . . [Erfurti] Typis Krischianis [1680]

 [20] p. 20 cm.   **[6481]**
 Diss.—Erfurt.

KORMARK, GEORG. *See* KORMART, Georg [*fl.* 1666-1668]

KORMART, GEORG [*fl.* 1666-1668] *praeses.* De spiritu animalium corporeo vero s. vitali . . . Lipsiae, Literis Ritzschianis [1666]

 [23] p. 19 cm.   **[6482]**
 Diss.—Leipzig (J. Schilling, *respondent*)

—Disputatio physica de elemento aquae Helmontii . . . Lipsiae, Literis Ritzschianis [1667]

 [12] p. 19 cm.   **[6483]**
 Diss.—Leipzig (D. Freywaldt, *respondent*)

KORNAX, MATHIAS. *See* CORNAX, Mathias [*d.* 1564]

KORNMANN, HEINRICH [*d. ca.* 1620] Opera curiosa in tractatus quatuor distributa, Quorum I. Miracula vivorum; II. Miracula mortuorum . . . III. Templum naturae historicum, in quo de natura & miraculis elementorum ignis, aeris, aquae et terrae disseritur. IV. Quaestiones enucleatae de virginum statu ac jure. Perquam diu a quam plurimis doctis et eruditis viris desiderata & expetita, nunc in lucem edita. Francofurti ad Moenum, Ex Officina Genschiana, 1694.

 [48], 295; [16], 472; 432, [16], 192 p. 17 cm.
            [6484]

—De miraculis vivorum; seu, De varia natura, variis singularitatibus, proprietatibus, affectionibus, mirandisque virtutibus, facultatibus & signis hominum vivorum, liber novus & singularis . . . Francofurti, Typis viduae Matthiae Beckeri, impensis Jacobi Fischeri, 1614.

 [40], 298 p. 17 cm.   **[6485]**

—Sibylla trygAndriana, seu, De virginitate, virginum statu & jure tractatus novus & jucundus, in quo ex jure naturali, divino, canonico et civili, scriptoribus ecclesiasticis & prophanis virginitatis status laudatur, virginum jura pertractantur . . . quaesita physica, medica, theologica & juridica accuratius & plenius resolvuntur . . . Francofurti, Typis Matthiae Beckeri, impensis Jacobi Fischeri, 1610.

 281, [6] p. 13 cm.   **[6486]**
 Imperfect: Linea amoris wanting.
 With this is bound: Meibom, J. H. De flagrorum usu in re medica et venerea, et lumborum renumque officio. Parisiis, 1792.

—[The same.] . . . Accessit noviter ejusdem authoris De linea amoris, annulo usitato, sponsalitio & signatorio tractatus absolutissimus. Francofurti, Apud haeredes Jac. Fischer, 1629.

 281, [6].; 244, [6] p. 15 cm. **[6487]**

Different setting of type.

"Linea amoris" and "De annulo triplici, usitato, sponsalitio, & signatorio tractatus" have half titles.

KORNMANN, JOHANNES JUSTUS [*fl.* 1685] *respondent. See* HOFFMANN, J. M., *praeses.* Dissertatio medica de anorexia. 1685.

KORNMESSER, JAKOB [*b.* 1636] *See* MARCH, K. Programma. 1665.

KORNTHAUER, JOB, *ed. See* PARACELSUS. De peste . . . tractatus. 1613.

Een **KORT** discours, om die geene, die 't lust reflexie te doen maken op 't leven, de siekte, en de dood. *See* BONTEKOE, C. Tractaat van het excellenste kruyd thee. 1679.

Een **KORTE** beschrijvinge van het wonderlijcke kruyt tobacco. 1623. *See* [CHUTE, A.]

KORTE en bondige verhandeling, van de voortteeling en t' kinderbaren met den aankleve van dien. 1695, 1699. *See* JANSONIUS, S.

KOSCHWITZ , DANIEL [*fl.* 1611–1616] *respondent.* Disputatio medica de haemorrhagia narium . . . Basileae, Typis Joh. Jacobi Genathii [1616]

[II] p.   22 cm.   [6488]

Diss. — Basel.

KOSCHWITZ, GEORGE DANIEL [*fl.* 1693] *comp. and tr. See* SCHRÖDER, J. Vollständige und nutzreiche Apotheke. 1693.

KOSMAS, *Saint. See* COSMAS, *Saint.*

KOVÁCS, GYÖRGY, *tatai* [*b.* 1645] Hercules vere cognitus, certus exul; id est, Epilepsiae vera dignotio, ac ejusdem certa curatio, libris duobus comprehensa . . . Lugduni Batavorum, Ex officina Arnoldi Doude, 1670.

[20], 152, [8] p.   13 cm.   [6489]

Imperfect: plate wanting.

— *respondent. See* REGIUS, H., *praeses.* Disputatio medica de renum et vesicae calculo. 1661.

KOVACS TATAI, GEORGIUS. *See* KOVÁCS, György, tatai [*b.* 1645]

KOZAK, JOHANN SOPHRON [1602–1685] Anatomia vitalis microcosmi in qua naturae humanę proprietates quas homo cum rebus extra se sitis communes habet, tum morborum origines, eorumque

legitimus curandi modus breviter & dilucide explicantur . . . [Bremae, Typis Bertholdi Villeriani] 1636.

[13], 269 (i.e. 271), [II] p.   20 cm.   [6490]

— Tractatus de haemorrhagia, partes duae: in prima, causae recensentur omnis generis haemorrhagiae; in secunda, omnium curandi rationalis methodus dictatur . . . Ulmae, Apud Balthasarum Kühnen, 1666.

[32], 692, [18] p.   17 cm.   [6491]

— Tractatus medicus de sale, ejusdemque in corpore humano resolutionibus salutaribus et noxiis . . . Francofurti, Prostat apud Balthasar Kühnen, 1663.

[30], 544, [7] p.   20 cm.   [6492]

Engraved title page.

Imperfect: lower part of title page wanting.

KOZERUS, AGAPETUS. *See* AUSTROPEDIUS, Agapetus Kozerus.

KRÄUTERMANN, VALENTIN, *pseud. See* HELL-WIG, Christoph von [1663–1721]

KRAFFT, JOHANN ANDREAS [*fl.* 1698] *praeses.* Dissertatio physica de objecto visus . . . Jenae, Typis Pauli Ehrichii [1698]

28 p.   19 cm.   [6493]

Diss. — Jena (C. H. Wentzel, *respondent*)

KRAFFT, THEOPHILUS. *See* CARRICHTER, B. Horn dess Heyls menschlicher Blödigkeit. 1673.

KRAFFTHEIM, JOHANN CRATO VON. *See* CRATO VON KRAFFTHEIM, Johann [1519–1585]

KRAFT, JOHANN. *See* CRATO VON KRAFFTHEIM, Johann [1519–1585]

KRAMER, DIETRICH VALENTIN [*fl.* 1692–1696] *respondent. See* SCHRADER, F., *praeses.* Disputatio medica inauguralis de idiosyncrasiis. 1696.

KRAPFF, JOHANN WOLFGANG [*fl.* 1607] *respondent. See* STUPANUS, J. N., *praeses.* Positiones iatricae de phrenitide. 1607.

KRAUSE, CHRISTOPH [*b.* 1662] *respondent. See* Fasch, A. H., *praeses.* Dissertationem inauguralem medicam de febre hectica . . . submittit. 1688.

— *See* FASCH, A. H. Augustini Henrici Faschii . . . Collegii Medici decani invitatio publica ad disputationem inauguralem de hectica. 1688.

KRAUSE, JOHANN JAKOB [*fl.* 1652] *respondent. See* PUFENDORFF, E., *praeses.* De temperamentis disquisitio. 1652.

KRAUSE, MICHAEL HEINRICH [*fl.* 1673] *respondent. See* REINHARD, J., *praeses.* Theranthropismus fictus. 1673.

KRAUSE, RUDOLPH WILHELM. *See* CRAUSE, Rudolf Wilhelm [1642–1718]

KRAUSOLDT, JOHANN ERNEST [*fl.* 1677–1678] *respondent. See* FASCH, A. H., *praeses.* Castoreum publico . . . examini committet . . . J. E. K. 1677; WEDEL, G. W., *praeses.* Disputationem medicam inauguralem de dentitione infantum . . . subjicit J. E. K. 1678.

KRAUSS, JOHANN PHILIPP [*fl.* 1692] *respondent. See* SCHELHAMMER, G. C., *praeses.* Dissertationem medicam inauguralem de tremore . . . submittit J. P. K. 1692.

KRAUSS, PETER [*fl.* 1602] *respondent. See* SCHRÖTER, J. F., *praeses.* Dysenteriae αποθεραπειαιατρικη. 1602.

KRAUSS, RUDOLF WILHELM. *See* CRAUSE, Rudolf Wilhelm [1642–1718]

KRAUSSOLD, ADAM FRIEDRICH [*fl.* 1669] *respondent. See* HUNDESHAGEN, J. C., *praeses.* Disputatio academica de sanguinis stillicidio. 1669.

KRECKE, ANTON [*fl.* 1656] *respondent. See* ZESCH, W., *praeses.* Disputationum physicarum de maximo et minimo rerum naturalium tertia et ultima. 1656.

KRECKLER, BALTHASAR [*fl.* 1649] *respondent. See* HOPP, J., *praeses.* Διάσκεψις φυσιολογικη και παθυλογικη ventriculi humani in theses redacta. 1649.

KREIENBERG, JUSTUS HEINRICH [*fl.* 1688–1690] *respondent. See* MEIBOM, H., *praeses.* Exercitatio medica inauguralis de venae sectionis in variolarum curatione usu. 1690; SCHRADER, F., *praeses.* Disputatio medica de hemicrania. 1690.

KREMER, ADAM FRIEDRICH [*fl.* 1680–*ca.* 1694] Heylsamer Brunn; oder, Kurtze Beschreibung, der gesunden mineralischen Wassern, welche in der Graffschafft Glatz, zu Oberthalheim . . . aus einem

. . . Felsen warm heraus fliessen . . . Wienn, Andreas Heyinger, 1694.

[4], 96 p.   front.   16 cm.   **[6494]**

—*respondent. See* KREMER, J. K., *praeses.* Disputatio medica de humoribus. 1680.

KREMER, JOHANN KONRAD [*fl.* 1680] *praeses.* Disputatio medica de humoribus . . . Viennae, Typis Joannis Christophori Cosmerovii [1680]

[34] p.   20 cm.   **[6495]**

Diss.—Vienna (A. F. Kremer, *respondent*)

KREPS, PETER [*fl.* 1678] *respondent. See* FRANCK VON FRANCKENAU, G., *praeses.* Satyrae medicae continuatio XV. de vitro et ὑαλοφαγοις von Glas-Frässern. 1678.

KRESS, SEBASTIAN [*fl.* 1682] *respondent. See* WINCKLER, F. C., *praeses.* Dissertatio inauguralis medica de plica. 1682.

KRETZSCHMAR, GOTTFRIED [*fl.* 1674] *respondent. See* MÜLLER, J. [*fl.* 1672–1679] *praeses.* Disputatio physica quaestionem utrum ex medulla spinae in homine mortuo serpens nascatur examinans. 1674.

KREUTTER, JOHANN ANDREAS [*fl.* 1657] *respondent. See* AMMANN, P., *praeses.* Quaestio physica. 1657.

KROKERIUS, PAUL. *See* CROQUERUS, Paulus [*fl.* 1616–1643]

KROKIER, PAWEL. *See* CROQUERUS, Paulus [*fl.* 1616–1643]

KRONLAND, JOHANN MARCUS MARCI. *See* MARCI VON KRONLAND, Johannes Marcus [1595–1667]

KRÜGENER, MICHAEL. *See* CRÜGENER, Michael [*fl.* 1648–1679]

KRÜGER, BARTHOLD. *See* KRUGER, Barthold [*b.* 1653]

KRÜGER, LEONHARD [*fl.* 1629–1638] *respondent. See* CONRING, H., *praeses.* Disputatio medica de scorbuto. 1671.

KRUGER, BARTHOLD [*b.* 1653] Anatomicus curiosus θεοδίδακτος; hoc est, Methodus secandi cadavera Hippocratica democritaea . . . Brunopoli, Literis Henrici Kesleri, 1700.

[8], 60, [8] p.   21 cm.   **[6497]**

—*respondent. See* FASCH, A. H., *praeses.* Dissertatio inauguralis medica de arthritide vaga scorbutica. 1683.

—*See* WEDEL, G. W. Decanus Facultatis Medicae Georgius Wolffgangus Wedelius . . . lectori benevolo S. P. D. 1683.

KRYT, HERPERT DE [*fl.* 1667] *respondent.* Disputatio medica inauguralis, de suppressione mensium . . . Ultrajecti, Ex officina Antonii Smytegelt, 1667.

[8] p. 20 cm. [6498]
Diss.—Utrecht.

KÜCHLER, ELIAS [*fl.* 1692] *respondent.* Dissertatio inauguralis medica, de cura palliativa . . . Erfordiae, Typis Joh. Henr. Groshii [1692]

32 p. 19 cm. [6499]
Diss.—Erfurt.

—*See* PETERMANN, A., *praeses.* De medicamentis alvum laxantibus. 1692.

KÜFFER, JOHANN [*fl.* 1606-1625] *respondent. See* STUPANUS, J. N., *praeses.* De morbo subitaneo. 1606.

KUEFFER, JOHANN [*fl.* 1637-1640] *respondent.* Disputatio medica inauguralis de erysipelate . . . Argentorati, Typis Johannis Reppii, 1640.

[21] p. 19 cm. [6500]
Diss.—Strasbourg.

—*See* SEBISCH, M. [1578-1674?] *praeses.* Examinis vulnerum partium dissimilarium pars I[-IV & ultima] 1636 [i.e. 1637]

KÜFFLER, JOHANN SIBERT [*fl.* 1616] *respondent. See* STUPANUS, E., *praeses.* Disputationum menstruarum medicarum exercitatio IIX. & ultima de virilium affectibus cognoscendis. 1616.

KÜHN, JOHANNES MICHAEL [*fl.* 1659] *respondent.* Disputatio medica inauguralis, de fluxu mensium nimio . . . Lugduni Batavorum, Apud Johannem Elsevirium, 1659.

[16] p. 19 cm. [6501]

KÜHN, LUCAS [*fl.* 1693] *respondent. See* VEHR, I., *praeses.* Diatriben inauguralem de minis medicis . . . offert L. K. 1693.

KUENBURG, MAXIMILIAN GANDOLPH. *See* GANDOLF, Maximilian, *count, Cardinal, Prince-Archbishop of Salzburg* [*d.* 1687]

KÜNNE, HEINRICH CHRISTOPH [*fl.* 1679] *respondent. See* RIVINUS, A. Q., *praeses.* Dissertatio medica de dyspepsia. 1679.

KÜRSNER, CHRISTIAN [*fl.* 1683-1685] *respondent. See* WALDSCHMIDT, J. J., *praeses.* Disputatio decima tertia de phthisi et empyemate. 1683 [and] Disputatio physica de causa partus monstrosi nuperrime nati. 1684 [and] Dissertatio medica de potu theae. 1685 [and] Dissertatio physica de primaevo et hodierno telluris statu. 1684.

KÜSTER, JOHANN [1614 *or* 15-1685] Affectuum totius corporis humani praecipuorum theoria et praxis, tabulis exhibitae. Non solum studiosis, operam medicinae daturis; sed & omnibus literatis ope medici indigentibus, maximae utilitati futuris. Accessit autoris . . . memoriae Caroli Gustavi, regis Sueciae . . . morbi & obitus relatio medica authore Johanne Costero . . . Francofurti, Apud Balthasar. Christoph. Wustium, sumptibus Ulrici Wetsteini, 1664.

[8], 399 p.; 16 p. 20 cm. [6502]

KUHL, JOHANN, *of Marburg, respondent.* Theses de risu, fletu, et locutione. *In* Goclenius, R. [1547-1628] Physiologia crepitus ventris. 1607.

KUHNE, JOHANNES [*fl.* 1663] *respondent.* Disputatio medica inauguralis, de phrenitide . . . Trajecti ad Rhenum, Ex officina Lucae de Vries, 1663.

[16] p. 20 cm. [6503]
Diss.—Utrecht.

KUNAD, ANDREAS [1602-1662] *praeses.* Disputatio inauguralis de confessione Petri et eam secuta Christi responsione, ex Matth. XVI, 13-19 adornata . . . defendet . . . D. IV Octobris, anno M DC LXII . . . Wittenbergae, Typis Christiani Schrödteri, 1680.

[48] p. 20 cm. [6504]
Diss.—Wittenberg, 1662 (J. C. Neander, *respondent*)

KUNAD, THEODOR [*fl.* 1681] *respondent. See* LOSS, J., *praeses.* Disputationem inauguralem erotomaniae seu amoris insani, theoriam & praxin pertractantem . . . submittit . . . T. K. 1681.

KUNCKEL, JOHANN [1630?-1703] Chymische Anmerckungen . . . darinn gehandelt wird von denen Principiis chymicis, Salibus Acidis und Alkalibus, fixis und volatilibus, in denen dreyen Regnis, minerali, vegetabili und animali; wie auch vom Geruch und Farben, &c. Mit Anhang einer chymischen Brille contra non-entia chym. . . . Wittenberg, In Verlegung Job Wilhelm Fincelii seel. Erben, druckts Christian Schrödter, 1677.

[7], 192 p. 15 cm. [6505]

Bound with Rummel, J. P. Medicina spagyrica. 1648.

—Chymischer Probier-Stein, de acido & urinoso, sale calid. & frigid. contra Herrn. Doct. Voigts, Spirit. vini vindicatum, an die weltberühmte Königl. Societät in England, als hierüber erbätene hohe Richter. Worbey angefüget die Epistola contra Spir. vini sine acido, so an Herrn D. Voigten abgelassen. Berlin, In Verlegung Rupert Völckers, 1686.

[252 +] p. 16 cm. [6506]

Signatures:) (8, A-M8, N6, A-B8.

Imperfect: C8, D7 at end wanting. Cf. Ferguson (A)

—Nützliche Observationes oder Anmerckungen, von der fixen und flüchtigen Saltzen, Auro und Argento Potabili, Spiritu Mundi und dergleichen . . . Hamburg, Auff Gottfried Schultzens Kosten, 1676.

[102] p. 17 cm. [6507]

KUNGLIGA COLLEGIUM MEDICUM, STOCKHOLM. See COLLEGIUM MEDICUM, Stockholm.

KUNRATH, KONRAD. See KHUNRATH, Konrad [*fl.* 1594–1604]

KUNTZ, JOHANN JAKOB [*fl.* 1683] *respondent.* Disputatio inauguralis medica de peste . . . Gissae, Ex Chalcographeo Acad. Kargeriano, 1683.

24 p. 19 cm. [6508]

Diss.—Giessen.

KUPITZ, ERDMANN [1668–1699] *respondent.* Dissertatio medica inauguralis de fluore albo . . . Altdorfii Noricorum, Typis Henrici Meyeri [1690]

20 p. 20 cm. [6509]

Diss. — Altdorf.

—See BRUNO, J. P., *praeses.* Αιγυογραφια. 1688.

KUPIZIUS, ERDMANNUS. See KUPITZ, Erdmann [1668–1699]

KUPPERHUSIUS, ANDREAS EPISCOPUS. See EPISCOPUS, Andreas [*fl.* 1626]

KURANUS. See KIRANUS, *King of Persia.*

KURSNER, CHRISTIAN [*fl.* 1684–1687] *respondent.* Diatriba inauguralis de purgantium de foro medico

proscriptione . . . Marburgi Cattorum, Typis Johannis Jodoci Kürsneri [1687]

32 p. 19 cm. [6510]

Diss. — Marburg.

KURTZ-VERFASTES Land-und Haus-Artzney-Büchlein, in welchem allerhand heilsame, an vielen Personen versucht- und bewehrt-befundene Artzney-Mittel . . . vorgestellet . . . Jetzo ganz neu heraus gegeben [n. p., 16–?]

192, [32] p. 16 cm. [6511]

Bound with Neu-vermehrtes . . . Aderlass-Büchlein. Nürnberg [ca. 1670]

KURTZE Beschreibung des heylsamen . . . Bronnens der Sahlbronnen. *See* THURNEISSER ZUM THURN, L. Zehen Bücher von kalten . . . Wassern. 1612.

KURTZE medicinalische Nachricht . . . wie sich die Gesunden zur Zeit der Sterbens-Lufft praeserviren . . . die Krancken aber curirt . . . werden sollen. Trier, Christoph Willhelm Reulandt, 1666.

60 p. 16 cm. [6512]

"Nothwendige Ordnung etc. welche auff gnädigste Verwillig- und Genehmhaltung ihrer churfürstl. Gnaden etc. Statthalter, Burgermeister, Scheffen, und Rath der Statt Trier, wegen der sterbender Lufft vorsorgentlich auffgerichtet . . .": p. 49–60.

KURTZE, nohtwendige Ordnung und Raht. 1609. *See* JULIUS UNIVERSITÄT, Helmstedt. Medizinische Fakultät.

KURTZE, und eigentliche Beschreibung, dess Ursprungs, Krafft, Nutzbarkeit unnd Gebrauchs dess . . . warmen Bads, zü Baden im Ergöuw . . . [n. p.] 1619.

broadside. 70 x 34 cm. [6513]

KURTZER Anhang, bestehend in einigen anatomischen Fragen, uber diejenigen Theile des menschlichen Cörpers, welche einem Chirurgo zu wissen . . . nöthig vorfallen . . . Nürnberg, In Verlegung Johann Ziegers und Georg Lehmanns, 1700.

[1], 154 p. plates. 17 cm. [6514]

—[The same.] *In* Jüngken, J. H. Chirurgia manualis. 1700.

KURTZER Bericht: der fürstlichen Württembergischen Hoff Medicorum. 1608. *See* GABELKOVER, O.

KURTZER Bericht; oder, Extract. 1680. *See* GLOGAU (FÜRSTENTUM) ORDINANCES, local laws, etc.

KURTZER Bericht und Ordnung. 1626. *See* UNIVERSITÄT WITTENBERG. Medizinische Fakultät.

KURTZER Bericht, wie die Artzneyen in der Apotheken angeordnet. 1607. *See* Universität Wittenberg. Medizinische Fakultät.

KURTZER Bericht, wie man sich in werender Pestilentz verwahren ... soll. 1629. *See* LÜBECK. Ordinances, local laws, etc.

KURTZER Bericht, wie sich die Gemain allhie, in Sterbens Läuffen mit ringen Mitteln ... verwahren solle. Augspurg, Gedruckt durch Andream Aperger, 1628.

[16] p. 16 cm. [6515]

Imperfect: margins trimmed.

Ein KURTZER Bericht, wie Terra Sigillata nützlich kan gebrauchet werden. [n. p.] 1602.

[7] p. 19 cm. [6516]

KURTZER, doch gründlicher Rath-und Unterricht. 1680. *See* BRUNSWICK (Duchy)

KURTZER, doch gründtlicher Unterricht wie man sich ... vor der Pestilentz bewahren sol. 1625. *See* Müller, J. [*fl.* 1611]

KURTZER, sehr nothwendig-und treuhertziger Bericht. 1679, 1680. *See* Kollegium der Aerzte, Regensburg.

KURTZER und einfältiger Bericht. *See* HALBERSTÄDTISCHES PEST-BEDENCKEN. 1680.

KURTZER Underricht in Sterbensläuffen. So wol für krancke Inficirte, als andere Personen ... mit angehenckter Praeservatif und nützlicher Vorsehung vor der Pestilentz. Durch dess ... Herrn Maximiliani Pfaltzgrafen bey Rhein ... Leib Medicos gestellt und auff newes recognosciert. Mit angehenckter ... Information ... durch Johann Fabern ...

Cölln, Gedruckt durch Petrum Cholinum, 1622.

153, [5] p. 17 cm. [6517]

Includes the text of Johann Faber's Kurtzer und nothwendiger Underricht.

KURTZER Unterricht vom Blut- oder Hoffgang. 1652. *See* UNIVERSITAS REGIA HAFNIENSIS. Facultas medica.

KURTZER Unterricht von Allerhandtmitteln, und Artzney. 1608. *See* HOHENLOHE (Grafschaft)

KURTZER, Unterricht von der jetzo herumbgehenden, und sich näher und näher annahenden ansteckenden Seuche und Pestilentz ... Aus hochfürstl. ... Verordnung in Marggraffthum Nieder Lausitz publiciret ... Berlin und Cölln, Rupertus Völcker, 1680.

[24] p. 14 cm. [6518]

KURTZER Unterricht, wie bey itzo herumb gehenden Fiebern, Gesunde und Krancke sich verhalten sollen, so wohl zur Praeservation als Curation dienlich ... Altenburg, Gedruckt von Gottfried Richtern, 1676.

[35] p. 20 cm. [6519]

KURTZER Unterricht, wie man sich für der giftigen anklebenden Seuche der Pestilentz ... bewahren ... solle. 1680. *See* BRUNSWICK (Duchy)

KUS, GEORG [*fl.* 1680-1682] *respondent. See* BORCH, O., *praeses.* Disputatio medica inauguralis de ascite. 1682.

—, *tr. See* BORCH, O. [Docimastice metallica. German.] 1680.

KUYL, NICOLAAS [*fl.* 1659] *respondent.* Disputatio medica inauguralis de arthritide ... Lugduni Batavorum, Ex officina Petri Leffen, 1659.

[8] p. 24 cm. [6520]

Diss. — Leyden.

KYPER, ALBERT. *See* KIJPER, Albert [1605?-1655]

KYRANUS. *See* KIRANUS, *King of Persia.*

L

L****.* *See* LUFNEU, Jacques [*fl.* 1697]

L., A. V., *Med. Doct. See* DISSERTATIO PHYSICO-MEDICA, DE FEBRIBUS. 1688.

L., B. *See* LEEMANN, Burkhard [1531-1613]

L., I. A. S., *ed. See* HYGIEIA. 1628; REGIMEN SANITATIS SALERNITANUM. MEDICINA SALERNITANA.

1605, 1611, 1612, 1622, 1624, 1628, 1638; Regimen sanitatis Salernitanum. Schola Salernitana. 1649, 1657, 1667, 1683.

L., J., *Gent. See* Lancaster, John [*fl. ca.* 1682]

L., J. H. D. M. *See* H., J., D. M. L.

L., L. M. S. *See* Schmuck, Martin [*d.* 1640?]

L., M. *See* Lister, Martin [1638?-1712]

L., M. B. *See* Linand, Barthélemy [*fl.* 1696-1697]

L., M. B. *See* Medicina animi in usum melancholicorum. 1685.

L., P. *See* Labbé, Pierre [1596-1678]

L., T. *See* Lodge, Thomas [1558?-1625]

L. L. M. C. *See* C., L. L. M.

L. N. M. E. M. *See* Moltke, Levin Nicolaus von [*d.* 1663]

LAAZ, Johann von [*fl.* 15th cent.] Tractatus . . . de lapide philosophorum Joannis de Lasnioro . . . 579-584 p., vol. 4. plate. 20 cm. (*In* Zetzner, Lazarus, *ed.* Theatrum chemicum. Argentorati, 1659-61) [6521]
Caption title.

LABACH, Leopold Albert [*b.* 1675] *respondent. See* Stahl, G. E., *praeses.* Dissertatio inauguralis medica de lapide manati. 1699 [and] Propempticon inaugurale de cornu cervi deciduo. 1699.

LABBÉ, P. L. *See* Labbé, Pierre [1596-1678]

LABBÉ, P. P. *See* Labbé, Pierre [1596-1678]

LABBE, Philippe [1607-1667] Bibliotheca bibliothecarum curis secundis auctior. Accedit Bibliotheca nummaria in duas partes tributa. I. De antiquis numismatibus. II. De monetis, ponderibus & mensuris. Cum Mantissa antiquariae supellectilis ex annulis, sigillis, gemmis, lapidibus, statuis, obeliscis, inscriptionibus, ritibus, similibusque, romanae praesertim antiquitatis monimentis collecta. . . . Ed. 2 auct., & meliori ordine disposita. Rothomagi, excudebat Thomas Maurry, impensis Ludovici Billaine, 1672.
16, 398 p. 18 cm. [6522]

LABBÉ, Pierre [1596-1678] Elogium funebre . . . domini D. Francisci Vautier. In Reflexions. 1652.

LA BELLIÈRE, Claude de, *sieur de la Nicolle* [*fl.* 1663-1664] La physionomie raisonnée; ou, Secret curieux, pour connoître les inclinations de chacun par les regles naturelles . . . Paris, Edme Couterot, 1664.
[24], 235, [50] p. 15 cm. [6523]

—[Italian tr.] La fisonomia con ragionamenti; ò, Lo specchio per vedere le passioni di ciascheduno . . . Parigi, Edmondo Couterot, 1664.
[24], 243, [55] p. 15 cm. [6524]

LA BESSÉE, Écuyer de duc de Bavière. *See* Solleysel, Jacques de [1617-1680]

LABIN, Heinrich [*fl.* 1700] *respondent. See* Klausing, H., *praeses.* Prima de motu corporum naturalium disputatio. 1700.

LA BOUTHIÈRE, George de [16th cent.] *tr. See* Aristoteles. Les problemes d'Aristote. 1618; 1683.

LA BREULLIE, Jean Louis de. Traicté de la contagion et de ses remedes . . . Geneve, Jaques de la Piere, 1641.
109 p. 15 cm. [6525]

LA BROSSE, Guy de [1586?-1641] De la nature, vertu, et utilité des plantes. Divisé an cinq livres . . . Paris, Rollin Baragnes, 1628.
[31], 849, [3] p. 18 cm. [6526]
Added engraved title page.
"Dessein d'un jardin royal pour la culture des plantes medicinales a Paris" (p. 681-828) has special title page.

—Description du Jardin royal des plantes medecinales, estably par le Roy Louis le Juste, à Paris. Contenant le catalogue des plantes qui y sont de present cultivées . . . Paris, 1636.
107, [1] p. plates. 23 cm. [6527]

LABROSSE, Joseph de. *See* Angelus de Sanctu Josepho, *Father* [1636-1697]

LA BRUNE, Jean de [*b. ca.* 1660] Methode que l'on pratique a l'hostel des Invalides pour guerir les soldats de la verolle [Paris, François Muguet, *ca.* 1685]
10, [4] p. 23 cm. [6528]
Caption title.

[**LA CALMETTE,** François de, *fl.* 1684] Riverius reformatus; sive, Praxis medica, methodo Riverianae non absimili . . . conscripta. Accesserunt Tractatus de morbis mulierum; de affectibus articulorum; de peste, & de febribus. Genevae, Apud Samuelem de Tournes, 1688.

[8], 529 (i.e. 527) p. 19 cm.   [6529]

Contents. — Liber primus [de morbis abdominis] — Liber secundus de morbis capitis et thoracis. — Liber tertius de morbis mulierum. — Tractatus de affectibus articulorum. — Tractatus de peste. — Tractatus de febribus.

—[The same.] ... Ed. priori Genevensi correctior: selectorum remediorum formulis: tum De morbis venereis tractatu: & Riverii Arcanis auctior. Lugduni, Apud Joannem Certe, 1690.

[16], 631 p. 18 cm.   [6530]

—[The same.] ... Ed. novissima priori multo accuratior; notis practicis singulis capitibus annexis, & novis aliquot ... tractatibus auctior. Genevae, Apud fratres de Tournes, 1696.

[12], 680 (i.e. 670) p. 18 cm.   [6531]

LA CHAMBRE, MARIN CUREAU DE. *See* CUREAU DE LA CHAMBRE, Marin [1593 *or* 4-1669]

LA CHARRIÈRE, JOSEPH DE [17th-18th cent.] Traité des operations de chirurgie: contenant leurs causes ... leurs signes, leurs simptomes & leur explication ... Et une Idée generale des playes ... Paris, Daniel Horthemees, 1690.

[16], 395, [1] p. 16 cm.   [6532]

Imperfect: p. 9-10 mutilated.
With this is bound Leclerc, C. G. L'ecole du chirurgien, 1684.

—[The same.] Nouvelles operations de chirurgie ... Paris, Daniel Horthemeis, 1692.

[23], 331 p. front. 14 cm.   [6533]

—[The same.] Traité des operations de chirurgie ... Paris, 1693.

[12], 406 p. 16 cm.   [6534]

—[The same.] ... 2. éd. corr. & augm. par l'auteur. Lyon, Antoine Perisse, 1699.

[8], 374, [2] p. 16 cm.   [6535]

—[English tr.] A treatise of chirurgical operations, after the newest, and most exact method founded on the structure of the parts ... To which is annex'd A general idea of wounds ... Translated into English by R. B. London, Dan. Brown, 1695.

[10], 345, [7] p. 16 cm.   [6536]

—[Italian tr.] *In* Guy de Chauliac. In maestro in chirurgia. 1697.

—*See* [Verduc, J. B.] Nouvelle methode d'operations de chirurgie. 1693.

LA CHASTRE, RENÉ DE. Le prototype ou tres parfait et analogique exemplaire de l'art chimicque a la phisique ou philosophie de la science naturelle. Contenant les causes principes & demonstrations scientifique de la certitude dudit art ... Paris, Jean Anthoine Joallin, 1620.

[8], 136, [14] p. 16 cm.   [6537]

LA CHÂTRE, RENÉ DE. *See* LA CHASTRE, René de.

LA CHAUME, *sieur de* [*fl.* 1679] Traité de medecine contenant la parfaite connoissance de l'homme, la sanguification au coeur, la circulation du sang, les causes de toutes sortes de fiévres ... Auxerre, François Garnier, 1679.

xv, [1], 288 p. 17 cm.   [6538]

Imperfect: p. 287-288 wanting; wormholes on p. 19-28.

—[The same.] ... Auxerre et Paris, Sebastien Cramoisy, 1680.

[xvi], 288 p. 17 cm.   [6539]

Errata: p. 287-288.
A reissue of the 1679 edition with new title page and p. 286 reset.

LACHMUND, FRIEDRICH [1635-1676] De ave Diomedea dissertatio, cum vera ejus effigie aeri incisa ... Amstelodami, Apud Andream Frisium, 1674.

52, [6] p. plates. 14 cm.   [6540]

Bound with Redi, F. Experimenta circa res diversas naturales. 1675.

—[The same.] *In* Redi, F. Opusculorum pars prior. 1685-1686 [v. 1 1686]

LA COLOMBIÈRE, MARC VULSON DE. *See* VULSON DE LA COLOMBIÈRE, Marc [*d.* 1658]

LA COUR, *sieur de, pseud. See* PINSONNAT, F.

LA COURVÉE, JEAN CLAUDE DE [*ca.* 1615-*ca.* 1664] De nutritione foetus in utero paradoxa ... Dantisci, Sumptibus Georgii Försteri, 1655.

[21], 254 p. 21 cm.   [6541]

Engraved title page.

—Discours sur la sortie des dens aux petits enfans, de la precaution, & des remedes, que l'on y peut apporter ... Varsaviae, Pierre Elert, 1651.

[8], 148, [10] p. 20 cm.   [6542]

—Ostentum; seu, Historia mirabilis trium ferramentorum notandae longitudinis ex insanientis dorso, & abdomine extractorum, qui ante menses decem ea voraverat . . . Parisiis, Apud Guilielmum Sassier, 1648.

36 p. 17 cm. [6543]

Bound with Wendelin, G. Pluvia purpurea Bruxellensis. 1647.

LA CROSE, JEAN DE. *See* CORNAND DE LA CROSE, Jean de [*d. ca.* 1705]

LACROZE, JEAN CORNAND DE. *See* CORNAND DE LA CROSE, Jean de [*d. ca.* 1705]

[LACTANTIUS, LUCIUS CAECILIUS FIRMIANUS] Phoenix atropicus de morte redux. Der wiederumb frischbelebte gebenedeyte philosophische Adrop, aus dem Grabe der Vergessenheit hervorgesucht . . . Aus arabisch-chaldaeisch-frantzösich- und lateinischer in hochteutscher Zungen beseelet und vorgestellet. [n. p.] 1681.

88 p. 14 cm. [6544]

LACUNA, ANDREAS. *See* LAGUNA, Andrés de [*d.* 1560]

LACY, NATHAN [*fl.* 1690–1697] Ad . . . principem Joannem Ernestum archiepiscopum Salisburgensem . . . comitem de Thunn . . . de . . . comitis Ferdinandi Caroli de Thunn . . . igneis tibialibus per Nathan Lacy . . . [Campidonum] Per Joannem Mayr, 1697.

36 p. 15 cm. [6545]

—De podagra . . . Venetiis, Apud Andream Poleti, 1692.

[10], 97 p. front. 19 cm. [6546]

—, *tr. See* LÉMERY, N. Corso di chimica. 1695, 1699, 1700.

LADEY, MARTIN [*fl.* 1678] *respondent. See* MEIBOM, H., *praes.* Disputatio medica inauguralis de febribus intermittentibus epidemicis. 1678.

LAELIUS, LUCIUS, *pseud. See* RECALCHI, Giulio [1552–1645]

LAERTIUS, DIOGENES. *See* DIOGENES LAERTIUS.

LAET, JOANNES DE [1593–1649] *ed. See* PISO, W. Historia naturalis Brasiliae. 1648; PLINIUS SECUNDUS, C. Historiae naturalis libri XXXVII. 1635.

LA FAUEUR. *See* MEBER, J. C. Anchora sauciatorum. 1687.

LA FIN, CHARLES DE. Sermo mirabilis; or, The silent language. Whereby one may learn . . . how to impart his mind to his mistress, or his friend, in any language . . . without the least noise, word or voice . . . The 3d ed., with additions. London, John Salusbury, 1696.

[1], 14 p. front., plates. 18 cm. [6547]

LA FONT, CHARLES DE [*d.* 1707] Dissertatio medica, de hydrope tympanite ubi tum genuinae ipsius causae ex recentiorum principiis deductae declarantur tum vera curandi methodus ex iisdem principiis desumpta, & experientiis innixa proponitur . . . Genevae, Sumptibus J. A. Chouët & D. Ritteri, 1697.

[16], 280, [4] p. 16 cm. [6548]

—Dissertationes duae medicae de veneno pestilenti, in quarum priori agitur de veneni pestilentis natura et causis . . . ubi etiam D. D. Thomae Willisii de veneni pestilentis natura opinio examinatur . . . In altera agitur de veneni pestilentis curatione . . . Avenione Ex typographia Petri Offray, 1670.

[8], 205, [3] p. 15 cm. [6549]

—[The same.] . . . Amstelodami, Apud Gerbrandum Schagen, 1671.

165, [9] p. 14 cm. [6550]

LA FONTAINE, JEAN DE [*b.* 1381] *See* JEAN DE LA FONTAINE [*b.* 1381]

LA FONTAINE, JEAN DE [1621–1695] Poëme du quinquina, et autres ouvrages en vers . . . Paris, Denis Thierry et Claude Barbin, 1682.

[4], 242 p. 17 cm. [6551]

LA FORGE, LOUIS DE [1632–1666] Traitté de l'esprit de l'homme, de ses facultez et fonctions, et de son union avec le corps. Suivant les principes de René Descartes . . . Paris, Michel Bobin & Nicolas Le Gras, 1666.

[56], 453, [2] p. 24 cm. [6552]

—[The same.] . . . Amsterdam, Abraham Wolfgang [1670]

[64], 462, [1] p. illus. 14 cm. [6553]

Errata: p. [1] at end.
Imprint supplied from Rahir, no. 2437 and Willems, no. 1834.

—[Latin tr.] Tractatus de mente humana, ejus facultatibus & functionibus, nec non de ejusdem unione cum corpore, secundum principia Renati Descartes ... Amstelodami, Apud Danielem Elzevirium, 1669.

[36], 224 p. illus. 22 cm. **[6554]**

Translated by Flayder. Cf. A. Chassagne. Louis De La Forge. Angers, 1938.

—[The same.] ... Bremae, Literis Arnoldi & Johannis Wesselii, prostant apud Johannem Wesselium, 1673.

[16], 224, [6] p. 20 cm. **[6555]**

—[The same.] ... Emendatus et auctus ... per J[ohann] F[lender] Amstelodami, Ex Typographia Blaviana, 1688.

[22], 241, [6] p. illus. 21 cm. **[6556]**

LA FORGE, LOUIS DE [1632–1666] *See* DESCARTES, R. L'homme ... et un traitté De la formation du foetus. 1664, 1677, 1680 [and] Opera philosophica. 1692 [and] Tractatus De homine, et De formatione foetus. 1677, 1686, 1692; [Dutch tr.] 1695.

LA FRAMBOISIÈRE, NICOLAS ABRAHAM DE. Les oeuvres ... Paris, Michael Sonnius, 1613.

[52], 1448 (i.e. 1442), [144] p. port. 23 cm. **[6557]**

Imperfect: portrait wanting, upper margins trimmed.

Includes: —La principauté. —Le gouvernement. —Les loix. —Les ordonnances. —La couronne. —Frambesariana gratiarum actio.

—Another issue, with imprint: Paris, Marc Orry, 1613. **[6558]**

Imperfect: upper margins trimmed.

—Les oeuvres ... oú sont ... descrites l'histoire du monde, la medicine, la chirurgie & la pharmacie, pour la conservation de la santé, & la guerison des maladies internes & externes ... Derniere ed. rev. corr. & augm. ... par l'autheur d'un VIII. tome. Lyon, Jean-Antoine Huguetan, 1644.

[40], 979, [82] p. 37 cm. **[6559]**

Contents as in the 1613 edition with the addition of Les clefs de la principauté de l'homme, Scholae medicae, and Advis ... pour la conservation de la santé.

—[The same.] ... Lyon, Pierre Compagnon, & Robert Taillandier, 1669.

[16], 977 (i.e. 979), [82] p. 38 cm. **[6560]**

Contents as in the 1644 edition.

—Another issue, with imprint: Lyon, Jean Certe, 1669. **[6561]**

Half title wanting?

—Opera medica. Quibus continentur I. Canones et consultationes medicinales ... II. Canones chirurgici ... III. Apologia pro veritate & innocentia medicamentorum chymicorum adversus criminatores. IV. Laurea academica Frambesariana. V. De praeservatione pestis. Francofurti, Apud Guilielmum Fitzerum, 1629.

[16], 12, 642, [6] p. 21 cm. **[6562]**

". . . De pestis curatione & praecautione libellus. Ed. ult. Francofurti, Apud Matthaeum Kempffer, impensis Wilhelmi Fitzerii, 1629" (12 p.) has special title page.

—Ad libros canonum medicinalium appendix. De arthritide. Parisiis, Apud Michaelem Sonnium, 1619.

95 p. 18 cm. **[6563]**

". . . Appendix [II] De medendis arthriticis" (p. [53]–80) has special title page.

—Canones et consultationes medicinales. Quibus recta medicinae faciendae via & ratio, praeceptis & exemplis perspicue demonstratur, Ed. ult. ab authore recognita & aucta. Parisiis, Apud Michaelem Sonnium, 1619.

[15], 162 (i.e. 164), [4] ll.; [8], 277, [3] p. port. 18 cm. **[6564]**

Part [1] has special title page: Canonum medicinalium libri tres. Part [2] has special title page: Consultationum medicinalium libri tres.

—De pestis curatione & praecautione libellus. Ed. ult. Parisiis, Apud Michaelem Sonnium, 1619.

[4], 12 p. 18 cm. **[6565]**

—L'estat des vertus de l'ame. *In* Marque, J. de. Methodique introduction a la chirurgie. 1680.

—Le gouvernement necessaire a chacun pour vivre longuement en santé. Avec Le gouvernement requis en l'usage des eaux minerals ... pour la guerison des maladies rebelles ... 3. ed. rev. & reformée par l'autheur. Paris, Marc Orry, 1608.

[16], 379, [17] p. port. 18 cm. **[6566]**

Imperfect: wormholes on p. 187–284.

—Idaea Frambesarianae academiae, in qua celebrentur, scholae artium ad humanitatem excolendam pertinentium, dialecticae, rethoricae, grammaticae. Scholae philosophicae cum ethicae ... tum physicae ... Scholae medicae ... Parisiis, Apud Michaelem Sonnium, 1619.

[16] p.   18 cm.   [**6567**]

—Les loix de medecine, pour proceder methodiquement a la guarison des maladies ... Paris, Michel Sonnius, 1608.

[32], 1034, [84] p.   port.   19 cm.   [**6568**]

Imperfect: p. 115-126, and sig. 4A8 (blank?) wanting. Wormholes on p. 71-72 and p. 747-912.

—Ordonnances sur la composition des medicamens, que les apothicaires doivent dispenser en leurs boutiques, reformees et illustrees ... Paris, Rolin Thierry, & Eustache Foucault, 1603.

192 ll.   17 cm.   [**6569**]

—Scholae medicae, ad canditatorum [sic] examen pro laurea impetranda subeundum. Quibus accessit Ambrosiopoea, eodem autore. Lugduni Batavorum, Ex officina Joannis Maire, 1628.

[11], 275 p.   13 cm.   [**6570**]

"... Ambrosiopoea, in qua elegantes medicamentorum praeparationes ... praescribuntur": p. [193]-275 has special title page.

—Scholae medicae, multo quam antehac ampliores ac locupletiores. In quibus de medicinae theoria & praxi acriter disputatur. Ad candidatorum examen pro laurea impetranda subeundum. Ed. 6 ... emend. ... auct., partim nova quaestionum variarum passim insertarum accessione partim examine quadruplici: Primo super anatomica administratione ... Secundo super actionibus, excrementis & habitu corporis ... Tertio super medicamentorum praeparandorum methodo duplici ... Quarto super symptomaton febres comitantium curatione ... Parisiis, Apud Joannem Jost, 1636.

759, [5] p.   15 cm.   [**6571**]

—Scholae medicae, ad candidatorum examen pro laurea impetranda subeundum. Huic editioni accessit, Examen practicum de recta curandarum febrium ratione, et Ambrosiopoea, eodem autore. Lugduni Batavorum, Ex officina Joannis Maire, 1640.

[11], 275 p.; 221, [14] p.   13 cm.   [**6572**]

"Ambrosiopoea ..." (p. [193]-275) and "Examen practicum ..." (part [2]) have special title pages.

—[The same.] ... Lugduni Batavorum, Ex officina Joannis Maire, 1647.

[12], 276 p.; 221, [14] p.   14 cm.   [**6573**]

Different setting of type.

LAGNEAU, DAVID [*ca.* 1590-1659] Harmonia seu consensus philosophorum chemicorum ...

718-804 p., vol. 4.   plate.   20 cm.   (*In* Zetzner, Lazarus, *ed.* Theatrum chemicum. Argentorati, 1659-61)   [**6574**]

Caption title.

—Traicté pour la conservation de la santé et sur la saignee de ce temps ... avec autres traictez ... *See* selon la doctrine des anciens medecins grecs, arabes, latins & françois. Augmenté d'un traicté de Galien, de l'alicement des malades. Apologie contre Jean Terud ... Examen du livre intitulé Medecin charitable. Traicté de la physiognomie, avec les figures propres, qui sont au nombre de 53 ... 3. ed. fort augm. ... Paris, Mathurin Henault, 1650.

[17], 834, [17] p.   front. (port.), illus., table.   24 cm.   [**6575**]

"Traitté de Galien, de l'alicement des malades" (p. 536-558) is a French translation of Imbrasius, of Ephesus De decubitu infirmorum ex mathematica scientia, translated by Justus Lagneau.
"Apologie contre Jean Fernel [et contre Terud]": p. 566-627.
"Examen du livre intitule medecin charitable a Paris [by Philbert Guibert]": p. 628-712.
"Responce faite a monsieur L'Aigneau [including the letter of Lagneau]": p. 716-720.

—, *tr. See* BASILIUS VALENTINUS. Les douze clefs de philosophie. 1660.

LAGNEAU, JUSTUS [*fl.* 17th cent.] *tr. See* LAGNEAU, D. Traicté pour la conservation de la santé. 1650.

LAGNEUS, DAVID. *See* LAGNEAU, David [*ca.* 1590-1659]

LA GRUE, JOANNES JOACHIMUS. *See* GRUE, Johann Joachim la [*fl.* 1682]

LA GRUE, PHILIPPE [17th cent.] *tr. See* MASSARD, J. Verscheide verhandelingen raakende de panacéen. 1687; SANTORIO, S. De ontdekte doorwaasseming des menschen lichaams. 1684.

LA GRUE, THOMAS [*fl.* 1661] *respondent.* Disputatio medica inauguralis de dysenteria ... Lugduni Batavorum, Ex officina Francisci Hackii, 1661.

[8] p.   19 cm.   [**6576**]

Diss. — Leyden.

LAGUNA, ANDRÉS DE [*d.* 1560] *comp. See* GALENUS. Epitome Galeni. 1604, 1643.

—, *ed.* and *tr. See* DIOSCORIDES, Pedanius, *of Anazarbos.* Acerca de la materia medicinal, y de los venenos mortiferos. 1677, 1695.

—*See* CARDANO, G. Contradicentium medicorum libri duo. 1607.

LAGUS, DANIEL [1618-1678] *praeses.* Disputatio publica de visu ... Regiomonti, Typis Laurentii Segebadii, 1638.

[16] p.   18 cm.   [6577]

Diss. — Königsberg (J. Michaelis, *respondent*)

LA HAYE, DE. *See* LA HAYE, François de [*fl.* 1689-1693]

LA HAYE, FRANÇOIS DE [*fl.* 1689-1693] Le medecin sincere, qui enseigne ... à guerir ... les maladies par des remedes doux, & faciles à composer. Il instruit aussi des vertus des metaux, des plantes, des animaux, & des eaux minerales ... Lyon, Aux dépens de l'auteur, & se vend chez Claude Carteron, 1691.

[33], 758, [58] p.   front. (port.)   18 cm.
[6578]

—[The same.] ... 2. ed. Lyon, Se vend a Paris, chés Marten [sic] Jouvenel et chés l'auteur, 1693.

[33], 758, [58] p.   front. (port.)   20 cm.
[6579]

A reissue of the 1691 edition, with new title page.

—[The same.] ... 2. ed. rev., corr., & augm. Lyon, Se vend a Paris, chez Laurent d'Houry, M.DC.LXCVII [i.e. 1697?]

[33], 758, [55] p.   front. (port.)   20 cm.
[6580]

Imperfect: Errata wanting.
A reissue of the 1691 edition with new title page.

LAHER, JOHANN VON [*fl.* 1670] *respondent.* Disputatio medica inauguralis de renum & vesicae calculo ... Basileae, Typis Jacobi Bertschii [1470] (i.e. 1670)

[35] p.   20 cm.   [6581]
Diss. — Basel.

LAHR, JOHANN VON DER [*fl.* 1662-1663] *respondent. See* CROCIUS, C. F., *praeses.* Disputatio medica de empyemate. 1662.

LAHR, PETER VON DER [*fl.* 1685-1687] *respondent.* Disputatio medica inauguralis de sterilitate ... Lugduni Batavorum, Apud Abrahamum Elzevier, 1687.

[28] p.   22 cm.   [6582]
Diss. — Leyden.

L'AIGNEAU, DAVID. *See* LAGNEAU, David [*ca.* 1590-1659]

L'AIGNEAU, JUSTUS. *See* LAGNEAU, Justus [*fl.* 17th cent.]

LAIRESSE, GÉRARD DE [1640-1711] *illus. See* BIDLOO, G. Anatomia humani corporis. 1685; [Dutch tr.] 1690; COWPER, W. The anatomy of humane bodies. 1698.

LAITAO, MANOEL. *See* LEYTAM, Manoel.

LAKENKOOPER, PIETER [*fl.* 1671] *respondent.* Disputatio medica inauguralis de hydrope ... Lugduni Batavorum, Apud viduam & heredes Joannis Elsevirii, 1671.

[16] p.   23 cm.   [6583]
Diss. — Leyden.

LAKIN, DANIEL [*fl.* 1635] A miraculous cure of the Prusian swallow-knife ... Together with the testimony of the king of Poland, of the truth of this wonderfull cure. Likewise the certificate of ... all the physitians of Leyden. Translated out of the Latin. Whereunto is added a treatise of the possibility of this cure ... As also a survay of the former translation, and censure of their positions ... London, I. Okes, 1642.

[15], 147 p.   front.   20 cm.   [6584]

LALLI, GIOVANNI BATTISTA [1572-1637] Franceide; evero, Del mal francese. Poema giocoso ... Foligno, Appresso Agostino Alterii, 1629.

235, [2] p.   14 cm.   [6585]

LALLI, GRANCHIO. Lettera piacevole di mastro Granchio Lalli [pseud.] ... a mastro Marforio [pseud.] in Roma ... Fiorenza, Accorto Sferzaimperiti, 1640.

[8] p.   22 cm.   [6586]

LAMAND, JEAN [*fl.* 1613-1614] *respondent.* Theses medicae de natura amoris et amantium amentium cura ... Basileae, Typis Joh. Jacobi Genathii, 1614.

[12] p.   20 cm.   [6587]
Diss. — Basel.

LA MARCHE, Marguerite Du Tertre de [1638-1706] Instruction familiere & trés-facile, faite par questions & résponses touchant toutes les choses principales qu'une sage-femme doit sçavoir pour l'exercice de son art. Composée par Marguerite du Tertre, veuve du sieur de La Marche . . . Paris, Ladite veuve de La Marche, 1677.

[11], 144, 31, [7] p.   17 cm.   **[6588]**

—Another issue, with date: 1627 (i.e. 1677).

[11], 144, 66, 31, [7] p.   17 cm.   **[6589]**

"Dissertation sur les accouchemens" (66 p., bound between text and index) has half title.

LA MARTINIÈRE, Pierre Martin de [1634-1690] Le chymique ingenu; ou, L'imposture de la pierre philosophale . . . Paris, L'auteur [not before 1669]

[4], 128 p.   15 cm.   **[6590]**

—[The same.] Tombeau de la folie. Dans lequel se void [sic] les plus fortes raisons que l'on puisse apporter pour faire connoître la realité & la possibilité de la pierre philosophale, & d'autres raisons & experiences qui en font voir l'abus & l'impossibilité . . . Paris, L'auteur [not before 1669]

[12], 128 p.   port.   15 cm.   **[6591]**

The preliminary matter is different, but the text is the same setting of type.

—Le naturaliste charitable, traittant des principes, des parties, des puissances . . . de la nature humaine . . . Avec un abregè des noms, causes, signes & accidens de cinq cens quatre-vingts dix maladies qui affligent le corps humain . . . Paris, L'auteur, 1666.

[13], 468, [11] p.   front. (port.)   16 cm.
          [6592]

—Traitté de la maladie venerienne de ses causes & des accidens provenans du mercure, ou vif argent . . . Paris, L'autheur, 1664.

167, [9] p.   11 cm.   **[6593]**

LAMBERMONTIUS, Ludovicus. Ἀκεστορίας Ἀνθολογια. Εἰτε συμπεροσματα τα ἐ ὁλης ἰατρικης τεχνης συνειλεγμενα. Quibus totius medicinae complexus sub intellectus aspectum ponitur . . . Londini, R. Nortonus, 1654.

[8], 38 p.   illus.   15 cm.   **[6594]**

LAMBERT, Antoine [fl. 1656-1677] Les commentaires . . . divisez en cinq parties . . . Marseille, Claude Garcin, 1662.

[16], 695, [5] p.   23 cm.   **[6595]**

Contents: —[1] Commentaire sur les ulceres malins. —[2] Commentaire sur la carie & corruption des os. —[3] Commentaire sur les fistules en general. —[4] Commentaire sur les fistules en particulier. —[5] Commentaire sur le chapitre general des Apostemes de Guidon. Items [2-3] and [5] have special title pages. The latter has date: 1663.

—[The same.] Les commentaries; ou, Les oeuvres chirurgicales . . . divisez en cinq parties . . . 2. ed. rev., corr. & augm. . . . Lyon, Pierre Compagnon, & Robert Taillandier, 1671.

[20], 692, [4] p.   23 cm.   **[6596]**

—[The same.] . . . 3. ed. rev., corr. & augm. . . . Marseille, Charles Brebion, 1677.

[12], 767, [17] p.   25 cm.   **[6597]**

Commentaire sur la carie, et corruption des os. Contenant plusieurs preceptes & enseignemens necessaires . . . pour la curation de la carie . . . Marseille, Claude Garcin, 1656.

[12], 290, [2] p.   18 cm.   **[6598]**

LAMBERT, Nicolas [fl. 1646] defendant. Factum, pour les sieurs conseillers de la chambre de ville de Nancy appellans de deux sentences des 30. aoust & 25. octobre 1646, en qualité d'administrateurs de l'Hospital de Mareuille dict des pestiferez renduës par les sieurs maistre Escheuin & Escheuins dudit Nancy. Contre noble Nicolas Lambert apoticaire, & maistre Estienne Tapissier procureur [sic] dudit Nancy . . . [Nancy? ca. 1647]

7 p.   21 cm.   **[6599]**

Caption title.

LAMBSPRINGK. De lapide philosophico . . .

765-774 p., vol. 3.   20 cm.   (In Zetzner, Lazarus, ed. Theatrum chemicum. Argentorati, 1659-61)   **[6600]**

Caption title.
Translated by Nicolas Barnaud.

—[The same.] . . . E Germanico versu Latine redditus, per Nicolaum Barnaudum . . . Francofurti, Apud Hermannum a Sande, 1677.

[337]-371 p.   illus.   22 cm.   (In Musaeum Hermeticum. Francofurti, 1678)   **[6601]**

LA MESNARDIÈRE, Hippolyte Jules Pilet de [1610-1663] Raisonnemens . . . sur la nature des esprits qui servent aux sentimens. Paris, Jean Camusat, 1638.

[21], 162, [20] p.   14 cm.   **[6602]**

LAMONIÈRE, JEAN DE [*d.* 1671] Observatio fluxus dysenterici Lugduni Gallo. populariter grassantis anno Domini 1625. & remediorum illi utilium ... In qua precipuae circa dysenteriae naturam, & curationem difficultates ... dissolvuntur. Lugduni, Sumptib. Bartholomaei Vincentii, 1626.

[24], 227, [11] p.   16 cm.   **[6603]**

LAMPADEM VITAE & MORTIS. 1678. *See* [BURGGRAV, J. E.]

LAMPE, HEINRICH [*fl.* 1695] *respondent.* Disputatio medica inauguralis de valetudine prospera & adversa ... Lugduni Batavorum, Apud Abrahamum Elzevier, 1695.

[20] p.   22 cm.   **[6604]**

Diss.—Leyden.

LAMPE, HERMANN [*fl.* 1693] *respondent.* Disputatio inauguralis medica de palpitatione cordis ... Duisburgi ad Rhenum, Apud Franconem Sas, 1693.

28 p.   20 cm.   **[6605]**

Diss.—Duisburg.

LAMPÉRIÈRE, JEAN DE [*fl.* 1620-1622] L'ombre de necrophore vivant chartier de l'Hostel Dieu. Au sieur Jouyse medecin deserteur de la peste, sur la sagesse de sa cabale, & autres grippes de son exament [sic] ... Rouen, David Ferrant, 1622.

[32], 295, [1] p.   16 cm.   **[6606]**

—Traité de la peste, de ses causes & de sa cure. Avec les moyens de s'en preserver & ses controverses sur ce sujet. Divisé en deux parties ... Rouen, David du Petit Val, 1620.

[15], 421, [7] p.   17 cm.   **[6607]**

—*See* JOUYSE, D. Examen du livre de Lamperiere. 1622.

LAMPUGNANI, AGOSTINO [*ca.* 1586-*ca.* 1666] La pestilenza seguita in Milano l'anno 1630 ... Milano, Carlo Ferrandi, 1634.

78, [4] p.   14 cm.   **[6608]**

Engraved title page.

LAMSWEERDE, JAN BAPTIST VAN [*fl.* 1657-*ca.* 1700] Chirurgiae, veteris ac modernae promptuarium tabulis viginti novem exornatum, instrumenta varia, eorumque, usum exhibentibus, nec non observa-

tionum medico-chirurgicarum centuria illustratum ... Amstelodami, Apud Joannem à Someren, 1672.

[4], 3-288, [11] p.   illus.   19 cm.   **[6609]**

—Consideratien en motiven dienende ter decisie ende ten voordeele van Dr. Joh. Baptista van Lamzweerde, tegens de heer Hooft-officier Hendrick Roeters. [Amsterdam] 1677.

14 p.   16 cm.   **[6610]**

—Deductie ... overgegeven aen de ... heeren van den Gerechte deser stadt Amsterdam, dienende tot justificatie van sijn tractaet, geintituleert, Geluckwenschingh den leden van ... Nil volentibus arduum ... Amsterdam, Hieronymus Sweerts [1677]

14 p.   16 cm.   **[6611]**

—Geluckwenschingh den Leden van de vergaderinghe, bekendt door den zinspreuck Nil volentibus arduum, gedaen over hunne crediteurschap van den desolaten boedel der medicijnen deses tijdts ... Amsterdam, Hieronymus Sweerts, 1677.

38, [2] p.   16 cm.   **[6612]**

—Historia naturalis molarum uteri, in qua de natura feminis, ejusque circulari in sanguinem regressu, accuratius disquiritur ... Lugd. Batav., Apud Petrum vander Aa, 1686.

[16], 341, (i.e. 337), [11] p.   plates.   17 cm.   **[6613]**

Added engraved title page.

—Respirationis Swammerdammianae exspiratio. Una cum anatomia neologices Joannis de Raei ... Quibus adjecta est utriusque philosophiae clavis, et mirabilis de carbonum, arenarum, & lapillorum excretione per alvum & vesicam, urinaeque vomitu historia ... Amstelodami, Ex officina Joannis à Someren, 1674.

[32], 352 p.   front., illus.   16 cm.   **[6614]**

—*respondent. See* DIEMERBROECK, I. VAN, *praeses.* Disputationis medicae de chymia. 1657; REGIUS, H., *praeses.* Disputationis medicae de chymia. 1657.

—, *ed. See* SCULTETUS, J. [1595-1645] Armamentarium chirurgicum. 1672, 1693.

—*See* BOSCH, P. van den. Antwoort ... op de toegift van Dr. Johan Baptista Lamsweerde. 1678; DORSCH-VLEGEL. 1677; HADDEN, J. van. Pleuris. 1660; HALLING, P. Bekentmakinge aen Doctor van Yperen.

1678; HARDER, J. K. Apiarium observationibus medicis centum. 1687.

LAMY, GUILLAUME [*fl.* 1650-1682] Discours anatomiques ... Avec des reflexions sur objections qu'on luy a faites contre sa maniere de raisonner de la nature de l'homme, & de l'usage des parties qui le composent. Et cinq lettres du mesme autheur, sur le sujet de son livre. Rouen, Jean Lucas, 1675.

[46], 180 p. 16 cm. [**6615**]

—[The same.] ... Rev. & augm. de toutes les plus curieuses découvertes des anatomistes modernes. Plusieurs lettres du mesme auteur, et ses reflexions sur ses discours. Bruxelle, Henry Fricx, 1679.

[12], 34, 345 (i.e. 343) p. 16 cm. [**6616**]

—[The same.] ... 2. ed. Bruxelles, & se vend a Paris, Chez Laurent d'Houry, 1685.

[12], 34, 4, 345 (i.e. 343) p. 16 cm. [**6617**]
Imperfect: 4 p. are from another edition.
A reissue of the 1679 edition with new title page.

—Dissertation sur l'antimoine ... Paris, Lambert Roulland, 1682.

50, [7], 183, [8] p. 15 cm. [**6618**]
Errata: p. [8]

—[The same.] Dissertation sur l'antimoine, dans laquelle la nature de ce mineral, & la cause de son principal effet sont clairement démontrez ... 2. ed. Paris, Laurent d'Houry, 1687.

50, [18], 183, [1] p. 15 cm. [**6619**]
Errata: p. [11]
A reissue of the 1682 edition with preliminary matter added.

—Explication mechanique et physique des fonctions de l'ame sensitive, ou des sens, des passions, et du mouvement volontaire. Discours sur la generation du laict. Dissertation contre la nouvelle opinion, qui prétend que tous les animaux sont engendrez d'un oeuf. Réponse aux raisons par lesquelles le sieur Galatheau prétend établir l'empire de l'homme sur tout l'univers ... Paris, Lambert Roulland, 1678.

[10], 316, [4] p. 15 cm. [**6620**]

—[The same.] ... Avec une addition curieuse ... 2. ed. Paris, Lambert Roulland, 1681.

[40], 460, [14] p. plates. 16 cm. [**6621**]

—[The same.] ... Et une description exacte de l'oreille. Nouv. ed. augm. ... Paris, Laurent d'Houry, 1687.

[40], 460, [14] p. plates. 16 cm. [**6622**]

Imperfect: last leaf (Approbation, p. [13]-[14] at end) wanting.
A reissue of the 1681 edition with new title page.

LAMY, HONORÉ. Abbregé chirurgical. Recueilly des plus doctes & renommez medecins & chirurgiens, tant anciens que modernes ... Paris, Anthoine Guedois, 1642.

10, 25-281, [4] p. 17 cm. [**6623**]

LAMY, JEAN [*fl.* 1617] *respondent.* Theses medicae de pleuritide ... Basileae, Typis Joh. Jacoby Genathii [1616]

[15] p. 19 cm. [**6624**]
Diss. — Basel, 1617.

LANAEUS, JOANNES. *See* LANAY, Jean [*d.* 1641]

LANAY, JEAN [*d.* 1641] Le triomphe de la moelle, pour duplique au Traité medullaire, ou replique de M. J. de Marque ... Paris, Martin Verac, 1609.

[5], 95 p. 18 cm. [**6625**]
Bound with Marque, J. de. Paradoxe; ou, Traicté medulaire. 1609.

—, *ed. See* HIPPOCRATES. Aphorismi ... Graece et Latine in novum ordinem digesti. 1628.

—*See* GORRIS, J. de [*fl.* 1572-1622] Opuscula quatuor, 1660; MARQUE, J. de. Paradoxe. 1609.

LANCASTER, JOHN [*fl. ca.* 1682] *tr. See* [CAPOA, L. di] The conclave of physicians. 1684 [and] The uncertainty of the art of physick. 1684.

LANCELLA, PIETRO JACOMO. Centuria de'secreti medicinali, politici, & naturali ... Venetia, Treuigi, & Padova, Nella stampa Camerale, 1616.

[16] p. 16 cm. [**6626**]

LANCETTA, TROILO [*fl.* 1630-1632] Di pestilenza commune a bruti, et di contaggio mortale dell'huomo ... Et appresso un dialogo, attinente alla missione di sangue col taglio della vena in ogni genere de mali. 2. impr. alla quale è stato aggiunto ... un 'altro dialogo del finimento naturale del contaggio ... Venetia, Guerigli, 1632.

[16], 131 p. 28 cm. [**6627**]

—Raccolta medica, et astrologica. Divisa in doi discorsi l'uno per Hippocrate contro Galeno, dell'abuso commune di cavar sangue col salasso nelle febri. L'altro per Hippocrate, & Aristotele contro li astrologhi giudiciarii, cosi in generale come per uso di medicina. A piedi dell'uno, & l'altro discorso si trovano annesse varie opportune considerationi delle medesime attinenze. Lootri Nacattel [pseud., i.e. Troilo Lancetta] compilatore, & conversore . . . Venetia, Li Guergli, 1645.

[16], 390 p.   22 cm.   **[6628]**

Includes excerpts from the works of Girolamo Cardano, Cesare Cremonini, Girolamo Fracastoro, and Prospero Marsiani.

—, ed. See CREMONINI, C. Tractatus tres. 1644.

LANCILLOTTI, CARLO [17th cent.] Opuscoli diversi . . . cioe' L'interprete chimico. Il trionfo del mercurio. Il chimico disuellato con aggiunta. Il giardino di vaghi fiori medicinali. Modona, Per il Sogliani [1677]

4 parts in 1 v.   15 cm.   **[6629]**

Each part has special title page dated 1677; printers vary: Per Viviano Soliani, and Per il Soliani.

The Giardino di vaghi fiori medicinali (part. [4]) is by Teresa Perillo Lancillotti.

—Farmaceutica antimoniale; overo, Trionfo dell'antimonio que si scorge il grave errore che commettono quelli, che cercano di alienarlo dal uso medico mentre, che col mezzo di molti gravi auttori si da à conoscere le sue eroiche virtudi, e si scopre li suoi rari arcani . . . Modona, Per gli eredi Soliani, 1683.

[1], 35, 287 p.   front., plates.   15 cm.   **[6630]**

Imperfect: plate opposite p. 282 wanting.

With this is bound *his* Farmaceutica mercuriale. 1683.

—Farmaceutica mercuriale; overo, Trionfo del mercurio nel quale si descrive li piu gravi autori, che di lui habbino scritto, e si da à conoscere al mondo se sia veleno ò nò, e se si deba accetare al uso medico ò rigetarlo . . . Modona, Per gli eredi Soliani, 1683.

8, 2, 209, [1] p.   15 cm.   **[6631]**

Imperfect: front. wanting.

Bound with *his* Farmaceutica antimoniale. 1683.

—Guida alla chimica che per suo mezzo conduce gl'affetionati alle operationi sopra ogni corpo misto animale, minerale, o vegetabile. Dimostrando come s'estraggono i loro sali, ogli, essenze, magisterii, mercurii, etc. con il modo di fare varii colori, belletti et altri rari secreti. Et in quest'ultima impr. ampliata di nuove aggiunte . . . Parte prima [-terza] Venetia, Nicolò Pezzana, 1674.

[10], 326, [18] p.   18 cm.   **[6632]**

—[The same.] . . . Venetia, Iseppo Prodocimo, 1697.

[24], 188 p.; [12], 126 p.; [16], 226 p.   plates.   14 cm.   **[6633]**

Parts 2 and 3 have special title pages.

—[Dutch tr.] De brandende salamander; ofte, Ontleedinge der chymicale stoffen . . . Item Den ontwaakten chymist, met een byvoegsel van de verikiesinge des vitriols . . . Uit het Italiaans vertaalt door Jacob Leeuw. Verciert met nooten van S[teven] B[lankaart] M.D. Amsterdam, Johannis ten Hoorn, 1680.

[24], 286 (i.e. 290) p.; [3], 38, [12] p.   17 cm.   **[6634]**

LANCILLOTTI, TERESA PERILLO [*fl.* 1677] See LANCILLOTTI, C. Opuscoli diversi. 1677.

LANCISI, GIOVANNI MARIA [1654–1720] See GENGA, B. Anatomia per uso et intelligenza del disegno. 1691.

LANCKISCH, FRIEDRICH VON [1618–1669] *praeses.* Δεκας θεωρηματων φυσικων de calico innato in genere . . . [Lipsiae] Literis Lanckischianis [1641]

[16] p.   19 cm.   **[6635]**

Diss.—Leipzig (T. Coler, *respondent*)

LANDENBERGER, JOHANN RUDOLPH [*fl.* 1555] *tr.* See [GESNER, K.] Köstlicher Artzneyschatz. 1608.

LANDRÉ, CHRISTOPHE [*fl.* 1545–ca. 1570] Oecoiatrie. *In* Alessio Piemontese, Les secrets. 16—, 1639, 1642, 1691, 1699.

LANDRINUS, CHRISTOPHORUS. See LANDRÉ, Christophe [*fl.* 1545–ca. 1570]

LANDTMAN, JACOB [*fl.* 1658–1659] Mis-geboorte of verhael van 't Abbekerker-wijf; haare drie miskramen; 't opgraven van drie miszelijcke poppen; haer vankenis; ondevraging; belijdenis; pijniging; verantwoording; en geheelen proceze; met alle d' advijsen van reghtsgeleerde, godts-geleerde, en de sententien daar op gevolgt . . . Hoorn, Hendrick Jansz. Marius [Ghedruckt by Abraham Jacobsz. vander Beeck] 1661.

[8], 135, [1] p.   15 cm.   **[6636]**

LANDULFO, CESARE [15th cent.] De febribus. *In* Gatinaria, M. De medendis humani corporis malis practica. 1604.

LANDULPHUS, BLASIUS CAESAR. See LANDULFO, Cesare [15th cent.]

LANFRANCO, OF MILAN [*fl.* 1290-1296] *See* VICARY, T. The English mans treasure. 1613, 1633, 1641 [and] The surgions directorie. 1651.

LANG, BERNHARD [*fl.* 1604-1609] *respondent.* Theses medicae de phthisi . . . Basileae, Typis Joannis Schroeteri [1609]

    [15] p. 20 cm.   [6637]
  Diss. — Basel.

LANG, JACOB AMBROSIUS [*fl.* 1686-1689] *respondent.* Dissertatio medica inauguralis, differentiam inter hominum morbos cum brutis communes, et proprios exhibens . . . [Altdorffii] Literis Henrici Meyeri [1689]

    20 p. 18 cm.   [6638]
  Diss. — Altdorf.

LANGE [*fl.* 1689] Traité des vapeurs où leur origine, leurs effets, et leurs remedes sont mécaniquement expliquez . . . Paris, Chez la veuve de Denis Nion [de l'imprimerie de la veuve d'Antoine Chrétien] 1689.

    16, 295, [1] p. 15 cm.   [6639]

— Trattato delli vapori, nel quale la loro origine, i loro effetti, & i loro rimedi sono mecanicamente spiegati . . . Parigi, Alvise Pavino, 1695.

    [24], 167 p. 15 cm.   [6640]

LANGE, CHRISTIAN [1619-1662] Opera omnia, tam olim sparsim edita, qual ἀνέκδοτα, quorum series suo quaeque loco videre est, nunc uno volumine edita, cum praefatione D. Georgii Franci . . . Francofurti ad Moenum, Sumptibus Georgii Henrici Oehrlingii, 1688.

    [19], 266, [10] p.; [8], 698, [18] p. 21 cm.
                          [6641]

  Added engraved title page.
  Part [1] has special title page: Miscellanea curiosa medica. Part [2] has special title page: Pathologia animata; seu Animadversiones in pathologiam spagiricam . . . Petri Johannis Fabri.
  Edited by Johann Centurio Macasius.

— Miscellanea curiosa medica, annexa disputatione de morbillis, quam prodromum esse voluit novae suae pathologiae animatae, itemque de elixir proprietatis, post autoris obitum conjunctim edita a Johanne Centurione Macasio . . . Lipsiae, Sumtibus Thomae Matthiae Göntzenii, literis Johannis-Erici Hahnii, 1669.

    [8], 162 (i.e. 172), [8] p. 20 cm.   [6642]

Dissertations — Leipzig

—*praeses.* Curationem calculi humani . . . p. p. Augustus Hauptmann . . . Lipsiae, Literis Quirini Bauchii [1652]

    [31] p. 19 cm.   [6643]
  A. Hauptmann, *respondent.*

— De genuino acidulas egranas salubriter usurpandi modo . . . Lipsiae, typis haeredum Timothei Hönii, 1651.

    [48] p. 19 cm.   [6644]
  A. Hauptmann, *respondent.*

— Disputatio inauguralis de malo literatis familiari, sive hypochondriaco . . . [Lipsiae] Literis Bauerianis [1658]

    [52] p. 20 cm.   [6645]
  A. G. Friderich, *respondent.*

— Disputatio medica de ambustionibus . . . Lipsiae, Literis Bauerianis [1658]

    [32] p. 20 cm.   [6646]
  P. Ammann, *respondent.*

— Disputationem medicam de morbo castrensi seu Hungarico . . . proponit Anton Marquart . . . Lipsiae, Typis Henningi Koleri, 1649.

    [24] p. 19 cm.   [6647]
  A. Marquart, *respondent.*

— Exercitationem medicam de cancro in genere . . . publice proponit Christophorus Beccerus . . . Lipsiae, Literis Christiani Michaelis [1661]

    [24] p. 19 cm.   [6648]
  C. Beccer, *respondent.*

— Faciem Hippocraticam levi penicillo adumbratam . . . publice sistit M. Heinricus-Andreas Mengering . . . [Lipsiae] typis haeredum Timothei Hönii [1651]

    [28] p. 19 cm.   [6649]
  H. A. Mengering, *respondent.*

— Generationem calculi humani . . . p. p. Augustus Hauptmann . . . Lipsiae, Impensis Henningi Schürerii, typis haeredum Timothei Hönii [1650]

    [24] p. 18 cm.   [6650]
  A. Hauptmann, *respondent.*

— Another issue, with Lector benvole [p. 25] added at end.

                          [6651]

—Medicam de lacte humano disquisitionem . . . examini sistit publico Fridericus Ortlob . . . Lipsiae, 1652.

    [32] p.   19 cm.   [6652]
F. Ortlob, *respondent.*

—[The same.] . . . Lipsiae, Typis Johannis Baueri, 1653
    [28] p.   19 cm.   [6653]
F. Ortlob, *respondent.*

—, *ed. See* KIRCHER, A. Scrutinium physicomedicum contagiosae luis. 1659, 1671.

LANGE, Christian Johann [1655-1701] Disputationem medicam de haemorrhagia . . . subjicit Christianus Johannes Lange . . . Lipsiae, Literis Johannis Georgii [1685]
    [20] p.   20 cm.   [6654]
Diss. pro loco—Leipzig (H. Siegfried, *respondent*)

—*praeses.* Disputatio inauguralis medica de morbis endemiis . . . Lipsiae, Typis Christoph. Fleischeri [1694]
    [40] p.   21 cm.   [6655]
Diss.—Leipzig (S. Veiel, *respondent*)

—Disputatio medica inauguralis de hydrope . . . Lipsiae, Literis, Joh. Heinrici Richteri [1695]
    [35] p.   19 cm.   [6656]
Diss.—Jena (G. Berggold, *respondent*)

—Dissertatio medica inauguralis de palpitatione cordis . . . Lipsiae, Literis Johann. Georg [1699]
    [28] p.   19 cm.   [6657]
Diss.—Leipzig (D. H. Weidemüller, *respondent*)

—Dissertatio medica inauguralis de remediis vulnerariis . . . Lipsiae, Typis Christoph. Fleischeri [1694]
    [36] p.   20 cm.   [6658]
Diss.—Leipzig (G. P. Ritter, *respondent*)

—Hominem aerometrum . . . in dissertatione publica considerandum . . . sistet . . . Gabriel Grosser . . . Lipsiae, Litteris Joh. Christoph Brandenburgeri [1694]
    [44] p.   20 cm.   [6659]
Diss.—Leipzig (G. Grosser, *respondent*)

—Valetudinarium gravidarum . . . Lipsiae, Literis Johannis Georgii [1696]
    [34] p.   19 cm.   [6660]
Diss.—Leipzig (J. G. Thamm, *respondent*)

—*respondent. See* BOHN, J., *praes.* Disputatio inauguralis de cephalalgia. 1680; RIVINUS, A. Q., *praeses.* Disputatio medica de acido ventriculi fermento. 1677.

—*See* AMMANN, P. Paulus Ammann . . . procancellarius. L. S. 1680.

LANGE, DANIEL [*fl.* 1606] *respondent. See* HORST, G. [1578-1636]. Σκεψις de naturali conservatione . . . cadaverum. 1608.

LANGE, JOHANN [*fl.* 1596-1604] De gemmarum natura. In Bacci, A. De gemmis et lapidibus pretiosis. 1603.

LANGE, JOHANN [*fl.* 1667-1696] *tr. See* BLEGNY, N. de. Monatliche neueröffnete Anmerckungen. 1680-1683; BOLNEST, E. Aurora chymica. 1675; BOYLE, *Hon.* R. Die lufftige Noctiluca. 1682; [CHAMBERLAYNE, J.] comp. Schatzkammer rarer und neuer Curiositäten. 1689; DIGBY, *Sir* K. Ausserlesene . . . chymische Experimente. 1684.

LANGE, JOHANN ERNST VON DER [*fl.* 1693] *respondent. See* WILDVOGEL, C., *praeses.* Dissertatio inauguralis juridica de jure embryonum von ungebohrner Kinder Rechte. 1693.

LANGE, JOHANN SIGISMUND [*fl.* 1684] *respondent. See* HARTMANN, P. J., *praeses.* Exercitationum anatomicarum in publicas lectiones de iis, quae contra peritiam veterum anatomicam afferuntur in genere, prima. 1684.

LANGE, JOHANNES [1485-1565] Epistolarum medicinalium volumen tripartitum, denuo recognitum, & dimidia sui parte auctum . . . Hanoviae, Typis Wechelianis, apud Claudium Marnium & haeredes Joann. Aubrii, 1605.
    [32], 1020, [1] p.   port.   19 cm.   [6661]
Preface by Nicolaus Reusner.

—[Adaptations.] *In* Mizauld, A. Opusculorum pars prima [-secunda] 1607.

—*See* DIOCLES CARYSTIUS. Aurea ad Antigonum regem epistola. 1607; SENNERT, D. De scorbuto tractatus. 1624.

L'ANGÉLIQUE, GILLES DE. La vraye pierre philosophale de medecine, heureusement trouvée par le moyen de l'alliance des sept planettes dominatrices, conservatrices, & protectrices des corps humains, verifiee par les ... effects miraculeux de la confection angelique ... Paris, Louys Boulanger, 1622.

    [23], 400, [18] p.   16 cm.   **[6662]**

Imperfect: wormholes on p. 349-384.

LANGELLOTT, JOËL [1617-1680] Epistola ad praecellentissimos naturae curiosos. De quibusdam in chymia praetermissis, quorum occasione secreta haud exigui momenti proque non-entibus hactenus habita, candide deteguntur ... Hamburgi, Apud Gothofredum Schultzen; Amsterodami, Apud Joannem Janssonium a Waesberge, 1672.

    32 p.   illus., plate.   16 cm.   **[6663]**

—*See* BECKE, D. von der. Epistola ad ... Joelem Langelottum. 1672; MEIBOM, H. De vasis palpebrarum novis epistola. 1666; PECHLIN, J. N. De aeris et alimenti defectu. 1676.

LANGELOTT, ADOLPH KUNRAD [*fl.* 1676] *respondent. See* PECHLIN, J. N., *praeses.* Exercitatio anatomico-medica de fabrica et usu cordis. 1676.

LANGENAUER, JOACHIM [*fl.* 1621] *respondent. See* SEBISCH, M. [1578-1674?] *praeses.* Disputatio de purgatione decima tertia. 1621 [and] Disputationes de recta ratione purgandi. 1621.

LANGERMANN, EBERHARD [*fl.* 1692-1694] *respondent. See* BOHN, J., *praeses.* Specimen tertium medicinae forensis. 1692.

LANGEWAGEN, NIKOLAUS [*fl.* 1691] *respondent.* Disputatio medica inauguralis de medicamentorum operationibus in genere ... Lugduni Batavorum, Apud Abrahamum Elzevier, 1691.

    [21] p.   22 cm.   **[6664]**

Diss. — Leyden.

LANGHAM, WILLIAM. The garden of health: containing the sundry rare and hidden vertues and properties of all kindes of simples and plants. Together with the manner how they are to bee used and applyed in medicine for the health of mans body ... The 2nd ed. corr. and amended. London, Thomas Harper, 1633.

    [8], 702, [66] p.   20 cm.   **[6665]**

STC 15196.

LANGHANS, GERHARD DANIEL [*fl.* 1694] *respondent.* Disputatio inauguralis medica de cardialgia ... Altdorfii, Henricus Meyer [1694]

    48 p.   20 cm.   **[6666]**

Diss. — Altdorf.

LANGHANS, MARTIN [*fl.* 1645] *respondent.* Disputatio medica inauguralis de paralysi ... Basileae, Typis Georgii Deckeri [1645]

    [11] p.   19 cm.   **[6667]**

Diss. — Basel.

LANGIUS, CHRISTIANUS. *See* LANGE, Christian [1619-1662]

LANGIUS, DANIEL. *See* LANGE, Daniel [*fl.* 1606]

LANGIUS, JOANNES. *See* LANGE, Johannes [1485-1565]

LANGLADE, SATURNIN [*fl.* 1685] *respondent. See* GAILLARD, J., *praeses.* Quaestiones medicae selectiores. 1685.

LANGLEY, THOMAS [*d.* 1581] *tr. See* [VERGILIUS, P.] A pleasant and compendious history.

LANGLEY, WILLIAM. *See* LANGLY, Willem [1616-1668]

LANGLI, WILLEM. *See* LANGLY, Willem [1616-1668]

LANGLY, WILLEM [1616-1668] De generatione animalium observationes. *In* Harvey, W. Observationes et historiae omnes & singulae e Guilielmi Harvei libello De generatione animalium excerptae. 1674.

LANGWEDEL, BERNHARD [1596-1656] Carolus Piso enucleatus; sive, Observationes medicae C. Pisonis certis conclusionibus physico-pathologicis comprehensae, rationibus firmis illustratae & in epitomen redactae, studio ac opera Bernhardi Langwedelii ... Hamburgi, Typis Jacobi Rebenlini, sumptibus Zachariae Hertelii, 1639.

    [15], 147, [1] p.   17 cm.   **[6668]**

—Colloquium Romano-Hippocraticum inter Marforium & Pasquinum patritios Romanos ... Lugduni Batavorum, Ex officina Joannis Maire, 1648.

    104 p.   14 cm.   **[6669]**

—, *ed. See* HIPPOCRATES. [Aphorismi. Latin] 1639.

LANI, GYÖRGY [1646–1688] *praeses.* Διάσκεψις philosophiae naturalis de unguento armario, quo vulnera longe absentium sine contactu sanantur ... Lipsiae, Typis Justini Brandii [1680]

[24] p. 20 cm. [6670]

Diss. — Leipzig (C. Schmer, *respondent*)

LA NOUE, FRANÇOIS DE, *Father* [*fl.* 1628] *See* GASSENDI, P. Epistolica exercitatio, in qua principia philosophiae Roberti Fluddi medici reteguntur. 1630.

LA NOUE, JEAN BAPTISTE DE [*fl.* 1660] *ed. See* CASTAIGNE, G. de, *Father.* Les oeuvres. 1661.

LANOVIUS, FRANCISCUS. *See* LA NOUE, François de, *Father* [*fl.* 1628]

LANSMAN, JAKOB [*fl.* 1692] *See* HOOGHT, E. van der. Omstandig bericht. 1693.

LANTANA, ERMETE FRANCESCO [*d. ca.* 1700] *See* ACTA NOVAE ACADEMIAE PHILEXOTICORUM NATURAE ET ARTIS. 1687.

LANTIN, JEAN BAPTISTE [1619–1695] *See* SAUMAISE, C. de. Claudii Salmasii Plinianae exercitationes in Caii Julii Solini Polyhistora. 1689.

LANZONI, GIUSEPPE [1663–1730] Additio ad Olai Borichi dissertationem de lapidum generatione in macro, & microcosmo. *In* Borch, O. Dissertatio de lapidum generatione. 1687.

—Animadversiones variae ad medicinam, anatomiam, & chirurgiam maxime facientes ... Ferrariae, Sumpt. & typis Theodori Schenck, 1688.

[16], 487, [25] p. 17 cm. [6671]

—Dell'uso delle ghirlande e degli unguenti ne' conuiti degli antichi ... Ferrara, Filoni, 1698.

[24], 108, [10] p. 16 cm. [6672]

—Dissertatio de lacrymis. Ferrariae, Ex Typographia Sancti Nicolai, 1692.

xv p. 20 cm. [6673]

—Dissertatio medica de clysteribus ... Ferrariae, Typis Hieronymi Filoni, 1691.

8 p. 31 cm. [6674]

—Dissertatio medica de febre quartana. Ferrariae, Typis Cong. Somaschae, opera Jo. Baptistae Occhi, 1691.

xv p. 21 cm. [6675]

—Tractatus de balsamatione cadaverum, in quo non tantum de pollinctura apud veteres; sed etiam de variis balsamandi cadavera modis apud recentes, multa curiosa breviter exponuntur. Ferrariae, Typis Antonii Carrarae, 1693.

100, [14] p. 15 cm. [6676]

—[The same.] ... Genevae, Apud J. A. Chouët & David Ritter, 1696.

92, [24] p. 16 cm. [6677]
—copy 2. 14 cm.

Imperfect: title page mutilated, imprint date trimmed.
With this are bound: Mapp, Marc. Historia exaltationis theriacarum in theriacum coelestem. 1695, Gehema J. A. a. Der wohlversuchte Feld-Medicus. 1689.

—*See* MØINICHEN, H. Observationes medico-chirurgicae. 1688, 1691.

LAPIS ANIMALIS MICROCOSMICUS. 1681. *See* DOLHOPFF, G. A., *comp.*

LA PUENTE, LUIS DE. *See* PUENTE, Luis de la, *Father* [1554–1624]

LA QUEUTE, CHARLES PASCAL, *vicomte de. See* PASCHAL, Charles, vicomte de La Queute [1547–1625]

LAREN ABRAHAM VAN [*b.* 1633] *tr. See* FEATLEY, J. Tranen eener barende-vrouwe. 1665; GODDELIJCKE VIERSCHARE, op-gheright, in 't haedt-huys, van 's menschen herte. 1665.

LARIZA, MIGUEL DE. *See* LERIZA, Miguel de.

LA ROCHE, JOHANN HEINRICH [*fl.* 1694–1695] *respondent. See* SCHRADER, F., *praeses.* Disputatio medica de vulnerum cura. 1695.

LAROUVIÈRE, JEAN [*fl.* 1699] Nouveau systême des eaux minerales de Forges, où l'on découvre ... quelle est la nature de ces eaux, & à quelles maladies elles conviennent ... Paris, Laurent d'Houry, 1699.

[24], 251 [1] p. plate. 17 cm. [6678]

LA RUE, FRANÇOIS [*ca.* 1520–1585] De gemmis. *In* Lemnius, L. Similitudinum ac parabolarum, quae in Bibliis ex herbis atque arboribus desumuntur, dilucida explicatio. 1608, 1626.

LA RUELLE, JEAN DE. *See* RUEL, Jean [1474?–1537]

LARVENBREGIUS, PETRUS. *See* LAUREMBERG, Peter [1585–1639]

LA SALLE, François de. *See* Monginot, François de [1569–1637]

LA SCALA, Domenico [1632–1697] Phlebotomia damnata ... sive, Anidii, Chrisippi-Cnidii, Aschlepiadis, Erasistrati, & Aristogenis contra sanguinis missionem doctrina e vetustatis tenebris in lucem ... revocata, & luculentius enucleata ... In qua singula rationum momenta, quae sanguinis eductioni adversantur, aequa veritatis lance expenduntur. Pavii, Ex typographia fratrum Sardi, 1696.

[16], 295 p.   21 cm.   **[6679]**

Imperfect: front. wanting.

Includes discussion of the works of Giovanni Alfonso Borelli, Walter Charleton, Jean Baptiste Helmont, Frans de Le Boë, and Thomas Willis.

—*See* Giorgi, M. Phlebotomia liberata. 1697.

LA SEINE, Petrus. *See* Lasena, Pietro [1590–1636]

LASENA, Pietro [1590–1636] Homeri nepentheis; seu, De abolendo luctu liber, in quinque divisus partes, quarum I. Parasceuastica de frugalitate. II. Historica de medicamentis. III. Allegorica de consolatione. IV. Anagogica de virtute. V. Symplerotica de avocamentis ... Lugduni, Sumpt. Ludovici Prost, haeredis Roville, 1624.

[16], 286, [18] p.   19 cm.   **[6680]**

LASHER, Joshua [1647–1729] Pharmacopoeus et chymicus, symmystae; seu, Pharmacopoeia chymica ... Londini, Tho. Speed, 1698.

[24], 223, [5] p.   16 cm.   **[6681]**

LASIUS, Johann Albert [*fl.* 1696] *respondent. See* Stahl, G. E., *praeses.* Dissertatio medica-practica, de αὐτοκρατία naturae. [n. d.]

LASIUS, Johannes Heinricus [*fl.* 1695] *respondent. See* Eysel, J. P., *praeses.* Dissertationem inauguralem de chiragra ... proponit J. H. L. 1695.

LASNIORO, Joannes de. *See* Laaz, Johann von [*fl.* 15th cent.]

LASSÉRÉ, Michel. *See* Chérubin d'Orléans, *Father* [1613–1697]

LATIMER, Thomas [*fl.* 1689] *See* Albinus, B. Inauguralis dissertatio medica de somnambulatione. 1689.

LATIOSO, Anselmo [17th cent.] In Hippocratis Aphorismos omnes perbreves commentarii. Eorum

in versus vernaculos versio ab ea certe, quae de Graeco habetur Latiali ex textu, atque excerptae omnes A. C. Celsi versiones, translationesve hic vero postpositae plerisque in aphorismis eisdem. Opus novum in libros octo divisum ... Anselmo Latioso ... auctore. Viterbii, Apud Petrum Martinellum, 1667.

[14], 542 p.   illus.   16 cm.   **[6682]**

Added engraved title page: Hippoc. Aphorism. omnium lib. VIII.

Includes the complete Latin version of the Aphorismi by Niccolò Leoniceno, with the 8th book by A. M. Brasavola, the version of Celsus when available, and the Italian verse paraphrase.

"Nova ... tabula ad dies in morbis natura enumerandos ... directa ... Anselmus Latiosus ... opusculum ..." (p. [481]–542) has special title page.

LATTER, Friedrich Wilhelm [*fl.* 1683] *respondent. See* Hartmann, P. J., *praeses.* Exercitationum anatomicarum ... de originibus anatomicae prima [-quarta] 1683.

LAUGIER, Jean François [*fl.* 1691] Traité des remedes vulneraires, dans lequel on explique leur nature ... avec la théorie des accidens qui se rencontrent dans les playes ... Lyon, Jean Certe, 1693.

[12], 494, [10] p.   16 cm.   **[6683]**

LAUNAY, de. *See* Launay, Albert Padioleau, *sieur de.*

LAUNAY, Albert Padioleau, sieur de. *tr. See* Hippocrates. Aphorismi. [Adaptations, etc. French]. 1642.

LAUNAY, Charles Denys de [*fl.* 1698–1725] Dissertation physique et pratique sur les maladies, et sur les operations de la pierre. Où l'on traite fort au long de sa formation & de la maniere la plus seure pour la tirer de la vessie ou de l'uretre ... Paris, Laurent d'Houry, 1700.

[38], 254 p.   16 cm.   **[6684]**

—Nouveau systeme concernant la generation, les maladies veneriennes et le mercure ... divisé en deux parties ... Paris, Estienne Michallet, 1698.

[28], 182, [6] p.   16 cm.   **[6685]**

LAUNAY, Jean Piochon de [1649–1701] Instructions necessaires pour ceux qui sont incommodés des décentes, avec quelques remarques sur le remede du roy, & sur les moyens qu'on peut prendre pour envoyer des bandages dans les provinces ... Paris,

Chez Laurent d'Houry [De l'imprimerie de Charles Coignard] 1690.

[16], 103 p. front., plates. 16 cm. [6686]

—Another issue. [6687]

Frontispiece, Approbation, etc. differ. Two leaves of dedicatory epistle inserted between sig. a1 and 2.

LAUREMBERG, Peter [1585-1639] Ἀνωνύμου εἰσαγωγη ἀνατομικη, anonymi philosophi antiquiss. isagoge anatomica. Nunc primum e sua bibliotheca edidit, & vertit Petrus Lauremberg. Hamburgi, Paulus Langius, 1616.

[8], 86, [1] p. 20 cm. [6688]

Imperfect: sheet H wrongly imposed.
Text in Greek and Latin.

—[The same.] . . . Nunc primum . . . edita . . . Lugduni-Batavorum, Sumptibus Joachimi Morsii. 1618.

[8], 87 p. 20 cm. [6689]

The text is a reissue of the 1616 edition.
With this is bound Maier, M. De circulo physico quadrato. 1616.

—Collegium anatomicum XII. disputationibus compraehensum & in Rostochiensium Academia propositum . . . Rostochii, Ex officina typographica haeredum Richelianorum, 1636.

[243] p. 20 cm. [6690]

Signatures: *², A-P⁴, Q², R-V⁴, X², Y-Z⁴, Aa-Bb⁴, Cc², Dd-Hh⁴, Ii².
Includes 83 leaves of manuscript: Liber de secretis, a collection of recipes.

—Deliria chymica. [n.p.] Excudebat Anton. Gunther. Billich, 1625.

95, [1] p. 16 cm. [6691]

—Pasicompse nova; id est, Accurata & curiosa delineatio pulchritudinis, qua tanquam in speculo ostenduntur notae & characteres, exactam pulchritudinem & formae elegantiam, cujusque membri in humano corpore, comitantes . . . Lipsiae, Ex Bibliopolio Hallervordiano, typis Ritzschianis, 1634.

[18], 152 p. 17 cm. [6692]

—Porticus Aesculapii; seu, Generalis artis medicae constitutio; in qua de medicinae genere, subjecto, fine, definitione, divisione, controversiae plaeraeque omnes examinantur . . . Rostochii, Typis Joachimi Pendani, prostat apud Joh. Hallervordium, 1630.

[1], 100 p. 20 cm. [6693]

—Copy 2. 19 cm.
With this is bound Sebisch, M. Disputationes de recta ratione purgandi. 1621.

—Procestria anatomica, in quibus proponuntur plaeraque quae ad generalem anatomiae et partium contemplationem attinent; quaedam etiam infimi ventris membra explicantur; et Andreae Laurentii Historia anatomica multis locis castigatur et corrigitur. Hamburgi, Apud Paulum Langium, 1619.

[1], 224 p. 19 cm. [6694]

Imperfect: title page mutilated.

—*See* LAUREMBERG, W. Epistolica dissertatio. 1623.

LAUREMBERG, Wilhelm [1547-1612] Epistolica dissertatio, curationem calculi vesicae continens; & Pet. Laurembergii Laurus Delphica, seu consilium, quo describitur methodus perfacilis ad medicinam. Wittebergae, Christianus Tham, 1623.

[1], 42, 49 p. 14 cm. [6695]

—*See* PAULLI, S. Quadripartitum botanicum de simplicium medicamentorum facultatibus. 1667.

LAURENBERG, Petrus. *See* LAUREMBERG, Peter [1585-1639]

LAURENDERIUS, Claudius Martinus. *See* Laurendière, Claude Martin de [*fl.* 1657]

LAURENDIÈRE, Claude Martin de [*fl.* 1657] ed. and *tr. See* CARDANO, G. Metoposcopia. 1658 [and] La metoposcopie. 1658.

LAURENS, André du. *See* Du Laurens, André [1558-1609]

LAURENS, Matthias Daniel [*fl.* 1689] *respondent. See* SCHULTZ, J., *praeses.* Disputatio juridica de contractu medici cum aegroto. 1689.

LAURENTI, Rodomonte [*fl.* 1649] De vitae humanae catastrophe ex pestilentia; seu, De pestis, pestiferęque febris essentia, pręcautione, atque curatione tractatus, in tres libros distributus . . . Pisauri, Typis Joannis Pauli de Gottis, 1649.

[24], 172, [28] p. 20 cm. [6696]

Errata: p. [27-28]

LAURENTIANUS, Laurentius. *See* LAURENZIANI, Lorenzo [*ca.* 1450-1502]

LAURENTIUS, Andreas. *See* Du Laurens, André [1558-1609]

LAURENTIUS, Antonius. *See* Lorenzini, Antonio [16th—17th cent.]

LAURENTIUS, Georgius Fridericus. *See* Lorenz, Georg Friedrich [1594-1673]

LAURENTIUS, Johann Christoph [*fl.* 1662] *respondent. See* Conradi, E., *praeses.* Ex physicis de aere. 1662.

LAURENTIUS, Johann Heinrich [*fl.* 1662-1669] *respondent. See* Friderici, J. A., *praeses.* Υοτερυδερίασις; sive, Uteri hydrops. 1669; Hentschel, S., *praeses.* Disquisitionem naturalem de asteria gemma . . . proponunt . . . Samuel Hentschel . . . & . . . Joh. Heinricus Laurentius. 1662.

LAURENZI, Rodomonte. *See* Laurenti, Rodomonte [*fl.* 1649]

LAURENZIANI, Lorenzo [*ca.* 1450-1502] *tr. See* Frigio, J. A. In magni Hippocratis Prognostica Jacobi Antonii Phrygii . . . explanatio. 1608; Lavelli, J. De pulsibus ad tyrones. 1602; Vega, C. de. Opera omnia. 1626.

LAURUS Batava in honorem . . . Henrici à Busch, cum . . . de delirio habita disputatione summis in medicina honoribus efferretur, decantata ab amicis . . . Lugduni Batavorum, Apud viduam & haeredes Johannis Elsevirii, 1668.

[8] p.   18 cm.   **[6697]**

LAUSITZ. *See* Lusatia, Lower.

LAUSNITZ. *See* Lusatia, Lower.

LAUTARET, D. T. de [*fl.* 1612-1620] Les merveilles des bains naturels et des estuves naturelles de la ville de Digne en Provence. Divisées en deux parties, la theorie & la practique. Avec un traicté de leurs serpents sans venim, et une sommaire description de tous autres . . . Aix, Jean Tholosan, 1620.

[15], 179 p.; [11], 151, [4] p.   17 cm.   **[6698]**
Part [2] has special title page: La practique des estuves des bains de Digne.

LAUTENBACH, Joseph [1568 *or* 9-1614] *ed.* Consilia medicinalia, cum mixtim praestantissimorum Italiae medicorum; tum seorsim Antonii Mariae Venusti . . . de gravissimis humani corporis malis curandis. Quibus accessere Julii Caesaris Claudini . . . Tractatus de natura & usu lactis & seri, thermarum, guaiaci ligni, sassafras, salsae parilliae . . .

Collecta, digesta, polita ac edita omnia a Josepho Lautenbachio . . . Francofurti, Ex officina typographica Wolfgangi Richteri, impensis Johannis Sartorii, 1605.

[12], 368, 284 p.   21 cm.   **[6699]**

—[The same.] Paradoxa medica; sive, Tractatus novi, singulares, absoluti de natura et usu thermarum, ligni guaiaci, sassafras, salsae parilliae . . . lactis & seri, aliorumque usu & frequentium & reconditorum, in variis, imo pene omnibus corporis humani morbis adhibendo: per diversas morborum, sive facti species, instar Consiliorum medicinalium conscripti, & editi a Julio Caesare Claudino . . . Francofurti, Apud Christ. Gerlach, 1660.

[8], 368, 284 p.   20 cm.   **[6700]**
A reissue of his Consilia medicinalia published in 1605; title page and preliminary matter reset, without the Dedicatio.

LAUTENSACK, Heinrich [1522-1568] Dess Circkelss und Richtscheyts, auch der Perspectiva, und Proportion der Menschen und Rosse, kurtze, doch gründtliche Underweisung, dess rechten Gebrauchs . . . Franckfurt am Mayn, Gedruckt bey Egenolff Emmel, in Verlegung Simonis Schambergers, 1618.

[4], 54 ll.   illus., plates.   31 cm.   **[6701]**

LAUTERBACH, Wolfgang Adam [1618-1678] *praeses.* Positiones juridicae de domiciliis pauperum, von Hospitälen . . . Tubingae, Typis excudebat Joachimus Hein [1676]

28 p.   19 cm.   **[6702]**
Diss.—Tübingen (J. Braun, *respondent*)

LAUTHIER, Honoratus Maria. *See* Lautier, Honoré Maria [*fl.* 17th cent.]

LAUTIER, Honoré Maria [*fl.* 17th cent.] Historiae inauditae rationes et mechanica [&] Responsio adversus medicum Massiliensem anonimum super Muscipontano prodigio. *In* Historia foetus Mussipontani. 1669.

—Prodigium . . . foetum humanum extra loco conceptum . . . Muscipontana exhibet civitas. *In* Sinibaldi, G. B. Geneanthropeiae. 1669.

LAUTITZ, Philipp Georg [*fl.* 1689] *respondent. See* Wedel, G. W., *praeses.* Dissertatio medica de morbis praecordialibus. 1689.

LAVAL, Antoine de. *See* Luynes, Louis Charles d'Albert, *Duc de* [1620-1690]

LAVATER, HEINRICH [1560-1623] Defensio medicorum Galenicorum adversus calumnias Angelii Salae . . . In qua superba ejus censura examinatur & confutatur . . . Hanoviae, Typis Thomae Willeriani, 1610.

95, [16] p.   17 cm.   [6703]

LAVATER, HENRICUS. *See* LAVATER, Johann Heinrich [1611-1691]

LAVATER, JOHANN HEINRICH [1611-1691] *praeses.* Σκιαγραφια θερμολογιας γενικης; seu, Adumbratio aquarum thermalium in genere consideratarum . . . Tiguri, 1667.

[14 +] p.   18 cm.   [6704]

Imperfect: all pages after p. [14] wanting.

Diss.—Zürich (J. H. Lavater, *fl.* 1667-1672, *respondent*)

—, *tr. See* FABRICIUS VON HILDEN, W. Opera. 1646, 1682.

LAVATER, Johann Heinrich [*fl.* 1667-1672] *respondent.* Theses inaugurales de 'εντεροπερισολη, seu intestinorum compressione . . . Basileae, Typis Jacobi Bertschii [1672]

[32] p.   19 cm.   [6705]

Diss.—Basel.

—*See* LAVATER, J. H. [1611-1691] *praeses.* Σκιαγραφια Θερμολογιας γενικης.

LAVATER, LUDWIG [1527-1586] De spectris, lemuribus et magnis atque insolitis fragoribus, variisque praefagitionibus, quae plerunque obitum hominum, magnas clades, mutationesque imperiorum praecedunt. Liber unus, in tres partes distributus . . . Ed. 2 . . . emend. Lugd. Batavorum, Apud Henr. Verbiest, [Ex typogr. Joh. Z. Baron] 1659.

[20], 245, [1] p.   14 cm.   [6706]

Added engraved title page.

LA VAUGUION, DE. Traité complet des operations de chirurgie . . . Paris, Estienne Michallet, 1696.

[48], 824, [8] p.   plates.   18 cm.   [6707]

—[The same.] . . . Paris, Barthelemy Girin, 1698.

[48], 824, [8] p.   plates.   18 cm.   [6708]

A reissue of the 1696 edition with new title page.

—[English tr.] A compleat body of chirurgical operations, containing the whole practice of surgery . . . Faithfully done into English. London, Henry Bonwick, T. Goodwin, M. Wotton, B. Took, and S. Manship, 1699.

[24], 447, [9] p.   20 cm.   [6709]

LAVAUS, G. [*fl.* 1697] Traité de la mauvaise articulation de la parole . . . Paris, Guillaume de Luyne, 1697.

[10], 151, [3] p.   16 cm.   [6710]

LAVELLI, JACOPO [1550-1627] De pulsibus ad tyrones, liber et Commentarii in primum librum Prognosticorum Hippocratis . . . Venetiis, Apud Jo. Baptistam Ciottum, 1602.

[4], 87 ll.; [4], 75, [1] ll.   20 cm.   [6711]

Part [2] has special title page. Colophon reads: Venetiis, Apud Marcum Antonium Zalterium, 1601.

Includes the Latin version of book 1 of Hippocrates' Prognostica translated by Lorenzo Laurenziani and the Latin text, with commentary, of Galen's De pulsibus ad tirones.

LA VIGNE, MICHEL DE [1588-1648] Diaeta sanorum; sive, Ars sanitatis. Studio Michaëlis de la Vigne authoris filii . . . Parisiis, Apud Gabrielem Targa, 1671.

[15], 128 p.   16 cm.   [6712]

LA VIGNE, MICHEL DE [*fl.* 1649-1704] *ed. See* LA VIGNE, M. de [1588-1648] Diaeta sanorum. 1671.

LA VILLE, DE [*fl.* 1677] *See* MALEBRANCHE, N. Treatise concerning the search after truth. 1694.

LAVINHETA, BERNARD DE. Opera omnia quibus tradidit artis Raymundi Lullii compendiosam explicationem, et ejusdem applicationem ad I. Logica. II. Rhetorica. III. Physica. IV. Mathematica. V. Mechanica. VI. Medica. VII. Metaphysica . . . Edente Johanne Henrico Alstedio. Opus . . . jam denuo recusum . . . Coloniae, Sumptibus Lazari Zetzneri, 1612.

[8], 668, [11] p.   illus.   19 cm.   [6713]

"Hortulus medicus . . . promens & proponens miracula medica . . . trium philosophorum celeberrimorum Raimundi Lullii, Joannis de Rupescissa, & Bernhardi de Lavineta . . . Nunc primum . . . exire jussus a Justo Hilario . . ." (p. [345]−443) has special title page.

LAVINIUS, WENCESLAUS [*fl.* 1580] Tractatus de coelo terrestri . . .

288-290 p., vol. 4.   20 cm.   (*In* Zetzner, Lazarus, *ed.* Theatrum chemicum. Argentorati, 1659-61)   [6714]

Caption title.

—[The same.] *In* [Eglinus Iconius, R.] Cheiragogia Heliana de auro philosophico necdum cognito. 1612.

LA VIOLETTE, JOSEPH DUCHESNE, *seigneur de.* *See* DUCHESNE, Joseph [*ca.* 1544–1609]

LAY, ANDREAS [*fl.* 1625] *respondent. See* SEBISCH, M. [1578–1674?] *praeses.* Exercitationes medicae. 1639.

LAZARI, DIONISIO DE [*fl.* 1606] Tractatulus de somniis . . . Venetiis, Ex Typographia Rampazettana, 1606.

[4], 70, [1] p. 18 cm. **[6715]**

LÁZARO GUTIÉRREZ, JUAN [*fl.* 17th cent.] Febrilogiae lectiones Pincianae, theoripracticum opus acroamaticum. Ad Hippocratis mentem, ad Galeni sensum; ad Avicennae judicium . . . Nunc primum prodit. Lugduni, Sumptibus Laurentii Anisson, 1668.

[8], 292, [11] p.; 56 p. 36 cm. **[6716]**

Part [2] has caption title: Appendix ad Febrilogiam, doloris diagnosim, prognosim, et curationem in communi, tum artem sphygmicam continens.

—Opusculum de fascino . . . Lugduni, Sumpt. Philip. Borde, Laur. Arnaud, & Cl. Rigaud, 1653. **[6717]**

— , *ed. See* MAROJA, C. Opera omnia medica. 1674, 1688.

LAZARUS, DYONISIUS. *See* LAZARI, Dionisio de [*fl.* 1606]

LEACHE, MIGUEL MARTINEZ DE. *See* MARTÍNEZ DE LEACHE, Miguel [*fl.* 1644–1652]

LEBENWALDT, ADAM VON [1624–1696] Land-Stadt- und Hauss-Artzney-Buch, in welchem angezeigt . . . wird, wie man denjenigen Kranckheiten, welche ein gantzes Land . . . anstecken, so dann durch Contagion . . . anderweitig fortgepflantzt . . . werden, als da seyn: die Pest . . . ungarische Kranckheit, rothe Ruhr . . . so wohl durch geringe als kostbare Mittel Widerstand thun könne . . . Samt einer Information, was zu solcher Contagions-Zeit, I. Status politicus und Land-Obrigkeiten, II. Status civilis oder Stadt-Obrigkeiten . . . zu thun haben. Dabey eine fünff-fache Cur zu finden . . . Nürnberg, In Verlegung Johann Christoph Lochners, 1695.

[24], 720, [31] p. plates. 34 cm. **[6718]**

—Sechstes Tractätl, von des Teuffels List und Betrug in der Waffen-Salben, und so genandten sympathetischen Pulver. Saltzburg, Johann Baptist Mayr, 1681.

[1], 198 p. 13 cm. **[6719]**

With this are bound *his*: Sibentes Tractätl, 1681; Achtes Tractätl, 1681.

—Sibentes Tractätl, von dess Teuffels List und Betrug in der Transplantation oder Uberpflantzung der Kranckheit. Saltzburg, Johann Baptist Mayr, 1681.

[1], 166 p. 13 cm. **[6720]**

Bound with *his* Sechstes Tractätl. 1681.

—Achtes Tractätl, von des Teuffels List und Betrug in Verführung der Menschen zur Zauberey . . . Saltzburg, Johann Baptist Mayr, 1681.

[3], 362 p. 13 cm. **[6721]**

Bound with *his* Sechstes Tractätl. 1681.

LE BEY, JEAN, *ed. and tr.* Recueil des secrets admirables, inventez et mis en oeuvre par des grands & signalez philosophes, astrologues & medecins, tant de Perse que d'Ethiopie. Recueillis & experimentez, & traduits de Latin en François, par moy Iean Le Bey . . . Grenoble, Pierre Verdier, 1637.

16 p. 16 cm. **[6722]**

LE BOË, FRANS DE [1614–1672] Totius medicinae idea nova; seu . . . Opera omnia . . . Pars prima [-secunda] Parisiis, Apud Fredericum Leonard, 1671.

[12], 454, [1] p.; [8], 344 p. 17 cm. **[6723]**

Part 2 has special title page.

Contents: Part 1: Instructiones medicinae.—Praxeos medicae. Liber I. Part 2: Praxeos medicae, liber II & III.—Disputationum medicarum I-IX.—De lue venerea.—De peste.—De chymia in genere.

—Opera medica, tam hactenus inedita, quam variis locis & formis edita . . . Amstelodami, Apud Danielem Elsevirium, et Abrahamum Wolfgang, 1679.

[8], 934, [26] p. 25 cm. **[6724]**

Imperfect: title page mutilated.

Contents.—Disputationum medicarum I-X.—De methodo medendi, liberi II.—Praxeos medicae idea nova, liberi III [&] Appendix.—Opuscula varia.

The Opuscula varia includes his Dictata ad Casparis Bartholini Institutiones anatomicas and Lucas Schacht's Oratio funebris in obitum . . . Francisci de Le Boe Sylvii.

—[The same.] ... Ed. alt. corr. & emend. Amstelodami, Apud Danielem Elsevirium, et Abrahamum Wolfgang, 1680.

[8], 934, [26] p.   24 cm.   [6725]

Imperfect: portrait wanting.

Different setting of type.

—[The same.] Opera medica; hoc est, Disputationum medicarum decas, Methodi medendi libri duo, Ideae novae praxeos medicae libri tres, ad eosque Appendix variaque alia Opuscula. Accessit huic editioni hactenus ineditum Collegium nosocomicum ab authore habitum, una cum Appendice de formulis quibusdam remediorum ad varios affectus ab eodem praescriptis ... Genevae, Apud Samuelem de Tournes, 1681.

[19], 747, [40] p.   port.   36 cm.   [6726]

—Another issue.   37 cm.   [6727]

Portrait differs.

—[The same.] ... Genevae, Apud Samuelem de Tournes, 1693.

[19], 747, [40] p.   port.   36 cm.   [6728]

Different setting of type.

—[The same.] Opera medica, tam hactenus inedita, quam variis locis & formis edita ... Ed. nova, cui accedunt Casus medicinales annor. 1659, 60, & 61, quos ex ore Cl. Sylvii calamo excepit Joachimus Merian ... Trajecti ad Rhenum, Apud Guillelmum van de Water, & Amstelodami, Apud Antonium Schelte, 1695.

[8], 934, [26] p.; 85, [9] p.   front. (port.) 25 cm.   [6729]

—[The same.] Opera medica, hoc est, Disputationum medicarum decas, Methodi medendi libri duo, Ideae novae praxeos medicae libri tres, ad eosque Appendix, variaque alia Opuscula. Accesserunt huic editioni hactenus inediti Casus medicinales annorum 1659, 60, & 61, quos ex ore Cl. Sylvii calamo excepit Joachimus Merian ... una cum Remediis Sylvianis; itemque Collegium nosocomicum ab authore habitum, una cum Appendice de formulis quibusdam remediorum ad varios affectus ab eodem praescriptis ... Venetiis, Apud Joannem Jacobum Hertz, 1697.

[20], 660, [36] p.   33 cm.   [6730]

Imperfect: worm holes on p. 33-66.

The Opuscula varia includes *his* Dictata ad Casparis Bartholini Institutiones anatomicas.

—[The same.] ... Ut & Collegium nosocomicum ab authore habitum, una cum formulis quibusdam Remediorum ad varios affectus ab eodem praescriptis. Quibus hac in editione accesserunt Casus medicinales, annor. M.DC.LIX, LX, & LXI, quos ex ore cl. authoris excepit Joachimus Merian ... Genevae, Fratres de Tournes, 1698.

[19], 747, [40], 67 p.   port.   35 cm.

[6731]

The Opuscula varia includes *his* Dictata ad Casparis Bartholini Institutiones anatomicas and Lucas Schacht's Oratio funebris in obitum ... Francisci de Le Boe Sylvii.

—Collegium medico-practicum dictatum 1660. Francofurti, Apud Thomam Matthiam Götzium, 1664.

[4], 113 p.   14 cm.   [6732]

Le Boë denies authorship of this work in the second preface of his A new idea of the practice of physick, London, 1675.

Bound with copy 2 of Regimen sanitatis Salernitanum. Schola Salernitana. 1667.

—De morbis infantum. *See his* Praxeos medicae liber quartus.

—[English tr.] Of childrens diseases, given in a familiar style for weaker capacities. With an apparatus or introduction explaining the authors principles; as also a treatise of the rickets, by R[ichard] G[ower] ... London, George Downs, 1682.

[22], 148, [2] p.   16 cm.   [6733]

—Disputationum medicarum pars prima; primarias corporis humani functiones naturales ... complectens. Amstelodami, Apud Johannem van den Bergh, 1663.

[56], 167 p.   13 cm.   [6734]

Contains 8 Leyden dissertations.

With this is bound *his* Disputatio medica de natura & usu succi pancreatici. 1664.

—Disputationum medicarum decas, primarias corporis humani functiones naturales, nec non febrium naturam ... complectens. Annexis 1. Epistola apologetica contra Antonium Deusingium. 2. De affectus epidemii, anno 1669, Leidae grassantis, causis naturalibus. 3. De hominis cognitione, binis orationibus. Omnibus ad Leidense exemplar fideliter conformatis. Ed. 3 ... Jenae, Impensis Joh. Fritschii, prodibat typis Joh. Gollneri, 1674.

[44], 408, p.   13 cm.   [6735]

The Epistola apologetica has special title page.

—Idea praxeos medicae. In tres libros divisae . . . Francofurti, Typis Hummianis, 1671.

    [8], 759, [24] p.   15 cm. .   **[6736]**

—Praxeos medicae idea nova liber primus, de affectibus naturales hominis functiones laesas vel constituentibus, vel producentibus, vel consequentibus. Lugduni Batavorum, Apud viduam Joannis Le Carpentier, 1671.

    23, [9], 980, [121] p.   14 cm.   **[6737]**
  "Index rerum locupletissimus a Martino Carceo . . . adornatus": [121] p.
  With this is bound Carceus, M. Index materiae medicae. 1671.

—[The same.] . . . Ed. alt. priore accuratior. Lugduni-Batavorum, Apud viduam Joannis Le Carpentier, 1672.

    24, [32], 980, [121] p.   14 cm.   **[6738]**
  Added engraved title page.
  A reissue with partly new, and partly reprinted preliminaries.

—[English tr.] A new idea of the practice of physic . . . The first book, of the diseases either constituting, producing or following the natural functions of man not in health . . . As also a new discovery of intermitting fevers, the yellow jaundice, and other diseases, never before discovered . . . Whereto is prefixed a preface written by Mar. Nedham. Translated . . . by Richard Gower. London, Brabazon Aylmer, 1675.

    [46], 511, [1] p.   front. (port.)   18 cm. **[6739]**

—*as subject. See* CARCEUS, M. Index materiae medicae. 1671.

—Praxeos medicae liber quartus, de morbis infantum, & aliis quibusdam memoratu dignis affectibus. Editus cura Justi Schraderi, M. D. Amstelodami, Apud Abrahamum Wolfgang, 1674.

    1214 p.   14 cm.   **[6740]**

—Verhandelinge van de pokken. *In* Blankaart, S. Venus belegert en ontset. 1684, 1688, 1696. [German tr.] 1689.

Dissertations—Leyden

—*praeses.* Disputatio medica de alimentorum fermentatione in ventriculo . . . Lugduni Batavorum, Apud Johannem Elsevirium, 1659.

    [8] p.   19 cm.   **[6741]**
  A. Quina, *respondent.*

—Disputatio medica de ischuria . . . Lugduni Batavorum, Apud viduam & haeredes Johannis Elsevirii, 1671.

    [12] p.   23 cm.   **[6742]**
  J. von Flammerdinge, *respondent.*

—Disputatio medica de natura & usu succi pancreatici . . . Lugd. Batav., Ex Officina Hackiniana, 1664.

    [2], 90 p.   plates.   13 cm.   **[6743]**
  R. de Graaf, *respondent.*
  Bound with *his* Disputationum medicarum pars prima. 1663.

—Disputatio medica de variis tabis speciebus . . . Lugduni Batavorum, Apud Johannem Elsevirium, 1661.

    [16] p.   20 cm.   **[6744]**
  R. Sibbald, *respondent.*
  Bound with Sibbald, *Sir* R. Phalainologia nova. 1692.

—Disputatio medica de vasis lymphaticis, & lympha . . . Lugduni Batavorum, Apud Johannem Elsevirium, 1661.

    [16] p.   19 cm.   **[6745]**
  C. Gottwaldt, *respondent.*

—Disputatio medica de venae-sectione, ejusque legitima administratione, in duas partes divisa . . . Lugduni Batavorum, Apud viduam & haeredes Johannis Elsevirii, 1671.

    [32] p.   20 cm.   **[6746]**
  J. Carolus, *respondent.*

—*See* DEUSING, A. Disquisitio anti-Sylviana de motu cordis et arteriarum. 1663 [and] Sylva-caedua cadens. 1664 [and] Sylva-caedua jacens. 1665 [and] *In* Sylvam echo; seu, Sylvius heuton-timoroumenos. 1663; DOLÄUS, J. Encyclopaedia chirurgica rationalis. 1689, 1690, 1695 [and] Encyclopaedia, medicinae theoretico-practica. 1684, 1686, 1688, 1690, 1691 [and] Opera omnia. 1695 [and] Systema medicinale, a compleat system of physick. 1686; ETTMÜLLER, M. Opera omnia theoretica et practica. 1685; GRUBE, H. De arcanis medicorum non arcanis commentatio. 1673; HOFMANN, C. Tractatus de usu lienis cerebri. 1682; LA SCALA, D. Phlebotomia damnata. 1696; LEICHNER, E. Epicrisis medico-analytica. 1676; PECHLIN, J. N. Jani Leoniceni Veronensis [pseud.] Metamorphosis. 1672, 1673; RAMBALDUS, J. Compendiaria tractatio de febris. 1689? SCHUYL, F. Pro veteri medicina. 1670; THIBAUT, P. Cours de chymie. 1674.

LE BON, JEAN [*d.* 1583?] Therapia puerperarum. *In* Houllier, J. De morbis internis libri II. 1603 [and] Omnia opera practica. 1623, 1635, 1664.

LE BOULANGER DE CHALUSSAY [1669-1672] Elomire hypocondre; ou, Les medecins vengez. Comedie . . . Paris, Charles de Sercy, 1670.

[8], 112 p.   14 cm.   [6747]

LEBRUN, JOHANN LUDWIG GREGOR [*fl.* 1698] *respondent. See* SPERLING, P. G., *praeses.* Disputatio inauguralis medica de haemoptysi. 1698.

LEBWALD VON LEBENWALD, ADAM. *See* LEBENWALDT, Adam von [1624-1696]

LE CERF, PIERRE THÉODORE [*fl.* 1682-1694] De febri Gallica tractatus. Francofurti, Apud Martin. Hermsdorff., typis Johannis Wustii, 1694.

[8], 31 p.   19 cm.   [6748]
Original date partly covered by label.

LECHEL, JOHANN [1634 or 5-1686] Warnung für dem unzeitigen . . . Aderlassen und Purgiren in giftigen . . . Flekk-und dergleichen Fiebern, wobey der Nutz des Schwitzens in angeregten Krankheiten deutlich gezeiget wird. Nebst warhafftigem Bericht von . . . Jeremias Liebens jüngster Krankheit . . . Braunschweig, Christoff-Friederich Zilliger, 1676.

[32] p.   18 cm.   [6749]

—*respondent.* Disputationem medicam inauguralem de lithiasi . . . publico examini . . . submittit Johannes Lechelius . . . Altdorffii, E chalcographeo Johannis Goebelii [1663]

32 p.   19 cm.   [6750]
Diss.—Altdorf.

—*See* FRÖLING, A., *praeses.* De qualitatibus primis dissertatio physica. 1658.

LECLERC, CHARLES GABRIEL [1644-1700?] L'appareil commode en faveur des jeunes chirurgiens . . . Paris, Jean Baptiste Delespine, 1700.

[16], 5-319, [1] p.   plates.   15 cm.   [6751]

—Another issue, with imprint: Paris, La veuve d'Estienne Michallet, 1700.   [6752]
Title page reset. Table and Privilege bound at end.

—L'ecole du chirurgien; ou, Les principes de la chirurgie francoise. Tirez de la connoissance du corps humain en toutes ses parties, de l'explication de ses maladies exterieures, & des operations pour les guerir

. . . Par G[abriel] C[harles] L[e] C[lerc] . . . Paris, Estienne Michallet, 1684.

[16], 138 (i.e. 140) p.   16 cm.   [6753]
Bound with La Charrière, J. de. Traité des operations de chirurgie. 1690.

—[English ed.] The compleat surgeon; or, The whole art of surgery explain'd in a most familiar method. Containing an exact account of its principles and several parts . . . To which is added, a chirurgical dispensatory . . . Written in French . . . and translated into English. London, M. Gillyflower, T. Goodwin, M. Wotton, J. Walthoe, and R. Parker, 1696.

[10], 341, 17 p.   16 cm.   [6754]
Imperfect: first preliminary leaf (blank?) wanting.

—[German tr.] Die . . . gefertigte vollkommene Chirurgie, oder: Wund-Artzney-Kunst, nach Innhalt ihrer Principiorum: der Osteologie, Myologie, menschlichen Zufällen, mit Application aller Gebände und Zubereitungen bey Brüchen und Verrenckungen; auch aller chirurgischen operationum, nebenst einer Pharmacie, und Methode, die mercurialische Panacée zubereiten. In das Teutsche übersetzt, und zum andern Mahle gedruckt. Dresden, Johann Jacob Winckler, 1699.

[11], 430, [18] p.   17 cm.   [6755]
Added engraved title page dated 1696.

—La medecine aisée, contenant plusieurs remedes faciles & expérimentez pour toute sorte de maladies internes & externes: avec une Petite pharmacie commode & facile à faire à toute sorte de personnes . . . Paris, Estienne Michallet, 1696.

[22], 376, 56 p.   17 cm.   [6756]

—[The same.] . . . Paris, Estienne Michallet, 1697.

[16], 360, 56 p.   16 cm.   [6757]

LE CLERC, DANIEL [1652-1728] Bibliotheca anatomica; sive, Recens in anatomia inventorum thesaurus locupletissimus . . . Adjecta est partium omnium administratio anatomica, cum variis earundem praeparationibus curiosissimis. Digesserunt, tractatus suppleverunt, argumenta . . . addiderunt Daniel Le Clerc & J. Jacobus Mangetus . . . Tomus primus [-secondus] Genevae, Sumptibus Joannis Anthonii Chovët, 1685.

2 v.   front., illus., plates.   38 cm.   [6758]

—Another issue. 37 cm.   [6759]

Different setting of type on p. [17] vol. 1.
Imperfect: front. and plate IV (vol. 1); plate LXXXII and LXXXIII (vol. 2) wanting.

—[The same.] ... Ed. 2, novis tractatibus, notis ac observationibus, tertia ad minimum parte, priore auctior ... Tomus primus [-secundus] Genevae, Sumptibus Johan. Anthon. Chouët & Davidis Ritter, 1699.

     2 v. illus., plates. 36 cm.   [6760]

—Histoire de la medecine ou l'on void l'origine & le progrés de cet art ... Par D[aniel] L[e] C[lerc] D. M. Geneve, J. A. Chouët & D. Ritter, 1696.

     [22], 694 p. 16 cm.   [6761]

Part 1 only.

—[English tr.] The history of physick, or, an account of the rise and progress of the art ... With remarks on the lives of the most eminent physicians. Written originally in French ... and made English by Dr. Drake and Dr. Baden ... London, D. Brown, A. Roper, T. Leigh and D. Midwinter, 1699.

     [22], 411 p. 20 cm.   [6762]

—*See* SCHELHAMMER, G. C. De lymphae ortu et lymphaticorum vasorum causis. 1683.

LE CLERC, ÉTIENNE [1599-1676] *ed. See* FOES, A. Oeconomia Hippocratis alphabeti serie distincta. 1662.

LECLERC, G. CHARLES. *See* LECLERC, Charles Gabriel [1644-1700?]

LECLERC, GABRIEL. *See* LECLERC, Charles Gabriel [1644-1700?]

LE CLERC, JEAN [1657-1736] Physica; sive, De rebus corporeis libri quinque, in quibus, praemissis potissimis corporearum naturarum phaenomenis & proprietatibus, veterum & recentiorum de eorum causis celeberrimae conjecturae traduntur ... Amstelodami, Apud Georgium Gallet, 1696.

     [24], 492, [4] p. 16 cm.   [6763]

LE CLERC, SÉBASTIEN [1637-1714] Discours touchant le point de veue, dans lequel il est prouvé que les choses qu'on voit distinctement, ne sont veuës que d'un oeil ... Paris, Thomas Jolly, 1679.

     [12], 86 p. illus. 16 cm.   [6764]

LE CLERCQZ, GABRIEL. Discursus succinctus phisico-medicus de morbis pauperum. Insulis, Ex officina Joannis Chrysostomi Malte, 1683.

     [10], 209, [1] p. 15 cm.   [6765]

Imperfect: sig. A1 wanting.

L'ÉCLUSE, CHARLES DE [1526-1609] Curae posteriores; seu, Plurimarum non ante cognitarum, aut descriptarum stirpium, peregrinorumque aliquot animalium novae descriptiones ... Accessit seorsim Everardi Vorstii ... Caroli Clusii vita & obitu oratio, aliorumque epicedia. [Lugduni Batavorum] In Officina Plantiniana Raphelengii, 1611.

     2 v. 23 cm.   [6766]

—Caroli Clusii ... Exoticorum libri decem, quibus animalium, plantarum, aromatum, aliorumque peregrinorum fructuum historiae describuntur. Item Petri Bellonii Observationes, eodem Carolo Clusio interprete ... [Lugduni Batavorum] Ex Officina Plantiniana Raphelengii, 1605.

     [16], 378, [9], 52, [42], 3-242, [1] p. illus. 36 cm.   [6767]

Pritzel 1760* (Antwerpiae)
Hunt 182.

—Caroli Clusii ... Rariorum plantarum historia ... Antwerpiae, Ex Officina Plantiniana, apud Joannem Moretum, 1601.

     [12], 364, cccxlviii, [11] p. illus., port. 37 cm.   [6768]

Engraved title page.
Portrait wanting.
"Honorii Belli ... ad Carolum Clusium aliquot epistolae, de rarioribus quibusdam plantis agentes" (p. [ccxcvii]-cccxiiii) has half title. "Epistola Thobiae Roelsii ad Carolum Clusium": p. cccxv-cccxx.
Pritzel 1759*
Hunt 180, variant state. Cf. M. Guédès. Notules de bibliographie botanique V. J. Soc. bibliog. nat. hist. vol. 6, pt. 3 (Oct. 1972) p. 174-175.

—, *tr. See* MONARDES, N. Ein nützlich und lustig Gespräche. 1615.

—*See* DODOENS, R. Cruydt-boeck. 1618, 1644; ORTA, G. d'. Histoire des drogues. 1602, 1619; [Italian tr.] 1605, 1616; RAY, J. Stirpium Europaearum extra Britannias nascentium sylloge. 1694; VORSTIUS, A. E. Oratio funebris in obitum ... Caroli Clusii. 1611.

L'ÉCLUSE, JULES CHARLES DE. *See* L'ÉCLUSE, Charles de [1526-1609]

LE COMTE, PIERRE [*fl.* 1617] Declaration . . . pour monstrer la fausseté de l'advis faict a messieurs les gens du Roy, sur la construction d'un theatre anatomique, par un qui a supprimé son nom . . . [Parisiis, 1617]

18 p.   22 cm.   [6769]

LE CONTE, JEAN [*fl.* 17th cent.] *tr. See* HELMONT, J. B. van. Les oeuvres. 1670, 1671.

LE CONTE, JOHANNES FRANCISCUS [*fl.* 17th cent.] Opuscula nova medica. Nunc primum edita . . . Francofurti & Lipsiae, 1690.

560, [22] p.   18 cm.   [6770]

LEDBERG, JACOB [1672-1731] Specimen physiologicum de coloribus . . . Hafniae, Literis Joh. Phil. Bockenhoffer [1690]

[2], 54 p.   18 cm.   [6771]

LEDDIN, JOHANN AUGUST [*fl.* 1689-1696] *respondent. See* VEHR, I., *praeses.* Disputationem inauguralem medicam, qua casus aegri sanguinam vomentis, resolutus sistitur . . . submittit J. A. L. . . . 1696.

LEDEL, SAMUEL [*d.* 1714] Grünbergischer Pest-Rath, allen verlangenden Ständen zur treuen Vorsorge fürgestellet . . . Züllichow, Michael Schwartzen, 1680.

[8], 57, [3] p.   18 cm.   [6772]

—*respondent. See* FRIDERICI, J. A., *praeses.* Dissertatio inauguralis medica de pica. 1668; GRUBE, H., *praeses.* Conflictus academicus de temperamento. 1666; SCHENCK, J. T., *praeses.* Dissertatio medica de phrenitide. 1667.

L'EDELPHE. *See* PLANIS CAMPY, David de [*b.* 1589]

LEDERER, JOHANN ERNST [*fl.* 1652-1654] *respondent.* Medica dissertatio de peste . . . Basileae, Typis Georgii Deckeri [1654]

[12] p.   20 cm.   [6773]
Diss. — Basel.

LEDESMA, ANTONIO COLMENERO DE. *See* COLMENERO DE LEDESMA, Antonio [16th-17th cent.]

LE DOUX, GASTON. *See* CLAVES, Gaston Le Doux, *known as* Gaston de [*b. ca.* 1530]

LEE, WILLEM VAN DER [*fl.* 1653] *respondent.* Disputatio medica inauguralis περὶ τῆς λευκοφλεγματιας . . . Lugduni Batavorum, Apud Johannem Meyer, 1653.

[12] p.   23 cm.   [6774]
Diss.—Leyden.

LEEMANN, BURKHARD [1531-1613] Instrumentum instrumentorum: horologiorum sciotericorum. Erstlich werdend gelehrt uffryssen die vier hauptsonnen Uhren ohne einiche Verenderung dess Circkels, ussgenommen was das Fundament anlagt. Darnach wie man durch diss nüw . . . Instrument, uffryssen möge, nit allein gemelte vier haupt, sonder allerley sort Sonnenuhren . . . nüwlich beschriben und Tag geben, durch B. L. Zürych, 1604.

9, [1] ll.   illus., plate.   20 cm.   [6775]
Bound with Bartisch, G. Warhafftige . . . Beschreibung. 1602.

LEENMANS, ANTON [*fl.* 1669] *respondent.* Disputatio medica inauguralis de dysenteria . . . Lugduni Batavorum, Apud viduam & haeredes Joannis Elsevirii, 1669.

[7] p.   23 cm.   [6776]
Diss.—Leyden.

LEEUW, ALARDUS DE [*fl.* 1687] *respondent.* Disputatio medica inauguralis, de convulsione . . . Trajecti ad Rhenum, Ex officina Francisci Halma, 1687.

14, [2] p.   22 cm.   [6777]

LEEUW, JACOB [*fl.* 1680] *tr. See* BROWNE, E. Naukeurige en gedenkwaardige reysen. 1682; Lancillotti, C. De brandende salamander. 1680.

LEEUWENHOEK, ANTHONY VAN [1632-1723] Ontdeckte onsigtbaarheeden. [Lugduni Batavorum: Cornelis Boutesteyn, Joh. Arnold. Langerack; Delft: Henrik van Kroonevelt, Andries Voorstad, Adriaan Beman] 1685-1718.

5 v.   illus., plates, port.   21 cm.   [6778]
Title from added engraved general title page.
Vols. 3 and 5 have added engraved title pages.
Dobell number of works: vol. 1: 8, 2, 5a, 6, 7, 9; vol. 2: 10a, 12, 13; vol. 3: 14, 15, 16; vol. 4: 18; vol. 5: 19. Items have special title pages.
In vol. 1, between the first and second part of no. 8, there is a later edition of Dobell 1 inserted, printed in Delft by Henrik van Kroonevelt in 1694, (10, 29–60 p.)
Imperfect: p. [1-2], 9-16 of part [1] and part [2] of vol. 1, no. 2, wanting.

—[The same.] ... Lugduni Batavorum, C. Boutesteyn [Joh. Arnold, Langerack; Delft: Henrik van Kroonevelt, Adriaan Beman] 1694-1718 [v. 1, 1696] 6 v. front. (port.), illus., plates. 21 cm. **[6779]**

General engraved title page.
Vols.4 and 6 have added engraved title pages.
Dobell number of works: vol. 1: 8a, 2a, 5b, 6a, 7a, 9a; vol. 2: 10b, 12a; vol. 3: 13, 14; vol. 4: 15, 16; vol. 5: 18; vol. 6: 19. Items have special title pages.
In vol. 1, between the first and second part of no. 8a, there is a later edition of Dobell 1 inserted, printed in Delft by Henrik van Kroonevelt in 1694, (10, 29-60 p.)
With vol. 6 of this is bound Bidloo, G. Brief ... aan Antony van Leeuwenhoek. 1698.

—Ondervindingen en beschouwingen der onsigbare geschapene waarheden, waar in gehandeld werd vande eyerstok ... Geschreven aande ... Koninklyke Societeit in Engeland ... Leyden, Daniel van Gaesbeeck, 1684.
[1], 21 p. illus. 20 cm. **[6780]**
Dobell 4.

—Anatomia et contemplatio nonnullorum naturae invisibilium secretorum comprehensorum epistolis quibusdam scriptis ad ... Societatis Regiae Londinensis Collegium ... Lugd. Batavorum, Apud Cornelium Boutesteyn, 1685.
78 p. illus. 19 cm. **[6781]**
Dobell 21.

—Anatomia; seu, Interiora rerum, cum animatarum tum inanimatarum, ope & beneficio exquisitissimorum microscopiorum detecta, variisque experimentis demonstrata, una cum discursu & ulteriore dilucidatione epistolis quibusdam ad ... philosophorum collegium datis comprehensa ... Lugduni Batavorum, Apud Cornelium Boutesteyn, 1687.
[8], 3-78, 258 (i.e. 260) p. illus., plates. 19 cm. **[6782]**

Added engraved title page: Epistolae ... 1685.
Imperfect: upper margin of title page trimmed.
Dobell 23.

—Continuatio epistolarum, datarum ad ... Regiam Societatem Londinensem ... Lugduni Batavorum, Apud Cornelium Boutestein, 1689.
[8], 124 p. illus., plates. 20 cm. **[6783]**
Dobell 24.

—[The same.] ... Ed. alt. Lugduni Batavorum, Apud Cornelium Boutestein, 1696.
[1], 124 p. illus., plates. 20 cm. **[6784]**
Dobell 24a.
Bound with *his* Arcana naturae. 1696.

—Arcana naturae detecta ... Delphis Batavorum, Apud Henricum a Krooneveld, 1695.
[9], 568, [14] p. front. (port.), illus., plates. 20 cm. **[6785]**
Added engraved title page.
Dobell 25.

—Another issue. **[6786]**
Pages 15-16 repeated; p. 16 has different setting of type; first two preliminary leaves reversed.

—Arcana naturae, ope & beneficio exquisitissimorum microscopiorum. Detecta, variisque experimentis demonstrata, una cum discursu & ulteriori dilucidatione; epistolis suis ad ... philosophorum collegium datis, comprehensa ... Ed. alt. Lugduni Batavorum, Apud Cornelium Boutestein, 1696.
[12], 58 (i.e. 64), 258 (i.e. 260) p. illus., plates. 20 cm. **[6787]**
Added engraved title page: Investigatio arcanorum.
Dobell 25a.
With this is bound *his* Continuatio epistolarum. 1696.

—Continuatio arcanorum naturae detectorum, qua continetur quicquid hactenus ab auctore lingua vernacula editum, & in linguam Latinam transfusum non fuit. Delphis Batavorum, Apud Henricum a Kroonevelt, 1697.
[1], 192, [8] p. plates. 20 cm. **[6788]**
Dobell 26.

—Observations sur le sang et sur le lait. *In* [Grew, N.] Recueil d'experiences et observations sur le combat, qui procede du mélange des corps. 1679.

—*See* BIDLOO, G. Brief ... aan Antony van Leeuwenhoek. 1698; HOOKE, R. Lectures and collections. 1678.

LE FEBVRE. *See* LE FÈVRE.

LEFER, DANIEL [*fl.* 1684] *respondent.* Disputatio inauguralis de ischuria ... Lugduni Batavorum, Apud Abrahamum Elzevier, 1684.
[16] p. 22 cm. **[6789]**
Diss.—Leyden.

LE FÈVRE, NICOLAS [*ca.* 1610–1669?] Traicté de la chymie. Tome premier [-second] . . . Paris, Thomas Jolly, 1660.

　　2 v. ([30], 510 p.; [3], 511–1092, [18] p.) plates. 18 cm. 　　　　　　　　　　　　　　　[6790]
First volume has added engraved title page.

　　—[The same.] . . . Corrigé de plusieurs fautes. Suivant la copie imprimé à Paris. Paris, Leyde, Arnoud Doude [Et se vendent chez Corneille Driehuysen] 1669.

　　2 v. ([66], 556 p.; [3], 557–1216, [21] p.) plates. 14 cm. 　　　　　　　　　　　　　　　[6791]
Added engraved title pages.

[English tr.] A compleat body of chymistry . . . comprehending in general the whole practice thereof, and teaching the most exact preparation of animals, vegetables and minerals, so as to preserve their essential vertues . . . Rendered into English by P. D. C. Esq. [i.e. Pierre de Cardonnel?] . . . Part. I. [-The second part] London, Printed by Tho. Ratcliffe for Octavian Pulleyn junior, 1664.

　　[12], 312, [7] p.; [1], 364, [8] p. plates. 21 cm. 　　　　　　　　　　　　　　　[6792]
Part 2 has special title page.

　　—[The same.] . . . With additions. London, Printed for O. Pulleyn junior, and sold by John Wright, 1670.

　　[12], 286, [6] p.; 320, [8] p. plates. 20 cm. 　　　　　　　　　　　　　　　[6793]
Part 2 has special title page and imprint: London, Printed by J. D. for John Wright, 1670.

　　—[German tr.] Neuvemehrter chymischer Handleiter, und guldnes Kleinod; das ist, Deutliche Unterweisung, wie man die von chymischer Wissenschafft ins gemein handelende Schrifften recht verstehen, und nach Ordnung der spagyrischen und apothekerischen Bereit-Kunst die darzu erforderte würckliche Operation gebührlich verrichten . . . müsse. Vormals . . . frantzösisch beschrieben . . . anjetzo aber . . . mit vielen spagyrischen Secreten . . . vermehret, worzu bey dieser neuen Edition noch kommt . . . Beschreib- und Erklärung der grossen Hertz-Stärckung dess Ritters Rawlichs . . . alles zum andernmal in den Druck gegeben worden von Joh. Hiskis Cardilucio . . . Nürnberg, In Verlegung Joh. Andreae Endters sel. Söhne, 1685.

　　[54], 1149, [19] p. plates. 17 cm. 　　[6794]
Added engraved title page: Chymisches Kleinod.

　　—Discours sur le grand cordial de Sr Walter Rawleigh . . . Londre, Octavian Pulleyn le jeune, 1665.

　　[15], 105 p. 15 cm. 　　　　　　　　　[6795]

　　—[English tr.] A discourse upon Sr. Walter Rawleigh's great cordial . . . Rendered into English by Peter Belon . . . London, Printed by J. F. for Octavian Pulleyn junior, 1664.

　　[18], 110 p. 16 cm. 　　　　　　　　　[6796]

　　—, *tr. See* BROWNE, *Sir* T. La religion du medecin. 1668.

　　—*See* DIGBY, *Sir* K. Medicina experimentalis Digbaeana. 1672–1676, 1687.

LE FÈVRE, TANNEGUY [1615–1672] *See* LUCRETIUS CARUS, Titus. De rerum natura libri sex. 1686.

LE GALLOIS, PIERRE [*fl.* 1672–1680] *ed. See* BOURDELOT, P. Conversations de l'Academie. 1672.

LEGANGER, IVARUS [*fl.* 1650] *respondent. See* BARTHOLIN, T., *praeses.* Collegii Anatomici disputatio quinta de epate et bilis receptaculis. 1650.

LEGATI, LORENZO [*d.* 1675] Museo Cospiano annesso a quello del famoso Ulisse Aldrovandi e donato alla sua patria dall'illustrissimo signor Ferdinando Cospi . . . march. di Petriolo . . . Descrizione di Lorenzo Legati . . . Bologna, Giacomo Monti, 1677.

　　[24], 532 p. illus., plates. port. 34 cm. 　　　　　　　　　　　　　　　[6797]

LE GIVRE, PIERRE [1618–1684] Le secret des eaux minerales acides . . . Avec les lettres de monsieur de Sartes . . . & de monsieur Cattier . . . qui combattent l'opinion de l'autheur, ausquelles il rêpond . . . Paris, Jean Ribou, 1667.

　　[20], 370, [1] p. 16 cm. 　　　　　　　[6798]

　　—[Latin tr.] Arcanum acidularum . . . Additae sunt epistolae multorum illustrium medicorum cum ejusdem responsis . . . Amstelodami, Apud Janssonio-Waesbergios, 1682.

　　[8], 366, [5] p. 13 cm. 　　　　　　　[6799]

　　—Traité des eaux minerales de Provins, contenant leur anatomie, la difference des fontaines, leurs proprietez . . . avec le regime de vivre qu'il faut observer en beuvant de ces eaux . . . Paris, Charles du Mesnil, 1659.

　　[13], 128 p. 18 cm. 　　　　　　　　　[6800]
Includes correspondence with Antoine de Sartes.

LE GRAND, Antoine [*d.* 1699] Curiosus rerum abditarum naturaeque arcanorum perscrutator; sive, Compendium rerum jucundarum, & memorabilium, in quo naturae arcana, multae rerum sympathiae & antipathiae, & auctoris observationes reserantur . . . Francofurti, 1681.

348, [31] p. 14 cm. [6801]

—Dissertatio de carentia sensus & cognitionis in brutis . . . Lugduni Batavorum, Apud Arnoldum Doude, et Felicem Lopez, 1675.

139, [5] p. 17 cm. [6802]

—[The same.] . . . Londini, Apud J. Martyn, 1675.

[9], 106 (i.e. 206), [10] p. 13 cm. [6803]

Errata: sig. A6.

—Historia naturae, variis experimentis & ratiociniis elucidata. Secundum principia stabilita in Institutione philosophiae edita . . . Londini, J. Martyn, 1673.

[24], 416, [15] p. front., illus. 18 cm. [6804]

—[The same.] . . . Norimbergae, Impensis Johannis Ziegeri, typis Christophori Gerhardi, 1678.

[14], 445, [18] p. front., illus. 17 cm. [6805]

—[The same.] . . . Ed. 2. priori auctior. Londini, Apud J. Martin, 1680.

[12], 431, [15] p. front. (port.), front., illus. 21 cm. [6806]

—[Philosophia veterum e mente Renati Descartes. English.] An entire body of philosophy, according to the principles of the famous Renate Des Cartes, in three books: I. The institution, in X. parts. . . . II. The history of nature . . . in IX. parts . . . III. A dissertation of the want of sense and knowledge in brute animals, in II. parts . . . Written originally in Latin . . . now . . . translated from the last corrections . . . and large additions of the author never yet published . . . By Richard Blome. London, Printed by Samuel Roycroft, and sold by Richard Blome, 1694.

[31], 403 p.; [3], 263 p. front., plates. 35 cm. [6807]

—*See* Rohault, J. Tractatus physicus. 1682.

LEHENHERR, Daniel [*fl.* 1685] *respondent.* Dissertatio medica inauguralis de vomitoriis . . . Basileae, Typis Jacobi Bertschii [1685]

[20] p. 19 cm. [6808]

Diss. — Basel.

LEHMAN, Samuel. Concentrirtes, das ist, von sehr vielen Polychrestis, Arcanen, Panaceen und raren Specificis welt-berühmter Medicorum practicorum, in die Enge verfassetes und zu genungsamer Beschützung und Unterhaltung menschlicher Gesundheit, in fünff Universal-Stücken, als I. Schweiss-oder Reise-Pillen, II. Brech-Pillen, III. Purgir-Pillen, IV. Güldene Ancker, V. Wunder-Pflaster betehendes Reise-Apothecklein . . . Lissa, Gedruckt durch Michael Bukken, 1679.

32 p. 21 cm. [6809]

LEHMANN, Christian Gottfried [*b.* 1674] *respondent. See* Wedel, G. W., *praes.* Dissertatio inauguralis medica de defectu lactis. 1699.

—*See* Slevogt, J. A. Decani Facultatis Medicae Jo. Hadriani Slevogtii . . . invitatio publica ad dissertationem inauguralem de defectu lactis. 1699.

LEHMANN, Christoph [*fl.* 1685] *respondent. See* Major, J. D., *praes.* Disquisitionem medicam . . . de moribundorum regimine, ubi incidenter quaedam de recte ferendis vulnerum judicis . . . habendam intimat . . . C. L. 1685.

LEHMANN, Gottlob [*fl.* 1698] *praeses.* De apotheosi naturae dissertationem priorem ex historia naturali . . . defendere constituit Gotthelf Schütze . . . Vitembergae, Stanno Hakiano [1698]

[16] p. 19 cm. [6810]

Diss. — Wittenberg (G. Schütze, *respondent*)

LEHMANN, Immanuel [*fl.* 1666] *respondent. See* Kirchmajer, S., *praes.* Exercitationem physicam de indiciis in inquisitione venarum metallicarum observandis . . . submittit . . . I. L. 1666.

LEHMANN, Joachim Gottlieb [*fl.* 1689-1691] *respondent. See* Berger, J. G. von, *praes.* Dissertationem inauguralem de ischuria . . . p. p. . . . J. G. L. 1691; *See* Bohn, J., *praes.* Disputatio physiologica. 1689.

LEHMANN, Johann Christian [1675–1739] *praeses.* Disputationem physicam de transmutationibus corporum extraordinariis . . . Joh. Christianus Lehmann . . . et . . . Andreas Bretag . . . exponent. Lipsiae, Stanno Christophori Fleischeri [1697]

[32] p.   20 cm.   **[6811]**

Diss. – Leipzig (A. Bretag, *respondent*)

—*respondent. See* Bohn, J., *praeses.* De medici officio dissertatio prima. 1697; Schamberg, J. C., *praeses.* Disputationem inauguralem medicam de peripneumonia . . . submittit . . . J. C. L. 1698.

LEHMANN, Johann Friedrich [*fl.* 1668–1672] *respondent. See* Rolfinck, W., *praeses.* Dissertatio medica inauguralis de catarrho ad nares. 1672.

LEHNE, Georg [*fl.* 1652] *respondent. See* Hoppius, C., *praeses.* Disputatio physica de principiis corporum naturalium. 1652.

Der LEIB- und Land-Medicus armer Leute. 1682. *See* Regnans, I., *ed.*

LEIBNIZ, Gottfried Wilhelm, *Freiherr von* [1646–1716] *See* Stisser, J. A. De variis erroribus. 1700.

LEICH Ordnung. *See* Nuremberg. Ordinances, local laws, etc. Verneuerte Leich Ordnung der Statt Nürmberg. 1625, 1662.

LEICHNER, Eckard [1612–1690] De generatione; seu, Propagativa animalium, plantarum & mineralium multiplicatione in genere exercitationes physicae anti-peripateticae XX. tredecim in Acad. Erfurtina antehac publice habitis disputationibus comprehensae, quarum postrema humanae animae traductionem adversus omnes contradicentium strophas . . . demonstrat . . . Erfurti, Typis Spangenbergicis, 1649.

[308] p.   20 cm.   **[6812]**

—De indivisibili & totali cujusque animae in toto suo corpore & singulis ejus partibus existentia, dissertatio tripartita . . . Erfurti, Impensis Johann Birckneri, typis Pauli Michaelis, 1650.

[142] p.   14 cm.   **[6813]**

—De motu sanguinis exercitatio anti-Harveiana. Arnstadiae, Impensis Johan. Birckneri, excusa typis Petri Smid, 1645.

[252] p.   14 cm.   **[6814]**

—De principiis medicis epistola apologetica ad illustre medicorum in Acad. Lipsiensi collegium, pro archeo synoptico contra pseudarchaeum syncopticum Pauli Ammanni scripta . . . Erffurti, Typis Kirschianis, 1675.

[2], 162, [1] p.   13 cm.   **[6815]**

—Epicrisis medico-analytica, super undecim dispp. medicis Francisci de Le Boe Sylvii. Erffurti, Typis Carol-Christiani Kirschii, 1676.

[42], 325, [4] p.   13 cm.   **[6816]**

Dissertations — Erfurt

—*praeses.* De calido innato exercitatio II . . . Erffurti, Typis Pauli Michaëlis, 1649.

[28] p.   19 cm.   **[6817]**

Signatures: ( )², C-E⁴.
Originally issued with Exercitatio I.
C. H. Wagner, *respondent.*

—De mensium suppressione dissertatio inauguralis . . . Erfordiae, Stanno Groschiano [1684]

[32] p.   19 cm.   **[6818]**

J. C. Altmann, *respondent.*

—Disputatio inauguralis medica, de cholera humida . . . [Erfurti] Stanno Hertziano [1670]

[32] p.   19 cm.   **[6819]**

J. A. Hermann, *respondent.*

—Disputatio medica inauguralis de dysenteria . . . Erfordiae, Stanno Kirschiano [1678]

[24] p.   19 cm.   **[6820]**

J. K. Westphal, *respondent.*

—Disputatio medica inauguralis de mania . . . Erffurti, Typis Kirschianis [1674]

[24]   19 cm.   **[6821]**

J. Z. Fürst, *respondent.*

—Dissertatio inauguralis, casum matronae hypochondriacae exhibens . . . Erfordiae, Typis Groschianis [1685]

24 p.   19 cm.   **[6822]**

J. C. Below, *respondent.*

—Dissertatio inauguralis medica de apoplexia . . . Erfordiae, Stanno Groschiano [1690]

28 p.   20 cm.   **[6823]**

J. Ziedler, *respondent.*

—Dissertatio inauguralis medica de catarrho . . . Erfordiae, Typis Johann-Henrici Groschii [1690]

16 p. 20 cm. [6824]

C. L. Reinesius, *respondent.*

—Dissertatio inauguralis medica de chlorosi . . . Erfordiae, Typis Joh. Henrici Groschii [1688]

24 p. 19 cm. [6825]

T. Altermann, *respondent.*

—Dissertationem de podagra . . . submittet Fridericus Cramer . . . Erfurti, Typis Kirschianis [1675]

[22] p. 18 cm. [6826]

F. Cramer, *respondent.*

—Dissertationem inauguralem de cancro . . . publico eruditorum examini sistit . . . Johannes Godofredus Schuckius . . . Erfordiae, Typis Johann-Henrici Groschii [1687]

22 p. 19 cm. [6827]

J. G. Schuck, *respondent.*

—Dissertationem inauguralem de . . . υστερομανια . . . offert . . . Johannes Unsenius . . . Erffurti, Literis Johannis Bernhardi Michaelis [1671]

28 p. 19 cm. [6828]

J. Unsen, *respondent.*

—Manus Dei funestissima, lues pestifera . . . Erfurti, Literis Kirschianis [1682]

[28] p. 19 cm. [6829]

J. Rösser, *respondent.*

—*respondent. See* SEBISCH, M. [1578-1674?] *praeses.* Collegii therapeutici disputatio I[-XIV] 1634 [i.e. 1635]

—*See* AMMANN, P. Consilium. 1693; VALENTINUS, J. Curriculum analyticum. 1673.

LEICKER, KARL JAKOB [b. 1663] *respondent. See* WEDEL, G. W., *praeses.* Disputatio medica inauguralis de bile ejusque morbis. 1689.

—*See* FASCH, A. H. Augustinus Henricus Faschius . . . Facultatis Medicae X. decanus S. P. D. benevolo lectori! 1689.

LEICKHER, CAROLUS JACOBUS. *See* LEICKER, Karl Jakob [b. 1663]

LEIDENFROST, JULIUS WERNER [*fl.* 1675] *See* SAGITTARIUS, C., *praeses.* De nudipedalibus veterum. 1675.

LEIGH, CHARLES [1662-1701?] Exercitationes quinque 1. De aquis mineralibus. 2. De thermis calidis. 3. De morbis acutis. 4. De morbis intermittentib. 5. De hydrope . . . Oxonii, Typis L. Lichfiel, impensis Ephr. Johnson & T. Bennet, 1697.

[16], 156 p. 19 cm. [6830]

—Phthisiologia Lancastriensis, cui accessit Tentamen philosophicum de mineralibus aquis in eodem comitatu observatis . . . Londini, Impensis Sam. Smith & Benj. Walford, 1694.

[9], 143, [1] p. 18 cm. [6831]

—*See* BOULTON, R. An examination of Mr. John Colbatch his books. 1699.

LEIPZIG. Ordinances, local laws, etc. Ordnung eines erbarn hochweisen Raths der Stadt Leipzig. Wessen sich ein jeder Bürger und Einwohner . . . der Stadt, so wol die jenigen, so auff die inficirten Häuser und kranck darnieder ligende Personen in Sterbensleufften bestellet, allenthalben verhalten sollen . . . [Leipzig] Michael Lantzenberger, 1607.

[62] p. 20 cm. [6832]

—Raths der Stadt Leipzig vor die Apotheken daselbst aussgerichtete und von Churf. Durchl. zu Sachsen . . . confirmirte Ordnung und Taxa. Leipzig, Verlegts Friedrich Lanckischens Erben [1689]

[5], 105, [5] p. 24 cm. [6833]

Added engraved title page.

LEIPZIG. Universität. *See* UNIVERSITÄT LEIPZIG.

LEIPZIGER Pest-Schade und Gottes Gnade; das ist, Nachricht von dem Anfange, Fortgange, Abnehmen, Cur und Beschaffenheit der bissher hin und wieder herumb gezogenen, und zu Leipzig auch besonders in verflossenen 1680 Jahre aussgestandenen pestilentzischen Seuche; worbey auch ein Abriss eines Schwitzkastens oder Stübgens . . . ist auffgesetzet . . . Leipzig, In Verlegung Gottfried Dehnens, Altenburg, Gedruckt bey Conrad Rügern, 1681.

[100] p. plate. 19 cm. [6834]

Preface by C. W. D., the author.

LEISNER, KARL CHRISTIAN [b. 1663] *respondent. See* WEDEL, G. W., *praeses.* Dissertatio medica inauguralis de circulatione sanguinis. 1696; WOLF, Jakob, *praeses.* Dissertatio medica de obesitate exsuperante. 1683.

—*See* SLEVOGT, J. A. Decani Facultatis Medicae Jo. Hadr. Slevogtii ... prolusio inauguralis de motore cordis. 1696.

LEISSNER, CAROLUS CHRISTIANUS. *See* LEISNER, Karl Christian [*b.* 1663]

LEITÃO, MANOEL. *See* LEYTAM, Manoel.

LEIVA Y AGUILAR, FRANCISCO DE. Desengaño contra el mal uso del tabaco; tocanse varias lecciones y tratanse al intento, muchas dudas: con resolución las nuevas, con novedad las antiguas ... Cordova, Por Salvador de Cea Tesa, 1634.

[8], 278, [18] ll.   20 cm.   **[6835]**

Imperfect: ll. 184 wanting.

[LE JEUNE DE BOULENCOURT] Description generale de l'hostel royal des Invalides établi par Louis le Grand dans la plaine de Grenelle près Paris. Avec les plans, profils & elevations de ses faces, coupes & appartemens. Paris, Chez l'auteur [De l'imprimerie de Gabriel Martin] 1683.

[8], 51 p.   front., plates.   45 cm.   **[6836]**

Espistre signed: L[e] J[eune] D[e] B[oulencourt]

LE LONG, MICHEL [*d.* 1642] *ed.* and *tr. See* HIPPOCRATES. Les sept livres d'Aphorismes. 1645; REGIMEN SANITATIS SALERNITANUM. Le regime de santé de l'Eschole de Salerne. 1633, 1637, 1643, 1649, 1660.

LE LORRAIN, PIERRE, *abbé de Vallemont. See* VALLEMONT, Pierre Le Lorrain, *abbé de* [1649-1721]

LE LORRAIN DE VALLEMONT, PIERRE. *See* VALLEMONT, Pierre Le Lorrain, *abbé de* [1649-1721]

LE LOYER, PIERRE, *sieur de La Brosse* [1550-1634] Discours, et histoires des spectres, visions et apparitions des esprits, anges, demons ... Divisez en huict livres ... Aussi est traicté des extases et ravissemens ... des magiciens & sorciers ... ensemble des remedes pour se preserver des illusions & impostures diaboliques ... Paris, Chez Nicolas Buon [Imprimer par Pierre Vitray & heureux Blanvilain] 1605.

[26], 976, [39] p.   25 cm.   **[6837]**

—A treatise of specters or straunge sights, visions and apparitions appearing sensibly unto men. Wherein is delivered, the nature of spirites, angels, and divels ... witches, sorcerers ... Newly done out of French ... London, Printed by Val. S. for Mathew Lownes, 1605.

[8], 145 ll.   20 cm.   **[6838]**

Imperfect: Errata (ll. [146]) wanting.

Translation of IIII. livres des spectres, by Zachary Jones. STC 15448.

LE MAIRE, ANTOINE [*fl.* 1684] *tr. See* KHUNRATH, K. Traité des vertus de l'esprit de sel philosophique. 1686.

LE MAISTRE, RODOLPHE [*d. ca.* 1632] Doctrina Hippocratis. Aphorismi: nova interpretatione ac methodo exornati. Leges medicinae. Arcana judicia. Limites hum[ani] partus. Patrocinium. Authore Rodolpho Magistro ... Parisiis, Excudebat Edmundus Martinus, cura & expensis authoris, 1613.

[20], 429 p.   15 cm.   **[6839]**

Pages [3-6], containing a French version of the dedicatory epistle to King Louis XIII, are printed on a fold inserted between title page and the Latin version.

Includes Greek and Latin texts of Hippocrates' Aphorismi and of the Hippocratic extracts in "Arcana judicia."

"Limites humani partus" and "Patrocinium" were published together in Nîmes in 1591 under title: De temporibus humani partus, Rodolphi Magistri ... liber ... Ejusdem Apologia medicinae.

—Another issue, with imprint: Parisiis, Ex Officina Nivelliana, apud Sebastianum Cramoisy, 1613.   **[6840]**

The title page is a cancel, with the spelling "autore" instead of "authore" in author statement.

—Another issue.   16 cm.   **[6841]**

The title page is a cancel, with slight typographical differences from that of the preceding issue.

Without p. [3-6] and [19-20]

—Le preservatif des fievres malignes de ce temps ... Paris, La vefue Abel L'Angelier, 1616.

7, 93, [1] p.   14 cm.   **[6842]**

LEMAÎTRE, RODOLPHE. *See* LE MAISTRE, Rodolphe [*d. ca.* 1632]

LEMBKA, MARTIN [*fl.* 1604] *respondent. See* STUPANUS, J. N., *praeses.* Theses cheirurgicae de ulceribus. 1604.

LEMBKEN, BURCHARD [*fl.* 1663] *respondent. See* TAPPE, J., *praeses.* Disputatio medica de apoplexia. 1663.

LEMCKE, CHRISTIAN [*b.* 1652] *respondent. See* HELWIG, C. Disputatio medica inauguralis de peste. 1682.

—*See* HELWIG, C. Programma, quo decanus Facultatis Medicae Christophorus Helwigius ... ad inauguralem de peste disputationem, quam ... Christianus Lemcke ... habebit ... invitat. 1682.

LÉMERY, NICOLAS [1645–1715] Cours de chymie, contenant la maniere de faire les operations qui sont en usage dans la medecine, par une methode facile. Avec des raisonnements sur chaque operation ... 2. ed., rev., corr. & augm. par l'autheur. Paris, Chez l'autheur, 1677 [De l'imprimerie de Jacques Langlois fils, 1676]

[30], 584, [15] p. 16 cm. **[6843]**

—[The same.] ... 3. ed. ... Paris, L'autheur, 1679.

[30], 659, [15] p. 17 cm. **[6844]**

—[The same.] ... 5. éd. ... Paris, Estienne Michallet, 1683.

[16], 632 p. illus. 20 cm. **[6845]**

—[The same.] ... 7. ed. ... Paris, Estienne Michallet, 1690.

[16], 768 p. front. (port.), illus., plates. 20 cm. **[6846]**

—[The same.] ... 8. ed. ... Paris, Estienne Michallet, 1693.

[16], 768 p. illus., plates. 19 cm. **[6847]**
Different setting of type.

—[The same.] ... 8. ed. ... Paris, Estienne Michallet, 1696.

[16], 836 p. front. (port.), illus., plates, table. 20 cm. **[6848]**

—[Latin tr.] Cursus chymicus continens modum parandi medicamenta chymica usitatoria brevi & facili methodo, una cum notis & dissertationibus super unamquamque praeparationem ... Ex ultima ed. Gallica Latine versus. A. I. C. De Rebecque ... Genevae, Apud Joannem Pictetum, 1681.

[10], 664, [14] p. 14 cm. **[6849]**

—[Dutch tr.] Het philosoophische laboratorium; of, Der chymisten stook-huis. Leerende op een korte en ligte wyse alle de gebruikelykste medicamenten op de chymische wyse bereiden; te gelyk met aanmerkingen en naukeurige redeneringen over yder preparatie in 't besonder ... Vertaalt na het laatste France exemplaar, en met noodige aanteikeningen verrijkt. Amsterdam, Jan ten Hoorn, 1683.

[8], 551, [8] p. front., plates. 17 cm. **[6850]**

—[English tr.] A course of chymistry. Containing an easie method of preparing those chymical medicins which are used in physick. With curious remarks and useful dicourses upon each preparation ... 2d ed. very much inlarged. Translated from the 5th ed. in the French, by Walter Harris ... London, Printed by R. N. for Walter Kettilby, 1686.

[27], 548, [16] p. plates. 20 cm. **[6851]**

—[The same.] ... 3d ed., translated from the 8th ed. in the French, which is very much enlarged beyond any of the former. London, Printed by R. N. for Walter Kettilby, 1698.

[23], 815, [15] p. plates. 20 cm. **[6852]**
Dedicatory epistle signed: James Keill.
Translated by Walter Harris.

—An appendix to A course of chymistry. Being additional remarks to the former operations. Together with the process of the volatile salt of tartar, and some other useful preparations. Writ in French ... Translated by Walter Harris ... London, Walter Kettilby, 1680.

[15], 140, [12] p. 17 cm. **[6853]**

—[German tr.] Cours de chymie; oder, Der vollkommene Chymist, welcher die in der Medicin gebräuchlichen chymischen Processe auff die leichteste und heilsamste Art machen lernt ... Aus der neunten frantzöischen [sic] Edition ... übersetzet. Dresden, Bey Johann Jacob Wincklern, 1698.

[24], 652 p.; 388, [96] p. plates. 17 cm. **[6854]**
Imperfect: sig.)(1 before Vorrede wanting.

—[Italian tr.] Corso chimico ... che contiene il modo di fare le operationi, che sono in uso nella medicina, con metodo facile, e ragionamenti sopra ciascuna operatione ... Tradotto dall'idioma francese nell'italiano da Claudio Francesco Jobelot ... 8. et ultima ed. Napoli, A spese del traduttore, 1695.

[24], 472, 273 (i.e. 257), [20] p. illus. 17 cm. **[6855]**

—[The same.] Corso di chimica ... Ch'insegna il modo di fare l'operationi, che sono usuali nella medicina con metodo facilissimo, et ragionamenti sopra ciascuna operatione. Tradotto dall'ultima editione francese da Nathan Lacy ... Torino, A spese di Gio. Giacomo Hertz in Venetia, 1695.

[24], 512 (i.e. 472), [16] p.   illus.   18 cm.

[6856]

—[The same.] ... Tradotto dall'ultima editione francese da Nathan Lacy ... Venetia, Gio. Giacomo Hertz, 1699.

[24], 12 (i.e. 472), [16] p.   illus.   17 cm.

[6857]

—[The same.] ... Aggiontovi nel fine li Segreti reconditi ò vero manipolazioni; ò siano chimiche invenzioni di Pietro Poterio ... Bologna, Giulio Borzaghi, 1700.

[16], 588 (i.e. 592), [18], 40 p.   illus.   15 cm.

[6858]

—[The same.] *In* Collegio dei fisici, Milan. Prospectus pharmaceutici ed. 2. 1698.

—Pharmacopée universelle, contenant toutes les compositions de pharmacie qui sont en usage dans la medecine, tant en France que par toute l'Europe ... Paris, Laurent d'Houry, 1697.

[16], 504, xxxii, 505–1050 (i.e. 1034), [38] p.   front. (port.)   26 cm.

[6859]

—Another issue, dated 1698.

[6860]

Without the portrait.

—Pharmacopoeia Lemeriana contracta: Lemery's Universal pharmacopoeia abridg'd, in a collection of recepe's and observations, compar'd with the London and with Bates's Dispensatories; and also, with Charas's Royal pharmacy. To which are added, some remedies recommended by the members of the French Royal Academy of Sciences, most collected out of the history of that society, lately published by John Baptista du Hamel. London, Walter Kettilby, 1700.

[12], 167, [1] p.   16 cm.

[6861]

With this is bound: Pechey, J. The London dispensary. 1694.

—Traité universel des drogues simples, mises en ordre alphabetique ... Ouvrage dépendant de la Pharmacopée universelle ... Paris, Chez Laurent d'Houry [De l'imprimerie de Denys Thierry] 1698.

[16], 838, [61] p.   27 cm.

[6862]

—*See* ÉMERY, *sieur d'*. Recueil de curiositez rares. 1674, 1676, 1681, 1684, 1685, 1688; [English tr.] 1685; Meber, J. C. Anchora sauciatorum. 1687.

LE MIRE, AUBERT [1573–1640] Illustrium Galliae Belgicae scriptorum icones et elogia ... Antverpiae, Apud Theodorum Gallaeum, 1608.

[58] ll.   56 ports.   29 cm.

[6863]

Engraved throughout.

LEMMEN, BALTHASAR [*fl.* 1695] *respondent.* Disputatio medica inauguralis de morbis castrensibus praecipuis ... Duisburgi ad Rhenum, Typis Johannis Sas, 1695.

26 p.   20 cm.

[6864]

Diss. — Duisburg.

LEMMENS. *See* LEMNIUS.

LEMMER, GREGOR VAN DEN [*fl.* 1693] *respondent.* Disputatio medico-practica inauguralis de purgantibus ... Lugduni Batavorum, Apud Abrahamum Elzevier, 1693.

[16] p.   22 cm.

[6865]

Diss. — Leyden.

LEMNIUS, GUILIELMUS [*ca.* 1530–1573] Emoot pestilentzie huru hwar och een menniskia sigh hålla skal, bådhe gamble och unge, rijke och fattige, til itt tiensteligit rådh och hielp, skriffuit genom Guilielmum Lemnium ... anno MDLXXII ... Stockholm, Hoos Ignatium Meurer, 1623.

[16] p.   19 cm.

[6866]

—*See* LEMNIUS, L. De termino vitae liber. 1639.

LEMNIUS, LEVINUS [1505–1568] De astrologia. *See his* Similitudinum ac parabolarum, quae in Bibliis ex herbis atque arboribus desumuntur, dilucida explicatio. 1608, 1626.

—De habitu et constitutione corporis, quam Graeci κρᾶσιν, Triviales complexionem vocant, libri II; omnibus quibus secunda valetudo curae est, apprime necessarii: ex quibus cuique proclive erit corporis sui conditionem, animique motus, ac totius conservandae sanitatis rationem ad amussim cognoscere ... Francofurti, Typis Nicolai Hofmanni, sumtibus Jonae Rhodii, 1604.

[16], 185 (i.e. 183), [9] p.   12 cm.

[6867]

With this is bound *his* Similitudinum ac parabolarum, quae in Bibliis ex herbis atque arboribus desumuntur, dilucida explicatio. 1608.

—[The same.] . . . Francofurti, Typis Nicolai Hofmanni, sumptibus haeredum Jacobi Fischeri, 1619.

[16], 185 (i.e. 183), [9] p. 13 cm. **[6868]**

Bound with *his* De miraculis occultis naturae. 1611.

—[English tr.] The touchstone of complexions: expedient and profitable for all such as bee desirous and carefull of their bodily health: containing most ready tokens, whereby every one may perfectly try, and thorowly know as well the exact state, habit, disposition, and constitution of his body outwardly: as also the inclinations, affections, motions, and desires of his minde inwardly. Written in Latine . . . and now Englished by T[homas] N[ewton] . . . London, Printed by E[lisabeth] A[llde] for Michael Sparke, 1633.

[8], 248, [10] p. 18 cm. **[6869]**

Signatures: A-2K⁴, 2L² (last leaf (blank) wanting)
STC 15458.

—De miraculis occultis naturae libri IIII. Item De vita cum animi et corporis incolumitate recte instituenda, liber unus. Illi quidem jam postremum emendati, & aliquot capitibus aucti, hic vero nunquam antehac editus . . . Francofurti, Typis Joannis Saurii, impensis Jacobi Fischeri, 1611.

[16], 582, [55] p. 13 cm. **[6870]**

Books 1-2 first published in 1559 under title: Occulta naturae miracula.

"Paraenesis, sive exhortatio ad vitam optime instituendam": p. 471-582.

With this is bound *his* De habitu et constitutione corporis. 1619.

—[The same.] . . . Francofurti, Typis excusi Wolfgangi Hofmanni, impensis haeredum Jacobi Fischeri, 1628.

[16], 582, [57] p. 13 cm. **[6871]**

Different setting of type.

With this is bound *his* Similitudinum ac parabolarum, quae in Bibliis ex herbis atque arboribus desumuntur, dilucida explicatio. 1626.

—De miraculis occultis naturae, libri IV. Ed. ult. prioribus emend. & corr. Lugduni Batav., Ex officina Johannis à Gelder, 1666.

[10], 638 p. 13 cm. **[6872]**

Without the Paraenesis.

—[English tr.] The secret miracles of nature: in four books . . . Treating of generation, and the parts thereof; the soul . . . of plants and living creatures; of diseases, their symptoms and cures, and many other rarities not treated of by any author extant . . .

Whereunto is added one book containing . . . rules how man shall . . . lead his life with health of body and mind . . . London, Printed by Jo. Streater, and sold by Humphrey Moseley, John Sweeting, John Clark and George Sawbridge, 1658.

[16], 398 p. plate. 28 cm. **[6873]**

Includes folded plate depicting London.
Imperfect: p. 387-390 wanting.
Translation of De miraculis occultis naturae and of Paraenensis; sive, Exhortatio ad vitam optime instituendam.

—A discoruse [sic] touching generation. Collected out of Laevinus-Lemnius . . . Fit for the use of physitians, midwifes, and all young married people. London, John Streater, 1667.

[12], 382 p. 13 cm. **[6874]**

Imperfect: p. 149-150 mutilated.
The first 16 chapters of Book 1 and scattered portions of the English translation of De miraculis occultis naturae.

—De termino vitae liber. Lugd. Bat., Ex officina Davidis Lopes de Haro, 1639.

[24], 143 p. 13 cm. **[6875]**

"De honesto animi et corporis oblectamento": p. [79]-136.
"Guilielmi Lemnii epistola ad Levinum Lemnium . . . qua obiter in dicat educationem in animis hominum plus efficere quam aeris ambientis, aut loci qualitatem": p. 137-143.

—Similitudinum ac parabolarum, quae in Bibliis ex herbis atque arboribus desumuntur, dilucida explicatio . . . Seorsum accesserunt De gemmis aliquot, iis praesertim quarum D. Joannes apostolus in sua Apocalypsi meminit: de aliis quoque, quarum usus hoc aevi apud omnes percrebuit, libri II. Auctore Francisco Rueo . . . Item Levini Lemnii De astrologia liber I. Francofurti, Apud Nicolaum Hoffmannum, impensis Jonę Rhodii, 1608.

[15], 288 p. 12 cm. **[6876]**

Bound with *his* De habitu et constitutione corporis. 1604.

[The same] . . . Francofurti, Typis Guolphg. Hofmanni, sumtibus haeredum Jacobi Fischeri, 1626.

[15], 288 p. 13 cm. **[6877]**

Bound with *his* De miraculis occultis naturae. 1628.

LE MOINE, ANTOINE [*fl.* 1662-1703] *ed. See* HIPPOCRATES. Hippocratis Coi, et Claudii Galeni . . . Opera. 1679.

LE MONNIER, LOUIS [*fl.* 17th cent.] Nouveau traité de la maladie venerienne . . . avec la plus seure & la plus facile methode de les guerir . . . Paris, Amable Auroy, 1689.

[24], 261 p. 16 cm. **[6878]**

—Traité de la fistule de l'anus ou du fondement ... dans lequel on expose ... les remedes pour la guerir, & les moyens de s'en preserver ... Paris, Chez Amable Auroy [De l'imprimerie de Laurent Rondet] 1689.

[34], 227 p.   16 cm.   [6879]

LE MORT, JACOB. *See* MORT, Jacob le [1650-1718]

LE MOULINET, NICOLAS, *tr. See* TOMAI, T. Abregé curieux, des plus beaux secrets de la nature. 1648.

LEMSE, LIEVEN. *See* LEMNIUS, Levinus [1505-1568]

LENCKE, CHRISTOPH [*fl.* 1666] Kurtzer und einfeltiger ... Bericht, wie man sich bey jetzt grassirenden Kranckheiten als weiss und rothen Ruhr ... verhalten sol ... Erffurdt, Gedruckt bey Johann Georg Hertzen [1666?]

[27] p.   19 cm.   [6880]

LENGERKEN, HERMANN VON [*fl.* 1676] *respondent. See* MAJOR, J. D., *praeses.* De aerumnis gigantum in negocio sanitatis. 1689.

LENIS, VINCENTIUS, *pseud. See* FROIDMONT, Libert [1587-1653]

LE NOBLE, CHARLES. *See* BARTHOLIN, T. Opuscula nova anatomica. 1670; HÉNAUT, G. de Clypeus. 1655.

LE NOIR, LOUIS [*fl.* 1646] *respondent. See* FORESTIER, J., *praeses.* Quaestio medica ... An contumacibus morbis ex stibio purgatio? 1646.

LENONIS Guillemei Scholae Parisiensis empirico-methodicae doctoris, et poste et fuste sublimis αποθεωσις ... Parisiis, 1654.

[8], 74 p.   22 cm.   [6881]
Dedicatory epistle signed by T.S.M.S.D.M.M., the author.

LENTEN, WILHELM VON [*fl.* 1682] *respondent. See* SAND, G., *praeses.* Dissertatio academica de incertitudine signorum conceptionis. 1682.

LENTHALL, WILLIAM [1591-1662] *See* PINDAR, M. A letter sent to the Honourable William Lenthall. 1644.

LENTILIUS, ROSINUS [1651-1733] Ad ... Ludovicum Christophorum Guckelinum ... de

hydrophobiae caussa et cura dissertatio ... Ulmae, Sumptibus Georgii Wilhelmi Kühnii, 1700.

[16], 56 p.   17 cm.   [6882]
Includes a case history described by Ludwig Christoph Guckelin.

—Miscellanea medico-practica tripartita. Quorum partibus prioribus continentur historiae, discursus, consilia, epistolae, ab auctore ad diversos, & a diversis ad ipsum exaratae ... Tertia autem tractatus & dissertationes virorum celeberrimorum inediti, cum sylloge medicamentorum ... Ulmae, Sumtibus Georgii Wilhelmi Kühnii, typis Ellae Kühnii, 1698.

[56], 648 (i.e. 654) p.; 336, [56] p.   illus., plate., port.   21 cm.   [6883]
Part 2 (p. [309]-648) and part 3 have special title pages.

—Τεχνημα πρακτικον; id est, Tabula consultatoria medica. Exhibens quaestiones maxime necessarias, aegrotis consilium exquirentibus a medico proponendas ... Praefixa vexatissimi problematis decisione: utrum & quei bonus theoreticus possit esse malus practicus? Ulmae, Sumptibus Georgii Wilhelmi Kühnii, typis haered. Christiani Balthasaris Kühnii, 1696.

[10], 83, [1] p.   plates.   17 cm.   [6884]

—*respondent.* Disputatio inauguralis medica de febre tertiana intermittente epidemia, praeterito vere septentrionem, subque ea Curlandiam infestante ... Altdorffii, Literis Henrici Meyeri [1680]

28 p.   20 cm.   [6885]
Diss.—Altdorf.

—*respondent. See* FRANCK VON FRANCKENAU, G., *praeses.* Disputatio physico-medica de saliva. 1673.

LENTNER, PANTALEON [*fl.* 1681] *respondent. See* HEINSIUS, U., *praeses.* Dissertatio historico-zoologica de alce. 1681.

LENTULUS, PAULUS [ca. 1560-1613] Historia admiranda, de prodigiosa Apolloniae Schreierae, virginis in agro Bernensi, inedia ... tribus narrationibus comprehensa, cui, ab eodem, complurium etiam aliorum, de ejusmodi prodigiosis inediis ... narrationes, & ... commentationes adjunctae ... Bernae Helvetiorum, Joannes le Preux, 1604.

[36], 211, [1] p.   plate.   21 cm.   [6886]
Part 1. No more appears to have been published.

LENTZ, JOHANN ANDREAS [*fl.* 1673] *respondent. See* WEDEL, G. W., *praeses.* Dissertatio medica de pleuritide. 1673.

LENZ, JOHANN BARTHOLOMÄUS [*fl.* 1699] *respondent. See* LENZ, J. L., *praeses.* Ex historia naturali de hominibus ad catadupa Nili obsurdescentibus. 1699.

LENZ, JOHANN LEONHARD [*d.* 1737] *praeses.* Ex historia naturali de hominibus ad catadupa Nili obsurdescentibus ... Wittebergae, Typis Christiani Schroedteri [1699]

    [17] p. 20 cm.   **[6887]**
    Diss. — Wittenberg (J. B. Lenz, *respondent*)

LEO, AFRICANUS. *See* LEO AFRICANUS, Joannes [16th cent.]

LEO, AMBROSIUS, *Nolanus. See* LEONE, Ambrogio [*d.* 1525]

LEO, BONCIUS, *ed. See* CAPIVACCIO, G. Medicina practica. 1601.

LEO, JOANNES, *Africanus. See* LEO AFRICANUS, Joannes [16th cent.]

LEO, JOHANN GEORG. *See* Löw, Johann Georg [1565-1610]

LEO, JOHN [*fl.* 1669] *respondent.* Disputatio medica inauguralis de epilepsia ... Lugduni Batavorum, Apud viduam & haeredes Joannis Elsevirii, 1669.

    [23] p. 20 cm.   **[6888]**
    Diss. — Leyden.

LEO AB ERLSFELDT, JOANNES FRANCISCUS. *See* LOEW VON ERLSFELD, Johann Franz, *Ritter* [1648-1725]

LEO AFRICANUS, JOANNES [16th cent.] Africae descriptio IX. lib. absoluta ... Lugd. Batav., Apud Elzevir, 1632.

    800, [16] p. 12 cm.   **[6889]**
    "... De Africae descriptione, pars altera ..." (p. [385]-800) has special title page.

LEÓN, ALVARO TENORIO DE. *See* TENORIO DE LEÓN, Alvaro [*fl.* 17th cent.]

LEÓN, ANDRÉS de [16th-17th cent.] Practico de morbo Gallico, en el qual se contiene el origen conocimiento desta enfermedad, y el mejor modo de curarla ... Valladolid, Luis Sanche, 1605.

    [12], 126, [2] ll. 21 cm.   **[6890]**

—Tratados de medicina, cirugia, y anatomia ... Valladolid, Luis Sanchez [1605]

    [8], 224 ll. 21 cm.   **[6891]**
    Imperfect: title page mutilated.

Imprint partly supplied from Palau 135083.
Libro quinto published separately in the same year.

LEÓN, FRANCISCO DE [*fl.* 17th cent.] Respuestas a las preguntas que me hizo el señor doct. D. Alonso Cornejo ... [Cadiz, 1699]

    7 p. 21 cm.   **[6892]**
    Caption title.

LEÓN, PEDRO LÓPEZ DE. *See* LÓPEZ DE LEÓN, Pedro [*fl.* 1578-1590]

LEÓN PINELO, ANTONIO. *See* LEÓN PINELO, Antonio Rodríguez de [*d.* 1660]

LEÓN PINELO, ANTONIO RODRÍGUEZ DE [*d.* 1660] Question moral si el chocolate quebranta el ayuno eclesiástico; tratase de otras bebidas y confecciones que se usan en varias provincias ... Madrid, Viuda de Juan Conçalez, 1636.

    [6], 122, [12] ll. 21 cm.   **[6893]**
    Engraved title page.

LEONARDI, CAMILLO [*fl.* 1496-1502] Speculum lapidum ... Cui accessit Sympathia septem metallorum ac septem selectorum lapidum ad planetas D. Petri Arlensis de Scudalupis ... Parisiis, Apud Carolum Sevestre, Davidem Gillium et Joannem Petitpas, 1610.

    [44], 499 (i.e. 451), [36] p. illus., ports. 18 cm.
                                        [6894]
    Engraved title page.
    The Sympathia septem metallorum has special title page.
    With this is bound Penot, B. G. De denario medico. 1608.

LEONE, AMBROGIO [*d.* 1525] *tr. See* JOANNES ACTUARIUS. De differentiis urinarum. 1688 [and] De urinis libri VII. 1670.

LEONE, GEORG. See Löw, Johann Georg [1565-1610]

LEONE, JOHANN GEORG. *See* Löw, Johann Georg [1565-1610]

LEONICENO, NICCOLÒ [1428-1524] *tr. See* ALBANESE, G. A. Aphorismorum Hippocratis expositio peripatetica. 1649; ARGENTERIO, G. Opera. 1606, 1610; CABOTIN, A. Commentaire en vers sur les Aphorismes d'Hypocrate. 1665; CARDILUCIUS, J. H., *ed.* and *tr.* Neuaufgerichtete Stadt- und Land-Apotheke. 1673-80; CELI, A. Antonini Caelii ... Introductio universalis ad medicam facultatem. 1618; CIGALINI, P. In Aphor. Hippocratis lib. primum et

secundum lectiones. 1653; FOUGEROLLES, F. de.
Methodus in septem Aphorismorum libros ab Hippocrate observata. 1612; GALENUS. [Ars medica] 1606,
1622, 1642, 1663; GENGA, B. In Hippocratis
Aphorismos. 1694, 1697; GHIRINZANA, L. In septem
libros Aphorismorum magni Hyppocratis . . .
animadversiones Hyppocraticae. 1649; HIPPOCRATES.
[Adaptations, etc. Latin] 1699 [and] [Aphorismi.
French] 1605, 1606, 162-?, 1620, 1627, 1628, 1646, 1660,
1666, 1671 [and] [Aphorismi. Greek and Latin] 1625,
1628, 1668 [and] [Aphorismi. Latin] 1610 [i.e. 1611],
1622, 1623, 1633, 1643, 1646, 1649, 1653, 1663; 1674, 1684.
LATIOSO, A. In Hippocratis Aphorismos . . . commentarii. 1667; MERCURIALE, G. In omnes Hippocratis Aphorismorum libros. 1619, 1621, 1631;
MORALIS, G. Commentaria in magni Hippocratis
Coi Aphorismos. 1648 [and] Enchiridium medicum.
1455 (i.e. 1655); NAVARRO, J. B. Commentarii ad
libros Galeni De differentiis febrium. 1651; OSORIO
Y PERALTA, D. Principia medicinae. 1685; ROSSELL,
J. F. Ad sex libros Galeni De differentiis. 1627; SAN-
TORIO, S. Commentaria in Artem medicinalem
Galeni. 1612, 1631 [and] Commentaria in primam sec-
tionem Aphorismorum Hippocratis. 1629 [and]
Opera omnia. 1660; SCHOLA MEDICA. 1682-84; TOZZI,
L. In Hippocratis Aphorismos commentaria. 1693.

LEONICENUS, JANUS, VERONENSIS. *See* PECHLIN,
Johann Nicolas [1644-1706]

LEONICENUS, NICOLAUS. *See* LEONICENO,
Niccolò [1428-1524]

LEONINI, JANI. *See* PECHLIN, Johann Nicolas
[1644-1706]

LEOPOLD, JOHANN [*fl.* 1614?] Quaestio tertia
continens Τὰ χειρονργουμενα περὶ ἀρθρων; hoc est,
Capita generalia de luxationibus ossium . . . Lipsiae,
Excudebat Laurentius Cober, 1614.
[24] p.   19 cm.   **[6895]**

LEOPOLD, JOHANN FRIEDRICH [*fl.* 1700] *respondent.* Dissertatio inauguralis medica de alce, magno
illo septentrionis animali, ejusque virtutibus . . .
Basileae, Typis Jacobi Bertschii [1700]
[42] p.   20 cm.   **[6896]**
Diss. — Basel

**LEOPOLDINA NATURAE CURIOSORUM
ACADEMIA.** *See* ACADEMIA NATURAE CURIOSORUM.

**LEOPOLDINISCH-CAROLINISCHE
DEUTSCHE AKADEMIE DER NATUR-
FORSCHER.** *See* ACADEMIA NATURAE CURIOSORUM.

LEOVITIUS, CYPRIANUS [*d.* 1574] De conjunctionibus magnis insignioribus superiorum
planetarum. *In* Goclenius, R. [1572-1621] Acroteleution astrologicum. 1618.

LE PAULMIER, PIERRE [1568-1610] Lapis
philosophicus dogmaticorum. Quo Paracelsista
Libavius restituitur, Scholae medicae Parisiensis
judicium de chymicis declaratur, censura in adulteria
& fraudes parachymicorum deffenditur . . . Adjecta
est Historia laeprosae mulieris persanatae. Parisiis,
Apud Davidem Doulceur, 1608.
[32], 160, [12] p.   18 cm.   **[6897]**

LE PAULMIER DE GRENTEMESNIL, JULIEN
[1520-1588] De morbis contagiosis libri septem . . .
Francofurti, Apud Claudium Marnium, & heredes
Joannis Aubrii, 1601.
[16], 552, [32] p.   18 cm.   **[6898]**

—[The same.]   . . . Hagae-Comitis, Ex
typographia Adriani Vlacq, 1664.
[16], 552, [31] p.   18 cm.   **[6899]**
Different setting of type.

—*See* ENCHIRIDION PRACTICUM MEDICO-
CHIRURGICUM. 1621, 1627, 1644; FERNEL, J. Universa
medicina. 1645, 1656, 1679.

LE PIPER, JOHANNES [*fl.* 1618-1621] *respondent. See*
HEURNE, O. van., *praeses.* Disputatio medica de
hydrope. 1621; VORSTIUS, A. E., *praeses.* Theses
medicae de melancholia. 1621

LE PIPRE, JOSEPH DE [*fl.* 1611] *respondent. See*
PETRAEUS, H., *praeses.* Disputatio medica de dieta.
1611.

LEPNER, FRIEDRICH [*d.* 1701] *praeses.* Disputatio
medica de catarrho . . . Regiomonti, Typis Paschalis
Mensenii, 1665.
[16] p.   19 cm.   **[6900]**
Diss. — Königsberg (C. Nitzschke, *respondent*)

—*respondent.* Disputatio medica inauguralis de
medicinae definitione, divisione & elementis . . .
Lugduni Batavorum, Apud viduam & haeredes
Johannis Elsevirii, 1662.
[16] p.   19 cm.   **[6901]**
Diss. — Leyden.

—*See* BECKHER, D. [1627-1670] *praeses.* Disputatio medica de epilepsia. 1661.

LE POIS, CHARLES [1563-1633] Discours de la nature, causes, et remedes, tant curatifs que preservatifs des maladies populaires accompagnees de dysenterie, & autres flus de ventre, & familiares aux saisons chaudes & seiches des années de semblable intemperature … Pont-a-Mousson, Sebastien Cramoisy, 1623.

134 p. 17 cm. [6902]

—Selectiorum observationum et consiliorum de praetervisis hactenus morbis affectibusque praeter naturam ab aqua, seu serosa colluvie & diluvie ortis liber singularis. Opus novitate et varietate doctrina utile juxta atque jucundum … Ponte ad Monticulum, Apud Carolum Mercatorem, 1618.

[28], 451 (i.e. 445), [4] p. 25 cm. [6903]

—[The same.] … Quod 2. hac ed., correctius multo … Lugduni Batavorum, E typographeo Francisco Hackii, 1650.

[32], 605, [25] p. 18 cm. [6904]

—*See* LANGWEDEL, B. Carolus Piso enucleatus. 1639.

—, *tr. See* MERCADO, L. Institutiones. 1625.

LE QUIN, ANTOINE [*b. ca.* 1657] Le chirurgien herniaire, contenant un nouveau traité des hernies ou decentes [sic] des femmes et des filles. Avec quelques observations sur la décente & chûte de la matrice … Paris, L'auteur et Laurent d'Houry, 1697.

[24], 131 p. 16 cm. [6905]

Original imprint partly covered by label.

LEQUIN, NICOLAS [*d.* 1688] Traité des hernies, ou des descentes, contenant les causes … remedes, & un avis aux hernieux, avec la maniere de bien faire & administrer les bandages d'acier, & de fil de fer … Paris, L'auteur, 1665.

[34], 112 p. 16 cm. [6906]

—[The same.] … Paris, L'auteur, 1685.
[32], 102, [3] p. illus. 17 cm. [6907]

—[The same.] … 2. ed. augmentée. Paris, Laurent d'Houry, 1690.

[32], 102, [3] p. illus. 17 cm. [6908]

A reissue of the 1685 edition with new title page.

LERA, MATHIAS DE. *See* LERA GIL DE MURO, Matías de [*fl.* 1657]

LERA GIL DE MURO, MATÍAS DE [*fl.* 1657] Practica de fuentes y sus utilidades, y modo de hazerlas y conservarlas con muchas advertencias muy importantes a la materia … Madrid, Pablo de Val, 1657.

[32], 215, [5] p. 21 cm. [6909]

Imperfect: p. [28] wrongly printed.

—[The same.] … [Madrid] Colegio Real de los Desamparados, a costa de Bernardo Sierra, 1671.

[20], 202, [4] p. 21 cm. [6910]

LERCHENFELDT, MAXIMILIEN [1606-1682] *praeses.* Disputatio philosophica de mutatione rerum naturalium … Ingolstadii, Typis Gregorii Haelini [1638]

[2], 14, [3] p. 19 cm. [6911]

Diss. — Ingolstadt (F. Mair, *respondent*)

LERIZA, MIGUEL DE. *See* ROMANO DE CÓRDOBA, A. Recopilacion de toda la theorica, y practica de cirugia. 1674.

LE ROY, HENRI. *See* REGIUS, Henricus [1598-1679]

LESCAUT, MICHEL. *See* SCOTT, Michael [1175?-1234?]

LESCELLIER, CHARLES. De febrium natura, differentiis, symptomatis, et causis paroxysmorum, libellus. Cui accesserunt quaestiones, ad praxim medicam, perutiles, ac necessariae, cum tractatu compendioso de causis, & signis urinarum, ac pulsuum … Ambiani, Ex typographia Jacobi Hubault, 1627.

[8], 220, [4] p. 17 cm. [6912]

LESCH, JOHANN GEORG [*fl.* 1685] *respondent. See* SCHRADER, F., *praeses.* Dissertatio physica de habitaculis animantium. 1685.

LESCHIUS, ESAIAS [*fl.* 1613-1614] *ed. See* REUSNER, H. Eygendtliche … Beschreibung dess … Badts zu Wembdingen. 1618.

LESCHIUS, JOHANNES GEORGIUS. *See* LESCH, Johann Georg [*fl.* 1685]

L'ÉSCLUSE, CHARLES DE. *See* L'ÉCLUSE, Charles de [1526-1609]

LESCURE, DE. *See* DELESCURE.

LESEYNA, Petrus. *See* Lasena, Pietro [1590-1636]

LESSIUS, Leonardus [1554-1623] Hygiasticon; seu, Vera ratio valetudinis bonae et vitae una cum sensuum, judicii, & memoriae integritate ad extremam senectutem conservandae … Subjungitur tractatus Ludovici Cornari … eodem pertinens, ex Italico … ab … Lessio translatus. Antverpiae, Ex Officina Plantiniana, apud viduam & filios Jo. Moreti, 1613

    [16], 108, [2] p. 18 cm.   **[6913]**

—[The same.] … Ed. 2. Antverpiae, Ex Officina Plantiana, apud viduam & filios Jo. Moreti, 1614.

    127 p. 17 cm.   **[6914]**

—[The same.] … Ed. 3. … Antverpiae, Ex Officina Plantiniana, apud Balthasarem Moretum, & viduam Joannis Moreti, & Jo. Meursium, 1623.

    132, [2] p. 18 cm.   **[6915]**

Imperfect: sheet H is misbound between sig. B4 and B5.

—[The same.] Novus annus incolumis et sanus; seu, Ars bene diuque valendi ac vivendi, quae consistit in diaeta sobria commendata olim perquam utili tractatu … Opusculo annexo … Ludovici Cornari … Graecii, Apud haeredes Widmanstadii, 1688.

    [12], 129 p. front. 13 cm.   **[6916]**

—[Dutch tr.] De schat der soberheit; of, Bequame middel tot onderhouding der gezonheit, en bewaring van de volkomenheit der zinnen, van't verstant, en van de geheugenis aan d'uitterste ouderdom … Met een Handeling van de nuttigheden van't sober leven, door Ludovicus Cornarus … beschreven. Uyt het Latijn vertaalt door J[an] H[endrik] G[lazemaker]. In deze laatste druk byna de helft vermeerdert, en uit het Italiaans vertaalt. Amsterdam, Pieter Arentsz, 1681.

    [22], 211, [3] p. 14 cm.   **[6917]**

Added engraved title page.

—[English tr.] Hygiasticon; or, The right course of preserving life and health unto extream old age. Together with soundnesse and integritie of the senses, judgement, and memorie. Written in Latine … and now done into English. The 2d ed. Cambridge [R. Daniel] 1634.

    [4], 210 p.; 70 p. 12 cm.   **[6918]**

Imprint partly supplied from STC.

Imperfect? First prelim. leaf wanting?

"To the reader" signed by T. S., the translator.

"A treatise of temperance and sobrietie. Written by Lud. Cornarus, translated … by Mr. George Herbert": 70 p.

STC 15520.

—[The same.] The temperate man; or, The right way of preserving life and health, together, with soundness of the senses, judgment, and memory unto extream old age. In three treatises. The first written by … Leonardus Lessius. The second by Lodowick Cornaro … The third by a famous Italian. Faithfully Englished. London, Printed by J. R. for John Starkey, 1678.

    [34], 168 p. 15 cm.   **[6919]**

—[French tr.] Deux traittez du regime de vivre pour la conservation de la santé du corps & de l'ame, jusques à une extreme viellesse. Traduction … du latin … par Sebastian Hardy … Paris, Guillaume Loyson, 1623.

    [8], 198, [2] p. 18 cm.   **[6920]**

—[The same.] Le vray regime de vivre pour la conservation de la santé du corps & de l'ame, & du parfait usage du jugement, de la memoire & de tous les sens jusqu'à une extreme viellese, sans l'usage d'aucune medecine … Ensemble un traitté de Louis Cornaro … sur le mesme sujet. Le tout traduit … par Sebastien Hardy … Rev., corr., & augm. d'annotations en marge, & de la vie admirable dudit Cornaro, et des tesmoignages des auteurs qui en ont parlé. Paris, Gervais Clousier, 1646.

    [12], 176 p.; 88 p. 18 cm.   **[6921]**

Part [2] has special title page: Trois discours nouveaux et curieux de Louis Cornaro … 1647.

—[German tr.] Kunst lang zu leben; oder, Ein bewehrtes Mittel, den menschlichen Leib in Gesundheit, auch ohne Verletzung der Sinnen, Verstands und Gedächtnuss biss auffs höchste Alter zu erhalten … In lateinischer Sprach beschrieben. Sampt einen Tractätlein Ludovici Cornari … von Nutzbarkeiten eines mässigen Lebens. Verteutschet durch Herrn P. A. V. Augspurg, Sebastian Hauser, 1697.

    66 (i.e. 90) p.; 38 p. 16 cm.   **[6922]**

[**LETI**, Gregorio, 1630-1701] Il puttanismo romano; ò vero, Conclave generale delle puttane della Corte; per l'elettione del nuovo pontefice. In Colonia [i.e. Amsterdam?] 1668.

    240 p. 14 cm.   **[6923]**

Preface signed A. D. A. S. [i.e. Gregorio Leti?]

A French translation, published in Cologne [i.e. Amsterdam] in 1670, gives as author Baldassare Sultanini, regarded by some authorities as the pseudonym of Gregorio Leti. Cf. N. Krivatsy. *Bibliography of the works of Gregorio Leti.* Oak Knoll Books. New Castle, Delaware. 1982. no. 163.

"Dialogo tra Pasquino, e Marforio sopra lo stesso sogetto del puttanismo": p. 109-240.

LETSCH, JOHANN GOTTLIEB [*fl.* 1696] *respondent. See* ALBINUS, B. Dissertatio medica inauguralis, de partu difficili. 1696 [and] De tabaco. 1695.

LETSCH, JOHANN THEOPHIL *See* LETSCH, Johann Gottlieb.

A LETTER concerning the present state of physick. 1665. *See* [MERRET, C.]

A LETTER sent to the Honourable William Lenthall. 1644. *See* PINDAR, M.

A LETTER to Mr. Henry Stubs concerning his Censure upon certain passages contained in the History of the Royal Society. London, Octavian Pullen, 1670.

    [1], 19 p.   21 cm.   **[6924]**

    Wing L1713B.

LETTERS to a sick friend, containing such observations as may render the use of remedies effectual towards the removal of sickness, and preservation of health. By J. M. London, Printed by J. A. for Thomas Parkhurst, 1682.

    [5], 250 p.   18 cm.   **[6925]**

LETTRE de M^r M*** ... a son ami. 1696? *See* MAURIN, J.

LETTRE par laquelle on fait connoistre le temps auquel il faut saigner. 1696? *See* [MAURIN, J.]

LETTRE philosophique. 1671. *See* [SENDIVOGIUS, M.]

LETUS, CALVIDIUS, *pseud. See* QUILLET, Claude [1602-1661]

LEUBIUS, WOLFGANG HEINRICH [*fl.* 1696] *respondent. See* PLANER, J. A., *praeses.* De nive dissertatio tertia. 1696.

LEUNCLAVIUS, JOHANNES [1533?-1593] *tr. See* ARTEMIDORUS DALDIANUS. Artemidori Daldiani & Achmetis Sereimi f. Oneirocritica. 1603.

LEUPOLD, ERDMANN [*b.* 1672] *respondent. See* WEDEL, G. W., *praeses.* Dissertatio medica inauguralis de sudore Anglico. 1697.

—*See* CRAUSE, R. W. Propemticum inaugurale de mathesi medico maxime necessaria. 1697.

LEURECHON, JEAN [1591-1670] Recreations mathematiques. *In* Mydorge, C. Examen du livre des Recreations mathematiques et de ses problemes en geometrie. 1638.

—[English tr.] Mathematicall recreations; or, A collection of many problems, extracted out of the ... philosophers, as secrets and experiments in arithmetick, geometry ... astronomie ... chemistry ... Written first in Greek and Latin, lately compil'd in French, by Henry Van Etten [pseud? i.e. Jean Leurechon?] and now in English ... Whereunto is added The description and use of the generall horologicall ring, and the double horizontall diall, invented and written by William Oughtred. London, William Leake, 1653.

    [38], 286, [1] p.; [16] p.   illus.   17 cm.

                                     [6926]

    Added engraved title page.

    Imperfect: sig. A8 (blank?) wanting; signatures of sheet A misbound.

    Part [1] is the translation by William Oughtred of Recréation mathematique.

    Part [2] has special title page: The description and use of the double horizontall dyall ... by W. O. ... 1652.

LE VASSEUR, LOUIS [*fl.* 1658-1674] De sylviano humore triumvirali, epistola ... Juxta exemplar Parisianum. [Leyden?] 1668.

    [4], 78 p.   14 cm.   **[6927]**

—*tr. See* GREW, N. Anatomie des plantes. 1675, 1679, 1685 [and] Recueil d'experiences et observations sur le combat, qui procede du mélange des corps. 1679.

—*See* SCHMITZ, J. A. Medicinae practicae compendium. 1666; SCHUYL, F. Pro veteri medicina. 1670.

LE VASSEUR DU VAUGOSSE, GILLES [*fl.* 1612] *respondent.* Suprema laurus medica ... Basileae, Typis Joannis Schroeteri, 1612.

    [8] p.   22 cm.   **[6928]**

    Caption title reads: Quaestio medica de purgatione ... utrum assumpto catharctico superdormire liceat?

    Diss. — Basel.

LEVENS, PETER [*fl.* 1552-1587] A right profitable books for all diseases; called, The path-way to health.

Wherein are to bee found most excellent and approved medicines of great vertue: as also notable potions and drinks, and for the distilling of divers precious waters, and making of oyles ... never before imprinted ... Now newly corr. and augm. ... London, Printed by John Beale for Robert Bird, 1632.

[2], 114, [3] ll.   17 cm.   [6929]

STC 15534

Imperfect: title page and leaves 6-7 mutilated, lower margins trimmed.

A page for page reprint of the "newly corrected and augmented" edition of 1597.

—[The same.] The path-way to health; wherein are to be found most excellent and approved medicins of great vertue, as also notable potions and drinks, with the art of distilling divers precious waters, for making oyles ... never before printed ... now newly corr. and augm. ... London, Printed for J. W. and sold by Charls Tyus, 1664.

[6], 380, [24] p.   15 cm.   [6930]

Imperfect: first prelim. leaf (blank?) wanting.

LEVI, PHILIPP [*fl.* 1684] *respondent.* Disputatio medica inauguralis de pleuritide ... Lugduni Batavorum, Apud Abrahamum Elzevier, 1684.

[12] p.   22 cm.   [6931]

LEVINS, PETER. *See* LEVÉNS, Peter [*fl.* 1552-1587]

LEVISTONIUS, JOANNES [*fl.* 1661] *respondent.* Disputatio medica inauguralis, de scorbuto ... Lugduni Batavorum, Apud Johannem Elsevirium, 1661.

[12] p.   21 cm.   [6932]

LEWENHAIMB, PHILIPP JAKOB SACHS *von. See* SACHS VON LEWENHAIMB, Philipp Jakob [1627-1672]

LEWENKLAIUS, JOHANNES. *See* LEUNCLAVIUS, Johannes [1533?-1593]

LEX talionis; sive, Vindiciae pharmacoporum; or, A short reply to Dr. Merrett's book. 1670. *See* [Stubbs, H.]

LEXICON HERODOTEUM. *See* HIPPOCRATES. Collected works [Greek and Latin] Tὰ εὑρισκόμενα. 1657, 1662.

LEYBURN, JOHN [1620-1702] *tr. See* DIGBY, *Sir* K. Demonstratio immortalitatis animae rationalis. 1664.

LEYDECKERS, REYNOUT [*fl.* 1689] *respondent.* Disputatio medica inauguralis de lumbricis ... Trajecti ad Rhenum, Ex officina Francisci Halma, 1689.

8, [4] p.   22 cm.   [6933]

Diss. — Utrecht.

LEYDEN. Ordinances, local laws, etc. Gildebrief, by die vande gerechte der stadt Leyden gemaect, verbetert ende vermeerdert, dienende tot onderhout van de conste, handelinghe, ende ouffeninghe vande chirurgie, mitsgaders vande barbiers ende andere, die gewoon zijn, in, ofte aen smenschen lichaem te practizeren ... [Leyden] Jay Claesz van Dorp, 1637.

[19] p.   21 cm.   [6934]

—Openen vande poorten om de vroevrouwen ... Is by die vande gerechte der stadt Leyden, syene ... geordonneert, op t verzouc vande ordinarijze vroevrouvvey in dienst ende eedt van dezer stede zijnde ... [Leyden] 1609.

[2] p.   21 cm.   [6935]

LEYDEN. Rijksuniversiteit. *See* RIJKSUNIVERSITEIT TE LEIDEN.

LEYDEN. Universiteit. *See* RIJKSUNIVERSITEIT TE LEIDEN.

LEYDINGER, PAULUS. *See* LEYTINGER, Paul [*fl.* 1629].

LEYS, LEONARD. *See* LESSIUS, Leonardus [1554-1623]

LEYSER, JOHANN. *See* LYSER, Johann [1631-1684]

LEYTAM, MANOEL. Pratica de barbeiros, em quatro tratados. Em os quaes se trata de como se ha de sangrar, & as cousas necessarias pera a sangria ... Coimbra, Manoel Rodrigues de Almeyda, 1693.

72 p.   15 cm.   [6936]

Die LEYTER der Philosophorum. *See* [MONTANOR, G. de]

LEYTINGER, PAUL [*fl.* 1629] *respondent. See* SEBISCH, M. [1578-1674?] *praeses.* Exercitationes medicae. 1639.

LEYTTERSPERGER, JOHANN GEORG [*fl.* 1632] *respondent. See* SEBISCH, M. [1578-1674?] *praeses.* Galeni Ars parva in disputationes triginta resoluta. 1633.

LEZIUS, CHRISTIAN RUDOLF [*fl.* 1687] *respondent.* See LIMMER, C. P., *praeses.* Collegii Physici disputatorii disputatio septima. 1687.

L'HOMMART, JACOB [*b.* 1666] *respondent.* See SCHELHAMMER, G. C., *praeses.* Dissertationem medicam inauguralem de paresi . . . publicae . . . disquisitioni sistit . . . 1693.

—*See* WEDEL, G. W. Propempticon inaugurale de faecula coa. 1693.

L'HONORÉ, GERMAIN [*fl.* 1672] Description d'un monstre dont une femme de la ville de Rouen accoucha le mois d'octobre 1672. Rouen, Antoine Maurry, 1673.

[6], 18 p.   illus.   25 cm.   **[6937]**

LIAGNO, TEODORO FILIPPO DI [*fl.* 17th cent.] Horarum fallax mors incertissima rerum attamen horarum cur tibi cura datur. Al' molto ill^re et ecc. s^re . . . Giovanni Fabro Lynceo philosopho, medico et semplista di sua sanita . . . [Romae? 1601?]

[1] p.   20 plates.   20 cm.   **[6938]**

Engraved title page.
Imperfect: lower part of title page trimmed.
Engravings of animals' skeletons with inscriptions.

LIBAU, ANDREAS. *See* LIBAVIUS, Andreas [*d.* 1616]

LIBAUTIUS, JOHANNES. *See* LIÉBAULT, Jean [*ca.* 1534-1596]

LIBAVIUS, ANDREAS [*d.* 1616] Alchymia . . . recognita, emendata, et aucta, tum dogmatibus & experimentis nonnullis; tum commentario medico physico chymico . . . Francofurti, Excudebat Joannes Saurius, impensis Petri Kopffii, 1506 (i.e. 1606)

[20], 196, [6] p.; [10], 402 p.; 192, [10] p.   illus.   35 cm.   **[6939]**

Parts [2] and [3] have special title pages: Commentariorum alchymiae . . . pars prima [-secunda]
Imperfect: first two leaves of each part mutilated.

—Praxis alchymiae; hoc est, Doctrina de artificiosa praeparatione praecipuorum medicamentorum chymicorum: duobus libris explicata: quorum primus de destillatione aquarum et oleorum . . . alter de lapide philosophorum agit . . . Uterque correctus, & declaratus . . . Annexus est libellus Jacobi Bessoni De absoluta ratione extrahendi olea & aquas e medicamentis simplicibus . . . Francofurti, Ex-

cudebat Joannes Savarius, impensis Petri Kopffii, 1604.

680, [20] p.   illus.   16 cm.   **[6940]**

Translated from the German by Leonhard Dold.

—Syntagmatis selectorum undiquaque et perspicue traditorum alchymiae arcanorum, tomus primus [-secundus] . . . Francofurti, Excudebat Nicolaus Hoffmannus, impensis Petri Kopffii, 1613-15 [v. 1, 1615]

2 v. in 1.   illus.   36 cm.   **[6941]**

Vol. 2 has title: Syntagmatis arcanorum chymicorum, ex optimis autoribus scriptis . . . collectorum tomus secundus . . . 1613.
With this is bound *his* Appendix necessaria Syntagmatis arcanorum chymicorum. 1615.

—Appendix necessaria Syntagmatis arcanorum chymicorum . . . In qua praeter arcanorum nonnullorum expositionem & illustrationem, quorundam item medicorum Hermeticorum, & mysticorum descriptionem, continentur defensiones geminae, primum eorum quae ab Henningo Scheunemano, & juniore Gramano sunt impugnata, postea quae in transmutatoria metallorum a Nicolao Guiberto . . . sunt attentata. Accesserunt I. Judicium breve de dea Hippocratis, seu Hygeia argentea (argentipara) Henningi Scheunemani . . . II. Schema medicinae Hippocraticae et Hermeticae . . . III. Examen philosophiae magicae Crollii; IV. Censura philosophiae vitalis Joannis Hartmanni . . . V. Admonitio de regulis novae rotae, seu harmonicae sphaerae Fratrum de Societate Rosae Crucis juxta famae editae indicem . . . Francofurti, Excudebat Nicolaus Hoffmannus, Impensis Petri Kopffii, 1615.

[12], 279, [11] p.; 306, [12] p.; 28 p.   36 cm.**[6942]**

Part [2] has special title page: Examen philosophiae novae, quae veteri abrogandae opponitur, in quo agitur de modo discendi novo; de veterum autoritate; de magia Paracelsi ex Crollio; de philosophia vivente ex Severino per Johannem Hartmannum; de philosophia harmonica magica Fraternitatis de Rosea Cruce.
Part [3] has title: Analysis confessionis Fraternitatis de Rosae Cruce.
Imperfect: title page wanting; supplied in photocopy.
Bound with *his* Syntagmatis selectorum . . . 1613-15.

Dissertations—Coburg

—*praeses.* De aquis pluviis, fontanis, fluviatilibus, stagnantibus etc. in colorem sanguinem, vel alium rubeum e solito transmutatis . . . Coburgi, Impressa a Justo Hauck [1609]

[19] p.   20 cm.   **[6943]**

A. Libavius [*fl.* 1609] *respondent.*

—De linguis originalibus Sacrae Scripturae, et antiquae versionis Latinae, quam ante annos circiter 46. Concilium Tridentinum authenticam esse jussit, fide, pars prima ... Coburgi, Justus Hauk [1609]
[20] p. 20 cm. [6944]
J. Hattenbach, *respondent.*

—De mundi corporumque mixtorum elementis, et principiis Platonicis, Aristotelicis, Hippocraticis, Hermeticis exercitatio physica ... Coburgi, Impressa a Justo Hauck [1608]
[40] p. 20 cm. [6945]
A. Theodoricus, *respondent.*

—De syrophoenissa haemorrhousa, Matth. IX, Marci 5, Lucae 8, et monumento Paneadis, seu Caesareae Philippi, apud Eusebium lib. 7, cap. 14 ... Coburgi, Justus Hauck, 1608.
[19] p. 20 cm. [6946]
J. Schnetter, *respondent.*

—De theriaca Andromachi senioris. Ex Mithridatio nata, & a temporibus Neronis principiis imperio Romano per Graecos & Latinos medicos celebrata, interque Arabum quoque medicamenta recepta, adeoque Hermeticis & dogmaticis, empiricisque familiari tractatus ... Coburgi, Typis Casparis Bertschii [1613]
[47] p. 21 cm. [6947]
J. Kesmann, *respondent.*

—Repetitio lectionum anatomicarum de spiritibus, humoribus, innato calido & facultatibus humanis ... [Coburgi] Justus Hauk, 1608.
[24] p. 20 cm. [6948]
M. Libavius, *respondent.*

—*See* FLUDD, R. Tractatus apologeticus integritatem Societatis de Rosea Cruce defendens. 1617; Le Paulmier, P. Lapis philosophicus dogmaticorum. 1608.

LIBAVIUS, ANDREAS [*fl.* 1609] *respondent. See* LIBAVIUS, A. [*d.* 1616] *praeses.* De aquis pluviis. 1609.

LIBAVIUS, MICHAEL [*fl.* 1608] *respondent. See* LIBAVIUS, A. [*d.* 1616] *praeses.* Repetitio lectionum anatomicarum de spiritibus ... facultatibus humanis. 1608.

LIBER de ponderibus & mensuris. *See* MESUË [924 or 5-1015] Opera. 1602, 1623.

LIBER pro recta administratione protomedicatus. 1666. *See* UNIVERSITÀ DI BOLOGNA. Collegio de medicina.

LIBERATI, LIBERATO [*fl.* 17th cent.] Podagra politica; seu, Tractatus podagricus, civili compositus doctrina, varia lectione & politicis sententiis refertus ... Noribergae, Litteris Michaelis Endteri, 1655.
[10], 304, [40] p. front. 14 cm. [6949]

—[The same.] ... Ed. alt. corr. & emend. Noribergae, Literis Michaelis Endteri, 1659.
[14], 305, [38] p. front. 14 cm. [6950]

LIBERATUS DE LIBERATIS. *See* LIBERATI, Liberato [*fl.* 17th cent.]

LIBRO de medicina llamado Thesoro de pobres. 1611. *See* JOHANNES XXI, *Pope.*

LICETI, FORTUNIO [1577-1657] Athos perfossus; sive, Rudens eruditus in Criomixi quaestiones de alimento dialogus prior, in quo montis Atho tetriores umbrae supra quadringentas, locutionem praesertim, & morum omne genus, necnon etiam variarum disciplinarum classem obtenebrantes, discutiuntur ... Patavii, Typis Paulli Frambotti, 1636.
[8], 185, [4] p. 22 cm. [6951]

—De anima ad corpus physice non propensa dialogus ... Utini, Typis Nicolai Schiratti, 1637.
[16], 356 p. 20 cm. [6952]
Added engraved title page.

—De anima subjecto corpori nil tribuente, deque seminis vita, & efficientia primaria in formatione faetus liber unus: in quo respondetur oppositionibus Ant. Ponce Sanctacrucii ... Patavii, Typis Varisci Variscii, 1631.
[8], 51, [5] p. 22 cm. [6953]
Signatures: B⁴, A-G⁴.

—De animarum coextensione corpori libri cuo, in quibus ex rei natura, consulto semper Aristotele, ostenditur animam tum vegetalem, tum sentientem, tum rationalem subdito sibi corpori toti coextendi ... nullamque animam in ulla viventis corporis particula, quantumuis principe, velut in suo domicilio, totam contineri, quicquid cum Platone plerique passim opinentur ... Patavii, Apud Petrum Bertellium, 1616.
78, [10] p. 20 cm. [6954]
Bound with Spiegel, A. van de. De lumbrico lato liber. 1618.

—De feriis altricis animae nemeseticae disputationes, in quibus encyclopediae, medicinae, philosophiae, celsiorisque sapientiae praesidio propulsantur ab olim culto mirabili mortalium jejunio vulgatae recens oppugnationes Asitiastis de Castro . . . Patavii, Typis Variscianis, 1631.

[8], 271, [16] p. illus. 22 cm.   [6955]

—De his, qui diu vivunt sine alimento libri quatuor, in quibus . . . de alimento, de alendi functione . . . disseritur; multa item Hippocratis, Platonis, Aristotelis, Galeni, Plinii, Celsi, & aliorum . . . theoremata illustrantur . . . Patavii, Apud Petrum Bertellium [Vicetiae, Typis Francisci Grossi, Patavii, praelo Gasparis Crivellarii] 1612.

[70], 199 p.; [1], 159 (i.e. 162), [2] p.   30 cm.   [6956]

Imperfect: title page and following leaf mutilated; wanting.

—De monstrorum caussis, natura, & differentiis libri duo . . . Patavii, Apud Casparem Crivellarium, 1616.

[16], 143, [25] p.   23 cm.   [6957]

—[The same.] . . . 2. ed. corr., auct. . . . Patavii, Apud Paulum Frambottum, 1634 [1633]

[16], 262, [26] p. illus. 20 cm.   [6958]

Added engraved title page.

—[The same.] De monstris. Ex recensione Gerardi Blasii . . . qui monstra quaedam nova & rariora ex recentiorum scriptis addidit. Ed. nov. . . . Amstelodami, Sumptibus Andreae Frisii, 1665.

[18], 316, [25] p. illus., plates. 21 cm.   [6959]

Added engraved title page.

"Appendix monstra quaedam nova, & rariora, cum satyro indico, & muliere cornuta, proponens" (p. [263–316]) has half title.

—[The same.] . . . Patavii, Apud haeredes Pauli Frambotti, 1668.

[14], 316, [25] p. illus., plates. 21 cm.   [6960]

Added engraved title page.

A reissue of the 1665 Amsterdam edition without the dedicatory epistle.

—De motu sanguinis, origine nervorum, cerebro leniente cordis aestum, imaginationis viribus, quarto-quaestis per epistolas clarorum virorum responsa

medico-philosophica . . . Utini, Ex typographia Nicolai Schiratti, 1647.

[8], 150 p. 21 cm.   [6961]

Includes correspondence with Sebastiano Baldo and Johann Vesling.

—De natura assistente dialogus: in quo late probatur nomen & rationem naturae proprie dictae convenire formis assistentibus, praesertimque summo Deo . . . Utini, Typis Nicolai Schiratti, 1637.

[16], 575, [1] p. 21 cm.   [6962]

Added engraved title page.

—De natura primo-movente libri duo: in quibus ex Aristotelis doctrina . . . ostenditur primi-moventis nomen & rationem proprie convenire finali caussae generatim, coelo seu mundo, intelligentiae cuique coelo assistenti, ac summo Deo: singulumque horum esse vere, dicique proprie naturam . . . Patavii, Typis Julii Crivellarii, 1634.

[16], 193, [7] p. 20 cm.   [6963]

—De ortu animae humanae libri tres . . . Ad Bartholomaeum Turrianum . . . Genvae, In aedibus Josephi Pavonii, 1602.

[16], 429, [33] p. 22 cm.   [6964]

—De perfecta constitutione hominis in utero liber unus . . . Patavii, Apud Petrum Bertellium, 1616.

119, [31] p. 20 cm.   [6965]

—De quaesitis per epistolas a claris viris responsa . . . Bononiae, Typis Nicolai Tebaldini, 1640.

[8], 325, [1] p. 21 cm.   [6966]

With this are bound his: De secundo-quaesitis per epistolas a claris viris . . . responsa. Utini, 1646; De tertio-quaesitis per epistolas clarorum virorum . . . responsa. Utini, 1646.

—De secundo-quaesitis per epistolas a claris viris, ardua, varia, pulchra, et nobilia queque petentibus in medicina, philosophia . . . & alio quovis eruditionum genere, responsa . . . Utini, Ex typographia Nicolai Schiratti, 1646.

[8], 389, [2] p. 21 cm.   [6967]

Bound with his De quaesitis per epistolas a claris viris responsa. Bononiae, 1640.

—De tertio-quaesitis per epistolas clarorum virorum, medicinalia potissimum, et aliarum disciplinarum arcana postulantium, responsa . . . Utini, Ex typographia Nicolai Schiratti, 1646.

[8], 236, [3] p. 21 cm.   [6968]

Bound with his De quaesitis per epistolas a claris viris responsa. Bononiae, 1640.

—De sexto-quaesitis, resurrectione multiplici, aenigmate mirabili, morborum enormi catastrophe, diaria phlebotomiam renuente, muliebri complexione calidiore virili, responsa ... Utini, Ex typographia Nicolai Schiratti, 1648.

[8], 209, [2] p.   21 cm.   [6969]

—De rationalis animae varia propensione ad corpus libri duo ... Patavii, Typis Paulli Frambotti, 1634.

[16], 118, [10] p.   21 cm.   [6970]

—De spontaneo viventium ortu libb. quatuor, in quibus de generatione animantium, quae vulgo ex putri exoriri dicuntur, accurate aliorum opiniones omnes ... examinantur ... Vicetiae, Ex typographia Dominici Amadei, apud Franciscum Bolzetam, 1618.

[6], 10, 323, [29] p.   31 cm.   [6971]

—De vita libri tres ... Genuae, Ex typographia Josephi Pavonii, 1606.

[16], 826, [34] p.   25 cm.   [6972]

Liber secundus and tertius have special title pages.
On title page of Liber secundus the original title vignette has been excised and replaced with one from another book.

—Mulctra; sive, De duplici calore corporum naturalium dialogus physico-medicus ... Utini, Ex typographia Nicolai Schiratti, 1636.

[4], 164 p.   22 cm.   [6973]

—Ψυχολογία ἀνθρωπίνη [sic]; sive, De ortu animae humanae libri III. In quibus multa arcana ac secreta naturae, tum de semine, tum de foetu, ut & assimilatione parentum & liberorum, panduntur ac revelantur ... Francofurti, Ex officina Joannis Saurii, 1606.

[16], 472, [45] p.   16 cm.   [6974]

Imperfect: p. [23–24] mutilated.

—Pyronarcha; sive, De fulminum natura deque febrium origine libri duo ... Patavii, Apud Crivellarum, 1634.

[8], 126, [12] p.   20 cm.   [6975]

—Ulysses apud Circen; sive, De quadruplici transformatione, deque varie transformatis hominibus dialogus ethico-physicus ... Utini, Ex typographia Nicolai Schiratti, 1636.

[8], 54, [2] p.   22 cm.   [6976]

—Verveceidos libri duo: in quibus Athos perfoditur, & Smilace coronatur ab Alumnis Adrastiae.

Collectore Conrado Van Roel [pseud., i.e. Fortunio Liceti] ... Ad Stephanum Rodericum Castrensem ... [Pisa] Oldenburgi [i.e. Pisae?] Apud successores Johannis Gutenbergii, 1636.

70 p.   15 cm.   [6977]

Spurious imprint. Cf. Weller.

—See BARTHOLIN, T. De armillis veterum schedion. 1676; NARDI, G. Apologeticon in Fortunii Liceti mulctram. 1638.

LICHTEN, ADAM [fl. 1599–1629] praeses. De melancholia, disputatio secunda, in qua de tertia melancholiae specie, quae ex hypochondriis originem ducit, agitur ... Helmaestadii, Ex typographeio Jacobi Lucii, 1609.

[24] p.   20 cm.   [6978]

Diss. —Helmstädt (C. Quartus, respondent)

—See also LUCHTEN, Adam (the same author).

LICHTNER, JOHANN CHRISTOPH [fl. 1653] De natura lucis exercitatio physica ... Lipsiae, Literis Lankisianis, imprimebat Christophorus Cellarius, 1653.

[24] p.   20 cm.   [6979]

Diss. pro loco—Leipzig.

LIDDEL, DUNCAN [1561–1613] Operum omnium iatro-Galenicorum, ex intimis artis medicae adytis, & penetralibus erutorum tomus unicus ... Repurgatus ... notatiunculis aliquot ... illustratus ... Opera ... Ludovici Serrani ... Lugduni, Sumptibus Antonii Chard, 1624.

[8], 473 p.; 308, [24] p.   26 cm.   [6980]

Imperfect: wormholes on p. [1–8], 1–28, and 213–304, part [1].

—Ars medica, succincte & perspicue explicata ... Hamburgi, Ex Bibliopolio Frobeniano, 1608.

[39], 868, [20] p.   17 cm.   [6981]

—[The same.] ... Alt. ed. emaculatior ... Hamburgi, Ex Bibliopolio Frobeniano, M. CD. XVII [1617]

[15], 868, [18] p.   17 cm.   [6982]

—[The same.] ... Ed. ejus ult. juxta exemplar, quod ipsemet auctor ante obitum ... correxerat et auxerat, recusa ... Accessit ejusdem Tractatus de dente aureo pueri Silesii contra Horstium; ex museo Joach. Morsii nunc primum prolatus. Hamburgi, Ex Bibliopolio Frobeniano, 1628.

[32], 826, [14] p.; 28 p.   17 cm.   [6983]

"Joannis Jessenii . . . historia de rustico Bohemo cultrivorace, Recusa ad exemplar Pragense . . . anno 1607" (p. 23-28, at end) has half title.

—Artis conservandi sanitatem libri duo, a . . . Doctore Liddelio defuncto delineati, atque opera & studio, D. Patricii Dunaei, M. D. ad colophonem perducti, & in apricum prolati. Aberdoniae, Excudebat Jacobus Brounus, 1651.

[16], 471, [1] p. 14 cm. [6984]

—De febribus libri tres . . . Hamburgi, Ex Bibliopolio Frobeniano [Excudebat Paulus Langius] 1610.

[16], 830, [2] p. 17 cm. [6985]

—praeses. Disputatio de apoplexia . . . Helmaestadii, Excudebat Jacobus Lucius, 1605.

[22] p. 20 cm. [6986]
Diss.—Helmstedt (J. Schulte, respondent)

LIEBAUD, JEAN. See LIÉBAULT, Jean [ca. 1534-1596]

LIÉBAULT, JEAN [ca. 1534-1596] ed. See HOULLIER, J. In Aphorismos Hippocratis commentarii. 1613, 1620, 1632, 1646, 1675.

—, tr. See GESNER, K. Quatre livres des secrets de medecine. 1628, 1643; MARINELLI, G. Les maladies des femmes. 1609, 1649.

LIEBAUT, JEAN. See LIÉBAULT, Jean [ca. 1534-1596]

LIEBE, GEORG HEINRICH [fl. 1700-1703] respondent. See SPERLING, P. G., praeses. Dissertatio medica inauguralis de vomitu simplici. 1700.

LIEBENFELDT, GUALTER AMBROSIUS WOLTER A. See WOLTER A LIEBENFELDT, Gualter Ambrosius [fl. 1666]

LIEBER, THOMAS. See ERASTUS, Thomas [1524-1583]

LIEBLER, THOMAS. See ERASTUS, Thomas [1524-1583]

LIEFMANN, FRIGYES [fl. 1696] respondent. See WEDEL, G. W., praeses. Dissertatio inauguralis medica de febri ephemera. 1696.

LIEGE, PIERRE [fl. 1695] respondent. See ALBINUS, B. Delineatio medica. 1695.

LIENBECK, HENNING [fl. 1700] Communication des Sympathetischen-Steins, ohne Einnehmung die Kranckheiten der Menschen durch application dessen in den Urin per sensibilem et insensibilem Transpirationem, zu curiren . . . Saalfeld, Johann Ritter [1700]

7 p. 18 cm. [6987]

LIEVENS, GERARD [fl. 1669] respondent. Disputatio medica inauguralis de syncope . . . Lugduni Batavorum, Apud viduam & haeredes Joannis Elsevirii, 1669.

[16] p. 23 cm. [6988]
Diss.—Leyden.

LIFES security. 1665. See [RAMESEY, W.]

LIGORIO, PIRRO [ca. 1510-1583] See MERCURIALE, G. De arte gymnastica. 1601, 1672.

LILIUM inter spinas.

323-333 p., vol. 6. 20 cm. (In Zetzner, Lazarus, ed. Theatrum chemicum. Argentorati, 1659-61) [6989]
Caption title.

LILLY, WILLIAM [1602-1681] See [GADBURY, J.] Philastrogus knavery epitomized. 1652.

LIMBORCH, GILBERT. See FUSCH, Gilbert [ca. 1504-1567]

LIMBORCH, GULIELMUS VAN [fl. 1693] Dodoneus cum Schrodero ambulans; sive, Breve utriusque compendium in quo mineralia, vegetabilia, animalia, virtutes, composita, et doses eorum exhibentur . . . Lovanii, Typis Guilielmi Stryckwant, 1693.

[196] p. 14 cm. [6990]

LIMMER, CONRAD PHILIPP [fl. 1685-1699]

Dissertations—Zerbst (Collegium Physicum)

—praeses. Collegii Physici disputatorii disputatio quarta. De atomis prima . . . Servestae, Joh. Ern. Bezelius [1687]

[4] p. 18 cm. [6991]
F. Encke, respondent.

—Collegii Physici disputatorii disputatio quinta. De atomis secunda . . . Servestae, Joh. Ern. Bezelius [1687]

[12] p. 18 cm. [6992]
J. R. Stubenrauch, respondent.

atomis tertia . . . Servestae, Joh. Ern. Bezelius [1687]
   [12] p. 18 cm.   **[6993]**
   F. C. Stannius, *respondent.*

—Collegii Physici disputatorii disputatio septima.
De vacuo, ejusque ridiculo metu . . . Servestae, Joh.
Ern. Bezelius [1687]
   [20] p. 19 cm.   **[6994]**
   C. R. Lezius, *respondent.*

—Collegii Physici disputatorii disputatio octava.
De corporis loco & spatio . . . Servestae, Joh. Ern.
Bezelius [1687]
   [8] p. 19 cm.   **[6995]**
   J. G. Raumer, *respondent.*

—Collegii Physici disputatorii disputatio nona. De
tempore . . . Servestae, Joh. Ern. Bezelius [1687]
   [8] p. 19 cm.   **[6996]**
   J. D. Cremer, *respondent.*

—Collegii Physici disputatorii disputatio decima.
De corpore raro & denso . . . Servestae, Joh. Ern.
Bezelius [1687]
   [16] p. 19 cm.   **[6997]**
   J. F. Müller, *respondent.*

—Collegii Physici disputatorii disputatio
duodecima. De corpore el vido, firmo, friabili et molli
. . . Servestae, Joh. Ern. Bezelius [1687]
   [24] p. 18 cm.   **[6998]**
   J. D. Appel, *respondent.*

—Collegii Physici disputatorii disputatio decima
tertia. De corpore humido & sicco . . . Servestae, Joh.
Ern. Bezelius [1687]
   [20] p. 19 cm.   **[6999]**
   C. F. Beerbalck, *respondent.*

—Disputatio chirurgico-medica de fonticulis in
qua irrationalis eorundem in vulgari medicorum
praxi usus ostenditur, nec non ex fabrica corporis
humani infallibiliter demonstratur . . . Servestae, Excudit Joh. Ernest. Bezelius [1687]
   [56] + p. 19 cm.   **[7000]**
   Imperfect: all after p. [56] wanting.
   C. G. Wenzlovius, *respondent.*

—Disputatio medico-physica de partu legitimo . . .
Servestae, Joh. Ern. Bezelius [1688]
   [40] p. 19 cm.   **[7001]**
   C. F. Beerbalck, *respondent.*

—Collegii Physici disputatorii disputatio sexta. De

—Disputatio physica extraordinaria de natura &
essentia mentis humanae . . . Servestae, Excudit Joh.
Ern. Bezelius [1687]
   [28] p. 19 cm.   **[7002]**
   N. Degen, *respondent.*

—Disputatio physica extraordinaria de sensibus internis . . . Servestae, Excudit Joh. Ern. Bezelius
[1695]
   [36] p. 19 cm.   **[7003]**
   J. C. Dares, *respondent.*

—Disputatio physica extraordinaria de unione
mentis humanae, cum corpore organico . . .
Servestae, Excudit Joh. Ern. Bezelius [1688]
   [32] p. 19 cm.   **[7004]**
   J. H. Stubenrauch, *respondent.*

—Disputatio physico-medica de monstroso abortu
Dessaviensi . . . Servestae, Joh. Ern. Bezelius [1694]
   [56] p. plate. 19 cm.   **[7005]**
   J. H. Graetz, *respondent.*

—Disputatio undecima de rarefactionis et condensationis aeris effectis in thermometris . . . Servestae,
Excudit Joh. Ern. Bezelius [1687]
   16 p. 18 cm.   **[7006]**
   C. Püschel, *respondent.*

—Dissertatio anatomica de cute, simulque insensibili transpiratione, sudoribus, pilis, et organo tactus . . . Servestae, Excudit Joh. Ern. Bezelius [1691]
   [18] p. 20 cm.   **[7007]**
   G. Günther, *respondent.*

Dissertation—Altdorf

—*respondent.* Disputatio medica inauguralis de
hydrophobia . . . Altdorffii, Literis Henrici Meyeri
[1688]
   12 p. 20 cm.   **[7008]**

LIMPRECHT, JOHANN ADAM [*fl.* 1672] *respondent.*
See BOHN, J., *praeses.* Exercitationum physiologicarum
prima . . . [-decima tertia] 1674?

LINACRE, THOMAS [*ca.* 1460-1524] *tr. See*
GALENUS. [Selected works. Latin] 1645.

LINAND, BARTHÉLEMY [*fl.* 1696-1697] Nouveau
traité des eaux minerales de Forges . . . Paris,

Laurent d'Houry, la veuve de Charles Coignard; Forges, Le sieur de la Cour, 1697.

[8], 135, [1] p. plate. 19 cm. [**7009**]

LINCK, JOHANN KARL [*fl.* 1685-1688] *respondent.* Casum medicum aegri epileptici ... publicae ... ventilationi subjiciet Joh. Carolus Linck ... [Altdorffii] Literis Henrici Meyeri [1688]

20 p. 20 cm. [**7010**]
Diss.—Altdorf

LINCKE, JOHANN JOACHIM [*fl.* 1678] *respondent. See* VEHR, I., *praes.* Dissertationem medicam inauguralem de soffocatione hysterica ... exhibet J. J. L. 1678.

LINDEMAN, JOHANN [1670-1700] *respondent. See* STAHL, G. E., *praes.* Disputatio inauguralis medica de morbo retrogrado. 1697.

LINDEN, JAN VAN DER [*fl.* 1633-1634] Cort verhael; oft, Tractaet vande contagieuse sieckte de peste ... Antwerpen, Guilliam Verdussen, 1634.

69, [1] p. 15 cm. [**7011**]
Imperfect: margins trimmed.

LINDEN, JOHANNES ANTONIDES VAN DER [1609-1664] De hemicrania menstrua, historia et consilium ... Lugduni Batavorum, Apud Johan. Elsevirium, 1660.

[24], 92, [4] p. 20 cm. [**7012**]

—De monstrosis vermibus, observatio rara. *In* Spiegel, A. van de. Opera quae extant, omnia. 1645.

—De scriptis medicis libri duo. Quibus praemittitur ... manuductio ad medicinam. Amstelredami, Apud Johannem Blaeu, 1637.

[48], 559, [24] p. 20 cm. [**7013**]

—[The same.] ... Ed. alt., auct. & emend. Amstelredami, Apud Johannem Blacu, 1651.

[16], 688, [28] p. 20 cm. [**7014**]

—[The same.] ... Ed. 3. & tertia auct. Amstelredami, Apud Joannem Blaeu, 1662.

[16], 755, [36] p. 20 cm. [**7015**]

—Dissertatio de lacte. *In* Deusing, A. De motu cordis et sanguinis. 1655.

—Historiae aegrotorum vigintiquinque ... [Leyden?] 1651.

[24] p. 13 cm. [**7016**]

—Lindenius renovatus; sive ... De scriptis medicis libri duo ... alphabetico hacque nova ... editione primum adornato ordine ... addita plurimorum authorum ... vitae curriculorum succincta descriptione ... continuati ... amplificati ... & ... purgati a Georg. Abrah. Mercklino ... Norimbergae, Impensis Johannis Georgii Endteri, 1686.

[23], 1097, [59] p.; [6], 160, [2] p. 22 cm. [**7017**]
Part 2 has special title page: Cynosura medica; sive, De scriptis medicis liber II.

—Another issue, with title page reset. [**7018**]
Imperfect: added engraved title page wanting.

—Manuductio ad medicinam. *In* Conring, H. In universam artem medicam singulasque ejus partes introductio. 1687.

—Medicina physiologica, nova curataque methodo ex optimis quinbusque auctoribus contracta, & propriis observationibus locupletata. Amstelaedami, Apud Joannem à Ravestein, 1653.

[8], 884 p. 21 cm. [**7019**]

—Medulla medicinae, partibus quatuor comprehensa. Tomus primus. Franekerae, Apud Uldericum Balck & Joh. Fabiani Deûring, 1642.

[15], 350 p.; 380 p. 15 cm. [**7020**]
Part 1 contains Manuductio ad medicinam. Editio tertia (p. [33]-142); and Medullae medicinae pars prima, physiologica (p. [143]-350) each with half title.

—Meletemata medicinae Hippocraticae. Lugduni Batavorum, Apud Gaasbekios, 1668.

[6], 399, [1] p. 19 cm. [**7021**]

—Selecta medica, et ad ea exercitationes Batavae. Lugduni Batavorum, Apud Johannem Elsevirium, 1656.

[12], 772, [56] p. 21 cm. [**7022**]
Contains fifteen passages in Greek with Latin translations (eleven from various Hippocratic works) and one in Latin, each with extensive commentary containing other excerpts.

—Another issue, with imprint: Amstelodami, Apud Ludovicum & Danielem Elsevirios, 1656.

[**7023**]

Dissertations — Leyden

—*praeses.* Hippocrates de circuitu sanguinis, exercitatio I. ... Lugduni Batavorum, Apud Johannem Elsevirium, 1659.

[8] p.   20 cm.   [7024]

T. Colbius, *respondent.*

—Hippocrates de circuitu sanguinis, exercitatio II. ... Lugduni Batavorum, Apud Johannem Elsevirium, 1659.

[8] p.   19 cm.   [7025]

N. A. Bartels, *respondent.*

—Hippocrates de circuitu sanguinis, exercitatio III. ... Lugduni Batavorum, Apud Johannem Elsevirium, 1659.

[8] p.   20 cm.   [7026]

A. Slingerlant, *respondent.*

—Hippocrates de circuitu sanguinis, exercitatio IV. ... Lugduni Batavorum, Apud Johannem Elsevirium, 1659.

[8] p.   20 cm.   [7027]

P. Hoffwenius, *respondent.*

—Hippocrates de circuitu sanguinis, exercitatio V. ... Lugduni Batavorum, Apud Johannem Elsevirium, 1660.

[8] p.   20 cm.   [7028]

H. Bailly, *respondent.*

—Hippocrates de circuitu sanguinis, exercitatio VI. ... Lugduni Batavorum, Apud Johannem Elsevirium, 1660.

[8] p.   20 cm.   [7029]

J. J. Wittig, *respondent.*

—Hippocrates de circuitu sanguinis, exercitatio VII. ... *Lugduni Batavorum, Apud Johannem Elsevirium,* 1660.

[8] p.   20 cm.   [7030]

P. Roosendael, *respondent.*

—Hippocrates de circuitu sanguinis, exercitatio VIII. ... Lugduni Batavorum, Apud Johannem Elsevirium, 1660.

[12] p.   20 cm.   [7031]

H. Meiling, *respondent.*

—Hippocrates de circuitu sanguinis, exercitatio IX. ... Lugduni Batavorum, Apud Johannem Elsevirium, 1660.

[12] p.   20 cm.   [7032]

—W. van den Hoorn, *respondent.*

—Hippocrates de circuitu sanguinis, exercitatio X. ... Lugduni Batavorum, Apud Johannem Elsevirium, 1600.

[12] p.   20 cm.   [7033]

A. Schonaeus, *respondent.*

—Hippocrates de circuitu sanguinis exercitatio XI. ... Lugduni Batavorum, Apud Johannem Elsevirium, 1660.

[12] p.   20 cm.   [7034]

A. a Mithoben, *respondent.*

—Hippocrates de circuitu sanguinis, exercitatio XII. ... Lugduni Batavorum, Apud Johannem Elsevirium, 1660.

[12] p.   20 cm.   [7035]

C. Pylius, *respondent.*

—Hippocrates de circuitu sanguinis, exercitatio XIII. ... Lugduni Batavorum, Apud Johannem Elsevirium, 1660.

[12] p.   20 cm.   [7036]

H. Nehtman, *respondent.*

—Mulieris colicae historia, lib. III. Epid. sect. II. aegr. IX. proposita, & exposita ... Lugduni Batavorum, Ex officina Francisci Hackii, 1652.

[18] p.   20 cm.   [7037]

Published also in Linden's Selecta medica, Lugduni Batavorum, 1656, p. 208-241, under title: Tisameni colica.

P. Caulier, *respondent.*

—*ed. See* CARDANO, G. De utilitate ex adversis capienda libri IV. 1648, 1672; CELSUS, A. C. De medicina libri octo. 1657, 1665, 1687; HARTMANN, J. Praxis chymiatrica. 1663; HIPPOCRATES. [Collected works. Greek and Latin] 1665. *See* COCCEJUS, J. Oratio. 1664.

LINDENER, KASPER. *See* LINDNER, Caspar [*d.* 1611]

LINDNER, CASPAR [*d.* 1611] *See* SCHOLTZ, L. Epistolarum philosophicarum: medicinalium, ac chymicarum ... volumen. 1610.

LINDNER, DANIEL [*fl.* 1669-1671] *respondent. See* ILMER, G., *praeses.* Dissertatio physico-philologica de tilia. 1669; ULMANN, D., *praeses.* Dissertatio physica de dracone volante. 1671.

LINE, FRANCIS. *See* HALL, Francis, *Father* [1595-1675]

LINEAE medicae, singulos per menses quotidie ductae ... anni M DC XCV [-M DCC] 1695-1700. *See* RIEDLIN, V.

LINEMANN, ALBERT [1603-1653] *praeses.* Disputatio psychologica ... de omni parte animae ... Regiomonti, Typis Johannis Reusneri, 1662.

[16] p.   18 cm.   **[7038]**

Diss.—Königsberg (H. Weghorst, *respondent*)

—Exercitatio philosophica visionis naturam physicis & opticis rationibus explicatam exhibens ... Regiomonti, Praelo Reusneriano, 1642.

[12] p.   18 cm.   **[7039]**

Diss.—Königsberg (B. Crusius, *respondent*)

L'INFERRIGNO, *pseud. See* ROSSI, Bastiano de [*fl.* 1585-1605]

LINGELSHEIM, GEORG MICHAEL [*fl.* 1596-1611] *See* BONGARS, J. Jacobi Bongarsii et Georgii Michaelis Lingelshemii epistolae. 1660.

LINSENBAHRT, ROSINUS LENTILIUS. *See* LENTILIUS, Rosinus [1651-1733]

LINSING, PETRUS [*fl.* 1688-1709] *respondent. See* WEINHART, F. K., *praeses.* Summa fundamentorum universae medicinae. 1688.

LINUS, FRANCISCUS. *See* HALL, Francis, *Father* [1595-1675]

LINYEROLA, ROCHO. *See* INSA, A. J. Officina medicamentorum. 1601 [i.e. 1603], 1698.

LIPEN, MARTIN [1630-1692] Bibliotheca realis medica, omnium materiarum, rerum, et titulorum, in universa medicina occurrentium ... Accedit index autorum copiosissimus ... Francofurti ad Moenum, Cura & sumptibus Johannis Friderici, prelo Johannis Nicolai Hummii, 1679.

[19], 492, [42] p.   36 cm.   **[7040]**
Added engraved title page.

LIPHIMEUS, SABALATHRUS. Warnung wider den Harn-Teuffel; das ist, Gründlicher Bericht, von dem Urin dess Menschen, unnd sonderlich wider diejenigen, so vorgeben, dass sie alle unnd jede Kranckheiten auss blosser Anschawung der Urin erkennen, urtheilen und curiren wollen ... Nürnberg, Gedruckt bey Simon Halbmayern, 1626.

75, [1] p.   17 cm.   **[7041]**

LIPPAY, JÁNOS [1606-1666] Posoni kert. Kiben minden kerti munkák, rendelések, virágokkal, veteményekkel, fákkal, gyümölcsökkel és kerti csömötékkel való baimlódások ... le-irattattanak ... Nagy Szombat, Az academiai bötükkel; Bécsbe, Cosmerovius Máthé, 1664-67.

[16], 148 p.; [16], 244 p.; [8], 302, [1] p. plates.   20 cm.   **[7042]**

Part 2 has special title page: Veteményes kert. Part 3 has special title page: Gyümölczös kert. Béczben, Cosmerovius Máté, 1667.
Imperfect: Part 3 bound before part 2; p. [1-16] and p. 241-244 of part 2 wanting.
Pagination partly supplied from Szinnyei.

LIPPE, H. D. *See* GREIFF, S. Wundartzeney. 1622.

LIPPOLDT, JOHANN GEORG [*fl.* 1693] *respondent. See* HEBENSTREIT, J. P., *praeses.* De remediis adversus locustas. 1693.

LIPSIUS, DAVID [*b.* 1578 or 9] Antipathiae singulares; sive, De naturali sed mirabili cibi et potus fastidio, odio, abstinentia dissertatio ... Jenae, Typis Johannis Gollneri, 1678.

22, [2] p.   20 cm.   **[7043]**

—Rahtschlag und Bericht wie bey denn Kindernn die anjetzo grassierende Blattern, beneden den Masern zuerkennen und zuheilen ... Erffurt, Gedruckt by Christoff Mehler, bey Sigismund Hoppfen zufinden, 1624.

73, [7] p.   20 cm.   **[7044]**

—Tractatus de hydropisis ejjusque specierum triplic. [sic] cognitione & curatione Galenico-spagyrica ... Adjectis auctarii loco capitibus Hubnerianis De morbis incurabilibus. [Erfurt?] Typis Wittelianis, 1624.

[2], 102 p.   20 cm.   **[7045]**

Imperfect: wormholes on p. 71-102.
The Capita de morbis incurabilibus is an Erfurt dissertation of 1591. Melchior Wedmann was respondent and Bartholomaeus Hubner acted as praeses.

—[The same.] ... Jenae, Typis Johannis Gollneri, 1678.

90, [5] p.   20 cm.   **[7046]**

LIPSIUS, JUSTUS [1547-1606] Diva Sichemiensis; sive, Aspricollis: nova ejus beneficia & admiranda. Antverpiae, Ex Officina Plantiniana, apud Joannem Moretum, 1605.

[8], 69, [10] p.   26 cm.   **[7047]**

—Het lof van den olyphant. *In* Veeler wonderens wonderbaarelijck lof. 1664.

LIPSTÖRP, GUSTAV DANIEL. *See* LIPSTORP, Gustav Daniel [1664-1689]

LIPSTORFF, HENRICUS. *See* LIPSTORP, Heinrich [1666-1701]

LIPSTORP, CHRISTOPH [1634-1690] Wolmeinendes Bedencken von der grassierenden Rohten Ruhr, mit beygefügten kurtzen Bericht von dem hitzigen, gifftigen Fieber, und wie man sich ... bewahren, oder da jemand damit behafftet würde, davon curieren könne. Stade, Caspar Holwein, 1676.

    [4], 60 p.   19 cm.   **[7048]**

—*respondent. See* SCHENCK, J. T., *praeses.* Disputatio dioptrico-anatomica de oculo. 1654.

LIPSTORP, GUSTAV DANIEL [1664-1689] *respondent.* Disputatio medica inauguralis de animalculis in humano corpore genitis ... Lugduni Batavorum, Apud Abrahamum Elzevier, 1687.

    [32] p.   21 cm.   **[7049]**
Diss.—Leyden.

—*respondent. See* ALBINUS, B. Dissertationem anatomico-medicam de poris humani corporis ... sistet ... G. D. L. ... 1685.

LIPSTORP, HEINRICH [1666-1701] *respondent.* Disputatio medica inauguralis de venae-sectionis usu & abusu ... Trajecti ad Rhenum, Ex officina Francisci Halma, 1693.

    15, [1] p.   20 cm.   **[7050]**
Diss.—Utrecht.

LIQUOR alchahest. 1675. *See* [STARKEY, G.]

LISCHKOW, SALOMON. *See* LISCOV, Salomon [1640-1689]

LISCHOVINI, ANDRÁS FERENCZ [*fl.* 1697-1703] *respondent. See* SANDEN, H. von, *praeses.* Dissertatio medica de molis. 1697.

LISCOV, SALOMON [1640-1689] *See* MÜHLMANN, J. Geistlicher Noth- und Todes-Schirm. 1680.

LISKOW, SALOMON. *See* LISCOV, Salomon [1640-1689]

L'ISLE, *le sieur de. See* SOREL, Charles [*ca.* 1602-1674]

LISLE, GUILLAUME DE. *See* INSULANUS MENAPIUS, Gulielmus [*d.* 1556]

LISSET-BENANCIO. *See* COLIN, Sébastien [1519?-1578?]

LIST, JOHANN JAKOB [*fl.* 1662] *respondent. See* PREGITZER, J. U., *praeses.* Exercitatio philosophica de affectibus appetitus sensitivi. 1662.

LISTEMANN, MAGNUS [*fl.* 1621] *respondent. See* AGER, N. Disputatio physica de somno. 1621.

LISTER, MARTIN [1638?-1712] Sex exercitationes medicinales de quibusdam morbis chronicis, quarum prima est, de hydrope; secunda, de diabete; tertia, de hydrophobia; quarta, de lue venerea; quinta, de scorbuto; sexta, de arthritide ... Londini, Impensis S. Smith & B. Walford, 1694.

    [16], 221, 48 p.   20 cm.   **[7051]**

—[The same.] ... Accessit G. G. L. Relatio ad inclytam Societatem Leopoldinam Naturae Curiosorum de novo antidysenterico ex America allato. Francofurti & Lipsiae, Sumptibus Gothofredi Freytagii, 1696.

    [16], 258, 38 p.   17 cm.   **[7052]**

—Octo exercitationes medicinales; quarum I. De hydrope. II. De diabete. III. De hydrophobia. IV. De lue venerea. V. De scorbuto. VI. De arthritide. VII. De calculo humano. VIII. De variolis. Alt. ed. ab auctore recognita, & non parum aucta. Londini, Apud Sam. Smith & Benj. Walford, 1697.

    [1], 348 p.   17 cm.   **[7053]**

—[The same.] ... Ed. ult. auct. & emend. Amstelodami, Apud Georgium Gallet, 1698.

    [8], 96 (i.e. 196), [4] p.   20 cm.   **[7054]**
With this are bound: Cole, W. Tractatus de secretione animali. 1698; Cole, W. Novae hypotheseos. 1698; Harris, W. De morbis acutis infantum. 1698.

—Conchyliorum bivalvium utriusque aquae exercitatio anatomica tertia. Huic accedit Dissertatio medicinalis de calculo humano ... Londini, Sumptibus authoris impressa, 1696.

    xliii, 173 p.; 51 p. plates.   21 cm.   **[7055]**
Part [2] has special title page.

—De fontibus medicatis Angliae, exercitatio nova & prior ... Juxta exemplar Eboracense. Francofurti

& Lipsiae, Sumptibus Johannis Grossii, literis Christiani Scholvini, 1684.

64 p. illus. 17 cm. [**7056**]

—[The same.] ... Ed. alt. auct. Londini, Walteri Kettilby, 1684.

[8], 104 p.; [11], 104 p. plate. 18 cm. [**7057**]

Part 2 has special title page: De fontibus medicatis Angliae exercitatio altera. Londini Typis R. E., impensis W. Kettilby, 1684.

—[The same.] Novae ac curiosae exercitationes & descriptiones thermarum ac fontium medicatorum Angliae ... Ed. ult. auct. & emend. Londini, [Typis R. E.] Impensis Walteri Kettilbi, 1686.

[12], 156 p. plate. 15 cm. [**7058**]

Added engraved title page: De thermis et fontibus medicatis Angliae.

A reprint of De fontibus medicatis Angliae with the addition of Exercitatio altera with special title page (p. [79])

—Another issue, with imprint: Lugd. Batav., Apud Petrum vander Aa, 1686. [**7059**]

—De morbis chronicis & De variolis. *In* Morton, R. Opera medica. 1696, 1697, 1699.

—Exercitatio anatomica. In qua de cochleis, maxime terrestribus & limacibus, agitur ... Londini, Sumptibus Sam. Smith & Benj. Walford, 1694.

[2], xi, 208 p. plates. 20 cm. [**7060**]

—Exercitatio anatomica altera, in qua maxime agitur de buccinis fluviatilibus & marinis. Ubi Aristotelis aliquot loca ab interpretum injuria ac errore vindicantur ... His accedit Exercitatio medicinalis de variolis. Londini, Sam. Smith & Benj. Walford, 1695.

[15], 267 p.; [1], 128 p. plates. 20 cm. [**7061**]

Part [2] has half title.

—Historiae animalium Angliae tres tractatus. Unus de araneis. Alter de cochleis tum terrestribus tum fluviatilibus. Tertius de cochleis marinis. Quibus adjectus est quartus de lapidibus ... ad cochlearum ... imaginem figuratis ... Londini, Joh. Martyn, 1678.

[7], 250, [1] p. plates. 21 cm. [**7062**]

Errata: p. [251]

The second book has special title page (p. [101]): Cochlearum Angliae et terrestrium et fluviatilium liber.

—A journey to Paris in the year 1698 ... London, Jacob Tonson, 1699.

[6], 245, [3] p. plates. 20 cm. [**7063**]

—[The same.] ... The 2d ed. London, Jacob Tonson, 1699.

[5], 245, [3] p. plates. 20 cm. [**7064**]

A reprint of the 1st edition, Errata corrected.

—Tractatus de quibusdam morbis chronicis, quorum I. est, de hydrope, II. de diabete, III. de hydrophobia, IV. de lue venerea, V. de scorbuto, VI. de artritide ... Genevae, Sumptibus Cramer & Perachon, 1696.

[8], 100 p. 22 cm. [**7065**]

—Tractatus de variolis variis historiis illustratus. Genevae, Sumptibus Cramer & Perachon, 1696.

40 p. 22 cm. [**7066**]

—, *ed.* and *tr.* *See* Goedaert, J. Of insects. 1682.

—, *ed. See* Goedaert, J. Johannes Goedartius De insectis. 1685.

LISTRIUS, GERARDUS [*fl.* 1513-1546] *ed. See* ERASMUS, D. Μωρίας ἐγκώμιον. 1676.

LITE, HENRY. *See* LYTE, Henry [1529?-1607]

LITTLETON, ADAM [1627-1694] Carmen elegiacum. *In* Hodges, N. Λοιμολογία, 1672.

—, *ed. See* HAMEY, B. Dissertatio epistolaris de juramento medicorum. 1693.

LIVINGSTONE, JOHN. *See* LEVISTONIUS, Joannes [*fl.* 1661]

LIZARAZO, PEDRO JERÓNIMO SÁNCHEZ DE. *See* SÁNCHEZ DE LIZARAZO, Pedro Jerónimo [*d.* 1614]

LIZZANUS, JOANNES ANDREAS [*fl.* 1700] Martinus in Trutina. *In* Celeberr. virorum apologiae pro R. D. Carolo Musitano. 1700.

LLERA, MATÍAS DE [*fl.* 1652-1666] Manus medica dextera quinque digitos continens, quorum primus disputationem in duos Galeni libros de febrium differentiis. Secundus librum, De curandi ratione per sanguinis missionem. Tertius, Controversias de purgatione ... Quartus, Tractatum de crisibus, et diebus decretoriis. Quintus ... Consultandi rationem proponit ... Caesar-Augustae, Apud Joannem de Ybar, 1666.

[44], 618, [1] p. front. (port.) 21 cm. [**7067**]

[**LLOYD**, DAVID, 1635-1692] Wonders no miracles; or, Mr. Valentine Greatrates [sic] gift of healing examined, upon occasion of a sad effect of his stroaking, March the 7. 1665 ... London, Sam. Speed, 1666.

[1], 46 p. 20 cm. [**7068**]

LLUELYN, MARTIN [1616-1682] *ed. See* BENNET, C. Tabidorum theatrum. 1656, 1665.

LLULL, RAMÓN. *See* LULL, Ramón [1232-*ca.* 1316]

L'OBEL, MATTHIAS DE [1538-1616] Diarium pharmacorum parandorum; Medicamenta composita; De succedaneis imitatione Rondeletii. *In* Cordus, V. Dispensatorium. 1627, 1651, [1652]; [Dutch ed.] 1632, 1656.

—In G. Rondelletii ... methodicam pharmaceuticam officinam animadversiones, quibus depravata & mutilata ex authoris mente corriguntur ... Accesserunt auctaria, in antidotaria vulgata censurae benevolae, & dilucidae simplicium medicamentorum explicationes, adversariorumque volumen ... cum Ludovici Myrei ... paragraphis utiliss. ... Londini, Excudebat praelum Thomae Purfootii, 1605.

[8], 156 p.; [15], 549 p. illus., plates. 29 cm.
[**7069**]

Mistakes in pagination.
Part [2] has special title page: Dilucidae simplicium medicamenorum [sic] explicationes, & stirpium adversaria ... Authoribus Petro Pena & Matthia de L'Obel ... Quibus accessit Altera pars ... opera ... Matthiae de L'Obel. Altera pars has half title.
"G. Rondelletii Tractatus de hydrope ... ejusdem ... Elephantiasis nova ... curandi ratio ... ": p. 542-549.
STC 19595.5.

—Another issue. [**7070**]

Mistakes in pagination corrected.

—Stirpium illustrationes. Plurimas elaborantes inauditas plantas, subreptitiis Joh. Parkinsoni rapsodiis (ex codice MS insalutato) sparsim gravatae. Ejusdem adjecta sunt ad calcem Theatri botanici à μαρτήματα. Accurante Guil. How ... Londini, Typis Tho. Warren, impensis Jos. Kirton, 1655.

[38], 170, [5] p. 20 cm. [**7071**]

—*See* PARKINSON, J. Theatrum botanicum. 1640.

LOBELIUS, MATTHIAS. *See* L'OBEL, Matthias de [1538-1616]

LOBKOWITZ. *See* ERBEN VON BRANDAU, Matthias [*fl.* 17th cent.]

LOCATELLI, GIOVANNI BATTISTA [*fl.* 1631] Della peste trattato ... Rovigo, Giacinto e Marin Bissuccio, 1631.

[8], 189, [7] p. 26 cm. [**7072**]

LOCATELLI, LODOVICO [*ca.* 1600-1657] Theatro d'arcani ... nel quale si tratta dell'arte chimica, & suoi arcani, con gli Afforismi d'Ippocrate commentati da Paracelso, & l'espositione d'alcune cifre, & caratteri oscuri de filosofi ... Milano, Gio. Pietro Ramellati, 1644.

[58], 456 p. illus. 18 cm. [**7073**]

Added engraved and woodcut title pages.
Imperfect: added engraved title page wanting.
"Espositione della prima divisione delli Afforismi d'Ippocrate, de prima sei della seconda, & delli nove ultimi della quarta divisione di Teofrasto Paracelso ... Di più un'altra espositione del primo Afforismo" (p. 308-402) includes the Latin text of the Aphorismi translated by Georg Forberger. The commentaries on books 1-2 of the Aphorismi are translated from Paracelsus' Erklärung über etliche Aphorismen des Hippokrates.
Sudhoff 361.

—[The same.] ... Venetia, Paolo Baglioni, 1667.

[16], 392, [22] p. diagr. 16 cm. [**7074**]

Some preliminary matter omitted.
Sudhoff 397.

LOCHNER, MICHAEL FRIEDRICH. *See* LOCHNER VON HUMMELSTEIN, Michael Friedrich [1662-1720]

LOCHNER VON HUMMELSTEIN, MICHAEL FRIEDRICH [1662-1720] *respondent.* De nymphomania historiam medicam ... in disputatione inaugurali publice defendet ... Mich. Fried. Lochner ... Altdorffii, Typis Henrici Meyeri [1684]

24 p. 22 cm. [**7075**]
Diss. — Altdorf.

LOCK, JOHN. *See* LOCKE, John [1632-1704]

LOCKE, JOHN [1632-1704] *See* BURTHOGGE, R. Of the soul of the world. 1699.

LOCQUES, NICOLAS DE [*fl.* 1664] Propositions touchant la physique resolutive ... Paris, Geoffroy Marcher, 1665.

[39] p. 19 cm. [**7076**]

—Les vertus magnetiques du sang, de son usage ... pour la guarison des maladies ... Paris, De l'imprimerie de Jacques le Gentil, et se vend chez l'autheur, 1664.

[16], 54, [2] p. 19 cm. [7077]

LOCQUET, JAN [*fl.* 1693] *respondent.* Disputatio anatomico-medica inauguralis de arteria hepatica ... Lugduni Batavorum, Apud Abrahamum Elzevier, 1693.

[24] p. 22 cm. [7078]
Diss.—Leyden.

LODETTI, GIOVANNI ANTONIO [*fl.* 1569] Dialogo de gl'inganni d'alcuni malvaggi speciali ... nel quale si scoprono molte frodi, che da detti speciali sono commesse, a pregiuditio si della vita de gli ammalati ... Padova, P. P. Tozzi, 1626.

69, [1] p. 15 cm. [7079]
Bound with Bovio, Z. T. Flagello de'medici rationali. 1626.

—Another issue.
69, [1] p. 15 cm. (Part [5] in Bovio, Z. T. Opere contra medici putaticii rationali. Padova, 1626) [7080]

—*See* COLIN, S. Declaratio fraudum et errorum apud pharmacopoeos commissorum. 1667, 1671.

LODGE, THOMAS [1558?-1625] A treatise of the plague, containing the nature, signes, and accidents of the same, with the ... cure of the fevers ... selected out of the writings of the best ... phisitians ... London, Edward White and N. L., 1603.

[86] p. 18 cm. [7081]
Signatures: A-K⁴, L³.
Imperfect: sig. L1 wanting; supplied in photocopy from Huntington Library.
STC 16676.

—, *tr. See* JOSEPHUS, F. The famous and memorable workes of Josephus. 1632.

LÖBER, CHRISTOPH HEINRICH [1634-1705] *praeses.* Disputatio physica de vita et morte ... Jenae, Literis Johannis Nisii, 1658.

[16] p. 20 cm. [7082]
Diss.—Jena (J. E. Stille, *respondent*)

LÖBER, VALENTINE [1620-1685] Anchora sanitatis, dialogice fabrificata. Cui annexa est Mantissa de venenis, et eorum antidotis ... Francofurti & Hamburgi, Impensis Joannis Naumanni & Georgii Wolffii, 1671.

239 p. 17 cm. [7083]

LOELIUS, JOHANN LORENZ [1641-1700] *respondent. See* ROLFINCK, W., *praeses.* Συξυτησις medica inauguralis de scorbuto. 1668; SENNERT, M., *praeses.* Disputatio physico-anatomica de sanguine. 1664.

LOENIUS, RUTGER [*d.* 1672] *ed. See* FERNEL, J. Pathologiae liber quartus De febribus. 1664.

LOESCHER, VALENTIN ERNST [1672-1749] *praeses.* Antisthenes; sive, Suspiciones opticae ... Vitembergae, Prelo Christiani Kreusigii [1698]

[28] p. 20 cm. [7084]
Diss.—Wittenberg (J. Praetorius, *respondent*)

LÖSEL, JOHANN [1607-1655] De podagra tractatus, morbi hujus indolem, & curam ... esponens. Rostochii, Sumptibus Joh. Hallerfordi, typis haeredum Richelianorum, 1638.

[4], 52 p. 20 cm. [7085]

—[The same.] ... Ed. 2. corr. & duplo auct. Accessit insuper Hieronymi Cardani ... Podagrae encomium. Lugduni Batavorum, Ex officina Joannis Maire, 1639.

382 p. 14 cm. [7086]

—Scrutinium renum in quo genuina renum fabrica, & actio, eorumque affectus ... explicantur. Additum est schema aberrantis structurae vasorum emulgentium & spermaticorum. Cum appendice observatorum in anatome corporis strangulati nuper administrata ... Regiomontani, Sumptibus Petri Hendelii, typis Reusnerianis, 1642.

[4], 67 p. illus. 21 cm. [7087]
Appendix has half title dated 1641.

LÖSER, JOHANN DIETRICH [*fl.* 1690] *respondent. See* FRANCK VON FRANCKENAU, G., *praeses.* Dissertatio inauguralis de hydrope ascite. 1690.

LÖW, ANDRÁS [*ca.* 1660-*ca.* 1710] *respondent. See* FASCH, A. H., *praeses.* Dissertatio medica inauguralis de morbo Hungarico. 1682; WEDEL, G. W., *praeses.* Dissertatio medica de lue venerea. 1682.

LOEW, JOHANN FRANZ. *See* LOEW VON ERLSFELD, Johann Franz, *Ritter* [1648-1725]

LÖW, JOHANN GEORG [1565-1610] *See* UEBELIN, S. Positiones physicae ωξὶ τῆς σηψεος. 1608.

LOEW VON ERLSFELD, JOHANN FRANZ, *Ritter* [1648-1725] Partus medicus multo labore a Leone in lucem editus; seu, tractatus novissimus de variolis et morbillis . . . Cui accessit Apodixis medica de morbis infantum . . . Norimbergae, Sumpt. Johannis Ziegeri & Georgii Lehmanni, 1699.

[12], 472, [14] p. 21 cm.   **[7088]**

LOEWENKLAU, JOHANN. *See* LEUNCLAVIUS, Johannes [1533?-1593]

LÖWENSTERN, JOHANN KUNCKEL VON. *See* KUNCKEL, Johann [1630?-1703]

LOF der medicine. 1641. *See* BEVERWIJCK, J. van.

LOFFHAGEN, GEORG [*fl.* 1694-1703] *respondent. See* SCHRADER, F., *praeses.* Disputatio medica de febre quartana. 1694.

LOFFREDO, FERRANTE, *marchese di Trivico* [16th cent.] L'antichità di Pozzuolo. *In* Bartoli, S. Breve ragguaglio. 1667.

LOGAN, GEORG ADAM [*fl.* 1691] *respondent. See* JACOBI, L. F., *praeses.* Disputatio medica de anima. 1691.

LOGES, JOHANN WOLFFGANG [*fl.* 1700-1703] *respondent. See* TRÜBE, G. T. Dissertatio historico-physica de mortus ex affectibus. 1700.

LOGORIUS, PYRRHUS. *See* LIGORIO, Pirro [*ca.* 1510-1583]

LOHDE, JOHANN [1619-1696] Historischer Discurs von Erfindung vieler guten Dinge, zu Hinbringung menschliches Lebens nötig und heilsam, benebenst . . . warhafftigern Berichte von dem schellendorffischen Heyl-Brunnen, zu Gutzschdorff bey Königsbrück gelegen . . . Freybergk, Gedruckt bey Georg Beuthern, 1647.

[107] p. illus. 20 cm.   **[7089]**

LOHEN, CHRISTOPHER A [*fl.* 1686] *respondent. See* BECKHER, D. C., *praeses.* Disputatio medica de salubri potu calidae. 1686.

LOHMEIER, PHILIPP [*d.* 1680] *praeses.* Exercitatio physica de fulmine . . . Rinthelii, Typis Godofr. Casp. Wächters [1676]

24 p. 19 cm.   **[7090]**
Diss.—Rinteln (J. A. Reuss, *respondent*)

LOHNER, BERNHARD [*fl.* 1675] *respondent. See* WEDEL, G. W., *praeses.* Disputatio medica inauguralis, de partu difficili. 1675.

LOHRMAN, GUSTAV [*fl.* 1664-1666] *respondent.* Disputatio medica inauguralis de hydrocephalo . . . Lugduni Batavorum, Ex officina Cornelii Driehuysen, 1666.

[12] p. 20 cm.   **[7091]**
Diss.—Leyden.

LOIECIUS, JOANNES [*fl.* 1607] *respondent.* De cardialgia conclusiones . . . Basileae, Typis Excertierianis, 1607.

[12] p. 20 cm.   **[7092]**
Diss.—Basel.

LOM, JOOST VAN. *See* LOMMIUS, Jodocus [*ca.* 1500-*ca.* 1564]

LOMAZZO, GIOVANNI PAOLO [1538-1600] Traicte de la proportion naturelle et artificielle des choses . . . Traduit d'italien . . . par Hilaire Pader . . . Tolose, Arnaud Colomiez, 1649.

[40], 91, [8] p. plates, port. 33 cm.

[7093]

Translation of the first book of the Trattato dell'arte della pittura . . . diviso in sette libri.

LOMBARD, KARL PHILIPP [*fl.* 1682-1688] *respondent.* Disputatio medica inauguralis de paralysi . . . Marburgi Catt., Typis Joh. Henr. Stockenii, 1686.

24 p. 19 cm.   **[7094]**
Diss.—Marburg.

—*See* DORSTEN, J. D., *praeses.* Exercitatio anatomica de monstro humano nupero. 1684; WALDSCHMIDT, J. J., *praeses.* Disquisitio medica de haemorrhagia narium. 1686.

L'OMBRE de necrophore vivant chartier de l'Hostel Dieu. 1622. *See* LAMPÉRIÈRE, J. de.

LOMELLINO, GIROLAMO VENEROSO. *See* VENEROSO LOMELLINO, Girolamo [1545-1625]

LOMM, JODOCUS. *See* LOMMIUS, Jodocus [*ca.* 1500-*ca.* 1564]

LOMMEN, JOSSE VAN. *See* LOMMIUS, Jodocus [*ca.* 1500-*ca.* 1564]

LOMMIUS, JODOCUS [*ca.* 1500-*ca.* 1564] Observationum medicinalium libri tres, quibus omnium morborum signa, & quae de his haberi possunt, praesagia, accuratissime pertractantur ... Ex musaeo Bernh. Rottendorff ... Francofurti, Impensis Johannis Davidis Zunneri, 1643.

[16], 290, [8] p. 17 cm. [7095]

Interleaved.

—[The same.] ... Nunc denuo editum cum praefatione Georgii Wolffgangi Wedelii. Francofurti & Lipsiae, Sumptibus Johan. Bielckii, 1688.

[32], 366, [10] p. 15 cm. [7096]

The LONDON almanack. For the year of our Lord, 1699. By William Salmon ... London, Printed by W. Horton for the Company of Stationers, 1699.

[48] p. 16 cm. [7097]

Sheet C bound before sheet A.

LONDON. Bridewell Hospital. *See* Bridewell Hospital, London.

LONDON. Christ's Hospital. *See* Christ's Hospital, London.

LONDON, Company of Parish Clerks. London's dreadful visitation; or, A collection of all the bills of mortality for this present year: beginning the 20th of December 1664, and ending the 19th. of December following; as also, The general or whole years bill ... London, E. Cotes, 1665.

[108] p. 23 cm. [7098]

LONDON. Corporation. Court of Common Council. The order of the hospitalls of K. Henry the viijth and K. Edward the vith, viz. St. Bartholomew's, Christ's, Bridewell, St. Thomas's. By the maior, cominaltie, and citizens of London, governeurs of the possessions, revenues and goods of the sayd hospitalls, 1557. [London, Samuel Pepys? not before 1690]

[115] p. 15 cm. [7099]

Preface signed by Goodfellow. John Goodfellow was town clerk from 1690–1700. Cf. Power, p. 108.

LONDON. Distillers. The distiller of London. *See* Mayerne, *Sir* T. T. de. The distiller of London. 1639, 1652.

LONDON. Ordinances, local laws, etc. Orders conceived and published by the Lord Mayor and Aldermen of the City of London, concerning the infection of the plague. London, James Flesher [1665]

15 p. 19 cm. [7100]

Signatures: A-B⁴.

Wing 0397.

Bound with another issue of Royal College of Physicians, London. Certain necessary directions. 1665.

LONDON. Parish Clerks' Company. *See* London. Company of Parish Clerks.

LONDON. Royal College of Physicians. *See* Royal College of Physicians, London.

LONDON. Royal Society. *See* Royal Society of London.

LONDON. St. Bartholomew's Hospital. *See* St. Bartholomew's Hospital, London.

LONDON. St. Thomas's Hospital. *See* St. Thomas's Hospital, London.

LONDON'S dreadful visitation; or, A collection of all the bills of mortality. 1665. *See* London. Company of Parish Clerks.

LONDRADA A PORTU AQUITANUS, Bernardus G. *See* Penot, Bernard Georges [*d.* 1617?]

LONER, Gabriel [*fl.* 1670-1672] *respondent. See* Rikemann, J., *praeses.* Ordinis et methodi cognoscendi praecavendi curandi ebrietatem. 1670; Rolfinck, W., *praeses.* Disputatio inauguralis medica de dysenteria maligna urbem Vinariensem depopulante. 1672.

LONG, Thomas [1621-1707] A review of Mr. Richard Baxter's life. Wherein many mistakes are rectified ... London, Printed by F. C. and sold by E. Whitlock, 1697.

[38], 274 p. 19 cm. [7101]

LONG-PRÉ, François de [*fl. ca.* 1628] *ed. See* Vigier, J. [*fl.* 1608?] Enchiridion anatomic. 1628.

LONGINUS, Caesar [*fl.* 1609-1614] *ed.* Trinum magicum; sive, Secretorum magicorum opus: continens 1. De magia naturali, artificiosa et superstitiosa disquisitiones axiomaticas. 2. Theatrum naturae, praeter curam magneticam & veterum sophorum sigilla et imagines magicas ... 3. Oracula Zoroastris, & mysteria mysticae philosophiae, Hebraeorum, Chaldaeorum, Aegyptiorum, Arabum, Persarum, Graecorum, Orphicorum, Pythagoricorum & Latinorum. Accessere nonnulla secreta secretorum

& mirabilia mundi . . . Francofurti, Ex officina typographica Antonii Hummii, 1616.

[20], 603 p. 14 cm. [7102]

Contents. — [1] Marci Antonii Zimarae Tractatus magicus. — [2] Appendix de mirandis quibusdam naturali magia factis operationibus. Ex. lib. 2. Mag. nat. Joan. Bapt. Port. — [3] Tractatus de vitutibus herbarum, lapidum et animalium, authore Alberto Magno. — [4] Commentatio de magnetica curatione vulnerum . . . Authore R[odolpho] G[oclenio] M.D. — [5] Logia; sive, Oracula Zoroastri, ex Platonicorum libris collecta.

The first tract is rather an anonymous treatise and not by Zimara. Cf. Thorndike, vol. 6, p. 601.

— [The same.] . . . Accessere nonnulla secreta secretorum & mirabilia mundi et Tractatus de proprii cujusque nati daemonis inquisitione . . . Francofurti, Sumptibus Jacobi Gothofredi Seyleri, 1673.

[24], 498 p. 14 cm. [7103]

LONICERUS, Adamus. *See* Lonitzer, Adam [1528–1586]

LONITZER, Adam [1528–1586] Kreuterbuch. Kunstliche Conterfeytunge der Bäume, Stauden, Hecken, Kreuter, Getreyde, Gewürtze . . . Sampt künstlichem und artlichem Bericht dess Distillierens. Item von fürnembsten Gethieren der Erden, Vögeln, unnd Fischen. Dessgleichen von Metallen, Ertze, Edelgesteinen, Gummi, und gestandenen Säfften. Jetzo auffs fleissigst zum letzten Mal von neuwem ersehen, und . . . gebessert . . . gemehret . . . Durch Adamum Lonicerum . . . Franckfort am Mayn, Getruckt durch Sigismundum Latomum, in Verlegung Vincentii Steinmeyers, 1604 [1603]

[12], ccclxxxii, [3] ll. illus. 32 cm. [7104]

Translation of *his* Naturalis historiae opus novum.

LOOM, Judocus van. *See* Lommius, Jodocus [ca. 1500–ca. 1564]

LOOSIUS, Joannes [*fl.* 1668] *respondent.* Disputatio medica inauguralis de phthisi . . . Trajecti ad Rhenum, Ex officina Antonii Smytegelt, 1668.

[11] p. 21 cm. [7105]

Diss. — Utrecht.

LOPEZ, Juan Joseph. *See* Trigo de Roxas, J. D. Memorial christiano. 1684.

LÓPEZ CORNEJO, Alonso [*fl.* 1699] Galeno ilustrado, Avicena explicado, y doctores sevillanos defendidos. Refutase la nueva con la antigua medicina, y manifiestase, que ni Hypocrates,

Galeno, Avicena, ni los practicos antiguos ignorarõ lo mas de lo moderno, y que de ellos se ha deducido, y trasladado lo mas util . . . Sevilla, Juan de la Puerta [1699?]

[46], 252, [51] p. 21 cm. [7106]

— *See* León, F. de. Respuestas a las preguntas que me hizo el señor doct. D. Alonso Cornejo. 1699.

LÓPEZ DE LEÓN, Pedro [*fl.* 1578–1590] Pratica y teorica de las apostemas . . . Questiones, y praticas de cirugia, de heridas, llagas, y otras cosas nuevas, y particulares . . . Primera [-segunda] parte . . . Sevilla, Luys Estupiñan, 1628.

[14], 370 ll. plates. 29 cm. [7107]

Imperfect: plates wanting.

— [The same.] . . . Calatayud, Joseph Vicente Mola [1697?]

[6], 388 (i.e. 405), [6] p. plates. 31 cm. [7108]

Imperfect: plates wanting, title page and last leaf mutilated.

LÓPEZ PINNA, Pedro [*b.* 1667] Tratado de morbo galico, en el qual se declara su origen, causas señales, pronosticos, y curacion . . . Sevilla, Juan Francisco de Blas, 1696.

[8], 182 (i.e. 180), [2] p. 20 cm. [7109]

LORENTZ, Justus [*fl.* 1673] *respondent. See* Roth, E. R. De velamine capitis virili exercitatio historica. 1673.

LORENZ, Georg Friedrich [1594–1673] Georgii-Friderici Laurentii Exercitationum in non nullos minus absolute veros Hippocratis Aphorismos, eorumque rationes, conscriptarum, pars prima. Hamburgi, Sumptibus autoris, typis Jacobi Rebenlini, 1647.

[56], 317, [3] p. port. 20 cm. [7110]

No more appears to have been published.

Includes Latin text of selected aphorisms, translated by Adolph Vorstius.

LORENZANO, Lorenzo. *See* Laurenziani, Lorenzo [ca. 1450–1502]

LORENZI, Lorenzo. *See* Laurenziani, Lorenzo [ca. 1450–1502]

LORENZINI, Antonio [16th–17th cent.] De risu, ejusque causis et effectis . . . libri duo. *In* Jossio, N. Tractatus novus . . . De voluptate et dolore. 1603.

LORENZINI, STEFANO [*fl.* 1678] Osservazioni intorno alle torpedini ... Firenze, L'Onofri, 1678.
    [8], 136 p. illus., plates. 25 cm. **[7111]**

LORENZO, ANDREA. *See* DU LAURENS, André [1558-1609]

LORICH, JOHANN WILHELM [*fl.* 1626] respondent. *See* CHARSTADIUS, V., *praeses.* Disputationum medicarum quarta de diaeta. 1626 [and] Disputationum medicarum nona de urina et pulsu. 1626.

LORME, CAROLUS DE. *See* DELORME, Charles [1584-1678]

LOSE, LAURENTIUS. *See* Loss, Laurentius [*fl.* 1679]

LOSEL, JOHANN. *See* LÖSEL, Johann [1607-1655]

LOSELLUS, GUILLELMUS. *See* LOYSEAU, Guillaume [*fl.* 1598-1617]

LOSEUS, STEPHAN [*fl.* 1634] respondent. *See* STUTHENIUS, G. Ψυχολογία; hoc est, Disquisitio physica de anima rationali. 1634.

LOSS, FRIEDRICH [*ca.* 1602-1680] Conciliorum; sive, De morborum curationibus. Liber posthumus ... Londini, Awnsham Churchill, 1684.
    [7], 295 p. 18 cm. **[7112]**

—[The same.] ... Lipsiae, Apud Maur. Georg. Weidmann, 1685.
    [8], 295 p. 18 cm. **[7113]**
Different setting of type.

—Observationum medicinalium libri quatuor ... Londini, Typis E. Flesher, & prostant apud Gualterium Kettilby, 1672.
    [14], 384 p. 16 cm. **[7114]**

—*See* ANIMADVERSIONS ON THE MEDICINAL OBSERVATIONS. 1674.

LOSS, HENRICUS [*fl.* 1600] respondent. *See* SIEGFRIED, J. Disputationum anatomicarum decima octava. 1600.

LOSS, JEREMIAS [1643-1684] Jeremias Lossius ... anat. et botanices prof. publicus ... S. P. D. lecturis. Wittebergae, Typis Christiani Schrödteri [1683]
    [8] p. 19 cm. **[7115]**
Program—Wittenberg (for G. E. Fromhold)

—*praeses.* De fermento ventriculi ... Jenae, Literis Krebsianis [1665]
    [24] p. 19 cm. **[7116]**
Diss.—Jena (J. C. Nettelbach, *respondent*)

Dissertations — Wittenberg
—*praeses.* Casum practicum de asthmate convulsio ... examini exponit Georgius Christianus Pfeifer ... Wittebergae, Typis Christiani Schrödteri [1676]
    [24] p. 19 cm. **[7117]**
G. C. Pfeifer, *respondent.*

—De glandulis in genere ... Wittenbergae, Typis viduae Augusti Brüningii [1682]
    [4], 20 p. 20 cm. **[7118]**
J. C. Below, *respondent.*

—Disputatio inauguralis medica de cancro mammarum ... Wittenbergae, Typis Christiani Schrödteri [1684]
    [64] p. 18 cm. **[7119]**
G. E. Fromhold, *respondent.*

—Disputatio inauguralis medica, de iliaca passione ... Wittenbergae, Typis describente Christiano Schrödtero [1682]
    [28] p. 19 cm. **[7120]**
V. H. Marold, *respondent.*

—Disputatio medica de salivae natura et usu ... Wittebergae, Typis Matthaei Henckelii [1677]
    [24] p. 20 cm. **[7121]**
G. Heydenreich, *respondent.*

—Disputationem de nuce vomica ... proponit Andreas Caspar Georgi ... Wittenbergae, Literis Johannis Wilkii [1683]
    [18] p. 20 cm. **[7122]**
Date altered by hand from MDCLXXXII to MDCLXXXIII.
A. C. Georgi, *respondent.*

—Disputationem inauguralem de lue venerea ... publicae eruditorum censurae subdit ... Joh. Georgius Rebentrost ... Wittenbergae, Typis Matthaei Henckelii [1683]
    [40] p. 20 cm. **[7123]**
J. G. Rebentrost, *respondent.*

—Disputationem inauguralem erotomaniae seu amoris insani, theoriam & praxin pertractantem ...

submittit M. Theodorus Kunadus ... Wittebergae, Literis Johannis Sigismundi Ziegenbeins [1681]

[42] p. 20 cm. [7124]

T. Kunad, *respondent.*

— Dissertatio inauguralis medica de inflammatione ... Wittenbergae, Typis Matthaei Henckelii [1683]

[30] p. 20 cm. [7125]

M. G. Ziegra, *respondent.*

— Dissertatio medica de glandulis in genere ... Wittebergae, Typis Martini Schultzii [1683]

[1], 20 p. 19 cm. [7126]

G. Pielow, *respondent.*

— Dissertatio medica de hydrophobia ... Wittebergae, Literis Brüningianis [1682]

[28] p. 20 cm. [7127]

G. F. Raussendorff, *respondent.*

— Dissertatione inaugurali morborum ab imaginatione ortorum, aliis idealium, ideam ... examini exponet publico M. Johann. Gerdes ... Wittenbergae, Literis Schrödteri, 1681.

[1], 44, [6] p. 20 cm. [7128]

J. Gerdes, *respondent.*

— Dissertationem medicam de arthritide ... publico ... examini exponit ... Martinus Tutius ... Wittenbergae, Typis viduae Augusti Brüningii [1683]

[32] p. 19 cm. [7129]

M. Tutius, *respondent.*

— Exercitatio anatomica de ovario humano ... Wittebergae, Christianus Schrödterus [1674]

[32] p. 20 cm. [7130]

G. Jachman, *respondent.*

— Another issue, with new title page dated 1675. [7131]

— Exercitatio pathologica de glandularum passionibus in genere ... Wittenbergae, Typis viduae Augusti Brünningii [1682]

[22] p. 20 cm. [7132]

G. E. Fromhold, *respondent.*

— Specimen academicum aegrum tertiana continua maligna laborantem sistens ... Wittenbergae, Typis Johannis Wilckii [1681]

[24] p. 20 cm. [7133]

H. V. Marold, *respondent.*

— *respondent. See* AMMANN, P., *praeses.* De ardore ventriculi. 1663; FRANCKENSTEIN, C. F., *praeses.* Academica de ephialte diatribe. 1663; SCHENCK, J. T., *praeses.* Thematum theoretico-practicorum de dolore capitis, sesqui-decas. 1665.

LOSS, LAURENTIUS [*fl.* 1679] Chirurgisches Hand-Büchlein, oder Erneurter Greif. Meiningen, Gedruckt bey Niclaus Hasserten [1682]

[14], 208 p. 14 cm. [7134]

Added title page.

With this are bound: *his* Pest-Barbierer. 1682; Approbirte Land- und Feld-Apothecken. 1690.

— Pest-Barbierer; oder, Wund-Artzt ... [Meiningen? Nikolaus Hassert?] 1682.

[57] p. 14 cm. [7135]

Bound with *his* Chirurgisches Hand-Büchlein. [1682]

LOSS, WOLFGANG [*fl.* 1592–1603] *praeses.* Themata de calculorenum et vesicae ... [Heidelbergae] Typis Voegelianis, 1603.

[10] p. 20 cm. [7136]

Diss. — Heidelberg (J. Barth, *respondent*)

LOSSAU, CHRISTIAN JOACHIM [*fl.* 1678] *See* ANDREAE, T. Disputatio. 1678.

LOTARIUS PHILOPONUS, *pseud. See* DU JON, François [1545–1602]

LOTH, GEORG [1579–1635] *praeses.* De urinis disputatio II. de urinarum judicio ... Regiomonti, Typis Laurenti Segebadii, 1623.

[12] p. 18 cm. [7137]

Diss. — Königsberg (A. Brunnmann, *respondent*)

— Kurtze Relation von einem, den 29 Maji ... abgeschluckten, und den 9 Julij allhie zu Königsbergk ausgezogenem Messer, nebenst dessen Conterfeyt und vorgenommenen Operation, und Curation ... Dantzig, Gedruckt bey Georg Rheten, zu Königsberg bey Peter Händeln zu finden, 1635.

[6], 44, [12] p. plate. 20 cm. [7138]

Preface signed by Daniel Beckher.

— *See* HEMSING, R. Non semel ilios vexata. 1635.

LOTH, GEORG [1623–1684] *respondent. See* SCHNEIDER, K. V., *praeses.* De pleuritide. 1648.

LOTICHIUS, JOHANN HEINRICH [1643–1693] *respondent. See* HECHLER, J. W., *praeses.* Disquisitio physica de noctambulis. 1682.

LOTICHIUS, JOHANN PETER [1598–1669] Consiliorum et observationum medicinalium libri VI, in quibus plerorumque corporis humani affectuum curationes, praesertim remedia euporista, ab ipsomet autore partim inventa, partim ab aliis ante experta ... proponuntur. Ulmae Suevorum, Impensis Joannis Gerlini, typis exscripsit Balthasar Kühne, 1664.

[16], 579, [10] p.   20 cm.   [**7139**]

—[The same.] ... Ed. 2. Ulmae Suevorum, Impensis Joannis Gerlini, 1658.

[16], 577 (i.e. 579), [10] p.   21 cm.   [**7140**]
Different setting of type.

—De bona mente oratio. Francofurti ad Moenum, Impensis Johannis Davidis Zunneri, 1643.

[1], 34 p.   20 cm.   [**7141**]
Bound with *his* De casei nequitia. 1643.

—De casei nequitia, tractatus medico-philologicus novus. Francofurti ad Moenum, Typis & sumptibus Johannis Friderici Weisii, 1643.

[14], 45 p.   20 cm.   [**7142**]
With this is bound *his* De bona mente oratio. 1643.

—De gummi (ut vocant) gotta laxativo Indico. In Dispensatorium chymicum. 1626.

—Gynaicologia; id est, De nobilitate & perfectione sexus feminei contra mastiges διασκεποις physica ... Rinthelii ad Visurgim, Petrus Lucius, 1630.

175, [1] p.   18 cm.   [**7143**]

—[German tr.] Gynaicologia; das ist, Grundunnd aussführlicher Discurs, von Perfection, und Fürtreffligkeiten, dess löblichen Frawenzimmers ... ubersetzt durch Joan. Tackium ... Franckfurt am Mayn, Getruckt bey Johann Friedrich Weissen, in Verlegung Philipps Jacobs Fischers, 1645.

[40], 187, [3] p.   front.   16 cm.   [**7144**]

—Paradoxon; sive, De febribus in genere dissertatio theorico-practica ... Accessit ejusdem Disputatio physica de dignitate & praestantia scientiae naturalis. Francofurti, Typis Caspari Rötelii, impensis Matthaei Meriani, 1627.

125, [1] p.   21 cm.   [**7145**]
The Disputatio physica has special title page.

LOTS, JOHANN HEINRICH [*fl.* 1671] *respondent. See* SIMON, J. G., *praeses.* Jura obstetricum. 1671.

LOUIS XIII, *King of France* [1601–1643] *See* LYONNET, R. Brevis dissertatio. 1647; Minaeus, F., *Father* [*fl.* 1622]

LOVE, JEREMIAH. Clavis medicinae; or, A new method of physick ... Likewise an excellent way to cure the gout, and to dissolve the stone ... London, Printed by J. R. for W. B., 1675.

[4], 59 p.   15 cm.   [**7146**]

—The practice of physick reformed, wherein is described the nature and cause of most diseases and the select way of cure for the same ... London, Henry Brome, 1675.

[4], 43 p.   15 cm.   [**7147**]
Imperfect: p. 34–42 mutilated.

LOVELL, ARCHIBALD [*fl.* 1677–1682] *tr. See* TOLET, F. A treatise of lithotomy. 1683.

LOVELL, ROBERT [1630?–1690] Παμβοτανολογία; sive, Enchiridion botanicum. Or a compleat herball ... Oxford, Printed by William Hall for Ric. Davis, 1659.

[84], 671, [1] p.   15 cm.   [**7148**]

—[The same.] ... The 2d ed. with many additions ... Oxford, By W. H. for Ric. Davis, 1665.

84, 675 (i.e. 673), [6] p.   16 cm.   [**7149**]
Imperfect: sig. A¹ mutilated.

—Πανξωορυκτολογία; sive, Panzoologicomineralagia. Or a compleat history of animals and minerals ... Oxford, Printed by Hen. Hall, for Jos. Godwin, 1661.

[96], 519 p.; [1], 152 (i.e. 154) p.   17 cm.
                                                [**7150**]

Part [2] has special page: Πανορυκτολογία; sive, Pammineralogicon. Or an universal history of minerales ... Oxford, Printed by W. Hall, for Joseph Godwin, 1661.

LOVER, REGNER DE [*fl.* 1687] *respondent.* Disputatio medica inauguralis, continens positiones ex universa medicina desumtas ... Trajecti ad Rhenum, Ex officina Francisci Halma, 1687.

8 p.   22 cm.   [**7151**]
Diss.—Utrecht.

A LOVER of the arts, *ed.* 1676. *See* BULLOKAR, J.

LOWE, PETER [1550?–1612?] A discourse of the whole art of chyrurgerie. Wherein is exactly set downe the definition, causes, accidents, prognostica-tions,and cures of all sorts of diseases ... Where-unto is added the rule of making remedies which chirurgions doe commonly use; with The Presages of divine Hyppocrates. The 2d ed.; corr. ... augm., and enl. by the author. London, Thomas Purfoot. 1612.

> [24], 446 (i.e. 447), [9] p.; [31] p.   illus.   20 cm.
> [7152]

Pages 125-126 are supplied from another copy.
STC 16870.

First published in 1597 under title: The whole course of chirurgerie. Cf. Finlayson, p. 31.

Part [2] has special title page: The Presages of ... Hippocrates ... translated by Peter Cole ... 1611.

—[The same.] ... The 3d ed.; corr. and much amended. London, Thomas Purfoot, 1634.

> [24], 447, [9] p.; [31] p.   illus.   20 cm.
> [7153]

Imperfect: p. 243-254 wanting; supplied in photocopy from the Yale Medical Library.

Part [2] has special title page.
STC 16871.

—[The same.] ... The 4th ed.; corr. and much amended. London, R. Hodgkinsonne, 1654 [i.e. 1655]

> [24], 487 p.   illus.   19 cm.   [7154]

Imperfect: p. 1-2, 25-26, and 33-34 mutilated.
"The Presages of divine Hippocrates" (p. 457-487) has special title page dated 1655.

LOWER, RICHARD [1631–1691] An appendix of the heart. *In* Browne, J. Myographia nova. 1697, 1698.

—Diatribae Thomae Willisii ... de febribus vin-dicatio adversus Edmundum de Meara ... Londini, Apud Jo. Martyn & Ja. Allestry, 1665.

> [15], 194, [1] p.   17 cm.   [7155]

Fulton(B) 2.
Errata: p. [195]

—[The same.] ... Amstelodami, Apud Gerbran-dum Schagen, 1666.

> 129 p.   15 cm.   [7156]

Fulton(B) 3.
Bound with copy 2 of Willis, T. Diatribae duae medico-philosophicae. 1663.

—Tractatus de corde. Item de motu & colore sanguinis et chyli in eum transitu ... Londini, Typis Jo. Redmayne, impensis Jacobi Allestry, 1669.

> [14], 220, [20] p.   plates.   17 cm.   [7157]

Imperfect: sig. A1 (blank) wanting.
Fulton(B) 4.

—[The same.] ... Amstelodami, Apud Danielem Elzevirium, 1669.

> [16], 232 p.   plates.   16 cm.   [7158]

Fulton(B) 6.

[The same.] ... Cui accessit dissertatio De origine catarrhi, in qua ostenditur illum non provenire a cerebro ... Ed. 3, & ultima. Amstelodami, Apud Danielem Elsevirium, 1671.

> [16], 237 p.   plates.   16 cm.   [7159]

Fulton(B) 8.

—[The same.] ... Ed. 4, ab authore jam postremo aucta & recognita. Londini, Typis M. C., impensis J. Martyn, 1680.

> [16], 175 p.   plate.   19 cm.   [7160]

Fulton(B) 9.

—[English excerpt.] *In* Fabricius von Hilden, W. Cista militaris. 1674.

—[French tr.] Traité du coeur, du mouvement et de la couleur du sang, et du passage du chyle dans le sang ... Traduit de Latin ... par M. ******. Paris, Estienne Michallet, 1679.

> [8], 237 p.   plates.   [7161]

Fulton(B) 17.

—*See* Vieussens, R. Réponse ... a trois lettres ... du sieur Chirac. 1698.

LOYDE, SAMUEL [*fl.* 1697] *respondent.* Disputatio medica inauguralis de pleuritide ... Trajecti ad Rhenum, Ex officina Francisci Halma, 1697.

> 23 p.   22 cm.   [7162]

Diss.—Utrecht.

LOYSEAU, GUILLAUME [*fl.* 1598-1617] Guillelmi Loselli ... De internorum externorumque ferme om-nium curatione libellus ... Burdigalae, Apud Gilber-tum Vernoy, 1617.

> [28], 246 p.   15 cm.   [7163]

Imperfect: wormholes on p. 221-246.

LUBBERT, JOHANN [*fl.* 1646-1655] *respondent.* Disputatio medica inauguralis, de podagra ac lue venerea ... Lugduni Batavorum, Apud Johannem Elsevirium, 1655.

> [18] p.   22 cm.   [7164]

Diss.—Leyden.
With this is bound Carmina gratulatoria. 1655.

—*See* Carmina gratulatoria, in honorem ... D. Johannis Lubberti. 1655.

LUBIENICIUS, STANISLAUS. *See* LUBIENIECKI, Stanislaw [1623-1675]

LUBIENIECKI, STANISLAW [1623-1675] *See* BARTHOLIN, T. De cometa. 1665.

LUBIENIESZKY DE LUBIENIETZ, STANISLAUS. *See* LUBIENIECKI, Stanislaw [1623-1675]

LUBIN, EILHARD [1565-1621] *ed.* and *tr.* Epistolae Hippocratis, Democriti, Heracliti, Diogenis, Cratetis, aliorumque ad eosdem. Nunc primum editae Graece simul ac Latine ... [Heidelbergae] Ex Officina Commeliniana, 1601.

     II, [1] p.; 12-95 (i.e. 97) ll.   18 cm.   **[7165]**

LUCAE, URBAN [*fl.* 1624] *respondent. See* BLUM, M., *praeses.* Positiones medicae de imbecillitate ventriculi. 1624.

LUCAN, MARTIN ECKHARD [*fl.* 1683] *respondent. See* WALDSCHMIDT, J. J., *praeses.* Disputatio physica de colore Aethiopium. 1683.

LUCAS, HEINRICH [*fl.* 1672] *respondent.* Disputatio medica inauguralis de suppressione mensium ... Duisburgi ad Rhenum, Apud Franconem Sas, 1672.

     [16] p.   20 cm.   **[7166]**
    Diss. — Duisburg.

LUCAS, JOHANN MATTHIAS [*fl.* 1686-1690] *praeses.* Disputatio medica inauguralis de palpitatione cordis ... Heidelbergae, Excudebat Joh. David. Bergmann [1686]

     16 p.   32 cm.   **[7167]**
    Diss. — Heidelberg (P. W. Virdung von Hartung, *respondent*)

—*See* JUANINI, J. B. Cartas escritas a los ... doctores ... Francisco Redi ... y ... Juan Mathias de Lucas. 1691.

LUCCA. Collegio de medici. *See* COLLEGIO DEI MEDICI, Lucca.

LUCERNE. Ordinances, local laws, etc. *See* NUTZLICHER UNND KURTZER BERICHT, REGIMENT UND ORDNUNG. 1611.

LUCHTEN, ADAM [*fl.* 1599-1629] Oratio Adami Luchtenii ... In qua tum de calumnia ipsa paucis disseritur, tum etiam de quibusdam calumniis ... in se jactis rationem reddit ... Helmaestadii, Typis Jacobi Lucii, impensis Samuelis Brehm, 1611.

     [78] p.   20 cm.   **[7168]**
    Includes Johannes Caselius' letter of 1611.

—*praes.* De melancholia, disputatio prima, in qua de melancholia cerebri primaria & ea quae fit per consensum totius, agitur ... Helmaestadii, Ex typographeio Jacobi Lucii, 1608.

     [19] p.   20 cm.   **[7169]**
    Diss. — Helmstädt (J. Husanus, *respondent*)

—*See also* Lichten, Adam (the same author).

LUCIANUS SAMOSATENSIS. *See* SENNERT, D. Practicae medicinae liber primus [-sextus] 1628-1635, 1629-36, 1632, 1636-54, 1653-62.

LUCIEN, *of Samosate. See* LUCIANUS SAMOSATENSIS.

LUCIUS, CASPAR. *See* LUTZ, Caspar [1555-1609]

LUCIUS, JODOCUS. *See* LUCIUS, Johannes Jodocus [1576-1613]

LUCIUS, JOHANNES JODOCUS [1576-1613] *praeses.* Disputatio medica de morborum natura et differentiis ... Heidelbergae, Typis Johannis Lancelloti [1608]

     8 p.   20 cm.   **[7171]**
    Diss. — Heidelberg (H. J. Fries, *respondent*)
    Author's presentation copy, unsigned.

LUCRETIUS CARUS, TITUS. De rerum natura libri sex. Quibus additae sunt conjecturae & emendationes Tan. Febri cum notulis perpetuis. Et praeterea Oberti Gifanii Vita Lucretii & De gente memmia ejusdem prolegomena ... Cantabrigiae, Ex officina Joann. Hayes, impensis H. Dickenson, 1686.

     [45], 454, [2] p.   17 cm.   **[7172]**

LUDEN, LORENZ [1592-1654] *praeses.* Disputatio physiologica de motu ... Gyphiswaldiae, Typis haeredum Johannis Albini, 1631.

     [12] p.   19 cm.   **[7173]**
    Dis. — Greifswald (A. Densov, *respondent*)

LUDERS, ANTON [*fl.* 1685] *respondent.* Disputatio medica de phthisi ... Lugduni Batavorum, Apud Abrahamum Elzevier, 1685.

     [12] p.   21 cm.   **[7174]**
    Diss. — Leyden .

—Disputatio medica inauguralis de rabie vulgo dicta hydrophobia ... Lugduni Batavorum, Apud Abrahamum Elzevier, 1685.

     [16] p.   22 cm.   **[7175]**
    Diss. — Leyden.

LUDKIN. *See* [Peachie, John] Some observations made upon the Calumba wood. 1694.

LUDOLPHUS, Verdemanus, *ed. See* Lull, R. Testamentum. 1663?

LUDWIG, Daniel [1625-1680] De pharmacia, moderno seculo applicanda, dissertationes III. Gothae, Apud Salomonem Reyherum, typis Reyherianis, exscrib. Joh. Mich. Schallio, 1671.
　　[8], 924 p. 13 cm. 　　　　　　**[7176]**

—[The same.] ... Ed. 2., cum augmento ... Gothae, Sumptibus Salomonis Reyheri, exscribebat Christoph. Reyherus, 1685.
　　[4], 749, 195, [70] p. front. (port.) 17 cm.
　　　　　　　　　　　　　　　　[7177]
　　Added engraved title page.

—[The same.] ... Ed. 2. Cum augmento ... Amstelaedami, Apud Joannem Wolters, 1688.
　　[23], 679, [41] p. front. (port.) 16 cm.
　　　　　　　　　　　　　　　　[7178]
　　Added engraved title page.

—[The same.] ... Huic editioni accessit praeter augmentum ... etiam praefatio nova Georgi Wolffgang. Wedeli. Hamburgi, Apud Henricum Schmidium, 1688.
　　[16], 415, 128, [48] p. 17 cm. 　　**[7179]**
　　Praefatio ad lectorem is the same as those in the 1671 and 1685 Gotha editions and in the 1688 Amsterdam edition.

—De volatilitate salis tartari dissertatio. Gothae, Impensis Salomonis Reyheri, exscrib. Joh. Mich. Schallio, 1667.
　　[4], 92, [1] p. 13 cm. 　　　　　**[7180]**
　　Errata: p. [1] at end.

—Ludovicus enucleatus ... et auctus. *See* König, E. Regnum vegetabile ... enucleatum. 1688.

—*See* Ettmüller, M. Opera medica theoretico-practica. 1696-1697 [and] Opera omnia. 1688 [and] Opera omnia medico-physica, theoretica et practica. 1700 [and] Opera pharmaceutico-chymica. 1686 [and] Operum omnium medico-phisicorum. 1690.

LUDWIG, Johann Georg [*fl.* 1696] *respondent. See* Wedel, G. W., *praeses.* Dissertatio inauguralis medica de febri maligna. 1696.

LÜBECK. Ordinances, local laws, etc. Eines ehrbarn Raths der Stadt Lübeck revidirte Pestord-

nung, sampt angehengtem Bericht, wie man sich in wehrender Pestilenz verwahren ... sol. Beneben der Taxa der Artzneyen, so auff der Apothecken verordnet. Lübeck, Valentin Schmalhertz, 1639.
　　[25] p. 19 cm. 　　　　　　　**[7181]**

—Kurtzer Bericht, wie man sich in werender Pestilentz verwahren ... soll, beneben der Taxa der Artzneyen, so auff der Apotheken verordnet ... Mit angehengtem eines ehrbaren Raths Mandat und Verordnung auff diese Zeit gerichtet. Lübeck, Gedruckt bey Samuel Jauchen s. Erben, 1629.
　　[16] p. 19 cm. 　　　　　　　**[7182]**

LÜBER, Thomas. *See* Erastus, Thomas [1524-1583]

LÜDDENS, Mumme [*fl.* 1682-1685] *respondent. See* Pechlin, J. N., *praeses.* Joh. Nicolai Pechlini ... historiam vulneris thoracici & in eam commentarium ... submittit. 1682.

LÜDER, Johannes Werner [*fl.* 1682] *respondent. See* Ursin, S. C., *praeses.* Quaestum meretricium, Germ. Hüren-Lohn. 1682.

LÜDER, Martin [*fl.* 1680-1684] *respondent. See* Schmid, J. A., *praeses.* Discursus physicus de lacrymis. 1680; Wedel, G. W., *praeses.* Dissertatio inauguralis medica de vitiis humorum morbificis. 1684.

LÜNEBURG. *See* Brunswick (Duchy). Kurtzer, doch gründlicher Rath- und Unterricht. 1680.

LUFFNEY. *See* Lufneu, Jacques [*fl.* 1697]

[**LUFNEU,** Jacques, *fl.* 1697] Ein Send-Schreiben, an Herrn B.*** [i.e. François Bayle] worin mit unmustösslichen Beweiss-Gründen dargethan wird, dass die sympathetische Würckungen nichtig und unmöglich seyen. Abgefasset von Herrn. L. *** ... [i.e. Jacques Lufnue] ... Auss dem Französischen ins Hochteutsche gebracht. Franckfurt am Mäyn, Im Verlag Georg Heinr. Oehrlings, 1700.
　　94 p. 17 cm. 　　　　　　　　**[7183]**

LUGE, Daniel [*fl.* 1693-1694] *respondent. See* Albinus, B. Exercitationem medicam de dysenteria ... submittit ... D. L. 1693.

LUIA, ELIAS [*fl.* 1624] *respondent.* Hydropiseos dignotio et curatio . . . Basileae, Typis Joan. Jacobi Genathii, 1624.

[12] p.   19 cm.   **[7184]**

Diss. — Basel.

Not in Husner.

LUIA, GOTTFRIED ADOLPH [*fl.* 1662] Disputatio medica inauguralis de elephantiasi Graecorum . . . Lugduni Batavorum, Apud Philippum de Cro-Y, 1662.

[16] p.   19 cm.   **[7185]**

Diss. — Leyden.

LULL, RAMÓN [1235–*ca.* 1316] Opera ea quae ad adinventam ab ipso artem universalem, scientiarum artiumque omnium brevi compendio, firmaque memoria apprehendendarum, locupletissimaque vel oratione ex tempore pertractandarum, pertinent. Ut et in eandem quorundam interpretum scripti commentarii . . . hoc demum tempore conjunctim emendatiora locupletioraque non nihil edita sunt. Accessit huic editioni Valerii de Valeriis . . . Aureum in artem Lulli generalem opus . . . Argentorati, Sumptibus haeredum Lazari Zetzneri, 1617.

[16], 1109, [41] p.   illus., tables.   19 cm.   **[7186]**

A reissue of the 1609 edition. Cf. Rogent and Duràn 180.

Partial contents. - Ars brevis (p. 1–42) - Ars magna et ultima (p. 218–663). - Henrici Cornelii Agrippae In Artem brevem Raymundi Lullii commentaria (p. 787–916). - Valerii de Valeriis Opus aureum in quo omnia breviter explicantur quae Raymundi Lullus tam in Scientiarum arbore quam Arte generali tradit (p. 968–1109).

—[The same.] . . . Ed. postrema. Argentorati, Sumptibus haeredum Lazari Zetzneri, 1651.

[16], 1109, [41] p.   illus., plates.   18 cm.   **[7187]**

Different setting of type.

Rogent and Duràn 233.

—Copy 2.   19 cm.

With this is bound: Alsted, J. Clavis artis Lullianae. 1652.

—Ars brevis. *In* Sánchez de Lizarazo, P. J. Generalis et admirabilis methodus. 1619.

—Ars magna. *See* ALSTED, J. H. Clavis artis Lullianae. 1652.

—Clavicula . . . quae & apertorium dicitur, in qua omnia quae in opere alchemiae requiruntur, aperte declarantur.

295–303 p., vol. 2.   20 cm.   (In Zetzner, Lazarus, ed. Theatrum Chemicum. Argentorati, 1659–61)   **[7188]**

Caption title.

—[The same.] *In* Broekhuizen, D. van. Secreta alchimiae magnalia D. Thomae Aquinatis. 1602.

—Elucidatio totius testamenti ad regem Odoardum . . . [&] . . . Compendium . . . de insula Majorcana in arte magna quo ad compositionem lapidis philosophorum.

139–150 p., and 165–174 p., vol. 3   17 cm.   (In Artis auriferae. Basileae, 1610)   **[7189]**

Caption title.

—[The same.] *In* Grasshoff, J. Ein philosophischer . . . Tractat. 1658.

—Libelli aliquot chemici. *In* his Testamentum. 1663?

—Opuscula philosophica quatuor, nunc primum in lucem data. I. Compendium artis alchimiae & naturalis philosophiae. II. De lapide & oleo philosophorum. III. Modus accipiendi aurum potabile. IV. Lapidarium, sive de lapidibus praetiosis.

77–120 p., vol. 3.   17 cm.   (In Artis auriferae. Basileae, 1610)   **[7190]**

Caption title.

—Praxis universalis magni operis ex tertia distinctione libri quintarum essentiarum . . .

165–166 p. vol. 3.   20 cm.   (In Zetzner, Lazarus, ed. Theatrum chemicum. Argentorati, 1659–61)   **[7191]**

Caption title.

—Testamentum . . . duobus libris universam artem chymicam complectens, & ejusdem Compendium animę transmutationis artis metallorum. Item, Testamentum novissimum, cum caeteris omnibus operibus quae in secunda parte libri continentur. Ultima ed. ex archetypis & exemplaribus fidelioribus ad unguem castigata, diligentia D. M. Rault . . . Juxta exemplaria Coloniae Agrippinae, Apud Joannem Birckmannum, 1573 [Rothomagi? 1663?]

355, [11] p.; [12], 393, [27] p.   illus., plates.   16 cm.   **[7192]**

Not in Rogent and Duràn.

Part 1 first issued by the same press in 1566. Present edition retains original dedication by Ludolphus Verdemanus, dated 22 Feb.

1566. Part 2, first issued in Basel in 1572, edited by Michael Toxites, under title: Libelli aliquot chemici.

Contents—pt. 1. Testamentum (Theorica, Practica); Compendium animae transmutationis artis metallorum.—pt. 2. Testamentum novissimum; Elucidatio Testamenti; Lux mercuriorum; Experimenta; Vade mecum; Compendium animae transmutationis artis metallorum [text varies somewhat from that in pt. 1]; Epistola accurtationis lapidis; Medicina magna; Lignum vitae, dialogus Raymundi Lullii [by Giovanni Bracesco] ex Italico in Latinum conversus.

—Theorica [&] Practica [&] . . . Compendium animae transmutationis artis metallorum . . .

1-194 p., vol. 4. illus., plates. 20 cm. (*In* Zetzner, Lazarus, *ed.* Theatrum chemicum. Argentorati, 1659-61) [7193]

Caption title.

—Tractatus brevis et eruditus, De conservatione vitae; item Liber secretorum seu quintae essentiae . . . Nunc primum in lucem editus. Argentorati, Impensis Lazari Zetzneri, 1616.

[8], III p. 17 cm. [7194]

The first work is a reprint of Libellus de conservatione vitae, published in Rome in 1516. The second work, often titled De secretis naturae, a Lullian version of De consideratione quintae essentiae by Joannes de Rupescissa, was first printed in Venice in 1514 with the Consilia of Giovanni Matteo Ferrari de Gradi.

Rogent and Duràn 64, 92, 179.

—Ultimum testamentum ad serenissimum Carolum regem [&] . . . Potestas divitiarum, in quo libro optima expositio testamenti Hermetis continetur.

1-76 p., vol. 3. 17 cm. (*In* Artis auriferae, Basileae, 1610) [7195]

Caption titles.

—*See* BELOT, J. Familieres instructions. 1624 [and] Les oeuvres. 1640, 1654; Bracesco, G. De alchemia. 1673; HOUPREGHT, J. F., comp. Aurifontina chymica. 1680; LAVINHETA, B. de Opera omnia. 1612; PARACELSUS. Of the chymical transmutation. 1657; SAUNDERS, R. Physiognomie. 1653, 1671; SUÁREZ DE FIGUEROA, C. Plaza universal de todas ciencias. 1629; VOGEL, E. Liber de lapidis physici conditionibus. 1659; WEIDENFELD, J. S. von. Four books . . . concerning the secrets of the adepts. 1685.

LUMBISANO, ORAZIO [*fl.* 1629] De feb. lib. III. In quibus de earundem essentia signis prognostico, & curatione agit. Amplius de peste feb. pest. curat. & praecaut. liber quartus. Item De terrae motu prout pestis causa est . . . disputatio unica. Neapoli, Ex typographia Matthaei Nuccii, 1629.

[12], 350, [2] p. 22 cm. [7196]

Errata: [2] p.

Imperfect: all after p. [352] wanting.

LUNARDI, CAMILLO. *See* LEONARDI, Camillo [*fl.* 1496-1502]

LUNGERSHAUSEN, JOHANN JAKOB [1665-1729] *praeses.* Disputatio physica de imitamentis naturae circa figuras . . . Jenae, Stanno Mulleriano [1698]

23, [1] p. 20 cm. [7197]

Diss.—Jena (A. Zinck, *respondent*)

LUNGWIZ, DAVID [*fl.* 1669-1672] *respondent.* Valetudo homo homini . . . Basileae, Literis Deckerianis [1672]

[16] p. 20 cm. [7198]

Diss.—Basel.

—*See* AMMANN, P., *praeses.* Theses medicae de lithiasi renum et vesicae. 1669.

LUPIN, WOLFFGANG DIETRICH [*b.* 1674] *respondent.* See SLEVOGT, J. A., *praeses.* Disputatio medica inauguralis de epilepsia infantili. 1696; WEDEL, G. W., *praeses.* Dissertatio medica de procidentia ani. 1696 [and] Exercitationum pathologico-therapeuticarum disputatio II. de inflammationibus. 1696 [and] Propempticum inaugurale de expectatione medica. 1696.

LUPIUS, JACOB [*fl. ca.* 1645] Schatzkammer der Natur: gründliche Erklärung dreyer grossen Geheimnüssen, und erstlichen, die Extractio der spiritualischen Mumiae des Menschen und anderer Thier . . . Zum andern, von dem grossen Mysterio magico, des Baums Erkentnüss Gutes und Böses . . . Zum dritten, Sonderbares jedoch naturliches Arcanum durch Traume etwas zu erfahren. Von newen ans Liecht gebracht . . . [Erfurt?] 1651.

75, [1] p. plates. 17 cm. [7199]

[LUPTON, THOMAS, *fl.* 1583] A thousand notable things of sundrie sorts: whereof some are wonderful, some strange, some pleasant, divers necessary, a great sort profitable, and many very precious . . . London, Printed by John Haviland, for Robert Bird, 1631.

[6], 336, [26] p. 16 cm. [7200]

Imperfect: p. [11-26] wanting.

STC 16961.

LUQUE, Cristóbal Francisco de [*fl.* 1682–1694] Apolineo caduceo haze concordia entre las dos opuestas opiniones, una que aprueba las consultas de los medicos para la curacion de las graves enfermedades, otra que las reprueba ... Sevilla, Lucas Martin de Hermosilla, 1694.

[40], 347 p.   21 cm.   **[7201]**

LUSART, Jan Babtista, *ed.* and *tr. See* Abercromby, D. De Spaanse pok-meester. 1691.

LUSATIA, Lower. *See* Kurtzer Unterricht von der jetzo herumbgehenden ... Pestilentz. 1680.

LUSCINIUS, Ottmar [1487?–1537?] *See* Mensa philosophica. 1602.

LUSITANO, Amato. *See* Amatus Lusitanus [1511–1568]

LUSITANO ZACUTO. *See* Zacutus, Abraham, Lusitanus [1575–1642]

LUSITANUS, Amatus. Amatus Lusitanus [1511–1568]

LUSITANUS, Dilectus. *See* Dilectus, Lusitanus [*fl.* 1642]

LUSSAULD, Charles [*fl.* 1648–1663] Apologie pour les medecins, contre ceux qui les accusent de deferer trop a la nature, & de n'avoir point de religion ... Paris, En la boutique de P. Rocolet, chez Damien Foucault, 1663.

[14], 187, [4] p.   15 cm.   **[7202]**

—Another issue: title page in different setting of type.   **[7203]**

LUTHER, Karl Friedrich [1663–1744] *respondent.* Theses medicas desumtas ex doctrina de viribus ... publice proponit Carolus Fridericus Luther. Erfordiae, Stanno Groschiano [1689]

[16] p.   19 cm.   **[7204]**

—*See* Bohn, J., *praeses.* Dissertationes chymicophysicae. 1685; Pauli, J. W. Disputatio medica de oedematis natura & cura. 1685.

LUTHER, Martin [1483–1546] *See* Goclenius, R. [1547–1628] Physiologia crepitus ventris. 1607; Paulinus, L., *Abp.* Loimoscopia. 1623; Zweyer vortrefflicher Theologen. 1680.

LUTZ, Caspar [1555–1609] Geistliche Apoteck, darauss zur Pestilentz unnd Sterbens Zeit allerhand Recipe und Antwort, auff allerley fürfallende Fäll and Fragen, zu nemmen seyn ... Franckfurt am Mayn, Gedruckt durch Wollfgang Richtern, in Verlegung Johannis Berneri, 1606.

184 p.   16 cm.   **[7205]**

—[The same.] Geistliche Apotecke, darauss zur gegenwettigen, auch Pestilentz und Sterbens-Zeit, allerhand Recipe und Antwort auff allerley vorfallende Fäll und Fragen, auch schöne Gebet und Seufftzer vor jeden Stand zunehmen seyn ... Franckfurt, Johann Georg Schiele, 1666.

[12], 249 p.   14 cm.   **[7206]**

Bound with Geist-reiches Donner und Wetter-Gebet-Büchlein. 1667.

LUTZ, Ludwig Heinrich [*fl. ca.* 1670] Ophiographia physico-chymico-medica; das ist, Eine Schlangen-Beschreibung, vermittelst deren man die wunderbahre Natur der Schlangen eigendtlich ergründen, und ... mancherley, sowohl galenisch als paracelsische edle Medicamenta zu der Menschen Wolfahrt leichtlich bereiten soll und könne ... Augspurg, Jacob Koppmayer, 1670.

[6], 128 p.   16 cm.   **[7206.1]**

LUTZEN, Ludovicus Henricus. *See* Lutz, Ludwig Heinrich [*fl. ca.* 1670]

LUX Orientalis; or, An enquiry into the opinion of the Eastern sages. 1662. *See* [Glanvill, J.]

LUYELACK, of t'samen-spraeck tusschen Wit en Swart. 1677. *See* Pijl, P.

LUYNES, Louis Charles d'Albert, *duc de* [1620–1690] *tr. See* Descartes, R. Les meditations metaphysiques. 1647.

LUYTS, Jan [1655–1721] *praeses.* Exercitatio philosophica, expendens, num consideratio finium in physica sit inutilis? ... Trajecti ad Rhenum, Ex officina Francisci Halma, 1689.

[16] p.   23 cm.   **[7207]**

Diss. — Utrecht (P. van Cleyburgh, *respondent*)

LYMBISANUS, Horace. *See* Lumbisano, Orazio [*fl.* 1629]

LYMBORH, Gilbertus. *See* Fusch, Gilbert [*ca.* 1504–1567]

LYNCKER, Nikolaus Christoph von [1643-1726] *praeses.* Disputatio inauguralis juridica de fatalibus ... Jenae, Stanno Nisiano [1678]

[83] p.   20 cm.   **[7208]**

Diss.—Jena (J. F. Herzog, *respondent*)

LYONNET, Robert [*fl.* 1629-1646] Brevis dissertatio de morbis haereditariis ... qua probatur, affectus morbosos quibuscum Ludovicos XIII rex Galliae ... conflictatus est, fuisse adventitios, non profectitios, non hereditarios. Parisiis, Apud Gasparum Meturas, 1647.

[16], 67 p.   22 cm.   **[7209]**

—Λοιμογραφια; seu, Reconditarum pestis, et contagii causarum curiosa disquisitio, ejusdemque methodica curatio. Lugduni, Sumptibus Claudii Prost, 1639.

[12], 362, [1] p.   18 cm.   **[7210]**

LYONS. Aumône générale. Institution de l'aumosne generale de Lyon, ensemble l'oeconomie & reglement qui s'observe dans l'hospital de Notre-Dame de la Charité, où sont les pauvres renfermez de ladite aumosne. Rev. & augm. de nouveau. 5. ed. Lyon, 1647.

[27], 126, [2] p.   plate.   23 cm.   **[7211]**

—[The same.] ... 6. ed. Rev. & augm. de nouveau. Lyon, 1662.

[12], 141, [2] p.   plate.   23 cm.   **[7212]**

LYONS. Collegium medicum. *See* Collège des médecins, Lyons.

LYONS. Hôpital de la charité. *See* Hôpital de la charité, Lyons.

LYONS. Hôpital de Nôtre-Dame de la charité. *See* Hôpital de la charité, Lyons.

LYONS. Hôstel-Dieu. *See* Hôtel-Dieu de Lyon.

LYONS. Ordinances, local laws, etc. L'ordre public pour la ville de Lyon, pendant la maladie contagieuse. Augmenté de plusieurs observations, & d'un traitté de la peste ... Lyon, Antoine Valançoe, 1670.

[14], 72 p.   24 cm.   **[7213]**

LYSECK, Johann Philipp de [*fl.* 1669-1673] Praeservativum pestilentiale; oder, Ausführlicher Bericht, wie man sich ... vor des Pestilentz praeserviren und fürsehen könne. Durch ... Mittel der Medicin, mit Hülff des astrologischen Verstands,

und Würckung der öbersten Cörper dess Himmels, in den untersten Leibern der Erden ... beschrieben ... Zu welchem Gebäw und Vormauer unterschiedlich metallischer Saltzstein, mineralischer Sulphur, oder Kalck, und mercurialisches Influenz-Wasser gehöret ... Straubing, Sumptibus Authoris bey Johann Chrysostomus Haan, 1673.

[7], 191, [3] p.   plate.   21 cm.   **[7214]**

Errata: [3] p.

Added title page: Speculum Salomonis; oder, Salomonischer Spiegel.

—[The same.] Propugnaculum contra pestem; oder, Vorbaw, wider die Pestilenz ... Neben Vorstellung dess salomonischen Spiegels, in welchem zusehen wie das new politische Wesen ... vergreiffen kan. Aus nevv politischer Sprach in die alt Teutsche versetzt ... Straubing, Johann Chrysostomus Haan [1674]

[8], 191, [3] p.   21 cm.   **[7215]**

An den Leser dated 1669.

A reissue, with reprinted preliminaries of the 1673 edition.

LYSER, Johann [1631-1684] Polygamia triumphatrix; id est, Discursus politicus de polygamia. Auctore Theophilo Aletheo [pseud., i.e. Johann Lyser] cum notis Athanasii Vincentii [pseud.] omnibus anti-polygamis ... opposita. Londini Scanorum, Sumtibus authoris post., 1682.

[10], 565, [32] p.   22 cm.   **[7216]**

LYSER, Michael [1626-1659] Culter anatomicus; hoc est, Methodus brevis, facilis ac perspicua artificiose & compendiose humana incidendi cadavera ... Hafniae, E chalcographeo Georgii Lamprechtii, 1653.

[31], 216 (i.e. 215), [1] p.   illus.   16 cm.   **[7217]**

—[The same.] ... 2. hac ed. observationibus nunnullis variorum aucta cum praefatione Th. Bartholini. Hafniae, Typis Matthiae Godicchenii, impensis Petri Haubold, 1665.

[32], 224 p.; 6, 231-100 (i.e. 300) p.   illus.   17 cm.   **[7218]**

"Observationes medicae, virorum clarissimorum Michaelis Lyseri, Henrici à Mönichen, Martini Bogdani, Jacobi Seidelii, è musaeo Th. Bartholini": p. 6, 231-100 (i.e. 300).

—[The same.] ... Accessit 3. huic ed. Caspari Bartholini Th. f. Administrationum anatomicarum specimen. Francofurti, Ex officina Haffniensi Petri Hauboldi, 1679.

[32], 237 p.; 76 p.   illus., plates.   17 cm.   **[7219]**

"Praefatio Th. Bartholini": p. [16–25]

"Observationes medicae virorum clarissimorum Michaelis Lyseri, Henrici à Moinichen, Martini Bogdani, Jacobi Seidelii, e musaeo Th. Bartholini . . . 1678" (p. [187]–237) has special title page.

Part [2] has special title page.

—*respondent. See* BARTHOLIN, T., *praeses.* De lacteis thoracicis in homine brutisque nuperrime observatis. 1652.

—*See* PECQUET, J. New anatomical experiments. 1653.

LYSIUS, HEINRICH [*fl.* 1624] *respondent. See* SENNERT, D., *praeses.* Hasce theses de febre quartana. 1624.

LYSSEL, ANDREAS. *See* EYSSEL, Andreas [*fl.* 1693–1694]

LYSTENIUS, JOHANN AUGUST [*fl.* 1680] *respondent. See* RIEMER, J., *praeses.* Dolos mulierum. 1680.

LYSTHENIUS, JOHANN FRIEDRICH [*fl.* 1661] *respondent. See* MOEBIUS, G., *praeses.* Dissertatio medica inauguralis de suffocatione uterina. 1661.

LYTE, HENRY [1529?–1607] *tr. See* DODOENS, R. A new herbal. 1619.

M

M***, *Docteur en médecine. See* OZON, Pierre [*fl.* 1689]

M***, *Monsieur. See* NOUVELLES OBSERVATIONS DE CHIRURGIE. 1700.

M*****, *Docteur en medecine. See* SAUVALLE [*fl.* 1682]

M******, *tr. See* LOWER, R. Traité du coeur. 1679.

M., A., *Med. of Trinity College near Dublin. See* MULLEN, Allen [*d.* 1690]

M., A. *See* A rich closet of physical secrets. 1652.

M., A. D., *tr. See* FERNEL, J. La pathologie, 1646, 1650, 1660.

M., A. F. *See* MARSIGLI, Antonio Felice [1649–1710]

M., D. H. *See* DESMARETS, Henri.

M., D. H. P. E. *See* HENRION, Denis [*d. ca.* 1640]

M., D. L. C. D. *See* LE CLERC, Daniel [1652–1728]

M., D. M. *See* MONTROEIL, DE, *ed.*

M., E. [*fl.* 1662] *ed. See* DEGRAVERE, J. Thesaurus remediorum. 1662.

M., E. *Med. D. See* MAYNWARING, Everard [1628–1699?]

M., G. *See* MARKHAM, Gervase [1568?–1637]

M., G., *ed. See* HERLS, C. Examen der chyrurgie. [n. d.]

M., G. A., *tr. See* BLANKAART, S. Neue und besondere Manier alle verstorbene Cörper. 1697.

M., H. T. P. R. *See* TENQUE, Jérôme [*d.* 1687]

M., J. *See* LETTERS to a sick friend. 1682.

M., J. *See* MICHAULT, Jean [1632–1694]

M., J., *ed. See* BOYLE, *Hon.* R. Experimenta et notae circa producibilitatem chymicorum principiorum. 1693.

M., J. B., *tr. See* DAELMANS, G. Die neu abgefaste Heyl-Kunst, auff den Grund Alcali und Acidi erbauet. 1694.

M., J. D. D. *See* CORTNUMM, Justus [*ca.* 1624–1675]

M., M. *See* MEAD, Matthew [1630?–1699]

M., M. I. S. R. D. *See* REFLEXIONS. 1652.

M., P., *Gent. See* [CHARLETON, W.] The Ephesian and Cimmerian matrons. 1668.

M., P. M. *See* TRAITÉ DES QUALITEZ DU KINKINA. P. M. M. 1685.

M., S., *ed. See* SYDENHAM, T. Processus integri in morbis fere omnibus curandis. 1693, 1694, 1695.

M., T. *See* MERRET, Christopher [1614–1695]

M., T., *tr. See* BACON, R. His discovery of the miracles of art. 1659.

M., T. S. M. S. D. M. *See* Lenonis Guillemei Scholae Parisiensis empirico-methodicae doctoris. 1654.

M., W. *See* The queens closet opened. 1658, 1674, 1683.

M. C. D. D. E. M. *See* Dellon, Gabriel [*b. ca.* 1649]

M. C. I. *See* I., M. C.

M. L. P. *See* Martin, Louis [*fl.* 1649]

MÅNSSON, Arvid [*fl.* 1637–1642] Practica, eller een liten doch nyttigh underwijssning, om åderlåtande, hwilka ådrer man for åtskillige siukdomar uplåta kan, begynnandes på hufwudet, och sedan nedher til fotterna ... Aff latiniska och tydska böcker in på wårt swenska tungemåål ... Stockholm, 1645.

    [10], 92, [2] p.   16 cm.   [7220]

MAAS, Friderich Otto [*fl.* 1678] *respondent. See* Johrenius, C., *praeses.* Disputatio inauguralis de pleuritide. 1678.

MAAS, Nikolaus Lorenz [*fl.* 1684] *respondent. See* Fasch, A. H., *praeses.* Dissertatio medica inauguralis de mola. 1684.

MACARONUS, Petrus. *See* Macherone, Pietro [*fl.* 1630]

MACASIUS, Johann Centurio [*fl.* 1660–1669] *praeses.* Disputatio medica de calculo renum ... [Lipsiae] Typis viduae Henningi Coleri [1666]

    [20] p.   20 cm.   [7221]

    Diss.—Leipzig (J. C. Hippius, *respondent*)

—, *ed. See* Lange, C. Miscellanea curiosa medica. 1669 [and] Opera omnia. 1688.

MACASIUS, Johann Georg [*d.* 1653] Promptuarium materiae medicae; sive, Apparatus ad praxin medicam, libris duobus adornatus ... Francofurti, Sumptibus Joannis Beyeri, 1654.

    [8], 378, [13] p.   17 cm.   [7222]

    Dedication signed by Johann Matthias Nester, the editor.

—[The same.] ... Nunc accurate revisum, variis arcanis ... auctum, & secunda vice cum appendice ... duarum observationum medicarum editum a D. Joh. Matthia Nestero ... Lipsiae, Sumptibus

Michaelis Russworm, literis Christiani Michaelis, 1677.

    [35], 974, [20] p.   16 cm.   [7223]

    Added engraved title page.

—*respondent. See* Schelhammer, C., *praeses.* Disputatio medica inauguralis de epilepsia. 1644.

MACASIUS, Paul [*fl.* 1607–1615] Von Natur, Krafft, Wirckung und Gebrauch des egrischen gebreuchlichen Sewrlings. Aus der andern lateinischen Edition ... ubersetzet ... Leipzig, Typis Grosianis [Gedruckt durch Justum Jasonium] 1616.

    [16], 143, [1] p.   16 cm.   [7224]

    Imperfect: title page mutilated.

    Translation of De acidularum Egranarum usualium.

—*respondent. See* Varus, A., *praeses.* Disputatio medica de venae sectione. 1607.

MACCARANI, Domenico [*fl.* 17th cent.] *ed. See* Santorelli, A. De sanitatis natura lib. XXIV. 1643.

MACCHELLI, Niccolò [1494?–1554] Tractatus methodicus, et omnibus numeris absolutus. De lue venerea, ejusque natura et caussis, et quae eam sequuntur, symptomatis, nec non singulorum curatione. Accesserunt disputationes medicae ... in quibus praeter rerum coelestium, terrestrium, & aquatilium tratationem, solidissime agitur de febris pestilentis cognitione & cura, authore Gerhardo Columba ... Francofurti, Excudebat Nicolaus Hoffmannus, impensis Joannis Jacobi Porssii, 1608.

    61, [6], 278, [16] p.   18 cm.   [7225]

—De morbo Gallico. *In* Columba, G. Disputationum medicarum de febris pestilentis cognitione. 1601.

MACCIONI, Girolamo [*fl.* 1631] Risposta ... al parere del. sig. Gasparo Marcucci intorno alla qualità del sapon molle, nella quale si dimostra con ragioni evidenti, la virtù del sapon sodo ... nell'espurgatione delle robbe infette, con l'attestatione delli signori Bernardino Vecoli, & Sebatiano Pessini, Fiorenza, Sermartelli, 1631.

    26, [2] p.   20 cm.   [7226]

    "Noi l'uffitio sopra le nuove arti della città di Lucca, dell'anno 1627 che siamo" ([2] p.) signed by Pompilio Minucciani.

MACCOLO, John. *See* Macolo, Joannes [*ca.* 1576–1622]

MACER. *See* Manitius, Samuel Gotthelf [*d.* 1698]

MACHAON II. *See* SORBAIT, Paul de [1624?-1691]

MACHARKYZUS, LAZARUS. *See* MARCQUIS, Lazarus [1574-1647]

MACHELLI, NICCOLÒ. *See* MACCHELLI, Niccolò [1494?-1554]

MACHERONE, PIETRO [*fl.* 1630] Responsa medica in quibus nonnulli morbi cum suis causis, & signis in examen adducuntur, multaque arduae questiones medicę, pertractantur ... Messanae, Tiyps [sic] R. C. Archiep., Apud Jo. Franc. Biancum, 1630.
    [8], 147 p.   21 cm.   **[7227]**
    Bound with Alaimo, M. A. Consultatio. 1632.

MACHFRED, ABRAHAM [*fl.* 1616] Tractatus de pestilitatibus; sambt, Gründlichem Bericht und Erklerung von den hifftigen pestilischen Ausgüssen der letzten Plagschalen des Zorns Gottes ... Auch von den natürlichen ... Schutz und Cur Mitteln beydes der innerlichen und eusserlichen Curation ... Lignitz, Gedruckt durch Nicolaum Schneider, 1618 [1619]
    [319] p.   18 cm.   **[7228]**

MACHIAVELLUS medicus; seu, Ratio status medicorum, secundum exercitium chymicum delineata, & in certas regulas redacta, atque ob usum, quem junioribus practicis praestat, publicae luci donata, a Philiatro [pseud.] Argentorati, 1698.
    [28] p.   20 cm.   **[7229]**
    Attributed to Jakob Barner. Cf. Waller 684.

—Another printing.   21 cm.   **[7230]**

MACHON II. *See* SOMMER, Johann Georg [1634-1705]

MACK, ANDREAS [*ca.* 1606-1683] *respondent. See* ROLFINCK, W., *praeses.* Decas thematum miscellaneorum. 1638.

MACK, JOHANN CHRISTIAN [1634-1701] *respondent. See* SCHENCK, J. T., *praeses.* Dissertatio physico medica de tribus coctionibus corporis humani. 1658.

MACKAILE, MATTHEW [*fl.* 1657-1696] The diversitie of salts and spirits mantained; or, The imaginary volatility of some salts and non-entity of the alcali ... by an onely lamp-furnace resolved into real improbability. By way of animadversions, upon Dr. D. C[oxe] his 3 papers, communicated to the R[oyal] S[ociety] and insert in the 9. vol. of the P[hilosophical] T[ransactions] Together, with a new system, of the order and gradation, in the worlds creation. As also, Scurvie alchymie discovered ... Aberdeen, John Forbes, 1683.
    [16], 145 (i.e. 144) p.   15 cm.   **[7231]**
    Scurvie alchymie discovered (p. [100]-145) has special title page.

—Moffet-well; or, A topographico-spagyricall description of the mineral wells, at Moffet in Annandale of Scotland. Translated, and much enlarged, by the author ... As also, The Oyly-well ... at St. Catharines Chappel in the paroch of Libberton. To these is subjoyned, a character of Mr. Culpeper and his writings ... Edinburgh, Robert Brown, 1664.
    196 p.   15 cm.   **[7232]**
    Imperfect: upper margins trimmed.
    "Culpeper's character" (p. [145]-196) has special title page.

MACOLO, JOANNES [*ca.* 1576-1622] Theoria chymica luis venereae quae hermeticae medicinae elementa pandit ... Florentiae, Apud heredem Christophani Marescoti, 1616.
    [8], 112 p.   17 cm.   **[7233]**

MCKULIO, JOHN. *See* MACOLO, Joannes [*ca.* 1576-1622]

MACLAEUS, JOHANNES [*fl.* 1632-1633] *respondent. See* SEBISCH, M. [1578-1674?] *praeses.* Galeni Ars parva in disputationes triginta resoluta. 1633 [and] Liber Galeni De tumoribus praeter naturam. 1633.

MACOPPE, ALESSANDRO KNIPS. *See* KNIPS-MACOPPE, Alessandro [1662-1744]

MADAI, DANIEL. *See* MÁDAY, Dániel [*fl.* 1699-1709]

MADATHANUS, HENRICUS. *See* MYNSICHT, Adrian von [1603-1638]

MÁDAY, DÁNIEL [*fl.* 1699-1709] *respondent. See* BARTHOLIN, C. [1655-1738], *praeses.* Dissertatio inauguralis medica de ascite hydrope. 1699.

MADEIRA ARRAIS, EDWARD. *See* MADEIRA ARRAIZ, Duarte [*d.* 1652]

MADEIRA ARRAIZ, DUARTE [*d.* 1652] Methodo de conhecer e curar o morbo gallico primeira parte ... Elargamente se trata do azougue, salsa parrilha, guaiacão, pao santo, raiz da China, & de todos os mais remedios desta enfermidade ... Lisboa, Antonio Rodriguez d'Abreu, a custa de Francisco de Sousa, 1674.

[24], 384, [22] p. 20 cm. [7234]
Part 1 only.

—Methodo de conhecer e curar o morbo gallico. Primeira, & segunda parte ... Lisboa, Antonio Craesbeeck de Mello, 1683.

[11], 236, [9] p.; [8], 220, [7] p. 28 cm.
[7235]
Imperfect: lower part of pages after p. 157 (part 2) mutilated.

—A physical account of the tree of life. *In* Bacon, R. The cure of old age. 1683.

MADEWEIS, FRIEDRICH [1648-1705] *praeses.* De filamentis d. Virginis, quae vulgo dicuntur der Sommer oder Marien-Garn ... Jenae, Stanno Nisiano, 1671.

[20] p. 20 cm. [7236]
Diss.—Jena (C. Häyner, *respondent*)

MADEWISIUS, FRIDERICUS. *See* MADEWEIS, Friedrich [1648-1705]

MADRID. HOSPITAL GENERAL. *See* HOSPITAL GENERAL DE MADRID.

MAENIUS, LORENZ [*fl.* 1619] *respondent. See* VARUS, A., *praeses.* Disputatio medica inauguralis de peripneumonia. 1619.

MAETS, CAREL LODEWIJK DE [*ca.* 1640-1690] Prodromus chemiae rationalis, ratiociniis philosophicis, observationibus medicis, &c. illustratae. Accedunt animadversiones in librum, cui titulus, Collectanea chymica Leidensia, id est Maetsiana, Marggraviana, Le Mortiana; opus, quoad excerpta Maetsiana, mutilum, multis mendis deturpatum, praecipuis suis ornamentis ... observationibus, destitutum ... Lugduni Batavorum, Apud Petrum de Graaf, 1684.

77 p. 19 cm. [7237]
Christopher Love Morley's Collectanea chymica Leydensia was published in the same year.

—*praeses.* Disputatio chemico-medica de calculo renum & vesicae ... Lugduni Batavorum, Apud Abrahamum Elzevier, 1686.

[12] p. 22 cm. [7238]
Diss.—Leyden (J. van de Velde, *respondent*)

—Disputatio medica de morbis soporosis ... Lugduni Batavorum, Apud Abrahamum Elzevier, 1687.

[20] p. 21 cm. [7239]
Diss.—Leyden.

—*See* MORLEY, C. L. Collectanea chymica Leydensia. 1684, 1693, 1696; [German tr.] 1696, 1700.

MAETS, CAROLUS DE. *See* MAETS, Carel Lodewijk de [*ca.* 1640-1690]

MÄTTIG, GREGOR [*fl.* 1607-1610] *respondent.* Discursus iatricus de febrium tecmarsi et curatione ... Basileae, Ex Officina Schroeteriana, 1610.

[28] p. 20 cm. [7240]

—*See* STUPANUS, J. N., *praeses.* Discursus medicus febrium naturam ac differentias ... explicans. 1609; RYFF, P. Gratiosus ... ordo medic. Basileens. 1610.

MÄYEN, PHILIPPUS. *See* MAY, Philippe [*fl.* 1665-1670]

MAFFEI, GIOVANNI PIETRO [*fl.* 1600-1603] *ed.* and *tr. See* FALLOPPIO, G. La chirurgia. 1603, 1647, 1675.

MAGALLOTI, JACOPO, *ed. See* COLLE, G. De omnibus malignis, et pestilentibus affectionibus, & earum medela. 1616.

MAGALOTTI, LORENZO, *conte* [1637-1712] *See* ACCADEMIA DEL CIMENTO, Florence. Essayes of natural experiments. 1684 [and] Saggi di naturali esperienze. 1667; REDI, F. Experimenta circa res diversas naturales. 1675 [and] Osservazioni intorno alle vipere. 1664, 1666, 1686, 1687.

MAGANZA, ALESSANDRO [1556-*ca.* 1630] *ed. See* MASSONIO, S. Archidipno. 1627.

MAGATI, CAESAR [1579-1647] De rara medicatione vulnerum; seu, De vulneribus raro tractandis, libri duo. In quibus nova traditur methodus, qua ... sanantur vulnera ... Permultaque explicantur Galeni, & Hippocratis loca eo spectantia. Haec autem duplici quaestione: I. Utrum melius sit vulnera quotidie solvere, ac procurare, an pluribus interjectis diebus. II. Utrum turundarum, & penicillorum usus in curatione vulnerum sit necessarius. Novum argumentum est ... vulnera tractantibus maxime fructuosum ... Venetiis, Apud Ambrosium, & Bartholomeum Dei, 1616.

[28], 122 (i.e. 202), [1] p.; [20], 121, [1] p. 33 cm.
[7241]

Part [2] has special title page: Liber secundus. In quo nova traditur methodus, ad vulnera particularia totius corporis cito, tute, & jucunde persananda. Cui juncta est Appendix de vulneribus tormento bellico inflictis.

—[The same.] . . . Accessit . . . Joannis Baptistae Magati Tractatus, quo rara vulnerum curatio defenditur contra Sennertum. Venetiis, Apud Jo. Jacobum Hertz, 1673.

    [8], 178 p.; [4], 172, [14] p. 34 cm.   **[7242]**

Part [2] has special title page: Liber secundus . . . cui juncta est Appendix de vulneribus tormento bellico inflictis . . . Opus . . . multo auctius, & emendatius.

Bound with Salius Diversus, P. In Avicennae librum tertium de morbis particularibus totius corporis. 1673.

—*See* Pisoni, A. Breve compendio. 1693.

MAGATI, Giovani Battista [*d.* 1658] *See* Magati, C. De rara medicatione vulnerum. 1673.

MAGINET, Pierre [*fl.* 1623] La theriaque francoise. Avec les vertus, et proprietez d'icelle selon Galien. Mises en vers francois . . . Dispensé publiquement à Salins par . . . Maginet, & Claude Thouverey freres Pharmaciens, en l'an 1623. Lyon, Barthelemy Vincent, 1623.

    90, [1] p. 17 cm.   **[7243]**

MAGINI, Giovanni Antonio [1555-1617] De astrologica ratione, ac usu dierum criticorum, seu decretoriorum; ac praeterea de cognoscendis & medendis morbis ex corporum coelestium cognitione. Opus duobus libris distinctum. Quorum primus complectitur Commentarium in Claudii Galeni librum tertium De diebus decretoriis. Alter agit De legitimo astrologiae in medicina usu. His additur De annui temporis mensura in directionibus, & de directionibus ipsis ex Valentini Naibodae scriptis . . . Venetiis, Apud haeredem Damiani Zenarii [Apud Bartholomęum Rodellam] 1607.

    [10], 120 (i.e. 118) p. illus. 23 cm.   **[7244]**

MAGINI, Giovanni Battista [17th cent.] De podagra brevis disceptatio, in qua morbi idea, causa, & curatio ab usu lactis sine aliis cibariis proponuntur . . . Romae, Fabius de Falco, 1670.

    51, [1] p. 15 cm.   **[7245]**

MAGIRUS, Johann [*d.* 1596] Anthropologia; hoc est, Commentarius eruditissimus in aureum Philippi Melanchthonis libellum De anima; completus & locupletatus opera Georgii Caufungeri . . . Francofurti, Prostat in officina Lichensi, excusus per Wolfgangum Richterum, sumtibus Conradi Nebenii, 1603.

    [36], 654, [18] p. 17 cm.   **[7246]**

Includes text on De anima.

Bound with *his* Physiologiae peripateticae libri sex. 1607.

—De memoria artificiosa libellus. Auctore Johanne Austriaco [pseud.] . . . Francofurti, Ex officina typographica Matthiae Beckeri, impensis Hieronymi Megiseri, 1603.

    93 p. 16 cm.   **[7247]**

—Kurtzer Unterricht, wie man sich für der Pestilentz und rother Ruhr . . . verwahren . . . und curieren könne . . . Marburg in Hessen, Salomon Schadewitz, 1666.

    [2], 30 p. 19 cm.   **[7248]**

—Physiologiae peripateticae libri sex, cum commentariis, in quibus praecepta illius perspicue eruditeque explicantur, & ex optimis quibusque peripateticae philosophiae interpretibus, Platone, Aristotele, Zabarella, Archangelo Mercenario, Thoma Erasto . . . & aliis disceptantur. Witebergae, Impensis Clementis Bergeri & Zachariae Schüreri, 1607.

    701 (i.e. 705), [15] p. 17 cm.   **[7249]**

With this is bound *his* Anthropologia. 1603.

—[The same.] . . . Accessit Caspari Bartholini . . . Enchiridion metaphysicum: ex philosophorum coryphaei Aristotelis, optimorumque ejus interpretum monumentis adornatum. Ed. 6. Wittebergensi melior & notis auctior . . . Francofurti, Impensis Petri Musculi & Ruperti Pistorii, e typographeo Matthiae Beckeri, 1610.

    666 p.; [4], 28, [13] p. 19 cm.   **[7250]**

Part [2] has special title page.

Dedication signed by Conradus Nebenius, the editor.

—[The same.] . . . Ed. 8. Wittenbergensi melior & notis auctior . . . Francofurti, Impensis Petri Musculi, excudebat Joannes Bringerus, 1616.

    666 p.; [4], 28, [13] p. 17 cm.   **[7251]**

Different setting of type.

—[The same.] . . . Ed. 7. [Witebergae] Impensis Clementis Bergeri, & Zachariae Schüreri, imprimebat Nicolaus Ball, 1618.

    [1], 846, [16] p.; [5], 34 p. 16 cm.   **[7252]**

Part [2] has special title page dated 1613.

—[The same.] . . . Londini, Apud Joannem Billium, 1619.

662 p.; [4], 28, [16] p. 17 cm.   [7253]

Part [2] has special title page dated 1618.

—[The same.] . . . Ed. 7. Wittenbergensi melior & notis auctior . . . Francofurti, Impensis Joannis Berneri, excudebat Joannes Nicolaus Stoltzenbergerus, 1619.

666 p.; [4], 28, [13] p. 18 cm.   [7254]

Part [2] has special title page dated 1619.

—[The same.] . . . Ed. ultima, infinitis mendis expurgata. Genevae, Apud Philippum Albertum, 1638.

665, [15] p.; 31, [1] p. 17 cm.   [7255]

Part [2] has half title.

—[The same.] . . . Quibus accessit Caspari Bartholini . . . Metaphysica major, scholiis insignibus illustrata, & ab ipso autore edita. Accessit denique Johannis Magiri De memoria artificiosa, liber singularis, in quatuor tractatus divisus. Omnia haec infinitis mendis repurgata, pluribus locis restituta, & jam denuo summa cum cura diligentiaque excusa. Cantabrigiae, Ex officina R. Danielis, 1642.

[8], 412, [4] p.; [2], 53 (i.e. 55), [1] p.; 26 p. 19 cm.   [7256]

Earlier editions of Bartholin's Metaphysica major were published under title: Enchiridion metaphysica.

—See FERNEL, J. Universa medicina. 1645, 1656, 1679.

MAGIRUS, JOHANNES GOTTFRIED [*fl.* 1698] *respondent.* Disputatio medica inauguralis de morbis complicatis . . . Trajecti ad Rhenum, 1698.

19 p. 20 cm.   [7257]

Diss. — Utrecht.

MAGISTER, RODOLPHUS. *See* LE MAISTRE, Rodolphe [*d. ca.* 1632]

MAGLIOCEA, MATTHIAS, *ed. See* POLVERINO, G. G. De curandis, juxta hodiernum usum, singulis humani corporis morbis. 1629, 1643.

MAGNALIA medico-chymica. 1676. *See* CARDILUCIUS, J. H., ed.

MAGNANI, NICCOLÒ [*fl.* 1630] *See* FLORENCE (City) Ordinances, local laws, etc. Instruzione del magistrato della sanità. 1630 [and] Ordini per la quarantena. 1630 [and] Proroga della quarantena. 1630.

MAGNASSIUS, JOSEPH DE. *See* SAINT-GERY, Joseph de [1590-1674]

MAGNEL, OLOF [*fl.* 1647] *respondent. See* UNON, O., *praes.* Generalis physiologiae ratio leviter libita. 1647.

MAGNEN, JEAN CHRYSOSTÔME [*fl.* 1646-1660] De manna. [n. p.] 1658.

[20], 100 p. 14 cm.   [7258]

—Exercitationes de tabaco . . . Ticini Regii, Apud Jo. Andream Magrium, 1648.

[16], 192 p. 22 cm.   [7259]

—[The same.] . . . [n. p.] 1658.

[24], 222 p. illus. 14 cm.   [7260]

—[The same.] De tabaco exercitationes quatuordecim . . . Ed. ult. a multis mendis repurgata. Hagae-Comitis, Ex typographia Adriani Vlacq, 1658.

24, 264 p. illus. 14 cm.   [7261]

—[The same.] De tabaco exercitationes quatuordecim. In quibus praeter historiam tabaci lectu jucundissimam, etiam herbae virtutes & vitia explicantur, ejusque usus ac abusus, et quantum in medicina valeat ostenditur. Amstelodami, Ex officina Henrici & Theodori Boom, 1669.

[24], 264 p. illus. 14 cm.   [7262]

Added engraved title page.

A reissue, with reprinted preliminaries, of the 1658 edition.

MAGNI, PIETRO PAOLO [16th-17th cent.] Discorsi . . . sopra il modo di sanguinare attaccar le sanguisughe, et le ventose, far le fregagioni, et vessicatorii a corpi humani. Di nuovo ristampato, ad istanza di Pietro Fetti . . . Roma, Jacomo Mascardi, 1613.

[4], 80 p. plates. 22 cm.   [7263]

Engraved title page.

Edited by Pietro Fetti.

—[The same.] . . . Di nuovo stampati, corretti & ampliati di utili avvertiments dal propria autore. Brescia, Bartholomeo Fontana [1618?]

[8], 88 p. illus., port. 21 cm.   [7264]

Engraved title page.

Imperfect: p. 5-12 wanting.

—[The same.] . . . Roma, Ad istanza di Jacomo Macuci, per Jacomo Mascardi [1626?]

[8], 71 p. illus., plates. 23 cm.   [7265]

Engraved title page.

—[The same.] . . . Bologna, Gio. Recaldini, 1674.
[19], 364 p. illus. 14 cm. [7266]
Imperfect: p. 301-304 mutilated.

—Discorso . . . sopra il modo di fare i cauterii, ò rottorii à corpi humani, nel quale si tratta de siti, ove si hanno da fare, de ferri che usar vi si debbono, del modo di tenergli aperti, delle legature, & delle palline, & dell'utilita che da essi ne vengono . . . Brescia, Bartolomeo Fontana, 1618.
[6], 82 p. illus., port. 22 CM. [7267]

MAGNOL, PIERRE [1638-1715] Botanicum Monspeliense; sive plantarum circa Monspelium nascentium index . . . Adduntur variarum plantarum descriptiones et icones. Cum appendice quae plantas de novo repertas continet, & errata emendat . . . Monspelii, Ex officina Danielis Pech, impensis Pauli Marret, 1686.
[16], 309 p. illus., plates. 18 cm. [7268]
With this is bound *his* Prodromus historiae generalis plantarum. 1689.

—Hortus regius Monspeliensis; sive, Catalogus plantarum quae in horto regio Monspeliensi demonstrantur . . . Accesserunt novae plurimarum plantarum cum suis iconibus, descriptiones . . . Monspelii, Apud Honoratum Pech, 1697.
[15], 209 p. plates. 19 cm. [7269]
Half title: Le jardin royal de Montpelier.

—Prodromus historiae generalis plantarum in quo familiae plantarum per tabulas disponuntur. Monspelii, Ex typographia Gabrielis & Honorati Pech, 1689.
[30], 79, [19] p. 18 cm. [7270]
Bound with *his* Botanicum Monspeliense. 1686.

—*See* RAY, J. Stirpium Europaearum extra Britannias nascentium sylloge. 1694.

MAGNUS, ALBERTUS. *See* ALBERTUS MAGNUS, *Saint, Bp. of Ratisbon* [1193?-1280]

MAGNUS, GEORG FRIEDRICH. *See* MAGNUS, György Frigyes [*fl.* 1665]

MAGNUS, GYÖRGY FRIGYES [*fl.* 1665] *respondent. See* ZIEGRA, C., *praeses.* Disputatio physica de magia. 1665.

MAHARKYZUS, LAZARUS. *See* MARCQUIS, Lazarus [1574-1647]

MAHEULT, MATHIEU [1630-1700] *See* POSTEL, N. Factum. 1685.

MAHEUST, MATTHIEU. *See* MAHEULT, Mathieu [1630-1700]

MAHLER, CHRISTOPH. *See* TINCTORIUS, Christoph [1604-1662]

MAI, JOHANN [*fl.* 1620] *respondent.* Themata inauguralia de cachexia . . . Basileae, Typis Johan. Jacobi Genathii [1620]
[17] p. 19 cm. [7271]
Diss.—Basel.

MAIER, JOHANN CHRISTOPH [*fl.* 1672-1680] *respondent.* Disputatio medica inauguralis de pernionibus . . . Altdorfii, Literis Henrici Meyeri [1680]
24 p. 19 cm. [7272]
Diss.—Altdorf.

—*See* BRUNO, J. P., *praeses.* Remorae ac impedimenta purgationis exercitationibus. 1672.

MAIER, MICHAEL [1568?-1622] Cantilenae intellectuales in tridas 9. distinctae, de phoenice redivivo, hoc est, medicinarum omnium pretiosissima, (quae mundi epitome & universi speculum est) non tam alta voce, quam profunda mente dictatae, & pro clave ternarum irreserabilium in chymia arcarum rationabilibus ministratae . . . Rostochii, Typis Mauritii Saxonis, prostat aput [sic] Johannem Hallerfordium, 1622.
[65] p. 14 cm. [7273]
In verse.

—Civitas corporis humani, a tyrannide arthritica vindicata; hoc est, Podagrae, chiragrae, et gonagrae . . . methodica curatio . . . Francofurti, Impensis Lucae Jennis, 1621.
216 p. 16 cm. [7274]

—De circulo physico, quadrato; hoc est, Auro, ejusque virtute medicinali, sub duro cortice instar nuclei latente, an & qualis inde petenda sit . . . Oppenheimii, Typis Hieronymi Galleri, sumptibus Lucae Jennis, 1616.
79 p. 20 cm. [7275]
Bound with Lauremberg, P. Ἀνωνυμον εἰσαγωγν ἀνατομιϰη. 1618.

—Lusus serius, quo Hermes sive Mercurius rex mundanorum omnium sub homine existentium, post longam disceptationem in concilio octovirali habitam, homine rationali arbitro, judicatus & constitutus est ... Oppenheimii, Ex chalcographia Hieronymi Galleri, sumptibus Lucae Jennis, 1616.

79 p.   20 cm.   [7276]

Title page with vignette.
Date altered by hand from 1616 to 1619.

—Secretioris naturae secretorum scrutinium chymicum, per oculis et intellectui accurate accommodata, figuris cupro ... incisa ... emblemata, hisque confines ... sententias, doctissimaque item epigrammata, illustratum ... Francofurti, Impensis Georgii Heinrici Oehrlingii, typo Johannis Philippi Andreae, 1687.

[8], 150 p.   illus.   21 cm.   [7277]

Imperfect: p. 87-88 mutilated.

—Subtilis allegoria super secreta chymiae ...

[701]-740 p.   22 cm.   (*In* Musaeum Hermeticum. Francofurti, 1678)   [7278]

—Themis aurea. The laws of the fraternity of the rosie crosse. Written in Latin ... and now in English ... Whereto is annexed an epistle to the fraternity in Latine, from some here in England. London, N. Brooke, 1656.

[30], 136 p.   illus.   15 cm.   [7279]

The letter in Latin is signed by Theodorus Verax [pseud., i.e. Clement Walker] and Theophilus Celnatus.

—Tractatus de volucri arborea, absque patre et matre, in insulis Orcadum, forma anserculorum proveniente; seu, De ortu miraculoso potius quam naturali vegetabilium, animalium, hominum & supranaturalium quorundam ... Francofurti, Typis Nicolai Hoffmanni, sumptibus Lucae Jennis, 1619.

180 p.   17 cm.   [7280]

Bound with *his* Verum inventum; hoc est, Munera Germaniae. 1619.

—, *ed.* Tripus aureus; hoc est, Tres tractatus chymici selectissimi, nempe I. Basilii Valentini ... Practica una cum 12. clavibus & appendice, ex Germanico; II. Thomae Nortoni ... Crede mihi seu ordinale ... nunc ex Anglicano manuscripto in Latinum translatum ... III. Cremeri ... Testamentum, hactenus nondum publicatum ... Francofurti, Ex chalcographia Pauli Jacobi, impensis Lugae Jennis, 1618.

196 p.   illus., port   20 cm.   [7281]

Each treatise has special title page.

—[The same.] ... Francofurti, Apud Hermannum a Sande, 1677.

[373]-544 p.   22 cm.   (*In* Musaeum Hermeticum. Francofurti, 1678)   [7282]

Each treatise has special title page.

—Verum inventum, hoc est, Munera Germaniae, ab ipsa primitus reperta ... & reliquo orbi communicata ... Francofurti, Typis Nicolai Hoffmanni, sumptibus Lucae Jennis, 1619.

[26], 11-249, [1] p.   17 cm.   [7283]

With this is bound *his* Tractatus de volucri arborea. 1619.

MAINARDES, Nicolo. *See* Monardes, Nicolás [*ca.* 1512-1588]

MAINVILLE, DE [*fl.* 1682] Du bonheur et du malheur du mariage, et des considerations qu'il faut faire avant que de s'y engager ... 2. ed. rev. corr. & augm, par l'auteur. Tome premier [-second] Paris, Amable Auroy, 1688.

2. v. in 1.   18 cm.   [7284]

MAINZ. Ordinances, local laws, etc. Reformatio, und ernewerte Ordnung deren Apotecken, und was sich die ordinarii Medici, Cheirurgi, Barbierer ... in der churfürstlichen Statt und Ertzstifft Meyntz hinfürter zuverhalten: sampt verordnetem Tax ... wie nemblich, und in was Werth alle Artzneyen durch die Apotecker hinfüre verkaufft ... werden sollen. Kürtzlich revidirt, und von newem wider auffgelegt ... Meyntz, Johann Albin, 1618.

8, 197, [6] p.   18 cm.   [7285]

The ordinance was issued by Johann Schweikard von Kronenberg, Abp. of Mainz.
Bound with Mercklin, B. Kurtzer verfasster Underricht. 1627.

—Tractätlein und kurtzer Bericht, wie man sich in Sterbens Läuffen verhalten ... vor dieser bösen Seucht, bewahren, und mit welchen Artzneyen dieselbige zu curiren sey ... Maintz, Johann Albin, 1606.

[24] p.   20 cm.   [7286]

MAIOLUS, Simon [*fl.* 1565-1597] Dies caniculares; hoc est, Colloquia tria et viginti physica, nova et penitus admiranda ... Quibus pleraque naturae admiranda, quae aut in athere fiunt, aut in Europa, Asia atque Africa, quin etiam in ipso orbe novo ... sunt, item mirabilia arte hominum confecta recensentur ... Ed. alt. priori auct. & corr. Moguntiae, Ex officina Joannis Albini, curante Joanni Theobal. Schönwetter & Conrado Meulio, 1607-[1612?]

4 v. in 3. 26 cm. [**7287**]

Vol. 2-4 have titles: Colloquiorum; sive, Dierum canicularium tomus secundus-tomus quartus. Imprint of vol. 2-3 reads: Helenopoli, Imp. Joh. Theo. Schönwetter poelo [sic] Richteriano. Vol. 4 has imprint: Helenopoli.

—[The same.] . . . Ed. nova. & caeteris auct. & corr. . . . Moguntiae, Apud Joh. Theobald. Schönwetter, cIɔ cI x [i.e. 1610]

[8], 558, [79] p. 25 cm. [**7288**]

Vol. 1 only.

MAIR, Franz [*fl.* 1638] *respondent. See* Lerchenfeldt, M., *praeses.* Disputatio philosophica de mutatione rerum naturalium. 1638.

MAISTERUS, Isaacus. *See* Meister, Isaak [*fl.* 1687]

MAISTRE, Rodolphe Le. *See* Le Maistre, Rodolphe [*d. ca.* 1632]

MAIUS, Heinrich. *See* May, Heinrich [1632-1696]

MAIUS, Johann. *See* Mai, Johann [*fl.* 1620]

MAIUS, Theodor. *See* Majus, Theodor [*fl.* 1610-1623]

MAIUS JOANNES BURCHARDUS. *See* Majus, Johann Burchard [1652-1726]

MAJERUS, Michael. *See* Maier, Michael [1568?-1622]

MAJOLI, Simon. *See* Maiolus, Simon [*fl.* 1556-1597]

MAJOR, Johann Daniel [1634-1693] Chirurgia infusoria, placidis cl. virorum dubiis impugnata, cum modesta, ad eadem, responsione. Kilonii, Sumptibus Joh. Lüderwald, imprimeb. Joach. Reumannus, 1667.

[8], 328, [1] p. illus. 20 cm. [**7289**]

—Consideratio physiologica occurrentium quorundam in nuper-editis epistolis duabus Dn. Franc. Jos. Burrhi, de cerebro & oculis, ad Dn. D. Th. Bartholinum scriptis. Kilonii, Literis Joachimi Reumanni [1669?]

[76] p. illus. 20 cm. [**7290**]

—De oraculis medicinae ergo quaesitis, et votivis convalescentium tabellis. *In* Sturm, S. Discursus. 1663.

—Deliciae hybernae; sive, Tria nova inventa medica . . . Kilonii, Typis Joachimi Reumanni, 1667.

[62] p. 29 cm. [**7291**]

Imperfect: sig. q2 (blank?) wanting.

—Dissertatio epistolica de cancris et serpentibus petrefactis ad Dn. D. Philippum Jacobum Sachs . . . cui accessit Responsoria dissertatio historico-medica ejusdem Philippi Jacobi Sachs à Lewenheimb . . . De miranda lapidum natura. Jenae, Sumpt. Esaiae Feligiebelii, 1664.

110, [1] p. 16 cm. [**7292**]

Errata: p. [III]

—Genius errans; sive, De ingeniorum in scientiis abusu dissertatio. Kiliae Holsatorum, Literis & sumptibus Joachimi Reumanni, 1677.

[350] p. illus. 21 cm. [**7293**]

Added engraved title page.

"Pestremo sequitur Benedicti Menzini . . . De literatorum hominum invidia, ad. Dn. Franciscum Redi, liber, Florentiae primum, anno 1675. nunc secundum editus, & genio erranti annexus ob affinitatem argumenti" (p. [287-314]) has half title.

—Historia anatomes Kiloniensis primae . . . Sub finem annexus est Catalogus scriptorum, successive inposterum ab autore edendorum. Kilonii, Literis Joachimi Reumanni, 1666.

26 p. illus. 36 cm. [**7294**]

Bound with copy 2 of Salvatico, B., *conte di.* Consiliorum et responsorum medicinalium centuriae quatuor. 1662.

—Historia anatomica calculorum, insolentioris figurae, magnitudinis ac molis, in renibus . . . J. Sperlingii, repertorum. Lipsiae, Impensis Johan. Barthol. Oehleri, excudebat Johan-Ericus Hahnius, 1662.

[28] p. illus. 21 cm. [**7295**]

—Memoriale anatomico-miscellaneum. Kilonii, Typis Joach. Reumanni, 1669.

[80] p. illus. 20 cm. [**7296**]

—Prodromus inventae a se chirurgiae infusoriae, sive, quo pacto agonizantes quidam, pro deploratis habiti, servari aliquandiu possint infuso in venam sectam liquore peculiari . . . Lipsiae, Typis Johannis Wittigau, 1664.

[2], 37 p. 16 cm. [**7297**]

—Disputationem medicam inauguralem de suppressione mensium ... habendam Joh. Daniel Maior ... quoscunque ... in gratiam candidati sui ... Caspari Merwiz ... invitat. Kiliae, Typis Joach. Reumanni, 1693.

[12] p.   20 cm.   [7298]

Program—Kiel (with vita of K. Merwitz)

Dissertations—Kiel

—*praeses*. De aerumnis gigantum in negocio sanitatis, disputationem medicam D. XVI M. Augusti M.DC.LXXVI ... habendam intimant praeses Joh. Dan. Major ... et respondens Hermannus de Lengerken ... Kiliae Holsatorum, Literis Joachimi Reumanni, 1689.

[96] p.   illus.   20 cm.   [7299]

Diss. 1676. H. von Kengerken, *respondent*.

—Disputatio medica inauguralis de amaurosi vel gutta serena ... Kiliae, Literis Joach. Reumanni, 1673.

[34] p.   20 cm.   [7300]

J. W. Schmidt, *respondent*.

—Disputatio medica inauguralis de malacia ... Kilonii, Typis Joachimi Reumanni, 1677.

[40] p.   20 cm.   [7301]

J. C. Tralles, *respondent*.

—Disputatio medica inauguralis de petechiis ... Kilonii, Literis Joachimi Reumanni, 1681.

31, [1] p.   20 cm.   [7302]

J. P. Förtsch, *respondent*.

—Disputatio medica inauguralis de tactis fulmine ... Kiliae Holsatorum, Joach, Reuman, 1673.

[32] p.   20 cm.   [7303]

J. J. Kisling, *respondent*.

—Disputatio medica inauguralis quam de usu et abusu mercurii in lue venerea ... defendendam suscipiet Joh. Nicolaus Schippel ... Kiliae, Literis Joach. Reumanni, 1673.

[44] p.   19 cm.   [7304]

J. N. Schippel, *respondent*.

—Disputationem anatomicam de sanguine peridromo ... intimant ... Joh. Daniel Major ... & ... Georgius Martinus Tatter ... Kiliae, Joach. Reumannus, 1673.

[28] p.   20 cm.   [7305]

G. M. Tatter, *respondent*.

—Disquisitionem medicam ... de moribundorum regimine, ubi incidenter quaedam de recte ferendis vulnerum judiciis ... habendam intimat ... Christophorus Lehmannus ... Kiliae-Holsatorum, Typis Joachimi Reumanni, 1685.

29 (i.e. 39), [1] p.   19 cm.   [7306]

C. Lehmann, *respondent*.

—Dissertationem medicam de febre artificiali ... pro virili tueri conabitur Andreas Cassius. Kilonii, Typis Joachimi Reumanni, 1666.

[20] p.   18 cm.   [7307]

A. Cassius, *respondent*.

—Positiones medicae variae earumque praecipuae de podagra ... Kiliae, Joachimus Reumann [1679]

[46] p.   19 cm.   [7308]

F. Hesporn, *respondent*.

—Theses medicae inaugurales de motu et sensu abolito in affectibus soporosis ... Kilonii, Typis Joachimi Reumanni, 1680.

[15] p.   20 cm.   [7309]

K. March, *respondent*.

—*See* Horst, J. D. Judicium de chirurgia infusoria Jo. Danielis Majoris. 1665; Jasolino, G. Collegium anatomicum. 1668; Morhof, D. G. Epistola de scypho vitreo. 1672.

MAJUS, Heinrich. *See* May, Heinrich [1632-1696]

MAJUS, Johann Burchard [1652-1726] *ed. See* Morhof, D. G. Dissertationes academicae & epistolicae. 1699.

MAJUS, Theodor [*fl.* 1610-1623] Ruhr Tractätlin. Worinnen aussführlich ... gehandelt wird von den jetzo grassierenden Hoffgang oder Durchlauff ... Magdeburg, Bey Johann Francken, 1623.

[48] p.   16 cm.   [7310]

—, *ed. See* Brian, T. Der englische Wahrsager aus dem Urin. 1693.

—*See* Columella, L. J. M. Agricultur; oder, Ackerbaw. 1612.

MAJUS, Tobias [1601-1632] *praeses*. Disputatio medica de catarrheumatismo in genere ... Wittebergae, Typis haeredum Christiani Tham, 1630

[23] p.   19 cm.   [7311]

Diss.—Wittenberg (W. Deichman, *respondent*)

MAKOWSKY, Samuel [*fl.* 1618–1633] *respondent.* Disputationem medicam de ephialte . . . publicae censurae committit Samuel Makowsky . . . die 30. Decembr. anno 1618. [Basel, 1618?]

[14] p.   20 cm.   [**7312**]

Signatures: q3–4, r⁴, s1.

MALACREDA, Andreas [*fl.* 1609–1610] *respondent.* *See* Stupanus, J. N., *praeses.* Σημειωτιces particularis cap. I. De affectibus. 1610.

—*See* Stupanus, J. N. Gratiosi medicorum Basiliens. collegii decreto 1610.

MALBEC DE TRESFEL, Jean [*fl.* 1668] *comp.* and *tr.* *See* Digby, *Sir* K. Recueil des remedes et secrets tirez des memoires de Mr. . . . Digby. 1669, 1684, 1689, 1700.

MALEBRANCHE, Nicolas [1638–1715] De inquirenda veritate libri sex, in quibus mentis humanae natura disquiritur . . . Ex ultima editione Gallica, pluribus illustrationibus ab ipso authore aucta, Latine versi. Genevae, Typis & sumptibus Societatis, 1690.

[41], 511, 143 p.   25 cm.   [**7313**]

"Illustrationes seu explicationes ad librum, De inquirenda veritate": 143 p.

—[English tr.] Treatise concerning the search after truth . . . To which is added the author's treatise of nature, and grace . . . Together with his answer to the animadversions upon the first volume: his defense against the accusations of Mʳ. De la Ville . . . All translated by T. Taylor . . . Oxford, Printed by L. Lichfield for Thomas Bennet, 1694.

[16], 172 (i.e. 174) p.; 10, 203 p.; 42 p.   illus.   34 cm.   [**7314**]

The last part has half title.

MALER, Ernest Christian [*fl.* 1692] *respondent.* Disputatio medica inauguralis de pica . . . Basileae, Typis Joh. Rudolphi Genathii [1692]

[16] p.   20 cm.   [**7315**]

Diss. — Basel.

MALER, Georg. *See* Pictorius, Georg [*ca.* 1500–1569]

MALESIEU, André, *tr.* *See* Gourmelen, É. Les oeuvres chirurgicales. 1647 [and] Le sommaire de toute la chirurgie. 1607.

MALEY, Johann Georg [*fl.* 1696] *respondent. See* Wedel, G. W., *praeses.* Diatribe medica exhibens aegrum memoriae debilitate laborantem. 1696.

MALFI, Tiberio [*fl.* 1626] Il barbiere . . . libri tre. Ne' quali si ragiona dell'eccellenza dell'arte, e de' suoi precetti. Delle vene, e regole d'aprirle. Dell'applicatione de' remedi chirurgici appartenenti al mestiere . . . Napoli, Ottavio Beltrano, 1626.

[24], 194 p.   illus., ports.   27 cm.   [**7316**]

Engraved title page.

—[The same.] Nuova prattica della decoratoria manuale, et della sagnia . . . divisa in libri tre. Nel primo de quali si spiegano gli ornamenti dell'arte del barbiere . . . Nel secondo si dimostra la piena anatomia delle vene . . . Nel terzo si da l'uso prattico delle sanguisughe, delle scarificationi . . . de vesicatorii . . . Napoli, Ottavio Beltrano, 1629.

[24], 194 p.   illus., ports.   26 cm.   [**7317**]

A reissue of the 1626 edition with new title page.

—[German tr.] Neue Anleitung zur Barbier- und Wund-Artzney-Kunst, in dreyen Büchern verabfasset; in deren erstem, von der Barbier-Kunst Lob, Würde und Vortrefflichkeit . . . im andern, von einer vollständigen Anatomie aller Blut-Adern, die der Aderlass unterworffen seyn . . . Im dritten, von Blut-Egeln, Fontanellen, Haarzügen, blasen-ziehenden Pflastern, und dergleichen, einem Wund-Artzt zuständigen Operationibus, mehr; aufs deutlichste . . . gehandelt wird . . . Mit einer . . . Vorrede, wie die Chirurgie gründlich zu studiren . . . sey? Nürnberg, In Verlegung Christoph Endters, 1676.

[18], lxxxiv, 484, [27] p.   front. (port.), illus., ports.   17 cm.   [**7318**]

Added engraved title page.

The preface is by Georg Abraham Mercklin.

MALLEOLUS, Benedictus [*fl.* 1620–1623] *respondent. See* Sebisch, M. [1578–1674?] *praeses.* Disputatio de alimentorum facultatibus quarta et ultima. 1620 [and] Disputatio de purgatione duodecima. 1621 [and] Disputationes de recta ratione purgandi. 1621 [and] Exercitationes medicae. 1639.

MALMUS, Gabriel [*fl.* 1654] *respondent. See* Friess, M. F., *praeses.* Dentes eruditorum limae ultra perpoliendos . . . subjicit . . . G. M. 1654.

MALPHIUS, Tiberius. *See* Malfi, Tiberio [*fl.* 1626]

MALPIGHI, MARCELLO [1628-1694] Opera omnia ... tomis duobus comprehensa ... Londini, Prostant apud Robertum Scott, 1686.

2 v. in 1. plates. 37 cm. **[7319]**

Added engraved title page.

Imperfect: Tabula VI of De ovo incubato wanting.

Vol. 2 has imprint: Londini, Typis M. F. impensis R. Littlebury, R. Scott, Tho. Sawbridge, & G. Wells, 1686. — Appendix (bound with vol. 2) has special title page with imprint: Londini, Impensis Roberti Scott, 1686.

Frati 2 (variant state)

—[The same.] ... Londini, Apud Robertum Littlebury, 1686-87 [v. 1, 1687]

2 v. in 1. plates. 37 cm. **[7320]**

Added engraved title page.

Appendix (bound with vol. 1) and vol. 2 are identical with vol. 2 of the Robert Scott edition.

Frati 2.

With this is bound *his* Opera posthuma. 1697.

—[The same.] ... Ed. nov. ... notis marginalibus ... adaucta ... emendata ... Lugduni Batavorum, Apud Petrum vander Aa, 1687.

2 v. in 1. plates. 24 cm. **[7321]**

Added engraved title page.

Imperfect: added engraved title page wanting.

Frati 3.

—Opera posthuma ... quibus praefixa est ejusdem vita a seipso scripta. Londini, Impensis A. & J. Churchill, 1697.

[2], 110 p.; 187, [1] p.; [2], 10 p. fronts. (port.), plates. 37 cm. **[7322]**

"Morborum exitialium tyrannica saevitia ... in medicam historiam redacta a Johanne Baptista Gyraldo" and "De structura glandularum conglobatarum ... epistola ... Londini, Apud Richardum Chiswell, 1697" have special title pages.

Imperfect: De structura glandularum conglobatarum ... epistola is misbound after first group of paging.

Frati 4.

Bound with Opera omnia. Londini, 1686-87.

—Opera posthuma. In quibus ... authoris vita continetur ... Supplementa necessaria, & praefationem addidit ... emendavit Petrus Regis ... Ed. ult. Amstelodami, Apud Georgium Gallet, 1698.

[14], 387 p. front., plates. 24 cm. **[7323]**

Frati 5 (variant state)

With this is bound another issue of Ruysch, F. Observationum anatomico-chirurgicarum centuria. 1691.

—Opera posthuma quibus praefationes, & animadversiones addidit, pluribusque in locis emendationes instituit Faustinus Gavinellus ... Ed. nov.

... Venetiis, Ex typographica Andreae Poleti, 1698.

[24], 334 p. plates., port. 40 cm. **[7324]**

Frati 6.

—Opera posthuma. In quibus ... authoris vita continetur ... Supplementa necessaria, & praefationem addidit ... emendavit Petrus Regis ... Ed. ult. ... Amstelodami, Apud Georgium Gallet, 1700.

[14], 387 p. front., plates. 25 cm. **[7325]**

A reissue of the 1698 Amsterdam edition.

Frati 8.

—Another issue, with imprint: Amstelodami, Apud Donatum Donati, 1700. Dedicatory epistle differs.

[7326]

Not in Frati.

—Anatome plantarum. Cui subjungitur Appendix, iteratas & auctas ejusdem authoris De ovo incubato observationes continens ... Londini, Impensis Johannis Martyn, 1675-79.

2 v. plates. 37 cm. **[7327]**

Each volume has added engraved title page.

Appendix has special title page dated 1675.

Imperfect: title page of volume 2 mutilated.

Frati 23.

—De externo tactus organo anatomica observatio ... Neapoli, Apud Aegidium Longum, 1665.

46 p. 14 cm. **[7328]**

Frati 14.

—De pulmonibus observationes anatomicae. *In* Bartholin, T. De pulmonum substantia. 1663.

Frati 11.

—De structura glandularum conglobatarum consimiliumque partium epistola ... Londini, Apud Richardum Chiswell, 1689.

[2], 36 p. 20 cm. **[7329]**

Frati 34.

—[The same.] ... Lugduni Batavorum, Apud Petrum van der Aa, 1690.

16 p. 24 cm. **[7330]**

Signatures: eG-eH⁴.

Frati 36.

—De viscerum structura exercitatio anatomica ... Accedit dissertatio ... De polypo cordis. Bononiae, Ex typographia Jacobi Monti, 1666.

[4], 172 p. 26 cm. **[7331]**

Frati 15.

—[The same.] . . . Londini, Typis T. R. Impensis Jo. Martyn, 1669.

[12], 180 p.   14 cm.   [**7332**]

Frati 17.

—[The same.] . . . Amstelodami, Apud Petrum le Grand, 1669.

[12], 168 p.   14 cm.   [**7333**]

Frati 18.

—Dissertatio epistolica de bombyce . . . Londini, Apud Joannem Martyn & Jacobum Allestry, 1669.

[9], 100 p.   plates.   23 cm.   [**7334**]

Preface signed by Henry Oldenburg, the editor.

Frati 20.

—[The same.] *See* AN ACCOMPT of some books. 1669.

—Dissertatio epistolica de formatione pulli in ovo . . . Londini, Apud Joannem Martyn, 1673.

[2], 42, [1] p.   plates.   23 cm.   [**7335**]

Frati 22.

Page [1] at end is the title page of his Dissertationes epistolicae duae.

—Epistolae anatomicae . . . Marcelli Malpighii et Caroli Fracassati . . . Amstelodami, Apud Casparum Commelinum, 1669.

[4], 260 p.   plates.   14 cm.   [**7336**]

Contents. By Marcello Malpighi: De cerebro. - De lingua. - De externo tactus organo. - De omento, pinguedine, et adiposis ductibus. By Carlo Fracassati: De lingua. - De cerebro. Items have half title pages.

Frati 19.

Bound with Case, J. [*fl.* 1680–1700] Compendium anatomicum. 1696.

—Another issue.   [**7337**]

Signature on p. 3 reads A3 instead of A2.

—Exercitationes de viscerum, nominatim pulmonum, hepatis, cerebri corticis, renum, lienis, structura, cum dissertatione De polypo cordis. Ed. alt. Jenae, Impensis Joh. Gollneri, 1677.

[10], 280, [46] p.   14 cm.   [**7338**]

Added engraved title page.

Frati 24.

Bound with copy 2 of Swalve, B. Querelae ventriculi renovatae. 1675.

—[The same.] Exercitationes de structura viscerum, nominatim hepatis, cerebri corticis, renum, lienis, cum dissertatione De polypo cordis, quibus accesserunt ob materiae vicinitatem . . .

epistolae duae De pulmonibus . . . Ed. alt. corr. Francofurti, Apud Augustum Boetium, 1678.

[10], 280, [50] p.   illus.   14 cm.   [**7339**]

Frati 25.

—[The same.] . . . Francofurti, et veneunt Monspelii, Apud Stephanum Marret, 1683.

[10], 254 p.   plates.   16 cm.   [**7340**]

Frati 28.

—[French tr.] Discours anatomiques sur la structure des visceres, sçavoir du foye, du cerveau, des reins, de la ratte, du polype du coeur, et des poulmons . . . Mis en françois par M. **** [i.e. Sauvalle] . . . Paris, Laurent d'Houry, 1683.

[18], 374, [2] p.   plates.   17 cm.   [**7341**]

Frati 29.

—[The same.] . . . 2. ed. Paris, Laurent d'Houry, 1687.

[18], 374, [2] p.; [1], 66 p.   plates.   17 cm.

[**7342**]

Part [2] has half title: "Nouvelle lettre . . . sur la structure des glandes conglobées, avec un Discours sur l'utilité du microscope."

A reissue of the 1683 edition with new title page and the addition of the Nouvelle lettre. The Discours sur l'utilité du microscope is by the younger Laurent Verduc.

Frati 33.

—Nouvelle lettre sur la structure des glandes conglobées. *See* BRUNET, C. Le progrès de la medicine. 1695.

—Opuscula anatomica . . . Bononiae, Typis Jacobi Montii, sumptibus Petri Botelli, 1680.

[8], 328 p.   plates.   15 cm.   [**7343**]

Frati 26.

—Praeclarissimo . . . viro D. Jacobo Sponio . . . Marcellus Malpighius S. P. . . . [London, Royal Society, 1684]

601–608 p.   23 cm.   [**7344**]

Caption title.

A letter from Malpighi to Spon, concerning a kidney of an unusual shape . . . taken out of the body of a man. Detached from Philosophical Transactions, 1684, vol. 14.

Frati 30.

With this are bound: *his* Praeclarissimo . . . viro D. Jacobo Sponio. [London, 1684] [Another letter]; An accompt of some books. [London, 1669]

—Praeclarissimo . . . viro D. Jacobo Sponio . . . Marcellus Malpighius S. P. . . . [London, Royal Society, 1684]

630–646 p.   23 cm.   [**7345**]

Caption title.

At end: Dabam Bononiae Calen. Novembris MDCLXXXI.
A letter from Malpighi to Spon, concerning the structure of the
womb. Detached from Philosophical Transactions, 1684, vol. 14.
Frati 31.

Bound with *his* Praeclarissimo ... viro D. Jacobo Sponio. [London, 1684] [Another letter]

— La structure du ver a soye, et de la formation
du poulet dans l'oeuf. Contenant deux dissertations
... mises en françois par *** docteur en medecine
[i.e. Sauvalle] Paris, Maurice Villery, 1686.

[4], 384, [10] p.   plates.   16 cm.   [**7346**]

"Dissertation ... touchant la maniere dont se forme le poulet
dans l'oeuf ..." (p. [305]-384) has half title.

Frati 32.

— *See* BAGLIVI, G. De praxi medica ad priscam
observandi rationem revovanda. 1699; FELIX, A.
Father. De ovis cochlearum epistola. 1684; HERFELT,
H. G. Philosophicum hominis, de corporis humani
machina. 1687; MARSIGLI, A. F. De ovis cochlearum
epistola. 1684 [and] Relazione del ritrovamento
dell'vova di chiocciole. 1683, 1695; VESLING, J. Syntagma anatomicum. 1666, 1677, 1696.

MALUICINUS, JULIUS. *See* MALVICINI, Giulio
[*fl.* 1682?]

MALVICINI, GIULIO [*fl.* 1682?] Utiles colectiones
medico phisicae ad medicinae inscios prolatae ...
Venetiis, Apud Combi, & La Noù, 1682.

[10], 444, [15] p.   front.   25 cm.   [**7347**]

MALYNES, GERARD DE [*fl.* 1586-1641] *See*
CHYMICAL, medicinal, and chyrurgical addresses.
1655.

MAN and woman their own doctor. 1676. *See*
PONTEOUS, doctor.

MAN, JAN DE [*fl.* 1671] *respondent.* Disputatio
medica inauguralis de catalepsi ... Lugduni
Batavorum, Apud viduam & haeredes Joannis
Elsevirii, 1671.

[9] p.   23 cm.   [**7348**]

Diss. — Leyden.

MANAGETTA, JOHANN WILHELM. *See* MANNAGETTA, Johann Wilhelm [1588-1666]

MANARDI, GIOVANNI [1462-1536] Ἰατρολογία επιστολική; sive, Curia medica ... viginti libris
epistolarum ac consultationum medicinalium adumbrata; nec non annotationibus & censuris ... in

Joannis Mesue simplicia & composita, adornata ...
tertio jam revisa ... emendata ... Hanoviae, Typis
Wechelianis, apud haeredes Joannis Aubrii, 1611.

[12], 432, [24] p.   35 cm.   [**7349**]

Edited by Peter Uffenbach.

— *See* MESÜE [924 or 5-1015] Opera. 1602, 1623.

MANCEBO, PETRUS. *See* MANCEBO AGUADO DE
MOLINA, Pedro [*fl.* 1618-1646]

MANCEBO AGUADO DE MOLINA, PEDRO
[*fl.* 1618-1646] De essentia, signis, causis, prognostico,
& curatione anginae, vulgo garrotillo, brevis tractatus
... Hispali, Rodriguez Gamarra, 1618.

[4], 36 ll.   21 cm.   [**7350**]

— Informe de como la enfermedad que padece en
el rostro, el ... Martin de Zañartu ... no es de la
que llama el vulgo, mal de San Lazaro ... Sevilla,
1646.

8, [1] p.   20 cm.   [**7351**]

— Libellus de melancholia hippochondriaca, in quo
usus chalybis impugnatur ... Sevilla, Simon
Fajardo, 1636.

[4], 23 ll.   21 cm.   [**7352**]

MANCINI, GIULIO [1558-1630] *ed. See* MERCURIALE, G. De morbis cutaneis. 1601.

MANCINI, JACOPO [*fl.* 1631] Practica visitandi infirmos, in duas partes divisa. In prima, nonnulla
dubia resolvuntur circa confessionem, communionem ... injuriarum, remissionem, ac denique irregularitatem ex mortis acceleratione, cum appendice ... In altera parte habentur monita scitu digna,
& alia contra insidias daemonum, cum precibus pro
iis adjuvandis, qui mortis in agone contendunt ...
Adjectae fuere elaboratae, ac selectiorum dubiorum
additiones ... a P. D. Laurentio Cutillo ... Et in
hac octava impressione plurimis supplementis, ac
duobus aliis tractatibus scilicet De praecendentia in
funebris associandis, aliisque processionibus servanda, & De quarta funerali sepulturae occasione
debita. Ab ... Laurentio Cutillo locupletata. Mercuriani, Apud Camillum Cavallum, 1642.

[16], 840, [56] p.   21 cm.   [**7353**]

Imperfect printing: p. 2-3 supplied in manuscript.
Part 2 has special title page (p. 685).

MANCINI, POLIZIANO [*fl.* 1602] *tr. See* FONSECA,
R. de. Del conservare la sanita. 1603.

MANCINUS, Julius. *See* Mancini, Giulio [1558-1630]

MANDA el Rey. *See* Portugal. Sovereigns, etc. [1621-1640] (Philip III). Manda el Rey. 1630.

MANDEVILLE, Bernard [1670?-1733] *respondent.* Disputatio medica inauguralis de chylosi vitiata . . . Lugduni Batavorum, Apud Abrahamum Elzevier, 1691.

    [12] p. 22 cm.   **[7354]**
Diss.—Leyden.

MANDIROLA, Agostino [17th cent.] Manuale de' giardinieri diviso in tre libri . . . Aggiuntovi il quarto libro, che dimostra le qualita . . . de' fiori descritti in questo volume. Venetia, Giacomo Zattoni, 1667.

    [12], 168 p. 16 cm.   **[7355]**

MANDRIOLA, Agostino. *See* Mandirola, Agostino [17th cent.]

MANDOSIO, Prospero [*ca.* 1648-1709] Θέατρον in quo maximorum Christiani orbis pontificum archiatros . . . spectandos exhibet. Romae, Typis Francisci de Lazaris, 1696.

    236 p. 23 cm.   **[7356]**

MANELFI, Giovanni [*fl.* 1618-1650] De febribus theoria . . . Romae, Sumptibus Joannis Manelphi, ex typographia Andreae Phaei, 1625.

    [31], 320 (i.e. 312) p. 23 cm.   **[7357]**
A part of this work (p. 60-145) appeared separately in 1623 under title: Prognostica in febribus in communi et ad mentem Hippocratis.

—De helleboro disceptatio . . . Romae, Apud haeredem Bartholomaei Zannetti, 1622.

    100 p. 17 cm.   **[7358]**

—Mensa Romana, sive, Urbana victus ratio . . . Romae, Typis & expensis Philippi de Rubeis, 1650.

    [12], 239, [19] p. 22 cm.   **[7359]**
Errata: p. [19]

Prognostica in febribus in communi, et ad mentem Hippocratis . . . Romae, Apud haeredem Bartholomaei Zannetti, 1623.

    184, [6] p. 13 cm.   **[7360]**

—[The same.] . . . In hac 2. ed. recognita, atque ampliata. Romae, Apud Manelphum Manelphium, sumptibus Jo. Baptistae Subissati, 1646.

    168, [6 +] p. 12 cm.   **[7361]**
Imperfect: all after p. [6] wanting.
Bound with Hippocrates. Aphorismi. Latin. 1646.

—Responsio brevis ad annotationes Prosperi Martiani . . . in commentationem Marsilii Cagnati . . . super aphorismo Concocta 22. lib. I. Hippocratis. Romae, Apud haeredem Bartholomaei Zannetti, 1621.

    [7], 71 p. 17 cm.   **[7362]**

—Tractatus de fletu, & lacrymis. Romae, Ex typographia Bartholomaei Zannetti, 1618.

    [8], 108, [18] p. 17 cm.   **[7363]**

—*See* Castelli, P. Epistola. 1622; Hippocrates. [Aphorismi. Latin] 1623., 1646., 1663; Marziani, P. Apologeticus liber. 1617.

MANELPHUS, Johannes. *See* Manelfi, Giovanni [*fl.* 1618-1650]

MANFREDI, Antonio [*fl. ca.* 1640] *See* Campi, B. Baldassari, e Michel Campi al sig. Antonio Manfredi . . . In dilucidotione, e confermatione maggiore di alcune cose state da noi dette nella risposta al sig. Gaspari medico. 1641; Castelli, P. Opobalsamum triumphans. 1640? Donzelli, G. Lettera familiare. 1643; Giaquinto, T. Ragguaglio primo- [secondo] venuto di Parnaso l'anno M.DC.XXXX. sopra il balsamo d'Arabia. 1640; Nemi, N. Imbiancatura di Nicolò Nemi da Novi. 1640; Panuzzi, F., ed. Francesco Panuzzi . . . a i lettori. 1640.

MANFREDI, Girolamo [*d.* 1492] Libro intitolato Il perche, tradotto di latino . . . Con mostrar le cagioni d'infinite cose, appartenenti alla sanità. Con la dichiaratione delle virtù d'alcune herbe. Di nuovo ristampata, & ripurgata . . . Venetia, I Guerra, 1607.

    [29], 314 p. 18 cm.   **[7364]**
First published in 1474 under title: Liber de homine.
Based largely on Aristotle's Problemata. Cf. Lawn, p. 112.

—[The same.] . . . Venetia, Lucio Spineda, 1613.

    [29], 313, [1] p. 16 cm.   **[7365]**

—[The same.] Il novo lume dell'arte; overo, Il perche, opera copiosa di varie cognitioni . . . Padova, I Gattella, 1667.

    [36], 311 p. 15 cm.   **[7366]**

—[The same.] . . . Padova, I Gattella, 1668.
[36], 311 p.   16 cm.   [**7367**]

Imperfect: p. [5–8] mutilated.
A reissue of the 1667 edition with date reset.

—[The same.] . . . Venetia, Steffano Curti, 1678.
369 p.   15 cm.   [**7368**]

MANFREDI, PAOLO [*d.* 1716] De nova et inaudita medico-chyrurgica operatione sanguinem transfundente de individuo ad individuum; prius in brutis, & deinde in homine Romae experta. Opusculum singulare . . . Romae, Typis Nicolai Angeli Tinassii, sumptibus Benedicti Carrarae, 1668.
32, [1] p.   plates.   22 cm.   [**7369**]

Errata: p. [33]

— Novae circa oculum observationes . . . Romae, Ex typographia Ignatii de Lazaris, 1674.
[11] p.   plates.   23 cm.   [**7370**]

The plate is dated 1673.

MANFRONCINI, GIOVANNI CESARE. *See* BERNARDI, F. L'ignoranza convinta. 1669.

MANGET, JEAN JACQUES [1652–1742] Bibliotheca medico-practica; sive, Rerum medicarum thesaurus cumulatissimus quo omnes prorsus humani corporis morbosae affectiones tum artem medicam in genere, tum chirurgicam in specie, spectantes ordine alphabetico explicantur . . . Tomus primus [-quartus] Genevae, Sumptibus Joannis Anthonii Chouët [et David Ritter] 1695–1697.
4 v.   36 cm.   [**7371**]

—, *comp. See* SCHRÖDER, J. Pharmacopoea Schrödero-Hoffmanniana illustrata et aucta. 1687.

—, *ed. See* BARBETTE, P. Medicinische, chirurgische und anatomische Schrifften. 1700 [and] Opera omnia medica et chirurgica. 1682, 1683, 1688 [and] La pratique de medecine. 1692; BONET, T. Sepulchretum. 1700; PIENS, F. H. Tractatus de febribus in genere. 1689; SCHMITZ, J. A. Medicinae practicae compendium. 1691.

— *See* [DUFOUR, P. S.] Novi tractatus de potu caphe; de Chinensium the; et de chocolata. 1699; LE CLERC, D. Bibliotheca anatomica. 1685, 1699; SCHELHAMMER, G. C. De lymphae ortu et lymphaticorum vasorum causis. 1683.

MANGETUS, JOHANNES JACOB. *See* MANGET, Jean Jacques [1652–1742]

MANGIN, CLÉMENT CYRIAQUE DE. *See* HENRION, Denis [*d. ca.* 1640]

MANGIN, PETRUS [*fl.* 1684] Neo-panacea adversus mortis & martis jacula divi Cosmas & Damianus annua panegyri honorati Pragae in Teynensi basilica . . . Pragae, Typis Catharinae Czernochianae viduae [1684]
[12] p.   20 cm.   [**7372**]

MANGOLDT, JOHANN GEORG [*fl.* 1672–1673] *respondent.* Theses medicae de catalepsi . . . Basileae, Apud Jacobum Werenfelsium [1673]
[8] p.   19 cm.   [**7373**]

Diss. — Basel.

— *respondent. See* BAUHIN, J. K., *praeses.* Dissertationem hancce de epilepsia . . . offert J. G. M. 1672.

MANIALD, ÉTIENNE [*fl.* 1574–1625] De partu prodigioso qui visus est in agro gradiniano juxta Burdigalam. Anno M. D. XCV. mense Augusto . . . Burdigalae, Apud S. Millangium, 1616.
16 p.   18 cm.   [**7374**]

—, *ed.* and *tr. See* HIPPOCRATES. [Selected works. Greek and Latin] Chirurgia. 1619.

MANITIUS, SAMUEL GOTTHELF [*d.* 1698] D. Samuelis Gotthilff Manitii Medicus hujus seculi; sive, Herma, tyroni medico expedissimam, qua ad veri medici requisita feliciter obtinenda, et miserias . . . declinandas, eundum, viam monstrans . . . Dresdae, Apud Joh. Jacob. Wincklerum, 1693.
[18], 17–287, [1] p.   17 cm.   [**7375**]

Imperfect: contains liber secundus only without the De miseriarum et contemptae medicinae causis (p. 1–17), and without the Errata.

—[The same.] D. Sempronii Gracchi Massiliensis [pseud.] Medicus hujus seculi; sive, Herma, tyroni medico expeditissimam, qua ad veri medici requisita felicirer [sic] obtinenda, & miserias . . . declinandas eundum, viam monstrans . . . Dresdae, Apud Joh. Jacob. Wincklerum, litteris Riedelianis, 1693.
[12], 330 p.; 287, [2] p.   17 cm.   [**7376**]

Errata: p. [2] at end.

— *respondent. See* SPERLING, P. G., *praeses.* Chymicam formicarum analysin . . . subjiciet S. G. M. 1689.

MANLIUS CONSTANTINOPOLITANUS. *See* MANLIUS, Arnold [*d.* 1607]

MANLIUS, ARNOLD [*d.* 1607] *See* SCHOLTZ, L. Epistolarum philosophicarum: medicinalium, ac chymicarum . . . volumen. 1610.

MANLIUS, GEORG [*fl.* 1603-1615] *respondent. See* MÖLLER, S., *praeses.* Themata medica de angina. 1603.

MANLOVE, TIMOTHY [1661 or 2-1669] *See* GILPIN, R. The comforts of divine love. 1700.

MANNAGETTA, JOHANN WILHELM [1588-1666] *praeses.* Disputatio medica, de purgandi ratione . . . Viennae Austriae, Typis Michaëlis Rictii [1632]

[20] p.   20 cm.   [7377]

Diss. — Vienna (G. Rinegger, *respondent*)

—Pest-Ordnung; oder, Der gantzen gemein nutzlicher Bericht und Gutacht, von der Eigenschafft und Ursachen der Pestilentz in genere . . . Auss dess . . . Herrn Joannis Guilielmi Mannagettae . . . Manuscriptis genommen; und durch den Herrn Paulum de Sorbait . . . revidirt, approbirt, vermehret . . . [Viennae] Johann Jacob Kürner, 1679.

[8], 180, [14] p.   21 cm.   [7378]

—[The same.] . . . Zum andern Mal aufgelegt und nachgedruckt. [Viennae?] 1680.

[6], 164, [4] p.   19 cm.   [7379]

MANNARINO, CATALDO ANTONIO [1568-1621] *See* FERDINANDI, E. Centum historiae. 1621.

MANNING, James [*fl.* 1604] A new booke, intituled, I am for you all, Complexions castle: as well in the time of the pestilence, as other times, out of the which you may learne your complexion, your disease incident to the same, and the remedies for the same . . . Cambridge, Printed by John Legat and sold by Simon Waterson, 1604.

[8], 40 p.   19 cm.   [7380]

STC 17257.

MANNIUS, VICTORIUS [*fl.* 1613] De balneis Sancti Cassiani tractatus tres in partes distribuitus . . . Senis, Apud Sylvestrum Marchettum, 1617.

[8], 82, [2] p.   20 cm.   [7381]

Errata: [2] p. at end.

MANNUCCI, VINCENZO [1586-1649] *ed. See* VITTORI, A. Medicae consultationes. 1640.

MANOLESSI, EMILIO MARIA [*fl.* 1660-1690] *ed. See* Relazione dell'esperienze fatte in Inghilterra. 1668.

MANSUETI, TESEO [16th-17th cent.] *tr. See* MARAFIOTI, G. Nova inventione et arte del ricordarsi. 1602.

MANSVELD, REGNER VAN [1639-1671] Petri ab Andlo [pseud.] . . . Animadversiones ad vindicias dissertationis quam Samuel Maresius edidit De abusu philosophiae Cartesianae. Lugduni Batavorum, Ex officina Felicis Lopez de Haro, 1671.

72 p.   20 cm.   [7382]

—Specimen confutationis dissertationis quam Samuel Maresius edidit De abusu philosophiae Cartesianae. Lugduni Batavorum, Ex officina Arnoldi Doude, 1670.

39 p.   20 cm.   [7383]

—Specimina bombomachiae Samuelis Maresii se defendentis clypeo orthodoxiae ceu vindiciis vindiciarum dissertationis De abusu philosophiae Cartesianae. Lugduni Batavorum, Ex officina Felicis Lopez de Haro, 1672.

26 p.   20 cm.   [7384]

—*See* DESMARETS, S. Samuelis Maresii Clypeus orthodoxiae. 1671 [and] Vindiciae dissertationis . . . De abusu philosophiae Cartesianae. 1670.

MANTEGARRIO, CIPRIANO [*fl.* 1613] *ed. See* GUARGUANTI, O. Responsa varia, ad varias aegritudines. 1613.

MANTEGARVIUS, CYPRIANUS. *See* MANTEGARRIO, Cipriano [*fl.* 1613]

MANTEL, JACQUES [*fl.* 1640-1642] Ἐπίϰϱασιο vindicata; seu, De vera et genuina ἐπιϰϱοσεως significatione dissertatio . . . [Parisiis] 1642.

46 p.   17 cm.   [7385]

—, *ed. See* RIOLAN, J. [1538?-1605?] Tractatus de febribus. 1640.

MANTUA, ITALY (CITY). **Ordinances, local laws, etc.** Il maestrato della sanità certificati noi dalli signori della sanità di Genova, Bologna, & Modona, & con la trasmissione de publici bandi, che nelli luoghi di Varsi, Castellaro, Brignano, Cela, Segno, e Cignolo . . . siano seguiti alcuni casi pestilentiali

... con la presente sospendiamo dal comertio di questa città ... [Mantova, 1639]

    broadside. 28 × 18 cm.   **[7386]**

Signed by Filippo Brondolo and others.

MANUALIS physici. *See* SANTORIO, S. Ars ... de statica medicina. 1670.

Le MANUEL du chirurgien d'armée; ou, L'art de guerir methodiquement les playes des arquebuzades, avec leurs accidens, expliquez suivant les principes de la nature. Accompagné d'un traité succint de l'anatomie conforme aux nouveautez du siecle. Par L.L.M.C. Paris, Maurice Villery, 1686.

    [28], 344 p. 17 cm.   **[7387]**

—[The same.] 2. ed., rev. & corr. Par L.L.M.C. Paris, Maurice Villery, 1693.

    [22], 348, [6] p. 16 cm.   **[7388]**

Imperfect: table partly bound at end. Last leaf of the table wanting.

MANZINI, CARLO ANTONIO [*d.* 1677] L'occhiale all'occhio dioptrica pratica ... dove si tratta della luce ... e de gli aiuti, che dare si possono à gli occhi ... Bologna, Per l'herede del Benacci, 1660.

    [12], 268, [4] p. illus., plate (port.) 21 cm.   **[7389]**

MAPHAEUS, JOHANNES PETRUS. *See* MAFFEI, Giovanni Pietro [*fl.* 1600-1603]

MAPP, MARC [1632-1701] Historia exaltationis theriacarum in theriacam coelestem hanc ipsam Dn. Friderico Strehlin ... dispensante, cum commendatione nobilissimi medicamenti proposita ... Argentorati, Impensis Joh. Frid. Spoor, 1695.

    [1], 70 p. 14 cm.   **[7390]**

Bound with copy 2 of Lanzoni, G. Tractatus de balsamatione cadaverum. 1696.

—Historia medica de acephalis ... Argentorati, Typis Joh. Friderici Spoor, 1687.

    [1], 30 p. plates. 20 cm.   **[7391]**

—Θερμοπόσια; seu, Dissertationes medicae duae de potu calido ... [Argentorati] Apud Joh. Frideric. Spoor & Reinhard. Waechtler, 1675.

    [1], 75 p. 19 cm.   **[7392]**

Dissertations — Strasbourg

—*praeses.* Disputatio de fistula genae terminata ad dentem cariosum ... Argentorati, Literis Joh. Friderici Spoor, 1675.

    28 p. 20 cm.   **[7393]**

J. K. Witzel, *respondent.*

—Copy 2.

Date has been altered by hand from December 1675 to 13 Januar. 1676.

—Disputationem medicam solennem de lue venerea ... submittit ... Johannes Casparus Sparr ... Argentorati, Typis Joh. Friderici Spoor, 1673.

    [4], 36 p. 19 cm.   **[7394]**

J. C. Sparr, *respondent.*

—Dissertatio medica de aurium cerumine ... Argentorati, Literis Joh. Friderici Spoor [1684]

    40 p. 19 cm.   **[7395]**

D. Meyer, *respondent.*

—Dissertatio medica de potu cafe ... Argentorati, Literis Joh. Friderici Spoor [1693]

    [2], 66 p. 19 cm.   **[7396]**

D. Wencker, *respondent.*

—Dissertatio medica de potu chocolatae ... Argentorati, Literis Joh. Friderici Spoor [1695]

    [1], 62 p. 19 cm.   **[7397]**

J. C. Huth, *respondent.*

—Dissertatio medica de potu thee ... Argentorati, Literis Joh. Friderici Spoor [1691]

    [2], 54 p. 19 cm.   **[7398]**

J. Heckheler, *respondent.*

—Dissertatio medica qua primarium catameniorum vitium, h. e. suppressionem ... disquisitioni submittit Johannes Joachimus Kast ... Argentorati, Typis Johannis Wilhelmi Tidemanni [1686]

    32 p. 20 cm.   **[7399]**

J. J. Kast, *respondent.*

—Quaestio medica physiologica de aquis, in quibus tempore gestationis foetus humanus quasi natat ... Argentorati, Literis Johannis Welperi [1685]

    [2], 30, [4] p. 19 cm.   **[7400]**

Imperfect: upper margins trimmed.

J. J. Espich, *respondent.*

—Theses botanicae et medicae de rosa de Jericho ... Argentorati, Literis Johannis Friderici Spoor [1700]

[2], 14 p.   20 cm.   [7401]

A. F. Mergiletus, *respondent.*

—Theses medicae de erysipelate ... Argentorati, Typis Johannis Friderici Spoor [1700]

[2], 18 p.   19 cm.   [7402]

G. B. Hofmann, *respondent.*

—Tractationis medicae de potu calido dissertatio altera ... Argentorati, Typis Joh. Friderici Spoor, 1673.

[2], 24, [1] p.   19 cm.   [7403]

J. U. Bix, *respondent.*

With this is bound Sebisch, J. A., praeses. Dissertatio solennis de instrumento olfactus. 1662.

—Ζητημάτων περι φυσωγ δεκας, h. e., De flatibus quaestiones decem ... Argentoratensis, Literis Georgii Andreae Dolhopffii, imprimebat Johannes Schütz [1675]

[2], 34 p.   19 cm.   [7404]

J. V. Scheid, *respondent.*

—*respondent.* Disputatio medica inauguralis de gurgulionis prolapsu ... Argentorati, Typis Eberhardi Welperi, 1660.

[23] p.   19 cm.   [7405]

—*See* Sebisch, M. [1578-1674?] *praeses.* Disputatio solennis de singultu. 1659.

MAPP, Marc [*fl.* 1687] *respondent. See* Scheid, J. V., *praeses.* De duobus ossiculis in cerebro humano mulieris apoplexia extinctae repertis. 1687.

MAPPUS, Marcus. *See* Mapp, Marc [1632-1701]

MARAFIOTI, Girolamo [16th-17th cent.] De arte reminiscentiae per loca, & imagines, ac per notas, & figuras in manibus positas ... Venetiis, Apud Jo. Baptistam Bertonum, 1602.

[8], 35 ll.   illus.   16 cm.   [7406]

Imperfect: wormholes on ll. [1]-10.

With this is bound *his* Nova inventione et arte del ricordarsi. 1602.

—Nova inventione et arte del ricordarsi, per luoghi, & imagini, & per segni, & figure poste nelle mani ... Tradotta di latino ... da D. Theseo Mansueti ... Vinegia, Giouan Battista Bertoni, 1602.

[7], 38 p.   16 cm.   [7407]

Bound with *his* De arte reminiscentiae per loca. 1602.

MARAIS, Pierre [*fl.* 1689-1741] *praeses.* Quaestio medica ... An dysentericis affectibus radix Brasiliensis? [Parisiis, Apud Franc. Muguet, 1690]

4 p.   25 cm.   [7408]

Diss.—Paris (L. de Vaux, *respondent*)

[**MARBECKE,** Roger, 1536-1605] A defence of tabacco, with a friendly answer to the late printed booke called Worke for chimny-sweepers, &c. ... London, Printed by Richard Field for Thomas Man, 1602.

70 p.   17 cm.   [7409]

Imperfect: upper margins trimmed.
STC 6468.
Arents 62.

MARBEEKE, Roger. *See* Marbecke, Roger [1536-1605]

MARCEL, Jean, *tr. See* Croll, O. La royalle chymie. 1627, 1634.

MARCEL DE BOULENE, J. *See* Marcel, Jean.

MARCELLIN, Pancrace, *ed. See* Mercuriale, G. In omnes Hippocratis Aphorismorum libros. 1621, 1631.

MARCELLINUS, Joannes Petrus Ayroldus. *See* Airoldi, Giovanni Pietro.

MARCELLUS EMPIRICUS. Vindiciano attributum carmen. *See* Celsus, A. C. De re medica libri octo. 1608, 1625.

MARCH, Kaspar [1629-1677] Programma quo ... decanus Caspar March ... ad disputationem inauguralem de fulmine tactis quam ... sub praesidio ... Joh. Danielis Majoris ... Johan Jacob Kisling ... habebit ... invitat. Kiliae, Literis Joachimi Reumanni [1673]

[8] p.   20 cm.   [7410]

Program—Kiel (with vita of J. J. Kisling)

—Programma quo ... decanus Caspar March ad disputationem inauguralem quam de affectione hypochondriac ... habebit ... Jacobus Kornmesser ... invitat. Rostochii, Typis Johannis Kilii [1665]

[8] p.   20 cm.   [7411]

Program—Rostock (with vita of J. Kornmesser)

MARCH, Kaspar [1654-1706] *See* Pechlin, J. N. Facultatis medicae ... decanus Joh. Nicolaus Pechlin ... ad audiendum theses de affectibus soporosis ... invitat. 1680.

MARCHAND, JOHANN JAKOB [*fl.* 1695] *respondent.*
See BERGER, J. G. von, *praeses.* Dissertatio solennis
de inflammatione. 1695; FRANCK VON FRANCKENAU,
G. In illustrissima Universitate Vitembergensi decani
Facult. medicae Georgii Franci de Frankenau ...
propempticon inaugurale de ψαμμισμῶ. 1695.

MARCHANT, JEAN [*fl.* 1666] De febre purpurata
hoc anno 1666 per Burgundiam grassante, deque
causa ejus proxima & vera curatione tractatus ...
Divione, Apud Petrum Palliot, & venundatur
Parisiis, Apud Heliam Josset, 1666.

    [12], 132 p.   16 cm.   [7412]

MARCHE, CASPAR. *See* MARCH, Kaspar.

MARCHETTI, DOMENICO DE [1626-1688]
Anatomia ... cui responsiones ad Riolanum ... in
ipsius animadversionibus contra Veslingium additae
sunt. Patavii, Apud Matthaeum Bolzettam [Apud Jo.
Baptistam Pasquatum] 1652.

    [10], 179, [2] p.   20 cm.   [7413]
    Added half title.

    —[The same.] ... Patavii, Apud Matthaeum
Cadorinum, 1654.

    [10], 179, [1] p.   port.   21 cm.   [7414]
    Added engraved title page.
    A reissue of the 1652 edition with title page and preliminary mat-
ters reset; without the colophon page.

    —[The same.] ... Ed. alt. Patavina correctior.
Hardevici, Ex officina Societatis typographica, 1656.

    [16], 289 (i.e. 291), [2] p.   14 cm.   [7415]
    Added title page.

    —[The same.] ... Ed. 3., Patavina correctior.
Lugduni Batavorum, Apud Cornelium Boutesteyn,
1688.

    [20], 292, [12] p.   15 cm.   [7416]
    Added engraved title page.

MARCHETTI, PIETRO DE [*ca.* 1589-1673] Observationum medico-chirurgicarum rariorum sylloge
... Patavii, Typis Matthaei de Cadorinis, 1664.

    [14], 188 p.   illus., port.   18 cm.   [7417]
    Added engraved title page.
    Imperfect: first preliminary leaf (blank?) wanting.

    —[The same.] ... Amstelodami, Ex officina Petri
le Grand, 1665.

    112 (i.e. 212) p.   plate.   14 cm.   [7418]
    Imperfect: p. 5-20 and plate wanting; p. 197-199 mutilated.

    —[The same.] ... Accesserunt aliquot observa-
tiones auctoris posthumae ... Patavii, Apud
Cadorinum, 1675.

    [16], 142 p.   illus.   17 cm.   [7419]
    Added engraved title page.
    Imperfect: plate wanting.

    —[The same.] ... Bononiae, Ex typographia de
Longhis, 1692.

    223 p.   illus.   14 cm.   [7420]
    Imperfect: plate wanting.

    —[German tr.] Seltzam-ausserlesen-medicinisch-
chirurgische Observationes; sambt einem Anhang,
von Geschwären und Fisteln dess Hindern, Mast-
Darms, und der Röhres im männlichen Glied ...
Aus der lateinischen in die teutsche Sprach
übersetzet. Nürmberg, In Verlegung Johann Daniel
Taubers, Druckts Christoff Gerhard, 1673.

    [7], 271, [17] p.   plate.   13 cm.   [7421]
    Added engraved title page.
    Imperfect: p. [6-9] and [14-17] mutilated.

    —*See* BONET, T., *ed.* Corps de medecine et de
chirurgie. 1679.

MARCHETTIS, DOMINICUS DE. *See* MARCHETTI,
Domenico de [1626-1688]

MARCHETTIS, PIERRE DE. *See* MARCHETTI,
Pietro de [*ca.* 1589-1673]

MARCHINI, FILIBERTO [1586-1636] Belli divini;
sive, Pestilentis temporis accurata, et luculenta
speculatio theologica ... philosophica ... Adictae
[sic] sunt etiam tum multorum tribunalium decisiones ... Florentiae, Ex Typographia Sermartelliana, 1633.

    [49], 310 p.; 63, [36] p.   port.   34 cm.

                                                        [7422]
    Added engraved title page.
    "Pars decima de temporali, et spirituali infectae urbis vel loci
regimine Panormitana, et Florentina praxis illa ab anno 1624. ad
1626. ista ab anno 1630. ad 1632 ... Accesserunt deinde tum praxis
Mediolanensis de anno 1576. ex Concilio V. provinciali excerpta
..." (p. [233-267]) has special title page.
    Part [2] has special title page: Philosophia de pestilentia pro-
blemata ... Adjectis etiam Thucydidis Graeci scriptoris De peste
Atheniensi, Procopii, & Evagrii de simili morbo historiis.

MARCI, JOANNES. *See* MARCI VON KRONLAND,
Johannes Marcus [1595-1667]

MARCI, JOHANNES MARCUS. *See* MARCI VON
KRONLAND, Johannes Marcus [1595-1667]

MARCI, Marc. *See* Marci von Kronland, Johannes Marcus [1595-1667]

MARCI, Philipp Mark [*fl*. 1666-1667] *respondent. See* Friderici, J. A., *praeses.* Consultatio medica de stupore manuum. 1667; Rolfinck, W., *praeses.* Dissertatio chirurgica inauguralis de scrophulis seu strumis. 1667.

MARCI VON KRONLAND, Johannes Marcus [1595-1667] Idearum operatricium idea; sive, Hypotyposis et detectio illius occultae virtutis, quae semina faecundat, & ex iisdem corpora organica producit . . . [Pragae, Typis Seminarii Archiepiscopalis] 1635.

[325] p. illus. 20 cm. [7423]
Engraved title page.
Signatures: []², (+)², (2+)¹, (3+)¹, A-Z⁴, 2A-2T⁴, 2U¹.
Errata: p. [351-352]

—Liturgia mentis; seu, Disceptatio medica, philosophica & optica de natura epilepsiae illius ortus & causis; deque symptomatis quae circa imaginationem & motum eveniunt . . . Opus posthumum. Cui accessit Tractatus medicus de natura urinae & Consilia tria medica . . . Ratisbonae, Sumptibus Joh. Conr. Emmrich, typis Augusti Hanckwitz, 1678.

[24], 166 p.; [1], 122, [27] p. 21 cm. [7424]
Edited by Jacobus Joannes Wenceslaus Dobrzensky.

—Copy 2.
With this are bound: another issue of Wille, J. V. [1651-1677] Tractatus medicus de morbis castrensibus internis. 1676; Sebisch, M. [1578-1674?]. Discursus medico-philosophicus de casu adolescentis. 1660.

—Philosophia vetus restituta . . . Pragae, Typis Academicis, 1662.

[21], 580, [4] p. 20 cm. [7425]
Engraved title page.
Errata: [4] p.

—Philosophia vetus restituta, partibus V. comprehensa, quarum I. De mutationibus, quae in universo fiunt. II. De partium universi constitutione. III. De statu hominis secundum naturam. IV. De statu hominis praeter naturam. V. De curatione morborum . . . Denuo recusa. Francofurti & Lipsiae, Sumptibus Christian Weidmanni, 1676.

[20], 580 p. plate. 22 cm. [7426]
Added engraved title page.
Different setting of type.

MARCQUIS, Guillaume [1604-1677] Decas pestifuga; seu, Decem quaestiones problematicae de peste, una cum . . . instructione purgandarum aedium infectarum . . . Antverpiae, Apud Caes. Joach. Trognaesium, 1627.

[16], 238, [1] p. 21 cm. [7427]
Bound with Fabricius von Hilden, W. Observationum & curationum chirurgicarum centuria V. 1627.

MARCQUIS, Lazarus [1574-1647] Volcomen tractaet van de peste . . . Vern. ende verm. In het welck distinctelijcker d'oorsaken de teeckenen der levende ende doode lichamen . . . Ende hoe de biechtvaders ende medicijns de inghefecteerde persoonen visiterende, sich van de contagie preserveren sullen. Antwerpen, Cesar Joachim Trognesius, 1636.

[8], 210, [5] p. 15 cm. [7428]

MARCUCCI, Gaspare [1624-1644] Quadripartitum melancholicum . . . quo variae quaestiones de melancholiae morbo . . . curatione habentur. Et plura de morbo hypocondriaco . . . innotescunt . . . Romae, Ex typographia Andreae Phaei, 1644.

[4], 306, [4] p. 26 cm. [7429]

—*See* Maccioni, G. Risposta. 1631.

MARENDA, Giampietro. *See* Merenda, Giovanni Pietro [*fl. ca.* 1544]

MARENGUS, Joannes Baptista. Palladis chymicae arcana detecta; sive, Mineralogia naturalis, & artificialis. In naturali ostenditur, quomodo a natura metalla in visceribus terrae generentur . . . Opus . . . in tres partes divisum. Auctoris nomen in hoc puro anagrammata delitescit Janus Gobrat sapiens manet [i.e. Joannes Baptista Marengus] Genevae, Typis Antonii Georgii Franchelli, 1674.

285, [2] p. 14 cm. [7430]

—[The same.] . . . Opus . . . in quo praecipue ostenditur modus efficiendi philosophorum lapidem, & multa alia lucrosa traduntur. 2. ed. . . . aucta . . . in duas partes divisa. Auctoris nomen in hoc puro anagrammate iterum delitescit. Janus Gobrat sapiens manet [i.e. Joannes Baptista Marengus] Genevae, Typis Antonii Georgii Franchelli, 1678.

426 p.; 355, [1] p. 15 cm. [7431]
Errata: [1] p.
Part 2 has special title page.

MARESCHAL, Anton Artus [*fl.* 1669] *respondent.* Disputatio medica inauguralis continens casum epilepticum ... Lugduni Batavorum, Apud viduam & haeredes Joannis Elsevirii, 1669.

[11] p. 23 cm. [7432]
Diss.—Leyden.

MARESCHAL, CLAUDE. Physiologie des eaux minerales de Vichy en Bourbonnois. Rev. corr. & augm. ... Moulins, Pierre Vernoy, 1642.

95 p. 16 cm. [7433]

MARESCHAL, PIERRE [*fl.* 1666] *respondent.* Disputatio medica inauguralis de peste ... Lugduni Batavorum, Ex officina Thomae Hoorn, 1666.

[15] p. 24 cm. [7434]
Diss.—Leyden.

Le **MARESCHAL** methodique. 1675. *See* [SOLLEYSEL, J. de]

MARESCOTTI, JACOPO ANTONIO. *See* MARIS-COTTUS, Jacobus Antonius.

MARESIUS, SAMUEL. *See* DESMARETS, Samuel [1599-1673]

MARETZ, SAMUEL NICOLAUS DES. *See* DES MARETZ, Samuel Nicolaus [*fl.* 1688]

MARFORIO, *pseud. See* LALLI, G. Lettera. 1640.

MARGGRAF, CHRISTIAN [1626-1687] Jacobi le Mort pseudochemici & ratiocinatoris dupondiarii ignorantia circa chemiam & universam scientiam naturalem ... Lugduni Batavorum, Apud Petrum de Graaf, 1687.

[11], 97 p. 18 cm. [7435]

—Materia medica contracta, exhibens simplicia & composita medicamenta officinalia ... munita viribus & dosibus, methodoque simplicia deligendi, praeparandi & componendi ... Lugduni Batavorum, Apud Arnoldum Duode, 1674.

[8], 252 p. 20 cm. [7436]
Imperfect: wormholes on p. 79-114.

—[The same.] ... Ed. 2 ab authore plurimum aucta ... Lugduni-Batavorum, Typis Johannis à Gelder, 1681.

[16], 280, [22] p. 21 cm. [7437]
Bound with *his* Prodromus medicinae practicae. 1673.

—[The same.] ... Ed. 2. ab autore plurimum aucta ... Amstelaedami, Apud Henricum Wetstenium, 1682.

[16], 280, [22] p. 20 cm. [7438]
A reissue of the 1681 Leyden edition with new title page and with the addition of errata on p. [2].

—Prodromus medicinae practicae dogmaticae & vere rationalis, superstructae circulari sanguinis motui, nec non principiis chemicis ac hypothesi Helmontianae & Sylvianae. Exhibens specimen methodi ... medendi plerisque corporis humani affectibus ope acidi & alcali. Sub tabellarum compendio primum propositus ... Lugduni Batavourm [sic] Ex officina Arnoldi Doude, 1673.

[4], 112 p. 21 cm. [7439]
With this is bound *his* Materia medica. 1681.

—[The same.] ... Lugduni Batavourm [sic], Ex officina Arnoldi Doude, 1674.

[4], 112 p. 19 cm. [7440]
A reissue of the 1673 edition with new date.

—[The same.] ... Ed. 2 ... auctior ... Lugduni Batavorum, Apud Cornelium Boutesteyn, 1685.

[28], 173, [7] p. 20 cm. [7441]
Added engraved title page.
"Vita Georgii Marggravii" p. [21-28]

—*respondent.* Disputatio medica inauguralis περι τω σπασμώ; seu, De convulsione ... Franekerae, Johannes Wellens, 1659.

[12] p. 19 cm. [7442]
Diss.—Franeker.

—*See* MORLEY, C. L. Collectanea chymica Leydensia. 1684, 1693, 1696; [German tr.] 1696, 1700; PECHEY, J. A plain introduction to the art of physick. 1697.

MARGGRAF, GEORG [1610-1644] Historia rerum naturalium Brasiliae libri octo. *In* Piso, W. Historia naturalis Brasiliae. 1648.

—Tractatus topographicus & meteorologicus Brasiliae, cum eclipsi solari. *In* Piso, W. De Indiae utriusque re naturali et medica libri quatuordecim. 1658.

—*See* BONDT, J. de. Oost-en West-Indische warande. 1694.

MARI, STEFANO [16th cent.] *See* FACIO, S. Paradoxes de la peste. 1620.

MARIA, *prophetess.* Practica . . . in artem alchimicam.

205-208 p., vol. 1   17 cm.   (*In* Artis auriferae. Basileae, 1610)   [**7443**]
Caption title.
Running title: Maria proph. ad Sarratant.

—[German ed.] Die Practica oder Ubung . . . in die löbliche Kunst der Alchemiae.

269-274 p., part 1.   19 cm.   (*In* Morgenstern, Philipp, *ed.* and *tr.* Turba philosophorum. Basel, 1613)
Caption title.   [**7444**]

—*See* ORTHELIUS. Explicatio verborum Mariae prophetissae. 1659.

MARIANUS SANCTUS BAROLITANUS. *See* SANTO, Mariano [*b. ca.* 1490]

MARIGNANO, GIAN GIACOMO DE' MEDICI, *marchio* [1495-1555] *See* PUTEANUS, E. Historiae Medicaeae libri duo. 1634.

MARIN, AEGIDIUS. De naturae humanae principiis; sive, De compositione hominis poema physiologicum. Statutis summis diorismis & theorematis physiologiae doctrinam, exquisitam atque solidam in universum explicans . . . Cui operi subjunguntur Regimen scholae Salerni metrorum structura exactiori expolitum, et methodus aphorismorum dispositiva scientifico ordine instituta. Parisiis, 1656.

[16], 58 p.; 50 p.   15 cm.   [**7445**]
Date altered by hand to 1676.
Imperfect: title page of part [2] wanting.

MARINELLI, CURZIO [*fl.* 1580-1615] De morbis nobilioris animae facultates obsidentibus libri tres . . . Quibus accedit liber patefaciens Galenum, & omnes alios . . . aut majorem partem eorum, quae de his morbis pronunciaverunt . . . Denique opusculum . . . continens nonnullas controversias, inconstantias, atque admirationes in dictis Galeni adinventas. Venetiis, Apud Juntas, 1615.

[15], 275 p.; [8], 72 p.   22 cm.   [**7446**]
Part [2] has special title page: De malis principem animam vexantibus ad mentem illorum, qui ante Galenum medicinam exercebant, liber unus.
"Controversiae inconstantiae, atque admirationes in dicti Galeni" (p. [51]-72, part [2]) has special title page.

MARINELLI, GIOVANNI [16th cent.] Commentaria . . . in lib. Hippocratis . . . Vincentiae, Sumptibus Francisci Lenii, & Orlandi Iadrae [Apud Jo. Petrum Joanninium] 1610.

[2], 140 ll.   33 cm.   (Vol. 2 *in* Hippocrates. Opera, quibus addidimus commentaria Joann. Marinelli. Vincentiae, 1610)   [**7447**]
A page for page reprint of the 1575 Venice edition.

—[The same.] . . . Venetiis, Apud Hieronymum & Alexandrum Polum, 1619.

[2], 140 ll.   34 cm.   (Vol. 2 *in* Hippocrates. Opera, quibus addidimus commentaria Joann. Marinelli. Venetiis, 1619)   [**7448**]
Different setting of type.

—[The same.] . . . Venetiis, Typis Abbundii Menafolii, 1679.

[2], 140 ll.   33 cm.   (Vol. 2 *in* Hippocrates. Opera, quibus addidimus commentaria Joan. Marinelli. Venetiis, 1679)   [**7449**]
Different setting of type.

—Le medicine partenenti all'infermità delle donne . . . Divise in tre libri . . . Nuovamente ristampate & con diligenza reviste & ricorrette . . . Venetia, Gio. Battista Bonfadino & compagni, 1610.

[24], 327 + ll.   15 cm.   [**7450**]
Imperfect: all after ll. 327 wanting.

—[French tr.] Les maladies des femmes & remedes d'ycelles, en trois livres . . . Traduicts en françois & amplifiés par M. Jean Liebaud . . . Et en ceste derniere edition, rev., corr. et augm. du tiers. Par Lazare Pe . . . Paris, J. Berjon, 1609.

[22], 863, [14] p.   illus.   17 cm.   [**7451**]
Issued also under title: Thresor des remedes secrets pour les maladies des femmes.

—[The same.] Trois livres des maladies et infirmitez des femmes. Pris du latin de M. Jean Liebaut . . . Rev., corr. & augm. en cette dernier impression. Rouen, Jean Berthelin, 1649.

[22], 924, [15] p.   illus.   17 cm.   [**7452**]
Preface by Lazare Pé[na], the editor.

—*See* HIPPOCRATES. [Collected works. Latin] Opera. 1610, 1619, 1679.

MARINGUE, JEAN BATISTE. *See* MARENGUS, Joannes Baptista.

MARINIS, DOMINICUS DE [*fl.* 1678] Dissertatio philosophico-medica de re monstrosa a Capuccino Pisauri per urinam excreta. Plura de sanguinis grumis, polypis, serpentibus, ac praecipue de vermibus in corpore humano procreatis non injucunda complectens ... Romae, Typis Jacobi Mascardi, 1678.

[18], 143, [1] p. 16 cm. [7453]

Includes a letter on the same subject by Alessandro Cocci.

MARIOTELLUS, Fulvius. *See* Mariottelli, Fulvio [1559–1639]

MARIOTTE, Edme [*ca.* 1620–1684] Lettres ecrites sur le sujet d'une nouvelle découverte touchant la veuë ... [Paris, Jean Cusson, 1682]

23 p. plate. 25 cm. [7454]

Caption title.

Includes a letter on the same subject by Claude Perrault.

—*See* [Perrault, C.] Description anatomique de divers animaux dissequez dans l'Academie royale des sciences. 1682.

MARIOTTELLI, Fulvio [1559–1639] Neopaedia; sive, Nova, aut inexplicata hucusque in discendis, atque docendis, methodi ratio ... Ex Platonis potissimum, atque Aristotelis principiis eruta ... Romae, Typis Jacobi Mascardi, 1624.

[15], 211, [1] p. 21 cm. [7455]

"Neopaediae medicina": p. 147–156.

MARIOTTI, Carlo [*fl.* 1654] De universarum febrium generibus tractatus ad Hippocratis, et Galeni mentem ... Cui ... opus de putredine, crisibus, diebus criticis, coctione, & cruditate, ac sanguinem emittendi tempore, purgandique in febribus corpora subnectitur ... Neapoli, Typis Camilli Cavalli, expensis Simonis, & Francisci Mansi, 1654.

[12], 334, [22] p. 31 cm. [7456]

MARISCOTTUS, Jacobus Antonius, *tr. See* Pleier, C. Medicus-criticus-astrologus. 1627.

MARIUS, Johann. J. F. Castorologia explicans castoris animalis naturam & usum medico-chemicum antidhac a Joanne Mario ... labori insolito subjecta, jam vero ejusdem auctoris & aliorum medicorum observationibus luculentis ineditis ... & propria experientia parili labore aucta a Joanne Franco ... Augustae Vindel., Typis Koppmayerianis, impensis vidua Theophili Goebelii, 1685.

[15], 223, [1] p. front., plate. 16 cm. [7457]

MARKAM, Gervase. *See* Markham, Gervase [1568?–1637]

MARKBEEKE, Roger. *See* Marbecke, Roger [1536–1605]

[**MARKHAM**, Gervase, 1568?–1637] Cheape and good husbandry for the well-ordering of all beasts, and fowles, and for the generall cure of their diseases. Contayning the natures, breeding ... and curing of the diseases of all manner of cattel ... shewing further, the whole art of riding great-horses ... Also, approved rules, for the cramming and fatting of all sorts of poultry ... Together with the use and profit of bees ... The 5th ed. London, Printed by Nicholas Okes for John Harison, 1631.

[26], 188 (i.e. 200) p. illus. 19 cm. [7458]

Imperfect: lower margin of title page trimmed.

STC 17339.

Poynter 34.5(b)

Also published as part [1] of *his* A way to get wealth. 1631.

—[The same.] ... Newly corrected ... with many ... additions. The 10th ed. London, Printed by W. Wilson, for George Sawbridge, 1660.

[10], 146, [10] p. illus. 18 cm. [7459]

Poynter 34.10

Also published as part [1] of *his* A way to get wealth. 1660.

—The English house-wife, containing the ... vertues which ought to be in a compleate woman. As her skill in physick, surgery, cookery ... Now the fifth time much augmented ... By G[ervase] M[arkham] London, Printed by Anne Griffin for John Harrison, 1637.

[10], 252 p. illus. 20 cm. [7460]

STC 17354.

Poynter 34.6.

Also published as part 3 of his A way to get wealth. 1638.

—[The same.] ... Now the eighth time much augmented ... London, George Sawbridge, 1675.

[8], 188 p. illus. 21 cm. [7461]

Poynter 34.13.

Also published as part 3 of his A way to get wealth, 1676.

—Markhams maister-peece. Contayning all knowledge belonging to the smith, farrier, or horseleech, touching the curing of all diseases in horses ... Being divided into two bookes ... Together with the true nature, use, and quality of every simple spoken of through the whole worke. Now the fifth time newly imprinted, corr. and augm. with above thirty new chapters, and above forty new medicines ... London, Nicholas and John Okes, 1636.

[13], 601 (i.e. 591), [12] p.   illus., plate.   19 cm.
[7462]

STC 17379.

Poynter 20.5.

Added engraved title page has imprint: London, Printed by Nicholas Okes, 1636.

"The second booke" has special title page (p. [233]).

An alternative title page, restored from fragments originally used in the binding, is inserted after the present title page. It has imprint: Imprinted at London by Nicholas and John Okes for John Smithwicke.

The Maister-peece is an expanded version of the veterinary book [VII] of the author's Cavelarice; or, The English horseman, first published in 1607. It is based almost entirely on Thomas Blundeville's The fower chiefyst offices belongyng to horseman-shippe (1st ed., 1565-66) Cf. Smith, v. 1, p. 262.

—[The same.] ... Now the sixt time newly imprinted, corr. and augm. ... London, John Okes, 1643 [i.e. 1644]

[15], 591, [21] p.   illus., plate.   20 cm.
[7463]

Poynter 20.6.

Added engraved title page dated 1644.

A reprint of the 1636 edition, with a postscript added (p. [593-600])

—[The same.] ... Now the seventh time newly imprinted, corr. and augm. ... London, William Wilson, 1651.

[15], 591, [21] p.   illus., plate.   19 cm.
[7464]

Imperfect: first preliminary leaf, p. 239-240, and plate wanting.

Poynter 20.7.

Added engraved title page.

—[The same.] Markham's master-piece revived ... Now the fifteenth time printed, corr. and augm. ... To which is added by way of appendix, The countrey-man's care for his other cattle ... And now in this impression is added the compleat jockey ... London, Printed by John Richardson for M. Wotton and George Coniers, 1694 [i.e. 1695]

[14], 394 p.; [1], 26 p., 49, [3] p.   illus.   20 cm.
[7465]

Poynter 20.15.

Added engraved title page: Markhams maister-peece ... 11th impression (without imprint).

The main work is a reprint of the 1644 edition.

"The second book" (p. [147]) has special title page.

"Appendix, containing the exacteth receipts for curing all diseases in oxen ..." ([1], 26 p.) has special title page with imprint: Lon-

don, Printed by Eliz. Holt for M. Wotton and George Coniers, 1695.

"The complete jockey, or The most exact rules and methods ... for the training up of race-horses ..." (49, [3] p.) has special title page with imprint: London, Printed in the year, 1695.

—See HALFPENNY, J. The gentleman's jockey. 1676.

MARKHAM, JERVIS. See MARKHAM, Gervase [1568?-1637]

MAROGNA, NICOLÒ. Commentarius in tractatus Dioscoridis, et Plinii de amomo. Basileae, Sumptibus Lazari Zetzneri, 1608.

[8], 75, [1] p.   illus.   20 cm.
[7466]

—See PONA, G. Monte Baldo descritto. 1617.

MAROJA, CIPRIANO [16th-17th cent.] Opera omnia medica tribus absoluta partibus, quarum I. Febrium naturam in communi, & in singulari, earumdemque ... curationem exhibet; cum brevi Tractatu de morbi Gallici ... curatione; & celebri Quaestione de partium materialium diversitate in mixtis. II. Praxim universalem de internorum morborum natura, & curatione complectitur ... III. Consultationes, observationes, & annotationes medicas continet ... Ed.alt. emend. ... Lugduni, Sumptibus Laurentii Arnaud, & Petri Borde, 1674.

[20], 632, [35] p.   37 cm.
[7467]

Preface signed by Juan Lázaro Gutiérrez, the editor.

—[The same.] ... Ed. alt. ... emend. ... Lugduni, Sumpt. Petri Borde, Joannis, & Petri Arnaud, 1688.

[20], 632, [35] p.   36 cm.
[7468]

Different setting of type.

MAROLD, HEINRICH VITUS [fl. 1681-1682] respondent. See LOSS, J., praeses. Disputatio inauguralis medica, de iliaca passione. 1682 [and] Specimen academicum aegrum tertiana continua maligna laborantem sistens. 1681.

MAROLD, JUSTINUS ORTOLPHUS. See MAROLT, Justin Ortolph [fl. 1669-1676]

MAROLDUS, ORTOLPHUS. See MAROLT, Ortolph [1526-1595]

MAROLT, JUSTIN ORTOLPH [fl. 1669-1676] Loemographia; oder, Pest-Discurs ... Nebst einer ... Pest-Ordonnance, darinnen zugleich die gründliche Praeservativ-und Curativ-Mittel dem gemeinen Nutzen zum besten treulich vorgestellet werden ... Schleusingen, Sebastian Göbel, 1680.

94, [2] p.   21 cm.   [7469]

—*respondent.* Dissertationem inauguralem de abortu per vomitum rejecto ... proponit Justinus Ortolphus Marold ... Altdorffii, Typis Johannis Henrici Schönnerstaedt [1669]

[1], 38 p.   20 cm.   [7470]

Diss.—Altdorf.

MAROLT, Ortolph [1526-1595] Practica medica ad omnis generis morbos feliciter curandos accommodata; nec non experimentis tum propriis, tum medicorum celeberrimorum familiaritate obtentis refertissima, in partes duas redacta ... Francofurti, Sumptibus Johannis Beyeri, 1650.

[4], 526, [22] p.   22 cm.   [7471]

MARONEA, Nicolaus. *See* Marogna, Nicolò.

MARQUARD, Antonius. *See* Marquart, Anton [*fl.* 1646-1650]

MARQUARD, Johann. Practica medicinalis ... nunc demum per P. U. in quatuor libros divisa, & ab omnibus mendis liberata. Huic in fine accesserunt Sebastiani Cortilionis ... Libri quinque institutionum chirurgicarum cum Practica chirurgica ejusdem quatuor libros continente. Francofurti, Typis Nicolai Hoffmanni, impensis Petri Musculi & Ruperti Pistorii, 1610.

[16], 705, [29] p.   17 cm.   [7472]

MARQUART, Anton [*fl.* 1646-1650] *respondent. See* HEILAND, M. De signaturis disputationem phytologicam pp. M. Michael Heiland, et Antonius Marquard. 1646; LANGE, C., *praeses.* Disputationem medicam de morbo castrensi seu Hungarico ... proponit A. M.; MICHAELIS, J., *praeses.* Morbos ab incantatione et veneficiis oriundos ... proponit ... A. M. 1650; MÖBIUS, G., *praeses.* De sterilitate sexus. 1650.

MARQUE, Jacques de [1569?-1622] Methodique introduction a la chirurgie. Extraict de bons autheurs, & divisée en deux parties ... Lyon, Claude Armand, dit Alphonse, 1628.

238 p.   15 cm.   [7473]

Imperfect: p. 5-8 wanting.
Bound with Guibert, P. Le medecin charitable. Lyon, 1626.

—[The same.] ... Rev. en cette derniere ed., corr. & enrichie d'annotations sur chaque chapitre. Et d'un Discours de la preseance contestee entre la diette, pharmacie, & chirurgie. Et d'un Sommaire des bandes & bandages. Paris, Jean Jost, 1639.

[20], 214, 23 (i.e. 24) p.; [1], 34, [2] p.   17 cm.   [7474]

Part [2] has half title.
"Paraphrase du Serment d'Hippocrate": p. [3-4]

—[The same.] ... Paris, Jean Jost, 1641.

[18], 214, 23 (i.e. 24), [1], 34, [2] p.   17 cm.   [7475]

Without the "Pharaphrase du Serment d'Hippocrate."
With this is bound: Bertrand, G. Les veritez anatomiques et chirurgicales. 1639.

—[The same.] ... Lyon, Pierre Baylly. 1647.

[24], 288 p.   15 cm.   [7476]

Added engraved title page.
"Paraphrase du Serment d'Hippocrate": p. [19-21]

—[The same.] ... Lyon, Jean Guillermet, 1652.
                                                       [7477]

"Paraphrase du Serment d'Hippocrate": p. [16]-[20]
Imperfect: p. [3] wrongly printed.

—[The same.] Oeuvres ... contenant sa Methodique introduction à la chirurgie ... ensemble son Traité des bandages en general ... avec le Sommaire desdits bandanges; et un Discours de la preseance. Nouv. ed. rev., corr. & augm. sur les manuscrits de l'autheur ... Paris, Jean Baptiste Loyson, 1662.

[22], 708 (i.e. 698), [6] p.   front. (port.) 20 cm.
                                                       [7478]

Without the "Paraphrase du Serment d'Hippocrate".
Discours sur la preseance signed by M.D.M. [i.e. M. de Montroeil] the editor.

—[The same.] Methodique introduction a la chirurgie. Tirée des bons autheurs, & divisée en deux parties ... Rev. en cette derniere ed., corr. & enrichie d'annotations sur chaque chapitre, et d'un Discours de la preseance contestée entre la diette, pharmacie, & chirurgie. Et d'un Sommaire des bandes & bandages. Paris, Jean d'Houry, 1674.

[22], 288 p.   16 cm.   [7479]

—[The same.] ... Rev., corr. & enrichie des doctes annotations de M. de Montroeil ... Et augm. en cette derniere ed. de plusieurs traitez, sçavoir de L'anatomie du corps humain; Des canons sur toute la chirurgie. D'un etat des versus [sic] de l'ame, com- posées par Monsieur de La Framboisiere ... D'un excélent abregé des bandes & bandages. Et d'un nouveau paraphrase, sur le Serment d'Hipocrate. Rouen, Chez Richard Lallemant [De l'imprimerie de Pierre Amiot] 1680.

> 5 parts in 1 v.   18 cm.   [7480]
> Parts [2-5] have special or half title pages.

—Paradoxe; ou, Traicté medulaire [sic] auquel est amplement prouvé contre l'opinion commune & vulgaire que la moelle n'est pas la nourriture des os. Rev. & amplifié de commentaires sur chacun chapitre, pour servir de replique à la responce de M. J. Lanay ... Paris, Catherine Niverd, 1609.

> [24], 238 (i.e. 234), [35] p.   18 cm.   [7481]
> With this is bound: Lanay, J. Le triomphe de la moelle. 1609.

—Traicté des bandages de la chirurgie ... Paris, La veufue Claude de Monstroeil [1618]

> [16], 430 p.   illus., port.   18 cm.   [7482]
> Engraved title page.
> Livre I.
> Imperfect: title page wanting; supplied in photocopy from Wellcome library.

—[The same.] ... Paris, Guillaume Loyson, 1631.

> [16], 430 p.   illus., port.   18 cm.   [7483]
> Engraved title page.
> Livre I.
> Different setting of type.

—See LANAY, J. Le triomphe de la moelle. 1609.

MARRA, PIO DELLA [fl. 1634] Opera pia per la salute del corpo humano ... Napoli, Il Beltrano, 1634.

> [20], 534, [14] p.   illus.   15 cm.   [7484]
> Engraved title page.

—Praxis methodica, et rationalis curandorum morborum omnium. In qua praeter remedia ... a Galeno, ab Hippocrate, & Avicenna desumpta, multa arcana medica continentur ... Neapoli, Apud Lazarum Scoriggium, expensis Dominici Vecchi, 1634.

> [16], 250, [14] p.   22 cm.   [7485]

MARRADÓN, BARTOLOMÉ [16th-17th cent.] See COLMENERO DE LEDESMA, A. Du chocolate. 1643; [DUFOUR, P. S.] De l'usage du caphé, du thé, et du chocolate. 1671. [and] DUFOUR, P. S. Traitez nouveaux & curieux de café, du thé et du chocolate.

1685, 1688, 1693; [Latin tr.] 1685, 1699; [German tr.] 1686, 1692.

The **MARRIAGES** of cousin Germans. 1673. See [DUGARD, S.]

MARSCHALCK, JOHANN [fl. 17th cent.] tr. See GLASER, C. Novum laboratorium medico-chymicum. 1677.

MARSHALL, WILLIAM [ca. 1621-1683] Philosophy delineated, containing a resolution of divers knotty questions upon suddry philosophical notions: viz. concerning the original of springs ... Of chymical multiplications or the increasing of quantity of liquors by distilation ... London, Obadiah Blagrave, 1678.

> [21], 237, [20] p.   plate.   17 cm.   [7486]
> Signature G7 (blank?) wanting.

MARSIGLI, ANTONIO FELICE [1649-1710] De ovis cochlearum epistola ad Marcellum Malpighium ... cum Joh. Jacobi Harderi ... epistolis aliquot, de partibus genitalibus cochlearum, generatione item insectorum ex ovo, ad praefatum abbatem, & D. Lucam Schröckium ... Augustae Vindelicorum, Sumptibus Theophili Goebelii, literis Leonhardi Zachariae, 1684.

> [10], 58 p.   plate.   16 cm.   [7487]
> Frati 161.

—Relazione del ritrovamento dell'vova di chiocciole di A[ntonio] F[elice] M[arsigli] in una lettera al sig. Marcello Malpighi ... Bologna, Eredi d'Antonio Pisarri, 1683.

> 83, [1] p.   plate.   16 cm.   [7488]
> Frati 159.

—[The same.] ... Roma, Domenico Antonio Ercole, 1695.

> 141 p.   plate.   16 cm.   [7489]
> "Riflessioni sopra la relatione del ritrouamento dell'vova di chiocciole di A[ntonio] F[elice] M[arsigli] ... inviate in una lettera ... da Godefrido Fulberti [pseud., i.e. Filippo Buonanni]" (p. [45]-141) has special title page.
> Frati 159.1.

MARSILI, ANTONIO FELICE. See MARSIGLI, Antonio Felice [1649-1710]

MARTEL, CLAUDIUS [fl. 1673] See PECHLIN, J. N. Jani Leoniceni Veronensis [pseud.] Metamorphosis. 1673.

MARTHE, SCÉVOLE DE SAINTE. See SAINTE-MARTHE, Scévole de [1536-1623]

MARTIALIS, MARCUS VALERIUS. *See* ZAROTTI, C. M. Valerii Martialis epigrammatum, medicae . . . considerationis enarratio. 1657.

MARTIANUS, FRANCISCUS. *See* MARZIANI, Francesco [*fl.* 1622]

MARTIANUS, PROSPER. *See* MARZIANI, Prospero [1567–1622]

MARTIN, BARTHÉLEMY [*b.* 1629] Dissertation sur les dents . . . Paris, Denys Thierry, 1679.

    [18], 136 p.   14 cm.   **[7490]**

—Traité de l'usage du lait . . . Paris, Denys Thierry, 1684.

    [12], 146, [7] p.   15 cm.   **[7491]**

MARTIN, BERNARDIN [*b.* 1629] *See* MARTIN, Barthélemy [*b.* 1629]

MARTIN, CLAUDE [*fl.* 1552–1554] *ed. See* GALENUS. [Selected works. French] 1605.

MARTIN, DAVID. *See* MARTINI, David [*fl.* 1673]

MARTIN, JEAN [*d.* 1609] Praelectiones in librum Hippocratis . . . De morbis internis . . . Editore M. Renato Morello . . . Parisiis, Apud Joan. Libert, 1637.

    [19], 473, [14] p.   23 cm.   **[7492]**

    Caption title: . . . Hippocratis De morbis internis, seu, Magnus liber de morbis.

    Includes Greek text and Martin's Latin translation of De internis affectionibus.

—Praelectiones in librum Hippocratis . . . De aere, aquis, et locis . . . Parisiis, Apud Mathaeum & Petrum Guillemot, 1646.

    [8], 164, [13] p.   23 cm.   **[7493]**

    Edited by René Moreau.

    Includes Greek text and Latin translation by Janus Cornarius.

—[The same.] . . . Parisiis, Apud Petrum Guillemot, 1655.

    [8], 164, [13] p.   24 cm.   **[7494]**

    A reissue of the 1646 Paris edition with new title page.

MARTIN, LOUIS [*fl.* 1649] L'Eschole de Salerne en vers burlesques. Et Poema macaronicum, de bello Huguenotico. Paris, Jean Henault, 1650.

    [21], 74, [2] p.   22 cm.   **[7495]**

    Added engraved title page: Lescolle de Salerne en vers burlesque, par L[ouis] M[artin] P[hysicien] . . .

Includes portions of the Latin text of the Regimen sanitatis Salernitanum.

    "Poema macaronicum, de bello Huguenotico" (p. 53–74) by Remy Belleau.

—[The same.] L'Eschole de Salerne, en suite le poeme macaronique. En vers burlesques. Paris, Antoine Rafflé [166–?]

    [1], 83 p.   15 cm.   **[7496]**

    Added engraved title page: Lescolle de Salerne en vers burlesque par L[ouis] M[artin] P[hysicien].

    Imperfect: p. 67–72 mutilated.

    Poème macaronique is a translation of Remy Belleau's Dictamen metrificum de bello Huguenotico.

—[The same.] . . . Paris, Jacques Le Gras, 1664.

    [11], 104 p.   1664.   **[7497]**

—[The same.] . . . Bordeaux, Claude Labottiere, 1697.

    [10], 73 p.   18 cm.   **[7498]**

MARTIN, MATTHÄUS. *See* MARTINI, Matthäus [*fl.* 1587–1624]

MARTINELLI, CECHINO [*fl.* 1604–1614] *ed. See* MOSTRAVERO, A. Risposta alle Considerationi d'Ottavio Campolongo. 1614 [i.e. 1615]

MARTINELLI, DOMENICO [*fl.* 1663–1669] Horologi elementari divisi in quattro parti . . . fatti con l'acqua . . . con la terra . . . con l'aria . . . col fuoco. Alcuni muti, & alcuni col suono . . . Venetia, Bortolo Tramontino, 1669.

    [16], 17–155, [4] p.   illus.   **[7499]**

    Sheet V in duplicate.

MARTINELLI, PAOLO [*fl.* 1604] *ed. See* COTUGNUS, J. Liber de abusu venae sectionis. 1604.

MARTINELLO, CECHINO. *See* MARTINELLI, Cechino [*fl.* 1604–1614]

MARTINEZ, MICHAEL. *See* MARTÍNEZ DE LEACHE, Miguel [*fl.* 1644–1652]

MARTÍNEZ DE LEACHE, MIGUEL [*fl.* 1644–1652] Discurso pharmaceutico, sobre los Canones de Mesue . . . Pamplona, Martin de Labàyen y Diego de Zabala. 1652.

    [27], 161 ll.   19 cm.   **[7500]**

    Imperfect: wormholes on ll. 160–161.

    Includes selected chapters from Mesüe's Canones generales.

MARTÍNEZ DE ZALDUENDO Y AGUIRRE, JOUAN [*fl.* 1696] Libro de los baños de arnedillo, y

remedio universal ... Pamplona, Francisco Antonio
de Neyra, 1699.

[20], 424 p.   21 cm.   [**7501**]

MARTINI, DANIEL [*fl.* 1696–1702] *respondent. See*
PETERMANN, A., *praeses.* Dissertatio medica de
enterocele. 1696.

MARTINI, DAVID [*fl.* 1673] Dissertatio medica de
natura acidi & alcali genuinarum sanitatis & morbi
causarum. Propter novitatem argumenti hac forma
recusa, in quibusdam locis aucta, ac a mendis
repurgata. Lugd. Batavorum, Apud Arnoldum
Duode, 1676.

[4], 50, [2] p.   16 cm.   [**7502**]

MARTINI, GREGORIUS [*fl.* 1617–*ca.* 1621] Commentatiuncula in libri qui inscribitur de chymicorum
cum Aristotelicis et Galenicis consensu ac dissensu
caput XI. quod est de principiis chymicorum. Trac-
tationem quaestionis: ansal sulphur, & mercurius sint
prima perfecte mixta ... Francofurti ad Oderam,
Typis Friderici Hartmanni, impensis Martini Guets,
1621.

[12], 243 p.   17 cm.   [**7503**]
With this is bound: Horst, G. Σκέψις de naturali conservatione
... cadaverum. 1608.

—*See* PANSA, M. Kurtze Defensionschrifft von der
Gicht. 1617.

MARTINI, HEINRICH [1615 *or* 6–1675] Anatomia
urinae Galeno-spagyrica. Ex doctrina Hippocratis &
Galeni nec non recentiorum, imprimis Theophrasti
Paracelsi, & Leonhardi Thrunheuseri, aliorumque
chymiatrorum principum scriptis adornata. Cui ac-
cessit ejusd. ars pronuntiandi ex urinis ... et
Caesaris Odoni De urinis libellus posthumus.
Francofurti, Sumpt. Georgii Fickwirti, 1658.

[28], 308 p.; [20] p.   table.   14 cm.   [**7504**]
Added engraved title page dated 1659.
Part [2] edited by Sebastian Scheffer has special title page.

—Anteambulo medicus; sive, Universitas artis
hebdomadali repraesentata in qua tota institutionum
doctrina compendiose traditur ... Bregae, Typis
Christoph. Tschorn, 1668.

[30], 470, [1] p.   15 cm.   [**7505**]
With this is bound: Conradt, I. Dissertatio ... de frigoris.
[Gedani] 1677.

MARTINI, HEINRICH [*fl.* 1672] *respondent. See*
GLASER, J. H., *praeses.* [Dissertatio casualis de caro
apoplexia terminato] 1672.

MARTINI, HENRICUS [*fl.* 1657] *respondent.*
Disputatio medica inauguralis, de pleuritide ...
Ultrajecti, Pro vidua Petri Baart, 1657.

[18] p.   20 cm.   [**7506**]
Diss.—Utrecht.

MARTINI, JAKOB [1570–1649] Dissertatio de peste
... Wittebergae, Ex officina Johannis Gormanni,
1613.

[36] p.   19 cm.   [**7507**]
Running title: Oratio de peste.

—*praeses.* Disputatio physica de animarum
humanarum origine ... Wittebergae, Ex officina
Johannis Matthaei, 1615.

[15] p.   19 cm.   [**7508**]
Diss.—Wittenberg (J. Ratichius, *respondent*)

MARTINI, JAKOB [*fl. ca.* 1632] *respondent. See*
FREITAG, J., *praeses.* Disputatio medica de morbis
substantię. 1632.

MARTINI, LODOVICO [*fl.* 1614] Brevi discorsi
della natura, & effetti de' bagni di Corsena di Lucca,
con alcuni necessarii avertimenti per quelli che
vogliono andare in detto luogo per recuperare la
sanita, et con i remedii à ciò appropriati ... Bologna,
Heredi di Gio. Rossi, 1614.

[24], 301, [2] p.   15 cm.   [**7509**]

MARTINI, MARTINO [1614–1661] *See* KIRCHER, A.
Magnes, 1643.

MARTINI, MATTHÄUS [*fl.* 1587–1624] De morbis
mesenterii abstrusioribus. In scholis medicorum
hactenus prętermissis, nec scriptis veterum illustratis.
Item Affectionum hypochondriacarum ... historia
& curatio. Halae-Saxonum, Apud Michaelem
Oelschlegelium, 1625.

[16], 486, [60] p.   17 cm.   [**7510**]

—[The same.] ... Lipsię, Sumptibus Casparis
Closemanni, 1630.

[16], 365, [41] p.   16 cm.   [**7511**]

—*See* SENNERT, D. De scorbuto tractatus. 1624
[and] Duo tractatus de dignotione & curatione scorbuti. 1624.

MARTINI, VALERIO [*fl.* 1628] Enchiridion in quo
de universa febrium, earumque symptomatum,
natura, cognitione, exactaque curatione agitur. Quod
in duas dividitur partes, cum multarum difficilium

quaestionum enodatione ... Venetiis, Apud Marcum Antonium Brogiollum, 1636.

[38], 263, [1] p.   21 cm.   [7512]

Added half title reads: Praxis medicae laconismi quibus enchiridion & opuscula insunt.

—Opuscula in quibus de vesicantium sinapismorum, cucurbitularum siccarum, ligaturae dolorificae frictionum lotionumque crurum, ac pedum recta administratione. Ac De asthmate et orthopnoea ... Atque De definitionis veneni pestilentis ... dilucidatione ... agitur ... Venetiis, Apud Marcum Antonium Brogiollum, 1636.

[18], 84 p.   22 cm.   [7513]

—Totius medicinae practicae exactissima collectio. In qua tria insunt promptuaria nempe, Promptuarium cujuslibet educationis sanguinis recte agendae; Promptuarium singulae vacuationis cacochymiae recte administrandae; Promptuarium cujuscunque cruditatis recte dignoscendae, recteque curandae. Ad quae accedit Certitudinis medicinae curiosa, & accurata constitutio ... [Venetiis, Apud Jo. Baptistam Combum, 1628]

4 parts in 1 v.   33 cm.   [7514]

Added engraved title page.
Each part has special title page.

MARTINIERE, DE LA. See LA MARTINIÈRE, Pierre Martin de [1634–1690]

MARTINO, PIERANTONIO. See CELEBERR. VIRORUM APOLOGIAE PRO R. D. CAROLO MUSITANO. 1700.

MARTINUS, BERNARDUS, BERENCLON DE. See BERENCLON, Bernardus Martinus de [fl. 1689–1695]

MARTINUS, JOHANNES [d. 1665] Etliche Gewissens-Fragen von der Pestilentz, auss der Heyligen Schrifft beantwortet; sampt Cypriani Tractat Von der Sterblichkeit oder von der Pest. Und Etlichen Gebätten ... Anfänglich gestellt in Nider-Deutsch durch Johannem Martinum ... Anjetzo aber ... in ... teutsche Sprach ... übersetzt durch Wolfgangum Christianum ... Bern, Georg Sonnleitner, 1668.

[54], 506, [22] p.; [1], 125 p.   18 cm.   [7515]

"... Cyprians ... Gedancken und ... Reden Von der Sterblichkeit oder von dem Sterbend oder Pestilentz ... Anfänglich verteutschet durch Adamum Olearium. Anjetzo aber ... ergäntzet und verbessert durch W[olfgangum] C[hristianum]" (p. [445]-506) has half title.

Part [2] has special title page: Etliche schöne und geistreiche Gebätte, für die Einfältigen in Pest-Zeiten sehr nutzlich zu gebrauchen. Auss dem Nieder-Teutschen ... übersetzt ... durch Wolffgang Christen.

MARTIUS, GALEOTTUS. See MARZIO, Galeotto [15th cent.]

MARTIUS, JEREMIAS [d. 1585] Curationes et observationes medica, medicae, e bibliotheca Georgii Hieronymi Velschii, cum ejusdem notis.

52, [8] p.   20 cm.   (Part [2] in Welsch, Georg Hieronymus. Sylloge curationum et observationum medicinalium. Aug. Vindel., 1667)   [7516]

Engraved title page.

—Another issue, with date changed to 1668.   [7517]

MARTIUS, JOHANN HEINRICH [d. 1709] respondent. See KIRCHMAJER, T., praeses. Dissertatio physica de virgula divinatrice. 1669.

MARTIUS, JOHANN NIKOLAUS [fl. 1700] respondent. Dissertatio inauguralis physico-medica de magia naturali, ejusque usu medico ad magice et magica curandum ... Erfordiae, Excudebat Joh. Henr. Grosch [1700]

44 p.   19 cm.   [7518]

Diss.—Erfurt.

MARTIUS, THEODOR [fl. 1696] respondent. See EYSEL, J. P., praeses. Dissertatio inauguralis medica, exhibens visionis statum naturalem et praeternaturalem. 1696.

MARTYN, JOHANNES ELIAS [fl. 1699] respondent. Disputatio medica inauguralis de scorbuto ... Lugduni Batavorum, Apud Abrahamum Elzevier, 1699.

[16] p.   22 cm.   [7519]

Diss.—Leyden.

MARUCCIUS, CASPAR. See MARCUCCI, Gaspare [fl. 1624–1644]

MARZIALE, MARCUS VALERIO. See MARTIALIS, Marcus Valerius.

MARZIANI, FRANCESCO [fl. 1622] See MARZIANI, P. Apologeticus liber. 1617.

MARZIANI, PROSPERO [1567–1622] Apologeticus liber in tres partes divisus, quae sunt Expositio, Annotatio, Antiparalogysmus. In quo praeter alia ad artem medicam necessaria purgationis, & venae sectionis usus juxta Germanam Hippocratis doctrinam explicatur . . . Romae, Ex typographia Gulielmi Facciotti, 1617.

[II], 84 p. 22 cm. [7520]

Imperfect: Expositio and Annotatio wanting.

Part [3] has special title page: Antiparalogismus ad ea quae exellentissimi DD. Aetius Cletus, et Joannes Manelphus scripsere contro Annotationem D. Prosperi Martiani, ad Marsilium Cagnatum. In quo Hippocratis auctoritate recentiorum medicorum abusus notantur circa venae sectionem, potissimum in pleuritidis curatione . . . Industria Francisci Martiani D. Prosperi filii . . . 1622.

—Brevis annotatio super expositionem aphorismi Concocta medicari M. Cagnati [as subject] See MANELFI, G. Responsio brevis ad . . . Prosperi Martiani. 1621.

—Hippocratis aphorismum XXII sectionis primae expositio, in quo universaliora praecepta continentur, quae ad purgationem rite perscribendam sunt necessaria, cui accesserunt alia duo loca obscuriora, alter ex libro primo morborum mulierum . . . alter ex VII. Epid. in cujus explicatione vera tum convulsionis, tum paralysis natura . . . demonstratur . . . Romae, Ex typographia Guileimi Facciotti, 1617.

[8], 61, [1] p. 23 cm. [7521]

—Magnus Hippocrates . . . notationibus explicatus . . . Romae, Typis Jacobi Mascardi, 1626.

[8], 618, [10] p. 33 cm. [7522]

With this is bound: Salius Diversus, P. Commentaria . . . in Hippocratis . . . De morbis libros IV. 1612.

—[The same.] . . . Venetiis, Apud Guerilios, 1652.

[8], 492, [8] p. 32 cm. [7523]

With this is bound: Valles, F. de, Commentaria in septem libros Epidemiorum. 1652 [i.e. 1653]

—[Excerpts.] See LANCETTA, T. Raccolta medica. 1645.

MARZIO, GALEOTTO [15th cent.] Della varia dottrina tradotto in volgare fiorentino per M. Francesco Serdonati con la giunta d'alcune brevi annotazioni . . . Fiorenza, Filippo Giunti, 1615.

[32], 469, [27] p. 17 cm. [7524]

Imperfect: title page mutilated.

MÁS, BERNARDO [fl. 1625] Orde breu, y regiment molt util, y profitos pera preservar, y curar de peste . . . Barcelona, Esteve Liberòs, 1625.

[8], 96 ll. 16 cm. [7525]

MĀSAWAIH al-MĀRDĪNĪ. See MESUË [924 or 5-1015]

MĀSAWAIH, YŪḤANNĀ IBN. See MESUË [d. 857]

MASCHOW, FRIEDRICH [fl. 1686] respondent. See VEHR, I., praeses. Dissertatio inauguralis medica de leucorrhoea. 1686.

MASCHURAT. See RENAUDOT, Théophraste [1584-1653]

MASIERO, FILIPPO. La chirurgia compendiata; overo, Instruzioni per il chirurgo in prattica . . . Venetia, Stefano Curti, 1688.

[32], 191 (i.e. 173), [3] p. front., illus. 19 cm. [7526]

Frontispiece reads: Il chirurgo in pratica.

—[The same.] . . . Accresciuta notabilmente dall'autore . . . & espurgata dagl'errori . . . 2. ed. Venetia, Steffano Curti, 1690.

[32], 416 p. front., illus. 19 cm. [7527]

—[The same.] . . . 3. ed. Venetia, Steffano Curti, 1698.

[32], 414 p. front., illus. 17 cm. [7528]

MASINUS, BERNARDINUS [fl. 1611] See REGGIO EMILIA (City) Ordinances, local laws, etc. Bando sopra la peste. 1611.

MASIUS, JOHANN [1613-1642] praeses. Decas positionum exhibens fabricam & usum oculi humani quam . . . examini subjiciunt . . . Johannes Masius . . . Georgius Hövell . . . Regiomonti, Typis haeredum Segebadii, 1639.

[16] p. 18 cm. [7529]

Diss.—Königsberg (G. Hövell, respondent)

—respondent. See TINCTORIUS, C., praeses. Generationem hominis ut & reliquorum animantium ex semine . . . subjiciet . . . Christophoro Tinctorio . . . J. M. 1637.

MASQUERIER, GUILIELMUS [fl. 1617] respondent. Theses inaugurales de medicina in genere . . . Lugduni Batavorum, Excudebat Georgius Abrahami a Marsse, 1617.

[8] p. 20 cm. [7530]

Diss.—Leyden.

MASSA, NICOLA [d. 1569] tr. See AVICENNA. Avicennae Arabum medicorum principis. 1608.

MASSARD, Jacques. Traité des panacées ou des remedes universels. Augmenté d'une seconde partie. Et d'un traité des abus de la medecine ordinaire. [Grenoble, L'auteur, 1681]

[24], 200 (i.e. 204), [2] p.; [12], 115 (i.e. 123), [4] p. fronts. 16 cm.   [7531]

Imperfect: wormholes on p. 35-96, part 2.

Title from half title; each part has special title page. Part [1]: Panacée, ou Discours sur les effets singuliers d'un remede . . . pour la guerison de la pluspart des longues maladies . . . Avec un traité d'Hypocrate de la cause des maladies, & de l'ancienne medecine, traduit en françois par l'auteur. Grenoble, L'auteur, 1679. Part 2: Seconde partie du traité des panacées ou des remedes universels. Avec un traité des abus de la medecine ordinaire . . . Et les avis de Vanhelmont sur la composition des remedes, traduits en françois par l'auteur. Grenoble, Chez P. Fremon, et se vendent chez Louis Nicolas, 1680.

Five leaves inserted after preliminaries in pt. [1] contain "Lettre de Monsieur de Blegny ecrite a M. Massard sur son traitté des panacées," dated Aug. 3, 1681, and "Extrait du Journal de Medecine du mois d'Aoust 1681," which notices the previous separate publication of the present volumes.

An enlarged edition, designated the second, was published in Amsterdam in 1686 under title: Divers traitez sur les panacées ou remèdes universels. Cf. BNC.

The treatise of Hippocrates (part [1], p. [153]-176) is a translation of De prisca medicina.

"Avis de [Jean Baptiste] Vanhelmont sur la composition des remedes" translated from "Pharmacopolium ac dispensatorium modernum" in his Ortus medicinae (Amsterdam, 1648)

—[Dutch tr.] Verscheide verhandelingen raakende de panacéen, ofte algemeene geneesmiddelen. Als meede de misslagen, die in de gemeene geneeskonst doorgaans begaan werden, met een nette vertaaling van Hippocrates aangaande de oorzaak der ziekten en van de oordeelen van van Helmont omtrent de samenvoeging der hulpmiddelen, en daar by noch eenige andere nutte redenen over verscheide ziekten . . . In't Nederduitsch overgebracht door Philippus de la Grue. Amsterdam, Aard Dirksz. Oossaan, 1687.

[8], 286, [2] p. 17 cm.   [7532]

Translation of Traité des panacées, based on the enlarged French edition, designated the second, published in Amsterdam in 1686. Cf. BNC; Bibl. Med. Neerland., p. 74.

Correspondence between Nicolas de Blegny and the author (letters dated Aug. 3–Sept. 24, 1681): p. 228-237.

MASSARIA, Alessandro [1510-1598] Opera medica: quibus methodus ac ratio cognoscendi et curandi totius humani corporis morbos, ad nativam genuinamque Hippocratis & Galeni mentem vere optimeque instituitur. Subjiciuntur tractatus quatuor utilissimi, De peste, De affectibus renum & vesicae,

De pulsibus, & De urinis: Consilium pro febre catarrhali cum totius macie, ventriculi imbecillitate, mesenterii obstructione, moestitia & vigiliis: Liber responsorum & consultationum medicinalium. Accedunt postremo disputationes duae, una De scopis mittendi sanguinem, altera De purgatione in principio morborum, quam excipit additamentum apologeticum ad priorem . . . Lugduni, Sumptibus Joannis-Amati Candy, 1634.

[8], 865 (i.e. 859), [34] p. 36 cm.   [7533]

"De collegiandi seu consultandi ratione, liber octavus": p. 487-490 [bis] on 2 leaves inserted after the original p. 490.

Collections containing nearly the same works were published under title: Practica medica.

—[The same.] . . . Ed. novissima a mendis expurgata. Lugduni, Sumptibus Laurentii Anisson, 1669.

[6], 860, [34] p. 36 cm.   [7534]

Imperfect? One preliminary leaf and one leaf at end (both blank?) wanting.

—Additamentum apologeticum. See Augenio, O. Epistolarum medicinalium tomi tertii. 1607.

—Disputationes duae. Una De scopis mittendi sanguinem, altera De purgatione principio morborum. Tertio editae, cum additamento apologetico ad priorem. Pars prima [-secunda] Lugduni, Sumptibus Laurentii Durand, 1622.

[23], 192 p.; [16], 288 p. 24 cm.   [7535]

Part 2 has special title page: Ad disputationem De scopis mittendi sanguinem additamentum apologeticum continens libros XI disputationes XI.

With this is bound *his* Liber responsorum et consultationum medicinalium. 1622.

—Libelli duo de pulsibus, & urinis. Nunc primum in lucem editi, ac diligenter emendati, ad communem medicinam facientium utilitatem. Quibus praeposuimus praefationem methodicam in morbis particularibus . . . Venetiis, Apud Robertum Meiettum, 1603.

[6], 51 p. 21 cm.   [7536]

Supplement the Practica medica, in later editions of which they were incorporated.

Dedication signed by Thomas Baglonius, the editor.

—Liber responsorum et consultationum medicinalium. Nunc primum collectus, & in lucem editus . . . Lugduni, Sumptibus Laurentii Durand, 1622.

100, [4] p. 24 cm.   [7537]

Running title: Consilia medica.

Also issued with the 1622 Lyons edition of his Practica medica, published by the same press.

Bound with *his* Disputationes duae. 1622.

—Practica medica; seu, Praelectiones academicae, continentes methodum ac rationem cognoscendi et curandi plerosque omnes totius humani corporis morbos, ad ... Hippocratis & ... Galeni mentem vere optimeque institutam ... Nunc primum ... publico ... commodo foras dantur abs Joanne Baumanno ... Francoforti, Sumptibus Nicolai Bassaei, typis Melchioris Hartmanni, 1601.

[16], 968, [28] p.   25 cm.   [7538]

Contents. — De affectibus capitis. — De affectibus thoracis. - De affectibus ventriculi, epatis, lienis, intestinorum.- De morbis mulierum. - De febribus. - De morbo Gallico. - De medicamentis purgantibus. - De collegiandi, seu co●sultandi ratione.

—Practica medica. In qua methodus accuratissima traditur, & cognoscendi, & rectissime curandi omnes humani corporis morbos, ad ... Hippoc. & Gal. mentem ... instituta. Cui recenter suis inserti locis ... conspiciuntur bini tractatus; De pulsibus quidem unus, De urinis vero alter; liber praeterea accessit renum & vesicae affectus omnes ... complectens. Appositi insuper praeter medicam in febre catarrali ... consultationem duo ... de peste fuerunt libelli ... Tarvisii, Sumptibus Jo. Baptistae Pulciani, 1607.

[34], 499, [1] p.; 51 p.   31 cm.   [7539]

Colophon: Tarvisii, Apud Evangelistam Deuchinum, 1606.

—[The same.] ... Jamvero in hac 3. et noviss. nostra impressione additus est Liber responsorum, & consultationum medicinalium ejusdem autoris ... Venetiis, Apud Trivisanum Bertolottum, 1613.

[31], 499, [4] p.; [51] p.; [4], 48 p.   31 cm.
                                               [7540]

Part [2]: De peste, has caption title; part [3]: Liber responsorum, has special title page.

—[The same.] ... 4. impressione ... Venetiis, Apud Trivisanum Bertolottum, 1618.

[27], 499, [1] p.; 51, [4] p.   31 cm.   [7541]

Imperfect: p. 239-240, and Liber responsorum, & consultationum medicinalium (48? p. at end) wanting.

—[The same.] ... 4. impressione ... Venetiis, Apud Joan. Antonium Julianum, 1622.

[27], 500 p.; [4], 51 p.; 48 p.   32 cm. [7542]

Imperfect: p. [1-2] of 3d group of paging (special title page?) wanting.

—[The same.] Practica medica; seu, Praelectiones academicae, continentes methodum ac rationem cognoscendi & curandi totius humani corporis morbos, ad ... Hippocratis & Galeni mentem vere optimeque institutam ... Accesserunt posteriori huic editioni Tractatus quatuor utilissimi, De peste, De affectibus renum & vesicae, De pulsibus, & De urinis. Necnon Liber responsorum & consultationum medicinalium ejusdem authoris. Annexum est pro exemplo Consilium pro febre catarrhali ... Lugduni, Sumptibus Laurentii Durand, 1622.

[16], 968, [27] p.; [1], 178, [11] p.; 100, [4] p.   24 cm.   [7543]

Parts 2 and 3 have special title pages.

—[The same.] ... Venetiis, Apud Baretium Baretium, 1642.

[27], 499 p.; [4], 51, [4], 48 p.   32 cm.
                                               [7544]

Part [3] has special title page.

A second "Index eorum quae in duobus de peste libris continentur" ([4] p.) of a different printing from that on p. [7-10] at the front of the volume, inserted after p. 499, preceding the text of the De peste.

—Tractatus quatuor utilissimi: quorum I est De peste. II. De affectibus rerum & vesicae. III. De pulsibus. IV. De urinis. Cui est annexum pro exemplo Consilium de febre catarrhali cum totius macie, mesenterii obstructione, moestitia & vigiliis. Nunc tandem post auctoris obitum ab haeredibus reperti, caeterisque ejusdem operibus adjuncti. Francofurti, Typis Matthiae Beckeri, impensis haeredum Nicolai Bassaei, 1608.

[21], 178 p.   24 cm.   [7545]

MASSELLA, BERNHARDT [*fl.* 1679] Bericht von der Pest; oder, Kurtze Instruction, wie man sich in contagiosischen Suchten, und absonderlich diss 1679. Jahrs hin- und wider grassierende Pest-Praeservative und Curative verhalten solle. An die Hochlöbl. Hn. Hn. Verordnete dises Ertzhertzogthumb Oesterreich ob der Enns, etc. Durch dero Ord. Physicum Seniorem in Lintz. [Lintz] Gedruckt by Joh. Jacob. Mayr, 1679.

[10], 103 p.   14 cm.   [7546]

Added engraved title page.

MASSON, MAGNUS [*fl.* 1681–1682] *respondent. See* HOFFMANN, J. M., *praeses.* Disputatio medica publica de carie ossium. 1681.

MASSONIO, Salvatore [1559-1629] Archidipno; overo, Dell'insalata, e dell'uso di essa, trattato nuovo ... Venetia, Marc'Antonio Brogiollo, 1627.

[16], 426, [2] p. 20 cm.   **[7547]**

Dedicatory epistle signed by Alessandro Maganza, the editor.

—Breve et utile discorso ... delle facolta et dell'uso dell'acque dell'antico bagno di Antredoco ... Napoli, Gio. Domenico Roncagliolo, 1621.

[8], 172, [3] p. 19 cm.   **[7548]**

Errata: p. [175]

MATAMOROS VÁZQUEZ GALLEGO, Benito [*fl.* 1622] Selectarum medicinae disputationum, tomus I. In quo praeter ea, quae de febrium theoria, coctione & putredine, & aliis ex professo disputantur; plura etiam alia difficillima ad utranque medicinae partem spectantia obiter disquiruntur ... Ursaonae, Apud Joannem Serrano de Vargas & Vreña, 1622.

[6], 2, 554 (i.e. 544), [36] p. 29 cm. **[7549]**

No more published.

Imperfect: p. 355-356 and 451-454 wanting; p. 261-264 and 455-458 mutilated.

MATENESIUS, Johann Friedrich [ca. 1580-1622] Critices Christianae libri duo de ritu bibendi super sanitate, pontificum ... ducum, magnatum amicorum, amicarum ... Coloniae, Sumptibus Conradi Butgenii, 1611.

[16], 189 p. 16 cm.   **[7550]**

Imperfect: p. 23-24 mutilated.

With this is bound *his* Syntagma criticum. 1612.

—Syntagma criticum. Nescis quid serus vesper vehat. De somno potuque Christianorum somnifero ... Coloniae, Sumptibus Conradi Butgenii, 1612.

[16], 101 p. 16 cm.   **[7551]**

Bound with *his* Critices Christianae. 1611.

MATERA, Eustazio da. *See* Eustazio da Matera [13th cent.]

MATHEMATICALL recreations. 1653. *See* [Leurechon, J.]

MATHENESIUS, Joannes Fridericus. *See* Matenesius, Johann Friedrich [*ca.* 1580-1622]

MATHESIUS, Daniel [*fl.* 1692] *respondent. See* Castanaeus, M., *praeses.* Pathologia generalis. 1692.

MATHEWS, Richard [*d. ca.* 1659] The unlearned alchymist his antidote; or, A more full and ample ex-planation of the use ... of my pill ... Togerher [sic] with A precious pearl in the midst of a dunghil, being a ... receit of Mr. Richard Mathew's pill ... presented to the world by Mris. Anne Mathews, amongst many sad complaints of wrongs done to her ... and her deceased husband ... London, Joseph Leigh, 1663.

[16], 157 p.; [1], 48, 204 (i.e. 194) p. 15 cm.   **[7552]**

Part [2] has special title page.
Imperfect: p. 1-150 of part 2 wanting.

—Copy 2.

Imperfect: 48 p. of part [2] bound before part [1]; p. [1-13] and p. 147-157 of part [1] wanting; p. [1], 25-28, 151-154 and 195-204 of part [2] wanting.

MATMAN, Rudolph [1566-1612] Tres capellae; sive, Admonitio ad Josephum Justum Burdonem [i.e. Joseph Juste Scaliger] Julii Caes. Burdonis f. Benedicti Burdonis n. [n. p.] 1608.

[2], 14 p. 20 cm.   **[7553]**

MATON, Pieter [*fl.* 1696] *respondent. See* Bidloo, G., *praeses.* Disputatio medica inauguralis de chlorosi. 1696.

MATTESILLANI, Giovanni Carlo [*b.* 1623] *ed. See* Claudini, G. C. [*d.* 1618] Empyrica rationalis libris VI. 1653.

MATTHAEI, Johann. *See* Matthaeus, Johann [1563-1621]

MATTHAEOLUS, Petrus Andreas. *See* Mattioli, Pietro Andrea [1500-1577]

MATTHAEUS, Johann [1563-1621] Centuria difficultatum medicarum tam jucundarum quam utilium, ex veterum & recentiorum medicorum libris erutarum, in quaestiones redactarum ... Herbornae Nassoviorum, Ex officina typographica Christophori Corvini, 1616.

[16], 304, [8] p. 18 cm.   **[7554]**

—Consilia medica diversorum auctorum ... Francofurti, E Collegio musarum Paltheniano, 1608.

[7], 143 p. 16 cm.   **[7555]**

—Discursus medicinalis, de febre pestilentiali, quae superioribus annis universam ferme Germaniam pervagata est. In quo ... demonstratur, sanguinis missionem pro curatione febrium pestilentialium pernitiosam esse ... Francofurti, Ex Officina Zachario Paltheniana, 1603.

    85 p. 17 cm.   **[7556]**

—Enodatio quaestionis: an armorum unguentum, ad curanda vulnera, nec visa nec tractata aliquid conferat.

    573–584 p. 21 cm. (*In* Theatrum sympatheticum auctum. Norimbergae, 1662)   **[7557]**
    Caption title.

—Quaestionum medicarum et jucundarum et lectu dignarum ac practico inprimis necessariarum enodatio scholastica ... Francofurti, Ex Officina Zachario-Paltheniana, 1603.

    [14], 143 p. 16 cm.   **[7558]**

—Rationalis et empirica thermarum marchicarum Badensium descriptio ... Ettlingae, Ex typographia Johannis Philippi Spiessii, 1606.

    [11], 107 p. 16 cm.   **[7559]**

—[The same.] ... Alt. auct. & emend. ed. ... Hanoviae, Typis & impensis Joannis Halbeii, 1608.

    [2], 122 p. 16 cm.   **[7560]**

—Speculum sanitatis: rerum non-naturalium, quas vocant, administrationem pro bona valetudine conservanda continens ... Accessit Hortulus medicus, simplicium medicamentorum qualitates ad certos gradus redactas ... Herbornae Nassoviorum, 1620.

    [11], 198, [10] p.; [10], 83 p. 18 cm. **[7561]**
    Part [2] has special title page.

MATTHAEUS, Philippus [1641–1690] *praeses.* Disputatio medica de chylo ... Franequerae, Johannes Gyselaar, 1681.

    16 p. 21 cm.   **[7562]**
    Diss. — Franeker (J. Acker, *respondent*)

—Disputatio medica de hydrope ascite ... Franekerae, Ex typographia Johannis Wellens, 1674.

    [16] p. 19 cm.   **[7563]**
    Diss. — Franeker (S. Blankaart, *respondent*)

—Disputatio medica de passione iliaca ... Ultrajecti, Ex officina Meinardi à Dreunen, 1669.

    [16] p. 23 cm.   **[7564]**
    Diss. — Utrecht (J. von Flammerdinge, *respondent*)

—Disputatio medica de scorbuto ... Ultrajecti, Ex officina Jacobi à Doeyenburgh, 1668.

    14, [1] p. 23 cm.   **[7565]**
    Diss. — Utrecht (C. Heidanus, *respondent*)

—Disputatio medica de variolis et morbillis ... Trajecti ad Rhenum, Typis Joannis ab Eede, 1667.

    [16] p. 23 cm.   **[7566]**
    Diss. — Utrecht (M. Várady, *respondent*)

MATTHAEUS, Theophil [*fl.* 1659] *respondent.* See Conring, H., *praeses.* Disputatio inauguralis medica de peste. 1659, 1678.

MATTHAEUS PLATEARIUS. See Platearius, Matthaeus [*d.* 1161?]

MATTHESILANUS, Joannes Carolus. *See* Mattesillani, Giovanni Carlo [*b.* 1653]

MATTHIAE, Daniel Meno. Experimentorum medico-chymicorum decades tres, in annum MDCLXXIX, LXXX, LXXXI. que lectori communicant arcanissimas chymicorum medicaminum praeparationes ... Adjiciuntur observationes miscellaneae chymicae, medicae, anatomicae ... Mantissae loco annectitur Disceptatio de reformandis pharmacopoliis, & rei medicae superfluae ... rejectione. Cui succedit Pharmacopoea Cracoviensis Johan. Woynae ... Francofurti, Impensis Johannis Justi Erythropyli, typis Joh. Andreae, 1683.

    147 p.; 109 p. plates. 14 cm.   **[7567]**
    Part [2] has caption title: Decas arcanorum medico-chymicorum. Wanting the Disceptatio de reformandis pharmacopoliis, and Pharmacopoea Cracoviensis.

MATTHIOLUS, P. *See* Mattioli, Pietro Andrea [1500–1577]

MATTHIS, Johann Konrad [*fl.* 1669] *respondent.* Disputatio inauguralis medica de mania ... Argentorati, Typis Johannis Welperi, 1669.

    30, [1] p. 20 cm.   **[7568]**
    Diss. — Strasbourg.

MATTIOLI, Pietro Andrea [1500–1577] Opera quae extant omnia; hoc est, Commentarii in VI. libros Pedacii Dioscoridis Anazarbei De medica materia ... a Casparo Bauhino ... post diversarum editionum collationem infinitis locis aucti ... Adjectis plantarum iconibus, supra priores editiones plus quam trecentis ... ad vivum delinatis. De ratione distillandi aquas ex omnibus plantis: et quomodo genuini odores in ipsis aquis conservari possint. Item, Apologia in Amatum Lusitanum, cum censura in ejusdem Enarrationes. Epistolarum medicinalium libri quinque. Dialogus De morbo Gallico . . . Ed. alt. Basileae, Sumptibus Joannis König [Typis exscripsit Joh. Rodolphus Genath] 1674.

[119], 1027 (i.e. 1029), [22] p.; 236, [6] p.   illus.
36 cm.   [**7569**]

Imperfect: sig. a6 wanting.
A reprint of the 1598 Frankfurt am Main edition.
Apologia adversus Amathum Lusitanum has special title page.
Includes the text of Dioscorides in Latin translation by Jean Ruel.

—[Commentarii. French tr.] Les commentaires . . . sur les six livres de Pedacius Dioscoride Anazarbeen, de la matiere medecinale. Traduits de latin en françois par M. Antoine du Pinet: et illustrez de nouveau, d'un bon nombre de figures; & augmentez en plus de mille lieux à la derniere edition de l'autheur, tant de plusieurs remedes & diverses sortes de maladies; comme aussi des distillations, & de la cognoissance des simples . . . Lyon, Pierre Rigaud, 1619.

[130], 606 (i.e. 619), [33] p.   illus., port.   36 cm.
[**7570**]

Includes the text of Dioscorides in French translation.
"Bref discours de la distillation des eaux": p. 600-606.

—Another issue, with imprint date changed to 1620.   [**7571**]

Imperfect p. 7-8 and 57-58 mutilated, portrait wanting.

—[The same.] . . . Lyon, Claude Rigaud & Claude Obert, 1627.

[130], 603 (i.e. 605), [33] p.   ports.   36 cm.
[**7572**]

"Bref discours de la distillation des eaux": p. 597-603.

—[The same.] . . . Lyon, La vefve de Claude Rigaud, & Pierre & Claude Rigaud fils, 1642.

[130], 605, [32] p.   illus., ports.   36 cm.[**7573**]

—[The same.] . . . Augmentez tant de plusieurs remedes à diverses sortes de maladies: comme aussi d'un Traité de chymie en abregé, pour l'analyse, tant des vegetaux que de quelques animaux & minearaux, par un docteur en medecine. Dern. ed., rev., corr. & mise dans un meilleur langage . . . Lyon, Jean-Baptiste de Ville, 1680.

[8], xcv, [15], 636, [33] p.   illus., port.   37 cm.
[**7574**]

—[German tr.] Kreutterbuch . . . Jetzt widerumb mit vielen schönen newen Figuren, auch nützlichen Artzeneyen, und andern guten Stücken, zum dritten Mal . . . gemehret und verfertigt durch Joachimum Camerarium . . . Franckfurt am Mayn [Gedruckt bey Nicolao Hoffman, In Verlegung Jacob Fischers] 1611.

[10], 460, [27] ll.   illus.   41 cm.   [**7575**]

Apparently reprinted from the Frankfurt am Main edition of 1586.
"A German translation by Georg Handsch of the botanical portion of Mattioli's Commentaries, without the text of Dioscorides, but having the Epistola nuncupatoria, in Latin, prefixed."—BM Nat. Hist. Cat.
"Von Distillier und Brennöfen. Ein kurtzer leichter Begriff und Unterricht künstliche Distillier und Brennöfen mit zugehörender Bereitschafft zu machen": leaves 456-460.

—[The same.] . . . Franckfurt am Mayn, Gedruckt bey Jacob Fischers s. Erben [Bey Wolffgang Hoffman] 1626.

[10], 460, [27] ll.   illus.   36 cm.   [**7576**]

Imperfect: title page and following 2 leaves mended.
Different setting of type.

—[The same.] Neu vollkommenes Kräuter-Buch, von allerhand Gewächsen der Baumen, Stauden und Kräutern, die in Teutschland, Italien, Franckreich, und is andern Orten der Welt herfür kommen. In welchem ohnzahlbare treffliche Artzneyen wider alle Kranckheiten, so wol der Menschen als dess Viehs, neben ihrem ordenlichen Gebrauch, beschrieben werden . . . Erstlich an das Tagliecht gegeben von . . . Pietro Andrea Matthiolo . . . zum 4. Mal . . . aussgefertiget durch . . . Joachimum Camerarium. Jetzund aber als ein neues Werck . . . mit den besten Hauss-Artzney-Mittlen . . . für innerliche und äusserliche Kranckheiten verbessert und vermehret von Bernhard Verzascha . . . Basel, Gedruckt bey Johann-Jacob Decker, in Basel bey Jeremiae Mitzen sel. Erben, in Franckfurt und Ambsterdam aber bey Heinrich Wettstein zu finden, 1678.

[12], 792, [77] p.   illus., port.   36 cm.
[**7577**]

Added engraved half title.
Imperfect: 6 leaves at end (sig. 4F 3-4 and 4G⁴ (last leaf; blank?) wanting; sig. 4F 3-4 supplied in photocopy from the National Agricultural Library.

—[The same.] Theatrum botanicum; das ist, Neu vollkommenes Kräuter-Buch, worinnen allerhand Erdgewächse der Bümen, Stauden und Kräutern . . .

vorgestellet sind . . . Erstens zwar an das Tagliecht gegeben von Herrn Bernhard Verzascha, anjetzo aber in eine gantz neue Ordnung gebracht, auch mehr als umb die Helffte vermehret und verbessert durch Theodorum Zvingerum . . . Basel, Gedruckt durch Jacob Bertsche, in Franckfurt zu finden bey Joh. Phillip Richtern, 1696.

[II], 995, [53] p.   port.   36 cm.   [7578]
Added engraved half title.

—[Italian tr.] I discorsi . . . ne i sei libri di Pedacio Dioscoride Anazarbeo della materia medicinale. Dal suo istesso auttore innanzi la sua morte ricorretti, et in più di mille luoghi aumentati . . . Venetia, Marco Ginami [Appresso Andrea Muschio] 1621.

[154], 843, [8] p.   illus.   33 cm.   [7579]
Includes the text of Dioscorides in Mattioli's Italian translation. "Del modo di distillare le acque di tutte le piante, et como vi si possino conservare i loro veri odori, & sapori": [8] p. at end.

—[The same.] . . . Venetia, Marco Ginammi, 1645.

[148] , 842, [9] p.   illus.   33 cm.   [7580]

—See BLAWEN, Andreas de. Epistola . . . ad Petrum Andream Matthiolium. 1661; SCHOLTZ, L. Consiliorum medicinalium . . . liber singularis. 1610.

MATTSPERGER, LUCAS [*fl.* 1618]. *See* SEBISCH, M. [1578-1674?] *praeses.* Disputatio de alimentorun facultatibus prima. 1618.

MAUBEC, DENYS DE, *sieur de Copponay.* Vertus et usage de la medecine universelle, de . . . Denis de Copponay de Grimaldy . . . avec un traité à l'avantage des vomitifs, soûtenu par les plus grands medecins de l'antiquité . . . Reimprimé pour la seconde fois . . . [Geneve? not before 1678]

96 p.   14 cm.   [7581]

MAUCHART, JOHANN DAVID [*fl.* 1691-1692] *respondent. See* CAMERARIUS, E. R., *praeses.* Disputatio inauguralis medica de febre tertiana maligna. 1692; ZELLER, J. G., *praeses.* Infanticidas non absolvit nec a tortura liberat nec respirationem foetus in utero tollit. 1691.

MAUCKISCH, JOHANN [*fl.* 1647] *praeses.* Aphorismi physici de pluvia . . . Lipsiae, Typis Henningi Cöleri [1647]

[20] p.   19 cm.   [7582]
Diss.—Leipzig (C. Funck, *respondent*)

MAUDEN, DAVID VAN [*d. ca.* 1612] Bedieninghe der anatomien, dat is: Maniere ende onderrichtinghe om perfectelijck des menschen lichaem t'anatomizeren, na de leeringhe Galeni, Vesallii, Faloppii ende Aranti, achtervolghende de figuren ende characteren oft letteren der Anatomie Vesalii en Valverde, van Plantino anno 1583 ende nu an. 1646 door Cornelis Danckertsz, int Nederlants ghedrukt . . . Amsterdam, Cornelis Danckertsz., 1646.

101, [2] p.   illus.   30 cm.   [7583]
Bound with Valverde, J. de. A. Vesalii en Valverda Anatomie. 1647.

[**MAUDUIT,** MICHEL, *Father,* 1644-1709] Dissertation sur la goutte, tant la chaude que la froide . . . 2. ed. rev. & augm. Paris, Laurent d'Houry, 1689.

[16], 188, 6 p.   17 cm.   [7584]
"Le remede du prieur de Cabriere, pour la guerison des décentes ou hernies": 6 p. at end.

—Dissertation sur la goutte. *See* [OZON, P.] Reponse a la dissertation sur la goutte [par M. Mauduit] 1690.

MAUL, JOHANN PHILIPP [*fl.* 1686] *respondent.* Disputatio medica inauguralis de abortu . . . Lugduni Batavorum, Apud Abrahamum Elzevier, 1686.

[16] p.   22 cm.   [7585]
Diss.—Leyden.

MAURER, JOSEPH. *See* MURER, Josias [1564-1630?]

MAURICE DE TOULON, *Father* [*d.* 1668] Le capucin charitable, enseignant la methode pour remedier aux grandes miseres que la peste a coûtume de causer parmy les peuples . . . Paris, La veuve Thierry, 1662.

[25], 407, [1] p.   front.   17 cm.   [7586]

—Trattato politico da pratticarsi ne' tempi di peste, circa gl'ordini communi, e particolari dell'infermarie, purgationi, e quarantene. Nel quale se risponde a chi contradice a' profumi. E si pondera la carità de' padri capuccini, mostrata verso gl'infetti l'anno 1656. e 57. Composta dal padre Mauritio de Tolone sacerdote capuccino . . . E tradotta da un religioso dell'istesso ordine. Genova, Pietro Giovanni Calenzani, 1661.

[16], 134 p.; [6], 3-129, [6] p.   front.   22 cm.   [7587]
Imperfect: sig. I4, part I (blank) wanting.
Part 2 has special title page.

MAURICEAU, François [1637-1709] Des maladies des femmes grosses et accouchees. Avec la ... méthode de les bien aider en leurs accouchemens naturels, & les moyens de remedier à tous ceux qui sont contre-nature, & aux indispositions des enfans nouveau-nés: ensemble une ... description de toutes les parties de la femme qui sont destinées à la generation ... Paris, Jean Henault, Jean d'Houry, Robert de Ninville, Jean Baptiste Coignara [Charles Coignard] 1668.

[26], 536 p. illus., port. 25 cm. [**7588**]
Added engraved title page.
Imperfect: p. 27-28 wanting.

—[The same.] Traité des maladies des femmes grosses, et de celles qui sont nouvellement aecouchées [sic], enseignant la ... methode pour bien aider les femmes en leurs accouchemens naturels, & les moyens de remedier à tous ceux qui sont contre nature, & aux indispositions des enfans nouveaux-nés; avec une description ... de toutes les parties de la femme qui servent à la generation ... 2. ed., corr. par l'auteur, & augm. ... de plus d'un tiers du discours, contenant toutes les plus particulieres observations touchant la pratique des accouchemens ... Paris, L'auteur, 1675.

[18], 501, [25] p. illus., port. 25 cm. [**7589**]
Imperfect: added engraved title page wanting.

—[The same.] ... 3. ed. ... Paris, L'auteur, 1681.
[17], 515, [21] p. illus., port. 26 cm. [**7590**]
Added engraved title page with title in Latin: De mulierum praegnantium, parturientium, et puerperarum morbis tractatus.

—[The same.] ... Derniere ed. ... [Lyon?] Suivant la copie imprimée a Paris, 1682.
[18], 437, [27] p. illus., plates, port. 22 cm. [**7591**]
Added engraved title page.
Probably one of the pirated editions published by "plusieurs libraires à Lyons," mentioned in the "Avertissement" in the author's Observations sur la grossesse et l'accouchement des femmes, Paris, 1695.

—Another issue, with imprint date changed to 1683. [**7592**]

—[The same.] ... *In* La Bibliotheque des acoucheurs et des sages-femmes. 1693.

—[The same.] ... 4. éd. ... Paris, Laurent d'Houry [Jean Anisson] 1694.

2 v. in 1 ([12], 555, [25] p.; [8], 572, [12] p.) front. (port.), illus. 26 cm. [**7593**]
Imperfect: p. 27-30 of v. [1] wanting.
Part [2] has special title page: Observations sur la grossesse et l'accouchement des femmes, et sur leurs maladies & celles des enfans nouveau-nez ... Paris, L'auteur, 1694. The two works were also issued separately.
"Aphorismes, touchant la grossesse, l'accouchement, les maladies, & autres dispositions des femmes" (pt. [1], p. 531-555) was also published separately in the same year.

—[Latin tr.] De mulierum praegnantium, parturientium, et puerperarum morbis tractatus; tradens ... methodum adjuvandi mulieres in partu naturali, & medendi cuilibet partui contra naturam, morbisque infantium recens-natorum; cum ... descriptione omnium mulieris partium generationi inservientium ... Parisiis, Apud auctorem, 1681.

[17], 358, [16] p. illus., port. 26 cm. [**7594**]
Added engraved title page.
Translated by the author from the 3d French ed., issued in the same year. Cf. Praefatio ad exteros.

—[Dutch tr.] Tractaet van de siektens der swangere vrouwen en der gene die eerst gebaert hebben. Aenwysende de rechte en ware manier om de vrouwen in hare natuurlyke baringen wel te helpen, de geboortens tegens de natuur te recht te brengen, en de siektens der jong-geborene kinderen te genesen ... Uit het Frans vertaelt. Amsterdam, Albert Magnus [1683?]

[16], 408, [23] p. illus., port. 21 cm. [**7595**]
Added engraved title page.
Translated from the 3d French ed. of 1681. Cf. Voor-reden.

—[English tr.] The accomplisht midwife, treating of the diseases of women with child, and in child-bed. As also, the best direction how to help them in natural and unnatural labours. With fit remedies for the several indispositions of new-born babes ... Written in French ... Translated, and enlarged with some marginal notes, by Hugh Chamberlen ... London, Printed by John Darby, and sold by Benjamin Billingsley. 1673.

[22], 437 (i.e. 439), [7] p. plates. 18 cm. [**7596**]
Imperfect: 2 plates wanting (one with 3 illus. at p. 158 and one depicting instruments at p. 285)
The "Traité anatomique des parties de la femme qui sont destinées à la generation" has not been translated in this edition, but was included in later English editions.
The translation, by the elder Hugh Chamberlen, has been erroneously attributed to his son of the same name.

—[The same.] The diseases of women with child, and in child-bed; as also the best means of helping them in natural and unnatural labours. With fit remedies for the several indispositions of new-born babes. To which is prefix'd an Anatomical treatise ... Written in French ... Translated by Hugh Chamberlen, M. D. The 3d ed., corr. London, Andrew Bell, 1697.

    xlvii, [1], 352 p. plates. 18 cm.   **[7597]**
"An anatomical treatise of the parts of a woman destin'd to generation": p. xv–xli.

—[German tr.] Tractat von Kranckheiten schwangerer und gebärender Weibs-Personen, in welchem beschrieben wird die warhafte und eigentliche Weise, wie denselben, so wol bey natürlicher als nicht natürlicher Gebärung beyzuspringen: auch der übeln Disposition und Beschaffenheit neugeborner Kindern zu helffen seye: samt einem ordentlichen Entwurff der weiblichen Geburtsgliedern ... Zum erstenmal ... auss dem Frantzösischen in das Teutsche übersetzet. Basel, Jacob Bertsche, 1680.

    [14], 34, 398 p. plates, port. 21 cm. **[7598]**
Added engraved title page.
Translated from the 2d French ed. of 1675. Cf. Des Verlegers Vorrede.

—[The same.] Der schwangern und kreistenden Weibs-Personen allerbeste Hülffleistung; das ist; Wahrer und gründlicher Bericht, wie denenselben, mit gutem und füglichem Vortheil, in ihrem sowol natürlichen, als unterweilen auch wider die Natur lauffenden Kind-haben glücklich beyzustehen. Ingleichem, was vor bewährte und hochstdienliche Mittel denen neugebornen Kindern, in ihren Unpässlichkeiten, zu gebrauchen; und dann, was es vor eine eigentliche Beschaffenheit mit denen zum Kinderzeugen gewidmeten Gliedern und Theilen der Weibs-Personen habe ... Erstesmals in französischer Sprache verfasset ... Nachmals aber, von einem Liebhaber der Arzney-Kunst, ins Teutsche übersetzet, und zum Druck befördert. Nürnberg, In Verlegung Johann Hofmanns Buch-und Kunsthändlers gedruckt bey Andreas Knorzen, 1681.

    [15], 607 p. plates, port. 17 cm.   **[7599]**
Added engraved title page.
Translated from the 1st French ed. of 1668.

—[Italian tr.] Trattato delle malattie delle donne gravide e delle infantate, che insegna il metodo ...

per aiutar le donne ne' parti naturali, ed il mezo di rimediare à que', che sono contro natura, ed a' fanciulli, che nascono; con una descrizione ... di tutte le parti della donna, che servono alla generazione ... Cologni, Gio. Luigi Du-Four, 1684.

    [12], 485 (i.e. 427), [1] p. illus. 22 cm.
                                     [7600]
Translated from the 2d French ed., 1675.

—Observations sur la grossesse et l'accouchement des femmes, et sur leurs maladies & celles des engans nouveau-nez. En chacune desquelles les causes & les raisons des principaux évenemens sont décrites & expliquées ... Paris, L'auteur, 1695.

    [8], 406, [9] p. 22 cm.   **[7601]**
Reprinted from the edition in larger format published in 1694 with his Traité des maladies des femmes grosses, et de celles qui sont accouchées, 4. éd., of which it formed vol. 2.

—*See* PEU, P. La pratique des acouchemens. 1694.

MAURICIUS, THEODOR [*fl.* 1677] *respondent. See* CRAUSE, R. W., *praeses.* Dissertatio medica inauguralis de cachexia. 1677.

MAURICK, WILLEM VAN [*fl.* 1657] *respondent.* Disputatio medica inauguralis, de epilepsia ... Trajecti ad Rhenum, Apud Johannem à Hulshuysen, 1657.

    [12] p. 20 cm.   **[7602]**
Diss.—Utrecht.

MAURIN, JEAN [*fl.* 1696] Lettre de M^r M*** docteur en medecine a son ami. Par laquelle on connoit les raisons qui ont engagé les anciens à n'admettre point de circulation du sang, & celles des novateurs à se détacher des sentimens des anciens. [Paris? 1696?]

    24 p. 15 cm.   **[7603]**
With this is bound *his* Lettre par laquelle on fait connoistre le temps auquel il faut saigner. [Paris? 1696?]

—Lettre par laquelle on fait connoistre le temps auquel il faut saigner & purger, & le nombre de ceux qui contredisent les medecins. [Paris? 1696?]

    30 p. 15 cm.   **[7604]**
Bound with *his* Lettre de M^r M*** ... a son ami. [Paris? 1696?]

MAURIN, RAPHAEL [*fl.* 1678–1700] *praeses.* Quaestio medica ... An subtilis materia cum aëre juncta aegrum sanat, & corpus animae domicilium conservat? [Parisiis, Apud Franciscum Muguet, 1700]

    4 p. 26 cm.   **[7605]**

Caption title.
Diss. — Paris (L. F. Dutal, *respondent*)

MAURITIUS, THEODORUS. *See* MAURICIUS, Theodor [*fl.* 1677]

MAURIZIO DA TOLONE. *See* MAURICE DE TOULON, *Father* [*d.* 1668]

MAURUS. *See* HRABANUS MAURUS, *Abp. of Mainz* [784?-856]

MAUSSAC, PHILIPPE JACQUES DE, *ca.* 1590-1650. Animadversiones. *In* Aristoteles. Περι ζωων ιστοριας ... Historia de animalibus. 1619.

— *See* HARPOCRATION, V. Λεξικὸν τῶν δέκα ῥητόρων ... Lexicon decem oratorum. 1683.

MAVIUS, ANDREAS VALENTIN [*fl.* 1665] *respondent.* *See* SCHMIDT, B., *praeses.* Exercitatio physiologica de hominis aetatibus. 1655.

MAVROCORDATOS, ALEXANDER [1641-1709] Pneumaticum instrumentum circulandi sanguinis; sive, De motu, & usu pulmonum ... Francofurti, Sumptibus Thomae Matthiae Götzii, 1665.

[8], 181, [2] p. 14 cm. [7606]

MAXIMILIAN GANDOLPH VON KUENBURG. *See* GANDOLF, Maximilian, *count, Cardinal, Prince-Archbishop of Salzburg* [*d.* 1687]

MAXIMUS VALERIUS. *See* STERRE, Dionysius van der [*d.* 1691]

MAXWELL, WILLIAM [*fl. ca.* 1676] De medicina magnetica libri III. In quibus tam theoria quam praxis continetur; opus novum ... ubi multa naturae secretissima miracula panduntur, spiritus vitalis operationes hactenus incognitae revelantur, totiusque hujus secretae artis fundamenta firmissimis rationibus experientia fultis ponuntur ... Edente Georgio Franco ... Francofurti, Sumptib. Joannis Petri Zubrodt, 1679.

[21], 200, [1] p. 15 cm. [7607]

Of the projected third book, "De dolore capitis", the author completed only one chapter (p. 191-200)

"De anima et spiritu universali & particulari aphorismi perutiles, quibus tota pene magia naturalis continetur": p. 167-189.

Bound with Theatrum sympatheticum. 1661.

— [German tr.] Drey Bücher der magnetischen Artzney-Kunst, worinnen so wol die Theorie als Practic, wie auch viel Neues ... und höchst,

Nützliches enthalten. So dann viel geheime Natur-Wunder geoffenbaret, die bisher unbekannte Würckungen des Lebens-Geistes entdecket ... An Tag gegeben ... durch Georgium Francken ... Anjetzo aber ... übersetzet von einem Liebhaber der Philosof. Franckfurt, Zu finden bey Joh. Ziegern, 1687.

[24], 282 (i.e. 280) p. 14 cm. [7608]

MAY, EDWARD [*fl.* 1633-1637] A most certaine and true relation of a strange monster or serpent found in the left ventricle of the heart of John Pennant ... London, George Miller, 1639.

[6], 40 p. 2 plates. 19 cm. [7609]

Imperfect: one plate wanting.
STC 17709.

MAY, HEINRICH [1632-1696] *praeses.* Disputatio medico-physiologica de calido innato et humido radicali ... Marpurgi Cattorum, Typis Salomonis Schadewitzii, 1674.

[14] p. 19 cm. [7610]

Diss. — Marburg (J. G. Winther, *respondent*)

— Disquisitio physica de animae rationalis ortu ... Marburgi Cattorum, Typis Salomonis Schadewitzii, 1676.

[12] p. 19 cm. [7611]

Diss. — Marburg (J. G. Heinius, *respondent*)

MAY, JOHANN BURCHARD. *See* MAJUS, Johann Burchard [1652-1726]

MAY, PHILIPPE [*fl.* 1665-1670] Chiromantia medica. Mitt einem Anhang von den Zeichen auff den Nägeln der Finger. Nebens einem Tractätlein von der Physiognomia medica. 's Graven-Haag, Levyn von Dyck, 1667.

[16], 158 p. plates. 15 cm. [7612]

— Another issue. [7613]

Erratum differs.

— [The same.] ... 's Graven-Haag, Levyn von Dyck, 1669.

[16], 158 p. plates. 15 cm. [7614]

Different setting of type.

— [The same.] ... Anjezo vermehret und durch Erfahrung noch deutlicher gemacht. Dressden, In Verlegung Andreae Löfflers, getruckt mit Seyfferts Schrifften, 1670.

[16], 208, [6 +] p. plates. 16 cm. [7615]

Imperfect: all after p. [6] at end wanting.

—[The same.] ... Mit einem Anhange von den Zeichen auff den Nägeln der Finger ... wie auch dessen noch nie in Druck gekommene Chiromantia curiosa ... An vielen Orten ... vermehret ... Dressden und Leipzig, Verlegts Johann Christoph Mieth, Druckts Christian Banckmann, 1691.

197, [9] p.   plates.   16 cm.   [7616]

—[French tr.] La chiromancie medicinale. Accompagnée d'un traité de La physionomie, & d'un autre des marques qui paroissent sur les ongles des doigts ... Traduit en françois par Philippe Henry Treuchses ... La Haye, Levijn van Dyck, 1665.

[14], 136 p.   plates.   15 cm.   [7617]

Imperfect: p. 79-80 mutilated.

—See HERLINUS, B. Consilium sanitatis. 1682.

MAY, THEODORUS. *See* MAJUS, Theodor [*fl.* 1610-1623]

MAYER, JOHANNES. *See* MARIUS, Johann.

MAYER, LUDWIG KASPAR [*fl.* 1693-1694] *respondent.* Prodromus de medicamentorum viperinorum usu ... [Altdorffii] Henricus Meyer [1694]

24 p.   20 cm.   [7618]

Diss. — Altdorf.

—*See* KIRCHMAYER, G. K., *praeses.* Metallo-metamorphosis. 1693.

MAYER, MARTIN [*fl.* 1624-1637] Kurtze Beschreibung dess egerischen Schleder-Sawerbrunnens, was vor Mineralien derselbe mit sich führe, was derselben Tugenden seyn, und auff was Weise derselbe recht zu gebrauchen seye. Nürmberg, Woffgang Endter, 1637.

[8], 170, [2] p.   13 cm.   [7619]

—[The same.] ... [Nürmberg? 1666?]

[8], 170 + p.   17 cm.   [7620]

Imperfect: title page, p. 161-162 and all after p. 170 wanting.
The text is of the same setting as the 1637 ed., the preliminaries are of a different setting of type.
Bound with Horst, J.D. Kurtze Beschreibung. 1659.

—[The same.] ... Welchen beygefüget ein besonder Tractätlein Von Natur, Krafft, Würckung und Gebrauch dess egerischen gebräuchlichen Säuerlings ... Nürnberg, In Verlegung Christoph Endters, 1667.

[8], 163, [3] p.; [6], 105, [2] p.   14 cm.
                                        [7621]

Part [2] has special title page.

—*respondent. See* SCHALLER, W., *praeses.* Sesquicenturia positionum medicarum de arthritide. 1625; SENNERT, D., *praeses.* Positiones medicae de singultu. 1624.

MAYER, MICHAEL VON. *See* MAIER, Michael [1568?-1622]

MAYERNE, LOUIS TURQUET DE [*ca.* 1550-1618] *tr.* *See* AGRIPPA VON NETTESHEIM, H. C. Paradoxe sur l'incertitude. 1603.

MAYERNE, *Sir* THÉODORE TURQUET DE [1573-1655] Opera medica, complectentia consilia, epistolas et observationes, pharmacopeam, variasque medicamentorum formulas. Duobus libris comprehensa, et jam in lucem edita, opera & cura Josephi Browne ... Londini, R. E., 1700.

[16], 400 p.; 222, [1], 142 p.   port.   42 cm.
                                        [7622]

—The distiller of London. Compiled and set forth by the speciall license and command of the Kings most excellent Majesty: for the sole use of the Company of Distillers of London. And by them to bee duly observed and practized. London, Richard Bishop, 1639.

[1], 67, [1] p.   plate.   27 cm.   [7623]

Jointly edited by *Sir* Théodore Turquet de Mayerne and *Sir* Thomas Cademan.
STC 16777.

—[The same.] The distiller of London: with the clavis to unlock the deepest secrets of that mysterious art. With many additions of the most excellent cordial waters which have been pen'd by our most able doctors and physicians ... London, Tho. Huntington and Wil. Nealand, 1652.

[22], 167 p.   15 cm.   [7624]

A reprint of the 1639 edition with the addition of "Choice cordial waters" (p. 71-167)

—Medicinal councels, or advices. Written originally in French ... Put out in Latine ... by Theoph. Bonetus, M.D. Englished by Tho. Sherley ... London, N. Ponder, 1677.

[14], 136, [7] p.   15 cm.   [7625]

Imperfect: title page and first preliminary leaf wanting.
With this is bound *his* A treatise of the gout. 1676.

—La pratique de medecine ... Avec Le regime des femmes grosses, et un traité de la goutte ... Lyon, Anisson & Posuel, 1693.

[12], 552, [43] p.   19 cm.   [7626]

Imperfect: title page mutilated.

—Praxeos Mayernianae in morbis internis praecipue gravioribus & chronicis syntagma, ex adversariis, consiliis ac epistolis ejus . . . concinnatum. Londini, Impensis Sam. Smith, 1690.

[24], 451, [20] p. 19 cm. [7627]

"Gualteri Charletoni M. D. Praeloquium": sig. A4-6.

Contents: I. De affectibus capitis. — II. De affectibus thoracis. — III. De affectibus abdominis.

—[The same.] Praxis medica: ad exemplar Londinense 1690. impressum, recusa. Cui accessit . . . libellus plane singularis, De cura gravidarum . . . Augustae Vindelicorum, Apud Laur. Kronicerum & haered. Theophili Göbelii, 1691.

[II], 606, [32], 56 p. 17 cm. [7628]

—Praxeos Mayernianae ex adversariis, consiliis ac epistolis ejus summa cura ac diligentia concinnatum syntagma alterum, quatuor tractatus continens: viz. I. De febribus, II. De morbis externis. III. De arthritide. IV. De lue venerea. Londini, Sam. Smith & Benj. Walford, 1695.

[7], 283, [5], 16 p. 20 cm. [7629]

—Tractatus de arthritide. Accesserunt ejusdem consilia aliquot medicinalia. Emittente Theoph. Boneto . . . Londini, Impensis Mosis Pitt [1676]

[6], 188, [13] p. 15 cm. [7630]

Imperfect: title page mutilated affecting imprint date.

Imprint date supplied from NUC.

"Consilium in epilepsia": p. 179-188.

Bound with Starkey, G. A brief examination. 1664.

—[English tr.] A treatise of the gout. Written originally in the French tongue . . . Englished . . . by Thomas Sherley . . . Whereunto is added, Advice about hypochondriacal-fits . . . London, D. Newman, 1676.

[14], 116, [4] p. 15 cm. [7631]

Bound with *his* Medicinal councels. 1677.

—, *ed. See* MOFFETT, T. Insectorum, sive minimorum animalium theatrum. 1634.

—*See* The compleat midwife's practice enlarged. 1663, 1697, 1698; [RIOLAN, J., 1580-1657] Apologia pro Hippocratis et Galeni medicina. 1603.

MAYERNE TURQUET, LOUIS DE. *See* MAYERNE, Louis Turquet de [*ca.* 1550-1618]

MAYERNE TURQUET, THÉODORE DE. *See* MAYERNE, *Sir* Théodore Turquet de [1573-1655]

MAYNWARING, EVERARD [1628-1699?] The efficacy and extent of true purgation . . . Distinguished from promiscuous evacuations; injuriously procured, and falsly reputed purging . . . London, D. Browne and R. Clavel, 1696.

[I], 34 p. 20 cm. [7632]

—The history and mystery of the venereal lues concisely abstracted and modelled . . . from serious strict perpensions, and critical collations of divers repugning sentiments . . . of . . . English, French, German . . . dissenting writers . . . With animadversions upon various methods of cure, practised in those several nations . . . London, J. M., 1673.

[8], 215 p. 18 cm. [7633]

—[Latin tr.] Historia et mysterium luis venereae; utrumque concise abstractum et formatum ex seriis perpensionibus & criticis collationibus diversarum repugnantium opinionum . . . medicorum Anglorum, Gallorum, Hispanorum . . . dissentientium scriptorum . . . una cum animadversionibus super diversas methodos curationum praedictis nationibus in usu . . . Francofurti & Hamburgi, Impensis Joannis Naumanni & Georgii Wolffii, 1675.

176 p. 17 cm. [7634]

Bound with copy 2 of Fedele, F. De relationibus medicorum libri quatuor. 1674.

—Ignota febris. Fevers mistaken, in doctrine and practice. Shewing how they assurge; and whereon they depend. Hinting the proper means of allay and extinction; adapt to the true notion thereof. By E[verard] M[aynwaring] Med. D. . . . [London, 1691?]

8 p. 22 cm. [7635]

Caption title.

—Ignota febris. Fevers mistaken in notion & practice. Shewing the frequent fatal consequents thereof . . . With remarks upon bleeding, blistering, juleps, and the Jesuit pouder, in fevers . . . London, Printed by J. Dawks and sold by D. Brown, 1698.

[4], 157, [I] p. 18 cm. [7636]

Imperfect: p. 45-46 mutilated.

—Medicus absolutus . . . the compleat physitian, qualified and dignified. The rise and progress of physick, historically, chronologically, and philosophically illustrated . . . London, 1668.

[22], 169, [4] p. port. 17 cm. [7637]

Imperfect: portrait wanting.

—The method and means of enjoying health, vigour, and long life. Adapting peculiar courses, for different constitutions, ages, abilities, valetudinary states ... and passions of mind ... London, Printed by J. M. for Dorman Newman, 1683.

[28], 211 p. 18 cm. [7638]

Published in 1669 as part [1] of Vita sana & longa.

—Monarchia microcosmi: The origin, vicissitudes, and period of vital government in man. For a farther discovery of diseases, incident to human nature ... London, John Everingham, 1692.

[1], 57 p.; 52 p.; 39 p.; 20, [5] p. 15 cm. [7639]

—Morbus polyrhizos et polymorphaeus. A treatise of the scurvy ... The 2d ed. rev. and enl. by the author ... London, Printed by J. D. for H. Broom, 1666.

[16], 134, [2] p. 16 cm. [7640]

"Antiscorbutick and catholick medicines ..." (p. [93]–134) has special title page dated also 1666.

—[The same.] ... The 3d impression with additions. Traversing some ... hypotheses of Dr. Willis upon the scurvy. With a considerable inquiry ... of tobacco, relating to this disease. London, G. Sawbridge, 1669.

[24], 230, [2] p. 17 cm. [7641]

—[The same.] ... With a true account of tobacco, relating to this disease. The 4th impr. corr. and augm. ... Whereunto is annexed Pharmacopoeia domestica. London, Printed by J. M. and sold by Peter Parker, 1672.

[7], 259, [2] p. front. (port.) 18 cm. [7642]

Pharmacopoeia domestica; sive, Repositorium Hippocraticum, has special title page (p. [239]).

—Another issue, with new title page dated 1679. [7643]

—The mystery of curing comprehensively, explained and proved, argumentatively & practically in three parts ... 2d impr., rev. and augm. .... London, W. Crook and J. Everingham, 1694.

[4], 28, 4 p. 22 cm. [7644]

—Nova medendi ratio, a short and easie method of curing. Exemplified by a ternary of radical medicines, universal in their respective classes, viz. purgation, transpiration, roboration. Compleating these three grand operations for cure in all diseases ... London, Printed by J. Dover for M. Speed, 1666.

[8], 34, [1] p. 20 cm. [7645]

—Pains afflicting humane bodies ... Shewing the tendency, of chronick, and acute diseases, for a seasonable prevention of fatal events. With a tract of issues and setons ... London, Henry Bonwicke, 1682.

[8], 229, [2] p. front. (port.) 19 cm. [7646]

—Praxis medicorum antiqua & nova: the ancient and modern practice of physick examined, stated, and compared ... With enforcing arguments for a return, and general conformity to the primitive practice ... London, Printed by J. M. and sold by T. Archer, 1671.

[2], 107, [1] p. 19 cm. [7647]

—A serious debate, and general concern, relating to health and sickness. By E[verard] M[aynwaring] Med. D. The 2d impression with a postscript ... [London, Thomas Basset and Thomas Horne, 1689]

8 p. 23 cm. [7648]

Caption title.
Imperfect: p. 7-8 mutilated.

—Solamen aegrorum, sive ternarius medicamentorum chymicorum ad omnes fere morbos curandum ... maxime deploratos & grandes, felicissime inventa remedia, in purgando, excudando, roborando, arcana in effectu potentissima ast mitissima in modo agendi ... Londini, Excusum per G. M. pro Gulielmo Crooke, 1665.

[15], 40, [8] p. 15 cm. [7649]

—Tabidorum narratio: a treatise of consumptions, scorbutick atrophies, tabes Anglica, hectick fevers, phthisicks, spermatick and venereous wasting. Radically demonstrating their nature and cures from vital and morbifick causes ... London, T. Basset, 1667.

[12], 107, [1] p. 15 cm. [7650]

—Tutela sanitatis; sive, Vita protracta. The protection of long life, and detection of its brevity, from diatetic causes and common customs ... With a treatise of fontinells or issues. Whereunto is annexed Bellum necessarium; sive, Medicus belligerans, the military or practical physitian reveiwing his armory

... London, Printed by Peter Lillicrap and sold by S. Thompson and T. Basset, 1664.

[24], 120 p. 16 cm.	[**7651**]

—Vita sana & longa. The preservation of health, and prolongation of life, proposed and proved ... London, J. D., 1669.

[8], 160 p.; 123, [3] p. 18 cm.	[**7652**]

Imperfect: portrait wanting; title page mutilated.

Part [1] published in 1683 under title: The method and means of enjoying health.

Part [2] has special title page: The pharmacopoeian physician's repository.

MAYOLUS, SIMON. See MAIOLUS, Simon [*fl.* 1565–1597]

MAYOW, JOHN [1640–1679] Tractatus quinque medico-physici. Quorum primus agit De sal-nitro, et spiritu nitro-aereo. Secundus De respiratione. Tertius De respiratione foetus in utero, et ovo. Quartus De motu musculari, et spiritibus animalibus. Ultimus De rhachitide ... Oxonii, E Theatro Sheldoniano, 1674.

[39], 335 p.; 152 p. front. (port.) plates. 19 cm.	[**7653**]

Imperfect: portrait wanting.

Part 2 has half title: Tractatus quartus.

Fulton(B) 108.

—[The same.] ... Opera omnia medico-physica, tractatibus quinque comprehensa ... Ed. nov. ... Hagae-Comitum, Apud Arnoldum Leers, 1681.

[8], 416, [23] p. plates. port. 17 cm.	[**7654**]

Fulton(B) 109.

—[De rachitide. English.] The mothers' family physician; or, The infants doctor. Being a discourse of the disease in children, commonly called the rickets ... to which is added a profitable Appendix touching weights, and measures used in the composition of medicines, and giving of medicinal doses ... Oxford, Printed by L. Litchfield for J. Cox, 1687.

[19], 100 p.; [1], 17, [11] p. plate. 15 cm.	[**7655**]

Fulton(B) 121.

—Tractatus duo quorum prior agit De respiratione: alter De rachitide ... Oxon., Excudebat Hen. Hall, impensis Ric. Davis, 1669.

[1], 108 p. plates. 16 cm.	[**7656**]

Tractatus secundus has special title page dated 1668.

Fulton(B) 105.

—[The same.] ... Lugd. Batavor., Apud Felicem Lopez de Haro, Cornelium Driehuysen, 1671.

[2], 57 p. plates. 16 cm.	[**7657**]

Bound with Bartholin, T. De hepatis exautorati desperata causa. 1666.

Fulton(B) 106.

MAYR, MARTIN. See MAYER, Martin [*fl.* 1624–1637]

MAYR, MICHAEL [*fl.* 1615] *respondent.* See MENZEL, A., *praeses.* Disputatio medica de dolore. 1615.

MAYSSONIER, PIERRE. See MEYSSONIER, Pierre.

MAZARIN, JULES, *Cardinal* [1602–1661] *See* LA JUSTE refutation. 1649.

MAZZA, ANTONIO [*fl.* 1681] Historiarum epitome de rebus Salernitanis, in quibus origo, situs ... Hippocraticum collegium, ac aliae res ad Salernitanam urbem spectantes dilucidantur ... Neapoli, Jo. Francisci Paci, 1681.

[12], 160, [15] p. front. 21 cm.	[**7658**]

Imperfect: frontispiece wanting.

MAZZA, NICOLÒ [*fl.* 1617] *See* VECOLI, B. Della preparazione della pietra lazzoli. 1617.

MEAD, MATTHEW [1630?–1699] An appendix to Solomon's prescription for the removal of the pestilence, enforcing the same from a consideration of the late dreadful judgement by fire ... By M[atthew] M[ead] [n. p.] 1667.

[1], 161 p. 18 cm.	[**7659**]

MEARA, DERMITIUS DE [*fl.* 1610] Pathologia haereditaria generalis. *In* Meara, E. de. Examen Diatribae Thomae Willisii ... de febribus. 1665, 1667.

MEARA, EDMUNDUS DE [*d.* 1680] Examen Diatribae Thomae Willisii ... de febribus. Cui accesserunt Historiae aliquot medicae rariores ... Londini, Typis J. Flesher, prostat venale apud Octav. Pulleyn juniorem, 1665.

[13], 240, [3] p.; [4] 241-315, [3] p. 17 cm.	[**7660**]

Added engraved title page.

Last leaf (blank) wanting.

Part [2] has special title page: Pathologia haereditaria generalis; sive, De morbis haereditariis tractatus spagyrico-dogmaticus ... authore Dermutio de Meara.

—[The same.] ... Amstelodami, Apud Gerardem Schagen, 1667.

233, [1] p. 15 cm.	[**7661**]

Added engraved title page.

"Pathologia haereditaria generalis; sive, De morbis haereditariis tractatus spagyrico-dogmaticus ... authore Dermutio de Meara" (p. [179]–233, [1]) has special title page.

—*See* LOWER, R. Diatribae Thomae Willisii. 1665, 1666.

MEARE. *See* [PEACHIE, John] Some observations made upon Molucco nutts. 1672.

MEBER, JOANNES CORNELIUS [*fl.* 1687] Anchora sauciatorum; hoc est, Liquor stypticus, sanguinem confestim, & moraculose sistens ... Accessere in hac nova ed. ... descriptiones aquarum stypticarum D. La Faeur, & D. L'Emery. Vratislaviae, Apud Joh. Adam. Kaestnerum, 1687.

    [8], 272 p.   16 cm.   [7662]

"Ad anchoram sauciatorum ... observationes ...": p. [113]–263.

MECHOV, WILHELM [*fl.* 1677] *respondent. See* MEIBOM, H., *praeses.* Consideratio medica. 1677.

MEDECIN chrestien et sans interest. Femmes en travail d'enfant. Paris, 1679.

    8 p.   24 cm.   [7663]

Caption title.

MEDECIJN-boeck. *See* ASSER, H. van. Myn Heer.

Le MEDECIN de soi-même. 1682, 1687, 1699. *See* [DEVAUX, J.]

Le MEDECIN des-interressé, ou l'on trouver a l'elite de plusieurs remedes infaillibles ... Le tout recueilly par les soins d'un docteur en medecine: il cite à chaque recepte les noms des medecins qui les ont données & éprouvées. Paris, Pierre Aubouyn, Pierre Emery, et Charles Clouzier, 1695.

    [16], 151, [1] p.   16 cm.   [7664]

Le MEDECIN et le chirurgien des pauvres. 1671. *See* [DUBÉ, P.]

Le MEDECIN reformé. Quatrain, au medecin charitable ... Faict par A. D. P. C. apotiquaire. [Paris?] 1623.

    8 p.   17 cm.   [7665]

In verse.

Bound with Guibert, P. Le medecin charitable. 1623.

La MEDECINE domestique, contenant Le gouvernement de la santé, L'apothiquaire, Le chirurgien, & Le medecin charitable. Avec une

Harangue de la goutee à messieurs ses hostes. Geneve, Jean Herman Widerhold, 1673.

    5 parts in 1 v.   18 cm.   [7666]

Each part has special title page.

With this is bound Beynon, Elias. Le samaritain charitable. [1673]

La MEDECINE pretendüe reformée. *See* BEZANÇON, G. de.

MEDELA medicorum; or, An enquiry into the reasons & grounds of the contempt of physicians. *See* STANES, W.

MEDICAEUS, Joannes Jacobus, Marchio Mariniani. *See* MARIGNANO, Gian Giacomo de' Medici, marchio [1495–1555]

MEDICAMEN spirituale contra pestem. *See* BONAVENTURA, *Saint, Cardinal.*

MEDICAMENTA militaria dogmatica. *See* RUMMEL, J. P. Opuscula chymico-magico-medica. 1635.

MEDICAMENTS for the poor. *See* PREVOST, J.

MEDICE cura teipsum; or, The apothecaries plea. 1671. *See* [STUBBS, H.]

MEDICI, GIAN GIACOMO DE'. *See* MARIGNANO, Gian Giacomo de' Medici, *marchio* [1495–1555]

I MEDICI alla censura. Tradotto dal francese dal sig. Constantin Belli. Lione, Gio. e Giacomo Anisson, e Gio Posuel, 1678.

    [10], 298 p.   15 cm.   [7667]

—[The same.] ... Milano, Ambrogio Ramellati, 1683.

    [8], 158 p.   15 cm.   [7668]

MEDICINA animi in usum melancholicorum, peregrinantium, et studiosorum praeparata. Continens quingentos sales atque facetias ... Opera & studio M.B.L. Germanopoli, 1685.

    [18], 362, [38+] p.   14 cm.   [7669]

Imperfect: all after p. [38] wanting.

MEDICINA corporis. *See* [TSCHIRNHAUS, E. W. von] Medicina mentis. 1687, 1695.

MEDICINA mentis. *See* [TSCHIRNHAUS, E. W. von] Medicina mentis. 1687, 1695.

MEDICINA SALERNITANA. *See* REGIMEN SANITATIS SALERNITANUM. Medicina Salernitana. 1605, 1611, 1612, 1622, 1624, 1628, 1638.

EL MEDICO caritativo. 1660? *See* [ZAQUIIAS, doctor]

MEDICOS Ordinarios der Statt Regensburg. *See* KOLLEGIUM DER AERZTE, Regensburg.

MEDICUS domesticus. *See* HYGIEIA. 1628.

MEDICUS INDICUS. *See* PEACHIE, John [*fl. ca.* 1683–*ca.* 1690]

MEDICUS legalis; oder, Gesetzmässige Bestell- und Ausübung der Artzney-Kunst worinn ... gezeiget wird wie das Artzney-Wesen dem gemeinen Besten gemäs nützlich einzurichten und gebührend zu bestellen sey. Jetzo zum andernmahl ... übersehen und ausgefertiget von C. B. B. M. D. Franckfurt und Leipzig, In Verlag Paul Zeisings in Helmstädt, 1696.

[8], 215, [1] p. 17 cm. [7670]

Vorrede signed: C.B.B.D.

MEDICUS politicus; dat is, Onderwys aan een jonger medicus, wegens de politike streeken; welke in de praktyk der medicynen ingerfloopen zyn. Amsterdam, Nicolaas ten Hoorn, 1700.

148, [2] p. 17 cm. [7671]

MEDICUS Romanus. 1681. *See* [BOECKELMANN, J. F.]

[**MEE,** *Dr.*] The character of a compleat physician, or naturalist. [London, 1680?]

8 p. 21 cm. [7672]

A reprint [?] of Wing M1613.

MEECKEREN, JOB VAN. *See* MEEKREN, Job van [1611?–1666]

MEEKREN, JOB VAN [1611?–1666] Heel- en genees- konstige aanmerkkingen ... Amsterdam, Casparus Commelijn, 1668.

[20], 495 (i.e. 497), [13] p. illus., front. 17 cm. [7673]

Imperfect? Sig. **[4] (blank?) wanting?

—[Latin tr.] Observationes medico-chirurgicae, ex Belgico in Latinum translatae ab Abrehamo Blasio ... Amstelodami, Ex officina Henrici & viduae Theodori Boom, 1682.

[16], 392, [5] p. illus. 17 cm. [7674]

Added engraved title page.

—[German tr.] Rare und wunderbare chyrurgisch-und beneesskünstige Anmerckungen ... Nürnberg, In Verlegung Paul Fürstens seel. Wittib und Erben, 1675.

[14], 537, [23] p. illus., front. 17 cm. [7675]

—*See* BECKE, D. von der. Dissertatio anatomico- practica de procidentia uteri. 1683.

MEEL, JOHANN CHRISTOPH. *See* MEELFÜHRER, Johann Christoph [1644–1708]

MEELFÜHRER, JOHANN CHRISTOPH [1644–1708] *respondent. See* ZIEGRA, C., *praeses.* De sympathia at- que antipathia rerum naturalium. 1663.

MEER, JAN VAN DER [*fl.* 1660] *respondent.* Disputatio medica inauguralis de fame canina ... Lugduni Batavorum, Apud Franciscum Moyaert, 1660.

[8] p. 22 cm. [7676]

Diss.—Leyden.

MEERSCHE, JASON VAN DER. *See* PRATENSIS, Jason [1486–1558]

MEGERLE, ULRICH. *See* ABRAHAM A SANCTA CLARA, *Father* [1644–1709]

MEGERLIN, AMADEUS [*fl.* 1663] *tr. See* SCULTETUS, J. [1595–1645] Wund-artzneyisches Zeug- Hauss. 1679.

MEGERLIN, CHRISTIAN ALBERT [*fl.* 1696] *respon- dent. See* CAMERARIUS, R. J., *praeses.* De diabete hypochondriacorum periodico. 1696.

MEGERLIN, JOHANN ULRICH. *See* ABRAHAM A SANCTA CLARA, *Father* [1644–1709]

MEGÍA, PEDRO. *See* MEXÍA, Pedro [1496?–1552?]

MEGISER, HIERONYMUS [*ca.* 1553–1618] *See* AR- NALDUS DE VILLANOVA. Omnia, quae exstant, opera chymica. 1603.

MEHUNG, JOANNES A. *See* JEAN DE MEUN [*d.* 1305?]

MEIBOM, DANIEL HEINRICH [*fl.* 1691–1697] *respon- dent. See* HOFFMANN, J. M., *praeses.* Exercitatio physiologicomedica de suturis cranii humani. 1691.

MEIBOM, HEINRICH [1555–1625] *ed. See* CORDUS, E. Opera poetica. 1614.

MEIBOM, HEINRICH [1638–1700] De medicorum historia scribenda epistola ad V. Cl. Georg. Hier.

Velschium ... Helmestadii, Typis Henningi Mulleri, 1669.

[16] p. 21 cm.   [7677]

—De vasis palpebrarum novis epistola ad V. Cl. D. Joelem Langellottium ... Helmestadii, Typis & sumptibus Henningi Mulleri, 1666.

[23] p. plate. 19 cm.   [7678]

—Epistola de longaevis ... Helmaestadii, Typis Henningi Mulleri, 1664.

[32] p. 19 cm.   [7679]

Dissertations — Helmstedt

—*praeses.* Consideratio medica veris morborumque vernalium et medendi rationis isto tempore instituendae ... Helmestadii, Typis Henrici Davidis Mulleri, 1677.

[40] p. 20 cm.   [7680]
W. Mechov, *respondent.*

—Disputatio inauguralis de suffocatione hysterica ... Helmestadii, Typis Georgii Wolfgangi Hammii [1684]

[48] p. 20 cm.   [7681]
K. B. Behrens, *respondent.*

—Disputatio medica de hernia ... Helmestadii, Apud Henricum Hessium [1686]

[24] p. 19 cm.   [7682]
F. Cellarius, *respondent.*

—Disputatio medica de variolis et morbillis ... Helmstadii, Literis Henrici Davidis Mülleri, 1676.

[44] p. 21 cm.   [7683]
M. Homeyer, *respondent.*

—Disputatio medica inauguralis de cardialgia ... Helmestadii, Typis Henrici Davidis Mülleri, 1679.

[24] p. 20 cm.   [7684]
T. Wilrich, *respondent.*

—Disputatio medica inauguralis de concoctione ventriculi laesa...Helmestadii, Typis Georg-Wolfgangi Hammii [1682]

[64] p. 20 cm.   [7685]
J. Schmied, *respondent.*

—Disputatio medica inauguralis de febribus intermittentibus epidemicis ... Helmestadii, Typis Henrici Davidis Mülleri, 1678.

[38] p. 20 cm.   [7686]
M. Ladey, *respondent.*

—Disputatio medica inauguralis de febribus malignis ... Helmestadii, Typis Henrici Davidis Mülleri, 1679.

[44] p. 20 cm.   [7687]
J. G. Schmiedt, *respondent.*

—Disputatio medica inauguralis de haemorrhoidibus ... Helmestadii, Typis Henningi Mulleri, 1670.

[36] p. 20 cm.   [7688]
P. C. Stockhausen, *respondent.*

—Disputatio medica inauguralis de leniorum medicamentorum eximio usu ... Helmestadii, Typis Georg-Wolfgangi Hammii [1692]

[40] p. 21 cm.   [7689]
B. D. Behrens, *respondent.*

—Disputatio medica inauguralis de lue venerea ... Helmstadii, Typis Georg-Wolfgangi Hammii [1682]

[40] p. 20 cm.   [7690]
A. W. Fischbeck, *respondent.*

—Disputatio medica inauguralis de oleorum stillatitiorum natura et usu in genere ... Helmestadii, Typis Henningi Mulleri, 1670.

[28] p. 19 cm.   [7691]
D. Kellner, *respondent.*

—Disputatio medica inauguralis de paracentesi in hydrope ... Helmestadii, Typis Jacobi Mülleri, 1670.

[23] p. illus. 20 cm.   [7692]
J. K. Axt, *respondent.*

—Disputatio medica inauguralis de sanguinis eductione ... Helmestadii, Typis Henrici Davidis Mulleri, 1674.

[32] p. 20 cm.   [7693]
J. G. Hieronymi, *respondent.*

—Disputatio medica inauguralis de spiritibus ex vegetabilibus per fermentationem paratis ... Helmestadii, Typis Henrici Davidis Mulleri, 1674.

[36] p. 20 cm.   [7694]
H. Erberfeldt, *respondent.*

—Disputatio medica inauguralis de suffusione ... Helmestadii, Typis Jacobi Mulleri, 1670.

[32] p. 21 cm.   [7695]
L. G. Rose, *respondent.*

—Disputatio medica inauguralis de ulcerum natura et curatione in genere . . . Helmestadii, Typis Henrici Davidis Mulleri, 1674.

[32] p.   20 cm.   **[7696]**

J. G. Alberti, *respondent.*

—Disputatio medica inauguralis de vomitu . . . Helmestadii, Typis Henrici Davidis Mulleri, 1678.

[40] p.   19 cm.   **[7697]**

A. H. Hellberg, *respondent.*

—Disputationem inauguralem medicam de haemorrhagia . . . publicae disquisitioni submittit Henricus Rademin . . . Helmestadii, Typis Georg-Wolfgangi Hammii [1684]

[40] p.   20 cm.   **[7698]**

H. Rademin, *respondent.*

—Dissertatio medica de aquae calidae potu . . . Helmestadii, Typis Georg-Wolfgangi Hamii [1689]

[36] p.   19 cm.   **[7699]**

B. D. Behrens, *respondent.*

—Dissertatio medica de atrophia . . . Helmestadii, Typis Henningi Mulleri, 1672.

[24] p.   21 cm.   **[7700]**

J. G. Hieronymi, *respondent.*

—Dissertatio medica de calculo renum . . . Helmestadii, Typis Henrici Davidis Mulleri [1679]

[48] p.   20 cm.   **[7701]**

J. N. Otto, *respondent.*

—Dissertatio medica inauguralis de laesionibus cranii a causa externa violenta . . . Helmestadii, Typis Henrici Davidis Mulleri, 1674.

[32] p.   18 cm.   **[7702]**

C. Richter, *respondent.*

—Dissertatio medica inauguralis de vulneribus lethalibus . . . Helmestadii, Typis Henrici Davidis Mulleri, 1674.

[40] p.   19 cm.   **[7703]**

J. A. Neukranz, *respondent.*

—[The same.] Dissertatio medica inauguralis de vulneribus lethalibus quam . . . subjicit . . . Johannes Antonius Neukranz . . . ad diem XVII Septembris CIƆIƆC LXXIV. Helmestadii, Typis Georgi-Wolfgangi Hammii, 1694.

[42] p.   20 cm.   **[7704]**

—Exercitatio anatomico-medica de valvulis seu membranulis vasorum earumque structura et usu . . . Helmestadii, Typis Georg-Wolfgangi Hammii [1682]

[44] p.   21 cm.   **[7705]**

J. G. Schmiedt, *respondent.*

Signatures: 1 leaf unsigned (A₁?),) (², A²⁻⁴, B-E⁴. Sig.)(, containing Meibom's epistle, appears to be an insert.

—Exercitatio medica de bubonibus . . . Helmestadi, Typis Jacobi Mulleri, 1671.

[32] p.   20 cm.   **[7706]**

H. S. Bergman, *respondent.*

—Exercitatio medica de cancro mammarum . . . Helmestadii, Typis Henrici Davidis Mülleri, 1673.

[35] p.   19 cm.   **[7707]**

J. S. Hecht, *respondent.*

—Exercitatio medica de cephalalgia . . . Helmestadii, Typis Henningi Mulleri, 1672.

[44] p.   19 cm.   **[7708]**

A. Homberg, *respondent.*

—Exercitatio medica de chylificatione . . . Helmestadii, Typis Henningi Mulleri, 1671.

[32] p.   18 cm.   **[7709]**

C. A. Conerding, *respondent.*

—Exercitatio medica de consuetudinis natura, vi, et efficacia ad sanitatem et morbum, ejusque in medendo observationis necessitate . . . Helmestadii, Typis haeredum Henrici Davidis Mulleri [1681]

[32] p.   19 cm.   **[7710]**

G. T. Spierman, *respondent.*

—Exercitatio medica de fluxu humorum ad oculos naturali et praeternaturali hujusque curatione . . . Helmstadii, Typis Georg-Wolfgangi Hammi [1687]

[24] p.   20 cm.   **[7711]**

A. U. Schwalenberg, *respondent.*

—Exercitatio medica de ossium constitutione naturali et praeternaturali . . . Helmestadii, Typis Henningi Mulleri, 1668.

[48] p.   20 cm.   **[7712]**

D. Kellner, *respondent.*

—Exercitatio medica de phthisi . . . Helmestadii, Typis Henrici Davidis Mülleri, 1675.

[35] p.   20 cm.   **[7713]**

H. C. Erythropilus, *respondent.*

—Exercitatio medica de phthisis curatione per lac ... Helmaestadii, Typis Georg-Wolfgangi Hammii [1687]

    [32] p.   20 cm.   **[7714]**

    C. Mente, *respondent.*

—Exercitatio medica de suppressione urinae ... Helmestadii, Typis Henrici Davidis Mulleri, 1676.

    [40] p.   19 cm.   **[7715]**

    J. A. Papke, *respondent.*

—Exercitatio medica de tumoribus pedum imprimis oedematosis ... Helmstadii, Typis Jacobi Mülleri, 1679.

    30, [2] p.   20 cm.   **[7716]**

    P. L. Petri, *respondent.*

—Exercitatio medica inauguralis de hydrope ascite ... Helmestadii, Typis Georgii Wolfgangi Hammii [1695]

    [56] p.   19 cm.   **[7717]**

    A. K. Schröder, *respondent.*

—Exercitatio medica inauguralis de venae sectionis in variolarum curatione usu ... Helmestadii, Typis Georgii-Wolfgangi Hammii [*ca.* 1690]

    [28] p.   18 cm.   **[7718]**

    J. H. Kreienberg, *respondent.*

—Exercitatio medico chirurgica de catheterismo ... Helmestadii, Typis Georg-Wolfgangi Hammii [1699]

    [28] p.   21 cm.   **[7719]**

    F. H. Grübeling, *respondent.*

—Theses medicae ex universa arte depromate ... Helmestadii, Typis Johannis Heitmulleri, 1668.

    [16] p.   21 cm.   **[7720]**

    H. K. Stisser, *respondent.*

—*respondent. See* Conring, H., *praeses.* Exercitatio philologico-medica. 1659; Tappe, J., *praeses.* Disputatio medica de hydrophobia. 1659. *ed. See* Cassiodorus Senator, F. M. A. Formula comitis archiatrorum. 1668; Kober, T. Observationum medicarum Castrensium Hungaricarum decades tres. 1685; Meibom, J. H. De cervisiis. 1668. *See* Boate, A. Observationes medicae de affectibus omissis. 1664; Meibom, J. H. De usu flagrorum. 1670.

MEIBOM, Johann Heinrich [1590-1655] De cervisiis potibusque & ebriaminibus extra vinum aliis commentarius. Accedit Adr. Turnebi libellus De vino. Helmestadii, Typis & sumptibus Johannis Heitmulleri, 1668.

    [192] p.   20 cm.   **[7721]**

    Edited by Heinrich Meibom.

—De flagrorum usu in re veneria & lumborum renumque officio, epistola ... Lugd. Batavorum, Ex Officina Elseviriana, 1643.

    48 p.   22 cm.   **[7722]**

—[The same.] ... Ed. 2. ... Lugd. Batavorum [1650?]

    48 p.   14 cm.   **[7723]**

    Different setting of type.

—[The same.] Thomae Bartholini, Joan. Henrici Meibomii, patris, Henrici Meibomi, filii, De usu flagrorum in re medica & veneria, lumborumque & renum officio. Accedunt de eodem renum officio Joachimi Olhafii & Olai Wormii Dissertatiunculae. Francofurti, Ex bibliopolio Hafniensi Danielis Paulli, 1670.

    144 p.   17 cm.   **[7724]**

    "Joachimi Olhafii & Olai Wormii Dissertatiunculae de usu renum, ex musaeo Th. Bartholini": p. [113]-144, has special title page with imprint: Francofurti, Ex Bibliopolio Paullino, 1670.

    Bartholin's work, De flagrorum usu medico (p. [3]-32) is an introductory epistle addressed to Heinrich Meibom, whose reply follows the text of J. H. Meibom's work, which was previously published under title: De flagrorum usu in re veneria & lumborum renumque officio.

—, *ed. See* Cassidorus Senator, F. M. A. Formula comitis archiatrorum. 1668; Hippocrates. Jusjurandum. 1643.

MEICHERNER, Matthias [*fl.* 1654] *respondent. See* Coler, M. C., *praeses.* Exercitatio physica de formis materialibus. 1654.

MEIER, Gerhard [1664-1723] *praeses.* Rationales de virginis partu cogitationes ... Hamburgi, Typis Conradi Neumanni [1695]

    [4], 24 p.   19 cm.   **[7725]**

    Diss.—Hamburg. Gymnasium (E. Ahrnds, *respondent*)

MEIER, Gottlob Friedlieb [*fl.* 1679] Oratio de origine et colore Aethiopum ... Francofurti cis Viadrum, Literis Christophori Zeitleri [1679?]

    [20] p.   19 cm.   **[7726]**

MEIER, HEINRICH LOHALM [*fl.* 1696] *respondent.* Disputatio medica inauguralis de animi, ejusque affectuum quoad valetudinem, impressionibus in corpus ... Lugduni Batavorum, Apud Abrahhamum Elzevier, 1696.

[15] p.   21 cm.   [7727]

Diss. — Leyden.

MEIER, HERMANN [*fl.* 1671] *respondent.* Disputatio inauguralis, de uxore virgine ... Basileae, Literis Deckerianis [1671]

[48] p.   20 cm.   [7728]

Diss. — Basel.

MEIER, MICHAEL. *See* MAIER, Michael [1568?-1622]

MEIER, SEBASTIAN [*fl.* 1648-1651] *respondent.* Disputatio medica inauguralis exhibens casum laborantis affectione hypochondriaca ... Lugduni Batavorum, Ex officina Francisci Hackii [1651]

[16] p.   19 cm.   [7729]

Imperfect: lower margin of title page trimmed.
Diss. — Leyden.

MEIGRET, LOUIS [16th cent.] *tr. See* DÜRER, A. Les quatre livres ... de la proportion des parties & pourtraicts des corps humains. 1613, 1614.

MEILING, HEINRICH [*fl.* 1660] *respondent. See* LINDEN, J. A. van der, *praeses.* Hippocrates de circuitu sanguinis, exercitatio VIII. 1660.

MEINEKE, DANIEL CHRISTOPH [*fl.* 1682-1683] *respondent. See* CRAUSE, R. W., *praeses.* Dissertationem medicam inauguralem de incubo ... submittit ... D. C. M. 1683; SCHELHAMMER, G. C., *praeses.* De peste. 1682.

MEINER, JOHANN GOTTLOB [*fl.* 1699] *respondent. See* TIMAEUS, G., *praeses.* Disputatio posterior, de metallurgia rerum gerendarum nervo. 1699.

MEISE, DAVID [*fl.* 1604] *respondent. See* BRENDEL, Z. [1553-1626] *praeses.* De pleuritide themata medica. 1604.

MEISNER, JOHANNES THEODOR [*fl.* 1688-1689] *respondent.* Disputatio medica inauguralis de febre catarrhali ... Trajecti ad Rhenum, Ex officina Francisci Halma, 1689.

[20] p.   18 cm.   [7730]

Imperfect: upper margins trimmed with possible loss of pagination.
Diss. — Utrecht.

—*See* BOHN, J., *praeses.* Dissertatio medica de atrophia in genere. 1688.

MEISNER, LORENTZ. Gemma gemmarum alchimistarum; oder, Erleuterung der parabolischen und philosophischen Schrifften fratris Basilii ... durch Laurentium Meisnerum ... Item, Ausslegung Rythmorum Basilii, von der Materia des Steins der Philosophen, gefertiget durch Conrad Schülern. Eissleben [Gedruckt durch Jacobum Gaubisch, Leipzig, In Vorlegung Jacob Apels] 1608.

[187] p.   illus.   17 cm.   [7731]

Part [2] has special title page: Gründliche Ausslegung und warhafftige Erklerung der Rythmorum ... Basilii Valentini ... Gefertiget durch Conrad Schülern.
Bound with Suchten, A. von. Mysteria gemina antimonii. 1675.

MEISSNER, CHRISTOPHER [*fl.* 1625] *respondent. See* SULTZBERGER, J. R., *praeses.* De cancro συζητησις medico-chirurgica. 1625.

MEISSNER, JOHANN THEODORUS. *See* MEISNER, Johannes Theodor [*fl.* 1688-1689]

MEISTER, ISAAK [*fl.* 1687] *respondent.* Dissertatio medica inauguralis de dysenteria ... Basileae, Typis Jacobi Bertschii [1687]

[20] p.   21 cm.   [7732]

Diss. — Basel.

MEJER, GERHARD. *See* MEIER, Gerhard [1664-1723]

MEJÍA, PEDRO. *See* MEXÍA, Pedro [1496?-1552?]

MELA, POMPONIUS. *See* VOSSIUS, I. Observationum ad Pomp. Melam appendix. 1686.

MELAMPUS. De divinatione per palpitationes. In Adamantius. La physionomie. 1635.

—De naevis corporis [Greek and Latin] *In* Cardano, G. Metoposcopia. 1658 and [Greek and French] La metoposcopie. 1658; [French] *In* Adamantius. La physionomie. 1635; [German] *In* Höchstfürtreflichtes chiromantisch-und physiognomisches Klee-Blat. 1695.

MELANCHTHON, PHILIPP [1497-1560] De anima. *In* Hygieia. 1628; Magirus, J. Anthropologia. 1603; Regimen sanitatis Salernitanum. De conservanda bona valetudine. 1607, 1619; Regimen sanitatis Salernitanum. Medicina Salernitana. 1605, 1611, 1612, 1622, 1624, 1628, 1638; Regimen sanitatis Salernitanum. Schola Salernitana. 1649, 1657, 1667, 1683; [Dutch tr.] 1658.

—*See* BEVERWIJCK, J. van. DD. virorum epistolae et responsa. 1665 [and] Epistolicae quaestiones, cum doctorum responsis. 1644; Gorris, P. de [*fl.* 1511] Formulae remediorum, quibus vulgo medici utuntur. 1612.

MELCHIN, JOHANN [*fl.* 1671] *respondent. See* HOFFMANN, C. Problema physicum. 1671.

MELCHIOR, EBERHARD. Anatomia hydrologica thermarum Wisbadensium ... das ist, Ausführlicher, genauer ursprünglicher Bericht und Cuhr-Buch, von Krafft und Würckung der Weltbekandten ... heylsamen Bäder zu Wissbaden ... Mayntz, Ludwig Bourgeat, 1697.
    [16], 10 (i.e. 108) p.   16 cm.   [**7733**]

—*See* SCHREY, C. H. Neugefaster ... wolckensteinischer Warmer-Bad- und Wasserschatz. 1696 [and] Thermarum contenta rejecta & retenta; das ist, Des uhralten-neugefassten Warmen-Bad -und Wasser-Schatzes. 1696.

MELCHIOR, PAUL [*fl.* 1675] *respondent.* Disputatio medica inauguralis, de morbo castrensi ... Gissae Hassorum, Typis Friderici Kargeri, 1675.
    50 (i.e. 48) p.   20 cm.   [**7734**]
Diss.—Giessen.

MELDER, CHRISTIAAN [*fl.* 1660-1663] *respondent.* Disputatio medica inauguralis, de diabete ... Trajecti ad Rhenum, Ex officina Jacobi à Doeyenburch, 1663.
    [10] p.   20 cm.   [**7735**]
Diss.—Utrecht.

—*See* BRUYN, J. de, *praeses.* Disputationis physicae de alitura pars sexta. 1660.

MELICH, GEORG [*fl.* 1575-1595] Avertimenti nelle compositioni de' medicamenti per uso della spetiaria, con una diligente esaminatione di molti simplici, tratta da più degni auttori ... Aggiuntovi un trattato delle mirabili virtù della theriaca, dell'eccellentissimo signor Oratio Guarguanti. Venetia, Giacomo Vincenti [1605]
    [16], 200 (i.e. 202) ll., 24 p.   20 cm.   [**7736**]
Guarguantis's Della theriaca has special title page dated 1605.

—[The same.] ... Et hora ristampati in miglior forma con aggionta di molte compositioni utili, e necessarie, raccolte da migliori antidotarii venuti in luce sino al presente ... da Alberto Stecchini ...

E nel fine il trattato delle virtù della theriaca dell'eccellentissimo signor Oratio Guarguante ... Venetia, Li Guerigli, 1648.
    [24], 344 p.   22 cm.   [**7737**]
Guarguanti's Della theriaca has caption title.

—[The same.] ... Venetia, Steffano Curti, 1678.
    [24], 343 p.   23 cm.   [**7738**]

—[Latin ed.] Dispensatorium medicum; sive, De recta medicamentorum ... parandorum ratione, commentarii ... in Latinum sermonem conversi, a Sam. Keller ... cui adjectum est Compendium medicinae practicae Franciscimariae de Tectoriis ... Francofurti, E Typographeo Paltheniano, 1601.
    [24], 647, [94] p.   13 cm.   [**7739**]
Last leaf (blank?) wanting.
The Compendium medicinae practicae has special title page (p. [621])

—*See* SGOBBIS DA MONTAGNANA, A. de. Nuovo, et universale theatro farmaceutico. 1667, 1682.

MELIPOT, NICOLAAS [*fl.* 1684] *respondent.* Dissertatio medica inauguralis de pleuritide ... Lugduni Batavorum, Apud Abrahamum Elzevier, 1684.
    [15] p.   22 cm.   [**7740**]
Diss.—Lyden.

MELLETIUS, GABRIEL, *ed. See* BONACCORSI, B. Praesidiorum descriptiones adversus pestiferam luem. 1630.

MELM, JOHANN KONRAD [1677-1714] *respondent. See* BARBECK, F. G., *praeses.* Disputatio medico-philosophica de generatione hominis. 1695.

MEMOIRES for a natural history of animals. 1687. *See* Académie royale des sciences, Paris.

MEMOIR'S [sic] for a natural history of animals. 1688. *See* ACADÉMIE ROYALE DES SCIENCES, Paris.

MEMOIRS for the ingenious. Containing several curious observations in philosophy, mathematicks, physick, philology, and other arts and sciences, in miscellaneous letters. By J. De La Crose, E. A. P. January, 1693 [-December 1693] To be continued monthly. Vol. I. ... London, H. Rhodes and J. Harris., 1693.
    [3], 389 (i.e. 413), [13] p.   illus., plates.   22 cm.
                           [**7741**]
Each month has special title page not included in the pagination.

MEMOIRS for the ingenious; or, The universal mercury; consisting of choice collections, and curious observations in history, philosophy, mathematicks, physick, philology, and other arts and sciences, in miscellaneous letters. By several hands. January, 1694. To be continued monthly. London, Randal Taylor, 1694.

    [6], 30 p. 19 cm. **[7742]**
Imperfect: lower margins trimmed, including part of imprint. Running title: The universal mercury.

A MEMORIAL for the learned; or, Miscellany of choice collections from most eminent authors, in history, philosophy, physick, and heraldry. By J. D. gent ... London, George Powell and William Powle, 1686.

    [24], 216 p. 18 cm. **[7743]**
The epistle dedicatory signed by Nahum Tate, the editor.

MEMORIE di diverse provisioni, et usi, praticati nella città di Palermo con occasione della peste gl'anni 1624, 1625, 1626. Modona, Giulian Cassiani, 1630.

    12, 9 p. 20 cm. **[7744]**

MÉNAGE, GILLES [1613-1692] See FABROT, C. A. Epistola ... de mutuo. 1645.

MENAGIUS, AEGIDIUS. See MÉNAGE, Gilles [1613-1692]

MENAPE, GUILLAUME. See INSULANUS MENAPIUS, Gulielmus [d. 1556]

MENAPIUS INSULANUS, GULIELMUS. See INSULANUS MENAPIUS, Gulielmus [d. 1556]

MENCEL, JOHANN [fl. 1613] Gründlicher Bericht und Ordnung, wie bey vorstehenden Sterbenssläufften die Gesunden für der abscheulichen Gifft-Seuche sich praeserviren, und die Krancken so damit angezündet worden, sich verhalten sollen, damit sie widerumb curiret und geheylet werden mögen ... Gross Glogaw, Gedruckt durch Joachimum Funck, 1613.

    [120] p. 19 cm. **[7745]**

MENCEL, PHILIPP. See MENZEL, Philipp [1546-1613]

MENDES, FERNANDO [d. 1724] Instrucçioens a quem houver de usar da agoa. In Azevedo, M. de. Father. Correcçam de abusos. 1690.

MENDOÇA P., ANTONIO DE. See MENDOZA P., Antonio de [fl. 1604]

MENDOZA P., ANTONIO DE [fl. 1604] See PORTUGAL. Sovereigns, etc. [1598-1621] (Philip II). Regimento dos medicos e boticarios. 1604.

MENGERING, HEINRICH ANDREAS [fl. 1649-1653] respondent. See LANGE, C., praeses. Faciem Hippocraticam levi penicillo adumbratum ... publice sistit M. H. A. M. 1651; MICHAELIS, J., praeses. Dissertatio inauguralis de quartana. 1652.

MENIŃSKI, FRANCISZEK [1623-1698] Thesaurus linguarum Orientalium Turcicae, Arabicae, Persicae, praecipuas earum opes a Turcis peculiariter usurpatas continens nimirum lexicon Turcico-Arabico-Persicum ... quarum quae Turcis usitatae aut communic usus sunt, Latine, Germanice, Italice, Gallice, Polonice ... explicantur & grammaticam Turcicam cum adjectis ad singula ejus capita praeceptis grammaticis Arabicae & Persicae linguae ... Ex ... Orientis authoribus collectum & in lucem editum opera, typis, & sumptibus Francisci a Mesgnien Meninski ... Viennae Austriae, 1680-1687

    2 v. in 5. 36 cm. **[7746]**
Vol. [2] has title: Complementum Thesauri linguarum Orientalium; seu, Onomasticum Latino-Turcico-Arabico-Persicum ... Viennae Austriae, 1687.

MENIOTIUS, ANTONIUS. See MENJOT, Antoine [ca. 1615-1696]

[MENJOT, ANTOINE, ca. 1615-1696] Febrium malignarum historia et curatio. Accesserunt dissertationes pathologicae, de rheumatismo, de bombis aurium, de catalepsi, de incubo, de spuria convulsione & spasmo cynico, de delirio in genere, de paraphrosyne, de furorore uterino. Parisiis, Apud Gasparum Meturas [Ex typis Petri Variquet] 1660.

    322, [4] p. 19 cm. **[7747]**
Author's presentation copy, signed.

—Febrium malignarum historia et curatio. Item dissertationes pathologicae de delirio in genere, de paraphrosyne, de furore uterino, de hydrophobia, de incubo, de catalepsi, de spuria convulsione & spasmo cynico, de catarrho, de rheumatismo, de mydriasi, de phthisi pupillae, de bombis aurium, de aphωnia, de voce depravata, rauca scilicet & clangosa, de mutitate & balbutie, de cholera, de dysenteria hepatica, de atrophia. Ed. alt. ... Parisiis, Apud Thomam Jolly, 1662.

    [8], 245, [3] p. 22 cm. **[7748]**

—[The same.] Febrium malignarum historia et curatio. Item dissertationes pathologicae in duas partes divisae. Quarum prior tertium jam editur, sed emendatior, multaque commentatione ac meditatione locupletior. Altera nunc primum in lucem prodit ... [Parisiis, Apud Sebastianum Cramoisy, et Sebast. Mabre-Cramoisy, 1665]

     [22], 775 p.   26 cm.   **[7749]**
Author's presentation copy, signed.

—[The same.] Febrium malignarum historia et curatio. Item Dissertationum pathologicarum pars prima [-tertia] ... Ed. 2. Parisiis, Apud Sebastianum Mabre-Cramoisy, 1674.

     3 parts in 2 vols.   24 cm.   **[7750]**
Added general half title.
Each part has special title page.
The main text of parts 1-2 is a reissue of the 1665 edition.

—*See* SCHMITZ, J. A. Medicinae practicae compendium. 1666, 1688, 1691.

MENNENS, GUILIELMUS [1525-1608] Aurei velleris; sive, Sacre philosophiae vatum selectae unicae, mysteriorumque ac Dei, naturae, et artis admirabilium, libri tres.

     240-428 p., vol. 5.   20 cm. (*In* Zetzner, Lazarus, *ed.* Theatrum chemicum. Argentorati, 1659-61)   **[7751]**
Caption title.

MENNI, JOHANN HEINRICH [*fl.* 1635] *ed. See* [TILEMANN, J.] Guldiner Apffel. 1635, 1666.

MENODOTUS, *pseud. See* BUDAEUS, Gottlieb [1664-1734]

MENON, DOMINIQUE. L'ecole de Salerne. Traduite de latin en françois, où chacun trouvera conformement à ses humeurs, la maniere de vivre, & se conserver long-temps dans une bonne & parfaite santé ... La Haye, Adrian Moetjens, 1695.

     24 p.   17 cm.   **[7752]**
Bound with Harvey, G. Ars curandi morbos expectatione. 1695.

MENSA philosophica; seu, Enchiridion, in quo de quaestionibus mensalibus, rerum naturis, statuum diversitate, variis & jucundis congressibus hominum philosophice agitur, in quatuor libros accurate distributum. Auctore Michaele Scoto ... Accessit libellus jocorum & facetiarum ... olim opera Othomari Luscinii ... concinnatus. Francofurti,

Typis Wolfgangi Richteri, sumptibus Nicolai Steinii, 1602.

     [24], 527 p.   13 cm.   **[7753]**
Variously attributed to Michael Scott and to Theobaldus Anguilbertus. Not to be confused with the Tractatus mensae philosophicae et responsorium curiosorum of Conradus, de Halberstadt. Cf. Lawn, p. 103-III, and Brunet, v. 3, cols. 1635-6.

MENSING, JOHANN. *See* MENSINGA, Johannes [1635-1698]

MENSINGA, JOHANNES [1635-1698] *See* MUNTING, A. Naauwkeurige beschryving der aardgewassen. 1696.

MENTE, CHRISTOPH [*fl.* 1687] *respondent. See* MEIBOM, H., *praeses.* Exercitatio medica de phthisis curatione per lac. 1687.

MENTZEL, JOHANN CHRISTIAN [*d.* 1718] *respondent. See* ALBINUS, B. Dissertatio de venenis. 1682.

MENUDIER, JEAN [*fl.* 1673-1690] *tr. See* GLASER, C. Chimischer Wegweiser. 1684.

MENZEL, ALBERT [*d.* 1632] *praeses.* Disputatio medica de dolore ... Ingolstadii, Ex typographeo Ederiano, apud Elisabetham Angermariam, viduam, 1615.

     [4], 13, [3] p.   21 cm.   **[7754]**
Diss. — Ingolstadt (M. Mayr, *respondent*)

—, *ed. See* MENZEL, P. Carminum ... libri quatuor. 1615.

MENZEL, PHILIPP [1546-1613] Carminum ... libri quatuor. Ed. alt. ... Ingolstadii, Ex Typographeo Ederiano, apud Elisabetham Angermariam, 1615.

     [40], 397, [11] p.   17 cm.   **[7755]**
"Oratio funebris, habita in tricesimo ... Philippi Menselii ... a Jacobo Reihing": p. [14-38]
Edited by Albert Menzel.

MENZIES, JOHN [1624-1684] A sermon, preached at the funeral of Sr. Alexander Fraiser ... principal physician to the king ... Edinburgh, Heir of Andrew Anderson, 1681.

     32 p.   18 cm.   **[7756]**

MENZINI, BENEDETTO [1646-1704] De literatorum hominum invidia liber. *In* Major, J. D. Genius errans. 1677.

MERBECK, ROGER. *See* MARBECKE, Roger [1536-1605]

MERBITZ, Johann Valentin [1650-1704] Biga disputationum physicarum quarum prima de infantibus suppositiis, vulgo Wechsel-Bälgen, altera de nymphis, Germanis Wasser-Nixen, incl. Facult. Philos. Lipsiens. indultu publice habitae a M. Joh. Valent. Merbitzio . . . jam vero ob exemplarium inopiam recusa . . . [Lipsiae] Sumtibus Johannis Christophori Mithii, typis Christophori Baumanni [1678]

    [56] p.   19 cm.   **[7757]**

— De varietate faciei humanae, discursus physicus. Appendicis loco accedent carmina figurata Rabani Mauri . . . Dresdae, Apud Mart. Gabrielem Hübnerum, typis viduae & haeredum Melchioris Bergenii, 1676.

    [17], 69, viii, [4] p.   plates.   20 cm.   **[7758]**

— *praeses.* Schediasma physicum de infantibus suppositiis, vulgo Wechselbälgen . . . Lipsiae, Typis Andreae Richteri [1671]

    [23] p.   20 cm.   **[7759]**
    Diss. — Leipzig (J. G. Jahn, *respondent*)

MERCADO, Luis [1525?-1611] Opera omnia in quatuor tomos divisa . . . Sedulo ac accurate relecta, emaculata, brevidus epitomis . . . donata, a Zacharia Palthenio . . . cum praefatione ac encomio Joannis-Hartmanni Beyeri . . . Francofurti, E Collegio Musarum Paltheniano, 1608.

    4 v.   36 cm.   **[7760]**
    Vol. 1-2 only. Contents. — v.1. 1. De constitutione corporis humani. 2. De sanitatis convervatione ac praecautione. 3. De morbis, eorum signis, caussis, symptomatibus, differentiis ac curatione. — v.2. 4. De recto praesidiorum artis medica usu. 5. De febrium essentia . . . 6. De pulsus arte & harmonia. 7. De morbi Gallici natura . . . 8. De morbis hereditariis.

— Opera omnia, in tres tomos divisa . . . Sedulo et accurate relecta, emaculata, brevibus epitomis . . . donata . . . Venetiis, Apud Bernardum Juntam, Joan, Bapt. Ciottu, & socios, 1609.

    [60], 875 p.   32 cm.   **[7761]**
    Vol. 1 only.

— Operum tomus primus [-quintus] . . . Relecti, emaculati, brevibus epitomis, ac indice locuplete donati, a Zacharia Palthenio . . . Cum praefatione ac encomio Joannis Hartmanni Beyeri . . . Francofurti, Typis Hartmanni Palthenii, sumptibus haeredum D. Zachriae Palthenii, 1614-1620 [v. 1, 1620; v. 2, 1619; v. 3-4, 1620; v. 5, 1614-15]

    5 v. in 2.   37 cm.   **[7762]**

Each part of vol. 5 has special title page.
Imperfect: Tomus quartus wanting. Pages 73-84 and 121-132 of Tomus quintus also wanting, supplied in photocopy from another issue in the library.
With vol. 5 are bound *his*: Institutiones ad usum & examen eorum. 1625; Institutiones chirurgicae. 1619.

— Another issue with different printers device at end. Part of Index reset.

                           [7763]
    Vol. 5 only.

— De mulierum affectionibus libri quatuor. Primus, de communibus mulierum passionibus disserit, secundus de virginum, & viduarum morbis, tertius, de sterilium, & praegnantium accidentibus, quartus, de puerperarum, & nutricum regimine . . . Venetiis, Apud Societatem Venetam, 1602.

    [20], 475 p.   21 cm.   **[7764]**
    Apparently based upon the edition printed in Venice in 1597 by Giovanii Guerigli, one of the members of the "Societas Veneta." His dedicatory epistle is here reprinted (p. [3-4])
    With this are bound: copy 2 of Grassi, Girolamo. Tractatus de tumoribus praeter naturam. Venetiis, 1562; copy 2 of Sassonia, E. Luis venereae perfectissimus tractatus. Patavii, 1597; Bauhin, K. Animadversiones in historiam generalem plantarum. 1601.

— [De natura et curatione pestis. Spanish.] Libro, en que se trata . . . la naturaleza, causas, providencia, y verdadera orden, y modo de currar la enfermedad vulgar, y peste que en estos años se ha divulgado por toda España. Puesto por . . . Mercado . . . en lengua vulgar, y traduzido del mismo que antes avia hecho en lengua latina, con cosas . . . añadidas, y un quinto tratado, en esta segunda impression. Y aora nuevamente impresso por mandado de los señores del Consejo. Madrid, Carlos Sanchez, 1648.

    [4], 128 ll.   15 cm.   **[7765]**
    A reprint of the enlarged "secunda impression" of 1599. The first edition, also printed in 1599, contained four tractates only.

— Institutiones ad usum & examen eorum, qui luxatoriam exercent artem . . . In quibus denique agitur de ossium fractura & curatione. Ex Hispanico idiomate in Latinum vertit Carolus Piso . . . Nunc primum in Germania e MS. . . . in lucem editae. Francofurti, Typis Hartm. Palthenii, Sumtibus haeredum D. Zachariae Palthenii, 1625.

    [8], 36 p.   illus.   37 cm.   **[7766]**
    Bound with vol. 5 of *his* Operum tomus primus [-quintus] 1614-15.

— Institutiones chirurgicae, in duos libros dissectae . . . nunc vero relectae, revisae, marginalibusque

. . . adornatae, primum in Germania editae . . . Francofurti ad Moenum, Ex officina Hartmanni Palthenii, sumptibus haeredum D. Zachariae Palthenii, p.m., 1619.

[8], 100, [6] p.   37 cm.   **[7767]**

Bound with vol. 5 of *his* Operum tomus primus [-quintus] 1614–15.

—Praxis medica, nunc primum hic in lucem edita: in quatuor partes divisa, I. De cognoscendis, & curandis internarum corporis humani partium affectibus. II. De morbi Gallici natura, causis, symptomatis, & therapia. III. De morbis haereditariis. IIII. De febrium essentia, differentiis, causis, signis, & cureatione . . . Omnes diligenter a mendis quibuscunque, ac erroribus . . . vindicati . . . Venetiis, Apud Bernardum Juntam, Joan. Bapt. Ciottum, & socios, 1608.

[12], 624, [67] p.   32 cm.   **[7768]**

—[The same.] Tomus secundus operum, quae nunc primum hic in lucem edita: in quattuor partes divisa . . . Venetiis, Apud Bernardum Juntam, Joan, Bapt. Ciottum, & socios, 1611.

[79], 624 p.   33 cm.   **[7769]**

Different setting of type.

MERCADO, MIGUEL. *See* MERCATI, Michele [1541–1593]

MERCATI, MICHELE [1541–1593] Instruccion sobre la peste . . . Traduxola de lengua toscana en castellana don Baltasar Vicente de Alhambra . . . [Zaragoza] Diego Dormer, 1648.

[32], 173, [11] p.   15 cm.   **[7770]**

Imperfect: title page mutilated, including imprint.

MERCATUS, LUDOVICUS. *See* MERCADO, Luis [1525?–1611]

MERCKEL, MARTIN [*fl.* 1688] *respondent. See* FRIDERICI, J. A., *praeses.* Dissertatio medica inauguralis de apoplexia. 1668; Rolfinck, W., *praeses.* Publicae . . . disquisitioni subjicit dissertationem hanc medico-chimicam de minera martis, M. M. 1668.

MERCKELL, JOHANN MATTHÄUS [*fl.* 1682] *respondent. See* ETTMÜLLER, M., *praeses.* Exercitatio medica sistens ideam praescribendarum formularum. 1682.

MERCKER, JOHANN [*fl.* 1619–1622] *respondent. See* SCHENCK, E., *praeses.* Disputatio medica inauguralis de pleuritide. 1619.

—*See* GREIFF, S. Wundartzeney. 1622.

MERCKLEIN, *See* MERCKLIN.

MERCKLIN, BARTHOLOME. Kurtzer verfasster Underricht, wie unnd wassen man sich bey disen so gefährlichen pestilentzischen Zuständen: zur Verhütung oder Praeservation zuhalten, und zu Curation solcher Seuchen brauchen soll . . . Dilingen, Getruckt bey Erhardt Lochnern, 1627.

[20] p.   18 cm.   **[7771]**

Imperfect: margins trimmed.

With this is bound Mainz. Ordinances, local laws, etc. Reformatio. 1618.

MERCKLIN, GEORG ABRAHAM [1644–1702?] Neu aussgefertigtes historisch-medicinisches Thier-Buch, in vier Theilen verabfasset; deren handelt I. Von vierfüssigen Thieren . . . II. Von Vögeln . . . III. Von Fischen . . . IV. Von allerley Ungezieffer, oder Gewürm, und kleinen zerkerbten Thierlein, so in der Medicin zu gebrauchen seyn. Enthaltende wider fast alle Krranckheiten und Leibes-Zufälle so wohl fremde, als eigene verschiedene heilsame Secreta und bewehrte Geness-Mittel . . . Nürnberg, In Verlegung Johann Ziegers, 1696.

[27], 732, [72] p.   plates.   17 cm.   **[7772]**

Added engraved title page.

—Sylloge physico-medicinalium casuum incantationi vulgo adscribi solitorum, maximeque prae caeteris memorabilium decurias VI. complectens . . . Cui loco mantissae accesserunt I. Quaestio solemnis: an monstrosa varia illa excreta revera in corpore fuerint, vel extrahantur? an vero praestigiae doemonis sint . . . II. Helmontii Tract. De receptis injectis . . . III. Laevin. Fischer. De morbis magice per sagas inductis naturaliter curandis. IV. Bartholom. Carrichteri Ratio medendi morbis ab incantatione dependentibus, nunc primum Latinitata donata. V. Collectanea & secreta myliana ad morbos magicos, maximam partem e Germanica in Latinam linguam translata, & nunc primum publicam in luce emissa . . . Norimbergae, Johannis Ziegeri & Georgii Lehmanni, 1698.

[44], 254, [12] p.   21 cm.   **[7773]**

—Tractatio med. curiosa, de ortu & occasu transfusionis sanguinis, qua haec, quae fit e bruto in brutum, a foro medico penitus eliminatur, illa quae e bruto in hominem peragitur, refutatur, & ista, quae ex homine in hominem exercetur, ad experientiae examen relegatur . . . Norimbergae, Sumptibus

Johannis Ziegeri, typis Christophori Gerhardi, 1679.

[27], 112, [4] p. 16 cm. **[7774]**

Added engraved title page.

—*respondent.* Prodromus palindromiae . . . Altdorphii, Typis viduae Joh. Leonhardi Winterbergeri [1670]

[16] p. 20 cm. **[7775]**

Diss. — Altdorf.

—, *ed. See* LINDEN, J. A. van der. Lindenius renovatus. 1686; PANDOLFINI, G. Tractatus de ventositatis spinae saevissimo morbo. 1674.

—*See* MALFI, T. Neue Anleitung zur Barbier- und Wund-Artzney-Kunst. 1676.

MERCKLIN, JOHANN ABRAHAM [1674-1720?] De feliciori nunc quam olim medicina diascepsis, plurima neotericorum inventa medica breviter complectens. Patavii, Ex typographia Sebastiani Spera, 1696.

[6], 32 p. 20 cm. **[7776]**

—*respondent.* Disputatio medica inauguralis de hydrope saccato . . . Altdorfii, Henricus Meyer [1695]

24 p. 20 cm. **[7777]**

Diss. — Altdorf.

MERCLIN, CHRISTOPH BARTHOLOMÄUS [*fl.* 1610] *respondent. See* CRÜGER, B., *praeses.* Disputatio medica septima. 1610.

MERCLIN, THEOPHILUS [*fl.* 1629] *respondent. See* SEBISCH, M. [1578-1674?] *praeses.* Exercitationes medicae. 1639.

MERCLINUS, GEORG ABRAHAM. *See* MERCKLIN, Georg Abraham [1644-1702?]

MERCURIALE, GIROLAMO [1530-1606] Tractatus varii de re medica, a variis medicis olim ex ipsius ore excepti, nunc vero, post eius obitum . . . evulgati . . . Atque hi omnes hac novissima editione suis propriis . . . indicibus . . . conlustrati. Lugduni, Sumptibus Antonii Pillehotte, 1618.

5 parts in 1 v. 24 cm. **[7778]**

Parts [2], [4] and [5] have half titles.

Contents. — De morbis muliebribus. — De puerorum morbis, cum Tralliani De lumbricis epistola (in Greek and Latin) & De venenosis, ac venenis opusculo (edited by Albertus Scheligius). — De peste, praesertim de Veneta, & Patavina. — De morbis cutaneis. — De excrementis.

—[The same.] . . . Lugduni, Sumptibus Antonii Pillehotte, 1623.

5 parts in 1 v. 24 cm. **[7779]**

Different setting of type.

—Opuscula aurea, & selectiora . . . Accedit novum Consilium de ratione discendi medicinam, aliasque disciplinas . . . Venetiis, Apud Juntas, & Baba, 1644.

[80], 492 p.; 101, [9] p. illus. 33 cm. **[7780]**

Dedicatory epistle by Francesco Baba, the editor.

Part [2] has half title: De pestilentia.

Contents. — De arte gymnastica, libri sex. — De morbis mulierum, libri quatuor. — De morbis puerorum, libri tres. — Variarum lectionum, libri sex. — Alexandri Tralliani Epistola de lumbrixis (in Greek and Latin). — De pestilentia lectiones. — De maculis pestiferis. — De hydrophobia. — De venenis, ac morbis venenosis.

—Commentarii eruditissimi, in Hippocratis Coï Prognostica, Prorrhetica, De victus rat. in morbis acutis, et Epidemicas historias. Quibus accessere tractatus luculentissimi, de hominis generatione, vino & aqua, balneisque Pisanis. A Marco Cornacchino . . . ex ore ipsius diligenter excepti, nunc primum in lucem editi . . . Francofurti, Typis Joannis Saurii, impensis Joannis Theobaldi Schönwetteri, 1602.

[6], 848, [22] p. 33 cm. **[7781]**

"Praelectiones . . . in Epidemicas Hippocratis historias" (p. 1-268) includes the Latin text of the case histories in books 1 and 3. The other commentaries do not include the Hippocratic texts.

Petrus de Wittendel edited the commentaries on Hippocrates' De victus ratione in morbis acutis.

—Consultationes, et responsa medicinalia tribus tomis comprehensa; postrema hac editione a Mundino Mundinio . . . exornata: addita Mercurialis Collegiandi (ut vocant) ratione . . . Venetiis, Apud Jacobum de Franciscis, 1604-20 [v. 1, 1620]

4 v. in 1. 33 cm. **[7782]**

Vols. 2 and 3, edited by Michele Colombo, are dated 1619. Vol. 4, edited by Gulielmus Athenius, has imprint: Venetiis, Apud Juntas, 1604.

Previously published under title: Responsorum et consultationum medicinalium tomus I [-VI]

—[The same.] . . . Venetiis, Apud Juntas, 1624-25.

4 v. in 1. 34 cm. **[7783]**

Different setting of type.

Imperfect: title page mutilated. Recto of 2d prelim. leaf mutilated, supplied in photocopy from the New York Academy of Medicine Library.

—De arte gymnastica libri sex, in quibus exercitationum omnium vetustarum genera, loca, modi, facultates, & quidquid denique ad corporis humani exercitationes pertinet, diligenter explicatur. Quarta editione correctiores, & auctiores facti . . . Venetiis, Apud Juntas, 1601.

[15], 308 (i.e. 326), [26] p. illus., 2 plans. 25 cm.
[7784]

Woodcut illustrations designed for the author by Pirro Ligorio and cut by Cristoforo Coriolani.

Mainly a page for page reprint of the 3d edition of 1587.

"Appendix ad caput antecedens [i.e. chap. II of book I] ubi iterum de accubitu, triclinio, & de Mariae Magdalenae historia tractatus": p. 65-76.

With this are bound his: De decoratione. 1601 (v. [2] of *his* De morbis cutaneis . . . De decoratione. 1601); Censura operum Hippocratis. Venetiis, 1585; De morbis puerorum. 1615; and De morbis muliebribus praelectiones. 1618.

—[The same.] . . . Ed. nov. aucta, emend. & figuris authenticis Christophori Coriolani exornata. Amstelodami, Sumptibus Andreae Frisii, 1672.

[10], 387, [41] p. illus., 5 fold. plates, 2 plans. 25 cm.
[7785]

Added engraved title page.

The woodcut illustrations, from the same blocks as those in the Giunta editions from 1573 to 1644, were designed for Mercuriale by Pirro Ligorio and cut by Cristoforo Coriolani. The plans are engraved after the original woodcuts. The engraved plates are newly added in this edition. Cf. editor's pref.

Edited by Andreas Frisius, the text based on the 1644 Giunta edition newly collated with several manuscript copies.

—Tractatus: De compositione medicamentorum, De morbis oculorum, & aurium. Ipso praelegente olim Patavii diligenter excepti. Et nunc primum a Michaele Columbo . . . editi . . . Venetiis, Apud Juntas, 1601.

2 parts in 1 v. 26 cm.
[7786]

Preface by Petrus de Wittendel, the editor.

First edited by Michele Colombo in 1590. Published in 1591 under title: De compositione medicamentorum tractatus . . . De oculorum et aurium affectibus praelectiones.

—De morbis cutaneis et omnibus corporis humani excrementis tractatus . . . Ex ore Hieronymi Mercurialis . . . excepti, atque in libros quinque digesti, opera Pauli Aicardii. Quibus accessit alius libellus De decoratione ex ejusdem Mercurialis . . . praelectionibus exceptus, & in capita redactus a Julio Mancino. Venetiis, Apud Juntas, 1601.

2 v. ([32], 210, [1] p.; [8], 44 ll.) 24 cm.
[7787]

Vol. [2], with title: De decoratione liber, is bound with *his* De arte gymnastica. 1601.

The two volumes were originally published separately in Venice in 1572 and 1585.

With vol. [1] is bound *his* De morbis muliebribus praelectiones. 1601.

—De morbis muliebribus praelectiones. Jam dudum a Gaspare Bauhino exceptae, ac paulo antea inscio autore editae: postremo vero per Michaelem Columbum ex collatione plurium exemplarium consensu auctoris locupletiores, & emendatiores factae. Quarta vero hac editione & auctiores, & castigatiores adhuc redditae . . . Venetiis, Apud Juntas, 1601.

[24], 236 p. 24 cm.
[7788]

Bound with vol. [1] of *his* De morbis cutaneis. 1601.

—[The same.] . . . Quinta hac editione . . . non solum auctae, & . . . emendatẹ, verum geminis indicibus . . . locupletissimis adornatae prodeunt . . . Venetiis, Apud Juntas, 1618.

[24], 236 p. 25 cm.
[7789]

Different setting of type.

Bound with *his* De arte gymnastica libri sex. 1601.

—De morbis puerorum tractatus locupletissimi . . . Ex ore . . . Hieronymi Mercurialis . . . excepti, atque in libros tres digesti: opera Johannis Chroscieyoioskii. Venetiis, Apud Juntas, 1601.

[14], 116 ll. 24 cm.
[7790]

—[The same.] . . . Venetiis, Apud Juntas, 1615.

[12], 116 ll. 25 cm.
[7791]

Different setting of type.

Bound with his De arte gymnastica. 1601.

—[German tr.] *In* Uffenbach, P. ed. and tr. Ein newes Artzney Buch. 1605.

—De pestilentia Hieronymi Mercurialis . . . lectiones habitae Patavii MCLXXVII. mense Januarii. In quibus de peste in universum, praesertim vero de Veneta, & Patavina . . . tractatur. Ejusdem Tractatus De masculis pestiferis, & De hydrophobia. Venetiis, Apud Juntas, 1601.

[3], 38, [5] ll.; 20 ll. 24 cm.
[7792]

Part [2] has special title page.

Edited by Hieronymus Zacchus.

—In omnes Hippocratis Aphorismorum libros praelectiones Patavinae. In quibus innumeri pene ipsius Hippocr. obscuriores loci, ac sententiae elucidantur, problemataque permulta obstrusiora facili methodo enodantur . . . Nunc primum a Maximiliano ipsius auctoris filio publici juris factum . . .

Bononiae, Apud Hieronymum Tamburinum, 1619.

[8], 830, [1] p.   32 cm.   [7793]

Includes the Latin text in Niccolò Leoniceno's version.

—[The same.] . . . In postrema hac editione opera
Pancracii Marcellini . . . notis marginalibus ditatae
. . . Lugduni, Sumptibus Antonii Pillehotte, 1621.

[7], 770 (i.e. 760), [43] p.   25 cm.   [7794]

—[The same.] . . . Denuo summa cum diligentia
& labore revisae & emendatae . . . Lugduni, Sumptibus Antonii Pillehotte, 1631.

[8], 770 (i.e. 760), [43] p.   24 cm.   [7795]

—In secundum lib. Epid. Hipp. praelectiones
Bononienses . . . Forolivii, Apud Cimattios, 1626.

[16], 314 p.   32 cm.   [7796]

Dedicatory epistle by Mercuriale Massimiliano.
Includes the Greek and Latin texts.

—Medicina practica; seu, De cognoscendis, &
curandis, omnibus humani corporis affectibus,
earumque causis indagandis, libri V. In Patavino
Gymnasio, olim ab ipso publice praelecti, & thesauri
instar a quibusdam hactenus reconditi, plurimorum-
que votis & desiderio summe expetiti: nunc autem
post obitum autoris . . . in lucem editi, studio &
opera, Petri de Spina . . . Francofurti ad Moenum,
In officina Joannis Theobaldi Schönwetteri, 1601.

[7], 652, [39] p.   32 cm.   [7797]

Imperfect: p. 305-312 wanting.

—[The same.] . . . Francofurti ad Moenum, *In* officina Joannis Theobaldi Schönwetteri, 1602.

[7], 594, [40] p.   33 cm.   [7798]

With this is bound: Fumanelli, Antonio . . . Opera multa.
Tiguri, 1557.

—[The same.] Praelectiones Patavinae. De
cognoscendis, et curandis humani corporis affectibus.
In quibus praeter alia, quae ad praxim exercendam
plurimum conferunt, & praeter variam eruditionem,
gravissimae quoque theoriae difficultates enodantur.
Nuper inscio, et tanquam mortuo authore editae,
nunc vero, tum ex diversis exemplaribus, eodem per-
mittente ac annuente, tum ex ipsiusmet ore praemon-
strante, atque dictante, recognitae, emendatae, & tertia parte auctae. Opera, ac studio Guglielmi Athenii
. . . Venetiis, Apud Juntas, 1603.

[34], 656 p.   36 cm.   [7799]

—[The same.] . . . In hacque postrema editione
summa cum diligentia expurgatae . . . Venetiis,

Apud Juntas, 1606.

[32], 644 p.   35 cm.   [7800]

—[The same.] . . . Et hac postrema editione
summa cum diligentia correctae, & genuino nitori
restitutae . . . Venetiis, Apud Juntas, 1617.

[28], 644 p.   35 cm.   [7801]

Different setting of type.

—[The same.] Medicina practica; seu, De
cognoscendis, discernendis, & curandis omnibus
humani corporis affectibus, earumque causis indagandis, libri. V. In Patavino Gymnasio, olim ab
ipso publice praelecti, & post obitum authoris . . .
in lucem editi, studio & opera, Petri de Spina . . .
Postrema editio a mendis repurgata, & elucidata.
Lugduni, Sumptibus Antonii Pillehotte, [Ex
typographia Claudii Cayne] 1617.

[8], 809, [54] p.   25 cm.   [7802]

Imperfect: p. [10-54] mutilated.

—[The same.] . . . Lugduni, Sumptibus Antonii
Pillehotte [Ex typographia Claudii Cayne] 1618.

[8], 809, [54] p.   25 cm.   [7803]

A reissue of the 1617 edition with new imprint and colophon.

—[The same.] . . . Lugduni, Sumptibus Antonii
Pillehotte, 1623.

[8], 809, [55] p.   24 cm.   [7804]

Different setting of type.

—[The same.] Praelectiones Patavinae, de
cognoscendis, et curandis humani corporis affectibus:
in quibus praeter alia, quae partim ad praxim in re
medica exercendam, partim ad uberiorem eruditionem comparandam plurimum conferunt, gravissimae quoque theoriae difficultates enodantur. Olim
inscio, et tanquam defuncto auctore editae, sed
postea cum ex diversis exemplaribus, eodem permit-
tente, ac annuente, tum ex ipsiusmet ore praemon-
strante, atque dictante, recognitae, emendatae, & tertia parte auctae, opera, ac studio Guglielmi Athenii
. . . et hac postrema editione summa cum diligentia
correctae, & genuino nitori restitutae . . . Venetiis,
Apud Juntas, 1627.

[28], 644 p.   32 cm.   [7805]

A reprint of the same publishers' edition of 1617.

—*as subject. See* MÜNSTER, J. Discussio. 1603.

—Tractatus: De maculis pestiferis. De hydrophobia. Ipso praelegente diligenter excepti, & nunc
primum editi. Venetiis, Apud Juntas, 1601.

20 ll. 24 cm. (Part [2] in *his* De pestilentia . . . De maculis pestiferis & De hydrophobia, 1601)

[7806]

—*See* SCHOLTZ, L. Epistolarum philosophicarum: medicinalium, ac chymicarum . . . volumen. 1610.

MERCURIALE, MASSIMILIANO. *See* MERCURIALE, G. In omnes Hippocratis Aphorismorum libros. 1619, 1621, 1631 [and] In secundum lib. Epid. Hipp. 1626.

MERCURIALIS, HIERONYMUS. *See* MERCURIALE, Girolamo [1530-1606]

MERCURIO, GIROLAMO [*d.* 1615] La commare o riccoglitrice dell'ecc^mo. s^r. Scipion Mercurii . . . Divisa in tre libri ristampata correta et accresciuta dall'istesso autore . . . Venetia, Gio. Bat. Ciotti, 1601.

[39], 356 p. illus. 21 cm. [7807]
Engraved title page.

—[The same.] . . . Milano, Gio. Batt. Bidelli, 1618. [48], 510 p. illus. 17 cm. [7808]

—[The same.] . . . Venetia, Gio. Bat. Ciotti, 1621. [36], 363 (i.e. 367) p. illus. 21 cm. [7809]
Engraved title page.
Books 2 and 3 have special title pages dated 1620.

—[The same.] . . . In questa ult. ed. corr. & accresciuta di due trattati; uno Del colostro, dove si tratta di diversi mali de i bambini . . . dell'eccellentiss. sig. Ezechiele di Castro . . . L'altro di un gravissimo autore, nel quale si risolvono alcuni dubi importanti circa il battesimo de i bambini, e si danno alcuni avisi spirituali molto à proposito per le parturienti . . . Verona, Francesco de' Rossi, 1642.

[24], 327 p.; 31, [4] p. illus. 21 cm. [7810]
Imperfect: added engraved title page wanting.
Part [2] has special title page.

—[The same.] . . . Verona, Francesco de' Rossi, 1645.

[24], 327, p.; 31, [4] p. illus. 21 cm.

[7811]
Imperfect: p. 177-184 wanting.
Part [2] has special title page.
Different setting of type.

—[The same.] . . . Venetia, Gio. Francesco Valvasense, 1680.

[24], 352 p. illus. 22 cm. [7812]

—[The same.] . . . Venetia, Gio. Francesco Valvasense, 1686.

[24], 350 p. illus. 21 cm. [7813]
Different setting of type.

—[German tr.] La commare dell Scipione Mercurio. Kindermutter oder, Hebammen Buch . . . Welches auss dem Italienischen in die hochteutsche Sprache versetzet, an vielen Orthen vermehret und . . . verbessert hat Gottfriedt Welsch . . . Leipzig, In Verlegung Timothei Ritzschens, gedruckt bey Quirino Bauchen, 1652.

[32], 844 (i.e. 836) p. plates. 20 cm. [7814]
Added engraved title page.
With this are bound: Boursier, Louise (Bourgeois). Hebammen Buch. [1628-48]; Boursier, Louise (Bourgeois). Schutzrede. 1629.

—[The same.] . . . Leipzig, In Verlegung Timothei Ritzschens, gedruckt bey Quirino Bauchen, 1653.

[30], 844 (i.e. 836) p. plates. 20 cm. [7815]
Imperfect: first prelim. leaf (engraved title page?) and p. 19-20 wanting.
A reissue of the 1652 edition with new title page and dedicatory epistle reset.

—[The same.] . . . Wittenberg, In Verlegung Tobiae Mevii sel. Erben, und Elerd Schumachers, druckts Matthaeus Henckel, 1671.

[31], 844 (i.e. 836) p. plates. 20 cm. [7816]
Added engraved title page.
Different setting of type.

—De gli errori popolari d'Italia, libri sette, divisi in due parti. Nella prima si trattano gl'errori, che occorrono in qualunque modo nel governo de gl'infermi . . . Nella seconda si contengono gl'errori quali si commettono nelle cause delle malattie . . . Dell'eccellentiss. sig. Scipione Mercurii . . . Venetia, Gio. Battista Ciotti, 1603.

[20], 395 (i.e. 406), [1] ll. 22 cm. [7817]
Part 2 has special title page (ll. [284])

—[The same.] . . . Verona, Francesco Rossi, 1645. [14], 592 p. 20 cm. [7818]
Part 2 has special title page (p. [425]).

—Another issue. [7819]
The preliminaries and Books 1-2 are of a different setting of type.

—[The same.] . . . Padova, Matteo Cadorino, 1658.

[12], 592 (i.e. 596) p. 21 cm. [7820]

Part 2 has special title page (p. [429]).

Part 2 is of the same setting as the 1645 ed., and has a new half title and a new title page inserted before the original title page, which has imprint: Verona, Francesco Rossi, 1645. Part 1 is a page for page reprint of the 1645 ed.

—[French tr.] Discours de l'origine, des moeurs, fraudes et impostures des ciarlatans, avec leur descouverte . . . Par I. D. P. M. O. D. R. Paris, Denys Langlois, 1622.

    [2], 51 (i.e. 49) p.   17 cm.   **[7821]**

Translation of chapter I–VIII, Book IV by I. D. P. M. O. D. R., presumably Jean Desgorris (i.e. Jean de Gorris) or Jean Duret. Cf. BNC.

—*See* ZECCHI, G. *In* primam D. Hipp. Aphorismorum sectionem . . . lectiones. 1629.

MERCURIO, SCIPIONE. *See* MERCURIO, Girolamo [*d.* 1615]

MERCURIUS botanicus. 1634. *See* JOHNSON, T.

MERCURIUS TRISMEGISTUS. *See* HERMES TRISMEGISTUS.

MERENDA, GIOVANNI PIETRO [*fl. ca.* 1544] *See* SCHOLTZ, L. Consiliorum medicinalium . . . liber singularis. 1610.

MERGILETUS, AUGUSTUS FRIDERICUS [*fl.* 1700–1701] *respondent. See* MAPP, M., *praeses.* Theses botanicae et medicae de rosa de Jericho. 1700.

MERIAN, JOACHIMUS [*fl.* 1659–1661] *See* LE BOË, E. de. Opera medica. 1695, 1697, 1698.

MERIAN, MATTHAEUS [1593–1650] *ed. See* BAUHIN, K. Vivae imagines. 1640.

MÉRINDOL, ANTOINE [1570–1624] Ars medica in duas partes secta, in qua non solum ea explicantur, quae ad medicinam discendam sunt necessaria, sed multa etiam, quae theologos & philosophos recreare valeant, continentur . . . Accessit . . . Exercitationum medicinalium decas unica. Aquis Sectiis, Typis Joannis Roize, 1633.

    [30], 419, [27] p.; [4], 153, [14] p.   front. (port.) 37 cm.   **[7822]**

Engraved title page.

Edited by Jacques Merindol.

—Selectae exercitationes VIII . . . Lutetiae Parisiorum, E typographia Edmundi Martini, 1617.

    [8], 215 p.   17 cm.   **[7823]**

Errata leaf pasted on blank p. [216]

Bound with copy 2 of Du Laurens, A. De crisibus liber tres. 1606.

MÉRINDOL, JACQUES [*fl.* 1631] *ed. See* MÉRINDOL, A. Ars medica in duas partes secta. 1633.

MERK, HEINRICH ANDREAS [*fl.* 1687] *respondent. See* WESTPHAL, J. C., *praeses.* De ventis. 1687.

MERK, MICHAEL [*fl.* 1622] *respondent. See* HORST, G., *praeses.* Theses medicae de venae sectione. 1622.

MERLET, JEAN [*fl.* 1654–1659] Opuscula medica duo: quorum unum est De cauteriis, alterum est Paradoxum de tussi. Parisiis, Apud Carolum Angot, 1659.

    76, [2] p.   15 cm.   **[7824]**

MERLIN. Allegoria . . . lapidis arcanum perfecte continens.

    252–254 p., vol. I.   17 cm.   (*In* Artis auriferae. Basileae, 1610)   **[7825]**

Caption title.

—[German ed.] [Die Allegoria . . . vom Geheimnuss dess Steins]

    340–344 p., part I.   19 cm.   (*In* Morgenstern, Philipp, *ed.* and *tr.* Turba philosophorum. Basel, 1613)   **[7826]**

Title from table of contents.

—*See* JĀBIR IBN ḤAIYĀN, al-Ṭarasūsi. Gebri . . . Summa perfectionis magisterii in sua natura. 1682.

MERMANN VON SCHÖNBURG, THOMAS [1547–1612] Consultationes ac responses medicae, a viris doctis hactenus diu multumque desideratissimae; nunc tandem opera et studio Francisci Ignatii Thiermairii . . . Ex variis manuscriptis . . . conquisitae, partim ex Germanico & Italico idiomate in Latinum versae, partim . . . annotationibus & remediis seccedaneis, auctae, in . . . libros octo distinctae . . . Ingolstadii, Typis & impensis Joannis Philippi Zinck, 1675.

    [32], 559, [13] p.   port.   29 cm.   **[7827]**

Added engraved title page.

Imperfect: p. 509 wrongly printed.

[MERRET, CHRISTOPHER, 1614–1695] The accomplisht physician, the honest apothecary, and the skilful chyrurgeon, detecting their necessary connexion, and dependance on each other. Withall a discovery of the frauds of the quacking empirick, the praescribing surgeon, and the practicing apothecary. Whereunto is added the physicians circuit, the history of physick, and a lash for Lex talionis . . . London, 1670.

 [7], 95 p. 20 cm.   **[7828]**
Wing 1835.
Attributed also to Gideon Harvey. Cf. BMC.
Lex talionis was written by Henry Stubbs.

—A collection of acts of Parliament, charters, trials at law, and judges opinions concerning those grants to the Colledge of Physicians London, taken from the originals, law-books, and annals . . . [London] 1660.

 [4], 135 p. 20 cm.   **[7829]**

[—] A letter concerning the present state of physick, and the regulation of the practice of it in this kingdom. Written to a doctor here in London . . . London, Jo. Martyn and Ja. Allestry, 1665.

 65 p. 19 cm.   **[7830]**
Signed at end by T. M.
Wing 1837.
"This work is attributed to Merret . . . but internal evidence makes this impossible"—R. S. Roberts. Jonathan Goddard. Medical History, vol. 8 (1964) p. 191.

—Pinax rerum naturalium Britannicarum, continens vegetabilia, animalia, et fossilia, in hac insula reperta inchoatus . . . Londini, Typis T. Roycroft, impensis Cave Pulleyn, 1667.

 [32], 223, [1] p. 16 cm. **[7831]**

—A short view of the frauds, and abuses committed by apothecaries, as well in relation to patients, as physicians, and of the only remedy thereof by physicians making their own medicines . . . London, James Allestry, 1669.

 53 p. 20 cm.   **[7832]**

—[The same.] . . . The 2d ed. more correct. London, James Allestry, 1670.

 78 p. 21 cm.   **[7833]**
Imperfect: p. 3-4 wanting.

—Some observations concerning the ordering of wines. *In* Charleton, W. Two discourses. 1669, 1675, 1692.

—*See* BOYLE, *Hon.* R. New experiments and observations touching cold. 1665, 1683; [STUBBS, H.] Lex talionis. 1670 [and] Medice cura teipsum; or, The apothecaries plea. 1671.

MERRYWEATHER, JOHN [*fl. ca.* 1644–*ca.* 1681] *tr. See* [BROWNE, *Sir* T.] Religio medici. 1644, 1652, 1665, 1677.

MERSENNE, MARIN, *Father* [1588-1648] *See* FLUDD, R. Medicina catholica. 1629-1631; GASSENDI, P. Epistolica exercitatio, in qua principia philosophiae Roberti Fluddi medici reteguntur. 1630.

MERTZ, JEREMIAS. *See* MARTIUS, Jeremias [*d.* 1585]

MERULA, PAULUS [1558-1607] Oratio posthuma, de natura Reip. Batavicae ex auctoris schedis descripta. Joachimus Morsius vulgavit. Lugduni Batavorum, Typis Jacobi Marci, 1618.

 [33] p. 21 cm.   **[7834]**
Imperfect: First preliminary leaf (blank?) wanting.

—*See* KIRCHMANN, J. In funere . . . Pauli . . . Merulae . . . oratio. 1672.

MERWITZ, KASPAR [*b.* 1658] *See* MAJOR, J. D. Disputationem medicam inauguralem de suppressione mensium . . . habendam J. D. M. . . . invitat. 1693.

MÉRY, JEAN [1645-1722] Observations sur la maniere de tailler dans les deux sexes pour l'extraction de la pierre, pratiquée par Frere Jacques. Nouveau systeme de la circulation du sang par le trou ovale dans le foetus humain, avec les réponses aux objections qui ont été faites contra cette hypothese . . . Paris, Jean Boudot, 1700.

 [19], 90 (i.e. 120), [14], ix, 187 p. illus., plates. 17 cm.   **[7835]**

—Another issue.

 [20], ix, [13], 90 (i.e. 120), 187 p. illus., plates. 16 cm.   **[7836]**
Imprint reads: Imprimé à Paris, et se vend à Amsterdam, chez Jean Louis Delorme, 1700.

—*See* [BRUNET, C.] Le progrès de la medecine. 1699; TAUVRY, D. Traité de la generation et de la nourriture du foetus. 1700.

MESGNIEN MENINSKI, FRANCISCUS A. *See* Meniński, Franciszek [1623-1698]

MESNARDIÈRE. *See* LA MESNARDIÈRE, Hippolyte Jules Pilet de [1610-1663]

MESSIA, PIETRO. *See* MEXÍA, Pedro [1496?-1552?]

MESSORIUS, BERNARDINUS [*fl.* 1626–1641] *See* COLLEGIO DEI MEDICI, Rome. Ordini. 1641.

MESTRAL, C. [*fl.* 1622] Dicours des escrouelles. Où est tres-doctement traicté le moyen de les discerner d'avec les autres maladies qui viennent au col ... Lyon, Pierre Drobet, 1622.

[14], 186 p. 17 cm. [7837]

MESUË [*d.* 857] APHORISMI. *In* Avicenna. Canticum principis ... de medicina. 1649.

—[The same.] *In* Hippocrates. [Aphorismi. French] 1605, 1606, 162-?, 1627, 1628, 1646, 1660, 1666.

—*See* SGOBBIS DA MONTAGNANA, A. de. Nuovo, et universale theatro farmaceutico. 1667, 1682.

MESUË [924 *or* 5-1015] Opera de medicamentorum purgantium delectu, castigatione, & usu, libri duo. Quorum priorem canones universales, posteriorem de simplicibus vocant. Grabadin, hoc est compendii secretorum medicamentorum, libri duo. Quorum prior Antidotarium, posterior de appropriatis vulgo inscribitur. Cum Mundini, Honesti, Manardi, & Sylvii in tres priores libros observationibus ... His accessere plantarum in libro simplicium descriptarum imagines ex vivo expressae. Atque item Joannis Costaei Annotationes ... Reliqua vero, quae cum Mesuae operibus exire solent, in aliud volumen conjecimus, quod nomine Supplementi in Mesuen inscriptum est. Quae omnia accuratissime hac postrema ed. prodeunt emendata ... expurgata. Venetiis [Apud Juntas] 1602.

[8], 252 ll.; [6], 278, [12] ll. illus. 34 cm. [7838]

Contents of the Supplementum (with special title page).— Abano, Pietro d'. Supplementum in secundum librum compendii Secretorum Mesuae.—Francesco di Piedimonte. Supplementum in secundum librum Secretorum remediorum Joannis Mesuae, quae vocant De appropriatis.—Nicolaus Salernitanus. Antidotarium Nicolai cum expositionibus & glossis ... magistri Joannis Platearii.—Saint-Amand, Jean de. Expositio ... supra Antidotarium Nicolai.—Gentile da Foligno. De proportionibus medicinarum.—[Anon.] Tractatus quid pro quo [&] Synonyma.—Abulcasis. Liber servitoris, id est liber 27. Bulchasim Benaberazerin, translatus a Simone Januensi interprete Abraham Judaeo Tortuosiensi.—Saladinus, Asculanus. Compendium aromatariorum.—Albengnefit Libellus in quo de simplicium medicinarum ... virtutibus ... pertractatur.—[Isidorus, Saint, Bp. of Seville] Apulei Liber de ponderibus, & mensuris, & signis cujuscunque ponderis [adapted from the Etymologiarum libri, book xvi, chap. 25–26]—Yā'kūb ibn Isḥāk ibn Ṣubbāh, Abū Yūsuf, al-

Kindī. De medicinarum compositarum gradibus investigandis. — Copho. Tractatus de arte medendi.

The works by Gentile da Foligno, 'Abd al-Raḥmān, Isidorus and Yā'kūb ibn Isḥāk were edited by Giovanni Battista Nicolini, Cf. edition of 1541.

—[The same.] ... Venetiis, Apud Juntas, 1623. [6], 252 ll.; [6], 278, [12] ll. illus. 36 cm. [7839]

Imperfect: ll. [12] wanting.
A reprint of the 1602 edition, without the dedicatory epistle.

—Canones generales. *In* Insa, A. J. Officina medicamentorum. 1698; Ranchin, F. Oeuvres pharmaceutiques. 1624, 1637.

—[Excerpts.] *In* Martínez de Leache, M. Discurso pharmaceutico, sobre los Canones de Mesue. 1652.

—De re medica libri tres. In Dubois, J. Jacobi Sylvii ... Opera medica. 1634, 1635.

—De simplicibus. *In* Ranchin, F. Oeuvres pharmaceutiques. 1624, 1637.

—[The same.] *See* MANARDI, G. Ἰατρολογία ἐπιστολική; sive, Curia medica. 1611.

—*See* CASTELLI, P. Discorso dell'eletuario rosato di Mesue. 1633.

La METALLIQUE transformation. Contenant trois anciens traictez en rithme françoise. A sçavoir, La fontaine des amoureux de science, autheur J. de La Fontaine. Les remonstrances de nature a l'alchymiste errant, avec la response dudict alchym. par J. de Mung. Ensemble un traicté de son Romant de la rose, concernant ledict art. Le sommaire philosophique de N. Flamel. Avec la deffense d'iceluy art, & des honestes personnages qui y vacquent, contre les efforts que J. Girard met à les outrager. Dern. ed. Lyon, Pierre Rigaud, 1618.

88 ll. 12 cm. [7840]

METHODE agreable et facile, pour avoir des fruicts és jardins. *See* GUIBERT, P. L'apotiquaire charitable. 1646.

METHODE asseurée. 1690. *See* ABERCROMBY, D.

METHODE facile pour la distribution des remedes des pauvres ... [Paris? 1678?]

4 p. 24 cm. [7841]

Caption title.

METHODE que l'on pratique a l'hostel des Invalides pour guerir les soldats de la verolle. *See* [LA BRUNE, J. de.]

METHODUS curandorum morborum mathematica. 1613. *See* GEUSS, W.

METZ, JOHANN ADAM [*fl.* 1667] *respondent. See* ZENTGRAF, J. J., *praeses.* Disputatio posterior de tactu regis Franciae. 1675.

METZGER, GEORG BALTHASAR [*d.* 1687] *praeses.* Fluxus et refluxus sanguinis; sive, Exercitationum medico-anatomicarum tertia, de sanguinis in circulum motu ... Giessae, Literis Caspari Vulpii, 1660.

    40 p. 19 cm.   [**7842**]
Diss. — Giessen (H. Rötel, *respondent*)

Dissertations — Tübingen

—*praeses.* Affectuum p. n. haereditariorum theoria ... Tubingae, Typis Gregorii Kerneri [*ca.* 1683]
    28 p. 20 cm.   [**7843**]
Zeller became M. D. in Tübingen in 1684. Cf. Hirsch.
J. G. Zeller, *respondent.*

—De aneurysmate, disputatio inauguralis medica ... Tubingae, Typis Joachimi Heinii, 1679.
    20 p. 21 cm.   [**7844**]
J. C. Cellarius, *respondent.*

—Disputatio inauguralis medica exhibens quaestiones nonnullas ex sectionis V. Aphorismorum Hippocraticorum Aph. XXXI, XXXII, XXXIII decerptas ... Tubingae, Typis Johann-Henrici Reisii [1671]
    8 p. 18 cm.   [**7845**]
Includes Greek and Latin texts of the three Aphorismi.
J. Wachter, *respondent.*

—Disputatio medica de fistulis ... Tubingae, Stanno Reisiano, 1682.
    [4], 20 p. 20 cm.   [**7846**]
J. M. Scultetus, *respondent.*

—Disputatio medica de tussi ... Tubingae, Joachimus Hein, 1676.
    [1], 22 p. 18 cm.   [**7847**]
J. U. Raith, *respondent.*

—Disputatio medica inauguralis de ictero albo virginum ... Tubingae, Literis Heinianis [1677]
    15 p. 19 cm.   [**7848**]
J. J. Kleinknecht, *respondent.*

—Disputatio medica inauguralis de sterilitate muliebri ... [Tubingae] Stanno Heiniano [1677]
    12 p. 22 cm.   [**7849**]
J. Francke, *respondent.*

—Disputatio medico anatomica de humoribus uteri ... Tubingae, Typis Johann-Henrici Reisii, 1677.
    20 p. 20 cm.   [**7850**]
J. H. Hiller, *respondent.*

—Dissertatio inauguralis medica de haemorrhoidum statu s. et p. n. ... Tubingae, Typis Johann-Henrici Reisii [1677]
    24 p. 20 cm.   [**7851**]
J. K. Härlin, *respondent.*

—Dissertatio inauguralis medica de podagra ... Tubingae, Ex Officina Reisiana, 1684.
    19 p. 20 cm.   [**7852**]
G. F. Raussendorff, *respondent.*

—Dissertatio medica inauguralis de acidulis ... Tubingae, Excudit Gregorius Kerner [1663]
    [4], 28 p. 20 cm.   [**7853**]
E. R. Camerarius, *respondent.*
With this is bound Eberhard-Karls-Universität Tübingen. Rector Academiae Tubingensis lect. ben. sal. [1695]

—Dissertationem inauguralem medicam de passione hysterica ... submittit Johann Fridericus Hellwag ... Tubingae, Typis Johann-Henrici Reisii [1677]
    16 p. 19 cm.   [**7854**]
J. F. Hellwag, *respondent.*

—Dissertationem medicam inauguralem de medicamentis sternutatoriis ... subjicit Johann-Henricus Hiller ... Tubingae, Typis Johann-Henrici Reisii, 1678.
    16 p. 19 cm.   [**7855**]
J. H. Hiller, *respondent.*

—Febris maligna petechialis ... Tubingae, Typis Johann-Henrici Reisii [1665]
    24 p. 19 cm.   [**7856**]
S. Braun, *respondent.*

—Historia anatomico-medica thymi ... Tubingae, Ex Officina Reisiana, 1679.
    12 p. 19 cm.   [**7857**]
J. K. Remmelin, *respondent.*

—Scrutinium λυθογενεσιας in humano corpore ex occasione singularis casus institutum . . . Tubingae, Typis Martini Rommeii, 1685.

19 p.   19 cm.   [7858]

J. U. Schmidlin, *respondent.*

—Σκιαγραφια suturarum cranii humani earumque veri usus . . . Tubingae, Typis Martini Rommeii, 1684.

14 p.   20 cm.   [7859]

C. Horlacher, *respondent.*

—Thesium chiriatricarum sylloge V, de fonticulis . . . Tubingae, Typis Johann-Henrici Reisii, 1675.

20 p.   19 cm.   [7860]

J. U. Raith, *respondent.*

—Thesium chiriatricarum sylloge VII & ultima, de vesicatoriis, . . . Tubingae, Literis Kernerianus [1679]

16 p.   21 cm.   [7861]

J. J. Schmidlin, *respondent.*

—Urocriterium brevibus thesibus exhibitum . . . Tubingae, Typis Johann-Henrici Reisii [1677]

8 p.   20 cm.   [7862]

J. Hafenreffer, *respondent.*

METZGER, GEORG FRIEDRICH [*fl.* 1692–1693] *respondent. See* CAMERARIUS, E. R., *praeses.* Disputatio medica de ozaena. 1692.

METZGER, JOHANN [*fl.* 1652] *respondent.* De lethargo. *In* Rolfinck, W., *praeses.* Methodus cognoscendi & curandi adfectus capitis particulares. 1653.

METZGER, KRISTÓF DÁNIEL [*fl.* 1685] *respondent.* Dissertationem inauguralem de lactatione . . . defendet Christophorus Daniel Mezger . . . Altdorffii, Literis Henrici Meyer [1685]

40 p.   19 cm.   [7863]

Diss. — Altdorf.

—*See* HOFFMANN, J. M., *praeses.* Dissertatio physiologico-pathologica de cuticula. 1685.

METZGER, MÁRTON KRISTÓF [1625–1690] *respondent. See* SEBISCH, M. [1578–1674?] *praeses.* Galeni quinque priores libri. 1651.

METZLER, JOHANN CHRISTOPH. *See* MEZLER, Johann Christoph [*fl.* 1692–1693]

MEULEN, JACOB VAN DER [*fl.* 1682] *respondent.* Disputatio medica inauguralis de inflammatione . . . Lugduni Batavorum, Apud Abrahamum Elzevier, 1682.

[12] p.   22 cm.   [7864]

Diss. — Leyden.

MEUN, JEAN CLOPINEL DE. *See* JEAN DE MEUN [*d.* 1305?]

MEUNG, JEAN DE. *See* JEAN DE MEUN [*d.* 1305?]

MEURER, FRIEDRICH [*fl.* 1619–1621] *respondent. See* KEST, F., *praeses.* Themata disputationis ordinariae de vertigine. 1621.

[**MEURISSE,** HENRI EMMANUEL, *d.* 1694] L'art de saigner, accommodé aux principes de la circulation du sang. Par un M^e chirurgien de Paris. Paris, Laurent d'Houry, 1686.

[21], 364, [4] p.   front., illus.   16 cm.   [7865]

Added engraved title page.

Imperfect: p. 293–294 mutilated.

[—] [The same.] . . . Où l'on explique toutes les circonstances qu'il faut observer pour bien faire la saignée . . . 2. ed. rev. & augm. par l'autheur. Paris, Chez Laurent d'Houry [De l'imprimerie de Charles Chenault, fils] 1689.

[21], 418, [4] p.   16 cm.   [7866]

Added engraved title page.

MEURS, JOHANNES VAN [1579–1639] Athenae Batavae; sive, De urbe Leidensi, & Academia, virisque claris, qui utramque ingenio suo, atque scriptis, illustrarunt, libri duo. Lugduni Batavorum, Apud Andream Cloucquim, et Elsevirios, 1625.

[44], 351 p.   illus., plates, ports.   21 cm.

[7867]

Engraved title page.

[—] Illustrium Hollandiae & Westfrisiae ordinum alma Academia Leidensis . . . Lugduni Batavorum, Apud Jacobum Marci, & Justum à Colster, 1614.

[54], 231 (i.e. 239) p.   illus., plate.   21 cm.

[7868]

Imperfect: p. 33–40 and p. 201–208 wanting.

Published also under titles: Illustris Academia Lugd.-Batava, 1613; and Athénae Batavae, 1625. Cf. Brunet.

Attributed also to Jan Janszn Orlers.

Edited by Andreas Cloucquius.

—Solon, sive, de ejus vita, legibus, dictis, atque scriptis, liber singularis. Hafniae, Apud Joach. Moltrenium, 1632.

[3], 127, [4] p.   19 cm.   [7869]

—, *ed. See* ANTIGONUS OF CARYSTUS. Historiarum mirabilium collectanea. 1619; PHLEGON OF TRALLES. Quae exstant, opuscula. 1620.

MEURS, JOHANNES VAN [*fl.* 1642] Arboretum sacrum; sive, De arborum, fruticum, & herbarum, consecratione, proprietate, usu ac qualitate, libri III. Lugduni Batavorum, Ex Officina Elseviriana, 1642.

[16], 140, [3] p.   15 cm.   [7870]

MEUVE, DE [*fl.* 1677] Dictionaire pharmaceutique; ou, Apparat de medecine, pharmacie et chymie ... Tiré & recueilli des meilleurs auteurs qui ont écrit de ces matieres ... 2. ed., rev., corr. & beaucoup augm. par l'autheur. Paris, Laurent d'Houry, 1689.

[8], 676, [32] p.   24 cm.   [7871]

Imperfect: p. 1-2 mutilated.

MEXÍA, PEDRO [1496?-1552?] De verscheyden lessen ... Waer inne beschreven worden de weerdichste geschiedenissen aller keyseren, coningen, ende loflycker mannen ... Hier zijn noch by gevoecht Seven verscheyden tsamensprekinghen: overgheset uyt den Fransoysche, in onse Nederduytsche tale. Amsterdam, Voor Pieter Jacobss. Paets [Ghedruckt by Paulus van Ravesteyn] 1617.

674, [11] p.; 168 p.   16 cm.   [7872]

Part [1] is the translation of his Silva de varia leccion, and part [2] (with half title) of his Los dialogos o coloquios.

MEY, HEINRICH. *See* MAY, Heinrich [1632-1696]

MEY, JOHANNES [*fl.* 1678-1681] *respondent. See* MUNNIKS, J., *praeses.* Disputatio medica.

MEY, JOHANNES DE [1617-1678] *ed. See* GOEDAERT, J. Metamorphosis et historia naturalis insectorum. 1667-70; [French tr.] 1700.

MEY, PHILIPP. *See* MAY, Philippe [*fl.* 1665-1670]

MEYEN, PHILIPPUS. *See* MAY, Philippe [*fl.* 1665-1670]

MEYER, ALBERT [*fl.* 1681] Dissertatio mathematica de observationibus aerometricis hactenus institutis & imposterum instituendis. Cum Appendice de moderno cometa. Kiliae Holsatorum,

Typis Joachimi Reumanni, 1681.

[48] p.   plate.   20 cm.   [7873]

MEYER, DAVID [*fl.* 1684] *respondent. See* MAPP, M., *praeses.* Dissertatio medica de aurium cerumine. 1684.

MEYER, HEINRICH [*fl.* 1639] *respondent. See* WELSCH, G. Anatome cerebri humani. 1639.

MEYER, JOHANN CONRAD [*fl.* 1678] *respondent.* Disputatio medica inauguralis, de phthisi ... Basileae, Typis Joh. Henrici Meyeri [1678]

[11] p.   19 cm.   [7874]

Diss.—Basel.

MEYER, JOHANN JAKOB [*fl.* 1625] *respondent. See* SEBISCH, M. [1578-1674?] *praeses.* Exercitationes medicae. 1639.

MEYER, PETER [*fl.* 1668] *praeses.* Disputationem physicam de anima, cum controversiis: 1. An anima sit hominis forma informans, an assistens? 2. An tres dentur in homine animae, an dola rationalis? 3. An anima hominis sit tota in toto corpore, & tota in qualibet parte? 4. An una anima humana sit melior altera? ... publice ventilandam exhibet ... Johannes Schwiger ... Rostochii, Typis Jacobi Richelii [1668]

[24] p.   20 cm.   [7875]

Diss.—Rostock (J. Schwiger, *respondent*)

MEYER, SEBASTIAN [*fl.* 1602-1603] Institutiones medicae primae. Omnes medicinae locos solidaque totius artis fundamenta, distincte, breviter, ordineque complectentes, quibusvis etiam literatis proficuae ... Frib. Brisgoiae, Martinus Böcklerus, 1603.

[12], 226 p.   13 cm.   [7876]

—Selectorum physicorum medicinalium, politicorum, aliorumque maxime memorabilium, exquisitorum, publicae privataeque foelicitati servientium sylloge prima ... Friburgi Brisgoiae, Ex typographeio Joannis Strasseri, 1617.

188 p.   14 cm.   [7877]

No more appears to have been published.

MEYR, SEBASTIAN. *See* MEYER, Sebastian [*fl.* 1602-1603]

MEYSSONERIUS, HIEREMIAS [*fl.* 1607] De peste libellus. In quo morbi essentia, causae, signa &

curatio, breviter pertractantur ... Avenione, I. Bramereau, 1607.

38, [1] p. 15 cm.   [7878]

With this are bound: Borgarucci, Prospero. De peste.Venetiis, 1565; Bruele, Gualtherus. Methodus ... pro cognitione ... pestis inserviens. Lugduni, 1586.

MEYSSONNIER, Lazare [1602–1672] La belle magie; ou, Science de l'esprit, contenant les fondemens des subtilitez & des plus curieuses & secretes connoissances de ce temps ... Lyon, Nicolas Caille, 1669.

[34], 542, [27] p. illus., plates. 15 cm.

[7879]

—Breviarium medicum, continens theoriae et praxeos medicae brevem summam, in quatuor sectiones, pro quatuor anni temporibus distributam ... Deinde Medicinae practicae Lazari Riverii ... compendium. Studio Bernhardi Verzaschae ... Lugduni, Sumptibus Laurenti Anisson, 1664.

[8], 56, 582, [34] p. 19 cm.   [7880]

—De abditis epidemion causis paraenetica velitatio ... Ad praecavendam & ... curandam luem pestiferam, cum caeteris malignis & popularibus febribus ... Lugduni, Sumptibus Petri Prost, 1641.

[8], 36 p. 23 cm.   [7881]

Bound with *his* Pentagonum philosoph.-medicum. 1639.

—Introduction à la belle magie. *In* Porta, G. B. della. La magie naturelle. 1678.

—Le medecin charitable abbregé. Pour guerir toutes sortes de maladies avec peu de remedes. Et L'almanach perpetuel ou Regime universel, dont ce sert celuy duquel le portrait est en la page cy-aprés pour son salut, sa santé, & celle de ses amis. 2. ed., rev., corr., & augm. ... Lyon [Chez Pierre Compagnon, de l'imprimerie de Marcelin Gautherin, 1668]

58, [1] p. port. 16 cm.   [7882]

"Sommaire des sentimens de M. L. Meyssonnier, extrait de ses oeuvres sur les cometes de 1664 & 1665": p. 52–57.

Bound (as issued) with Hippocrates. Les aphorismes. 1668.

—[The same.] *In* Hippocrates [Aphorismi. French] 1684.

—Nova, et arcana doctrina febrium. Quam ex sectione vivorum & mortuorum animalium, analysi quae fit ignis & aquae beneficio, omnium propemodum seculorum observatione historica-medica

corporum, morborum, et remediorum ... concinnavit ... Lugduni, Sumptibus Petri Prost, 1641.

[12], 105, [7] p. 23 cm.   [7883]

Bound with *his* Pentagonum philosoph.-medicum. 1639.

—Pentagonum philosoph.-medicum; sive, Ars nova reminiscentiae. Cum institutionibus philosophiae naturalis, & medicinae ... et clave ... omnium arcanorum naturalium macrocosmi & microcosmi traditorum, vel scriptorum ... Lugduni, Sumptib. Jacobi & Petri Prost, 1639.

[20], 104, [11] p. illus. 23 cm.   [7884]

With this are bound *his*: De abditis epidemion causis. 1641; Nova, et arcana doctrina febrium. 1641.

—La poudre de sympathie. *In* Digby, Sir K. Demonstratio immortalitatis animae rationalis. 1664.

—Theorie de la medecine. *In* Guyon, L., *sieur de la Nauche.* Le miroir de la beauté. 1643, 1664, 1671, 1673, 1678.

—, *ed. and tr. See* Hippocrates. Les aphorismes. 1668, 1684

—*See* Duchesne, J. La pharmacopée des dogmatiques reformee. 1648; Guy de Chauliac. Les fleurs de Guidon. 1673.

MEYSSONIER, Pierre, *ed. See* Wecker, J. J. Les secrets et merveilles de nature. 1620, 1627, 1699.

MEZEREY, Pierre Du. *See* Du Mezerey, Pierre.

MEZGER, Christoph Daniel. *See* Metzger, Kristóf Dániel [*fl.* 1685]

MEZGER, Georg Balthasar. *See* Metzger, Georg Balthasar [*d.* 1687]

MEZGER, Martinus Christophorus. *See* Metzger, Márton Kristóf [1625–1690]

MEZLER, Johann Christoph [*fl.* 1692–1693] *respondent. See* Spina, D. de., *praes.* Disputatio medica de venenis. 1692.

MICALORI, Biagio [17th cent.] Tractatus de coeco, surdo, et muto ... in quo ipsorum miseria, quid scire, atque addiscere possint, quos contractus celebrare ... et plura alia hujuscemodi ... discutiuntur ... Venetiis, Apud Guerilios, 1646.

[8], 152, [21] p. 23 cm.   [7885]

Errata: p. [21]

Imperfect: title page mutilated.

MICCINI, GIACOMO. *See* MICCIONI, Giacomo [*fl.* 1656–1657]

MICCIONI, GIACOMO [*fl.* 1656–1657] Previdenza, e providenza de' dolori articolari e podagrici ... Perugia, Sebastiano Zecchini, 1657.

[4], 91, [1] p. 22 cm. [7886]

MICHAEL SCOTUS. *See* SCOTT, Michael [1175?–1234?]

MICHAEL, GREGORIUS. *See* MICHAELIS, Gregorius [1625–1686]

MICHAEL, JAKOB [*fl.* 1613] Εξεζασις physica, de fontibus et fluminibus ... [Jenae] Typis Johannis Weidneri [1613]

[16] p. 19 cm. [7887]

Diss. pro loco — Jena (J. Assing, *respondent*)

MICHAELI, PIETRO DE. *See* BAIRO, Pietro [1468–1558]

MICHAELIS, B. J. *See* PORTATILE MEDICUM. 1680.

MICHAELIS, GREGORIUS [1625–1686] *ed. See* GAF-FAREL, J. Curiositez inouyes. 1676.

MICHAELIS, JOHANN [1606–1667] Opera medico-chirurgica quotquot innotuerunt omnia. Ejus nempe I. Praxis clinica generalis ad Jonstoni ideam occupata circa affectus corporis humani ... II. Praxis clinica specialis ... III. Apparatus formularum, seu annotationes in Morellum de praescriptione formularum. IV. Ordo visitandi officinas ... V. Clavis ad authoris polychresta ... Norimbergae, Sumptibus Johannis Hofmanni, typis Johannis Michaelis Spörlini, 1688.

[14], 647 (i.e. 747), [26] p. front. 22 cm. [7888]

—Opera quotquot haberi potuerunt omnia. I. Praxis clinica ad Jo. Jonstoni ideam comparata. II. Apparatus medicamentarius ad P. Morelli methodum praescribendi formulas remediorum. III. Animadversiones in Joh. Schroederi pharmacopoeiam. IV. Notationes ad Guerneri Rolfincii chymiam. V. Officinas pharmaceuticas visitandi ratio. VI. Medicamentorum familiar. syllabus. Ed. alt. ... repurgata et ... locupletata ... Norimbergae, Sumptibus haered, Johannis Hoffmanni, 1698.

[24], 728, [23], 103, [5] p. front. 22 cm. [7889]

—Dissertatio pharmaceutico-therapeutica de natura tincturae bezoardicae D. Johannis Michaelis cum Appendice ... de mistura simplici, his praefixae sunt epistolae honorariae nonullorum veteranorum medicorum. Opera et studio ... Godofredi Schultzii ... Hall. Saxon., Sumtibus Simon. Joh. Hubneri, literis Christiani Michaelis, 1678.

[4], 197, [2] p. 17 cm. [7890]

Dissertations — Leipzig

—*praeses.* Anatomiam martis; seu, Dissertationem medico-chymicam de ferro ... subjicit Elias Schmidt ... [Lipsiae] Johannes Bauer [1658]

[60] p. 19 cm. [7891]

E. Schmidt, *respondent.*

—De apoplexia disputationem inauguralem ... submittit Martinus Fridericus Friess ... [Lipsiae] Literis Bauerianis [*ca.* 1657]

[44] p. 20 cm. [7892]

M. F. Friess, *respondent.*

—De morbo malo; sive, De peste ... Lipsiae, Typis Gregorii Ritzschii [1638]

[40] p. 19 cm. [7893]

A. Rivinus, *respondent.*

—Diatriben medicam de asthmate ... submittit ... M. Florianus Gerstmann ... Lipsiae, Literis Bauerianis, 1656.

[28] p. 18 cm. [7894]

F. Gerstmann, *respondent.*

—Disputatio inauguralis ... de paresi, vel paralysi ex colica ... Lipsiae, Literis Johannis Baueri [1660]

[32] p. 20 cm. [7895]

P. Ammann, *respondent.*

—Disputatio medica de rosa ... Lipsiae, Ex Officina Bauchiana [1655]

[20] p. 19 cm. [7896]

J. Strauch, *respondent.*

—Disputatio medica inauguralis, de morbis metallariorum ... Lipsiae, Quirinus Bauch [1652]

[28] p. 18 cm. [7897]

L. Ursin, *respondent.*

—Disputatio medica inauguralis de pica ... Lipsiae, Typis haered. Frid. Lanckisch, 1638.

[27] p. 18 cm. [7898]

Imperfect: title page mutilated.

H. Boezo, *respondent.*

—Disputationem de phthisi . . . subjicit Gabriel Clauderus . . . Lipsiae, Excudebat Johannes Wittigau [1658]

[62] p. 19 cm. [7899]

G. Clauder, *respondent.*

—Disputationem inauguralem de philtris . . . subjicit . . . Gabriel Clauderus . . . Lipsiae, Excudebat Johannes Wittigau [1661]

[24] p. 18 cm. [7900]

G. Clauder, *respondent.*

—Dissertatio inauguralis de quartana . . . Lipsiae, Literis Quirini Bauchii [1652]

[40] p. 19 cm. [7901]

H. A. Mengering, *respondent.*

—Morbos ab incantatione et veneficiis oriundos . . . proponit . . . Anton Marquart . . . [Lipsiae] Typis haeredum Timothei Hönii, 1650.

[56] p. 19 cm. [7902]

Interleaved.
Imperfect: title page mutilated.
A. Marquart, *respondent.*

—Themata miscellanea, in disputationem medicam solennem proposita . . . Lipsiae, Johan Albertus Mintzelius, 1636.

[20] p. 19 cm. [7903]

A. Gantzland, *respondent.*

—, ed. *See* CROLL, O. Basilica chymica. 1635, 1643, 1658; HEER, H. de. Observationes medicae oppido rarae. 1645.

—*See* BIERLING, C. G. Thesaurus theoretico-practicus. 1695; DRAWITZ, J. Bericht und Unterricht von der Kranckheit des schmertz-machenden Scharbocks. 1658, 1671; HARTMANN, J. Praxis chymiatrica. 1633, 1634, 1639, 1682; HOFFMANN, F. [1626–1675] Clavis pharmaceutica Schröderiana. 1675, 1681 [and] Opus de methodo medendi. 1668; HORLACHER, C. Allgemeine Schatz-Kammer. 1694; SCHRÖDER, J. Trefflich-versehene medicin-chymische Apotheke. 1685; SCHULTZ, G. Scrutinium cinnabarinum. 1679?

MICHAELIS, JOHANN [*fl.* 1634] *respondent. See* BECKHER, D., *praeses.* Disputatio physica de lachrymis. 1634; LAGUS, D., *praeses.* Disputatio publica de visu. 1638.

MICHAELIS, JOHANN MARTIN [*fl.* 1682–1688] *respondent. See* SPENER, J. J., *praeses.* De magnete errores variorum. 1688.

MICHAELIS, JOHANNES [*fl.* 1676] *respondent. See* BORCH, O., *praeses.* Dissertatio medica inauguralis de apoplexia. 1676.

MICHAELIS, JUSTUS CONRADUS. *See* CORTNUMM, Justus [*ca.* 1624–1675]

MICHAELIS, PHILIPPUS. *See* SCHOLTZ, L. Consiliorum medicinalium . . . liber singularis. 1610.

MICHAELIUS, JOANNES [1578–1651] De oculo; seu, De natura visus libellus. Accedunt Dialogus de aeternitate, & quaedam Poëmatia ejusdem auctoris. Dordrechti, Excudebat Henricus Essaeus, 1645.

[16], 84, [22] p.; [148] p. 15 cm. [7904]

Part [2] has half title.

—[The same.] Oculi fabrica, actio, usus; seu, De natura visus libellus. Lugduni Batavorum, Apud Franciscum Moyaert, 1651.

[15], 84, [22] p.; [148] p. 15 cm. [7905]

Part [2] has half title.

—Another issue, with imprint: Lugduni Batavorum, Ex officina Davidis Lopez de Haro, 1651.

[7906]

MICHAELIUS HORNANUS, JOHANN. *See* MICHAELIUS, Joannes [1578–1651]

MICHALORIUS, BLASIUS. *See* MICALORI, Biagio [17th cent.]

MICHAULT, JEAN [1632–1694] Le barbier medecin; ou, Les fleurs d'Hypocrate. Dans lequel la chirurgie a repris la queuë du serpent . . . Par I. M. D. V. C. A. P. Paris, Jean Guignard, 1672.

[52], 475, [1] p. illus., plate. 16 cm. [7907]

Attributed to Jean Michault. Cf. Pauly, col. 664.

MICHELET, HONORÉ [*fl.* 1695] *respondent. See* THOMASSEAU, J., *praeses.* Quaestio medica . . . An ab exlege inspirati aëris motu, febres? 1695.

MICHELSPACHER, STEFFAN. *See* SPACHER, Stephan Michael [*fl.* 1614–1619]

MICHON, PIERRE. *See* BOURDELOT, Pierre [1610–1684 or 5]

MICONE, FILIPPO. *See* ANTERO MARIA DA SAN BONAVENTURA [1620–1686]

MICRER. *See* MICRERIS.

MICRERIS. Tractatus Micreris suo discipulo Mirnefindo.

90-101 p., vol. 5   20 cm.   (*In* Zetzner, Lazarus, *ed.* Theatrum chemicum. Argentorati, 1659-61)

Caption title.   [7908]

MIDDELHUISEN, JAN [*fl.* 1669] *respondent.* Disputatio medica inauguralis de lactis generatione laesa ... Lugduni Batavorum, Apud viduam & haeredes Joannis Elsevirii, 1669.

[16] p.   23 cm.   [7909]

Diss. — Leyden.

[**MIDGLEY**, ROBERT, 1653-1723] A new treatise of natural philosophy, free'd from the intricacies of the schools. Adorned with many curious experiments both medicinal and chymical, as also with several observations useful for the health of the body. London, Printed by R. E. for J. Hindmarsh, 1687.

[II], 342, [3] p.   16 cm.   [7910]

The **MID-WIVES** just complaint, and, divers other welaffected gentlewomen both in city and country, shewing to the whole Christian-world, the just cause of their long-sufferings in these distracted times, for want of trading ... Which sad complaint was tendered to the house on Tuesday, Septemb. 22. 1646 ... London, T. S., 1646.

[I], 6 p.   19 cm.   [7911]

MIEDES, BERNARDINO GÓMEZ. *See* GÓMEZ MIEDES, Bernardino [1521-1589]

MIJL, ABRAHAM VAN DER. *See* MYL, Abraham van der [1563-1637]

MIJN heer. *See* ASSER, H. van. Myn Heer.

MILAN. Collegium physicorum. *See* COLLEGIO DEI FISICI, Milan.

MILAN (DUCHY) **Laws, statutes, etc.** Sospensione della città di Granoble, e di Gap, L'avviso c'hanno ricevuto li SS. presidente, e conservatori della sanita dello stato di Milano, che nelle città di Granoble, e di Gap situate nel Delfinate, si sia dichiarato il mal contagioso a segno d'haver obligato li SS. della città di Torino, a sospender il commercio della loro giurisditione con dette città ... Milano, Giulio Cesare Malatesta [1664]

broadside.   36 x 26 cm.   [7912]

—*See* SETTALA, L. De peste. 1622.

MILAN. OSPEDALE MAGGIORE. *See* OSPEDALE MAGGIORE DI MILANO.

MILAN. Tribunale della sanità. *See* TRIBUNALE DELLA SANITÀ DI MILANO.

MILIUS, ABRAHAMUS. *See* MYL, Abraham van der [1563-1637]

MILLER, GEORG ULRICH [*fl.* 1683] *respondent.* Dissertatio inauguralis de dolore nephritico ... Basileae, Typis Jacobi Bertschii [1683]

[16] p.   19 cm.   [7913]

Diss. — Basel.

MILLER, LUDWIG [1654-1690] *respondent.* Disputatio inauguralis medica de varicibus ... Altdorffii, Literis Schönnerstaedtianis [1680]

24 p.   19 cm.   [7914]

Diss. — Altdorf.

—*See* BRUNO, J. P., *praeses.* Disputatio physiologica. 1680.

MILLI, GIULIO. *See* MILLO, Giulio.

MILLIET DE CHALES, CLAUDE FRANÇOIS. *See* CHALES, Claude François Milliet de, *Father* [1621-1678]

MILLO, GIULIO. Naturae morbos decernentis arcanum opus. Nova collustratum lucerna, ac duobus libris comprehensum. Quorum alter continet ea, quae universim ad crises faciunt: alter Coacas Hipp. & sigillatim morborum omnium enarrat eventa ... Venetiis, Typis Ginammeis, 1654.

[35], 610 (i.e. 600) p.   plate.   23 cm.   [7915]

The second book (p. [171]-610) contains the Latin text of Hippocrates' Coacae praenotiones (generally following Janus Cornarius' version) with commentary.

MINADOI, GIOVANNI TOMMASO [*ca.* 1540-1615] De arthritide liber unus ... Patavii, Apud Franciscum Bolzettam, ex typographia Laurentii Pasquati, 1602.

[4], 82 ll.   21 cm.   [7916]

Bound with *his* De variolis et morbillis liber unicus. 1603.

—De variolis et morbillis liber unicus ... Patavii, Apud Franciscum Bolzettam, ex typographia Laurentii Pasquati, 1603.

[4], 66 ll.   21 cm.   [7917]

With this is bound *his* De arthritide liber unus. 1602.

—Medicarum disputationum liber primus ... Tarvisii, Apud Angelum Mazzolinum, 1610.

[8], 126 (i.e. 128), [12] ll.   26 cm.   [7918]

Imprint date MDCX may be misprint for MDXC, the colophon date. Dedicatory epistle is dated 1590.

No more appears to have been published.

Contents. — De sudore sanguineo. — De adaequato indicante venae sectionis. — De injucunditate in curationibus devitanda. — De cucurbitulis corneis, ustione, et aurium scarificatu. — Quod liber Ad Thrasybulum . . . Galenicus fuerit. — Quid magis pro aquarum correctione praestet coctio, an sublimatio. — De adaequato subjecto facultatis anatomicae.

MINAEUS, Franciscus, *Father* [*fl.* 1622] Justa Ludovici Justi adversus injustam novatorum rebellionem defensio . . . Parisiis, Ex officina C. Morelli, 1622.

95, [1] p.   16 cm.   **[7919]**

Bound with copy 2 of Goclenius, R. Mirabilium naturae liber. 1625.

MINDERER, Raymund [*ca.* 1570–1621] Aloedarium marocostinum. Augustae Vindelicorum [Apud Christoph. Mangium] 1616.

[26], 135 (i.e. 235), [7] p.   16 cm.   **[7920]**

Engraved title page.

— [The same.] . . . Cum annexis Compositionibus aliquot magistratibus medicis autoris, quas lux prius non viderat, nunc . . . in lucem datis . . . Augustae Vindelicorum, Typis Andreae Apergeri, sumptibus Sebastiani Mylii, 1622.

[33], 308, [8] p.; [1], 53 p.   14 cm.   **[7921]**

Part [2] has special title page.

— De calcantho seu vitriolo. Ejusque qualitate, virtute, ac viribus, nec non medicinis ex eo parandis. Disquisitio iatrochymica . . . Augustae Vindelicorum, Apud Saram Mangin viduam, 1617.

[1], 22, 113, [5] p.   21 cm.   **[7922]**

— De pestilentia liber unus, veterum et neotericorum observatione constans . . . [Augustae Vindelicorum, 1608]

[34], 386 (i.e. 384) p.   16 cm.   **[7923]**

Engraved title page.

Imprint supplied from Linden.

— [The same.] . . . Curae secundae. [Augustae Vindelicorum, Apud Andream Aperger, 1619]

[16], 402, [30] p.; [94] p.   16 cm.   **[7924]**

Engraved title page.

". . . In librum De pestilentia appendix, febrium pestilentium, causonidum, maculosarum . . . cognitionem, causas, curationemque perfunctoriam comprehendens . . . ": [94] p.

— Medicina militaris; das ist, Gemeine Handstücklein zur Kriegs-Artzney gehörig . . . Sampt angehengtem rätlichen Gutachten, die jetzt schwebende und unter den Soldaten mehrentheils

grassirende Sucht betreffend . . . Augspurg, Gedruckt durch Andream Aperger, 1623.

389, [53] p.   14 cm.   **[7925]**

Imperfect: p. 219–220 mutilated; wormholes throughout.

— [The same.] Medicina militaris; seu, Libellus castrensis . . . Id est: Gemaine Handstücklein zur Kriegs-Artzney gehörig . . . Ingolstadt, Wilhelm Eder, 1632.

[9], 232, [7] p.   16 cm.   **[7926]**

— [The same.] Medicina militaris; das ist, Gemeine Handstücklein zur Kriegs-Artzney gehörig . . . Sampt angehengtem räthlichen Gutachten, die jetzt schwebende und unter den Soldaten mehrentheils grassirende Sucht betreffend . . . Nürnberg, Gedruckt bey Jeremia Dümlern [not before 1633]

383, [71] p.   14 cm.   **[7927]**

Jeremias Dümler printed from 1633 to 1652 in Nuremberg. Cf. Benzing (A).

— [The same.] Neu-verbesserte Kriegs-Artzney; das ist, Wol-erfahrne und gemeine Hand-Stücklein der edlen Artzney-Kunst . . . Samt angehängtem rähtlichen [sic] Gutachten, von der schwebenden Soldaten-Sucht . . . Nürnberg, In Verlegung Johann Andreas Endters, und Wolffgang, dess Jüngern, seel. Erben, 1667.

394, [86] p.   14 cm.   **[7928]**

— [English tr.] Medicina militaris: or, A body of military medicines experimented . . . Englished out of High-Dutch. London, Printed by William Godbid, and sold by Moses Pitt, 1674.

[1], 152, [12] p.   18 cm.   **[7929]**

Issued also with Barbette, Paul. Thesaurus chirurgiae: the chirurgical & anatomical works. London, 1676, 1687.

— Threnodia medica; seu, Planctus medicinae lugentis . . . [Augustae Vindelicorum, Andreas Aperger] 1619.

[48], 597, [18] p.   16 cm.   **[7930]**

Engraved title page.

— *See* Verbezius, D. Pro Raymundi Mindereri . . . disquisitione iatrochymica de chalcantho. 1626.

MINEUS, Franciscus. *See* Minaeus, Franciscus, *Father* [*fl.* 1622]

MINGELOUSAULX, Simon [*fl.* 1637–*ca.* 1668] *ed.* and *tr. See* Guy de Chauliac. La grande chyrurgie. 1672, 1683.

MINI, Paolo [1642-1693] Medicus igne, non cultro necessario anatomicus, disquisitio ... Venetiis, Apud Joannem Franciscum Valvasensem, 1678.

[20], 169, [1] p. 23 cm. [**7931**]
Errata: p. [1] at end.

MINNER, Johann Christoph [*fl.* 1700] *respondent. See* Vater, C., *praeses.* Dissertatio solennis de pulmonum vomica. 1700.

MINNITI, Francesco. Armonia astro-medico-anotomica; o' sia, Colleganza degl'astri con il microcosmo, e di questo con i vegetabili, con un'appendice della nautica, ed in calce un raccolto di arcani esperimentati ... Furto all'otio di Z. C. Francesco Minniti ... Venetia, Gio. Francesco Valvasense, 1690.

24 p. illus. 23 cm. [**7932**]
Identical in contents with Daniel Ricco's Ristretto anatomico. The illustration has movable parts.

MINOT, Jacques [*fl.* 1684-1691] De la nature et des causes de la fievre, avec quelques experiences sur le quinquina, & des reflexions sur l'action de ce remede ... Paris, Robert Pepie, 1684.

[16], 176 p. 15 cm. [**7933**]

—De la nature et des causes de la fiévre, du legitime usage de la saignée & des purgatifs. Avec des experiences sur le quinquina, & des réfléxions sur les effets de ce remede ... Paris, Laurent d'Houry, 1691.

[8], 360, [24] p. 17 cm. [**7934**]

MINUCCIANI, Pompilio [*fl.* 1627] *See* Maccioni, G. Risposta. 1631.

Les MIRACLES de la nature en la guerison de toutes sortes de maladies. 1660. *See* Mouteau, P.

MIRAEUS, Aubertus. *See* Le Mire, Aubert [1573-1640]

MIRAVAL, Blas Alvarez. *See* Alvarez Miraval, Blas [*fl.* 1597-1598]

MIRÓ, Juan de Vidós y. *See* Vidós y Miró, Juan de [*fl.* 1674-1699?]

MIRUS, Adam Erdmann [1656-1727] *praeses.* Disputatio physica de monstris ... Wittenbergae, Imprimebat Matthaeus Henckelius [1681]

[16] p. 20 cm. [**7935**]
Diss. —Wittenberg (J. H. Fischer, *respondent*)

—Erotema physicum an & quomodo sol calefaciat? ... Wittenbergae, Matthaeus Henckelius [1684]

[16] p. 20 cm. [**7936**]
Imperfect: title page and p. [9-12] mutilated.
Diss. —Wittenberg (B. Bartsch, *respondent*)

MISALDUS, Antonius. *See* Mizauld, Antoine [*d.* 1578]

MISANDER, *pseud. See* Adami, Johann Samuel [1638-1713]

MISAURUS, Philander. *See* Philander Misaurus.

MISCELLANEA. *See* [Temple, *Sir* W., bart.]

MISCELLANEA curiosa medico-physica. *See* Miscellanea curiosa; sive Ephemeridum medico-physicarum Germanicarum.

MISCELLANEA curiosa; sive, Ephemeridum medico-physicarum Germanticarum ... decuriae 1, annus 1-9/10, 1670-1678/79; decuriae 2, annus 1-10, 1682-91; decuriae 3, annus 1-9/10, 1694-1705. Lipsiae [etc.] Sumpt. Viti Jacobi Trescheri, typis Johannis Baueri [etc.] 1670-1706.

24 v. in 13. illus., plates, port. 20 cm. [**7936.1**]
Title varies: 1670-1675/76, Miscellanea curiosa medico-physica.
Decuriae I-II have separate index volume.
Some volumes issued in revised editions.
Separately paged supplements accompany most volumes.
Issued under earlier names of the Deutsche Akademie der Naturforscher: 1670-1686, Academia Naturae Curiosorum; 1687-1691, Academia Imperialis Leopoldina Naturae Curiosorum; 1694-1706, Academia Caesareo-Leopoldina Naturae Curiosorum.
Superseded by Academiae Caesareae: Leopoldino Carolinae Naturae Curiosorum ephemerides.

—Another printing.
8 v. in 5.
Decuria 1, annus 1, 3-7, 9-10 only.
All of the volumes are of different editions than those in the preceding set. Some of the supplements differ.

MISCELLANEA medico-physica Academiae Naturae Curiosorum Germaniae [Annus primus]. *In* quibus plurimae et novae observationes, medicae, chirurgicae, anatomicae, therapeuticae, physicae, chymicae, & botanicae, continentur ... Parisiis, Apud Ludovicum Billaine [Typis Theodoricianis] 1672.

[12], 335 (i.e. 327) p. plates. 24 cm. [**7937**]

MISIATRUS, PHILANDER. *See* PHILANDER MISAURUS.

MISLER, JOHANN JAKOB [*fl.* 1678-1680] *respondent.* Disputatio inauguralis medica de visus statu naturali et praeternaturali ... Gissae, Ex Chalcographia Academ. Kargeriana, 1680.

    [4], 48 p. 19 cm.   **[7938]**
    Diss. — Giessen.

MISOCAPNUS. *See* EVERARD, G. De herba panacea. 1644.

MISOCOLO, EURETA, *pseud. See* PONA, Francesco [1594-1652]

MISSIONS faites en Bretagne l'an 1676. Extrait d'une lettre ... [n. p., 1676?]

    7 p. 24 cm.   **[7939]**
    Caption title.

MISSIVE, Aen D. Balthazar Bekker. 1692. *See* [SCHUTS, J.]

MITHOBEN, AXELIUS A [*fl.* 1660] *respondent. See* LINDEN, J. A. van der, *praeses.* Hippocrates de circuitu sanguinis exercitatio XI. 1660.

MITTENDORF, BERNHARD [*fl.* 1661] *respondent. See* NOTTNAGEL, C. *praeses.* Disputatio physico-mathematica de ventis insolentibus. 1661.

MITTLACHER, ZACHARIAS [*fl.* 1675] *respondent. See* SCHNEIDER, K. V., *praeses.* Disputatio inauguralis de partu difficili. 1675.

MITZEL, JOHANN [1642-1677] *praeses.* Dissertatio juridica de testimonio foeminarum, quam ... sub praesidio ... Johannis Mitzelii ... sistit Georg. Plene ... ad d. 13. Jul. anno 1687 [i.e. 1677?] Regiomonti, Typis Friderici Reusneri [1677?]

    [32] p. 21 cm.   **[7940]**
    Johann Mitzel died October 8, 1677. Cf. Jöcher, vol. 3, p. 562. Friedrich Reusner died in April 1678. Cf. Benzing (A), p. 247-7.

MIZALDUS, ANTONIUS. *See* MIZAULD, Antoine [*d.* 1578]

MIZAULD, ANTOINE [*d.* 1578] Opusculorum pars prima [-secunda] ... Parisiis, Apud Claudium Morellum, 1607.

    2 v. in 1. 18 cm.   **[7941]**
    Imperfect: printer's device excised from title page of "Alexikepus."
    Part 1 is made up of 3 sections, part 2 of 5 sections, each of which has special title page and separate foliation, and reprints an earlier separate edition by the same publisher.

    Contents: — Pars 1. [1] Hortorum secreta, cultus & auxilia (followed by De hortensium aborum insitione, Dendranatome, and De hominis symmetria, as published by the same press in 1575); [2] Alexikepus; [3] Artificiosa methodus comparandorum hortensium fructuum. — Pars 2. [1] Memorabilium ... centuriae novem; [2] Harmonia superioris naturae mundi & inferioris (title page dated 1598); [3] Paradoxa rerum coeli (title page dated 1598); [4] Opusculum de sena; [5] Dioclis Carystii ... Aurea ad Antigonum regem epistola (followed by Arnaldi a Villa-nova ... Consilium ad regem Aragonum, de salubri hortensium usu, and the adaptations from Johannes Lange entitled "De syrmaismo" and "An caseus edendo sit salubris," which were all published together in a single volume by the same press in 1572).

    — Centuriae IX. memorabilium, utilium, ac jucundorum in aphorismos arcanorum omnis generis locupletes, perpulcre digestae ... Accessit his Appendix nonnullorum secretorum experimentorum, antidotorumque contra varios morbos, tam ex libris manuscriptis quam typis excusis, collecta. Seorsum excusa, Harmonia coelestium corporum & humanorum ... Item, Memorabilium aliquot naturae arcanorum sylvula ... Francofurti, Ex officina typographica Nicolai Hoffmanni, 1613.

    [32], 443, [1] p. 12 cm.   **[7942]**
    Centuriae IX was first published in Paris in 1566 under title: Memorabilium ... centuriae IX. The Appendix (p. [211]-267) is the work of Wilhelm Antonius. Memorabilium aliquot ... silvula (p. [269]-355, with special title page) first appeared in Paris in 1554. Harmonia coelestium corporum et humanorum (p. 357-443, with special title page) was first published in Paris in 1555.

    — Alexikepus; seu, Auxiliaris et medicus hortus rerum variarum & secretorum remediorum accessione locupletatus ... Parisiis, Apud Claudium Morellum, 1607.

    [12], 107, [5] ll. 18 cm. (Section [2] in *his* Opusculorum pars prima, Parisiis, 1607) **[7943]**
    Imperfect: title page mutilated, section bearing printer's mark cut away.

    — [French tr.] Le jardin medecinal ... enrichi de plusieurs secrets & remedes ... Ville-Franche, Jean Arnaud, 1605.

    276, [8] p. 18 cm.   **[7944]**
    Signatures: p^{3-8}, q-z^8, A-I^8.
    Translations, by André Caille, of Alexikepus and Artificiosa methodus comparandorum hortensium fructuum, being parts 3-4 of the author's opuscula published in Cologne in 1576 under title: Historia hortensium quatuor opusculis methodicis contexta.

    — [German tr.] Artztgarten, von Kreutern so in den Gärten gemeinlichen wachsen, und wie man durch dieselbigen allerhand Kranckheiten und

Gebrechen eylendts heilen soll. Item ein Artzbüchlin, newe und wunderbare Weiss begreiffend wie man allerley Frücht, Gartenkräuter, Wurtzel, Beer und Trauben artznen soll, dass man dieselb zum Purgieren möge brauchen. Auch ein schöne Weiss und Kunst mancherley Wein zu machen, sampt einer Erzehlung etlicher geartzneten Wein, so für allerhand Kranckheiten nutzlich seind ... Erstlich in Latein aussgangen, jetzund aber newlich verteutscht durch Georgen Henisch von Bartfeld ... Basel, In Verlegung Ludwig Königs, 1616.

[12], 382 (i.e. 302), [6] p ; [1], 109 p. 16 cm.
[7945]

Imperfect: pages [5-6] of Artztgarten, 5-8 of Artzbüchlin wanting.

Artzbüchlin has half-title.

Translations of Alexikepus and Nova et mira artificia comparandorum fructuum. These translations were published separately in Basel in 1575 and 1574, respectively.

—Artificiosa methodus comparandorum hortensium fructuum, olerum, radicum, uvarum, vinorum, carnium & jusculorum, quae corpus clementer purgent, & variis morbis, absque ulla noxa, & nausea, blande succurrant ... Parisiis, Apud Claudium Morellum, 1607.

[8], 39 ll. 18 cm. (Section [3] in his Opusculorum pars prima, Parisiis, 1607)   **[7946]**

—[French tr.] *In his* Le jardin medecina. 1605.

—Harmonia superioris naturae mundi et inferioris; una cum admirabili foedere & sympatheia rerum utriusque ... Parisiis, Ex officina Fed. Morelli, 1598.

[8], 36 ll. 18 cm. (Section [2] in his Opusculorum pars secunda. Parisiis, 1607)   **[7947]**

First published in Paris in 1577.

"Erasmi Roterodami, De varia rerum omnis generis sympathia & antipathia, dialogus pulcher & eruditus": ll.29-36.

—Mizaldus redivivus; sive, Centuriae XII memorabilium ... in aphorismos arcanorum omnis generis locupletes ... digestae, partim ab Antonio Mizaldo ... partim ex aliis ... auctoribus excerptae. Ed. nov. in decem capita ... distributa. Noribergae, Impensis Johannis Zigeri, typis Andreae Knorzii, 1681.

[7], 486, [22] p. 14 cm.   **[7948]**

Added engraved title page.

—Nova et mira artificia comparandorum fructuum. German.] *In his* Artztgarten. 1616.

—Opusculum de sena, planta inter omnes, quotquot sunt, hominibus beneficentissima & saluberrima ... Accessit Proclus De arcanis naturae. Parisiis, Apud Claudium Morellum, 1607.

18, [1] ll. 18 cm. (Section [4] in his Opusculorum pars secunda, Parisiis, 1607)   **[7949]**

A page for page reprint of the same publisher's edition of 1572, but without the list of the author's works at the end.

—Paradoxa rerum coeli ... Parisiis, Ex officina Fed. Moreli, 1598.

36 ll. 18 cm. (Section [3] *in his* Opusculorum pars secunda, Parisiis, 1607)   **[7950]**

—Le traité du sené. *In* Guibert, P. [L'apothiquaire charitable. ca. 1640] [and] Le medecin charitable. 1645 [and] Les oeuvres charitables. 1632, 1633, 1636, 1639, 1640, 1641, 1645, 1647, 1649, 1653, 1656, 1657, 1660, 1670, 1674, 1678; [Latin tr.] 1649.

—, *tr. See* DIOCLES CARYSTIUS. Aurea ad Antigonum regem epistola. 1607; HYGIEIA. 1628; REGIMEN SANITATIS SALERNITANUM. Medicina Salernitana. 1605, 1611, 1612, 1622, 1624, 1628, 1638 [and] Schola Salernitana. 1649, 1657, 1667, 1683.

MOCCA, CESARE [*fl. ca.* 1599] Consilia medicinalia multis praestantissimis remediis insignita, in quibus vera consultandi methodus explendescit ... Taurini, Apud Jacobum Lazaronum, & Umbertinum Merulum, 1620.

[8], 221, [6] p. 21 cm.   **[7951]**

—Discorsi preservativi e curativi della peste, col modo di purgare le case, & robbe appestate ... Torino, & Bologna, Presso Clemente Ferroni, ad instanza di Giorgio Vagnoni, 1630.

68, [4] p. 20 cm.   **[7952]**

Dedicatory epistle signed by Gio. Francesco Zavatta, the editor.

"Instruttione circa il purgar le robbe, e case de gl'appestati": p. 66-68.

MOCHA, CAESAR. *See* MOCCA, Cesare [*fl. ca.* 1599]

MOCHINGER, GEORG [*fl.* 1618-1629] Compendium institutionum medicarum. Danielis Sennerti ... disputationibus XVII in ... Academia Lipsiensi propositum ... Multo quam antea emendatior ... Parisiis, Apud Antonium de Sommavilii, 1631.

[7], 532, [12] p. 14 cm.   **[7953]**

—*praeses.* Sesqui-decas thematum medicorum miscellaneorum ... publicae ... ventilationi subjicit

Henricus Rupitzius ... Lipsiae, Excudebat Fridericus Lanckisch [1629]

[16] p. 20 cm.   **[7954]**

Diss. — Leipzig (H. Rupitz, *respondent*)

MOCHINGER, JAKOB [*fl.* 1651] *respondent. See* ROLFINCK, W., *praeses.* Disputatio medica de catarrho. 1651.

MODENA (DUCHY) **Laws, statutes, etc.** Bando, provvisioni, et ordini per conservazione della sanità, che per Dio gratia si gode intiera in questa città, e ducato ... Modana, Per gli eredi di Giuliano Cassiani, 1682.

broadside. 49 x 36 cm.   **[7955]**

Imperfect: mutilated.

MODENA, Ordinances, local laws, etc. Bandi, provigioni, et ordini, publicati in Modona per occasione di contagio. Principiando nel fine dell'anno 1629. sino per l'anno 1631 ... Modona, Giulian Cassiani, 1632.

[2], 64, [8] p. illus. 31 cm.   **[7956]**

— Bando per causa di contagio, et introduttione dell'uso delle fedi di sanità ... Modona, Giulian Cassiani [1634]

broadside. 41 x 28 cm.   **[7957]**

— Bando per causa di peste ... Modona, Giulian Cassiani, 1630.

broadside. 40 x 28 cm.   **[7958]**

— Bando per causa di peste ... Modona, Giulian Cassiani [1634]

broadside. 40 x 28 cm.   **[7959]**

— Bando per occasione di contagio ... Modona, Stamperia ducale [1639]

broadside. 37 x 28 cm.   **[7960]**

— Grida sopra la custodia delle porte della città di Modana ... Modana, Andrea Cassiani, 1657.

broadside. 50 x 38 cm.   **[7961]**

— Grida sopra l'espurgatione della città per conservatione della sanità ... Modona, Giulian Cassiani [1629]

broadside. 39 x 29 cm.   **[7962]**

— Grida sopra il sepelire le bestie morte, e non vender, e comprar bestie malate ... Modona, Giulian Cassiani [1634]

broadside. 40 x 28 cm.   **[7963]**

— Provigioni, et ordini per conservatione della publica salute per tener lontani i pericoli di contagio ... Modana, Gli eredi di Giuliano Cassiani, 1679.

broadside. 43 x 29 cm.   **[7964]**

— Tassa delle robbe medicinali tanto semplici quanto composte ad uso di ... città di Modana, et suo distretto. Dall'illustrissima communità, e dall'eccellentissimo Collegio de signori medici con l'intervento delli eletti del Collegio de spetiali, con ogni cautezza esattamente revista, & approvata il presente anno 1677. Modana, Vivano Soliani, 1677.

36 p. front. 29 cm.   **[7965]**

MODO d'adoperare l'orvietano contra veleni vivi, e morti. *See* TUSCANY. Laws, statutes, etc. Bando contro a chl [sic] fraudolentemente dispenserà l'orvietano di Francesco di Jacopo Sozzi. 1639.

MÖBIUS, FRIEDRICH TOBIAS [*fl.* 1667-1672] *respondent. See* THOMASIUS, J. [1622-1684] *praeses.* De transformatione hominum in bruta dissertationem philosophicam ... subjicit ... F.T.M. 1673.

MÖBIUS, GOTTFRIED [1611-1664] Anatomia camphorae, ejus originem, qualitates, praeparationes chimicas, ac vires, quas in omnibus fere totius humani corporis morbis instar panaceae cujusdam praestat, nec non in aliis rebus usum succincte exhibens ... Jenae, Impensis Joh. Ludovici Neunhahnii, charactere Sengenwaldiano, 1660.

[8], 104 p. 21 cm.   **[7966]**

Bound with *his* Epitome institutionum medicarum. 1663.

— Epitome institutionum medicarum, ex neotericorum fundamentis ... adornata ... Jenae, Typis, & impensis Samuelis Krebsii, 1663.

[14], 738, [16] p. 21 cm.   **[7967]**

Imperfect: engraved title page wanting.

With this are bound: *his* Anatomia camphorae. 1660; Kerger, M. De fermentatione liber. 1663.

— Fundamenta medicinae physiologica, in quibus origo, & natura medicinae, doctrina de animae facultatibus, spiritibus ac temperamento ... ventilantur ... Jenae, Impensis Johannis Ludovici Neuenhahns, typis Caspari Freyschmidii, 1661.

[6], 608 p. port. 20 cm.   **[7968]**

— Copy 2. front. (port)

Imperfect: title page mutilated.

With this is bound Rolfinck, W. Ordo et methodus medicinae specialis commentatoriae ὡς ἐν γένει. 1665.

—[The same.] . . . Prodeunt tertium . . . cum nova praefatione Georgii Wolfgangi Wedelii . . . Francofurti & Lipsiae, Impensis Augusti Boetii, typis Christophori Fleischeri, 1678.

[10], 608, [46] p. port. 21 cm.   **[7969]**

—Synopses epitomes institutionum medicinae . . . concinnatae . . . Jenae, Typis & impensis Samuelis Krebsii, 1662.

[1], 33 double ll. 30 cm.   **[7970]**

Printed on inside of double leaves (37 × 30 cm.).

Dissertations—Jena

—*praeses.* De natura et usu clysterum saluberrimo, disputatio medica . . . Jenae, E chalcographeo Joh. Christ. Weidneri, 1649.

[44] p. 19 cm.   **[7971]**

S. H. Cravelius, *respondent.*

—De sterilitate sexus utriusque disputationem inauguralem . . . p. p. Anton. Marquart . . . [Jenae] E calcographeo Georgii Segenwaldi [1650]

[44] p. 19 cm.   **[7972]**

A. Marquart, *respondent.*

—Discursus inauguralis de legitimo venaesectionis usu . . . Jenae, Excudebat Johannes Nisius [1654]

[16] p. 20 cm.   **[7973]**

C. Funcke, *respondent.*

—Disputatio inauguralis medica de dolore capitis . . . Jenae, Literis Johannis Nisii, 1653.

[40] p. 18 cm.   **[7974]**

J. C. Frommann, *respondent.*

—Disputatio inauguralis medica de epilepsia . . . Jenae, Literis Caspari Freyschmids, 1659.

[1], 83, [3] p. 18 cm.   **[7975]**

T. Bussius, *respondent.*

—Disputatio inauguralis medica de scirrho lienis . . . Jenae, Charactere Sengenwaldiano, 1655.

[32] p. 19 cm.   **[7976]**

F. Gerber, *respondent.*

—Disputatio medica de bilis natura ejusque usu nobilissimo . . . Jenae, Typis Steinmannianis, 1644.

[23] p. 19 cm.   **[7977]**

J. M. Nester, *respondent.*

—Disputatio medica de tertiana intermittente . . . Jenae, Typis Johan. Christoph. Weidneri, 1641.

[16] p. 19 cm.   **[7978]**

G. C. Wolff, *respondent.*

—Disputatio medica dogmaticorum, nec non Hermeticorum fundamentis illustrata de phrenitide . . . Jenae, E chalcographeo Blasii Lobensteins, 1647.

[28] p. 19 cm.   **[7979]**

G. P. Klug, *respondent.*

—Disputatio medica inauguralis de variolis et morbillis . . . Jenae, E typogr. Johannis Nisii, 1653.

[44] p. 19 cm.   **[7980]**

W. Prenke, *respondent.*

—Dissertatio inauguralis medica de pleuritide . . . [Jenae] Literis Johannis Nisii, 1656.

[1], 42 p. 19 cm.   **[7981]**

P. J. Caleni, *respondent.*

—Dissertatio medica de chylificatione seu coctione prima . . . Jenae, Typis Georgii Sengenwaldts & Caspari Freyschmieds, 1645.

[26] p. 20 cm.   **[7982]**

C. Aussfeldt, *respondent.*

—Dissertatio medica inauguralis de ardore ventriculi . . . Jenae, Typis Sengenwaldianis [1660]

[1], 21, [1] p. 19 cm.   **[7983]**

G. Förster, *respondent.*

—Dissertatio medica inauguralis, de epilepsia . . . Jenae, Typis Samuelis Krebsii [1664]

[32] p. 19 cm.   **[7984]**

B. Chiliani, *respondent.*

—Dissertatio medica inauguralis de febre petechiali . . . Jenae, Typis Johannis Nisii, 1658.

60 p. 19 cm.   **[7985]**

J. Rhetius, *respondent.*

—Dissertatio medica inauguralis de suffocatione uterina . . . Jenae, Typis Johann. Nisii, 1661.

[28] p. 19 cm.   **[7986]**

Imperfect: p. [27–28] mutilated.

J. F. Lysthenius, *respondent.*

—Institutionum medicarum disputatio decima de usu hepatis et bilis . . . [Jenae] Charactere Freyschmidiani, In fLorente ACaDeMIa IenensI [1654]

[52] p. 19 cm.   **[7987]**

G. Clauder, *respondent.*

—Institutionum medicarum disputatio decima quarta de usu partium genitalium in foeminis . . . Jenae, Charactere Freyschmidiano, 1658.

[58] p. 19 cm.   **[7988]**

J. A. Bossert, *respondent.*

MÖBIUS, JOHANN [*fl.* 1671] *respondent. See* POSNER, C., *praeses.* Disputatio physiologica de respiratione. 1671.

MÖBIUS, PAUL CHRISTOPH [*fl.* 1671] *respondent. See* SCHENCK, J. T., *praeses.* Dissertatio inauguralis medica de catalepsi. 1671.

MÖGLING, JOHANN BURCKHARD [*fl.* 1679] *respondent. See* CAMERARIUS, E. R., *praeses.* Disputatio inauguralis medica de ictero. 1679.

MÖGLING, JOHANN LUDWIG [*fl.* 1608-1655] De inconsiderato acidularum usu . . . Tubingae, Typis Theodorici Werlini, 1615.

    [2], 57 p. 16 cm.   **[7989]**

    —*praeses.* Lanx satura rerum medicarum . . . disputatio gradualis . . . Tubingae, Typis Theodorici Werlini, 1622.

    [8], 154, [1] p. 18 cm.   **[7990]**
    Diss.—Tübingen (F. Monavius, *respondent*)

    —Problemata practica publica de scurbuto [sic] . . . Tubingae, Typis Theodorici Werlini, 1620.

    [1], 14 p. 18 cm.   **[7991]**
    Diss.—Tübingen (B. Reyhing, *respondent*)

MÖGLING, JOHANN LUDWIG [*fl.* 1662-1685] *praeses.* Exercitatio physica de inferno naturali, aliisque huic cognatis specubus . . . Tubingae, Literis Johann Henrici Reisii, 1685.

    20 p. 19 cm.   **[7992]**
    Diss.—Tübingen (J. M. Brigel, *respondent*)

    —Vigilia . . . Tubingae, Joachimus Hein, 1672.

    24 p. 19 cm.   **[7993]**
    Diss.—Tübingen (G. Wachter, *respondent*)

MÖHRING, Paul Heinrich [*fl.* 1667] *respondent. See* VOIGT, G., *praeses.* Disputatio physica de amore ovis et lupi. 1667.

MÖINICHEN, ERICUS A. SEE MØINICHEN, Erik [1672-1728]

MØINICHEN, ERIK [1672-1728] *respondent. See* SEERUP, G. N., *praeses.* Triumphus lithargyriatorum. 1700.

MØINICHEN, HENRIK [1631-1709] Observationes medico-chirurgicae, missae ad Thomam Bartholinum, nunc a Josepho Lanzono . . . adauctae. Quibus accessere Arnoldi Bootii & aliorum med. doctorum Observationes . . . Ferrariae, Sumptibus & typis Hieronymi Filoni, 1688.

    [8], 78, 72, [21] p. 15 cm.   **[7994]**
    Errata: p. [21]

    —[The same.] Observationes medico-chirurgicae, cum annotationibus Josephi Lanzonii . . . Dresdae, Sumptib. Gottofr. Kettneri, Typis Ridelianis, 1691.

    [12], 95, [11] p. 14 cm.   **[7995]**

    —*See* LYSER, M. Culter anatomicus. 1665, 1679.

MOELLENBROCK, VALENTIN ANDREAS [*d.* 1675] Cochlearia curiosa . . . Lipsiae, Sumptib. Joh. Grossii & socii, typis Christophori Uhmanni, 1674.

    [12], 140, [20] p. 17 cm.   **[7996]**
    Bound with *his* De varis. 1672.

    —[English tr.] Cochlearia curiosa; or, The curiosities of scurvygrass. Being an exact scrutiny and careful description of the nature and medicinal vertue of scurvygrass. In which is exhibited to publick use the most and best preparations of medicines, both Galenical and chymical . . . in which the plant, or any part thereof is imployed . . . Englished by Tho. Sherley . . . London, Printed by S. and B. Griffin, for William Cademan, 1676.

    [15], 195, [28] p. front., 4 fold. plates. 17 cm.
                               [7997]
    Imperfect: front. and p. 17-32 wanting.

    —De varis, seu arthritide vaga scorbutica tractatus . . . Lipsiae, Sumpt. haered. Gothofredi Grossii, typis Christiani Michaëlis, 1663.

    [16], 167, [9] p. 17 cm.   **[7998]**
    With this is bound copy 3 of Brucaeus, Heinrich. De scorbuto propositiones. [n. p.] 1589.

    —[The same.] . . . Ed. alt. auct. & emend. . . . Lipsiae, Sumptib. Joh. Grossii & socii, typis Christiani Michaelis, 1672.

    [14], 284, [65] p. 17 cm.   **[7999]**
    With this is bound *his* Cochlearia curiosa. 1674.

    —*praeses.* Disputatio medica de peste . . . Erfurti, Typis Pauli Michaëlis, 1654.

    [16] p. 20 cm.   **[8000]**
    Diss.—Erfurt (G. Eichelborn, *respondent.*)

    —Disputationum medicarum de ventriculo secunda . . . Erfurti, Typis Pauli Michaëlis, 1656.

    [20] p. 18 cm.   **[8001]**
    Diss.—Erfurt (C. Zeumer, *respondent*)

—*See* DORNCREILIUS, T. Medulla totius praxeos medicae aphoristica. 1656.

MOELLER, DANIEL WILHELM. *See* MOLLER, Daniel Wilhelm [1642-1712]

MÖLLER, FRIEDRICH [*fl.* 1607-1652] Observatio singularis et rara de partu 173. dierum vivo, qui legitimus in foro judiciali competente, postquam per integrum decennium de illo controversia fuit agitata, declaratus, cujus rationes ex solidis naturae fundamentis plenius deduxit ... Cüstrini, Typis Christophori Sönniken, & impensis Georgii Dennewitzen, 1662.

    [10], 86 p. 14 cm.   [8002]

—*respondent. See* MÖLLER, S., *praeses.* Themata de dysenteria. 1607

MÖLLER, GEORG CHRISTOPH [*fl.* 1688-1700] *praeses.* Disputatio physico-medica de saccharo ... Gissae, Literis Henningi Mülleri [1698]

    32 p. 19 cm.   [8003]
  Diss.—Giessen (J. A. Höcher, *respondent*)

MÖLLER, JACOB [*fl.* 1691] Discursus duo philologico-juridici, prior de cornutis, posterior de hermaphroditis, eorumque jure, uterque ex jure divino, canonico, civili ... congestus ... Francofurti, Typis Christoph. Andreae Zeitleri, 1692.

    [8], 214 p. 18 cm.   [8004]

MÖLLER, JOHANN [*fl.* 1648] *respondent. See* EICHSTÄD, ` ., *praeses.* Disputatio generalis de osteologia humana. 1648.

MÖLLER, JOHANN GEORG [*fl.* 1695] *respondent. See* SLEVOGT, J. A., *praeses.* Diatribe physiologica de affectibus animi. 1695.

MÖLLER, PETER [1628-1680] *praeses.* Historia chirurgica rarior de ventositate spinae ... Regiomonti, Typis Friderici Reusneri [1673]

    [24] p. illus. 19 cm.   [8005]
  Diss.—Königsberg (J. G. Pötter, *respondent*)

MÖLLER, SEBASTIAN [*d.* 1609]

Dissertations—Frankfurt an der Oder

—*praeses.* Disputatio medica de phthisi ... [Francofurti] Typis Sciurinis [1603]

    [12] p. 20 cm.   [8006]
  M. Weinrich, *respondent.*

—Themata de dysenteria, et colore colico ... respondebunt M. Fridericus Mollerus ... Henricus Cunitius ... Godfrid Schmol ... Franciscus Omichius ... Francofurti Marchionum, Ex officina typographia Joannis Eichorn, 1607.

    [30] p. 19 cm.   [8007]
  H. Cunitz, F. Möller, F. Omich, G. Schmol, *respondents.*

—Themata medica de angina ... Francofurti, Typis Sciurianis [1603]

    [8] p. 20 cm.   [8008]
  G. Manlius, *respondent.*

—Theses medicae de vertigine ... Francofurti, Typis Sciurinis, 1602.

    [12] p. 20 cm.   [8009]
  C. Schobart, *respondent.*

MÖNCH, MARTIN [*fl.* 1681] *respondent. See* RUROCK, J. C., *praeses.* Disputatio medica de haemorrhoidibus. 1680.

MOENE DE GRIMALDI, DENIS, *seigneur de Copponay. See* COPPONAY DE GRIMALDY, Denis de [*ca.* 1623-1717]

MOENICHEN, ERIC. *See* MØINICHEN, Erik [1672-1728]

MOFFAT, THOMAS. *See* MOFFETT, Thomas [1553-1604]

MOFFETT, THOMAS [1553-1604] De jure et praestantia chemicorum medicamentorum ... [&] Epistolae quinque medicinales.

    70-108 p., vol. 1. 20 cm. (*In* Zetzner, Lazarus, *ed.* Theatrum chemicum. Argentorati, 1659-61)   [8010]
  Caption titles.

—Healths improvement; or, Rules comprizing and discovering the nature, method, and manner of preparing all sorts of food used in this nation ... Corr. and enl. by Christopher Bennet ... London, Tho. Newcomb for Samuel Thomson, 1655.

    [7], 296 p. 20 cm.   [8011]

—Insectorum, sive minimorum animalium theatrum: olim ab Edoardo Wottono, Conrado Gesnero, Thomaque Pennio inchoatum, tandem Tho. Moufeti ... opera ... concinnatum, auctum, perfectum ... Londini, Thom. Cotes, 1634.

    [20], 326 (i.e. 316), [4] p. illus. 30 cm.
                              [8012]

Edited by *Sir* Théodore Turquet de Mayerne.

—Another issue. [8013]

Imprint differs: Londini, Ex officina typographica Thom. Cotes, et venales extant apud Guiliel. Hope, 1634.

—Another issue. 32 cm. [8014]

Imprint differs: Londini, Ex officina typographica Thom. Cotes, et venales extant apud Benjam. Allen, 1634.

—[English tr.] The theater of insects. *In* Topsell, E. The history of four-footed beasts and serpents. 1658.

—*See* SCHOLTZ, L. Epistolarum philosophicarum: medicinalium, ac chymicarum ... volumen. 1610.

MOGEN, PHILIPP WILHELM [*fl.* 1694] *respondent.* Dissertatio inauguralis medica de colica ... [Altdorffii] Typis Henrici Meyeri [1694]

32 p. 20 cm. [8015]

Diss.—Altdorf.

MOGROBESIUS, TURIBIUS ALPHONSUS. *See* MOGROVEJO, Toribio Alfonso de, *Saint* [1538-1606]

MOGROVEJO, TORIBIO ALFONSO DE, *Saint* [1538-1606] *See* CATHOLIC CHURCH. *Congregatio Sacrorum Rituum.* Contregatione Sacrorum Rituum ... Beatificationis, & canonizationis ... Turibii Alphonsi Mogrobesii, 1675.

MOHR, NICOLAS CONRAD [*fl.* 1678] *respondent. See* JOHRENIUS, C., *praeses.* De affectione hypochondriaca diatribe. 1678.

MOHY, HENRI [*fl. ca.* 1620-1650] Pulvis sympatheticus, quo vulnera sanantur absque medicamenti ad partem affectam applicatione, & superstitione; Galenicarum, Aristotelicarumque rationum cribro eventilatus. [n. p.] 1639.

34, [1] p. 20 cm. [8016]

Last line on p. 8 pasted in.
Bound with Plemp, V. F. Animadversio. 1642.

—[The same.] ... Ed. nova. [Bruxellis? 1640?]
72 p. 15 cm. [8017]

Imprint supplied from BMC.
"Nicolai Papinii ... Brevis & accuratior pulveris sympathici praeparandi & applicandi methodus ...": p. 57-72.

—[The same.]
[165]-176 p. 21 cm. (*In* Theatrum sympatheticum auctum. Norimbergae, 1662) [8018]

Half title.
Without Papin's tract.

—*as subject. See* DEUSING, A. *In* Sympathetici pulveris examen. 1662.

—Tertianae crisis. Qua DD. Petri Barbae ... praxis curandae tertianae, & V. F. Plempii ... animadversio discutitur, ac legitima demum tertianae curatio exponitur. [n. p., 1642?]

15 p. 20 cm. [8019]

Caption title.
Bound with Plemp, V. F. Animadversio. 1642.

MOHYUS, ERYCIUS. *See* MOHY, Henri [*fl. ca.* 1620-1650]

MOINE, ANTOINE LE. *See* LE MOINE, Antoine [*fl.* 1662-1703]

MOIX, JOAN RAPHEL [*fl.* 1587-*ca.* 1612] Methodi medendi per venae sectionem morbos muliebres acutos libri quatuor. Quibus succedit spicilegium eorum, qua a variis sunt scripta de curandi ratione per venae sectionem febres, quas humor putrescens accendit ... Coloniae Allobrogum, Apud Philippum Albertum, 1612.

[31], 1189, [205] p. 18 cm. [8020]

Imperfect: wormholes on p. 931-942 and 1101-1138; signatures of sheets 4A and 4E interposed.

MOL, PIETER [*fl.* 1668] *respondent.* Disputatio medica inauguralis de suffusione ... Lugduni Batavorum, Apud viduam & haeredes Joannis Elsevirii, 1668.

[12] p. 24 cm. [8021]

Diss.—Leyden.

MOLANUS, JOHANN HEINRICH [*fl.* 1674] *respondent. See* SCHWELING, J. E., *praeses.* Sol obscuratus. 1674.

MOLCKENBOUR, GERARD [*fl.* 1685] *respondent.* Disputatio medica inauguralis, de ictero flavo ... Harderovici, Apud Albertum Sas, 1685.

[16] p. 22 cm. [8022]

Diss.—Harderwijk.

MOLIMBROCHIUS, ANDREAS VALENTINUS. *See* MOELLENBROCK, Valentin Andreas [*d.* 1675]

MOLINA, FRANCISCO JUAN. *See* INSA, A. J. Officina medicamentorum. 1601 [colophon: 1603], 1698.

MOLINAEUS, JOANNES. *See* DESMOULINS, Jean [1530-1620?]

MOLINARIIS, SIMON DE [*fl.* 1663-1672] Ambrosia Asiatica seu, De virtute, & usu herbae the sive cia. Nec non de modo adhibendae, & praeparandae ejus potionis juxta regulas bene medendi ... Genvae, Typis Antonii Georgii Franchelli, 1672.
    227 p. 14 cm.   **[8023]**
  Imperfect: title page and p. 225-227 mutilated.

MOLINES, ALLAN. *See* MULLEN, Allen [*d.* 1690]

MOLINES, WILLIAM. *See* MOLINS, William [*fl.* 1648-1680]

MOLINETTI, ANTONIO [*d.* 1675] Dissertationes anatomicae, et pathologicae de sensibus, & eorum organis. Patavii, Ex typographia Matthaei Bolzetta de Cadorinis, 1669.
    [8], 116 p. plates. 20 cm.   **[8024]**
  Added engraved title page.

— Dissertationes anatomico-pathologicae quibus humani corporis partes accuratissime describuntur morbique singulas divexantes explicantur ... Venetiis, Apud Paulum Balleonium, 1675.
    [8], 338 p. illus., plate, table. 25 cm.
                             [8025]

MOLINETTI, MICHELANGELO [1645?-1714?] Indicantur lectiones quas, Deo dante in universam humani corporis fabricam ... In celeberrimo Patavino theatro ... habebit ad annum 1690 ... [Patavii, Apud Cadorinum, 1640 (i.e. 1690?)]
    4 p. 23 cm.   **[8026]**
  Caption title.

— *See* GODI, G. C. Lucubratiunculae ... a Michaele Angelo Molinetto. 1686.

MOLINEUX. *See* MOLYNEUX, William [1656-1698]

MOLINIUS, ANTONIUS. *See* DU MOULIN, Antoine [*b. ca.* 1510]

MOLINS, WILLIAM [*fl.* 1648-1680] Μυσκοτομια; or, The anatomical administration of all the muscles of an humane body, as they arise in dissection. As also an analitical table, reducing each muscle to his use and part ... London, Printed by John Field for Edward Husband, 1648.
    [13], 111 p. 15 cm.   **[8027]**
  Interleaved. Ink drawing illustrating text on leaf following p. 4.

— [The same.] *In* Browne, J. A compleat treatise of the muscles. 1681, 1683, 1697, 1698; [Latin tr.] 1684, 1687, 1694.

MOLK, LEVIN-NICOLAS DE. *See* MOLTKE, Levin Nicolaus von [*d.* 1663]

MOLITOR, JOHANNES HORATIUS [*fl.* 1676] Tractatus de thermis artificialibus septem mineralium planetarum, in quo ... quaestiones celebres thermas nostras attingentes solvuntur, ac quomodo corpus ante usum illarum praeparandum explicatur ... Jenae, Excudebat Samuel Krebs, 1676.
    [22], 72, [26] p. 14 cm.   **[8028]**
  Imperfect: all after p. [26] wanting.
  Bound with Wedel, G. W. Theoremata medica. 1677.

MOLL, NIKOLAUS [*fl.* 1653] *respondent. See* ROLFINCK, W., *praeses.* Disputatio medico-chirurgica inauguralis de vulneribus. 1653.

MOLLER, DANIEL [*fl.* 1605] *respondent. See* POLL, M., *praeses.* De spiritibus corporis humani. 1605.

MOLLER, DANIEL WILHELM [1642-1712] *praeses* Disputationem circularem de Onuph. Panvinio ... ingredietur Leonhardus Reuterus ... [Altdorffii] Cattiero Henrici [1697]
    24 p. 20 cm.   **[8029]**
  Diss. — Altdorf (L. Reuter, *respondent*)

MOLLER, FRIEDRICH [*fl.* 1625] *respondent. See* SENNERT, D., *praeses.* Positiones medicae de colica. 1625.

MOLLER, JACOB. *See* MÖLLER, Jacob [*fl.* 1691]

MOLLER, Károly Otto [1670-1747] *respondent.* Dissertatio inauguralis medica de divino in medicina ... [Altdorffii] Literis Henrici Meyeri [1696]
                             [8030]
  Diss. — Altdorf.

MOLLERUS, FRIDERICUS. *See* MÖLLER, Friedrich [*fl.* 1607-1652]

MOLLERUS, SEBASTIANUS. *See* MÖLLER, Sebastian [*d.* 1609]

MOLTKE, LEVIN NICOLAUS VON [*d.* 1663] *See* BROWNE, *Sir* T. Religio medici cum annotationibus. 1652, 1665, 1677.

MOLYNEUX, WILLIAM [1656-1698] Dioptrica nova. A treatise of dioptricks, in two parts. Wherein the various effects and appearances of spherick glasses ... together with their usefulness in many concerns of humane life, are explained ... London, Benj. Tooke, 1692.
    [14], 301, [2] p. plates. 24 cm.   **[8031]**

MONARDES, Nicolás [*ca.* 1512-1588] Delle virtu del tabaco, e sue grandissime, e meravigliose operationi ... Venetia, Leonardo Pittoni, 1689.

34, [2] p.   plate.   16 cm.   [8032]

Translation of Del tabaco y de sus grandes virtudes, originally published in the second part of his Cosas que se traen de las Indias Occidentales.

— [Dos libros, el uno trata de todas la cosas que traen de nuestras Indias Occidentales, que sirven al uso de medicina. Italian] *In* Orta, G. d'. Dell'historia de i semplici aromati. 1605, 1616.

— Ein nützlich und lustig Gespräche, von Stahl und Eisen. Darinnen dieser Metallen Würdigkeit und Artzney Tugenden angezeiget werden. Erstlich in spannischer Sprache geschrieben, von dem ... Nicolao Monardo, und ... in die Lateinische gebracht, durch ... Carolum Clusium, jetzo aber ... in unsere deutsch Sprache versetzt. Sampt einem andern Tractätlin von dem Schnee und Eyss ... vermehrt, durch Jeremiam Gesnerum ... Leipzig, Bey Abraham Lamberg, in Verlegung Johan Eyerings und Johan Perferts, Buchhandler in Bresslaw, 1615.

[10], 123 p.   19 cm.   [8033]

Translation of Dialogo del hierro, y de sus grandezas and Libro de la nieve y del modo de enfriar con ella, originally published with the third part of his Cosas que se traen de las Indias Occidentales.

— [Primera y segunda y tercera partes de la historia medicinal de las cosas que se traen de nuestras Indias Occidentales que sirven en medicina. French] *In* Orta, G. d'. Histoire des drogues. 1602, 1619.

— *See* EVERARD, G. Panacea. 1659; L'ÉCLUSE, C. de. Caroli Clusii ... Exoticorum libri decem. 1605; WITTICH, J. Bericht von den wunderbaren bezoardischen Steinen. 1612.

MONATLICHE neueröffnete Anmerckungen. 1680-1683. *See* BLEGNY, N. de.

MONAU, FRIEDRICH VON. *See* MONAVIUS, Friedrich [1592-1659]

MONAU, PETER. *See* MONAVIUS, Petrus [1551-1588]

MONAVIUS, FRIDERICUS JAC. F. *See* MONAVIUS, Friedrich [1592-1659]

MONAVIUS, FRIEDRICH [1592-1659] Bronchotome: nimirum gutturis artificiose aperiendi ἐγχ-

εἴρησις, cum appendice gemina tam elenchi affectuum ocularium hecatontadem ipsam excedentis, quam hypotyposeos febrium omnium ... [Königsberg] Typis Johannis Reusneri, 1644.

[8], 56 p.   illus., table.   20 cm.   [8034]

— *respondent, See* CRÜGER, B., *praeses.* Disputatio medica quarta. 1610; MÖGLING, J. L. [*fl.* 1608-1655] *praeses.* Lanx satura rerum medicarum. 1622.

—, *ed. See* PREVOST, J. De compositione medicamentorum libellus. 1649.

MONAVIUS, PETRUS [1551-1588] *See* SCHOLTZ, L. Consiliorum medicinalium ... liber singularis. 1610 [and] Epistolarum philosophicarum: medicinalium, ac chymicarum ... volumen. 1610.

MONCONYS, BALTHASAR DE [1611-1665] Voyages ... divisez en V. tomes. Où les sçavans trouveront un nombre infini de nouveautez, en machines de mathematique, experiences physiques ... outre la description de divers animaux & plantes rares, plusieurs secrets inconnûs pour le plaisir & la santé ... Paris, Pierre Delaulne, 1695.

5 v. in 4.   plates.   18 cm.   [8035]

Vol. 1 has added engraved title page.

MONDEVILLE, HENRI DE [14th cent.] *See* VICARY, T. The English mans treasure. 1613, 1633, 1641 [and] The surgions directorie. 1651.

MONDINI, MONDINO [*fl.* 1609-1631] Ad disputationem de genitura. Additamentum apologeticum in quo Aemilii Parisani opinionem de seminis a toto proventu, & de stygmatum causis ab omni probabilitate alienam esse sustinetur ... Venetiis, Apud Evangelistam Deuchinum, 1625.

[8], 131 p.   21 cm.   [8036]

— De genitura pro Galenicis adversus Peripateticos & nostrae aetatis philosophos, ac medicos disputatio. In qua nova praesertim dogmata spectantia ad fortuum generationem ... refelluntur. Nec non animatio seminis adversus recentiores ... defenditur ... Venetiis, Apud Evangelistam Deuchinum, 1622.

[20], 360 p.   21 cm.   [8037]

—, *ed. See* MERCURIALE, G. Consultationes. [1604-20], 1624-25.

— *See* HOFMANN, C. De generatione hominis. 1629; SARRATI, A. Apologia. 1631.

MONDINO DEI LUZZI [*d.* 1326] *See* MESUË [924 *or* 5-1015] Opera. 1602, 1623.

MONDSCHNEIDER, JOHANNES DE. *See* MONTE-SNYDER, Johannes de [*fl.* 17th cent.]

MONEGLIA, GIOVANNI ANDREA. *See* MONIGLIA, Giovanni Andrea [1624-1700]

MONGINOT, FRANÇOIS DE [1569-1637] Secrets polydaedales contre la peste . . . Paris, Georges Lombard, 1606.

96 (i.e. 83), [1] p. 17 cm. [8038]

—Traitté de la conservation et prolongation de la santé . . . Paris, N. Bourdin & L. Perier, 1635.

[II], 141, [2] p. 13 cm. [8039]

[**MONGINOT**, FRANÇOIS, *the younger*] Traité de la guérison des fiévres par le quinquina. Lyon, Guillaume Barbier, 1679.

[4], 74 p. 15 cm. [8040]

—[The same.] . . . De la guerison des fievres par le quinquina. Paris, René Guignard, 1680.

146, [2] p. 16 cm. [8041]

—[The same.] . . . 4. ed., rev. & augm. Lyon, Antoine Briasson, 1681.

[4], 140, [2] p. 15 cm. [8042]
Title page is a cancel.

—[The same.] 4. ed., rev. & augm. . . . Paris, René Guignard, 1683.

[1], 141, [1] p. 17 cm. [8043]

—[The same.] . . . 4. ed., rev. & augm. Paris, Robert Pepie, 1688.

[4], 140, [2] p. 16 cm. [8044]

—[Latin tr.] *In* [Nigrisoli, F. M.] *ed.* Febris china chinae expugnata. 1687, 1700.

MONGIO, GIOVANNI PAOLO, [16th cent.] *ed. See* AVICENNA. Avicennae Arabum medicorum principis. 1608.

MONHEMIUS, FRANCISCUS [*fl.* 17th cent.] *respondent. See* HORST, G. [1578-1636] Ἐξετάσεων παθολογικῶν. 1629 [and] Prognosis febrium. 1622.

[**MONIGLIA**, GIOVANNI ANDREA, 1624-1700] Celer excursus in librum . . . Hippocratis de decenti ornatu . . . Florentiae, Apud Caesarem de Bindis, 1700.

54, [1] p. 22 cm. [8045]

Errata: p. [55]
Bound with *his* De aquae usu medico. 1700.

—De aquae usu medico in febribus . . . Florentiae, Apud Vincentium Vangelisti, 1684.

[3]-341 p. 19 cm. [8046]
Author's presentation copy, unsigned.

—[The same.] . . . Florentiae, Apud Caesarem de Bindis, 1700.

159, [1] p. 22 cm. [8047]
Errata: p. [160]
With this is bound *his* Celer excursus. 1700.

—Risposte . . . alle repliche voarcadumiche del sig. dottore Innocenzio Valentini. [Florentiae, Badia, 1663]

[5], 3-116 p. 20 cm. [8048]

—*See* Bertini, A. F. Risposta apologetica. 1700; RAMAZZINI, B. Risposta. 1682.

MONMOUTH, HENRY, *2nd Earl of* [1596-1661] *tr. See* SENAULT, J. F. The use of passions. 1671.

MONNIER, I. L. [*fl.* 1666] Le cabinet secret des grands preservatifs & specifiques propres, contre la peste, fievres pestilentielles, pourpres, petites verolles, & toutessortes de maladies contagieuses . . . Paris, Philippe d'Arbisse, 1666.

[8], 95, [1] p. 17 cm. [8049]

MONQUENTIN, PETRUS LEONARDUS DE. Thermologia Badavino-Austriaca; das ist, Kurtze . . . Beschreibung der Natur . . . des heylsamen Badwassers zu Baden alhie in Nider Oesterreich . . . Regenspurg, Christoff Fischer, 1651.

[109] p. 14 cm. [8050]

MONSCHEIN, JOHANN WOLFFGANG [*fl.* 1700] *respondent. See* JOHRENIUS, C., *praeses.* Dissertatio solennis de epilepsia. 1700.

Mʳ de***. *See* FRÉMONT D'ABLANCOURT, Nicolas [1625?-1693]

MONSIEUR Scharxl; oder, Kurtzweilige Zeit-Vertreibung in der Bad- und Saur-brunnen-Cur, den lang-weiligen Brüdern die eintringende melancholische Fausen auf ein angenehme Weis zu underbrechen. Worinn obgedachtens Monsieur närrischer und seltsamer Lebens-Wandel mit sehr nutzlichen schönen Discursen . . . undermenget wird. Herausgegeben bey dem G'sund-Brunnen zu Cucurbita . . . [n. p.] 1699.

[10], 297 p. front. 17 cm. [8051]

MONT-SAINCT, Thomas [*fl.* 1604–1617] Histoire miraculeuse des eaux rouges comme sang, tombees dans la ville de Sens & és environs, le jour de la grand feste Dieu derniere, 1617 . . . Paris, Sylvestre Moreau, 1617.

    [8] p.   17 cm.   **[8052]**

MONTAGNANA, Bartolomeo. Selectiorum operum Bartholomaei Montagnanae . . . in quibus ejusdem Consilia, variique tractatus alii . . . continentur, liber unus & alter . . . revisi, relecti, locupletati, a Petro Uffenbachio . . . [Francofurti] Prodeunt e Paltheniano musarum Francofurtensium Collegio, 1604.

    [7], 1309, [13] p.   34 cm.   **[8053]**
    With this is bound (as issued?) Cermisone, A. Consilia medicinalia. 1604.

MONTAIGNE, Michel Eyquem de [1533–1592] Lof der genees-konste. *In* Beverwijck, J. van. Wercken der genees-konste. 1664, 1672.

    — *See* Beverwijck, J. van. Lof der medicine; ofte, Genees-konste. 1641, 1647.

MONTALBANI, Marcantonio. *See* Fratta e Montalbano, Marcantonio della, marchese [1635–1695]

MONTALBANI, Ovidio [1601–1671] Eticofisiologia; overo, Discorso delle naturalezze morali. Colle astrologiche temporaneità prevedute dell'anno MDCLXIV . . . Bologna, Giacomo Monti, 1663.

    56 p.   21 cm.   **[8054]**

    — Il pestifugo Esculapio; cioè, Regole più sicure per iscampare da ogni contagioso pericolo; considerationi di Gio. Antonio Bumaldi [pseud., i.e. Ovidio Montalbani] . . . Bologna, Giacomo Monti, 1656.

    32 p.   21 cm.   **[8055]**

    — *ed. See* Aldrovandi, U. Dendrologiae naturalis . . . libri duo. 1668.

MONTALTE, Louis de, *pseud. See* Pascal, Blaise [1623–1662]

MONTANI, Giuseppe [*fl.* 1679] *See* Moro, G. Anotomia ridotta all'uso de' pittori. 1679.

MONTANO. Benito Arias. *See* Arias Montanus, Benedictus [1527–1598]

[**MONTANOR**, Guido de, *fl. ca.* 1400] Scala philosophorum . . .

71–III p., vol. 2.   17 cm.   (*In* Artis auriferae. Basileae, 1610)   **[8056]**
    Caption title.
    Attributed to Guido de Montanor. Cf. Ferguson (A). Vol. 2, p. 100.

    [—German tr.] Die Leyter der Philosophorum.

    94–154 p., part 2.   19 cm.   (*In* Morgenstern, Philipp, *ed.* and *tr.* Turba philosophorum. Basel, 1613.)   **[8057]**
    Caption title.

    —Guidonis Magni de Monte . . . Tractatulus seu descriptio philosophici adrop. Quaenam sit ejus species, & quomodo debeat elaborari, & praeparari.

    543–568 p., vol. 6.   20 cm.   (*In* Zetzner, Lazarus, *ed.* Theatrum chemicum. Argentorati, 1659–61)   **[8058]**
    Caption title.

MONTANUS, Benedictus Arias. *See* Arias Montanus, Benedictus [1527–1598]

MONTANUS, Comes. *See* Monte, Conte da [*d.* 1587]

MONTANUS, Joannes Baptista. *See* Monte, Giovanni Battista da [1498–1551]

MONTANUS, Robert [*fl.* 1624–1632] Diaetema; sive, Salubris victus ratio novo-antiqua . . . Accessit ejusdem Nutritio foetus utero matris . . . demonstrata. Ed. 2. Lovanii, Apud Everardum de Witte, 1640.

    [8], 30 (i.e. 330) p.   16 cm.   **[8059]**

MONTANUS, Thomas. *See* Berghe, Thomas van den [1615–1685]

MONTE, Conte da [*d.* 1587] *See* Hofmann, C. Animadversiones in Com. Montani . . . De morbis. 1641.

MONTE, Giovanni Battista da [1498–1551]. [Selections] *In* Bertocci, A. Methodus curativa. 1608.

    —*See* Bertocci, A. Methodus curativa. 1608; Solenander, R. Consiliorum medicinalium . . . sectiones quinque. 1609.

MONTE, Guido Magnus de. *See* Montanor, Guido de [*fl. ca.* 1400]

MONTE, Petrus de. *See* Bairo, Pietro [1468–1558]

MONTE CUBITI, Vigilantius de. *See* Vigilantius de Monte Cubiti, *pseud.*

MONTE-MELLINI, Niccoló [*fl.* 17th cent.] Problema fatto da Anton Francesco Bertini ... risoluto ... Lucca, Per i Marescandoli, 1700.

10 p.   22 cm.   [8060]

[**MONTE-SNYDER,** Johannes de, *fl.* 17th cent.] Commentatio de pharmaco catholico; quomodo nimirum istud in tribus illis naturae regnis, mineralium, animalium, ac vegetabilium, reperiendum ... Insuper qualiter per idipsum (supple menstruum) alias fixum illud indestructibile aurum, redigendum sit in verum & inculpatum aurum potabile ... E Germanismo in Latinismum trajecta ... Amstelodami, Apud Elizeum Weyerstraten, 1678.

80 p.   16 cm.   [8061]

—Tractatus de medicina universalis; das ist, Von der Universal-Medicin, wie nemlich dieselbe in denen dreyen Reichen der Mineralien, Animalien und Vegetabilien zu finden ... auch wie ... das fixe unzerstörliche Gold in ein warhafftes Aurum Potabile zu bringen ... lässet ... Anjetzo wiederum zum Druck befördert, und mit einer kurtzen gründlichen Erklärung, auch beygrfügeten Spagyrischen Grund-Regeln illustriret. Durch A. Gottlob B. Franckfurt am Mayn, In Verlegung Georg Heinrich Oeberlings [not before 1678]

176 p.   16 cm.   [8062]
Imperfect: lower margin of title page trimmed affecting imprint.

—[Latin tr.] *In* Reconditorium ac reclusorium opulentiae sapientiaeque numinis mundi magni. 1666.

MONTECUCCOLI, Carlo, *conte* [1592–1611] *See* Polemo, A. Fisonomia. 1623, 1626; Porta, G. B. della. Della fisionomia dell'huomo. 1644.

MONTECUCCOLI, Francesco, *conte, tr. See* Polemo, A. Fisonomia. 1623, 1626; Porta, G. B. della. Della fisionomia dell'huomo. 1644.

MONTEMAYOR, Cristóbal [16th–17th cent.] Medicina y cirugia de vulneribus capitis ... Valladoli, Juan Godinez de Milli, 1613.

[8], 192, [5 +] ll.   illus.   15 cm.   [8063]
Imperfect: title page mutilated; all after ll. [5] at end, wanting.

—[The same.] ... Va añadido el Tratado de Amato Lusitano, de heridas de cabeça, ult. impr. ...

Zaragoça, Por Juan de Ybar, a costa de Matias de Lizau, 1664.

[8], 156, [2] ll; 68 ll.   15 cm.   [8064]
Dedicatory epistle signed by Sebastian de Gallego, the editor. Part [2] has caption title: Dialogo en el qual se trata de las heredias de cabeça con el casco descubierto ... compuesto por ... Amato Lusitano ... traduzido de Latin ... por Geronimo de Virues.

MONTEUX, Hierosme de. *See* Monteux, Jérôme de [*fl.* 1518–1559]

MONTEUX, Jérôme de [*fl.* 1518–1559] Practica medica a doctis viris diu desiderata, & nunc primum in lucem edita, in sex partes divisa. 1. De profligandis humani corporis morbis particularibus. 2. De deprehendendis, & expurgandis febribus. 3. De curandis infantium morbis ... 4. De chirurgicis auxiliis ad effectus, qui repentinam exigunt curationem. 5. De tuenda sanitate ... 6. Compendium curatricis scientiae, & de purgatione juxta doctrinam ... Venetiis, Apud Variscos, 1626.

[36], 200, 339 p.   21 cm.   [8065]

MONTFAUCON DE VILLARS, Nicolas Pierre Henri, *abbé de. See* Villars, Nicolas Pierre Henri de Montefaucon [*ca.* 1635–1673]

MONTI, Domenico. Modo di adoperare il pretioso oglio de filosofi, inventato da Bartolomeo Bonfante ... Roma, Bologna & Genova, Vincenti [16 —]

broadside.   21 x 15 cm.   [8066]

MONTI, Giovanni Battista. *See* Monte, Giovanni Battista da [1498–1551]

MONTI, Horazio [*fl.* 1627] Trattato della missione del sangue. Contro l'abuso moderno dove si dimostra in quant'errore siano quelli, che lo cavano in gran quantità, & in tutte le febbre putride. Aggiunto un trattato della consuetudine, con il modo di governare l'eserciti e naviganti, e dell'infermità loro, e loro curazione ... Pisa, Lionardo Zeffi, 1627.

[14], 100, [11] p.   22 cm.   [8067]

MONTIA, Antonius Maria. *See* Monza, Antonio Maria [*fl.* 17th cent.]

MONTIGNY, Jean de [*fl.* 1648?] *ed. See* Fierabras, H. La vraye methode de la parfaicte chirurgie de fierabras. 1648.

MONTPELLIER, FRANCE. Université. Faculté de médecine. *See Université de Montpellier. Faculté de médecine.*

MONTPELLIER, FRANCE. **Université de médecine.** *See* UNIVERSITÉ DE MONTPELLIER. Faculté de médecine.

MONTROEIL, DE. *See* MARQUE, J. de. Methodique introduction a la chirurgie. 1680.

MONTUUS, HIERONYMUS. *See* MONTEUX, Jérôme de [*fl.* 1518-1559]

MONZA, ANTONIO MARIA [*fl.* 17th cent.] La medicina difesa ... Crema, Giacomo Marchetti, 1655.

    [15], 52, [3] p.   24 cm.   **[8068]**

MOOR, BARTHOLOMAEUS DE [1649-1724] Cogitationum de instauratione medicinae, ad sanitatis tutelam, morbos profligandos, nec non vitam prorogandam, libri tres. Amstelaedami, Gerardus Borstius, 1695.

    [32], 440, [2] p.   plates.   17 cm.   **[8069]**
Added engraved title page.
Errata: [2] p.

    —*respondent.* Disputatio medica inauguralis de suffocatione hypochondriaca ... Lugduni Batavorum, Apud viduam & haeredes Joannis Elsevirii, 1669.

    [20] p.   23 cm.   **[8070]**
Diss. — Leyden.

MORA, GIACOPO. *See* MORO, Giacopo.

MORABEAU, FRANCOIS MARIE DE, *tr. See* HIPPOCRATES. [Prognostica. French] 1645.

MORAEUS, FRANCISCUS [*fl.* 17th cent.] Opus de maligna febre paroxisante, divisum in tres tractatus, consultationes, et ... observationes continens ... Venetiis, Apud Paulum Baleoneum, 1669.

    [12], 302 p.   23 cm.   **[8071]**

    —[The same.] De maligna febre paroxisante opus consultationes et ... observationes continens. Francofurti, Sumptibus Joh. Petri Zubrodt, typis Pauli Hummii, 1670.

    [16], 412 p.   14 cm.   **[8072]**

MORAEUS, RENATUS. *See* MOREAU, René [1587-1656]

MORALES, GEORGIO. *See* MORALIS, Georgius [*fl.* 1648-1655]

MORALIS, GEORGIUS [*fl.* 1648-1655] Commentaria in magni Hippocratis Coi Aphorismos ... Venetiis, Apud Paulum Baleonium, 1648.

    [16], 410 (i.e. 408), [24] p.   23 cm.   **[8073]**
Covers books 1-2 only. Apparently no more published. Includes the Latin text in two versions: the "vulgata" (i.e. Niccolò Leoniceno's) and that of Anuce Foes.

    —Enchiridium medicum, ethicum, et theologicum; sive magni Hippocratis Coi Aphorismorum sect. VII. In quibus, facta sacrarum sententiarum ad Aphorismos collatione, brevissima elicitur methodus, dignoscendarum, praesagiendarum, & curandarum animi simul, atque corporis aegritudinum ... Venetiis, Apud Juntas, 1455 (i.e. 1655)

    [60], 546 (i.e. 536), [16] p.   15 cm.   **[8074]**
Includes Latin text of the Aphorismi, translated by Niccolò Leoniceno.
Errata on final leaf.

    —Manuductio ad universam Aphorismorum doctrinam ... Venetiis, Apud Guerilios, 1653.

    [16], 130, [27] p.   17 cm.   **[8075]**
Running title: Manuductio ad Aphoristicam Hippocratis doctrinam.

    — ed. *See* HIPPOCRATES. [Aphorismi. Latin] 1653.

MORAND, ANTOINE [*fl.* 1633-1646] *ed. See* FREY, J. C. Opuscula varia. 1646.

MORATO ROMA, FRANCISCO. *See* ROMA, Francisco Morato [1588-1668]

MORATTI, PIETRO [*fl.* 1630] Racconto de gli ordini e provisioni fatte ne' lazaretti in Bologna, e suo contado in tempo del contagio dell'anno 1630 ... Bologna, Presso Clemente Ferroni, ad instanza di Bartolomeo Cavalieri, & Cesare Ingegnieri, 1631.

    [7], 124 p.   21 cm.   **[8076]**

MORBUS EPIDEMIUS ANNI 1643. 1643. *See* [GREAVES, *Sir* E.]

MORDICUS, GULIDEOLUS, *tr. See* GANIVET, J. Amicus medicorum. 1614; PLEIER, C. Medicus-criticus-astrologus. 1627.

MORE, HENRY [1614-1687] *See* BOYLE, *Hon.* R. Tracts ... containing new experiments touching the relation betwixt flame and air. 1672; BROWNE, *Sir* T. Pseudodoxia epidemica [German tr.] 1680; BUTLER, J. Ἁγιαστϱολογία. 1680; GLANVILL, J. Saducismus triumphatus. 1681, 1700; STUBBS, H. A censure upon certain passages contained in the history of the Royall Society. 1671; STURM, J. C. Collegium experimentale. 1676; VAUGHAN, T. The man-mouse taken in a trap. 1650.

MORE, SIR THOMAS [1478-1535] *See* ERASMUS, D. Μωρίας ἐγκώμιον. 1676.

MOREAU, FRANÇOIS. *See* MORAEUS, Franciscus [*fl.* 17th cent.]

MOREAU, JACQUES [1647-1729] Traité chimique de la veritable connoissance des fievres continues, pourprées, et pestilentes, et des moyens de les guerir ... conformement à la doctrine practique d'Hypocrate & de Gallien ... Dijon, Jean Ressaryre, 1683.

[59], 263 p. 16 cm. **[8077]**

—[The same.] De la veritable connoissance des fievres continues, pourprées, et pestilentes, et des moyens de les guerir ... conformement à la doctrine pratique d'Hippocrate & de Galien ... Dijon, & se vend a Paris, Laurent d'Houry, 1685.

[60], 263 p. front. (port.) 16 cm. **[8078]**
A reissue, with new title page, of the 1683 Dijon edition.

MOREAU, JEAN BAPTISTE [*fl.* 1648] *respondent. See* GUILLEMEAU, C., *praeses.* Question cardinale a disputer aux escholes de medecine. 1648.

MOREAU, RENÉ [1587-1656] De missione sanguinis in pleuritide. *In* Brissot, P. Apologetica disceptatio. 1622.

—Epistola exegetica de affecto loco in pleuritide, ad ... Baldum Baldium ... Parisiis, Apud Sebastianum Cramoisy, 1641.

51, [1] p. 17 cm. **[8079]**
Bound with (as issued?) Baldi, B. De loco affecto in pleuritide disceptatio. 1640.

—[The same.] *In* Baldi, B. De loco affecto in pleuritide disceptationes. 1643.

—*ed., tr. See* COLMENERO DE LEDESMA, A. Du chocolate. 1643.

—, *ed. See* DUBOIS, J. Jacobi Sylvii ... Opera medica. 1634, 1635; FEYNES, F. Medicina practica. 1650; MARTIN, J. Praelectiones in librum Hippocratis ... De morbis internis. 1637; REGIMEN SANITATIS SALERNITANUM. Schola Salernitana. 1625, 1672.

—*See* BAILLOU, G. de. Consiliorum medicinalium libri II. 1635-*1636;* 1635-1649; BARTHOLIN, T. De angina puerorum ... epidemica. 1646; PARDOUX, B. Bartholomaei Perdulcis ... Universa medicina. 1630, 1640, 1649, 1650.

MOREL, FÉDÉRIC [1558-1630] *ed.* and *tr. See* HIPPOCRATES. [De medicamentis purgatoriis] 1617; THEOPHILUS PROTOSPATHARIUS. Ἰατροσοφιότον περι οὔρων. Iatrosophistae de urinis lib. singularis. 1608.

MOREL, JEAN [1593-1668] De febre purpurata, epidemia, & pestilenti, quae ab aliquot annis in Burgundiam & omnes ferè Galliae provincias misere debacchatur medica dissertatio ... Lugduni, Sumpt. Jo. Antonii Huguetan, 1641.

[12], 132 p. 17 cm. **[8080]**

MOREL, PIERRE. Methodus praescribendi formulas remediorum ... Cum annexo Systemate materiae medicae, methodo medendi, & formulis medicamentorum praescribendis accomodato. Coloniae Allobrogum, Apud Jacobum Chouët, 1639.

[23], 254 p.; 150 p. 17 cm. **[8081]**
Part [2] has half title.

—[The same.] Formulae remediorum studio & opera Jo. Jacob à Brunn ... Cujus accedit Systema materiae medicae ... Patavii, Typis Pauli Frambotti, 1647.

[23], 296 p.; 187 p. 17 cm. **[8082]**
Part [2] has special title page dated 1646.
Imperfect: p. 83-187 of part [2] ink stained affecting pagination and text.

—[The same.] Methodus praescribendi formulas remediorum ... Cum annexo Systemate materiae medicae, methodo medendi, & formulis medicamentorum praescribendis accommodato. Genevae, Apud Petrum Chouët, 1650.

[23], 252 p.; 150 p. 16 cm. **[8083]**
Part [2] has half title.
Interleaved.

—[The same.] Formulae remediorum. Studio & opera Joan. Jacob. à Brunn ... Cujus accedit Systema materiae medicae ... Lugduni, Sumptibus Petri Rigaud, 1657.

[24], 306, [8], p.; 197, [4] p. 15 cm. **[8084]**
Part [2] has special title page.

—[The same.] Methodus praescribendi formulas remediorum. Cum adjuncto Materiae medicae systemate. Aucta, variisque modis illustrata à Gerardo Leon. Blasio ... Amstelodami, Apud Aegidium Jansonium Valckenier, 1659.

[47], 623, [13] p.   table.   14 cm.   [8085]
Added engraved title page.

—[The same.] ... Nunc pro 2. ed. recensita a Gerardo Blasio ... Amstelodami, Apud Casparum Commelinum, 1665.

[36], 578, [6] p.   14 cm.   [8086]
Added engraved title page.

—[The same.] ... Tertium recensita, acuta, illustrata a Gerardo Blasio ... Amstelodami, Apud Henr. & Theod. Boom, 1680.

[20], 578 p.   14 cm.   [8087]
Added engraved title page.

[—English tr.] The expert doctors dispensatory. The whole art of physick restored to practice. The apothecaries shop, and chyrurgions closet open'd; wherein all safe and honest practices are maintained and dangerous mistakes discovered ... To which is added by Jacob a Brunn ... a compendium of the body of physick ... London, N. Brook, 1657.

[28], 471, [9] p.   front.   17 cm.   [8088]
Imperfect: frontispiece wanting.
"The physicall magazeen; or, A systeme of the matter of physick ... by Doctor Jacob A Brunn" (p. [281]-471) has special title page.
Edited by Nicholas Culpeper.

—Systema parascevasticum ad praxin, materiae medicae sylvam complectens, et rationem praescribendi ipsam in formulas secundum leges pharmaciae & normam practicandi Monspelii usitatam ... Nunc primum studio ... alterius medici, ex manuscriptis in lucem prodit. Genevae, Apud Jacobum Chouët, 1628.

323, [4] p.   17 cm.   [8089]
Bound with Varanda, J. de Formulae remediorum. 1620.

—See Ettmüller, M. Opera omnia. 1688 [and] Operum omnium medico-phisicorum. 1690; Michaelis, J. Opera. 1688, 1698.

MORELLO, FRANCESCO [*fl.* 17th cent.] Medicinale patrocinium in sanguinis circulationem ... Neapoli, Ex Officina Bulifoniana, 1678.

72 p.   22 cm.   [8090]

MORELLUS, FEDERICUS. *See* MOREL, FÉDÉRIC [1558-1630]

MORELLUS, FRANCISCUS. *See* MORELLO, Francesco [*fl.* 17th cent.]

MORELLUS, JOANNES, *Cabilonensis. See* MOREL, Jean [1593-1668]

MORELLUS, RENATUS. *See* MOREAU, René [1587-1656]

MORENU BONUS, JOSEPH [*fl.* 1669] *respondent.* Disputatio medica inauguralis de peripneumonia ... Lugduni Batavorum, Apud viduam & haeredes Joannis Elseverii, 1669.

[15] p.   23 cm.   [8091]
Diss.—Leyden.

MORÉRI, LOUIS [1643-1680] Le grand dictionaire historique; ou, Le mélange curieux de l'histoire sacrée et profane ... 6. éd. ... Autrecht, Halma & Van de Water, 1692.

4 v.   38 cm.   [8092]
Added engraved title page.

MORERY, LOUYS. *See* MORÉRI, Louis [1643-1680]

MORESCOTTUS, ALFONSUS [*fl.* 1367-1383?] Compendium medicinae totius; in quo de complexionum arcanis indiciis, morborum praecipuorum causis, prognosticis & signis, deque fabrica receptorum breviter tractatur ... Additis Formulis remediorum Petri Gorraei ... Herbornae Nassoviorum, 1604.

399, [9] p.   14 cm.   [8093]
Imperfect: wormholes on p. 3-8.
The work by Pierre de Gorris (p. [295]-378) was edited by his son Jean.
"Doctrinae et praecepta quaedem ex probatissimis quibusque medicis desumpta ...": p. 379-399.

MORGENSTERN, JOHANN ERNST [*fl.* 1670] *respondent.* Disputatio medica inauguralis de podagra ... Lugduni Batavorum, Apud viduam & haeredes Joannis Elseverii, 1670.

[12] p.   23 cm.   [8094]
Diss.—Leyden.

MORGENSTERN, PHILIPP, *ed.* and *tr.* Turba philosophorum; das ist, Das Buch von der güldenen Kunst, neben andern Authoribus, welche mit einander 36. Bücher in sich haben. Darinn die besten ... Philosophi zusammen getragen, welche Tractiren alle einhellig von der Universal Medicin, in zwey

Bücher abgetheilt . . . Jetzund newlich . . . an Tag geben . . . Basel, In Verlegung Ludwig Königs, 1613.

[14], 560 p.; [6], 455 p. illus. 19 cm.   **[8095]**

Imperfect: first preliminary leaf (blank?) of part 1, and last leaf (blank?) of part 2 wanting.

Part 2 has special title page: Das ander Theil der güldinen Kunst . . . Basel, Johann Schröter, 1613.

The German translation of the first two volumes of Auriferae artis (1572) and Artis auriferae (1610).

Analysed in part. For full contents see J. Ferguson (A) Vol. 2, p. 107.

MORGUES, MICHEL. *See* MOURGUES, Michel, *Father* [1650–1713]

MORHOF, DANIEL GEORG [1639–1691] Dissertationes academicae & epistolicae . . . Accessit autoris vita . . . et praefatio Joannis Burchardi Maji . . . Hamburgi, Sumptu Gottfredi Liebernickel, 1699.

[8], 143, [6], 616, [42] p. front. (port.), illus. 22 cm.   **[8096]**

—Epistola de scypho vitreo per centum humanae vocis sonum rupto ad . . . Johannem Danielem Majorem . . . Kilonii, Imprimebat Joachimus Reuman, 1672.

[51] p. 20 cm.   **[8097]**

—Stentor Ύαλοκλαστης; sive, De scypho vitreo per certum humanae vocis sonum fracto . . . dissertatio . . . Ed. alt. . . . auct. Kilonii, Literis & sumptibus Joachimi Reumanni, 1683.

247 (i.e. 246), [2] p. illus. 19 cm.   **[8098]**

—[Dutch tr.] . . . Brief, over het breecken van een glase roemer door seecker menschelijck geluyt, geschreven in het Latijn . . . en in onse Nederduytse taale overgebraght door D.P. Amsterdam, Jacobus Lemmers, 1672.

78 p. 16 cm.   **[8099]**

Added engraved title page.

—*praeses.* Dissertatio de paradoxis sensuum . . . Kilonii Literis Joachimi Reumanni [1676]

[30] p. 19 cm.   **[8100]**

Diss. – Kiel (A. Plomann, *respondent*)

—Another issue, with added text on last page.   **[8101]**

—[The same.] . . . Kilonii, Literis Joachimi Reumanni [1685]

[40] p. 22 cm.   **[8102]**

—Princeps medicus . . . disquisitioni publicae exhibitus a Reimaro Nicolao Stapeln . . . Rostochii, Typis Johannis Kilii, 1665.

[44] p. 19 cm.   **[8103]**

Diss. – Rostock (R. N. Stapel, *respondent*)

—*See* HANNEMANN, J. L. Ovum Hermetico-Paracelsico-Trismegistum. 1694.

MORI, GIACOPO. *See* Moro, Giacopo.

MORICEAU, FRANCESCO. *See* Mauriceau, François [1637–1709]

MORIENUS. Liber de compositione alchemiae, quem edidit Morienus Romanus, Calid regi Aegyptiorum, quem Robertus Castrensis de Arabico in Latinum transtulit.

3–37 p., vol. 2. 17 cm. (*In* Artis auriferae. Basileae, 1610)   **[8104]**

Caption title.

—[German tr.] Das Buch von der Zurichtung der güldinen Kunst, welches Morienus Romanus hat lassen aussgehen an den Calid der egypter König, welches Robertus Castrensis auss dem Arabischen in Latein bracht hat.

[3]–44 p., part 2. 19 cm. (*In* Morgenstern, Philipp, *ed.* and *tr.* Turba philosophorum. Basel, 1613)   **[8105]**

Caption title.

MORISON, ROBERT [1620–1683] Plantarum umbelliferarum distributio nova, per tabulas cognationis et affinitatis ex libro naturae observata & detecta . . . Oxonii, E. Theatro Sheldoniano, 1672.

[47], 91, [27] p. illus., port. 41 cm.   **[8106]**

—, *ed. See* BOCCONE, P. Icones & descriptiones rariorum plantarum Siciliae. 1674.

—*See* KÖNIG, E. Regni vegetabilis pars altera. 1696.

MORLAND, *Sir* SAMUEL, *bart.* [1625–1695] *See* WEPFER, J. J. Observationes anatomicae. 1675, 1681.

MORLEY, CHRISTOPHER LOVE [*b. ca.* 1646] *ed.* Collectanea chymica Leydensia, id est, Maëtsiana, Margraviana, Le Mortiana. Scilicet trium in Academia Lugduno-Batava facultatis chimicae . . . professorum . . . qui isthaec discipulis suis . . . non solum ostenderunt, verum etiam suis verbis dictarunt

... Lugduni Batavorum, Apud Henricum Drummond, sumptibus J. A. de la Font, 1684.

[32], 506, [21] p.   21 cm.   [8107]

—[The same.] ... Olim trium in Academia Lugduni-Batava facultatis chymicae ... professorum ... qui isthaec discipulis suis ... non solum ostenderunt, verum etiam suis verbis dictarunt ... Nunc autem plurimis novis ... experimentis ... aucta, meliorem in ordinem redacta ... per Theodorum Muykens ... Lugduni Batavorum, Sumptib. Cornelii Boutesteyn & Frederici Haaring, 1693.

[48], 587, [37] p.   18 cm.   [8108]
Added engraved title page.

—[The same.] ... Olim publice & privatim in Academia Lugduno-Batava chymiam profitentium, ac docentium.

[4], 228, [10] p.   20 cm.   (Part [4] *in* Mort, Jacob le. Chymiae verae nobilitas. Lugduni Batavorum, 1696)   [8109]

—[German tr.] Collectanea chymica Leydensia; oder Ausserlesene mehr als 700 chymische Processe welche von Hn. Maetsio Margravio und le Mortio ... dictirt worden. Vor diesen von Hn. Christoph Ludwig Morleii ... zusammen getragen, in Ordnung und ans Licht bracht, nachmahls durch Hn. Theodorum Muyckens ... vermehret ... nun aber ... ins Teutsche übersetzt ... Jena, Henr. Christoph Cröker, 1696.

[7], 724 (i.e. 732) p.   18 cm.   [8110]
Added engraved title page.

—[The same.] ... Ed. 2. Jena, Henrich Christoph Cröker, 1700.

[7], 785, [43] p.   17 cm.   [8111]
Added engraved title page.

—[The same.] *See* MAETS, C. L. de. Prodromus chemiae rationalis. 1684.

—De morbo epidemico, tam hujus, quam superioris, anni, id est, 1678, & 1679, narratio ... Cui accessit ... Lucae Schacht ... de eodem morbo ad auctorem epistolica narratio ... Londini, Impensis Johannis Gay, 1680.

[15], 139, 145-206 p.   15 cm.   [8112]
"Appendix. Proprii morbi narratio": p. 145-206.

MORO, ALESSANDRO [*fl. ca.* 1664-1670] *See* REDI, F. Experimenta circa res diversas naturales. 1675

[and] Lettera ... sopra alcune opposizioni fatte alle sue Osservazioni intorno alle vipere. 1670, 1685, 1687.

MORO, GIACOPO. Anotomia ridotta all'uso de' pittori, e scultori ... Vinegia, Gio. Francesco Valvasense, 1679.

23, 25, [2] p.   illus., plates.   47 cm.   [8113]
Dedicatory epistle signed by Giuseppe Montani.
Illustrations based on the Vesalian plates.
Cushing VI.D.-18a.

MORONE, MATTIA [1594-1646] Directorium medico-practicum; sive, Index praeternaturalium affectuum cum simplicium, tum complicatorum, de quibus peculiares extant gravissimorum virorum consultationes, epistolae, responsiones, observationes, historiae, &c. medicis, praesertim tyronibus, quae consimilibus in casibus imitentur exempla praemonstrantes ... Lugduni, Sumpt. Joannis-Antonii Huguetan, patris & filii, 1647.

[16], 400 p.   18 cm.   [8114]
A subject index to works mainly of the late 16th and early 17th centuries, preceded by an "Index auctorum" (bibliography) p. [9-15]

—[The same.] ... Lugduni, Sumpt. Joan. Ant. Huguetan, & Marci Ant. Ravaud, 1650.

[24], 523 p.   19 cm.   [8115]
Preface signed by Joannes Gulielmus Gerardus, the editor.
A reprint of the first edition of 1647, with a revised "Index auctorum et librorum" (p. [17-22]) and a new "Index onomasticus, earum ... affectionum praeter naturam, maleque affectarum partium nomina ordine alphabetico collecta exhibens" (p. 401-523)

—[The same.] ... Jam primum in Germania editi, variisque auctorum exemplis aucti. Opera & studio Sebastiani Schefferi D. Francofurti ad Moenum, Sumptibus viduae Joannis Godofredi Schönwetteri, typis Matthaei Kempfferi, 1663.

[24], 494 (i.e. 492), [15] p.   22 cm.   [8116]
Contains new works not analyzed in the 1647 edition, and a new "Index ... affectus simplices & comitatos universaliores ... comprehendens."

MOROVELLI DE LA PUEBLA, FRANCISCO [1575-1649] Advierte con novedad las causas y efetos deste veneno que se teme de Milan ... [Sevilla, 1631]

[19] p.   19 cm.   [8117]
Caption title.
Imperfect: upper margins of p. [3-4] trimmed.
"Respuesta a lo que quatro medicos de Sevilla an publicado despues de escrito este papel ... En Sevilla en 15. de enero de 1631. annos": p. [13-19]
Palau 183229 (Variant state.)

MORRIS, SAMUEL [*b. ca.* 1643] *respondent.* Disputatio medica inauguralis de catarrho ... Lugduni Batavorum, Apud viduam & haeredes Joannis Elsevirii, 1668.

[12] p. 24 cm. [8118]

Diss. — Leyden.

MORSIUS, JOACHIM [1593–1642?] *ed. See* BARONIO, C., *Cardinal.* Epistola. 1619; DUYCK, F. Comparatio elegans venatoris et amatoris. 1619; FIORDIBELLO, A., *Bp.* Panegyricus Carolo V. Rom. imperatori dictus. 1619; LAUREMBERG, P. Ἀνώνυμον εἰσαγωγη ἀνατομικη. 1616, 1618; MERULA, P. Oratio posthuma. 1618. SCALIGER, J. C. Epistola duo lectu dignissima. 1619; SCALIGER, J. J. Loci cujusdam Galeni difficillimi explicatio. 1619; [THORIUS, R.] Medici Londinensis eximii. 1619.

—*See* LIDDEL, D. Ars medica. 1628.

MORT, JACOB LE [1650–1718] Chymiae verae nobilitas & utilitas, in physica corpurculari, theoria medica, ejusque materia et signis, ad majorem perfectionem deducendis. Comprehendens opera ejus omnia, hucusque typis commissa, quibus seorsim excusa collectanea, Maetsiana & Martgraviana, bibliopolae subjunxerunt. Lugduni Batavorum, Apud Cornelium Boutesteyn, Fredericum Haaring, 1696.

4 parts in 1 v. 20 cm. [8119]

Parts [2] and [3] have half titles; part [4] has special title page.

—Chymia, rationibus et experimentis auctioribus, iisque demonstrativis superstructa in qua malevolorum calumniae modeste simul diluuntur ... Lugduni Batav., Apud Petrum vander Aa, 1688.

[36], 365, [63] p. 17 cm. [8120]

Added engraved title page.
Bound (as issued?) with *his* Pharmacia. 1688.

—Fundamenta nov-antiqua theoriae medicae, ad naturae operas revocata. Superstructa fluido corporum exercitio, humanam machinam afficienti. Chymiae nobilioris, hoc est, physicae antiquae experientia suffulta. Lugduni-Batavorum, Apud Jordanum Luchtmans, 1700.

[38], 444, [47] p. 17 cm. [8121]

—Idea actionis corporum, motum intestinum praesertim fermentationem delineans. Lugd. Batav., Apud Fredericum Haaring, 1693.

[8], 172 + p. 14 cm. [8122]

Imperfect: all after p. 172 wanting.

—Pharmacia & Chymia medico physica, rationibus et experimentis instructa. Lugduni Batavorum, Apud Petrum vander Aa, 1684.

2 parts in 1 v. 17 cm. [8123]

Engraved title page.
Each part has special title page.

—Pharmacia, rationibus et experimentis auctioribus instructa methodo Galenico-chymica adornata ... Lugduni Batav., Apud Petrum vander Aa, 1688.

[14], 255, [35] p. 17 cm. [8124]

Added engraved title page.
With this is bound (as issued?) *his* Chymia. 1688.

—*See* MARGGRAF, C. Jacobi le Mort ... ignorantia circa chemiam & universam scientiam naturalem. 1687; MORLEY, C. L. Collectanea chymica Leydensia. 1684, 1693, 1696, 1700.

MORTO, VIVO. Accademico incognito. *See* VIVO MORTO, Accademico della Crusca.

MORTON, CHARLES [*ca.* 1660–1731] *respondent.* Disputatio medica inauguralis de corde ... Lugduni Batavorum, Apud Abrahamum Elzevier, 1683.

[12] p. 22 cm. [8125]

Diss. — Leyden.

MORTON, RICHARD [1637–1698] Opera medica, in tres tomos distributa. I. De phthisi. II. De morbis universal. acutis. III. De febribus inflammatoriis. Ed. ult. emend. Amstelodami, Apud Donatum Donati, 1696.

3 v. in 1. front. (port.), plates. 20 cm. [8126]

Imperfect: portrait wanting.

—[The same.] ... Venetiis, Typis Hieronymi Albrizzi, 1696.

3 v. in 1. 23 cm. [8127]

Imperfect: sig. a8 wanting; text supplied in manuscript.

—Opera medica, quorum posthac extat elenchus ... Accedunt insigniores tractatus Martini Lister De morbis chronicis, & Gualteri Harris De morbis acutis infantum. Lugduni, Anisson & Posuel, 1696.

[36], 535 (i.e. 531), [37] p.; [4], 98, [2] p.; 48 p. table. 25 cm. [8128]

Imperfect: title page mutilated affecting date.
Parts [2] and [3] have half titles.

—Opera medica quibus additi fuere tractatus sequentes I. Gualt. Harris De morbis acutis infantum.

II. Gul. Cole Novae hypotheseos, ad explicanda febrium intermittentium symptomat & typos excogitatae hypotyposis &c. III. Ejusd. De secretione animali. IV. Mart. Lister. De morbis chronicis. V. Ejusdem De variolis. VI. Thomae Sydenham Processus integri in morbis fere omnibus curandis cum Tract. de phthisi nunquam antehac edito ... Genevae, Cramer & Perachon, 1696.

9 parts in 1 v. front. (port.), tables. 22 cm. **[8129]**

Each part has special title page.

—Opera medica ... Editio recens, cui accedunt insigniores tractatus Martini Lister De morbis chronicis, & De variolis; Gulielmi Cole, De febribus, ac De secretione animali; Gualteri Harris De morbis infantum; et Thomae Sydenham Processus in morbis, ac De phthisi. Lugduni, Sumptibus Anisson & Posuel, 1697.

6 parts in 1 v. 24 cm. **[8130]**

Each part has half title.

—Opera medica, in quatuor tomos distributa. Quibus additi tractatus sequentes I. Gualt. Harris De morbis acutis infantum. II. Gul. Cole Novae hypotheseos, ad explicanda febrium intermittentium symptomat. & typos excogitatae hypotyposis &c. III. Ejusdem De secretione animali. IV. Mart. Lister De morbis chronicis. V. Ejusdem De variolis. Ed. ult. emend. ... Amstelodami, Apud Donatum Donati, 1699.

4 v. in 2. front. (port.), tables. 21 cm. **[8131]**

Parts I.-IV, of vol. 4 (Appendix ad ... Opera medica) have special title pages.

—Phthisiologia; seu, Exercitationes de phthisi tribus libris comprehensae ... Londini, Impensis Samuelis Smith, 1689.

[23], 411, [1] p. 19 cm. **[8132]**
Errata: p. [1] at end.

—[The same.] ... Francofurti & Lipsiae, Apud Georg. Wilh. Kühnen, 1691.

[24], 455 p. 14 cm. **[8133]**

—[English tr.] Phthisiologia; or, A treatise of consumptions ... Translated from the original. London, Sam. Smith and Benj. Walford, 1694.

[9], 360, [16] p. front. (port.) 20 cm. **[8134]**

—Πυρετολογία; seu, Exercitationes de morbis universalibus acutis ... Londini, Impensis Samuelis Smith, 1692.

[80], 430, [18] p. plates. 20 cm. **[8135]**

—Πυρετολογίας, pars altera; sive, Exercitatio de febribus inflammatoriis universalibus ... Londini, Sam. Smith & Benj. Walford, 1694.

[48], 511, [16] p. 20 cm. **[8136]**

MOSAN, Jacob, *tr. See* Wirsung, C. The general practise of physicke. 1605, 1617, 1654.

—*See* Wolff, H. Beschreibung des mineralischen Brunnen. 1609.

MOSDORFF, Johann Gottfried [*fl.* 1690] *respondent. See* Wedel, G. W., *praeses.* Dissertatio medica inauguralis de febre intermittente. 1690.

MOSE, James. *See* Mosan, Jacob.

MOSER, Bartholomaeus [*fl.* 1645] *ed. See* Bacon, F., *viscount St. Albans.* Historia vitae et mortis. 1645.

MOSER, Franz Ludwig [*fl.* 1694] *respondent. See* Amling, J. Theses inauguralis. 1694.

MOSIS, Johann Konrad [*fl.* 1696] *respondent. See* Eglinger, N., *praeses.* Exercitatio chirurgico-medica de fracturis. 1696.

MOSSA, Pedro Aquenza y. *See* Aquenza y Mossa, Pedro [*fl.* 1696–1726]

MOSSEDER, Johann Jakob [*fl.* 1692] *respondent.* Disputatio inauguralis medica de deliquio animi ... Argentorati, Literis Georgii Andreae Dolhopffii [1692]

[40] p. 19 cm. **[8137]**
Diss. — Strasbourg.

MOSTRAVERO, Asdrubale. Risposta alle Considerationi d'Ottavio Campolongo ... intorno alla compositione della teriaca ... Ravenna, Per li Stampatori Camerali, 1614 [i.e. 1615]

75 p. 18 cm. **[8138]**
Dedicatory epistle dated: 1615.
Edited by Cechino Martinelli.
Bound with Campolongo, O. Considerationi ... intorno alla theriaca. 1614 [1615]

MOTHE, Paulus [*d.* 1670] *See* Paulli, S. Παρεκβασις; seu, Digressio de vera, unica, & proxima causa febrium. 1660, 1678.

MOUCHES a miel ... Autre avis. Messieurs les cures, qui voudront avoir ce livre, gratuitement, Les remedes de la part du roy ... Paris, La veuve Denis Langlois, 1680.

2 p. 24 cm. [8139]

Caption title.
Publisher's announcement.

MOUFET, THOMAS. *See* MOFFETT, Thomas [1553-1604]

MOULIN, ALLEN. *See* MULLEN, Allen [d. 1690]

MOULIN, ANTOINE DU. *See* DU MOULIN, Antoine [b. ca. 1510]

MOULINET, NICOLAS LE. *See* LE MOULINET, Nicolas.

MOULTON, THOMAS [*fl.* 1540?] The compleat bone-setter: wherein the method of curing broken bones, and strains, and dislocated joynts ... is fully demonstrated. Whereunto is added The perfect oculist, and The mirrour of health, treating of the pestilence, and all other diseases ... Also, the acute judgement of urines ... Revised, Englished and enlarged by Robert Turner ... London, Printed by J. C. for Martha Harison, 1656.

[18], 3-175 p. 14 cm. [8140]

— [The same.] The compleat bone-setter enlarged: being the method of curing broken bones, dislocated joynts and ruptures ... To which is added, The perfect oculist, The mirrour of health, The judgement of urines, treating of the pestilence and all other diseases ... Englished and enlarged by Robert Turner Med. The 2d ed. London, Nath. Crouch, 1666.

[14], 3-681 (i.e. 168) p. front. (port.) 15 cm. [8141]

MOURGUES, MICHEL, *Father* [1650-1713] *See* RECUEIL des plus beaux secrets de medicine. 1695.

MOUSIN, JEAN [1573-1645] Discours de l'yvresse, et yvrongnerie. Auquel les causes, nature, & effects ... sont amplement deduictz, avec la guerison & preservation d'icelle. Ensemble la maniere de carousser, & les combats Bacchiques des anciens yvrongnes ... Toul, Sebastien Philippe, 1612.

[23], 390 p. 17 cm. [8142]

MOUTEAU, PHILIPPE [*fl.* 1655] Les miracles de la nature en la guerison de toutes sortes de maladies.

Par l'usage des eaux minerales de Bourbon Lancy ... Chalon, Philippe Tan, 1660.

37 p. 15 cm. [8143]

MOUTEAU, PIERRE. *See* MOUTEAU, Philippe [*fl.* 1655]

MOXIUS, JOANNES RAPHAEL. *See* MOIX, Joan Raphel [*fl.* 1587-ca. 1612]

MOYANO, JUAN. *See* MOYANO DE MEDINA, Juan [*fl.* 17th cent.]

MOYANO DE MEDINA, JUAN [*fl.* 17th cent.] *See* TENORIO DE LEÓN, A. Atomos que nuevamente se han descubierto con las luzes de Apolo. 1650.

MUCHE, CHRISTIAN [*fl.* 1652-1653] *respondent.* De phrenitide. *In* ROLFINCK, W., *praeses.* Methodus cognoscendi & curandi adfectus capitis particulares. 1653.

MUDDYCLIFT, JOHN [*fl.* 1670] *respondent.* Disputatio medica inauguralis, de apoplexia ... Trajecti ad Rhenum, Ex officina Henrici Versteegh, 1670.

[12] p. 20 cm. [8144]

Diss. — Utrecht.

MÜHLEMANN, JOHANN. *See* MÜHLMANN, Johann [1573-1613]

MÜHLMANN, JOHANN [1573-1613] Geistlicher Noth- und Todes-Schirm; oder, Die gewisseste Hülffe, und bewehrteste Artzeney wider die schädliche Seuche der Pestilentz ... genommen auss dem 91. Psalm ... Mit sonderbaren Gebeten und Liedern vermehret von M. Salomon Liscovio ... [Leipzig] Zu finden bey Christoff Klingern, 1680.

[16], 224 p.; 80, 86, [14] p. 15 cm. [8145]

Added engraved title page.
Part [2] has special title page: Frommer Christen Fast-Buss- und Bet-täglich allerbeste Erquickstunden.

MÜHLPFORT, JOHANN ADOLPH [*fl.* 1694] *respondent.* *See* VATER, C., *praeses.* Dissertationum physiologicarum quinta qua motus animalis e fundamentis genuinis erutus. 1694.

MÜHLPFORT, JOHANN JUSTIN [*fl.* 1671] *respondent.* Dissertatio inauguralis juridica circa morbum et curam aegrotorum ... Argentorati, Typis Johannis Welperi, 1671.

51 p. 19 cm. [8146]

Diss. — Strasbourg.

MÜLLER, ACHATIUS [*fl.* 1689-1690] *respondent. See* VEHR, I., *praeses.* Dissertatio medica inauguralis de astrobolismo. 1690.

MÜLLER, ANDREAS CHRISTOPH [*fl.* 1660-1670] *respondent. See* SCHNEIDER, K. V., *praeses.* Paralysin . . . solenni disputationi submittit . . . A. C. M. 1670; SENNERT, M., *praeses.* Disputatio anatomica de intestinis. 1664.

MÜLLER, BALTHASAR [*fl.* 1664] Ein neuer nützlicher und bewährter Tractat, von rechtem wahren Gebrauch Natur, Krafft und Vermögen der gemeinsten und gebräuchlichsten als 147. distilirten Wasser. Wie dieselbe von den edelsten und fürtreflichsten Kräutern, itzo gemeiniglich von fleissigen Haushaltern, nicht allein bereit und ausgebrant, sondern auch von männiglichen vor allerhand innerliche und eusserliche Leibes Gebrechen gleich einer Haus Apotheken können dienstlich genützet und gebrauchet werden, alles aus langwiriger Erfahrung, auch von berühmten und erfahrnen Medicis approbiret und bewehrt befunden . . . Budissin, In Verlegung Bartholom. Kretzschmars, Zittau, Druckts Johann Caspar Dehne, 1664.

    [7], 80, [9] p.   17 cm.   **[8147]**

    Bound with Arnaldus, de Villanova. Practica medica . . . 1619.

MÜLLER, BERNHARD [*fl.* 1619] *respondent.* Disputatio de plantarum cognitione medico necessaria . . . Basileae, Typis Joh. Jacobi Genathii, 1616.

    [8] p.   22 cm.   **[8148]**

    Diss. — Basel.

MÜLLER, BONAVENTURA [*fl.* 1686-1689] *respondent. See* BOHN, J., *praeses.* Dissertatio medica de inflammatione. 1686; FASCH, A. H., *praeses.* Specimen inaugurale medicum de morbillis. 1689.

MÜLLER, GOTTFRIED ERNST [1678-1747] Dissertatio physica de saltu naturae . . . Lipsiae, Literis Johannis Andreae Zschauens [1699]

    [24] p.   19 cm.   **[8149]**

    Diss. — Leipzig (G. A. Jenichen, *respondent*).

MÜLLER, GOTTFRIED WILHELM [*fl.* 1698] *respondent. See* HOFFMANN, F. [1660-1742] *praeses.* Dissertatio inauguralis medica de mechanica operandi ratione medicamentorum. 1698.

MÜLLER, GOTTFRIEDT [*fl.* 1650] *respondent. See* SPERLING, J. *praeses.* Dissertatio physica de sanguine. 1650.

MÜLLER, HIERONYMUS [*fl.* 1674] *respondent. See* STURM, J. C., *praeses.* De clepsydrarum . . . phaenomenis & effectibus. 1674.

MÜLLER, JAKOB [1594-1637] *praeses.* Disquisitio medica φυσιολογικὴ calidi innati et influentis . . . Marpurgi, Typis Casparis Chemlini, 1627.

    [4], 59 p.   20 cm.   **[8150]**

    Diss. — Marburg (E. Jordan, *respondent*).
    Bound with Horst, Gregor. Dissertationes medicae tres. 1627.

    — *respondent. See* HORST, G. [1578-1636] *praeses.* De natura motus animalis. 1617.

MÜLLER, JEREMIAS [1666 *or* 69-1747] *respondent. See* WALDSCHMIDT, W. U., *praeses.* Dissertatio inauguralis medica de usu & abusu potus thee in genere praecipue vero in hydrope. 1692 [and] Dissertatio medica, de ignorantia et nequitia empiricorum. 1692.

    — *See* WALDSCHMIDT, W. U. Facultatis Medicae . . . decanus Wilhelmus Huldericus Waldschmiedt . . . ad audiendam dissertationem inauguralem de usu & abusu potus thee quam . . . submittet . . . J. M. . . . invitat. 1692.

MÜLLER, JOHANN [*fl.* 1611] Kurtzer, doch gründtlicher Unterricht wie man sich . . . vor der Pestilentz bewahren sol . . . Nebest einem Appendice, wie man die Gemach, darin die Krancken gelegen, und gestorben sein, sampt ihrem Gerethe, das sie gebraucht haben, wieder reinigen sol . . . Berlin, Gedruckt durch George Rungern, in Verlegung Martin Enthen, 1625.

    [54] p.   20 cm.   **[8151]**

MÜLLER, JOHANN [1598-1672] *praeses.* Στοιχειολογία disputatio III de aqua . . . Wittebergae, Typis Johannis Gormanni, 1622.

    [16] p.   19 cm.   **[8152]**

    Diss. — Wittenberg (J. Gloger, *respondent*)

MÜLLER, JOHANN [*fl.* 1672-1679]

    Dissertations — Wittenberg

    — *praeses.* Disputatio physica de corporum defunctorum operationibus . . . Wittebergae, Typis Matthaei Henckelii [1679]

    [28] p.   19 cm.   **[8153]**

    J. G. Bierling, *respondent.*

    — Disputatio physica da lapide fulminari . . . Wittenbergae, Typis Joh. Borckardi, excud. Simon Lieberhirt [1679]

    [16] p.   19 cm.   **[8154]**

    S. Hommel, *respondent.*

—Disputatio physica de notis & figuris infantum, ab imaginatione matrum ortis ... [Witebergae] Typis Matthaei Henckelii [1677]

[16] p. 18 cm. [8155]

G. Brüschmann, *respondent.*

—[The same.] ... [Wittebergae] Typis Matthaei Henckelii, 1681.

[16] p. 20 cm. [8156]

A reprint of the 1677 edition.

—Disputatio physica de tarantula ... Wittebergae Literis Christiani Schrödteri [1676]

[16] p. 19 cm. [8157]

C. F. Braun, *respondent.*

—Disputatio physica quaestionem utrum ex medulla spinae in homine mortuo serpens nascatur examinans ... Wittebergae, Typis Johannnis Haken [1674]

[16] p. 20 cm. [8158]

G. Kretzschmar, *respondent.*

MÜLLER, JOHANN [*b.* 1666] *respondent. See* CRAUSE, R. W., *praeses.* Disputatio medica inauguralis de diabete. 1692.

—*as subject. See* WEDEL, G. W. Propempticon inaugurale de suspendio virginum milesiarum. 1692.

MÜLLER, JOHANN [*b.* 1667] *respondent. See* FASCH, A. H., *praeses.* Specimen inaugurale medicum de febre amatoria. 1689; PETERMANN, A., *praeses.* Disputatio medica de ephialte seu incubo. 1688.

—*as subject. See* FASCH, A. H. Augustinus Henricus Faschius ... Facultatis Medicae X. decanus S. P. D. benevolo lectori! 1689.

MÜLLER, JOHANN CHRISTIAN [*fl.* 17th cent.] Praxis medica imperfecta; sive, Fundamentorum medicorum disputabilitas, quam brevissimis hisce lineis adumbrare, imprimis vero horum omnium sententiam a nobilissimo Bisioli ... expetere voluit ... Parmae, Ex typographia Alberti Pazzoni, & Pauli Montii sociorum, 1696.

43, [1] p. 17 cm. [8159]

MÜLLER, JOHANN CHRISTOPH [*fl.* 1686-1687] *respondent. See* VESTI, J., *praeses.* Disputatio physicomedica de pulvere sympathetico. 1687 [and] Dissertatio medica de mictione cruenta. 1686.

MÜLLER, JOHANN FRIEDRICH [*fl.* 1687] *respondent. See* LIMMER, C. P., *praeses.* Collegii Physici disputatorii disputatio decima. 1687.

MÜLLER, JOHANN GERHARD [*fl.* 1691] *respondent. See* MÜLLER, Peter, *praeses.* De verbis minitantibus von Drau-Worten. 1691.

MÜLLER, JOHANN HEINRICH [*fl.* 1648] *respondent. See* WALTHER, J., *praeses.* Disputatio physica de lapidibus in genere. 1648.

MÜLLER, JOHANN JULIUS [*fl.* 1664] *respondent. See* TAPPE, J., *praeses.* Disputatio medica inauguralis de arthritide. 1664.

MÜLLER, JOHANN KASPAR. *See* MULLER, Johann Kaspar [*b.* 1675]

MÜLLER, JOHANN LUDWIG [*b.* 1669] *respondent. See* WEDEL, G. W., *praeses.* Dissertatio inauguralis de morbis tartareis. 1695 [and] Propempticum inaugurale de nummis pileatis. 1695.

MÜLLER, JOHANN PAUL. *See* MULLERUS, Joannes Paulus [*fl.* 1643-1649]

MÜLLER, JOHANN SIGFRID [*fl.* 1676-1678] *respondent. See* BROTBECK, J. K., *praeses.* Dissertatio medica de pica. 1676.

MÜLLER, JOHANN ULRICH [*fl.* 1654] *respondent.* Disputatio inauguralis medica de mania seu insania ... Argentorati, Typis Eberhardi Welperi, 1654.

[23] p. 19 cm. [8160]

Diss. — Strasbourg.

MÜLLER, JOHANN ULRICH, [*fl.* 17th cent.] *ed. & tr. See* SCHRÖDER, J. Trefflich-versehene medicin-chymische Apotheke. 1685.

MÜLLER, JOHANN WILHELM [*fl.* 1692] *respondent. See* ZELLER, J. G., *praeses.* Vita humana ex fune pendens. 1692.

MÜLLER, LUDWIG. *See* MILLER, Ludwig [1654-1690]

MÜLLER, PETER [1640-1696] De annulo pronubo, vulgo, Vom Jaworts- oder Trau-Ring Hypomnema, cui accessit De modo ac usu computationis graduum dissertatio. Ed. 3. Jenae, Typis & sumtibus Johannis Jacobi Bauhoferi, 1680.

[1], 108 (i.e. 110) p. 20 cm. [8161]

—De osculo sancto commentatio. Jenae, Typis Bauhoferianis, 1675.

[8], 62 p.   20 cm.   [8162]

—*praeses.* De verbis minitantibus von Drau-Worten ... Jenae, Typis Nisianis [1691]

40 p.   21 cm.   [8163]

Diss. — Jena (J. G. Müller, *respondent*)

—Dissertatio de hierologia; seu, Benedictione sacerdotali in matrimonii negotio usitata, von priesterlicher copulation oder Einsegnung angehender Eheleute ... quam ... ad d. 18 Mai. 1678 ... proponit Johann Samuel Stehelin ... Ed. 4. Jenae, Typis Gollnerianis, 1694.

72 p.   21 cm.   [8164]

Diss. — Jena, 1678 (J. S. Staehelin, *respondent*)

—Dissertatio de jocalibus vom Weiber-Schmuck ... Jenae, Literis Müllerianis, 1686.

[60] p.   21 cm.   [8165]

Diss. — Jena (K. Creutzing, *respondent*)

MÜLLER, PHILIPP [1585-1659] Miracula chymica et misteria medica. Libris quinque enucleta ... [Wittebergae] Ex typographia Laurentii Seuberlichs, sumptibus Clementis Bergeri, 1611.

[23], 189 (i.e. 191) p.   illus.   13 cm.   [8166]

—[The same.] ... Ed. 2. ... Accesserunt his: I. Tyrocinium chymicum. 2. Novum lumen chymicum ... [Wittebergae] Impensis Clementis Bergeri, 1614.

[22], 190, 151-493, [4] p.   illus.   14 cm.   [8167]

The Tyrocinium chymicum is by Jean Béguin and the Novum lumen chymicum by Michael Sendivogius.

—[The same.] ... Ed. 3. ... [Wittebergae] Impensis Clementis Bergeri, 1616.

[22], 190, [151-493], [4] p.   illus.   14 cm.   [8168]

Interleaved.
Different setting of type.

—[The same.] ... Ed. 4. ... Wittebergae, Sumptibus Clement Bergeri, typis Johannis Haken, 1623.

[22], 109 (i.e. 192), 151-493, [4] p.   illus.   14 cm.   [8169]

Different setting of type.

—Miracula chymica, et mysteria medica. Libris quinque enucleata ... Parisiis, Apud Melchiorem Mondiere, 1644.

[22], 191 p.   illus.   14 cm.   [8170]

—[The same.] ... Accesserunt his, 1. Tyrocinium chymicum. 2. Novum lumen chymicum ... Amstelodami, Apud Aegidium Janssonium Valkenier, 1656.

[20], 379, [3] p.   14 cm.   [8171]

Added engraved title page.

—Miracula chymica et mysteria medica libris quinque enucleata ... Ex recensione Gerardi Blasii ... Amstelodami, Apud Aegidium Jansonium Valckenier, 1659.

[22], 140 p.   illus.   14 cm.   [8172]

Added engraved title page.

MUELLER, SAMUEL [*fl. ca.* 1687] Vade-Mecum botanicum; oder, Beyträgliches Kräuter-Büchlein, darinnen der vornehmsten und in der Artzney-Kunst gebräuchlichsten Kräuter und Bewächse ... vorgestellet werden ... Ins Teutsche versetzet. Deme beygefügt Der curiöse Medicus und Chirurgus. Franckfurt und Leipzig, Johann Christoph Mieth, 1687.

3 parts in 1 v.   front., illus.   17 cm.   [8173]

Part [2] has special title page: Vade-Mecum curiosum medicum et chirurgicum ... Dresden, In Verlegung Johann Christoph Miethens, 1687. Part [3] has special title page: Urin-und Hauss-Artzney-Büchlein.

MÜLLER, THEOPHIL [*fl.* 1670-*ca.* 1675] Kurtzer jedoch nützlicher Bericht von etlichen Winter-Kranckheiten, woher dieselbigen entstehen, und auff was Art und Weise solche zu curiren sind, insonderheit wie die Fontanellen in Kopffschmertzen, Schwindel und Schlag sollen eingebracht, unterhalten und gehandelt werden ... Franckfurt und Leipzig, 1687.

110 p.   17 cm.   [8174]

—*respondent.* Dissertatio medica inauguralis de aegro agonizante ... Altdorffii, Typis Henrici Meyeri [1675]

48 p.   20 cm.   [8175]

Diss. — Altdorf.

—*See* ETTMÜLLER, M., *praeses.* Dissertatio medica de medicis balneis artificialibus. 1672 [and] Exercitium medicum de medicis balneis artificialibus quam ... subjiciet T. M. 1672.

MÜLLER, VITUS [1561-1627] *praeses.* Aristotelis De longitudine et brevitate vitae, liber per quaestiones et theses breves expositus . . . Tubingae, Typis Johannis Alexandri Cellii, 1617.

[2], 36 p.   16 cm.   [8176]

Diss.—Tübingen (I. Brunner, *respondent*)

MÜLLER, Wilhelm [*fl.* 1680–1684] *respondent. See* Wedel, G. W., *praeses*. Dissertatio medica de pernionibus. 1680 [and] Dissertatio medica inauguralis de convulsione. 1684.

MÜLLER À LOWENSTEIN, Friedrich, *pseud. See* Spaenholz, N.

MÜLMANN, Johann. *See* Mühlmann, Johann [1573–1613]

MÜLMANN, Paul [*fl.* 1630] *praeses*. Disputatio physica de insomnii . . . Lipsiae, Typis haeredum Lambergianorum, 1630.

[15] p.   18 cm.   [8177]

Diss.—Leipzig (A. Gruningk, *respondent*)

MÜLPFORT, Johann Justin. *See* Mühlpfort, Johann Justin [*fl.* 1671]

MÜNCER, Paul [1590–1633] Lib. II. von den gifftigen Fiebern und der Pest, so wol ihren bösen Zufällen, also geschrieben, dass ein jeder dieselben leicht erkennen . . . und . . . curiren könne . . . Leipzig, Bey Abraham Lamberg, in Verlegung Johan Eyerlings seligen Erben, und Johan Perferts [Druckts Andreas Mamitzsch] 1621.

[62], 506, [6] p.   17 cm.   [8178]

Imperfect: p. [49–50] mutilated.

—*respondent*. XL contradictiones quibus ratio & curatio morborum occultorum παχυλῶς delineata . . . Basileae, Typis Joh. Jacobi Genathii, 1616.

[20] p.   22 cm.   [8179]

Diss.—Basel.

MÜNDERERUS, Raymundus. *See* Gockel, E. Enchiridion medico-practicum de peste. 1669.

MÜNSTER, Johann [1571–1606] Discussio eorum quae ab Abrahamo Schopffio . . . in Generalis suae, omnium praesidiorum medicorum, universalium & topicorum, disquisitionis, libri tertii, sectione quarta, cum de aliis quibusdam ad purgandi negotium spectantibus theorematis, tum vero maxime de purgatione principio morborum instituenda, contra magnum illud magni Hippocratis 1. Aphor. 22. oraculum scripta sunt. Quibus duae accesserunt, ejusdem argumenti, appendices: una, contra

Hieronymum Capovacceum. Altera, contra Hieronymum Mercurialem. Autore Joanne Munstero . . . Francofurti, Typis Joachimi Bratheringii, impensis Joan. Spiessii & Joan. Lud. Bitschii, 1603.

[8], 326, [2] p.   16 cm.   [8180]

Errata: [2] p. at end.

Bound with copy 2 of Hafenreffer, S. Raphael artem medicam explanans. 1629.

—*See* Trincavelli, V. Controversiarum medicinalium practicarum libre quinque. 1617.

MÜNSTER, Johann Ludwig [*fl.* 1623] *respondent. See* Sebisch, M. [1578–1674?] *praeses*. Exercitationes medicae. 1639.

MÜNTZER, Paul. *See* Müncer, Paul [1590–1633]

MÜRICK, Johannes [*fl.* 1675] *respondent. See* Norcopensis, A., *praeses*. Disputatio philosophica de somniis. 1675.

MUFFET, Thomas. *See* Moffett, Thomas [1553–1604]

MUHAMMAD IBN AHMAD, Abū al-Walīd, *called* Ibn Rushd. *See* Averroës [1126–1198]

MUHAMMAD IBN ZAKARĪYĀ, Abū Bakr, al-Rāzī [865–925] Liber nonus ad Almansorem. *In* Giachini, L. In nonum librum Rasis . . . ad Almansorem . . . de partium morbis eruditissima commentaria. 1622.

—[The same, *as subject.*] *See* Rolfinck, W., *praeses*. Epitome methodi cognoscendi & curandi particulares corporis affectus. 1655, 1675.

MUIKERS, Theodor. *See* Muykens, Theodor [1665–1721]

MUIS, Joannes. *See* Muys, Jan [*b.* 1654]

MUL, Johan [*fl.* 1694] *respondent*. Disputatio medica inauguralis de fluore albo . . . Lugduni-Batavorum, Apud Abrahamum Elzevier, 1694.

[24] p.   19 cm.   [8181]

Diss.—Leyden.

MULLEN, Allen [*d.* 1690] An anatomical account of the elephant accidentally burnt in Dublin . . . in the year 1681 . . . Together with A relation of new anatomical observations in the eyes of animals

. . . By A[llen] M[ullen] . . . London, Sam. Smith, 1682.

> 72, [4] p.   plates.   21 cm.   **[8182]**
>
> The second treatise has special title page.

MULLER, CHRISTIAN [*fl.* 1661] *praeses*. Exercitatio anthropologica de cute . . . Lipsiae, Literis Johann-Erici Hahnii [1661]

> [28] p.   19 cm.   **[8183]**
>
> Diss. — Leipzig (C. H. Kauderbach, *respondent*)

MULLER, JEREMIAS. *See* MÜLLER, Jeremias [1666 *or* 69–1747]

MULLER, JOANNES. *See* MÜLLER, Johann [*b.* 1667]

MULLER, JOHANN [*fl.* 1632] *praeses*. Ἀνθρωποψυχολογίας διάσκεψις secunda de corpore ejusque partibus similaribus & dissimilaribus in genere . . . Lipsiae, Excudebat Gregorius Ritzsch, 1632.

> [8 +] p.   20 cm.   **[8184]**
>
> Imperfect: all after p. [8] wanting.
>
> Diss. — Leipzig (A. Cademan, *respondent*)

MULLER, JOHANN JAKOB [*fl.* 1676] *respondent. See* SCHNEIDER, K. V., *praeses*. Disputatio medica de spasmorum subjecto. 1676.

MULLER, JOHANN KASPAR [*b.* 1675] *respondent. See* SLEVOGT, J. A., *praeses*. Polypos capitis . . . exponit J. C. M. 1699; WEDEL, E. H., *praeses*. Dissertatio anatomico-medica de peritonaeo. 1696.

— *See* SLEVOGT, J. A. Decani Facultatis Medicae Jo. Hadriani Slevogtii . . . prolusio de polypodio ad dissertationem inauguralem de polypis capitis. 1699.

MULLER, JOHANNES JAKOB [*fl.* 1682] *respondent*. Disputatio medica inauguralis, de hydrope . . . Ultrajecti, Typis Appelarianis [1682]

> [16] p.   19 cm.   **[8185]**
>
> Imperfect: lower margin of title page trimmed; imprint date may read 1682.
>
> Diss. — Utrecht.

MULLERUS, GOTTFRIDUS ERNESTUS. *See* MÜLLER, Gottfried Ernst [1678–1747]

MULLERUS, JACOBUS. *See* MÜLLER, Jakob [1594–1637]

MULLERUS, JOANNES PAULUS [*fl.* 1643–1649] *respondent. See* TAPPE, J., *praeses*. Disputatio medica de phrenitide. 1643.

MULLINS, JAMES, *physician*. Some observations made upon the Cylonian plant. Shewing its . . . virtues against deafness. Written by a physitian to the Honourable Esq. Boyle. London, 1695.

> 8 p.   19 cm.   **[8186]**
>
> Letter signed: James Mullins.
>
> Attributed also to John Pechey.
>
> Wing M3060.

MULTIBIBUS, BLASIUS. Jus potandi; oder, Zech Recht. Darinnen von Ursprung, Gebräuchen, unnd Solenniteten, so wol auch von der Antiquitet, Effect und Wirkung dess Zechens und Zutrinckens . . . discurrirt wird. Durch Blasium Multibibum [*pseud.*] . . . Auss Lateinischer in deutsche Sprache gebracht, per . . . Joannam Elisabetham de Schwinutzki . . . [n. p.] Der HIrsch woLL aVsseM BrVnne sprVng [1616]

> [48] p.   18 cm.   **[8187]**
>
> Translation of Disputatio inauguralis theoretica practica jus potandi breviter adumbrans.

MUNCH, ERIK [*fl.* 1686] *respondent. See* GLUD, S. P. Quinque sensus exteriores eorumque organa vera. 1686.

MUNDANUS, THEODORUS [*fl.* 1684] *See* DICKINSON, E. Edmund Dickinson . . . De chrysopoeia. 1687? [and] Epistola . . . ad Theodorum Mundanum. 1686.

MUNDAY, HENRY. *See* MUNDY, Henry [1623–1682]

MUNDINIUS, MUNDINUS. *See* MONDINI, Mondino [*fl.* 1609–1731]

MUNDINUS DE LENTIIS. *See* MONDINO DEI LUZZI [*d.* 1326]

MUNDIUS, HENRICUS. *See* MUNDY, Henry [1623–1682]

MUNDT, HENRICUS. *See* MUNDY, Henry [1623–1682]

MUNDY, HENRY [1623–1682] Opera omnia medico-physica, tractatibus tribus comprehensa, de aere vitali, de esculentis, de potulentis. Una cum appendice de parergris in victu ut chocolata, coffe, thea, tabaco &c. Lugd. Batav., Apud Petrum vander Aa, 1685.

> [22], 362 p.   19 cm.   **[8188]**

—Novum physicae hodiernae lumen quo mira jucundaque de aere vitali, esculentis, potulentis ac de parergis in victu inaudita propalantur ... Lipsiae, Apud Johannem Justum Erythropilum; Jenae, Typis Nisianis, 1685.

[4], 496,[28] p. 14 cm. [8189]

MUNG, Jean de. *See* Jean de Meun [*d.* 1305?]

MUNIERUS, Joannes Alcidius [*fl.* 1650] *ed.* De venis tam lacteis thoracicis, quam lymphaticis. Sylloge anatomica ... Genuae, Typis & impensis Benedicti Guaschi, 1654.

[24], 224, [1] p. plates. 15 cm. [8190]

Imperfect: Errata wanting.

"Joannis Pecqueti ... Experimenta nova anatomica ...": p. 1-77; "Thomae Bartholini ... De lacteis thoracicis ...": p. [79]-168; "Thomae Bartholini ... Vasa lymphatica ...": p. [171]-[209]; "Jo. Alcidii Munieri ... Auctoriolum in quo celeberrimorum aliquot virorum sententiae de lacte, et lacteis in thorace recensentur": p. 211-224.

MUNNICKS, Johannes. *See* Munniks, Johannes [1652-1711?]

MUNNIKS, Johannes [1652-1711?] Cheirurgia, ad praxin hodiernam adornata, in qua veterum pariter, ac neotericorum dogmata dilucide exponuntur. Trajecti ad Rhenum, Ex officina Francisci Halma, 1689.

[12], 507, [4] p. 21 cm. [8191]

Added engraved title page: Praxis cheirurgica.

—De re anatomica liber. Trajecti ad Rhenum, Apud Antonium Schouten, 1697.

[24], 239, [17] p. front. 20 cm. [8192]

—[The same.] Anatomia nova qua juxta neotericorum inventa tota res anatomica breviter & dilucide explicatur. Ed. nov. ... Lugduni, Sumptibus Jacobi Tenet, 1699.

[15], 229, [11] p. front., plates. 19 cm. [8193]

—Dissertatio de urinis, earundemque inspectione. Trajecti ad Rhenum, Typis Rudolphi a Zyll, 1674.

[20], 75 p. 14 cm. [8194]

—[The same.] Tractatus de urinis, earundemque inspectione. Ed. alt. auct. & emend. Trajecti ad Rhenum, Typis Rudolphi a Zyll, 1683.

[16], 64 p. 16 cm. [8195]

—*praeses.* Disputatio medica continens casum anatomicum de admirando dextrae tubae uterinae hydrope ... Ultrajecti, Ex officina Arnoldi ab Eynden, 1678.

[12] p. plate. 21 cm. [8196]

Diss. — Utrecht (J. Mey, *respondent*)

—*respondent.* Disputatio medica inauguralis, de fluore muliebri ... Trajecti ad Rhenum, Typis Gysberti à Zyll, 1670.

[12] p. 20 cm. [8197]

Diss. — Utrecht.

—*See* Bruyn, J. de, *praeses.* Disputatio physica de alitura foetus in utero. 1670.

—*as subject. See* Guenellon, P. Epistolica dissertatio, de genuina medicinam instituendi ratione. 1680.

MUÑOZ, Alfonso, *sangrador del rey. See* Tamayo, A. de. Tratados breves de algebra. 1621.

MUÑOZ Y PERALTA, Juan [*fl.* 17th cent.] Escrutinio phisico medico de un peregrino especifico de las calenturas intermitentes, y otros achaques, motivado de un libro que escrivia el Dr. D. Joseph Colmenero ... Sevilla, Juan de la Puerta, 1699.

[20], 67 p. 21 cm. [8198]

Imperfect: sig 2 wanting; title page mutilated.

MUNSTER, Johann. *See* Münster, Johann [1571-1606]

MUNTING, Abraham [1626-1683] De vera artiquorum herba Britannica, ejusdemque efficacia contra stomacaccen seu scelotyrben ... dissertatio historico-medica ... Amstelodami, Apud Hieronymum Sweerts, 1681.

[28], 231 p.; 33, [19] p. plates, port. 21 cm. [8199]

Added engraved title page.

Imperfect: title page mutilated affecting date of imprint.

Part [2] has special title page: Aloidarium; sive, Aloës mucronato folio Americanae majoris, aliarumque ejusdem speciei historia ... 1680.

—[The same.] Dissertatio historico medica, de vera herba Britannica. Adjuncta est ejusdem Aloidarum historia. Amstelodami, Apud Johannem Wolters, 1698.

[18], 231 p.; 33, [19] p. plates. 20 cm. [8200]

A reissue of the 1681 edition, with preliminary matters partly reset.

—Naauwkeurige beschryving der aardgewassen, waar in de ... aart en ... eigenschappen der boomen, heesters, kruyden, bloemen ... neevens derzelver ... aanwinning, en ... genees-krachten ... beschreeven worden ... Nu eerst nieuwelijks uitgegeeven ... Leyden, Pieter vander Aa; Utrecht, Francois Halma, 1696.

[40] p. 929 col., [64] p. plates. 40 cm.

[8201]

Added half title, and added engraved title page.
"Joh. Mensingaes Lykreden op 't afsterven ... Abraham Munting ... Uit het Latijn ... vertaald door P. Rabus": p. [23-33]

—[The same.] Waare oeffening der planten ... Amsterdam, Jan Rieuwertsz, 1672.

[74], 652 (i.e. 667), [38] p. plates. 21 cm.

[8202]

Added engraved title page.
Without Johannes Mensinga's Lykreden.

MURALT, JOHANN CONRAD VON [1673-1732] *respondent.* Dissertationem inauguralem de iliaca passione ... publico ventilandam sistit ... Basileae, Ex officina typograph. Emanuelis & Joh. Georgii Regum [1693]

[48] p. 19 cm.   **[8203]**

Diss. — Basel.

—*See* WELSCH, C. L., *praeses.* Compendiosam naturalis hominis status historiam ... publico eruditorum examini subjiciunt ... C. L. W. ... et ... J. C. de M. 1692.

MURALT, JOHANNES VON [1645-1733] Anatomisches Collegium in welchem alle und jede Theile des menschlichen Leibes zusamt denen Kranckheiten und Zufällen welchen sie unterworffen, nach ihren aus den neuesten Lehr-Sätzen untersuchten Ursachen und bewährt darwider befundenen Artzney-Mitteln beschrieben worden. Mit einer Erklärung der fürnehmsten in Artzney gebräuchlichen Kräuter vorgetragen zu Zürch, auf einer löblichen Gesellschafft zum Schwartzen Garten ... Nürnberg, In Verlegung Wolfgang Moritz Endters 1687.

[25], 775, [89] p. front. (port.) 17 cm.

[8204]

Added engraved title page.

—Chirurgische Schrifften, in sich haltend I. Eine kurtze ... Auläitung zur Wund-Artzney ... II. Chirurgische Handgriffe ... III. Merckwürdige chirurgische Geschichte und Anmerckungen mit ... Zugaben ... von ... Lucas Schröcken ... und ...

Emanuel König ... Sammt einer wohlbewährten Feldschärer-kunst ... Basel, In Verlag Emanuel und Joh. Georg Königen, 1691.

[32], 894, [33] p. front. (port.) 18 cm.

[8205]

—Exercitatio anatomica de experimentis novissime factis ... Monspelii, Apud Danielem Pech [1670]

[13] p. 22 cm.   **[8206]**

—Hippocrates Helveticus; oder ... Eydgnössische Stadt-Land-und Hauss Artzt, in welchem eine klare und wahrhaffte Beschreibung innerlicher Gebrechen und Kranckheiten des menschlichen Leibs ... nach den besten Grundsätzen der Heil-Kunst enthalten ... Basel, In Verlag Emanuel und Johann Georg Königen, 1692.

[32], 1046, [24] p. front. 18 cm.   **[8207]**

—Vade mecum anatomicum; sive, Clavis medicinae, pandens experimenta de humoribus, partibus, et spiritibus ... Tiguri, Typis Davidis Gessneri [1677]

[26], 593, [17] p. 14 cm.   **[8208]**

Added engraved title page.

—*respondent. See* BAUHIN, J. K., *praeses.* Consultatio medica de angina [1667]

—*See* PEYER, J. K. Parerga anatomica et medica septem. 1681.

MURATORI, FRANCESCO [1659-1630] Scelta, compendio, et raccolta d'alcuni medicamenti rationali, quali tanto ne' nobili, quanto ne' poveri possono valere à curare il presente male contagioso in qual si voglia persona; raccolti e composti dall'eccellentissimi ... Francesco Muratori ... Tomaso Ciani [et al.] ... Bologna, Per l'herede del Benacci, 1630.

[4], 36 p. 20 cm.   **[8209]**

MURER, JOSIAS [1564-1630?] *illus. See* CASSERIO, G. De vocis auditusque organis historia anatomica. 1601.

MURICK, JOHANNES. *See* MÜRICK, Johannes [*fl.* 1675]

MURILLO, GERÓNIMO [16th cent.] *tr. See* GALENUS. [Selected works. Spanish] 1624, 1651; HOULLIER, J. Tratado de la materia de cirurgia. 1624, 1651.

MURILLO, Thomas a. *See* Murillo Velarde y Jurado, Tomás [*fl.* 1650-1673]

MURILLO JURADO, Thomas. *See* Murillo Velarde y Jurado, Tomás [*fl.* 1650-1673]

MURILLO VELARDE Y JURADO, Tomás [*fl.* 1650-1673] Novissima, verifica, et particularis hypochondriacae melancholiae curatio, et medela ... Lugduni, Sumptibus Claudii Bourgeat, 1672.

    [72], 320, [26 +] p.   16 cm.   **[8210]**

Imperfect: all after p. [26] at end, wanting.

—Resolucion philosophica, y medica, muy util para medicos, y philosophos, del verdadero temperamento, frio, y humedo de la nieve, en que se trata de sus utilidades, y danos; y se responde a un tratado, que defiende que la nieve tiene sequedad a predominio ... Madrid, Julian de Paredes, 1667.

    [6], 35, [1] ll.   20 cm.   **[8211]**

—Tratado de raras, y peregrinas yervas, que se han hallado en esta corte, y sus ... virtudes, y la diferencia que ay entre el antiguo abrotano, y la natural, y legitima planta buphthalmo y unas anotaciones a las yerbas mandragoras, macho, y hembra ... Madrid, Francisco Sanz, 1674.

    [12], 50 ll.   illus.   20 cm.   **[8212]**

MURRAY, Patrick [*d.* 1671?] *See* Balfour, *Sir* A. Letters writen to a friend. 1700.

MUSA, Antonio [1500-1555] *See* Brasavola, Antonio Musa [1500-1555]

MUSAEUM Hermeticum reformatum et amplificatum, omnes sopho-spagyricae artis discipulos ... erudiens, quo pacto ... lapidis philosophici medicina ... inveniri & haberi queat. Continens tractatus chimicos XXI ... In gratiam filiorum doctrinae, quibus Germanicum idioma ignotum est, Latina lingua ornatum. Francofurti, Aud Hermannum a Sande, 1678.

    [12], 863, [1] p.   illus., plates.   22 cm.   **[8213]**

Added engraved title page.

Each tract (except the fifth) has special title page or half title. Many are dated 1677.

Ferguson (A) Vol. 2, p. 120.

MUSAEUS, Johann Theodor [*b.* 1677] *respondent. See* Slevogt, J. A., *praeses.* De paracentesi thoracis et abdominis. 1697.

—*See* Slevogt, J. A. Decani Facultatis Medicae Jo. Hadriani Slevogtii ... prolusio inauguralis de

scarificatione hydropicorum remedio paracentesis succedaneo. 1697.

MUSCOV, Heinrich Ernst [*fl.* 1687-1689] *respondent. See* Vater, C., *praeses.* Disquisitionem physico-medicam de vermibus intestinorum ... instituet H. E. M. 1687.

MUSCULUS, Balthasar Justus [*fl.* 1685] Specimen inaugurale de pleuritidis natura et cura ... Erfordiae, Typis Groschianis [1685]

    36 p.   19 cm.   **[8214]**

Diss. — *Erfurt* (J. A. Kiesewetter, *respondent*)

MUSEUM Regalis Societatis; or A catalogue & description of the natural and artificial rarities belonging to the Royal Society. 1681. See Royal Society of London.

MUSITANO, Carlo [1635-1714] Chirurgia theoretico-practica; seu, Trutina chirurgico-physica in IV. tomos divisa ... Coloniae Allobrogum, Sumptibus Cramer & Perachon, 1698.

    4 v. in 1.   port.   23 cm.   **[8215]**

Imperfect: portrait wanting.

Edited by Giuseppe Musitano.

Contents—v. 1. De tumoribus.—v. 2. De ulceribus.—v. 3. De vulneribus.—v. 4. De lue venerea.

—Opera medica chymico-practica; seu, Trutina medico-chymica, in III. partes divisa. Omnia juxta recentiorum philosophorum principia, & medicorum experimenta excogitata, & adornata ... Coloniae Allobrogum, Sumptibus Chouet, G. de. Tournes, Cramer, Perachon, Ritter & S. de Tournes, 1700.

    3 parts in 2 v.   port.   24 cm.   **[8216]**

Parts [2-3] have special title pages. Contents. — pt. [1] Trutina medica. — pt. [2] Pyretologia; sive, Tractatus de febribus. — pt. [3] Pyrotechnia sophica.

With vol. 2 is bound: Celeberr. virorum apologiae pro R. D. Carolo Musitano. Kruswick, 1700.

—[De lue venerea. Italian] Del mal francese libri quattro ... Tradotti dalla lingua latina nell'idioma italiano da Giuseppe Musitano ... Neapoli, Giacinto Pittante, 1697.

    [8], 324, [4] p.   illus.   17 cm.   **[8217]**

—Pyrotechnia sophica rerum naturalium ... Ubi rerum omnium principiis vestigatis, reliquisque chymici apparatus expensis, singulorum corporum ex triplicato naturae regno, vegetantium nempe, mineralium, & animalium principia, genesis, dotes, praeparationes, usus, & dosis ignis artificio . . . explorantur . . . Neapoli, Ex typographia Antonii Gramignani, 1683.

[8], 452, [12] p.   22 cm.   [8218]
Imperfect: wormholes throughout.

—Trutina medica antiquarum, ac recentiorum disquisitionum gravioribus de morbis habitarum, in qua rationibus, & experimentis undequaque conquisitis, quae ex Hippocrate, Galeno, Paracelso, Van-Helmontio, omnibusque neotericis dogmata accepimus, ad examen revocantur exactissime . . . Quibus omnibus . . . peculiares conjecturae de unoquoque morbo, & complura medicamenta chymiae ductu noviter confecta, longoque usu firmata accesserunt . . . Venetiis, Typis Johannis Petri Foresti, 1688.

[24], 441, [3] p.   20 cm.   [8219]
Imperfect: p. 89-96 and 361-368 wanting. Duplicates of p. 177-184 bound in place of p. 361-368.

—*See* Celeberr. virorum apologiae pro R. D. Carolo Musitano. 1700.

MUSITANO, GIUSEPPE, *ed. See* MUSITANO, C. Chirurgia theoretico-practica. 1698.

—, *tr. See* MUSITANO, C. Del mal francese libri quattro. 1697.

MUTONI, NICCOLÒ [*fl.* 1552] Μιθριδατειοτεχνια; hoc est, De mithridatii legitima constructione Nicolai Mutoni collectanea . . . emaculata, annotationibus atque controversiis . . . locupletata, & in publicum novissime producta; cum auctario gemino: quorum prius exhibet Ἀχρόαμα medico-philosophicum, de opii usu . . . posterius Διατριβὴν de opobalsamo . . . per Michaelem Döringium . . . Jenae, Typis Johannis Beitmanni, impens. haered. Johannis Eyringii, & Johannis Perferti, 1620.

3 parts in 1 v.   16 cm.   [8220]
Parts [2] and [3] have special title pages.

MUYEN, JAN VAN [*fl.* 1685] *respondent.* Disputatio medica inauguralis de phthisi . . . Lugduni Batavorum, Apud Abrahamum Elzevier, 1685.

[12] p.   22 cm.   [8221]
Diss. — Leyden.

MUYKENS, THEODOR [1665-1721] *ed. See* MORLEY, C. L. Collectanea chymica Leydensia. 1693; [German tr.] 1696, 1700.

MUYS, JAN [*b.* 1654] Podalirius redivivus; sive, Dialogus inter Podalirium & Philiatrum. In quo juxta normam philosophiae solidioris, multa medicochirurgica . . . examinantur. Lugd. Batav., Apud Petrum vander Aa, 1686.

[16], 137 p.   14 cm.   [8222]
Imperfect: first preliminary leaf wanting.

—Praxis chirurgia rationalis; seu, Observationes chirurgicae secundum solida verae philosophiae fundamenta resolutae. Decas prima [-secunda] Lugd. Batavor., Apud Petrum vander Aa, 1683.

[24], 84 p.; [4], 44 p.   14 cm.   [8223]
Added engraved title page.

—[The same.] . . . Quinque decades. Decas I [-VII] Lugd. Batav., Apud Petrum vander Aa, 1685-90.

2 v. in 1. ([20], 318 p.; [16], 28, [1], 78 (i.e. 58), 16 p.)   16 cm.   [8224]
Added engraved title page.

—[The same.] . . . Decades duodecim. Amstelaedami, Apud Joannem Wolters, 1695.

[10], 419, [8] p.   illus., plate.   17 cm. [8225]
Added engraved title page.

—[Dutch tr.] Redelyke heelkonstoeffening; of, Heelkonstige aenmerkingen na de vaste gronden der waerachtige filozofie opgelost . . . vertaelt door David van Hoogstraten. Het eerste [-vijfde] tiental Rotterdam, Fransois van Hoogstraten, 1684.

1 v. illus.   16 cm.   [8226]
Various pagings.
Decas III-IV and Decas V. have special title pages dated 1685.

—[English tr.] A rational practice of chyrurgery; or, Chyrurgical observations resolved according to the solid fundamentals of true philosophy . . . In five decades . . . London, Printed by F. Collins for Sam. Crouch, 1686.

[16], 248 p.   front., illus.   17 cm.   [8227]
To the reader, signed by J. W.

—[German tr.] Der treu-gesinnete Samaritter; das ist . . . Vernünfftige Praxis der Wund-Artzney. Oder fünff Abhandlungen, nach denen festen Gründen, der neuen wahren Philosophie erkläret. Anjetzo von vielen . . . Fehlern geläutert, und mit zwey neuen ins Teutsche übersetzten Abhandlungen vermehret denen, oben-gedachten Autoris sogenandte

Podalirius redivivus ... beygefüget ist. Berlin, In Verlegung Rupert Völckern, 1694.

[24], 456, [47] p. illus. 16 cm. [8228]

Decas I-VII.

—, *ed. See* BARBETTE, P. Chirurgia. 1693.

MYDORGE, CLAUDE [1585-1647] Examen du livre des Recreations mathematiques et de ses problemes en geometrie, mechanique, optique, & catoptrique. Où sont aussi discutées & restablies plusieurs experiences physiques y proposées ... Paris, Rolet Boutonne, 1638.

[16], 280 p.; 63 p.; [1], [65]-106, [9] p.; 39 p. illus. 18 cm. [8229]

Part [1] includes the text of Jean Leurechon's Recreations mathematiques, originally published under the pseudonym of Hendrik van Etten.

La seconde and Troisieme partie have special title pages.

Nottes sur les recreations mathematiques ... par D. H. P. E. M. [i.e. Denis Henrion] at end, has special title page.

MYE, FREDERIK VAN DER [*fl. ca.* 1625] De arthritide, & calculo gemino tractatus duo. In quibus universa horum morborum essentia, causae ... curatio, secundum Hippocratis, & Galeni mentem dilucidissime explicantur. Una cum disputatione phylosophica, de lapidum generatione. Ejusdem Historia medica. Hagae-Comitum, Apud Arnoldum Meuris, 1624.

[156] p. 20 cm. [8230]

—De morbis et symptomatibus popularibus Bredanis tempore obsidionis, et eorum immutationibus pro anni victusque diversitate, deque medicamentis in summa rerum inopia adhibitis, tractatus duo. Ejusdem dissertationes duae medicophysicae, de contagio, & cornu monocerotis quondam in aquis circa Bredam reperto. Antverpiae, Ex Officina Plantiniana Balthasaris Moreti, 1627.

[8], 160, [3] p. 19 cm. [8231]

MYL, ABRAHAM VAN DER [1563-1637] De origine animalium, et migratione populorum ... Ubi inquiritur, quomodo quaque via homines caeteraque animalia terrestria provenerint, & post deluvium in omnes orbis tarrarum partes & regiones pervenerint ... Genevae, Apud Petrum Columesium, 1667.

68 p. 15 cm. [8232]

—[German tr.] Merckwürdiger Discurss von dem Ursprung der Thier, und Ausszug der Völcker. In welchem nachgeforschet wird, wie und auff was

Weise, so wohl die Menschen, als auch alle Thier dess gantzen Erd-Kreyss anfänglich entsprungen, und nach der Sündflut, in alle vier Theil der Welt ... kommen seyen ... Auss dem Lateinischen, in die teutsche Sprach versetzet, und mit vielen ... Anmerckungen ... vermehret, durch Joh. Christoph Bitterkraut ... Salzburg, Johann Baptist Mayr, 1670.

[16], 400, [36] p. 14 cm. [8233]

Added engraved title page.

MYLE, AEGIDIUS VAN DER [*ca.* 1594-1652] *See* TIMAEUS VON GÜLDENKLEE, B. Baldassaris Timaei von Guldenklee ... epistolae et consilia. 1665.

MYLIUS, IMMANUEL [*fl.* 1624] *respondent. See* INNICHENHÖFER, H., *praeses.* Υπνολογια; sive Tractatus jucundus physiologicus. 1624.

MYLIUS, JAKOB [*d.* 1682] *praeses.* Diatribe physica de dracone volante et igne fatuo ... Lipsiae, Excudebat Quirinus Bauch [1653]

[16] p. 19 cm. [8234]

Diss.—Leipzig (B. Praetorius, *respondent*)

MYLIUS, JOHANN DANIEL [*b.* 1585 *or* 6] Opus medico-chymicum: continens tres tractatus sive basilicas: quorum prior inscribitur Basilica medica; secundus Basilica chymica; tertius Basilica philosophica. Francoffurti, Apud Lucam Jennis, 1618-30.

2 v. illus., plates, port. 20 cm. [8235]

Vol. 1 contains the first three books of Basilica medica; and the first four books of Basilica chymica with special title page.

Vol. 2 has title: Operis medico-chymici pars altera. Qua continentur tres libri posteriores Basilicae chymicae, ut & Basilica philosophica, perfecta, in libros tres distributa ... 1620. "Tractatus secundi, seu, Basilicae chymicae, liber septimus: De animalibus", "Tractatus III. seu, Basilica philosophica", and the index, have special title pages dated 1620, 1618, 1630, respectively.

—Antidotarium medico-chymicum reformatum: continens quatuor libros distinctos. Quorum I. Generaliora in pharmaciam requisita explicat. II. Tractat de quibusdam exoticis in nostris Basilicis omissis. III. Tradit praecepta Galenic. & chymicorum de praeparatione medicamentorum. IV. Resolvit formas & dividit medicamenta tam Galen. quam chymicorum. Francofurti, Sumptibus Lucae Jennis, 1620.

[12], 1044, [71] p. port. 20 cm. [8236]

—Complementum operis medico-chymici, continens tres tractatus sive Basilicas. Quorum prior inscribitur Basilica medica, contines III. libros de medicina antique Hippocratica. Secundus inscribitur Basilica chymica, contines libros septem de metallis mineralibus, vegetabilibus & animalibus. Tertius Basilica philosophica, tractat de medicina universali, chymicorum instrumnetis & obscuritatibus. Francofurti, Impensis Lucae Jennis, 1620

    1 v. plates. 20 cm.   **[8237]**

Various pagings.

Imperfect: books 1 and 2 of Basilica medica, books 1 and 7 of Basilica chymica, book 1 of Basilica philosophica and the index wanting.

—Pharmacopoeae spagyricae; sive, Practicae universalis Galeno-chymicae liber secundus . . . Cui accessit Marci Antonii Cornacchini . . . Methodus hactenus incognito modo, cito & chymice curandi affectiones corporis, ab humoribus copia vel qualitate peccantibus geritae . . . Francofurti, Impensis Theobaldi Schönwetteri, 1628.

    [21], 896 p. 18 cm.   **[8238]**

Liber II. only.

—, ed. *See* BURNET, D. Iatrochymicus. 1616, 1621.

MYLIUS, KONRAD CHRISTIAN [*fl.* 1667–1671] *respondent.* Disputatio medica inauguralis de pernione . . . Lugduni Batavorum, Apud viduam & haeredes Joannis Elsevirii, 1671.

    [24] p. 19 cm.   **[8239]**

Diss.—Leyden.

—*See* VOGLER, V. H., *praeses.* Disputatio medica de tussi. 1667.

MYLIUS, WILLEM [*fl.* 1698] *respondent.* Disputatio anatomico-medica inauguralis de glandulis . . . Lugduni Batavorum, Apud Abrahamum Elzevier, 1698.

    [32] p. 22 cm.   **[8240]**

Diss.—Leyden.

MYLNES, RICHARD [*fl.* 1609] *respondent.* Theses medicae de febris hecticae tum cognitione, tum curatione . . . Basileae, Typis Joan. Jacobi Genathii, 1609.

    [12] p. 20 cm.   **[8241]**

Diss.—Basel.

MYN Heer. *See* ASSER, H. van.

MYNSICHT, ADRIAN VON [1603–1638] Aureum seculum redivivum, cum nunc iterum apparuit, suaviter floruit, & odoriferum aureumque semen peperit. Carum pretiosumque illud semen omnibus verae sapientiae & doctrinae filiis monstrat & relevat Hinricus Madathanus [pseud.] Francofurti, Apud Hermannum a Sande, 1677.

    [53]–72 p. 22 cm. (*In* Musaeum Hermeticum, Francofurti, 1678)   **[8242]**

—Hadriani à Mynsicht, aliàs Tribudenii . . . Thesaurus medico-chymicus; hoc est, Selectissimorum pharmacorum conficiendorum secretissima ratio. Propria laborum experientia, multiplici & felicissima praxi confirmata & antea nunquam edita . . . Cui in fine adjunctum est Testamentum Hadrianeum, de aureo philosophorum lapide . . . Hamburgi Ex Bibliopolio Frobeniano, 1631.

    [28], 304 (i.e. 404) p. port. 20 cm. **[8243]**

—[The same.] Thesaurus et armamentarium medico-chymicum. In quo selectissimorum contra quosvis morbos pharmacorum conficiendorum secretissima ratio aperitur, una cum eorumdem virtute, usu, & dosi. Cui in fine adjunctum est Testamentum Hadrianeum de aureo philosophorum lapide. Lugduni, Sumpt. Joan. Antonii Huguetan, 1641.

    [40], 490, [68] p. 17 cm.   **[8244]**

—[The same.] . . . Lubecae, Sumptibus Henrici Schernwebel, et typis Valentini Schmalhertzii, 1646.

    [43], 24, [44], 95, 532 p. front. (port.). 20 cm.   **[8245]**

Added engraved title page.

—[The same.] . . . Rothomagi, Sumptibus Joannis Berthelin, 1651.

    [40], 490, [67] p. 17 cm.   **[8246]**

A reprint of the 1641 Lyons edition.

—[The same.] . . . Lubecae, Impensis Augusti Johannis Beckeri, typis haeredum Schmalhertzianorum, 1662.

    [12], 532, [50], 24 p. port. 20 cm. **[8247]**

Imperfect: portrait and added engraved title page wanting.

—[The same.] . . . Ed. nov. Lugduni, Apud Jacobum Faeton, 1664.

    [32], 490, [67] p. 18 cm.   **[8248]**

A reprint of the 1641 Lyons edition.

—[The same.] . . . Ed. 2 emend. Lugduni, Sumptib. Joannis Antonii Huguetan & Guillelmi Barbier, 1670.

    [40], 490, [67] p. 19 cm.   **[8249]**

Different setting of type.

—[The same.] . . . Francofurti, Impensis & typis Balthas. Christoph. Wustii, 1675.

[15], 525 (i.e. 522), [54], 22 p. front. (port.) 18 cm. [8250]

Added engraved title page.

—[The same.] . . . Ed. 3. emend. Venetiis, Apud Combi & La Nou, 1696.

[32], 490, [46] p. 17 cm. [8251]

—[English tr.] Thesaurus & armementarium medico-chymicum; or, A treasury of physick. With the most secret way of preparing remedies against all diseases . . . Written originally in Latine . . . and . . . rendred into English by John Partridge . . . London, Printed by J. M. for Awnsham Churchill, 1682.

[15], 377, [34] p. port. 18 cm. [8252]

Imperfect: portrait wanting.

—[German tr.] Medicinisch-chymische Schatz- und Rüst-Kammer; das ist, Eine sonderbahre Art und Weiss, wie man die ausserlesenste und geheimste Arzney-Mittel, wider allerley Kranckheiten und Zustände dess menschlichen Leibs . . . verfertigen soll . . . Anfangs von dem Authore in lateinischer Sprache geschrieben; anjetzo aber . . . in unsere teutsche Mutter-Sprach übersetzt . . . von einem eiferigen Liebhaber der edlen Medicin . . . Stuttgart, In Verlegung Joh. Gottfried Zubrodts, Gedruckt bey Melchior Gerhard Lorbern, 1686.

[16], 663, [85] p. 17 cm. [8253]

—[The same.] . . . Offenbach am Mäyn, Verlegts Philibert Brunn und Augustus Metzler, Druckst Bonaventura de Launoy, 1695.

[16], 663, [85] p. 17 cm. [8254]

With this is bound Becher, J. J. Medicinische Schatz-Kammer. 1700.

MYREUS, LUDOVICUS. See L'OBEL, M. de. In G. Rondelletii . . . methodicam pharmaceuticam officinam animadversiones. 1605.

MYSTERIA physico-medica. 1681. See [KIRANUS, King of Persia]

MYSTERIUM occultae naturae. See GRASSHOFF, J. 1661.

N

N., I. See LA VERGE DE JACOB. 1693.

N., M. See NEDHAM, Marchamont [1620-1678]

N., N. See BERTINI, Anton Francesco [1658-1726]

N., N., tr. See [CUSANI, R.] Il Galenista confuso. 1697.

N., N. de [fl. 1696] See ILLUSTRISSIMI SIGNORI. 1669.

N., R. C. P. R. See CANTEREL, Robert.

N., S. T. D., tr. See HÖCHSTFÜRTREFLICHTES CHIROMANTISCH-UND PHYSIOGNOMISCHES KLEE-BLAT. 1695.

N. N. See SCHUTS, Jacobus [fl. 1682-1692]

N.P.D.M. See P., N., D. M.

NABOD, VALENTINUS. See NAIBOD, Valentin [d. 1593]

NABOTH, MARTIN [1675-1721] respondent. See SCHAMBERG, J. C. Disputationem medicam de respiratione laesa. 1693.

NACATTEL, LOOTRI. See LANCETTA, Troilo [fl. 1630-1632]

NACHTIGALL, OTTMAR. See LUSCINIUS, Ottmar [1487?-1537?]

NAEVIUS, CASPAR. See NEEFFE, Kaspar [ca. 1514-1580]

NAEVIUS, JOHANNES. See NEEFFE, Johann [1499-1574]

NAGELIUS, BARTHOLOMAEUS [fl. 1642] respondent. See SEBISCH, M. [1578-1674?] praeses. Disputatio de variolis et morbillis prima [-sexta & ultima] 1642.

NAIBOD, VALENTIN [d. 1593] See MAGINI, G. A. De astrologica ratione. 1607.

NAIRONI, ANTONIO FAUSTO [1635 or 6-1707] De saluberrima potione cahue; sue, Cafe nuncupata discursus . . . Romae, Typis Michaelis Herculis, 1671.

57 p. 14 cm. [8255]

NAIRONUS, FAUSTUS. See NAIRONI, Antonio Fausto [1635 or 6-1707]

NALDI, MATTEO [*d.* 1682] Aphorismorum Hippocratis explanatio auctore Matthia Naldio ... Romae, Typis Ignatii de Lazaris, 1657.

[16], 2, 226, [14] p.   26 cm.   **[8256]**

Covers book 1 only. Includes Greek and Latin text.

—Παμφιλία mundi universi amicitia, cui dissidentes philosophorum opiniones conciliantur, & parantur ex re medica amicitiae, & praesertim conjugiis conducentia formositas, & foecunditas ... Senis, Apud Bonettos, typis Publicis [apud Herculem de Goris] 1647.

[13], 5-7, [8], 396, [1] p.   front.   22 cm.
    [8257]

—Regole per la cura del contagio ... Roma, Mascardi, 1656.

[4], 81 p.   23 cm.   **[8258]**

—Rei medicae prodromi praecipuorum physiologiae problematum tractatus quibus peripateticae doctrinae nova traditur etymologia, & quaestiones de primo cognito: de coeli corruptibilitate ... &c. enodantur; et ostenditur Aristotelem ... caeteris philosophis ethnicis Christianae religioni propiora sapuisse, miraque ingenii sublimitate animorum non solum immortalitatem docuisse, sed etiam caelorum creationi & eorundem animorum reditui protulisse non repugnantia ... Romae, Ex typographia Ignatii de Lazaris, 1682.

[3] 519 p.   illus., plates.   34 cm.   **[8259]**

NANCY. Chambre de ville. *See* LAMBERT, N., defendant. Factum, pour les sieurs conseillers de la chambre de ville de Nancy appellans de deux sentences. 1647.

NANCY. Ordinances, local laws, etc. Articles concernants ce que les commissaires des quartiers doibuent faire en temps de soubçon de maladie contagieuse. Nancy, Anthoine Charlot, 1631.

[7] p.   24 cm.   **[8260]**

NANTES BARRERA, OLIVA SABUCO DE. *See* SABUCO DE NANTES BARRERA, OLIVA [1562-1622?]

NAPLES. Deputati per la sanità. *See* CONSULTA DE MEDICI per preservarsi da mali correnti nella città di Napoli. 1656.

NARDI, FILIPPO [*fl. ca.* 1655] *See* NARDI, G. Noctes geniales. 1656.

NARDI, GIOVANNI [*ca.* 1580–*ca.* 1655] Apologeticon in Fortunii Liceti mulctram, vel de duplici calore. [Florentiae, Typis Amatoris Massae, & soc., 1638]

[1], 537, [7] p.   24 cm.   **[8261]**

—De prodigiosis vulnerum curationibus.

605-608 p.   21 cm.   (*In* Theatrum sympatheticum auctum. Norimbergae, 1662)   **[8262]**

Caption title.

—Lactis physica analysis ... [Florentiae, Typis Petri Nestii, 1634]

[16], 342, [18] p.   23 cm.   **[8263]**

Engraved title page.

—Noctes geniales ... Annus primus. Bononiae, Typis Jo. Baptistae Ferronii, 1656.

[12], 748, [40] p.   22 cm.   **[8264]**

Edited by Elias Schottelius.

Dedicatory epistle signed by Filippo Nardi, the author's son.

—*See* PANUZZI, F., *ed.* Francesco Panuzzi ... a i lettori. 1640.

A NARRATIVE of the late extraordinary cure wrought ... upon Mrs. Eliz. Savage. (lame from the birth) without the using of any natural means ... With an appendix, attempting to prove, that miracles are not ceas'd. London, John Dunton and John Harris, 1694.

46, [3] p.   18 cm.   **[8265]**

NASTURTIUS, PHILO, *pseud. See* SPAENHOLZ, N.

NATHUSIUS, ELIAS [*fl.* 1651] *respondent. See* OHEIM, J. P. Theses physicae de qualitatibus occultis in genere. 1651.

NATURA exenterata. 1655. *See* PHILIATROS.

NATURAL history of the passions. 1674. *See* [CHARLETON, W.]

NATURE'S cabinet unlock'd. 1657. *See* BROWNE, *Sir* T.

NAUDÉ, GABRIEL [1600-1653] Apologie pour tous les grands personnages qui ont esté faussement soupçonnez de magie ... Paris, François Targa, 1625.

[24], 615 (i.e. 649), [23] p.   18 cm.   **[8266]**

Imperfect: p. 209-210 mutilated.

—[English tr.] The history of magick by way of apology, for all the wise men who have unjustly been reputed magicians . . . Englished by J. Davies. London, John Streater, 1657.

[16], 306 p.   17 cm.   [8267]

—[The same, *as subject*] *See* CHEVANES, J. de. L'incredulité sçavante. 1671.

—Quaestio iatrophilogica. An magnum homini, a venenis periculum? Romae, Ex typographia Gulielmi Facciotti, 1632.

29 p.   18 cm.   [8268]

With this are bound *his*: Quaestio quarta iatrophilologica. 1635; Quaestio tertia iatrophilologica. 1634; Questio secunda iatrophilologica. 1634.

—Questio secunda iatrophilologica. An vita hominum hodie quam olim brevior? Caesenae, Ex typographia Josephi Nerii, 1634.

27 p.   18 cm.   [8269]

Bound with *his* Quaestio iatrophilologica. 1632.

—Quaestio tertia iatrophilologica. An matutina studia vespertinis salubriora. Patavii, Ex typographia Julii Crivellarii, 1634.

[8], 45, [1] p.   18 cm.   [8270]

Bound with *his* Quaestio iatrophilologica. 1632.

—Quaestio quarta iatrophilologica. An liceat medico fallere aegrotum? Romae, Ex typographia Jacobi Facciotti, 1635.

51, [1] p.   18 cm.   [8271]

Bound with *his* Quaestio iatrophilologica. 1632.

—Πέντας quaestionum iatro-philologicarum. I. An magnum homini a venenis periculum? II. An vita hominum hodie quam olim brevior? III. An matutina studia vespertinis salubriora? IV. An liceat medico fallere aegrotum? V. De fato & fatali vitae termino. Genevae, Apud Samuelem Chouët, 1647.

[8], 332, [4] p.   18 cm.   [8272]

—Vita Cardani. *In* Cardano, G. Opera omnia. 1663.

—*See* CARDANO, G. De propria vita liber. 1654; GASSENDI, P. Viri illustris Nicolai Claudii Fabricii de Peiresc . . . vita. 1655; PARDOUX, B. Bartholomaei Perdulcis . . . *In* Jac. Sylvii anatomen et in lib. Hippocratis De natura humana commentarii. 1643; RIOLAN, J. [1538?–1605?] In artem parvam Galeni commentarius. 1631; RORARIO, G. Quod animalia bruta ratione utantur melius homine. 1654.

NAURATH, MARTIN [*d.* 1679 *or* 80] Tractatus politico-juridicus ad usum horum temporum accommodatus, de vita et morte hominis . . . Accesserunt . . . additamenta miscellanea practica . . . Gissae Hassorum, Ex officina Jac. Gotofr. Seyler, 1673.

[16], 456, [24] p.   17 cm.   [8273]

Added engraved title page has imprint: Franckfurt, Sumptibus Jacobi Gottofriedi Seileri, 1673.

NAVARRO, JUAN BAUTISTA [*b.* 1558] Commentarii ad libros Galeni De differentiis febrium, De pulsibus ad tyrones, & spurium De urinis . . . In hac ultima editione, addita est Anachaephaleosis librorum Galeno de crisibus. Barcinonae, Ex typographia Elenae Deu viduae, 1649.

[8], 507, [12] p.   15 cm.   [8274]

Imperfect: wormholes on p. 413–454.
Includes short portions of the Galenic texts.

—[The same.] . . . Valentiae, Ex typographia Lucae Fuster, expensis Laurentii Cabrera, 1651.

[6], 619 (i.e. 617), [7] p.   15 cm.   [8275]

Imperfect: first preliminary leaf (blank?) wanting.
Includes considerable portions of the Galenic texts in the translation of Herman Croeser (De pulsibus ad tirones), Niccolò Leoniceno (De differentiis febrium) and Josephus Struthius (De urinis).

NAVARRO, JUAN DE DIOS HUARTE. *See* HUARTE DE SAN JUAN, JUAN [1529?–1588]

NEANDER, JOHANN [*ca.* 1596–*ca.* 1630] Antiquissimae et nobilissimae medicinae natalitia, sectae earumque placita: tum ejus catacrypses ac instauratores; & . . . propagatores cum historiis eorum, vitis ac scriptis . . . Adita est . . . De medicina Hermetica & Paracelsica . . . dissertatio. Bremae, Typis Johannis Wesselii, 1623.

[36], 368, [23] p.   19 cm.   [8276]

Imperfect: sig. (*) 3–4 wanting.

—Tabacologia; hoc est, Tabaci, seu nicotianae descriptio medico-cheirurgico-pharmaceutica: vel ejus praeparatio & usus in omnibus corporis humani incommodis . . . Lugduni Batavorum, Ex officina Isaaci Elzevirii, 1622.

[40], 256, [3] p.   illus.   23 cm.   [8277]

Errata: p. 255–6.

—[The same.] ... Lugduni Batavorum, Ex officina Isaaci Elzeviri, 1626.

[38], 256 p. illus. 22 cm. [8278]

Engraved title page.
Errata: p. 255-6.
Mainly a reissue of the 1622 edition.

—[The same.] *In* Everard, G. De herba panacea. 1644.

—[French tr.] Traicté du tabac; ou, Nicotiane, panacee, petun: autrement herbe a la reyne, avec sa preparation & son usage, pour la plus part des indispositions du corps humain ... Composé premierement en latin ... & mis de nouveau en françois, par I[acques] V[eyras] ... Lyon, Barthelemy Vincent, 1626.

[8], 342 p. plates. 18 cm. [8279]

—[Excerpts. English]. *In* Everard, G. Panacea. 1659.

NEANDER, Josias Christoph [*fl.* 1655?-1662] *respondent. See* Kunad, A., *praeses.* Disputatio inauguralis de confessione Petri et eam secuta Christi responsione. 1680.

NEAPOLITANISCHER Zorn-Spiegel dess grossen und gerechten Gottes, nebenst Beschreibung der ... Haupstadt Neapolis ... und darauff ihr ... erschröcklichen Pestilentz. Mit angehängter Verzeichniss vieler von etlich hundert Jahren her vorgangener grossen Pest, Städt- Land- und Welt-Sterben ... [n. p.] 1656.

[31] p. 18 cm. [8280]

NEBEL, Daniel [1664-1733] *praeses.* Exercitationum anatomicarum prima anatomes praeliminaria et partes corporis humani vulgo dictas similares plerasque sistens ... Marburgi Catorum, Typis haered. Joh. Jococi Kürsneri [1696]

[2], 32 p. 19 cm. [8281]

Imperfect: all after p. 32 wanting.
Diss.—Marburg (J. G. Dexbach, *respondent*)

—*respondent. See* Franck von Franckenau, G., *praeses.* Agonismata physico-medica sexta vice. 1682.

NEBENIUS, Conrad [*fl.* 1600] *ed. See* Magirus, J. Physiologiae peripateticae libri sex. 1610, 1616, 1618, 1619, 1638, 1642.

NECCER, Karl Ludwig [*fl.* 1691] *respondent. See* Albinus, B. Dissertatio inauguralis de fame canina. 1691.

NEDHAM, Marchamont [1620-1678] Medela medicinae. A plea for the free profession, and a renovation of the art of physick, out of the noblest ... writers ... The author, M[archamont] N[edham] med. Londinens. ... London, Richard Lownds, 1665.

[23], 516 p. 17 cm. [8282]

—[The same, *as subject.*] *See* Sprackling, R. Medela ignorantiae. 1665; Twysden, J. Medicina veterum vindicata. 1666.

—*See* Bolnest, E. Medicina instaurata. 1665; Castle, G. The chymical Galenist. 1667; Le Boë, F. de. A new idea of the practice of physic. 1675.

NEEDHAM, Walter [1631?-1691?] Disquisitio anatomica de formato foetu ... Londini, Typis Gulielmi Godbid, prostanque venales apud Radulphum Needham, 1667.

[24], 205, [15] p. plates. 17 cm. [8283]

Imperfect: p. 123-124 mutilated.

—Another issue. 18 cm. [8284]

Page [5] numbered 199.

—[The same.] ... Ed. alt. priori emend. Amstelodami, Apud Petrum Le Grand, 1668.

[20], 234 p. plates, tables. 13 cm. [8285]

NEEFFE, Johann [1499-1574] *See* Scholtz, L. Consiliorum medicinalium ... liber singularis. 1610; Sennert, D. De febribus libri IV. 1628, 1633, 1641, 1653.

NEEFFE, Kaspar [*ca.* 1514-1580] *See* Scholtz, L. Consiliorum medicinalium ... liber singularis. 1610.

NEESSEN, Johannes. *See* Neeffe, Johann [1499-1574]

NEFE, Caspar. *See* Neeffe, Kaspar [*ca.* 1514-1580]

NEFE, Johann. *See* Neeffe, Johann [1499-1574]

NEGRISOLI, Franciscus Maria. *See* Nigrisoli, Francesco Maria [1648-1727 *or* 8]

NEHEMIAS, Abraham [*fl.* 1591] Methodus medendi universalis, per sanguinis missionem, et purgationem, in libros duos divisa ... Accessit De tempore aquae frigidae in febribus ardentibus ad satietatem exhibendae, liber unus. 3. ed. ... Venetiis, Apud Joannem Baptistam Ciottum, 1604.

[7], 83, [12] p. 21 cm. [8286]

With this is bound Cesalpino, A. De metallicis libri tres. 1602.

NEHMITZ, WILHELM HEINRICH [*fl.* 1698] *respondent. See* Vehr, I., *praeses.* Disputatio inauguralis medica de affectione marmorea. 1698.

NEHTMAN, HERMANN [*fl.* 1660] *respondent. See* LINDEN, J. A. van der, *praeses.* Hippocrates de circuitu sanguinis, exercitatio XIII. 1660.

NEITHARDT, PETER [*fl.* 1681] *respondent.* Disputatio inauguralis medica de tributo lunari foeminarum intercepto, in certo quodam casu . . . Altdorfii, Literis Henrici Meyeri [1681]

    12 p.   21 cm.   **[8287]**
    Diss. — Altdorf.

NEMESIUS, BP. *of Emesa.* Περὶ φύσεως ἀνθρώπον βιβλίον ἑν . . . De natura hominis liber unus, denuo recognitus, & manuscriptorum codicum collatione in integrum restitutus, annotationibusque insuper illustratus. Oxonii, E Theatro Sheldoniano, 1671.

    [16], 345, [5], 42 (i.e. 50) p.   20 cm.
                             [8288]
    Text in Greek and Latin.
    Translation by Saint Gregorius Nazianxenus; edited by John Fell, bishop of Oxford.

—[English tr.] The nature of man . . . Written in Greek . . . Englished and divided into sections, with briefs of their principall contents: by Geo. Wither. London, Printed by M. F. for Henry Tauton, 1636.

    [44], 660 p.   15 cm.   **[8289]**
    Imperfect: first preliminary leaf wanting.

NEMI, NICOLÒ [*fl. ca.* 1640] Imbiancatura di Nicolò Nemi da Novi. Data ad un certo libro di Stefano di Gaspara . . . Fatta da esso control il vero opobalsamo operato dal Manfredi, & dal Panutio, in fare le loro theriache. [Torino, Giacomo Sarcina, 1640]

    [8] p.   22 cm.   **[8290]**
    Caption title.

NEODORPIUS, GERARDUS [*fl.* 1631] *respondent. See* BURGERSDIJCK, F. P., *praeses.* Collegium physicum. 1642.

NEOVIN, OTTON JEAN MICHEL [*fl.* 1682] *respondent. See* SCHMID, J. A., *praeses.* Coecus de colore judicans. 1682.

NEPITA, ANTONIO DE [*fl.* 1668] *respondent. See* BOHN, J., *praeses.* Exercitationum physiologicarum prima . . . [-decima tertia] 1674?

NERI, FILIPPO, *Saint. See* FILIPPO NERI, *Saint* [1515-1595]

NERIS, THOMAS DE [*fl.* 1622] De Tyburtini aeris salubritate commentarius . . . Romae, Apud Alexandrum Zannettum, 1622.

    [16], 110, [1] p.   plate.   16 cm.   **[8291]**

NERVIUS, VALERIUS [*fl.* 1624?] *ed. See* CASTRO, E. R. de. Tractatus de complexu morborum. 1624.

NESCHULITZ, LAZAR [*fl.* 1614] *respondent.* Theses de febre hectica . . . Basileae, Typis Joan. Jacobi Genathii [1614]

    [12] p.   21 cm.   **[8292]**
    Diss. — Basel.

NESSEL, DANIEL [1644-1699] *respondent. See* RACHEL, S., *praeses.* Dissertatio moralis de principiis actionum humanarum. 1660.

NESSEL, EDMOND [*ca.* 1658-1731] Traité des eaux de Spa avec une analyse d'icelles, leurs vertus et usage . . . Spa, J. Salpeteur; et Liege, La vefue d'Adrien Brixhe, 1699.

    [6], 116 p.   plates.   15 cm.   **[8293]**
    With this is bound: Sandberg, J. H. Essai sur les eaux minérales ferrugineuses de Spa. Liege, 1780.

NESTER, JOHANN [1596-1662] *See* REINESIUS, T. Epistolarum ad Nesteros, patrem et filium conscriptarum farrago. 1670.

NESTER, JOHANN MATTHIAS [1622-1679] *respondent. See* MÖBIUS, G., *praeses.* Disputatio medica de bilis natura ejusque usu nobilissimo. 1644; ROLFINCK, W., *praeses.* Disputatio medica inauguralis περι ἀνορεξιας. 1649.

—, *ed. See* MACASIUS, J. G. PROMPTUARIUM MATERIAE MEDICAE. 1654, 1677; REINESIUS, T. Epistolarum ad Nesteros, patrem et filium conscriptarum farrago. 1670.

NESTER, KARL FRIEDRICH [*b.* 1662] *respondent. See* WEDEL, G. W., *praeses.* Disputationem inauguralem medicam de colica scorbutica . . . submittit C. F. N. 1688.

—*See* WEDEL, G. W. Propempticon inaugurale de morbo crasso Hippocratis. 1688.

NESTOR, *pseud. See* WELSCH, Georg Hieronymus [1624-1677]

NETHERLANDS (United Provinces, 1581–1795) **Laws, Statutes, Etc.** Reglement ende ordre, van de hoogh mogende heeren Staten generael der vereenighde Nederlanden, tot voorkominge ende redres van sieckten, onder 's landts militie, in het leger ende elders. 's Graven-Hage, Jacobus Scheltus, 1673.

[8] p. 20 cm. **[8294]**

NETTELBACH, Johann Christian [*fl.* 1665–1667] *respondent. See* Loss, J., *praeses.* De fermento ventriculi. 1665; Schneider, K. V., *praeses.* Disputationem inauguralem de epilepsia . . . submittit J. C. N. 1667.

NETTESHEIM, Heinrich Cornelius Agrippa von. *See* Agrippa von Nettesheim, Heinrich Cornelius [1486–1535]

NEU ausführlich und wohl gegründetes Aderlass-Büchlein. 1700. *See* [Pansa, M.]

NEU-ERFUNDENE mathematische Curiositäten. 1695. *See* Alencé. J. d'.

NEU-VERMEHRTES und verbessertes Aderlass-Büchlein; das ist, Ein astronomischer Grund und Bericht, vom Aderlassen, Schrepfen, und Baden, zu Erhaltung menschlicher Gesundheit, und Verlängerung dess Lebens . . . Nürnberg, Bey Johann Andreae, und Wolffgang Endter dess Jüngern sel. Erben [*ca.* 1670]

144, [8] p. illus., plate. 16 cm. **[8295]**

Imperfect: title page and last leaf mutilated.

With this are bound: Horlacher, C. Die höchstschädliche Würckung des Aderlassens. 1691; Aletophilus, J. M. Unvorgreiffliches Bedencken. 1691; Kurtz-verfastes Land- und Haus-Artzney-Büchlein [16–?]

NEUBAUR, Heinrich [*fl.* 1686] *respondent. See* Schrader, F., *praeses.* Disputatio medica inauguralis lympham et glandulas pathologice considerans. 1686.

NEUBERGER, Johann Christoph [*fl.* 1665–1669] *respondent. See* Rolfinck, W., *praeses.* Ordinem et methodum cognoscendi et curandi ileum . . . submittit . . . J. C. N. 1669; Thymius, A., *praeses.* Magni Hippocratis Coi Aphorismi XLV. sectionis VI. ulcerum antiquorum statum et prognosin continentis, resolutio. 1665.

NEUBICH, Johann Christoph [*fl.* 1689–1691] *respondent. See* Wedel, G. W., *praeses.* Dissertatio medica de similitudine morborum. 1689.

NEUBIG, Joannes Christophorus. *See* Neubich, Johann Christoph [*fl.* 1689–1691]

NEUCRANTZ, Paul [1605–1671] De harengo exercitatio medica, in qua principis piscium exquisitissima bonitas summaque gloria asserta & vindicata . . . Lubecae, Literis Gothofredi Jegeri, sumptibus Joachimi Wildii bibliopol. Rostoch., 1654.

83, [5] p. 19 cm. **[8296]**

—De purpura liber singularis, in quo febrium malignarum natura & curatio proponitur . . . Lubecae, Literis Gothofredi Jegeri, prostat apud Henricum Schernwebelium, 1648.

[8], 552, 22, [2] p. 20 cm. **[8297]**

—[The same.] . . . Francofurti & Lubecae, Sumpt. Augusti Johannis Beckeri, 1660.

[8], 552, 22, [2] p. 20 cm. **[8298]**

A reissue of the 1648 edition with new title page and dedicatory epistle.

NEUCRANZ, Zacharias. *See* Neukrantz, Zacharias [*fl.* 1676]

NEUE Infections-Ordnung. [1680?] *See* Austria. Sovereign, 1658–1705 (Leopold I).

NEUENHAHN, Johann Ludwig [*fl.* 1674–1685] Nostri notitiam esse viam ad Dei cognitionem, in anatome cadaveris foeminei chirurgico-practica ostenditur: cui literarum atque anatomiae fautores humanitus adesse gestit . . . Meiningae, Literis Hassartinis, 1682.

[8] p. 19 cm. **[8299]**

—*respondent.* Dissertatio medica inauguralis carcinomatis malignitatem ejusque curam exhibens . . . Altdorfii, Typis Henrici Meyeri [1685]

[16] p. 21 cm. **[8300]**

Diss. — Altdorf.

—, *respondent. See* Wedel, G. W., *praeses.* Dissertatio medica de scabie. 1674.

NEUES Viehe Büchlein, darinnen die Beschreibung, wie auch die meisten Kranckheiten und darwider dienende Artzneyen der Rinder, Schafe, Ziegen, Schweine, Hunde, Hühner, Gänse, Enden und Tauben zu finden. Männiglichen, insonderheit aber den Haussvätern zu Nutz mit Fleiss colligirt, und beschrieben [n. p.] 1677.

123, [5] p. illus. 17 cm. **[8301]**

NEUKRANTZ, Zacharias [*fl.* 1676] *respondent.* *See* Ettmüller, M., *praeses.* Abstrusum respirationis humanae negotium. 1676.

NEUKRANZ, Johann Anton [*fl.* 1674–1698] *respondent. See* Meibom, H., *praeses.* Dissertatio medica inauguralis de vulneribus lethalibus. 1674, 1694.

NEUMANN, Caspar [1648–1715] *praeses.* ... Judicium discursu physico explicatum ... Jenae, Typis Bauhoferianis [1678]

    [32] p.   20 cm.   **[8302]**
   Diss.—Jena (G. C. Eckelt, *respondent*)

NEUMANN, Gottfried [*fl.* 1652] *respondent. See* Pufendorff, E., *praeses.* De sanguine et ejus motus dissertatio. 1652.

NEUSE, Johann Georg [*fl.* 1685] *respondent. See* Wedel, G. W., *praeses.* Dissertationem medicam inauguralem de melancholia ... subjicit J. G. N. 1685.

NEVYE, Jan [*fl.* 1662] *respondent.* Disputatio medica inauguralis de nutritione ... Lugduni Batavorum, Apud Franciscum Moyaert, 1662.

    [12] p.   23 cm.   **[8303]**
   Diss.—Leyden.

A NEW and needful treatise of wind offending mans body. 1676. *See* Feyens, J.

A NEW method of curing the French-pox, written by an eminent French author. Together with the practice and method of Monsieur Blanchard, as also Dr. Sydenham's judgement on the same. To which is added Annotations and observations by William Salmon ... London, John Taylor and Thomas Newborough, 1690.

    [8], 256, 36 p.   16 cm.   **[8304]**
   "Some curious problems: in which the finest questions ... concerning the venereal distemper, are resolved ... By the same author. 1689" (p. [105]–161) and "Mr. Stephen Blankards's practice relating to the venereal distemper ... 1689" (p. [163]–256) have special title pages.
   Sydenham's contribution called for on the title page does not seem to have been included.

A NEW treatise of natural philosophy. 1687. *See* [Midgley, R.]

NEWCASTLE, Margaret (Lucas) Cavendish, *duchess of* [1624?–1674] Grounds of natural philosophy: divided into thirteen parts: with an appendix containing five parts. The 2d ed., much altered from the first, which went under the name of Philosophical and physical opinions ... London, A. Maxwell, 1668.

    [12], 311 p.   32 cm.   **[8305]**

  —The worlds olio ... London, J. Martin and J. Allestrye, 1655.

    [14], 216, [3] p.   28 cm.   **[8306]**

NEWCOME, Henry [1650–1713] The compleat mother; or, An earnest perswasive to all mothers ... to nurse their own children ... London, J. Wyat, 1695.

    [4], 112 p.   16 cm.   **[8307]**

NEWTON, *Sir* Isaac [1642–1727] *See* Briggs, W. Nova visionis theoria. 1685.

NEWTON, Thomas [1542?–1607] *tr. See* Lemnius, L. The touchstone of complexions. 1633.

NEYDECKER, Johann [*fl.* 1631] *ed. See* Stainer, B. Gerocomicon. 1631.

Le NEZ pourry de Theophraste Renaudot. [not before 1644] *See* [Patin, G.]

NFERIGNO, *accademico della Crusca. See* Rossi, Bastiano de [*fl.* 1585–1605]

NICANDER, *pseud. See* Screta, Heinrich [1637–1689]

NICANDER, *of Colophon.* Alexipharmaca. *In* Gorris, J. de [1505–1577] Opera. Definitionum medicarum libri XXIIII. 1622.

  —Theriaca. *In* Gorris, J. de [1505–1577] Opera. Definitionum medicarum libri XXIIII. 1622.

NICAUD, Robert [1643] Historia memorabilis foeminae Montelucianae bis triennio per hypochondria parientis ... Parisiis, Apud Petrum de Bresche, 1644.

    14 p.   19 cm.   **[8308]**

NICCOLÒ DA LONIGO. *See* Leoniceno, Niccolò [1428–1524]

NICEPHORUS, *Saint, patriarch of Constantinople. See* Artemidorus Daldianus. Artemidori Daldiani & Achmetis Sereimi f. Oneirocritica. 1603.

NICODEMO, Francesco, *comp. See* Toppi, N. Biblioteca napoletana. Addizioni. 1683.

NICODEMO, Lionardo, *comp. See* Toppi, N. Biblioteca napoletana. Addizioni. 1683.

NICOLAI, CHRISTOPH [1618-1662] *praeses.* Disputatio medica, de pernicioso Paracelsistarum hoplochrismate . . .

624-649 p. 21 cm. (In Theatrum sympatheticum auctum. Norimbergae, 1662) [**8309**]

Caption title.

Diss. — Altdorf, 1662 (J. Bürlein, *respondent*)

NICOLAI, HALVARD [*fl.* 1678] *respondent. See* BARTHOLIN, C. [1655-1738], *praeses.* Positiones anatomicae. 1678.

NICOLAI, HEINRICH [*fl.* 1675] *respondent.* Disputatio inauguralis medica de vulneribus sclopetorum . . . Argentorati, Typis Johannis Welperi [1675]

[4], 40 p. 20 cm. [**8310**]

Diss. — Strasbourg.

NICOLAI, NICOLAUS CASPAR [*fl.* 1676] *respondent. See* ADLUNG, J. C., *praeses.* Miraculosa . . . piscina. [1676]

NICOLAUS LEONICENUS. *See* LEONICENO, Niccolò [1428-1524]

NICOLAUS, PRAEPOSITUS SALERNITANUS. *See* NICOLAUS SALERNITANUS [12th cent.]

NICOLAUS SALERNITANUS [12th cent.] *See* MESUË [924 *or* 5-1015] Opera. 1602, 1623.

NICOLAUS, DANIEL [*fl.* 1692] *respondent. See* ALBINUS, B. Dissertatio inauguralis medica, de mania. 1692.

NICOLINI, GIOVANNI BATTISTA [*fl.* 1527] *ed. See* MESUË [924 *or* 5-1015] Opera. 1602, 1623.

NICOLLINUS, JOANNES BAPTISTA. *See* NICOLINI, Giovanni Battista [*fl.* 1527]

NICQUET, HONORAT [1585-1667] Physiognomia humana libris IV. distincta. Ed. 1. Lugduni, Sumptib. haered. Petri Prost, Philippi Borde, & Laurentii Arnaud, 1648.

[16], 320, [23] p. 23 cm. [**8311**]

NIEDERLAUSITZ. *See* LUSATIA, Lower.

NIEMAND, HIERONYMUS [*fl.* 1673-1676] *respondent.* Disputatio medica inauguralis de suffusione . . . Argentorati, Typis Joh. Friderici Spoor, 1676.

[2], 26 p. 20 cm. [**8312**]

Diss. — Strasbourg.

— *See* STRAUSS, L., *praeses.* Physicarum quaestionum decas de elementis. 1673.

NIEREMBERG, JUAN EUSEBIO [1595-1658] Historia naturae . . . libris XVI. distincta. In quibus rarissima naturae arcana . . . etiam cum proprietatibus medicinalibus, describuntur . . . Accedunt de miris & miraculosis naturis in Europa libri duo: item de iisdem in terra Hebraeis promissa liber unus. Antverpiae, Ex Officina Plantiniana Balthasaris Moreti, 1635.

[8], 502, [104] p. illus. 35 cm. [**8313**]

NIESIUS, BENJAMIN. *See* NIESS, Benjamin [*fl.* 1670-1674]

NIESS, BENJAMIN [*fl.* 1670-1674] *respondent.* Disputatio medica inauguralis de elephantiasi, seu lepra Arabum . . . Argentorati, Typis Johannis Welperi [1673]

28 p. 20 cm. [**8314**]

Diss. — Strasbourg.

NIETNER, JOHANN GOTTFRIED [*fl.* 1694] *respondent. See* EYSEL, J. P., *praeses.* Disputationem anatomico-medicam de glandularum natura et usu . . . exponet J. G. N. 1694.

NIETO DE VALCÁRCEL, JUAN [*fl.* 1681-1685] Disputatio epidemica. Teatro racional, donde desnuda de la verdad se presente al examen de los ingenios. Thesis en que se ventila el uso de los alexifarmacos sudorificos, en el principio de las malignas del año de 84 . . . Valencia [1685]

[14], 280, [1] p. 21 cm. [**8315**]

Errata: p. [281]

NIETSCH, ANDREAS. *See* NITZSCH, Andreas [*fl.* 1630-1631]

NIEU licht der apotekers en distilleerkonst. 1657, 1662, 1667. *See* PHARMACIA Galenica & chymica.

NIEULANDT, PIETER [*fl.* 1660] *respondent.* Disputatio medica inauguralis, de mola uteri . . . Ultrajecti, Ex officina Jacobi à Doeyenburch, 1660.

[8] p. 20 cm. [**8316**]

Diss. — Utrecht.

NIEUSTADT, PIETER RUTGERSZ. VAN, *ed. See* GUY DE CHAULIAC. De chirurgije. 1646.

— *tr. See* PIGRAY, P. Kort begryp. 1662.

NIFO, Agostino [*ca.* 1473-1545?] De auguriis, libri II. nec non De diebus criticis, liber I. nunc denuo excusi, et ... repurgati. His accesserunt Uraniae divinatricis, quoad Astrologiae generalia, libri II. jam primo in lucem evolantes, alas suppeditante Rodolpho Goclenio ... Marpurgi, Typis Pauli Egenolphi, 1614.

    [8], 143, 150 p.   20 cm.   **[8317]**

NIGER HAPELIUS, Nicolaus. *See* Eglinus Iconius, Raphael [1559-1622]

NIGRISOLI, Francesco Maria [1648-1727 *or* 8] Dell'anatomia chirurgica delle glandole di Francesco Maria Giglio [pseud.] ... Parte prima [-seconda] ... Ferrara, Per l'erede di Giulio Bulzoni Giglio, 1681-82.

    2 v.   21 cm.   **[8318]**

[—] *ed.* Febris china chinae expugnata; seu, Illustrium aliquot virorum opuscula, quae veram tradunt methodum, febres china chinae curandi ... Collegit, argumenta, notas, observationes addidit med. Ferrariensis. Ferrariae, Typis Bernardini Pomatelli, 1687.

    xvi, 204 p.   plates.   22 cm.   **[8319]**
    Contains Latin translations of four treatises, previously published in French.

    Contents. — Remedium Anglicum pro curatione febrium a Nicolao de Blegny. — De febrium curatione per usum quinquinae auctore D. Monginot. — Hippocrates de curatione febrium per usum chinae chinae auctore D. Raymundo Restaurando. — Observationes de febribus, & febrifugis habitae a clarissimo viro I. S. D. M. L. [i.e. Jacobo Sponio doctore medico Lugdunensi]

     — [The same.] ... Ed. alt. ab auctore recognita, emendata, plurimisque observationibus aucta. Ferrariae, Apud Lilium, 1700.

    [24], 329, [2] p.   plates, port.   21 cm.
                                  [8320]
    Contents as in the 1687 Ferrara edition.

NIGRISOLI, Girolamo [1620-1689] Progymnasmata in quibus novum praesidium medicum appositio videlicet hirudinum internae parti uteri in puerperii, & mensium suppressione exponitur ... de vena in febribus malignis secanda disseritur ... Salisburgi, Sumpt. Joannis Baptistae Mayer, 1689.

    197 p.   22 cm.   **[8321]**
    Imperfect: sheets A–B wanting; last leaf (blank?) wanting; wormholes throughout.

EL NIGROMANTICO de suplicio severo. 1670. *See* Pérez de Castro, J.

NIHUS, Barthold, *Bp. of Myra* [1589-1657] *See* Bartholin, T. De cruce Christi hypomnemata IV. 1670.

NIJLANDT, P. *See* Nylandt, Petrus.

NIKANDER, *of Colophon. See* Nicander, *of Colophon.*

NIMPTSCH, Ulrich Sigismund [1672-1726] *respondent.* Disputatio inauguralis medica de ἀγρυπνία; sive, Vigilia praenaturali ... [Altdorffii] Literis Henrici Meyeri [1697]

    24 p.   19 cm.   **[8322]**
    Diss. — Altdorf.

     — *See* Detharding, G., *praeses.* Exercitatio anatomico-physiologica de fontanella infantum. 1695.

NIPHUS, Augustinus. *See* Nifo, Agostino [*ca.* 1473-1545?]

NITNER, Andreas [*fl.* 1669] Vom Spiritu Mundi, oder Edlen Krafft-Wasser; erörtherte und erklährte vorheissene sechzehen Fragen ... Leipzig, Bey Johann Grossen und Consort, gedruckt bey Christian Michaeln, 1669.

    [1], 70 p.   20 cm.   **[8323]**

     — *See* Cramer, C., *praeses.* Specimen inaugurale de spiritu mundi Nitneriano ... subjicit G. A. U. 1680.

NITSCHKE, Eliasz [1644-1711] *respondent.* Disputatio medica inauguralis de custode errante Helmontii, sive productione muci depravata ... Lugduni Batavorum, Apud viduam & haeredes Joannis Elsevirii, 1670.

    [23] p.   23 cm.   **[8324]**
    Diss. — Leiden.

     — *See* Bohn, J., *praeses.* Exercitationum physiologicarum prima ... [-decima tertia] 1674?

NITSCHKE, Eliasz Gotfryd [1676-1718] *respondent.* Disputatio medica inauguralis de calculo renum ... Lugduni Batavorum, Apud Abrahamum Elzevier, 1700.

    [46] p.   19 cm.   **[8325]**
    Diss. — Leyden.

NITSCHKI, Eliasz Gittfried. *See* Nitschke, Eliasz Gotfryd [1676-1718]

NITSCHMANN, Samuel. *See* Coryli, Samuel [*fl.* 1693-*ca.* 1726]

NITZEN, ERNST [*fl.* 1615–1617] *respondent*. De principalibus τῶν ἀρχῶν μορίων affectibus quaestiones varias . . . Basileae, Per Joan. Jacobum Genathium [1617]

[24] p. 19 cm. [8326]

Diss. — Basel.

NITZSCH, ANDREAS [*fl.* 1630–1631] *respondent*. *See* SEBISCH, M. [1578–1674?] *praeses*. Exercitationes medicae. 1639 [and] Libri sex Galeni De morborum differentiis. 1632.

NITZSCHKE, CHRISTIAN [*fl.* 1665–1670] *respondent*. *See* BECKHER, D. [1627–1670] *praeses*. Disputatio medica de intestinorum vermibus. 1666; LEPNER, F., *praeses*. Disputatio medica de catarrho. 1665; SENNERT, M., *praeses*. Disputatio inauguralis . . . casum geminum lactis e vena aperta educti tractans. 1670.

NOBEL, JEAN, *pseud*. *See* LE BON, Jean [*d.* 1583?]

NOBILISSIMI signiori, questo, e il vero ritrato di un giovine con due teste, che si puó chiamare l'ottava maraviglia del mondo avendo l'istesse teste ochi bocca denti, e capelli, et e batezate tutte due con nome diferente, ciove la maggiore Giacomo et la minore Matteó cosa di grand.^mo stupore degna d'esserveduta da ogni persona e si conduce a casa de cavaglieri per maggior comodo delle nobilita lovo. Venetia, 1695.

broadside. 28 x 19 cm. [8327]

Engraved title.

NOCERA, GIUSEPPE [*b.* 1643] Opus medicophysicum contemplativum in quo variae medentum sectae circa phlebotomiam & pharmaciam discutiuntur. Systema de febribus nondum clare divulgatum juxta Democriti & Epicuri dogmata novis rationibus & experimentis propugnatur. Messanae, Typis Vincentii de Amico, 1695.

[II], 444, [25] p. 16 cm. [8328]

NOËL, FRANÇOIS. *See* SILATAN, François [*fl.* 1655?]

NOËL DE PIVIER, NICOLAS BENJAMIN. *See* PIVIER, Nicolas Benjamin Noël de [*fl.* 1691]

NOHTWENDIGER Unterricht, wie der gifftigen anklebenden Seuche der Pestilentz . . . curiren sey. 1680. *See* BRUNSWICK (Duchy)

NOLA, FRANCESCO [*fl.* 1620] De epidemio phlegmone anginoso grassante Neapoli . . . Venetiis,

Ex typographica officina Jo. Baptistae Ciotti, 1620.

77, [2] p. 21 cm. [8329]

NOLANUS, AMBROSIUS LEO. *See* LEONE, Ambrogio [*d.* 1525]

NOLL, HENRICUS. *See* NOLLE, Heinrich [*fl.* 1612–1619]

NOLLE, HEINRICH [*fl.* 1612–1619] De generatione rerum naturalium liber ex vero naturae lumine in gratiam sincerioris philosophiae studiosorum confirmatus . . . Francofurti, E Collegio Musarum Paltheniano, 1615.

[129]–151 p. 16 cm. (Part [2] in *his* Systema medicinae Hermeticae generale, Francofurti, 1613) [8330]

—Naturae sanctuarium; quod est, Physica Hermetica . . . ad promovendam rerum naturalium veritatem . . . & admirandorum secretorum in naturae abbysso latentium philosophica explicatione . . . in undecim libris tractata . . . Sub finem duae appendices, quarum I. Pansophiae fundamentum, & II. Philosophiam Hermeticam de lapide philosophorum quatuor tractatibus antehac editis, jam vero recognitis & auctis comprehensam explicat, annexae sunt. Praeterea etiam Remora studii medici . . . adjecta est, & errores medicorum multorum inibi delucide deteguntur. Francofurti, Typis Nicolai Hoffmanni, sumptibus Jonae Rosae, 1619.

838, [12] p. 18 cm. [8331]

—Systema medicinae Hermeticae generale, in quo I. Medicinae verae fundamentum, II. Sanitis conservatio, III. Morborum cognitio, & curatio . . . explicantur . . . Francofurti, Prostat in Francoforti Paltheniana, 1613.

151 p. 16 cm. [8332]

—Theoria philosophiae Hermeticae, septem tractatibus, quorum primus est; I. Verus Hermes. II. Porta Hermeticae sapientiae. III. Silentium Hermeticum. IV. Axiomata Hermetica. V. De generatione rerum naturalium. VI. De regeneratione rerum naturalium & VII. De renovatione . . . Hanoviae, Apud Petrum Antonium, 1617.

[4], 119 p. 16 cm. [8333]

Two dedicatory leaves inserted at front.
Imperfect: margins of [4] p. trimmed.

—Verae physices compendium novum, in sincerioris philosophiae studiosorum gratiam conscriptum, & in lucem editum ... Steinfurti, Excudit Theoph. Caesar, prostat apud Joan Carolum Unckel, 1616.

[16], 112 p.   16 cm.   [8334]

NOLLENS, CASPAR [*fl.* 1630] *tr. See* CABROL, B. Het anatomiicke A. B. C. 1630; FABRICIUS, H., ab Aquapendente. De chirurgicale operatien. 1630.

NOLLIUS, HENRICUS. *See* NOLLE, Heinrich [*fl.* 1612-1619]

NONIUS PINCIANUS, FERDINANDUS. *See* NÚÑEZ DE GUZMÁN, Fernando [16th cent.]

NONNIUS, ALVARUS. *See* NUÑEZ, Alvaro [16th cent.]

NONNIUS, LUDOVICUS [*ca.* 1555-1645?] Diaeteticon; sive, De re cibaria libri IV. Antverpiae, Apud Petrum & Joannem Belleros, 1627.

[32], 638, [1] p.   16 cm.   [8335]
Errata: p. [639]

—[The same.] ... 2. ed. et auctior. Antverpiae Ex officina Petri Belleri, 1645.

[24], 526, [1] p.   20 cm.   [8336]
Engraved title page.

—[The same.] ... Nunc primum lucem vidit. Antverpiae, Ex officina Petri Belleri, 1646.

[24], 526, [1] p.   19 cm.   [8337]
Engraved title page.
A reissue of the 1645 edition, with an altered title page, and a royal privilege dated 1644 added on p. [8]

—Ichtyophagia; sive, De piscium esu commentarius. Antverpiae, Apud Petrum & Joannem Belleros [1616]

[16], 176, [16] p.   17 cm.   [8338]
Imperfect: title page mutilated including date of imprint.

NONNUS, LUDOVICUS. *See* NONNIUS, Ludovicus [*ca.* 1555-1645?]

NOODIGHE op-rechtinghe van't Collegie der Medecyne. 1660. *See* COLLEGIE DER MEDECYNE, Brussels.

NORCOPENSIS, ANDREAS [*fl.* 1673-*ca.* 1693] *praeses.* Disputatio philosophica de somniis ... Holmiae, Typis Nicolai Wankivii, 1675.

[64] p.   15 cm.   [8339]
Diss.—Uppsala (J. Mürick, *respondent*)

NORR, ERHARDT [*fl.* 1676] Chirurgischer Wegweiser: allen Angehenden, so zur Wund-Artzney-Kunst zu gelangen Begierde haben, in neun Haupt-Theilen, gesprächsweis: sampt einem Vocabulario aller Namen ... vorgezeiget ... Nürnberg, In Verlegung Johann Hoffmann, gedruckt bey Johann-Philipp Miltenberger, 1677.

846, [40] p.   14 cm.   [8340]
Title on p. 9. Half title on p. 1 reads: Erhard Norren Chirurgisches Hand-Büchlein.

—[The same.] ... Nürnberg, In Verlegung Johann Hoffmanns, gedruckt bey Joh. Christoff Frisch, 1697.

[47], 660 p.   14 cm.   [8341]

NORTHUSANUS, JOHANNES FRIDERICUS. *See* FRIDERICI, Johannes [*fl.* 1656]

NORTON, SAMUEL [1548-1604?] Mercurius redivivus; seu, Modus conficiendi lapidem philosophicum tam album, quam rubeum e mercurio ... Nunc vero editus opera & studio Edmundi Deani ... Cui accessit modus faciendi utrumque fermentum tam album e luna, sive argento, quam rubeum e sole, sive auro ... Francofurti, Typis Caspari Rötelii, impensis Guilielmi Fitzeri, 1630.

20 p.   illus.   23 cm.   [8342]

—Metamorphosis lapidum ignobilium in gemmas quasdam pretiosas; seu, Modus transformandi perlas parvas, et minutulas, in magnas & nobiles; ac etiam construendi carbunculos artificiales, aliosque lapides pretiosos, naturalibus praestantiores ... nunc vero editus diligentia Edmundi Deani ... Cui accessit modus componendi electrum artificiale ... cum indicatione electri naturalis & metallici, veteribus prorsus incogniti ... Francofurti, Typis Caspari Rötelii, impensis Guilielmi Fitzeri, 1630.

12 p.   illus.   23 cm.   [8343]

—Saturnus saturatus dissolutus, et coelo restitutus; seu, Modus componendi lapidem philosophicum tam album, quam rubeum e plumbo; ac etiam eadem methodo e Jove, sive stanno ... Nunc vero edente Edmundo Deano ... Cui accessit accurtatio operis Saturni, una cum modo extrahendi Arg. vivum e plumbo. Accessit praeterea tractatus parvus de metho [sic] philosophorum in opere Saturni secundum Georgium Riplaeum auctus, & emendatus; una cum accuratione Riplaeana mercurii sublimati emendata etiam, & auctiore reddita ... Francofurti, Typis

Joan-Nicolai Stoltzenbergeri, impensis Guilielmi Fitzeri, 1630.

24 p. illus. 23 cm. [8344]

—Venus vitriolata, in elixer conversa; nec non Mars victoriosus, seu elixerizatus; sive, Modus conficiendi lapidem philosophicum tam e venere, sive cupro, quam a marte, sive chalybe . . . nunc vero editus studiis, & diligentia Edmundi Deani . . . Francofurti, Typis Caspari Rötelii, impensis Guilielmi Fitzeri, 1630.

16 p. illus. 23 cm. [8345]

—See VIGILANTIUS DE MONTE CUBITI, ed. and tr. Dreyfaches hermetisches Kleeblat. 1667.

NORTON, THOMAS [fl. 1477] Ordinall of alchemie. In Ashmole, E. Theatrum chemicum Britannicum. 1652.

—Tractatus chymicus. In Maier, M. Tripus aureus. 1618, 1677.

NOTABEL arrest van't Parlement 's Hoffs van Grenoble, gegeven tot profijt van eene joffrou, over de gheboorte van eene van hare soonen, geschiet vier jaren naer d'absentie van haren man, sonder eenighen man bekent te hebben. Achtervolghende het rapport in't voorsz Hoff ghedaen by verscheyden doctoren inde medicijnen tot Montpelier, mitsgaders vroe-vrouwen, matronen ende andere persoonen van qualiteyt. 's Graven-Hage, Ludolph Breeckevelt, 1637.

[8] p. 20 cm. [8346]

NOTHWENDIG- und nützlicher Unterricht. 1682. See SAXONY. Laws, statutes, etc.

NOTHWENDIG- und nützlicher Unterricht . . . vor die bestellten Wehemütter . . . im Fürstenthumb Gotha. See GOTHA (Fürstentum)

NOTHWENDIGER Bericht. 1632? See EISENMENGER, J. C.

NOTOMIE di Titiano. 1670. See [VESALIUS, A.]

NOTTNAGEL, CHRISTOPH [1607–1666] praeses. Disputatio physico-mathematica de ventis insolentibus & inprimis eo, qui circa proxime praeteritum IX Decemb. totam ferme Europam perflasse creditur. Cum appendice de recenti cometa . . . Wittebergae, Ex Ergasterio Henckeliano, 1661.

[48] p. 19 cm. [8347]

Diss.—Wittenberg (B. Mittendorff, respondent)

NOTTNAGEL, CHRISTOPH [fl. 1669] respondent. See KIRCHMAJER, T., praeses. Elegantissimum ex phisicis thema de hominibus apparenter mortuis . . . sistent . . . T. K. . . . et C. N. 1669, 1700.

NOTWENDIGER Unterricht. 1680. See BRUNSWICK (Duchy)

NOUVEAU cours de medecine, ou selon les principes de la nature & des mécaniques, expliqués par Messieurs Descartes, Hogelande, Regius, Arberius, Villis . . . & par d'autres: on aprend le cors de l'homme, avec les moiens de conserver la santé, & de chasser les maladies. Paris, François Clousier & Pierre Aubouyn, 1669.

[6], 728, [8] p. 16 cm. [8348]

Includes "La physique d'uzage" published in Paris in 1664. Translated by D. R.

Attributed to Louis Henry Rouvière by BNC based on Barbier, p. 883, vol. 3, but M. Bouvet denies this attribution. Cf. his Les Rouvière. Paris. Société d'Histoire de la Pharmacie, 1959, p. 5.

—[The same.] . . . Paris, La veuve Jean d'Houry & Laurent d'Houry, 1683.

[6], 728, [8] p. 16 cm. [8349]

A reissue of the 1669 edition with new title page.

NOUVEAU traitté du pourpre, de la rougeole et petite verole. 1688. See PORCHON, A.

NOUVEAUX secrets rares et curieux. 1660. See ERRESALDE, P.

NOUVEL avis utile. Dans la boutique du libraire, au Bon Pasteur . . . à Paris . . . on y donne à lire gratuitement . . . Paris [16--]

1 p. 24 cm. [8350]

Caption title.

NOUVELLE osteologie. 1689. See [VERDUC, J. B.]

NOUVELLES conjectures sur les organes des sens où l'on propose un nouveau sistéme d'optique. 1687. See BRUNET, C.

NOUVELLES observations de chirurgie, suivant l'opinion des modernes. Par Monsieur M***. Trevoux, Par les soins du Sieur Ganeau, et se vendent a Lyon, chez Hilaire Baritel, 1700.

[8], 566, [60] p. illus. 16 cm. [8351]

Running title: Observations de chirurgie.

NOVA praxis medica de morbis mulierum. 1698. See PICCOFONCCI, G.

NOVAE hypotheseos de pulmonum motu, et respirationis usu specimen. Lugduni Batavorum, Ex officina Felicis Lopez, 1671.

20 p. 16 cm. [8352]

NOVAE regulae sanitatis medico-physicae; sive, Disputationes inaugurales de esculentis et poculentis. 1657. *See* Weis- et Rothwein de Rebensafft, J.

NOVARINUS, ANTONIUS. Anatomia curiosa; das ist ... Wahrhafftige Beschreibung, und vortreffliche Vorstellung ... von dess Menschen ... Ursprung ... Ferner von allen eüserlich- und innern Glidern ... discurriret würd ... Franckfurt, Frantz Mayer, 1681.

[1], 103 p. 30 numbered tables. 33 cm. [8353]

Running title reads: Wahrhafftige Beschreibung und Anatomi aller Glieder menschlichen Cörpers.

—[The same.] ... Erster Theil [Anderer Theil] Rotenburg, Noah von Millenau, 1682.

[1], 109, [2] p.; [1], 103 p. illus., plates, tables. 31 cm. [8354]

The Erster Theil is a reissue of the 1681 Rothenburg edition.
Anderer Theil has special title page: Chirurgia curiosa; oder, Neues Feld- und Stadt Buch bewehrter Wundt-Artzney.
Text of Anatomia curiosa has running title: Wahrhafftige Beschreibung und Anatomi aller Glieder menschlichen Cörpers. The text of Chirurgia curiosa has running title: Feldt und Stadtbuch, Bewerter Wundartznei.
Imperfect: a number of plates and "Tables" wanting. The chirurgical and anatomical plates and "Tables" are in most cases misbound without regard to which part they belong. The title page of Erster Theil (Anatomia curiosa) is followed by the text of Anderer Theil (Chirurgia curiosa). After the title page of Anderer Theil is the text of Erster Theil.

NOVI tractatus de potu caphe; de Chinensium the; et de chocolata. 1699. *See* [DUFOUR, P. S.]

NOVUM laboratorium medico-chymicum. 1677. *See* GLASER, C.

NOVUM lumen chemicum. 1678. *See* [SENDIVOGIUS, M.]

NOVUM lumen chirurgicum extinctum; or, Med. Colbatch's New light of chirurgery put out. Wherein the dangerous and uncertain woundcuring of the pretending med. and the base imposture of his quack medicines, are impartially examin'd ... By W. W. surgeon, London, Andrew Bell, 1695.

[4], 64 p. 15 cm. [8355]

NOZET, JOANNES JACOBUS [*fl.* 1688] *See* PIENS, F. H. Tractatus de febribus in genere. 1689.

NUCIUS, LAURENS. Een schoon tractaet, van alderhande paerden, om te leeren kennen de natuere ende eijghenschap derselver: ende welcke de schoonste, beste, sterckste ende cloeckste zijn ... Uijt het Italiaensch verduijtscht. Noch Een cleijn tractaetjen van veelderleij dieren ... Dordrecht, Peeter Verhaghen, 1622.

[5], 87 (i.e. 88), [2] p. 21 cm. [8356]

"Een cleijn tractaetjen" has special title page.

NUCK, ANTON [1650–1692] Adenographia curiosa et uteri foeminei anatome nova. Cum epistola ad amicum, De inventis novis ... Lugduni Batavorum, Apud Jordanum Luchtmans, 1691.

[16], 152, [27] p. plates. 17 cm. [8357]

Added engraved title page.

—[The same.] ... Accedit in hac nova editione Dissertatio anatomico-medica inauguralis, de motu bilis circulari ejusque morbis, olim publice proposita a ... Mauritio van Reverhorst ... Lugduni Batavorum, Apud Jord. Luchtmans, 1696.

[16], 152, [27] p.; 64 p. plates. 17 cm. [8358]

Added engraved title page dated 1697.

—De ductu salivali novo, saliva, ductibus oculorum aquosis, et humore oculi aqueo. Lugduni Batavorum, Apud Petrum vander Aa, 1685.

[12], 175, [17] p. plates. 14 cm. [8359]

Added engraved title page dated 1686.

—[The same.] Sialographia et ductuum aquosorum anatome nova, priori auctior & emendatior. Accedit Defensio ductuum aquosorum, nec non Fons salivalis novus, hactenus non descriptus ... Lugduni Batavorum, Apud Petrum vander Aa, 1690.

[16], 158, [16] p. plates. 16 cm. [8360]

Added engraved title page.
Errata on p. [16] at end.

—[The same.] ... Lugduni Batavorum, Apud Jordanum Luchtmans, 1695.

[16], 158, [16] p. illus. 17 cm. [8361]

Added engraved title page dated 1696.
A reprint of the 1690 edition without the Errata.

—Defensio ductuum aquosorum, cui accedunt, Solutionum apologeticarum eversiones, editae per

Mauritium van Reverhorst ... Lugd. Bat., Apud
Jordanum Luchtmans, 1691.

    32 p. 16 cm.   **[8362]**

  A reply to Chrouet's criticism of Nuck's De ductu salivali novo,
saliva, ductibus oculorum aquosis, et humore oculi aqueo.

  Bound with Goodschalk, D. Prodromus de ossium tum generatione, tum corruptione interna. 1691.

— Operationes & experimenta chirurgica, edita per
J[ohann] T[iling] ... Lugduni Batavorum, Apud
Cornelium Boutesteyn, 1692.

    [8], 170, [6] p. plates. 16 cm.   **[8363]**

  Added engraved title page.
  Imperfect: plates wanting.

— [The same.] ... Edita per Johannis Tilingii ...
Lugduni Batavorum, Apud Cornelium Boutesteyn,
1696.

    [8], 170, [6] p. plates. 17 cm.   **[8364]**

  Added engraved title page.
  Different setting of type.

— [The same.] ... Juxta exemplar Lugdun.
Batav. Jenae, Apud Henric. Christoph. Cröckerum,
1698.

    [8], 129, [7] p. illus. 16 cm.   **[8365]**

— *respondent.* See SCHACHT, L., *praeses.* Disputatio
medica de rabie hydrophobica. 1676.

— See CAMERARIUS, E. Dissertationes tres. 1694;
CHROUET, W. Dissertatio medico-physica. 1688, 1691.

NÜSCHELER, HANS JAKOB [1551–1620] *tr. See*
GESNER, K. Köstlicher Artzneyschatz. 1608.

NUESCHLER, JOHANN JACOB. *See* NÜSCHELER,
Hans Jakob [1551–1620]

NÜSSLER, JOHANN GOTTLOB [1664–1711] *respondent.*
Disputatio medica inauguralis, de dolore colico ...
Trajecti ad Rhenum, Ex officina Francisci Halma,
1688.

    24 p. 22 cm.   **[8366]**
  Diss. — Utrecht.

NÜSSLER, WILHELM [*fl.* 1680] *praeses.* Dissertatio
physica de anima brutorum ... Wittebergae, Imprimebat Matthaeus Henckelius [1680]

    [14] p. 20 cm.   **[8367]**
  Diss. — Wittenberg (S. Gross, *respondent*)

NÜTZLER, GUILIELMUS. *See* NÜSSLER, Wilhelm
[*fl.* 1680]

NUGAE venales; sive, Thesaurus ridendi & jo-
candi. Ad gravissimos severissimosque viros, patres
melancholicorum conscriptos. Ed. ult. auct. & corr.
[n. p.] Prostant apud Neminem; sed tamen Ubique,
1689.

    [4], 323 (i.e. 325) p. front., plate. 14 cm.
                                 [8368]

  "Pugna porcorum per P. Porcium [pseud., i.e. Johannes Placen-
tius] ... Niverstadii, Apud Casparum Myrrheum Melchiorem
Thureum, & Balthasarum Aureum, 1689" (p. [237]–252) has special
title page.

NUISEMENT, CLOVIS HESTEAU, *baron. See*
HESTEAU, Clovis, *sieur de Nuisement* [*fl.* 1578–1594]

NUISEMENT, JACQUES DE. *See* HESTEAU, Clovis,
sieur de Nuisement [*fl.* 1578–1594]

NUNES, AMBRÓSIO [1529 *or* 30–1611] Tractado
repartido en cinco partes principales, que declaran
el mal que significa este nombre peste con todas sus
causas, y señales prognosticas, y indicativas del mal,
con la preservacion, y cura ... Coimbra, Diogo
Gomez Loureyro [Manoel D'Araujo] 1601.

    [12], 123, 60, [4] ll. 21 cm.   **[8369]**

NÚÑEZ, ALFONSO [*b.* 1559] Assertio judicii
Ludovici Septalii ... De margaritis nuper ex India
allatis ... Mediolani, Apud Jo. Baptistae Bidellium,
1620]

    30 p. 22 cm.   **[8370]**

— See CHIFFLET, J. J. Acia Cornelii Celsi propriae
significationi restituta. 1633.

NUÑEZ, ALVARO [16th cent.] *See* ARCEO, F. De
recta curandorum vulnerum ratione. 1658 [and] Kort-
bondige, ende rechte middel, en kunst. 1667.

NÚÑEZ, AMBROSIO. *See* NUNES, Ambrósio [1529
or 30–1611]

NÚÑEZ, FRANCISCO [16th cent.] Libro del parto
humano, en el qual se contienen remedios muy utiles
y usuales para el parto dificultoso de las mugeres,
con otros muchos secretos a ello pertenecientes, y a
las enfermedades de los niños ... Madrid, Por
Tomas Junti, a costa de Juan Antonio Tauàno, 1621.

    [4], 93, [3] ll. illus. 16 cm.   **[8371]**

— [The same.] *In* Ayala, G. de. Principios de
cirugia. 1693.

NUÑEZ, Luis. *See* Nonnius, Ludovicus [*ca.* 1555–1645?]

NÚÑEZ DE ACOSTA, Duarte [*fl.* 1653–1681] Clava de Alcides, con que se desbaratan propugnaculos tan ruidosos en la apariencia, como vanos en la contextura. Muestrase quan en vano se ha pretendido la concordia en las dos opiniones del sitio de las sangrias … [Xerez? Diego Perez de Estupiñan? not before 1655]

[4], 67 (i.e. 70) ll.   20 cm.   [8372]
Palau 196936.1.

—Tratado practico del uso de las sangrias assi en las enfermedades particulares, como en las calenturas. Explicase el artificio methodico de la via racional, con que Galeno procede, y los demas authores assi antiguos, como modernos en la determinacion de las sangrias, y contra la nueva opinion … Xerez, Diego Perez de Estupiñan, 1653.

[4], 73 ll.   20 cm.   [8373]
Imperfect: ll. 73 wanting.

NUÑEZ DE CORIA, Francisco [16th cent.] *See* Nuñez, Francisco [16th cent.]

NÚÑEZ DE GUZMÁN, Fernando [16th cent.] *See* Plinius Secundus, C. Naturalis historiae, tomus primus [-tertius] 1668–1669.

NUNNEZ, Louis. *See* Nonnius, Ludovicus [*ca.* 1555–1645?]

NUOVA, et vera relatione del morbo contagioso successo in Vienna, & in altre parti l'anno 1679. Milano, Piacenza, Parma, & Modona, Per gli heredi Soliani [1680?]

4 p.   20 cm.   [8374]

NUREMBERG. Collegium der Aerzte. *See* Kollegium der Aerzte, Nuremberg.

NUREMBERG. Collegium Medicum. *See* Kollegium der Aerzte, Nuremberg.

NUREMBERG. Hospital zum Heiligen Geist. *See* Hospital zum Heiligen Geist, Nuremberg.

NUREMBERG. Ordinances, local laws, etc. Eines wol edlen, bestrengen, fürsichtig, und hochweisen Rahts, der Stadt Nürnberg, Ordnung, wie es bey denen anderwärts leider! sehr einreissenden ansteckenden Kranckheiten zu halten, damit bey hiesiger Stadt und Landschafft … noch

ferners reiner, und gesunder Lufft erhalten, und solches Ubel abgewendet werden möge. [Nuremberg] Michael Endter, 1679.

[11] p.   19 cm.   [8375]
"Decretum in Senatu, den 6. Octob. A. 1679."

—Verneuerte Gesetz, Ordnung und Tax eines edlen, ehrnuesten fürsichtigern und weissen Raths, dess Heÿ. Reichs Statt Nürmberg, dem Collegio Medico: den Apoteckern und andern angehörigen daselbsten gegeben. Anno M.DC.XXIV. [Nürmberg, Bey Simon Halbmayern zu finden, 1624]

[63] p.   20 cm.   [8376]
Engraved title page.
"Decretum in Senatu 7 April. 1624."
"Valor sive taxatio medicamentorum tam simplicium quam compositorum, quae in officinis pharmaceuticis, inclytae Reipubl. Noribergensis prostant, alphabetico ordine conscripta, &c.": p. [30–63]
With this is bound the 1700 Nuremberg edition.

—[The same.] Verneuerte Gesetz und Ordnung eines hoch edlen und hochweisen Raths, des Heiligen Reichs Stadt Nürnberg, dem Collegio Medico, den Apotheckern, und andern angehörigen daselbst gegeben. [Nürnberg] Balthasar Joachim Endter, 1700.

[24] p.   20 cm.   [8377]
"Decretum in Senatu, 22. Junii, 1700."
This edition lacks the "Valor sive taxatio medicamentorum".
Bound with the 1624 Nuremberg edition.

—Verneuerte Leich Ordnung der Statt Nürmberg. Nürnberg, Gedruckt bey Balthasar Scherffen, 1625.

[10] p.   22 cm.   [8378]

—Verneuerte Leich-Ordnung, wie es mit denenselben, allhie in der Stadt Nürnberg … und auf dem Land dess gantzen nürnbergischen Gebiets, gehalten werden solle. [Nürnberg] Michael Endter, 1662.

[16] p.   19 cm.   [8379]

NUREMBERG. Stadtmagistrat. *See* Hoffmann, M. Kurtzer … Bericht. 1680.

NUSSER, Franz [*fl.* 1628] *respondent.* *See* Wangnereck H., *praeses.* Conclusiones philosophicae ex libris De generatione [Aristotelis] 1628.

NUSSLER, Johann Gottlob. *See* Nüssler, Johann Gottlob [1664–1711]

NUTZLICHE, bewehrte und an vilen öffters probierte Hauss-Mittel. 1665. *See* [BREM, W. S.]

NUTZLICHER unnd kurtzer Bericht, Regiment und Ordnung, in pestilentzischen Zeiten zu gebrauchen, auss Befelch der ... Herrn Schultheissen und Rachts der catholischen Statt Lucern ... nach eines jeden Person, Vermögen, Stand und Gelegenheit, gericht, und auff das einfältigest und deutlichest gestellt und beschrieben ... Widerumb ernewert ... München, Getruckt bey Anna Bergin Wittib, 1611.

    [1], 40, [1] p.   21 cm.   **[8380]**

   A word for word reprint of the 1594 edition.

   Attributed to Renward Cysat and Lorenz Hager. Cf. B. Brunner-Wildisen. Medizinisches aus den Schrifften des R. Cysat. Zürich, Juris Druck und Verlag, 1980, p. 14, 73.

Ein NUTZLICHES HAND-BÜCHLEIN, darinnen allerhand Artzneyen für den gemeinen Mann, der in der Eyl die Apotheck (oder im Gut nicht vermag) und hiemit ihme selbsten mit geringem Kosten zu Hulff kommen kan. Fleissig corrigiert, und mit viel Stücken gebessert. Colmar, Johann-Jacob Decker, 1684.

    240, [5] p.   illus.   16 cm.   **[8381]**

   Imperfect: title page mutilated.

   Running title: Von gemeiner Hauss-Artzney.

   Also published in Colmar in 1684 under title: Hauss Apoteck; oder, Ein gemein nützliches Haussartzney Büchlein.

NUYSEMENT, JACQUES. *See* HESTEAU, Clovis, *sieur de Nuisement* [*fl.* 1578-1594]

NYLAND, PETER. *See* NYLANDT, Petrus.

NYLANDT, PETRUS. De Nederlandtse herbarius of kruydt-boeck, beschryvende de geslachten, gedaente, plaetse, tijt ... en medicinael gebruyck van alderhande boomen, heesteren ... kruyden en planten, die in de Nederlanden ... gevonden ... Als mede de uytlandtsen of vreemde droogens ... in de apothekers winckels gebruyckt worden. Uyt verscheyde druydt-beschrijvers, tot nut van alle natuur-kunders ... apothekers, chirurgijns ... beschreven ... Amsterdam, Door Marcus Doornick [Gedruckt by Daniel Bakkamude] 1670.

    [8], 342, [24] p.   illus.   20 cm.   **[8382]**

   —[The same.] ... Amsterdam, Michiel de Groot, 1682.

    [8], 342, [24] p.   illus.   21 cm.   **[8383]**

A reissue of the 1670 edition with new imprint and without the colophon.

   Bound with 't Vermakelijck landt-leven. Amsterdam, 1686.

   —De medicyn-winckel. *In* 't Vermakelijck landt-leven. 1686.

   —Den naerstigen byen-houder. *In* 't Vermakelijck landt-leven. 1686.

   —Den verstandigen hovenier. *In* 't Vermakelijck landt-leven. 1686.

NYMANN, GREGOR [1594-1638] De apoplexia tractatus, in quo hujus gravissimi morbi tum curatio, tum ab illo praeservatio perspicue proponitur, clareque demonstratur ... Wittebergae, Typis Jobi Wilhelmi Fincelii, impensis Pauli Helwigii, 1629.

    [32], 369, [15] p.   port.   19 cm.   **[8384]**

   —[The same.] ... Ed. 2. Wittebergae, Typis & sumptibus haeredum Jobi Wilhelmi Fincelii, 1670. [Wittebergae, Typis Jobi Wilhelmi Fincelii, 1629]

    [30], 369, [15] p.   19 cm.   **[8385]**

   Imperfect: wormholes on first 30 leaves.

   A reissue of the 1629 edition with new title page.

   —Dissertatio de vita foetus in utero, qua luculenter demonstratur, infantem in utero non anima matris, sed sua ipsius vita vivere ... Witebergae, Impensis Pauli Helwigi, 1628.

    [8], 70 p.   20 cm.   **[8386]**

   —[The same.] ... Lugduni Batavorum, Ex officina Davidis Lopes de Haro, 1644.

    [7], 87 p.   14 cm.   **[8387]**

   Imperfect: Last leaf (blank?) wanting.

   "Adriani Spigelii ... epistola de incerto tempore partus": p. 63-87.

   —[The same.] De vita foetus in utero. In Plazzoni, F. De partibus generationi inservientibus. 1644, 1664.

   —*praeses.* Disputatio medica de apoplexia ... Wittebergae, Typis Johannis Matthei, 1619.

    [68] p.   19 cm.   **[8388]**

   Diss. — Wittenberg (M. Blum, *respondent*)

   —*See* WINCKLER, D. Animadversiones. 1630.

NYMANN, HIERONYMUS [1554 *or* 5-1594] *See* TANDLER, T. Dissertationes physicae-medicae. 1613.

O

O., A., *ed. See* The experienc'd farrier. 1691/2.

O., W. *See* OUGHTRED, William [1575–1660]

OBEL, MATTHIAS DE L'. *See* L'OBEL, Matthias de [1538–1616]

OBELE, JOHANN GEORG [*fl.* 1618–1620] *respondent. See* HORST, G. [1578–1636] Disputatio de morbis puerorum. 1618; SCHENCK, E., *praeses.* De crisibus. 1620.

OBERMEYER, GERMAN [1588–1655] *respondent. See* FRÖLICH, J. H., *praeses.* Σημειωτιχὴ φοιβεία paradoxis & heterodoxis . . . D. Felicis Plateri . . . adornata. 1612.

OBERNDÖRFER, Johann [*fl.* 1584–1621] The anatomyes of the true physition, and counterfeit mounte-banke: wherein both of them, are graphically described, and set out in their right, and orient colours. Published in Latin by John Oberndorff . . . and translated into English by F[rancis] H[erring], fellow of the Coll. of Physitions in London. Hereunto is annexed: A short discourse, or discovery of certaine stratagems, whereby our London-empericks, have bene observed strongly to opugne, and oft times to expunge their poor patients purses. London, Arthur Johnson, 1602.

     [12], 43 p.   19 cm.   **[8389]**

Imperfect: upper margins trimmed.
STC 18759.
Translation of De veri et falsi medici agnitione.
The translator is also the author of the discourse (p. 23–43) with caption title: A discovery of certaine stratagems.

—[The same.] Beware of pick-purses; or, A caveat for sick folkes to take heede of unlearned phisitions, and unskilfull chyrurgians. By F[rancis] H[erring] doctor in physick. London, 1605.

     [12], 43 p.   19 cm.   **[8390]**

A reissue of the 1602 edition with new title page.
STC 18759.5.

—Descriptio morbi Ungarici; das ist, Warhafftige und eigendliche Erklärung der genanten ungarischen Kranckheit . . . Franckfort am Mayn, In Verlegung Jacob Fischers seeligen Erben, 1620.

     276 p.   20 cm.   **[8391]**

—*See* STROBELBERGER, J. S. Tractatus novus. 1620.

OBERNDORFFER, JOHANN. *See* OBERNDÖRFER, Johann [*fl.* 1584–1621]

OBEZ, SCIPIONE, *pseud. See* BERNARDI, Florio [17th cent.]

OBICIUS, HIPPOLYTUS. *See* OBIZZI, Ippolito [*fl.* 1605–1612]

OBIZZI, IPPOLITO [*fl.* 1605–1612] Apologia, ad serenissimum Venetiarum principem Marcum Antonium Memo. Venetiis, Apud Franciscum Rampazettum, 1612.

     20 ll.   20 cm.   **[8392]**

Includes letters written to Bernardinus Caius.

—De multiplici in medicina abusu. Tractatus ubi difficultates majores ad praxim artis spectantes discussae habentur huic alia ejusdem authoris opuscula medica de recte medicinam faciendam addita sunt . . . Vicentiae, Sumptibus Roberti Meietti, 1618.

     [32], 104, 55, 43, p.   24 cm.   (Part [2] in his Iatrastronomicon. Vicentiae, 1618)   **[8393]**

"... Advesus vesicantia reprobantes decem decisiones ...": 55 p.; "... Consilia medicinalia ...": p. 1–33; "... Commentarius in duos primos Hippocratis Aphorismos": p. 34–43.
Imperfect: Liber de utilitate astrologiae pro medicinae usu, wanting. Cf. BNC.

—De nobilitate medici contra illius obtrectatores, dialogus tripertitus. In quo . . . comprobatur medicum jurisprudente esse nobiliorem; postea de omnibus scientis, artibusque . . . compendiosus habetur tractatus . . . Venetiis, Apud Robertum Meiettum, 1605.

     [32], 237 p.   21 cm.   **[8394]**

Imperfect: last leaf (blank?) wanting.

—[The same.] . . . Moguntiae, Ex officina typographica Joannis Albini, 1619.

     [14], 389, [25] p.   17 cm.   **[8395]**

Imperfect: outer margins trimmed on p. 374 and 386; wormholes on p. 169–176; p. 250 mutilated.

—Iatrastronomicon varios tractatus medicos, & astronomicos ad rectum medendi usum pernecessarios complectens. Quibus additus est De multiplici abusu in medicina utilis tractatus, aliaque medica opuscula quorum omnium elenchum sequens pagina dabit ... Vicentiae, Apud Jacobum Violatum, 1618.

[38], 93, 95, 30 p.; [32], 104, 55, 43 p. illus. 24 cm. [8396]

Contents of part [1] — Tractatus apologeticus adversus astrologiam pro medicinae usu rejicientes. — Commentarius in Galeni librum tertium De diebus decretoriis. — Appendix, quae a Julio Cesare Claudino contra astrologos scripta sunt. — Astronomicarum praedictionum ... liber. — Brevis cosmologia ad mundi cognitionem. — De mutationis temporum ratione tractatulus.

— Staticomasti. *See* SANTORIO, S. Ars Sanctorii Sanctorii ... de statica medicina. 1624, 1634, 1642, 1657, 1664, 1670, 1690 [and] Medicina statica; or, Rules of health. 1676 [and] Opera omnia. 1660 [and] Science de la transpiration; ou, Medecine statique. 1694.

OBREGÓN, BERNARDINO DE [1540-1599] Instruccion de enfermeros para aplicar los remedios a todo genero de enfermedades, y acudir à muchos accidentes, que sobrevienen en ausencia de los medicos. Compuesto por los hermandos de la Congregacion del hermano Bernardino de Obregon, en el Hospital General de Madrid, y agora nuevamente por el hermano Andres Fernandez ... corregido, y emendado ... Zaragoça, 1664.

[8], 220, [8] p.; [4], 92, [3] p. 15 cm. [8397]

Part [2] has a special title page: Tratado de lo que se ha de hazer con los que están en el articulo de la muerte, sacado de diversos libros espirituales.

OBSEQUENS, JULIUS. De prodigiis liber; cum annotationibus Joannis Schefferi ... Accedit Conr. Lycosthenis supplementum obsequentis. Amstelaedami, Apud Henricum & Theodorum Boom, 1679.

[16], 156, [32] p. [8398]

Added engraved title page.
Imperfect: Conrad Lycosthenes' Supplementum wanting.

OBSERVATIONES anatomicae. 1673. *See* COLLEGIUM PRIVATUM AMSTELODAMENSE.

OBSERVATIONS both historical and moral upon the burning of London. 1667. *See* Rege Sincera.

OBSERVATIONS de chirurgie. *See* Nouvelles observations de chirurgie. 1700.

OBSERVATIONS de medecine. 1689. *See* BETBEDER, P.

OBSERVATIONS et histoires chirurgiques tirées des oeuvres de quatre excellens medecins. *See* BONET, T., *ed.* Corps de medecine et de chirurgie. 1679.

OBSERVATIONS et histories chirurgiques tirées des oeuvres latines. *See* BONET, T., *ed.* Corps de medecine et de chirurgie. 1679.

OBSERVATIONS sur les fievres et les febrifuges. 1681. *See* SPON, J.

OBSERVATIONUM chymico-physico-medicarum curiosarum. *See* STAHL, G. E. Georgii Ernesti Stahl ... Observationum chymico-physico-medicarum curiosarum. 1698.

OBSERVATIONUM selectarum ad rem litterariam spectantium tomus I [-X] Halae Magdeburgicae, Prostat in Officina Libraria Rengeriana, 1700-1705.

II v. 18 cm. [8399]

Vols. 1-2, 6-8 and II (Additamentum) only.

OBSOPAEUS, JOHANNES. *See* OPSOPÄUS, Johannes [1556-1596]

OCCHI RIZETTI, GIROLAMO [*d.* 1659] De pestilentibus, ac venenosis morbis. Libri quator ... His accessit De febribus malignis vulgaribus, tractatio ... Brixiae, Apud Jo. Baptistam Gromii, 1650.

[20], 284 p. 26 cm. [8400]

OCCLERIO, PIETRO FRANCESCO [*fl.* 1592-1613] *ed.* *See* HIPPOCRATES. [Aphorismi. Latin.] 1610 [i.e. 1611], 1622, 1649, 1663, 1674, 1684.

OCCO, ADOLF [1524-1606] *See* SCHOLTZ, L. Epistolarum philosophicarum: medicinalium, ac chymicarum ... volumen. 1610.

OCHLITIUS, SAMUEL. *See* OCHLIZ, Samuel [*fl.* 1665-1666]

OCHLIZ, SAMUEL [*fl.* 1665-1666] *respondent. See* ROLFINCK, W., *praes.* Ordo et methodus medicinae specialis commentatoriae ... dissertatio quinta. 1665; SCHENCK, J. T., *praes.* Dissertationem inauguralem de passione hypochondriaca ... submittit ... S. O. 1666.

OCHO, GIROLAMO. *See* OCCHI RIZETTI, Girolamo [*d.* 1659]

OCHUS, HIERONYMUS. *See* OCCHI RIZETTI, Girolamo [*d.* 1659]

OCIORUS, TARQUINIUS. *See* SCHNELLENBERG, Tarquinius [*fl.* 1546]

OCKEL, Christian [1671-1706] *respondent. See* Hoffmann, F. [1660-1742] *praeses.* Dissertatio inauguralis physico-medica de potentia ventorum in corpus humanum. 1700.

OCKERS, Gysbert [*fl.* 1664] *respondent.* Disputatio medica inauguralis de quartana intermittente ... Lugduni Batavorum, Ex officina Jacobi Voorn, 1664.

     [II] p.   23 cm.   **[8401]**
    Diss.—Leyden.

OCLERIUS, Petrus Franciscus. *See* Occlerio, Pietro Francesco [*fl.* 1592-1613]

O'CONNOR, Bernard. *See* Connor, Bernard [1666?-1698]

OCYORUS, Tarquinius. *See* Schnellenberg, Tarquinius [*fl.* 1546]

ODDI, Marco degli [1526-1591] *ed. See* Oddi, O. degli. Expositio. 1607.

ODDI, Oddo degli [1478-1558] Expositio, in librum Artis medicinalis Galeni. Nunc primum in lucem edita, et castigata laboribus ... Marci Oddi ... Brixiae, Ex typographia Comini Praesenii, ad instantiam Francisci Lennii, 1607.

     [35], 501 p.   tables.   22 cm.   **[8402]**
    Bound with Casserio, G. Tabulae anatomicae LXXIIX. 1632.

ODDONE, Cesare [*d.* 1571] De urinis libellus. *In* Martini, H. Anatomia urinae Galeno-spagyrica. 1658.

ODERUS, Wilhelmus [*fl.* 1657] *respondent. See* Bartholin, T., *praeses.* De usu thoracis partiumque ineo contentarum dissertatio anatomica. 1657.

ODHELIUS, Ericus E. [1661-1704] *respondent. See* Bilberg, J., *praeses.* Specimen cogitationum de magnetismis rerum. 1683; Bohn, J., *praeses.* Dissertationes chymico-physicae. 1685.

ODOMARUS. Practica magistri Odomari ad discipulum. [&] Historia antiqua de antiqua de argento in aurum verso.

     166-172 p.   vol. 3.   20 cm. (*In* Zetzner, Lazarus, *ed.* Theatrum chemicum. Argentorati, 1659-61)
                               [8403]
    Caption titles.

ODONUS, Caesar. *See* Oddone, Cesare [*d.* 1571]

O'DOWDE, Thomas [*fl.* 17th cent.] *See* Trye, Mrs. M. Medicatrix. 1675.

ODRY, Guilielmus, *ed.* and *tr. See* Hippocrates. Aphorismorum Hippocratis textus. 1634.

O'DWYER, Joannes [*b. ca.* 1620] Querela medica; seu, Planctus medicinae modernae status ... Montibus, Ex officina Aegidii V. Havart, 1686.

     [37], 312, [2] p.   15 cm.   **[8404]**
    Errata: [2] p.

OECONOMIA animalis ad circulationem sanguinis breviter delineata. 1685. *See* [Craanen] T.

OEHMB, Karl [1653-1706] *respondent. See* Bohn, J., *praeses.* Dissertatio medica de catarrhis. 1675 [and] Exercitationum physiologicarum prima ... [-decima tertia] 1674?

OEHME, Carl. *See* Oehmb, Karl [1653-1706]

OELER, Johann Ulrich [*fl.* 1662-1681] Vincetoxicum löimicum; das ist, Kurtzer Discurs, wie sich in der allergefährlichsten Seuch der Pestilentz, wol zu praeserviren, und glücklich zu curiren ... Augspurg, In Verlegung Gottlieb Göbels, gedruckt bey Johannes Schönigk, 1671.

     93 p.   14 cm.   **[8405]**

—Vincetoxicum loimicum correctius; das ist, Kurtze Beschreibung, wie man sich in der höchst tödlichen Seuch der Pest ... gewiss zu praeserviren und glücklich zu curiren ... Augspurg, In Verlegung Gottlieb Göbels, gedruckt bey Leonhard Zacharias, 1681.

     [26], 82 p.   14 cm.   **[8406]**
    Between the title page and sig. A2, six leaves are inserted including second title page with imprint: Augspurg, In Verlegung dess Authoris ... 1681.

—Another issue. 13 cm.   **[8407]**
    Sig.) (⁶ not present.

—*respondent.* Disputatio medica inauguralis, exhibens problemata medica miscellanea ... Argentorati, Typis Eberhardi Welperi, 1663.

     [20] p.   19 cm.   **[8408]**
    Diss.—Strasbourg.

—Disputatio solennis de morbis novis ... Argentorati, Typis Eberhardi Welperi, 1662.

     32 p.   19 cm.   **[8409]**
    Diss.—Strasbourg.

OELHAF, Joachim [1570–1630] De usu renum endoxa paradoxa. *In* Meibom, J. H. De usu flagrorum. 1670.

OELHAF, Peter [1599–1654] *praeses.* Dissertatio physico-medica de morbis totius substantiae in genere, & in specie de contagio, singulari eorundem causa ... Regiomonti, Excusa typis Laurentii Segebadii [1625]

[20] p. 19 cm. **[8410]**

Diss.—Königsberg (S. Peltz, *respondent*)

OERTEL, Johann Gottfried [*fl.* 1700–1704] *respondent. See* Brendel, A., *praeses.* De Homero medico. 1700.

ÖSLER, Philipp [*b.* 1654] *respondent. See* Helwig, C. Disputatio inauguralis medica de pleuritide. 1686.

—*See* Helwig, C. Programma, quo decanus Facultatis Medicae Christophorus Helvigius ad inauguralem disputationem, quam de pleuritide ... subjiciet ... Philippus Ösler ... invitat. 1686.

ÖSTREICHER, Sebastian. *See* Austrius, Sebastianus [*d.* 1550]

OF absolute rest in bodies. *See* Boyle, Hon. R. Certain physiological essays and other tracts. [1668]–1669.

OF the usefulnesse of naturall philosophy. *See* Boyle, Hon. R. Some considerations touching the usefulnesse of experimental naturall philosophy. 1663.

OFFENBACH, Peter. *See* Uffenbach, Peter [1566–1635]

OFFENEY, Johann Wilhelm [*fl.* 1697] *respondent. See* Schmid, J. A., *praeses.* Dux foemina facti haereseos vel autor vel fautor. 1697.

OFFICINA chymicha formacium, vasorum, ac instrumentorum. *In* A Puteo, Z. Clavis medica rationalis spagyrica. 1612.

OFFREDI, Paul [1582–1618] In librum Aphorismorum Hippocratis commentaria aphoristica, ad methodum analyticam redacta. Cum Graeco textu, Latinaque ejus interpretatione ... Nunc primum in lucem edita. Aureliae Allobrogum, Petrus de la Roviere, 1606.

[12], 365, [1] p. 14 cm. **[8411]**

O'GLACAN, Nial [*fl.* 1629–1655] Nellani Glacani ... Cursus medicus. Libris XIII. propositus et in

tres tomos divisus. Quorum primus continet physiologiam ... alter pathologiam ... tertius denique semeiotica ... Bononiae, Sumptibus Sebast. Combi, & Joan. Lanou, 1655.

3 v. in 2. 24 cm. **[8412]**

—Tractatus de peste; seu, Brevis, facilis, & experta methodus curandi pestem. Authore ... Nellano Glacan ... Tolosae, Typis Raym. Colomerii, 1629.

[16], 58 (i.e. 258) p. 15 cm. **[8413]**

OGLE, Luke, *Esq. See* Mandeville, Bernard [1670?–1733]

OGLE, Nicholas [*b.* 1670 *or* 71] *respondent.* Disputatio medica inauguralis, de asthmate ... Trajecti ad Rhenum, Ex officina Francisci Halma, 1696.

16 p. 21 cm. **[8414]**

Diss.—Utrecht.

OGLERIUS, Petrus Franciscus. *See* Occlerio, Pietro Francesco [*fl.* 1592–1613]

OHEIM, Benedikt [*fl.* 1617] *respondent. See* Arnisaeus, H., *praeses.* Theses medicas de hydropum essentia. 1617.

OHEIM, Johann Philipp [1631–1697] Theses physicae de qualitatibus occultis in genere ... [Lipsiae] Typis haeredum Timothei Hönii [1651]

[16] p. 19 cm. **[8415]**

Diss.—Leipzig (E. Nathusius, *respondent*)

OHEIMB, Carl. *See* Oehmb, Karl [1653–1706]

OHM, Wilhelm [*fl.* 1681] *respondent. See* Winckler, F. C., *praeses.* Disputatio medica, de ea melancholiae specie. 1681.

OHMB, Carl. *See* Oehmb, Karl [1653–1706]

OLDEKOP, Justus [1597–1667] *See* Schmidts, M. Acten gemässe relatio facti & juris. 1664.

OLDEKOP, Magnus Petrus [*fl.* 1687] *respondent. See* Hoffmann, F. [*fl.* 1687] *praeses.* Disputatio physica, de imaginationis natura ejusque viribus. 1687.

OLDENBORCH, Johann Erik [*fl.* 1672] *respondent. See* Bohn, J., *praeses.* Exercitationum physiologicarum prima ... [-decima tertia] 1674?

OLDENBURG, Henry [1615?–1677] *ed. See* Malpighi, M. Dissertatio epistolica de bombyce.

1669; REDI, F. Opuscoli vari. 1675 [and] Osservazioni intorno alle vipere. 1687.

OLDENBURG, JOHANN [*fl.* 1642] *respondent. See* GARPIUS, P., *praeses.* Disputatio physica de anima. 1642.

OLEARIUS, ADAM [*ca.* 1600–1671] *tr. See* MARTINUS, J. Etliche Gewissens-Fragen von der Pestilentz. 1668.

OLEARIUS, JOHANN [1611–1684] Thaumatologia. Die grossen Wunder der göttlichen Allmacht, welche an dem weitberühmten Carls-Bade . . . täglich zu verspüren . . . Hall in Sachsen, Gedruckt bey Christoff Salfelden, 1668.

    [64] p.   16 cm.   **[8416]**

—*praeses.* De mantice cometica dissertatio theologica . . . Lipsiae, Literis Christiani Michaelis [1681]

    [76] p.   20 cm.   **[8417]**
    Diss.—Leipzig (A. Rancke, *respondent*)

—*See* STOCKMANN, E. Hodegeticum pestilentiale sacrum. 1667, 1681.

OLHAFIUS, PETRUS. *See* OELHAF, Peter [1599–1654]

OLIMART, ANTON HEINRICH [*fl.* 1694] *respondent.* Disputatio medica inauguralis de apoplexia . . . Duisburgi ad Rhenum, Apud Franconem Sas, 1694.

    24 p.   20 cm.   **[8418]**
    Diss.—Duisburg.

OLIPHANT, CHARLES [*d.* 1719] A short discourse, to prove the usefulness of vomiting in fevers, by plain reasoning and the authority of the best physicians, ancient and modern . . . Edinburgh, Thomas Carruthers, 1699.

    [6], 14 p.   16 cm.   **[8419]**
    Imperfect: title page mutilated.

—*See* An answer to the pretended refutation of Dr. Olyphant's defence. 1699; BROWN, A. The epilogue. 1699; A refutation of Dr. Olyphant's Defence of his Short discourse. 1699.

OLITZSCH, THEODOR [*fl.* 1672] *respondent. See* AMMANN, P., *praeses.* Disputatio inauguralis medica. 1672.

OLIVER, JOHN [*fl. ca.* 1663] A present to be given to teeming women, by their husbands or friends; con-

taining scripture-directions for women with-child, how to prepare for the hour of travel . . . London, Printed by A. Maxwell for Tho. Parkhurst, 1669.

    [28], 168 p.   16 cm.   **[8420]**

OLIVER, THOMAS. *See* OLIVIERI, Tommaso [*fl.* 1645]

OLIVERI, TOMMASO. *See* OLIVIERI, Tommaso [*fl.* 1645]

OLIVIERI, ASCANIO [*fl.* 1576] Elettuarii contra la peste preservativi, e curativi . . . Bologna, Herede del Benacci, 1630.

    broadside.   28 x 20 cm.   **[8421]**
    Bound with *his* Secreto preservativo. 1630.

—Secreto preservativo, & curativo dalla peste . . . [Bologna, Herede del Benacci, 1630]

    [4] p.   20 cm.   **[8422]**
    With this is bound *his* Elettuarii contra la peste. 1630.

OLIVIERI, TOMMASO [*fl.* 1645] Nocturna contemplatio supra febrem de marema Liguriae nautarum horridum flagellum . . . Genuae, Ex typographia Petri Joannis Calenzani 1645.

    46, [1] p.   22 cm.   **[8423]**

OLLIVIER, L. [*fl.* 1629] Traicté des maladies des reins, et de la vessie, contenant la cure de la pierre & gravelle . . . De plus quelques histoires remarquables sur ce sujet. Avec un inventaire des plus celebres personnages qui ont illustré la medecine, depuis Apollo jusques à present. Rouen, Pierre Maille, 1631.

    [15], 215, [7] p.   17 cm.   **[8424]**

OLMO, MARC'ANTONIO. Marci Antonii Ulmi Patavini . . . Physiologia barbae humanae, in tres sectiones divisa . . . in quarum prima declarantur nonnulla ad barbae naturam pertinentia. In altera opiniones Chrysippi, Diogenis . . . Galeni, Arabum, & Latinorum, praesertim J. Caesaris Scaligeri . . . considerantur. In tertia proponit autor . . . opinionem suam . . . Bononiae, Apud Joannem Baptistam Bellagambam, 1602.

    [20], 72, 81–317, [1] p.   33 cm.   **[8425]**

—[The same.] . . . Ed. alt. Cui . . . jam primum accessit Appendix historica, & symbolica barbae humanae . . . Bononiae, Apud Joannem Baptistam Bellagambam, impensis Gasparis Bindoni, 1603.

    [20], 317, [1] p.   illus.   29 cm.   **[8426]**
    "Appendix": p. 73–79.
    Mainly a reissue of the 1602 edition.

—Marci Antonii Ulmi Patavini ... Uterus muliebris; hoc est, De indiciis cognoscendi temperamenta uteri, vel partium genitalium ipsius mulieris. Liber unus ... Graecorum, Arabum, & Latinorum testimonia ad hanc doctrinam pertinentia ... Bononiae, Apud Joannem Baptistam Bellagambam, 1601.

[50], 235 p. 20 cm. [8427]

—Copy 2.

Bound with *his* Opinio. Mutinae, 1599.

OLPIUS, JOHANN [*fl.* 1628] *respondent.* Disputatio medica de natura, causis, signis, differentiis & curatione humoris melancholici ... Marpurgi Cattorum, Ex officina typographica Casparis Chemlini, 1628.

[16] p. 18 cm. [8428]

Diss. — Marburg.

OLSCHLEGEL, NICOLAUS [*fl.* 1607] *See* KNOBLOCH, T., *praeses.* Disputationes anatomicae. 1608, 1612.

OLYPHANT, DR. *See* OLIPHANT, Charles [*d.* 1719]

OMATI, STANISLAO [*fl.* 1674-1675] Antilogia apologetica ... contro all'Apologia del. sig. Filippo Trombetti ... Piacenza,Gio. Bazachi, 1677.

[20], 536 p. 21 cm. [8429]

—*See* TROMBETTI, F. Apologia ... contro una lettera del sig. Stanislao Omati 1674 [and] La bilancia nella quale si librano autorità. 1682.

O'MEARA, DERMOD. *See* MEARA, Dermitius de [*fl.* 1610]

O'MEARA, EDMUND. *See* MEARA, Edmundus de [*d.* 1680]

OMEIS, MAGNUS DANIEL [1646-1708] *praeses.* Dissertatio de eruditis Germaniae mulieribus ... [Altdorfii] Literis Henrici Meyeri [1688]

24, [4] p. 19 cm. [8430]

OMICH, FRANZ [*fl.* 1603-1636] *respondent. See* HORST, G. [1578-1636] Σκεψις. 1606, 1608; MÖLLER, S., *praeses.* Themata de dysenteria. 1607; SENNERT, D., *praeses.* De methodo medendi disputatio X, de revulsione et derivatione. 1604.

OMIUS, SIMON. *See* OOMIUS, Simon [1628-1706]

ONEIDES, MARTIN [*fl.* 1680] *respondent.* Disputatio medica chirurgica inauguralis de hernia

uterina ... Lugduni Batavorum, 1680.

[16] p. 21 cm. [8431]

Imperfect: title page and p. [7-8] wanting.
Title from caption title.
Diss. — Leyden.

ONESTI, CRISTOFORO DEGLI. *See* HONESTIS, Christophorus de [*d.* 1392]

ONUPHRIIS, FRANCESCO DE. *See* HONUPHRIIS, Franciscus de [*fl.* 1691]

OOMIUS, SIMON [1628-1706] Des heeren verderflicke pyl; ofte, Twee boeken van de pest, in dewelcke alles, 't geen tot dese stoffe behoort, kortelick en klaerlick, tot noodige onderrichtinge, waerschouwinge, en vertroostinge, is verhandelt ... Achter aen is ... gevoegt een Tractaetken van de goddelicke voorsienigheydt ... Amsterdam, Willem van Beaumont, 1665.

[64], 536, [26] p. 17 cm. [8432]

Added engraved title page.
The second treatise has special title page.

OOSTEE, BALDUIN VAN [*fl.* 1658] *respondent.* Disputatio medica inauguralis, de anasarca ... Ultrajecti, Ex officina Cornelii Noenaert, 1658.

[8 +] p. 20 cm. [8433]

Imperfect: p. [8] mutilated; all after p. [8] wanting.
Diss. — Utrecht.

OOSTEE, JOHANNES VAN [*fl.* 1700] *respondent.* Disputatio medica inauguralis, de paralysi ... Trajecti ad Rhenum, Ex officina Guilielmi vande Water, 1700.

14, [2] p. 23 cm. [8434]

Diss. — Utrecht.

OOSTERDIJK SCHACHT, HERMANNUS [1672-1744] *respondent.* Disputatio medica inauguralis, de melancholia hypochondriaca ... Lugduni Batavorum, Apud Abrahamum Elzevier, 1693.

[23] p. 22 cm. [8435]

Diss. — Leyden.

OOSTWOUDT, JAN [*fl.* 1694] *respondent.* Disputatio medica inauguralis de fame canina ... Lugduni Batavorum, Apud Abrahamum Elzevier, 1694.

[12] p. 22 cm. [8436]

Diss. — Leyden.

OPALA, ADAM [*fl.* 1619-1620] *respondent. See* SEBISCH, M. [1578-1674?] *praeses.* Disputatio de purgatione secunda. 1620 [and] Disputatio de venae sectione vigesima sexta. 1620 [and] Disputationes de recta ratione purgandi. 1621.

OPENEN vande poorten om de vroevrouwen. 1609. *See* LEYDEN. Ordinances, local laws, etc.

Les **OPERATIONS** de chirurgie. 1691, 1693. *See* [VERDUC, J. B.]

OPHOVEN, GEORGE AB [*fl.* 1674] *respondent. See* SENGUERDIUS, W., *praeses.* Disputationum physicarum selectarum decima quae est de rabie canum prior. 1674.

OPMEER, T. PETRI AB [*fl.* 1621] *respondent.* Disputatio medica inauguralis de peripneumonia . . . Lugduni Batavorum, Ex officina Jacobi Marci, 1621.
　　[8] p.　19 cm.　　　　　　**[8437]**
　　Diss. — Leyden.

OPPERDOES, PIETER [*fl.* 1693] *respondent.* Disputatio medica inauguralis de hydrophobia . . . Lugduni Batavorum, Apud Abrahamum Elzevier, 1693.
　　[16] p.　18 cm.　　　　　　**[8438]**
　　Diss. — Leyden.

OPSOPÄUS, JOHANNES [1556–1596] *tr. See* ARTEMIDORUS DALDIANUS. Artemidori Daldiani & Achmetis Sereimi f. Oneirocritica. 1603; HIPPOCRATES. [Selected works. Greek and Latin] 1607, 1627.

OPSOPÄUS, SIMON [1576–1619] *praeses.* Medicam de phrenitide συϛησιν . . . proponit M. Philippus Werner . . . Heidelbergae, Typis Johannis Lancelloti, 1614.
　　20 p.　18 cm.　　　　　　**[8439]**
　　Diss. — Heidelberg (P. Werner, *respondent.*)

OPSOPOEUS. *See* OPSOPÄUS.

OPUSCULA mythologica physica et ethica. 1688. *See* GALE, T., ed.

OPUSCULA nova anatomica. 1680. *See* CELLIER, A., *ed.*

ORATIO in laudem medicinae. 1662. *See* VERMEIREN, N.

ORCHAMUS, JANUS, *pseud. See* VORST, Johannes [1623–1676]

The **ORDER** of the hospitalls of K. Henry the

viijth. Not before 1690. *See* LONDON. Corporation. Court of Common Council.

ORDERS conceived and published by the Lord Mayor and Aldermen of the City of London. 1665? *See* LONDON. Ordinances, local laws, etc.

ORDERS thought meet by His Maiestie, and his Privie Councell. 1625, 1629. *See* GT. BRIT. Privy Council.

ORDINI appartenenti al governo dell'Hospitale grande di Milano. 1642. *See* OSPEDALE MAGGIORE DI MILANO.

ORDINI per la quarantena. 1630. *See* FLORENCE (City) Ordinances, local laws, etc.

ORDNUNG eines erbarn hochweisen Raths der Stadt Leipzig. 1607. *See* LEIPZIG. Ordinances, local laws, etc.

ORDONNANCES de la police generalle tenue en Parlement en la Chambre Sainct Louys. 1623. *See* FRANCE. Parlement (Paris)

ORDONNANCES sur la composition des medicamens. 1603. *See* LA FRAMBOISIÈRE. N. A. de.

ORDONNANTIE vande vroedschap der stadt Utrecht. 1655; 1679. *See* UTRECHT. Ordinances, local laws, etc.

ORDONNANTIE, waer nae de doctoren in de medicijne binnen de stadt Utrecht practiferende. 1655. *See* UTRECHT. Ordinances, local laws, etc.

ORDONNANTIEN ende statuten, gemaeckt by heer ende weth der stadt Gendt. 1685? *See* GHENT. Ordinances, local laws, etc.

L'**ORDRE** public pour la ville de Lyon. *See* LYONS. Ordinances, local laws, etc.

ORELL, HERMANN D' [*fl.* 1669] *respondent.* Disputatio medica inauguralis continens casum de asthmate . . . Lugduni Batavorum, Apud viduam & haeredes Joannis Elsevirii, 1669.
　　[20] p.　19 cm.　　　　　　**[8440]**
　　Diss. — Leyden.

ORIBASIUS. In Aphorismos Hippocratis commentaria hactenus non visa, Joannis Guinterii Andernaci . . . industria velut e profundissimis tenebris eruta, et nunc primum in medicinae

studiosorum utilitatem aedita. Patavii, Typis Matthaei Cadorini, 1658.

[20], 273, [2] p.   15 cm.   [8441]

Added engraved title page.

Imperfect: p. 166 mutilated.

First published in Paris in 1533 under title: Commentaria in
Aphorismos Hippocratis.

Includes Latin text of the Aphorismi.

—[Collecta medicinalia. Books 43, 45. French.
1634] *In* Guidi, G. [*ca.* 1500-1569] Les anciens et
renommés autheurs de la medecine & chirurgie. 1634.

ORLERS, Jan Janszn [1570-1646] *See* [Meurs, J.
van, 1579-1639] Illustrium Hollandiae & Westfrisiae
ordinum alma Academia Leidensis. 1614.

ORLIX, Petr d' *See* Dorlix, Petr

OROBIO À CASTRO, Moses [*fl.* 1678] *respondent.*
Disputatio medica inauguralis de hydrope ...
Lugduni Batavorum, Apud viduam & heredes
Johannis Elsevirii, 1678.

[14] p.   22 cm.   [8442]

Diss. —Leyden.

OROLOGIO, Jacopo Dondi dall'. *See* Dondi
dall' Orologio, Jacopo [*ca.* 1293-1359]

ORSINI, Fulvio [1529-1600] *See* Faber, Johannes.
In imagines illustrium ex Fulvii Ursini bibliotheca
... commentarius. 1606.

ORSINI, Giovanni. *See* Ursinus, Joannes [16th
cent.]

ORTA, Garcia d' [1501 *or* 2?-1568] [Coloquios dos
simples, e drogas he cousas mediçinais da India.
French] Histoire des drogues, espiceries, et de certains medicamens simples, qui naissent és Indes, tant
Orientales que Occidentales, divisée en deux parties.
La premiere composée de trois livres: les deux
premiers de M. Garcie du Jardin, & le troisiesme de
M. Christophle de la Coste. La seconde composée
de deux livres de M. Nicolas Monard, traittant de
ce qui nous est apporté des Indes Occidentales, autrement appellées les Terres Neuves. Le tout fidelement
translaté en nostre vulgaire françois sur la traduction latine de Clusius: par Anthoine Colin ... & par
luy augm. de plusieurs figures. Lyon, Jean Pillehotte,
1602.

[16], 711 (i.e. 722), [29] p.   illus.   17 cm.

[8443]

Books 1 and 2 of the Monardes item have special title pages not
included in the paging.

Traicté de Christophle de la Coste ... des drogues &
medicamens qui naissent aux Indes (p. [343]-501) is a translation
and abridgement of Tractado de las drogas y medicinas de las Indias Orientales.

Histoire des simples medicamens apportés des terres neuves,
desquels on se sert in la medicine, par Nicolas Monard (p. 503-711
(i.e. 722)) is a translation of Primera y segunda y tercera partes
de la historia medicinal de las cosas que se traen de nuestras Indias Occidentales que sirven en medicina.

—[The same.] Histoire des drogues, espiceries, et
de certains medicamens simples, qui naissent és Indes & en l'Amerique, divisé en deux parties. La
premiere comprise en quartre livres: les deux
premiers de Me. Garcie du Jardin, le troisiesme de
Me. Christophle de la Coste, & le quatriesme de
l'Histoire du baulme adjoustee de nouveau en ceste
2. éd.: où il est prouvé, que nous avons le vray
baulme d'Arabie, contre l'opinion des anciens &
modernes. La seconde composee de deux livres de
Maistre Nicolas Monard, traictant de ce qui nous est
apporté de l'Amerique ... 2. éd. rev. & augm. Lyon,
Jean Pillehotte, 1619.

4 parts in 1 v.   illus.   18 cm.   [8444]

Parts [2-4] have special title pages.

Contents as in the 1602 edition with the addition of Histoire du
baulme, par Prosper Alpin, which is a translation of De balsamo
dialogus.

—Another issue, with title page reset.

[8445]

—[Italian tr.] Dell'historia de i semplici aromati,
et altre cose che vengono portate dall'Indie Orientali pertinenti all'uso della medicina. Di don Garzia
dal'Horto ... con alcune brevi annotationi di Carlo
Clusio. Parte prima divisa in quattro libri. Et due
altri libri parimente di quelle cose che si portano
dall'Indie Occidentali; con un trattato della neve &
del bever fresco, di Nicolò Monardes ... Hora
tradotti dalle loro lingue nella nostra italiana da m.
Annibale Briganti ... Venetia, L'herede di Girolamo
Scotto, 1605.

[31], 525 p.   illus.   17 cm.   [8446]

Della historia de i semplici, aromati, livro terzo-quarto, da Nicolò
Monardes (p. 258-380) is a translation of Dos libros, el uno trata
de todas las cosas que traen de nuestras Indias Occidentales, que
sirven al uso de medicina ... El otro libro, trata de dos medicinas
maravillosas que son contra todo veneno, la piedra bezaar, y la
yerva escuerçonera.

Delle cose che vengono portate dall'Indie Occidentali, pertinenti
all'uso della medicina, parte seconda, da Nicolò Monardes

(p. 386-525) is a translation of Segunda parte del libro, de las cosas que se traen de neustras Indias Occidentales, que sirven al uso de medicina.

—[The same.] ... Venetia [Giovanni Salis] 1616. [32], 525, [1] p. illus. 16 cm.   **[8447]**
Different setting of type.

—See BONDT, J. de. De medicina Indorum lib. IV. 1642 [and] Oost- en West-Indische warande. 1694 [and] Oost-Indische warande. 1673; L'ÉCLUSE, C. de. Caroli Clusii ... Exoticorum libri decem. 1605; PISO, W. De Indiae utriusque re naturali et medica libri quatuordecim. 1658; WITTICH, J. Bericht von den wunderbaren bezoardischen Steinen. 1612.

ORTEL. *See* ORTHELIUS.

ORTEL, STEPHAN [*fl.* 1629] *respondent. See* SCHMALTZ, Q., *praeses.* Theses medicae, de colica. 1629.

ORTELIUS, ANDREAS. *See* ORTHELIUS.

ORTHELIUS. Commentatio in epistolam Joh. Pontani de lapide ph.
489-496 p., vol. 6. 20 cm. (*In* Zetzner, Lazarus, *ed.* Theatrum chemicum. Argentorati, 1659-61)   **[8448]**
Caption title.

—Orthelius commentator in Novum lumen chymicum Michaelis Sendivogii ... [&] Epilogus et recapitulatio ... in Novum lumen chymicum Sendivogii.
397-458 p., vol. 6. illus. 20 cm. (*In* Zetzner, Lazarus, *ed.* Theatrum chemicum. Argentorati, 1659-61)   **[8449]**
Caption titles.

—Discursus ... de ... epistola Andreae de Blawen.
470-474 p., vol. 6. 20 cm. (*In* Zetzner, Lazarus, *ed.* Theatrum chemicum. Argentorati, 1659-61)   **[8450]**
Caption title.

—Explicatio verborum Mariae prophetissae.
480-487 p., vol. 6. 20 cm. (*In* Zetzner, Lazarus, *ed.* Theatrum chemicum. Argentorati, 1659-61)   **[8451]**
Caption title.

ORTHOLANUS. *See* HORTULANUS.

ORTIZ DE LA LAGUNA, GABRIEL [*fl.* 1634] Responde al doctor Simon Ramos ... a un papel que embiò contra el doctor Caldera ... Lisboa, Horge Rodriguez, 1634.
12 ll. 19 cm.   **[8452]**
Imperfect: upper margins trimmed.

ORTLOB, FRIEDRICH [*fl.* 1653] *respondent. See* LANGE, C., *praeses.* Medicam de lacte humano disquisitionem ... examini sistit publico F. O. 1652, 1653.

ORTLOB, JOHANN CHRISTOPH [1676-1751] De principiis physicorum non apodicticis ... Lipsiae, Literis Christiani Goezii [1700]
[24] p. 18 cm.   **[8453]**
Diss. pro loco—Leipzig.

ORTLOB, JOHANN FRIEDRICH [1661-1700] Historia partium et oeconomiae hominis secundum naturam; sive, Dissertationes anatomico-physiologicae, in Academia Lipsiensi publice ventilatae ... Lipsiae, Apud Joh. Frider. Gleditsch, 1697.
[9], 7, 296, [20] p. plate. 21 cm.   **[8454]**
Includes 37 Leipzig dissertations by 13 authors.

—De rhachitide ... Lipsiae, Literis Johannis Georgii [1687]
[20] p. 20 cm.   **[8455]**
Diss. pro loco—Leipzig (G. C. Habermass, *respondent*)

—Palaestram medicam; sive, Exercitium disputatorium, quo praecipua oeconomiae animalis secundum naturam capita, XXXIII dissertationibus comprehensa publice ventilabuntur ... Lipsiae, Typis Christiani Goezii [1694]
[8] p. 19 cm.   **[8456]**
Program—Leipzig.

Dissertations—Leipzig
—*praeses.* Analogiam nutritionis plantarum & animalium ... exponet ... Christiano Schmeer ... Lipsiae, Typis Christiani Götzii [1683]
[16] p. 19 cm.   **[8457]**
C. Schmeer, *respondent.*

— Ἀντίπραξιν partium oeconomiae animalis legibus minus conformen ... [Lipsiae] Literis Goezianis [1693]
[24] p. 19 cm.   **[8458]**
F. W. Klose, *respondent.*

—Disputatio inauguralis de dentitione puerorum difficili . . . Lipsiae, Literis Christoph. Fleischeri [1694]

[24] p. 22 cm.					**[8459]**

C. G. Finger, *respondent.*

—Disputatio inauguralis de pleuritide . . . [Lipsiae] Literis Goezianis [1696]

[28] p. 19 cm.					**[8460]**

J. A. Beer, *respondent.*

—Disputatio inauguralis medica de rheumatismo . . . [Lipsiae] Typis Goezianis [1696]

[32] p. 20 cm.					**[8461]**

H. H. Helcher, *respondent.*

—Disputatio medica inauguralis de ictero . . . Lipsiae, Typis Immanuelis Titii [1695]

[24] p. 20 cm.					**[8462]**

J. C. Emmerich, *respondent.*

—Dissertatio medica de hydrae in hypochondriis nidulantis origine, indole, antidoto . . . Lipsiae, Typis Joh. Heinrici Richteri [1696]

[46] p. 19 cm.					**[8463]**

B. Gullmann, *respondent.*

—Dissertatio medica de tono & atonia . . . Lipsiae, Literis Gözianis [1700]

[24] p. 20 cm.					**[8464]**

C. M. Adolphi, *respondent.*

—Exercitatio medico-chirurgica, de vesicatoriis . . . Lipsiae, Typis Goezianis [1696]

[32] p. 20 cm.					**[8465]**

J. A. Beer, *respondent.*

—Exercitium anatomico-physiologicum, integrum χοληποιησεως negotium examinans . . . exponit Joh. Christoph. Schroeerus . . . [Lipsiae] Typis Christiani Goezii [1691]

[28] p. 20 cm.					**[8466]**

J. C. Schröer, *respondent.*

—Scrutinium recidivarum . . . Lipsiae, Typis Immanuelis Titii [1696]

[36] p. 19 cm.					**[8467]**

A. Hoffmann, *respondent.*

—*respondent. See* ALBINUS, B. Disputatio medica. 1681 [and] Dissertationem diaeteticam de affectibus animi . . . submittet . . . J. F. O. 1690; BOHN, J., *praeses.* Dissertationes chymico-physicae. 1685; FRIESS, M. F., *praeses.* De salivatione. 1684.

ORVILLE, PETER FRIEDRICH D' [*fl.* 1684] *respondent.* Disputatio medica inauguralis continens theoriam morborum soporosorum . . . Lugduni Batavorum, Apud Abrahamum Elzevier, 1684.

[27] p. 22 cm.					**[8468]**

Diss. — Leyden.

ORTLOB, KARL [1628–1678] *respondent. See* POMARIUS, S. De generatione aequivoca disputatio physica. 1650.

ORTLOP, CAROLUS. *See* ORTLOB, Karl [1628–1678]

ORTOLANUS. *See* HORTULANUS.

ORTULANUS. *See* HORTULANUS.

OSANN, ANDREAS WILHELM [*fl.* 1662–1665] *respondent. See* FRIDERICI, J. A., *praeses.* Dissertatio inauguralis medica, de δυστοκία naturali. 1665; ROLFINCK, W., *praeses.* Disputatio medica de mola. 1662.

OSCHWALD, JOHANN JAKOB [*fl.* 1687] *respondent.* Disputatio inauguralis medica de παιδαρθροκακη . . . Basileae, Literis Joh. Ludovici Koenig & Johannis Bradmylleri [1687]

[20] p. 20 cm.					**[8469]**

Diss. — Basel.

With this is bound: Flores poetici. Basileae [1687]

—*See* FLORES POETICI. 1687.

OSENBRUCK, GEORG THEODOR [*fl.* 1672] *respondent.* Disputatio medica inauguralis de suffocatione hypochondriaca & uterina . . . Lugduni Batavorum, Apud viduam & haeredes Joannis Elsevirii, 1672.

[34] p. 19 cm.					**[8470]**

Diss. — Leyden.

OSIANDER, JOHANNES CHRISTOPHORUS [*fl.* 1623] *respondent. See* SEBISCH, M. [1578–1674?] *praeses.* Exercitatio medica. 1623 [and] Exercitationes medicae. 1639.

OSIANDER, LUCAS [1571–1638] De igne philosophico. *In* Resch, J. U. Osiandrische Experiment von Sole. 1659.

OSLEVIUS, CAROLUS [*fl.* 1583–1584] *See* SCHOLTZ, L. Epistolarum philosophicarum: medicinalium, ac chymicarum . . . volumen. 1610.

OSORIO Y PERALTA, DIEGO. Principia medicinae, epitome, et totius humani corporis fabrica seu ex microcosmi armonia divinum, germen ... Mexici, Apud heredes viduae Bernardi Calderon, 1685.

    [6], 104 (i.e. 105) ll. illus. 21 cm.   **[8471]**

Medina. La imprenta en México, no. 1354.

Contents. — Anothomia. — Tractatus unicus de partibus. — Tractatus de crisibus. — Breve discurso conque preuba ... que la enfermedad, que ha padecido el muy Rdo. P. Fr. Fernando de la Purificacion ... no es. ni ha sido lepra, ò mal del Señor San Lazaro. — Anothomia (Spanish version of the first work) — Hippocratpis [sic] Aphorismata, fideliter deprompta ex versione Leoniseni [sic] veriori. — Tabula in qua omnes [Hippocratis] Aphorismi consiliantur cum morbis in particulari.

OSPEDALE DI MON'AGNESA, Siena. *See* Riforma dell ospedale detto di Mon'Agnesa. 16 — ?

OSPEDALE DI SAN GIACOMO IN AUGUSTA, Rome. Statuti del venerabile Archiospidale di San Giacomo in Augusta, nominato dell'incurabili di Roma. [Roma] Appresso gli Stampatori Camerali, 1659 [1658]

    [1], 80, [3] p.   24 cm.   **[8472]**

Engraved title page.

OSPEDALE MAGGIORE DI MILANO. Ordini appartenenti al governo dell'Hospitale grande di Milano, e di tutti gli altri hospitali à questo uniti. Con le instrutioni di tutti gli officiali, & ministri suoi di nuovo riformati. Milano [Gio. Battista, & Giulio Cesare Malatesta, 1642]

    [8], 174 (i.e. 180) p.   26 cm.   **[8473]**

OSSEQUENTE, Giulio. *See* Obsequens, Julius.

OSSORIO Y PERALTA, Diego. *See* Osorio y Peralta, Diego.

OSSORIUS ET PERALTA, Didacus. *See* Osorio y Peralta, Diego.

OSTENFELD, Christen [1619-1670] *praeses.* Exercitationum de medicinae fundamentis prodromus ... Hafniae, Literis Petri Morsingii, 1656.

    [50] p.   18 cm.   **[8474]**

Diss. — Copenhagen (D. Jersin, *respondent*)

OSTENS, Gisbert [*fl.* 1696] *respondent.* Disputatio medica inauguralis de hydrope ascite ... Lugduni Batavorum, Apud Abrahamum Elzevier, 1696.

    [19] p.   23 cm.   **[8475]**

Diss. — Leyden.

OSTERICHER, Sebastian. *See* Austrius, Sebastianus [*d.* 1550]

OSVALD, Johann Jacob. *See* Oschwald, Johann Jacob [*fl.* 1687]

OSWALD, Johann Jacob. *See* Oschwald, Johann Jacob [*fl.* 1687]

OSWALD, Johann Wolfgang [1662-1738] *respondent. See* Sturm, J. C., *praeses.* Destinatum prolixiori tractatui argumentum de respiratione ὡς ἐν συνοψει hic ... exponunt ... J. C. S. et J. W. O. 1686.

OTHO, Georg Andreas [*fl.* 1698] *respondent.* Dissertatio inauguralis medica de podagra ... Duisburgi ad Rhenum, Typis Johannis Sas, 1698.

    28 p.   20 cm.   **[8476]**

Diss. — Duisburg.

OTT, Johann Heinrich [*fl.* 1666] *respondent. See* Bauhin, H., *praeses.* Theses ... de diaeta sanorum. 1666.

OTT, Johannes [1639-1717] *respondent.* Dissertatio inauguralis de propriorum oculorum defectibus ad leges mechanices revocatis ... Basileae, Apud Jacobum Werenfelsium [1671]

    [4], 20 p.   18 cm.   **[8477]**

Diss. — Basel.

— *See* Wepfer, J. J. Observationes anatomicae. 1675, 1681.

OTTO, Georg Friedrich [*fl.* 1700] *respondent. See* Hoffmann, F. [1660-1742] *praeses.* Dissertatio inauguralis chirurgico-medica de membris fractis. 1700.

OTTO, Johann Georg [*fl.* 1690] *respondent.* Disputatio medica inauguralis περὶ ἐιλεοῦ; sive, De passione iliaca ... Argentorati, Literis Joh. Friderici Spoor [1690]

    [2], 30 p.   20 cm.   **[8478]**

Diss. — Strasbourg.

OTTO, Johann Sebastian [*fl.* 1663-1664] *respondent. See* Sebisch, M. [1578-1674?] *praeses.* Disputatio medica solennis. 1663.

OTTO, Justus Nikolaus [*fl.* 1676-1679] *respondent. See* Meibom, H., *praeses.* Dissertatio medica de calculo renum. 1679; Posner, C., *praeses.* Dissertatio physica de foetuum in uteris vita. 1676.

OTTO, Sigismund Gabriel [*fl.* 1672] *respondent.* Disputatio medica inauguralis de ictero flavo ... Lugduni Batavorum, Apud viduam & haeredes Joannis Elsevirii, 1672.

[12] p.   20 cm.   **[8479]**

Diss. — Leyden.

OTTONIS, Jacobus [*fl.* 1624] *See* Freitag, J. De opii natura. 1632.

OUGHTRED, William [1575-1660] *See* [Leurechon, J.] Mathematicall recreations. 1653

OVERBEKE, Aernout van [1632-1674] Extract van 't Kennip-zaat ... Gedruckt in Japan aen den Leysten Dam. [Amsterdam? not before 1663]

broadside.   40 x 26 cm.   **[8480]**

In verse.

OVERCAMP, Heydentrijk. *See* Overkemp, Heydentryk [1651?-1692 *or* 3]

OVERDATZ, Louis [1618-1682] Kort verhael van de peste, met hare genees-middelen ... Brussel, Jan Mommaert, 1668.

[16], 87 p.   15 cm.   **[8481]**

OVERKAMP, Heydentryk [1651?-1692 *or* 3] Alle de medicinale, chirurgicale en philosophische werken ... Erste deel. Bestaande in de nieuwe beginzelen tot de genees-en heel-konst ... Nevens een Verklaring over de doorwazeming van Sanctorium, en nader onderzoek over 't II. deel der wysbegeerte, van R. des Cartes. Amsterdam, Jan teen Hoorn, 1694.

2 parts in I v.   illus., port.   22 cm.   **[8482]**

"Nader verklaringe, over de ontdeke doorwaasseming ... van Sanctorius" and "... Tweede deel. Der chirurgie ... Nevens een klaare verhandeling van de pokken en haar geneezing" have special title pages.

—Nieuw gebouw der chirurgie of heel-konst, getimmert op de nieuwe beginselen vande genees en heel-konst ... Door klare en onderscheydene beginselen, over een stemmende met die van Renatus des Cartes. Nevens een brief over dit werk, van Cornelis Bontekoe ... Amsterdam, Jan ten Hoorn, 1682.

[24], 459, [1] p.   port.   16 cm.   **[8483]**

—[German tr.] Neues Gebäude der Chirurgie, gezimmert nach den neuen principen der Medicin ... Durch klare und unterschiedene Principia, so übereinkommen mit den Renatus des Cartes, nebenst einem Brieff über das Werck von Cornelius Bontekoe. Alles aus denen Holländischen in das Hochteutsche übergesetzet durch D. Johann Schreyern ... Leipzig, Johann Friedrich Gleditsch, 1689.

[46], 908, [28] p.   front. (port.)   17 cm.

[8484]

—[The same.] Neu erfundene Heyl-Kunst, oder Chirurgia, auf die Lehr-Sätze Renatus Des Cartes gegründet ... Nebenst einem Brieff über diss Werck von Cornelius Bontekoe. Aus dem Holländischen ins Hochteutsche übergesetzet und verbessert von D. J[ohann] S[chreyer] Zum andernmal in Druck befördert. Leipzig, Joh. Friedrich Gleditsch, 1692.

[46], 900, [74] p.   front. (port.)   18 cm.

[8485]

—Oeconomia animalis; oder, Gründlicher Unterricht, von der Geburt-Nahrung und Wachsthum des Menschen. Worbey unterschiedene uber Speiss und Tranck, auch andere zum Leben nöthige Dinge, vorfallende curieuse Fragen nach den Lehrsätzen Renatus des Cartes erörtert werden. Erstlich ... in Holländischen beschrieben; jetzo ins Hochdeutsche zusammen gezogen von D. Johann Schreyern ... Leipzig, In Verlegung Joh. Friedrich Gleditsch, 1690.

[30], 431, [17] p.   front. (port.)   18 cm.

[8486]

—Reden, over het leven en de doot van de heer Cornelis Bontekoe ... Amsterdam, Thimotheus ten Hoorn, 1685.

[7], 32 p.   22 cm.   **[8487]**

OVERSCHIE, Adrian [*fl.* 1699] *respondent.* Disputatio medica inauguralis de phthisi ... Lugduni Batavorum, Apud Abrahamum Elzevier, 1699.

[28] p.   22 cm.   **[8488]**

Diss. — Leyden.

OVID. *See* Ovidius Naso, Publius.

OVIDIUS NASO, Publius. *See* Faber, Johannes. De nardo et epithymo adversus Josephum Scaligerum. 1607.

OVIEDO, Luís de [*fl.* 1580-*ca.* 1617] Methodo de la coleccion y reposicion de las medicinas simples, de su correccion y preparacion ... Va añadido en algunos lugares el tercer libro, y todo el quarto libro: en que se trata de la composicion de los unguentos, cerotos, y emplastos, que estan en uso, y las recetas ... Madrid, Luis Sanchez, 1622.

[8], 524, [36] p.   30 cm.   **[8489]**

Edited by Gregorio Gonzalez.

—[The same.] ... Madrid, Melchor Alvarez. 1692.

[8], 524, [36] p. 30 cm. **[8490]**

A reprint of the 1622 edition, with new preliminary matter.

OWEN, JOHN [1560?-1622] *See* REGIMEN SANITATIS SALERNITANUM. Schola Salernitana. 1649, 1657, 1667, 1683.

OXFORD UNIVERSITY. *See* UNIVERSITY OF OXFORD.

P

P., A. *See* PITFIELD, Alexander [1659?-1728]

P., A. *See* PORCHON, A.

P., D., *tr. See* MORHOF, D. G. Brief. 1672.

P., F., *ed. See* WINSTON, T. Anatomy lectures at Gresham Colledge. 1659.

P., G. *See* PLATTES, Gabriel [*fl.* 1638-1643]

P., H. S. [*fl.* 1682] *ed. See* POMPEJUS, N. Praecepta chiromantica. 1682.

P., I. M. D. V. C. A. *See* MICHAULT, Jean [1632-1694]

P., J. *See* PRIMROSE, James [1592-1659]

P., M. G. *See* PURMANN, Matthias Gottfried [1649-1711]

P., M. L. *See* MARTIN, Louis [*fl.* 1649]

P., N., *D. M., tr. See* GRAAF, R. de. Histoire anatomique des parties genitales. M.DC. LXCIX (i.e. 1699?)

P., N. D. S. *See* D., N., B. P.

P., N. O. *See* PAULONI, Nicolò Orfeo [1653-1721]

P., R. *See* PEMELL, Robert [*d.* 1653]

P., R. *See* PLOT, Robert [1640-1696]

P., R. *See* PUGH, Robert [1609-1679]

P., S. *See* PARKER, Samuel, *Bp. of Oxford* [1640-1688]

P., T. *See* PEUCER, Tobias [*fl.* 1690-1691]

P., T. *See* WOOLLEY, Hannah [*fl.* 1670]

P.M.T.Ph.C. *See* T., P. M. [*fl.* 1688]

OYLIME, *doctor. See* [ZAQUIIAS, doctor] El medico caritativo. 1660?

[**OZON,** PIERRE, *fl.* 1689] Response a la dissertation sur la goutte [par M. Mauduit]. Par M*** Docteur en Medecine. Paris, Daniel Horthemels, 1690.

[16], 294, [1] p. 17 cm. **[8491]**

PAAW, Petrus. *See* PAUW, Pieter [1564-1617]

PACICHELLI, GIOVANNI BATTISTA [1641-1702] Chiroliturgia; sive, De varia, ac multiplici manus administratione. Lucubrationes juridico-philologicae ... Coloniae Agrippinae, Typis Wilhelmi Friessem, 1673.

[12], 155, [12] p. 20 cm. **[8492]**

First and last sheets imperfectly bound.

PACK, CHR. *See* PACKE, Christopher [*fl.* 1670-1711]

PACKE, CHRISTOPHER [*fl.* 1670-1711] Mineralogia: or, An account of the preparation, manifold vertues and uses of a mineral salt, both in physick and chyrurgery ... To which is added, A short discourse of the nature and uses of the sulphurs of minerals and metals in curing the most chronical and pertinacious diseases. London, D. Newman, 1693.

[2], 65, [1] p. 16 cm. **[8493]**

—, *ed.* and *tr. See* GLAUBER, J. R. The works. 1689.

—, *ed. See* COUCH, R. Praxis catholica. 1680.

—, *tr. See* GRAAF, R. de. De succo pancreatico. 1676.

PADER, HILAIRE [1607-1677] *tr. See* LOMAZZO, G. P. Traicte de la proportion naturelle et artificielle des choses. 1649.

PADIOLEAU, ALBERT, *sieur de Launay. See* LAUNAY, Albert Padioleau, *sieur de.*

PADOANO, HELIDAEO [*d.* 1576] Processus, curationes & consilia in curandis particularibus morbis, quae prosperos habuerunt eventus ... Nunc primum in publicum edita a Johanne Wittichio ... Lipsiae,

Sumptibus Nicolai Nerlichii [Michael Lantzen-berger] 1607.

[20], 318, [15] p. port. 19 cm.   **[8494]**

—See SCHOLTZ, L. Consiliorum medicinalium ... liber singularis. 1610.

PADOVANI, ELIDEO. *See* PADOANO, Helidaeo [*d.* 1576]

PADOVANI, FABRIZIO [16th cent.] De morbis in quibus praesentaneis uti convenit remediis. *In* Seidel, B. Liber, morborum incurabilium causas ... ex-plicans. 1662.

PADUA. REALE UNIVERSITÀ DEGLI STUDI. *See* UNIVERSITÀ DI PADOVA.

PADUA UNIVERSITÀ. *See* UNIVERSITÀ DI PADOVA.

PADUANIUS, FABRITIUS. *See* PADOVANI, Fabrizio [16th cent.]

PAEANTIUS, ALEXANDER. *See* BENEDETTI, Alessandro [*d.* 1512]

PAËPP, JOHANN [*d.* 1613] Artificiosae memoriae fundamenta, ex Aristotele, Cicerone, Thoma Aquinate, aliisque praestantissimis doctoribus petita, figuris, interrogationibus, ac responsionibus clarius quam unquam antehac demonstrata ... Lugduni, Sumptibus auctoris, apud Bartholomaeum Vincentium, 1619.

[24], 120 p. illus., plates, tables. 15 cm.   **[8495]**

Bound with Ravelli, F. M. Ars memoriae. 1617.

—Εισαγωγη; seu, Introductio facilis in praxim ar-tificiosae memoriae ... Lugduni, Sumptibus auc-toris, apud Bartholomaeum Vincentium, 1618.

[23], 102 p. plates. 15 cm.   **[8496]**

Bound with Ravelli, F. M. Ars memoriae. 1617.

—Vita M. Tullii Ciceronis in annos distincta, ac in epitomen secundum artem mnemonicam redacta ... cui adjuncti sunt catalogi pontificum & im-peratorum a mendis purgati, qui typographorum in-curia in Schenckelio detecto irrepserant. Lugduni, sumptibus auctoris, apud Bartholomaeum Vincen-tium, 1618.

45, [1] p. 15 cm.   **[8497]**

Bound with Ravelli, F. M. Ars memoriae. 1617.

PAGET, NATHAN [1615-1679] Bibliotheca medica, viri clarissimi Nathanis Paget, M. D., cui adjiciun-tur quamplurimi alii libri theologici, philosophici, &c.; quorum omnium auctio habebitur Londini, ad insigne Pelicani in vico vulgo dicto Little-Britain 24 die Octobris 1681. Per Gulielmum Cooper bibliopolam. London [1681]

[4], 52 p. 25 cm.   **[8498]**

PAGGI, CARLO ANTONIO [*fl.* 17th cent.] Enchiri-dion medico-astro-chymicum; universam medicinae theoriam complectens ... Ulyssipone, Ex proelo An-tonii Craesbeeck a Mello, 1664.

[16], 426, [13] p. 20 cm.   **[8499]**

ΠΑΙΔΩΝ νοσήματα; or, Childrens diseases. 1664. *See* [STARSMARE, J.]

Le **PALAIS** des curieux. 1660. *See* VULSON DE LA COLOMBIÈRE, M.

PALLADIUS, RUTILIUS TAURUS AEMILIANUS. *See* COLUMELLA, L. J. M. Agricultur; oder, Ackerbaw. 1612.

PALLADIUS IATROSOPHISTA. De febribus concisa synopsis. Interprete Joanne Chartier ... Parisiis, Apud Jacobum Senlecam, 1646.

[6], 46, [1] p. plate. 25 cm.   **[8500]**

In Greek and Latin.

—Scholia in Hippocratis De fracturis. *In* HIP-POCRATES. [Collected works. Greek and Latin] Τὰ εὑρισκόμενα. 1621, 1624, 1657, 1662.

PALLIERIO, PAULO FRANCISCO. De vera lactis genesi, & usu, disquisitio medico anatomica multa nova ad Hippocratis mentem complectens. Genuae, Ex typographia Jo. Ambrosii de Vincentiis, 1663.

[24], 145, [10] p. 19 cm.   **[8501]**

PALMARIUS, JULIUS. *See* Le PAULMIER de Grentemesnil, Julien [1520-1588]

PALMARIUS, PETRUS. *See* Le PAULMIER, Pierre [1568-1610]

PALMEIRO, ANTOINE. *See* PALMIERI, Antonio [1630-1711]

PALMER, JOSUA [*fl.* 1681-1683] *respondent.* Disputatio medica inauguralis de medicamentorum sudoriferorum natura, operatione, & usu ... Lugduni Batavorum, Apud Abrahamum Elzevier, 1682.

[16] p.   22 cm.   [8502]

Diss. — Leyden.

PALMERIUS, ANTONIUS. *See* PALMIERI, Antonio [1630-1711]

PALMIERI, ANTONIO [1630-1711] *See* HIPPOCRATES. [Aphorismi. Adaptations, etc. Latin] 1699.

PALMIERI, LORENZINO. Perfette regole, et modi di cavalcare ... et insieme si tratta della natura de' cavalli; si propongono le loro infermità; e s'additano gli rimedi per curarle ... Venetia, Barezzo Barezzi, adistanza di Paolo Frambotto, 1625.

[8], 112 p.   plate.   22 cm.   [8503]

Added engraved title page, dated 1626.

PALTHENIUS, ZACHARIAS [1570-1615] *ed. See* MERCADO, L. Opera omnia. 1608 [and] Operum tomus primus [-quintus] 1614-1620; PARACELSUS. Operum medico chimicorum. 1603-1605; RIOLAN, J. [1538?-1605?] Opera cum physica, tum medica. 1611.

—*See* SEIDEL, B. Liber, morborum incurabilium causas ... explicans. 1662.

PALUDANO, ANTONIO [*fl.* 1631?] *respondent. See* BURGERSDIJCK, F. P., *praeses.* Collegium physicum. 1642.

PAMAN, HENRY [1626-1695] *See* SYDENHAM, T. Epistolae responsoriae duae. 1680, 1683.

PAMIO, TEOFILO, *pseud. See* MONIGLIA, Giovanni Andrea [1624-1700]

PANAROLI, DOMENICO [1587-1657] Abuso nel governo de i putti ... Roma, Domenico Marciani, 1642.

16 p.   16 cm.   [8504]

—Iatrologismi, sive, Medicae observationes, quibus additus est in fine Plantarum amphitheatralium catalogus. Romae, Typis Dominici Marciani, 1643.

[10], 74 (i. e. 75), [11] p.   17 cm.   [8505]

—Iatrologismorum; seu, Medicinalium observationum pentacostae quinque ... in calce adduntur opuscula ... Romae, Apud Franciscum Monetam, 1652.

[46], 445, [15] p.   plates, port.   21 cm.

[8506]

Added engraved title page.

Partial contents: De simplicium cognitione medico necessaria; Plantarum amphitheatralium catalogus; Chamaeleo examinatus; Arcanorum fasciculus I; Arcanorum fasciculus II.

With this is bound Wolf, Ido. Observationum chirurgico-medicarum libri duo. Quedlimburgi, 1704.

—[The same.] ... Hanoviae, Typis Johannis Aubry, sumptibus Johannis Bayeri, 1654.

[24], 226 (i. e. 227), [8] p.   illus.   21 cm.

[8507]

PANATI. *See* PANUTIO, Vincenzo [*fl. ca.* 1640]

PANCIROLI, GUIDO [1523-1599] Rerum memorabilium; sive, Deperditarum pars prior [-liber secundus] Comentariis illustrata, et locis prope innumeris postremum aucta, ab Henrico Salmuth ... Francofurti, Sumptibus Godefridi Schonwetteri, 1646.

[8], 349, [23] p.; 313, [17] p.   21 cm.   [8508]

Engraved title page.

The second part completed by Heinrich Salmuth.

PANCKOW, THOMAS [1622-1665] Herbarium; oder, Kräuter- und Gewächs Buch, darinn so wol einheimische als aussländische Kräuter zierlich und eigentlich abgebildet zufinden ... Ubersehen ... vermehret ... und ... verbessert durch Bartholomaeum Zornn. Cölin an der Spree, Georg Schultze, 1673.

[20], [198], 425 p.   1536 woodcuts.   20 cm.

[8509]

Added engraved title page.

Nissen 1485, Pritzel 6919.

Illustrations originally made by Peter Holzmeyer for Leonhard Thurneisser zum Thurn's Historia und Beschreibung, published in Berlin, 1578.

PANCOVIUS, THOMAS. *See* PANCKOW, Thomas [1622-1665]

PANDOLFINI, GIUSEPPE. Tractatus de ventositatis spinae saevissimo morbo; de quo nihil fere Graeci, & paucissima Arabes, Latinique conscripsere; revisus, correctus & annotationibus, novisque cum propriis tum alienis observationibus e variorum authorum monumentis erutis illustratus & ad hodierna medicine principia accommodatus a Georgio Abrahamo Merclino ... Noribergae, Apud Johannis Andreae & Wolffgangi Endteri junioris haeredes, 1674.

[36], 520, [32] p.   14 cm.   [8510]

PANICELLI, CARLO [*fl.* 1629] Trattato de gl'effetti maravigliosi delle carni di vipere . . . Fiorenza, Simone Ciotti, 1630.

[7], 103, [8] p.   19 cm.   **[8511]**

PANIZZOLA, FRANCESCO [*fl.* 1657] *ed. See* BOLZETTA, A. De affectionibus cordis tractatus. 1657.

PANRING, JOHANN HEINRICH [*fl.* 1687–1689] *respondent. See* HARTMANN, P. J., *praeses.* Exercitationum anatomicarum in publicas lectiones de iis, quae contra peritiam veterum anatomicam afferuntur in genere, secunda. 1687.

PANSA, MARTINUS [*b. ca.* 1580] Aureus libellus de proroganda vita, in quo causae longioris ac brevioris vitae exquisite describuntur, & quanam diaeta, quibusque medicamentis tam vulgaribus, quam pretiosis & arcanis vita longa sit comparanda, evidentissime ac fidelissime monstratur . . . Lipsiae, Impensis Thomae Schüreri, 1615–16.

3 parts in 1 v.   16 cm.   **[8512]**
Part 4, published in 1620, wanting.

—[German excerpts.] Köstlicher und heilsamer Extract der gantzen Artzneykunst, darinnen kürtzlich die Ursachen des . . . Lebens, und allerhand Kranckheiten menschliches Leibes beschrieben . . . Leipzig, In Vorlegung Henning Grossens des Jüngern, 1618.

[23], 381 (i.e. 385), [5] p.   16 cm.   **[8513]**

—Bad Ordnung; das ist, Kurtzer und allgemeiner Bericht von den Warmen Bädern und ihren Eigenschafften . . . Leipzig, Bey Abraham Lamberg, In Vorlegung Johann Enrings seligen Erben und Johann Perferts [Typis Lambergianis, gedruckt durch Johann Glück] 1618.

[13], 143, [1] p.   15 cm.   **[8514]**

—Consilium antinephriticum; das ist, Ein heylsamer Rathschlag vom Lendenstein, darinnen zwar kürtzlich jedoch gar deutlich und gnugsam angezeiget wird was der Lendenstein sey, woraus er erwachse und wie man ihn recht erkennen auch glücklich vertreiben sol . . . Leipzig, In Verlegung Henning Grossen des Jüngern, 1615.

[24], 272 (i.e. 262), [1] p.   16 cm.   **[8515]**
With this is bound *his* Consilium antipodagricum. 1613.

—Consilium antipestiferum; das ist, Ein getrewer Rath in gefehrlichen und gifftigen Sterbens-Leufften oder Pestilentzseuche . . . Leipzig, Gedruckt bey

Valentin am Ende, In Vorlegung Thomae Schürers, 1614.

3 v. in 1.   20 cm.   **[8516]**

—Consilium antipodagricum; das ist, Ausführlicher Bericht darinnen verfast ob das Zipperlein eine heilbare Kranckheit sey oder nicht; was der Ursprung und Ursach desselbigen seyn, wie man sich darvor hüten und praeserviren; dessgleichen durch was Mittel es beydes zu vertreiben und auch zu lindern . . . Leipzig, In Verlegung Thomae Schürers, 1613.

[16], 237, [1] p.   16 cm.   **[8517]**
Bound with *his* Consilium antinephriticum. 1615.

—[The same.] . . . Leipzig, In Verlegung Thomae Schürers s. Erben, 1615–17 [v. 1, 1617]

2 v. in 1.   16 cm.   **[8518]**
Vol. 2 has title: Consilium antipodagricum secundum speciale; das ist, Der andere Rathschlag vom Zipperlein.
The text of vol. 1 is a reissue of the 1613 edition.

—[The same.] . . . Leipzig, In Verlegung Thomas Schürers und Matthiae Götzens s. Erben, 1663.

[16], 237 p.   17 cm.   **[8519]**
A reprint of the 1613 edition.

[—] Appendix consilii antipodagrici specialis darinnen X consilia specialissima . . . Leipzig, In Verlegung Zacharias Schürers des Jungern und Matthias Görzens, 1625.

[28], 303 p.   16 cm.   **[8520]**
Engraved title page.

—Consilium evacuatorium; das ist, Ein nützlicher Rathschlag vom Purgieren, darinnen anfänglich die Störer, Pfuscher, und losen Fischer in der Artzneykunst purgieret, taxiret, unnd aussgemustert werden; und ferner der rechte Gebrauch des Purgierens eröffnet, und nach allen umbständen beschrieben wird . . . Sampt vier und zwantzig disputierlichen Fragen von dieser Materia . . . Leipzig, In Verlegung Henning Grossen des Jüngern, 1615.

[24], 369 (i.e. 383) p.   16 cm.   **[8521]**
Imperfect: p. 143–144 wanting.
Bound with *his* Consilium phlebotomicum. [1615]

—Consilium phlebotomicum; das ist, Ein gantz newes, ausführliches und wolgegründetes Aderlassbüchlein, darinnen angezeiget wird was vom Aderlassen und Schrepffen eigentlich zuhalten:

dessgleichen wenn wie und an welchen Orten des Leibes die Adern und Haut in- und ausserhalb der Leibsgebrechen fruchtbarlich zu öffnen seyen ... Sampt 50. zu Ende angehengten schonen Fragen vom Blut und Blutlassen ... Leipzig, In Verlegung Henning Grossen des Jüngern [Gedruckt bey Lorentz Kober, 1615]

[24], 382 (i.e. 380), [1] p. illus. 16 cm.

[8522]

With this is bound *his* Consilium evacuatorium. 1615.

—[The same.] Neu ausführlich und wohl gegründetes Aderlass-Büchlein, worinnen angezeiget wird was vom Aderlassen und Schrepffen eigendlich zu halten, desgleichen wann, wie und an welchen Orten des Leibes die Adern und Haut, in und ausserhalb des Leibes Gebrechen fruchtbarlich zu öffnen seyn ... Sampt funfftzig Fragen von Blud-Aderlassen und Schrepffen ... Schneeberg, Bey Michael Jammerten, 1700.

[22], 382 (i.e. 380) p. 16 cm.   [8523]

A reprint of the 1615 edition without the colophon.

—Güldenes Kleinod menschlicher Gesundheit: darinnen die Lehr von des menschen Gesundheit als welche unter andern Gütern und Kleinodien dieser Welt das allerfürtrefflichste ist weitleufftig erkläret ... Leipzig, In Verlegung Zachariae Schürers und Matthiae Götzen, 1626.

[42], 879 (i.e. 881), [7] p. 20 cm.   [8524]

Imperfect: engraved title page and title in red and black wanting.

—Kurtze Beschreibung dess Carolsbades, so nahe beym Städlein Ellnbogen in Böhmen gelegen: wie man sich darinnen zuverhalten habe, wann unnd zu was Kranckheiten es gut sey, auch was man für Remedia darbey könne gebrauchen ... Darneben auch die Beschreibung dess Wiesenbades zu befinden ... S. Annenbergk, Gedruckt bey Christian Behm, in Verlegung Tobiae Ecksteins, 1609.

2 parts in 1 v. 15 cm.   [8525]

—Kurtze Defensionschrifft von der Gicht ... wider D. Gregorii Martinii zu Wolaw aussgesprengte Schmehekarte, so er nennet Discursum philosophico-medicum ... [n. p.] 1617.

[38] p. 16 cm.   [8526]

Bound with *his* Kurtzer und sehr nothwendiger Bericht von den gifftigen Fiebern. 1618.

—Kurtzer Bericht von der Colica oder Darmgrimmen, darinnen von dieser Kranckheit Eigenschafft, Sitz, Zeichen und Ursachen: dessgleichen von derselben künfftigen Gefahr, auch wie man sich mit guter Diaet darvor praeserviren ... erkleret ... Leipzig, In Verlegung Henning Grossen des Jüngern [Vorrede 1618]

148 p.; [12], 104 p. 16 cm.   [8527]

"Kurtzer Bericht von der Melancholeykranckheit" ([12], 104 p.) has half title.

—Kurtzer Bericht von der Schwindsucht, darinnen der Ansitz mancherley Arten, Beschreibung und Ursachen der Schwindsucht; dessgleichen wann diese Kranckheit zu curiren, und von rechter Praeservation, Curation und Inhibition derselben ... fleissig erkleret wird ... Leipzig, Gedruckt durch Lorentz Kober, in Verlegung Henning Grossen des Jüngern, 1618.

[16], 172, [1] p. 16 cm.   [8528]

Bound with *his* Kurtzer und sehr nothwendiger Bericht von den gifftigen Fiebern. 1618.

—Kurtzer und sehr nothwendiger Bericht von den gifftigen Fiebern, welche Malignae genennet werden, darinnen klärlich angezeiget wird die Natur und Eigenschafft dieser Fieber ... Leipzig, Gedruckt durch Lorentz Kober, in Vorlag Henning Grossen des Jüngern, 1618.

[16], 120 p. 16 cm.   [8529]

With this are bound *his*: Kurtze Defensionschrifft von der Gicht. 1617; —Kurtzer Bericht von der Schwindsucht. 1618.

—Pharmacotheca publica et privata. Das ist: Stadt-, Hoff- und Haussapothecke ... Leipzig, In Vorlegung Henning Grossen des Jüngern s. Erben, gedruckt bey Johann Glück, 1622.

4 parts in 1 v. port. 19 cm.   [8530]

Imperfect: leaf preceding title page and p. 133-136 of part 3 wanting.

Imprint varies: Th. 3-4, Gedruckt durch Justum Jansonium Danum, in Verlegung Henning Grossen des Jüngern seligen Erben.

Parts [2] and 3 have special title pages.

—*respondent.* Theses de generali pestis natura, praeservatione et curatione ... Basileae, Typis Johannis Schroeteri, 1606.

[24] p. 19 cm.   [8531]

Diss. — Basel.

PANTALEON, *pseud.* See GASSMANN, Franz.

PANTELIUS, MICHAEL [1665-1699] *praeses.* Disputatio medico-chymica de mercurio, et ejus in usu medico operandi ratione . . . Regiomonti, Typis Reusnerianis [1698]

16 p.   19 cm.   [8532]

Diss. — Königsberg (D. P. Vasmar, *respondent*)

PANTEO, Giovanni Agostino. *See* Pantheo, Giovanni Agostino [*fl. ca.* 1517-1535]

PANTHAEUS, Joannes Augustus. *See* Pantheo, Giovanni Agostino [*fl. ca.* 1517-1535]

PANTHEO, Giovanni Agostino [*fl. ca.* 1517-1535] Ars et theoria transmutationis metallicae cum voar-chadumia, proportionibus, numeris, & iconibus rei accommodis illustrata . . .

459-549 p., vol. 2 illus.   20 cm.   (*In* Zetzner, Lazarus, *ed.* Theatrum chemicum. Argentorati, 1659-61)   [8533]

Caption title.

PANTHOT, Jean Baptiste [*ca.* 1640-1707] Let-tre . . . écrite a . . . Gui Crescent Fagon . . . sur la maladie extraordinaire dont feu M. Jean De-Rhodes . . . est decedé le 13. Avril 1695 . . . [Lyon? 1695?]

13 p.   22 cm.   [8534]

—Reflections sur l'estat present des maladies, qui regnent dans la ville de Lyon, dans ce royaume, & en diverses parties de l'Europe, depuis la fin de l'an-née derniere 1693 jusques à present . . . Lyon, Jac-ques Guerrier, 1695.

[28], 114 p.   15 cm.   [8535]

—Traité des dragons et des escarboucles . . . Lyon, Thomas Amaulry, 1691.   [8536]

PANUTIO, Vincenzo [*fl. ca.* 1640] *See* Castelli, P. Opobalsamum triumphans. 1640?; Donzelli, G. Lettera familiare. 1643; Giaquinto, T. Ragguaglio primo -[secondo] venuto di Parnaso l'anno M.DC.XXXX. sopra il balsamo d'Arabia. 1640; Nemi, N. Imbiancatura di Nicolò Nemi da Novi. 1640; Panuzzi, F., *ed.* Francesco Panuzzi . . . a i lettori. 1640.

PANUZZI, Francesco [*fl. ca.* 1640] *ed.* Francesco Panuzzi . . . a i lettori. Eccovi . . . la traduttione di latino in volgare di due lettere sopra il balsamo del quale fù composto Theriaca da Antonio Manfredi, & Vincenzo Panuzzi . . . stampate nel fin dell'opera fatto sopra la medema materia dal signor Baldo Baldi . . . [Roma, Lodovico Grignani, 1640]

[8] p.   22 cm.   [8537]

Contains Giovanni Nardi's letter written to Paolo Zacchia and Baldo Baldi, and Johann Vesling's letter addressed to Baldo Baldi.

PANUZZI, Vincenzo. *See* Panutio, Vincenzo [*fl. ca.* 1640]

PANVINIO, Giacomo. *See* Panvinio, Onofrio [1530-1568]

PANVINIO, Onofrio [1530-1568] *See* Moller, D. W., *praeses.* Disputationem circularem de Onuph. Panvinio . . . ingredietur Leonhardus Reuterus. 1697.

PAOLINI, Fabio. *See* Paulinus, Fabius [*d.* 1605]

PAOLONI, Niccolo Orfeo. *See* Pauloni, Nicolò Orfeo [1653-1721]

PAPA, Giuseppe del [1648 *or* 9-1735] Della natura dell'umido e del secco, lettera all'illustrissimo sig. Francesco Redi . . . Firenze, Vincenzo Vangelisti, 1681.

220 p.   plates.   24 cm.   [8538]

—Lettera intorno alla natura del caldo e del freddo, scritta all'illustrissimo sig. Francesco Redi . . . Firenze, Francesco Liui, 1674.

250 p.   16 cm.   [8539]

—[The same.] Della natura del caldo e del freddo; lettera all'illustriss. sig. Francesco Redi . . . scritta nel 1674. 2. impr. Firenze, Piero Matini, 1690.

[1], 152 p.   25 cm.   [8540]

With this is bound (as issued?) *his* Lettera nella quale si discorre se il fuoco e la luce sieno una cosa medesima. 1690.

—Lettera nella quale si discorre se il fuoco e la luce sieno una cosa medesima, scritta nel 1675 all'illustriss. sig. Francesco Redi . . . 2. impr. Firenze, Piero Matini, 1690.

[2], 30 p.   25 cm.   [8541]

Bound with (as issued?) *his* Della natura del caldo e del freddo. 1690.

PAPAFAVA, Roberto [*fl.* 1636] Syrinx physiologica . . . compacta et publicae disputationis flatibus ad veritatis concentum exposita . . . Patavii [Apud Paullum Frambottum] 1636.

[12], 3-71 p.   21 cm.   [8542]

Signatures: A⁶, A⁴-I⁴.
Imperfect? p. 1-2 wanting?
Engraved title page.

PÁPAI PÁRIZ, Ferenc [1649-1716] Pax corporis; az az, Az emberi testnek belsö nyavalyáinak okairól, fészkeiröl, s'-azoknak orvoslásának módgyáról való tracta ... Mágyar nyelven másodszor ki adott ... Löcsén, Brewer Samuel, 1692.

[16], 339, [5] p. 16 cm. [8543]

— *respondent.* Disputatio inauguralis tribus consiliis medicis absoluta ... Basileae, Typis Joh. Rodolphi Genathii [1674]

[20] p. 19 cm. [8544]

Diss. — Basel.

PAPE, ANDREAS [*fl.* 1610] *respondent. See* STUPANUS, J. N., *praeses.* Σημειωτιces particularis cap. I. De affectibus. 1610.

PAPE, JOHANN [1558-1622] *See* RECORDE, R. The urinal of physick. 1651, 1665.

PAPIN, DENIS [1647-1714] La maniere d'amolir les os, et de faire cuire toutes sortes de viandes en fort peu de temps, & à peu de frais ... Paris, Estienne Michallet, 1682.

[12], 164, [11] p. plates. 16 cm. [8545]

— [The same.] ... Nouv. ed., rev. & augm. d'une 2. partie. Amsterdam, Henry Desbordes, 1688.

2 parts in 1 v. plates. 15 cm. [8546]

Part 2 has special title page: Continuation du digesteur; ou, Maniere d'amolir les os.

— [English ed.] A new digester or engine for softning bones, containing the description of its make and use in ... cookery ... chymistry, and dying ... London, Printed by J. M. for Henry Bonwicke, 1681.

[7], 54 p. plates. 23 cm. [8547]

With this is bound *his* A continuation of the new digester. 1687.

— A continuation of the new digester of bones: it's improvements and new uses ... Together with some improvements and new uses of the air-pump ... London, Joseph Streater, 1687

[7], 123, [1] p. plates. 23 cm. [8548]

Bound with *his* A new digester. 1681.

PAPIN, NICOLAS [*d.* 1653?] De pulvere sympathico dissertatio. Lutetiae, Apud Simeonem Piget, 1647.

[14], 40 p. 17 cm. [8549]

— [The same.] ... Lutetiae, Apud Simonem Piget, 1650.

[14], 40 p. 17 cm. [8550]

Different setting of type.
Bound with [Cattier, I.] Divers traictez. Paris, 1651.

— [The same.] ... Patavii, Typis Matthaei Cadorini, 1654 [i. e. 1655]

[12], 48 p. 16 cm. [8551]

Added half title. Added engraved title page dated 1655.

— [The same.] ... Rothomagi, Sumptibus Joannis Berthelin, 1650 [i. e. 1656?]

[8], 43 p. 16 cm. [8552]

Dedicatory epistle, dated Jan. 1, 1656, signed: Joannes Baptista Pasquati.

— [The same.] *In* Theatrum sympatheticum. 1660, 1661.

— [The same.] ... 143-164 p. 21 cm. (*In* Theatrum sympatheticum auctum. Norimbergae, 1662) [8553]

Caption title.

— [Dutch ed.] Theatrum sympateticum; ofte, Wonder-tooneel des natuers verborgentheden zijnde een noodigh vervolgh op de oratie van den Heere ... Digby ... Werdende hier in eerst te recht gheleert de bereydinghe des poeders de sympathie, ende desselfs ghebruyck in verscheyde soorten van wonden ... Uyt de Latijnsche gheschriften van ... Nicolai Papinii, ende Sylvestri Rattray. Getranslateert door I[ohannes] C[asteleyn] Haerlem, Joannes Casteleyn 1662.

[7], 30 p. 19 cm. [8554]

Bound with Digby, Sir K. D'eminente oratie. 1661.

— [The same.] *In* Theatrum sympatheticum auctum. 1681, 1697.

— La poudre de sympathie, deffendue contre les objections de M[r] Cattier, medecin du roy ... Paris, Simeon Piget, 1651.

[8], 56 p. 17 cm. [8555]

A defense of the author's De pulvere sympathico dissertatio, 1647, against the views expressed in Isaac Cattier's De la poudre de sympathie, 1650, which Papin considered to be an attack on his earlier work, although Cattier, in his Response à Monsieur Papin, 1651, protests that he had not been aware of Papin's work when he prepared his Discours.
Bound with [Cattier, I.] Divers traictez. 1651.

— *See* CATTIER, I. Divers traictez. 1651; DIGBY, *Sir* K. Discours fait en une celebre assemblée. 1673, 1681; MOHY, H. Pulvis sympatheticus. 1640?

PAPIUS. *See* PAPE.

PAPIUS AHALSOSSA. *See* PAPE, Johann [1558-1622]

PAPKE, JOHANN ALBERT [*fl.* 1676] *respondent. See*
CONRING, H., *praeses.* Disputatio medica inauguralis
de peripneumonia. 1676; MEIBOM, H., *praeses.* Exercitatio medica de suppressione urinae. 1676.

PARACELSUS [1493-1541]
Collected works are placed first;
other works are arranged according to Sudhoff.

—Erster [-zehender] theil der Bücher und Schriff-
ten . . . jetzt auffs new . . . an Tag geben: durch
Joannem Huserum Brigosium . . . Franckfort am
Meyn, Gedruckt bey Joh. Wechels Erben, 1603.
     10 parts in 3 vols.   illus., table.   25 cm.
                                                        [8556]
     Imperfect: title page of part 8 (vol. 3) wanting.
     Sudhoff 254-255.
     Each part has separate title page. Parts 1-[2] have continuous
     pagination. Part 5 includes commentaries on a number of Hip-
     pocrates' Aphorismi, taken from books 1-2 and 4 (p. 81-104).

—Opera Bücher und Schrifften . . . mit . . . ihren
. . . eigener handgeschriebenen Originalien colla-
cioniert, vergliechen, verbessert und durch Joannem
Huserum Brisgoium . . . in Truck gegeben. Jetzt von
newem . . . ubersehen, auch mit etlichen bisshero
unbekandten Tractaten gemehrt . . . Strassburg, In
Verlegung Lazari Zetzners, 1603.
     2 v. in 1.   illus., tables.   35 cm.   **[8557]**
     Sudhoff 256-257.
     Based on the 1589-1590 Huser edition.

—[The same.] . . . Strassburg, In Velegung [sic]
Lazari Zetzners seligen Erben, 1616.
     [12], 1127, [53] p.   tables.   34 cm.   **[8558]**
     Vol. 2 wanting.
     Sudhoff 300.
     Reprint of 1603 ed.

—Operum medico chimicorum; sive, Paradox-
orum, tomus genuinus primus [-undecimus] . . .
Recenter Latine factus . . . Francofurto, A Collegio
Musarum Palthenianarum, 1603-1605.
     11 v. in 4.   illus., ports.   25 cm.   **[8559]**
     Sudhoff 259-263, 269-274.
     Edited by Zacharias Palthenius.
     Translation based on the 1589-1590 Huser edition.
     With vol. 4 of this is bound *his* Bertheonea. 1603

—Opera omnia medico-chemico-chirurgica, tribus
voluminibus comprehensa. Ed. novissima et emendatissima, ad Germanica & Latina exemplaria accuratissime collata: variis tractatibus & opusculis . . .
locupletata . . . Volumen primum [-tertium]

Genevae, Sumptibus Joan. Antonii, & Samuelis De
Tournes, 1658.
     3 v.   port (front.), illus.   34 cm.   **[8560]**
     Sudhoff 381-383.
     Edited by Friedrich Bitiskius.

—La grand chirurgie . . . trad. en francois de la
version latine de Josquin d'Alhem . . . par Claude
Dariot . . . Plus, un Discours de la goutte & causes
d'icelle, avec sa guerison. Item: III traictez de la
preparation des medicamens . . . Nouvellement
reveu & mis en lumiere par ledit Dariot. 2. ed. Lyon,
Antoine de Harsy, 1603.
     14, [1], 301, [7] p.; 207 p.; 51 p.   illus., tables.   25
cm.   **[8561]**
     Sudhoff 253.
     "Trois discours (i.e traictez) de la preparation des medicamens"
     and "Discours de la goutte," both by Claude Dariot, have special
     title pages.
     "La Grand Chirurgie" is a translation of Paracelsus' Grosse Wun-
     darzney, published in 1573.

—Chirurgische Bücher und Schrifften . . . jetzt
auffs new auss den originalen . . . Handschrifften . . .
an Tag geben . . . sambt einem Appendice etlicher
nutzlicher Tractat . . . Durch Johannem Huserum
. . . Strassburg, In Verlegung Latzari [sic] Zetzners,
1605.
     [16], 680, [42], 115, [7] p.   illus., port.   33 cm.
                                                        [8562]
     Sudhoff 267.
     Ander-, Dritter-, Vierdter Theil and Appendix have special ti-
     tle pages.
     Based on the 1589-1590 Huser edition.

—La grand chirurgie . . . trad. en francois de la
version latine de Josquin d'Alhem . . . par Claude
Dariot . . . Plus, un Discours de la goutte & causes
d'icelle, avec sa guerison. Item: III traitez de la
preparation des medicamens . . . 3. ed. Montbeliart,
Jaques Foillet, 1608
     [16], 280, [6] p.; 51 p.; 162 (i.e. 192) p.   illus.,
tables.   18 cm.   **[8563]**
     Sudhoff 279.
     "Trois Discours de la preparation des medicamens" and "Discours
     de la goutte" have special title pages.

—Bertheonea; sive, Chirurgia minor. Cum tractatibus ejusdem: De apostematibus, syronibus &
nodis. De cutis apertionibus. De vulnerum &
ulcerum curis. De vermibus, serpentibus, ac maculis

a nativitate ortis ... Francofurti, Prostat Paltheniano, 1603.

    [4], 327 (i.e. 227), [12] p.   25 cm.   **[8564]**
Sudhoff 258.
Bound with vol. 4 of *his* Operum medico-chimicorum. 1603–1605.

—Zween underschiedene Tractat: I. Von dess
Harns und Puls Urtheil ... II. Von den Gradibus
unnd Compositionibus der Recepten und natürlichen
Dingen ... Auss dem fünfften und siebendem Theyl
seiner Operum in quarto zu Basel getruckt von ...
I. C. K. Chirurgo A. R. durch einem Magistirum
... zu verteutschen verordnet ... und nun erst lateinischer Sprachen unerfahrnen zum besten in offentlichen Truck publicieret durch Benedictum
Figulum [i.e. Benedict Toepfer] ... Strassburg, In
Verlegung Lazari Zetzners, 1608.

    303 p.   tables.   17 cm.   **[8565]**
Sudhoff 285.
Translation of De urinarum, and De gradibus, as published in
Johan Huser's edition, Bücher und Schrifften, 1589–1590.

—Dat secreet der philosophien, inhoudende
hoemen alle aertsche dingen, gelijck als alluyn, solfer,
coperroot ende diergelijcken bereyden sal ende
gebruycken ... Altesamen getogen wt die boecken
Paracelsi, door ... Philippus Hermanni ... Leyden,
Uldrick Cornelissz ende Joris Abramsz, 1612.

    [3], xxvii, [2] ll. illus. 15 cm.   **[8566]**
Sudhoff 292.
The book is really by the alleged compiler, Hermanni, who has
used Paracelsus' name to boost his own work. Cf. Sudhoff 31.
Bound with Follinus, H. Den Nederlandtsche sleutel. 1613.

—De peste ... tractatus, so er an die Statt Störtz-
zingen geschrieben ... cum commentariis Jobi
Kornthaueri ... Oppenheim, Gedruckt bey
Hieronymo Gallern, in Verlegung Johan-Theodor de
Bry, 1613.

    123 p.   table. 20 cm.   **[8567]**
Sudhoff 293.

—Chirurgische Bücher und Schrifften ... jetzt
auffs new auss den originalen ... Handschrifften ...
an Tag geben ... sambt einem Appendice etlicher
nutzlicher Tractat ... Durch Johannem Huserum
Brisgoium ... Strassburg, In Verlegung Lazari Zetzners S. Erben, 1618.

    [12], 795, [39] p. illus., port. 31 cm.
                                        [8568]
Sudhoff 302.
Ander-, Dritter-, Vierdter Theil and Appendix have special title
pages.
Imperfect: p. 737–738 wanting.

—Philosophia de limbo, aeterno perpetuoque
homine novo secundae creationis ex Jesu Christo ...
Publicirt durch Joannem Staricium ... Magdeburg,
Johan Francken, 1618.

    [24], 159 p. 19 cm.   **[8569]**
Sudhoff 303.

—Theophrastische Practica; das ist, Ausserlesene
Theophrastische Medicamenta, beneben eigentlicher
Beschreibung derer Praeparation: auch richtigem
Nutz und Gebrauch, weyland durch Herren Gerhard
Dorn, in lateinischer Sprache beschrieben, ins
Teutsch versetzt, und nunmehr in Druck befördert
durch Michaelem Horingium ... [Halle] Gedruckt
bey Peter Schmidt, in Vorlegung Michael
Oelschlägels, 1618.

    [8], 491 (i.e. 493), [11] p. 15 cm.   **[8570]**
Sudhoff 305.
Translation of Fasciculus Paracelsicae medicinae.

—La petite chirurgie; autrement ditte, La ber-
theonee ... Plus les traittez du mesme autheur, des
apostemes syrons ou noeuds, des ouvertures du cuir,
des ulceras, des vers, serpens, taches ou marques qui
viennent de naissance, & des contractures ... Avec
notes ... par Daniel du Vivier ... Paris, Oliver de
Varennes, 1623.

    [52], 752 p. 18 cm.   **[8571]**
Translation of *his* Chirurgia minor, published in Frankfurt in
1603.
Sudhoff 323; Sudhoff(B) 520.

—Clavis; oder, Das zehende Buch der Archidox-
en ... Wie auch desselben Manualis Aussanlegung,
sampt noch andern vortrefflichen grossen Arcanis.
Biss anhero noch in grosser Geheimb gehalten,
nunmehr aber ... ans Tagelicht gegeben, durch
Joann. Staricium ... Magdeburg, Bey Johann
Francken, 1624.

    [68] p. 19 cm.   **[8572]**
Sudhoff 328.
"Ausslegung des Manuals ... Paracelsi" has special title page
(p. [29])
The text is different from the tenth book published in the 1570
Strasbourg edition of the Archidoxa.

—De kleyne chirurgie, ende, 't Gast-huys boeck
... Nu eerst uyt den Hoodh-duytsche in onse
Nederlandsche sprake over-geset, door M. Everaert
B[ruggeling] Utrecht, Amelis Janssz, 1629.

    [184, 64] p. 15 cm.   **[8573]**
Signatures: A–P⁸, Q⁴.
Sudhoff 332.

A translation of Drei Bücher von Wunder und Schaden, first published in 1563, reprinted from edition published in Antwerp by Hans de Laet, 1568

—Coelum philosophorum sive Liber vexationum. *In* Glauber, J. R. Operis mineralis. 1651. Sudhoff 366.

—One hundred and fourteen experiments and cures, of . . . Theophrastus Paracelsus. Whereunto is added certain excellent works, by B. G. a Portu Aquitano [i.e. B. G. Penot] Also certain secrets of Isaac Hollandus, concerning the vegetall and animal work. Likewise the Spagyrick antidotary for gunshot, by Josephus Quirsitanus [i.e. Duchesne] London, G. D[awson] 1652.

[12], 75 p. vol. 4. 19 cm. (*In* Fioravanti, Leonardo. Three exact pieces . . . Whereunto is annexed Paracelsus his One hundred and fourteen experiments . . . London, 1652) **[8574]**
Sudhoff 370.
Reprint of the edition published in London in 1596, but without J. Hester's dedication to Sir Walter Raleigh.

—Dispensatory and chirurgery; the Dispensatory contains the choisest of his physical remedies; and all that can be desired of his Chirurgery, you have in the Treatises of wounds, ulcers, and aposthumes. Faithfully Englished by W. D. [i.e. William Dugard?] London, Printed by T. M. for Philip Chetwind, 1656.

[24], 407 p. 14 cm. **[8575]**
Sudhoff 376.

—Of the chymical transmutation, genealogy and generation of metals & minerals; also, Of the urim and thummim of the Jews; with, an Appendix of the vertues and use of an excellent water made by Dr. Trigge. The 2d part of the mumial treatise [of Tentzelius], whereunto is added, Philosophical and chymical experiments of . . . Raymond Lully . . . Transl. . . . by r. Turner . . . London, Rich. Moon and Hen. Fletcher, 1657.

[8], 166 p. 17 cm. **[8576]**
Sudhoff 379.
"Philosophical and chymical experiments, London, James Cottrel, 1657" (p. [35]-166) has special title page.

—Archidoxis, comprised in ten books, disclosing the genuine way of making quintessences, arcanums, magisteries, elixirs, &c. Together with his books, Of renovation and restoration . . . And finally his seven books, Of the degrees and compositions of receipts, and natural things . . . Englished, and published by

J[ohn] H[arding] . . . London, Printed for W. S., and sold by Thomas Brewster, 1660.
[8], 158, [2], 171, [1] p. 15 cm. **[8577]**
Sudhoff 392.

—Another issue, with imprint: London, Printed for W. S., and sold by Samuel Thompson, 1661.
Title page reset: varies. **[8578]**
Sudhoff 393.

—Another issue, with imprint: London, Printed for Lodowick Lloyd, 1663.
Title page reset: varies. **[8579]**
Sudhoff 395.

—Erklärung über etliche Aphorismen des Hippokrates. Italian. *In* Locatelli, L. Theatro d'arcani . . . nel quale si tratta dell'arte chimica. 1644, 1667.
Sudhoff 361, 397.

—Liber de occulta philosophia. Auss einem uhralten Tractat wegen seiner einhabenden Hochwichtigkeiten von neuem hervor gebracht, und . . . zum offenen Druck befördert von einem unbekanten Philosopho. [n. p.] 1686.
[2], 86 p. 13 cm. **[8580]**
Sudhoff 420.
A reprint of the last treatise in *his* Archidoxa . . . von Heymligkeiten der Natur, published in 1570 and edited by Michael Toxites.

—[Excerpts] *In* Burggrav, J. E. Biolychnium. 1611; Dolhopff, G. A., comp. Lapis animalis microcosmicus. 1681 [and] Lapis vegetabilis. 1681; Glauber, J. R. Miraculum mundi; oder, Ausführliche Beschreibung der wunderbaren Natur. 1653; Penot, B. G. [Quaestiones tres de corporali mercurio] 1659.

—[Vita] *See* JOHNSON, W. Lexicon chymicum. 1660, 1678.
Sudhoff 391, 409.

—*See* CARDILUCIUS, J. H., ed. Magnalia medicochymica. 1676; CONRING, H. De Hermetica . . . medicina liber unus. 1648 [and] De Hermetica . . . medicina libri duo. 1669 [and] CROLL, O. Philosophy reformed & improved. 1657; DÖRING, M. De medicina et medicis adversus iatromastigas et pseudiatros libri II. 1611; DOLÄUS, J. Encyclopaedia chirurgica rationalis. 1689, 1690, 1695 [and] Encyclopaedia, medicinae theoretico-practicae. 1684, 1686, 1688, 1690, 1691 [and] Opera omnia. 1695 [and]

Systema medicinale, a compleat system of physick. 1686; DORN, G. [Clavis totius philosophiae chemisticae. 1659.]; Fioravanti, L. Three exact pieces of Leonard Phioravant. 1652; GLAUBER, J.R. The works. 1689; GOCKEL, E. Enchiridion medicopracticum de peste. 1669; GREIFF, S. Wundartzeney. 1622; GREMBS, F. O. Arbor integra et ruinosa homminis. 1657; 1671; HEADRICH, J. Arcana philosophica; or, Chymical secrets. 1697; HÉRY, T. de. La methode curatoire de la maladie venerienne. 1634; HESTER, J. The secrets of physick and philosophy. 1633; KHUNRATH, H. De igne magorum philosophorumque secreto externo. 1608; LIBAVIUS, A. [d. 1616] Appendix necessaria Syntagmatis arcanorum chymicorum. 1615; PARTLIZ, S. A new method of physick. 1654; POPPE, J. Thesaurus medicinae. 1628 [and] Von der gifftigen epidemischen Hauptkranckheit. 1623 [and] Von der Wassersucht und dero Zufällen. 1623; RHENANUS, J. Solis e puteo emergentis. 1613; ROLFINCK, W. Ordo et methodus cognoscendi & curandi febres generalis. 1658; SENDIVOGIUS, M. A new light of alchymie. 1650, 1674; SENNERT, D. De chymicorum cum Aristotelicis et Galenicis consensu ac dissensu liber. 1629, 1655; SØRENSEN, P. Idea medicinae philosophicae. 1660; SUCHTEN, a. von. Chymische Schrifften. 1680; TENTZEL, A. Medicina diastatica. 1629, 1666.

A PARADOX. *See* LESSIUS, L. The temperate man. 1678.

PARAVICINO, FABRIZIO [*ca.* 1631-1695] Abuso de medici nel medicare gl'absenti infermi . . . Milano, Carlo Federico Gagliardi, 1694.

95 p.   19 cm.   [8581]

PARAVICINO, GIOVANNI PIETRO [*fl.* 1648] Avertimenti sopra li bagni del Masino, overo di S. Martino per valersene internamente, & esternamente . . . Milano, Gio. Pietro Cardi, 1649.

[50], 308, [2] p.   13 cm.   [8582]

— Assertiones in usu aquarum thermalium Masini Sancti Martini in Valletellina . . . Novocomi, Ex officina Pauli Antonii Caprani, 1678.

44 p.   14 cm.   [8583]

Extract from *his* Avertimenti sopra li bagni del Masino. 1649.

PARCOV, FRANZ [1560-1611] *praeses.* De angina . . . Helmaestadii, Ex officina typographica Jacobi Lucii, 1610.

[20] p.   20 cm.   [8584]

Diss. — Helmstedt (G. Hurlebusch, *respondent*)

PARDO, JERÓNIMO [*fl.* 1661-1688] Tratado del vino aguado, y agua envinada, sobre el Aforismo 56. de la seccion 7. de Hipocrates . . . Valladolid, Valdivielso, 1661.

[44], 145, [20] p.   21 cm.   [8585]

PARDOUX, BARTHÉLEMY [1545-1611] Bartholomaei Perdulcis . . . Ars sanitatis tuendae. Parisiis, Apud Ludovic. Boullenger & Joannem Becodianum, 1637.

[20], 239 p.   15 cm.   [8586]

Edited by Guillaume Sauvageon.

First published in 1630 as Book 4 of Pardoux's Universa medicina.

—Bartholomaei Perdulcis . . . In Jac. Sylvii anatomen et in lib. Hippocratis De natura humana commentarii nunc primum prodeunt ex bibliotheca Gabrielis Naudaei. Parisiis, Apud Herveum du Mesnil & Olivarium de Varennes, 1643.

[4], 56 p.   24 cm.   [8587]

Bound with Cabrol, Barthélemy. Ἀλφαβητον ἀνατομιχον; hoc est, Anatomes elenchus. 1604.

—Bartholomaei Perdulcis . . . Universa medicina, ex medicorum principum sententiis consiliisque collecta, a Renato Charterio . . . emendata, digesta, ac in lucem primum edita. Adjecta est Bartholomaei Perdulcis vita . . . Parisiis, Apud Mathurinum Henault, 1630.

[32], 943 (i.e. 944), [28] p.   25 cm.   [8588]

Vita of Pardoux by René Moreau.

Book 7, Ars chirurgica, by Étienne Gourmelen, was originally published in Paris, in 1580.

—[The same.] . . . Ed. 2., studio & opera G. Sauvageon . . . Aggregati . . . ex autoris autographo, aucta, & ubique emendata. Cui etiam accessit De morbis animi liber. Parisiis, Apud Olivarium de Varennes, 1640.

[26], 944, [28] p.; [12], 73, [1] p.   23 cm.   [8589]

Part [2] De morbis animi has special title page with imprint: Parisiis, Ludovic. Boullenger, 1639.

—[The same.] . . . Ed. postrema . . . Lugduni, Sumptibus Jacobi Carteron, 1649.

[24], 944, [27] p.; [10] p. 72 p.   24 cm.   [8590]

De morbis animi has special title page.

—[The same.] . . . Lugduni, Typis Simonis Rigaud, 1650.

[30], 944, [27] p.; [4], 71, [1] p.   24 cm.   [8591]

Different setting of type.

De morbis animi has special title page.

PARÉ, Ambroise [1510?–1590] Les oeuvres ... Divisees en vingt-neuf livres. Avec les figures & portraicts, tant de l'anatomie que des instruments de chirurgie, & de plusieurs monstres. 7. ed. Rev. & augm, en divers endroicts. Paris, Nicolas Buon, 1614.

[26], 1228, [113] p.   port.   37 cm.   **[8592]**

Doe 35.

The book was presented to Gilbert Breschet [1784–1845] in 1806 in the name of Emperor Napoleon I by his minister of interior as first prize in surgery at the medical school of Paris.

—[The same.] ... 8. ed. Rev. & corr. en plusieurs endroicts, & augm. d'un fort ample Traicté des fiebures, tant en general qu'en particulier, & de la curation d'icelles, nouvellement treuvé dans les manuscrits de l'autheur. Avec les portraicts & figures tant de l'anatomie que des instruments de chirurgie, & de plusieurs monstres. Paris, Nicolas Buon, 1628.

[25], 1320, [113] p.   illus., ports.   35 cm.   **[8593]**

Added engraved title page.

Doe 37.

—[The same.] ... Lyon, La vefve de Claude Rigaud et Claude Obert, 1633.

[24], 986 (i.e. 988), [107] p.   illus., ports.   38 cm.   **[8594]**

Doe 38.

—[The same.] ... Lyon, La vefve de Claude Rigaud, & Pierre Rigaud fils, 1641.

[24], 846 (i.e. 854), [80] p.   illus., ports.   36 cm.   **[8595]**

Doe 41.

—[The same.] ... Avec les voyages qu'il a faits en divers lieux: et les pourtraits & figures, tant de l'anatomie que des instruments de chirurgie, & de plusieurs monstres. Lyon, Pierre Rigaud, 1652.

[24], 846 (i.e. 854), [80] p.   illus., ports.   35 cm.   **[8596]**

Doe 42.

Imperfect: signature [é6] and p. [75–76] wanting.

Different setting of type.

—[The same.] ... 12. ed. rev. ... Lyon, Jean Gregoire, 1664.

[16], 852, [74] p.   illus., ports.   38 cm.   **[8597]**

Doe 43.

—[The same.] ... 13. ed. ... Lyon, Pierre Valfray, 1685.

[12], 808, [60] p.   illus., ports.   37 cm.   **[8598]**

Doe 44.

—[Dutch tr.] De chirurgie, ende alle de opera ofte wercken van Mr. Ambrosius Paré ... Nu eerst uyt de Fransoysche, in onse gemeyne Nederlantsche sprake, ende uyt de 4. ed. ... overgheset ... door D. Carolum Battum ... Amsterdam, Hendrick Laurenszoon, 1615.

[16], 940, [10] p.   illus.   35 cm.   **[8599]**

Imperfect? last leaf (blank?) wanting.

Doe 60.

—[The same.] ... Rotterdam, De weduwe van Matthijs Bastiaensz, 1636.

[16], 940, [12] p.   illus.   32 cm.   **[8600]**

Doe 63.

Different setting of type.

—[The same.] ... Amstelredam, J. J. Schipper, 1649.

[12], 940, [11] p.   illus.   33 cm.   **[8601]**

Doe 65.

Different setting of type.

—[The same.] ... Amstelredam, Jan Fredericksz Stam, 1655.

[12], 940, [11] p.   illus.   33 cm.   **[8602]**

Doe 67.

Different setting of type.

—[English tr.] The workes of ... Ambrose Parey translated out of Latine and compared with the French by Th. Johnson ... London, Th. Cotes and R. Young, 1634.

[14], 487, 553–1083, 1093–1173, [22] p.   illus., ports.   34 cm.   **[8603]**

Signatures: 1 leaf unsigned, C^2, A^4, B–$2S^6$, $2T^4$, 3A–$4V^6$, 4X–$4Y^4$, $4Z^6$, 5A–$5E^6$, $5F^4$, 5G–$5H^6$.

Engraved title page.

Doe 51.

—[The same.] ... Whereunto are added three tractates out of Adrianus Spigelius of the veines, arteries, & nerves ... London, Printed by Richard Cotes and Willi Dugard and sold by John Clarke, 1649.

[22], 388, 773 (i.e. 787), [8] p.; [4], 50, [1] p.   illus., ports.   34 cm.   **[8604]**

Imperfect: p. 593–594 wanting; 2 lines of text cut from p. 733–734.

Doe 52.

Engraved title page.

"'Αγγειολογία: or, A description of the vessels in the body of man ... translated out of the anatomie of Adrianus Spigelius [by J. G.]" has special title page and separate paging.

—[The same.] ... London, Printed by E. C. and sold by John Clarke, 1665.

[20], 778 (i.e. 764) p.; [4], 50, [14] p. illus., ports. 33 cm. **[8605]**

Imperfect: 6th prelim. leaf, p. 97-520, 681-682, 685-686, and last leaf (sig. 4G6) wanting.

Engraved title page.

Doe 53.

—[The same.] ... London, Printed by Mary Clark, and sold by John Clark, 1678.

[20], 713 p.; [4], 44, [17] p. illus., ports. 38 cm. **[8606]**

Doe 54.

—[German tr.] Wundt Artzney, oder Artzney Spiegell ... Von Petro Uffenbach ... auss der lateinischen Edition Jacobi Guillemeau ... in die teutsche Sprach ... gesetzt ... Franckfurt am Mayn, Gedruckt bey Zacharia Palthenio, in Verlegung Peter Fischers s. Erben, 1601.

[16], 1239, [16] p. illus., ports. 34 cm. **[8607]**

Imperfect: p. 949-972, 1127-1128, 1217-1218, 1221-1222 wanting.

Doe 56.

—[The same.] ... Nun zum andernmal in Truck verfertiget und an vielen Orten verbessert ... Franckfurt am Mayn, Gedruckt bey Caspar Rötell, in Verlegung Jacob Fischers s. Erben, 1635.

[16], 984, [31] p. illus., ports. 35 cm. **[8608]**

Doe 57.

—See CROOKE, H. Μικροκοσμογραφία. A description of the body of man. 1631 [and] Σωματογραφια ανθρωπινη; or, A description of the body of man. 1616, 1634; GOURMELEN, É. Les oeuvres chirurgicales. 1647; UFFENBACH, P. Thesaurus chirurgicae. 1610.

PARENT, ABRAHAM [*fl.* 1651-1655] Anatomisch vertoon van het ghehoor by ... Louys de Bils ... aen ons onderschreven [i.e. Abraham Parent and Laurens Jordaen] gedaen, ende in dese by-gaende plaetjens den liefhebbers ghemeyn ghemaeckt. Brugghe, Lucas vanden Kerchobe, 1655.

7 p. illus. 20 cm. **[8609]**

—See BILS, L. de. Specimina anatomica. 1661; RAEDT, F. de. Anatomische beschrijvinge van een wanschepsel. 1659.

PARENT, DANIEL [*fl.* 1675] *respondent.* Disputatio medica inauguralis de apoplexia ... Lugduni

Batavorum, Apud viduam & heredes Johannis Elsevirii, 1675.

[12] p. 22 cm. **[8610]**

Diss. – Leyden.

PARERE dell'almo Collegio de Spetiali di Napoli. 1640. *See* COLLEGIO DEGLI SPEZIALI, Naples.

PARIGI, LORENZO [*fl.* 1616-1618] Dialogo primo [-terzo] sopra alcune cose di medicina, alla state appartenenti ... Firenze, Zanobi Pignoni, 1618.

16 p.; 17 p.; 23 p. 22 cm. **[8611]**

Parts 2 and 3 have special title pages.

PARIS. Assemblée charitable. *See* ASSEMBLÉE CHARITABLE À PARIS.

PARIS. Bureau d'adresse. CONFÉRENCES. *See* CONFERENCES DU BUREAU D'ADRESSE, Paris.

PARIS. Collège des maîtres chirurgiens jurés. *See* COLLÈGE DES MAÎTRES CHIRURGIENS JURÉS DE PARIS.

PARIS. Faculté de médecine. *See* UNIVERSITÉ DE PARIS. FACULTÉ DE MÉDECINE.

PARIS. Hôpital général. *See* HÔPITAL GÉNÉRAL, Paris. L'Hospital general de Paris. 1676.

PARIS. Université. FACULTÉ DE MÉDECINE. *See* UNIVERSITÉ DE PARIS. Faculté de médecine.

PARISIANO, EMILIO [1567-1643] Lapis Lydius de diagphragmate ad Joh. Riolan. *See* RIOLAN, J. [1580-1657] Opera anatomica vetera. 1650 [and] Opuscula anatomica nova. 1649.

—Nobilium exercitationum libri duodecim, de subtilitate ... Accessit Par & sanius judicium, de seminis a toto proventu, ac de stigmatibus. Venetiis, Apud Evangelistam Deuchinum, 1623-33.

[26], 678 (i.e. 684), [4] p. illus., port. 32 cm. **[8612]**

Imperfect: 9 preliminary leaves including half title, prefatory note, privilege, laudatory poems, portrait; and at end: Syllabus auctorum and indexes for p. 1-566 wanting.

Special title page dated 1633 (with dedicatory epistle) inserted between p. 566 and 567 reads: Par et sanius judicium de seminis a toto proventu ac de stigmatibus.

—[The same.] ... [Pars una]-quarta. Venetiis, Apud Evangelistam Deuchinum, 1623-43.

4 v. ([26], 566, [30] p.; 521, [25] p.; [6], 208 p.; [12], 60, [12], 39, [4] p.) illus., port. 32 cm. **[8613]**

Vol. 2 has title: Pars altera De diaphragmate singularis certaminis lapis Lydius ... Venetiis, Apud Marcum Antonium Bregiolum, 1635. "De cordis et sanguinis motu singularis certaminis lapis Lydius. Ad Guilielmum Harveum" (p. [383]-521) with half title, includes the text, almost complete, of William Harvey's De motu cordis with Parisano's commentary.

Vol. 3 has title: Pars tertia. De seminis a toto proventu, de principiis generationis, singularis certaminis lapis Lydius ... De visione ... Venetiis, Apud Junctas, 1638. The "De visione" mentioned on the title page does not seem to have been included.

Vol. 4 has half title: Pars quarta. Microcosmi salus cosmica subtilitas. [Liber unus]-secundus. [Venetiis, Apud heredes Joan. Salis, 1643]

—Oratio. In hominis et anatomes laudem Venetiis publice habita ad augustissimum medicorum Venetum collegium. Venetiis, Aere Bartholomei Magni, 1612.

10 l.   21 cm.   [8614]

—See ENT, Sir G. Apologia pro circuitione sanguinis. 1685 [and] Opera omnia medico-physica. 1687; HARVEY, W. De motu cordis. 1639, 1674; MONDINI, M. Ad disputationem de genitura. 1625.

PARISH CLERKS' COMPANY, London. See LONDON. Company of Parish Clerks.

PARISI, LORENZO. See PARIGI, Lorenzo [fl. 1616-1618]

PARISI, PIETRO [d. 1620] Aggiunta a gli Avvertimenti sopra la peste ... per l'occasione della peste de Malta gli anni del sig. 1592, 1593, infino all'anno 1603 ... Con un breve Discorso sopra il medicamento di vino & oglio per guarire ogni sorte di ferite ... Palermo, Gio. Antonio de Franceschi, 1603.

[8], 202, [49] p.   22 cm.   [8615]

—Brief discours du docteur Pierre Paris ... touchant le medicament du vin & de l'huile, pour guarir toutes sortes de blessures. Trad. de nouveau en françois. Paris, François Jacquin, 1607.

[28], 49 p.   17 cm.   [8616]

Translation of Breve discorso sopra il medicamento di vino e olio, first published in Palermo, in 1603.

Dedicatory epistle signed by the translator, F. P. P. R.

PARISIENSIS, CHRISTOPHORUS. See CHRISTOPHORUS PARISIENSIS [13th cent.]

PARISIUS [fl. 1620] Consilia medicinalia de conservanda sanitate, et proprie corporum, quorum caput & stomachus ab aequali, ad intensam declinant humiditatem ... Auctore D. Aparisiis, Neapolitano.

Edinburgi, Excudebat Thomas Finlason, 1620.

[8], 48 p.   illus.   20 cm.   [8617]

"Rationes brevissimae contra antimonium" (p. [34]-48) has half title.

STC 698a.

PÁRIZ, FERENC, pápai. See PÁPAI PÁRIZ, Ferenc [1649-1716]

PARKER, SAMUEL, Bp. of Oxford [1640-1688] See FAIRFAX, N. A treatise of the bulk and selvedge of the world. 1674.

PARKINSON, JOHN [1567-1650] Paradisi in sole paradisus terrestris; or, A garden of all sorts of pleasant flowers which our English ayre will permitt to be noursed up ... together with the right orderinge, planting & preserving of them and their uses & vertues ... [London, Humfrey Lownes and Robert Young] 1629.

[12], 612 [16] p.   illus., port.   32 cm.   [8618]

Engraved title page.
Hunt 215.
Henrey, v. 1, no. 282.
STC 19300.

—[The same.] ... The 2d impr. much corr. and enl. London, Printed by R. N., and sold by R. Thrale, 1656.

[12], 612, [16] p.   illus.   32 cm.   [8619]

Added engraved title page.
Imperfect: title page wanting.
Different setting of type.
Hunt 267.

—Theatrum botanicum: the theater of plants; or, An herball of a large extent ... distributed into sundry classes or tribes, for the more easie knowledge of the many herbes of one nature and property, with the chief notes of Dr. Lobel, Dr. Bonham, and others inserted therein ... London, Tho. Cotes, 1640.

[16], 1756 (i.e. 1746), [2] p.   illus.   35 cm. [8620]

Added engraved title page.
Imperfect: sig. 7H6-7I6 wanting.
Hunt 235.
STC 19302.

—See L'OBEL, M. de. Stirpium illustrationes. 1655.

PARMA, IPPOLITO. Praxis chirurgica, in qua omnes operationes ex usu artis ad caput spectantes, delucide & exquisite ad mentem Hippocr. describuntur, nec non & ejusdemmet Hippocratis libellus De capitis vulneribus commentariis illustratur . . . Venetiis, Apud Evangelistam Deuchinum & Joan. Baptistam Pulcianum. 1608.

[16], 166 p.   16 cm.   [8621]

Includes Latin text of the De capitis vulneribus in Janus Cornarius' translation.

PARMAN, NIKOLAUS [*fl.* 1618] *respondent.* Problemata medica . . . Basileae, Typis Joan. Jacobi Genathii [1618]

[8] p.   22 cm.   [8622]

Diss. — Basel.

Le PARNASSE assiegé; ou, La guerre declarée entre les philosophes anciens & modernes. Lyon, Antoine Boudet, 1697.

[14], 140, [8] p.   14 cm.   [8623]

The permit is granted to Sieur F. A. D. M.

PAROLINI, ANTONIO MARIA [*d.* 1588] Trattato della peste . . . Diviso in tre parti: Nella prima si tratta della natura, cause, e segni della peste. Nella seconda del preservarsi dalla peste. Nella terza della curatione d'essa . . . Ferrara, Francesco Suzzi, 1630.

[7], 82, [1] p.   20 cm.   [8624]

PARR, THOMAS [1483?-1635] *See* BETTS, J. De ortu et natura sanguinis. 1669.

PARRA Y AREVALO, ALFONSO GOMEZ DE LA. *See* GÓMEZ DE LA PARRA Y ARÉVALO, Alfonso [*fl.* 1621]

PARRUCCA, RAINERO. *See* PERUCA, Rainero [*fl.* 1652]

PARTENIO, FRANCESCO, *pseud. See* ROCCO, Michele [*fl.* 1646]

PARTHON, GUILLAUME [*fl. ca.* 1657] *ed. See* THÉVENIN, F. Les oeuvres. 1658, 1669, 1691.

PARTICULARE ex universali; oder, Kurtzer Entwurff einer sonderbahren Artzney, so auch in denen gefährlichsten Kranckheiten Wunder thut, deren hoch-ansehnlichen dess H. Röm. Reichs Academicorum Naturae Curiosorum, wie auch gesamten der grösten Kunst besitzern, und Liebhabern Judicio unterworffen. Von einem der die That eines wahren Philosophi mit Namen führet. Augsburg, Joh. Schönig, 1677.

131, [1] p.   15 cm.   [8625]

PARTIUM humani corporis, quae sine anatome sub sensu cadunt, icnographia [sic], et nominatio . . . Bononiae, Typis Josephi Longi, 1673.

broadside.   54 x 39 cm.   [8626]

PARTLICIUS, SIMEON. *See* PARTLIZ, Simeon [*fl.* 1620-1624]

PARTLIZ, SIMEON [*fl.* 1620-1624] Medici systematis harmonici, in quo nova plane et artificiosa discendae et exercendae medicinae methodus, per praecepta brevia traditur, canones selectos illustratur, commentaria dilucida explicatur . . . Francofurti, Sumptibus Danielis & Davidis Aubriorum & Clementis Schleichii, 1625.

[16], 299, [14] p.   tables.   15 cm.   [8627]

—[English tr.] A new method of physick; or, A short view of Paracelsus and Galen's practice, in 3 treatises: I. Opening the nature of physick and alchymy; II. Shewing what things are requisite to a physician and alchymist; III. Containing an harmonical systeme of physick. Trans. . . . by Nicholas Culpeper . . . London, Printed by Peter Cole and sold by S. Howes, J. Garfield and B. Westbrook, 1654.

[17], 548 (i.e. 348) p.   14 cm.   [8628]

Imperfect: sig. A3-4 and B1 wanting? p. 53-60, 101-102 wanting.

—Officiarium magistratus, medicorum, amicorum; pictura justitiae, Aesculapi, amicitiae . . . Erfurti, Typis Philippi Witelli, impens. Johan. Birckneri [1624]

[3], 45 p.   illus.   12 cm.   [8629]

PARTRIDGE, JOHN [1644-1715] *tr. See* MYNSICHT, A. von. Thesaurus & armamentarium medicochymicum. 1682.

PASCAL, BLAISE [1623-1662] Traitez de l'equilibre des liqueurs, et de la pesanteur de la masse de l'air. Contenant l'explication des causes de divers effets de la nature qui n'avoient point esté bien connus jusques ici, & particulierement de ceux que l'on avoit attribuez à l'horreur du vuide. Par monsieur Pascal. Paris, Guillaume Desprez, 1663.

[28], 232, [7] p.   illus., plates.   15 cm.

[8630]

PASCAL, JACQUES [*fl.* 1607] Traicté contenant la pharmacie chymique, ou spagyrique, avec la Galenique, ou ordinaire; ensemble, la Demonstration des abus qui se commettent sur les principaux medicamens officinaux de l'apothicaire ordinaire; &, le Catalogue des medicamens à eux necessaire ... Lyon, Louys Vivian, 1633.

[48], 330, [3] p. table. 17 cm.   [8631]

Previously published under title: Discours contenant la pharmacie chymique.

PASCAL, JEAN [17th–18th cent.] La nouvelle découverte, et les admirables effets des fermens dans le corps humain, expliquez par des experiences & des raisonnemens tres solides ... Paris, Edme Couterot, 1681.

[24], 334 p. port. 15 cm.   [8632]

— Traité des eaux de Bourbon l'Archambaud selon les principes de la nouvelle physique ... Paris, Claude Jombert, 1699.

[14], 373, [5] p. plate. 16 cm.   [8633]

Original imprint covered with slip cancel.

PASCAL, PIERRE [fl. 1626–1630] Praxis medicinae de febribus. In qua methodo facillima dilucidissima-que omnium febrium cognitio & curatio traditur ... Lugduni Batavorum, Ex officina Joannis Maire, 1631.

181, [1] p. 17 cm. (Part [2] Bruele, Gualtherus. Praxis medicinae theorica et empirica familiarissima ... Lugduni Batavorum, 1647)   [8634]

— respondent. Disputatio medica inauguralis de febre vulgo ardente dicta ... Basileae, Typis Johan. Jacobi Genathii [1626]

[15] p. 18 cm.   [8635]

Errata: p. [15]
Diss. — Basel.

PASCALIUS, CAROLUS. See PASCHAL, Charles, vicomte de La Queute [1547–1625]

PASCH, GEORG [1661–1700] De novis inventis: quorum accuratiori cultui facem praetulit antiquitas, tractatus secundum ductum disciplinarum, facultatum atque artium in gratiam curiosi lectoris eoncinnatus. Ed. 2. ... Lipsiae, Sumptibus haeredum Joh. Grossi, 1700.

[20], 812, [125] p. front. 21 cm.   [8636]

Previously published in Kiel, in 1695, under title Schediasma de curiosa hujus seculi inventis.

— praeses. Dissertationem physicam de brutorum sensibus atque cognitione ... publice opponet ...

Jo. Jacobo Stolterfoht ... Wittenbergae, Typis C. Fincelii [1686]

[32] p. 19 cm.   [8637]

Diss. pro loco — Wittenberg (J. J. Stolterfoht, respondent)

PASCH, JOHANN [1661–1709] praeses. Gynaeceum doctum ... dispicit Joh. Andreas Planerus ... Wittenbergae, Typis Matthaei Henckelii [1686]

[64] p. 19 cm.   [8638]

Diss. — Wittenberg (J. A. Planer, respondent)

PASCHA, NIKOLAUS BENEDICT [1643–1704] praeses. Disputatio physica de quaestione an Esau fuerit monstrum ... Wittebergae, Literis Wendianis excudebat Daniel Schmatz, 1672.

[16] p. 19 cm.   [8639]

Diss. — Wittenberg (M. Pohl, respondent)

PASCHAL, CHARLES, vicomte de La Queute [1547–1625] Oratio pro medico. In Hafenreffer, S. Raphael artem medicam ... informans. 1622, 1629, 1642.

PASCHALIS, PETRUS. See PASCAL, Pierre [fl. 1626–1630]

PASCHALIUS, MICHAEL JOANNES. See PASCUAL, Miguel Juan [fl. 1532]

PASCHETTI, BARTOLOMEO [fl. 1578–1616] Del conservare la sanità, et del vivere de' Genovesi ... Libri tre: ne' quali si tratta di tutte le cose appartenenti alla conservatione della sanità di ciascuno in generale, & in particolare degli huomini, & donne genovesi ... Genova, Giuseppe Pavoni, 1602.

[16], 439 p. 21 cm.   [8640]

PASCOLI, ALESSANDRO [1669–1757] Il corpo-umano; o, Breve storia, dove con nuovo metodo si descrivono in compendio tutti gli organi suoi, e i loro principali ufizi ... Perugia, Constantini, si vende in Venetia presso Andrea Poletti, 1700.

[22], 339, [1], lxxxviii p. illus., port. 22 cm.   [8641]

With this is bound (as issued?) Baglivi, G. De fibra motrice et morbosa. 1700.

— Delle febbri teorica e pratica. Secondo il nuovo sistema, ove il tutto si spiega, per quanto è possibile, ad imitazion de'geometri ... Si aggiungono in fine alcuni Discorsi in forma di lettere, per chiarezza maggiore di quanto precedentemente si disse. Perugia, Constantini, 1699.

[8], xx, 240 p.; [2], 94 p. 21 cm.   [8642]

Part [2] has special title page.

—*See* BAGLIVI, G. De fibra motrice et morbosa. 1700.

PASCUAL, MIGUEL JUAN [*fl.* 1532] Praxis medica. *In* Pereda, P. P. Scholia in Michaelis Joannis Paschasii medici Methodum curandi. 1602, 1630, 1664.

—, *tr. See* VIGO, G. de. Teorica y pratica en cirugia. 1627.

PASQUAL, MIGUEL JUAN. *See* PASCUAL, Miguel Juan [*fl.* 1532]

PASQUALE, CARLO. *See* PASCHAL, Charles, vicomte de La Queute [1547–1625]

PASQUALE, NICOLO [17th cent.] A' posteri della peste di Napoli, e suo regno nell'anno 1656 ... Napoli, Luc'Antonio di Fulco, 1668.

[8], 72 p.   22 cm.   [**8643**]

PASQUALI, CARLO. *See* PASCHAL, Charles, vicomte de La Queute [1547–1625]

PASQUALI, GIOVAN NICCOLÒ ALIDOSI. *See* ALIDOSI, Giovanni Niccolò Pasquali [1570–1627]

PASQUATI, JOANNES BAPTISTA [*fl.* 1656] *ed. See* AVICENNA. Quarti libri canonis fen prima de febribus. 1659 [1660]; PAPIN, N. De pulvere sympathico dissertatio. 1650 [i.e. 1656?]

PASQUILLE-MAKERS hekel, anders genaemt, een samenspraeck tusschen de duyvel en de doodt. Amsterdam [1678]

15, [1] p.   16 cm.   [**8644**]

PASSALO. *See* BOVIO, Z. T. Melampigo. 1617, 1626.

PASSAU, DIOCESE. Abgetrocknete Thränen. Das ist: Von der wunderthätigen zähe-trieffenden Bildnus der gnaden-reichen Gottes-Gebährerin, so zu Pötsch in Ober-Hungarn anno 1696, den 4. Monats-tag Novembris an beeden Augen zu weinen angefangen, und folglich (die Aussetzungen behgerechnet) biss 8. December geweinet. Lob- Preiss- Danck- und Lehr Discursen, durch fünf und dreyssig ... Symbolen: So dann auch verschiedenen Predigten, so in dem uralten Passauerischen Gottes-Haus in Wien ... vorgetragen worden. Zusamm gezogen durch hochwürdig und hochgelehrte Subjecta Passauerischer Dioeces ... Nürnberg und Franckfurt, Johann Christoph Lochner, 1698.

[40], 456, 104, [14] p.   illus.   20 cm. [**8645**]

PASSERA, FELICE [1610–1702] Il nuovo tesoro degl'arcani farmacologici galenici, & chimici, ò spargirici ... divisa in tre libri ... Venetia, Giovanni Parè, 1688.

[8] p., 865 col., [1] p.; [4] p., 688 col., [28] p.   illus., tables.   34 cm.   [**8646**]

Book 3 (second group of paging) has special title page, dated 1689.

—Practica universale nella medicine, overo annotationi sopra tutte le infermità più particolari, che giornalmente sogliono avvenire ne corpi humani ... divisa in quattro libri ... Milano, Carlo Antonio Malatesta, 1693.

[8], 442 p.; 40 p.   illus.   34 cm.   [**8647**]

Part [2] "Libro quarto, nel qual si tratta de' veleni in generale, et in particolare del morso del cane rabbioso", has half title.

PASTOR, GENESIUS. *See* PASTOR DE GALLEGO, Ginés [*fl.* 1624]

PASTOR DE GALLEGO, GINÉS [*fl.* 1624] Brevis epitome valde utilis ad praedicendum futura in morbis acutis ... Oriolae, Apud Augustinum Martinez, 1624.

[32], 169, [6] p.   16 cm.   [**8648**]

PATERNO, BERNARDINO [d. 1592] *See* SCHOLTZ, L. Consiliorum medicinalium ... liber singularis. 1610.

PATIN, CHARLES [1633–1693] De febribus ... Patavii, Ex typographia Petri Antonii Brigoncii, 1686.

[2], 313–318 p.   23 cm.   [**8649**]

—De febribus oratio, habita in Archi-Lycaeo Patavino, die 4. Nov. 1677. Patavii, Typis Petri Mariae Frambotti, 1677.

[2], 35–40 p.   24 cm.   [**8650**]

Signature: A⁴.

Bound with *his* De optima medicorum secta. 1676.

—De morbis capitis ... Patavii, Ex typographia Seminarii, 1689.

[2], 465–470 p.   23 cm.   [**8651**]

—De optima medicorum secta, oratio inauguralis habita in Archi-Lycaeo Patavino, die 8. Nov. 1676. Patavii, Typis Petri Mariae Frambotti, 1676.

[2], 19–24 p.   24 cm.   [**8652**]

With this is bound *his* De febribus oratio. 1677.

—Dissertatio therapeutica de peste, habita in Archi-lyceo Patavino ... Augustae Vindelicorum, Typis Koppmayerianis, excudi curabat Theophilus Göbelius, 1683.

61, [1] p.   19 cm.   [**8653**]

—Luem veneream non esse morbum novum. Oratio habita in Archi-lyceo Patavino, die 5. Novembris, 1687 . . . Patavii, Ex typographia Seminarii, 1687.

[2], 357-362 p.   23 cm.   **[8654]**

Signature: A⁴.

—Lyceum Patavinum; sive, Icones et vitae professorum Patavii, MDCLXXXII publice docentium. Pars prior, theologos, philosophos & medicos complectens. Patavii, Typis Petri Mariae Frambotti, 1682.

[1], 137 p.   front., illus., ports.   25 cm.

[8655]

No more published.

—Quatre relations historiques . . . Basle, 1673.

[8], 3-336 p.   front., port., plates.   16 cm.

[8656]

Imperfect: portrait and map wanting.

—[English tr.] Travels thro' Germany, Bohemia, Swisserland, Holland, and other parts of Europe: describing the most considerable citys, and the palaces of princes, together with historical relations and critical observations upon ancient medals and inscriptions . . . Made English . . . London, A. Swall and T. Child, 1697.

[7], 334, [2] p.   port. (front.), plates.   17 cm.

[8657]

Added engraved title page.

—Troisiesme relation . . . Strasbourg, 1672.

107 p.   illus.   14 cm.   **[8658]**

—Quod medicus debeat esse πολμαθηος. Oratio habita in Archi-lyceo Patavino, die 3. Novembris, 1684 . . . Venetiis, Typis Io. Francisi Valvasensis, 1684.

[2], 193-198 p.   23 cm.   **[8659]**

Signature: A⁴.

—Vanam esse astrologiam medico plane indignam. Oratio habita in Archi-lyceo Patavino, die III. Novembris, 1690 . . . Patavii, Typis Seminarii Patavini, 1690.

[2], 481-486 p.   23 cm.   **[8660]**

Signature: A⁴.

—ed. See ERASMUS, D. Μωρίας ἐγκώμιον. 1676.

—See KNIPS-MACOPPE, A. De aortae polypo epistola medica. 1693.

PATIN, GUY [1601-1672] Lettres choisies . . . Dans lesquelles sont contenuës plusieurs particularités historiques, sur la vie & la mort des savans de ce siècle, sur leurs ecrits, & sur plusieurs autres choses curieuses depuis l'an 1645 jusqu'en 1672. Francfort, J. L. Du-Four, 1683.

[20], 522 p.   port.   15 cm.   **[8661]**

Added engraved title page.

—[The same.] . . . Paris, Jean Petit, 1685.

[22], 499 p.   port.   14 cm.   **[8662]**

Added engraved title page with portrait wanting.

—[The same.] . . . Augmentées de plus de 300 lettres dans cette derniére edition; & divisées en trois volumes. Volume I. Cologne, Pierre du Laurens, 1692.

[21], 328 p.   port.   17 cm.   **[8663]**

Vols. 2 and 3 wanting.

Added engraved title page.

[—] Le nez pourry de Theophraste Renaudot, grand gazettier de France, et espion de Mazarin . . . Avec sa vie infame et bouquine, recompensée d'une verole euripienne . . . [n. p., not before 1644]

6 p.   22 cm.   **[8664]**

Attributed to Guy Patin. Cf. BNC.

—, ed. See DU LAURENS, A. Andreae Laurentii . . . Opera omnia. 1628; HOFMANN, C. Apologiae pro Galeno. 1668; RIOLAN, J. [1580-1657] Opera anatomica vetera. 1650; SENNERT, D. Opera omnia in tres tomos distincta. 1641.

—See HIPPOCRATES. [Selected works. Greek and Latin] Aphorismi Graeco-Latini e regione. 1631.

PATRIARCHA, ANNIBALE [fl. 1630] Modo et ordine ch'hà tenuto, e tiene . . . per la quale si sente haver sanato, & sana tanti amalati di contaggio . . . Bologna, Nicolò Tebaldini, 1630.

21, [1] p.   21 cm.   **[8665]**

PATRICIUS, FRANCISCUS. See PATRIZI, Francesco [1529-1597]

PATRIZI, FRANCESCO [1529-1597] tr. See HERMES TRISMEGISTUS. Sesthien boecken. 1652.

PAUER, JOHANN [fl. 1693] respondent. Dissertationem . . . inauguralem de scirrho mammarum . . . submittet Johannes Pauer . . . [Altdorffii] Literis Henrici Meyeri [1693]

[32] p.   20 cm.   **[8666]**

Diss.—Altdorf.

PAUL D'ÉGINE. *See* PAULUS AEGINETA.

PAULI, AUGUST CHRISTIAN [*fl.* 1691] *respondent. See* BERGER, J. G. von, *praes.* Positiones physiologicas de homine . . . p. p. 1691.

PAULI, JOHANN WILHELM [1658–1723] Disputatio medica de oedematis natura & cura . . . Lipsiae, Literis Johannis Georgii [1685]

[16] p.   20 cm.   [8667]

Diss. pro loco — Leipzig (K. F. Luther, *respondent*)

—*praes.* Diatriben inauguralem medicam de anorexia . . . submittit Johann. Benjamin Glado . . . Lipsiae, Literis Krügerianis [1696]

[28] p.   21 cm.   [8668]

Diss. — Leipzig (J. B. Glado, *respondent*)

—Disputatio inauguralis medica de dolore capitis . . . Lipsiae, Typis Immanuelis Titii [1697]

[44] p.   20 cm.   [8669]

Diss. — Leipzig (B. Bullmann, *respondent*)

—Disputatio medica inauguralis de medicamentorum delectu . . . Lipsiae, Typis Christoph. Fleischeri [1694]

[24] p.   20 cm.   [8670]

Diss. — Leipzig (C. S. Quellmaltz, *respondent*)

—*respondent. See* AMMANN, P., *praes.* Dissertationem inauguralem de ictero . . . sistit. 1681; BOHN, J., *praes.* Dissertationes chymico-physicae. 1685; ETTMÜLLER, M. *praes.* Exercitationem therapeuticam de praecipitantium vero usu feroque abusu . . . exponunt. 1681.

PAULI, MICHAEL [*fl.* 1679–1681] *respondent.* Disputatio inauguralis physico-medica de calido innato seu spiritu corporis vitali . . . Basileae, Typis Jacobi Bertschii [1681]

[23] p.   20 cm.   [8671]

Diss. — Basel.

—*See* SCHNEIDER, K. V., *praes.* Disputatio medica de sanguine. 1679.

PAULI, SIMON. *See* PAULLI, Simon [1603–1680]

PAULINI, KRISTIAN FRANTZ. *See* PAULLINI, Christian Franz [1643–1712]

PAULINUS, FABIUS [*d.* 1605] Praelectiones Marciae; sive, Commentaria in Thucydidis Historiam, seu narrationem de peste Atheniensium. Ex ore Fabii

Paulini . . . excepta et edita . . . Venetiis, Apud Juntas, 1603.

[44], 600 p.   23 cm.   [8672]

Includes excerpts from Thucydides, in Greek and Latin.

—, *ed. See* AVICENNA. Avicennae Arabum medicorum principis. 1608; GALENUS. Opera ex octava Juntarum editione. 1609, 1625.

—*See* ARGENTERIO, G. Opera. 1610; VESALIUS, A. Anatomia. 1604.

PAULINUS, LAURENTIUS, *Abp.* [1565–1646] Loimoscopia; eller, Pestilentz speghel. Thet är, andeligh och naturligh underwiisning, om pestilentzies beskriffwelse, orsaker, praeserwatiiff, läkedomar och befriielser . . . sampt timmeligha wälfärdz och ewigha saligherz befordring. Widh ändan ärtilfadt D. D. Mart. Lutheri Grundryke underwissning om pestilentziske förwarningar . . . Strängnäs, Aff Olog Olofzson enaeo, 1623.

[8], 123 (i.e. 124), [2] ll.   20 cm.   [8673]

PAULLI, JACOB HENRIK [1637–*ca.* 1702] Anatomiae Bilsianae anatome, occupata inprimis circa vasa meseraica & labyrinthum in ductu rorifero. Accessit . . . Jo. Jac. Wepferi De dubiis anatomicis epistola, cum responsione. Argentorati, Apud Simonem Paulli, 1665.

128 p.   plates.   16 cm.   [8674]

—*praes.* Anatome anatomiae Bilsianae, imprimis circa vasa meseraica uti & labyrinthum in ductu rorifero occupata . . . Hafniae, Literis Henrici Gödiani [1663]

[4], 52 p.   plates.   18 cm.   [8675]

Diss. — Copenhagen (C. Friese, *respondent*)

—*See* VESLING, J. Syntagma anatomicum. 1666, 1677, 1696.

PAULLI, SIMON [1603–1680] Commentarius de abusu tabaci Americanorum veteri, et herbae thee Asiaticorum in Europa nova . . . Argentorati, Sumptibus authoris filii Simonis Paulli, 1665.

[11], 56, [2], 58–61 ll.   port., plates.   21 cm.
                                              [8676]

Sabin 59223.

—[The same.] . . . Ed. 2. priori auct. & corr. Argentorati, Sumptibus authoris filii Simonis Paulli, 1681.

[60], 87, [12] p.   illus., plates, port.   21 cm.
                                              [8677]

Sabin 59223.

"Historia vitae et mortis . . . Simonis Paulli" by Hans Bagger, on p. [29-46]

List of the author's works published by his son, p. [47-48]

—De anatomiae origine. *In* Casserio, G. Julii Casserii . . . Anatomische Tafeln, 1656, 1683.

—Epistola votiva ad Johannem Valentinum Willium. [Hafniae, 1676]

[8] p.   19 cm.   **[8678]**

—Flora danica; det er, Dansk urtebog; udi huilcken . . . icke aleeniste Urternis historiske beskrifvelse, krafter, oc virckninger, med zijrligste figurer andragis: men endocsaa laegedomme til alle siugdomme gafnlige, korteligen oc klarligen antegnis: saa af den er baade en urtebog oc laegebog . . . Kiøbenhafn, Melchior Martzan, 1648.

[37], 393 (i.e. 948), [92] p.; 383, [2] p.   illus., plates, port.   20 cm.   **[8679]**

Added engraved title page.

The second part (illustrations) was printed in Antwerp in 1647 by Balthasar Moretus.

Imperfect: plate facing sig. 6B2 wanting, supplied in photocopy. Pritzel 6993.

Nissen 1497.

The pagination of the text corresponds with that of the illustrations.

—Oratio introductoria . . . cum Galenum De ossibus, ad sceleton, publice in Collegio Finckiano esset interpretaturus . . . [Hafniae] Typis Henrici Crusii, prostat apud Jo. Moltken [1641]

[48] p.   19 cm.   **[8680]**

Imperfect: lower margins of p. [1-4] mutilated.

—Παρεκβασις; seu, Digressio de vera, unica, & proxima causa febrium . . . Francofurti, Sumptibus Thomae Matthiae Götzii, 1660.

[16], 144 p.   23 cm.   **[8681]**

"Appendix, seu Historica relatio de periculissimo . . . casu, ad . . . Johannem Riolanum . . . anno 1652 . . . missa a Simone Paulli . . . cui jam accessit Pauli Moth . . . Casus chirurgicus . . . descriptus. Ed. 2. castigatior" (p. [III]-144) has special title page.

—[The same.] . . . Argentorati, Sumptibus auctoris filii, 1678.

26, [2], 187, [1] p.   port., illus.   20 cm.
                                                    [8682]

Second edition, edited by Johannes Hardovicus Hampe.

The Appendix (p. [141]-163) has special title page.

—Quadripartitum, de simplicium medicamentorum facultatibus . . . Rostochii, Ex Bibliopolio Hallervordiano, 1640.

1 v.   19 cm.   **[8683]**

Various pagings.

A reissue of the 1639 edition with a new title page.

". . . Oratio . . .", at end, has special title page, with imprint: Rostochii, Apud Johan. Hallervordium.

—[The same.] Quadripartitum botanicum de simplicium medicamentorum facultatibus . . . Additis dosibus purgantium . . . Argentorati, Impensis auth. fil. Simonis Paulli, 1667.

62, [2], 690 p.   illus.   21 cm.   **[8684]**

Added engraved title page.

"Appendix, continens D. Simonis Paulli Orationem . . . anno 1634 . . . Ut & ejusdem Programma . . . anno 1665 . . . Nec non . . . Guil. Laurenbergii Botanothecam" (p. [609]-660) has special title page.

—*See* BORCH, O. Dissertationem hanc inauguralem de malo hypochondriaco . . . submittit . . . S. P. . . . 1676.

PAULLINI, CHRISTIAN FRANZ [1643-1712] De asino liber historico-physico-medicus, ad normam . . . Academiae Caes. Leopoldinae Nat. Curios. scriptus . . . Francofurti ad Moenum, Impensis Joh. David. Zunneri, 1695.

[45], 281, [7] p.   16 cm.   **[8685]**

Added engraved title page has title: Onographia curiosa.

—De jalapa liber singularis, secundum leges & methodum . . . Academiae Leopoldinae Naturae Curios. scriptus . . . Francofurti ad Moenum, Impensis Friderici Knochii, 1700.

[17], 417, [5] p.   19 cm.   **[8686]**

Added engraved title page.

—Flagellum salutis; das ist, Curieuse Erzählung, wie mit Schlägen allerhand schwere, langweilige, und fast unheylbare Kranckheiten offt, bald und wohl curiret worden . . . Franckfurt am Mäyn, In Verlegung Friederich Knochens, 1698.

[25], 158, [4] p.   16 cm.   **[8687]**

Added engraved title page.

—Heilsame Dreck-Apotheke, wie nemlich mit Koth und Urin fast alle, ja auch schwerste gifftige Krankheiten . . . curirt worden . . . Franckfurt am Mayn, In Verlegung Friedrich Knochens, 1696.

[1], 268, [4] p.   17 cm.   **[8688]**

Added engraved title page.

—[The same.] Neu-vermehrte heilsame Dreck-Apotheke . . . Ubermals bewährt und nun zum dritten Mal um ein Merckliches vermehrt, und verbessert . . . Franckfurt am Mayn, Zu Verlegung Friedrich Knochens, druckts Peter Begereiss, 1699.

[36], 420, [4] p.   18 cm.   **[8689]**

Added engraved title page.

—Lagographia curiosa; seu, Leporis descriptio, juxta methodum & leges . . . Academiae Leopoldinae nat. curios adornata . . . Augustae Vindelicorum, Impensis Laur. Kronigeri & Theoph. Goebelii haeredum, typis Joh. Jacob Schönigii, 1691.

[31], 408, [4] p.   15 cm.   **[8690]**

Added engraved title page.

—Lycographia; seu, De natura & usu lupi, libellus physico-historico-medicus, ad normam . . . Academiae Lepoldinae scriptus . . . Francofurti ad Moenum, Impensis Joh. David. Zunneri, 1694.

[16], 214, [4] p.   front.   17 cm.   **[8691]**

Imperfect: frontispiece wanting.

—Observationum medico-physicarum decades duae. Norimbergae, 1689.

54 p.   19 cm.   **[8692]**

Imperfect: sig. A1-2 wanting; sig. H2-4 wanting(?)

—Sacra herba; seu, Nobilis salvia, juxta methodum et leges . . . Academiae Naturae Curiosorum descripta, selectisque remediis, et propriis observationibus conspersa . . . Augustae Vindelicorum, Impensis Laur. Kronigeri, & Theoph. Goebelii haeredum, typis Caspari Brechenmacheri [1688]

[15], 414, [10] p.   16 cm.   **[8693]**

Added engraved title page.

—Talpa, juxta methodum & leges . . . Academiae Leopoldinae descripta, variisque observationibus & curiositatibus conspersa. Francofurti & Lipsiae, Sumpt. Joh. Christiani Wohlfarti, 1689.

[1], 214 p.   14 cm.   **[8694]**

Added engraved title page.

—, tr. See AMMANN, P. Medicina critica. 1677, 1693.

—See REISKE, J. Ad . . . Chr. Franc. Paullini . . . epistola. 1685.

PAULMIER DE GRENTEMESNIL, JULIEN LE. See LE PAULMIER DE GRENTEMESNIL, Julien [1520-1588]

PAULONI, NICOLÒ ORFEO [1653-1721] See SCARAMUCCI, G. B. De motu, et circuitu sanguinis. 1677.

PAULSEN, STATIUS GOTTFRIED [*fl.* 1698] respondent. See WEDEL, E. H., *praeses.* Dissertatio medica de ephemera. 1698.

PAULUCCI, GIOVANNI BATTISTA [*fl.* 1643] See DONZELLI,G. Lettera familiare. 1643.

PAULUS AEGINETA. De chirurgia. *In* Dalechamps, J. Chirurgie françoise. 1610.

—*See* ROLFINCK, W. Liber de purgantibus vegetabilibus. 1667.

PAULUS, GEORGIUS [*fl.* 1605] respondent. See KECKERMANN, B., *praeses.* Cursus philosophici disputatio XIX. De homine. 1605.

PAUVRES. *See* ASSEMBLÉE CHARITABLE À PARIS.

PAUVRES . . . Liste des 40. hospitaux generaux établis par des missionaires . . . [Paris?] 1680.

8 p.   20 cm.   **[8695]**

Caption title.

PAUW, PIETER [1564-1617] Observationes anatomicae selectiores, jam primum editae, curante Th. Bartholino. Hafniae, Literis Petri Morsingii [1656]

45, [2] p., vol. 1   17 cm.   (*In* Bartholin, Thomas. Historiarum anatomicarum rariorum centuria I-VI. Hafniae, 1645-61)   **[8696]**

—Primitiae anatomicae. De humani corporis ossibus. Lugduni Batavorum, Ex officina Justi à Colster, 1615.

[16], 188, [3] p.   plates.   20 cm.   **[8697]**

Leaf of dedicatory verse (signed .**V) and errata leaf at end.

—[The same.] . . . Amstelreodami, Apud Henricum Laurentii, 1633.

[16], 172 p.   illus., plates.   20 cm.   **[8698]**

—Succenturiatus anatomicus. Continens commentaria in Hippocratem, De capitis vulneribus. Additae in aliquot capita libri VIII C. Celsi explicationes . . . Lugduni Batavorum, Apud Jodocum à Colster, 1616.

[24], 270 p.; [2], 128 p.   illus., plates, port.   20 cm.   **[8699]**

Imperfect: p. 57-64 wanting.

"A. Cornelii Celsi De re medica liber octavus; ejus priora quatuor capita commentariis illustrata" has special title page.

Includes Greek and Latin text of Hippocrates' De capitis vulneribus.

With this is bound: Cornarius, Diomedes. Consiliorum medicinalium . . . tractatus. Lipsiae, 1599.

—Tractatus de peste, cum Henrici Florentii ad singula ejusdem Tractatus capita additamentis. Lugduni Batavorum, Ex officina Abrahami Commelini [Typis Wilhelmi Christiani] 1636 [pref. 1637] [24], 188, [2] p. 12 cm. **[8700]**

Dedicatory epistle, by Henricus Florentius, dated 1637.

—*praeses.* Propositiones medicae-chirurgicae de capitis vulneribus ... Lugduni Batavorum, Excudebat Henricus Ludovici ad Haestens, 1615. [10] p. 19 cm. **[8701]**

Diss. — Leyden (L. Ernon, *respondent*)

—*ed. See* CELSUS, A. C. De re medica liber octavus. 1616; HEURNE, J. van. Institutiones medicinae. 1609, 1611, 1627, 1638; VESALIUS, A. Epitome anatomica. 1616.

PAUWELSZOON, JAN, *tr. See* GERSDORFF, H. von. Chirurgia. 1605; RULAND, M. [1532-1602] Empirica. 1660.

PAWIUS, PETRUS. *See* PAUW, Pieter [1564-1617]

PAYER, JÁNOS LIPOT. Ex universa medicina aphorismi duodeni, annexis sex tabulis de natura humana, ejusdemque substantia et accidentiis ... Wien, Typis Joannis Georgii Schlegel, 1700. [12] p. 19 cm. **[8702]**

PAYNE, KAREL [*fl.* 1655] *respondent.* Disputatio medica inauguralis de hydrope ascite ... Lugduni Batavorum, Ex officina Francisci Moyardi, 1655. [12] p. 22 cm. **[8703]**

Diss. — Leyden

PAYNELL, THOMAS [*fl.* 1528-1567] *tr. See* REGIMEN SANITATIS SALERNITANUM. Regimen sanitatis Salerni; or, The Schoole of Salernes regiment of Health. 1617, 1634, 1649.

PAZ, FRANCISCO DE [*d.* 1640] *See* CHIFFLET, J. J. De morte ... D. Francisci de Paz. 1640.

PÉ, LAZARE. *See* PÉNA, Lazare [*d.* 1653]

PEACHEY, JOHN. *See* PECHEY, John [1655-1716]

[PEACHIE, JOHN, *fl. ca.* 1683–*ca.* 1690] Some observations made upon the Angola seed: shewing its ... virtue in curing all distempers of the eyes. Written by a doctor of physick in the countrey to Dr. Goddard, one of the Royal Society at London, anno 1660. London, 1682. 7 p. 19 cm. **[8704]**

This and the succeeding works entered under Peachie have been attributed also to John Pechey. Wing P926.

[—] Some observations made upon the banellas, imported from the Indies: shewing their ... virtues in curing melancholly and distraction. Written by a physitian in the countrey to Dr. Allen, one of the Royal Society at London. London, 1694. 8 p. 19 cm. **[8705]**

Wing P927.

[—] Some observations made upon the Barbado seeds, shewing their ... virtue in curing dropsies. Written by a physitian in the countrey to Sir George Ent at London. London, 1694. 7 p. 19 cm. **[8706]**

Wing P928.

[—] Some observations made upon the Bengala bean, imported from the Indies: shewing its ... virtues in curing all sorts of hemorrages, and particularly spitting of blood. Written by a doctor of physick in the countrey to one of his patients in London. [London?] 1694. 7 p. 19 cm. **[8707]**

Wing P929.

[—] Some observations made upon the Bermudas berries: imported from the Indies: shewing their ... virtues in curing the green-sickness. Written by a doctor of physick in the countrey to the Honourable Esq. Boyle. London, 1694. 7 p. 19 cm. **[8708]**

Wing P930.

[—] Some observations made upon the blatta Bizantina, shewing its ... virtues in curing asthmas, and shortness of breath. Written by a doctor of physick in the countrey to Dr. Meverell at London. London, 1694. 8 p. 19 cm. **[8709]**

Wing P931.

[—] Some observations made upon the Brasillian root, called ipepocoanha: imported from the Indies: shewing its ... virtue against vomiting and loosness. Written by a physitian in the countrey [i.e. John Peachie? or John Griffith?] to the president of the Colledge of Physitians in London. London, 1682. 7 p. 19 cm. **[8710]**

Wing G2003A

[−] Some observations made upon the Calumba wood, otherwise called Calumback: imported from the Indies: shewing its . . . virtues in curing the gout, and easing all sorts of rheumatical pains. Written by a doctor of physick in the countrey [i.e. John Peachie? or Ludkin?], to the president of the Colledge of Physicians in London. London, 1694.

    7 p. 19 cm.   **[8711]**
    Wing L3458 (1682 ed.)

[−] Some observations made upon the herb called perigua, imported from the Indies: shewing its . . . virtues in curing the diabetes. Written by a Dr. of physick in the countrey [i.e. John Peachie?] to Dr. Burwell, president of the Colledge of Physitians at London. London, 1694.

    7 p. 19 cm.   **[8712]**
    Wing P932.

[−] Some observations made upon the herb cassiny; imported from Carolina: shewing its . . . virtues in curing the small pox. Written by a physitian in the countrey to Esq. Boyle at London. London, 1695.

    8 p. 19 cm.   **[8713]**
    Wing P933.

[−] Some observations made upon the Malabar nutt, imported from the Indies: shewing its . . . virtues in curing the kings-evil, beyond anything yet found out. Written by a doctor of physick in the countrey to his friend in London, troubled with that distemper. London, 1694.

    7 p. 19 cm.   **[8714]**
    Wing P934.

[−] Some observations made upon the Maldiva nut; shewing its . . . virtue in giving an easie, safe and speedy delivery to women in child-bed. Written by a physitian in the countrey to Dr. Hinton at London, 1663. London, 1694.

    7 p. 19 cm.   **[8715]**
    Wing P935.

[−] Some observations made upon the Mexico seeds, imported from the Indies: shewing their . . . virtue against worms in the bodies of men, women, and children. Written by a countrey physitian to Dr. Burwell, president of the Colledge of Physitians in London. London, 1695.

    7 p. 19 cm.   **[8716]**
    Wing P936.

[−] Some observations made upon Molucco nutts, imported from the Indies: shewing their . . . virtues in curing the collick, rupture, and all distempers proceeding from the wind. Written by a doctor of physick in the countrey [i.e. John Peachie? or Meare?], to Dr. Castle, one of the Royal Society in London. [London?] 1672.

    7 p. 19 cm.   **[8717]**
    Wing M1578.

[−] Some observations made upon the root called casmunar, imported from the East-Indies: shewing its nature and vertues above any other as yet written of, in curing apoplexies, convulsions, palsies, lethargies, tremblings, fitts of the mother, giddiness in the head, and all distempers of the brain and nerves. Published by a doctor of physick in Glocestershire Lonlon [sic] Reprinted in the year 1693.

    8 p. 19 cm.   **[8718]**
    Wing P937.

[−] Some observations made upon the root called nean, or ninsing, imported from the East-Indies. Shewing its . . . virtue, in curing consumptions, ptissicks, shortness of breath, distillation of rhume . . . Published by a doctor of physick in York-shire [i.e. John Peachie? or Robert Wittie?], in a letter to Mr. Colwell, a member of the Royal Society, 1680. London, Printed for the author [1680?]

    7 p. 19 cm.   **[8719]**
    Wing P937A.

[−] Some observations made upon the root called serapias, or salep, imported from Turkey. Shewing its . . . virtues in preventing womens miscarriages. Written by a doctor of physick in the countrey to his friend in London. [London?] 1694.

    7 p. 19 cm.   **[8720]**
    Wing P938.

[−] Some observations made upon the Russia seed, shewing its . . . virtues in curing the rickets in children. Written by a doctor of physick in the countrey to Esq. Boyle at London, 1674. London, 1694.

    8 p. 19 cm.   **[8721]**
    Wing P938A.

[−] Some observations made upon the serpent stones, imported from the Indies: shewing their . . . virtues in curing malignant spotted feavers. Written by a countrey physitian to Dr. Burwell, president of the Colledge of Physitians in London. London, 1694.

8 p.   19 cm.   [8722]

Wing P939.

[—] Some observations made upon the Virginian nutts, imported from the Indies: shewing their . . . virtue against the scurvy. Written by a doctor of physick in the countrey to Dr. Croon, one of the Royal Society in London, 1681. London, 1682.

7 p.   19 cm.   [8723]

Wing P940.

[—] Some observations made upon the wood called lignum nephriticum, imported from Hispaniola; shewing its . . . virtues in dissolving the stone in the reins and bladder, helping the strangury, and stoppings in the water, and easing all pains proceeding from thence, &c. Written by a doctor of physick in the countrey to the president of the Colledge of Physicians in London. [London?] 1694.

8 p.   19 cm.   [8724]

Wing P941.

The PEARLE of practice. *See* The QUEENS closet opened. 1658, 1675, 1683.

PEARSE, JAMES [*fl.* 1678] *See* YONGE, J. Currus triumphalis. 1679.

PEARSON, JOHN, *Bp. of Chester* [1613?-1686] Expositio symboli apostolici, juxta editionem Anglicanam quintam, in linguam Latinam translata . . . Francofurti ad Viadrum, Sumptibus Jeremiae Schrey & haeredum Henrici Joannes Meyeri, 1691.

[13], 699, [44] p.   front. (port.)   21 cm.

[8725]

A translation by S. J. Arnold of An exposition of the creed, 5th edition, published in London in 1683. Cf. Lowndes, p. 1811.

PECCANA, ALESSANDRO [*fl.* 1627] Del bever freddo libro uno, con Problemi intorno alla stessa materia . . . Verona, Angelo Tamo [1627]

[24], 128 (i.e. 124), [1] p.   22 cm.   [8726]

"Problemi" (p. [75]-128) has special title page.

PECCETTI, FRANCESCO [*fl.* 1616] Cheirurgia . . . in qua omnia, tam ad hujus artis theoriam, guam praxim spectantia traduntur . . . in quatuor libros digesta . . . Quorum in primo agitur de tumoribus . . . In secundo de vulneribus . . . In tertio eadem ratione, & in ordine de ulceribus. In quarto . . . de

fracturis . . . Florentiae, Apud Jo. Donatum, & Bernardinum Junctas, & socios, 1616.

[8], 616, [19] p.   34 cm.   [8727]

— [The same.] . . . Tidini Regii, Apud haeredes Caroli Francisi Magrii, 1697.

[8], 654, [17] p.   35 cm.   [8728]

PECHEY, JOHN [1655-1716] A collection of chronical diseases, viz. the colick, the bilious colick, hysterick diseases, the gout, and the bloody urine from the stone in the kidnies . . . London, Printed by J. R., and sold by Henry Bonwicke, 1692.

[8], 152 p.   17 cm.   [8729]

"The first chapter is taken from Riverius, the other from the worthy Dr. Sydenham's works." Cf. Preface.

— Collections of acute diseases. Taken from the best authors . . . The first part contains all that . . . Dr. Sydenham has written of the small pox and measles . . . London, Printed by F. C. and sold by Henry Bonwicke, 1687.

[6], 8, 101, [9] p.   17 cm.   [8730]

— The compleat herbal of physical plants. Containing all such English and foreign herbs, shrubs and trees, as are used in physick and surgery . . . Also directions for making compound-waters, syrups . . . and other sorts of medicines. Moreover, the gums, balsams . . . and the like . . . sold by apothecaries and druggists, are added . . . and their virtues and uses are fully described . . . London, Printed for Henry Bonwicke, 1694.

[8], 349, [32] p.   17 cm.   [8731]

Pritzel 7845.

— A general treatise of the diseases of infants and children. Collected from the best practical authors . . . London, R. Wellington, 1697.

[24], 160, [8] p.   16 cm.   [8732]

— The London dispensatory, reduced to the practice of the London physicians. Wherein are contain'd the medicines, both Galenical and chymical, that are now in use. Those that are out of use, are omitted: and such as are in use, and not in the Latin copy, are added; with vertues and doses . . . London, Printed by F. Collins, for J. Lawrence, 1694.

[24], 187, [5] p.   16 cm.   [8733]

Bound with Lémery, N. Pharmacopoeia Lemeriana contracta. 1700.

—A plain introduction to the art of physick, containing the fundamentals, and necessary preliminaries to practice ... To which is added, the Materia medica contracted. And alphabetical tables of the vertues of roots, barks ... Also a collection of choice medicines chymical and Galenical. Together with a different way of making the most celebrated compositions in the apothecaries shops ... London, Henry Bonwicke, 1697.

[16], 390, [1] p. 20 cm.   **[8734]**

"The second part ... Materia medica contracted, was chiefly collected from Etmuller and Marggravius. Lastly, I have added, Marggrav's Shopcompositions ..." Cf. Preface.

—Promptuarium praxeos medicae; seu, Methodus medendi, praescriptis celeberrimorum medicorum Londinensium concinnata, et in ordinem alphabeticum digesta ... Londini, Impensis Henrici Bonwicke, 1693.

[4], 272, [1] p. 14 cm.   **[8735]**
Errata at end.

—[The same.] ... Juxta exemplar Londinense. Amstelodami, 1694.

[1], 302, [10] p. front. 14 cm. **[8736]**

—The store-house of physical practice, being a general treatise of the causes and signs of all diseases afflicting human bodies. Together with the shortest, plainest and safest way of curing them ... To which is added ... several choice forms of medicines used by the London physicians ... London, Henry Bonwicke, 1695.

[8], 1-320, 355-544, [2] p. 20 cm. **[8737]**

—, *ed. See* THE COMPLEAT MIDWIFE'S PRACTICE ENLARGED. 1697, 1698.

—, *tr. See* SYDENHAM, T. The whole works. 1696, 1697.

—*See* MULLINS, J., *physician.* Some observations made upon the Cylonian plant. 1695; [PEACHIE, J.] Some observations. 1682.

PECHLIN, JOHANN NICOLAS [1644-1706] Jani Philadelphi [pseud.] Consultatio desultoria de optima Christianorum secta, et vitiis pontificiorum. Prodromus religionis medici. Patavii, 1688.

[6], 119 p. 16 cm.   **[8738]**
Attributed to Sir Thomas Browne by Jöcher, v. 1, p. 1407. Keynes(B) p. 240.

—De aeris et alimenti defectu, et vita sub aquis, meditatio ad ... Joelem Langelottum ... Kilonii, Impensis Gothofredi Schultzen, prostat & Amsterodami apud Janssonio Waesbergios, 1676.

183, [1] p. 16 cm.   **[8739]**

—De habitu & colore Aethiopum, qui vulgo nigritae, liber ... Kilonii, Literis ac impensis Joach. Reumanni, 1677.

208 p. 16 cm.   **[8740]**

—De purgantium medicamentorum facultatibus exercitatio nova.Lugd. Batav. & Amstelod., Apud Danielem, Abrahamum & Adrianum à Gaasbeek, 1672.

[32], 515 p. plates, tables. 16 cm. **[8741]**
Added engraved title page.

—Jani Leoniceni Veronensis [pseud.] Metamorphosis Aesculapii & Apollinis Pancreatici. Gratianopoli, Apud Orlandum Bon-Tempi, 1672.

[8], 125 p. 17 cm.   **[8742]**
Fictitious imprint. Lugduni Batavorum, Apud Philippum Bonum. Cf. Weller, vol. 1, p. 275.
A satire on the works of Frans de Le Böe and Reinier de Graaf.
Bound with Brunner, J. C. Experimenta nova circa pancreas. 1683.

—[The same.] ... Lugd. Batavorum, Apud Philippum Bonum, 1673.

[8], 125 p. 17 cm.   **[8743]**
A reissue of the 1672 edition, with new title page.

—Another issue with new title page: ... Editio altera duabus epistolis Cl. Martelli & J. Leoniceni auctior

[8], 125, [20] p. 16 cm.   **[8744]**
Letters added at end (20 p.) have special title page: Claudii Martelli epistola ad Janum Leonicenum Veronensem de nupera metamorphosi.

—Observationum physico-medicarum libri tres, quibus accessit, Ephemeris vulneris thoracici & in eam commentarius. Hamburgi, Ex Officina Libraria Schultziana, 1691.

[23], 544 p.; 68, [2] p. front., plates. 21 cm.
           [8745]
Part [2] has half-title.

—Theophilus Bibaculus; sive, De potu theae dialogus. Kilonii & Francofurti, Impensis Johannis Sebastiani Riechelii, 1684.

[8], 103 p. 19 cm.   **[8746]**

With this are bound: Tappe, J. Oratio de tabaco. 1660; Auff- und zugemachte Schnupff Tabacks Büchse. [1694?]

—Another issue, with place of printing: Francofurti.

[8747]

Programs — Kiel

—Facultatis Medicae ... decanus Joh. Nicolaus Pechlin ... ad audiendum theses de affectibus soporosis, quas ... sub praesidio ... Joh. Danielis Maioris ... examini exhibebit ... Caspar March ... invitat. Kilonii, Literis Reumannianis [1680]

[8] p.　20 cm.　　　　　　　　　　[8748]

With vita of K. March.

—Facultatis Medicae decanus Johannes Nicolaus Pechlin ... ad disputationem inauguralem de vulneribus sclopetorum in genere quam ... submittit Georg. Jacobus Blank ... officiose invitat. Kiloni, Joachimus Reuman [1674]

[8] p.　19 cm.　　　　　　　　　　[8749]

With vita of G. J. Blank.

Dissertations — Kiel

—praeses. Disputatio medica inauguralis de epilepsia & specificis contra eam ... Kilonii, Typis Joach. Reumanni, 1678.

40 p.　18 cm.　　　　　　　　　　[8750]

G. M. Tatter, respondent.

—Disputatio medica inauguralis de haemorrhagia narium ... Kilonii, Literis Joach. Reumanni, 1680.

32 p.　20 cm.　　　　　　　　　　[8751]

G. Brasch, respondent.

—Disputatio medica inauguralis de phrenitide ... Kilonii, Joachimus Reumann [1681]

51, [1] p.　20 cm.　　　　　　　　[8752]

H. C. Esmarch, respondent.

—Disputatio medica inauguralis de vulneribus sclopetorum in genere ... Kilonii, Joach. Reumannus [1674]

[36] p.　19 cm.　　　　　　　　　[8753]

G. J. Blank, respondent.

—Exercitatio anatomico-medica de fabrica et usu cordis ... Kilonii, Literis Joachimi Reumanni, 1676.

62, [2] p.　19 cm.　　　　　　　　[8754]

A. C. Langelott, respondent.

—Joh. Nicolai Pechlini ... historiam vulneris thoracici & in eam commentarium ... submittit Mummius Lüddens ... Kilonii, Literis Joachimi Reumanni [1682]

[70] p.　19 cm.　　　　　　　　　[8755]

M. Lüddens, respondent.

—respondent. Disputatio medica inauguralis de apoplexia ... Lugduni Batavorum, Apud viduam & haeredes Joannis Elsevirii, 1667

[20] p.　19 cm.　　　　　　　　　[8756]

Diss. — Leyden.

—See HAMMEN, L. von. De herniis dissertatio academica. 1681.

PECQUET, JEAN [1622-1674] Experimenta nova anatomica, quibus incognitum hactenus chyli receptaculum & ab eo per thoracem in ramos usque subclavios vasa lactea deteguntur. Ejusdem Dissertatio anatomica de circulatione sanguinis, et chyli motu. Accedunt clarissimorum virorum perelegantes ad authorem epistolae. Parisiis, Apud Sebastianum Cramoisy et Gabrielem Cramoisy, 1651.

[12], 108 p.　illus.　19 cm.　　　[8757]

—[The same.] ... Juxta exemplar Parisiis impressum. Hardervici, Apud Joannem Tollium, 1651.

[22], 204 p.　plates.　13 cm.　　[8758]

—[The same.] In Munierus, J. A., ed. De venis tam lacteis thoracicis. 1654.

—[The same.] In Hemsterhuis, S. Messis aurea triennalis. 1654, 1659.

—[The same.] ... Huic secundae editioni, quae emendata est ... accessit De thoracicis lacteis dissertatio, in qua Jo. Riolani responsio ad eadem experimenta nova anatomica refutatur ... Sequuntur gratulatoriae clarissimorum vivorum ... ad authorem epistolae, quibus & adjungitur brevis destructio, seu litura responsionis Riolani ad ejusdem Pecqueti experimenta. Parisiis, Ex Officina Cramosiana, 1654.

[16], 252, [2] p.　illus.　20 cm.　[8759]

Errata: [2] p.

—[The same.] ... Amstelaedami, Apud Aegidium Janssonium Valkenier, 1661.

[22], 204 p.　plates.　14 cm.　　[8760]

A reprint of the 1651 Harderwijk edition.

With this is bound Diemerbroeck, I. van. Disputationum practicarum pars prima & secunda. 1664.

—[The same.] . . . Ed. alt. Amstelaedami, Apud Franciscum vander Plaats, 1700.

[22], 204 p. 14 cm.   [8761]

A reissue of the 1661 edition with title page and preliminaries reset.

—[English tr.] New anatomical experiments . . . By which the hitherto unknown receptacle of the chyle, and the transmission from thence to the subclavial veins by the now discovered lacteal chanels of the thorax, is plainly made appear in brutes. As also an anatomical dissertation of the motion of blood and chyle. Together with the further description of the same lacteal chanels newly discovered in the body of man as well as brutes. Being an anatomical historie, publickly propos'd by Thomas Bartoline . . . To Michael Lysere, answering. London, Printed by T. W. for Octavian Pulleyn, 1653.

[12], 177 p.; [4], 127 p. illus., plates. 15 cm.
[8762]

Imperfect: sig. A2 and plate opposite p. 40, first group of paging, wanting.

Thomas Bartholin's Anatomical history, second group of paging, has special title page, with imprint: London, Printed by Francis Leach for Octavian Pulleyn, 1653.

—See BARTHOLIN, T. Opuscula nova anatomica. 1670; HÉNAUT, G. de. Clypeus. 1655; [PERRAULT, C.] Description anatomique de divers animaux dissequez dans l'Academie royale des sciences. 1682.

PECQUET, R. Discours ou il est succinctement traicté de la lepre & de la peste . . . Amiens, Jacques Hubault, 1626.

56 p. 16 cm.   [8763]

PEDRO HISPANO. See JOHANNES XXI, Pope [d. 1277]

PEDRO JULIÃO. See JOHANNES XXI, Pope [d. 1277]

PEERS, RICHARD [1645-1690] tr. See WOOD, A. à. [Historia et antiquitates Universitatis Oxoniensis. 1674]

PEGANIUS, CHRISTIAN, psued. See KNORR VON ROSENROTH, Christian [1636-1689]

PEICHEL, CHRISTIAN [fl. 1686] respondent. See VEHR, I., praeses. Disputatio inauguralis, de hydrope sicco. 1686.

PEIRCE, ROBERT. See PIERCE, Robert [1622-1710]

PEIRESC, NICOLAS CLAUDE FABRI DE [1580-1637] See GASSENDI, P. Viri illustris Nicolai Claudii Fabricii de Peiresc . . . vita. 1655.

PEIRESKIUS, NICOLAUS CLAUDIUS FABRICIUS DE. See PEIRESC, Nicolas Claude Fabri de [1580-1637]

PEIRESO, NICOLAUS CLAUDIUS FABRICIUS DE. See PEIRESC, Nicolas Claude Fabri de [1580-1637]

PEIRUIS DES AMBIES, DE. Le medecin sincere, qui apres avoir enseigné que la veritable medecine, bien loin d'approuver la multiplicité des remedes, demand que l'usage en soit tres-moderé, en montre clairement, & en peu de mots, la pratique. Marseille, Charles Brebion, 1675.

[16], 118 p. 15 cm.   [8764]

PELAEUS, JULIANUS. See PELEUS, Julianus [d. ca. 1625]

PELECYUS, JOHANN, Father [1545-1623] De humanorum affectuum, morborumque cura. Libri duo . . . Monachii, Ex formis Bergianis [apud viduam], impensis Joannis Hertsroy, 1617.

[24], 373, [26] p. 13 cm.   [8765]

PELÉE, JULIEN. See PELEUS, Julianus [d. ca. 1625]

PELETARIUS, JACOBUS. See PELETIER, Jacques [1517-1582]

PELETIER, JACQUES [1517-1582] De conciliatione locorum Galeni. In Cardano, G. Contradicentium medicorum libri duo. 1607.

PELEUS, Julianus [d. ca. 1625] Quaestio nobilissima, de solutione matrimonii ex causa frigoris publice tractata & judicata . . . Parisiis, Apud Claudium Morellum, 1602.

39 p. 18 cm.   [8766]

With this is bound copy 1 of his Quaestio singularis. 1602.

—Copy 2. 17 cm.

Bound with Roulliard, Sébastien. Capitulaire auquel est traicté qu'un homme nay sans testicules apparens . . . est capable des oeuvres du mariage. Paris, 1600.

—Quaestio singularis, de solutione matrimonii ob defectum testium non apparentium in senatu tractata & judicata . . . Parisiis, Apud Claudium Morellum, 1602.

83 p. 18 cm.   [8767]

Bound with copy 1 of his Quaestio nobilissima. 1602.

—Copy 2.   18 cm.

Bound with Roulliard, Sébastien. Capitulaire auquel est traicté qu'un homme nay sans testicules apparens . . . est capable des oeuvres du mariage. Paris, 1600.

[**PELLEGRINI**, BONAVENTURA] Secreti nobilissimi dell'arte profumatoria. Ne quali si insegna a fare ogli, acque, paste, balle, moscardini, uccelletti, paternostri, e tutta l'arte intiera come si ricerca, si nella città di Napoli, come in Roma, in Venetia, & in molte città d'Italia . . . Bologna, Giovanni Recaldini, 1672.

[4], 224 p.   illus.   14 cm.   [8768]

PELLETIER, JACQUES. *See* PELETIER, Jacques [1517–1582]

PELLETIER, NICOLAS [*fl.* 1672–1675] *praeses.* Quaestio medica . . . An magnis lienibus ferrum. [Parisiis, Apud Franciscum Muguet, 1675]

4 p.   25 cm.   [8769]

Dis. — Paris (F. Girard, *respondent*)

—*respondent. See* FARCY, D. de, *praeses.* Quaestio medica . . . An paralysi sudorifica? 1674.

PELLICINI, ANTONIO. Discorso sopra de mali contagiosi pestilenziali . . . Fiorenza, Zanobi Pignoni, 1630.

86 p.   16 cm.   [8770]

PELLISSON-FONTAINER, PAUL [1624–1693] *See* BEARN [France] Relations envoyées a Monsieur Pelisson. 1680.

PELSHOFER, JOHANN GEORG [1599–1637] *praeses.* Dissertatio . . . de Paracelsistarum unguento armario . . .

[705]–722 p.   21 cm.   (*In* Theatrum sympatheticum auctum. Norimbergae, 1662)   [8771]

Caption title.
Diss. — Wittenberg (H. Wecker, *respondent*)

—*respondent. See* SENNERT, D., *praeses.* De ileo theses disputationis medicae. 1622.

— *ed. See* BÉGUIN, J. Tyrocinium chymicum. 1643, 1650, 1659, 1669; HARTMANN, J. Opera omnia medicochymica. 1684, 1694 [and] Tractatus physico-medicus, de opio. 1635.

PELTRE, JAKOB [*fl.* 1645] *respondent. See* SEBISCH, M. [1578–1674?] *praeses.* Disputatio de naturalibus facultatibus prima [-octava & ultima] 1644 [i.e. 1645]

PELTZ, SIMON [*fl.* 1625] *respondent. See* OELHAF, P., *praeses.* Dissertatio physico-medica de morbis totius substantiae in genere. 1625.

PELTZER, JOHANN BAPTISTA [*fl.* 1698] *respondent.* Disputatio medica inauguralis de vermibus intestinorum . . . Duisburgi ad Rhenum, Typis Johannis Sas, 1698.

36 p.   20 cm.   [8772]

Diss. — Duisburg.

PEMELL, ROBERT [*d.* 1653] De morbis capitis; or, Of the chief internal diseases of the head . . . by R[obert] P[emel] . . . London, Philemon Stephens, 1650.

[14], 141 p.   14 cm.   [8773]

—De morbis puerorum; or, A treatise of the disease of children; with their causes, signs, prognosticks, and cures . . . London, Printed by J. Legatt, for Philemon Stephens, 1653.

[4], 58, [2] p.   18 cm.   [8774]

Signatures: A², 3G³⁻⁸, 3H–3K⁸. (Part [3] in his Tractatus de simplicium medicamentorum. London, 1652)

—Πτωχοφαρμακον; seu, Medicamen miseris, or, Pauperum pyxidicula salutifera. Help for the poor, collected for the benefit of such as are not able to make use of physitians and chirurgians, or live remote from them. Also an appendix concerning letting blood in the small pox . . . London, Printed by J. L. for Philemon Stephens, 1650.

[6], 70, [4] p.   15 cm.   [8775]

—[The same.] . . . London, Philemon Stephens, 1653.

[6], 70, [4] p.   15 cm.   [8776]

Different setting of type.

—Tractatus de simplicium medicamentorum facultatibus. A treatise of the nature and qualities of such simples as are most frequently used in medicines . . . To which is added: many compound medicines for most diseases . . . Together with the explanation of all hard words or termes of art . . . London, Printed by M. Simmons, for Philemon Stephens, 1652.

3 parts in 1 v.   20 cm.   [8777]

Various pagings.
Errata at end of part [1]
Part 2 has special title page with imprint: London, Printed by J. Legatt for Philemon Stephens, 1653.
Part [3] has special title page: De morbis puerorum. London, Printed by J. Legatt, for Philemon Stephens, 1653.

—Another issue, with new title page.

[8778]

Imperfect: signatures of sheet 3F misbound.
Parts [1] and 2 only.

PEMMEL, Robert. *See* Pemell, Robert [*d.* 1653]

PEÑA, Antonio de Fuente da. *See* Fuente la Peña, Antonio de, *Father* [*fl.* 1676]

PÉNA, Lazare [*d.* 1653] *ed. See* Marinelli, G. Les maladies des femmes. 1609, 1649.

PENA, Pierre [*fl.* 1535-1605] *See* L'Obel, M. de. In G. Rondelletii ... methodicam pharmaceuticam officinam animadversiones. 1605.

PENES NOS UNDA TAGI. *See* Espagnet, Jean d' [17th cent.]

PENICHER, Louis [*fl.* 1698] Collectanea pharmaceutica; seu, Apparatus ad novam pharmacopoeam ... Parisiis, Apud Stephanum Michallet, 1695.
[16], 217, [22] p.   27 cm.   [8779]

—Traité des embaumemens selon les anciens et les modernes. Avec une description de quelques compositions balsamiques & odorantes ... Paris, Barthelmy Girin, 1699.
[24], 315, [3] p.   16 cm.   [8780]

PENNY, Thomas [*d.* 1589] *See* Moffett, T. Insectorum, sive minimorum animalium theatrum. 1634.

PENOT, Bernard Gabriel. *See* Penot, Bernard Georges [*d.* 1617?]

PENOT, Bernard Georges [*d.* 1617?] De denario medico, quo decem medicaminibus, omnibus morbis internis medendi via docetur. Cui plures alii tractatus additi sunt ... Bernae Helvetiorum, Excudebat Joannes le Preux, 1608.
[2], 203, [3] p.   18 cm.   [8781]
"Johannis Isaaci Hollandi, De tribus ordinibus elixiris & lapidis theoria": p. 163-203.
Bound with Leonardi, C. Speculum lapidum. 1610.

—Epistola.
364-367 p., vol. 4.   20 cm.   (*In* Zetzner, Lazarus, *ed.* Theatrum chemicum. Argentorati, 1659-61)
[8782]
Running title.

—[Quaestiones tres de corporali mercurio, an arte ex corporibus perfectis extractus, suo corpori commixtus faciat ad generationem lapidis physici, sicut est quorundam firma opinio] [&] [Quinquaginta septem canones de opere physico, quibus ars dilucidior fit] [&] [Vera mercurii ex auro extractio cum sua historia] [&] Chrysorrhoas; sive, De arte chemica dialogus ...
129-150 p., vol. 2.   20 cm.   (*In* Zetzner, Lazarus, *ed.* Theatrum chemicum. Argentorati, 1659-61)
[8783]

Titles supplied from table of contents, except the last item.
Contains selections from Paracelsus's De usu antimonii and De podagra. Cf. Sudhoff 238 and Duveen, p. 464.

—Tractatus varii, de vera praeparatione et usu medicamentorum chymicorum nunc primum editi, authore et collectore Bernardo G. Penoto à Portu S. Mariae Aquitano ... Editio tertia prioribus emendatior. Ursellis, Ex officina Cornelii Sutorii, sumtibus Joane Rhodii, 1602.
256 p.   17 cm.   [8784]

Imprint on title page appears to have been altered by inserting a second I between C and I.
"Quartus et ultimus tractatus de quarundam herbarum salibus" (p. [211]-256) has special title page. Date of imprint 1601.

—[Selections.] ...
592-682 p., vol. 1.   20 cm.   (*In* Zetzner, Lazarus, *ed.* Theatrum chemicum. Argentorati, 1659-61)
[8785]
Caption title.

—, *ed. See* Aegidius de Vadis. Dialogus. [1659]; Claves, G. Le D., *known as* Gaston de. Apologia chrysopoeiae et argyropoeiae, adversus Thomam Erastum. 1602 [and] Philosophia chymica. 1612; Fioravanti, L. Three exact pieces of Leonard Phioravant. 1652; Paracelsus. One hundred and fourteen experiments and cures. 1652; Tancke, J. Viro nobilissimo ... Dn. Bernhardo G. Penoto ... S. P. Epistola. 1659.

PENUTI. *See* Panutio, Vincenzo [*fl. ca.* 1640]

PERALTA, Diego Osorio y. *See* Osorio y Peralta, Diego.

PERALTA BARNUEVO ROCHA Y BENAVIDES, Pedro de [1663-1743] *See* Rivilla Bonet y Pueyo, J. de. Desvios de la naturaleza. 1695.

PERCIS, HELIOPHILUS A. *See* EGLINUS ICONIUS, Raphael [1559-1622]

PERDU, BENOÎT [1615-1694] Statera sanguinis; sive, Disceptatio de saphenae sectione in febribus tum in viris, tum in praegnantibus. Et de quibusdam aliis casibus. Tornaci, Typis viduae Adriani Quinque, 1668.

[16], 86 p.   18 cm.   **[8786]**

Errata slip mounted on p. [78]
"Corollarium de pestis modernae remedio": p. 79-86.

PERDULCIS, BARTHOLOMAEUS. *See* PARDOUX, Barthélemy [1545-1611]

PEREDA, PEDRO PABLO [16th cent.] Scholia in Michaelis Joannis Paschasii medici Methodum curandi, omnibus medicinam exercentibus maxime utilia ... Venetiis, Apud Societatem Venetam, 1602.

[16], 213 (i.e. 232) ll.   17 cm.   **[8787]**

Contains the text of Pascual's Praxis medica; sive, Methodus curandi, with Pereda's commentary.

—[The same.] In Michaelis Joannis Paschalis Methodum curandi scholia. Addita in extremo operis Disputatio medica, an cannabis, & aqua, in qua mollitur, possint aërem inficere. Opus recens recognitum ... Ed. nov. Lugduni, Sumptibus Jacobi Cardon, 1630.

[8], 212, [8] ll.   19 cm.   **[8788]**

—[The same.] ... Ed. nov., accessit Chymica appendix, authore Car. Sponio ... Lugduni, Sumptibus Laurentii Anisson, 1664.

[16], 635, [17] p.   19 cm.   **[8789]**

PEREIRA, BENITO [*ca.* 1535-1610] De magia, de observatione somniorum et de divinatione astrologica libri tres. Adversus fallaces, et superstitiosas artes. Coloniae Agrippinae, Apud Joannem Gymnicum, 1612.

324, [8] p.   14 cm.   **[8790]**

Bound with Cardano, G. De propria vita liber. 1654.

PERERIUS, BENEDICTUS. *See* PEREIRA, Benito [*ca.* 1535-1610]

PEREYRA, BENITO. *See* PEREIRA, Benito [*ca.* 1535-1610]

PÉREZ, ANTONIO [16th cent.] Summa, y examem [sic] de cirugia, de lo mas necessario que en ella se contiene. Con breves exposiciones de algunas sentencias de Hipocrates, y Galeno ... Valencia, Por Silvestre Esparsa, a costa de Benito Durand, 1634.

[8], 88, [8] ll.   15 cm.   **[8791]**

"Aphorismos de cirugia ... de Hipocrates ... Traduzidos de lengua latina en nuestro vulgar castellano, por ... Antonio Perez": [8] ll. at end.

PÉREZ CASCALES, FRANCISCO [*fl.* 1576-1611] Liber de affectionibus puerorum, una cum tractatu de morbo illo vulgariter garrotillo appellato, cum duabus quaestionibus. Altera, de gerentibus utero rem appententibus denegatam. Altera vero de fascinatione ... Matriti, Apud Ludovicum Sanches, 1611.

[8], 129 (i.e. 131), [2] ll.   20 cm.   **[8792]**

PÉREZ DE BUSTOS, DIEGO [*fl.* 17th cent.] Tratado breve de flobotomia ... Barcelona, Pablo Campins [1627]

[16], 60 p.   illus.   15 cm.   **[8793]**

PÉREZ DE CASTRO, JERÓNIMO [*fl.* 1670] El nigromantico de suplicio severo. Le dedica a las memorandas cenizas de la flor de la andante cavalleria ... el nunca assazmente celebrado, protocavallero Don Quixote de La Mancha ... Barcelona, Murillo, 1670.

[4], 92 ll.   15 cm.   **[8794]**

PÉREZ DE TABORA, FRANCISCO. Tratado contra el abuso de sangrar siempre del tovillo en todas enfermedades universales, y particulares de partes superiores ... Sevilla, Tomás López de Haro [1682]

[12], 192 p.   21 cm.   **[8795]**

PÉREZ RAMÍREZ, LUIS [*fl.* 17th cent.] *See* TENORIO DE LEÓN, A. Atomos que nuevamente se han descubierto con las luzes de Apolo. 1650.

The PERFECT and compleat bel-man. 1666. *See* HORN, H.

Περὶ πολυπαιδίας. 1695. *See* [DUGARD, S.]

PERIANDER *pseud. See* LOCHNER VON HUMMELSTEIN, Michael Friedrich [1662-1720]

Il PERICOLO dimostrato, e'l niente annichilato ... [Ancona, Stamperia camerale, 1696]

[4] p.   29 cm.   **[8796]**

Caption title.

PERIUS, JACOBUS, *ed. See* SETTALA, L. Animadversionum, et cautionum medicarum libri novem. 1650.

PERLA, Francesco. De orientali opobalsamo nuper in theriacae confectione adhibito, et inter Romanos medicos controverso, historica & physica dissertatio. Romae, Ex typographia Ludovici Grignani, 1641.

[8], 214, [25] p.   14 cm.   **[8797]**

—, *ed. See* Hippocrates. [De locis in homine. Latin. 1638.]

PERLINUS, Hieronymus [*fl.* 1610–1612] Binae historiae; seu, Instructiones medicae, physiologicae, pathologicae, pathologicae, et therapeuticae . . . in partes tres divisa . . . Ed. nova, aucta et castigata. Hanoviae, Typis Wechelianis, apud haeredes Joannis Aubrii, 1613.

155 p.   24 cm.   **[8798]**

"De alexiteriis et alexipharmacis commentariolus": p. 72–86; "De morte, caussa graviditatis abortus vel partus medica . . . disputatio": p. 87–155. Items have half titles.

—Declamatio adversus morborum contagionem hujusque auctores & fautores, imo seculum in parte; seu, Praeludium in ejusdem auctoris tres de contagionibus, ac morbis contagiosis contra vulgarem & communem opionionem libros, in quattuor capita divisum . . . Hanoviae, Typis Wechelianis, apud haeredes Joannis Aubrii, 1613.

34, [16] p.   24 cm.   **[8799]**

[PERRAULT, Claude, 1613–1688] Description anatomique d'un cameleon, d'un castor, d'un dromadaire, d'un ours, et d'une gazelle. Paris, Frederic Leonard, 1669.

120 p.   plates.   26 cm.   **[8800]**

Attributed to Claude Perrault by Barbier, vol. 1, col. 889.

[—] Description anatomique de divers animaux dissequez dans l'Academie royale des sciences. Accompagnez de leurs squelet, et representez en figures gravées. Avec les observations faites en leur dissection. 2. ed., augmentée d'une decouverte particuliere touchant la veüe. Paris, Laurent d'Houry, 1682.

120 p.; 27 p.   illus., plates.   25 cm.   **[8801]**

Imperfect: p. 1–2 of part [2] wanting.

Part [1] is a reissue with new title page of Perrault's Description anatomique d'un cameleon . . . Paris . . . 1669.

Part [2] contains letters of Edme Mariotte and Jean Pecquet.

—*See* Académie royale des sciences, Paris. Memoires for a natural history of animals. 1687 [and] Memoir's [sic] for a natural history of animals. 1688;

Mariotte, E. Lettres ecrites sur le sujet d'une nouvelle découverte touchant la veuë. 1682.

PERRAULT, François [1572–1657] The devill of Mascon; or, A true relation of the chiefe things which an uncleane spirit did, and said at Mascon in Burgundy, in the house of Mr Francis Perreaud . . . Published in French . . . and now made English . . . Oxford, Printed by Hen. Hall, for Rich. Davis, 1658.

[28], 46, [3] p.   14 cm.   **[8802]**

Fulton(A) 200.

Letter from Robert Boyle to the translator, Pierre Du Moulin, p. [3–5]

A translation of part [2] of the author's Demonologie, previously published in Geneva, in 1653.

PERRE, Wouter van den [*fl.* 1633] Pest-boeck; ofte, Remedien teghen de pestilentiale cortse, ende om de contagieuse sieckte te ghenesen, met haer symthomatha, ende ghe experimenteerde recepten, midisgaders voor de pocxkens ende maeselen der jonghe kinderen . . . Uyt diversche autheuren . . . Antwerpen, Hendrick Aertssens, 1633.

[8], 112, [7] p.   16 cm.   **[8803]**

PERREAU, Jacques [*fl.* 1654] Rabbat-ioye de l'antimoine triomphant; ou, Examen de l'antimoine justifié de M. Eusebe Renaudeot, &c. . . . Paris, Caspar Meturas, 1655.

[59], 288, [10], 84, [6] p.   24 cm.   **[8804]**

Apparently a reissue of the 1654 edition with new title page mounted on the original.

PERREAUD, François. *See* Perrault, François [1572–1657]

PERSEUS. *See* Scholz, Johann [1621–1687?]

PERSIKE, Andreas [*fl.* 1673] *respondent. See* Rolfinck, W., *praeses.* Specimen hocce inaugurale de siti immoderata . . . submittit. 1673.

PERSIO FLACCO, Aulo. *See* Persius Flaccus, Aulus.

PERSIUS, Philippus [1569–1644] Kurtzer und klarer Bericht: wie man sich zu Zeiten der Pestilentz, und andern in Oesterrich, gewöhnlichen Seuchen; als, Ungrischen [sic] Kranckheit, Rhur, Peteckien, Breun, Kindsblattern und Flecken, und was sonst mehr denen anhängig, verhatten, dieselben sampt ihren Ursachen recht erkennen, sich dafür vorsehen und bewahren solle . . . Auss Befelch der löblichen

Ständt dess Ertz-Hertzogthumbs ob der Ennss, und zum andern Mal übersehen, corrigirt und verbessert ... Anjetzo aber wider auffs new auffgelegt und ubersehen. Lintz, Maria Kürnerin, Wittib, 1649.

[2], 205, [9] p.   15 cm.   **[8805]**

PERSIUS FLACCUS, AULUS. Persio tradotto in verso sciolto e dichiarato da Francesco Stelluti ... Roma, Giacomo Mascardi, 1630.

[24], 218, [20] p.   illus., port.   22 cm.   **[8806]**

Engraved title page.

Latin text and Italian translation of the Satires on facing pages, with commentary below.

"Vita di Persio": p. [11-16]

PERTSCH, STEPHAN KASPAR [1660-1717] *respondent*. Disputatio inauguralis de phthisi ... Argentorati, Literis Johannis Welperi [1685]

[16] p.   20 cm.   **[8807]**

Diss. — Strasbourg.

—*See* RIVINUS, A. Q., *praeses*. Dissertatio medica de asthmate. 1684.

PERUCA, Rainero [*fl.* 1652] Apologia de medici ... in riposta d'altra di Rafaello Carrara [pseud.] intitolata Le confusioni de medici, nella quale, confutate le ragioni aversarie, prova non esservi errore, ne inganno ne medici. Milano, Lodovico Monza, 1655.

[32], 160 p.   15 cm.   **[8808]**

PERUCCI, FRANCESCO [*d.* 1647] Pompe funebri di tutte le nationi del mondo, raccolte dalle storie sagre, e profane ... in questa 2. impr. reviste, e con somma accuratezza da molti errori e spurgate, e corrette. Verona, Francesco Rossi [1646]

[16], 146, [1] p.   illus.   17 x 23 cm.   **[8809]**

PERUCHIO, DE. La chiromance, la physionomie, et la geomance, avec la signification des nombres, & l'usage de la roüe de Pytagore ... Paris, Louis Billaine, 1663.

[16], 343 p.   illus., plates, tables.   24 cm.

[8810]

Caillet 8555.

PERUGIA. Magnifica arte delli spetiali. Tariffa et prezzi da vendere, & apprezzare le robbe, e mercantie delle spetiarie di Perugia, e suo contado. Constituita, & ordinata dalla Magnifica arte delli spetiali di detta città, comminciando adi primo di Maggio

1683. [Perugia, Per gli heredi di Alessandro Petrucci, 1619]

[32] p.   21 cm.   **[8811]**

Maggio 1683 added on title page by hand.

Prices after each item listed by hand.

Imperfect: top margin shaved, affecting text.

PERUGINO, LUDOVICO AURELI. *See* AURELI, Lodovico, *Father* [*d.* 1637]

PESCHINUS, CYPRIANUS [*fl.* 1626] Christlicher Bericht von Sterbensläufften, darinnen vermög göttlichen Worts ... was die Plage der Pestilentz sey ... Aus den Schrifften etlicher fürtreflichen und hochgelarten Theologen aussgezogen ... Lignitz, Fürstl. Druckerey, 1626.

[164] p.   19 cm.   **[8812]**

PESSERL, JONAS [*fl.* 1602-1605] *respondent. See* SENNERT, D., *praeses*. De methodo medendi disputatio VIII, de humorum coctione et praeparatione. 1604.

PESSINA, SEBASTIANO. *See* PISSINI, Sebastiano [*fl.* 1609-1654]

PEST-BESCHRIJVING, waer in naukeurigh de naeste oorzaeke der peste onderzocht, en haere grondige genezing, in verscheyde geneeskundige aenmerkingen, voorgestelt wort. Uyt verscheyde ervaerene artzen, als Diemerbroek, Tomas Willis, Deuzing, Barbette, &c. By een verzamelt door Dr. H. S. Amsterdam, Abram Witteling, 1664.

[1], 142 p.   16 cm.   **[8813]**

With this is bound (as issued?) Deusing, A. Twee diepzinnige en heilzame onderzoekingen nopende de pest. 1664.

—Another issue, with new title page: De pest, naaukeurig onderzocht, grondigh geneezen, en volmaakter als oit beschreven ... Amsterdam, Jan van Duisbergh, 1664.

[8814]

PESTIS vera, et nova idea in duas partes digesta. Quarum prior aphorismos de natura, essentia, causa; & origine pestis posterior eam depellendi, & extinguendi methodum infallibilem, in paucas regulas ex diffusiori ejus historia contractam, continet. Wratislaviae, In Officina Baumanniana, typis exprimebat Joannes Jankius [1699?]

31 p.   16 cm.   **[8815]**

Johann Jancke printed in Breslau from 1699. Cf. Benzing (A)

PETAU, DENIS [1583-1652]. *See* CARRANZA, A. Diatriba. 1628 [and] Tractatus novus ... de partu naturali et legitimo. 1629, 1630.

PETAVIUS, DIONYSIUS. *See* PETAU, Denis [1583-1652]

PETER, CHARLES [*fl.* 1665-1695] A description of the venereal disease: declaring the causes, signs, effects and cure thereof. With a discourse of the most wonderful antivenereal pill ... London, Printed for the author, 1675.

    16 p. 16 cm.   **[8816]**
    Imperfect: margins shaved.

—Observations on the venereal disease, with the true way of curing the same ... London, Printed by D. Mallet, and sold by the author, 1686.

    76 p. 14 cm.   **[8817]**
    Date changed by pen to 1693.

—New observations on the venereal disease, with the true way of curing the same. The 2d ed., corr. and enl. ... London, Printed by S. D. and D. N., and sold by the author, 1695.

    [8], 132 (i.e. 136) p. 15 cm.   **[8818]**

PETER, JOHN [*fl.* 1677-1683] A philosophical account of this hard frost. From whence is rationally concluded what effects it may probably have upon humane bodies, as to health and sickness ... With cautionary directions for the prevention of such distempers as are likely to be the natural consequence ... London, Sam. Smith, 1684.

    [2], 10 p. 20 cm.   **[8819]**

—A treatise of Lewisham (but vulgarly called Dulwich) Wells in Kent. Shewing the time and manner of their discovery, the minerals with which they are impregnated, the several diseases experience hath found them good for; with directions for the use of them, &c. ... London, Printed by Tho. James for Sam. Tidmarsk, 1681.

    [24], 88 p. 14 cm.   **[8820]**

PETERMANN, ANDREAS [1649-1703]

Dissertations — Leipzig

—*praeses.* De medicamentis alvum laxantibus ... Lipsiae, Typis John. Christoph. Brandenburgeri [1692]

    [16] p. 19 cm.   **[8821]**
    E. Küchler, *respondent.*

—Disputatio medica de ephialte seu incubo ... Lipsiae, Typis Christophori Fleischeri [1688]

    [40] p. 18 cm.   **[8822]**
    J. Müller, *respondent.*

—Disputatio medica de pleuritide ... Lipsiae, Typis Christiani Banckmanni [1690]

    [22] p. 19 cm.   **[8823]**
    D. K. Köster, *respondent.*

—Dissertatio medica de enterocele ... Lipsiae, Typis Christoph. Fleischeri [1696]

    [28] p. 20 cm.   **[8824]**
    D. Martini, *respondent.*

—Dissertatio physiologica de visu ... Lipsiae, Literis Christophori Guntheri [1690]

    [20] p. 19 cm.   **[8825]**
    M. G. Schuster, *respondent.*

—Dissertationem medicam de gonorrhoea ... exponit Tobias Peucer ... [Lipsiae] Typis Justi Reinholdi [1690]

    [20] p. 20 cm.   **[8826]**
    T. Peucer, *respondent.*

—Scrutinium icteri ex calculis vesiculae fellis occasione casus cujusdam singularis ... Lipsiae, Excudebat Christoph. Fleischerus [1696]

    [40] p. 20 cm.   **[8827]**
    J. G. Albrecht, *respondent.*

—*respondent.* Dissertatio medica inauguralis de nutritione integra servanda abolitaque reparanda ... Altdorffii, Typis Henrici Meyeri [1672]

    28 p. 19 cm.   **[8828]**
    Diss.—Altdorf.

— *See* SIEGEMUND, J. D. Wider Herrn D. Andreae Peterman ... von ihm also-genante gründliche Deduction vieler Handgriffe. 1692.

PETERMANN, DANIEL [*fl.* 1669-1677] *praeses.* Disputationem de glacie ... exponit Gottfried Schmied ... Lipsiae, Coberianis [1670]

    [20] p. 20 cm.   **[8829]**
    Diss.—Leipzig (G. Schmied, *respondent*)

PETERS, FRANZ [*fl.* 1663-1669] *respondent. See* SCHENCK, J. T., *praeses.* Disputationem medicam inauguralem de imbecillitate ventriculi ... publico sistit examini ... F. P. 1669; STRAUSS, L., *praeses.* Disputatio physico-medica de potu coffi. 1666.

PETERS, PETRUS [*fl.* 1679] *respondent.* Disputatio medica inauguralis de diarrhoea ... Lugduni Batavorum, Apud viduam & heredes Johannis Elsevirii, 1679.

[16] p. 22 cm. **[8830]**

Diss. — Leyden.

[PETERSEN, JOHANN WILHELM, 1649-1727] Elegia propemptica cum ... domini Dn. Joannis Tackii, medici consummatissimi filius aemulus ... Dn. Ludovicus Christianus Tackius ... discederet, ad contestandem veteris amicitiae fidem fusa & transmissa ab ejus commensalibus. Gissae-Hassorum, Literis Friderici Kargeri, 1675.

[8] p. 20 cm. **[8831]**

PETIT, PIERRE [1617-1687] De lacrymis libri tres. Parisiis, Apud Claudium Cramoisy, 1661.

[15], 212 (i.e. 221), [17] p. 18 cm. **[8832]**

—De motu animalium spontaneo liber unus, in quo partim Aristotelis de hujus motus principio sententia illustratur, partim nova musculorum motus ratio indagatur. Parisiis, E typographia Claudii Cramoisy, 1660.

176, [3] p. 17 cm. **[8833]**

—De natura & moribus anthropophagorum dissertatio. Trajecti ad Rhenum, Ex officina Rudolphi a Zyll, 1688.

152 p. 19 cm. **[8834]**

Bound with *his* Homeri nepenthes. 1698.

—Homeri nepenthes; sive, De Helenae medicamento luctum, animique omnem aegritudinem abolente, & aliis quibusdam eadem facultate praeditis, dissertatio. Trajecti ad Rhenum, Ex officina Rudolphi a Zyll, 1689.

[30], 159 p. 19 cm. **[8835]**

Sig. xx8 (blank) wanting.

—Another issue, with imprint: Trajecti ad Rhenum, Apud Franciscum Halmam, 1698.

[8836]

Title page and preliminary matter reset.
With this is bound *his* De natura & moribus anthropophagorum. 1688.

—Miscellanearum observationum libri quatuor, nunquam antehac editi. Trajecti ad Rhenum, Typis Rudolphi a Zyll, 1682.

[16], 308, [25] p. 20 cm. **[8837]**

PETIT DOUXCIEL, ANCELME [*fl.* 1648] Speculum physionomicum ... Langres, Paris, L'autheur, Gervais Clousier, 1648.

[12], 184 p. port., plates. 20 cm. **[8838]**

PETRAEUS, HENRICUS [1589-1620] Encheiridion cheirurgicum: Handbüchlein oder kurtzer Begriff der Wundartzney ... Auss den aller besten und bewehrtesten Scribenten zusammen gezogen, verdeutschet, und in X. Tractätlein ... verfertiget ... Marpurg, Paul Egenolph, 1617.

[16], 293 p. plates. 21 cm. **[8839]**

—[The same.] Encheiridion cheirurgicum; das ist, Kurtzer Bericht oder Handbuch der Kunst der Wundartzney. Item, Guilielmi Fabritii Hildani Tractat vom heissen und kalten Brandt. Auff das Neu revidirt und verbessert ... Nürnberg, Abraham Wagenmann [1625]

[16], 959, [14] p. illus., plates. 16 cm. **[8840]**

—*praeses.* Agonismata medica Marpurgensia, dogmatica juxta & hermetica I. De aphaeresi, seu evacuatione universali, disputationes V. II. Disputationes miscellaneae XV ... III. His accessit ogdoas disp. med. inauguralium ... Adjectae sunt ad calcem assertiones & quaestiones de genuina febris Ungaricae natura, & cura multis hactenus incognita. Marpurgi Cattorum, Excudebat Paulus Egenolphus, 1618.

[16], 419 p. 19 cm. **[8841]**

Contains 29 Marburg dissertations.

—Nosologia harmonica dogmatica & hermetica: dissertationibus quinquaginta in celeberrima Academia Mauritiana ... Tomus primus [-secundus] ... Marpurgi Cattorum, Typis Pauli Egenolphi, 1615.

2 v. 21 cm. **[8842]**

Contains 52 Marburg dissertations, enumerated in the Index-Catalogue, 1st ser., vol. 10.

—Copy 2.

Vol. 1 only.
With this is bound Brendel, J. P. Consilia medica. 1615.

—Disputatio medica de dieta, sive sex rebus non naturalibus ... Marpurgi Hessorum, Paulus Egenolphus, 1611.

[16] p. 19 cm. **[8843]**

Diss. — Marburg (J. de Le Pipre, *respondent*)

—Disputatio medica de natura, differentiis, usuque partium in genere . . . Marpurgi Cattorum, Excudebat Paulus Egenolphus, 1615.

[8] p.   20 cm.   [8844]

Diss. — Marburg (H. Goeddaeus, *respondent*)

—Disquisitio hermetica de origine formarum e seminio virtute plastica instructo, omnibus in rerum naturalium jucunda cognitione, & fructuosa applicatione sincere versantibus physicis, ac medicis summa necessaria . . . Marpurgi Cattorum, Typis Pauli Egenolphi, 1612.

[26] p.   20 cm.   [8845]

Diss. — Marburg (H. U. Grob, *respondent*)

PETRAEUS, Peter Paul. *See* Petreus, Petrus Paulus.

PETREIUS, Nicolas [1500-1568] *tr. See* Hippocrates. [Collected works. Latin] Opera. 1610, 1619, 1679 [and] [Collected works. Greek and Latin] Τὰ εὑρισκόμενα. 1657, 1662; Stefani, G. In Hippocratis Coi libellum De hominis structura commentarius. 1633.

PETREIUS, Petrus Paulus. *See* Petreus, Petrus Paulus.

PETREJUS, Henricus. *See* Petraeus, Henricus [1589-1620]

PETREO, Nicola. *See* Petreius, Nicolas [1500-1568]

PETREUS, Petrus Paulus. Musaeum Travaginianum; seu, Hermeticorum medicamentorum, quae in . . . Francisci Travagini musaeo elaborata reperiuntur, elenchus, ubi eorumdem virtutes, doses, cautelae, & usus clare designantur, cura, & studio . . . Venetiis, Apud Jo. Jacobum Hertz, 1679.

[36], 141 p.   plates.   16 cm.   [8846]

Imperfect: plates wanting.

PETRI, Georg Christoph, von Hartenfels. *See* Petri von Hartenfels, Georg Christoph [1633-1718]

PETRI, Georg Heinrich [*fl.* 1667] *respondent. See* Zentgraf, J. J., *praeses*. Disputatio prior de tactu regis Franciae. 1675.

PETRI, Johann [*fl.* 1661] *respondent.* Disputatio medica inauguralis de febri quartana exquisite intermittente . . . Altdorffii, Typis Georgii Hagen [1661]

[23] p.   19 cm.   [8847]

Imperfect: wormholes throughout.
Diss. — Altdorf.

PETRI, Peter Lambert [*fl.* 1679] *respondent. See* Meibom, H., *praeses*. Exercitatio medica de tumoribus pedum imprimis oedematosis. 1679.

PETRI VON HARTENFELS, Georg Christoph [1633-1718] Pestis tela praevisa; das ist, Nützliche Anleitung, wie bey diesen besorglichen Zeiten Reiche und Arme vor der abscheulichen Seuche der Pestilentz durch bewährte Schutz-Mittel sich bewahren . . . und retten könne . . . Erffurt, Benjamin Hempel, 1682.

[22], 168 p.   14 cm.   [8848]

— شوک مبارک Asylum langventium; seu, Carduus sanctus, vulgo benedictus . . . Jenae, Impensis Viti Jacobi Trescheri, typis Johannis Nisii, 1669.

252, [20] p.   illus.   16 cm.   [8849]

Dissertations — Erfurt

—*praeses*. Diatribe inauguralis medica de suffocatione uterina . . . Erfordiae, Typis Joh. Georgi Hertzii [1672]

[28] p.   20 cm.   [8850]

J. J. Gotter, *respondent*.

—Disputatio inauguralis medica de febre petechiali . . . Erfordiae, Stanno Groschiano [1691]

[24] p.   19 cm.   [8851]

G. E. Wirth, *respondent*.

—Disputatio inauguralis medica, de morbo comitiali . . . Erffordiae, Stanno Groschiano [1688]

28 p.   19 cm.   [8852]

D. C. Völcker, *respondent*.

—Disputatio inauguralis medica, de phlegmone . . . Erfordiae, Typis Joh. Henrici Groschii [1690]

32 p.   20 cm.   [8853]

J. C. Adami, *respondent*.

—Disputatio inauguralis medica, de strangulatione a vaporibus externis . . . [Erfordiae] Ex officina Joh. Heinr. Groschii [1693]

[16] p.   19 cm.   [8854]

G. Schultz, *respondent*.

—Disputatio medica inauguralis virginem chlorosi . . . Erffurti, Typis Joh. Henr. Groschii [1693]

[16] p.   20 cm.   [8855]

C. von Hellwig, *respondent*.

—Dissertatio inauguralis medica, de dolore hypochondriaco . . . Erfordiae, Stanno Groschiano [1691]

    28 p.   20 cm.   **[8856]**

  M. G. Schuster, *respondent.*

—Dissertatio inauguralis medica de febre hectica . . . Erfurt, Stanno Kirschiano [1679]

    [28] p.   19 cm.   **[8857]**

  C. Schuchmann, *respondent.*

—Dissertatio medica inauguralis de anorexia seu apositia, Germanice Unlust zum Essen . . . Erfordiae, Typis Joh. Henr. Groschii [1692]

    36 p.   20 cm.   **[8858]**

  C. Gehrig, *respondent.*

—Dissertationem inauguralem de abortu . . . submittit Christianus Heinricus Weber . . . Erfordiae, Charactere Kirschiano [1678]

    [28] p.   19 cm.   **[8859]**

  C. H. Weber, *respondent.*

—Ignem microcosmicum, qui Graecis, καυσος, Latinis, febris ardens, Germanis, das hitzige Fieber, vocantur . . . pro licentia . . . Submittit Bernhardus Herlinus . . . Erffurti, Literis Joh. Georg. Hertzii [1670]

    [24] p.   20 cm.   **[8860]**

  B. Herlinus, *respondent.*

PETROGONE, Vincenzo. *See* Petrone, Vincenzo di [d. 1655]

PETRONE, Vincenzo di [d. 1655] Literarium duellum inter Salernitanos, et Neapolitanos medicos . . . in quo de intestinorum phlegmone controvertitur casus. Una cum Michaelis Rocci . . . Apologia. Et alio ejusdem auctoris literario addito De hepatis inflammatione duello . . . Venetiis, Apud Bertanos, 1647.

    [8], 144 p.   22 cm.   **[8861]**

PETRUCCI, Giuseppe [d. 1680] Prodomo apologetico alli studi chircheriani. Opera di Gioseffo Petrucci . . . nella quale . . . si dá prova dell'esquisitio studio ha tenuto il . . . padre Atanasio Chircher, circa il credere all'opinioni degli scrittori . . . e particolarmente intorno a quelle cose naturali dell'India, che gli furon portate, ò referte da'quei, che abitarono quelle parti. Amsterdam, Presso li Janssonio-Waesbergi, 1677.

    [16], 200 p.   illus., plates.   24 cm.   **[8862]**

  Added engraved title page.

PETRUCCI, Tommaso [1648–*ca.* 1711] Spigilegium anatomicum. *In* Cellier, A., *ed.* Opuscula nova anatomica. 1680.

PETRUS ARLENSIS DE SCUDALUPIS. *See* Leonardi, C. Speculum lapidum. 1610.

PETRUS DE ABANO. *See* Abano, Pietro d' [1250–1315?]

PETRUS DE SILENTO. Opus . . .

    985–997 p., vol. 4.   20 cm. (*In* Zetzner, Lazarus, *ed.* Theatrum chemicum. Argentorati, 1659–61)   **[8863]**

  Caption title.

PETRUS DE ZALENTO. *See* Petrus de Silento.

PETRUS DRASENSIS. *See* Petrus Dresdensis [d. 1440]

PETRUS DRESDENSIS [d. 1440] *See* Thomasius, J. [1622–1684] *praeses.* Dissertatio historica de Petro Dresdensi. 1678.

PETRUS HISPANUS. *See* Johannes XXI, *Pope* [d. 1277]

PETRUS JULIANES. *See* Johannes XXI, *Pope* [d. 1277]

PETRUS LUSITANUS. *See* Johannes XXI, *Pope* [d. 1277]

PETRUS PADUANENSIS. *See* Abano, Pietro d' [1250–1315?]

PETRUS VON LISSABON. *See* Johannes XXI, *Pope* [d. 1277]

PETTY, Sir William [1623–1687] An essay concerning the multiplication of mankind: together with another essay . . . concerning the growth of the city of London . . . 2. ed. rev. and enl. . . . London, Mark Pardoe, 1686.

    [1], 50 p.   16 cm.   **[8864]**

  Imperfect: upper margins trimmed.
  A reprint of Another essay.
  Keynes(C) 26.

—Five essays in political arithmetick, viz. I. Objections from the city of Rey in Persia, and from Monsr Auzout, against two former essays, answered . . . II. A comparison between London and Paris . . . III. Proofs that at London . . . there live about 696 thousand people. IV. An estimate of the people in London, Paris, Amsterdam ... V. Concerning Holland ... London, Henry Mortlock, 1687.

[8], 51 (i.e. 102) p.   16 cm.   **[8865]**

In French and English.
Keynes(C) 31.

—Observations upon the cities of London and Rome ... London, Henry Mortlocke and J. Lloyd, 1687.

[2], 4 p.   16 cm.   **[8866]**

Keynes(C) 28.
Bound (as issued) with *his* Two essays. 1687.

—Political arithmetick; or, A discourse concerning the extent and value of lands, people, buildings ... As the same relates to every country in general, but more particularly to the territories of His Majesty of Great Britain, and his neighbours of Holland, Zealand, and France ... London, Robert Clavel and Hen. Mortlock, 1691.

[21], 117, [3] p.   18 cm.   **[8867]**

Keynes(C) 35.

—Two essays in political arithmetick, concerning the people, housing, hospitals, &c. of London and Paris ... London, J. Lloyd, 1687.

[5], 21, [1] p.   16 cm.   **[8868]**

Keynes(C) 28.
With this is bound (as issued) *his* Observations. 1687.

—*See* GRAUNT, J. Natural and political observations. 1662, 1665, 1676.

PETZ, GEORG SIGISMUND [*fl.* 1674] *respondent.* De phthisi disputatio medica inauguralis ... Altdorfii, Typis Henrici Meyeri [1674]

24 p.   20 cm.   **[8869]**

Diss.—Altdorf.

PETZ, WILHELM CHRISTOPH PAUL [*fl.* 1699] *respondent. See* SLEVOGT, J. A., *praeses.* Aegram lochiorum fluxu nimio vel potius haemorrhagia uteri laborantem ... exponet W. C. P. P. 1699.

PETZOLD, JUSTINUS [*fl.* 1581] *See* SCHOLTZ, L. Epistolarum philosophicarum: medicinalium, ac chymicarum ... volumen. 1610.

PEU, PHILIPPE [1623–1707] La pratique des acouchemens ... Paris, Jean Boudot, 1694.

[24], 613, [1] p.   front. (port.), plates.   18 cm.
                                              [8870]

Imperfect: frontispiece misbound after title page.

—Another issue.

[24], 613, [1] p.; 15 p.; 114, [2] p.   20 cm.
                                              [8871]

Imperfect? sheet á bound before sheet a.

Includes Avertissement de M. Mauriceau, Réponse a l'Avertissement [de M. Mauriceau], (second group of paging); and Réponse de Mr. Peu aux Observations ... de Mr. Mauriceau (third group of paging).

Mauriceau's Avertissement originally formed p. [5–6] of his Observations (Part [2] of Traité des maladies des femmes grosses, 4. ed.) published in Paris in 1694.

—Another issue.   20 cm.   **[8872]**

A reissue of the enlarged 1694 edition with original imprint covered by label: Paris, Nicolas le Clerc, 1726.

PEUCER, TOBIAS [*fl.* 1690–1691] *respondent. See* PETERMANN, A., *praeses.* Dissertationem medicam de gonorrhoea ... exponit ... T. P. 1690.

—, *tr. See* BLANKAART, S. Collectanea medico-physica. 1690; SOLINGEN, C. Embryulcia. 1693.

PEUSCHEL, JOHANN FRIEDRICH [*fl.* 1667] *respondent. See* HUNDESHAGEN, J. C., *praeses.* Disputationem meteorologicam de ventis ... examini subjiciet ... J. F. P. 1667.

PEYER, HANS CONRAD *See* PEYER, Johann Konrad [1653–1712]

PEYER, JOHANN KONRAD [1653–1712] Exercitatio anatomico-medica de glandulis intestinorum, earumque usu & affectionibus, cui subjungitur Anatome ventriculi gallinacei ... Scafhusae, Impensis Onophrii a Waldkirch, typis Alexandri Riedingii, 1677.

[28], 136 p.   plates.   16 cm.   **[8873]**

"Anatome ventriculi gallinacei" (p. 97–136) has half-title.

—[The same.] ... Amstelaedami, Apud Henricum Weststenium, 1681.

[28], 136 p.   plates.   16 cm.   **[8874]**

A reissue of the 1677 edition with new title page.

—Merycologia; sive, De ruminantibus et ruminatione commentarius ... Basileae, Apud Joh. Ludovicum Koenig & Joh. Brandmyllerum, 1685.

[8], 288, [34] p.   plates.   20 cm.   **[8875]**

—Methodus historiarum anatomico-medicarum exemplo ascitis, vitalium organorum vitio, ex pericardii coalitu cum corde nati illustrata ... Parisiis, Apud Lambertum Roulland, 1678.

[22], 166 p.   15 cm.   **[8876]**

—Parerga anatomica et medica septem, ratione ac experientia parentibus concepta & edita. Genevae, J. Herman. Widerhold, 1681.

    [40], 202 p. plates. 18 cm.   **[8877]**

Contents.—Exercitatio anatomico medica prima, de glandulis intestinorum. Adjecta est Anatome ventriculi gallinacei, editio altera priore correctior.—Exercitatio anatomico-medica II. De glandulis intestinorum, quae nunc primum priori auctarii vice accedit; and letters addressed to J. v. Muralt, C. Spon, and J. J. Harder, and their answers.

Items have half titles.

—Schediasma de pancreate et ejus usu. *In* Brunner, J. C. Experimenta nova circa pancreas. 1683.

—*praeses*. Meditatio de valetudine humana ... Basileae, Typis Jacobi Bertschii, 1681.

    [12] p. 19 cm.   **[8878]**

—*See* HARDER, J. J. Paeonis [pseud.] et Pythagorae [pseud., i.e. J. C. Peyer] Exercitationes anatomicae. 1682 [and] Prodromus physiologicus. 1679.

PEYMA, JOHANN IGNATIUS WORP BEINTEMA VAN. *See* WORB, Johan Ignaz [*b.* 1666]

PEYSSONEL, JEAN DE [*fl.* 1660] De temporibus humani partus, juxta doctrinam Hippocratis, tractatus. Lugduni, Sumptib. Joan. Ant. Huguetan, & Marci-Anton. Ravaud, 1665.

    [8], 86 (i.e 88) p. illus. 16 cm.   **[8879]**

Imperfect: movable parts of the diagram on the leaf between pages 58 and 59 wanting.

Includes extracts in Greek and Latin from various Hippocratic works, especially the De septimestri partu.

—Another issue, with the imprint date altered to 1666.   **[8880]**

Diagram with movable parts on leaf between pages 58 and 59.

—[The same.] *In* Barra, P. De veris terminis partus humani libri tres ex Hippocrate. 1666.

PEZ, WILHELM CHRISTOPH PAUL [*b.* 1674] *See* WEDEL, G. W. Propemticum inaugurale de ramo aureo Virgilii II. 1700.

PEZEL, CHRISTOPH [1539-1604] Praecepta genethliaca; sive, De prognosticandis hominum nativitatibus commentarius eruditissimus, in quo non solum astrologiae praecepta & certa istius fundamenta demonstrantur, verum etiam varii casus, historiae, eventus & exempla lepidissima proponuntur ... Francofurti, Typis Wolfgangi Richteri,

impensis Johan. Theobaldi Schonwetteri & Cunradi Meulii, 1607.

    [8], 227 p. illus., tables. 20 cm.   **[8881]**

PEZOLD, CASPAR [1666-1715] *respondent. See* CRAUSE, R. W., *praeses*. Disputatio inauguralis medica de phrenitide. 1689; WEDEL, G. W. Propempticon inaugurale de morbo hiobi. 1689.

PEZOLD, JOHANN CHRISTOPH [*fl.* 1695-1699] *respondent. See* HOFFMANN, F. [1660-1742] *praeses*. Dissertatio inauguralis medico-practica, de pleuritide. 1699; VATER, C., *praeses*. De mercurialibus medicamentis. 1695 [and] Rationes et curationes dolorum. 1696.

PEZOLD, KARL FRIEDRICH [1675-1731] *praeses*. Dissertationem philologico-physico-historicam de memoria memorabili ... submittit ... Johannes Georgius Pielz ... Lipsiae, Literis Brandenburgerianis [1699]

    [32] p. 20 cm.   **[8882]**

Diss.—Leipzig (J. G. Pielz, *respondent*)

PEZOLDUS, JUSTINUS. *See* PETZOLD, Justinus [*fl.* 1581]

PEZZINI, SEBASTIANO. Del modo di purgare le case e robbe infette, e sospette. Relatione ... fatta di ordine del Collegio de Medici ... Lucca, Ottaviano Guidoboni, 1631.

    [1], 7-44 p. 20 cm.   **[8883]**

Imperfect: p. 41-44 mutilated.

PFANN, JOHANN [*fl.* 1626-*ca.*1670] Biblische Emblemata und Figuren welche in den zweyen verneurten Stuben dess Hospitals zum Heiligen Geist in Nûrmberg allen Krancken zu sondern Trost anstatt der Schrifft sind vorgemalet worden. In Küpffer gestochen ... [Nürnberg] 1626.

    [5], 16 plates. 19 cm.   **[8884]**

Engraved title page.

Has additional half title: Aigentlicher Abriss der neuen im Spital aufgehengten Tafeln.

Imperfect: plates [2-5] bound between plates 8 and 9.

PFANNER, JOHANN [*fl.* 1628] De generali morborum curatione, & curationibus insolitis, prodigiosis, ipsaque armorum inunctione dissertationes tres ... Basileae, Apud Ludovicum Regem [1628?]

    79 p. 16 cm.   **[8885]**

PFAUTZ, CHRISTOPH [1645-1711] *praeses*. Dissertatio historico-physica, de fluxu sanguinis e corpore occisi ad praesentiam occisoris . . . Lipsiae, Typis Joh. Wittigau, 1664.

[32] p.   19 cm.   [8886]

Diss. — Leipzig (C. Blauschmied, *respondent*)

PFAUTZ, ERHARD [*fl.* 1662] *respondent.* *See* SCHWENCK, J. S., *praeses.* Decuria positonum physicarum. 1662.

PFAUZIUS, ERHARDUS. *See* PFAUTZ, Erhard [*fl.* 1662]

PFEIFER, GEORG CHRISTIAN [*fl.* 1672-1677] *respondent. See* LOSS, J., *praeses.* Casum practicum de asthmate convulsio . . . examini exponit . . . G. C. P. 1676; SENNERT, M., *praeses.* Disputatio inauguralis medica de dysenteria. 1677.

PFEIFFER, ANDREAS [*fl.* 1653] *respondent.* De convulsione. *In* Rolfinck, W., *praeses.* Methodus cognoscendi & curandi adfectus capitis particulares. 1653.

PFEIFFER, AUGUST [1640-1698] Christognosia orthodoxa; oder, Nach Anleitung S. Johannis und Pauli deutlich gewiesene christliche Wissenschafft von Christo nebst denen Lineamenten oder Entwurff und Inthalt unsers christl. evangelischen Glaubens-Bekäntnisses der augspurgischen Confession . . . Leipzig, Bey Christian Michaeln, 1682.

[12], 91 p.   21 cm.   [8887]

—Passions-Register; oder, Das Leiden und Sterben unsers Heylands Jesu Christi nach seinen vornehmsten Stücken . . . aus dem XXII. Psalm Davids gezogen . . . [Leipzig] Zum Drucke befordert von Christian Michaelis, 1682.

76, [4] p.   21 cm.   [8888]

—Salve Lipsiacum, bestehend in einer Gast-Predigt, darinnen instrumentum pacis conjugalis, der Ehe-Friedens-Schluss; und in einer Anzugs-Predigt, darinnen idea pastoris conscientiosi, das Muster eines gewissenhafften Predigers . . . [Leipzig] Zum Druck befördert von Christian Michaelis, 1682.

68, [2] p.   21 cm.   [8889]

PFEIFFER, GEORGIUS CHRISTIANUS. *See* PFEIFER, Georg Christian [*fl.* 1672-1677]

PFEIFFER, JOHANN [1606-1667] *praeses.* Disputatio physica de primis qualitatibus elementorum,

quatenus considerantur in perfecte mixtis . . . Lipsiae, Typis exscribebat Gregorius Ritzsch, 1629.

[11] p.   18 cm.   [8890]

Diss. — Leipzig (J. Dreyscherff, *respondent*)

PFEIFFER, JOHANN PHILIPP [1645-1695] *praeses.* Dissertatio philologica, de cura virginum apud veteres, prima . . . Regiomonti, Typis Friderici Reusneri [1672]

[31] p.   20 cm.   [8891]

Diss. — Königsberg (C. Rahnisch, *respondent*)

PFEIFFER, SALOMON. *See* TRISMOSIN, Salomon, *pseud.?*

PFEIFFER, SIEGMUND AUGUST [*fl.* 1690-1719] *respondent. See* STOLTERFOHT, J. J., *praeses.* Physiologia in nuce. 1697.

PFEIL, JOHANN [*d.* 1544] *See* SCHOLTZ, L. Consiliorum medicinalium . . . liber singularis. 1610.

PFENDLER, HEINRICH [*fl.* 1616] *respondent. See* STUPANUS, E., *praeses.* Τοῦ κατὰ την καρδίαν παλμὸν διαγνώσεώς τε καὶ Θεραπείας διάσκεψις. 1616.

PFENDTNER, EMERICUS [*fl.* 1689-1691] Oesterreicherischer Galenus; das ist, Lob-Leich- und Ehren-Predig . . . dess . . . Herrn, Pauli de Sorbait . . . den 10. Maii anno 1691. Wienn, Leopold Voight [1691?]

[54] p.   19 cm.   [8892]

PFEYL, JOHANN. *See* PFEIL, Johann [*d.* 1544]

PFISTER, ALEXANDER [*fl.* 1689] *respondent.* Disputatio inauguralis medico-chirurgica de νδροσαρκοηλη . . . Basileae, Typis Jacobi Bertschii [1689]

[26] p.   19 cm.   [8893]

Diss. — Basel.

—*See* HARDER, J. J. Alexander Pfisterus. 1689.

PFITZER, JOHANN NICOLAUS [1634-1674] Vernünfftiges Wunden-Urtheil, wie man nemlich von allen Wunden dess menschlichen Leibs gründlichen Bericht, ob solche gefährlich, tödtlich, oder nicht vor Gericht und anderswo ertheilen möge . . . Nürnberg, In Verlegung Johann Andreae Endter und Wolfgang dess Jüngern sel. Erben, 1668.

[24], 192 p.   14 cm.   [8894]

—Zwey sonderbare Bücher, von der Weiber Natur, wie auch deren Gebrechen und Kranckheiten ... Sampt einem Anhang von den Zufällen und Kranckheiten der Kinder ... Nürnberg, In Verlegung Johann Andreae und Wolfgang Endters dess Jüngern Sel. Erben, 1673.

[56], 336, [8], 337–760, [16] p.   17 cm.   **[8895]**

Das andere Buch has special title page.

—[The same.] ... Anjetzo mit curieusen und aus denen neuesten Authorn gezogenen Erfind- und Anmerckungen bereichert und vermehrt. Altdorff, Gedruckt bey Heinrich Meyern, in Verlegung Wolfgang Moritz Endters, 1691.

[56], 404, [8], 405–856, [24] p.   17 cm.   **[8896]**

Das andere Buch has special title page, dated 1692.

—*respondent.* Disputatio inauguralis medica de variolis et morbillis ... Argentorati, Typis Johannis Goebelii [1660]

43 p.   19 cm.   **[8897]**

Diss. — Strasbourg.

PFITZER, JOHANN PHILIPP [*fl.* 1634] *respondent.* Disputatio inauguralis theorico-practica de phthisi ... Argentorati, Typis haeredum Pauli Ledertz, 1634.

[17] p.   19 cm.   **[8898]**

Diss. — Strasbourg.

PFIZER, JOHANN NICOLAUS. *See* PFITZER, Johann Nicolaus [1634–1674]

PFUNDT, EHRENFRIED [*fl.* 1673–*ca.* 1685] *respondent. See* SIEGFRIED, C. E. [*fl.* 1673] *praeses.* Disputatio physica de magnete. 1673.

PHAEDRO, GEORGIUS, Rhodochaeus. *See* FEDRO VON RODACH, Georg [16th cent.]

PHAEDRON, MAGNUS GEORG DE GELEINEN. *See* FEDRO VON RODACH, Georg [16th cent.]

PHAÉTON. *See* SCARAMUCCI, Giovanni Battista [1650–*ca.* 1710]

PHALAIA tripartita. *See* RUMMEL, J. P. Opuscula chymico-magico-medica. 1635.

PHARMACIA Galenica & chymica; dat is, Apotheker ende alchymiste ofte distilleer-konste ... Door een liefhebber der selver konste. Amsteldam, Johannes van Ravesteyn, 1657.

[8], 460, [12] p.   illus.   17 cm.   **[8899]**

Added engraved title page reads: Nieu licht der apotekers en distilleerkonst.

—[The same.] Pharmacia Galenica & chymica; dat is, De vermeerderde ende verbeterde apotheker en alchymiste licht ende distilleer-konst ... Doorgaens op't nieuw by den autheur oversien, en verrijckt met een kort Examen der chirurgie, benevens een tractaet van de kennisse der droogen. 4. druck. Amstelredam, Johannes van Ravesteyn, 1662.

[16], 460, [12] p.   front., illus.   17 cm.   **[8900]**

Imperfect: Examen de chirurgie, and Tractaet van de Kennisse der drooghen wanting.

The main text is a reissue of the 1657 edition.

—[The same.] ... En verrijckt met een vermeerderde Examen der chirurgie, benevens een tractaet van de kennisse der drooghen. Antwerpen, Reynier Sleghers, 1667.

[16], 466, [21] p.; 70, [2] p.   illus.   16 cm.   **[8901]**

Different setting of type.

—[German tr.] Neues Liecht vor die Apothecker, wie selbige nach den Grund-Regeln der heutigen Destillir-Kunst ihre Artzeneyen zubereiten sollen. Mit einigen Anmerckungen vermehret und verbessert durch die ... Herren Sylvius, Willis, Blanckart, und andere. Nebenst einem Anhange von denen Irrthümern, so bey Bereitung der Medicamenten vorzugehen pflegen, des Herrn Anton de Heidens ... Aus dem Holländischen ... übergesetzet von D. J[ohann] S[chreyer] Leipzig, Johann Friedrich Gleditsch, 1690.

[10], 780, [32] p.   front., illus.   17 cm.   **[8902]**

—[The same.] ... Leipzig, Thomas Fritsch, 1700.

[1], 673, [27] p.   front., illus.   17 cm.   **[8903]**

A reprint of the 1690 Leipzig edition without Johann Schreyer's dedicatory epistle.

PHARMACOPOEA AMSTELREDAMENSIS, senatus auctoritate munita. Amstelredami, Apud Guilielmum & Johannem Blaev, 1636.

[12], 126, [6] p.   24 cm.   **[8904]**

Originally compiled by members of the Collegium Medicum of Amsterdam.

—[The same.] ... Amstelaed., Sumpt. Henr. Wetstenii [1639?]

133, [11] p.   12 cm.   **[8905]**

"Extractum ex statutis Amstelredamensibus": p. 7–8, dated 1636 and 1639.

—[The same.] . . . Ed. 6. Amstelaedami, Apud Joannem Blaeu, 1660.

134, [10] p. 11 cm.   [8906]

"Extractum ex statutis Amstelredamensibus": p. 7-8, dated 1636 and 1639.

—[English tr.] Pharmacopoea Belgica; or, The Dutch dispensatory, revised and confirmed by the Colledge of Physitians at Amsterdam . . . Whereunto is added, The compleat herbalist, being a physicall discourse of all common herbs and fruits . . . Together with many excellent receipts . . . Rendred into English [by John Rouland] . . . London, Printed by E. C. for Edw. Farnham and Robert Horn, 1659.

[8], 428 p. 17 cm.   [8907]

Translation with commentary.

"The small herbalist, or book of plants . . . new printed and enlarged" (p. [181]-354) has special title page.

PHARMACOPOEA auctior, et correctior, jussu . . . Senatus Bruxellensis edita, opera & studio sex Collegii Medici assessorum . . . Bruxellae, Apud Petrum Hacquebaut, 1671.

[12], 237, [11] p. 32 cm.   [8908]

Added engraved title page.

PHARMACOPOEA CATHALANA. 1686. *See* Alós, J.

PHARMACOPOEA HAGIENSIS communi Collegii Medici ejusdem loci opera adornata. Hagae Comitum, Apud Joannem Tongerloo, 1659.

[15], 108, [12] p. 22 cm.   [8909]

—Another printing.

[12], 122, [10] p. 14 cm.   [8910]

PHARMACOPOEA HARLEMENSIS senatus auctoritate munita. Harlemi, Apud Wilh. van Kessel, et Amstelodami, Apud Joannem ten Hoorn, 1693.

[24], 113, [12] p. illus. 14 cm.   [8911]

PHARMACOPOEA LUGDUNENSIS. Lugduni, Apud viduam Thomae Soubrom, 1628. [Lyon, Jean Jacquemetton, 1627]

[24], 112, 72, [16] p. 23 cm.   [8912]

PHARMACOPOEA PERSICA ex idiomate Persico in Latinum conversa . . . Opus missionariis, mercatoribus . . . accedunt in fine specimen notarum in Pharmacopoeam Persicam . . . Lutetiae Parisiorum, Typis Stephani Michallet, 1681.

[6], 56, [8], 370, [27] p. 20 cm.   [8913]

Errata: p. [27]

Translated by Angelus de Sanctu Josepho.

PHARMACOPOEA, sive dispensatorium COLONIENSE jussu, et authoritate S. PQ. Agrippinensis, revisum et auctum labore . . . Petri Holtzemii . . . Coloniae, In officina Birckmannica [1628]

[12], 103, [8] p.; [15] p. illus. 30 cm.   [8914]

Engraved title page.

The "Decreta et statuta . . . senatus Coloniensis, medicos, pharmacopoeos, & chirurgos concernentia" (15 p. at end) is dated 1628.

PHARMACOPOEA ULTRAJECTINA, senatus auctoritate edita & munita. Trajecti ad Rhenum, Typis Gisberti à Zyll, & Theodori ab Ackersdyck, 1656.

[18], 104, [6] p. 22 cm.   [8915]

PHARMACOPOEIA AMSTELREDAMENSIS [English tr.] See Pharmacopoea Belgica. 1659.

PHARMACOPOEIA AUGUSTANA. Jussu et auctoritate amplissimi senatus a Collegio Medico rursus recognita, ac elaboratior, et auctior, nunc sextum in lucem emissa. Augustae Vindelicorum [Excudebat Christoph. Mangus, prostant apud Joannem Krugerum] 1613.

[8], 23, 298, [46] p. tables. 31 cm. [8916]

Engraved title page.

"Amplissimi Senatus Augustani decretum medicos chirurgos et pharmacopoeos concernens . . . 1613": p. [17-19]; "Taxa seu pretium medicamentorum . . . Reip. Aug. Vindel . . ." (p. [21-46]) has half title.

—[The same.] . . . Nunc septimum in lucem emissa. Augustae Vindelicorum [Ex officina typographica Andreae Apergeri, prostant apud Joannem Krugerum] 1622.

[8], 23, 298, [54] p. tables. 30 cm. [8917]

Engraved title page.

Different setting of type.

—Pharmacopoeia Augustana auspicio amplissimi senatus cura octava Collegii Medici recognita Hippocratica et Hermetica mantissa locupletata. Augusta, 1643.

[16], 83, 795, [91] p. tables. 17 cm. [8918]

Engraved title page.

—Animadversiones in Pharmacopoeiam Augustanam et annexam ejus mantissam cum Dispensatorio novo Joannis Zwelfer . . . [Noribergae?] Sumptibus authoris, 1652.

2 parts in 1 v. 32 cm.   [8919]

Imperfect: last leaf (blank?) of part [2] wanting.

Engraved title page.

Part [1] has special title page: Animadversiones in Pharmacopoeiam Augustanam et annexam ejus mantissam; sive, Pharmacopoeia Augustana reformata ... Nunc primum in lucem edita opera & studio Joannis Zwelfer ...

Part [2] has special title page: Pharmacopoeia regia; seu, Dispensatorium novum ... authore Joanne Zwelfer ...

The 1667 and 1675 Nuremberg editions by Michael and Johann Friedrich Endter used the same engraved title and similar type face.

—Pharmacopoeia Augustana reformata, et ejus mantissa. Cum Animadversionibus Joannis Zwelferi ... Annexa ejusdem autoris Pharmacopoeia regia. Goudae, Sumptibus Wilhelmi Verhoeven, 1653.

[16], 917, [19] p.   18 cm.   [8920]

Added engraved title page.

Pharmacopoeia regia ... has special title page.

With this is bound: Zwelfer, J. Appendix ad Animadversiones in Pharmacopoeiam augustam ... 1658.

—Animadversiones in Pharmacopoeiam Augustanam, ejusque mantissam, tertium revisae. Cum Appendice annexa. Quibus accessit Pharmacopoeia regia nova locupletata & absolutae. Adjecta Mantissa spagyrica. Cura Joannis Zwelferi. [Noribergae, Sumtibus Michaelis & Johan. Friderici Endterorum, 1667-68]

3 v. in 1.   illus.   34 cm.   [8921]

Engraved title page. The Animadversiones has special title page and the Appendix ad animadversiones has half title.

The Pharmacopoeia regia has engraved and special title pages, both dated 1668. The Mantissa spagyrica has caption title.

With this is bound (as issued?) Zwelfer, J. Discursus apologeticus. 1668.

—[The same.] ... [Noribergae, Sumtibus Michaelis & Johan. Friderici Endterorum, 1675].

3 v. in 2.   illus.   33 cm.   [8922]

Different setting of type.

With volume 2 of this is bound (as issued?) Zwelfer, J. Discursus apologeticus. 1675.

—Pharmacopoeia Augustana reformata cum ejus mantissa & appendice, simul cum animadversionibus, authore Joanne Zwelfer. Cui annexa est ejusdem authoris Pharmacopoeia regia ut & Mantissa spagyrica. Accessere etiam huic editioni bini Discursus apologetici contra Otth. Tachenium & Francisc. Verny. Dordrechti, Apud Vincentium Caimax, 1672.

[8], 876, [36] p.; [8], 66, [2] p.; [8], 239 p.   illus.   21 cm.   [8923]

Added engraved title page.

Items have special title pages.

—Pharmacopoeia Augustana renovata et aucta ... Augustae Vindelicorum, Typis Joh. Jacobi Schönigii, 1684.

[18], 337, [14], 47 p.   tables.   34 cm.   [8924]

Added engraved title page.

Preface by Lucas Schroeck.

"Illustrissimi Senatus Augustani decretum medicos, chirurgos, et pharmacopoeos concernens ... 1684": p. [13-15]; "Taxa, sive pretium medicamentorum ... in officinis pharmaceuticis Augustanis usualium": 47 p. at end.

—[The same.] ... Augustae Vindelicorum, Apud Laurentium Kronigerum & haeredes Theophili Göbelii, 1694.

[20], 343, [14], 47 p.   tables.   33 cm.   [8925]

Added engraved title page.

PHARMACOPOEIA Holmiensis Galenochymica complectens compositiones apprime necessarias, usibus hodiernis destinatas; earumque conficiendi modos. Holmiae, Joh. G. Eberdt, 1686.

[12], 173, [9] p.   front.   20 cm.   [8926]

Imperfect: frontispiece wanting.

Edited and compiled by J. M. Rothloeben for the Collegium medicum, Stockholm.

PHARMACOPOEIA Lemeriana contracta. 1700. *See* Lémery, N.

PHARMACOPOEIA Londinensis. *See* CULPEPER, Nicholas. Pharmacopoeia Londinensis. 1653, 1654, 1659, 1665, 1669, 1672, 1675, 1679, 1683, 1695.

PHARMACOPOEIA Londinensis, in qua medicamenta antiqua et nova usitatissima, sedulo collecta, accuratissime examinata, quotidiana experientia confirmata describuntur ... Revisa, denuo recusa, emendatior, auctior. Ed. 5. Opera Medicorum Collegii Londinensis ... London, John Marriott, 1639.

[38], 200, [6] p.   29 cm.   [8927]

Engraved title page.

STC 16776.

According to the printer's note to the reader (last page), the book was printed in 1638. Imprint date on engraved title page appears to have been changed to 1639.

PHARMACOPOEIA Londinensis collegarum hodie viventium studiis ac symbolis ornatior. Londini, Typis G. Du-gard impensis Stephani Bowteii, 1650.

[14], 212, [8] p.   29 cm.   [8928]

Engraved title page.

—[The same.] ... Londini, 1662.

[18], 371, [21] p.   13 cm.   [8929]

—[The same.] Collegii Regalis Londini. Londini, Impensis Tho. Newcomb, Tho. Basset, Joh. Wright, & Ric. Chiswel, 1677.

[18], 208, [6] p.   plate.   33 cm.   [8930]

Added engraved title page.

PHARMACOPOEIA Regia. *See* PHARMACOPOEIA augustana. 1652, 1667-68, 1675.

PHARMACOPOEIA Regia. *See* PHARMACOPOEIA augustana reformata cum ejus mantissa & appendice. 1672.

PHARMACOPOEIAE Collegii Regalis Londini remedia, succincte descripta; atque serie alphabetica ita digesta ... Cura J[ames] S[hipton] ... Londini, Typis Tho. Newcomb, prostant venales apud Joh. Martin, Tho. Basset, Hen. Brome, Joh. Wright, & Rich. Chiswel, 1678.

141, [1] p.   15 cm.   [8931]

—[The same.] ... Ed. altera priori castigatior & auctior. Huic annexus est Catalogus simplicium ... Accessit in calce Manuale ad forum: nec-non Pinax posographicus. Cura Ja. Shipton ... Londini, T. Basset, R. Chiswell, & S. Smith, 1689.

[3], 164, 54, [1] p.; [1], 24 p.   14 cm.   [8932]

The "Manuale ad forum" has special title page.

—[The same.] ... Ed. 3., prioribus emendatior & auctior. Huic insuper adjiciuntur Pharmaca nonnulla in usu hodierno apud medicos Londinenses. Accessit item in calce Prosodia medica ... Cura Ja. Shipton ... Londini, Impensis R. Chiswell, S. Smith, B. Walford, N. Wotton, G. Conyers, W. Battersby, 1699.

[3], 104 p.; 101, [3] p.   15 cm.   [8933]

Part [2] has caption title.

"Manuale ad forum ... nec-non Pinax posographicus ..." (p. [57]-91) has special title page.

—[English tr.] Pharmacopoeia Londinensis; or, The new London dispensatory. In six books. Translated into English ... Together with several choise medicines added by the author. As also, The praxis of chymistry ... By William Salmon ... London, Thomas Dawks, 1678.

[16], 896 p.   20 cm.   [8934]

—[The same.] ... The 2d ed., corr. and amended ... by William Salmon ... London, Th. Dawks,

Th. Basset, Jo. Wright, and Ri. Chiswell, 1682.

[16], 877 (i.e. 909), [2] p.   19 cm.   [8935]

The Table of diseases (p. 865 (i.e. 897)-[909]) has caption title.

—[The same.] ... The 3d ed., corr. and amended. By William Salmon ... London, Printed for Thomas Dawks, Tho. Bassett, and Richard Chiswell, 1685.

[16], 877 (i.e. 909), [2] p.   18 cm.   [8936]

A reprint of the 1682 edition.

Imperfect: lower margins trimmed.

—[The same.] ... The 4th ed., corr. and amended. By William Salmon ... London, Printed for T. Bassett, R. Chiswell, M. Wotton, G. Conyers, A. and I. Dawks; and by Awnsham and John Churchill, 1691.

[16], 887 (i.e. 909), [2] p.   18 cm.   [8937]

Different setting of type.

—[The same.] ... The 5th ed., corr. and amended. By William Salmon ... London, Printed by J. Dawks. for T. Bassett, R. Chiswell, M. Wotton, G. Conyers, and J. Dawks, 1696.

[16], 887 (i.e. 909), [2] p.   19 cm.   [8938]

Different setting of type.

The PHARMACOPOEIAN physician's repository. In Maynwaring, E. Vita sana & longa. 1669.

PHARMACOPOEIAS

—1601. *See* MELICH, G. Dispensatorium medicum.

—1604. *See* SANTINI, G. Ricettario medicinale.

—1605. *See* MELICH, G. Avertimenti nelle composizioni de' medicamenti per uso della spetiaria.

—1608. *See* RENOU, J. de. Institutionum pharmaceuticarum. 1608.

—1612. *See* BAUDERON, B. Paraphrase sur la pharmacopee (also Pharmacopee de Bauderon).

—1615. *See* RENOU, J. de. Dispensatorium medicum.

—1623. *See* RENOU, J. de. Dispensatorium medicum.

—1624. *See* RENOU, J. de. Le grand dispensaire medicinal.

—1626. *See* RENOU, J. de. Le grand dispensaire medicinal.

—1627. *See* BAUDERON, B. Paraphrase sur la pharmacopee (also Pharmacopee de Bauderon).

—1628. *See* ZIEGLER, A. Pharmacopoea spagyrica.

—1631. *See* MYNSICHT, A. von. Hadriani à Mynsicht.

—1637. *See* RENOU, J. de. Le grand dispensaire medicinal.

—1637. *See* SADLER, J. Praxis medicorum.

—1638. *See* UNIVERSITÉ DE PARIS. Faculté de médecine. Codex medicamentarius.

—1639. *See* UNIVERSITÉ DE PARIS. Faculté de médecine. Codex medicamentarius.

—1640. *See* BAUDERON, B. Paraphrase sur la pharmacopee (also Pharmacopee de Bauderon).

—1641. *See* MYNSICHT, A. von. Thesaurus et armamentarium medico-chymicum.

—1641. *See* SCHRÖDER, J. Pharmacopoeia medico-chymica.

—1644. *See* BAUDERON, B. Paraphrase sur la pharmacopee (also Pharmacopee de Bauderon).

—1645. *See* RENOU, J. de. Dispensatorium medicum.

—1645. *See* UNIVERSITÉ DE PARIS. Faculté de médecine. Codex medicamentarius.

—1646. *See* MYNSICHT, A. von. Thesaurus et armamentarium medico-chymicum.

—1648. *See* MELICH, G. Avertimenti nelle composizioni de' medicamenti per uso della spetiaria.

—1649. *See* SCHRÖDER, J. Pharmacopoeia medico-chymica.

—1650. *See* BAUDERON, B. Paraphrase sur la pharmacopee (also Pharmacopee de Bauderon).

—1651. *See* HORST, J. D. Pharmacopoeia Galeno-chemica.

—1651. *See* MYNSICHT, A. von. Thesaurus et armamentarium medico-chymicum.

—1655. *See* BAUDERON, B. Paraphrase sur la pharmacopee (also Pharmacopee de Bauderon).

—1655. *See* SAINT GERMAIN, C.de. Le medecin royal.

—1656. *See* SCHRÖDER, J. Pharmacopoeia medico-chymica.

—1657. *See* RENOU, J. de. A medicinal dispensatory.

—1657. *See* SADLER, J. Enchiridion medicum: an enchiridion of the art of physick.

—1662. *See* MYNSICHT, A. von. Theasurus, et armamentarium medico-chymicum.

—1662. *See* SCHRÖDER, J. Pharmacopoeia medico-chymica.

—1663. *See* BAUDERON, B. Paraphrase sur la pharmacopee (also Pharmacopee de Bauderon).

—1664. *See* MYNSICHT, A. von. Theasurus et armamentarium medico-chymicum.

—1665. *See* SCHRÖDER, J. Pharmacopoeia medico chymica.

—1667. *See* SGOBBIS DA MONTAGNANA, A. de. Nuovo, et universale theatro farmaceutico.

—1668. *See* SAINT GERMAIN, C. de. Le medecin royal.

—1670. *See* MYNSICHT, A. von. Thesaurus et armamentarium medico-chymicum.

—1672. *See* BAUDERON, B. Paraphrase sur la pharmacopee (also Pharmacopee de Bauderon).

—1672. *See* SCHRÖDER, J. Pharmacopoeia medico-chymica.

—1675. *See* MYNSICHT, A. von. Theasurus, et armamentarium medico-chymicum.

—1677. *See* SCHÖNFELD, P. J. Synopsis medica super Pharmacopoeiam Augustanam pro praecipuis humani corporis affectibus.

—1677. *See* SCHRÖDER, J. Pharmacopoeia medico-chymica.

—1678. *See* MELICH, G. Avertimenti nelle composizioni de' medicamenti per uso della spetiaria.

—1679. *See* INSULAE CEYLONIAE thesaurus medicus.

—1679. [*See* Sirena, F. L'arte dello spetiale.]

—1680. *See* SIRENA, F. L'arte dellos spetiale.

—1681. *See* BAUDERON, B. Paraphrase sur la pharmacopee (also Pharmacopee de Bauderon).

—1681. *See* SCHRÖDER, J. Pharmacopoeia medico-chymica.

—1682. *See* MYNSICHT, A. von. Thesaurus & armamentarium medico-chymicum.

—1682. *See* SGOBBIS DA MONTAGNANA, A. de. Nuovo, et universale theatro farmaceutico.

—1683. *See* SALMON, W. Doron medicum.

—1684. *See* MORLEY, C. L. Collectanea chymica Leydensia.

—1686. *See* ALÓS, J. Pharmacopoea Cathalana.

—1686. *See* MYNSICHT, A. von. Medicinisch-chymische Schatz- und Rüst-Kammer.

—1687. *See* SCHRÖDER, J. Pharmacopoeia Schrödero-Hoffmanniana illustrata et aucta.

—1688. *See* BATE, G. Pharmacopoeia Bateana.

—1688. *See* SALMON, W. Doron medicum. 1688 [and] Phylaxa medicina: a supplement to the London-dispensary.

—1689. *See* SAINT GERMAIN, C. de. The royal physician.

—1691. *See* BATE, G. Pharmacopoeia Bateana.

—1692. *See* ZWELFER, J. Königliche Apotheck.

—1693. *See* MORLEY, C. L. Collectanea chymica Leydensia.

—1693. *See* SALMON, W. Seplasium. The compleat English physician.

—1693. *See* SCHRÖDER, J. Vollständige und nutzreiche Apotheke.

—1694. *See* BATE, G. Pharmacopoeia Bateana. [English tr.]

—1694. *See* PECHEY, J. The London dispensatory.

—1695. *See* LE MEDECIN DES-INTERRESSÉ.

—1695. *See* MYNSICHT, A. von. Medicinisch-chymische Schatz- und Rüst-Kammer.

—1695. *See* PENICHER, L. Collectanea pharmaceutica.

—1696. *See* MORLEY, C. L. Collectanea chymica Leydensia.

—1696. *See* MYNSICHT, A. von. Thesaurus et armamentarium medico-chymicum.

—1697. *See* LÉMERY, N. Pharmacopée universelle.

—1698. *See* BATE, G. Pharmacopoeia Bateana. [Dutch tr.]

—1698. *See* LASHER, J. Pharmacopoeus et chymicus, symmystae.

—1698. *See* LÉMERY, N. Pharmacopée universelle.

—1698. *See* SCHRÖDER, J. La pharmacopée raisonée.

—1700. *See* BATE, G. Pharmacopoeia Bateana. [English tr.]

—1700. *See* LÉMERY, N. Pharmacopoeia Lemeriana contracta.

—1700. *See* MORLEY, C. L., *ed.* Collectanea chymica Leidensia.

—1700. *See* SPINA, D. de. Manuale sive lexicon pharmaceutico-chymicum.

BELGIUM (BRUSSELS)—1671. *See* PHARMACOPOEA AUCTIOR.

FRANCE (LYONS)—1627. *See* PHARMACOPOEA LUGDUNENSIS.

GERMANY (AUGSBURG)—1613. *See* PHARMACOPOEIA AUGUSTANA.

—1622. *See* PHARMACOPOEIA AUGUSTANA.

—1643. *See* PHARMACOPOEIA AUGUSTANA.

—1652. *See* PHARMACOPOEIA AUGUSTANA.

—1653. *See* PHARMACOPOEIA AUGUSTANA REFORMATA.

—1667-68. *See* PHARMACOPOEIA AUGUSTANA. Animadversiones in Pharmacopoeiam augustanam.

—1672. *See* PHARMACOPOEIA AUGUSTANA reformata cum ejus mantissa & appendice.

—1675. *See* PHARMACOPOEIA AUGUSTANA. Animadversiones in Pharmacopoeiam augustanam.

—1684. *See* PHARMACOPOEIA AUGUSTANA.

—1694. *See* PHARMACOPOEIA AUGUSTANA.

—(BRANDENBURG)—1698. *See* DISPENSATORIUM BRANDENBURGICUM.

—(COLOGNE)—1628. *See* PHARMACOPOEA, sive dispensatorium Coloniense.

—(NUREMBERG)—1666. *See* DISPENSATORIUM PHARMACORUM OMNIUM.

—GT. BRIT. (LONDON)—1639. *See* PHARMACOPOEIA LONDINENSIS.

—1650. *See* PHARMACOPOEIA LONDINENSIS.

—1662. *See* PHARMACOPOEIA LONDINENSIS.

—1677. *See* PHARMACOPOEIA COLLEGII REGALIS LONDINI.

—1678. *See* PHARMACOPOEIAE COLLEGII REGALIS LONDINI REMEDIA.

—1678. *See* PHARMACOPOEIA LONDINENSIS.

—1682. *See* PHARMACOPOEIA LONDINENSIS.

—1685. *See* PHARMACOPOEIA LONDINENSIS.

—1689. *See* PHARMACOPOEIAE COLLEGII REGALIS LONDINI remedia.

—1691. *See* PHARMACOPOEIA LONDINENSIS.

—1696. *See* PHARMACOPOEIA LONDINENSIS.

—1699. *See* PHARMACOPOEIAE COLLEGII REGALIS LONDINI remedia.

—ITALY (BOLOGNA)—1641. *See* UNIVERSITÀ DI BOLOGNA. Collegio de medicina. Antidotarium Bononien: a Medicinae Collegio nuperrime auctum et emendatum.

—1674. *See* UNIVERSITÀ DI BOLOGNA. Collegio de medicina. Antidotarium Bononien: a Medicinae Collegio nuperrime auctum et emendatum.

—1674. *See* UNIVERSITÀ DI BOLOGNA. Collegio de medicina. Antidotarium Bononiense novissimum.

—(FLORENCE)—1623. *See* RICETTARIO FIORENTINO.

—NETHERLANDS (AMSTERDAM)—1636. *See* PHARMACOPOEA AMSTELREDAMENSIS.

—1639?. *See* PHARMACOPOEA AMSTELREDAMENSIS.

—1659. *See* PHARMACOPOEA AMSTELREDAMENSIS.

—1659. *See* Pharmacopoea Amstelredamensis [English tr.] PHARMACOPOEA BELGICA.

—(HAARLEM)—1693. *See* PHARMACOPOEA HARLEMENSIS senatus auctoritate munita.

—(HAGUE)—1659. *See* PHARMACOPOEA HAGIENSIS communi Collegii Medici ejusdem loci opera adornata.

—(UTRECHT)—1656. *See* PHARMACOPOEA ULTRAJECTINA.

—SWEDEN (STOCKHOLM)—1686. *See* PHARMACOPOEIA HOLMIENSIS.

PHELTEN, JAN [*fl.* 1684] *respondent.* Disputatio medica inauguralis de hydrope ascite . . . Lugduni Batavorum, Apud Abrahamum Elzevier, 1684.

[20] p.   22 cm.   **[8939]**

Diss.—Leyden.

PHELTEN, PIETER [*fl.* 1660] *respondent.* Disputatio medica inauguralis de febre ardente, seu causo . . . Ultrajecti ad Rhenum, Ex officina Adriani van Dam, 1660.

[12] p.   20 cm.   **[8940]**

Diss.—Utrecht.

PHILADELPHUS, JANUS, *pseud. See* PECHLIN, Johann Nicolas [1644–1706]

PHILALETHA, *pseud. See* PHILALETHES, Eirenaeus.

PHILALETHA, *anonymus, pseud. See* PHILALETHES, Eirenaeus.

PHILALETHA, EUGENIUS, *pseud. See* VAUGHAN, Thomas [1622–1666]

PHILALETHA, EYRAENEUS, *pseud. See* PHILALETHES, EIRENAEUS.

PHILALETHES, AEYRENAEUS, *pseud. See* PHILALETHES, EIRENAEUS.

PHILALETHES, EIRENAEUS. (Works entered under this pseudonym have been variously attributed to George Starkey, Thomas Vaughan, and John Winthrop.)

—Arcanuum liquoris immortalis ignis-aquae; seu alkahest. Ab Eirenaeo Philaletha [pseud.] The secret of the immortal liquor called alkahest, or ignis-aqua. [Latin and English] *In* Collectanea chymica. 1684.

—Anonymi Philalethae, *pseud.* . . . De liquore alcahest. *In* Wirdig, S. Nova medicina spirituum. 1673, 1688.

— Enarratio methodica trium Gebri medicinarum, in quibus continetur lapidis philosophici vera confectio. Autore anonymo sub nomine Aeyrenaei Philalethes ... Amstelodami, Apud Danielem Elsevirium, 1678.

222, [2] p.   17 cm.   **[8941]**

"Vade-mecum philosophicum; sive, Breve manuductorium ad campum Sophiae ... Auctore Agricola Rhomaeo, horum arcanorum vere adepto ..." (p. [189]-222) has half title.

— Introitus apertus, ad occlusum regis palatium. Authore anonymo Philaletha [pseud.] ...

[647]-699 p.   22 cm.   (*In* Musaeum Hermeticum. Francofurti, 1678)   **[8942]**

— [English tr.] Secrets reveal'd; or, An open entrance to the shut-palace of the king; containing, the greatest treasure in chymistry, never yet so plainly discovered. Composed by ... Eyraeneus Philaletha Cosmopolita [pseud.] ... London, Printed by W. Godbid for William Cooper, 1669.

[30], 120, [6] p.   17 cm.   **[8943]**

— [German tr.] Der vortreffliche Tractat und Hauptschlüssel aller Hermetischen Schrifften genannt: Introitus apertus ad occlusum regis palatium, das ist; Offenstehender Eingang zu dem vormals verschlossenen Königlichen Pallast. Nach dem Manuscript verteutschet [by Johannes Hiskias Cardilucius] ...

[297]-399 p. (*In* Cardilucius, Johannes Hiskias. Magnalia medico-chymica. Nürnberg, 1676)   **[8944]**

— Ripley reviv'd; or, An exposition upon Sir George Ripley's hermetico-poetical works ... Written by Eirenaeus Philalethes [pseud.] ... London, Printed by Tho. Ratcliff and Nat. Thompson for William Cooper, 1678.

1 v.   18 cm.   **[8945]**

Various pagings.

Added engraved title page.

Contents. — [1] An exposition upon Sir George Riple'ys [sic] Epistle to King Edward IV. — [2] An exposition upon Sir George Ripley's Preface. — [3] An exposition upon the first six gates of Sir George Ripley's Compound of alchymie. — [4] Experiments for the preparation of the sophick mercury. — [5] A breviary of alchemy, or a commentary upon Sir George Ripley's Recapitulation. — [6] An exposition upon Sir George Ripley's Vision.

Items [1-4] are the sheets of the 1677 printings, with general title page and preliminary matter added. Items [1-3], paged continuously, have special title pages dated 1677. Item [4] has half title and separate pagination. Items [5-6] each with separate pagination, have special title pages dated 1678.

[—] Tres tractatus de metallorum transmutatione ... Incognito auctore. Adjuncta est Appendix medicamentorum antipodagricorum & calculifragi. Qua omnia ad bonum publicum promovendum nunc primum in lucem edi curavit Martinus Birrius ... apud quem medicamenta ista reperiuntur. Amstelodami, Apud Johannem Janssonium à Waesberge, & viduam Elizei Weyerstraet, 1668.

[15], 110 p.   17 cm.   **[8946]**

Imperfect? portrait wanting?

— Philalethae Tractatus tres. I. Metallorum metamorphosis. II. Brevis manuductio ad rubinum coelestem. III. Fons chymicae veritatis.

[741]-814 p.   22 cm.   (*In* Musaeum Hermeticum. Francofurti, 1678)   **[8947]**

— [English tr.] Three tracts of the great medicine of philosophers for humane and metalline bodies. I. Intituled, Ars metallorum metamorphoseos. II. Brevis manuductio ad rubinum coelestem. III. Fons chymicae philosophiae. All written in Latine by Eirenaeus Philalethes [pseud.] ... Translated into English ... London, T. Sowle, [1694]

[28], 186 p.   17 cm.   **[8948]**

Tracts [II] and [III] have special title pages.

— *See* CARDILUCIUS, J. H., *ed.* Magnalia medicochymica. 1676.

PHILALETHES, EIRENAEUS PHILOPONOS, *pseud.* *See* STARKEY, George [1627-1665]

PHILALETHES, EUDOXUS, *pseud. See* DONZELLINI, Girolamo [*d.* 1588]

PHILALETHES, EUGENIUS, *pseud. See* VAUGHAN, Thomas [1622-1666]

PHILANDER, *pseud. See* In speculo teipsum contemplare Dr. Black. 1692.

PHILANDER MISAURUS. The honour of the gout; or, A rational discourse ... By way of a letter to an eminent citizen ... London, A. Baldwin, 1699.

[4], 61, [5] p.   15 cm.   **[8949]**

PHILANDER MISIATRUS. *See* PHILANDER MISAURUS.

PHILANDER, EUGENIUS, *pseud. See* GUIDOTT, Thomas [1638-1706]

PHILANTHROPOS, EUGENIUS [*fl.* 1665] *ed.* Dr. Trigg's secrets, arcana's & panacea's approved by his long ... practice, whereby he wrought such wonderfull cures ... Now after death to fulfill his request published as a legacy to his patients. By Eugenius Philanthropos. London, Printed by R. D. for Dixy Page, 1665.

[8], 160 + p.   15 cm.   **[8950]**

Imperfect: p. 71-74, 113-126 and all after p. 160 wanting.

PHILARETES. *See* BONTEKOE, Cornelis [1640?-1685]; FRANCK VON FRANCKENAU, Georg Friedrich [1669-1732]

PHILARETES, TANTARARA, TANTARARA, SPITTLEFIELD, *pseud.* Culpeper revived from the grave, to discover the cheats of that grand impostor call'd aurum potabile. Wherein is declared the grand falsities thereof and abuses thereby. Published to undeceive the people, and to stop the violent current of such a mischievous designe. [London] 1655.

[1], 6 p.   19 cm.   **[8951]**

Imprint partly supplied from Wing C7565.
Imperfect: outer and lower margins trimmed.

PHILARETUS *pseud. See* THEOPHILUS PROTOSPATHARIUS [7th cent.]

PHILARETUS, GILBERTUS, *pseud. See* FUSCH, Gilbert [*ca.*1504-1567]

PHILASTROGUS knavery epitomized. 1652. *See* [GADBURY, J.]

PHILELEUTHERUS TIMARETES. *See* ALMELOVEEN, Theodoor Jansson van [1657-1712]

PHILIATER, *pseud. See* MACHIAVELLUS MEDICUS. 1698.

PHILIATROS. Natura exenterata; or, Nature unbowelled by the most exquisite anatomizers of her. Wherein are contained ... receipts, fitted for the cure of all sorts of infirmities ... Collected ... by several persons of quality ... whose names are prefixed to the book ... Whereunto are annexed many ... inventions ... London, H. Twiford, G. Bedell and N. Ekins, 1655.

[6], 369 (i.e. 469), [30] p.   front. (port.)   18 cm.
                                         [8952]

Preface signed: Philiatros.
Second copy of portrait mounted at end.

PHILIATRUS. *See* PHILIATER, *pseud.*

PHILIATRUS, EUONYMUS, *pseud. See* GESNER, Konrad [1516-1565]

PHILIP of Tripoli. *See* PHILIPPUS TRIPOLITANUS [13th cent.]

PHILIPPE, JOHANN DAVID [*fl.* 1686] *respondent.* Meditatio de catalepsi ... Basileae, Typis Jacobi Bertschii, 1686.

[12] p.   20 cm.   **[8953]**

Diss. — Basel.

PHILIPPES, JEAN [*d.* 1622] De l'excellence de l'homme et de sa naissance ... Paris, Francois Jaquin, 1603.

[16], III, 76 p.   14 cm.   **[8954]**

Engraved title page.

PHILIPPUS CLERICUS. *See* PHILIPPUS TRIPOLITANUS [13th cent.]

PHILIPPUS NERIUS, *Saint. See* FILIPPO NERI, *Saint* [1515-1595]

PHILIPPUS TRIPOLITANUS [13th cent.] *See* STEFANI, G. In Aristotelis libellum de conservatione sanitatis. 1637

PHILOCHEMICUS, *pseud. See* EGLINUS ICONIUS, Raphael [1559-1622]

PHILOCHIMICO, *pseud. See* MENUDIER, Jean [*fl.* 1673-1690]

PHILOCOPHUS; or, The deafe and dumbe mans friend. 1648. *See* [BULWER, J.]

PHILOCTETES, EYRENEUS. Philadelphia; or, Brotherly love to the studious in the hermetick art. Wherein is discovered the principles of hermetick philosophy, with much candor and plainness. Written by Eyreneus Philoctetes [pseud.] ... [London] T. Sowle, 1694.

[32], 70 p.   13 cm.   **[8955]**

Imperfect: p. 49-50 mutilated.
"To the studious reader" subscribed by Philomathes (p. [18]); "To his respected ... friend" signed by Philetaeros (p. [32]). "Written in the year 1691" (p. 70).
Wing (S 5282) lists this work among the Philalethes tracts under George Starkey, but Wilkinson (Ambix, XII, 1, 1964, p. 33) shows this to be a confusion of pseudonyms.

PHILODUSUS, JANUS, *pseud. See* HEINSIUS, Daniel [1580-1655]

PHILOLOGUS, JONAS, *pseud. See* GUINTERIUS, Joannes, Andernacus [1505-1574]

PHILOMANTHES, *pseud. See* IN SPECULO TEIPSUM CONTEMPLARE DR. BLACK. 1692.

PHILOMUSUS, *pseud. See* GUIDOTT, Thomas [1638–1706]

PHILOMUSUS, ANONYMUS. *See* CARRICHTER, Bartholomäus [1507–1573]

PHILOPONUS, LOTARIUS, *pseud. See* DU JON, François [1545–1602]

Het **PHILOSOOPHISCHE** laboratorium. 1683. *See* LÉMERY, N.

PHILOSOPHIA mathematica. 1693. *See* WEIGEL, E.

The **PHILOSOPHICAL** epitaph of W[illiam] C[ooper] 1673–75. *See* COOPER, W.

PHILOSOPHICAL transactions. *See* Royal Society of London.

La **PHILOSOPHIE** naturelle restablie en sa pureté. 1651. *See* [Espagnet, Jean d']

PHILOTHEUS. *See* THEOPHILUS PROTOSPATHARIUS [7th cent.]

PHINELLUS, PHILIPPUS. *See* FINELLA, Filippo [*b. ca.* 1585]

PHIORAVANTI, LEONARDO. *See* FIORAVANTI, Leonardo [1517–1588]

PHLEGON OF TRALLES [*fl.* 2d cent.] Quae exstant, opuscula. Joannes Meursius recensuit, & notas addidit. Lugduni Batavorum, Apud Isaacum Elzevirium, 1620.

    [8], 190 p. 19 cm.   **[8956]**

  "De rebus mirabilibus liber" (p. [1]-101); "De longaevis libellus" (p. [103]-133); "De Olympiis fragmentum" (p. [135]-147); "Joannis Meursii . . . notae" (p. [149]-173) have half titles.

  Contains Greek texts with Latin translations by Gulielmus Xylander.

PHLEGON, PUBLIUS AELIUS. *See* PHLEGON OF TRALLES [*fl.* 2d cent.]

PHOCAE maris anatome in Academia Kiloniensi suscepta. 1699? *See* [SCHELHAMMER, G. C.]

PHOENIX atropicus de morte redux. 1681. *See* [LACTANTIUS, L. C. F.]

The **PHOENIX** of these late times; or, The life of Mr. Henry Welby, Esq., who lived at his house in Grub-street forty foure yeares, and in that space, was never seene by any . . . With some new epitaphs by those who formerly knew that gentleman . . . London, Printed by N. Okes, and sold by Richard Clotterbuck, 1637.

    [46] p. front. (port.) 18 cm.   **[8957]**

  STC 25227.

PHRIGIUS, JACOPUS ANTONIUS. *See* FRIGIO, Jacopo Antonio [*fl.* 1608]

PHRIGIUS, PETRUS FRANCISCUS. *See* FRIGIO, Pietro Francesco [1586 *or* 7–1659]

PHRISIUS, JAN PAUWELSZOON. *See* PAUWELSZOON, Jan.

PHRYGIUS, JACOBUS ANTONIUS. *See* FRIGIO, Jacopo Antonio [*fl.* 1608]

PHRYGIUS, PETRUS FRANCISCUS. *See* FRIGIO, Pietro Francesco [1586 *or* 7–1659]

PHYSICA naturalis rotunda visionis chemicae cabalisticae.

    344–381 p., vol. 6. 20 cm. (*In* Zetzner, Lazarus, *ed.* Theatrum chemicum. Argentorati, 1659–61)   **[8958]**

  Caption title.

  Running title: Cabala chemica.

A PHYSICAL dictionary; or, An interpretation of such crabbed words . . . as are derived from the Greek or Latin, and used in physick, anatomy, chirurgery, and chymistry. With a definition of most diseases incident to the body of man; and a description of the marks and characters used by doctors in their receipts. Published for the more perfect understanding of Mr. Tomlinson's translation of Rhaenodaeus Dispensatory . . . London, Printed by G. Dawson, for John Garfield, 1657.

    [58] p. 28 cm.   **[8959]**

  Bound with Renou, J. de. A medicinal dispensatory. 1657.

PHYSICK for families. 1669. *See* WALWYN, W.

PHYSICORUM COLLEGIO CIVITATIS MEDIOLANI. *See* COLLEGIO DEI FISICI, Milan.

PHYSIOLOGUS, PHILOTHEOS. *See* TRYON, Thomas [1634–1703]

La **PHYSIQUE** d'uzage. *See* ARBERIUS.

PIACENZA. Laws, Statutes, etc. Grida di diversi capi concernenti la sanità, & sospensione delle città di Bergamo, & Vercelli con suoi territorii, & altri luoghi, & bando d'alcuni luoghi nel Cremasco . . . Piacenza, Giacomo Ardizzoni [1630]

broadside. 55 x 43 cm.   **[8961]**

PIAZZA, CARLO BARTOLOMEO [1632-1713] Opere pie di Roma, descritte secondo lo stato presente . . . Roma, Per Gio. Battista Bussotti, 1679.

[24], 788 p. 20 cm.   **[8962]**

PIAZZA, MATTEO [*fl.* 1629-1631] Prattica per espurgare le case, et robbe infette, e sospette di contagio . . . Bologna, L'herede del Benacci, 1630.

12 p. 20 cm.   **[8963]**

PIAZZA, PIETRO [1606-1678] Breve et utile discorso di chirurgia . . . Roma, Per il success. al Mascardi, ad instanza di Gregorio, e Giovanni Andreoli, 1669.

80 p. 20 cm.   **[8964]**

—[The same.] *In* Salvi, T. Il chirurgo. 1650, 1669, 1688.

PIAZZI, MATTEO. *See* PIAZZA, Matteo [*fl.* 1629-1631]

PICCART, MICHAEL [1574-1620] Oratio academica de praestantia cognitionis. Habita publice . . . MDCXIII. Altorfii, E typographeo Cunradi Agricola [1613]

[28] p. 20 cm.   **[8965]**

—Oratio academica qua Altorfinam Norimbergensium Academiam metu luis per contagium invectae dilabentem, cum bono et propitio Deo revocavit restituitque. Habita ibidem . . . anni MDCXII. Altorfii, Apud Cunradum Agricolam [1612]

[24] p. 20 cm.   **[8966]**

PICCINETTI, DOMENICO [*fl.* 1619] *tr. See* CASTELLANI, G. M. Filactirion della flebotomia. 1619.

PICCIOLI, ANTONIO, *da Cento* [17th cent.] Technae iatricae, sive artis medicinalis libri tres. Quibus, quaecumque ad dignoscendas, curandasque omnes humani corporis aegritudines perquiruntur, brevi, facilique methodo explanantur. Accessit ejusdem De medicamentis, quae in medendo maximè usu veniunt, libellus. Venetiis, Apud Joannem Viezzerum, 1664.

[16], 177 (i.e. 199), [3] p. port. 30 cm.
                    [8967]

PICCOFONCCI, GASPARO. Nova praxis medica de morbis mulierum, cum exacta medicamentorum notabilium expositione . . . auctore Gasparo Piccofoncci [pseud.] Venetiis, Sumptibus Josaph Mariae Ruinetti, 1698.

[8], 270 p. 22 cm.   **[8968]**

"De medicamentis usualibus" (p. [183]-270) has half title.

PICCOLOMINEUS, SEXTILIUS. *See* PICCOLOMINI, Sestilius [*fl.* 1601]

PICCOLOMINI, SESTILIUS [*fl.* 1601] *See* [CYNTHIUS, C.] Disputationes medicae de natura atque facultatibus ligni sancti. 1602.

PICHON, PIERRE [*fl.* 1673] Quaestiones medicae duodecim. Ab . . . Michaele de Chicoynfau [sic] [et al.] . . . propositae . . . pro regia professione vacante pro [sic] obitum . . . Gaspari Fesquet . . . quas . . . propugnabit . . . Petrus Pichon . . . Monspelii, Apud Danielem Pech, 1673.

[4], 21, [2] p. 23 cm.   **[8969]**

Thèse de concours—Montpellier.

PICHTEL, BALTHASAR JOHANN [*fl.* 1656-1659] *praeses.* Disputatio physica de speciebus sensibilibus . . . Wittenbergae, Typis Johannis Röhneri, 1659.

[16] p. 18 cm.   **[8970]**

Diss.—Wittenberg (C. Elliger, *respondent*)

PICKHARD, MICHAEL. *See* PICCART, Michael [1574-1620]

PICO DELLA MIRANDOLA, GIOVANNI FRANCESCO [1470-1533] Opus aureum de auro tum aestimando, tum conficiendo, tum utendo, ad conjugem.

312-377 p., vol. 2. 20 cm. (*In* Zetzner, Lazarus, *ed.* Theatrum chemicum. Argentorati, 1659-61)   **[8971]**

Caption title.

PICOT, CLAUDE [*d.* 1668] *See* DESCARTES, R. Les passions de l'ame. 1649.

PICTORIUS, GEORG [*ca.* 1500-1569] Sanitatis tuendae methodus. *In* Regimen sanitatis Salernitanum. De conservanda bona valetudine. 1607, 1619 [and] Scola Salernitana. 1630, 1662, 1666, 1677.

PIDOUX, BARTHÉLEMY. *See* PARDOUX, Barthélemy [1545-1611]

PIDOUX, François [1586–1662] De febre purpurea. Augustoriti Pictonum, Sumptibus Jul. Thoreau & Jean. Fleuriau, 1656.

[8], 101, [1] p.   19 cm.   [8972]

PIELAT, Barthélemy [*fl.* 1671] tr. See Insulae Ceyloniae thesaurus medicus. 1679.

PIELOW, Georg [*fl.* 1683] respondent. See Loss, J., *praeses.* Dissertatio medica de glandulis in genere. 1683.

PIELZ, Johann Georg [*fl.* 1699] respondent. See Pezold, K. F., *praeses.* Dissertationem philologico-physico-historicam de memoria memorabili . . . submittit . . . J. G. P. 1699.

PIENS, Franciscus Hadrianides [*fl.* 1669] Tractatus de febribus in genere & specie ex veterum ac recentiorum scriptis perpensus; seu, Febris heautontimorumenos . . . Neomagi Batavorum, Ex officina Reineri Smetii, 1669.

[16], 279 p.; 285, [14] p.   plate.   16 cm.
                                              [8973]
Added engraved title page.
Part [1] has colophon: Enchusae, Ex typographeia Egberti vanden Hooff, 1665.

—[The same.] . . . Ed. nov. Notis, observationibus, opusculis integris & remediis quibusdam selectioribus, a Joh. Jacobo Mangeto, adjectis multo auctior. Coloniae Allobrogum, Apud Samuelem de Tournes, 1689.

[32], 824 p.   plate.   22 cm.   [8974]
". . . Observationes selectiores a . . . Nozet . . . communicatae": p. 792–824.
With notes by H. Screta and J. Jones.

PIERCE, Robert [1622–1710] Bath memoirs; or, Observations in three and forty years practice, at the Bath, what cures have been there wrought, (both by bathing and drinking these waters) by God's blessing, on the directions of Robert Peirce . . . a constant inhabitant in Bath, from the year 1653 to this present year 1697. Bristol, H. Hammond, 1697.

[32], 399, [2] p.   plate.   18 cm.   [8975]
Errata at end.
Part 2, p. [247]–399, has special title page, with imprint: Bristol, Printed by and for W. Bonny and H. Hammond, 1697.

PIERER, Georg Peter [1646–1685] De natta dissertatiuncula medica . . . Argentorati, Literis Joh. Wilhelmi Tidemanni, 1669.

[13], 84 (i.e. 70) p.   front.   14 cm.   [8976]
Bound with Gans, J. L. Coralliorum historia. 1669.

PIERIO VALERIANO, Bolzano. See Valeriano Bolzani, Giovanni Pierio [1477–1560]

PIERIUS, Joannes. See Valeriano Bolzani, Giovanni Pierio [1477–1560]

PIERRE, Petrus de la. See Peters, Petrus [*fl.* 1679]

PIETRAGRASSA, Bartolomeo [*fl.* 1649] Politica medica per il governo conservativo del corpo humano. Divisa in due trattati. Nell'uno si discorre d'alcune cose proemiali, nell'altro dell'aria. Con la cui salutare dispositione si mantiene la sanita . . . Pavia, Gio. Andrea Magri, 1650.

[28], 496, [23] p.   31 cm.   [8977]
Added engraved title page.
Colophon: Pavia, Gio. Andrea Magri, 1649.

PIETRE, Jean [d. 1666] respondent. See Biard, G., *praeses.* Quaestio medica. 1647.

PIETRE, Simon [*fl.* 1614] praeses. Quaestio medica . . . An ourethrae angustiis nocent καθαιρετικὰ? Ed. 2. [Parisiis? 1647]

2 p.   24 cm.   [8978]
Diss. — Paris, 1614 (N. Rousseau, *respondent*)

PIETRO ANTONIO BONI, of Ferrara. See Boni, Pietro Antonio, of Ferrara.

PIETRO D'ABANO. See Abano, Pietro d' [1250–1315?]

PIGNOCATTI, Francesco. See Venturini, A. Le medecine che da tutti gl'animali si può cavar à beneficio dell' huomo. 1654, 1672, 1674.

PIGNORIA, Lorenzo [1571–1631] De servis, et eorum apud veteres ministeriis, commentarius. In quo familia, tum urbana, tum rustica, ordine producitur & illustratur. Augustae Vindelicorum, Ad insigne pinus, 1613.

[12], 280 p.; [10] p.   illus.   20 cm.   [8979]
"Antonii Velseri ad Hieronymum Fabrum medicum, De zeta & zetario; sive, Diaeta et diaetario, epistola . . . Frisingae, 21 Maii, 1604": [1–7] p. at end.

PIGRAY, Pierre [1532?–1613] La chirurgie tant theorique que pratique . . . Rev., corr. et augm. par l'autheur. 2. ed. [Paris] Marc Orry, 1604.

[8], 712 (i.e. 714), [38] p.   16 cm.   [8980]
Engraved title page.
Imperfect: p. 1–2 wanting.

—[The same.] Epitome des preceptes de medecine et chirurgie avec ample declaration des remedes propres aus maladyes . . . Parisiis, Apud Marcum Orry, 1609.

[8], 764, [41] p. port. 18 cm. **[8981]**
Engraved title page.

—[The same.] . . . Rouen, Adrien Ovyn, 1615.

[48], 764, [2] p. 17 cm. **[8982]**
Different setting of type.

—[The same.] . . . Rouen, Jean Berthelin, 1625.

[47], 764, [2] p. 18 cm. **[8983]**
Different setting of type.
With this is bound Gelee, T. L'anatomie françoise. 1630.

—[The same.] . . . Epitome des preceptes de medecine et chirurgie. Contenant plusieurs enseignemens & remedes necessaires aux maladies du corps humain . . . Rev. & augm. en ceste derniere ed. de divers chapitres. Lyon, Jean Aymé Candy, 1628.

[47], 764, [2] p. port. 18 cm. **[8984]**
Different setting of type.

—[The same.] . . . Rev. & augm. en cette derniere ed. de divers chapitres. Lyon, La vefue de Claude Rigaud, & Philippes Bordes, 1637.

[8], 764, [41] p. port. 18 cm. **[8985]**
Different setting of type.

—[The same.] Epitome des preceptes de medecine et chirurgie. Avec ample declaration des remedes propres aux maladies . . . Rouen, Louys du Mesnil, 1638.

[56], 764, [2] p. 17 cm. **[8986]**

—[The same.] . . . Rouen, Daniel Loudet, 1642.

[44], 764 p. 17 cm. **[8987]**
Different setting of type.

—[The same.] Epitome des preceptes de medecine et chirurgie. Contenant plusieurs enseignemens & remedes, necessaires aux maladies du corps humain . . . Rev. & augm. en cette derniere ed. de divers chapitres. Lyon, Jean Huguetan, 1643.

[8], 764, [34] p. 17 cm. **[8988]**
Different setting of type.

—[The same.] Epitome des preceptes de medecine et chirurgie. Avec ample declaration des remedes propres aux maladies . . . Rouën, David Berthelin, 1666.

[56], 764, [2] p. 18 cm. **[8989]**
Different setting of type.

—Another issue, with imprint: Rouën, Jacques Besongne, 1666.

[8990]

—[The same.] . . . Rouen, Pierre Amiot, 1672.

[56], 764, [2] p. 17 cm. **[8991]**
Imperfect: 2d prelim. leaf and p. 355-356 mutilated.
Different setting of type.

—[The same.] Epitome des preceptes de medecine et chirurgie, contenant plusieurs enseignemens & remedes necessaires aux maladies corps humain . . . Rev. & augm. en cette derniere ed. de divers chapitres. Lyon, Jean Baptiste de-Ville, 1673.

[8], 764 (i.e. 762), [37] p. 17 cm. **[8992]**

—[The same.] Epitome des preceptes de medecine et chirurgie. Avec ample declaration des remedes propres aux maladies . . . Rouen, François Vaultier, 1681.

[56], 764, [2] p. 18 cm. **[8993]**
Different setting of type.

—[The same.] Epitome des preceptes de medecine et chirurgie, contenant plusieurs enseignemens & remedes necessaires aux maladies du corps humain . . . Rev. & augm. en cette derniere ed. de divers chapitres. Lyon, Antoine Beaujollin, 1682.

[12], 623 (i.e. 633), [33] p. 19 cm. **[8994]**

—[Latin tr.] Chirurgia cum aliis medicine partibus juncta . . . Parisiis, Apud Marcum Orry, 1609.

II, [1], 771 + , [1] p. port. 18 cm. **[8995]**
Engraved title page.
Imperfect: all after p. [772] wanting.

—Another printing.

II, [1], 768, [34] p. 18 cm. **[8996]**

—[The same.] Epitome praeceptorum medicinae chirurgiae. Cum ampla singulis morbis convenientium remediorum expositione . . . Parisiis, Apud viduam Marci Orry, 1612.

II, [1], 771, [33] p. port. 18 cm. **[8997]**
Engraved title page.

—[Dutch tr.] Kort begryp, van de genees ende heelkonst . . . Met een wijdtloopige verklaringe der genees-middelen, tot yder sieckten behoorende. Overgeset door Pieter Rutgersz. van Nieustadt . . . 3. druck, oversien ende verbetert. Amsterdam, De weduwe van Theunis Jacobsz., 1662.

[12], 450, [10] p. 19 cm. **[8998]**

PIHRINGER, Krisztián [1641-1694] *praeses.* Disputatio physica de monstro ... Wittebergae, Ex offic. typogr. Michaelis Wendt, 1664.

[18] p.   19 cm.   [8999]

Diss. — Wittenberg (R. G. Bürger, *respondent*)

PIJL, Paul [*fl. ca.* 1677] Den aftocht ter eeren van de krakkeelende doctoren en chirurgijns van Amsterdam, over het verschil tusschen den ... Bonaventura van Dortmont ... Fredericus Ruysch, met zijn vroet-meester Andries Boeckelman ... Amsterdam, Autheur, 1677.

24 p.   16 cm.   [9000]

— Luyelack, of t'samen-spraeck tusschen Wit en Swart; anders genaemt antwoort aen den auteur van den Aftoch: Ter eeren de krakkelende doctoren en chirurgijns van Amsterdam. Valschelijk uytgegeven op de naem van Mr. Paulus Pyl ... Amsterdam, 1677.

65 (i.e. 63) p.   16 cm.   [9001]

PIKER, Christian [*fl.* 1692] *respondent.* Disputatio medica inauguralis de haemorrhoidibus ... Lugduni Batavorum, Apud Abrahamum Elzevier, 1692.

[23] p.   19 cm.   [9002]

Diss. — Leyden.

PILES, Roger de [1635-1709] Abregé d'anatomie, accommodé aux arts de peinture et de sculpture ... Mis en lumiere par François Tortebat [pseud.] ... Paris, Tortebat, 1667.

[26] p. incl. 12 plates.   47 cm.   [9003]

Plate B and Privilege dated 1668.

Cushing VI.D.25.

The illustrations reproduce plates from Vesalius' Fabrica and the Epitome.

PILET DE LA MESNARDIÈRE, Hippolyte Jules. *See* La Mesnardière, Hippolyte Jules Pilet de [1610-1663]

PILIEU, Julien. *See* Peleus, Julianus [*d. ca.* 1625]

PILLING, Johann Georg [*b.* 1672] *respondent. See* Slevogt, J. A., *praeses.* Disputatio medica inauguralis de sudoribus. 1697.

— *See* Slevogt, J. A. Decani Facultatis Medicae Jo. Hadriani Slevogtii ... prolusio inauguralis de publicis utriusque Americae sudatoriis. 1693.

PILLING, Johann Peter [*fl.* 1687] *respondent. See* Boess, D., *praeses.* Specimen pathologico-therapeuticum de plica. 1687.

PILLING, Matthias Zacharias [*fl.* 1665-1674] Kurtze Beschreibung des zu Ronneburg ... entsprungenen mineralischen Wassers, von dessen Halt, Krafft und Wirckung ... Altenburg, Johann Michael [1667?]

64 p.   16 cm.   [9004]

Imprint partially supplied from W. T. von Renz. Balneologische Bibliothek. Frankfurt am Main, 1900.

— *respondent. See* Rolfinck, W., *praeses.* Dissertatio medica de vertigine. 1665.

PIMBIOLO DEGLI ENGELFREDDI, Annibale Domenico [*d.* 1731] Synopsis, praelectionum de morbis a corde infra quorum praestantiores meditatione complectetur allabentis litterarii hujus anni curriculo ... [Patavii, Typis Petri Mariae Frambotti, 1682?]

[4] p.   23 cm.   [9005]

Caption title.

PIMBIOLUS, Annibal Dominicus. *See* Pimbiolo degli Engelfreddi, Annibale Domenico [*d.* 1731]

PINAEUS, Antonius. *See* Du Pinet, Antoine, *sieur de Noroy* [1515?-1584?]

PINAEUS, Severinus. *See* Pineau, Séverin [*d.* 1619]

PINCIANUS, Ferdinandus. *See* Núñez de Guzmán, Fernando [16th cent.]

PINCKER, Christian Friedrich [*fl.* [1689-1691] respondent. Disputatio medica inauguralis de haemorrhoidibus ... Lugduni Batavorum, Apud Abrahamum Elzevier, 1691.

[16] p.   19 cm.   [9006]

Diss. — Leyden.

— *See* Rivinus, A. Q., praeses. Dissertatio medica de dubio medicamentorum effectu. 1689.

PINDAR, Martin [*fl.* 1644] A letter sent to the Honourable William Lenthall ... Speaker of the House of Commons, wherein is truely related the great victory obtained by Gods blessing, by the Parliaments army, against the Kings forces, neer

Newbery, on Sunday the 27. of this present October ... London, Edw. Husbands, 1644.

[8] p.   19 cm.   **[9007]**

Signed by M. Pindar and others.

PINEAU, SÉVERIN [*fl.* 1619] De integritatis & corruptionis virginum notis: de graviditate & partu naturali mulierum. Ludov. Bonacioli ... Enneas muliebris ... Fel. Plateri ... De origine partium, earumque in utero conformatione. Pet. Gassendi De septo cordis pervio, observationes ... Lugduni-Batavorum, Apud Franciscos Hegerum & Hackium, 1639.

[8], 183 p.; [1], 272, [40] p.   illus., plates.   13 cm.   **[9008]**

Added engraved title page.

Part [2] has half title: De faetus formatione.

— [The same.] De integritatis et corruptionis virginum notis ... V. Melchioris Sebizii De notis virginitatis ... Lugduni-Batavorum, Apud Franciscum Hegerum, 1640.

[8], 183 p.; [1], 310, [40] p.   illus., plates.   13 cm.   **[9009]**

Added engraved title page, dated 1641.

— [The same.] ... Lugduni-Batavorum, Apud Franciscum Hegerum, 1641.

182 p.; [1], 298, [40] p.   illus., plates.   13 cm.   **[9010]**

Added engraved title page.

— [The same.] ... Lugduni-Batavorum, Apud Franciscum Moyaert, 1650.

182 p.; [1], 338 p.   illus., plates.   14 cm.   **[9011]**

Added engraved title page.

— [The same.] ... Amstelodami, Apud Joannem Ravesteinium, 1663.

394, [36] p.   illus., plates.   14 cm.   **[9012]**

Added engraved title page.

— [The same.] ... Ed. 3 auctior & correctior. Francofurti & Lipsiae, Apud Christophor. Wohlfart, 1690.

[7], 210 p.; 348, [44] p.   illus.   14 cm.   **[9013]**

Added engraved title page, dated 1689.

— Opusculum physiologum et anatomicum. *In* Boursier, L. (Bourgeois). Hebammen Buch. 1628-48, 1644-52.

PINEDO, MOSES DE [*fl.* 1685] *respondent.* Disputatio medica inauguralis de dysenteria vera ... Lugduni Batavorum, Apud Abrahamum Elzevier, 1685.

[20] p.   22 cm.   **[9014]**

Diss. — Leyden.

PINELLI, GIOVANNI VINCENZO [1535-1601] *See* GUALDO, P. Vita Joannis Vincentii Pinelli. 1607.

PINELLI, GIROLAMO. *See* PINNELLI, Girolamo.

PINELO, ANTONIO LEON DE. *See* LEÓN PINELO, Antonio Rodríguez de [*d.* 1660]

PINELO, ANTONIO RODRÍGUEZ DE LEÓN. *See* LEÓN PINELO, Antonio Rodríguez de [*d.* 1660]

PIÑERO, JUAN BAPTISTA. Concordia de la controversia sobre el sitio de la sangria, en los principios de las enfermedades ... Proponese quando se deve sangrar del tovillo, y quando del braço: explicando con novedad util algunas doctrinas antiguas ... Sevilla, Francisco Ygnacio de Lyra, 1655.

24 ll.   19 cm.   **[9015]**

— Propugnaculo de la Concordia, sobre la controversia del sitio de la sangria, en los principios de las enfermedades superiores ... contiene dos cartas: la primera es de un moderno ... ingenio, en la qual procura desvanecer el vero fundamento de la referida Concordia ... la segunda es respuesta del doctor Don Juan Baptista Piñera a la referida carta ... Ezija, Juan Malpartida de las Alas, 1659.

[44] p.   19 cm.   **[9016]**

Upper margins trimmed.

PINNA, PEDRO LOPEZ. *See* LÓPEZ PINNA, Pedro [*b.* 1667]

PINNELL, HENRY [*fl.* 1656] *ed.* and *tr. See* CROLL, O. Philosophy reformed & improved. 1657.

PINNELLI, GIROLAMO. Theoricae, ac practicae medicinae aphorismorum libri VIII ... Senis, Apud Silvestrum Marchetum, 1617.

256 p.   15 cm.   **[9017]**

[PINSONNAT, FRANÇOIS] Regime de santé pour, se procurer une longue vie & une vieillesse heureuse ... Contre un livre intitulé Le medecine de soymême [by J. Devaux] Par le sieur D. L. C. [pseud.] Paris, Maurice Villery, 1686.

[24], 146 p.   16 cm.   **[9018]**

PINTIANUS, FERDINANDUS. *See* NÚÑEZ DE GUZMÁN, Fernando [16th cent.]

PINTO, CELLINI. Compendioso trattato sopra'l male della peste e contagio sua preservatione e cura. Parte prima [-quarta] . . . Bracciano, Andrea Fei, 1632.

[28], 747 p.   16 cm.   [9019]

Imperfect: title page and preliminary matter for parte terza and parte quarta misbound at front.

Each part has special title page.

PIPERNO, PIETRO [*fl.* 1624-1634] De magicis affectibus horum dignotione, praenotione, curatione, medica, stratagemmatica, divina, plerisque curationibus electis. & De nuce Beneventana maga . . . Omnibus scientiis opera ornata nova. [Neap., Ex typ. Jo. Dominici Roncalioli, 1634-1635]

[8], 1-168, [16], 169-208 p.; 24 p.   21 cm.

[9020]

Part 2 has special title page with imprint: Neapoli, Typis Jo. Dominici Montanari, 1635.

—[The same.] De effectibus magicis libri sex ac De nuce maga Beneventana liber unicus . . . Neap., Per Franciscum Hieronymum Colligni, 1647.

[1], 168, 85 (i.e. 55), [5] p.   20 cm.   [9021]

Imperfect: title page mutilated.

—Medicae petrae . . . Divisae in duobus trinis. Primus habet petras tres. I. De cognitione aeris in communi, & Beneventani. II. De regimine aeris Beneventani, & similis. III. De quibusdam antidotis pro vita. Secundus vero alias tres. I. De mutatione aeris. II. De regimine anni scalaris. III. De natatione in coi, ac de fluviis Beneventanis . . . Neapoli, Ex typographia Aegidii Longhi, 1624.

[40], 159 p.; [15], 64 p.   15 cm.   [9022]

Part 2 has special title page.

PIPRE, JOSEPHUS DE LE. *See* LE PIPRE, Joseph de [*fl.* 1611]

PIRCKHEIMER, WILIBALD [1470-1530] Apologia; seu, Laus podagrae . . . Ambergae, Ex Typographeo Forsteriano, 1610.

[1], 32 p.   20 cm.   [9023]

—[The same.] *In* Admiranda rerum admirabilium encomia. 1666, 1677; Argumentorum ludicrorum et amoenitatum scriptores varii. 1623; Dissertationum ludicrarum et amoenitatum. 1638.

—[Dutch tr.] Apologie of verantwoordingh van 't podagra. *In* Veeler wonderens wonderbaarelijck lof. 1664.

—Elegia in obitum Alberti Dureri. *In* Dürer, A. Beschryvinghe . . . van de menschelijcke proportion. 1622.

PIRRONE, CARLO GIOVANNI. *See* CAROLUS JOANNES A JESU [1640-1686]

PISANELLI, BALDASSARE [*fl.* 1559-1583] Trattato della natura de' cibi, et del bere . . . Nel quale non solo tutte le virtù, & vitii di quelli minutamente si palesano, ma anche i rimedii per correggere i loro difetti copiosamente s'insegnano . . . Trevigi, Angelo Reghettini, 1611.

[8], 182, [1] p.   16 cm.   [9024]

—[The same.] . . . Ridotto . . . & aggiontovi di molte dotte, & belle annotationi sopra ogni capo dal sig. Francesco Gallina . . . Di nuovo ristampata, & . . . ricorretta. Torino, 1612.

[15], 383 p.   13 cm.   [9025]

—[The same.] . . . Venetia, Pietro Miloco, 1619.

[8], 182, [2] p.   15 cm.   [9026]

A reprint of the 1611 edition with similar title.

—[The same.] *In* Benzi, U. Regolle della sanità. 1620.

—[The same.] . . . Venetia, Ad instanza del Turrini, 1649.

184, [8] p.   15 cm.   [9027]

—[The same.] . . . Venetia, Francesco Ginami, 1659.

184, [6] p.   16 cm.   [9028]

Different setting of type.

—[Latin tr.] De esculentorum potulentorumque facultatibus. Liber unus. Laconica quidem, et varia jucundaque, medica & historica eruditione refertus. Ex Italico . . . scripto nunc primum in Latinam linguam conversus ab Arnoldo Freitagio . . . Genevae, Apud Philippum Albert [1620]

320, [8] p.   12 cm.   (Part [2] *in* Baricelli, G. C. Hortulus genialis . . . Genevae, 1620)   [9029]

—[The same.] De alimentorum facultatibus libellus aureus. Bruxellis, Typis Francisci Foppens, 1662.

[4], 398 (i.e. 298), [5] p.   14 cm.   [9030]

PISCINARIUS, Joannes. *See* Wier, Johann [1515–1588]

PISO, Carolus. *See* Le Pois, Charles [1563–1633]

PISO, Homobonus. *See* Pisoni, Omobono [*ca.* 1664–1748]

PISO, Willem [1611–1678] De Indiae utriusque re naturali et medica libri quatuordecim ... Amstelaedami, Apud Ludovicum et Danielem Elzevirios, 1658.

[24], 327, [5] p.; 39 p.; 226, [2] p. illus. 35 cm.   [**9031**]

Engraved title page.
Each part has half title.
Contents.—Gulielmi Pisonis ... I. De aëribus, aquis, & locis. II. De natura & cura morborum, occidentali Indiae, imprimis Brasiliae, familiarium. III. De animalibus ... IV. De arboribus ... V. De noxiis & venenatis ... VI. Mantissa aromatica & c. Posita post Bontii tractatus. — Georgii Margravii ... I. Tractatus topographicus & meteorologicus Brasiliae ... II. Commentarius de Brasiliensium & Chilensium indole ac lingua &c. — Jacobi Bontii ... I. De conservanda valetudine. II. Methodus medendi. III. Observationes in cadaveribus. IV. Notae in Garciam ab Orta. V. Historia animalium. VI. Historia plantarium, Quibus sparsim inservit G. Piso annotationes & additiones ...

—Historia naturalis Brasiliae ... Lugdun. Batavorum, Apud Franciscum Hackium et Amstelodami, Apud Lud. Elzevirium, 1648.

[12], 122, [2] p.; [8], 293, [7] p. illus. 40 cm.   [**9032**]

Engraved title page.
Part [2] has half title.
Contents.—Guilielmi Pisonis ... De medicina Brasiliensi libri quatuor: I. De aëre, aquis, & locis. II. De morbis endemiis. III. De venenatis & antidotis. IV. De facultatibus simplicium. Et Georgii Marcgravii de Liebstad ... Historiae rerum naturalium Brasiliae, libri octo: quorum Tres priores agunt de plantis. Quartus de piscibus. Quintus de avibus. Sextus de quadrupedibus & serpentibus. Septimus de insectis. Octavus de ipsa regione, & illius incolis. Cum appendice de Tapuyis, et Chilensibus. — Joannes de Laet ... in ordinem digessit & annotationes addidit, & varia ab auctore omissa supplevit & illustravit.

—Tractatus de aeribus, aquis, & locis in Brasilia. *In* Baerle, K. van. Rerum per octennium in Brasilia. 1660.

—*See* Bondt, J. de. Oost-en West-Indische warande. 1694; Steno, N., *Bp.* De musculis et glandulis observationum specimen. 1664, 1683.

PISONI, Alessandro [*d.* 1702] Breve compendio dell'opinione di Cesare Magatto intorno al modo di medicare rare volte le ferite ... Cremona, Lorenzo Ferrari, 1693.

46, [1] p.   15 cm.   [**9033**]

PISONI, Omobono [*ca.* 1664–1748] Cruentum periculum ... in quo cubiti phlebotomia tali sectioni praefertur contra sectatores Arabum: et sanguinis missio in febribus contra Helmontium asseritur. Cremonae, Typis Laurentii Ferrarii, 1695.

[12], 168 p.   17 cm.   [**9034**]

—Dissertatio de usu vesicantium in febri maligna ... Cremonae, Typis Laurentii Ferrarii, 1694.

[12], 65, [6] p.   16 cm.   [**9035**]

—Ultio antiquitatis in sanguinis circulationem. Hoc est opusculum ... in quo sanguinis circulatio antiquis ignota a recentioribus inventa refellitur. Cremonae, Ex typographia Laurentii Ferrarii, 1690.

107, [5] p.   18 cm.   [**9036**]

PISSINI, Sebastiano [*fl.* 1609–1654] De cordis palpitatione cognoscenda, & curanda libri duo ... Francofurti, Apud Claudium Marnium & heredes Joannis Aubrii, 1609.

193, [23] p.   17 cm.   [**9037**]

—De diabete dissertatio ... Accessit ejusdem Epistola de cordis polypo ... Mediolani, Ad instantiam & sumptus haered. Jo. Baptistae Bidelli, 1654.

[12], 132 p.   21 cm.   [**9038**]

The Epistola de polypo cordis has half title (p. [119]).

—*See* Maccioni, G. Risposta. 1631.

PISSPEN, Jacob Daniel. *See* Jacob Da[niel vo]n Pisspen, auss dem Land Lünenburg ... [n. d.]

PISTORIUS, Johann [1546–1608] Consilium antipodagricum; sive, Dissertatiuncula brevis de arthritide morbo pertinacissimo moletissimo ac dolorifico ... Das ist: Kurtzer und gründlicher Bericht, von der sehr beschwerlichen und unleidlichen schmertz-hafften Kranckheit der Glieder-Sucht, Zipperlein oder Podagra ... Halberstadt, In Verlegung Henrici Praetorii, 1659.

[12], 88 p.   19 cm.   [**9039**]

Colophon: Quedlinburg, Johann Ockeln, 1659.

—Daemonomania Pistoriana. Magica et cabalistica morborum curandorum ratio ... Cum Antidoto prophylactico Jacobi Heilbronneri ... Lavingae, Typis Palatinis, 1601.

[52], 134 p.   16 cm.   [**9040**]

PISTORIUS, JOHANN PHILIPP [*fl.* 1684] *respondent.*
Decreto ... Ordinis Asclepiadei ... casum viri colico dolore laborantis ... examini submittit Johannes Philippus Pistorius ... Giessae, Typis Henningi
Mülleri [1684]

   16 p. 19 cm.   **[9041]**
  Diss.—Giessen.

PITCAIRNE, ARCHIBALD [1652-1713] Apollo
staticus; or, The art of curing fevers by the staticks
... now made English by a well-wisher to the
mathematicks ... Edinburgh, Printed by J. W. and
sold at James Wardlaw's shop, 1695.

   [8], 24 p. 16 cm.   **[9042]**

—Dissertatio, de legibus historiae naturalis. Edinburgi, Typis Joannis Reid, & sumptibus Thomae
Carruthers, 1696.

   94, [2] p. 16 cm.   **[9043]**

—Oratio, qua ostenditur medicinam ab omni
philosophorum secta esse liberam, habita Lugduni-
Batavorum die 26. Aprilis MDCXCII ... Lugduni-
Batavorum, Apud Abrahamum Elzevier, 1692.

   32 p. 23 cm.   **[9044]**

—[The same.] ... Edinburgi, Typis Joannis Reid,
& sumptibus Thomae Carruthers, 1696.

   23 p. 16 cm.   **[9045]**

—*praeses.* Dissertatio de caussis diversae molis qua
fluit sanguis per pulmonem natis & non natis ...
Lugduni Batavorum, Apud Abrahamum Elzevier,
1693.

   [26] p. 22 cm.   **[9046]**
  Diss. — Leyden (J. Johnston, *respondent*)

—Dissertatio de motu sanguinis per vasa minima
... Lugduni Batavorum, Apud Abrahamum
Elzevier, 1693.

   [24] p. 24 cm.   **[9047]**
  Diss. — Leyden (G. Hepburne, *respondent*)

—*See* BELLINI, L. Opuscula aliquot ad Archibaldum Pitcarnium. 1695, 1696; [EIZAT, *Sir* E.]
Apollo mathematicus. 1695.

PITFIELD, ALEXANDER [1659?-1728] *See*
ACADÉMIE ROYALE DES SCIENCES, Paris. Memoires for
a natural history of animals. 1687 [and] Memoir's [sic]
for a natural history of animals. 1688.

PITHOPAEUS, CHRISTOPHORUS. *See* PITHO-
POEIUS, Christoph [*fl.* 1563-1569]

PITHOPOEIUS, CHRISTOPH [*fl.* 1563-1569] *See*
SCHOLTZ, L. Epistolarum philosophicarum:
medicinalium, ac chymicarum ... volumen. 1610.

PITHOPOEUS, WILHELM. Vincedoxicum; das
ist, Wie man sich wider hefftige ... Kranckheit der
Pestilentz oder Infection, und auch wider alles Gifft
und Vergeben ... curiren könne. Sampt einem Antidotario ... Nürnberg, Gedruckt bey Christoph
Endtern, 1674.

   [36], 143 p. 16 cm.   **[9048]**
  Signatures: Gg–Qq^8, R^4.
  Imperfect: sign. Nn$^{1-3,\ 6-8}$, Pp$^{1,\ 7-8}$, Qq^1 wanting.
  Part [2] of Franz Ritter's Astronomia inferior, published in
Nuremberg, in 1674.
  First published in Kempten in 1611.

PITISCUS, SAMUEL [1636-1727] *ed. See* SAUMAISE,
C. de. Claudii Salmasii Plinianae exercitationes in
Caii Julii Solini Polyhistora. 1689.

PITOPOEIUS, CHRISTOPHERUS. *See* PITHO-
POEIUS, Christoph [*fl.* 1563-1569]

PITORIUS, PEREGRINUS. *See* PITTORE, Pellegrino
[17th cent.]

PITTON, JEAN-SCHOLASTIQUE [1621-1689] Les
eaux chaudes de la ville d'Aix ... Aix, Charles
David, 1678.

   [18], 213, [8] p. 18 cm.   **[9049]**

PITTON DE TOURNEFORT, JOSEPH. *See*
TOURNEFORT, Joseph Pitton de [1656-1708]

PITTORE, GIORGIO. *See* PICTORIUS, Georg [*ca.*
1500-1569]

PITTORE, PELLEGRINO [17th cent.] Opobalsami
Romani censura ... Cum appendice contra
Castellum pro theriacis Venetis ... Venetiis, Per
Gulielmum Oddonum, 1642.

   [16], 86 p. 15 cm.   **[9050]**
  Engraved title page.

PIUS Papa IV. Confirmatio privilegiorum Collegii Medicorum urbis. 1675? *See* CATHOLIC CHURCH.
Pope, 1559-1565 (Pius IV)

PIUS Papa V. Ad perpetuam rei memoriam. 1675.
See CATHOLIC CHURCH. *Pope,* 1566-1572 (Pius V)

PIVATI, AGOSTINO [1644?-1695] Syntagma
praelectionum Augustini Pivati ... Venetiis, Typis
Jacobi Ferretti, 1689.

   8 p. 23 cm.   **[9051]**

Date altered by hand from M.DC.LXXXVII to M.DC.LXXXVIIII.

Imperfect: p. 3-6 wanting, but supplied in manuscript.

PIVIER, NICOLAS BENJAMIN NOËL DE [*fl.* 1691] *respondent. See* ALBINUS, B. Dissertatio inauguralis de tarantismo. 1691.

PIZZUTO, PAOLO [*d.* 1684] *ed. See* SICILY, Protomedico. Constitutiones. 1657.

PLACCIUS, JOHANNES [1605-1656] *respondent. See* ROLFINCK, W., *praeses.* Disputatio medica de dolore capitis. 1629.

PLACE, FRANCIS [1647-1728] *See* GOEDAERT, J. Of insects. 1682.

PLACENTINUS, JULIUS. *See* CASSERIO, Giulio [1561?-1616]

PLACENTIUS, JOANNES LEO. *See* PLACENTIUS, Johannes [1500?-1550?]

PLACENTIUS, JOHANNES [1500?-1550?] *See* NUGAE venales. 1689.

PLACHET, JOHANN [*fl.* 1633] *praeses.* Disputatio medica de lue, nunc passim saeviente, Ungarica dicta ... Tubingae, Typis Eberhardi Wildii junioris, 1633.
[1], 23, [1] p. 19 cm. **[9052]**
Diss. — Tübingen (J. Wolffgang, *respondent*)

PLACITUS, *Sextus Papyriensis. See* COLUMELLA, L. J. M. Agricultur; oder, Ackerbaw. 1612.

PLANÇON, GUILLAUME. *See* PLANCY, Guillaume [1514-*ca.*1568]

PLANCUS, HEINRICH [*fl.* 1631-1635] *respondent. See* VARUS, A., *praeses.* Disputatio inauguralis medica de dysenteria. 1635.

PLANCY, GUILLAUME [1514-*ca.* 1568] *ed.* and *tr. See* GALENUS. [In Hippocratis Aphorismos. Greek and Latin] In Aphorismos Hippocratis commentaria. 1633.

—*ed. See* FERNEL, J. Universa medicina. 1602, 1607, 1610, 1602-15, 1619, 1627, 1637, 1638, 1644, 1645, 1656, 1679.

—*tr. See* HIPPOCRATES. [Aphorismi. French] 1645 [and] [Aphorismi. Adaptations, etc. Latin] 1647, 1669; HOULLIER, J. In Aphorismos Hippocratis commentarii. 1613, 1620, 1632, 1646, 1675.

—*See* FERNEL, J. Pharmacia. 1605.

PLANER, ANDREAS [*fl.* 1620] *respondent. See* WEIGANMAIER, J. B., *praeses.* Disputatio physica de nutritione. 1620.

PLANER, ANDREAS [*fl.* 1685-1686] *respondent. See* CAMERARIUS, E. R., *praeses.* Indicatio symptomatum. 1686.

PLANER, JOHANN ANDREAS [*d.* 1714] *praeses.* De nive dissertatio secunda ... Vitembergae, Prelo Christiani Kreusigii [cI vI cc] [i.e. 1695]
[16] p. 19 cm. **[9053]**
Diss. — Wittenberg (C. Schmeltzer, *respondent*)

—De nive dissertatio tertia ... Vitembergae, Prelo Martini Schultzii [1696]
[20] p. 19 cm. **[9054]**
Diss. — Wittenberg (W. H. Leubius, *respondent*)

—De nive dissertatio quarta ... Vitembergae Prelo Christiani Kreusigii [1696]
[20 +] p. 19 cm. **[9055]**
Imperfect: lower margin of p. [20] trimmed; all after p. [20] wanting.
Diss. — Wittenberg (B. Siber, *respondent*)

—*respondent. See* PASCH, J., *praeses.* Gynaeceum doctum ... dispicit J. A. P. 1686; SEBISCH, M. [1578-1674?] *praeses.* Galeni quinque priores libri. 1651.

PLANETEN-BUCH. *See* DAS GROSSE PLANETEN-BUCH. [not before 1694]

PLANIS CAMPY, DAVID DE [*b.* 1589] Les oeuvres ... contenant les plus beaux traictez de la medecine chymique que les anciens autheurs ont enseigné ... Rev., corr. par l'autheur avant son deceds & augm. de plusieurs traictez non imprimez. Paris, Estienne Danguy, 1646.
[16], 752 (i.e. 746) p. illus. 34 cm. **[9056]**

—Bouquet composé des plus belles fleurs chimiques. Ou, Ajencement des préparations, & expériences és plus rares secrets, & médicamens pharmaco chimiques; prins des mineraux, animaux, & végétaux. Le tout par une methode très-facile, & non commune aux chimiques ordinaires ... Paris, Pierre Billaine, 1629.
[32], 1005, [2] p. illus., port. 18 cm. **[9057]**
Added engraved title page.
Errata at end.

—Discours de la phlebotomie ou est monstré en bref, les deux temps d'icelle, à sçavoir le temps d'eslection: & le temps de necessité ... Plus un traitté des crises, où il est monstré comme l'on s'abuze au jugement d'icelles, ne cognoissant le mouvement des astres ... Paris, Jeremie Perier & Abdias Buisard, 1621.

164,[2] p.   17 cm.   [9058]

Imperfect? p. [1–2] (engr. title page?) wanting?
With this is bound his La petite chirurgie. 1621.

—Generale instruction et tres-asseurée methode qu'il faut tenir en la consulte des maladies ... Paris, Denys Moreau, 1644.

[24], 132 (i.e. 136) p.   port.   18 cm.   [9059]

Dedication signed by Pierre de Planis Campy, the editor.

—L'Hydre morbifique exterminee par l'Hercule chimique; ou, Les sept maladies tenües pour incurables jusques à present, renduës guerissables par l'art chimique medical. Où est traicté briefvement de leur definition, causes, differences, signes, pronostic & cure. Le tout selon l'ancienne & moderne medecine ... Paris, Hervé du Mesnil, 1628.

[48], 576 p.   port.   18 cm.   [9060]

Imperfect: 1st leaf (engraved title page) and 9th leaf (portrait) wanting.

—L'Ouverture de l'escolle de philosophie transmutatoire metallique; ou, La plus saine et veritable explication & consiliation de tous les stiles desquels les philosophes anciens se sont servis en traictant de l'oeuvre physique ... Paris, Charles Sevestre, 1633.

[36], 185, [3] p.   port.   18 cm.   [9061]

Added engraved title page.
Imperfect: all pages after 184 wanting.

—La petite chirurgie chimique medicale. Ou est traicté amplement de l'origine des maladies & curation d'icelles ... Paris, Jeremie Perier, & Abdias Buissart, 1621.

[14], 333 (i.e. 323), [3] p.   17 cm.   [9062]

Bound with his Discours de la phlebotomie. 1621.

—[The same.] La chirurgie chimique medicale ... Avec le Discours de la phlebotomie, où est monstré, en bref les deux temps d'icelle. Plus le traitté des crises ... Rouen, Jacques Caillöué, 1642.

[14], 333 (i.e. 323), [1] p.; [3]–147, [1] p.   illus.   17 cm.   [9063]

Part [2] has special title page.

—Traicté de la vraye unique, grande, et universelle medecine des anciens; dite des recens, or potable. Ouvrage autant enrichi des passages de l'Escriture saincte, tesmoignage des SS. Peres, exemples des Hebreux, & des cabalistes philosophes hermetiques, que de la doctrine receuë en l'escolle ... Paris, François Targa, 1633.

[28], 163, [1] p.   port.   17 cm.   [9064]

"Addition a L'or potable, contenant le grand miroir de la nature" (p. [115]–163) has half title.

—Traicté des playes faites par les mousquetades. Ensemble la vraye methode de les guerir. Avec la refutation des erreurs, qui s'y commettent, tant en leur theorie, que practique ... Paris, Nicolas Bourdin, 1623.

12, [4], 271 (i.e. 281), [2] p.   illus.   18 cm.
                                              [9065]

—La verolle recogneue, combatue et abbatue sans suer, & sans tenir chambre, avec tous ses accidens. Le tout selon l'ancienne & moderne medecine. Où est adjousté L'antidotaire venerien, dans lequel sont contenus plusieurs medicamens, preparez chimiquement, pour la parfaicte curation de ceste maladie ... Paris, Nicolas Bourdin, 1623.

7, [23], 189 (i.e. 187), [3] p.   17 cm.   [9066]

PLANIS CAMPY, Pierre de, *ed. See* Planis Campy, D. de. Generale instruction. 1644.

PLANTIUS, Gulielmus. *See* Plancy, Guillaume [1514–*ca.* 1568]

PLAT, Gabriel. *See* Plattes, Gabriel [*fl.* 1638–1643]

PLAT, *Sir* Hugh [1552–1611?] The jewel house of art and nature: containing divers rare and profitable inventions, together with sundry new experiments in the art of husbandry. With divers chymical conclusions concerning the art of distillation ... Whereunto is added, A rare and excellent discourse of minerals, stones, gums, and rosins ... by D. B. Gent. [i.e. Arnold Boate] London, Elizabeth Alsop, 1653.

[8], 232 p.   illus.   19 cm.   [9067]

Imperfect: p. 175 burned, affecting text.
"An additional discourse of several sorts of stones" (p. 217–232) by D. B. and the editorship of the entire work are attributed to Arnold de Boate. Cf. *Dict. Nat. Biog.*

—Sundry new, and artificial remedies against famine. *In* Collectanea chymica. 1684.

PLATEARIUS, Matthaeus [*d.* 1161?] *See* Mesuë [924 *or* 5-1015] Opera. 1602, 1623; Salmon, W. Iatrica. 1681, 1684, 1694.

PLATER. *See* Platter.

PLATO. Timaeus [Selections] *In* Restaurand, R. Monarchia microcosmi, Hippocratis magni, Platonis et Aristotelis insperato foedare restituta. 1657.

—*See* Conring, H. De sanguinis generatione, et motu naturali. 1646; Stefani, G. Hippocratis Coi theologia. 1638.

PLATO, *chemist.* [Platonis Libri quartorum; seu Stellici cum commento Hebuhabes Hamed, explicati ab Hestole ...]

101-185 p., vol. 5. 20 cm. (*In* Zetzner, Lazarus, *ed.* Theatrum chemicum, Argentorati, 1659-61) **[9068]**

Title from table of contents.

PLATON I. *See* Faber, Johann Matthias [*d.* 1702]

PLATT, *Sir* Hugh. *See* Plat, *Sir* Hugh [1552-1611?]

PLATT, Thomas [*fl. ca.* 1670-1673] *See* Redi, F. Opuscoli vari. 1675 [and] Osservazioni intorno alle vipere. 1687.

PLATTER, Felix [1536-1614] De corporis humani structura et usu libri III. Tabulis methodice explicati, iconibus accurate illustrati ... Basileae, Apud Ludovicum König, 1603.

[7], 197, [3] p.; [1], 50, [1] ll. plates. 29 cm. **[9069]**

Froben press mark at end of first group of paging.

"Liber tertius" (2nd group of paging) has special title page, and consists of 50 engraved plates with accompanying letterpress. The plates are for the most part reduced copies of those in Vesalius. Cf. author's letter to the reader, and Cushing. Hamden, 1962, p. 97-98.

—Felix Platerus ... decreto, die Martis, qui octavus Maii erit, proximo, candidatis quatuor subscriptis, ob doctrinam & eruditionem in celeberrimis Germaniae, Belgii, Italiae, Galliae, academiis, diutino studio ... comparatam ... commendatis ... Hermanno Solenandro ... Johanni ab Heimbach ... Thomae Carbasio ... Andreae Schifnero ... discussuris. I. An pulmones solum fuga vacui, vel etiam propriis viribus in respiratione moveantur? II. An calculi in homine ex pituita vel sero suam trahant originem? III. An aer cordis refrigerii tantum, vel

etiam majoris utilitatis causa inspiretur? IIII. An aurum in cordis virium reparatione eas praestet facultates, quae illi assignantur? Doctoratus in arte medica insignia dignitatemque collaturus ... invitat ... Basileae, Typis Joannis Jacobi Genathii [1610] broadside. 22 x 36 cm. **[9070]**

Bound with Stupanus, J. N. Positiones iatricae de phrenitide. 1607.

—Felix Platerus ... decreto die Jovis, qui quartus Januarii erit, proximo candidatis quinque subscriptis ob doctrinam & eruditionem in celeberrimis Germaniae & Italiae academiis diutino studio comparatam ... commendatis ... Gregorio Schönio ... Nicolao Heinio ... Paulo Hepnero ... Joan. Bechtoldo Rivio ... Sigismundo Rüdelio ... discussuris an humor crystallinus, visionis: tympanum, auditus: lingua, gustus: nares, olfactus: cutis, tactus: primaria sint instrumenta, sensus hosce quinque percipientia? Doctoratus in medica arte insignia dignitatemque ... collaturus omnes ... academiae cives ... invitat ... Basileae, Typis Joan. Jacobi Genathii, 1610.

broadside. 23 x 36 cm. **[9071]**

Bound with Schön, G. Theses hasce chirurgico-medicas de fonticulis ... proponit. 1609.

—A golden practice of physick. In five books, and three tomes ... Full of proper observations and remedies: both of ancient and modern physitians ... By Felix Plater ... and R. W. [i.e. William Rowland?] Abdiah Cole ... Nich. Culpeper ... Unto which is added two ... treatises ... London, Peter Cole, 1662.

[8], 688 p.; [2], 75, [1], 87, [1] p. 29 cm. **[9072]**

Imperfect: p. 141-148 wanting, supplied in photocopy from Yale University library.

Part [2] has special title page: Two treatises. The first of the veneral pocks ... The second ... of the gout ... By Daniel Sennert ... Nicholas Culpeper ... Abdiah Cole ... 1660.

"To the reader" signed by Felix Plater (the younger) and Abdiah Cole.

—Observationum, in hominis affectibus plerisque, corpori & animo, functionum laesione, dolore, aliave molestia & vitio incommodantibus, libri tres ... Basileae, Impensis Ludovici König, typis Conradi Waldkirchii, 1614.

[48], 845 p. 19 cm. **[9073]**

—[The same.] . . . Secunda nunc vice typis mandati . . . ad autographum plurimis in locis emendati, Medicamentorum in opere non descriptorum . . . locupletiores. Opera & studio Felicis Plateri, Felicis . . . nepotis . . . Basileae, Impensis Ludovici König, 1641.

[48], 912, [108] p.   18 cm.   **[9074]**

—[The same.] Observationum . . . libri tres totidem praxeos ejus tractatibus, indole & methodo respondentes, atque affectuum corporis & animi . . . tertia nunc vice typis mandati . . . nova insuper, Fel. Plateri . . . nep. Selectiorum observationum mantissa, locupletati. Opera & studio Francisci Plateri . . . Basileae, Typis & impensis Joh. Ludovici König & Johannis Brandmylleri, 1680.

[40], 894, [106] p.; 114, [6] p. 18 cm.   **[9075]**
Part [2] has special title page.

—Praxeos seu, de cognoscendis, praedicendis, praecavendis, curandisque affectibus homini incommodantibus tractatus [primus - secundus] . . . Basileae, Typis Conradi Waldkirchii, 1602-1603.

2 v.   19 cm.   **[9076]**

—[The same.] . . . Tractatus [primus -tertius] . . . Basileae, Typis Conradi Waldkirchii, 1609.

3 v.   19 cm.   **[9077]**

—[The same.] Praxeos medicae tomi tres . . . Quibus accessit Quaestionum medicarum paradoxarum et endoxarum centuria posthuma, studio & opera Thomae Plateri . . . Nunc primum in lucem edita. Basileae, Impensis Ludovici Regis, typis Joannis Schroeteri, 1625.

4 v. in 1.   25 cm.   **[9078]**
The Quaestionum medicarum paradoxarum et endoxarum centuria posthuma has special title page.

—[The same.] Praxeos medicae opus, quinque libris adornatum & in tres tomos distinctum . . . 3. hac ed. . . . locupletatum, & . . . emendatum a Felice Platero . . . Fel. nep. Huic accessit, ejusdem Quaestionum medicarum paradoxarum & endoxarum, centuria posthuma, opera primum Thomae Plateri . . . edita, nunc ab eodem nep. Th. fil. revisa & recusa. Basileae, Impensis Emanuelis König, typis viduae Joh. Jac. Genathii, 1656.

3 v. in 1.   25 cm.   **[9079]**

—Quaestionum medicarum paradoxarum & endoxarum, juxta partes medicinae dispositarum, cen-

turia posthuma: opera Thomae Plateri . . . nunc primum edita. Basileae, Impensis Ludovici Regis., 1625.

[15], 277, [8] p.   17 cm.   **[9080]**

—[The same.] . . . 3. ed. Parisiis, Apud Joannem Jost, 1639.

[23], 344, [10] p.   15 cm.   **[9081]**

—*praes.* De febrium malignarum curatione in genere disputatio . . . Basileae, Typis Johannis Schroeteri, 1607.

[31] p.   20 cm.   **[9082]**
Diss. — Basel (M. Döring, *respondent*)

—Disputatio medica de mola matricis . . . Basileae, Typis Joannis Schroeteri [1607]

[8] p.   20 cm.   **[9083]**
Diss. — Basel (G. Hebenstreit, *respondent*)

—Theses medicae de ἀπεψία, seu concoctionis defectu . . . Basileae, Typis Joan. Jacobi Genathii, 1609.

[8] p.   20 cm.   **[9084]**
Diss. — Basel (J. Zehner, *respondent*)

—Theses miscellae . . . Basileae, Typis Johan. Jacobi Genathii [1612]

[20] p.   19 cm.   **[9085]**
Diss. — Basel, 1605 (J. H. Frölich, *respondent*)

—*See* BONET, T., *ed.* Corps de medecine et de chirurgie. 1679; PINEAU, S. De integritatis & corruptionis virginum notis. 1639, 1640, 1641, 1650, 1663, 1690; RULAND, M. [1532-1602] Experimental physick. 1662.

PLATTER, FELIX [1605-1671] *ed. See* PLATTER, Felix [1536-1614] Observationum . . . libri tres. 1641, 1680 [and] Praxeos medicae opus. 1656.

—*See* PLATTER, FELIX [1536-1614] A golden practice of physick. 1662.

PLATTER, FRANZ [1645-1711] *respondent.* Dissertatio physico-medica de tarantismo . . . Basileae, Ex Typographia Deckeriana [1669]

[42] p.   19 cm.   **[9086]**
Diss. — Basel.

—*See* EGLINGER, S., *praeses.* [De]lienter[ico] et coeliac[o] affect[u] delineat[io]. 1667; PLATTER, Felix [1536-1614] Observationum . . . libri tres. 1680.

PLATTER, THOMAS [1547–1628] *ed. See* PLATTER, F. [1536–1614] Praxeos medicae tomi tres. 1625, 1656 [and] Quaestionum medicarum. 1625, 1639.

PLATTES, GABRIEL [*fl.* 1638–1643] *See* CHYMICAL, medicinal, and chyrurgical addresses. 1655.

PLATZ, ABRAHAM CHRISTOPH [*fl.* 1673] *respondent. See* DRECHSSLER, J. G., *praeses.* Disputatio II. de metallorum transmutatione. 1673.

PLATZ, HIERONYMUS [*fl.* 1625] *respondent. See* SEBISCH, M. [1578–1674?] *praeses.* Exercitationes medicae. 1639.

PLAZZONI, FRANCESCO [*d.* 1622] De partibus generationi inservientibus libri duo ... Patavii, Ex typogr. Laur. Pasquati, 1621.
 [8], 158, [1] p. 21 cm. **[9087]**

—[The same.] ... Item Gregorii Nymmani, De vita foetus in utero, dissertatio. Lugduni Batavorum, Ex officina Davidis Lopes de Haro, 1644.
 [8], 184 p.; [7], 87 p. 13 cm. **[9088]**
 Added engraved title page.
 Part [2] has special title page.
 "Adriani Spigelii ... Epistola de incerto tempore partus": p. 63–87, part 2.

—[The same.] ... Item Arantii De humano foetu libellus. Item Gregorii Nymmani De vita foetus in utero, dissertatio. Lugduni Batavorum, Ex officina Felicis Lopez de Haro, 1664.
 [8], 184 p.; 50 p.; [8], 84 p. 13 cm. **[9089]**
 Added engraved title page.
 Parts [2] and [3] have special title pages.
 "Adriani Spigelii ... Epistola de incerto tempore partus" (p. 61–84 of part [3]) has caption title.
 With this is bound Deusing, A. Vindiciae foetus. 1664.

—De vulneribus sclopetorum ... Venetiis, Apud Robertum Meglietum [Ex typographia Georgii Valentini] 1618.
 [16], 174, [18] p. 20 cm. **[9090]**

—[The same.] ... Patavii, Apud Franciscum Bolzettam, 1643.
 [8], 174, [21] p. 19 cm. **[9091]**

—[French tr.] Traité des blesseures et playes faites par armes a feu, vulgairement dites playes d'arquebusades ... Corr. & augm. de plusieurs remedes ... Mis en françois par Pierre Dailly ... Paris, André Boutonné, 1668.
 [22], 418 (i.e. 416) p. 15 cm. **[9092]**

A PLEASANT and compendious history of the first inventers and instituters of the most famous arts. *See* [VERGILIUS, Polydorus]

PLEIER, CORNELIUS [*fl.* 1617–1627] Medicus-criticus-astrologus, ex veteribus iatromathematicis productus ... Noribergae, Sumptibus & typis Simonis Halbmayeri, 1627.
 237, [1] p. illus. 13 cm. **[9093]**
 "Astrologia Hippocratis, de significatione morborum, mortis & vitae, secundum motum lunae ... & positus planetarum, Gulideolo interprete prisco" and "Astrologia Galeni, Jacobo Antonio Mariscotto ... interprete" (in parallel columns): p. III–199. These are variant versions of the Prognostica de decubitu ascribed to Imbrasius of Ephesus.

PLEMP, VOPISCUS FORTUNATUS [1601–1671] Animadversio in veram praxim curandae tertianae propositam a ... Petro Barba ... Lovanii, Typis ac sumptibus Jacobi Zegeri, 1642.
 49 p. 20 cm. **[9094]**
 Imperfect: p. 3–4 wanting.
 With this are bound: Mohy, H. Tertianae cirsis [1642?]; Soers, M. Stricturae. 1642; Mohy, H. Pulvis sympatheticus. 1639; Helmont, J. B. van. Propositiones. 1634; Barba, P. Vera praxis. [n.d.]

—Antimus Conygius Peruviani pulveris febrifugi defensor repulsus. *In* Fabri, H. Pulvis Peruvianus. 1655.

—De togatorum valetudine tuenda commentatio ... Bruxellis, Typis Francisci Foppens, 1670.
 [19], 338, [26] p. 21 cm. **[9095]**

—Fundamenta medicinae ad scholae acribologiam aptata. Ed. altera recognita, interpolata, aucta. Accessit Danielis Vermostii ... Breve apologema pro authore adversus dicteria & ineptias cujusdam Κηπουρον [A. Kijperi] Louvanii, Typis ac sumptibus viduae Jacobi Zegers, 1644.
 [10], 383 p. plate, port. 33 cm. **[9096]**
 Part [2] has special title page.
 "Danielis Vermostii Responsio ad confutationem Apologematis" (p. 371–383) has caption title.
 With this is bound *his* Ophthalmographia. 1648.

—[The same.] ... Ed. 3 ... Item doctorum aliquot in Academia Lovaniensi virorum judicia de philosophia Cartesiana. Lovanii, Typis ac sumtibus Hieronymi Nempaei, 1654.
 [4], 427 p. illus. 33 cm. **[9097]**

—Loimographia; sive, Tractatus de peste ... Amstelodami, Apud Joannem Ravestinium, 1664.
 [8], 36 p. 20 cm. **[9098]**

—Ophthalmographia; sive, Tractatio de oculi fabrica, actione, & usu praeter vulgatas hactenus philosophorum ac medicorum opiniones . . . Amsterodami, Sumptibus Henrici Laurentii, 1632.

    [20], 340, [2] p. 21 cm.   **[9099]**
Errata at end.

—[The same.] . . . Ed. altera. Cui praeter alia accessere affectionum ocularium curationes . . . Lovanii, Typis ac sumptibus Hieronymi Nempaei, 1648.

    [15], 240 p. 33 cm.   **[9100]**
Bound with *his* Fundamenta medicinae. 1644.

—[The same.] . . . Ed. 3. Recognita & aucta. Cui praeter alia accessere Gerardi Gutischovii Animadversiones in Ophthalmographiam ad easque responsio. Lovanii, Typis ac sumptibus Hieronymi Nempaei, 1659.

    [5], 299, [8] p. illus. 32 cm.   **[9101]**

—Verhandelingh der spieren. By de welcke aenghewesen wort, wat in hun onnaeturige toevallen en te voorsegghen en te hant-wercken staet . . . Amstelredam, Jacob Aertsz. Colom, 1630.

    [8], 228 p. 14 cm.   **[9102]**

—[The same.] . . . Dordrecht, Gedruckt by Hendrick van Esch, voor Pieter Loymans, ende Maerten de Bot, 1645.

    [6], 176 p. 16 cm.   **[9103]**
Bound with Beverwijck Jan van. Heel-konste. 1645.

—, *ed.* and *tr. See* AVICENNA. Canon medicinae interprete & scholiaste Vopisco Fortunato Plempio. 1658.

—, *tr. See* CABROL, B. Ontleeding des menschelycken lichaems. 1633, 1648.

—*See* ARBERIUS. La physique d'uzage. 1664; BALDI, S. Anastasis corticis Peruviae. 1663; BEVERWIJCK, J. van. Wercken der genees-konste, 1664, 1672; BLASIUS, G. Impetus Jacobi Primirosii . . . in Vop. Fort. Plempium . . . retusus a Gerardo Leon. Blasio. 1659; GRAAF, R. de. Partium genitalium defensio. 1673; KIJPER, A. Anthropologia corporis humani. 1660 [and] Institutiones physicae. 1647; MOHY, H. Tertianae crisis. 1642?; NOUVEAU COURS DE MEDECINE. 1669, 1683; SOERS, M. Stricturae in ceritum quemdam Eburonem inconditum blateronem controversiae de curanda tertiana inter D. D. Petrum Barbam et V. F. Plempium. 1642.

PLENE, GEORG [1677?] *respondent. See* MITZEL, J., *praeses.* Dissertatio juridica de testimonio foeminarum. 1677?

PLESSEUS, CAROLUS ARTURUS. *See* DU PLESSIS, Charles Arthur [*b. ca.* 1592]

PLESSIS, CAROLUS ARTHURUS. *See* DU PLESSIS, Charles Arthur [*b. ca.* 1592]

PLEYER, CORNELIUS. *See* PLEIER, Cornelius [*fl.* 1617–1627]

PLINIUS SECUNDUS, C. Historiae naturalis libris XXXVII. Lugduni Batavorum, Ex Officina Elzeviriana, 1635.

    3 v. port. 13 cm.   **[9104]**
Vol. 1 has engraved title page.
Vol. 2–3 have title: . . . Naturalis historiae, tomus secundus [-tertius]
Edited by Joannes de Laet.

—Naturalis historiae, tomus primus [-tertius] Cum commentariis & adnotationibus Hermolai Barbari, Pintiani, Rhenani, Gelenii, Dalechampii, Scaligeri, Salmasii, Is. Vossii, & variorum . . . Item Joh. Fr. Gronovii Notarum liber singularis . . . Lugd. Batav., Roterodami, Apud Hackios, 1668–69 [v. 1, 1669]

    3 v. 21 cm.   **[9105]**
Each volume has added engraved title page, dated 1669.
"De C. Plinii Secundi patria, a Paulo Cigalino . . . lectio prima [-altera]": vol. 1, p. 1–80.

—[Dutch excerpts.] . . . Boecken ende schriften, in vier deelen onderscheyden: het eerste tracteert van de natuer, aert ende eyghenschap aller creaturen ofte schepselen Godes. Als namentlijck, van de menschen . . . Het tweede: van de viervoetighe dieren . . . Het derde van de vogelen . . . Oock van de uitrenne kruyp ende wormen, als slangen, etc. . . . Het vierde, van de visschen . . . Nu nieuwelijck uyt den Hoochduycsche in onse nederlantsche sprake overgeset, ende met schoone figuren verciert. Campen, Arent Benier, voor Hendrick Laurentsz., [1644?]

    [8+], 512 p.; 93, [5] p. illus. 19 cm. **[9106]**
Incomplete. Pages after [p. 8] wanting.
Pages 57–64 bound before p. 49–56 in second group of paging.
Translation of extracts from books 7–11 of the Historia naturalis, with the addition of selections from other writers.

—[English excerpts.] The historie of the world. Commonly called, The naturall historie of C. Plinius

Secundus. Translated into English by Philemon Holland ... Londini, Impensis G. B., 1601.

2 v. in l.   35 cm.   **[9107]**

Title page of vol. 1 is a cancel.

Title page of vol. 2 has imprint: London, Printed by Adam Islip, 1601.

STC 20029.5.

—[The same.] ... London, Printed by Adam Islip, 1634.

2 v. in l.   34 cm.   **[9108]**

Title page of vol. 1 is a cancel.

STC 20030.

—[Spanish tr.] Historia natural ... traducida por ... Geronimo de Huerta ... Y ampliada por el mismo, con escolios y anotaciones, en que aclara lo oscuro y dudoso, y añade lo no sabido hasta estos tiempos ... Madrid, Luis Sanchez [Juan Goncalez] 1624–29.

2 v.   illus., plates, port.   30 cm.   **[9109]**

Imperfect: outer margins of p. 1–21, vol. 2, trimmed.

—*See* HOFMANN, C. Variarum lectionum lib. VI. 1619; MAROGNA, N. Commentarius in tractatus Dioscoridis, et Plinii de amomo. 1608; PONA, G. Monte Baldo descritto. 1617; SAUMAISE, C. de. Claudii Salmasii Plinianae exercitationes in Caii Julii Solini Polyhistora. 1689; SENNERT, D. De scorbuto tractatus. 1624.

PLOEGH, CORNELIS [1624?–1696?] *See* Rouwklachten over de dood van den eerwaarden ... Cornelis Ploegh. 1696.

PLOHR, JOHANN ANDREAS [*fl.* 1698–1699] *respondent. See* WERNHER, J. B., *Freiherr von, praeses.* Disputationem physicam de saporibus eorumque differentiis ... publico ... examini exponit ... J. A. P. 1698.

PLOMANN, ANDREAS [*fl.* 1676] *respondent. See* MORHOF, D. G., *praeses.* Dissertatio de paradoxis sensuum. 1676, 1685.

PLOT, ROBERT [1640–1696] The natural history of Oxford-shire, being an essay toward the natural history of England. By R[obert] P[lot] ... Printed at the Theater in Oxford, and are to be had there. And in London at Mr. S. Millers, 1677.

[10], 358, [12] p.   plates, map.   33 cm.   **[9110]**

Errata: p. [1] at end.

Imperfect: plate 14 wanting.

—The natural history of Stafford-shire ... Oxford, Printed at the Theater, 1686.

[16], 450, [14] p.   plates, map.   36 cm.   **[9111]**

Plate 32 misbound before plate 26.

PLUMIER, CHARLES [1646–1704] Description des plantes de l'Amerique ... Paris, Imprimerie royale, 1713 [i.e. 1693]

[8], 94, [9] p.   98 plates.   43 cm.   **[9112]**

Colophon: Paris, Imprimerie royale, par les soins de Jean Anisson.

PODAGRA politica. 1659. *See* LIBERATI, L.

POETON, EDWARD [*fl.* 1630] *ed. See* BONHAM, T. The chyrurgians closet. 1630.

PÖTTER, JOHANN GEORG [*fl.* 1673] *respondent. See* MÖLLER, P., *praeses.* Historia chirurgica rarior de ventositate spinae. 1673.

POHL, MARTIN [*fl.* 1672] *respondent. See* PASCHA, N. B., *praeses.* Disputatio physica de quaestione an Esau fuerit monstrum. 1672.

POIRIER, LOUIS [*d.* 1718] *praeses.* Quaestio medica ... An dysenteriae, mochlica purgatio? [Parisiis, Apud Franciscum Muguet, 1695]

4 p.   25 cm.   **[9113]**

Diss.—Paris (D. Tauvry, *respondent*)

POISSON, JOANNES [*fl.* 1681] *respondent. See* SORAND, F., *praeses.* Quaestio medica ... An calculus a caseo? 1681.

POLAND. Sovereign, 1632–1648 (Wladislas IV) *See* LAKIN, D. A miraculous cure of the Prussian swallow-knife. 1642.

POLÁNI, JÁNOS [*fl.* 1642] *praeses.* Discursus de origine animae rationalis ... Regiomonti, Praelo Reusneriano, 1642.

[16] p.   18 cm.   **[9114]**

Diss.—Königsberg (G. Wolffgang, *respondent*)

POLEMANN, JOACHIM [*fl.* 1659] Novum lumen medicum. In welchem die vortrefliche und hochnötige Lehre des hochbegabten Philosophi Helmontii, von dem hohen Geheimnüs des Sulphuris Philosophorum ... erkläret wirdt ... Amsterdam, Bey Henrico Betkio, 1659.

[6], 182 p.   12 cm.   **[9115]**

—[The same.] ... Amsterdam, Bey Henrico Betkio, 1660.

[6], 245 p. 13 cm.   **[9116]**

—[The same.] ... Amsterdam, Kosten Wilhelm Welmsonii und Leipzig bey Joh. Herbord, 1699.

[6], 245 p. 14 cm.   **[9117]**

Different setting of type.

With this is bound De viribus & usu auri & argenti. 1699.

—[Latin tr.] Novum lumen medicum de mysterio sulphuris philosophorum ...

600-674 p., vol. 6. 20 cm. (*In* Zetzner, Lazarus, *ed.* Theatrum chemicum. Argentorati, 1659-61)

                               [9118]

Caption title.

POLEMO, ANTONIUS [*ca.* 88-145] Fisonomia di Polemone tradotta di Greco in Latino dall'illustrissimo signor co. Carlo Montecuccoli, con annotationi del medemo; et poscia di Latino fatta volgare dal co. Francesco suo fratello. Padova, Pietro Paolo Tozzi, 1623.

40 p. 23 cm. (Part [3] in Fisonomia naturale di Gio. Battista dalla Porta, Giovanni Ingegnieri [e] Polemone. 1622)   **[9119]**

"Regole delle forme humane secondo la Fisonomia del medesimo Polemone, tradotte dal medesimo Carlo Montecuccoli": p. 35-40.

This text, attributed to Antonius Polemo, is the forgery of the Byzantine period. Cf. Foerester (which prints all the extant texts) and Pauly-Wissowa, v. 21, col. 1345-1348.

—[The same.] ... Padova, Pietro Paolo Tozzi, 1626.

32 p. 21 cm.   **[9120]**

Bound with Porta, G. B. della. Della fisonomia dell'huomo. Padova, 1627.

—[The same.] *In* Porta, G. B. della. Della fisionomia dell'huomo ... Aggiontavi la Fisionomia naturale di monsignor Giovanni Ingegnieri, Polemone ... Venetia. 1644, 1668.

—[French tr.] *In* Adamantius. La physionomie. 1635.

POLIDORO VERGILIO. *See* VERGILIUS, Polydorus [*d.* 1555]

POLISIUS, GOTHOFREDUS SAMUEL [*fl.* 1658-1661] *respondent.* De metallis imperfectis duris duobus, ferro et cupro. *In* Rolfinck, W., *praeses.* Dissertationes chimicae sex de tartaro. 1660, 1679.

POLITIANUS, ANGELUS. *See* POLIZIANO, Angelo [1454-1494]

POLITIUS, ANTONINUS [*fl.* 1613-1625] De febribus pestilentialibus pestis a menominatis cum bubonibus carbunculis & aliis pravis synthomatibus grassantibus per fel: urbem Panormi die 16. Junii 7. indictionis 1624. consultatio ... Panormi, Apud Angelum Orlandi, 1625.

68 p. 20 cm.   **[9121]**

POLIZIANO, ANGELO [1454-1494] *tr. See* ARISTOTELES. Aristotelis, aliorumque philosophorum, ac medicorum problemata. 1631.

POLL, MICHAEL [*fl.* 1603-1605] *praeses.* De spiritibus corporis humani ... [Francofurti ad Oderam?] Typis Voltzianis, 1605.

[8] p. 19 cm.   **[9122]**

Diss. — Frankfurt an der Oder (D. Moller, *respondent*)

POLLIO, JOACHIM [1602-1656] *praeses.* Disputatio physica de insomniis ... Lipsiae, Typis exscribebat Georgius Liger, 1626.

[16] p. 18 cm.   **[9123]**

Diss. — Leipzig (L. Pollio, *respondent*)

POLLIO, LUCAS [1605-1643] *respondent. See* POLLIO, J., *praeses.* Disputatio physica de insomniis. 1626.

POLLMAR, CHRISTOPH FRIEDRICH [*fl.* 1671-1672] *respondent. See* FRIDERICI, J. A., *praeses.* Dissertatio medico-chirurgica de gangraena et sphacelo. 1671.

POLLONI, NICOLÒ ORFEO. *See* PAULONI, Nicolò Orfeo [1653-1721]

POLNER, ZACHARIAS [*fl.* 1627-1628] *respondent. See* SENNERT, D., *praeses.* Disputatio medica de cardialgia. 1627.

POLVERINO, GIOVANNI GIROLAMO [*fl.* 1586-1589] De curandis, juxta hodiernum usum, singulis humani corporis morbis, opus; sive, Praxis accurata brevi, dilucida, et absoluta methodo explicata, ac tradita. In hac 2. ed. ab authore ipso diligentissime recognita, & locupletior facta ... Venetiis, Apud Jac. Ant. Somaschum & Paulum Venturium, 1605.

[8], 536 p. 22 cm.   **[9124]**

—[The same.] ... 5. ed. ... Neapoli, Apud Lazarum Scoriggium, sumptibus Jo. Dominici Montanarii, & Jo. Antonii Farina, 1629.

[8], 215 p.; 57, [1] p. 29 cm. **[9125]**

Part [2] has caption title: Joannis Hieronymi Pulverini ... De curandorum febrium methodica, & plena ratio, per Matthiam Maglioccam ... nunc primo publicae utilitati imposita ... Correpta [sic] ac expurgata ... a Jo. Bernardino Corbiserio ...

—[The same.] De singulis humani corporis juxta hodiernum usum, curandis morbis medica praxis, accurata ... & absoluta methodo explicata, ac tradita. Cui novissime accessit ejusdem auctoris methodica, & plena ratio juxta eundem hodiernum usum de curandis febribus per Matthiam Maglioccam ... publicae utilitati impertita ... Correcta ... ac quam pluribus additionibus donata a Jo. Berardino Corbiserio ... Neapoli, Apud Camillum Cavallum, 1643.

[8], 215, 57, [1] p. 30 cm. **[9126]**

Different setting of type.

—[The same.] Medicina practica, morborum; tam universalium, quam particularium, accuratam plenamque curationem continens. Ed. 7. Ex recensione Gerhardi Blasii ... Lugduni Batavorum, Ex officina Francisci Hackii, 1649.

[16], 747, [15] p. 19 cm. **[9127]**

POLYBIUS, *of Cos. See* POLYBUS.

POLYBUS. De salubri victus ratione privatorum. *In* Gorris, P. de [*fl.* 1511] Formulae remediorum, quibus vulgo medici utuntur. 1612.

POLYDORE, VERGIL. *See* VERGILIUS, Polydorus [*d.* 1555]

POLYGAMIA triumphatrix. 1682. *See* LYSER, J.

POMARIUS, PETRUS. *See* VALENTINUS, Petrus Pomarius.

POMARIUS, SAMUEL [1624–1683] De generatione aequivoca disputatio physica ... [Wittenbergae] Typis Michaelis Wendt [1650]

[44] + p. 19 cm. **[9128]**

Imperfect: all after p. [44] wanting.
Diss. pro loco—Wittenberg (K. Ortlob, *respondent*)

Dissertations — Wittenberg

—*praeses.* De modo visionis disputatio secunda ... [Wittenbergae] Typis Michaelis Wendt [1650]

[20] p. 20 cm. **[9129]**

J. Scheffrichius, *respondent.*

—De modo visionis disputatio tertia ... [Wittenbergae] Typis Michaelis Wendt [1650]

[24] p. 20 cm. **[9130]**

C. Bohemus, *respondent.*

—De modo visionis disputatio quarta, eademque ultima ... [Wittenbergae] Typis Michaelis Wendt [1650]

[24] p. 20 cm. **[9131]**

F. Hoffmann, *respondent.*

—De noctambulis disputatio prior ... [Wittenbergae] Typis Johannis Röhneri [1649]

[24] p. 18 cm. **[9132]**

J. Fabiger, *respondent.*

—[The same.] De noctambulis disputatio prior, quam ... ad D. XXIIX Septembris, A. C. cIɔ. Iɔc. xlix disquisitionis sistunt publicae ... Ed. 4. Witienbergae, Typis Christiani Schrödteri, 1686.

[24] p. 20 cm. **[9133]**

Diss.—1649 (J. Fabiger, *respondent*)

—De noctambulis disputatio posterior ... [Wittenbergae, 1650]

[32] p. 20 cm. **[9134]**

Signatures: D-G⁴.
J. Schultz, *respondent.*

—Another issue, with textual changes on title page.

[9135]

POMET, PIERRE [1658–1699] Histoire generale des drogues, traitant des plantes, des animaux, & des mineraux ... avec un discours qui explique leurs differens noms, les pays d'où elles viennent, la maniere de connoître les veritables d'avec les falsifiées, & leurs proprietez, où l'on découvre l'erreur des anciens & des modernes ... Paris, Jean-Baptiste Loyson, et Estienne Ducastin, 1694.

[12], 304 (i.e. 336) p.; 108 p.; 116, [37] p. illus., plate, port. 39 cm. **[9136]**

Pages 233i–264xxxii inserted between p. 232 and 233 of part 1.
Imperfect: plate wanting; sheet B of part 1 wanting; p. 96–97 of part 3 misbound after p. 98.
Appendix at end.

—[The same.] Le marchand sincere; ou, Traite general des drogues simples et composees. Renfermant dans les trois classes des vegetaux, des animanx [sic], & des mineraux; tout ce qui est l'objet de la physique, de la chimie, de la pharmacie ... Paris, L'auteur, 1695.

[12], 264, 233-304, 108, 116, [37], 16 p. illus., plates, port. 40 cm.   **[9137]**

Added half title reads: Histoire generale des drogues.

POMEY, François Antoine [1618-1673] Indiculus universalis, rerum fere omnium, quae in mundo sunt, scientiarum item, artiumque nomina, apte, breviterque colligens ... Lyon, Antoine Molin, 1667.

[24], 276 p. 16 cm.   **[9138]**

POMMEREAU, E. *See* POMMEREAU, Edmond [*fl.* 1676]

POMMEREAU, Edmond [*fl.* 1676] Traité des eaux mineralles; ou, La nouvelle fontaine de Saint Gordon, avec une pathologie chimique des fiévres, & un discours raisonné sur la maladie du tems ... Orleans, La veuve, François Boyer, & Jean Boyer, 1676.

[18], 269, [5] p. 15 cm.   **[9139]**

POMMEREAU, Étienne. *See* POMMEREAU, Edmond [*fl.* 1676]

POMPEJUS, Nicolaus [1591?-1659] Praecepta chiromantica ... praelecta olim ab ipso, anno Christianorum 1653^tio, jam vero recognita, descripta, figurisque ligno incisis aucta. Hamburgi, Sumptibus Zachar. Hertelii & haeredum Matth. Weyrauchii, typis v. Rebenlinianis, 1682.

[12], 163 (i.e. 164), [4] p. illus., plates. 16 cm.   **[9140]**

Errata at end.
Edited by H. S. P.

PONA, Carlo [*fl.* 1641] *ed.* and *tr. See* PONA, F. Dell'anello fisico. 1641, 1680.

PONA, Francesco [1594-1652] L'Amalthea; overo, Della pietra belzoar orientale, dialogo primo [-secundo] ... Venetia, Lorenzo Griffo, 1626.

38 p. 19 cm.   **[9141]**

Dialogo secondo has special title page: Il lince; overo, Della pietra bezoar orientale.

—Dell'anello fisico; overo, Del ristretto dell'arte medica ... Tradottione, & ampliatione di Carlo Pona ... Verona, Bartolomeo Merlo, 1641.

[16], 259, [5] p. 22 cm.   **[9142]**

—[The same.] ... Venetia, Per Iseppo Prodocimo, 1680.

[24], 320 p. 15 cm.   **[9143]**

—Physicum annulum; seu, Medicae artis breviarium ... [Veronae, Merulus, 1638]

[8], 81, [1] p. 21 cm.   **[9144]**

Engraved title page.

—Ferdinando Quarto ... prodentiam medicam ... d. d. ... Venetiis, Apud Franciscum Baba, 1650.

131, [5] p. 14 cm.   **[9145]**

Errata: p. [5].
With this are bound: Schoppe, K. De paedia humanarum ac divinarum literarum. 1647; Schoppe, K. Consultationes, 1636.

—Trattato de' veleni, e lor cura ... Verona, Bortolamio Merlo, 1643.

[8], 96 p. 22 cm.   **[9146]**

—*tr. See* PONA, G. Monte Baldo descritto. 1617.

PONA, Giovanni [*fl.* 1595-1623] Del vero balsamo de gli antichi commentario ... sopra l'Historia di Dioscoride. Nel quale si prova, che solo l'opobalsamo Arabico è il legitimo; e s'esclude ogn'altro licore, abbracciato sotto nome di balsamo dagli antidoti ... Venetia, Roberto Miglietti [Appresso Barezzo Barezzi] 1623.

[8], 54, [2] p. plates. 22 cm.   **[9147]**

—Monte Baldo descritto ... in cui si figurano, & descrivono molte rare piante de gli antichi, da' moderni fin' hora non conosciute. Et due Commenti del ... Nicolo Marogna ... sopra l'amomo de gli antichi; per Francesco Pona dal Latino tradotti ... Venetia, Roberto Meietti, 1617.

[16], 248, [15] p.; 132 p. illus. 22 cm.   **[9148]**

Errata at end of part 1.
Part [2] has special title page: Commentario ne' trattati di Dioscoride, & di Plinio dell'amomo.

—Plantae, seu simplicia, ut vocant, quae in Baldo monte, et in via ab Verona ad Baldum reperiuntur ... Antverpiae, Ex Officina Plantiniana, Apud Joannem Moretum, 1601.

[cccxxi]-cccxlviii p. illus. 37 cm. (In L'Écluse, Charles de. Caroli Clusii ... Rariorum plantarum historia. Antverpiae, 1601)   **[9149]**

PONCE DE SANTA CRUZ, Alfonso [*fl. ca.* 1600] *See* PONCE DE SANTA CRUZ, Antonio.

PONCE DE SANTA CRUZ, Antonio [*d. ca.* 1650] Opuscula medica, et philosophica ... Quae continent 1. Disputationes in primam primi Avicennae. 2. De Hippocratica philosophia. 3. De pulsibus. 4. ... Alphonsi de Sanctacruce, diu desideratum, modo filii sui opera in lucem editum, De melancholia inscriptum libellum. Matriti, Apud Thomam Juntam, vendese en casa de Geronimo de Courbes, 1624.

4 parts in 1 v.   31 cm.   **[9150]**

Parts [2-4] have special title pages with imprint: Matriti, Apud Thomam Juntam, 1622.

"Tassa" for the 4 works, dedicatory epistle, and colophon dated 1622.

Special title page of part [3]: Exactissimae disputationes de pulsibus, quibus Galeni et Avicennae doctrina philosophice perpenditur.

Imperfect: part [4] precedes part [3]

A reissue, with title page, of the 1622 edition of the works, published without a general title. Cf. C. Pérez Pastor 1878; and Palau 231048.

Part [2] includes Latin text of book 1 of Hippocrates' De victus ratione.

Bound with Savonarola, G. M. Practica major. Venetiis, 1560.

—De impedimentis magnorum auxiliorum, in morborum curatione. Lib. III ... Matriti, Ex Typographia Regia, 1629.

[6], 208, [3] p.   21 cm.   **[9151]**

—[The same.] ... secundis curis emendatiores e museo Petri A Castro ... Patavii, Typis Pauli Frambotti, 1652.

[20], 451, [1] p.   14 cm.   **[9152]**

Errata: p. [452]

—[The same.] ... in hac ultima impressione annotationibus quibusdam illustratum opus ... Valencia, Heredero de Benito Macè, acosta de Claudio Macè, 1695.

[8], 372, [9] p.   16 cm.   **[9153]**

—Praelectiones Vallisoletanae, in librum magni Hipp. Coi De morbo sacro. Auctore D. Antonio Ponze Sancta Cruz ... Matriti, Apud viduam Ludovici Sanchez, 1681.

[12], 188 p.   30 cm.   **[9154]**

Includes Latin text of De morbo sacro.

—*See* FEYENS, T. Pro sua de animatione foetus tertia die opinione. 1629; LICETI, F. De anima subjecto corpori nil tribuente. 1631.

PONSARD, François. Traicté de l'election et choix des lieux salubres; pour la construction des bastimens; tant en la situation terrestre que celeste, selon la doctrine des anciens & modernes ... Paris, 1617.

[8], 31, [2] p.   24 cm.   **[9155]**

PONTANUS, Johannes [*d.* 1572] Epistola, in qua de lapide, quem philosophorum vocant, agitur.

734-743 p., vol. 3.   20 cm. (*In* Zetzner, Lazarus, *ed.* Theatrum chemicum. Argentorati, 1659-61)   **[9156]**

Caption title.

—[The same.]

487-489 p., vol. 6.   20 cm. (*In* Zetzner, Lazarus, *ed.* Theatrum chemicum. Argentorati, 1659-61)   **[9157]**

Caption title.

—*See* GLAUBER, J. R. De tribus lapidibus ignium secretorum. 1667; ORTHELIUS. Commentatio in epistolam Joh. Pontani de lapide ph. 1659; RANTZAU, H. De conservanda valetudine. 1601; THOR, G., astromagus. Cheiragogia heliana. 1659; WITTICH, J. Consilia. 1604.

PONTANUS A BRAITENBERG, Georgius Bartholdus [*d.* 1616] *ed. See* BARTHOLOMAEUS ANGLICUS. De genuinis rerum coelestium. 1601.

PONTE, Luigi da. *See* PUENTE, Luis de la, *Father* [1554-1624]

PONTEOUS, *Doctor.* Man and woman their own doctor; or, A salve for every sore. Being a book full of rare receipts for the most dangerous distempers incident to the bodies of men, women, and children ... Gathered out of the library of ... Docter Ponteous ... With six ... receipts for all sorts of cattle whatsoever ... London, L. White, 1676.

8 p.   19 cm.   **[9158]**

Imperfect: margins trimmed.

PONZE SANCTA CRUZ, Antonius. *See* PONCE DE SANTA CRUZ, Antonio [*d. ca.* 1650]

The POORE-MANS plaster-box. 1634. *See* [HAWES, R.]

POORT, Henricus van, *tr. See* HIPPOCRATES. [Adaptations, etc. Latin] Aphorismi. 1657.

POPP, Johannes. *See* POPPE, Johann [*b.* 1577]

POPPE, Johann [*b.* 1577] Chymische Medicin, von dem Nutz und Gebrauch der distillierten Oelen,

Extracten, Quintis essentiis ... zu allerley ... Artzneyen ... zu gebrauchen: sampt der Praeparation und chymischen Zubereitung ... beschrieben ... Franckfurt am Mayn, In Verlegung Daniel und David Aubrii und Clemens Schleichen, 1625.

[14], 523, [5] p.   16 cm.   [9159]

—De pestilitate; das ist, Von dem Ursprung der Pestilentz und derselben eygentlichen Cur ... Franckfurt am Mayn, Bey Daniel und David Aubrii und Clement Schleichen, 1625.

202 p.   16 cm.   [9160]

—Kurtzes Handbüchlein und Experiment. Vieler Artzeneyen, von allerhandt Thieren, Gewürmen, von Vögeln und von Fischen. Auch von Gewächsen, Steinen, Mineralien ... worzu dieselbigen Nutz, und in der Artzney zugebrauchen sindt ... Franckfurt am Mayn, In Verlegung Daniel und David Aubrii und Clemens Schleichen, 1625.

221, [9] p.   16 cm.   [9161]

—Thesaurus medicinae; oder, Chymischer Artzney Schatz ... Alles auss eigener erfahrner Heimligkeit, oder auss andern bewehrten Autoribus, fürnemlich auss Theophrasto, zusammen gelesen ... Leipzig, In Vorlegung Zachariae Schürers und Matthiae Götzen, 1628.

[16], 812 p.   port.   20 cm.   [9162]

—Von der gifftigen epidemischen Hauptkranckheit, oder pestilentzischem Gallenfieber; sampt andern Kranckheiten und Zufällen, so aus dem Haupt entspringen, als da ist der Schlag, hinfallende Sucht ... und dergleichen: beneben deroselben Curation und Heilung &c. dessen Fundamenta ... aus dem Paracelso, Arnoldo de Villa Nova, und andern bewärten Philosophis zusammen getragen ... [Leipzig] In Verlegung Thomae Schürers s. Erben, Gedruckt bey Friederich Lanckisch, 1623.

[16], 127 p.   16 cm.   [9163]
With this is bound *his* Von der Wassersucht. 1623.

—Von der Wassersucht und dero Zufällen. Item von der Steinkranckheit, des Sandes, Griesses, Lenden und Blasensteines, auch aller derer Steinkranckheiten, so unter die tartarischen Flüsse gerechnet werden. Wie man diese Kranckheiten erkennen, curiren, und all Medicamenta, so von Autore selbsten probiret ... darzu praepariren soll. Aus dem Paracelso, und andern fürnemen Autoribus

zusammen getragen ... Leipzig, In Verlegung Thomae Schürers s. Erben, 1623.

[166] p.   16 cm.   [9164]
Bound with *his* Von der gifftigen epidemischen Hauptkranckheit. 1623.

—*See* AGRICOLA, J. Deutlich- und wolgegründeter Anmerckungen über die chymische Artzneyen. 1686.

POPPIUS, HAMERUS. Basilica antimonii, in qua antimonii natura exponitur et ... remediorum formulae, quae pyrotechnica arte ex eo elaborantur, quam accurate traduntur ... Francofurti, Apud Antonium Hummium, 1618.

50 p.   21 cm.   [9165]

—[The same.] *In* Hartmann, J. Praxis chymiatrica. 1639, 1682.

POPPO, JOHANN GABRIEL [*fl.* 1689] *respondent. See* SCHAMMEL, J. M., *praeses.* Disputationem physicam de aquae marinae salsugine ... proponunt ... J. G. P. 1689.

PORCHON, ANT. Nouveau traitté du pourpre, de la rougeole et petite verole, de leur nature & de leurs remedes. Avec un traitté de la douleur nephretique, de la pierre des reins, & de la vessie, des remedes qui soulagent, qui s'opposent à sa formation, & qui contribuënt le plus à sa guerison. Paris, Maurice Villery [De l'imprimerie de Charles Coignard] 1688.

[12], 287 p.   15 cm.   [9166]
Dedicatory letter signed A. Porchon.

—Les regles de la santé; ou, Le veritable regime de vivre, que l'on doit observer, dans la santé, & dans les maladies. Avec une table alphabetique de tous les alimens, tirez des plantes & des animaux, dont l'usage est ordinaire. Par A[nt.] P[orchon] docteur en medecine ... Lyon, Rolin Glaize, 1692.

[10], 166 p.   15 cm.   [9167]

PORCIUS, PUBLIUS, *pseud. See* PLACENTIUS, Johannes [1500?-1550?]

PORDAGE, SAMUEL [1633-1691?] *tr. See* WILLIS, T. Practice of physick. 1684 [and] The remaining medical works. 1681.

PORPHYRIUS. Περὶ ἀποχῆς ἐμψυχων βιβλία τεσ —σαρα ... De non necandis ad epulandum animantibus libri IIII. Ejusdem selectae brevesque sententiae ducentes ad intelligentiam rerum, quae mente noscuntur. E Graeco exemplari facta versione Latina, scholiis & praefationibus illustrata per F. de Fogerolles ... Lugduni, Sumptibus Claudii Morillon, 1620.

[72], 464, [8] p. 19 cm. **[9168]**

Text in Greek and Latin, in parallel columns.

PORRAL, CLAUDE [*fl.* 1578–1579] *ed. See* ARANZI, G. C. In librum Hippocratis De vulneribus capitis commentarius. 1639.

PORT, FRANÇOIS DU. *See* DUPORT, François [1548–1624]

PORT, HENRICUS VAN. *See* POORT, Henricus van.

PORTA, CASPAR. Medicina brevis, exhibens hominis machinam, ejusque morbum, morbique curationem paucis iisque selectis & rite paratis medicaminibus instituendam ad mentem neotericorum. Lugduni Batavorum, Typis Frederici Haaring, 1688.

96, [8] p. plates. 17 cm. **[9169]**

PORTA, GIOVANNI BATTISTA DELLA [1535?–1615] Ars reminiscendi ... Neapoli, Apud Joan. Baptistam Subtilem, 1602.

[4], 42 p. illus. 18 cm. **[9170]**

—Coelestis physiognomoniae libri sex ... Unde quis facile ex humani vultus extima inspectione, poterit ex conjectura futura praesagire. In quibus etiam astrologia refellitur, & inanis, & imaginaria demonstratur. Neapoli, Ex typographia Jo. Baptistae Subtilis, 1603.

[8], 191 (i.e. 187) p. illus. 26 cm. **[9171]**

—[The same.] Physiognomoniae coelestis libri sex. Rothomagi, Sumptibus Joannis Berthelin, 1650.

[12], 154 p. 20 cm. **[9172]**

With this is bound *his* De humana physiognomonia. 1650.

—[Italian tr.] Della celeste fisonomia ... libri sei. Nei quali ributtata la vanità dell'astrologia giudiciaria, si dà maniera di essattamente conoscere per via delle cause naturali tutto quello, che l'aspetto, la presenza, & le fattezze de gl'huomini possono fisicamente significare, e promettere ... Padova, Pietro Paolo Tozzi, 1616.

[12], 144, [3] p. illus., port. 23 cm. **[9173]**

Bound with *his* Della fisonomia dell'huomo. 1615.

—[The same.] ... Opera nuova ... Padova, Pietro Paolo Tozzi, 1622.

[12], 147 p. illus., port. 23 cm. (Part [4] *in* Fisonomia naturale di Gio: Battista dalla Porta, Giovanni Ingegnieri [e] Polemone. 1622) **[9174]**

—[The same.] ... Padova, Pietro Paolo Tozzi, 1627.

[12], 147 p. illus., port. 21 cm. **[9175]**

Different setting of type.
Bound with (as issued) *his* Della fisonomia dell'huomo. 1627.

[—De chirophysionomia. Italian.] Della chirofisonomia; overo, Di quello parte della humana fisonomia, che si appartiene alla mano, libri due ... tradotti da un manoscritto latino dal signor Pompeo Sarnelli ... Contro i chiromanti impostori, che con vane osservationi havevano sporcato questa scienza, la quale si mostra fondata sopra naturali congetture. Nap[oli] Antonio Bulifon, 1677.

[25], 167, [13] p. plate. 15 cm. **[9176]**

Inserted after the printed title page is an engraved title page with title: Chirofisonomia.
The Latin original was apparently never published.
"Vita di Gio: Battista della Porta Napolitano scritta da Pompeo Sarnelli": p. [13–25]

—De distillatione lib. IX. Quibus certa methodo, multiplicique artificio, penitioribus naturae arcanis detectis, cujuslibet mixti in propria elementa resolutio, perfecte docetur. Romae, Ex typographia Rev. Camerae Apostolicae, 1608.

[20], 154, [6] p. illus., port. 22 cm. **[9177]**

—[The same.] ... Nunc primum in Germania typis evulgati ... Argentorati, Sumptibus Lazari Zetzneri, 1609.

[16], 149, [10] p. port., illus. 20 cm. **[9178]**

—[German tr.] Ars destillatoria; das ist, Die edele und in aller Welt geliebte Kunst zu destilliern. Welche nicht allein einen newen und zuvor unbekannten Methodum und Weg allerley Kräuter, Wurtzeln, Blumen, Samen, Metall, Edelgestein und dergleichen ... zu destilliern ... in sich begreifft: sondern auch alle Heimlichkeiten der Natur zuerkündigen, und alle vermischte Sachen in ihre ... Elementen zu resolviren, verständtlich und in einer feinen Kürtze unterweist ... In lateinischer Sprach ... beschrieben: folgents in unsere hochteutsche Sprach ubersetzt ... Franckfurt am Mayn, Getruckt bey Johann Bringern, 1611.

[12], 174, [7] p. illus. 21 cm. **[9179]**

Translated by Peter Uffenbach.

—De furtivis literarum notis vulgo De ziferis libri quinque. Altero libro superaucti, & quamplurimis in locis locupletati ... Neapoli, Apud Joannem Baptistam Subtilem, 1602.

[12], 314 (i.e. 226) +, [2] p.   illus.   30 cm.

[9180]

Signatures: a⁶, A-2F⁴.
Imperfect: all pages between p. 314 and last leaf wanting.

—De humana physiognomonia ... libri IV. Qui ab extimis, quae in hominum corporibus conspiciuntur signis, ita eorum naturas, mores & consilia (egregiis ad vivum expressis iconibus) demonstrant, ut intimos animi recessus penetrare videantur ... Nunc ab innumeris mendis, quibus passim Neapolitana scatebat editio, emendati, primumque in Germania in lucem editi ... Ursellis, Typis Cornelii Sutorii, sumptibus Jonae Rosae fr., 1601.

[16], 534, [57] p.   illus., plates.   19 cm.   **[9181]**

For the most part, contents are identical, page for page, with those of the edition published in Hanau in 1593. The corrigenda of the earlier edition are corrected.

—[The same.] ... Ed. postrema ·iori correctior ... Francofurti, Apud Nicolaum Hoffmannum, impensis haeredum Jacobi Fischeri, 1618.

[12], 402, [42] p.   illus.   20 cm.   **[9182]**

—[The same.] ... Ed. postrema priori correctior ... Rothomagi, Sumptibus Joannis Berthelin, 1650.

[12], 403, [41] p.   illus.   20 cm.   **[9183]**

Different setting of type.
Bound with *his* Physiognomoniae coelestis libri sex. 1650.

—[French tr.] La physionomie humaine ... Divisée en quatre livres. Enrichie de quantité de figures tirées au naturel, ou par les signes exterieurs du corps, on voit si clairement la complexion, les moeurs, & les desseins des hommes, qu'on semble penetrer jusques au plus profond de leurs ames. Oeuvre d'une singuliere erudition ... Nouvellement traduite du latin en françois par le sieur Rault ... 2. ed. Rouen, Jean & David Berthelin, 1660.

[16], 572 (i.e. 570), [32] p.   illus.   18 cm.

[9184]

Leaves paged 165-166, 235-236, and 281-282 are cancels; fragments of the original leaves (used in the binding) are inserted in pocket.

—[Italian tr.] Della fisonomia dell' huomo ... libri sei. Tradotti di latino in volgare, e dall'istesso auttore accresciuti di figure, & di passi necessarii à diverse parti dell'opera: et hora in quest'ultima editione migliorati in più di mille luoghi, che nella stampa di Napoli si leggevano scorettissimi, & aggiontavi la Fisonomia naturale di monsignor Giovanni Ingegneri. Vicenza, Pietro Paolo Tozzi, 1615.

[8], 219 (i.e. 217), [5] ll.; 60, [4] p.   illus., ports.   23 cm.   **[9185]**

The Fisionomia by Ingegneri has special title page and separate paging.
With this is bound *his* Della celeste fisonomia. 1616.

—[The same.] ... 3. ed. ... Padova, Pietro Paolo Tozzi, 1622.

[8], 222 ll.; 64 p., illus., ports.   23 cm. (Part [1-2] *In* Fisonomia naturale di Gio: Battista dalla Porta, Giovanni Ingegneri [e] Polemone. 1622)   **[9186]**

Ingegneri's Fisionomia naturale has special title page, dated 1623, and separate paging.
Reprint of the same publisher's edition issued in Vicenza in 1615, with a new dedication by the publisher, dated 1622.

—[The same.] ... 4. ed. Padova, Pietro Paolo Tozzi, 1627.

[8], 222 ll.; 64 p.   illus., ports.   21 cm.   **[9187]**

Imperfect: leaves 113 and 120 wanting.
Ingegneri's Fisionomia naturale has special title page dated 1626.
Reprint of the "terza editione," 1622 with the old dedication slightly changed and redated 1 Jan. 1627.
With this are bound (as issued): Polemo, A. Fisonomia. 1626; Porta, Giovanni Battista della. Della celeste fisonomia. 1627.

—Della fisonomia di tutto il corpo humano del s. Gio. Battista della Porta ... libri quattro, ne' quali si tratta di quanto intorno a questa materia n' hanno Greci, Latini, e gli Arabi scritto. Hora brevemente in tavole sinottiche ridotta et ordinata da Francesco Stelluti ... Roma, Vitale Mascardi, 1637.

[8], 155, [3] p.   24 cm.   **[9188]**

Engraved title page.

—Della fisonomia dell'huomo ... libri sei. Tradotti dal Latino, e dallo stesso authore accresciuti di figure, e di passi necessarii à diverse parti dell'opera. Aggiontavi la Fisonomia naturale di monsignor Giovanni Ingegnieri, Polemone, e la Celeste [fisonomia] dello stesso Porta. In questa quinta, & ultima impressione migliorati in più di due mila luoghi ... et aggiontovi il Discorso di Livio Agrippa sopra la natura, e complessione humana et il Discorso de' nei di Lodovico Settali ... Venetia, Christoforo Tomasini, 1644.

[12], 570 (i.e. 568), [4] p.   illus., ports.   23 cm.   **[9189]**

Items have half titles.
The work here attributed to Antonius Polemo is the forgery of the Byzantine period. The Italian version was translated by conte

Francesco Montecuccoli from the Latin version made by his brother, conte Carlo Montecuccoli, from the original Greek.

De i nei is a translation by G. A. Biffi of Settala's De naevis, which was published in Milan in 1606 and 1628.

—[The same.] La fisonomia dell'huomo, et la Celeste [fisonomia] . . . libri sei. Tradotti di Latino in volgare, & hora in questa settima, & ultima impressione ricorretta, & postovi le figure à propri suoi luoghi. Con la Fisonomia naturale di monsignor Giovanni Ingegnieri, di Polemone, di Adamantio, & il Discorso di Livio Agrippa sopra la natura, & complessione, humana, con il Trattato di nei di Lodovico Settali . . . Aggiontovi da nuovo la Metoposcopia di Ciro Spontone. Venetia, Nicolò Pezzana, 1668.

[8], 591 (i.e. 579) p. illus., port. 23 cm.
[9190]
Items have half titles.
The work of Adamantius is not present.

Differs from the 5th edition (Venice, 1644) in the omission of the publisher's dedication and that of Porta to Cardinal d'Este, and in the addition of the tract by Spontone, followed by a group (p. 578–591) of 5 anonymous works: Discorso sopra il nascimento dell'huomo, e della donna. Fisonomia dell'huomo, e della donna, scielta da piu gravi auttori. Modo per saper conoscere quant'anni può vivere la persona. Delli nei dalla faccia. Dell'indole, che per l'aspetto, presenza e fattezza de gli huomini, si puo giudicare gli eventi loro.

—Magiae naturalis libri viginti. Ab ipso quidem authore adaucti, nunc vero ab infinitis, quibus editio illa scatebat mendis, optime repurgati: in quibus scientiarum naturalium divitiae & deliciae demonstrantur . . . Rothomagi, Sumptibus Joannis Berthelin, 1650.

[14], 662 p. illus. 19 cm.
[9191]

—[The same.] . . . Amstelodami, Apud Elizeum Weyerstraten, 1664.

[16], 670, [22] p. illus. 14 cm.
[9192]
Added engraved title page.

—Magiae naturalis libri IV. *In* Longinus, C. ed. Trinum magicum. 1616, 1673.

—[English tr.] Natural magick . . . In twenty books . . . Wherein are set forth all the riches and delights. Of the natural sciences. London, Printed for John Wright, 1669.

[6], 409, [6] p. illus. 28 cm.
[9193]
Signatures: []¹, C², D–3I⁴.

—[French tr.] La magie naturelle divisée en quatre livres . . . Contenant les secrets & miracles de nature,

et nouvellement, l'Introduction à la belle magie. Par Lazare Meysonnier . . . Lyon, Simon Potin, 1678.

[12], 406 (i.e. 396), 25, 2–6, [18] p. 15 cm.
[9194]

Meyssonier's L'introduction à la belle magie (25 p., with special title page bearing imprint, Lyon, Claude Langlois, 1678, and special dedication) was originally prepared as an introduction to a new edition of the French version of Porta's Magia naturalis.

"Divers secrets mis en lumiere par Toussaint Bourgeois": p. 391–406.

"Plusieurs beaux secrets, mis en lumiere par E[stienne] Telam": p. 2–6 at end.

—[German tr.] Magia naturalis; oder, Haus-Kunst- und Wunder-Buch. Zu erst . . . lateinisch beschrieben . . . nunmehr aber . . . durch alle zwantzig Bücher gantz aufs neu in die hochteutsche Sprache übersetzet; von allen Fehlern . . . gereiniget; in gewisse mit Zahlen unterschiedene Absätze abgetheilet; mit deutlichen teutschen Kunst-Reimen gezieret; an Figuren gebessert, mit shönen Kupfern geschmücket; mit nothwendigen Anmerckungen und Auflösungen der darinn enthaltenen Rätzel, wie auch vielen neuen ungemeinen guten chymischen und andern Stücken vermehret . . . und in zweyen Theilen, deren das erste, die ersten sieben; das andre die letzten dreyzehen Bücher in sich enthält, heraus gegeben durch Christian Peganium [pseud.] sonst Rautner [pseud.] [i.e. Christian Knorr von Rosenroth] genannt. Nürnberg, In Verlegung Johann Ziegers [etc., etc.] 1680.

2 v. illus., port. plates. 17 cm. **[9195]**
Vol. 2 wanting.
Vol. 1 has added engraved title page, with author's portrait.
"Chymische Zugabe": p. [77–114] at end of v. 1.

—Phytognomonica . . . octo libris contenta; in quibus nova, facillimaque affertur methodus, qua plantarum, animalium, metallorum; rerum denique omnium ex prima extimae faciei inspectione quivis abditas vires assequatur. Accedunt ad haec confirmanda infinita propemodum selectiora secreta . . . Nunc primum ab innumeris mendis, quibus passim Neapolitana editio scatebat, vindicata; cum . . . indice locupletissimo. Francofurti, Apud Nicolaum Hoffmannum, impensis Jonae Rhodii, 1608.

[16], 539 p. illus. 20 cm. **[9196]**
Pasted to front flyleaf is an engraved portrait (from another book) with legend: Joan. Baptista Imperialis.

Except for the index, a page for page reprint of the edition published in Frankfurt in 1591.

—[The same.] . . . Rothomagi, Sumptibus Joannis Berthelin, 1650.

[16], 605 (i.e. 603) p. illus. 19 cm. **[9197]**

—Pneumaticorum libri tres. Quibus accesserunt Curvilineorum elementorum libri duo. Neapoli, Apud Jo. Jacobum Carlinum, 1601.

2 v. illus. 19 cm. **[9198]**

Vol. [2], "Curvilineorum elementorum libri duo" wanting. Imperfect: p. 55-69 of vol. 1 mutilated.

—[Italian tr.] I tre libri de' spiritali . . . cioè, D'inalzar acque per forza dell'aria. Napoli, Gio. Jacomo Carlino, 1606.

98, [1] p. illus. 21 cm. **[9199]**

Translated by Juan Escrivano, with additions received orally from the author.

—Vita. *In his* Della chirofisonomia. 1677.

—*See* SALA, A. Processus . . . de auro potabili. 1630.

PORTA, ULRICH. *See* GABELKOVER, O. Kurtzer Bericht: der fürstlichen Württembergischen Hoff Medicorum. 1608, 1626.

PORTAIL, CLAUDE, *See* PORTAL, Paul [1630-1703]

PORTAL, PAUL [1630-1703] La pratique des accouchemens soutenue d'un grand nombre d'observations . . . Paris, De l'imprimerie de Gabriel Martin, et se vend chez l'auteur, 1685.

[21], 368 p. front. (port.), plates. 20 cm. **[9200]**

—[The same.] *In* La bibliotheque des accoucheurs et des sages-femmes. 1693.

—[Dutch tr.] De practyk der vroed' meesters, en vroed' vrouwen; of, De wyse van een vrouw' te helpen in haar kinderbaren. Bekragtigt met een groot getal aanmerkingen . . . Uyt de Franse in de Nederduytse tale overgeset . . . Amsterdam, Timotheus ten Hoorn, 1690.

[23], 342, [7] p. front. (port.), plates. 20 cm. **[9201]**

Translation by Pieter Adriaansz, Gomer van Bortel, and Pieter Guenellon.

PORTATILE medicum; seu, Regularum pharmaceuticarum atque chymicarum centuria in usum non solum studiosorum medicinae, sed & pharmacopaeorum collecta atque in hunc ordinem con-gesta cui in fine modus, B. Michaelis &c. Pharmacopolia visitandi, adjunctus est, apprime utilis iis potissimum, quibus onus hoc imponitur, a J. H. D. M. L. [n. p.] 1680.

48 p. 14 cm. **[9202]**

"Regulae circa modum pharmacopolia visitandi observandae a B. J. Michaele . . . Auditoribus suis olim dictatae": p. [33]-43, has half title.

PORTIGLIOTTO, CARLO GIUSEPPE. *See* GERENZANO PORTIGLIOTTO, Carlo Giuseppe [1644-1722]

PORTIUS, AEMILIUS. *See* PORTUS, Aemilius [1550-1614 *or* 15]

PORTIUS, JOHANN DAVID. *See* PORZ, Johann David [*fl.* 1672-1679]

PORTIUS, LUCAS ANTONIUS. *See* PORZIO, Luca Antonio [1637-1715]

PORTU AQUITANO, BERNARDUS GEORGIUS a. *See* PENOT, Bernard Georges [*d.* 1617?]

PORTUGAL, Sovereign [1598-1621] (Philip II). Regimento dos medicos a boticarios . . . Eu el Rey . . . ordenou que . . . ouvesse sempre na Universidade de Coimbra trinta estudantes Christãos velhos . . . que estudassem medicina, & cirurgia . . . [Lisbon, 1604]

10, [5] p. 31 cm. **[9203]**

Caption title.
Signed by Fernao Marecos Botelho and Antonio de Mendoza P.

PORTUGAL. Sovereign [1621-1640] (Philip III). Manda el Rey . . . que se lancem logo pregões pellos lugares costumados nesta cidade, nas quaes se declare, que alem do que le tem declarado, & publicado nos que estão publicados . . . Lisboa, 1630.

broadside. 28 x 20 cm. **[9204]**

PORTUS, AEMILIUS [1550-1614 or 15] *See* HIPPOCRATES. [Collected works. Greek and Latin] Tὰ εὑρισκόμενα. 1621, 1624,1657, 1662.

PORTUS, FRANCISCUS. *See* DUPORT, François [1548-1624]

PORTZ, PIETER DE [*fl.* 1698] *respondent.* Dissertatio medica inauguralis de fermentatione & effervescentia in corpore humano . . . Lugduni Batavorum, Apud Abrahamum Elzevier, 1698.

[22] p. 24 cm. **[9205]**

Diss.—Leyden.

PORTZIUS, Johann David. *See* Porz, Johann David [*fl.* 1672-1679]

PORZ, Johann David [*fl.* 1672-1679] Demonstratio brevis medico chyrurgica de tumoribus et in specie de παιδαρθροκακη. Vel tumore spina ventosa dicto ex acido & alcali tanquam principiatis novis eruta, causis ex illis inventis, ut & modo agendi deprompta ac experientia multiplici anatomica comprobata ... Adjunctam epistolam apologeticam ad ... Barnerum in fine opusculi hujus conspicient L. B. Leovardiae, Apud Heronem Nautam, 1679.

[12], 132 p. 14 cm. [9206]

Imperfect: p. [7-8] torn, affecting text.
Letter signed Johannes Germanus.

PORZIO, Luca Antonio [1637-1715] De militis in castris sanitate tuenda. Oder, Von dess Soldaten im Läger Gesundheit Behaltung ... Viennae Austriae, Typis apud haeredes Viviani, 1685.

[12], 373, [3] p. plate. 14 cm. [9207]

Text in Latin.

—Del sorgimento de' licori nelle fistole aperte d'ambidue gli estremi, et intorno à molti corpi, che tocchino la loro soperficie ... Vinezia, 1667.

[4], 108 p. plates. 20 cm. [9208]

—Dissertationes variae. Venetiis, Sumptibus Combi, & Lanovii, 1684.

[8], 152, [1] p. 17 cm. [9209]

Contents. — De difficultate medicinae. — De aere artificiali flammae & animalibus mortifero. — De rarefactionum natura. — An frigidi sit condensare, & calidi rarefacere.

—Erasistratus; sive, De sanguinis missione ... Venetiis, Apud Nicolaum Pezzana, 1683.

[16], 398, [17] p. 15 cm. [9210]

"Apologia Galeni qua praecipue sit manifestum secundum Galeni regulas rare venas esse secandas": p. 328-398.
Contains quotations from the works of Erasistratus, Galenus, Jean Baptiste van Helmont, and Thomas Willis.

—In Hippocratis librum De veteri medicina ... paraphrasis. Extant alia ... Romae, Typis Angeli Bernabò, 1681.

[6], 205, [16] p. plate. 15 cm. [9211]

The first work is "une traduction trés libre où l'auteur a introduit quelques développements." Cf. Littré.
Contents. — In Hippocratis De veteri medicina [i.e. De prisca medicina] paraphrasis. — Fons Jovis, fons Solis, Padi fons, aliique similes. — Epistola de incremento, sive generatione metallorum. — Dissertatio logica. — Epistola Urbani Davisii de fontium atque fluminum origine.

—*See* Aquenza y Mossa, P. De sanguinis missione. 1696.

POSNER, Caspar [1626-1700] Γενεανθρωπολόγια; sive, Generationis humanae operum naturalium maxumi secundum varias veterum, recentiorum atque novissimorum opiniones ac observationes descriptio succinctis tabulis in usum lectionum academicarum adornata ... Jenae, Sumtibus Tobiae Oehrlingii, typis Johannis Jacobi Bauhoferi, 1692.

[37] ll. 44 cm. [9212]

Dissertations — Jena

—*praeses.* De causarum generibus, inquantum sub physicam cadunt ... Jenae, Prelo Nisiano, 1656.

[28] p. 20 cm. [9213]

W. H. Amthor, *respondent.*

—De manna ... Jenae, Literis Johannis Nisii [1677]

[16] p. 18 cm. [9214]

P. Fritsch, *respondent.*

—Diatribe academica de longaevitate hominum ... Jenae, Stanno Nisiano, 1673.

[56] p. 20 cm. [9215]

J. H. Vultejus, *respondent.*

—Diatribe physica de virunculis metallicis ... Jenae, Literis Krebsianis, 1662.

[32] p. 20 cm. [9216]

M. Dachselt, *respondent.*

—Disputatio physica de ignibus lambentibus ... Jenae, Literis Jochann Zach. Nisii [1686]

[32] p. 19 cm. [9217]

J. C. Vulpius, *respondent.*

—Disputatio physica de morte ... Jenae, Prelo Nisiano, 1659.

[40] p. 18 cm. [9218]

T. Rollius, *respondent.*

—Disputatio physica de ordine partium in compositione ac formatione corporis animalium ... Jenae, Prelo Joannis Nisii, 1668.

[118] p. 20 cm. [9219]

C. Richter, *respondent.*

—Disputatio physica de principatu partium ... Jenae, Prelo Nisiano, 1663.

[52] p. 18 cm. [9220]

H. Köhn, *respondent.*

—Disputatio physica de principiis generationis atque nativitatis humanae ... Jenae, Prelo Jo. Nisii, 1672.

[108] p.   18 cm.   [**9221**]

J. F. Gieseler, *respondent.*

—Disputatio physiologica de respiratione ... Jenae, Literis Johannis Jacobi Bauhoferi, 1671.

[32] p.   20 cm.   [**9222**]

J. Möbius, *respondent.*

—Dissertatio academica de somniis vigilantium ... Jenae, Literis Bauhoferianis [1670]

[24] p.   18 cm.   [**9223**]

C. Hermann, *reespondent.*

—Dissertatio physica de animae adcessu in generatione hominis quando hic fiat cumprimis secundum sententiam Aristotelis ... [Jenae] Stanno Joann. Zachariae Nisii [1688]

[64] p.   20 cm.   [**9224**]

G. E. Ising, *respondent.*

—Dissertatio physica de calido innato viventium, cumprimis vero animalium perfectiorum ... Jenae, Charactere Samuelis Krebsii, 1663.

[72] p.   19 cm.   [**9225**]

J. G. Elsner, *respondent.*

—Dissertatio physica de foetuum in uteris vita ... Jenae, Prelo Johannis Nisii [1676]

[84] p.   20 cm.   [**9226**]

J. N. Otto, *respondent.*

—Dissertatio physica de igne ... Jenae, Typis Johannis Jacobi Krebsii [1696]

16 p.   19 cm.   [**9227**]

J. A. Wedel, *respondent.*

—Dissertatio physica de viventibus mobilibus a seipsis secundum sententiam Aristotelis aliorumque veterum & contra modernam scholam Cartesianam ... Jenae, Typis Pauli Ehrichii, 1697.

32 p.   20 cm.   [**9228**]

N. Zurner, *respondent.*

—, *respondent.* See Rolfinck, W., *praeses.* Methodi cognoscendi et curandi adfectus particulares capitis. 1652, 1653.

P[OST] S[criptum] of, na-courier, van de Tweede missive aen Dr. Balthasar Bekker ... zoo voor als tegen sijn E. uytgegeven: ook met een om voor te komen alle verkeerde bevattingen, die Ericus Walten in sijn Brief aen den grave van Portland, tracht in te boesemen. 's Gravenhage, Meyndert Uytwerf, 1692.

16 p.   20 cm.   [**9229**]

Linde 175.

POST, Johann. *See* Posthius, Johannes [1537-1597]

POSTEL, Guillaume. *See* Potel, Guillaume [*fl.* 1596-1623]

POSTEL, Johann [*fl.* 1682] *respondent. See* Seligmann, G. F., *praeses.* Sciagraphiam virium imaginationis ... publice exhibebit J. P. 1682.

POSTEL, Nicolas [*fl.* 1675-1685] Factum pour maistre Nicolas Postel ... contre ... Mathieu Mahuelt, Jean-Baptiste Calart, & Pierre du Mezerey ... intimés. Ou dissertation sur les peripneumonies d'hyver, pour servir d'apologie à la these composée par ledit sieur Postel. Contre la censure des intimés, & du sieur Puylon ... [Cadomi?] 1685.

[45], 222 p.   15 cm.   [**9230**]

Imperfect: p. 219-222 torn, affecting text.
"Quaestio medica ... in Scholis Medicorum ... Cadomensis Academiae ... praeside ... Nicolao Postel ... proponebat Ludovicus Barasin ... 17. Martii ... M.DC.LXXXV": p.[18-28]
Includes French translation of Quaestio medica.

—Oratio ... cum enarrationem libri Galeni De inaequali intemperie solenniter auspicaretur ... [Cadomi? 1675?]

46 p.   23 cm.   [**9231**]

Caption title.

—*praeses.* Quaestio medica ... in Scholis Medicorum ... Cadom. Academiae ... praeside M. Nicolao Postel [proponebat Ludovicus Barasin ... 10 Martii ... M.DC.LXXXV] ... Cadomi, Apud Joannem Cavelier, 1685.

7 p.   22 cm.   [**9232**]

Diss.—Caen (L. Barasin, *respondent*)

POSTH, Erasme [1582-1618] *respondent.* Theses medicae de podagra ... Basileae, Typis Joan. Jacobi Genathii, 1613.

[11] p.   20 cm.   [**9233**]

Diss.—Basel.

POSTHIUS, Johannes [1537-1597] *tr. See* Israeli, I. Thesaurus sanitatis. 1607.

POTAGES. [Pour les pauvres gens] *See* Assemblée charitable à Paris.

POTEL, Guillaume [*fl.* 1596-1623] Traicté de la peste advenue en ceste ville de Paris, l'an mil 1596, 1606, 1619. Et 1623, avec les remedes . . . Paris, Nicolas Callemont, 1624.

[12], 55 p.; 128 p. 16 cm. **[9234]**

Imperfect: sig. Al (part 1) wanting; all pages before p. 11 (part 2) wanting.

Part 2 has special title page: Discours des malades epidemiques, dated 1623.

POTERIE, Pierre de la. *See* Potier, Pierre [*fl.* 1609-1643]

POTERIUS, Petrus. *See* Potier, Pierre [*fl.* 1609-1643]

POTIER, Pierre [*fl.* 1609-1643] Libri duo de febribus, Insig. curat. & sing. obser. centuriae tres, & Pharmacopoea spagirica. Bononiae, Typis Jacobi Montii, 1643.

1 v. port. 24 cm. **[9235]**

Various pagings.

Engraved title page.

Half title: Petri Poterii Opera.

—Opera omnia medica, et chymica. Lugduni, Sumpt. Joan. Antonii Huguetan, 1645.

[12], 792, [44] p. 19 cm. **[9236]**

—[The same.] . . . Adjecta est doctissima dissertatio Petri Guissonii . . . de tribus principiis chemicis et nova recentiorum medendi methodo. Francofurti, Apud Wilh. Richardum Stockium, 1666.

[12], 24 p.; 752, 32 p. 19 cm. **[9237]**

"Petri Guissonii . . . Epistolica dissertatio de anonymo libello (circa abbreviatum verae medicinae genus) ubi potissimum eventilatur principiorum chymicorum hypothesis" (24 p.) has special title page.

—[The same.] . . . Cum annotationibus et additamentis utilissimis pariter ac curiosis Friderici Hoffmanni filii . . . Accessit nova doctrina de febribus, ex principiis mechanicis solidè deducta . . . Francofurti ad Moenum, Impensis Friderici Knochii, 1698.

[14], 882, [26] p. port. 22 cm. **[9238]**

—Insignes curationes, et singulares observationes centum. In quibus varia morborum genera, eorum egregia propriaque remedia therapeuticaque ratio explicantur. Coloniae Agrippinae, Apud Matthaeum Schmitz, 1616.

158, [7] p. 13 cm. **[9239]**

Imperfect: title page mutilated.

—[The same.] Insignium curationum, & singularium observationum centuria prima [et secunda] In quibus varia morborum genera, eorum egregia propriaque remedia therapeuticaque ratio explicantur . . . Bononiae, Typis Nicolai Tebaldini, sumptibus Marci Antonii Berniae, 1622.

2 v. 19 cm. **[9240]**

Vol. 1 only.

—[The same.] Insignes curationes, et singulares observationes centum. In quibus varia morborum genera, eorumque propria & appositissima remedia therapeuticaque ratio explicantur. Accesserunt Henrici Cornelii Agrippae . . . Contra pestem antidoton haud vulgare. Itemque Consilium contra diarrhoeam . . . Coloniae Agrippinae, Matthaeus Smitz, 1625.

2 v. in 1. 14 cm. **[9241]**

Vol. 2 has title: Insignium curationum et singularium observationum centuria secunda.

—Pharmacopoea spagirica . . . Bonon. [Typis Nicolai Tebaldini?] 1622.

[31], 280 p. 19 cm. **[9242]**

Engraved title page.

—Pharmacopoea spagirica, tertia parte aucta . . . 3. ed. Bononiae, Ex typographia Jacobi de Monte & Caroli Zeneri, 1635.

[19], 387 (i.e. 427), [29] p. illus., port. 23 cm. **[9243]**

—*See* Dispensatorium chymicum. 1626; Ettner, J. C. von. Manes Poteriani, i.d. Petri Poterii . . . Inventa chymica. 169-?, 1700.

POTINIUS, Conrad [*d.* 1640] Prognosticum divinum; das ist, Ein göttlich Prognosticum darinnen Gott viel Wunders ankündiget. 1. In einem Wunderkinde. 2. Noch in einer Wundergebuhrt. 3. Als auch in sieben Wundergesichten . . . Bremen, Georg Martens, 1629.

[16], 67 (i.e. 63) p. illus. 19 cm. **[9244]**

La **POUDRE** de sympathie. 1658. *See* Belin, J. A.

[**POULAIN DE LA BARRE**, François, 1647-1723] De l'egalité des deux sexes, discours physique et moral, où l'on voit l'importance de se défaire des préjugez. Paris, Jean Du Puis, 1676.

[16], 221, [2] p. 14 cm. **[9245]**

The privilege is granted to "sieur P."

[—] De l'excellence des hommes, contre l'egalité des sexes. Paris, Jean du Puis, 1675.
>2 v. in 1.   14 cm.   **[9246]**

[—] Another printing.
>529 (i.e. 329), [5] p.   15 cm.   **[9247]**

POURRET, Petrus [*fl.* 1660] *See* Tardy, C. An morbi omnes a vitiato circulari motu sanguinis? 1660?

POUTSMA, Tammer [*fl.* 1666] *respondent.* Disputatio medica inauguralis de phthisi ... Lugduni Batavorum, Apud Philippum de Cro-Y, 1666.
>[12] p.   24 cm.   **[9248]**
>Diss. — Leyden.

POW-ELLUS, Petrus [*fl.* 1660] *respondent.* Disputatio medica inauguralis de pleuritide ... Lugduni Batavorum, Ex officina Francisci Hackii, 1660.
>[8] p.   21 cm.   **[9249]**
>Diss. — Leyden.

POWER, Henry [1623-1668] Experimental philosophy, in three books: containing new experiments microscopical, mercurial, magnetical. With some deductions, and probable hypotheses, raised from them, in avouchment and illustration of the now famous atomical hypothesis ... London, T. Roycroft, for John Martin and James Allestry. 1664.
>[23], 193, [1] p.   illus., plate.   21 cm.   **[9250]**
>Books [2] and [3] have special title pages, with imprint: London, 1663.
>"Subterraneous experiments; or, Observations about cole-mines" (p. [171]-181) has half title.
>Errata: p. [1] at end.

POWER, Thomas [*fl.* 1678-1699] *See* Ανθολογια; seu, Selecta quaedam poemata Italorum. 1684.

POYNEL, Thomas. *See* Paynell, Thomas [*fl.* 1528-1567] Pr., Doctor. *See* Primrose, James [1592-1659]

PRAAT, Jason de. *See* Pratensis, Jason [1486-1558]

A PRACTICAL and short discourse of stoving and bathing. *See* Cocke, T. Kitchin-physick. 1676.

The PRACTICE of lights. *See* Collectanea chymica. 1684.

PRADE, Jean Le Royer, sieur de [*fl.* 1640-1685] Discours du tabac, ou il est traité particulierement du tabac en poudre. Par le Sr Baillard [pseud.] Paris, Martin le Prest, 1668.
>[24], 125, [19] p.   illus.   17 cm.   **[9251]**

—[The same.] Histoire du tabac, ou il est traité particulierement du tabac en poudre ... Paris, Le Prest, 1677.
>[34], 172, [6] p.   port., plates.   16 cm.   **[9252]**

—[The same.] ... Avec des raisonnemens physiques sur les vertus & sur les effets de cette plante, & de ses divers usages dans la medecine. Par le sieur Baillard [pseud.] Paris, Jean Jombert, 1693.
>[24], 125, [19] p.   illus.   17 cm.   **[9253]**
>A reissue of the 1668 edition with new title page.

PRAESERVATIO corporum sanorum. *See* Castelli, P. Illustrissimis senatoribus ... Petrus Castellus Romanus foelicitatem. [1648]

PRAESERVATIVUM universale naturale. 1679. *See* Dobrzensky, J. J. W.

PRAETORIUS, Benjamin [*fl.* 1653-ca. 1664] *respondent. See* Mylius, J., *praeses.* Diatribe physica de dracone volante et igne fatuo. 1693.

PRAETORIUS, Daniel [*fl.* 1699-1701] *respondent. See* Wedel, G. W., *praeses.* Dissertatio medica de varice. 1699.

PRAETORIUS, Johann [1630-1680] Ludicrum chiromanticum Praetorii; seu, Thesaurus chiromantiae ... Lipsiae, Impensis Johannis Bartholom. Oehleri; Jenae, Litteris Caspari Freyschmidii, 1661.
>[3], 36, [11], 301-340 p.; [1], 1-156 p., 157-190 ll., 215-10026 (i.e. 1026) p.   illus., table.   21 cm.   **[9254]**
>Added engraved title page.
>Part [2] has special title page: ... Metoscopia; seu, Prosopomantia ...
>"Chiromantia Roberti Fludtii": ll. 157-190.

PRAETORIUS, Johann [*fl.* 1698] *respondent. See* Loescher, V. E., *praeses.* Antisthenes. 1698.

PRAETORIUS, Johann Friedrich [*fl.* 1693] *respondent. See* Albinus, B. Disputatio solennis medica de vomica pulmonum. 1693.

PRAETORIUS, Wesselus [*fl.* 1631] *respondent. See* Burgersdijck, F. P., *praeses.* Collegium physicum. 1642.

PRAEVOTIUS. *See* Prevost.

PRANGE, CHRISTIAN [*fl.* 1693] *respondent. See* HEBENSTREIT, J. P., *praeses.* De locustis. 1693.

PRAT, ABRAHAM DU. *See* DU PRAT, Abraham

PRAT, ELLIS. *See* BRUGIS, T. Vade mecum. 1681, 1689.

PRATENSIS, JASON [1486-1558] De arcenda sterilitate, et progignendis liberis, liber unus . . . Amstelaedami, Sumptibus Joannis Blaeu, 1657.

[12], 216 p. 13 cm. **[9255]**

—De pariente et partu liber . . . Amstelaedami, Typis Joannis Blaeu, 1657.

[4], 110, [2] p. 13 cm. **[9256]**

—De uteris libri duo . . . in quibus . . . naturalium rerum & historiarum supellectilem invenies. Amstelaedami, Sumptibus Joannis Blaeu, 1657.

[16], 297 p. 14 cm. **[9257]**

La PRATIQUE des estuves des bains de Digne. *See* LAUTARET, D. T. de. Les merveilles des bains naturels . . . de Digne en Provence. 1620.

PRATIS, JASON a. *See* PRATENSIS, Jason [1486-1558]

PRATO, FRANCESCO MARIA [*d. ca.* 1678] Nicander, doctoris Francisci Mariae Prati ad judicatum utriusque magnae curiae, proprio motu . . . comitis Castrilli, assumpti, sive Gestorum per ipsum in eo subeundo munere, ac in cadaverum humatione crassante peste in florentissima civitate Neapolis de anno 1656 . . . [Naples? 1659]

[113] p. 30 cm. **[9258]**

PRATT, E. *See* PRAT, Ellis.

PRAXIS chymiatrica rationalis. *See* CHEMIA RATIONALIS rationibus philosophicis. 1687.

PRĘCLARA res est, quae ex opere, quod quis didicit, proficiscitur oratio. 1688. *See* BORROMEO, A.

PREDIGER, GEORG KONRAD [*fl.* 1626] *respondent. See* CHARSTADIUS, V., *praeses.* Disputationum medicarum quinta de morbo. 1626 [and] Disputationum medicarum undecima de methodo medendi in specie. 1626.

PREEST, ROBERT. *See* PRIEST, Robert [*ca.* 1550-*ca.* 1590]

PREGITZER, JOHANN ULRICH [1611-1672] *praeses.* Exercitatio philosophica de affectibus appetitus

sensitivi . . . Tubingae, In officia Werliniana [1662]

16 p. 19 cm. **[9259]**

Diss.—Tübingen (J. J. List, *respondent*)

PREISS, CHRISTOPH ROMAN [*fl.* 1693] *respondent. See* HARDT, F. C., *praeses.* Porositatis omnibus in corporibus adsertio. 1693.

PRENKE, WILHELM [*fl.* 1651-1653] *respondent. See* MÖBIUS, G., *praeses.* Disputatio medica inauguralis de variolis et morbillis. 1653; ROLFINCK, W., *praeses.* Methodus cognoscendi & curandi adfectus capitis particulares. 1653.

PRENNER, SEBASTIAN, *ed. See* DAS GROSSE PLANETEN-BUCH. [not before 1694]

PRETTEN, JOHANN RAPHAEL [*fl.* 1684-1689] *respondent. See* BERGER, J. G. von, *praeses.* Exercitationem inauguralem de polypo cordis . . . p. p. J. R. P. 1689; WOLF, Jakob, *praeses.* Disputatio seu judicium medicum de cerevisia Numburgensi. 1684.

PREUDHOMME, ROBERT [*fl.* 1639-1669] *tr. See* CONTI, L. Discours philosophiques. 1678.

PREUSS, MAXIMILIAN [*ca.* 1652-*ca.* 1719] *respondent. See* ETTMÜLLER, M., *praeses.* Parva magnorum morborum initia. 1676.

PREVOST, JEAN [1585-1631] Tractatus, de remediorum cum simplicium tum compositorum materia: cui annexa est Joannis Stephani . . . Cosmetice. Medicina pauperum, sive De remediis facile parabilibus. De venenis et alexipharmacis. De signis. De compositione medicamentorum . . . Francofurti ad Moenum, Apud Joannem Beyerum, 1656.

[96], 1170 p. 14 cm. **[9260]**

Imperfect: p. 264-270 mutilated.

Added engraved title page: Opera medica posthuma.

Printer's error: 12 pages of text between pages 456 and 457 omitted.

—[The same.] . . . [&] Selectiora remedia . . . Hanoviae, Apud Wilhelmum Reichardum Stockium, 1666.

[96], 1170 p.; [4], 200, [12] p. 14 cm. **[9261]**

Half-title: Opera medica posthuma.

The main text is a reissue of the 1656 edition.

—De compositione medicamentorum libellus: iterum editus cura Friderici Monavii . . . Rintelii, Typis Petri Luel, 1649.

[16], 136 p. 14 cm. **[9262]**

—Johannis Prevotii Artem componendi medicamenta genuinae restitutam integritati exhibet Adolphus Storck. Amstelodami, Apud Danielem Elzevirium, 1665.

[8], 184 p.   14 cm.   **[9263]**

A revision of De compositione medicamentorum libellus.

—De compositione medicamentorum tractatus posthumus . . . Ab ejusdem filiis Jo. Baptista, et Theob. summa diligentia ex proprio autographo desumptus, & in lucem editus . . . Patavii, Typis Matthaei Bolzzettae de Cadorinis, 1666.

[12], 230, [10] p.   15 cm.   **[9264]**

Bound with *his* De urinis. 1667.

—De remediorum cum simplicium, tum compositorum materia . . . Venetiis, Apud Bertanos, 1640.

[24], 470 (i.e. 480) p.   15 cm.   **[9265]**

"Cosmetices particula obiter adjecta a Joanne Stephano": p. 461–470.

—De urinis tractatus posthumus . . . Ab ejusdem filiis Jo. Batista, et Theob. summa diligentia ex proprio autographo desumptus & in lucem editus . . . Patavii, Typis Matthẹi Bolzzettae de Cadorinis, 1667.

[12], 166, [1] p.   15 cm.   **[9266]**

Added engraved title page.

With this is bound *his* De compositione medicamentorum. 1666.

—Hortulus medicus selectioribus remediis; ceu, Flosculis versicoloribus refertus. Authore Jo. Praevotio . . . Plantatio tertia . . . Patavii, Typis Matthaei Bolzetta de Cadorinis, 1666.

[14], 162, [10] p.   14 cm.   **[9267]**

Added engraved title page.

Imperfect: title page mutilated.

Edited by the author's sons, Jean Baptiste and Thibaut Prevost. Previously published in Frankfurt in 1659 under title: Selectiora remedia multiplici usu comprobata.

—[The same.] . . . Ed. 4. . . . Patavii, Typis Jacobi de Cadorinis, 1681.

[12], 162, [6] p.   14 cm.   **[9268]**

Added engraved title page.

The main text is reprinted from the 3d ed., and bears as running title the original title (abbreviated): Selectiora remedia.

With this is bound: Tilemann, J. Experimenta circa veras, & irreducibiles auri solutiones. 1669.

—Medicina pauperum ac ejusdem De venenis ac eorundem alexipharmacis opusculum. Francofurti, Sumptibus Johannis Beÿeri, 1641.

377 (i.e. 383) p.   13 cm.   **[9269]**

Engraved title page.

—[The same.] Medicina pauperum, cum Censu venenorum & alexipharmacorum. Quibus accessit De medicamentorum materia tractatus . . . Lugduni, Sumptib. Petri Ravaud, 1643.

[8], 718 (i.e. 720), [14] p.   15 cm.   **[9270]**

—[The same.] Medicina pauperum. Sive, De remediis facile parabilibus. Tractatus posthumus. Huic pauperum thesauro adjungitur ejusdem auctoris libellus aureus De venenis. Ed. 3. emendatissima; ex proprio authographo desumpta. Venetiis, Apud Turrinum, 1654.

[24], 346 p.; [2], 73, [9] p.   12 cm.   **[9271]**

"De venenis et alexipharmacis compendiosa tractatio ([2], 73 p. at end) has special title page.

—[The same.] Medicina pauperum; mira serie continens remedia ad aegrotos cujuscunque generis persanandos aptissima, facile parabilia, extemporanea, & nullius, vel perexigui sumptus. Huic pauperum thesauro adjungitur ejusdem auctoris libellus aureus De venenis. Lugduni, Sumptibus Pauli Frambotti, 1660.

[10], 332, [2], 70, [16] p.   14 cm.   **[9272]**

Part [2] has special title page dated 1659.

—[The same.] Medicina pauperum; sive, De remediis facile parabilibus. Tractatus posthumus. Huic pauperum thesauro adjungitur ejusdem auctoris libellus aureus De venenis. Ed. 4. emendatissima; ex proprio authographo desumpta. Venetiis, Apud Stephani Curtii, 1679.

[12], 245 p.; [2], 53, [8] p.   15 cm.   **[9273]**

Part [2] has special title page.

[—English tr.] Medicaments for the poor; or, Physick for the common people. Containing, excellent remedies for most common diseases, incident to mans body; made of such things as are common to be had in almost every country in the world: and are made with little art, and smal charge . . . Hereunto is added an excellent book, called Health for the rich and poor, by diet without physick. The 2d ed. By Nich. Culpeper . . . London, Peter Cole, 1662.

[24], 388 (i.e. 288) p.; [6], 41 p.   17 cm.

[9274]

Part [2]: Health for the rich and poor, by dyet, without physick ([6], 41 p. at end) has special title page dated 1656.

—[The same.] . . . In two books, I. Containing excellent remedies for most common diseases, incident to mans body; made of such things as are common to be had in almost every countrey in the world; and are made with little art, and small charge. First written in Latin ... Translated into English, with additions. Secondly, Health for the rich and poor, by diet, without physick. By Nich. Culpeper ... London, Printed by John Streater, for George Sawbridge, 1670.

[8], 135 p.   18 cm.   **[9275]**

—[French tr.] La medecine des pauvres. Où sont contenus les remedes a toutes maladies, aages & temperamens de chaque personne, lesquels se peuvent preparer à peu de frais, en tous lieux, & en toutes saisons par toutes personnes ... Paris, Gervais Clousier, 1646.

[24 +], 259 p.   18 cm.   **[9276]**

Imperfect: Catchword on p. [24] ("Privilege") does not carry over to p. [1].

—*See* CULPEPER, N. Two books of physick. 1656; GOCKEL, E. Enchiridion medico-practicum de peste, 1669.

PREVOST, JEAN BAPTISTE, *ed. See* PREVOST, J. De compositione medicamentorum tractatus. 1666 [and] De urinis tractatus. 1667 [and] Hortulus medicus selectioribus remediis. 1666.

PREVOST, THIBAUT [*fl.* 1666] *ed. See* PREVOST, J. De compositione medicamentorum tractatus. 1666 [and] De urinis tractatus. 1667 [and] Hortulus medicus selectioribus remediis. 1666.

PREVOTIUS, JOHN. *See* PREVOST, Jean [1585-1631]

PREZ, JACOBUS DE. *See* DES PREZ, Jacques [*fl.* 1677-1695]

PRICKIUS, NICOLAUS [*fl. ca.* 1652] *respondent. See* DEUSING, A. Idea doctrinae de febribus. 1655.

PRIEST, ROBERT [*ca.* 1550–*ca.* 1590] *tr. See* GERARD, J. The herball: or, Generall historie of plantes. 1633, 1636.

PRIMIROSIUS, JACOBUS. *See* PRIMROSE, James [1592-1659]

PRIMEROSE, JAMES. *See* PRIMROSE, James. [1592-1659]

PRIMROSE, JAMES [1592-1659] Animadversiones in theses, quas pro circulatione sanguinis in Academia Ultrajectensi D. Henricus Le Roy ... disputandas proposuit.

14-30 p., part [2]   20 cm. (*In* Recentiorum disceptationes de motu cordis. Lugduni Batavorum, 1647)   **[9277]**

Caption title.

—Antidotum adversus Henrici Regii ... venentam spongiam; sive, Vindiciae animadversionum. Lugduni Batavorum, Ex officina Joannis Maire, 1644.

51 p.   20 cm.   **[9278]**

Published also as part [3] in Recentiorum disceptationes de motu cordis, sanguinis, et chyli in animalibus. Lugduni Batavorum, 1647.

—Ars pharmaceutica methodus brevissima de eligendis & componendis medicinae. Amsteledami, Apud Joannem Janssonium, 1651.

[1], 272, [9] p.   13 cm.   **[9279]**

[—De calice ex antimonio sive stibio. English] The antimoniall cup twice cast; or, A treatise concerning the antimoniall cup, shewing the abuse thereof. First written in Latine ... in consideration of a small pamphlet set forth by the founder of the cup. Translated into English by Robert Wittie ... London, B. A[lsop] and T. Fawcet, 1640.

[4], 34 (i.e. 30), [1] p.   14 cm.   **[9280]**

Signatures: A-D⁴, E².

STC 20383.

The original Latin text was printed as Caput LV of Book 4 of his De vulgi erroribus in the editions of 1658 and 1668.

—De febribus libri quatuor. In quibus plurimi veterum, & recentiorum errores declarantur & refelluntur. Plurima nova & paradoxa continentur. Roterodami, Ex officina Arnoldi Leers, 1658.

[8], 443 (i.e. 459) p.   20 cm.   **[9281]**

Bound with *his* De mulierum morbis. 1655.

—De mulierum morbis et symptomatis libri quinque. In quibus plurimi tum veterum, tum recentiorum errores breviter indicantur & explicantur ... Roterodami, Ex officina Arnoldi Leers, 1655.

[8], 390, [6] p.   20 cm.   **[9282]**

With this is bound *his* De febribus. 1658.

—De vulgi in medicina erroribus libri quatuor ... Londini, Apud B[ernard] A[lsop] & T[homas] F[awcet] pro H. Robinsonio, 1638.

[16], 431 (i.e. 427) p.   14 cm.   **[9283]**

STC 20384.

—[The same.] ... Amstelodami, Apud Joannem Janssonium, 1639.

5, [7], 237 p.   13 cm.   **[9284]**

—[The same.] . . . Amstelodami, Apud Joannem Janssonium, 1644.

3, [9], 237 p.　13 cm.　　　　　　[9285]
Different setting of type.

—[The same.] . . . Ab auctore recensiti & plus quam tertia parte aucti. Roterdami, Ex officina Arnoldi Leers, 1658.

[20], 561, [1] p.　14 cm.　　　　[9286]

—[The same.] . . . Lugduni, Apud Jacobum Faeton, 1664.

[16], 448 p.　18 cm.　　　　　　[9287]

—[The same.] . . . Ed. postrema, prioribus emendatior. Roterodami, Ex officina Arnoldi Leers, 1668.

[20], 561, [1] p.　14 cm.　　　　[9288]
A reprint of the 1658 edition.

—[English tr.] Popular errours. Or, The errours of the people in physick, first written in Latine by . . . James Primrose . . . To which is added by the same authour his verdict concerning the antimoniall cuppe. Translated into English by Robert Wittie . . . London, Printed by W. Wilson for Nicholas Bourne, 1651.

[23], 461, [13] p.　18 cm.　　　　[9289]
Added engraved title page.

—[French tr.] Traité de Primerose sur les erreurs vulgaires de la medecine avec des additions tres-curieuses, par M. de Rostagny . . . Lyon, Jean Certe, 1689.

[28], 860 p.　19 cm.　　　　　　[9290]

—[German tr.] In Scharff, B. Unvorgriefliche Gedancken von . . . magnetischen Curen. 1700.

—Enchiridion medicum; sive, Brevissimum medicinae systema . . . Amstelodami, Apud Joannem Janssonium, 1650.

[1], 223, [3] p.　13 cm.　　　　[9291]

—Enchiridion medicum practicum. Complectens omnium morborum communium & particularium naturam, causas, signa & curationem. Amstelodami, Apud Joannem Janssonium, 1654.

[3], 232, [4] p.; 364, [12] p.　13 cm.　[9292]
Part 2 has half title: . . . De morbis a capite ad pedes.

—Exercitationes, et animadversiones in librum, De motu cordis, et circulatione sanguinis. Adversus

Guilielmum Harveum . . . Londini, Gulielmus Jones, pro Nicolao Bourne, 1630.

[11], 108 p.　19 cm.　　　　　　[9293]
STC 20385.

—[The same.] In Harvey, W. De motu cordis. 1639, 1647.

—Partes duae de morbis puerorum . . . Roterodami, Ex officina Arnoldi Leers, 1659.

[1], 125 p.　14 cm.　　　　　　[9294]

—See BLASIUS, G. Impetus Jacobi Primirosii . . . in Vop. Fort. Plempium . . . retusus a Gerardo Leon. Blasio. 1659; DRAKE, R. Contra animadversiones Jac. Primrosii. 1647; REGIUS, H. Spongia, qua eluuntur sordes animadversionum, quas Jacobus Primirosius . . . edidit. 1647; ROSS, A. Arcana microcosmi. 1652.

The **PRINCIPLES** of the chymists of London stated. 1676. See [Society of Apothecaries of London]

PRISCIANUS, THEODORUS [*fl.* 5th cent.] See THEODORUS, *medicus.* Diaeta. 1632.

PRISCO, GIUSEPPE [*fl.* 1700] Nuncius Parnassius. *In* CELEBERR. VIRORUM APOLOGIAE pro R. D. Carolo Musitano. 1700.

PRISGUS, JOSEPHUS. See PRISCO, Giuseppe [*fl.* 1700]

PRIVIGYEI, MIKLÓS [*fl.* 1694] See ALBINUS, B. Dissertationem chirurgico-medicam de paronychia . . . publicae . . . indagationi permittet M. P. 1694.

PRIVILEGIUM comitatus palat., & militiae auratae a Ferdinando III. Romanorum imperatore. 1653. See FERDINAND III, *Emperor of Germany.*

PROBLEMATA physica et medica. 1677. See [BAYLE, F.]

PROBST, ANDREAS [*fl.* 1638–1640] *respondent.* See CONRING, H., *praeses.* Disputatio medica de apoplexiae natura causis. 1640 [and] Disputatio philosophica ac medica de terris. 1678.

PROBUS HETEROPOLITANUS, *pseud.* See LE BON, Jean [*d.* 1583?]

PROCACCINI, CALISTO [*fl.* 1587–1617] Liber, qui dicitur medicus, ad tyrones non minus utilis, quam curiosus cupidis litterarum. Romae, Ex typographia Spadae, apud Stephanum Paulinum, 1617.

[8], 244, [3] p.   23 cm.   [9295]

Errata: p. [3] at end.

A PROCLAMATION declaring His Majesties pleasure touching orders to be observed for prevention of dispersing the plague. 1636. *See* GT. BRIT. *Sovereign* [1625-1649] (Charles I)

A PROCLAMATION for restraint of unnecessarie resorts to the court. 1625. *See* GT. BRIT. *Sovereign* [1625-1649] (Charles I)

A PROCLAMATION for the adjournement of part of Trinitie terme. 1625. *See* GT. BRIT. *Sovereign* [1625-1649] (Charles I)

A PROCLAMATION for the better ordering of those who repair to the court. 1662. *See* GT. BRIT. *Sovereign* [1660-1685] (Charles II)

A PROCLAMATION prohibiting the keeping of Bartholomew faire. 1636. *See* GT. BRIT. *Sovereign* [1625-1649] (Charles I)

A PROCLAMATION to prohibit the keeping of this next Sturbridge faire. 1636. *See* GT. BRIT. *Sovereign* [1625-1649] (Charles I)

PROCLUS, DIADOCHUS. *See* PROCLUS LYCIUS, *surnamed* Diadochus.

PROCLUS LYCIUS, *surnamed* DIADOCHUS. *See* MIZAULD, A. Opusculum de sena. 1607.

PROCOPIUS, *of Caesarea. See* MARCHINI, F. Belli divini; sive, Pestilentis temporis accurata. 1633.

PRODROMUS religionis medici. *See* PECHLIN, J. N. Jani Philadelphi [pseud.] Consultatio desultoria de optima Christianorum secta. 1688.

PROFIUS, GOTTLIEB [*fl.* 1677-1682] *respondent. See* WEDEL, G. W., *praeses.* Dissertatio medica inauguralis de chorea S. Viti. 1682.

LE PROGRÈS de la medecine. 1698, 1699. *See* [BRUNET, C.]

PROLUSIONES apologeticae approbatorum stibii, adversus authorem libelli infandi, qui inscribitur Pithoegia ... Parisiis, Apud Joannem Henault, 1654.

62 p.   22 cm.   [9296]

Bound with [Blondel, F., 1609?-1682] Alethophanis archiatri ad Jacobum Thevartum. 1655.

PROMPTUARIUM Hippocratis in locos communes ordine alphabetico, nec sine compendio digestum. 1683. *See* HIPPOCRATES. [Adaptations, etc. Latin.] 1683.

PROPERTIUS, SEXTUS AURELIUS. *See* FABER, Johannes. De nardo et epithymo adversus Josephum Scaligerum. 1607.

Les PROPORTIONS du corps humain. *See* [AUDRAN, G.]

PROPOSITIONS concerning optic-glasses. 1679. *See* [WALKER O.]

PROROGA della quarantena. 1630. *See* FLORENCE (City) Ordinances, local laws, etc.

PROSPECTUS pharmaceuticus. 1668, 1698. *See* COLLEGIO DEI FISICI, Milan.

PROST, J., *tr. See* DIEMERBROECK, I. van. L'anatomie du corps humain. 1695.

PROTIMUS, MELIPPUS, *pseud. See* PLEMP, Vopiscus Fortunatus [1601-1671]

PROVANCHÈRES, SIMÉON DE [*ca.* 1540-1617] Discours sur l'inappetence d'un enfant de Vauprofonde confins de Sens, qui n'abeu ny mangé depuis sept mois ... Sens, George Niverd, 1611.

23 p.   16 cm.   [9297]

Supplemented by additional discourses in later editions: 2d ed. (discourses 1-2) 1612; 3d ed. (discourses 1-3) 1615; 4th ed. (discourses 1-4, under title: Histoire de l'inappetence d'un enfant de Vauprofonde prez Sens) 1616.

—Histoire de l'inappetence d'un enfant de Vauprofonde prez Sens, de son desistement de boire & de manger quatre ans unze mois, & de sa mort ... 4. ed. augm. par l'autheur d'un quatriesme discours. Sens, George Niverd, 1616.

48 ll.   17 cm.   [9298]

"Cinquième discours apologétique ... d'un enfant de Vauprofonde" was published separately in 1617.

—, ed. and *tr. See* FERNEL, J. La chirurgie. 1667.

—, ed. *See* AUGENIO, O. Epistolarum et consultationum medicinalium prioris tomi libri XII. 1602.

—, *tr. See* TAGAULT, J. La chirurgie. 1629, 1645.

—*See* COLLECTANEA DE DIUTURNA GRAVIDITATE. 1662; ROUSSET, F. Exsectio foetus vivi ex matre viva sine alterutrius vitae periculo. 1601.

PROVIGIONI, et ordini per conservatione della publica salute. 1679. *See* MODENA. Ordinances, local laws, etc.

PROVISIONE de mol. mag. sig. uffitiali della sanita. 1616. *See* FLORENCE (CITY) Magistrato di sanità.

PRUECKELIUS, JOANNES PETRUS. *See* PRÜKKEL, Johann Peter [*fl.* 1658-1676]

PRÜKKEL, GEORG. Foetus posthumus, oder, Bericht von dem grausamen Reissen und Grimmen im Leibe, Colica genant, was von solchen Schmertzen zu wissen nützlich, auch bey dessen Cur, Zufällen und Praeservirung meist zu beobachten nothwendig erfodert werde . . . An Tag gegeben von Johann Peter Prükkeln . . . Jena, Bey Johann Jacob Bauhofern, 1676.

[8], 188 p.   21 cm.   **[9299]**

PRÜKKEL, JOHANN PETER [*fl.* 1658-1676] Kurtzes Bedencken uber die Seuche, welche sich drey Herbst nacheinander in dem so genandten Dorff Ober-Oppurg eingefunden . . . Regenspurg, Paulus Dallnsteiner, 1675.

[40] p.; [64] p.   21 cm.   **[9300]**

Part [2] has half title: Notae, Cicero in oratore. In poetis non Homero soli locus est, nec Aristotelem in philosophia deteruit a scribendo amplitudo Platonis . . .

With this is bound *his* Panacea microcosmica. 1676.

—Panacea microcosmica ostendens breviter usum partium humani corporis medicum . . . Ratisbonae, Literis Pauli Dalnsteineri, 1676.

[10] p.; [11] p.   21 cm.   **[9301]**

Part [2] has half title: Imago pacis. Ad Cornel. Taciti Annalem I. Cap. X.

Bound with *his* Kurtzes Bedencken uber die Seuche. 1675.

—*respondent. See* FRIDERICI, J. A., *praeses.* Scrutinium hydrocephali. 1669; ROLFINCK, W., *praeses.* Dissertationem de variolis . . . proponit . . . J. P. P. 1658.

—, *ed. See* PRÜKKEL, G. Foetus posthumus. 1676.

PRUGGMAYR, MARTIN MAXIMILIAN [*fl.* 1687] Scrutinium philosophicum de vero elixire vitae; seu, Genuino auro potabili philosophico, quo non solum omnes humani corporis morbi quondam sanabantur,

verum & immunda, ac leprosa corpora metallorum curabantur . . . Salisburgi, Sumptibus Joannis Baptistae Mayr, Typographi Aulico-Academici, 1687.

[30], 146, [6] p.   16 cm.   **[9302]**

Imperfect: outer margins of p. [1]-8, [17], 19-23 trimmed.

With this is bound Struve, Ernst Gotthold. Paradoxum chymicum sine igne. Jenae [1715?]

PRYNNE, WILLIAM [1600-1669] Healthes sicknesse; or, A compendious and briefe discourse; proving, the drinking and pledging of healthes, to be sinfull, and utterly unlawfull unto Christians . . . London, 1628.

[31], 86 p.   18 cm.   **[9303]**

STC 20462.

PSICHHOLTZ, BARTHOLOMEUS [*fl.* 1604-1606] *respondent. See* SENNERT, D., *praeses.* De caussis morborum disputatio altera. 1605 [and] De methodo medendi disputatio IV, de causus morborum. 1604.

PUEBLA, FRANCISCO MOROVELLI DE. *See* MOROVELLI DE LA PUEBLA, Francisco [1575-1649]

PUENTE, LUIS DE LA, *Father* [1554-1624] Tesoro nascosto nelle infermità, e ne' travagli . . . Tradotto dal Castigliano . . . dal. P. Cammillo Maria Rinaldi . . . Roma, Domenico Ant. Ercole, 1690.

xxix, [1], 375, [1] p.   16 cm.   **[9304]**

Added engraved title page.

A translation of Modo breve de ayudar a ben morir, first published in Tortosa, in 1636.

PUERARI, DANIEL [1621-1692] *ed. See* BURNET, *Sir* T. Thesaurus medicinae practicae. 1678, 1687.

—*See* BARTHOLIN, T. De flammula cordis epistola. 1667.

PUEYO, JOSÉ DE RIVILLA BONET Y. *See* RIVILLA BONET Y PUEYO, José de.

PUFENDÖRFFER, ESAIAS. *See* PUFENDORFF, Esaias [1628-1689]

PUFENDORFF, ESAIAS [1628-1689] *praeses.* De igne nativo disquisitio . . . Lipsiae, Exscribebat Henningus Colerus [1650]

[20] p.   19 cm.   **[9305]**

Diss.—Leipzig (A. Calisius, *respondent*)

—De sanguine et ejus motus dissertatio . . . [Lipsiae] Johannes Bauerus [1652]

[24] p.   19 cm.   **[9306]**

Diss.—Leipzig (G. Neumann, *respondent*)

—De temperamentis disquisitio . . . Lipsiae, Apud Johannem Bauerum [1652]

[16] p.   19 cm.   **[9307]**

Diss.—Leipzig (J. J. Krause, *respondent*)

PUGH, ROBERT [1609–1679] Bathoniensium et Aquisgranensium thermarum comparatio variis adjunctis illustrata. R[obert] P[ugh] Epistola . . . Londini, J. Martyn, 1676.

[5], 96, [9] p.   15 cm.   **[9308]**

PUJASOL, ESTEVAN [*fl.* 1622–1637] El sol solo, y para todos sol, de la filosofia sagaz, y anotomia de ingenios . . . Barcelona, Pedro La Cavalleria, 1637.

[8], 118, [8] p.   illus.   21 cm.   **[9309]**

PULVERINUS, JOANNES HIERONYMUS. *See* POLVERINO, Giovanni Girolamo [*fl.* 1586–1589]

PURMANN, MATTHIAS GOTTFRIED [1649–1711] Ausführlicher Unterricht, und Anweisung wie die Salivation-Cur . . . auffs beste und sicherste vorzunehmen . . . Liegnitz, In Verlag Michael Rohrlachs [1692?]

[109] p.   illus.   17 cm.   **[9310]**

—Grosser und gantz neugewundener Lorbeer-Krantz; oder, Wund-Artzney, in III. Theil und 127. Capittel abgetheilet . . . Franckfurth und Leipzig, In Verlegung Michael Rohrlachs, gedruckt bey Joh. Christoph Brandenburgern, 1692.

[30], 784 p.; 296, [56] p.   front. (port.), plates.   21 cm.   **[9311]**

Added engraved title page.
Part 3 has half title.

—Herausgegebene chirurgia curiosa . . . Alles in drey Theil und 73. Capitel abgetheilet, und mit vielen . . . Kupffer-Tabellen . . . versehen. Franckfurt und Leipzig, In Verlegung Michael Rohrlachs seel. Wittib und Erben [Jena, Gedruckt bey Paul Ehrichen] 1699.

[16], 746, [48] p.   plates.   20 cm.   **[9312]**

Imperfect: sig. 5G⁴ (blank?) wanting.
With this is bound *his* Curiöse chirurgische Observationes. Franckfurth und Leipzig, 1710.

—Kurtze, doch gründliche, Anweisung, wie man alle Arten der bösen und gifftigen pestilentzischen Drüsen, Beulen, Carbunckel und Apostemata, nach deren Ursprung und Ansehen, recht erkennen und

. . . fundamentaliter curiren könne . . . von M. G. P. [n. p.] 1686.

68 p.   17 cm.   **[9313]**

—Copy 2.

With this is bound Der vollkommene und wolerfahrne Wundarzt. 1687.

—Der rechte und warhafftige Feldscher; oder . . . Feldschers-Kunst. Worinnen kürtzlich, doch grundrichtig gewiesen wird, wie man alle Verletzungen des gantzen menschlichen Leibes . . . vollkömmlich erkennen . . . können . . . Franckfurt und Leipzig, Michael Rohrlach, 1690.

[32], 480, [24] p.   17 cm.   **[9314]**

Added engraved title page.

PURPAN, PONTIUS FRANCISCUS, *ed. See* CODEX MEDICAMENTARIUS. 1648.

PURPIUS, ADAM [*fl.* 1669–1679]

Dissertations — Wittenberg

—*praeses.* De sede vitae in calido innato dissertatio . . . Wittebergae, Typis Michaelis Meyeri [1671]

[16] p.   18 cm.   **[9315]**

Imperfect: uper margins trimmed.
W. D. Walther, *respondent.*

—Exercitatio academica prior de causis laboranti naturae obstetricantibus . . . Wittebergae, Typis Michaelis Wendt, 1669.

[16] p.   19 cm.   **[9316]**

J. C. Adlung, *respondent.*

—Exercitatio academica posterior de causis laboranti naturae obstetricantibus . . . Wittebergae, Literis Michaelis Wendt, 1669.

[16] p.   19 cm.   **[9317]**

J. C. Adlung, *respondent.*

—Humanae nutritionis rationem . . . [Wittenbergae] Literis Wendianis, excudebat Daniel Schmatz [1672]

[16] p.   18 cm.   **[9318]**

F. Geitzinger, *respondent.*

—Reserata geocosmi majestas, per XII exercitationes physicas, quarum primam . . . submittet . . . Christian Ehrenfried Winzer . . . Wittebergae, Typis Michaelis Wendt, 1669.

[16] p.   19 cm.   **[9319]**

C. E. Winzer, *respondent.*

—*respondent. See* SENNERT, M., *praeses.* Disputationem inauguralem de lue venerea . . . proponit M. A. P. 1679.

The PURPLE island; or, The isle of man. 1633. *See* FLETCHER, P.

PUSCHEL, CHRISTIAN [*fl.* 1687] *respondent. See* LIMMER, C. P., *praeses.* Disputatio undecima de rarefactionis et condensationis aeris effectis in thermometris. 1687.

PUT, HENDRIK VAN DER. *See* PUTEANUS, Erycius [1574–1646]

PUTEANUS, ERYCIUS [1574–1646] Comus; sive, Phagesiposia cimmeria somnium. 2. . . . ed. Lovanii, Typis Gerardi Rivii, 1611.

    [1], 204, [1] p. 16 cm.   **[9320]**

—Historiae Medicaeae libri duo: res . . . circa Lacum Larium a Jo. Jacobo Medicaeo gestae. Accedit Galeatii Capellae De bello Mussiano liber singularis. Antverpiae, Typis Joannis Cnobbari, 1634.

    [4], 161, [2] p. port. 11 cm.   **[9321]**
  "Anacephalaeosis libri I[-II]": p. 142–158.

—[The same.] *See* [Charleton, W.] The Ephesian and Cimmerian matrons. 1668.

—Ovi encomium, quo summum & unicum naturae miraculum describitur . . . Monaci, Ex formis Bergianis, apud viduam; impensis Raphaelis Sadleri, 1617.

    120 p. 14 cm.   **[9322]**
  With this is bound Goclenius, R. [1572–1621] Tractatus de magnetica. 1610.

PUTEANUS, GUILHELMUS. *See* DUPUIS, Guillaume [*fl.* 1536–1551]

PUTEANUS, PETRUS [*fl.* 1662] *respondent.* Disputatio medica inauguralis de scorbuto . . . Lugduni Batavorum, Ex officina Francisci Moyardi, 1662.

    [16] p. 21 cm.   **[9323]**
  Diss.—Leyden.

PUTEO, ZACCHARIAS A [*fl.* 1611] *See* A PUTEO, Zaccharias [*fl.* 1611]

PUTHMAN, EVERT [*fl.* 1593] Puthmans manuael; oft, Cleyn pest-boecxken . . . Van nieus

oversien, vermeerdert, ende gecorriegert. Amstelredam, Cornelis Claesz, 1603.

    [72] p. 16 cm.   **[9324]**
  With this is bound Blasius, G. Pest-geneesing. 1663.

—[The same.] Putmans manuael; dat is, Een kleyn pest-boecxken . . . Ende nu van nieus wat gecozrigeert ende vermeerdert. door Abraham Lenertsz. Vrolingh . . . Zaerdam, Heyndrick Jacobsz. Soet [1646?]

    [8], 72, [8] p. 15 cm.   **[9325]**

—*See* VROLINGH, A. L. Matroosen gesontheyt. 1680.

IL PUTTANISMO romano. 1668. *See* [LETI, G.]

PUTTE, HENDRIK VAN DER. *See* PUTEANUS, Erycius [1574–1646]

PUTTEN, HENDRIK VAN DER. *See* PUTEANUS, Erycius [1574–1646]

PUY, HENRI DU. *See* PUTEANUS, Erycius [1574–1646]

PUYLON, CLAUDE [*fl.* 1660–1696] *praeses.* Quaestio medica . . . An chronicorum morborum medicina, in alimento? [Parisiis, Apud Franciscum Muguet, 1695]

    8 p. 24 cm.   **[9326]**
  Diss.—Paris (P. Hecquet, *respondent*)

—Quaestio medica . . . An conformatio temperiei nota. [Parisiis, Ex typographia Francisci Muguet, 1670]

    4 p. 26 cm.   **[9327]**
  Caption title.
  Diss.—Paris (A. de Sainct-Yon, *respondent*)

—*respondent. See* BRAYER, N., *praeses.* Quaestio medico. 1670.

PUYLON, DENIS [*fl.* 1670–1685] *ed. See* UNIVERSITÉ DE PARIS. Faculté de médicine. Statuts de la Faculté de medecine en l'Université de Paris. 1672.

—*See* POSTEL, N. Factum. 1685.

PYL, PAULUS. *See* Pijl, Paul [*fl. ca.* 1677]

PYLIUS, CHRISTIANUS [*fl.* 1660] *respondent. See* LINDEN, J. A. van der, *praeses.* Hippocrates de circuitu sanguinis, exercitatio XII. 1660.

PYRMONTANUS, JOHANN. *See* FEUERBERG, Johann [*fl.* 1556?]

PYROPHILUS, J. A. *See* AstelL, James [17th cent.]

PYRRHO, *of Elis. See* Sextus Empiricus. Opera. 1621.

PYTHAGORAS. *See* Averroës. Averroeana: being a transcript of several letters from Averroes. 1695.

PYTHAGORAS, *pseud. See* Peyer, Johann Konrad [1653-1712]

Q

QUADRAMIO, Evangelista. *See* Quattrami, Evangelista [*fl.* 1586-1597]

QUADRANI, Francesco. *See* Quattrami, Evangelista [*fl.* 1586-1597]

QUARTUS, Christoph [*fl.* 1605-1609] *respondent. See* Lichten, A., *praeses.* De melancholia. 1609.

QUATRAMIO, Evangelista. *See* Quattrami, Evangelista [*fl.* 1586-1597]

QUATROUX, Isaac, *Brother* [*fl.* 1671] Traité de la peste, contenant sa definition, ses especes & differences ... Ensemble la difference qui est entre le pourpre, la petite verole, & la peste ... Avec quelques discours sur leurs causes, signes, accidens, & les remedes ... Paris, Edme Couterot, 1671.

[22], 194, [14] p. 19 cm. [**9328**]

QUATTRAMI, Evangelista [*fl.* 1586-1597] Tractatus brevis de praeservatione & curatione pestis. F. Evangelistae Quattrammi ... Romę olim ante XXX. annos editus. Jam vero ex Italico Latinus, opera & studio And. Hiltebrandi ... Lipsiae, Impensis Eliae Rehefeldii & Johannis Grosii [Typis Augustini Jungii, excudebat Andreas Oswald] 1618.

[6], 94, [1] p. 16 cm. [**9329**]

QUECCIUS, Gregor [1596-1632] Anatomiae philologicae pars prima continens discursus philologicos de nobilitate et praestantia hominis contra iniquos conditionis humanae aestimatores ... Noribergae, Typis & sumptibus Simonis Halbmayeri, 1632.

[36], 552, [44] p. 20 cm. [**9330**]

No more published. Cf. Jöcher.

—*respondent.* Disputatio inauguralis de variolis et morbillis ... Basileae, Typis Joh. Jacobi Genathii [1620]

[40] p. 18 cm. [**9331**]

Diss. — Basel.

The **QUEENS** closet opened. Incomparable secrets in physick, chyrurgery, preserving, candying, and cookery; as they were presented unto the queen ... The 4th ed. corr. with many additions ... Transcribed ... by W. M. ... London, Nathaniel Brooks, 1658.

[10], 300, [23] p.; 123, [17] p. front. (port.) 15 cm. [**9332**]

Part [1] has running titles: "The pearle of practice" and "A queens delight."

Part [2] has special title page: The compleat cook.

—[The same.] ... Corrected and revised, with ... additions ... London, Printed for Nath. Brooke and sold by Tho. Guy, 1674.

3 parts in 1 v. front. (port.) 16 cm. [**9333**]

Various pagings.

Part [1] has running title: The pearl of practice.

Part [2] has special title page dated 1675: A queens delight; or, The art of preserving, conserving, and candying.

Part [3] has special title page dated 1675: The compleat cook: expertly prescribing ... wayes ... for dressing of flesh and fish, ordering of sauces or making of pastry.

Letter to the reader signed W. M.

—[The same.] ... London, Obadiah Blagrave, 1683.

3 parts in 1 v. 15 cm. [**9334**]

Various pagings.

A reprint of the 1674 edition.

A QUEENS delight. *See* The queens closet opened. 1658, 1675, 1683.

QUELLENBURGH, Henricus [*fl.* 17th cent.] *respondent. See* Bruyn, J. de, *praeses.* Disputatio physica, qua rationes pro formis substantialibus adferri solitae expenduntur. 1657.

QUELLMALTZ, Christian Samuel [*fl.* 1694] *respondent. See* Pauli, J. W., *praeses.* Disputatio medica inauguralis de medicamentorum delectu. 1694.

QUERCETANUS, Josephus. *See* Duchesne, Joseph [*ca.* 1544-1609]

QUERCETANUS, Nicolas. *See* Chesneau, Nicolas [*ca.* 1601–*ca.* 1680]

QUERCETANUS redivivus. 1648, 1679. *See* Duchesne, J.

QUESTEL, Kaspar [*fl.* 1678–1687] Dissertatio academica de pulvinari morientibus non subtrahendo, von Abziehung der sterbenden Hauptküssen, ex moralibus, divinis, juris item ac artis medicae principiis methodice proposita, et exemplis rarioribus illustrata ... Jenae, Typis ac sumtibus Johannis Gollneri, 1678.

[8], 54, [16] p.   20 cm.   [9335]

—[The same.] ... ed. alt. variis accessionibus utilissimis auctior. Jenae, Typis ac sumtibus Johannis Gollneri, 1683.

[8], 53, [16] p.   20 cm.   [9336]
Different setting of type.

QUESTIER, Georges. De naturalibus et legitimis matrimonii dissolvendi causis, medica decisio ... Rothomagi, Apud Thomam Ovin, 1660.

[4], 90 p.   17 cm.   [9337]

A QUESTION. Why dead bodies bleed in the presence of their murtherers. 1640. *See* Conferences du Bureau d'Adresse, Paris.

QUEUTE, Charles Paschal, *vicomte de la. See* Paschal, Charles, *vicomte de La Queute* [1547–1625]

QUEYRATS, Ludovicus. Tractatus de vulneribus capitis ... Tolosae, Apud Arnaldum Colomerium, 1657.

[7], 237, [1] p.   18 cm.   [9338]

QUILLET, Claude [1602–1661] Calvidii Leti [pseud.] Callipaedia; seu, De pulchrae prolis habendae ratione. Poema didacticon ad humanam speciem belle conservandam apprime utile. Lugduni Batavorum, Parisiis, Apud Thomam Jolly, 1655.

56 p.   21 cm.   [9339]

With this is bound Fronteau, J. Dissertatio I. philologica. 1651.

—[The same.] ... Cum uno et altero ejusdem authoris carmine. Parisiis, Apud Thomam Joly, 1656.

[16], 94, [2] p.   19 cm.   [9340]
"... In obitu Petri Gassendi ... encomium" (p. [89]–94) has half title.

QUINA, Abraham [*fl.* 1659–1660] *respondent.* Disputatio medica inauguralis de medicina ... Lugduni Batavorum, Ex officina Danielis & Abrahami à Gaasbeek, 1660.

[8] p.   18 cm.   [9341]
Diss. — Leyden.

—*See* Le Boë, F. de., *praeses.* Disputatio medica de alimentorum fermentatione in ventriculo. 1659.

QUIÑONES, Juan de [*d. ca.* 1650] Al illustrissimo ... Señor Don Fray Antonio de Sotomayor, confessor de ... Felipe IIII ... Madrid, 1632?

21 ll.   20 cm.   [9342]
Caption title.
"Discurso sobre la sangre menstrua de los Judios a proposito del Auto da Fe celebrado el 4 de Julio de 1632, en el que entre otros reos lo fué el Judio Francisco de Andrada, aquejado de este mal." Cf. Palau 245386.

QUINTAL, Henrique do. Guia de sangradores ordenada ... Lisboa, Joam da Costa, 1669.

79 p.   15 cm.   [9343]

QUINTIANO, Antonio da [*fl.* 1668] Il mele granato succo medicinale, diviso in due parti. Nella prima si tratta di tutte le conditioni delle febri, e de polsi. Nella seconda si contengono molti ... secreti per la conservatione de corpi humani ... Venetia, Francesco Valvasense, 1668.

[36], 434 p.   15 cm.   [9344]

—[The same.] ... 2. impr. Venetia, Steffano Curti, 1675.

420 p.   17 cm.   [9345]

QUIRSITANUS, Josephus. *See* Duchesne, Joseph [*ca.* 1544–1609]

QUONIAM lumen est Deus illustrans omnia, omnia eodem perfundit. 1689. *See* Borromeo, A.

R

R., A. *See* Read, Alexander [1586?–1641]

R., A. *See* Rosa, Andreas [*b.* 1665]

R., D. *See* Rouvière, Henry Louis de [*d.* 1712 *or* 13]

R., D. [*fl. ca.* 1660] *tr. See* Arberius. La physique d'uzage. 1664; Nouveau cours de medecine. 1669, 1683.

R., E., *Gent. See* THE EXPERIENCED FARRIER. 1678, 1691/2.

R., F. P. P. [*fl.* 1607] *tr. See* PARISI, P. Brief discours. 1607.

R., I. D. P. M. O. D., *tr. See* [MERCURIO, G.] Discours de l'origine, des moeurs, fraudes et impostures des ciarlatans. 1622.

R., J. *See* ROGERS, John [1627-1665?]

R., J., *M.D. See* ROWLAND, John, M. D.

R., J. P. C., *tr. See* SALA, A. Anatomia vitrioli. 1617.

R., M. A., *tr. See* SALA, A. Tractatus duo. 1608, 1649.

R., R. *See* RESTAURAND, Raymond [1627-1682]

R., T. *See* RANDOLPH, Thomas [1605-1635]

R., W. *See* [RAMESEY, W.] Lifes security. 1665.

R., W. *See* RAND, William [*fl.* 1656]

R., W. *See* RUMSEY, Walter [1584-1660]

R. P. *See* PUGH, Robert [1609-1679]

RAABE, JACOB JODOCUS [1629-1708] *praeses.* Exercitatio medica casum practicum exponens . . . Jenae, Typis Johannis Nisii, 1656.

[16] p. 20 cm.   [**9346**]
Diss. — Jena (G. C. Amman, *respondent*)

—Exercitatio medica theorico-practica περι της αίμοπτυσεος seu sanguinis sputo . . . Jenae, Excudebat Samuel Krebsius [*ca.* 1660]

[28] p. 19 cm.   [**9347**]
Diss.—Jena (J. P. Deissler, *respondent*)

—*respondent. See* SCHENCK, J. T., *praeses.* Medicochirurgicam disserationem de fistularum vera natura & recta ratione curandarum . . . submittit . . . J. J. R. 1656.

RABANUS MAURUS. *See* HRABANUS MAURUS, *Abp. of Mainz* [784?-856]

RABUS, PETRUS [1660-1702] *tr. See* MUNTING, A. Naauwkeurige beschryving der aardgewassen. 1696.

RACCOLTA di avvertimenti & raccordi per conoscer la peste. 1630, 1682. *See* VENICE (Republic, to 1797) Magistrato della sanità.

RACCOLTA di tutti li bandi, ordini, e provisioni fatte per la città di Bologna. *See* BOLOGNA. Ordinances, local laws, etc.

RACHAIDIBI. *See* KHĀLID IBN YAZĪD, al-Umawi.

RACHEL, SAMUEL [1628-1691] *praeses.* Dissertatio moralis de principiis actionum humanarum . . . Helmestadii, Typis Henningi Mulleri, 1660.

[32] p. 20 cm.   [**9348**]
Diss.—Helmstedt (D. Nessel, *respondent*)

RADEMIN, HEINRICH [*fl.* 1684] *respondent. See* MEIBOM, H., *praeses.* Disputationem inauguralem medicam de haemorrhagia . . . submittit . . . H. R. 1684.

RAEDT, FRANCISCUS DE [*fl.* 1656-1659] Anatomische beschrijvinge van een wanschepsel, geboren op de Elderschans buyten aerdenburg, ontleet, door . . . Louis de Bils . . . briefs-gewyse gesonden door . . . F. de Raet aen A. Parent . . . Middelburgh, Henrick Smidt, 1659.

16 p. plates. 20 cm.   [**9349**]

—*respondent.* Disputatio medica inauguralis, de phtisi . . . Ultrajecti, Ex officina Johannis à Waesberge, 1656.

[8] p. 20 cm.   [**9350**]
Diss.—Utrecht.

—*See* BILS, L. de. Specimina anatomica. 1661.

RAEI, JOHANNES DE [1618-1702] *praeses.* Disputatio philosophica qua quaeritur, quo pacto anima in corpore moveat & sentiat . . . Lugduni Batavorum, Apud viduam & haeredes Johannis Elsevirii, 1663.

[8] p. 25 cm.   [**9351**]
Diss.—Leyden (L. van Gaesbeeck, *respondent*)

—*See* CASSIUS, A. De triumviratu intestinali. 1669; LAMSWEERDE, J. B. van. Respirationis Swammerdammianae exspiratio. 1674.

RAESVELT, THOMAS LUDOLPHUS [*fl.* 1687] *respondent.* Disputatio inauguralis medica, de melancholia . . . Trajecti ad Rhenum, Ex officina Francisci Halma, 1687.

8 p. 22 cm.   [**9352**]
Diss.—Utrecht.

RAET, FRANCISCUS DE. *See* RAEDT, Franciscus de [*fl.* 1656-1659]

RAFFAELLO, FRANCESCO DI. Trattato delle virtu et proprieta dell'olio quint'essenza, & vero balsamo, che si cava dal rosmarino ... Roma, Perugia, Ristampato in Siena, Matteo Florimi, 1610.

22, [2] p.   15 cm.   [9353]

RAGAZZINA, FRANCESCO FERDINANDO. La medicina posta all'essame nel tribunale della verità. Discorso apologetico diviso in due trattati ... Nel primo de' quali ... delle febri, e de li cordiali ... Nel secondo de' narcotici ... Brescia, Policreto Turlino, 1693.

43, 328 (i.e. 330) p.   front., illus.   25 cm.
[9354]

Additional page at end of part 1, numbered 171, inserted.
Edited by Pietro Comi.
Errata on p. 7-13, first group of paging, corrected by slips pasted over misprints.

RAGUAGLIO, della peste. 1658. *See* COLANTONIO, G.

RAGUSEO, GIORGIO [*ca.* 1579-1622] Epistolarum mathematicarum; seu, De divinatione, libri duo ... His accessit ejusdem autoris Disputatio de puero, & puella, qui superioribus annis Patavii, occasione magni cujusdam incendii, e ruinis extracti atque ... revixisse putantur. Parisiis, Sumptibus Nicolai Buon, 1623.

[8], 643, [33] p.   18 cm.   [9355]
Edited by Charles Annibal Fabrot.

RAHN, MARTIN [*fl.* 1682] *respondent.* Positiones inaugurales de morbillis ... proponit Martinus Rahn ... Altdorfii, Literis Henrici Meyeri [1682]

20 p.   19 cm.   [9356]
Diss. — Altdorf.

RAHNISCH, CHRISTOPH [*fl.* 1672] *See* PFEIFFER, J. P., *praeses.* Dissertatio philologica. 1672.

RAHTS zu Halberstadt abgefassete Apotheken-Ordnung und revidirte Taxa. 1697. *See* HALBERSTADT. Ordinances, local laws, etc.

RAICUS, JOHANN [*d.* 1631] Tractatus de podagra medico-kimicus. Francofurti, In officina Danielis & Davidis Aubriorum & Clementis Schleichii, 1621.

[24], 54 p.   16 cm.   [9357]

—*praeses.* De phthisi ex tartaro, ut frequentiore disputatio publica ... Upsaliae, Excudebat Eschillus Matthiae, 1628.

[58] p.   18 cm.   [9358]
Diss. — Uppsala (O. J. Bååk, *respondent*)

RAIDA, BALTHASAR [*fl.* 1614-1624] *praeses.* Disputatio medica de apoplexia ... Bremae, E typographeo Johannis Wesselii, 1617.

18, [2] p.   20 cm.   [9359]
Diss. — Bremen (J. Danielis, *respondent*)

RAIDIUS, BALTHASAR. *See* RAIDA, Balthasar [*fl.* 1614-1624]

RAINSSANT, NICOLAS [*fl.* 1663-1699] *praeses.* Quaestio medica ... Est-ne optima vivendi lex sua unicuique consuetudo? [Lutetiae, Josephus Thomasseau, 1676]

4 p.   25 cm.   [9360]
Diss. — Paris (J. Thomasseau, *respondent*)

RAITH, JOHANN KONRAD [*fl.* 1692] *respondent. See* CAMERARIUS, R. J., *praeses.* Dissertatio physica de elementis. 1692.

RAITH, JOHANN ULRICH [*fl.* 1675-1676] *respondent. See* METZGER, G. B., *praeses.* Disputatio medica de tussi. 1676 [and] Thesium chiriatricarum sylloge V. de fonticulis. 1675.

RAIUS, JOANNES. *See* RAY, John [1627-1705]

RALEIGH, Sir WALTER [1552?-1618] *See* DIGBY, Sir K. Medicina experimentalis Digbaeana. 1672-1676, 1687; LE FÈVRE, N. Discours sur le grand cordial de Sr Walter Rawleigh. 1665 [and] A discourse. 1664.

RALL, GEORG FRIEDRICH [*d.* 1670] De generatione animalium disquisitio medico-physica in qua ... D. D. Guilielmi Harvei & Anton. Deusingii sententia a nuperis Jani Orchami [pseud.] instantiis vindicatur, ipsumque generationis opus juxta recentiorum observata succincte exponitur. Stetini, Typis Michaelis Höpfneri, impensis Melchioris Klosemanni Jun. bibliopol. Francofurt. [1669?]

[24], 379 (i.e. 377), [2] p.   14 cm.   [9361]

RAM, PIETER DE [*fl.* 1668] *respondent.* Disputatio medica inauguralis de angina ... Lugduni Batavorum, Apud viduam & haeredes Joannis Elsevirii, 1668.

[8] p.   23 cm.   [9362]
Diss. — Leyden.

RAM, RUDOLF [*fl.* 1678] *respondent.* Disputatio medica inauguralis de fluxu foemineo ... Franequerae, Ex officina Johannis Gyselaer, 1678.

[16] p.   21 cm.   **[9363]**

Diss. — Franeker.

RAMAZZINI, BERNARDINO [1633-1714] De constitutione anni M. DC. LXXXX. ac de rurali epidemia, quae Mutinensis agri, & vicinarum regionum colonos graviter afflixit, dissertatio ... Mutinae, Typis haeredum Juliani Cassiani, 1690.

88 p.   23 cm.   **[9364]**

"De constitutione anni M. DC. LXXXXI. apud Mutinenses dissertatio ... Mutinae, Typis haeredum Cassiani, 1691" (p. [53]-88) has special title page.

— De fontium Mutinensium admiranda scaturigine tractatus physico-hydrostaticus ... Mutinae, Typis haeredum Suliani, 1691.

87 p.   plate, table.   21 cm.   **[9365]**

— De morbis artificum diatriba ... Mutinae, Typis Antonii Capponi, 1700.

viii, 360 p.   18 cm.   **[9366]**

— Exercitatio iatropologetica ... seu, Responsum ad scripturam quandam ... Annibalis Cervii ... Mutinae, Apud Demetrium Dignum, 1679.

17, [1] p.   26 cm.   **[9367]**

— Risposta ... alla terza censura dell'eccellentiss. sig. dottore Gio. Andrea Moneglia. Modana, Eredi di Viviano Soliani, 1682.

70 p.   30 cm.   **[9368]**

— *See* ARIOSTO, F. De oleo montis Zibinii. 1698.

RAMBALDI, ANGELO [*fl.* 1690] Ambrosia arabica, overo della salutare bevanda cafe ... Bologna, Longhi, 1691.

69 p.   14 cm.   **[9369]**

RAMBALDUS, JOSEPH [*fl.* 1689] Compendiaria tractatio de febris quidditate juxta veterum, & recentiorum placita ... Accessit Responsum consultationi P.M.T. Ph.C. Genuae, Typis Antonii Georgii Franchelli [1689?]

[8], 163 p.   14 cm.   **[9370]**

"De quidditate febris juxta placita Sylvii, et Galeni" (p. [76]-142) has special title page.

Imperfect: p. 1-2 wanting.

RAMELIN, JEAN. *See* REMMELIN, Johann [1583-1632]

RAMELOV, MATTHIAS [*fl.* 1642-1651] *respondent.* See SEBISCH, M. [1578-1674?] *praeses.* Disputatio de variolis et morbillis prima [-sexta & ultima] 1642.

RAMESEY, WILLIAM [*b.* 1626 *or* 7] Ελμινθολογια; or, Some physical considerations of the matter, origination, and several species of wormes ... London, Printed by John Streater, for George Sawbridge, 1668.

[4], 9, 364 (i.e. 374), [1] p.   front. (port.), plate.   17 cm.   **[9371]**

— Θανασιμα, και δηαητηρια, Tractatus de venenis; or, A treatise of poysons; their sundry sorts, names, natures and virtues, with their severall symptomes, signes, diagnosticks, prognosticks, and antidotes ... London, Printed by S. G. for D. Pakeman, 1661.

[32], 239, [16] p.   15 cm.   **[9372]**

— [The same.] Lifes security; or, A phylosophical and physical discourse; shewing the names, natures, & vertues of all sorts of venomes and venemous things ... And the remedy for the cure of any poyson by them ... As it was humbly tendred ... about four years ago; and now anno dom. 1665. published ... By W. R. ... London, 1665.

[63], 239, [16] p.   15 cm.   **[9373]**

Imperfect: margins trimmed.

RAMIREZ, GASPAR BRAVO DE SOBREMONTE. *See* BRAVO DE SOBREMONTE RAMIREZ, Gaspar [1603-1683]

RAMÍREZ, LUIS. *See* PÉREZ RAMÍREZ, Luis [*fl.* 17th cent.]

RAMÍREZ DE CARRIÓN, MANUEL [1584-1650] Maravillas de naturaleza, en que se contienen dos mil secretos de cosas naturales ... Recogidos de la leccion de diversos ... autores ... Montilla, Juan Batista de Morales, 1629.

[6], 146 (i.e. 144) ll.   19 cm.   **[9374]**

Imperfect: ll. 113-116 misbound between ll. 140 and ll. 143 (i.e. ll. 141).

RAMÓN LULL. *See* LULL, Ramón [1232-*ca.* 1316]

RAMOS, SIMÓN [*fl.* 1606-1634] *See* ORTIZ DE LA LAGUNA, G. Responde al doctor Simon Ramos ... a un papel que embiò contra el doctor Caldera. 1634.

RAMPALLE, sieur de [*d. ca.* 1660] *tr. See* RONPHYLE. La chyromantie naturelle de Ronphile. 1653, 1665; [German tr.] *In* Höchstfürtreflichtes chiromantisch- und physiognomisches Klee-Blat. 1695.

RAMSAY, Charles Aloysius [*fl.* 1689] *tr. See* Digby, *Sir* K. Medicina experimentalis Digbaeana. 1672–1676, 1687.

RAMSAY, William. *See* Ramesey, William [*b.* 1626 *or* 7]

RAMSAY, William. *See also* Ramsye, William.

RAMSEY, *Judge. See* rumsey, Walter [1584–1660]

RAMSYE, William. Conjugium conjurgium; or, Some serious considerations on marriage. Wherein (by way of caution and advice to a friend) its nature, ends, events, concomitant accidents, etc. are examined by William Seymar Esq. [pseud.] . . . London, Allen Bancks, 1673.

[48], 153 p. 15 cm. **[9375]**

Imperfect: upper margins trimmed.

RANCHIN, François [1564–1641] Opuscula medica . . . publici juris facta, cura & studio Henrici Gras . . . Lugduni, Apud Petrum Ravaud, 1627.

[22], 731, [31] p. 26 cm. **[9376]**

First gathering: t. p., ã2, ã3, [2d] ã2, unsigned leaf.
Signature ã3, supplied in photocopy, contains an epistle by Henri Gras addressed to the author. Conjugate leaf of ã3 wanting.
Contents. — Apollinare sacrum; De Monspeliensis Universitatis origine, progressu, administratione & celebritate. — In Hippocratis Jusjurandum commentarius (with Greek and Latin texts). — Pathologia universalis. — Tractatus de morbis puerorum. — Tractatus de morbis virginum. — Gerocomia, seu Tractatus de morbis senum. — Tractatus de morbis subitaneis. — Tractatus de curatione morborum, qui purgationem comitantur, aut consequuntur. — Tractatus de consultationibus medicis.

—Opuscules; ou, Traictés divers et curieux en medecine . . . Lyon, Pierre Ravaud, 1640.

[40], 824 p. 18 cm. **[9377]**

Contents. — De la peste. — L'histoire de la peste qui affligea Montpellier és années 1629 & 1630. — De la lepre. — De la verole. — Des accidens de la poste. — Des accidens de la gehenne. — De la cruentation des corps morts. — De la nature & propriétés des cerfs. — De la therebentine.

—Oeuvres pharmaceutiques . . . Assavoir, un traicté general de la pharmacie. Ensemble en docte commentaire sur les quatre theoremes & canons de Mesuè. Avec deux . . . traictez, l'un des simples medicamens purgatifs, & l'autre des venins . . . Lyon, Pierre Ravaud, 1624.

[36], 980, [19] p. 17 cm. **[9378]**

Includes Latin text of Mesuë's Canones generales and a paraphrastic commentary on his De simplicibus.
"Traicté des venins. Dicté a Montpellier aux compagnons pharmaciens, par M. François Ranchin": p. [809]-980.

—[The same.] . . . Rouen, Romain de Beauvais, 1637.

[32], 850 (i.e. 879), [16] p. 17 cm. **[9379]**

Imperfect: title page mutilated.

—Questions en chirurgie, sur les oeuvres de maistre Guy de Gauliac, divisées en trois parties . . . Rev., cor., & parfaicte de nouveau par l'autheur. Paris, Marc Orry, 1604.

2 v. ([36], 626, [12] p.; [31], 761, [15] p.) 18 cm. **[9380]**

"Seconde et troisieme partie" has special title page.

—[The same.] Questions françoises, sur toute la chirurgie de M. Guy de Gauliac, divisée en trois parties . . . Derniere ed. rev. & corr. . . . Lyon, Simon Rigaud, 1627.

[16], 552 (i.e. 554), [22] p.; [8], 691, [29] p. 19 cm. **[9381]**

"Seconde, & troisieme partie" has special title page.

—[The same.] . . . Rouen, Jacques Besongne, 1628.

[15], 554, [21] p.; [8], 691, [29] p. 18 cm. **[9382]**

"Seconde, & troisime partie" has special title page.
Different setting of type.

—[Dutch tr.] Heelkonstige geschillen, wegens de werken van Meester Guido de Gauliac, geschift in drie deelen . . . Beschreven in 't Frans . . . En nu vertaalt door Aarnout van Wymis . . . Amsterdam, Jacob Benjamin, 1662.

[8], 358 p.; [4], 466, [8] p. 19 cm. **[9383]**

"Het tweede en derde deel" has special title page dated 1661.

—Tractatus duo posthumi: I. De morbis ante partum, in partu, & post partum. II. De purificatione rerum infectarum post pestilentiam. Lugduni, Sumptibus Petri Ravaud, 1645.

[16], 320 p. 18 cm. **[9384]**

RANCKE, Andreas [*fl.* 1681] *respondent. See* Olearius, J., *praeses.* De mantice cometica dissertatio theologica. 1681.

RAND, William [*fl.* 1656] *tr. See* Riolan, J. [1580–1657] A sure guide. 1657, 1665, 1671.

[**RANDOLPH**, Thomas, 1605-1635] Cornelianum dolium. Comoedia lepidissima, optimorum judiciis approbata, & theatrali coryphoeo, nec immerito, donata, palma chorali apprime digna. Auctore, T. R. . . . Londini, Apud Tho. Harperum, et vaeneunt per Tho. Slaterum, & Laurentium Chapman, 1638.

[19], 142, [2] p.   15 cm.   [**9385**]

Added engraved title page.

Imperfect: sig. G^I and G^{I2} interchanged.

STC 20691.

RANGO, Conrad Tiburtius [1639-1700] De capillamentis seu vulgo parucquen, liber singularis. Magdeburgi, Sumptibus Tobiae Schröteri, imprimebat Johannes Müllerus, 1663.

[2], 254 p.   14 cm.   [**9386**]

RANGO, Tiburtius. See Rango, Conrad Tiburtius [1639-1700]

RANNUTIO, Arragoni. See Arragoni, Rannutio.

RANTZAU, Henrik [1526-1598] Henrici Rantzovii De conservanda valetudine liber, in privatum liberorum suorum usum ab ipso conscriptus, ac editus, a Dethlevo Silvio . . . In quo de diaeta, itinere, annis olimactericis, & antidotis praestantissimis, brevia & utilia praecepta continentur. 5. ed., auctior & emendatior. Seorsim accessit Gulielmi Grataroli . . . De literatorum, & eorum qui magistratum gerunt, conservanda valetudine. Liber. Francofurti, Typis Nicolai Hofmanni, sumtibus Jonę Rhodii, 1604.

239 p.   13 cm.   [**9387**]

"Guilielmi Grataroli . . . De memoria reparanda" (p. [192]-239) has special title page.

Reprint of the 1596 Frankfurt edition.

—[The same.] . . . 6. ed., auctior & emendatior . . . Francofurti, Typis Nicolai Hofmanni, sumptibus haeredum Jacobi Fischeri, 1617.

239 p.   13 cm.   [**9388**]

"Guilielmi Grataroli . . . De memoria reparanda" (p. [193]-239) has special title page.

Different setting of type.

—[The same.] In Hygieia. 1628; Regimen sanitatis Salernitanum. The Englishmans doctor. 1624.

—[German tr.] De conservanda valetudine; das ist, Von Erhaltung menschlicher Gesundheit . . . Vor dieser Zeit von . . . Heinrich Rantzau . . . in Latein gebracht, jetzt aber gantz trewlich verdeutscht, zum

Andernmal ubersehen, und mit vielen herzlichen Experimentlein . . . vermehret. Darbey auch zwey nützliche Tractetlein von der erschrecklichen Seuche der Pestilenz, des . . . Johannis Pontani verzeichnet, desgleichen ein kurtzer Extract Johannis Wittichii De peste . . . Durch Johannem Wittichium . . . [Heidelberg?] Typis Voegelinianis, 1601.

[24], 263; [63] p.   20 cm.   [**9389**]

Published in Heidelberg? Cf. Benzing (A), p. 185.

Contents as in the 1587 Leipzig edition.

RAOUL, Jean, ed. and tr. See Guy de Chauliac. Les fleurs du grand Guidon. [n.d.], 1646, 1660, 1673, 1693.

RAPAERTIUS, Petrus [fl. 1606] See Stull, J. Medendi practica generalis. 1606.

RAPHAEL, Solomon, pseud. See rummel, Johann Pharamund [fl. 1630-1648]

RAPHELENGIEN, Franciscus [1539-1597] See Dodoens, R. Cruydt-boeck. 1618, 1644.

RAPHELENGIEN, Justus [d. 1628] ed. See Dodoens, R. Cruydt-boeck. 1618, 1644.

RAPIN, médecin de Dijon [fl. 1682] See Dissertation sur les ulceres des reins et de la vessie. 1685.

RAPP, Johann Konrad [fl. 1681] respondent. See Winckler, F. C., praeses. Disputatio inauguralis medica de dysenteria. 1681.

RAPPORT de l'ouverture du corps de feu Madame. See Boursier, L. (Bourgeois). Fidelle relation de l'accouchement. 1627

RAS, Ernestus, ed. See Hippocrates. [Aphorismi. Dutch.] 1665.

RASIS. See Muḥammad ibn Zakarīyā, Abū Bakr, al-Rāzi [865-925]

RASOR, Johann Konrad [fl. 1669-1675] respondent. Disputatio medico-chirurgica inauguralis de ophthalmia una cum fistula lacrymali . . . Lugduni Batavorum, Apud viduam & heredes Johannis Elsevirii, 1675.

[16] p.   19 cm.   [**9390**]

Diss.—Leyden.

—See Sebisch, J. A., praeses. Disputatio cheirurgica de tumoribus praeter naturam in genere. 1669.

RASPANUS, FABRITIUS, *ed. See* AVICENNA. Avicennae Arabum medicorum principis. 1608.

RASPE, GOTTFRIED [*d.* 1633] Disputatio decimanona, de visu et auditu ... Lipsiae, Gregorius Ritzsch [1628]

[16] p.   18 cm.   **[9391]**
Diss.—Leipzig (C. Göbel, *respondent*)

RASPIUS, GOTFRIDUS. *See* RASPE, Gottfried [*d.* 1633].

RAST, GEORG [1651-1729] *praeses.* Ebrietas medice considerata ... Regiomonti, Typis Friderici Reusneri haeredum [1682]

[32] p.   20 cm.   **[9392]**
Diss. pro loco—Königsberg (C. R. Hertz, *respondent*)

RATHS DER STADT LEIPZIG ... ORDNUNG UND TAXO. 1689. *See* LEIPZIG. Ordinances, local laws, etc.

RATICHIUS, JAKOB [*fl.* 1615] *respondent. See* MARTINI, J., *praeses.* Disputatio physica de animarum humanarum origine. 1615.

RATISBON. COLLEGIUM MEDICUM. *See* KOLLEGIUM DER AERZTE, Regensburg.

RATTA, GIOVANNI ANTONIO. Breve descrizione del corpo umano e dell'uso delle sue parti ... Roma, Per il Buagni, 1700.

[14], 140, [8] p.   front.   15 cm.   **[9393]**

RATTO, GIUSEPPE [16th cent.] *See* FACIO, S. Paradoxes de la peste. 1620.

RATTRAY, SYLVESTER [*fl.* 1650-1666] Aditus novus ad occultas sympathiae et antipathiae causas inveniendas: per principia philosophiae naturalis, ex fermentorum artificiosa anatomia hausta, patefactus ... Glasguae, Andreas Anderson, 1658.

[16], 135 p.   15 cm.   **[9394]**
First prelim. leaf (p. [1-2]) blank except for a capital A near the center of the recto.
According to James Finlayson (Janus, 5. année, 1900, p. 569) the first medical work printed in Glasgow.

—[The same.] ... Tubingae, Impensis Johannis Henrici Reisii, 1660.

216 p.   13 cm.   **[9395]**
Imperfect: p. 167-170 wanting.

—[The same.]
[1]-71 p.   21 cm. (*In* Theatrum sympatheticum auctum. Norimbergae, 1662)   **[9396]**
Caption title.

—*See* PAPIN, N. Theatrum sympateticum. 1662; THEATRUM SYMPATETICUM. Dutch. 1697.

RATZENBERGER, MATTHÄUS [1501-1559] *See* SCHOLTZ, L. Consiliorum medicinalium ... liber singularis. 1610.

RAU, JOHANN JACOB [1668-1719] Responsio ad qualemcunque defensionem Frederici Ruischii, quam haud ita pridem edidit, pro septo scroti. In qua hujus litis anatomicae detegitur origo ... Adjuncta est hujus calci auctoris epistola. Amstelaedami, Apud Janssonio-Waesbergios, 1699.

[1], 14, [6] p.   plates.   22 cm.   **[9397]**

—Another issue, with date changed to 1700.
                                               [9398]
Imperfect: [6] p. (plates with text) wanting.

RAUCHWOLFF, LEONHARD. *See* RAUWOLFF, Leonhard [*d.* 1596]

RAULT [*fl.* 1659-ca. 1673] *tr. See* DIGBY, *Sir* K. Discours fait en une celebre assemblée. 1673, 1681; PORTA, G. B. della. La physionomie humaine. 1660.

RAULT, D. M., *ed. See* LULL, R. Testamentum. 1663?

RAUMBURGER, ANTON [*fl.* 1697] *respondent.* Disputatio inauguralis medica exhibens puerulum rhachitide detentum ... Gissae Hassorum, Typis Henningi Mülleri [1697]

[4], 24 p.   22 cm.   **[9399]**
Diss.—Giessen.

—*See* VALENTINI, M. B., *praeses.* Disputatio medico-chirurgica. 1697.

RAUMER, JOHANN GEORG [*fl.* 1687] *respondent. See* LIMMER, C. P., *praeses.* Collegii Physici disputatorii disputatio octava. 1687.

RAUSSENDORFF, GEORG FRIEDRICH [*fl.* 1682-1684] *respondent. See* LOSS, J., *praeses.* Dissertatio medica de hydrophobia. 1682; METZGER, G. B., *praeses.* Dissertatio inauguralis medica de podagra. 1684.

RAUTNER, CHRISTIAN, *pseud. See* KNORR VON ROSENROTH, Christian [1636-1689]

RAUWOLFF, LEONHARD [*d.* 1596] A collection of curious travels & voyages. In two tomes. The first containing Dr. Leonhart Rauwolff's Itinerary into the Eastern countries ... Translated from the high Dutch by Nicholas Staphorst. The second taking in many parts of Greece, Asia minor, Egypt ... from the observations of Mons. Belon, Mr. Vernon, Dr. Spon, Dr. Smith, Dr. Huntington, Mr. Greaves, Alpinus, Veslingius, Thevenot's Collections, and others. To which are added, three catalogues of such trees, shrubs, and herbs as grow in the Levant. By John Ray ... London, S. Smith and B. Walford, 1693.

[31], 396 (i.e. 380) p.; [1], 186 (i.e. 184) p.; 45, [3] p.   illus.   19 cm.   **[9400]**

Part [3] has half title: Stirpium orientalium rariorum catalogi tres.

Part 1 is a translation of Aigentliche Beschreibung der Raiss, so er vor diser Zeit gegen Auffgang inn die Morgenländer, published in Lauingen, in 1583.

The first issue of 1693. Cf. Keynes (F) 92.

RAVE, ERNESTUS REGNERUS [*fl.* 1695] *respondent.* Disputatio medica inauguralis de hydrope in genere ... Trajecti ad Rhenum, Ex officina Francisci Halma, 1695.

[16] p.   24 cm.   **[9401]**

Diss. — Utrecht.

RAVEAU, NICOLAS [*fl.* 1675] *See* BACHOT, E. Vesperiae et pileus doctoralis. 1675.

RAVELINGEN, FRANS VAN. *See* RAPHELENGIEN, Franciscus [1539-1597]

RAVELINGEN, JOOST VAN. *See* RAPHELENGIEN, Justus [*d.* 1628]

RAVELLI, FRANCESCO MARTINO. Ars memoriae: hactenus ab ejus primo autore, hujusce secundo quidem incognito, ita obscure studio tradita, ut legere nedum intelligere quis posset jam vero in gratiam et usum juventutis explicata, exemplis aucta ... Francofurti, Typis Nicolai Hoffmanni, sumptibus Joann. Theodorici de Bry, 1617.

710 (i.e. 107), [5] p.   15 cm.   **[9402]**

With this are bound; Paëpp, J. Artificiosae memoriae fundamenta. 1619; Paëpp, J. Εισαγωγη; seu, Introductio. 1618; Paëpp, J. Vita M. Tullii Ciceronis. 1618.

RAVELLY, JEAN. Dissertation sur la nature des cours de ventre, et sur les remedes qu'on y peut apporter ... Paris, Jean d'Houry, 1677.

[12], 142 p.   16 cm.   **[9403]**

—Traité de la maladie da la rage ... Metz, Jean Collignon, 1696.

[12], 92 (i.e. 192) p.   15 cm.   **[9404]**

RAVENS, JOANNES ARNOLDSZ. *See* CORVINUS, Johannes Arnoldi [*ca.* 1582-1650]

RAVENSTEIN, ADRIAN. *See* RAVESTEIN, Adrian [*fl.* 1651]

RAVESTEIN, ADRIAN [*fl.* 1651] *ed. See* CASTELLI, B. Lexicon medicum Graeco-Latinum. 1651, 1657, 1664, 1665, 1669, 1685.

RAVESTEYN, JOANNES VAN [1618-1681] *ed. See* JOEL, F. [1510-1570] Opera medica. 1663.

RAWLEIGH, WALTHER. *See* RALEIGH, *Sir* Walter [1552?-1618]

RAWLEY, WILLIAM [1588?-1667] *ed. See* BACON, F., *viscount St. Albans.* History naturall and experimentall. 1638 [and] Operum moralium et civilium tomus. 1638 [and] Sylva sylvarum. 1627, 1658, 1664, 1676.

RAWLIN, THOMAS [1569-1613] Admonitio pseudochymicis; seu, Alphabetarium philosophicum ... in quo D. D. Antonii Aurum potabile obiter refutatur, & genuina veri auri potabilis ... praeparatio proponitur ... Londini, Ed. Allde [1610?]

[14], 42 p.   19 cm.   **[9405]**

STC 20768.

RAWOLFF, LEONHARD. *See* RAUWOLFF, Leonhard [*d.* 1596]

RAY, JOHN [1627-1705] Catalogus plantarum Angliae, et insularum adjacentium: tum indigenas, tum in agris passim cultas complectens ... Londini, Typis E. C. & A. C., impensis J. Martyn, 1670.

[22], 358, [1] p.   16 cm.   **[9406]**

Errata: p. [359]

First preliminary leaf (blank) wanting.

Keynes(F) 7.

—[The same.] ... Ed. 2., plantis circiter quadraginta sex, & observationibus aliquam multis auctior ... Londini, Typis Andr. Clark, impensis Joh. Martyn, 1677.

[28], 311, [15] p.   plates.   16 cm.   [**9407**]
Keynes(F) 8.

—De variis plantarum methodis dissertatio brevis. In qua agitur I. De methodi origine & progressu. II. De notis generum characteristicis. III. De methodo sua in specie. IV. De notis quas reprobat & rejiciendas censet D. Tournefort. V. De methodo Tournefortiana. Londini, S. Smith & B. Walford, 1696.

[13], 48 p.   20 cm.   [**9408**]
Keynes(F) 99.
Bound with *his* Synopsis methodica stirpium Britannicarum. 1696.

—Historia plantarum species hactenus editas aliasque insuper multas noviter inventas & descriptas complectens. In qua agitur primo de plantis in genere, earumque partibus, accidentibus & differentiis; deinde genera omnia tum summa tum subalterna ad species usque infimas, notis suis certis & characteristicis definita, methodo naturae vestigiis insistente disponuntur ... Tomus primus [-secundus] Londini, Typis Mariae Clark, prostant apud Henricum Faithorne, 1686-1688.

2 v.   illus.   38 cm.   [**9409**]
Keynes(F) 48-49.

—Methodus plantarum nova, brevitatis & perspicuitatis causa synoptice in tabulis exhibita ... Londini, Impensis Henrici Faithorne & Joannis Kersey, 1682.

[24], 166, [34] p.   front., plate.   17 cm.   [**9410**]
Keynes(F) 40.

—Observations topographical, moral, & physiological; made in a journey through part of the Low-countries, Germany, Italy and France: with A catalogue of plants not native to England, found spontaneously growing in those parts, and their virtues ... Whereunto is added A brief account of Francis Willughby ... his voyage through a great part of Spain. London, John Martyn, 1673.

[15], 499 p.; [7], 115 p.   illus., plates, port.   19 cm.   [**9411**]
Part [2] has special title page: Catalogus stirpium in exteris regionibus a nobis observatarum, quae vel non omnino vel parce admodum in Anglia sponte proveniunt. Londini, Typis Andreae Clark, impensis J. Martyn, 1673.
Keynes(F) 21.

—Stirpium Europaearum extra Britannias nascentium sylloge. Quas partim observavit ipse, partim e Car. Clusii Historia, C. Bauhini Prod. & cat. Bas., F. Columnae Ecphrasi, Catalogis Hollandicar. A. Commelini, Altorfinarum M. Hofmanni, Sicularum P. Bocconi, Monspeliensium P. Magnoli collegit Joannes Raius. Adjiciuntur Catalogi rariorum Alpinarum & Pyrenaicarum, Baldensium, Hispanicarum Grisleii, Graecarum & Orientalium, Creticarum, Aegyptiacarum aliique: ab eodem ... Londini, Sam. Smith & Benj. Walford, 1694.

[28], 45-220, 225-400 p.; 45, [3] p.   front. (port.)   19 cm.   [**9412**]
Keynes(F) 97.

—Synopsis methodica animalium quadrupedum et serpentini generis ... Praemittuntur nonnulla De animalium in genere, sensu, generatione, divisione, &c. ... Londini, S. Smith & B. Walford, 1693.

[16], 336, [8] p.   front. (port.)   20 cm.   [**9413**]
Keynes(F) 91. (Without the errata slip mounted on the verso of the title page.)
With this is bound *his* Methodus insectorum. Londini, 1705.

—Synopsis methodica stirpium Britannicarum, tum indigenis, tum in agris cultis, locis suis dispositis, additis generum characteristicis, specierum descriptionibus, & virium epitome. Ed. 2. ... Accessit ... Aug. Rivini Epistola ad Joan. Raium de methodo: cum ejusdem responsoria, in qua D. Tournefort Elementa botanica tanguntur. Londini, S. Smith & B. Walford, 1696.

[38], 346, [22] p.; 55, [1] p.   20 cm.   [**9414**]
Keynes(F) 55.
Addition to errata pasted on last page.
With this is bound *his* De variis plantarum methodis. 1696.

—Three physico-theological discourses, concerning I. The primitive chaos, and creation of the world. II. The general deluge ... III. The dissolution of the world ... 2. ed. corr. ... enl. ... London, Sam. Smith, 1693.

[24], 162, [8], 163-406, [2] p.   plates.   19 cm.   [**9415**]
Keynes(F) 82.

—, *ed. See* RAUWOLFF, L. A collection of curious travels & voyages. 1693.

—*See* KÖNIG, E. Regni vegetabilis pars altera. 1696.

RAYGER, FERDINAND [*fl.* 1655] *respondent. See* SEBISCH, J. A., *praeses.* Dissertatio anatomica de jecore. 1655.

RAYGER, KÁROLY [1641-1707] *respondent.* Dissertatio medica inauguralis de salivae natura et vitiis . . . Argentorati, Literis Georgii Andreae Dolhopffii, 1667.

[28] p. 19 cm. **[9416]**

Diss. — Strasbourg.

—*See* SEBISCH, J. A., *praeses.* Dissertatio medica de inedia. 1664.

—, *ed. See* SPINDLER, P. Observationum medicinalium centuria. 1691.

RAYGER, KÁROLY [1675-1731] *respondent.* Dissertatio inauguralis medica de labrosulcio, seu cheilocace . . . [Altdorffii] Cattitero Henrici Meyeri [1698]

36 p. 20 cm. **[9417]**

Diss. — Altdorf.

—*See* HOFFMANN, J. M., *praeses.* Exercitatio anatomico-physiologica de fluidorum catholicorum foetus motu. 1695.

RAYMUNDUS LULLIUS. *See* LULL, Ramón [1232-*ca.* 1316]

RAYNALDE, THOMAS [*fl.* 1540-1555] *See* [ROESLIN, E.] The birth of mankinde. 1604, 1613, 1626, 1634, 1654.

RAYNAUD, FRANÇOIS. Traité des fievres malignes et pourprées; dans lequel on propose un systéme nouveau sur la nature de ces mêmes fiévres, qui explique mécaniquement tous les symptomes; d'où resulte la maniere précise de les guérir, non pas par l'usage de la saignée, des acides & de la glace, mais par celui des diaphorétiques, ou remedes propres à faire transpirer . . . Carpentras, Barthelemy Ravase, 1695.

[20], 276 p. 15 cm. **[9418]**

Imperfect: sig. āii-āiii wanting?

—[The same.] . . . Brusselle, François Foppens, 1695.

[6], 165, [2] p. 15 cm. **[9419]**

RAYNAUD, THÉOPHILE, *Father* [1587-1663] De incorruptione cadaverum, occasione demortui foeminei corporis post aliquot secula incorrupti, nuper refossi

carpentoracti . . . Ed. alt., emaculata, & aucta. Arausioni, Typis Eduardi Rabani, 1651.

[19], 324, [11] p. 18 cm. **[9420]**

—De martyrio per pestem ad martyrium improprium, & proprium vulgare comparato, disquisitio theologica . . . Lugduni, Sumpt. Jacobi Cardon, 1630.

[16], 633, [15] p. 18 cm. **[9421]**

—De ortu infantium contra naturam, per sectionem caesaream, tractatio . . . Accessit discussio erroris popularis, de communione pro mortuis. Lugduni, Sumpt. Gabr. Boissat [Ex typographia Claudii Cayne] 1637.

[24], 398, [17] p. 18 cm. **[9422]**

RAZENBERGER, MATTHAEUS. *See* RATZENBERGER, Matthäus [1501-1559]

al-RĀZĪ. *See* MUHAMMAD IBN ZAKARĪYĀ, ABŪ BAKR, al-Rāzī [865-925]

RAZZENBERG, MATTHAEUS. *See* RATZENBERGER, Matthäus [1501-1559]

READ, ALEXANDER [1586?-1641] The workes . . . Containing I. Chirurgicall lectures of tumors and ulcers. II. A treatise of the first part of chirurgery . . . and the methodicall doctrine of wounds. III. A treatise of all the muscles of the body of man . . . Published in his lifetime in severall treatises, and now in one volume, corrected and amended. The 2d ed. London, Printed by E. G. for Richard Thrale, and sold by John Clarke, 1650.

[8], 270 p.; [10], 206 p.; [4], [8] p. 23 cm. **[9423]**

Parts 2 and 3 have special title pages.

—[The same.] . . . The 3rd ed. London, Printed by E. T. for Richard Thrale, 1659.

[12], 524 (i.e. 520), [8] p. 19 cm. **[9424]**

Imperfect? p. 277-280 wanting? (error in pagination?); leaves of sheet 3y wrongly inserted.

"A treatise of the first part of chirurgery . . . containing the methodicall doctrine of wound" (p. [275]-485) and "A treatise of all the muscles of the whole body" (p. [487]-524 (i.e. 520), [1-8]) have special title pages.

—The chirurgicall lectures of tumors and ulcers. Delivered on Tusedayes appointed for these exercises, and keeping of their courts in the Chirurgeans

Hall these three yeeres last past, viz. 1632, 1633, and 1634 ... London, Printed by J. H[aviland] for Francis Constable and E. B[ush] 1635.

[14], 334 p.   19 cm.   **[9425]**
STC 20781.

—Chirurgorum comes; or, the whole practice of chirurgery. Begun by ... Dr. Read; continued and completed by a member of the College of Physicians in London ... London, Printed by Edw. Jones for Christopher Wilkinson, 1687.

[26], 714 p.   plate.   20 cm.   **[9426]**

"An appendix concerning chirurgeon-reports before a magistrate, upon their view of a wounded person" (p. 415-473) is a summary of Fortunato Fidele's De relationibus medicorum, published in Palermo in 1602.

"Chapt. XLII. Of lithotomy, or cutting for the stone" (p. 626-643) is a close paraphrase of Joannes Groeneveld's Διθολογια' A treatise of the stone and gravel, published in London in 1677.

"The practice of chirurgery. Part IV. Book VIII. Of supplying defects in the body" (p. 645-704) is a summary of Book 2 of Gaspare Tagliacozzi's De curtorum chirurgia per insitionem, published in Venice in 1597.

—The manuall of the anatomy; or, Dissection of the body of man ... Enlarged this present yeer 1642, and more methodically digested into 6 books ... London, Printed by R. Bishop, for Francis Constable, 1642.

[11], 246 (i.e. 446), [12] p.   plates.   15 cm.
                                               [9427]

Added engraved title page.
Imperfect: plates 1 and 2 wanting, supplied in photocopy from the New York Academy of Medicine Library.

—[The same.] ... The 5th ed. ... London, Printed by S. Griffin, for Richard Thrale, 1655.

[11], 446, [12] p.   plates.   15 cm.   **[9428]**
Added engraved title page.

—Most excellent and approved medicines & remedies for most diseases ... incident to man's body, lately compiled and extracted out of the originals ... By A[lexander] R[ead] Doctor in physick deceased. And since revised by an able practitioner ... London, Printed by J. C. for George Latham junior, 1652.

[16], 144 p.   15 cm.   **[9429]**
Dedicatory epistle signed: T. A.

A treatise of the first part of Chirurgerie ... Containing the methodical doctrine of wounds, delivered in lectures in the Barber-Chirurgeons Hall, upon Tuesdayes ... London, Printed by John Haviland for Francis Constable, 1638.

[8], 247 p.   17 cm.   **[9430]**

Imperfect: margins trimmed: p. 25-72, and 105-128 wanting, supplied in photocopy from the New York Academy of Medicine Library.
STC 20786.

—, ed. See [CROOKE, H.] Σωματογραφια ανθρωπινη; or, A description of the body of man. 1616, 1634.

—See WOOD, O. An alphabetical book of physicall secrets. 1639, 1653.

READ, R., Dr., ed. See WECKER, J. J. Eighteen books of the secrets of art & nature. 1661.

READ, THOMAS. See RHAEDUS, Thomas [d. 1624]

READE, Dr. See READ, R., Dr.

REAL crida y edicte. 1630. See VALENCIA. Laws, statutes, etc.

REALE Università degli studi, PADUA. See UNIVERSITÀ DI PADOVA.

REALIZIONE del ritrovamento dell'vova di chiocciole. 1683. See MARSIGLI, A. F.

REBELLO, PEDRO JULIÃO. See JOHANNES XXI, Pope [d. 1277]

REBENTROST, JOHANN GEORG [fl. 1683] respondent. See LOSS, J., praeses. Disputationem inauguralem de lue venerea ... publicae eruditorum censurae subdit ... J. G. H. 1683; THILE, J., praeses. Disputatio medico-chymica. 1683.

REBEQUE, JACQUES-CONSTANT DE. See CONSTANT DE REBEQUE, Jacob de [1635-1730]

REBHOLD, CHRISTIAN. See REHEBOLD, Christian [b. ca. 1625]

REBUFFI, PIERRE [1487-1557] Tractatus de sententiis praejudicialibus. In Sordi, G. P. Tractatus de alimentis plenissimus ... in quo universa alimentorum materia. 1613.

RECALCHI, GIULIO [1552-1645] De febre typhode tractatus ... Ferrariae, Apud Josephum Gironum, 1638.

[4], 107, [35] p.   16 cm.   **[9431]**

RECCHI, Nardo Antonio, *ed. See* Hernández, F. Rerum medicarum Novae Hispaniae thesaurus. 1628, 1651.

RECENTIORUM disceptationes de motu cordis, sanguinis, et chyli, in animalibus ... Lugduni Batavorum, Ex officina Joannis Maire, 1647.

[8], 267, 84, [4] p.; 240 p.; 51 p.; [8], 104, [8] p. illus., plates. 20 cm. **[9432]**
9 works in 4 parts.
Keynes(D) 6.

RECHENBERG, Adam [1642-1721] *praeses.* De gemmis errores vulgares ... Lipsiae, Typis Christophori Fleischeri [1687]

[32] p. 20 cm. **[9433]**
Diss. — Leipzig (J. J. Spener, *respondent*)

— De mundi anima dissertatio philosophica ... Lipsiae, Literis Christiani Scholvini [1678]

[24] p. 20 cm. **[9434]**
Diss. — Leipzig (J. D. Güttner, *respondent*)

RECHPERGER, Guilielmus [*fl.* 1636] *praeses.* Disputatio medica [de scorbuto] ... Viennae Austriae, Gregorius Gelbhaar, 1636.

[19] p. 21 cm. **[9435]**
Diss. — Vienna (P. H. Sprenger, *respondent*)

Eine RECHTE warhaffte Abcontrofactur eines wunderbarlichen Geschöpffs Gottes einer Jungfrauern ... im Ostfriessland den 12. Stemb. ... 1596 geboren ... Magdalena Emohne ... Prag, 1616.

[2] p. illus. 32 cm. **[9436]**

RECHTENBACH, Polycarp Michael [*fl.* 1673] *respondent. See* Drechssler, J. G., *praeses.* Dissertatio historico-physica de sermone brutorum. 1673.

RECHZINNIG oordeel over de twee bordeelsdeunen, gevelt door een onpartydig liefhebber der waarheyt ... Amsterdam, Gedruckt in de Pars van Eer, 1678.

[8] p. 16 cm. **[9437]**

RECIT de ce qui s'est passé en l'establissement des Hospitaux de Saint Louis & de S. Roch de la ville de Roüen. 1654. *See* Rouen.

RECK, Jacob [*fl.* 1685] *respondent.* Disputatio medica inauguralis de angina ... Lugduni Batavorum, Apud Abrahamum Elzevier, 1685.

[16] p. 22 cm. **[9438]**
Diss. — Leyden.

RECONDITORIUM ac reclusorium opulentiae sapientiaeque numinis mundi magni, cui deditur in titulum Chymica vannus, obtenta quidem & erecta auspice mortale coepto; sed inventa proauthoribus immortalibus adeptis ... Amstelodami, Apud Joannem Janssonium à Waesberge, & Elizium Weyerstraet, 1666.

392 (i.e. 294) p.; [2], 76, [1] p. front., illus. 21 cm. **[9439]**
Imperfect: frontispiece wanting; supplied in manuscript.
Commentatio de pharmaco catholico ([2], 76, [1] p.) is a translation of the treatise by Johannes de Monte-Snyder titled: Von der universal medicin.

RECORD, Robert. *See* Recorde, Robert [1510?-1558]

RECORDE, Robert [1510?-1558] The urinal of physick ... Whereunto is added an ingenious treatise concerning physicians, apothecaries and chyrurgians, set forth by a dr. in Queen Elizabeths dayes. With a translation of Papius Ahalsossa concerning apothecaries confecting their medicines ... London, Gartrude Dawson, 1651.

[19], I-III, [11] p.; [9], 123-243, [5] p. illus. 14 cm. **[9440]**
"The urinall of physick" (p. I-III) has running title: The judiciall of urine.
"A detection of some faults in unskilful physitians, ignorant ... apothecaries, and unknowing ... chirurgians. Written by a doctor of physick ... And also a translation of Papius concerning apothecaries ... London, G. D., 1651" (second group of paging) has special title page, and preface signed W. I.
"A translation of Papius concerning apothecaries" (p. 185-243) is a translation of Pape's Tractatus de medicamentorum praeparationibus, published in Wittenberg in 1612.

— [The same.] ... London, G. D., 1665.

[20], [1]-III, [3] p.; [8], 123-237, [5] p. illus. 15 cm. **[9441]**
Different setting of type.
"A detection of some faults in unskilful physitians, ignorant ... apothecaries, and unknowing ... chirurgians. Written by a doctor of physick ... And also a translation of Papius, concerning apothecaries ... London, G. Dawson, 1662" (second group of paging) has special title page.

RECTOR Academiae Tubingensis lect. ben. sal. 1695. *See* Eberhard-Karls-Universität Tübingen.

RECTORIUS, Livonius [*fl.* 1593-1594] De lapidis renum, ac vesicae affectione curatione ... Florentiae, Ex typographia Francisci Honuphrii, 1666.

[11], 9-74, [1] p. illus. (port.) 22 cm. **[9442]**
Edited by Agostino Coltellini.

RECUEIL des plus beaux secrets de medecine, pour la guerison de toutes les maladies, blessures, & autres accidens qui surviennent au corps humain . . . Comme aussi plusieurs secrets curieux sur d'admirables effects de la nature & de l'art. Avec un Traité des plus excellens preservatifs contre la peste . . . & toutes sortes de maladies contagieuses. Le toute experimenté, recueilli, & donné au public par une personne trés-habile & charitable. Divisé en deux parties. Paris, Thomas Guillain, 1695.

    [1], 406, [23] p. front. 17 cm.   **[9443]**

Attributed to Michel Mourgues by BMC.

"Nouveau recueil de secrets curieux, d'admirables preservatifs . . ." (p. [354]-406) has half title.

RECUEIL d'experiences et observations sur le combat. 1679. *See* [GREW, N.]

REDI, FRANCESCO [1626-1697] Esperienze intorno a diverse cose naturali, e particolarmente a quelle, che ci son portate dall'Indie . . . scritte in una lettera al . . . Atanasio Chircher . . . Firenze, All'insegna della nave, 1671.

    [6], 152 p. plates. 24 cm.   **[9444]**

  —[The same.] . . . Firenze, Piero Matini, 1686.

    [6], 122 p. plates. 28 cm.   **[9445]**

  —[The same.] . . . Napoli, Giacomo Raillard, 1687.

    [12], 125, [2] p. plates. 17 cm.   **[9446]**

With this is bound (as issued?) *his* Osservazioni intorno alle vipere. 1687.

  —[Latin tr.] Experimenta circa res diversas naturales, speciatim illas, quae ex Indiis adferuntur. Ex Italico Latinitate donata. Amstelodami, Sumptibus Andreae Frisii, 1675.

    [4], 193, [15] p.; III, [9] p.; 72 p. plates. 14 cm.   **[9447]**

Added engraved title page.

Part [2] has half title: Observationes de viperis. Scriptae literis ad . . . Laurentium Magalotti . . . Ex Italica in Latinam translata.

Part [3] has half title: Epistola . . . scripta ad D. Alexandrum Morum, & D. Abbatem Bourdelot . . . Ex Italica in Latinam translata.

". . . Observationes, circa illas guttulas & fila ex vitro . . . ex. MS. Italico Latinitate donata": p. [53]-72 of part [3]

With this is bound Lachmund, F. De ave Diomedea dissertatio. 1674.

  —Esperienze intorno alla generazione degl'insetti . . . scritte in una lettera all'illustrissimo signor Carlo Dati. Firenze, All'insegna della stella, 1668.

    [6], 228 p. illus., plates. 23 cm.   **[9448]**

  —[The same.] . . . 3. impr. Firenze, Francesco Onofri, 1674.

    [1], 136 p. plates. 24 cm.   **[9449]**

  —[The same.] . . . Napoli, Giacomo Raillard, 1687.

    [14], 195 p. illus., plates. 17 cm.   **[9450]**

Imperfect: p. [15-16] wanting?

  —[The same.] . . . 5. impressione. Firenze, Piero Matini, 1688.

    [6], 176, [1] p. illus., plates. 24 cm.   **[9451]**

  —[Latin tr.] Experimenta circa generationem insectorum ad . . . Carolum Dati. Amstelodami, Sumptibus Andreae Frisii, 1671.

    [12], 230 (i.e. 330), [18] p. plates. 13 cm.   **[9452]**

Added engraved title page.

  —Lettera intorno all'invenzione degli occhiali scritta . . . all' . . . Paolo Falconieri. Con aggiunta in questa nuova impressione. Firenze, Piero Matini, 1690.

    15 p. 25 cm.   **[9453]**

  —Lettera . . . sopra alcune opposizioni fatte alle sue Osservazioni intorno alle vipere. Scritta alli signori Alessandro Moro e Abate Bourdelot . . . Firenze, Nella stamperia della stella, 1670.

    47, [1] p. 24 cm.   **[9454]**

  —[The same.] . . . Firenze, Piero Matini, 1685.

    31, [1] p. 24 cm.   **[9455]**

Bound with *his* Osservazioni intorno alle vipere. 1686.

  —Opuscoli vari . . . [Firenze, Piero Matini, *ca.* 1675]

    23, 8 p. 21 cm.   **[9456]**

  —Opusculorum pars prior; sive, Experimenta circa generationem insectorum . . . Accedit J. Frid. Lachmund De ave Diomedea dissertatio. Amstelaedami, Apud Henricum Wetstenium, 1685-1686 [v. 1, 1686]

    2 v. illus., plates. 14 cm.   **[9457]**

Each vol. has added engraved title page.

Vol. 2 has title: Experimenta circa varias res naturales, speciatim illas quae ex Indiis afferuntur, and also contains Observationes de viperis, Epistola de quibusdam objectionibus contra suas De viperis observationes, and Observationes circa illas guttulas & filia ex vitro.

—Observazioni . . . intorno agli animali viventi che si trovano negli animali viventi. Firenze, Piero Matini, 1684.

[7], 253 (i.e. 244) p. front. (port.) plates. 24 cm.   [9458]

Imperfect: frontispiece wanting.

—[The same.] . . . Napoli, Giacomo Raillard, 1687.

[12], 216 p. plates. 17 cm.   [9459]

Imperfect: p. [11-12] wanting.

—Osservazioni intorno alle vipere . . . scritte in una lettera all'illustriss. signor Lorenzo Magalotti . . . Firenze, All'insegna della stella, 1664.

91, [4] p. 22 cm.   [9460]

Errata: p. [95]
Prandi 2. (The second issue of 1664.)

—[The same.] . . . Paris, Olivier de Varennes, 1666.

[1], 62 p. 16 cm.   [9461]

—[The same.] . . . Firenze, Piero Matini, 1686.
66 p. 24 cm.   [9462]

With this is bound *his* Lettera . . . sopra alcune opposizioni fatte alle sue Osservasioni intorno alle vipere. 1685.

—[The same.] . . . Napoli, Giacomo Raillard, 1687.

[12], 240 (i.e. 140) p. 17 cm.   [9463]

Imperfect: p. [11-12] wanting.

Includes also: — Lettera . . . sopra alcune opposizioni fatte alle sue Osservazioni intorno alle vipere. Scritta alli signori Alessandro More e Abate Bourdelot (p. 65-94); — Osservazioni . . . intorno a quelle gocciole, e fili di vetro, che rotte in qual si sia parte, tutte quante si stritolano (p. 97-106); — Esperienze fatte . . . intorno a quell'acqua . . . che stagna subito tutti quanti i flussi di sangue, che sgorgan da qual si sia parte del corpo (p. 107-115); — Lettera intorno all'invenzione degli occhiali scritta . . . all'illustrissimo signore Paolo Falconieri (p. [116]-124); — Esperienze . . . intorno a' sali fattizi (p. [125]-234 (i.e. 134)); — Lettera d'alcune sperienze intorno al veleno delle vipere, scritta al . . . Arrigo Oldenburg . . . dal . . . Tomaso Platt . . . Estratta dal XII Giornale de letterati di Roma dell'anno 1673 (p. 235-240 (i.e. 135-140)). Except the last one all items have half titles.

Bound with (as issued?) *his* Esperienze intorno a diverse cose naturali. 1687.

—*See* BONOMO, G. C. Osservazioni intorno a' pellicelli del corpo umano; BOURDELOT, P. Recherches et observations sur les viperes. 1671; CALDESI, G. B. Osservazioni anatomiche. 1687; CHARAS, M. Nouvelles experiences sur la vipere. 1669; HONUPHRIIS, F. de. Abortus bicorporeus monoceps.

1691; JUANINI, J. B. Cartas escritas a los . . . doctores . . . Francisco Redi . . . y . . . Juan Mathias de Lucas. 1691; MAJOR, J. D. Genius errans. 1677; PAPA, G. del. Della natura del caldo e del freddo. 1690 [and] Della natura dell'umido e del secco. 1681 [and] Lettera intorno alla natura del caldo e del freddo. 1674 [and] Lettera nella quale si discorre se il fuoco e la luce sieno una cosa medesima. 1690; SAN GALLO, P. P. da. Experienze intorno alla generazione delle zanzare. 1679.

REENBERG, FRANZ [*fl.* 1683] *respondent. See* BORCH, O., *praeses.* Dissertatio medica inauguralis de morbis soporosis comate somnolento. 1683.

REEVE, RICHARD [1642-1693] *tr. See* WOOD, A. à [Historia et antiquitates Universitatis Oxoniensis. 1674]

REFLEXIONS de M. I. S. R. D. M. sur l'epitaphe de Mr Vautier, composé par le P. l'Abbé. Paris, 1652.

[1], 26 p. 23 cm.   [9464]

REFORMATIO, und ernewerte Ordnung. *See* MAINZ. Ordinances, local laws, etc.

REFORMATION; oder, Ernewerte Ordnung der Statt Franckfurt am Mayn, die Pflege der Gesundtheit betreffendt. 1628, 1656, 1687. *See* FRANKFURT AM MAIN. Ordinances, local laws, etc.

A REFUTATION of Dr. Olyphant's Defence of his Short discourse of the usefulness of vomiting in fevers . . . Edinburgh, Printed by J. W. for John Vallange, 1699.

19 p. 15 cm.   [9465]

REGAZZOLA, GIOVANNI BERNARDO. *See* FELICIANUS, Joannes Bernardus [*ca.* 1490–*ca.* 1552]

REGE SINCERA. Observations both historical and moral upon the burning of London, September 1666. With an account of the losses. And a most remarkable parallel between London and Mosco, both as to the plague and fire . . . By Rege Sincera [pseud.] London, Printed by Thomas Ratcliffe, and are to be sold by Robert Pawlet, 1667.

[4], 36 p. 17 cm.   [9466]

REGEMANN, JOHANN GOTTFRIED [*fl.* 1697] *respondent. See* EYSEL, J. P., *praeses.* Disputatio inauguralis medico chirurgica de herniis. 1697.

REGEMORTER, Ahasuerus. *See* Regimorter, Assuerus [1614-1650]

REGENSBURG. Collegium Medicum. *See* Kollegium der Aerzte, Regensburg.

REGGIO EMILIA (City) **Ordinances, local laws, etc.** Bando sopra la peste . . . Nomi delle città e luoghi banditi . . . Reggio, Flavio e Flaminio Bartoli, 1611.

    broadside.   36 x 25 cm.   **[9467]**

Dated 9 January.
Signed Paulus Scaruffius.

—Bando in occasione di peste . . . Reggio, Flavio e Flaminio Bartoli, 1611.

    broadside.   30 x 20 cm.   **[9468]**

Dated 29, 30 & 31 January.
Signed Paolo Scaruffi.

—Bando sopra la peste . . . Seguono i nomi d'i luoghi, che con la presente grida si bandiscono . . . Reggio, Flaminio e Flavio Bartoli, 1611.

    broadside.   31 x 21 cm.   **[9469]**

Dated 5 August.
Signed Bernardinus Masinus.

—Bando per occasione di sospetto di peste . . . Reggio, Flaminio Bartoli, 1629.

    broadside.   31 x 22 cm.   **[9470]**

Dated 13 December.
Signed Alfonso Bertollotti.
Imperfect: upper corner torn, affecting coat of arms.

—Bando in occasione di peste . . . Reggio, Flaminio Bartoli, 1630.

    broadside.   30 x 22 cm.   **[9471]**

Dated 15 and 16 April.
Signed Giulio Rolli.

—Bando in occasione di peste . . . Reggio, Flaminio Bartoli, 1630.

    broadside.   31 x 21 cm.   **[9472]**

Dated 16 and 17 April.
Signed Giulio Rolli.

—Sospensione per occasione di peste . . . Luoghi banditi . . . Reggio, Flaminio Bartoli, 1636.

    broadside.   29 x 19 cm.   **[9473]**

Dated 14 August.
Signed Domenico Grandi.

REGGIUS, Honorius, *pseud. See* Horn, Georg [1620-1670]

REGIA ACADEMIA DI FRANCIA PITTURA E SCULTURA, Rome. *See* Académie de France à Rome.

REGIA ACADEMIA HAFNIENSIS. *See* Universitas Regia Hafniensis. Facultas medica.

REGIME de santé. *See* [Pinsonnat, F.]

Le REGIME de santé de l'Eschole de Salerne. 1633, 1637, 1643, 1649, 1660. *See* Regimen sanitatis Salernitanum. French.

REGIMEN SANITATIS SALERNITANUM

—De conservanda bona valetudine, opusculum scholae Salernitanae, ad regem Angliae, cum Arnoldi Novicensis . . . enarrationibus . . . novissime impressis, & auctis per Joan. Curionem, & ab erroribus, accuratissimè repurgatis, & vindicatis . . . Venetiis, Apud Lucium Spinedam, 1607

    [12], 271, [4] ll.   14 cm.   **[9474]**

"De oratione victus salutaris post incisam venam, & emissum sanguinem, & Armatum epigramma Anastasii": ll. 248; "Victus, et cultus ratio, exposita . . . versibus per Joachimum Camerarium": ll. 248-249; "Loci aliquot [Philippi Melancth.] De moderatione cibi & potus, item somni & vigilarum: ll. 249-251; "Polybius [i.e. Hippocrates] De salubri victus ratione privatorum. Joanne Guinterio Andernaco interprete": ll. 251-254; "Sanitatis tuendae methodus . . . carmine elegiaco per D. Georgium Pictorium . . . conscripta": ll. 254-271.

—[The same.] . . . Venetiis, Apud Petrum Milocum, 1619.

    [12], 271, [4] ll.   14 cm.   **[9475]**

Different setting of type.

—Medicina Salernitana; id est, Conservandae bonae valetudinis praecepta, cum . . . Arnoldi Villanovani in singula capita exegesi, per Joannem Curionem recognita & repurgata. Nova ed. melior, & aliquot medicis opusculis . . . auctior . . . Francofurti, Excudebat Joannes Saurius, impensis Vincentii Steinmeieri, 1605.

    [32], 478, [1] p.   13 cm.   **[9476]**

"Emissi sanguinis observatio ex Joannis Fernelii Vacuandi ratione, cap. 20": p. 402-405; "Dioclis Carystii . . . Aurea ad Antigonum Asiae regum epistola . . . e Graeco Latine reddita, per Antonium Mizaldum": p. 406-412; "De salubri diaeta incerti autoris liber, Hippocrati quondam falso adscriptus. Jano Cornario . . . interprete Argumentum in librum sequentem Joan. Culm. Gepping": p. 413-420; "De ratione victus salutaris post incisam venam & emissum sanguinem, ad Armatum epigramma Anastasii": p. 421; "Victus et cultus ratio exposita . . . versibus, per Joachimum

Camerarium": p. 421-423; "Loci aliquot Philippi Melancht. in lib. De anima, de moderatione cibi & potus, item somni & vigiliarum": p. 423-426; "Nonulla de regimine sanitatis juxta sex res non naturales, placita ex Hippocratis & Galenis libris desumpta ... per D. Joannem Katzchium ... jam olim edita, sed recens a variis mendis repurgata per I. A. S. L.": p. 427-478.

The last item is extracted from Joannes Katzschius' De gubernanda sanitate secundum sex res non naturales, first published in Leipzig in 1549.

—[The same.] ... Duaci, Ex officina Joannis Bogardi, 1611.

[16], 479 p.   12 cm.   [9477]

Imperfect: p. 323-334 and 355-366 wanting.

—[The same.] ... Francofurti, Excudebat Joannes Saurius, impensis Vincentii Steinmeyeri, 1612.

[32], 478, [1] p.   13 cm.   [9478]

—[The same.] ... Monspessuli, Apud Franciscum Chouët, 1622.

[32], 478 p.   13 cm.   [9479]

Different setting of type.

—Another issue, with imprint: Genevae, Apud Petrum Albertum, 1622.

[32], 478 p.   12 cm.   [9480]

—[The same.] ... Antverpiae, Apud Petrum & Joannem Belleros, 1624.

[8], 487 p.   11 cm.   [9481]

—Another issue, with imprint: Duaci, Ex officina Joannis Bogardi, 1624.

                                                [9482]

—[The same.] ... Francofurti, Excudebat Matthaeus Kempffer, impensis Vincentii Steinmeyeri, 1628.

[32], 478, [1] p.   13 cm.   [9483]

—[The same.] ... Genevae, Apud Jacobum Stoër., 1638.

[32], 478 p.   12 cm.   [9484]

Imperfect: outer margins of p. [27-30] trimmed affecting text. Different setting of type.

—[The same.] Schola Salernitana; sive, De conservanda valetudine praecepta metrica. Autore Joanne de Mediolano hactenus ignoti [sic] Cum ... Arnoldi Villanovani in singula capita exegesi. Ex recensione Zachariae Sylvii ... Nova ed., melior & aliquot medicis opusculis auctior ... Roterodami, Ex officina Arnoldi Leers, 1649.

[48], 519 (i.e. 517), [11] p.   front.   14 cm.

                                                [9485]

Contents as in the previous editions of Medicina Salernitana, with additions of "P. Scriverii Saturnalia, continuentia usum & abusum tabaci" (p. 501-516); "Ex Casparis Barlaei Epigrammatis Aenigmaticis" (p. 518); "Ex Hugonis Grotii Epigrammatis" (p. 519)

With this is bound Follinus, J. Synopsis tuendae ... valetudinis. 1646.

—[The same.] ... Roterodami, Ex officina Arnoldi Leers, 1657.

[46], 517, [11] p.   front.   13 cm.   [9486]

Imperfect: p. 499-504 wanting; p. 131-134 mutilated affecting text.

—[The same.] ... Roterodami, Ex officina Arnoldi Leers, 1667.

[46], 517, [10] p.   front.   13 cm.   [9487]

Different setting of type.
—Copy 2.   14 cm.

With this are bound: Hofmann, C. Tractatus tres de usu lienis ... cerebri ... et de ichoribus. [1664?]; Le Boe, Frans de. Collegium medico-practicum. 1664.

—[The same.] ... Hagae-Comitum, Ex officina Arnoldi Leers, 1683.

[32], 512, [8] p.   14 cm.   [9488]

—Schola Salernitana; hoc est, De valetudine tuenda, opus nova methodo instructum, infinitis versibus auctum, commentariis Villanovani, Curionis, Crellii & Costansoni illustratum. Adjectae sunt animadversiones novae & copiosae Renati Moreau ... Parisiis, Sumptibus Thomae Blasii, 1625.

[16], 52, 795, [20] p.   plate.   18 cm.   [9489]

—[The same.] ... Lutetiae Parisiorum, Apud Lud. Billaine, 1672.

[48], 828 (i.e. 826), [22] p.   plate.   19 cm.
                                                [9490]

—[Dutch tr.] Schoola Salernitana bestaende in reghelen tot behoudenis der gesontheydt. Eertijts in 't Latijn beschreven vande hoog-geleerde doctooren, der Salernitaanse Schole ... En nu met seer profijtelicke uyt-leggingen van andere geleerde mannen verrijckt. Vertaelt door J. G. [i.e. Jan Hendrik Glazemaker] Amsterdam, By Cornelis Jansz. [Gedruckt by Gabriël à Roy] 1658.

[6], 394, [7] p.   14 cm.   [9491]

Added engraved title page.
Includes a translation of the commentary of Arnaldus de Villanova.
"Eenige plaetsen van Philippus Melanton, in sijn boeck van de ziele; van de matigheydt van spijse en dranck, als mede van slapen en waken": p. 384-388; "De verklaringe van Guinterius Joann. Andemacus over Polybius [i.e. Hippocrates] van een gesonde maniere des levens voor particuliere personen": p. 388-394.

—[The same.] ... Den 2. druk, van veel fauten verbetert. Amsterdam, Jan Hendriksz., 1658.

[6], 394, [7] p.   14 cm.   [9492]

Different setting of type.

—[English] The Englishmans doctor; or, The schoole of Salerne; or, Physicall observations for the perfect preserving of the body of man in continuall health. London, John Helme and John Busby, junior, 1608.

[43] p.   16 cm.   [9493]

Translated, in verse, by Sir John Harington.
STC 21606.

—[The same.] ... London, John Helme, 1609.

[43] p.   14 cm.   [9494]

A reprint of the 1608 edition.
Imperfect: first and last leaf (blank) wanting.
STC 21607.

—[The same.] ... Whereunto is adioyned Precepts for the preservation of health. Written by Henricus Ronsovius for the private use of his sons. And now published for all those that desire to preserve their bodies in perfect health. Translated by Sir John Harington. London, Printed by A. M. for Thomas Dewe, 1624.

[8], 43 (i.e. 35) p.; [4], 48 p.   14 cm. [9495]

Imperfect: margins cropped.
Part [2] has special title page: De valetudine conservanda; or, The preservation of health; or, A dyet for the healthfull man. Collected out of Henricus Ronsovius ... and now published ... By S. H. ... London, Printed by August Mathewes for Thomas Dewe, 1624. The special dedication is signed "S.H."
STC 21609.

—Regimen sanitatis Salerni. The Schoole of Salernes most learned and juditious directorie, or methodicall instructions, for the guide and governing the health of man ... Perused, and corrected from many great and grosse imperfections, committed in former impressions: with the comment, and all the Latine verses reduced into English, and ordered in their apt and due places. London, Imprinted by Barnard Alsop, and sold by John Barnes, 1617.

[4], 207 (i.e. 208), [11] p.   19 cm.   [9496]

Text in Latin and English verse, translated by Philemon Holland.
The commentary is a translation by Thomas Paynell of the original commentary of Arnaldus de Villanova.
STC 21603.

—[The same.] Regimen sanitatis Salerni; or, The Schoole of Salernes regiment of health. Contayning most learned and judicious directions and instructions, for the guide and government of mans life ... Reviewed, corrected, and inlarged with a commentary ... Whereunto is annexed, a necessary discourse of all sorts of fish, in use among us, with theyr effects, appertayning to the health of man. London, B. Alsop and T. Fawcet, 1634.

[8], 200 (i.e. 218), [13] p.   18 cm.   [9497]

Imperfect: first prelim. leaf (blank except for signature mark) wanting.
STC 21604.

—[The same.] ... Reviewed, corrected, and inlarged with a commentary ... By P[hilemon] H[olland] ... Whereunto is annexed, a necessary discourse of all sorts of fish, in use among us, with their effects appertaining to the health of man. As also, now, and never before, is added certain precious and approved experiments for health, by a right honorable and noble personage. London, B. Alsop, 1649.

[4], 206, [12], 207-220, [3] p.   18 cm. [9498]

Dedication signed: H.H. [i.e. Henry Holland]
A reprint of the 1617 edition.

—[French tr.] Le regime de santé de l'Eschole de Salerne. Traduit et commenté par M. Michel Le Long ... Avec l'Epistre de Diocle Carystien, touchant les presages des maladies à Antigon Roy d'Asie, & le Serment d'Hippocrate, mis de prose en vers françois par le mesme. Paris, Nicolas & Jean de La Coste, 1633.

[15], 700, [16] p.   16 cm.   [9499]

Includes the Latin text of the Regimen sanitatis, with translation in verse.

—[The same.] ... 2d ed., rev., corr., & augm. ... Paris, Nicolas & Jean de La Coste, 1637.

[16], 705, [43] p.   18 cm.   [9500]

—[The same.] ... 3. ed. Paris, Nicolas & Jean de La Coste, 1643.

[16], 705, [42] p.   18 cm.   [9501]

Different setting of type.

—[The same.] ... 4. ed. Paris, Nicolas et Jean de La Coste, 1649.

[16], 705, [42] p.   18 cm.   [9502]

Different setting of type.

—[The same.] L'Escole des medecins de Salerne
… Enrichie de plusieurs beaux & doctes discours,
sur les choses naturelles, non naturelles, & contre
nature. Et sur les proprietez des medicaments …
Augm. de l'epistre que Diocle Carystien … envoya
a Antigon roy d'Asie … Traduit du grec en francois; & illustré des commentaires de M. Michel Le
Lond … Rouen, Clement Malassis, 1660.

[16], 605 (i.e. 603), [43] p.   17 cm.   **[9503]**

"Le serment d'Hippocrate mis en vers": p. [11-13], last group of
paging.

—[Italian tr.] Scola Salernitana per acquistare, e
custodire la sanità, tradotta fedelmente dal verso
latino in terza rima piacevole volgare dall'incognito
academico Vivo Morto. Aggiontivi i Discorsi della
vita sobria del signor Luigi Cornaro … Venetia,
Carlo Brogiollo, 1630.

9, 2-120 p.   16 cm.   **[9504]**

"Altre regole per conservare la sanità tradotte per il medesimo
autore dal verso elegiaco latino di Giorgio Pictorio": p. 33-68.
"Discorsi della vita sobria" (p. [69]-120) has special title page.

—[The same.] … Venetia, Gio. Pietro Brigonci,
1662.

[8], 120 p.   16 cm.   **[9505]**

Different setting of type.

—[The same.] … Venetia, Gio. Pietro Brigonci,
1666.

[8], 120 p.   17 cm.   **[9506]**

Different setting of type.

—[The same.] … Venetia, Benedetto Miloco,
1677.

[8], 120 p.   16 cm.   **[9507]**

Imperfect: p. 35-36 mutilated.
Different setting of type.

—*See* DU FOUR DE LA CRESPELIÈRE. Commentaire
en vers françois, sur l'Ecole de Salerne. 1671; HYGIEIA.
1628; MARIN, A. De naturae humanae principiis.
1656; MARTIN, L. L'Eschole de Salerne. 1650, 166-?,
1664, 1697; MENON, D. L'ecole de Salerne. 1695.

REGIMORTER, ASSUERUS [1614-1650] *See*
GLISSON, F. De rachitide. 1650, 1660, 1671, 1682;
[English tr.] 1668.

RÉGIS, PIERRE DE [1656-1726] *ed. See* MALPIGHI,
M. Opera posthuma. 1698, 1700.

REGISTER der boeckjens, rakende het verschil
tusschen Dr. Bonaventura van Dortmont, en Mr.

Andries Boeckelman … [Amsterdam, Leyden,
Haarlem, Utrecht, 1677-1678]

Various pagings.   16 cm.   **[9508]**

Contains 40 pamphlets, entered separately in the catalogue. For
titles, see Index-catalogue, 1. ser., v. 2 (1881) p. 202-203.
Imprints have in many cases been supplied from Catalogus. Vol.
1, p. 35-36.

REGIUM cor, cono, ac pineae nuci haud absimile, iram nutriens. 1687. *See* BORROMEO, A.

REGIUS, HENRICUS [1598-1679] Fundamenta
medica. Ultrajecti, Apud Theodorum Ackersdy-
dium, 1647.

[19], 281, [1] p.   21 cm.   **[9509]**

Errata: p. [1] at end.
Bound with *his* Fundamenta physices. 1646.

—[The same.] Medicinae libri IV. Ed. 2., priore
locupletior & emendatior. Trajecti ad Rhenum,
Typis Theodori ab Ackersdijck, & Gisberti a Zijll,
1657.

[36], 676 p.   20 cm.   **[9510]**

"Henrici Regii … Praxis medica …" (p. [281]-676) has special
title page, and includes theses for which Regius was praeses.
"Renatus des Cartes, in epistola ad P. Dinetum; quae responsi-
oni ad septimas objectiones est addita": p. [11]

—[The same.] Medicina, et Praxis medica,
medicationum exemplis demonstrata. Ed. 3,
prioribus multo locupletior & emendatior. Trajecti
ad Rhenum, Ex officina Theodori ab Ackersdijck,
1668.

[43], 155 (i.e. 355), [1] p.; [8], 439, [1] p.   20
cm.   **[9511]**

—[The same.] *In* Craanen, T. Observationes. 1689
[and] Opera omnia. 1689.

—Fundamenta physices. Amstelodami, Apud
Ludovicum Elzevirium, 1646.

[16], 306, [1] p.   illus.   21 cm.   **[9512]**

Errata: p. [1] at end.
Includes illustrations based on Descartes' Principia philosophiae
and Specimina philosophiae.
With this is bound *his* Fundamenta medica. 1647.

—[The same.] Philosophia naturalis. Ed. 2, priore
multo locupletior, & emendatior. Amstelodami,
Apud Ludovicum Elzevirium, 1654.

[47], 442 p.   illus., port.   21 cm.   **[9513]**

—[The same.] Philosophia naturalis; in qua tota rerum universitas, per clara & facilia principia, explanatur. Amstelaedami, Apud Ludovicum & Danielem Elzevirios, 1661.

[44], 523, [1] p. illus., plates, port. 21 cm. [9514]

—Spongia, qua eluuntur sordes animadversionum, quas Jacobus Primirosius ... adversus theses pro circulatione sanguinis in Academia Ultrajectina disputatas nuper edidit.

139–166 p., part [2] 20 cm. (*In* Recentiorum disceptationes de motu cordis. Lugduni Batavorum, 1647) [9515]

Caption title.

—*praeses.* Disputatio medica de renum et vesicae calculo ... Ultrajecti, Ex officina Meinardi à Dreunen, 1661.

[20] p. 18 cm. [9516]

Diss. — Utrecht (Tatai G. Kovács, *respondent*)

—Disputationis medicae de chymia, pars posterior ... Trajecti ad Rhenum, Typis Gisberti à Zijll & Theodori ab Ackersdijck, 1657.

[10] p. 20 cm. [9517]

Diss. — Utrecht (J. B. van Lamsweerde, *respondent*)

—*See* BROEN, J. Animadversiones medicae. 1695; NOUVEAU COURS DE MEDECINE. 1669, 1683; PRIMROSE, J. Animadversiones. 1647 [and] Antidotum adversus Henrici Regii ... venentam spongiam. 1644.

REGIUS, HONORIUS, *pseud. See* HORN, Georg [1620–1670]

REGIUS, ZACHARIAS [*ca.* 1660–1692] Morborum princeps: sive, Meditationes de natura et cura pestis ... Brigae, Exprimebat Johannes Christophorus Jacobi, 1680.

[13], 248 p. 16 cm. [9518]

Imperfect: upper margins trimmed.
Errata: p. [13]

—*respondent. See* CRAANEN, T., *praeses.* Disputatio medica de calculo renum & vesicae. 1676.

REGLEMENS de la conduite des hôpitaux du diocese de Besançon. 1697. *See* BESANÇON, France. Diocese.

REGLEMENS que le roy veut estre executez dans l'Hôpital General de Paris. 1684. *See* FRANCE. Sovereigns, etc. [1643–1715] (Louis XIV)

REGLEMENT de la cour. 1699. *See* FRANCE. Laws, statutes, etc.

REGLEMENT ende ordre, van de hoogh mogende heeren Staten generael der vereenighde Nederlanden. 1673. *See* NETHERLANDS (United provinces, 1581–1795) Laws, statutes, etc.

REGLEMENT politic sur l'ayde et subvention des pauvres malades de peste. 1627. *See* SENS. LAWS, STATUTES, ETC.

REGLEMENT pour la pharmacie. 1690? *See* HÔTEL-DIEU DE LYON.

Les REGLES de la santé. 1692. *See* PORCHON, A.

REGNANS, IGNAZ, *ed.* Der Leib- und Land-Medicus armer Leute. Wie dieselbigen ... mit ... probirten Hauss-Mitteln ohne sonderliche Kosten ihr Leben und Gesundheit erhalten können ... Von einem alten erfahrnem fürstl. Leib-Medico zusammen getragen, und aus dessen verlassenen Manuscripts ausgesuchet und in Druck befördert, durch Ignatium Regnantem ... Merseburg, Zu finden bey Christian Forbergern, 1682.

[22], 935 p. front. 14 cm. [9519]

REGNANTIUS, IGNATIUS. *See* REGNANS, Ignaz.

REGNERUS, ERNESTUS. *See* RAVE, Ernestus Regnerus [*fl.* 1695]

REGOLATIONE de pretii delle cose medicinali semplici. 1696. *See* VERONA (CITY) ORDINANCES, local laws, etc.

REGOLE osservate da PP. Theatini di Palermo in S. Gioseffo nel tempo del contagio. 1624? *See* THEATINES. Congregazione di Palermo.

Een REGT bescheyt, geschreven door een Hollander en Vrieseman, in 't twist-jaar der medicijnen tot Amsterdam. [Amsterdam] Gedrukt met een instrument van Mr. Andries Boekelman, by Jan Olofsz. Hortulanus [1678]

7 p. 16 cm. [9520]

REGULUS, JOANNES FRIDERICUS [*fl.* 1621] *respondent. See* SEBISCH, M. [1578–1674?] *praeses.* Disputatio de purgatione undecima. 1621 [and] Disputationes de recta ratione purgandi. 1621.

[REHEBOLD, CHRISTIAN, *b. ca.* 1625] Salomon & Marcolphus Justiniano-Gregoriani; hoc est,

Sapida, ac insipida, sana, atque insana, nimirum theologica; juridica ... medica ... collecta, ac nunc primum edita, autore Δ.X.Δ ... Francofurti & Dresdae, Apud Christianum Bergen, 1678.

[10], 126 p. 17 cm. [9521]

Bound with Elsholtz, J. S. Anthropometria. 1663.

REHEFELD, JOHANN [*ca.* 1590-1648] Medicinalischer Anschlag vornemlich gerichtet auff das einfältige und haussarme der Stadt Erffurt zugehörige Landvolck; wie ... sich dasselbe zwar durch schlechte ... jedoch aber bewehrte Artzney vor der Pestseuche behüten ... kan ... Zum andern Mahl publicirt ... [Erffurdt] Gedruckt bey Christoff Mechler, in Verlegung Johannis Birckners, 1626.

[31] p. 20 cm. [9522]

—*praeses.* Exercitatiuncula posterior de lipyriae cura ... Erffurti, Ex academico Dedekindi typographeo, 1636.

[8] p. 18 cm. [9523]

Diss. — Erfurt (J. B. Tagius, *respondent*)

REHM, JOHANN CHRISTOPH [1627-1693] Kurtzer Unterricht wie man sich bey denen jetzigen gefährlichen Läufften, wegen besorglich-einschleichender pestilentialischen Seüche ... nicht nur allein praeserviren und verwahren, sondern auch ... curiren und heilen soll ... Onolzbach, Gedruckt bey Jeremias Kretschmann, 1679.

93 p. 14 cm. [9524]

Interleaved.

REHME, AMBROS [*fl.* 1684] *respondent. See* WEDEL, G. W., *praeses.* Disputatio inauguralis medica de ophthalmia. 1684.

REHME, JOHANN CHRISTOPH [*fl.* 1664-1679] *respondent.* Disputatio medica de pleuritide ... Basileae, Typis Joh. Jacobi Deckeri [1664]

[28] p. 22 cm. [9525]

Diss. — Basel.

REICH, JOHANN JAKOB [*fl.* 1695] *respondent. See* STAHL, G. E., *praeses.* Disputationem inauguralem de passionibus animi corpus humanum varie alterantibus ... submittit J. J. R. 1695.

—*See* STAHL, G. E. Propempticon inaugurale, de συνεργεια naturae in medendo. 1695.

REICHARD, CHRISTOPH [*fl.* 1672] *respondent. See* SCHRÖTER, E.F., *praeses.* Dissertationem de stylo curiae. 1688.

REICHE, GOTTFRIED [*fl.* 1660] *respondent. See* BECKER, J. Dissertationem meteorologicam de grandine ... submittunt M. J. B ... & ... G. R. 1660.

REICHEL, JOHANNES KARL [*fl.* 1699] *respondent.* Dissertatio medica inauguralis de haemoptysi ... Trajecti ad Rhenum, Ex officina Guilielmi vande Water, 1699.

14 p. 20 cm. [9526]

Diss. — Utrecht.

REICHELT, JULIUS [1637-1719] Exercitatio, de amuletis, aeneis figuris illustrata. Argentorati, Apud Joh. Frid. Spoor, & Reinhard, Wechtler, 1676.

[6], 94 p. plates. 21 cm. [9527]

REICHENBACH, JOHANNES GLOGERIUS. *See* GLOGER, Johann [*fl.* 1622]

REICHENOW, GEORG LEBERECHT [*fl.* 1680] *respondent.* Disputatio medica inauguralis de χλώρωσι, seu morbo virgineo ... Lugduni Batavorum, Apud viduam & haeredes Johannis Elsevirii, 1680.

[16] p. 20 cm. [9528]

Diss. — Leyden.

REICHHELM, JEREMIAS GOTTLIEB [*fl.* 1694-1702] *respondent. See* WERCKMEISTER, F. H., *praeses.* Disputatio medica de absoluta lethalitate vulneris arteriae magnae. 1694.

REID, ALEXANDER [1586?-1641] *See* READ, Alexander [1586?-1641]

REID, THOMAS. *See* RHAEDUS, Thomas [d. 1624]

REIES FRANCO, GASPAR DOS. *See* REYES FRANCO, Gaspar de los [*fl.* 1658]

REIFF, WALTHER HERMANN. *See* RYFF, Walther Hermenius [d. 1548]

REIHING, JACOB [1577 or 9-1628] *See* MENZEL, P. Carminum ... libri quatuor. 1615.

REIMAN, JOHANNES BAPTISTA [*fl.* 1613] *ed. See* BAUDIS, J. Zwey Tractätlein von der Pest. 1613.

REIN, JOHANN DAVID [*fl.* 1681] *respondent.* Dissertatio inauguralis medica περι της γυναικαγονιας ... Argentinae, Literis Johannis Friderici Spoor [1681]

[1], 34 p. 20 cm. [9529]

Imperfect: p. 33—34 misbound before p. 1.

Diss. —Strasbourg.

REINECCIUS, JOHANN PAUL [*fl.* 1676] *respondent. See* WOLF, J. [*fl.* 1673-1680] *praeses.* Disputationem physicam evolventem qu. num daemon cum sagis generare possit ... submittit J. P. R. 1676.

REINERS, Hendrik [*fl.* 1686] *respondent.* Disputatio medica inauguralis, continens varias, ex singulis medicinae partibus desumptas, positiones ... Ultrajecti, Ex officina Francisci Halma, 1686.

    10, [2] p. 22 cm.   **[9530]**
Diss. — Utrecht.

REINES, Thomas. *See* Reinesius, Thomas [1587-1667]

REINESIUS, Christoph Ludwig [*fl.* 1690] *respondent. See* Leichner, E., *praeses.* Dissertatio inauguralis medica de catarrho. 1690.

REINESIUS, Johann Moritz [*d.* 1680] Wolgemeintes Consilium Medicum, wie ... die Stadt Magdeburg, gegen bevorstehende Gefahr der pestilentzialischen Seuche ... sich in Verfassung setzen, und, wie insonderheit ein jeder Hausswirth, sich und die Seinigen mit bewehrter Artzeney vor dieselbe verwahren und ... davon wieder befreyen könne ... Magdeburg, Verlegt von Johann Lüderwaldten und gedruckt bey Johann Daniel Müllern, 1680.

    [2], 68 (i.e. 70), [2] p. plate. 20 cm.**[9531]**

—*respondent. See* Conring, H., *praeses.* Commentariolum in Cl. Galeni lib. XIII. 1663.

REINESIUS, Thomas [1587-1667] Ad viros clariss. D. Casp. Hoffmannum. Christ. Ad. Rupertum ... epistolae. Lipsiae, Sumptibus Johannis Scheibii, imprimebat Johannes Bauerus, 1660.

    [10], 681, [11] p. illus., tables. 21 cm.
                                    [9532]
With this is bound *his* Variarum lectionum libri III. 1640.

—Epistolarum ad Nesteros, patrem et filium conscriptarum farrago: in qua varia medica et philologica lectu jucunda continentur: antehac a B. authore numquam edita. Lipsiae, Sumptibus Schüreri Götzianorum haeredum et Joh. Fritschii, 1670.

    [8], 112 p. 20 cm.   **[9533]**
Edited by Johann Matthias Nester.

—Variarum lectionum libri III. priores. In quibus de scriptoribus sacris & profanis classicis plerisque differetur ... Altenburgi, Otto Michael, 1640.

    [20], 694, [62] p. 21 cm.   **[9534]**

Bound with *his* Ad viros clariss. D. Casp. Hoffmanum. Christ. Ad. Rupertum ... epistolae. 1660.

—, *ed. See* Fedele, F. Schola jure-consultorum medica. 1679.

REINHARD, Georg Michael [*fl.* 1700] *respondent.* ... De tussi ... [Altdorffii] Literis Henrici Meyeri [1700]

    24 p. 19 cm.   **[9535]**
Diss. — Altdorf.

REINHARD, Johann [1645-1691] *praes.* Theranthropismus fictus ... Wittebergae, Excudebat Johannes Borckardi, 1673.

    [16] p. 19 cm.   **[9536]**
Diss. — Wittenberg (M. H. Krause, *respondent*)

REINHARD, Johann Christoph. *See* Reinhart, Hans Christoff [*fl.* 1608-1611]

REINHARD, Johann Georg [*fl.* 1653] Oratiunculam medicam, de quaestione: an sit doctus medicus felici praeferendus? ... Repraesentat, ac typis exscribi curat Johann-Georg Reinhard ... Lipsiae, Literis Ritzschianis, 1653.

    [8] p. 19 cm.   **[9537]**

REINHARD, Johann Simeon [*fl.* 1688-1692] *respondent. See* Berger, J. G. von, *praeses.* Dissertationem inauguralem de suppressione catameniorum ... exhibet ... J. S. R. 1692; Bohn, J., *praeses.* Dissertationem medicam de vomitu ... exhibet ... J. S. R. 1688.

REINHART, Hans Christoff [*fl.* 1608-1611] Der gülden Gesundbrunnen. Zu unerschöpfflicher Wolfart, in Basilii Valentini Schrifften, Schlüsseln, und Capitteln geschöpffet, und ... geleitet und entblösset ... Hall, Gedrukt durch Erasmum Hynitzsch, in Verlegung Joachimi Krüsicken, 1611.

    [60] p. 16 cm.   **[9538]**

REIS TAVARES, Manuel dos. *See* Reys Tavares, Manuel dos [*fl.* 1667]

REISEL, Salomen [1625-1702] *respondent. See* Sebisch, M. [1578-1674?] *praeses.* Galeni quinque priores libri. 1651.

REISING, Johann Benjamin [*fl.* 1680] *respondent. See* Ziegra, C. S., *praeses.* Disputatio physica de morte plantarum. 1680.

REISKE, JOHANN [1641-1701] Ad . . . Chr. Franc. Paullini . . . de morbo Jobi difficillimo periscylacismo Graeco nec non canibus inter numos ac inscriptiones veteres receptis epistola. Helmstadii, Typis Georg Wolfgangi Hammii, 1685.

[24] p. 20 cm. **[9539]**

—De glossopetris Lüneburgensibus ad . . . Joh. Georg. Hieronymi . . . epistolica commentatio . . . Lipsiae, Sumtu Joh. Georg. Lipperi, 1684.

56 p. plate. 20 cm. **[9540]**

REITMEYER, GEORG [*fl.* 1666-1673] *respondent. See* BRUNO, J. P., *praeses.* Disquisitionem medicam de medicamentorum facultatibus . . . examini subjicit G. R. 1670.

RELATIONI di varie pesti in Italia sin'all'anno corrente 1630. Con tutti li segni di quelle, e rimedii esperimentati nella vera cura, e preserva. Con il modo di purgar le robbe, e case infette, mandate da varii medici assistenti in detta cura. Stampate per ordine del magistrato della sanità in Venetia e ristampate in Napoli . . . Napoli, Appresso Ottavio Beltrano, si vendeno nella libraria d'Andrea Paladino, 1631.

[8], 63, [1] p. 20 cm. **[9541]**

RELAZIONE dell'esperienze fatte in Inghilterra, Francia, ed Italia intorno alla celebre, e famosa transfusione del sangue per tutto maggio 1668 . . . La maniera di facilmente pratticarla ne gli huomini . . . con nuova esperienza in un cane vecchio . . . Bologna, Manolessi, 1668.

[4], 74, [1] p. plate. 21 cm. **[9542]**
Imperfect: plate wanting.
Edited by Emilio Maria Manolessi.

RELIGIO medici. 1642, 1644. *See* [BROWNE, *Sir* T.]

RELOU, CHRISTOPH [*fl.* 1661-1664] *respondent. See* ROLFINCK, W., *praeses.* Dissertatio medica inauguralis, de febre petechiali. 1664.

REMEDE universel pour les pauvres gens et leur bestiaux . . . 9. ed. rev. & augm. de nouveau. Paris, La veuve Denis Langlois, 1681.

4 p. 24 cm. **[9543]**
Caption title.

Les REMEDES des maladies du corps humain. *See* [SAINT HILAIRE, *sieur de.*] L'anatomie du corps humain, avec maladies. 1680, 1684-85.

REMEDES des pauvres. 1679? *See* FALAISE, Normandie. Religieuses hôpitalieres.

REMEDES pour les pauvres gens. 1678. *See* TRÉGUIER, France (Diocese) Bishop.

REMEDES. Pour les pauvres gens. [1677]. *See* ASSEMBLÉE CHARITABLE À PARIS.

REMEDES pour les pauvres gens de la campagne, & pour leurs bestiaux, qui coûtent peu . . . Avec privilege, & l'exhortation de l'Assemblée generale du Clergé de France, du 17. Novembre 1670. à tous les eveques du royaume, pour établir la distribution de ces remedes dan les paroisses de leur dioceses . . . 6. ed. Paris, Denys Langlois, 1672.

56 p. 22 cm. **[9544]**

REMEDIE voor de brandende kreeft. 1683. *See* VALCKENIER.

REMEDIE voor den desolaten boedel, der medicijne deses tijds; Uytgesproken van Doctor over het pesthuis, en Apoteker in het gasthuis . . . Amsterdam, Pieter Schijn [1677]

29 p. 16 cm. **[9545]**

REMEDIEN tegen de peste; oft, Verscheyden korte onderwijsen . . . Brugghe, Nicolaes Breyghel, 1632.

24 p. 15 cm. **[9546]**

REMELIN, JOHANNES ANASTASIUS. *See* REMMELIN, Johannes Anastasius [*fl.* 1644]

REMI, NICOLAS [1530-1612] Daemonolatria; oder, Beschreibung von Zauberern und Zauberinnen . . . Erster Theil. Der ander Theil hält in sich . . . Historien von des Teuffels Hinterlist, Betrug, Falschheit und Verführungen, an, bey und umb den Menschen . . . Mit einem Anhange . . . Hamburg, Gedruckt bey Thomas von Wiering; sind auch zu Franckf. und Leipz. bey Zacharias Hertelnzu bekommen, 1693.

[10], 288 p.; [8], 544, [16] p.; 96 p. front., plates. 17 cm. **[9547]**
Part 2 has special title page and frontispiece.
Part 3 has half title: Der Gespensten Bauckel-Wercks . . . worinnen enthalten, viele . . . Gespensten und Erscheinungen. Aus vielen Büchern zusammen gebracht.
A translation of Daemonolatreiae, published in Lyons in 1595.

[REMMELIN, JOHANN, 1583-1632] [Catoptrum microcosmicum.] Visio prima [-tertia] Τοῦ *κατόπτρου μιϰροϰοσμιϰου* absolutam admirandae partium hominis creaturarum divinarum praestantissimi fabricae eximio artificio sculptam structuram revidendam exhibentis: cum enarratione historica brevi at perspicua et explicationis & indicis vice addita ... J[ohann] R[emmelin] inventor, L[ucas] K[ilian] sculptor ... [Augspurg?] Stephan Michelspacher, 1613.

3 plates. 58 cm. **[9548]**

Place of publication from W. Pfeilsticker. Johannes Rümelin. (Sudhoff's Archiv für Geschichte der Medizin. v. 22 (1929) p. 180)

Unauthorized edition of Catoptrum microcosmicum; incorrectly attributed to Stephan Michael Spacher, the publisher. Cf. Choulant-Frank, p. 232-233.

[—] Elucidarius tabulis synopticis, microcosmici laminis incisi aeneis, admirandam partium hominis ... fabricam repraesentantis catoptri, litteras & characteres explicans, ex Pinace microcosmographico eidem catoptro ac historica ... Enarratio addito, exscriptus et nunc primum ... publicae datus divulgatusque à Stephano Michelspachero ... [Augspurg] Sumptibus Stephani Michelspacheri] 1614.

II, [I] ll. 22 cm. **[9549]**

Unauthorized edition of the explanation of the plates of the author's Catoptrum microcosmicum. Cf. Bibl. Osler.

Bound with *his* Pinax microcosmographicus [Augspurg] 1615.

[—] Pinax microcosmographicus; hoc est, Admirandae partium hominis creaturarum divinarum praestantissimi universarum fabricae, historica brevis at perspicua enarratio, microcosmico tabulis sculpto aeneis catoptro incidissimo explicationis vice addita, impensisque maximis Stephani Michelspacheri ... [Augspurg, Sumptibus Stephani Michelspacheri] 1615.

[4], 30, [4] ll. 22 cm. **[9550]**

Unauthorized edition of the text to accompany the author's Catoptrum microcosmicum. Cf. Bibl. Osler.

With this is bound *his* Elucidarius. [Augspurg] 1614.

—Catoptrum microcosmicum, suis aere incisis visionibus splendens, cum historia, & pinace, de novo prodit ... Augustae Vindelicorum, Typis Davidis Francki, 1619.

[2], 27 (i.e. 25), [I] p. illus., port. 47 cm. **[9551]**

Imperfect: p. 9-10 (including "Visio ... prima") wanting.

Engraved title page.

Remmelin's own corrected edition. Cf. Choulant-Frank, p. 232.

[—] Pinax microcosmographicus, in quo certissimum anatomiae compendium proponitur. Auctore Stephano Michaele Spachero ... in usum medicorum, chirurgorum, ac pharmacopaeorum conscriptus. Et nunc in maternam nostram linguam translatus, & artificiose sculptus, a Cornelio Danckero ... D'ontlegingh des kleyne werelds; ofte, Een konstige vertoningh van alle de deelen van 't menschelicke lichaem ... Amsterdam, Cornelis Danckersz, 1645.

[7] p. plates. 48 cm. **[9552]**

Text in Latin and Dutch translation.

—Catoptrum microcosmicum, suis aere incisis visionibus splendens cum historia, & pinace, de novo prodit ... Francofurti ad Moenum, Sumptibus ac typis heredum Antonii Hummen, 1660.

27 (i.e. 25), [I] p. illus. 48 cm. **[9553]**

Engraved title page.

A reprint of the 1619 edition.

—Another issue, with imprint: Ulmae Suevorum, Sumptibus Johannis Görlini, 1660. **[9554]**

—[Dutch tr.] *See* Pinax microcosmographicus. 1645.

—[English tr.] A survey of the microcosme; or, The anatomie of the bodies of man and woman, wherein the skin, veins, nerves, muscles, bones, sinews and ligaments thereof are accurately delineated, and so disposed by pasting, as that each part of the said bodies both inward and outward are exactly represented ... By Michael Spaher ... and Remilinus. Englished by John Ireton ... London, Joseph Moxon, 1675.

[II] p. illus. 40 cm. **[9555]**

—[German tr.] Kleiner Welt Spiegel; das ist, Abbildung Göttlicher Schöpffung an dess Menschen Leib, mit beygesetzter schrifftlicher Erklärung ... Auss ... lateinischem Exemplar, in die teutsche Sprach ubersetzet, durch M. Johannem Ludovicum Remmelinum ... Ulm, Gedruckt durch Johann Ulrich Schönigk, in Verlag Johann Remmelins, 1632.

[2], 22 p. illus., port. 45 cm. **[9556]**

Colophon: Gedruckt zu Augspurg, durch Johann Ulrich Schönigk, in Verlag Johann Remmelin in Ulm, Buchhändlers, 1632.

Labels, formerly covering original imprint and colophon but now mounted on fly leaves, read: Ulm, In Verlegung Johann Gerlin, 1639 (imprint); and, Ulm, In Verlegung Johann Gerelins ... 1639 (colophon).

—[The same.] . . . Ulm, Gedruckt durch Johann Schultes, in Verlegung Johann Görlin, 1661.

[1], 22 p.   illus.   49 cm.   [9557]

Colophon: Gedruckt zu Augspurg, durch Johann Schultes, in Verlegung Johann Gorlin, Burger und Buchhändlers in Ulm . . . 1661.

Imperfect: p. 19-20 (including "Das dritte Gesicht") wanting.

REMMELIN, JOHANN KONRAD [*fl.* 1679-1681] *respondent. See* CAMERARIUS, E. R., *praeses.* Dissertatio medica inauguralis de palpitatione cordis. 1681; Metzger, G. B., *praeses.* Historia anatomico-medica thymi. 1679.

REMMELIN, JOHANN LUDWIG [*fl.* 1631] *tr. See* REMMELIN, J. Kleiner Welt Spiegel. 1632, 1661.

REMMELIN, JOHANNES ANASTASIUS [*fl.* 1644] *respondent. See* SEBISCH, M. [1578-1674?] *praeses.* Disputatio de naturalibus facultatibus prima [-octava & ultima] 1644 [i.e. 1645]

REMMIUS FLAVIANUS. *See* FLAVIANUS, Remmius.

REMY, NICOLAS. *See* REMI, Nicolas [1530-1612]

RENALDINUS, CAROLUS. *See* RINALDINI, Carlo [1615-1698]

RENAUDOT, EUSÈBE [*d.* 1679] L'antimoine justifié et l'antimoine triomphant; ou, Discours apologetique faisant voir que la poudre; & le vin emetique & les autres remedes tirés de l'antimoine ne sont point veneneux . . . Avec leurs preparations . . . tant de la pharmacie, que de la chymie . . . Paris, Jean Henault [1653]

[20], 396 (i.e. 398), [1] p.   22 cm.   [9558]

Imperfect: wormholes on p. 25-86.

Errata: p. [1] at end.

[—] A general collection of discourses, of the virtuosi of France, upon questions of all sorts of philosophy, and other natural knowledg . . . Render'd into English by G. Havers . . . London, Thomas Dring and John Starkey, 1664.

[15], 580 p.   30 cm.   [9559]

A translation of the first hundred conferences of the "Recueil général des questions traictées ès conférences du Bureau d'adresse" compiled by Théophraste and Eusèbe Renaudot and published under title "Première [-quatriesme] Centurie des questions traitées ez conférences du Bureau d'adresse."

With this is bound *his* Another collection of philosophical conferences. 1665.

—Another collection of philosophical conferences of the French virtuosi, upon questions of all sorts: for the improving of natural knowledg . . . Render'd into English, by G. Havers . . . & J. Davies . . . London, Thomas Dring and John Starkey, 1665.

[15], 496 p.   30 cm.   [9560]

A translation of 240 conferences of the "Recueil général des questions traictées ès conférences du Bureau d'adresse."

Bound with *his* A general collection of discourses. 1664.

—*See* HIPPOCRATES. [Collected works. French] 1697; PERREAU, J. Rabbat-ioye de l'antimoine triomphant. 1655.

RENAUDOT, THÉOPHRASTE [1586-1653] *ed. See* CONFERENCES DU BUREAU D'ADRESSE, Paris. A question. Why dead bodies bleed in the presence of their murtherers. 1640; [RENAUDOT, E.] A general collection of discourses of the virtuosi of France. 1664 [and] Another collection of philosophical conferences of the French virtuosi. 1665.

—*See* CHYMICAL, medicinal, and chyrurgical addresses. 1655; [PATIN, G.] Le nez pourry de Theophraste Renaudot. 1644; RIOLAN, J. [1580-1657] Curieuses recherches sur les escholes en medecine de Paris. 1651.

RENEAULME, PAUL DE [1560?-1624] Ex curationibus observationes quibus videre ets [sic] morbos tuto cito & jucunde posse debellari: si praecipue Galenicis praeceptis chymica remedia veniant subsidio . . . Parisiis, Apud Adrianum Beys, 1606.

[32], 152, [5] p.   16 cm.   [9561]

Imperfect: [32] p. wanting; supplied in photocopy from New York Academy of Medicine library.

RENGER, JOHANN FRIEDRICH [*fl.* 1676] *respondent.* Disputatio medica inauguralis de scirrho lienis . . . Altdorfii, Literis Henrici Meyeri [1676]

35 p.   18 cm.   [9562]

Diss. — Altdorf.

RENNER, FRANZ [*fl.* 1554-1571] Ein köstlich und bewärtes Artzney Buchlein aller innerunnd eusserlichen Artzney, wider die abschewliche Kranckheit der Frantzosen und Lähmung: auch vor alle andere Seuchten, so auss dieser Kranckheit erfolgen . . . Amberg, Michael Forster, 1609.

[11], 300 p.   illus.   20 cm.   [9563]

RENODAEUS, JOANNES. *See* RENOU, Jean de [*fl.* 1608]

RENOU, Jean de [*fl.* 1608] Institutionum pharmaceuticarum. Libri quinque quibus accedunt De materia medica. Libri tres. Omnibus succedit Officina pharmaceutica, sive Antidotarium ab eodem autore commentariis illustratum ... Parisiis, Apud viduam Gulielmi de la Nouë et Dionys. de la Nouë, 1608.

    10, [16], 195, 257, 40 p.; [24], 320, 24 p. port. 23 cm. **[9564]**

  Engraved title page.

  Part [2] has special engraved title page.

  Imperfect: p. 9-10, [1-6] of preliminary matter, and portrait wanting.

—[The same.] Dispensatorium medicum ... Quibus accessit Josephi Quercetani ... Pharmacopoea dogmaticorum restituta. Item Nicolai Epiphanii ... Empirica nunc e manuscripto luci data. Hac editione omnia jam denuo revisa ... Francofurti, Apud Paulum Jacobi, impensis Joannis Theobaldi Schönwetteri, 1615.

    [42], 538, [30] p.; [8], 229, [10] p.; 90, [13] p. 21 cm. **[9565]**

  Part [2] has special title page.

—[The same.] ... Nunc cum triplice indice editum. Coloniae Allobrogum, Ex typographia Jacobi Stoer, 1623.

    [80], 1115, [50] p. 18 cm. **[9566]**

  Imperfect: Signatures of sheet + + + + + wrongly imposed. Without the works of Duchesne and Epiphanius.

—[The same.] ... Genevae, Ex typographia Jacobi Stoer, 1645.

    [80], 1115, [50] p. 17 cm. **[9567]**

  Different setting of type.

—[English tr.] A medicinal dispensatory, containing the whole body of physick ... In five books of philosophical and pharmaceutical institutions; three books of physical materials Galenical and chymical. Together with a ... pharmacopoea or apothecaries shop ... And now Englished and revised, by Richard Tomlinson ... London, Printed by Jo. Streater and Ja. Cottrel, and sold by John Garfield, 1657.

    [51], 1-216 p.; [7], 217-472 p.; [8], 471-2, 481-738, [23] p. front. 28 cm. **[9568]**

  Imperfect: frontispiece and vertical half-title wanting.

  With this is bound A physical dictionary. 1657.

—[French tr.] Le grand dispensaire medicinal. Contenant cinq livres des institutions pharmaceutiques. Ensemble trois livres de la matiere medicinale.

Avec une pharmacopoee, ou antidotaire fort accompli ... Traduict ... par Mr. Louys de Serres ... Lyon, Pierre Rigaud, & associez, 1624.

    [24], 982, [18] p. 25 cm. **[9569]**

  Added engraved title page reads: Les oeuvres pharmaceutiques.

—[The same.] Les oeuvres pharmaceutiques ... Augm. d'un tiers en cette 2. ed. par l'auteur; puis traduittes ... & mises en lumiere par M. Louis de Serres ... Lyon, Chez Antoine Chard [Imprimé par Pierre Colombier] 1626.

    [28], 467 p.; [1], 468-762, [22] p. illus., plates. 36 cm. **[9570]**

  Imperfect: first preliminary leaf wanting.

  "Boutique pharmaceutique, ou Antidotaire" (second group of paging) has special title page.

—[The same.] ... Lyon, Nicolas Gay, 1637.

    [28], 467 p.; [2], 468-762, [22] p. illus., plates. 36 cm. **[9571]**

  Different setting of type.

—*See* HORST, J. D. Pharmacopoeia Galeno-chemica. 1651; A physical dictionary. 1657.

RENZ, Benedict [*fl.* 1692] *respondent*. Disputatio medica inauguralis de hypercatharsi ... Basileae, Typis Joh. Rudolphi Genathii [1692]

    [36] p. 21 cm. **[9572]**

  Diss. — Basel.

REPONSE a la dissertation sur la goutte. 1690. *See* [Ozon, P.]

REPONSE a un censeur. Paris?, *ca.* 1672.

    [2], 23 p. 22 cm. **[9573]**

  "Histoire de la maladie, & de la mort de Madame de Morangis, tirée des Conversation Academiques de M^r l'Abé Bourdelot": p. 21-22.

RESCH, Johann Ulrich [*b. ca.* 1589] Osiandrische Experiment von Sole, Luna & Mercurio ... Mit angehängtem ... Tractätlein, De igne philosophico ... Auch Historien warhoffter Verwandlung der Metallen in Gold und Silber. Item, wie man sich vor Betriegeren hüten soll, sammt andern ... Observationen und Explicationen, colligirt und practicirt durch Joan Ulrich Reschen ... Nürnberg, Bey Johann Andreas und Wolffgang Endters dess Jüngern sel. Erben, 1659.

    [8], 327 p. 16 cm. **[9574]**

  "Caput III. De igne philosophico. D. D. Luc. Osiand. indagatio de igne philosophico moderando pro solutione debita acquirenda" has caption title.

"Caput X. De historiis transmutationis metallorum. Kurtzer Bericht ... dass die Alchimey, oder ... Goldmacher-Kunst, ein sonderbarer Geschenck Gottes, und derentwegen mehr als gewiss und warhafftig. Von ... Ewald von Hohelande [i.e. Theobaldus van Hoghelande?] beschrieben. In Teutsch versetzt durch J[oachim] T[ancke] P[oeseos] D[octor] anno 1604" has half title.

RESERIUS, HORATIUS [*fl.* 1556-1558] *See* SCHOLTZ, L. Consiliorum medicinalium ... liber singulares. 1610.

RESOLUTIE VANDE ED. GROOT MOG. heeren staten van Hollandt ende West-Vrieslandt. 1664. *See* HOLLAND (Province) Laws, statutes, etc.

RESPONSE au Medecin reformé. Quatrain a l'apoticaire DesPeCé [i.e. A.D.P.C.] [Paris?] 1623.
7 p.   17 cm.   **[9575]**
In verse.
Bound with Guibert, P. Le medecin charitable. 1623.

RESTAURAND, RAYMOND [1627-1682] Exercitatio medica de usu vini emetici in curatione febrium malignarum ad mentem Hippocratis. Adjuncta est oeconomia physiologicorum Hippocratis. Parisiis, Apud Joannem Dupuis, 1662.
[9], 96, 10 p.   15 cm.   **[9576]**
"Lectori" (2d-4th prelim. leaves) signed: R[aymond] R[estaurand]
"Magni Hippocratis Coi ... physiologica. Operis oeconomia" (10 p. at end) was also published under title: Magnus Hippocrates ... redivivus. Tomus primus: physiologica continens.

—Hippocrate de l'usage du boire a la glace, pour la conservation de la santé ... Lyon, Germain Nanty, 1670.
[16], 88, [1] p.   16 cm.   **[9577]**

—[The same.] ... Rev., corr., & augm. par l'hauteur, en cette 2. ed. Pezenas, Jean Martel, 1677.
[20], 131, [2] p.   15 cm.   **[9578]**

—Hippocrate de l'usage du china-china, pour la guerison des fiévres. Par M^r M^e R[aymond] R[estaurand] D. M. ... Lyon, Esprit Vitalis, 1681.
[16], 135 p.   15 cm.   **[9579]**

—[Latin tr.] *In* [Nigrisoli, F.M.] *ed.* Febris china chinae expugnata. 1687, 1700.

—[Italian tr.] Ippocrate dell'uso della kinakina per la guarigione delle febbri ... Aggiuntovi il segreto della rotture. Opera portata dal francese in italiano à beneficio publico ... Parma, Alberto Pazzoni, e Paolo Monti, 1695.
[14], 95 p.   15 cm.   **[9580]**

Dedicatory preface signed by the translator: Carlo Richany. "Rimedio dell'abbate di Cabrieres, per le rotture": p. 89-95.

—Hippocrates de inustionibus, sive fonticulis. Opus historiis medicis refertum, & in praxi utilissimum ... Adjuncta est Oeconomia physiologicorum Hippocratis redivivi. Lugduni, Apud Spiritum Vitalis, 1681.
[12], 323, [4] p.; II p.   17 cm.   **[9581]**
"Magnus Hippocrates Cous, medicorum omnium facile princeps, redivivus. Tomus primus; physiologica continens ... Autore R[aymond] R[estaurand] ..." (II p. at end) has special title page.

—Hippocrates de natura lactis, et de hujus usu in curationibus morbum ... Ed. 2. ab erroribus expurgata. Lugduni, Apud Spiritum Vitalis, 1682.
214 (i.e. 204) p.   15 cm.   **[9582]**
Includes selections from various works of Hippocrates in Latin.

—Monarchia microcosmi, Hippocratis magni, Platonis et Aristotelis insperato foedere restituta. In tres partes divisa. Quarum prima, commentarium continet in Hippocratis magni librum De corde: altera, in varios textus ex libro primo De victus ratione, ejusdem authoris: tertia, divini Platonis mentem, ex ejus Timaeo depromptam. Quibus, prostrata triplicis spiritus tyrannide, & sanguinis circulatione, animantis cor, supremo, partium corporis, & omnium functionum imperio redintegratur ... [Lyons?] 1657.
[44], 101 p.; [1], 72 p.; [4], 26 p.   24 cm.   **[9583]**

Includes Latin text of Hippocrates' De corde, selections from book one of his De victus ratione, and selections from Plato's Timaeus.

—*See* [GRAINDORGE, A.] In fictilem figuli exercitationem de principiis foetus. 1658.

REUDEN, MICHAEL [*b. ca.* 1571] Bedencken ob und wie die Artzneyen, so durch alchimistische Kunst bereitet werden, sonderlich vom Vitriol, Schwefel, Antimonio Mercurio, und dergleichen fruchtbarlich zugebrauchen sein ... Mit einer kurtzen Vorrede von dem Unterschied der hermetischen und galenischen Medicin Joachimi Tanckii ... Leipzig, In Verlegung Johan Rosen [Gedruckt bey Michael Lantzenberger] 1605.
[23], 101, [1] p.   17 cm.   **[9584]**

—*respondent.* De cardialgia theses medicas ... Jenae, Ex officina Christophori Lippoldi [1602]
[8] p.   20 cm.   **[9585]**
Diss.—Jena.

REUS, ABRAHAM DE [*fl.* 1668-1672] *respondent.*
Disputatio medica inauguralis de bulimo, seu appetentia canina ... Lugduni Batavorum, Apud viduam & haeredes Joannis Elsevirii, 1672.
　[26] p.　22 cm.　　　　　　**[9586]**
　Diss. — Leyden.

REUS, JOHANN [*fl.* 1698] *respondent.* Dissertatio medica inauguralis de apoplexia ... Lugduni Batavorum, Apud Abrahamum Elzevier, 1698.
　[30] p.　23 cm.　　　　　　**[9587]**
　Diss. — Leyden.

REUSNER, HIERONYMUS [*b.* 1558] Curationes et observationes medicae, e bibliotheca Georgii Hieronymi Velschii, cum ejusdem notis.
　109, [17] p.　20 cm.　(Part [5] in Welsch, Georg Hieronymus. Sylloge curationum. Aug. Vindel., 1667)　　　　　　**[9588]**
　Half title.

— Another issue. Sylloge curationum has title page dated 1668.　　　　　　**[9589]**

— Diexodicarum exercitationum liber de scorbuto. German. *In* Uffenbach, P., ed. and tr. Ein newes Artzney Buch. 1605.

— Eygendtliche unnd gründtliche Beschreibung dess uhralten heylsamen minerischem Badts zu Wembdingen ... In Truck gegeben, durch Esaiam Leschium ... Neuburg, Lorentz Danhauser, 1618.
　192 p.　16 cm.　　　　　　**[9590]**

— *See* JOANNES ACTUARIUS. De urinis libri VII. 1670.

REUSNER, NIKOLAUS [1545-1602] *See* LANGE, J. Epistolarum medicinalium volumen tripartitum. 1605.

REUSS, JOHANN ALBERT [*fl.* 1676] *respondent. See* LOHMEIER, P., *praeses.* Exercitatio physica de fulmine. 1676.

REUTER, LEONHARD [*fl.* 1697] *respondent. See* MOLLER, D. W., *praeses.* Disputationem circularem de Onuph. Panvinio ... ingredietur I. R. 1697.

REUTER, SIMON [*fl.* 1683] *respondent. See* ALBINUS, B. Disputatio medica inauguralis de sterilitate. 1693.

REVERHORST, MAURITS VAN [1666-1722] *respondent.* Dissertatio anatomico medica inauguralis de motu bilis circulari, ejusque morbis ... Lugduni

Batavorum, Apud Abrahamum Elzevier, 1692.
　[2], 25, [7] p.　illus.　21 cm.　　**[9591]**
　Diss. — Leyden.

— [The same.] *In* Nuck, A. Adenographia curiosa. 1696.

— [The same.] ... Lugduni Batavorum, Apud Jord. Luchtmans, 1696.
　64, [8] p.　17 cm.　　　　　　**[9592]**
　"Joachimi Targiri animadversio Dissertationem anatomico-medicam de motu bilis circulari Mauritii van Reverhorst ... Apud Cornelium Willegardium bibliopolam Dordracenum": [8] p.
　Bound with Blasius, G. Ontleeding des menschelyken lichaems. 1675.

— Solutionum apologeticarum eversiones. *In* Nuck, A. Defensio ductuum aquosorum. 1691.

REVIDIRTE ORDNUNG. *See* BRANDENBURG (Electorate) Laws, statutes, etc.

REWINKEL, GERARD [*fl.* 1652] *respondent.* Disputatio medica inauguralis de apoplexia ... Lugduni Batavorum, Apud Davidem Lopez de Haro, 1652.
　[12] p.　22 cm.　　　　　　**[9593]**
　Diss. — Leyden.

REYERSSEN, JOHANNES [*fl.* 1662] *respondent.* Dissertatio medica inauguralis de crisibus ... Lugduni Batavorum, Ex officina Salomonis Wagenaer, 1662.
　[16] p.　22 cm.　　　　　　**[9594]**
　Diss. — Leyden.

REYES FRANCO, GASPAR DE LOS [*fl.* 1658] Elysius jucundarum quaestionum campus, omnium literarum amoenissima varietate refertus. Medicis imprimis, tanquam in quo luxuriantis naturae spectatissimi flores erumpant, & admiranda illius opera contemplentur, maxime delectabilis ... Bruxellae, Typis & sumptibus Francisci Vivien, 1661.
　[28], 746, [59] p.　35 cm.　　　**[9595]**

— [The same.] ... Francofurti ad Moenum, Sumptibus haered. Johannis Beyeri, 1670.
　[39], 1263, [95] p.　22 cm.　　　**[9596]**

REYHER, SAMUEL [1635-1714] Dissertatio de aere ... Kiliae, Imprimebat Joach. Reuman, 1670.
　[84] p.　illus.　20 cm.　　　　**[9597]**

REYHING, BONAVENTURA [*fl.* 1620] *respondent. See* MÖGLING, J. L. [1608–1655] *praeses.* Problemata practica publica de scurbuto [sic] 1620.

REYMANN, JOHANN GOTTLOB [*fl.* 1697] *respondent. See* VESTI, J., *praeses.* Disputatio inauguralis medica, qua hectica cardiaca . . . examini submittitur a J. G. R. 1697.

REYNOLDES, THOMAS. *See* RAYNALDE, Thomas [*fl.* 1540–1555]

REYNOLDS, EDWARD, *Bp. of Norwich* [1599–1676] A treatise of the passions and faculties of the soule of man . . . London, R. H. for Robert Bostock, 1640.

[19], 553 (i.e. 497) p. 20 cm. **[9598]**

Imperfect: first preliminary leaf (portrait?) wanting.

—[The same.] . . . London, Printed by F. N. for Robert Bostock and George Badger, 1650.

[18], 553 (i.e. 497) p. 20 cm. **[9599]**

Different setting of type.

REYS TAVARES, MANUEL DOS [*fl.* 1667] Controversias philosophicas, et medicas. Ex doctrina de febribus . . . Communi censurę mittit judicandas. Ulyssipone, Ex typographia Joannis a Costa, 1667.

[11], 330 (i.e. 430) p. 20 cm. **[9600]**

Includes commentaries on the works of Avicenna, Galenus, Pedro Garcia Carrero and Tomás Rodrigues da Veiga.

REYSINGH, JOHANN HENNEMANN [*d.* 1614] Idaea loimodes, in qua salubres . . . in praesentissima luis pestiferae contagie praeservandi curandique, rationes ac media . . . suggeruntur . . . Nunc primitus . . . in lucem producta. Francofurti, Typis Antonii Hummii, impensis Martini Gnisen & Davidis Molleri, 1615.

[5], 75 p. 20 cm. **[9601]**

RHABANUS MAURUS. *See* HRABANUS MAURUS, *Abp. of Mainz* [784?–856]

RHAEDUS, THOMAS [*d.* 1624] *See* BARCLAY, W. Judicium. 1620.

RHAZES. *See* MUḤAMMAD IBN ZAKARĪYĀ, Abū Bakr, al-Rāzī [865–925]

RHEAD, ALEXANDER. *See* READ, Alexander [1586?–1641]

RHEBOLD, CHRISTIAN. *See* REHEBOLD, Christian [*b. ca.* 1625]

RHEINHART, HANS CHRISTOFF. *See* REINHART, Hans Christoff [*fl.* 1608–1611]

RHEMUS, JOHANN CHRISTOPH. *See* REHME, Johann Christoph [*fl.* 1664–1679]

RHENANUS, JOHANN [*fl.* 1610] Solis e puteo emergentis; sive, Dissertationis chymiotechnicae libri tres. In quibus totius operationis chymicae methodus practica: materia lapidis philosophici, & nodus [sic] solvendi ejus, operandique, ut & clavis operum Paracelsi, qua abstrusa explicantur deficientia supplentur. Cum praefatione chymiae veritatem asserente. Francofurti, Impensis Antonii Hummi, 1613.

[23], 80 (i.e. 78) p.; 31 p.; 24 p. illus., table. 21 cm. **[9602]**

Parts 2 and 3 have special title pages.
Bound with Burggrav, J. E. Introductio in vitalem philosophiam. 1643.

—*See* PLINIUS SECUNDUS, C. Naturalis historiae, tomus primus [-tertius] 1668–1669.

RHETIUS, ANDREAS CHRISTIAN [*fl.* 1698] *respondent. See* STAHL, G. E., *praeses.* Disputatio medica inauguralis de morbis habitualibus. 1698.

—*See* STAHL, G. E. Propempticon inaugurale quis bonus theoreticus, malus practicus. 1698.

RHETIUS, JEREMIAS [*fl.* 1655–1658] *respondent. See* MÖBIUS, G., *praeses.* Dissertatio medica inauguralis de febre petechiali. 1658.

RHIJNE, WILLEM TEN [1647–1700] Dissertatio De arthritide; Mantissa schematica; De acupunctura, et orationes tres, I. De chymiae ac botaniae antiquitate et dignitate. II. De physiognomia; III. De monstris . . . Londini, R. Chiswell, 1683.

[46], 334 p. front. (port.), plates. 20 cm. **[9603]**

Imperfect: frontispiece, and plates 2 and 4 wanting.

—Meditationes in magni Hippocratis textum xxiv De veteri medicina. Quibus traduntur brevis πνευματολογία, succincta φυτολογία, intercalaris χυμολογία &c. Cum additamento & variis hinc inde laciniis de salium &c. figuris. Lugd. Batavorum, Apud Johannem à Schuylenburgh, 1672.

[22], 387, [29] p. front., plate. 14 cm. **[9604]**

Errata: p. [28–29]

—Copy 2.

Imperfect: front. and plate wanting.

With this are bound: Wedel, G. W. Specimen experimenti chimici novi, de sale volatili plantarum. 1672; Hesteau, Clovis, sieur de Nuisement. Tractatus de vero sale secreto philosophorum, 1671.

—Verhandelinge van de Asiatise melaatsheid, na een naaukeuriger ondersoek, ten dienste van het gemeen . . . Amsterdam, Abraham van Someren, 1687.

[18], 181 p.   17 cm.   **[9605]**

RHIJNE, WILLEM TEN [1647-1700] Chineese en Japanse wijze om allerlei ziekten door het branden van moxa en het steken met een goude naald zekerlijk te genesen. In Blankaart, S. Verhandelinge van het podagra en vliegende jicht. 1684; [German tr.] 1690, 1692.

RHODA, FRIEDRICH WILHELM VON [1671-1723] *respondent. See* CRAUSE, R. W., *praeses*. De opisthotono dissertationem inauguralem . . . submittit . . . F. W. R. 1696; WEDEL, G. W., *praeses*. Dissertatio medica de acidulis. 1695.

—*See* WEDEL, G. W. Propempticum inaugurale de morbo nabalis. 1696.

RHODE, AMBROSIUS [1605-1696] Disputationes supra Ideam medicinae philosophicae Petri Severini . . . Quibus loca illius libri obscura & difficilia il-lustrantur, adversarii refutantur, & multi discursus . . . deprompti moventur . . . Hafniae, Sumptibus authoris, typis Salomonis Sartorii, 1643.

[19], 214, [1] p.   20 cm.   **[9606]**

Errata: p. [1] at end.

RHODE, JOHAN. *See* RODE, Johan [1587-1659]

RHODIANUS. *See* JĀBIR IBN ḤAIYĀN, al-Ṭarasūsī. Gebri . . . Summa perfectionis magisterii in sua natura. 1682.

RHODION, EUCHARIUS. *See* ROESLIN, Eucharius [d. 1526]

RHODIUS, AMBROSIUS. *See* RHODE, Ambrosius [1605-1696]

RHODIUS, JOHANNES. *See* RODE, Johan [1587-1659]

RHODOCH, FEDRO VON. *See* FEDRO VON RODACH, Georg [16th cent.]

RHODOCHAEUS, PHAEDRUS. *See* FEDRO VON RODACH, Georg [16th cent.]

RHODOKANAKIS, CONSTANTINE [1635-1689] Alexicacus; spirit of salt of the world . . . long look'd for, and now philosophically prepared and purified . . . 7th ed. enlarged with testimonies, adver-tisements, and rare medicaments . . . London, W. G., 1670.

[4], 24 p.   18 cm.   **[9607]**

RHOMAEUS, AGRICOLA. Vade-mecum philosophicum. *In* Philalethes, E. Enarratio methodica trium Gebri medicinarum. 1678.

RHOSITHINAS, PETRUS. *See* ROSTINIO, Pietro [16th. cent.]

RHUMELIUS. *See* RUMMEL.

RHYAKINUS, *pseud. See* RIVINUS, Andreas [*ca.* 1601-1656]

RHYNE, WILHELM TEN. *See* RHIJNE, Willem ten [1647-1700]

RHYTMI de lapide philosophorum. *See* SUMMA rhytmorum Germanicorum de opere universali ex coelo soloque prodeunte. 1661.

RHYTMI parvi Germanici. *See* SUMMA rhyt-morum parvorum Germanicorum. 1661.

RICANI, CARLO [*fl.* 1695] *tr. See* LES ADMIRABLES qualitez du kinkina. La kinakina, e le di lei stupende qualita. 1694; RESTAURAND, R. Ippocrate dell'uso della kinakina. 1695.

RICARDUS, PARISIENSIS [*d.* 1252] Libellus utilissimus Περὶ χημείας cui titulum fecit, Correc-torium [&] Libellus alius Περὶ χημείας utilissimus, et rerum metallicarum cognitione refertissimus, Rosarius minor inscriptus, incerti quidem, sed harum tamen rerum non imperiti auctoris.

385-422 p., vol. 2.   20 cm. (*In* Zetzner, Lazarus, *ed.* Theatrum chemicum. Argentorati, 1659-61)   **[9608]**

Caption titles.

RICCO, DANIEL [*fl.* 1690] Ristretto anotomico; o sia, Aleanza de gl'astri, con l'huomo, e vegetabili. Fatica laboriosa de' medici, e chirurghi primati di Spagna . . . donato all' Hospitale di Madrid . . .

Venetia, Brescia, Milano, Marc'Antonio Pandolfo Malatesta [1690?]

20 p.　front.　23 cm.　　　　**[9609]**

Identical in contents with Francesco Minniti's Armonia astro-medico-anatomica, published in Venice in 1690.

RICETTARIO fiorentino, di nuovo illustrato. [Firenze, Pietro Cecconcelli] 1623.

[10], 296, [46] p.　illus.　33 cm.　　**[9610]**

Engraved title page.

Part 1 has caption title: Del ricettario dell'arte, et universita de' medici, e speziali della citta di Firenze.

A reprint of the 1597 edition.

First published in 1498 under title: Nuovo receptario. Titles of later editions vary: Ricettario dell'arte, Ricettario medicinale, Ricettario utilissimo.

—[The same.] . . . [Firenze, Nella stamperia di S. A. Sereniss. per Vincenzio Vangelisti, e Pietro Matini] 1670.

[6], 281, [46] p.　illus.　34 cm.　**[9611]**

Engraved title page.

A revised version of the 1623 edition.

—[The same.] . . . [Firenze, Nella stamperia di S. A. S. per Gio. Filippo Cecchi] 1696.

[6], 331 p.　illus.　38 cm.　　**[9612]**

Engraved title page.

—*See* SANTINI, G. Ricettario medicinale. 1604.

A RICH closet of physical secrets, collected by the elaborate paines of four severall students in physick, and digested together; viz. The child-bearers cabinet. A preservative against the plague and small pox. Physicall experiments presented to our late Queen Elizabeths own hands. With certain approved medicines, taken out of a manuscript . . . and supplied with some of his own experiments, by a late English doctor. London, Printed by Gartrude Dawson, and sold by [William Nealand? 1652]

[8], 71 p.; [6], 65 p.; 97-66 (i.e. 146), [14] p.　19 cm.　　　　　　　　　　　　　**[9613]**

Imperfect: [14] p. at end wanting.

Imprint lacks William Nealand's name.

Letters to the reader signed A. M.

"Thus farre Doctor Edwards doctor in physick and chirurgery": p. 104.

Part 2 has special title page: A treatise concerning the plague and the pox.

A RICH storehouse or treasurie for the diseased . . . First set foorth for the benefit and comfort of the poorer sort of people . . . By G. W[ateson] And now

sixtly augm. and inl. by A. T. . . . London, Ralph Blower, 1616.

[14], 176 (i.e. 145) ll. illus. 19 cm.　**[9614]**

STC 23609.

—[The same.] . . . Now seventhly augm. and inl. by A. T. . . . London, Printed by Richard Badger, for Philemon Stephens and Christopher Meredith, 1630.

[24], 317, [1] p.　19 cm.　　**[9615]**

Imperfect: p. 95-96 imperfectly printed, affecting text.

STC 23610.

—Another issue, with imprint dated 1631.

[9616]

Colophon: London, Printed by Richard Badger, for Philemon Stephens and Christopher Meredith, 1630.

Interleaved.

STC 23611.

—[The same.] . . . The 8th ed., augm. and enl., by D. B. London, John Clowes, 1650.

[24], 274 (i.e. 280) p.　18 cm.　**[9617]**

Imperfect: sig. A¹ (blank?), A⁴ wanting; sig.*⁴ misbound; lower margins trimmed; p. 245-274 mutilated.

RICHANY, CARLO. *See* RICANI, Carlo [*fl.* 1695]

RICHARDSON, EDWARD [*b. ca.* 1617] *respondent.* Disputatio medica inauguralis de dolore nephritico . . . Lugduni Batavorum, Apud viduam & haeredes Johannis Elsevirii, 1664.

[8] p.　24 cm.　　　　**[9618]**

Diss.—Leyden.

RICHARDUS, ANGLICUS. *See* RICARDUS, Parisiensis [*d.* 1252]

RICHELMANN, JOHANN ERNST [*fl.* 1683] *respondent. See* KEMPER, T., *praeses.* Dissertatio anatomico-medica de valvularum in corporibus hominis et brutorum natura. 1683.

RICHIER, JOHANN [*fl.* 1682-1683] *respondent. See* FRANCK VON FRANCKENAU, G., *praeses.* Disputatio medica inauguralis de risu sardonio. 1683 [and] Satyrae medicae, continuatio XVIII. 1682.

RICHMAN, JOHANN [*fl.* 1667] *respondent. See* ROLFINCK, W., *praeses.* Ordo et methodus cognoscendi praecavendi. 1667.

RICHTER, CHRISTIAN [*fl.* 1668-1674] *respondent. See* MEIBOM, H., *praeses.* Dissertatio medica inauguralis de laesionibus cranii a causa externa violenta. 1674; POSNER, C., *praeses.* Disputatio physica de ordine partium in compositione ac formatione corporis animalium. 1668.

RICHTER, CHRISTIAN [*fl.* 1678] *respondent. See* RIVENUS, A. Q., *praeses.* Dissertatio medica de sangvificatione. 1678.

RICHTER, CHRISTIAN ALBERT [*b.* 1674] *respondent. See* STAHL, G. E., *praeses.* Disputatio medica inauguralis, quae exhibet venaesectionis patrocinium. 1698 [and] Dissertatio medica qua temperamenta physiologico-physiognomico-pathologico-mechanice enucleantur. 1698.

—*See* STAHL, G. E. Propempticon inaugurale de commotionibus sanguinis activis et passivis. 1698.

RICHTER, CHRISTIAN FRIEDRICH [*fl.* 1671] *respondent. See* FRIDERICI, J. A., *praeses.* Disputationem inauguralem de cardialgia ... publicae ... censurae exponit ... C. F. R. 1671.

RICHTER, CHRISTOPH [*fl.* 1669-1671] *respondent. See* Friderici, J. A., *praeses.* Dissertationem medicam de vertigine ... submittit ... C. R. 1669.

RICHTER, CHRISTOPH [*fl.* 1691] *respondent. See* VESTI, J., *praeses.* Disputatio inauguralis medica de anorexia. 1691.

RICHTER, CHRISTOPH FRIEDRICH [*fl.* 1697-1707] *respondent. See* BOHN, J., *praeses.* De medici officio dissertatio quarta. 1699.

RICHTER, CHRISTOPH HEINRICH [*fl.* 1698] *respondent. See* COLER, J. A., *praeses.* Ex mechanicis de vesica. 1698.

RICHTER, ERNST EUSEBIUS [*fl.* 1683-1737] Dissertatio inauguralis medica, casum de chlorosi ... Gissae, Literis Kargerianis [1683]

    16 p.   18 cm.   [9619]
Diss.—Giessen.

RICHTER, FRANZ [*fl.* 1624] *respondent. See* INNICHENHÖFER, H., *praeses.* Ὑπνολογια; sive, Tractatus jucundus physiologicus. 1624.

RICHTER, JOHANN [*b.* 1652] *respondent. See* STAHL, G. E., *praeses.* Dissertatio medica inauguralis de calculorum generatione. 1699.

—*See* STAHL, G. E. Propempticon inaugurale de empeiria. 1699.

RICK, THEODORUS. *See* RYCKE, Theodor [1640-1690]

RICOME, LAURENS [1654-1711] Quaestiones medico-chymico-practicae duodecim ab ... Michaele de Chicoyneau [et al.] ... propositae ... pro regia chymiae professione vacante ... per obitum ... Arnaldi Fonsorbe ... quas ... propugnabit ... Laurentius Ricome ... Monspelii, Apud Honoratum Pech, 1696.

    22 p.   22 cm.   [9620]
Thèse de concours—Montpellier.

RIDDERUS, FRANCISCUS [1620-1683] Historisch sterf-huys; ofte, t' Samen-spraeck uyt ... historien over allerley voorval ontrene siecke en stervende ... Den 3. druck. Amsterdam, Michiel de Groot, 1678.

    487, [1] p.   14 cm.   [9621]
Added engraved title page.

RIDER, CARDANUS, *ed. See* RIDERS (1677.) British Merlin. 1677.

RIDER, HUGH. *See* RYDER, Hugh [*fl.* 1673-1697]

RIDERS (1677.) British Merlin: bedeckt with many delightful varieties, and useful verities ... With notes of husbandry, physick fayrs, & marts ... Made and compiled for the benefit of his country, by Cardanus Riders. London, Tho. Newcomb, for the Company of Stationers, 1677.

    [48] p.   14 cm.   [9622]

RIDEUX, PIERRE [*d.* 1707] Quaestiones medico-chymico-practicae duodecim ab ... Michaele Chicoyneau ... propositae ... pro regia chymiae professione vacante per obitum ... Arnaldi Fonsorbe ... quas ... propugnabit ... Petrus Rideu ... Monspelii, Apud Honoratum Pech, 1697.

    [5], 21 p.   22 cm.   [9623]
Thèses de concours—Montpellier.

RIDLEY, HUMPHREY [1653-1708] The anatomy of the brain. Containing its mechanism and physiology; together with some new discoveries and corrections of ancient and modern authors upon that subject. To which is annex'd a particular account of animal functions and muscular motion ... London, Sam. Smith and Benj. Walford, 1695.

    [15], 200, [24] p.   plates.   20 cm.   [9624]
Illustrated by William Cowper.

RIEDLIN, Veit [1628-1668] Observationum medicarum centuriae tres. Editae ab auctoris filio Vito Riedlino ... Augustae Vind., Apud Laurentium Kronigerum, & haeredes Theoph. Göbelii, typis viduae Leonh. Zachariae, 1691.

[20], 264 p.; [12], 233, [31] p.; 265-475, [17] p. plate. 14 cm. **[9625]**

—*respondent. See* Sebisch, M. [1578-1674?] *praeses.* Galeni quinque priores libri. 1651.

RIEDLIN, Veit [1656-1724] Lineae medicae, singulos per menses quotidie ductae ... anni M DC XCV [-M DCC] ... Augustae Vindelicorum, Impensis Laurenti Kronigeri, & haered. Theophili Göbelii, typis Antonii Nepperschmidii, 1695-1700.

6 v. in 10. 17 cm. **[9626]**

Each volume has added engraved title page.
Vols. [5] and [6] were printed by Johann Christopher Wagner.
Inserted in vol. [6], facing p. 1011, is an engraved title page, "Anatomia nova rationalis."

—Observationum medicarum centuria. Anno ... M. DC. LXXXII. Augustae Vindelicorum, Impensis Theophili Göbelii, typis Joh. Jacobi Schönigkii, 1682.

[24], 233, [31] p. plate. 13 cm. **[9627]**

—, *ed. See* Riedlin, V. [1628-1668] Observationum medicarum centuriae tres. 1691.

RIEDMILLER, Hieronymus [*fl.* 1628] *respondent. See* Wangnerick, H., *praeses.* Conclusiones philosophicae ex libris De generatione [Aristotelis] 1628.

RIEL, Kristoph Fridrich. *See* Rüel, Christopher Friedrich [*fl.* 1681]

RIEMER, Johann [1648-1714] Vitia virtuosa sexus feminini ex dolis bellis et duellis mulierum historico et politico filo contexta ... Weissenfelsae, Sumptibus Christophori Enoch Buchta, excudebat Johannes Brühl, 1680.

[8] p. 19 cm. **[9628]**

—*praeses.* Bella mulierum ... Weissenfelsae, Literis Johannis Brühlii [*ca.* 1680]

[40] p. 19 cm. **[9629]**

Diss.—Weissenfels. Gymnasium (J. C. Frauendorff, *respondent*)

—Dolos mulierum ... publicae ventilationi subjicient praeses Johannes Riemer ... et respondens

Johannes Augustus Lystenius ... Weissenfelsae, Literis Johannis Brühlii [1680]

[84] p. 19 cm. **[9630]**

Diss.—Weissenfels. Gymnasium (J. A. Lystenius, *respondent*)

—Duella mulierum ... Weissenfelsae, Literis Johannis Brühlii [1680]

[24] p. 19 cm. **[9631]**

Diss.—Weissenfels, Gymnasium (S. Carpzov, *respondent*)

RIEROS, Juan Sorapan. *See* Sorapán de Rieros, Juan [*fl.* 1615-1638]

RIESNER, Johann Andreas [*fl.* 1696-1699] *respondent. See* Winther, J. G., *praeses.* Diatribam hanc medicam hydropem ascitem examinantem censurae sistit J. A. R. 1699.

RIETMAKERS, Hubert Arnold [*fl.* 17th cent.] Tractatus de nephritico dolore; in quo essentia, differentiae, causae, signa, & curatio calculi & arenularum explanantur ... Lovanii, Apud Henricum Hastenium, 1622.

78, [2] p. 18 cm. **[9632]**

Errata: p. [2] at end.

RIETMANN, Ulrich [*fl.* 1620-1621] *respondent. See* Sebisch, M. [1578-1674?] *praeses.* Disputatio de purgatione sexta. 1621 [and] Disputatio de venae sectione vigesima septima. 1620 [and] Disputationes de recta ratione purgandi. 1621.

RIFFUS, Gualtherius Hermenius. *See* Ryff, Walther Hermenius [*d.* 1548]

RIFORMA dell ospedale detto di Mon'Agnesa ... [Siena? 16—?]

46 p. 20 cm. **[9633]**

Caption title.
Dedicated to Ferdinando Medici, granduca di Toscana.

RIGAULT, Nicolas [1577-1654] *ed.* and *tr. See* Artemidorus Daldianus. Artemidori Daldiani & Achmetis Sereimi f. Oneirocritica. 1603.

—*See* Kirchmann, J. De funeribus Romanorum libri quatuor. 1672.

RIGHI, Alessandro [*fl.* 1630] Historia contagiosi morbi, qui Florentiam populatus fuit anno 1630 ... Florentiae, Typis Francisci Honufrii, 1633.

[16], 236, [1] p. 20 cm. **[9634]**

RIGIUS, Heino [*fl.* 1649] *respondent.* Decas thesium inauguralium de affectione hypochondriaca

... Lugduni Batavorum, Ex officina Jacobi Lauwijck, 1649.

 [12] p.　20 cm.　　　　　　　　**[9635]**
Diss.—Utrecht.

RIGOGOLI, LATTANZIO. *See* SANLORINI, A. La polvere schernita. 1654.

RIJKSUNIVERSITEIT TE LEIDEN. *See* MEURS, J. van [1579–1639] Athenae Batavae. 1625 [and] Illustrium Hollandiae & Westfrisiae ordinum alma Academia Leidensis. 1614.

—Anatomisch Kabinet. *See* BLANCKEN, G. Catalogus antiquarum et novarum rerum ex longe dissitis terrarum oris congestis. 1700; [VOORN, J.] Catalogus antiquarum et novarum rerum ex longe dissitis terrarum oris. 1690?

—Faculteit der Medicijn. Attestatie, 1679. *See* ANTWOORD op seker boekjen, rakende de genesinge van een hooft-wonde. 1687.

RIJNE, WILLEM TEN. *See* RHIJNE, Willem ten [1647–1700]

RIKEMANN, JOHANN [*fl.* 1669–1689] *praeses*. Ordinis et methodi cogniscendi praecavendi curandi ebrietatem et inde ortam crapulam editio secunda ... Jenae, Stanno Johannis Jacobi Bauhoferi [1670]

 [1], 49, [3] p.　19 cm.　　　　　　**[9636]**
Diss.—Jena (G. Loner, *respondent*)

—Satyriasin et priapismum publicae philiatrorum disquisitioni ... Jenae, Ex officina Samuelis Krebsii, 1670.

 52, [4] p.　20 cm.　　　　　　　　**[9637]**
Diss.—Jena (J. Eschenbach, *respondent*)

RIMPAU, SIGMUND CHRISTIAN [*fl.* 1698] *respondent*. *See* SCHRADER, F., *praeses*. De regularum sanitatis prudenti applicatione dissertatio. 1698.

RINALDI, CAMILLO MARIA, *Father* [1631–1700] *tr*. *See* PUENTE, L. de la, *Father*. Tesoro nascosto nelle infermità. 1690.

RINALDI, GIOVANNI DE'. Il mostruosissimo mostro ... Diviso in due trattati. Nel primo de' quali si ragiona del significato de' colori. Nel secondo si tratta dell' herbe, & fiori. Di nuovo ristampato, & con somma diligenza corretto ... Venetia, Ghirardo, & Iseppo Imberti, 1626.

 78, [1] ll.　14 cm.　　　　　　　　**[9638]**

RINALDINI, CARLO [1615–1698] Pagina, summatim exhibens ea, de quibus ipse in suis praelectionibus est acturus, dum labente anno Aristotelis primum, & secundum De anima subtilissimos libros interpraetabitur. Prolegomena in quibus 1. Explicatur quae sit horum librorum cum praecedentibus connexio. Et quem in physiologia locum, hoc opus De anima, obtineat. 2. Quae subjecta materies. 3. Quae tandem divisio ... [Patavii, Typis seminarii, 1689]

 xi p.　23 cm.　　　　　　　　　　**[9639]**
Caption title.
Pages v-viii in duplicate.

RINCIO, CESARE [*d.* 1580] *See* CENTORIO DEGLI HORTENSII, A. I cinque libri de gli avvertimenti, ordini, gride, et editti: fatti ... in Milano. 1631.

RINDFLEISCH, DANIEL. *See* BUCRETIUS, Daniel [*d.* 1631]

RINEGGER, GEORG [*fl.* 1632] *respondent*. *See* MANNAGETTA, J. W., *praeses*. Disputatio medica, de purgandi ratione. 1632.

RINGELMAN, JOHANN LUDOLPH [*fl.* 1664] *respondent*. *See* ROLFINCK, W., *praeses*. Diatribe inauguralis medica. 1664.

RINGELSTEIN, JOHANN ADOLF [*fl.* 1625] *See* DUCHESNE, J. Diaeteticon polyhistoricum. 1625.

RINGMACHER, DANIEL [1662–1728] Dissertationem de variis philosophorum circa principia corporum naturalium, praessertim viventium, placitis ... p. p. ... M. Daniel Ringmacher ... respondente Joh. Adamo Glasero ... Lipsiae, Typis Joh. Christoph. Brandenburgerii [1688]

 68 p.　20 cm.　　　　　　　　　**[9640]**
Diss. — Leipzig (J. A. Glaser, *respondent*)

RINVILLUS, BRISTOLLENSIS, *pseud*. *See* NORTON, Samuel [1548–1604?]

RIO, MARTIN ANTOINE DEL. *See* DEL RIO, Martin Antoine [1551–1608]

RIOLAN, JEAN [1538?–1605?] Opera cum physica, tum medica, authoris postrema manu exarata & exornata ... Cui accessit Anatomia Joannis Riolani filii ... Francofurti, Apud D. Zachariam Palthenium, 1611.

 [16], 567, [15] p.　port.　33 cm.　　**[9641]**
A reprint of the 1610 Paris edition, edited by the author's son. Provided with a new index by the publisher. Cf. dedicatory epistle, signed: Zacharias Palthenius ... librarius.

The "Anatome Joannis Riolani filii" (p. 439-567) had been published in Paris in 1608 under title: Schola anatomica.

—Opera medica. Tam hactenus edita quam postuma, authoris postrema manu exarata & exornata. Quibus universam medicinam fideliter & accurate descripsit atque illustravit. Parisiis, Ex Officina Plantiniana, apud Hadrianum Perier, 1619.

3 v. in 1.   18 cm.   [9642]

Vols. [2-3] dated 1681.

The three works were issued separately by Perier in 1618.

Contents.—Universae medicinae compendium.—Ars bene medendi.—Chirurgia. Ed. 3., ab authore aucta & recognita.

—Ars bene medendi . . . Parisiis, In Officina Plantiniana, Apud Hadrianum Perier, 1601.

[8], 210 (i.e. 211), [1] ll.   17 cm.   [9643]

—[The same.] . . . Parisiis, Ex Officina Plantiniana, Apud Hadrianum Perier, 1618.

[15], 740, [12] p.   19 cm.   [9644]

With this is bound *his* Chirurgia.

—[The same.] . . . Artis bene medendi methodus generalis . . . Hac postrema editione aucta, plurimisque mendis vindicata. Parisiis, Apud Ludovicum Boullenger, 1638.

[12], 158, [9] p.; [10], 7-628 (i.e. 584), [20] p.   18 cm.   [9645]

Part [2] has special title page: Artis bene medendi methodus particularis.

—[English tr.] *In* Vaughan, W. Directions for health. 1626, 1633.

—Artis medicinalis, theoricae & practicae sejunctim hactenus multoties excusae, systema, ab Emmanuele Stupano . . . hac forma adornatum, recognitum & studiosissime emendatum. Basileae, Sumptibus Ludovici Regis, 1629.

2 v. in 1.   17 cm.   [9646]

Vol. [1] was first published in 1598 under title: Universae medicinae compendia.

Vol [2] with title "Morborum curandorum ratio generalis particularis" was also published separately under title: Ars bene medendi.

—Chirurgia. [Lipsiae] Impensis Henrici Osthausii [Lipsiae, Excudebant haeredes Francisci Schnelbolzii, typis haeredum Beyeri] 1601.

[6], 175, [1] p.   15 cm.   [9647]

Edited by Johann von Jessen.

—[The same.] . . . Ed. 3, ab authore aucta & recognita. Parisiis, Ex Officina Plantiniana, Apud

Hadrianum Perier, 1618.

[7], 159 p.   19 cm.   [9648]

Edited by Johann von Jessen.

Bound with *his* Ars bene medendi. 1618.

—[The same.] . . . Parisiis, Apud Ludovicum Boullenger, 1638.

157, [10] p.   17 cm.   [9649]

Edited by Johann von Jessen.

With this is bound *his* Tractatus de febribus. 1640.

—[French tr.] Chirurgie . . . Traduite en françois. Avec un traité des maladies veneriennes & la methode pour en guerir. Par Monsieur B******* D. M. Paris, La Boutique de Langelier, chez René Guignard, 1669.

[16], 266 (i.e. 264), 38 p.   16 cm.   [9650]

Dedicatory epistle by the translator signed: J. B.

"Traité des maladies veneriennes": 38 p. at end.

—In artem parvam Galeni commentarius. Ex bibliotheca G. Naudaei. Pariis, Dionysius Langlaeus, 1631.

[12], 162 p.   13 cm.   [9651]

—Praelectiones in libros physiologicos & De abditis rerum causis; cum brevibus scholiis ejusdem auctoris. Accesserunt opuscula quaedam philosophica . . . Parisiis, Ex Officina Plantiniana, apud Hadrianum Perier, 1601.

240 p.; 250, [1] p.   18 cm.   [9652]

The "Praelectiones in libros physiologicos" were first published collectively in 1588 under title: In libros Fernelii . . . physiologicos . . . commentarii.

The commentary on the De abditis rerum causis was published separately in 1598 under title: Ad libros Fernelii De abditis rerum causis . . . commentarius.

—Tractatus de febribus. Ex bibliotheca Jacobi Mantelli ejusdem professionis & ordinis. Parisiis, Apud Ludovicum Boullenger, 1640.

[16], 39, [7] p.   17 cm.   [9653]

Bound with *his* Chirurgia. 1638.

—Universae medicinae compendium . . .

[10], 340 p.   18 cm.   (Vol. 1 *in* his Opera medica, Parisiis, 1619)   [9654]

Caption title.

—[The same.] . . . Parisiis, Apud Simonem Perier, 1626.

[12], 348 p.   15 cm.   [9655]

—*See* BAYLEY, W. Two treatises concerning the preservation of eie-sight. 1616; DALECHAMPS, J. Chirurgie françoise. 1610.

RIOLAN, Jean [1580-1657] Opera anatomica vetera, recognita, & auctiora ... Lutetiae Parisiorum, Sumptibus Gaspari Meturas, 1650.

[28], 872, 56 p.   38 cm.   **[9656]**

"Anthropographiae liber primus [-septimus]": p. 1-425.

"In librum Galeni De ossibus, ad tyrones Commentarius ... Simiae osteologia ... Osteologia ex Hippocratis libris eruta, collecta, & in ordinem digesta" (p. [427]-538); "Opuscula anatomica nova" (p. 539-842); and "Spongia alexiteria, adversus ... Aemilii Parisiani, sive responsio ad singulare certamen de diaphragmate" (p. [843]-869) have half titles.

"Rarae observationes anatomicae" (p. 870-872) has caption title.

Edited by Guy Patin.

—Animadversiones in Syntagma anatomicum Joannis Veslingii. *See* Marchetti, D. de. Anatomia. 1652, 1654, 1656, 1688.

—Anthropographia. Ex propriis, & novis observationibus collecta, concinnata ... Parisiis, Ex Officina Plantiniana, Apud Hadrianum Perier, 1618.

[46], 666 p.; [5], 101, [3] p.   18 cm.   **[9657]**

Part [2] has half title: Anatomica. Humani foetus historia. Adjectae sunt viventis animalis observationes anatomicae.

—Anthropographia, et Osteologia. Omnia recognita, triplo auctiora, & emendatiora, ex propriis, ac novis cogitationibus, & observationibus ... [Francofurti] Prostant in officina Bryanae, 1626.

[74], 938, [60] p.   24 cm.   **[9658]**

Imperfect? Added engraved title page and portrait wanting?

"Osteologia novantiqua ex recentiorum et veterum anatomicorum praeceptis. In qua continentur Isagoge de ossibus, cum osteologia infantis ... In librum Galeni De ossibus ad tyrones Commentarius ... Simiae osteologia, ut discrimen ossium hominis & simiae innotescat. Osteologia ex Hippocratis libris eruta, collecta, & in ordinem digesta" (p. [671]-922) has half title.

—[French tr.] Les oeuvres anatomiques ... reveuës & augmentees d'une cinquiesme partie en ceste edition. Tome premier [-second] ... Le tout rangé, corrigé, divisé, noté & mis en françois par M. Pierre Constant ... Paris, Denys Moreau, 1628-29 [v. 1, 1629]

2 v. in 1.   24 cm.   **[9659]**

Imperfect: preliminary matter of v. 1 misbound; cancel and original half of privilege present.

Added engraved title page.

[—] Apologia pro Hippocratis et Galeni medicina adversus Quercetani [pseud., i.e. Joseph Duchesne] Librum de priscorum philosophorum verae medicinae materia, praeparationis modo atque in curandis morbis praestantia. Accessit censura scholae Parisiensis. Parisiis, Ex Officina Plantinia, Apud Hadrianum Perier, 1603.

63 (i.e. 93) p.   15 cm.   **[9660]**

Variously ascribed to the younger Jean Riolan, and to Sir Théodore Turquet de Myerne. Cf. BMC, BNC.

—[The same, *as subject.*] *See* Duchesne, J. Jos. Quercetani ... Ad veritatem hermeticae medicinam. 1604, 1605; [English tr.] 1605.

[—] Brevis excursus in battologiam Quercetani [pseud., i.e. Joseph Duchesne] quo alchymiae principia funditus diruuntur, & artis vanitas demonstratur. Accessit censura Scholae Parisiensis. Parisiis, Ex Officina Plantiniana, Apud Hadrianum Perier, 1604.

180 p.   14 cm.   **[9661]**

—[The same, *as subject.*] *See* Duchesne, J. Jos. Quercetani ... Tetras gravissimorum totius capitis affectum. 1617.

—Censura demonstrationum Harveti pro veritate alchymiae ... Parisiis, Ex Officina Plantiniana, Apud Hadrianum Perier, 1606.

84 p.   15 cm.   **[9662]**

A reply to Israel Harvet's Demonstratio veritatis doctrina chymicae which censured Riolan's Comparatio veteris medicinae cum nova, published in Paris in 1605.

Bound with Glisson, F. Tractatus de ventriculo et intestinis. 1677.

—Comparatio veteris medicinae cum nova. *See* Harvet, I. Demonstratio veritatis doctrinae chymicae. 1605.

—Curieuses recherches sur les escholes en medecine de Paris, et de Montpelier, necessaires d'estre sçeuës, pour la conservation de la vie. Par un ancien docteur en medecine de la Faculté de Paris. Paris, Gaspar Meturas, 1651.

[14], 291, [11] p.   17 cm.   **[9663]**

"Additions au discours precedent" and "Additions au texte de ce discours": [11] p. at end.

In part a reply to the attacks of Théophraste Renaudot on the Faculté de médecine of Paris.

—De monstro nato Lutetiae anno Domini. 1605. disputatio philosophica ... Parisiis, Apud Olivarium Varennaeum, 1605.

[3], 28 ll. plates.   17 cm.   **[9664]**

Three of the four plates issued originally in other works.

With this is bound Histoire d'un homme monstreux, qui pesoit 640. [n. p., 1750?]

[—] Discours sur les hermaphrodits. Où il est demonstré contre l'opinion commune, qu'il n'y a point de vrays hermaphrodits. Paris, Pierre Ramier, 1614.

    [8], 136 p. 18 cm.   **[9665]**

—Encheiridium anatomicum, et pathologicum, in quo ex naturali constitutione partium, recessus à naturali statu demonstratur ... Parisiis, Apud Gasparum Meturas, 1648.

    [27], 618, [16] p. 14 cm.   **[9666]**

—Copy 2. 14 cm.

With this is bound Harvey, W. Exercitatio anatomica de circulatio sanguinis. 1650.

—[The same.] ... Lugduni Batavorum, Ex officina Adriani Wyngaerden, 1649.

    [20], 410, 417-471, [72] p. plates. 19 cm.

                                  [9667]

Added engraved title page.

—[The same.] ... Ed. 4., renovata, illustrata, variis tractatibus locupletata, & emendata ... Parisiis, Apud Casparum Meturas, 1658.

    [32], 610, [64] p. front. (port.) 17 cm.

                                    [9668]

In addition to the contents of the 1649 edition, includes his: Commentatio adversus novum de venis lacteis commentum; — Additamentum, in quo declaratur Riolani judicium generale, de motu sanguinis in brutis, & homine; —De unguibus; —De pilis; —De valvulis venarum; —Tractatus de anatome pneumatica; —Caroli Arturi Plessi ... Observatio.

—[The same.] ... Ed. nova, emendatior, & variis tractatibus aliis auctior ... Ed. 2. Francofurti, Sumtibus Augusti Boetii, bibliopolae Gothani, 1677.

    2 parts in 1 v. plates. 18 cm.   **[9669]**

Added engraved title page.
Pt. [2] has half-title: Opuscula quaedam physiologico-medica.

—[English tr.] A sure guide; or, The best and nearest way to physick and chyrurgery ... Being an anatomical description of the whole body of man, and its parts ... Englished by Nich. Culpeper ... and W[illiam] R[and]. London, Peter Cole, 1657.

    [12], 288 (i.e. 240), [60] p. plates. 28 cm.

                                    [9670]

Imperfect: sheet B wanting; supplied in photocopy from New York Academy of Medicine Library. Title label "Culpepers six books of physick and chyrurgery" bound at front.

—[The same.] ... London, Peter Cole, 1665.

    [10], 288 (i.e. 240), [62] p. plates. 28 cm.

                                    [9671]

The text is of the same setting as the 1657 edition.
Sheet inserted before plates reads: The use of the letters and figures, directing to the twenty four tables ...
Bound with Bartholin, T. Anatomy. 1665.

—[The same.] ... The 3rd ed., corr. and amended. Englished by Nicholas Culpeper ... and W[illiam] R[and] ... London, Printed by John Streater, and sold by George Sawbridge, 1671.

    [8], 288 (i.e. 240), [58] p. plates. 29 cm.

                                    [9672]

Different setting of type.

—Another issue.   **[9673]**

Imperfect: plate 23 wanting.
The explanations of the tables reset.

—[French tr.] Manuel anatomique et pathologique; ou, Abregè de toute l'anatomie, & des usages que l'on en peut tirer pour la connoissance, & pour la guerison des maladies ... Nouv. ed. corr. & augm. de la sixiéme partie, sur les memoires & livres imprimez de l'autheur. Paris, Gaspar Meturas, 1661.

    [48], 779 p. port. 16 cm.   **[9674]**

Imperfect: port. wanting.
Translation by François Sauvin.
Contents as in 1658 Latin edition, except that De valvulis venarum is not present.

—[The same.] ... Lyon, Antoine Laurens, 1672.

    [47], 779 p. 16 cm.   **[9675]**

Different setting of type.

—Incursionum Quercetani [pseud., i.e. Joseph Duchesne] depulsio ... Parisiis, Ex Officina Plantiniana, Apud Hadrianum Perier, 1605.

    [1], 66, [2] p. 15 cm.   **[9676]**

Apparently a reply to Joseph Duchesne's Ad Brevem Riolani excursum brevis incursio.
"Scholae Parisiensis de Quercetano judicium" (p. [67-68]) is dated April 18, 1604 and signed: G. Heron decanus.
Bound with Glisson, F. Tractatus de ventriculo et intestinis. 1677.

—Opuscula anatomica nova. Quae nunc primum in lucem prodeunt. Instauratio magna physicae & medicinae per novam doctrinam de motu circulatorio sanguinis in corde. Accessere Notae in Joannis Wallaei duas epistolas de circulatione sanguinis ... Animadversiones in Historiam anatomicam Andreae Laurentii. In Theatrum anatomicum Caspari Bauhini. In librum anatomicum de fabrica humana Andreae Spigelii. Ad institutiones anatomicas Caspar Bartholini. Ad anatomica Caspari Hofmanni. In Syntagma anatomicum Joannis Veslingii. In tractatum de diaphragmate Aemilii Parisiani. De monstro nato Lutetiae, liber jampridem editus. Londini, Typis Milonis Flesher, 1649.

[4], 536 p. 19 cm. [9677]

"Quaestio medica, quodlibetariis disputationibus mane discutienda in scholis medicorum" (p. 1-19) and "Probationes theseos. circulationis sanguinis primus author & inventor Harveus" (p. 20-145) have caption titles.

—Opuscula nova anatomica, judicium novum de venis lacteis tam mesentericis quam thoracicis, adversus Th. Bartholinum. Lymphatica vasa Bartholini refutata. Animadversiones secundae ad anatomiam reformatam Bartholini. Ejusdem Dubia anatomica de lacteis thoracicis resoluta. Hepatis funerati & ressuscitati vindiciae ... Parisiis, Apud viduam Mathurini du Puis, 1653.

[16], 58 p.; [8], 113, [1] p. 18 cm. [9678]

"Animadversiones secundae, ad anatomiam reformatam Thomae Bartholini ..." (second group of paging) has special title page.
"Commentatio adversus novum de venis lacteis commentum" (p. 99-113) has caption title.
With this is bound (as issued?) Bartholin, T. De lacteis thoracicis. 1653.

—Osteologia ex veterum et recentiorum praeceptis descripta. In qua continentur: Isagogica de ossibus tractatio, cum osteologia infantium usque ad septennium, per Joannem Riolanum. Claudii Galeni liber De ossibus ad tyrones. Et in eundem librum, Jacobi Sylvii ... commentarius. Joannis Riolani ... explanationes apologeticae, pro Galeno adversus novitios & novatores anatomicos. Simiae osteologia, sive ossium hominis & simiae comparatio. Osteologia ex Hippocratis libris eruta, collecta, & in ordinem digesta. Parisiis, Ex officina Adriani Perier, 1614.

[8], 574 p. 18 cm. [9679]

"Osteologia ex veterum et recentiorum praeceptis descripta" (with running title: Isagocica tractatio) and "Claudii Galeni liber de ossibus ad tyrones" have special title pages dated 1613. "Osteologia corporis humani, ex Hippocrate collecta" has half title.

—Schola anatomica novis et raris observationibus illustrata. Cui adjuncta est accurata foetus humani historia ... Parisiis, Apud Alrianum Perier, 1608.

[6], 369, [1] p. 18 cm. [9680]

Imperfect: title page mutilated.

—[The same.] ... Postrema editio prioribus auctior & emendatior ... Genevae, Sumptibus Joannis Celerii, 1624.

[6], 369 p. 16 cm. [9681]

Different setting of type.

RIOLAN, JEAN [1580-1657] See BARTHOLIN, T. Defensio vasorum lacteorum et lymphaticorum adversus Joannem Riolanum. 1655 [and] Opuscula nova anatomica. 1670; [CATTIER, I.] Seconde apologie. 1653; HARVET, I. Animadversiones. 1604; HARVEY, W. Exercitatio anatomica. 1650; PAULLI, S. Παρεκβασις; seu, Digressio de vera, unica, & proxima causa febrium. 1660, 1678; PECQUET, J. Experimenta nova anatomica. 1654; SCHLEGEL, P. M. De sanguinis motu commentatio. 1650; SEGER, G. Triumphus et querimonia cordis. 1661.

RIPAMONTI, GIUSEPPE [1573-1643] De peste quae fuit anno MDCXXX. Libri V. Desumpti ex annalibus urbis quos LX. decurionum autoritate scribebat. [Mediolani, Apud Malatestas] 1641.

[12], 411, [1] p. 23 cm. [9682]

Engraved title page.

RIPENHAUSEN, OTTO ARNOLD [fl. 1687-1688] respondent. See SCHRADER, F., praeses. Exercitatio academica de insipidorum efficacia. 1687.

RIPLEY, GEORGE [d. 1490?] The bosome-book. In Collectanea chymica. 1684.

—Compound of alchemie. In Ashmole, E. Theatrum chemicum Britannicum. 1652.

—Duodecim portarum axiomata philosophica.

110-123 p., vol. 2 20 cm. (In Zetzner, Lazarus, ed. Theatrum chemicum. Argentorati, 1659-61)

[9683]

Caption title.
Running title: Axiomata philosophica.

—[Excerpts.] In Dolhopff, G. A., comp. Lapis animalis microcosmicus. 1681.

—See CHYMICAL, medicinal, and chyrurgical addresses. 1655; HOUPREGHT, J. F., comp. Aurifontina chymica. 1680; NORTON, S. Saturnus saturatus dissolutus. 1630; PHILALETHES, E. Ripley reviv'd. 1678; SALMON, W. Medicina practica. 1692.

RIST, JOHANNES [1607-1667] Philosophischer Phoenix. In Feyens, T. Zwölff Bücher von der Wund-Arzney-Kunst. 1675.

RITTER, FRANZ [d. 1641] See PITHOPOEUS, W. Vincedoxicum. 1674.

RITTER, GEORG PAUL [fl. 1694] respondent. See LANGE, C. J., praeses. Dissertatio medica inauguralis de remediis vulnerariis. 1694.

—*See* RIVINUS. A. Q. L. S. D. Facultatis Medicae ... procancellarius, Augustus Quirinus Rivinus. 1694.

RITTER, JOHANN JAKOB [*b.* 1662] *respondent.* Disputatio inauguralis medica de arthritide ... Basileae, Typis Jacobi Werenfelsii [1682]

[39] p.   21 cm.   **[9684]**
Diss.—Basel.

RITTER, JOHANN KARL [*fl.* 1691] *respondent. See* FRIESE, F., *praeses.* Dissertationem physicam de curiosa et superstitiosa rusticorum physica ... submittit ... 1691.

RITTERSHAUSEN, KONRAD [1560-1613] Fama de pestilentia Altorfina ... Witebergae, Typis Meisnerianis, 1606.

[8] p.   19 cm.   **[9685]**

RITZ, JOHANN [*fl.* 1690] *respondent.* Disputatio medica inauguralis de hydrope ascite ... Basileae, Typis Jacobi Bertschii [1690]

[24] p.   21 cm.   **[9686]**
Diss.—Basel.

RIVERIUS reformatus. 1688, 1690, 1696. *See* [La CALMETTE, F. de]

RIVERIUS, LAZARUS. *See* RIVIÈRE, Lazare [1589-1655]

RIVET, ANDRÉ [1572-1651] Meditation sur le Pseaume XCI pour servir d'antidote contre la peste, & de precaution contre tous dangers. Avec une lettre ... sur la question, s'il est loisible en temps de peste de s'efloigner des lieux infectez ... Queuilly, Jacques Caillové, 1638.

[8], 187 (i.e. 183) p.   14 cm.   **[9687]**

—*See* BÈZE, T. de. De pestis contagio & fuga dissertatio. 1636; Variorum tractatus theologici de peste. 1655.

RIVEYRON, LOUIS, *Father* [*fl.* 1641] Secrets, et moyens faciles pour conserver le bestail du mal contagieux, & de la cure d'iceluy ... par l'ordre de messieures les capitouls de Tolose. Tolose, J. Boude, 1641.

15 p.   20 cm.   **[9688]**

RIVIÈRE, DAVACH DE LA. *See* DAVACH DE LA RIVIÈRE, Jean [*fl.* 1696]

RIVIÈRE, GUILLAUME [1655-1734] Quaestiones medico-chymico-practicae duodecim ab ... Michaele de Chicoyneau [et al.] ... propositae ... pro regia chymiae professione vacante per obitum Arnaldi Fonsorbe ... quas ... propugnabit ... Guillelmus Riviere ... Monspelii, Apud Honoratum Pech, 1696.

26 p.   22 cm.   **[9689]**
Thèse de concours—Montpellier.

RIVIÈRE, LAZARE [1589-1655] Opera medica universa: quibus continentur I. Institutionum medicarum, libri quinque. II. Praxeos medicae, libri septemdecim. III. Observationum medicarum, centuriae quatuor. Quibus accedunt Observationes variae ab aliis communicatae: itemque Observationes infrequentium morborum. Omnia ab ipsomet auctore ultimo revisa ... Lugduni, Sumptibus Antonii Cellier, 1663.

[10], 186, [10] p.; [8], 348, [25] p.; [4], 143, [5] p.   38 cm.   **[9690]**
Imperfect: first leaf (half-title?) wanting.
"... Praxis medica cum theoria. Ed. nova ..." (second group of paging) has special title page.
"... Observationum medicarum, et curationum insignium centuriae quatuor ..." (third group of paging) edited by Siméon Jacoz has special title page.

—[The same.] ... Ed. ultima auctior et correctior. Francofurti, Sumptibus Johannis Petri Zubrodt, typis Pauli Humii, 1669.

[5], 700 (i.e. 701), 39 p.   35 cm.   **[9691]**
Edited by Johann Daniel Horst.

—[The same.] ... Quibus accedunt Observationes variae ab aliis communicatae: itemque Observationes infrequentium morborum. Omnia ab ipsomet auctore ultimo revisa, emaculata, locupletata ... Lugduni, Sumptibus Antonii Cellier, patris & filii, 1672.

3 parts in 1 v.   front. (port.)   37 cm. **[9692]**
Parts [2] and [3] have special title pages, that to part [2] dated 1671.
Part [2] edited by Siméon Jacoz.

—[The same.] ... cum Observationibus rarioribus, ab aliis communicatis. Ed. ultima, auctior et correctior, adornata a Joh. Daniele Horstio ... nunc denuo recusa. Ex recensione Joannis Jacobi Döbelii ... Francofurti, Sumptibus Joannis Petri Zubrodt, 1674.

[8], 194, [6] p.; [1], 195-554, [1] p.; [1], 555-700, 39 p.   front. (port.)   39 cm.   **[9693]**

—[The same.] ... Quibus accedunt Observationes variae ab aliis communicatae: itemque Observationes infrequentium morborum. Ac denique ipsissima Arcana Riverii plene revelata. Omnia non tantum ab ipsomet authore ultimo revisa, emaculata, locupletata; sed etiam a Johanne Daniele Horstio, adornata, necnon a Joh. Jacobo Doebelio recensita ... Lugduni, Sumpt. Joannis-Antonii Huguetan, & soc., 1679.

[14], 604, [35] p. port. 36 cm. **[9694]**

Imperfect: portrait wanting.

—[The same.] ... cum Observationibus rarioribus, ab aliis communicatis. Adornata a Joh. Daniele Horstio, ed. novissima, auctior, et correctior, cui praefatus est Jacobus Grandius ... Accesserunt in Riverii Institutiones utiles anonymi animadversiones, & supplementa. Venetiis, Apud Julianos, 1686.

[12], 590 (i.e. 574), [30] p. 32 cm. **[9695]**

—[The same.] ... Venetiis, Typis Stephani Curti, 1687.

[12], 319 (i.e. 315); 292 p. 33 cm. **[9696]**

Imperfect: p. 97-98 of Institutiones medicae mutilated.

—[The same.] ... Quibus accedunt Observationes variae ab aliis communicatae: itemque Observationes infrequentium morborum. Ac denique ipsissima Arcana Riverii plene revelata. Omnia non tantum ab ipsomet authore ultimo revisa, emaculata, locupletata; sed etiam a Joanne Daniele Horstio adornata, necnon a Joh. Jacobo Doebelio recensita ... Lugduni, Apud Joannem-Henricum Huguetan, 1690.

[16], 604, [35] p. 37 cm. **[9697]**

—[The same.] ... Lugduni, Sumptibus Anisson, & Joannis Posüel, 1698.

[8], 604, [35] p. 37 cm. **[9698]**

Different setting of type.

—[The same.] ... cum Observationibus rarioribus, ab aliis communicatis. Adornata a Joh. Daniel Horstio, ed. novissima, auctior et correctior; cui praefatus est Jacobus Grandius. Accesserunt in Riverii Institutiones, utiles anonymi animadversiones, & supplementa ... Venetiis, Apud Jo. Baptistam Indrich, 1700.

[12], 590 (i.e. 574), [30] p. 33 cm. **[9699]**

Imperfect: first prelim. leaf (half-title?) wanting.

—Institutionum medicinae libri quinque. Universam medicinam; nempe, physiologiam, pathologiam, semeioticem, hygieinen, & terapeuticen docentes. Lypsiae, Apud Matthiam Trinkber, 1655.

[15], 815 p. tables. 18 cm. **[9700]**

Imperfect: tables facing p. 210 and 296 wanting.

—Another issue, with date changed to 1657. **[9701]**

Imperfect: table facing p. 284 wanting.

—[The same.] Institutiones medicae, in quinque libros distinctae, quibus totidem medicinae partes, physiologia, pathologia, semeiotice, hygieine, & therapeutice dilucide explicantur ... Lugduni, Sumptibus Antonii Cellier, 1656.

[16], 535 (i.e. 533), [2] p. port., tables. 23 cm. **[9702]**

—[The same.] ... Hagae-Comitis, Ex typographia Adriani Vlacq, 1657.

[14], 582 (i.e. 580) p. port., tables. 18 cm. **[9703]**

—[The same.] ... Hagae-Comitis, Ex typographia Adriani Vlacq, 1662.

[14], 582 (i.e. 580) p. tables. 18 cm. **[9704]**

Different setting of type.

—[The same.] ... Lugduni, Sumpt. Antonii Cellier, patris & filii, 1672.

[16], 535 (i.e. 533), [19] p. front. (port.), tables. 24 cm. **[9705]**

—[English tr.] The universal body of physick, in five books; comprehending the several treatises of nature, of diseases and their causes, of symptomes, of the preservation of health, and of cures. Written in Latine ... Exactly translated into English by William Carr ... London, Philip Briggs, 1657.

[18], 417 (i.e. 387), [1] p. tables. 29 cm. **[9706]**

—Institutiones, Observationes, et Praxis medicae. [Venetiis, Apud Franciscum Brogiollum, 1663-64] [part 1, 1664]

[12], 159, [9] p.; 443, [21] p. 32 cm. **[9707]**

Title from general half title.

"... Institutionum medicarum. Libri quinque. Universam medicinam; nempe, physiologiam, pathologiam, semeioticem, hyeienen, & therapeuricen docentes ..." (first group of paging); "Observationum medicarum, et curationum insignium centuriae tres ... necnon centuria quarta ... Simeonis Jacoz ... in lucem denuo edita . . ." (p. 1–[140]); and " . . . Praxis medica cum theorica. Ed. postrema . . .": (p. [141]–443) have special title pages.

Observationes medicae edited by Siméon Jacoz.

—[The same.] . . . [Venetiis, Apud Franciscum Brogiollum, 1674]

[12], 159, [9] p.; 443, [21] p.   37 cm.   **[9708]**

Different setting of type.

—Methodus curandarum febrium. Lutetiae Parisiorum, Sumptibus Olivarii de Varennes, 1645.

[7], 247 p.   17 cm.   **[9709]**

Published in 1653 and subsequently, as Liber 17 of *his* Praxis medica cum theoria.

—[The same.] . . . Lutetiae Parisiorum, Sumptibus Olivarii de Varennes, 1648.

[7], 247 p.   16 cm.   **[9710]**

Different setting of type.

—[The same.] . . . Goudae, Typis Gulielmi vander Hoeve, 1649.

[7], 166 p.   17 cm.   **[9711]**

Bound with *his* Praxis medica. 1649.

—[The same.] . . . Hagae Comitis, Sumptibus Adriani Vlacq, 1651.

[7], 166 p.   19 cm.   **[9712]**

Different setting of type.
Bound with *his* Praxis medica. 1651.

—Observationes medicae et curationes insignes. Quibus accesserunt, Observationes ab aliis communicatae. Parisiis, Apud Sebastianum Piquet, 1646.

[12], 253 (i.e. 255), 110, [2] p.   24 cm.   **[9713]**

—[The same.] . . . Londini, Typis Milonis Flesher, 1646.

[8], 451, [4] p.   19 cm.   **[9714]**

—[The same.] . . . Delphis, Sumptibus Adriani Vlacq, 1651.

[8], 394 (i.e. 404), [4] p.   19 cm.   **[9715]**

Bound with *his* Praxis medica. 1651.

—[The same.] . . . Hagae-Comitum, Apud Adrianum Vlacq, 1656.

[6], 371, [7] p.   18 cm.   **[9716]**

Imperfect: p. 185–186 wanting.
With this is bound *his* Observationum medicarum . . . centuria quarta. 1659.

—Another printing.   20 cm.   **[9717]**

Differs only in the setting of type from the other edition printed by Vlacq in the same year.
With this is bound *his* Observationum medicarum . . . centuria quarta. 1662.

—[The same.] Observationum medicarum, & curationum insignium centuriae tres, quibus accesserunt Observationes ab aliis communicatae: necnon Centuria quarta, post obitum authoris in ejus musaeo reperta; & cura ac diligentia Simeonis Jacoz . . . in lucem nunc primum edita, cum Observationibus morborum infrequentium, anonymi cujusdam, inter ejus scripta repertis. Lugduni, Sumptibus Antonii Cellier, 1659.

[8], 311, [9] p.   23 cm.   **[9718]**

—Observationum medicarum, & curationum insignium centuria quarta, post obitum authoris in ejus musaeo reperta; & cura ac diligentia Simonis Jacoz . . . in lucem nunc primum edita, cum Observationibus morborum infrequentium, anonymi cujusdam, inter ejus scripta repertis. Hagae-Comitum, Apud Adrianum Vlacq, 1659.

[8], 102, [2] p.   18 cm.   **[9719]**

Bound with *his* Observationes medicae. 1656.

—[The same.] . . . Hagae-Comitum, Apud Adrianum Vlacq, 1662.

[8], 102, [2] p.   20 cm.   **[9720]**

Different setting of type.
Pages of final signature wrongly imposed.
Bound with another printing of *his* Observationes medicae. 1656.

—[French tr.] Les observations de medecine de Lazare Riviere . . . qui contiennent quatre centuries de guerisons tres-remarquables: ausquelles on a joint des Observations qui luy avoient êté communiquées. Le tout mis en françois par M. F. Deboze . . . Lyon, Jean Certe, 1680.

[14], 823, [89] p.   19 cm.   **[9721]**

—[The same.] . . . 2. ed., rev. & corr. sur le latin. Lyon, Jean Certe, 1688.

[14], 742, [82] p.   19 cm.   **[9722]**

—[The same.] . . . 2. ed., rev. & corr. sur le latin. Lyon, Jean Certe, 1694.

[14], 742, [80] p.   19 cm.   **[9723]**

Different setting of type.
Imperfect: p. 207–208 wanting; p. [743–744] mutilated.

—Praxis medica. Ed. 2., ab authore aucta & correcta. Lutetiae Parisiorum, Sumptibus Olivarii de Varennes, 1644–45.

2 v. in 1.   18 cm.   **[9724]**

—[The same.] . . . Ed. postrema emendatior. Goudae, Typis Gulielmi vander Hoeve, 1649.

2 v. in 1.   17 cm.   **[9725]**

Vol. 1 has added engraved title page.

Imperfect: p. 157-180 in vol. 1 mutilated.

With this is bound *his* Methodus curandarum febrium. 1649.

—[The same.] ... Ed. postrema emendatior. Hagae Comitis, Sumptibus Adriani Vlacq, 1651.

    2 v. in 1. 19 cm.   **[9726]**

Vol. 1 has added engraved title page.

With this are bound *his* Methodus curandarum febrium. 1651; Observationes medicae & curationes insignes. 1651.

—[The same.] ... Ed. 8. Integra morborum theoria, & quamplurimis remediis selectissimis locupletata. Lugduni, Sumpt. Joannis-Antonii Huguetan, & Marci-Antonii Ravaud, 1653.

    2 v. front. (port.) 18 cm.   **[9727]**

Vol. 1 only.

Imperfect: index wanting.

—Praxis medica cum theoria. Ed. 9. ... Lugduni, Sumpt. Joannis-Antonii Huguetan, & Marci-Antonii Ravaud, 1657.

    [12], 365, [24] p. front. (port.) 36 cm.

                                       [9728]

—[The same.] ... Ed. 9., integra morborum theoria, & quamplurimis remediis ... locupletata. Hagae-Comitis, Apud Adrianum Vlacq, 1658.

    2 v. 18 cm.   **[9729]**

Added engraved title page with date altered by hand from 1651 to 1658.

A reprint of the 1651 edition.

—[The same.] ... Ed. ultima ... Lugduni, Sumpt. Joannis-Antonii Huguetan, & Marci-Antonii Ravaud, 1660.

    2 v. front. (port.) 19 cm.   **[9730]**

Vol.1 only.

Imperfect: p. 261 mutilated.

—[The same.] ... Ed. 10., integra morborum theoria, & quamplurimis remediis selectissimis locupletata. Hagae-Comitis, Apud Adrianum Vlacq, 1664.

    2 v. 19 cm.   **[9731]**

Imperfect: first preliminary leaf (half-title?) wanting.

—[The same.] ... Ed. novissima ... [Lugduni, Sumpt. Joannis-Ant. Huguetan, 1674]

    2 v. front. (port.) 18 cm.   **[9732]**

Imperfect: title page of vol. 1 mutilated.

—[Abridgments, etc.] Medicina practica in succinctum compendium redacta studio & sumptibus Bernhardi Verzaschae. Basileae, Typis Jacobi Werenfelsi, 1663.

    [24], 582, [27] p. port. 18 cm.   **[9733]**

Half title: Riverius contractus.

Errata: p. [27]

—[English tr.] The practice of physick, in seventeen ... books ... by N. Culpeper, A. Cole and W. Rowland. Being chiefly a translation of the works of L. Riverius ... with these books is bound a Physical dictionary explaining hard words ... London, Peter Cole, 1655.

    [16], 645 (i.e. 517) p.; [17] p. front. (ports.) 29 cm.   **[9734]**

Imperfect: title page wanting.

Title supplied from BMC.

Part [1] has special title page: The compleat practice of physick, in eighteen several books ... The eighteenth book is a physical dictionary, explaining hard words.

Part [2] has special title page: A physical dictionary.

—[The same.] The practice of physick, wherein is plainly set forth, the nature, cause, differences, and several sorts of signs: together with the cure of all diseases in the body of man. With many additions in several places never printed before ... Written in Latin, and in English, By Lazarus Riverius ... Nicholas Culpeper ... Abdiah Cole ... and W[illiam] R[owland] ... There is now added An alphabetical table of diseases. Also the Idea of practical physick in twelve books. And four other books; 1. Of natural phylosophy. 2. Of chyrurgery in six parts. 3. Of the whores pox. 4. Of the gout. All in two volums. By Daniel Sennertus, John Johnston, and Abdiah Cole ... London, Peter Cole, 1658-61 [v. 1, 1661]

    2 v. in 1. 29 cm.   **[9735]**

Contains none of the titles listed on title page after An alphabetical table of diseases.

Added special title page: The rationall physitian's library ... Partly collected out of the best authors ... and partly from Dr. Rason, and Experience ... by Abdiah Cole ... W. R. and Nich. Culpeper ... London, Printed by Peter Cole and Edward Cole ... 1661.

Vol. [2] has title: Four books ... unto which is added, a fift book, being Select medicinal counsels of John Fernelius ... All Englished by Nicholas Culpeper ... London, Printed by Peter Cole ... 1658.

—[The same.] The practice of physick, in seventeen several books. Wherein is plainly set forth, the nature, cause, differences, and several sorts of signs; together with the cure of all diseases in the body. By

Nicholas Culpeper ... Abdiah Cole ... and William Rowland ... Being chiefly a translation of the works of ... Lazarus Riverius ... To which are added Four books containing five hundred and thirteen observations of famous cures. By the same author. And a fifth book of Select medicinal counsels. By John Fernelius. With ... a physical dictionary, explaining the hard words used in these books. London, Printed by John Streater, and sold by George Sawbridge, 1672.

    [12], 645 (i.e. 517), [12], 463 (i.e. 363), [32] p. front. (ports.) 30 cm.   **[9736]**

—[The same.] ... London, George Sawbridge, 1678.

    [12], 645 (i.e. 517), [12], 463 (i.e. 363), [32] p. front. (ports.) 31 cm.   **[9737]**
    Different setting of type.

—[French tr.] La pratique de medecine avec la theorie ... Traduite nouvellement en François par M. F. Deboze ... Tome premier [-second] Lyon, Jean Certe, 1682.

    2 v.   19 cm.   **[9738]**

—*See* CRISTINI, B., *ed.* Arcana Lazari Riverii. 1676, 1696; [Excerpts.] 1680.

—*See* [La CALMETTE, F. de] Riverius reformatus. 1688, 1690, 1696; MEYSSONNIER, L. Breviarium medicum. 1664; PECHEY, J. A collection of chronical diseases. 1692; RULAND, M. [1532-1602] Experimental physick. 1662.

RIVILLA BONET Y PUEYO, JOSÉ DE. Desvios de la naturaleza; o, Tratado de el origen de los monstros. A que va anadido un compendio de curaciones chyrurgicas en monstruosos accidentes ... Lima, En la Imprenta Real por Joseph de Contreras y Alvarado impressor, 1695.

    [22], 116 (i.e. 118) ll.   plates.   21 cm.   **[9739]**
    Binder's error: leaves 9-10 duplicated.
    Attributed also to P. J. de Peralta Barnuevo Rocha y Benavides. Cf. Palau.

RIVINUS, ANDREAS [*ca.* 1601-1656] *praeses.* Δευτέραι φροντίδες φιλοσοφικώτεραι, de aestu marino, ejusque variis causis & inde manantibus speciebus ... [Lipsiae] Excudebant haered. Timothei Hönii [1649]

    [38] p.   19 cm.   **[9740]**
    Diss.—Leipzig (J. Knoblauch, *respondent*)

—*respondent. See* MICHAELIS, J., *praeses.* De morbo malo. 1638.

—*See* ASCLEPIADEA SACRA. [1638]; KIRANUS, *King of Persia.* Moderante auxilio redemptoris supremi, Kirani Kiranides. 1638, 1681; [English tr.] 1685.

RIVINUS, ANDRES BACHMANN. *See* RIVINUS, Andreas [*ca.* 1601-1656]

RIVINUS, AUGUSTUS QUIRINUS [1652-1723] Dissertatio de Lipsiensi peste anni 1680. Lipsiae, Apud Laur. Sig. Cornerum [1681?]

    [8], 136 p.   17 cm.   **[9741]**
    Dedicatio dated 1681.

—Lectorem benevolum ad orationem sub auspicium professionis suae ... majoris principium habendam ... invitat D. Augustus Quirinus Rivinus. [Lipsiae, 1691]

    [8] p.   20 cm.   **[9742]**

Programs — Leipzig

—Facultatis Medicae in Academia Lipsiensi p. t. procancellarius, Augustus Quirinus Rivinus ... L. S. D. [Lipsiae, Typis Christoph. Fleischeri, 1694]

    [8] p.   20 cm.   **[9743]**
    For diss. of C. F. Zimmermann.

—L. S. D. Facultatis Medicae ... procancellarius, Augustus Quirinus Rivinus ... [Lipsiae, Typis Christoph. Fleischeri, 1694]

    [8] p.   20 cm.   **[9744]**
    For diss. of G. P. Ritter.

—L. S. D. Facultatis Medicae ... pro-cancellarius, Augustus Quirinus Rivinus ... [Lipsiae, Literis Goezianis, 1696]

    [8] p.   19 cm.   **[9745]**
    With vita of J. A. Beer.

—L. S. D. Facultatis Medicae ... procancellarius, Augustus Quirinus Rivinus ... [Lipsiae, 1696]

    [8] p.   19 cm.   **[9746]**
    With vita of J. G. Thamm.

—L. S. D. Facultatis Medicae ... procancellarius Augustus Quirinus Rivinus ... [Lipsiae, Literis Immanuelis Titii, 1697]

    [8] p.   19 cm.   **[9747]**
    For diss. of B. Gullmann.

—L. S. D. Facultatis Medicae . . . procancellarius Augustus Quirinus Rivinus . . . [Lipsiae, Literis Johann Georg, 1699]

[8] p. 20 cm. [9748]

With vita of D. H. Weidemüller.

Dissertations—Leipzig

—*praeses*. Disputatio inauguralis de situ aegrorum commodo . . . Lipsiae, Literis Christiani Scholvini [1700]

[20] p. 20 cm. [9749]

C. H. Erndl, *respondent*.

—Disputatio medica de acido ventriculi fermento . . . Lipsiae, Apud Nicolaum Zibium [1677]

[16] p. 19 cm. [9750]

C. J. Lange, *respondent*.

—Disputatio medica, in qua agrestis vitae sanitas . . . exhibetur a Joh. Christoph. Caesare . . . Lipsiae, Literis Joh. Georg [1677]

[16] p. 20 cm. [9751]

J. C. Caesar, *respondent*.

—Disputationem inauguralem medicam de frigoris damno . . . submittit Johann Adam Kirch . . . Lipsiae, Typis Joh. Heinrici Richteri [1696]

[36] p. 19 cm. [9752]

J. A. Kirch, *respondent*.

—Dissertatio de spiritu hominis vitali . . . Lipsiae, Literis Johannis Georgii [1681]

[72] p. 19 cm. [9753]

J. K. Glaser, *respondent*.

—Dissertatio medica de asthmate . . . Lipsiae, Literis Johannis Georgii [1684]

[16] p. 19 cm. [9754]

S. K. Pertsch, *respondent*.

—Dissertatio medica de dubio medicamentorum effectu . . . Lipsiae, Typis Christophori Guntheri [1689]

[20] p. 18 cm. [9755]

C. F. Pincker, *respondent*.

—Dissertatio medica de dyspepsia . . . Lipsiae, Apud Nicolaum Zibium [1679]

[16] p. 20 cm. [9756]

H. C. Künne, *respondent*.

—Dissertatio medica de febribus malignis . . . Lipsiae, Literis Johannis Georgii [1684]

[16] p. 20 cm. [9757]

P. Hille, *respondent*.

—Dissertatio medica de ischuria . . . [Lipsiae] Literis Johann. Georg [1682]

[16] p. 20 cm. [9758]

J. S. Kiessling, *respondent*.

—Dissertatio medica de sangvificatione . . . [Lipsiae] Literis Johannis Georgii [1678]

[20] p. 20 cm. [9759]

C. Richter, *respondent*.

—Dissertatio medica de thoracis empyemate . . . Lipsiae, Literis Johannis Georgii [1686]

[16] p. 20 cm. [9760]

D. Kinner, *respondent*.

—Dissertatio physiologica de bile . . . Lipsiae, Literis Johannis Georgii [1679]

[16] p. 19 cm. [9761]

J. E. Heimburger, *respondent*.

—[The same.] . . . quam . . . d. 30. Maji M. DC LXXIX . . . proponit J. E. Heimburger . . . Lipsiae, Impensis Nicolai Scipionis recusa 1688.

[16] p. 20 cm. [9762]

J. E. Heimburger, *respondent*.

—Dissertatio physiologica de nutritione . . . Lipsiae, Literis Joh. Georg [1678]

[32] p. 20 cm. [9763]

J. S. Kiessling, *respondent*.

—Dissertatio physiologica de visu . . . Lipsiae, Literis Johannis Georgii [1686]

[20] p. plate. 21 cm. [9764]

S. Hahn, *respondent*.

—Dissertatio therapeutica de medicamentorum proprietatibus . . . Lipsiae, Typis Christiani Goezii [1692]

[24] p. 20 cm. [9765]

S. Veiel, *respondent*.

—Dissertationem medicam inauguralem de cholera . . . exponet Abraham Hoffmann . . . Lipsiae, Typis, Joh. Wilhelmi Krügeri [1698]

[24] p. 19 cm. [9766]

A. Hoffmann, *respondent*.

—Dissertationem therapeuticam de remediis antepilepticis . . . submittit . . . Caspar Wendeland . . . Lipsiae, Typis Christophori Fleischeri [1692]

[16] p. 19 cm. [9767]

K. Wendeland, *respondent*.

—Exercitatio medica de febribus intermittentibus
... Lipsiae, Literis Joh. Georg [1683]

[32] p.   19 cm.   **[9768]**

D. H. Kellner, *respondent.*

—Medicum inculpatum ... sistit Christianus
Bukky ... Lipsiae, Literis Christoph. Fleischeri
[1699]

[19] p.   19 cm.   **[9769]**

C. Bukky, *respondent.*

—Medicum superstitiosum ... examini sistit
Godofredus Klaunig ... Lipsiae, Typis Christoph.
Fleischeri [1698]

[28] p.   20 cm.   **[9770]**

G. Klaunig, *respondent.*

—*respondent. See* Conring, H., *praeses.* Dissertationem inauguralem de diabete ... proponet ...
A. Q. R. 1676.

—*See* Ray, J. Synopsis methodica stirpium Britannicarum. 1696.

RIVINUS, Florens. *See* Rivinus, Quintus Septimus Florens [1651-1713]

RIVINUS, Quintus Septimus Florens [1651-1713]
Schediasma de noctu lucentibus ... Lipsiae, Literis
Joh. Georg [1673]

[12] p.   19 cm.   **[9771]**

Diss.—Leipzig (J. G. Böhme, *respondent*)
Author's presentation copy, signed.

RIVIUS, Gualtherius Hermenius. *See* Ryff,
Walther Hermenius [d. 1548]

RIVIUS, Joannes Bechtold [*fl.* 1609-1610] *respondent.* Themata medica de pleuritide ... Basileae,
Typis Joan. Jacobi Genathii, 1609.

[22] p.   20 cm.   **[9772]**

Diss.—Basel.

—*See* Stupanus, J. N., *praeses.* Σημειωτιces particularis cap. I. De affectibus. 1610.

—*See* Platter, F. [1536-1614] Felix Platerus ...
decreto. 1610.

RIZ, Christian Gottlob [*fl.* 1700] *respondent. See*
Berger, J. G. von, *praeses.* Dissertatio solennis de
haemorrhoidibus. 1700.

RIZ, Jacob [*fl.* 1700] *respondent.* Dissertatio medica
inauguralis, quam de foetoribus humani corporis

viventis cognoscendis et curandis tractantem quidem,
sed minime tamen foetentem ... proponit Jacobus
Rizius ... Basileae, Typis Jacobi Bertschii [1700]

[16] p.   19 cm.   **[9773]**

Diss.—Basel.

ROBERG, Lars [1664-1742] *praeses.* Dissertatio
medica de thermis ... [Upsaliae, 1699]

[4], 28 p.   plate.   21 cm.   **[9774]**

Diss.—Uppsala (C. Rockmann, *respondent*)

—Dissertatio medica varios effluviorum effectus
breviter ostendens ... Upsaliae, Henricus Keyser
[1699]

[4], 30 p.   20 cm.   **[9775]**

Diss.—Uppsala (G. Holsten, *respondent*)

ROBERT OF CHESTER [*fl.* 1141-1150] *tr. See*
Morienus. Liber de compositione alchemiae. 1610;
[German tr.] 1613.

ROBERTI, Jean, *Father* [1569-1651] Goclenius
heautontimorumenos; id est, Curationis magneticae,
& unguenti armarii ruina, Ipso Rodolpho Goclenio
juniore, nuper parente, & patrono; nunc cum sigillis,
& characterib. magicis, ultro proruente ... Et
Goclenii magneticam synarthrosin meram
ἀνάϙθϙωσιν esse ostendit ... Luxemburgi, Excudebat Hubertus Reulandt, 1618.

[48], 356, [4] p.   16 cm.   **[9776]**

—Tractatus novi de magnetica vulnerium curatione, autore D. Rodolpho Goclenio ... brevis
anatome ... [&] Goclenius heautontimorumenos; id
est, Curationis magneticae, & unguenti armarii ruina
...

[226]-236 and [309]-456 p.   21 cm.   (*In*
Theatrum sympatheticum auctum. Norimbergae,
1662)   **[9777]**

—*See* Goclenius, R. [1572-1621] Synarthrosis
magnetica. 1617 [and] Tractatus de manetica [sic]
vulnerum curatione. 1662; Helmont, J. B. van. De
mag[netica] vulnerum curatione. 1662.

ROBERTUS RETENENSIS. *See* Robert of
Chester [*fl.* 1141-1150]

ROBLEDO, Diego Antonio de [*fl.* 17th cent.]
Compendio cirurgico, util, y provechoso a sus pro-
fesores ... 2. imp. corr., y enmend. por su autor;

y añadidos quatro tratados . . . Madrid, Mateo de Llanos y Guzman, 1687.

[8], 478 + p.   30 cm.   [**9778**]

Imperfect: all after p. 478 wanting.

ROCAMORA, Isaac de [*fl.* 1693] *respondent.* Disputatio medica inauguralis de diabete . . . Trajecti ad Rhenum, Ex officina Francisci Halma, 1693.

10, [2] p.   21 cm.   [**9779**]

Diss. — Utrecht.

ROCCA, Bartolommeo della. *See* Cocles, Bartolommeo della Rocca, *known as* [1467-1504]

ROCCA, Michele. *See* Rocco, Michele [*fl.* 1646]

ROCCIO, Giovanni Vittorio. *See* Rossi, Gian Vittorio [1577-1647]

ROCCO, Michele [*fl.* 1646] *See* Petrone, V. di. Literarium duellum inter Salernitanos, et Neapolitanos medicos. 1647.

ROCHA Y BENAVIDES, Pedro de Peralta Barnuevo. *See* Peralta Barnuevo Rocha y Benavides, Pedro de [1663-1743]

ROCHAS, Henry de [*fl.* 1619-1648] Examen ou raisonnement sur l'usage de la saignée. Avec une parfaite cognoissance des facultez & vertus du sang, & des autres humeurs. La philosophie hermetique, ou confection d'une medecine corrective . . . Paris, L'autheur, 1644.

109, [3] p.   17 cm.   [**9780**]

—Notabilia excerpta. De thermis et acidulis artificialibus. Ex daubus editionibus authoris cujusdam Gallici, quarum tituli hi sunt; Primae; Ieurage [sic] anatomie spagiiriques des eaus mineralles . . . 1637. Secundae: La phiisique demonstrativa . . . 1642. Prioris quidem Germanice alterius & posterioris autem Latine versa ac reddita a Philaletha Anonymo [pseud., i.e. Tobias Ludwig Kolhans] [n. p.] 1663.

[46] p.   16 cm.   [**9781**]

Dedicatory epistle signed A. V. V. V.

—Nouvelles demonstrations, pour cognoistre la cause des fiévres intermitantes & continuës, dysenteries . . . & tout autre flux de ventre. Avec un ample & asseuré prognostic sur chacune d'icelles, & les remedes specifiques pour leur guerison . . . Paris, L'autheur, 1645.

[23], 112 p.   17 cm.   [**9782**]

—La physique reformée, contenant la refutation des erreurs populaires, et le triomphe des veritez philosophiques. La genealogie des elemens, & des principes, l'origine, & les operations de la nature, en la generation & production des animaux, vegetaux, & mineraux . . . Paris, L'autheur, 1648.

[8], 567 p.   23 cm.   [**9783**]

—Traicté des observations nouvelles et vraye cognoissance des eaux mineralles . . . ensemble de l'esprit universel . . . Paris, L'autheur, 1634.

[4], 302 (i.e. 272) p.   16 cm.   [**9784**]

—La vraye anatomie spagyrique, des eaux mineralles, et de toutes les choses qui les composent . . . Livre premier [-second] Paris, L'autheur, 1636.

[1], 16, 302 (i.e. 272) p.; [16], 180 p.   17 cm.   [**9785**]

Vol. 1 is a reissue of *his* Traicté des observations nouvelles.

—[Latin tr.] Tractatus de observationibus novis et vera cognitione aquarum mineralium et de illarum qualitatibus & virtutibus antehac incognitis: item de spiritu universali . . . Anno 1634. Gallice scriptus, nunc vero in Latinam linguam translatus . . .

716-772 p., vol. 6.   20 cm.   (*In* Zetzner, Lazarus, *ed.* Theatrum chemicum. Argentorati, 1659-61)   [**9786**]

Caption title.

ROCHE, Joannes Henricus la. *See* La Roche, Johann Heinrich [*fl.* 1694-1695]

ROCHETAILLADE, Jean de. *See* Joannes de Rupescissa [*fl.* 1328-1365]

ROCHLIZ, Samuel [*fl.* 1680-1685] *respondent. See* Fasch, A. H., *praeses.* Dissertatio medica inauguralis, spicilegium pestis exhibens. 1685.

ROCKMAN, Carl [*fl.* 1699] *respondent. See* Roberg, L. Dissertatio medica de thermis. 1699.

RODARGIRUS, Lucas. Pisces zodiaci inferioris; vel, De solutione philosophica. Cum aenigmatica totius lapidis epitome . . . [&] . . . Chymia compendiaria, ad Johannem Riturum.

723-765 p., vol. 5.   20 cm.   (*In* Zetzner, Lazarus, *ed.* Theatrum chemicum. Argentorati, 1659-61)   [**9787**]

Caption titles.

RODE, Johan [1587-1659] De acia dissertatio ad Cornelii Celsi mentem. Patavii, Typis Pauli Frambotti, 1639.

[29], 197 p. illus., plates. 23 cm. **[9788]**

—[The same.] De acia dissertatio ad Cornelii Celsi mentem qua simul universa fibulae ratio explicatur, secundis curis ex autographo autoris auctior & emendatior, cum judiciis doctorum edita a Th. Bartholino. Accedit De ponderibus et mensuris ejusdem autoris dissertatio, & Vita Celsi. Hafniae, Typis Matthiae Godicchenii, sumptibus Petri Hauboldi, 1672.

[26], 218, [23] p.; 71 p. front. (port.), illus., plates. 21 cm. **[9789]**

Part 2 has special title page.

—[The same.] Antiquitates philosophicae, medicae & chirurgicae, a summis viris Cornelio Celso & Johanne Rhodio, maximo cum labore erutae dissertationibus quibusdam De acia pondere & mensuris ... multorum rogatu ab interitu & oblivione revocatae per V. J. B. T. [i.e., Thomas Bartholin?] Londini Scanorum, 1691.

[20], 218, [24] p. illus., plates. 20 cm. **[9790]**

Imperfect: sig. A²⁻⁴ (dedication) wanting; part [2] (De ponderis & mensuris) wanting.

A reissue of sheets B-Gg of the 1672 edition of *his* De acia, with new title page, and last page of the index reset.

—Analecta et notae in Ludovici Septalii Animadversiones et cautiones medicas. *In* Settala, L. Animadversionum et cautionum medicarum libri IX. 1652.

—Mantissa anatomica ad Thomam Bartholinum. Hafniae, Typis Henrici Gödiani, impensis Petri Hauboldi, 1661.

32 p. 16 cm. **[9791]**

Issued also as part 2 of Thomas Bartholin's Historiarum anatomicarum ... centuria V. & VI., published in Copenhagen in 1661.

—Introductio ad medicinam. *In* Conring, H. In universam artem medicam singulasque ejus partes introductio. 1687.

—Observationum medicinalium centuriae tres. *In* Borel, P. Historiarum et observationum medicophysicarum centuriae IV. 1676.

—*ed. See* Frigimelica, F. De balneis metallicis artificio parandis. 1659, 1679.

—*See* Castelli, B. Amaltheum Castello-Brunonianum; sive, Lexicon medicum. 1700; Celsus, A. C. De medicina libri octo. 1687; Scribonius Largus. Compositiones medicae. 1655.

RODERICUS A VEIGA, Thomas. *See* Rodrigues da Veiga, Tomás [1513-1579]

RODERICUS CASTRENSIS, Stephanus. *See* Castro, Estevão Rodrigues de [1559-1637?]

RODIGAST, Samuel [*fl.* 1678-1679] *praeses.* Disquisitio physica, de calore nivis ... Jenae, Typis Johannis Wertheri [1678]

[36] p. 20 cm. **[9792]**

Diss.—Jena (J. N. Trombsdorff, *respondent*)

RODOCHS, Johann Christian [*fl.* 1684] *tr. See* Blankaart, S. Von Würckungen derer Artzneyen in dem menschlichen Leibe. 1690.

—*See* Blankaart, S. Schau-Platz der Raupen. 1690; Schouten, W. Verletzter Kopff. 1695.

RODOMONTE, Lorenzo. *See* Laurenti, Rodomonte [*fl.* 1649]

RODRIGO DE CASTRO, Esteban. *See* Castro, Estevão Rodrigues de [1559-1637?]

RODRIGO DE RAMOS, Simón. *See* Ramos, Simón [*fl.* 1606-1634]

RODRIGUES, João de Castello Branco. *See* Amatus Lusitanus [1511-1568]

RODRIGUES DA VEIGA, Tomás [1513-1579] Practica medica. Cui accessit ejusdem auctoris tractatus de fontanellis, & cauteriis. Opus posthmum [sic] nunc primum in lucem editum. Ulyssipone, Ex typographia Joannis a Costa senioris, sumptibus Josephi Ferreira, 1668.

[7], 351 p. 20 cm. **[9793]**

—*See* Reys Tavares, M. dos. Controversias philosophicas, et medicas. 1667.

RODRIGUES DE CASTRO, Estevam. *See* Castro, Estevão Rodrigues de [1559-1637?]

RODRÍGUEZ, Félix Julián [*d.* 1693] Praxis medica Valentina, in gratiam tyronum scripta; in tres libros digesta ... Valentiae, Typis Hieronymi Vilagrasa, 1671.

[24], 605 p. 19 cm. **[9794]**

RODRÍGUEZ CARDOSO, Fernando. *See* Cardoso, Fernando Rodriguez [*d.* 1608]

RODRIGUEZ DE CASTELLO BRIANCO, João. *See* Amatus Lusitanus [1511–1568]

RODRIGUEZ DE CASTRO, Esteban. *See* Castro, Estevão Rodrigues de [1559–1637?]

RODRÍGUEZ DE LEÓN PINELO, Antonio. *See* León Pinelo, Antonio Rodríguez de [*d.* 1660]

RODRIGUEZ DE PEDROSA, Luis [*fl.* 1666] Selectarum philosophiae et medicinae difficultatum, quae a philosophis vel omittuntur, vel negligentius examinantur. Tomus primus ... Salmanticae, Ex officina Melchioris Estevez, 1666.
    [20], 396, [47] p. 29 cm.   **[9795]**
  No more appears to have been published.

RODRÍGUEZ GUERRERO, Diego. [Quod febris intermittens possit esse pestilents] Doctoris Didaci Roderici Guerrero ad ... doctorem, Joannem de Spinosa praeceptorem suum. Hispali, Joannes Leonius, 1603.
    [42] p. 20 cm.   **[9796]**
  Title supplied from running title.

RÖBER, Paul Philipp [*fl.* 1656] *respondent. See* Sperling, J., *praeses.* Θανατολογὶα; sive, Disputatio philosophica de morte. 1656.

RÖDER, Johann [*fl.* 1669–1675] *respondent. See* Frommann, J. C., *praeses.* Exercitationis medicae prioris de haemorrhoidibus. 1669; Wedel, G.W., *praeses.* Disputatio medica, aegram dysentericam sistens. 1675.

ROEL, Conradus van, *pseud. See* Liceti, Fortunio [1577–1657]

ROELS, Tobias [*d.* 1602] *See* L'Écluse, C. de Caroli Clusii ... Rariorum plantarumm historia. 1601.

RÖHRENSEE, Christian [1641–1713] *praeses.* Propositas theses physicas defendendas suscipit M. Christoph. Jacobus Wächtler ... Vitembergae, Praelo viduae Matthaei Henckelii [1191]
    [4] p. 19 cm.   **[9797]**
  Diss.—Wittenberg (C. J. Wächtler, *respondent*)

RÖMANISCH-KAISERLICHE AKADEMIE DER NATURFORSCHER. *See* Academia Naturae Curiosorum.

ROEMER, Ole. *See* Rømer, Ole Christensen [1644–1710]

RØMER, Ole Christensen [1644–1710] *praeses.* Rector Regiae Universitatis Hafniensis Dn. Olaus Rømer ... L. S. [Hafniae, 1693]
    broadside. 30 × 38 cm.   **[9798]**
  Program—Copenhagen (with vita of A. Kahle)

RÖPER, Johann Nikolaus [*fl.* 1694–1697] *respondent. See* Hoffmann, F. [1660–1742] *praeses.* Dissertatio inauguralis medico-chirurgica. 1697 [and] Dissertatio medica de imaginatione. 1694; Werckmeister, F. H., *praeses.* Dissertatio medica de imaginatione. 1694.

ROESCHEL, Johann Baptista [1652–1712] *praeses.* Disputationem physicam primam de fontium origine ... submittit ... Petrus Hermannus ... [Vitembergae] Litteris Fincelianis [1700]
    [16] p. 19 cm.   **[9799]**
  Diss.—Wittenberg (P. Hermann, *respondent*)

—Paradoxorum physicorum dodecas ... Vitembergae, Typis Christiani Kreusigii [1699]
    [20] p. 20 cm.   **[9800]**
  Diss.—Wittenberg (A. G. Stübner, *respondent*)

RÖSELER, Jakob [*fl.* 1654] *respondent. See* Conring, H., *praeses.* Disputatio medica inauguralis de pleuritide. 1654.

ROESENBOSCH, Hendrik [*fl.* 1689] *respondent.* Disputatio medica inauguralis, de pleuritide ... Trajecti ad Rhenum, Ex officina Frnacisci Halma, 1689.
    12 p. 22 cm.   **[9801]**

RÖSER, Jakob [*fl.* 1673] *respondent. See* Wedel, G. W., *praeses.* Dissertatio medica de epilepsia. 1673.

RÖSER, Johann [*fl.* 1688–1692 *respondent. See* Winther, J. G., *praeses.* De admirando illo affectu catalepsi. 1692 [and] Sermo physicus de sermone seu loquela. 1688.

ROESER, Johann Georg [1659–1715] *praeses.* Dissertatio physica, quam de venenis recensebit ... Wittenbergae, Literis Christiani Schrödteri [1687]
    [1], 26 p. 20 cm.   **[9802]**
  Diss.—Wittenberg (K. C. Kirchmajer, *respondent*)

[**ROESLIN,** Eucharius, *d.* 1526] [Der swangern Frauwen und Hebammen Rosengarten. Dutch] Het kleyn vroetwijfs-bock; ofte, Vermeerderden Roosengaert, van de bevruchte vrouwen, en hare secreten, ontfanginge, baringe vrouwen en mannen raedt te geven die onvruchtbaer zijn: alle sieckten der swangere vrouwen (oock als sy in barens-noodt ende van kinde gelegen zijn) te remedieren. Vele ge-experimenteerede remedien voor voesters, kinderen, ende wat daer aen kleeft ... Item, noch van menigerhande toevallende sieckten der nieuw-geboren kinderkens, en hoe men die te hulpe komen sal. Amsterdam, Michiel de Groot, 1667.

    61, [3] ll., 48 p. illus. 15 cm.   **[9803]**

    Imperfect: ll. 1-8 mutilated..

Daniels, C. E. and Moes, E. W. Eucharius Röslins Rosengarten. Centralblatt für Bibliothekswesen, XVI (1899) p. 123 no. 20.

   —[The same.] ... Amsterdam, Michiel de Groot [ca. 1670]

    60, [4] ll., 48 p. illus. 15 cm.   **[9804]**

    Imprint partly supplied from Nederlandsche Maatschappij tot Bevordering der Geneeskunst. Catalogus. 1930, p. 336.

    Imperfect: ll. 11-14 wanting.

    Different setting of type.

    Daniels and Moes, no. 21.

   —[The same.] ... Amsterdam, Gysbert de Groot, 1685.

    128, 48 p. illus. 15 cm.   **[9805]**

    Daniels and Moes, no. 22.

   [—English tr.] The birth of mankinde; otherwise named, The womans booke. Set foorth in English by Thomas Raynalde ... and by him corr., and augm. ... London, Thomas Adams [1604]

    [8], 204 p. illus. 19 cm.   **[9806]**

    STC 21161.

    Translation of Roeslin's Rosengarten with added material, by Raynalde, Cf. J. W. Ballantyne, "The Byrth of Mankynde", London [1907]

   —[The same.] ... London, Thomas Adams [1613]

    [8], 204 p. illus. 20 cm.   **[9807]**

    Different setting of type.

    STC 21162.

    With this is bound Guillimeau, J. Childbirth; or, The happy deliverie of women. 1612.

   —[The same.] ... London, Printed for A. H[ebb] and sold by James Boler, 1626.

    [8], 204 p. illus. 19 cm.   **[9808]**

    Imperfect: p. 33-34 mutilated, affecting text.

    Different setting of type.

    STC 21163.

   —[The same.] ... London, Printed for A. H[ebb] and sold by John Morret, 1634.

    [8], 204 p. illus. 18 cm.   **[9809]**

    STC 21164.

   —[The same.] ... The 4th ed. corr. and augm. London, J. L., Henry Hood, Abel Roper, and Richard Tomlins, 1654,

    [7], 193 (i.e. 195) p. illus. 19 cm.   **[9810]**

    Includes the addition of "Directions for the nursing of children, and how to choose a good nurse", p. 191-193 (i.e. 193-195)

RÖSSEL, PAUL [*fl.* 1617] *praeses.* Disputatio physica de unione animae rationalis cum corpore ... Wittebergae, Ex officina Johannis Matthaei, 1617.

    [20] p. 19 cm.   **[9811]**

    Diss.—Wittenberg (J. J. Firnhaber, *respondent*)

RÖSSER, JACOB [*fl.* 1682] *respondent. See* LEICHNER, E., *praeses.* Manus Dei funestissima, lues pestifera. 1682.

RÖSSLIN, EUCHARIUS. *See* ROESLIN, Eucharius [*d.* 1526]

ROET, ISAAC [*fl. ca.* 1666-1667] Pestis adumbrata in libris V. aphorismorum ... Intercessit etiam pestis a pestilenti febre differentia ... Londini, J. H. pro S. Thomson, 1666.

    [6], 74 p. 16 cm.   **[9812]**

RÖTEL, HIERONYMUS [*d.* 1676] *respondent. See* MET-ZGER, G. B., *praeses.* Fluxus et refluxus sanguinis. 1660.

RÖTENBECK, JOHANN [1606-1634] Berichtvom Schorbock, dem gemeinen Mann zum besten zusammen getragen ...

    [121]-254 p. 14 cm. (*In* Viel-vergröster und hellerpolirter Schorbocks-Spiegel. Nürnberg, 1659)
    [9813]

    Half title.

   —Speculum scorbuticum ... in zweyen unterschiedlichen Tractätlein verfasset ... Nürnberg, 1633.

    [1?], 112 p.; 68 + p. 17 cm.   **[9814]**

    Imperfect: title page wanting; all pages after p. 68 of part [2] wanting; p. 15—16 of part [1] misbound before p. 3(?)

    Title and imprint supplied from BMC.

    Part [1] has half title: Bericht vom Schorbock; dem gemeinen Mann zum besten zusammen getragen und beschrieben durch Johann Rötenbeck.

    Part [2] has half title: Kurtzer und nontwendiger Bericht von der ... Kranckheit, dem Schorbock. Manniglich zur Nachricht gestellet von Caspar Horn.

   —*respondent.* Alvi astrictio in theses contracta ... Altdorphii, E typographia Balthasaris Scherffii [1630]

    [12] p. 19 cm.   **[9815]**

    Diss.—Altdorf.

—*respondent. See* SEBISCH, M. [1578-1674?] *praeses.* Exercitationes medicae. 1639.

RÖTENBECK, JOHANN GEORG [*fl.* 1669-1676 *respondent.* Disputatio medica inauguralis de sudore praeternaturam . . . Altdorffii, Literis Henrici Meyeri [1676]

40 p. 20 cm. **[9816]**

Diss. — Altdorf.

ROETERS, HENDRICK. *See* LAMSWEERDE, J. B. van. Consideration en motiven dienende ter decisie ende ten voordeele van Dr. Joh. Baptista van Lamzweerde. 1677.

ROGERI, GIOVANNI GIACOMO. *See* ROGGERI, Giovanni Giacomo [17th cent.]

ROGERS, GEORGE [1618-1697] Oratio anniversaria, habita in Theatro Collegii Medicorum Londinensium, decimo octavo die Octob. . . . 1681 in commemorationem beneficiorum a Doctore H arveio . . . eidem college praestitiorum . . . Necnon & Oratio in Gymnasio Patavino habita prid. cal. Maii an. MDCXLVI . . . Londini, Benj. Tooke, 1682.

[7], 42 (i.e. 44) p. 21 cm. **[9817]**

ROGERS, JOHN [1627-1665?] Analecta inauguralia; sive, Disceptationes medicae . . . Necnon diatribae discussoriae de quinque corporis humani concoctionibus, potissimumque de pneumatosi ac spermatosi . . . Londini, E. C. pro H. Eversden, 1644.

[96], 499, [363]-740, [2] p. 18 cm. **[9818]**

"Oratiuncula anthropologica ex Ἀνθρωποφύης ᾽απακριβῶς explorandae gratia comparata; ordin. Acad. Ultrajectin. . . . 1662" (p. 1-60) has half title, and includes "De ratione evacuandi, aphorismi sequentis & Hippocratis τοῦ ἀρχιάτου explicatio", with texts of selected aphorisms in Greek.

"Disputatio medica inauguralis in apoplexiam . . . Ed. 2. . . ." (p. [61]-82); "Diatribae . . . de pneumatosi . . . Lib. II" (p. [83]-499); and "Diatribae . . . de spermatosi . . . Lib. III" (p. [363]-740) have special title pages.

Catchword "Cap." at end of preliminary matter, p. [96], does not carry over.

Errata: [2] p.

ROGGERI, GIOVANNI GIACOMO [17th cent.] Catalogo delle piante native del suolo Romano. *In* Donzelli, G. Teatro farmaceutico dogmatico, e spagirico. 1681, 1686, 1696.

ROHAULT, JACQUES [1620-1675] Tractatus physicus Gallice emissus et recens Latinitate donatus,

per Th. Bonetum . . . Cum animadversionibus Antonii Le Grand. Londini, G. Wells & A. Swalle, 1682.

[47], 253, 289, [2] p. plates. 19 cm. **[9819]**

ROHR, PHILIPP [*fl.* 1672-1679] *praeses.* Dissertatio historico-philosophica de masticatione mortuorum . . . Lipsiae, Typis Michaelis Vogtii [1679]

[24] p. 19 cm. **[9820]**

Diss. — Leipzig (B. Frizschius, *respondent*)

ROLAND, JACQUES, *sieur de Belebat* [*fl.* 1625-1630] Aglossostomographie; ou, Description d'une bouche sans langue. Laquelle parle et faict naturellement toutes ses autres fonctions . . . Saumur, Pour Claude Girard et Daniel de l'Erpiniere [De l'imprimerie de Jean Lesnier, & Isaac Desbordes] 1630.

[24], 79, [1] p. 15 cm. **[9821]**

ROLANDER, LAURENTIUS PETRUS. *See* ROLANDUS, Laurentius Petrus [*fl.* 1631].

ROLANDO OF PARMA. *See* also CAPELLUTI, Rolando [*b. ca.* 1430]

ROLANDUS, LAURENTIUS PETRUS [*fl.* 1631] *respondent. See* BURGERSDIJCK, F. P., *praeses.* Collegium physicum. 1642.

ROLFINCK, WERNER [1599-1673] Chimia in artis formam redacta, sex libris comprehensa. Jenae, Samuel Krebs, 1661.

[16], 443, [11] p. table. 20 cm. **[9822]**

—Dissertatio de hepate, ex veterum & recentiorum, propriisque observationibus concinnata, et ad circulationem accommodata. Jenae, Typis Georgii Sengenwaldi, 1653.

[64] p. 19 cm. **[9823]**

—Dissertationes anatomicae methodo synthetica exaratae, sex libris comprehensae . . . Noribergae, Michael Endterus, 1656.

[40], 1303 p. 21 cm. **[9824]**

Added engraved title page.

With this is bound *his* Ordo et methodus generationi dicatarum partium. 1664.

—Epitome methodi cognoscendi & curandi particulares corporis affectus secundum ordinem Abubetri Rhazae ad regem Mansorem libro nono, Hippocraticis, Paracelsicis & Harveanis principiis illustratae & recognitae, philiatrorum in gratiam adornata & exscripta. Jenae, Literis Johannis Nisii, 1655.

[16], 384 (i.e. 396) p. 21 cm. **[9825]**

Includes extensive quotations in Greek with Latin translations, from the works of Aretaeus Trallianus, Galen and Hippocrates.

Bound with *his* Ordo et methodus medicinae specialis consultatoriae ὡς ἐν ἀτομω. 1669.

—[The same.] . . . Editione hac secunda . . . cum nova praefatione & recensione Georgii Wolfgangi Wedelii . . . Jenae, Impensis Joh. Birckneri, Typis Johannis Nisii, 1675.

[18], 396, [16] p.   front. (port.).   21 cm.

[9826]

—Wernerus Rolfinck . . . fabricae humani corporis studiosos salutat anatomen a calumniis defendit, eosque ad demonstrationem admirandae hujus structurae perhummaniter invitat. Jenae, Typis viduae Tobiae Steinmanni, 1632.

[16] p.   20 cm.

[9827]

—Liber de purgantibus vegetabilibus, sectionibus XV absolutus . . . Jenae, Impensis Johan. Ludovici Neuenhahnii, typis Johannis Wertheri, 1667.

[24], 454, [6] p.   19 cm.

[9828]

Includes quotations in Arabic and Greek, with Latin translations, including Avicenna, Dioscorides, and Paulus Aegineta.

—Ordo et methodus cognoscendi & curandi febres generalis. Hippocraticis, Paracelsicis, Harveanis, et Helmontianis principiis illustrata, Jenae, Samuel Krebs, 1658.

[8], 437 p.   20 cm.

[9829]

Copy 2.

With this is bound Stisser, J. A. Febrium intermittentium. Brunsvigae, 1687.

—Ordo et methodus generationi dicatarum partium, per anatomen, cognoscendi fabricam, liber unus . . . Jenae, Samuel Krebs, 1664.

[16], 214, [14] p.   21 cm.

[9830]

Bound with *his* Dissertationes anatomicae methodo synthetica exaratae. 1656.

—Ordo et methodus medicinae specialis commentatoriae ὡς ἐν γενει . . . Jenae & Francofurti, Apud Thomam Matthiam Goetzenium, curabat Samuel Krebs, 1665.

[36], 1069 (i.e. 1001), [41] p.   21 cm.   [9831]

Dedicatory epistle and laudatory poem inserted between sheet a and A.

—Another issue.

[12], 1069 p.   20 cm.

[9832]

Imperfect: p. 935–1069 wanting.

Without the insertions.

Bound with copy 2 of Möbius, G. Fundamenta medicinae physiologica. 1661.

—Ordo et methodus medicinae specialis commentatoriae, ὡς ἐν ειδει cognoscendi & curandi dolorem capitis . . . Jenae, Johannes Nisius, 1671.

[8], 245, [11] p.   19 cm.

[9833]

—Ordo et methodus medicinae specialis consultatoriae ὡς ἐν ἀτομω, continens consilia medica . . . Jenae, Excudebat Samuel Kregs, impensis Urbani Spaltholzii, 1669.

[32], 62 (i.e. 962), [22] p.   21 cm.

[9834]

Errata: p. [21–22] at end.

With this are bound *his* Epitome methodi cognoscendi & curandi particulares corporis. 1655; Schenck, J. T., *praeses.* De sero sanguinis. 1655.

Dissertations—Jena

—*praeses.* Dissertationes chimicae sex de tartaro, sulphure, margaritis, perfectis metallis duobus auro et argento, antimonio, et imperfectis metallis duris duobus ferro et cupro. Jenae, Literis Krebsianis, 1660.

1 v.   20 cm.

[9835]

Various pagings.

Each dissertation has special title page. *Respondents:* H. Andreae, E. B. Frosten, C. Gigas, G. S. Polisius, T. Rollius, J. G. Sommer.

—[The same.] . . . Jenae, Literis Krebsianis, 1679 excusae.

1 v.   20 cm.

[9836]

Various pagings.

Each dissertation has special title page.

Imperfect: Dissertatio chimica tertia, quarta and quinta wanting. *Respondents:* H. Andreae, E. B. Frosten, C. Gigas, G. S. Polisius, T. Rollius, J. G. Sommer.

—Methodus cognoscendi & curandi adfectus capitis particulares . . . Hippocraticis, Paracelsicis, ac Harvejanis principiis illustrata, dissertationibus duodecim explanata . . . Jenae, Expressit Johannes Nisius, 1653.

Various pagings.   20 cm.

[9837]

Each dissertation has special title page.

Respondents: C. Posner, no. 1; C. Muche, no. 2; J. Metzger, no. 3; G. Walter, no. 4; F. Gerstmann, no. 5; H. C. Ehrlich, no. 6; W. Prenke, no. 7; F. Gerber, no. 8; J. G. Dornau, no. 9; C. Funcke, no. 10; A. Pfeiffer, no. 11; A. Wansleben, no. 12.

Individual dissertations—Jena

—Ad chimiam in artis formam redactam, illustrandam breves notae, publicae ventilationi expositae . . . a Luca Schröckio . . . Jenae, Ex officina Samuelis Krebsii, 1669.

[16] p.   19 cm.

[9838]

L. Schroeck, *respondent.*

—Αγωνισμα iatrikon de hydrope ... Jenae, E Chalcographeo Wertheriano, 1667.

[56] p. 18 cm. [9839]

J. A. Euth, *respondent.*

—Casus practicus medicus, proponens aegram phthisicam ... Jenae, Typis Samuelis Krebsii [1664]

[20] p. 19 cm. [9840]

J. C. Seminarius, *respondent.*

—Commentarius in Hippocratis primum libri Aphorismum ... Jenae, Literis Krebsianis, 1662.

[8], 32 p. 20 cm. [9841]

J. A. Clotz, *respondent.*

—De ichore ulcerum seroso, Gliedwasser ... Jenae, Literis Steinmannianis, 1642.

[54] p. 20 cm. [9842]

J. Drawitz, *respondent.*

—De inundatione microcosmi, disputationem inauguralem ... P. P. Gottfried Walter. [Jena] Ex officina Freyschmidiana, 1652.

64, [2] p. 20 cm. [9843]

G. Walter, *respondent.*

Imprint partly supplied from Benzing (A).

—De phthisi disputationem inauguralem ... submittit ... Christophorus Knauth ... Jenae, Typis Samuelis Krebsii, 1664.

[56] p. 19 cm. [9844]

C. Knauth, *respondent.*

—Decas thematum miscellaneorum ... Jenae, Typis Ernesti Steinmanni, 1638.

[40] p. 18 cm. [9845]

A. Mack, *respondent.*

—Diatribe inauguralis medica ... Jenae, Typis Samuelis Krebsii [1664]

[128] p. 19 cm. [9846]

Imperfect: title page mutilated.

J. L. Ringelman, *respondent.*

—Discursus medicus de vertiginis διαγνωσει, προγνωσει, και θεραπεια [sic] ... Jenae, Literis Samuelis Krebsii, 1659.

48, [3] p. 19 cm. [9847]

J. F. Bollmann, *respondent.*

—Disputatio inauguralis de catarrho ... Jenae, Ex Officina Steinmanniana, 1637.

[16] p. 19 cm. [9848]

A. Birnbaum, *respondent.*

—Disputatio inauguralis de pleuritide ... Jenae, Ex Officina Steinmanniana [1638]

[16] p. 19 cm. [9849]

J. S. Albinus, *respondent.*

—Disputatio inauguralis de scorbuto ... Jenae, Typis Blasii Lobensteins, 1648.

[28] p. 21 cm. [9850]

L. Blumentrost, *respondent.*

—Disputatio inauguralis medica de dysenteria maligna urbem Vinariensem depopulante ... Jenae, Characteribus Johannis Jacobi Bauhoferi, 1672.

[39] p. 19 cm. [9851]

G. Loner, *respondent.*

—Disputatio inauguralis medica de phrenitide ... Jenae, Typis Johannis Nisii [1672]

[44] p. 19 cm. [9852]

J. F. Held, *respondent.*

—Disputatio inauguralis medica de plica Polonica ... [Jenae] Typis Johannis Nisii, 1658.

[1], 22 p. 19 cm. [9853]

C. E. Taube, *respondent.*

—Disputatio inauguralis medica de podagra ... Jenae, Typis Krebsianis [1672]

[24] p. 20 cm. [9854]

J. Eschenbach, *respondent.*

—Disputatio medica de catarrho ... Jenae, Literis Georgii Sengenwaldi, 1651.

[24] p. 19 cm. [9855]

J. Mochinger, *respondent.*

—Disputatio medica de dolore capitis ... Jenae, Typis Steinmannianis, 1629.

[12] p. 18 cm. [9856]

Diss.—Jena (J. Placcius, *respondent*)

—Disputatio medica de febre maligna ... Jenae, Typis Lobensteinianis [1642]

[24] p. 19 cm. [9857]

J. Volck, *respondent.*

—Disputatio medica, de febris malignae natura et curatione ... Jenae, Typis Blasii Lobensteins, 1638.

[20] p. 20 cm. [9858]

A. Haberkorn, *respondent.*

—Disputatio medica de melancholia ... Jenae, Sub calcographeo Tobiae Steinmanni, 1629.

[16] p. 19 cm. [9859]

J. K. Horn, *respondent.*

—Disputatio medica de mola ... Jenae, Typis Johannis Jacobi Bauhöfferi [1662]
[32] p. 19 cm.   **[9860]**
A. W. Osann, *respondent.*

—Disputatio medica de strangulatione uteri ... Jenae, Typis Johannis Wertheri [1672]
[44] p. 20 cm.   **[9861]**
J. G. Grübel, *respondent.*

—Disputatio medica inauguralis, de Χλωρωσει, seu foedis virginum coloribus ... Jenae, Aere Krebisno, 1665.
[44] p. 20 cm.   **[9862]**
J. N. Ewaldt, *respondent.*

—Disputatio medica inauguralis de dysenteria ... [Jenae] Stanno Caspari Freyschmidii, 1651.
[44] p. 18 cm.   **[9863]**
F. Hoffmann, *respondent.*

—Disputatio medica inauguralis de hydrope ascite ... Jenae, Typis Samuelis Krebsii [1672]
[28] p. 20 cm.   **[9864]**
C. H. Ruperti, *respondent.*

—Disputatio medica inauguralis de salivatione ... Jenae, Literis Wertherianis [1670]
32 p. 19 cm.   **[9865]**
J. J. Hager, *respondent.*

—Disputatio medica inauguralis περι ἀνορεξιας seu, De inappetentia ventriculi ... Jenae, E Calcographeo Lobensteiniano, 1649.
[32] p. 19 cm.   **[9866]**
J. M. Nester, *respondent.*

—Disputatio medico-chirurgica inauguralis de vulneribus ... Jenae, E typogr. Johannis Nisii, 1653.
[24] p. 18 cm.   **[9867]**
N. Moll, *respondent.*

—Disputationem hanc inauguralem de partu difficili ... ventilandam dabit Alhardus Hermannus Cummius ... Jenae, Typis Samuelis Krebsii [1664]
[84] p. 20 cm.   **[9868]**
A. H. Cummius, *respondent.*

—Dissertatio chirurgica inauguralis de scrophulis seu strumis ... Jenae, Literis Johannis Wertheri, 1667.
30, [2] p. 19 cm.   **[9869]**
P. M. Marci, *respondent.*

—Dissertatio de chylo et sanguine ... Jenae, Expressit Christianus Laurentius Kempff, 1652.
[35] p. 20 cm.   **[9870]**
J. G. Dornau, *respondent.*
Imperfect: wormholes on p. [13–35]

—Dissertatio inauguralis medica de pollutione nocturna ... Jenae, Typis Joh. Jac. Krebsii [1667]
[56] p. 20 cm.   **[9871]**
G. W. Wedel, *respondent.*

—Dissertatio inauguralis medica, qua ... apoplexiam ... offert disquisitioni M. Johann Arnoldus Friderici ... Jenae, E Chalcographeo Krebsiano, 1661.
[32] p. 18 cm.   **[9872]**
J. A. Friderici, *respondent.*

—Dissertatio inauguralis medica, qua ... catarrhum suffocativum ... proponit ... Wilhelmus Heinricus Schwartz ... Jenae, Johannis Nisii [1655]
23, [1] p. 20 cm.   **[9873]**
W. H. Schwartz, *respondent.*

—Dissertatio medica de chylificatione laesa ... Jenae, Literis Johannis Nisii, 1663.
[68] p. 20 cm.   **[9874]**
H. Schröder, *respondent.*

—Dissertatio medica de dysenteria ... [Jenae] Typis Johannis Wertheri, 1667.
[32] p. 20 cm.   **[9875]**
J. G. Gerlach, *respondent.*

—Dissertatio medica de partu difficili ... Jenae, Typis Johannis Wertheri [1666]
[4], 36, [4] p. 20 cm.   **[9876]**
J. A. Harssleben, *respondent.*

—Dissertatio medica de phthisi ... Jenae, Typis Wertherianis [1667]
46, [2] p. 19 cm.   **[9877]**
J. Schlegel, *respondent.*

—Dissertatio medica de tussi ... Jenae, Literis Johannis Nisii, 1663.
40 p. 19 cm.   **[9878]**
G. W. Wedel, *respondent.*

—Dissertatio medica de vertigine ... Jenae, Typis Johannis Wertheri, 1665.
74 p. 20 cm.   **[9879]**
M. Z. Pilling, *respondent.*

—Dissertatio medica inauguralis de catarrho ad nares, fauces & pulmones ad normam recentiorum dogmatum ... Jenae, Typis Samuelis Krebsii [1672]

[27] p. 19 cm. [9880]

J. F. Lehmann, *respondent.*

—Dissertatio medica inauguralis, de dolore colico ... Jenae, Typis Samuelis Krebsii [1660]

[36] p. 18 cm. [9881]

H. Andreae, *respondent.*

—Dissertatio medica inauguralis, de febre petechiali ... Jenae, Literis Nisianis [1664]

[64] p. 18 cm. [9882]

C. Relou, *respondent.*

—Dissertatio medica inauguralis de pleuritide ... Jenae, Typis Johannis Nisii [1671]

[32] p. 19 cm. [9883]

G. Handel, *respondent.*

—Dissertatio medica sistens aegrum laborantem febre tertiana intermittente scorbutica ... Jenae, Typis Johannis Wertheri [1669]

[32] p. 20 cm. [9884]

G. Schultz, *respondent.*

—Dissertatio practica de curatione hydropis ascitis, potissimum de παρα ἀκεντησι, agens ... Jenae, Typis Johannis Nisii [1668]

40 p. 20 cm. [9885]

B. Simon, *respondent.*

—Dissertationem de variolis ... proponit Johann. Petrus Prückelius ... Jenae, Typis Georgii Stengenwaldii [1658]

[50] p. 19 cm. [9886]

J. P. Prükkel, *respondent.*

—Dissertationem hanc inauguralem de affectu hypochondriaco ... submittit Henricus Cellarius ... Jenae, Typis Johannis Jacobi Bauhoferi, 1671.

[4], 28 p. 19 cm. [9887]

H. Cellarius, *respondent.*

—Dissertationem inauguralem de tertiana intermittente ... proponit ... Johannes Georgius Trott ... In Athenae Salano, Typis Krebsianis, 1662.

[48] p. 19 cm. [9888]

J. G. Trott, *respondent.*

—Exercitatio medica de genuina calculorum in humano corpore praecipue renibus et vesica generatione, nec non eorum signis & remediis ... Jenae,

Apud Georgium Sengenwald, 1664.

[4], 100 p. 20 cm. [9889]

A reissue of the 1663 edition with new title page. Cf. BMC. J. C. Jehring, *respondent.*

—Hoc cardialgiae scrutinium ... exponit Johann. Georgius Trumphius ... Jenae, Stanno Krebsiano, 1667.

[2], 73, [5] p. 19 cm. [9890]

J. G. Trumph, *respondent.*

—Ἰχνογράφημα theoretico-practicum de pyretologia in genere ad legem κυκλοφορίας αἱματικῆς conformatum ... Jenae, Literis Wertherianis, 1666.

[2], 24, [2] p. 20 cm. [9891]

J. L. Fabri, *respondent.*

—Methodi cognoscendi et curandi adfectus particulares capitis, ... Hippocraticis, Paracelsicis ac Harvejanis principiis illustratae dissertatio prima, de dolore capitis ... Jenae, Stanno Steinmanniano, expressit Christianus Laurentius Kempff, 1652.

[42] p. 19 cm. [9892]

C. Posner, *respondent.*

—Non ens chimicum, mercurius metallorum et mineralium ... Jenae, Johannes Wertherus [1670]

[1], 24, [2] p. 20 cm. [9893]

D. G. Waldburger, *respondent.*

—Another issue, with preliminary material added.

[8], 24 p. 19 cm. [9894]

—Ordinem et methodum cognoscendi et curandi ileum ... submittit Johannes Christophorus Neubergerus ... Jenae, Literis Samuelis Krebsii [1669]

[32] p. 19 cm. [9895]

J. C. Neuberger, *respondent.*

—Ordo et methodus cognoscendi & curandi maniam ... Jenae, Literis Krebsianis [1666]

68 p. 18 cm. [9896]

J. W. Faust, *respondent.*

—Ordo et methodus cognoscendi praecavendi, curandi ebrietatem, et inde ortam crapulam ... Jenae, Stanno Samuelis Krebsii, 1667.

[1], 42, [3] p. 20 cm. [9897]

J. Richman, *respondent.*

—Ordo et methodus medicinae specialis commentatoriae ... dissertatio quinta ... Jenae, Literis Krebsianis, 1665.

[4], 128 (i.e. 127) - 143 (i.e. 158) p.   19 cm.
[9898]

Signatures: [A]², R¹⁶.
S. Ochliz, *respondent.*

—Phrenitidem publico ... subjicit Henricus Schaevius ... Jenae, Excudebat Georgius Sengenwaldus, 1650.

[8] p.   19 cm.   **[9899]**

H. Schaeve, *respondent.*

—Publicae ... disquisitioni subjicit dissertationem hanc medico-chimicam de minera martis, Martinus Merckel ... Jenae, Literis Wertherianis, 1668.

[2], 27, [3] p.   19 cm.   **[9900]**

M. Merckel, *respondent.*

—Specimen hocce inaugurale de siti immoderata ... submittit ... Andreas Persike ... Jenae, Aere Samuelis Krebsii, 1673.

[24] p.   19 cm.   **[9901]**

A. Persike, *respondent.*

—Specimen inaugurale de dolore capitis, secundum ordinem & methodum medicinae specialis commentatoriae ... Jenae, Typis Samuelis Krebsii [1668]

[1], 22 p.   19 cm.   **[9902]**

C. Sörgel, *respondent.*

—Συζυτησις medica inauguralis de scorbuto ... Jenae, E chalcographeo Johannis Nisii [1668]

98, [6] p.   20 cm.   **[9903]**

J. L. Loelius, *respondent.*

—Σεα μισοπτωχος vulgo medicorum opprobrium podagra ... Jenae, Literis Samuelis Krebsii [1663]

[56] p.   20 cm.   **[9904]**

A. H. Fasch, *respondent.*

—*tr. See* BRENDEL, Z. [1592-1638] Chimia in artis formam redacta. 1641, 1671.

—*See* BECHER, J. J. Experimentum chymicum novum. 1671; ELSHOLTZ, J. S. Destillatoria curiosa. 1674; HORNE, J. van. Μικροκοσμος. 1675; MICHAELIS, J. Opera. 1698; SCHENCK, J. T., *praeses.* Guerneri Rolfincii ... Epitomes methodi cognoscendi & curandi affectus corporis humani particulares. 1655.

ROLLI, GIULIO [*fl.* 1630] *See* REGGIO EMILIA (City) Ordinances, local laws, etc. Bando in occasione di peste. 1630.

ROLLIUS, THEODORUS [*fl.* 1659-1663] *respondent.* De metallis perfectis auro & argento. *In* Rolfinck, W., *praeses.* Dissertationes chimicae sex de tartaro. 1660.

—*See* POSNER, C., *praeses.* Disputatio physica de morte. 1659.

ROMA, ANTONIO DE [*fl. ca.* 1667] *ed. See* ROMA, F. de. Consultationes medico-chirurgicae. 1669.

ROMA, FRANCISCO DE [*d. ca.* 1667] Consultationes medico-chirurgicae ... Opus posthumum ... Neapoli, Apud Novellum de Bonis, 1669.

[19], 380, [20] p.   33 cm.   **[9905]**

Edited by Antonio and Gennaro de Roma.

ROMA, FRANCISCO MORATO [1588-1668] Luz da medicina pratica racional, e methodica, guia de infermeiros, directorio de principiantes ... Coimbra, Manoel Rodrigues d'Almeyda, 1686.

[16], 428 p.   19 cm.   **[9906]**

—[The same.] ... Coimbra, Joam Antunes, 1700 [i.e. 1701]

[16], 419, [11] p.   21 cm.   **[9907]**

Privileges dated 1700 and 1701.

ROMA, GENNARO DE [*fl. ca.* 1667] *ed. See* ROMA, F. de Consultationes medico-chirurgicae. 1669.

ROMAIN, ADRIEN. *See* ROOMEN, Adriaen van [1561-1615]

ROMANO DE CÓRDOBA, ALONSO. Recopilacion de toda la theorica, y practica de cirugia ... Aora nuevamenta lleva añadido un Tratado del modo de curar carnosidades, y callos de la via de la orina de Miguel de Leriza ... Zaragoça, Herederos de Diego Dormer, acosta de Antonio Cabeças, 1674.

[8], 231 p.   16 cm.   **[9908]**

ROMANUS, ADRIANUS. *See* ROOMEN, Adriaen van [1561-1615]

ROMANUS, EGIDIUS. *See* COLONNA, Egidio [1247?-1316]

ROMANUS, PAUL FRANZ [*d.* 1675] *praeses.* [Diatribes juridicae de medico] Lipsiae, Literis Johannis Georgii [1670]

[32] p.   20 cm.   **[9909]**

Title from p. [3]
Diss.—Leipzig (M. Kegel, *respondent*)

ROMANUS, Wilhelm [*ca. 1644–1688*] *respondent.*
Disputatio inauguralis juridica de amore . . . Lipsiae,
Typis Johannis Georgii [1668]

[30] p.   20 cm.   **[9910]**
Diss. — Leipzig.

ROMATET, Charles [*fl. 1625–1635*] Crisiologia
medica; sive, Doctrina de morborum judicationibus,
in duos libellos divisa, quorum alter est de crisibus,
alter vero de diebus criticis. Ed. 2. . . . Accessit huic
secundae editioni luculentus De peste tractatus . . .
Parisiis, Apud Nicolaum Gasse, 1635.

[14], 128 p.; [1], 109, [11] p.   17 cm.   **[9911]**
Imperfect: special title page of part 2 wanting.
Includes extracts from Galenus and Hippocrates.

ROME (City) Académie de France. *See*
Académie de France à Rome.

ROME (City) Arciospedale di San Giacomo in
Augusta. *See* Ospedale di San Giacomo in Augusta,
Rome.

ROME (City) Collegio de' medici. *See* Collegio
dei medici, Rome.

ROME (City) Igreja e Hospital de Santo
António da Nação Portuguesa. *See* Igreja e
Hospital de Santo António da Nação Portuguesa.

ROME (City) Ordinances, local laws, etc.
Bando per causa di contagio . . . Roma & Perugia,
Sebastiano Zecchini, 1656.

broadside.   32 × 23 cm.   **[9912]**
Signed: G. Card. Sacchetti.

ROME (City) Ospedale di San Giacomo in
Augusta. *See* Ospedale di San Giacomo in Augusta,
Rome.

ROMEL, Peter. See Rommel, Peter [1643–1708]

ROMEO, Lorenzo [*fl. 1623*] Desengaño del abuso
de la sangria, y purga . . . Tarragona, Gabriel Roberto, 1623.

[16], 165, [5] ll.   15 cm.   **[9913]**

ROMER, Ole. *See* Rømer, Ole Christensen
[1644–1710]

ROMERUS, Oleaus. *See* Rømer, Ole
Christensen [1644–1710]

ROMIEU, Pierre. Traité de la nature et proprieté
des eaux minerales, & bains acides, nouvellement

découverts prés d'un lieu nommé Vendres . . . avec
la maniere d'en pratiquer l'usage. Perpignan, La
vefve de Jean Figuerola, 1683.

[5], 34 + p.   19 cm.   **[9914]**
Imperfect: mutilated, all pages after p. 34 wanting; missing text
supplied by pen.

ROMMEL, Peter [1643–1708] Discursus physico-
medicus, de foetibus leporinis, extra uterum repertis; aliisque tam de leporibus, quam etiam de conceptione extra-uterina raris & curiosis . . . Ulmae,
Typis haered. Christiani Balthas. Kühn, 1680.

15 p.   20 cm.   **[9915]**

—Der grausame, von Gott verhengte, und im
Finstern schleichende, doch zimlich entdeckte
Meuthel-Mörder; das ist, Gründlicher Bericht von
der Pest . . . Franckfurt, Verlegts Matth. Wagner,
drukts Joh. Andrea, 1680.

[1], 236 p.   front.   17 cm.   **[9916]**

ROMMEL, Theodor Renatas [*fl. 1690–1692*] *respondent. See* Wedel, G. W., *praeses.* Dissertatio inauguralis medica, de amarorum natura & usu. 1692
[and] Dissertatio medica de insomniis. 1690.

ROMPEO, Christian Constantino. *See* Rumpf,
Christiaan Constantijn [1633–1706]

ROMPF, Christian Constantin. *See* Rumpf,
Christiaan Constantijn [1633–1706]

RONDELET, Guillaume [1507–1566] Methodus
curandorum omnium morborum corporis humani,
in tres libros distincta. Ejusdem De dignoscendis
morbis. De febribus. De morbo Italico. De internis
& externis. De pharmacopolarum officina. De fucis.
Omnia nunc in lucem Castigatius edita. Lugduni,
Apud Joannem Lertout, 1601.

[16], 1277 p.   17 cm.   **[9917]**

—[The same.] . . . [Genevae] Apud Jacobum
Stoer, 1609.

[16], 1277 p.   18 cm.   **[9918]**
Different setting of type.

—[The same.] Opera omnia medica, nunc ab infinitis quibus antehac scatebant mendis, studio &
opera J . Croqueri . . . repurgata, & in gratiam
medicinae studiosorum nitori suo restituta . . .
Geneva, Stephanus Gamonetus, 1619.

[15], 1277 p.   18 cm.   **[9919]**
Contents. — Methodus curandi morbos. — De dignoscendis morbis. — De curandis febribus. — De morbo Italico. — De medicamentis

internis. — De medicamentis externis. — Pharmacopolarum officina. — Tractatus de fucis.

Different setting of type.

—[The same.] ... Ed. postrema, aliquot opusculis hujus authoris nondum antehac editis aucta ... Genevae, Apud Petrum & Jacobum Chouët, 1620.

[16], 87, [1] p.; 1277 p. 18 cm. **[9920]**

A reissue of the 1619 editon with the addition of his Introductio ad praxim; Tractatus de urinis; Consilia.

—[The same.] ... [Genevae] Apud Petrum & Jacobum Chouët, 1628.

[16], 1359 p. 17 cm. **[9921]**

[The same.] Opera omnia medica. Studio & labore J. Croqueri ... Genevae, Sumptibus Leonardi Chouët & socii, 1685.

[16], 1359 p. 17 cm. **[9922]**

Seemingly a reissue of the 1628 editon with new title page and preliminary matter reset.

—Dispensatorium seu pharmacopolarum officina. *See* L'Obel, M. de. *In* G. Rondelletii ... methodicam pharmaceuticam officinam animadversiones. 1605.

—Tractatus de urinis. Ante hac non editus. Francofurti, Impensis haeredum Nicolai Bassaei, 1610.

[1], 138 p. 13 cm. **[9923]**

—*See* CORDUS, V. Dispensatorium. 1627, 1651 [1652]; GESNER, K. Historiae animalium liber primus [-liber V]. 1617-1621 [v. 1, 1620]; SCHOLTZ, L. Consiliorum medicinalium ... liber singularis. 1610.

RONDINELLI, FRANCESCO [1589-1665] Relazione del contagio stato in Firenze l'anno 1630. e 1633. Con un breve ragguaglio della miracolosa immagine della Madonna dell'Impruneta ... Fiorenza, Gio. Batista Landini, 1634.

[16], 284, [4] p. 23 cm. **[9924]**

"Canzone dei sig. Francesco Rovai, nella quale si loda la pietà del serenissimo granduca di Toscana": p. [5-12]

"Al serenissimo Ferdinando II granduca di Toscana, per la liberazione di Firenze dalla peste. Panegirico di Mario Guiducci ..." (p. [106]-139) has half title.

RONPHILE. *See* RONPHYLE.

RONPHYLE. La chyromantie naturelle de Ronphile [pseud?]. Lyon, Antoine Jullieron, 1653.

[16], 78 p. illus. 15 cm. **[9925]**

Dedicatory epistle signed by Rampalle, the translator.

—[The same.] ... Paris, J. Baptiste Loyson, 1665.

[16], 78 p. illus. 15 cm. **[9926]**

Blank leaf following page 78 wanting.

Different setting of type.

—[German tr.] *In* Höchstfürtreflichtes chiromantisch- und physiognomisches Klee-Blat. 1695.

RONS, BOUDEWIJN. *See* RONSSE, Boudewijn [1525-1597]

RONSOVIUS, HENRICUS. *See* RANTZAU, Henrik [1526-1598]

RONSS, BAUDOUIN VAN. *See* RONSSE, Boudewijn [1525-1597]

RONSSAEUS, BALDUINUS. *See* RONSSE, Boudewijn [1525-1597]

RONSSE, BOUDEWIJN [1525-1597] *See* SENNERT, D. De scorbuto tractatus. 1624.

ROOMEN, ADRIAEN VAN [1561-1615] *praeses.* Disceptatio anatomica de partibus thoracis earumque convenienti administrandi ratione ... Wiceburgi, Typis Georgii Fleischmanni, 1602.

[4], 37 (i.e. 34), [1] p. 19 cm. **[9927]**

Diss. — Würzburg (K. Fridericus, *respondent*)

—Disputatio anatomica de partibus corporis nutritioni dicatis, earumque administrandi ratione ... Wirceburgi, Typis Georgii Fleischmanni, 1603.

[4], 63 p. 19 cm. **[9928]**

Diss. — Würzburg (J. K. Burckhard, *respondent*).

ROONHUYSE, HENDRICK VAN [1625-1672] Genees en heel-konstige aanmerkingen ... Amsteldam, De weduwe van Theunis Jacobsz Lootsman, 1672.

[16], 251, [5] p. illus. 17 cm. **[9929]**

Added engraved title page has title: Heel-konstige aenmerckingen. Amsterdam, 1672.

With this is bound (as issued) *his* Heel-konstige aanmerkkingen ... betreffende de gebreekken der vrouwen. 1672.

—Heel-konstige aanmerkkingen ... betreffende de gebreekken der vrouwen. Amsterdam, De weduwe van Theunis Jacobsz, 1663.

[16], 244, [4] p. illus. 17 cm. **[9930]**

Added engraved title page.

—[The same.] ... De 2. druk, met verscheyde nieuwe stoffen, en geneesmiddelen vermeerdert.

Amsterdam, De weduwe van Theunis Jacobsz, 1672.
[16], 184, [8] p. illus. 17 cm. [9931]
Added engraved title page.
Bound (as issued) with *his* Genees en heel-konstige aanmerkingen. 1672.

— [English tr.] Medico-chirurgical observations. *In* Busschof, H. Two treatises. 1676.

— [German tr.] Historischer Heil-Curen in zwey Theile verfassete Anmerckungen: deren erster Theil allerhand, an Manns- und Weibspersonen, sich ereignende . . . Gebrechen, zusamt denen darwider geordneten Artzneymitteln . . . der andere aber die . . . Gebrechen der schwangern, und anderer Weiber . . . vorstellet . . . In unsere hochteutsche Mutter-Sprach . . . übersetzet . . . Nürnberg, In Verlegung Michael und Johann Friederich Endtern, 1674.
[13], 235, [7] p. plates. 16 cm. [9932]
Added engraved title page.

— *See* BECKE, D. von der. Dissertatio anatomico-practica de procidentia uteri. 1683.

ROOS, THEODOR [*fl.* 1688] *respondent.* Disputatio medica inauguralis, de febre tertiana intermittente . . . Trajecti ad Rhenum, Ex officina Francisci Halma, 1688.
12 p. 22 cm. [9933]
Diss. — Utrecht.

ROOSENDAEL, PETRUS [*fl.* 1660] *respondent. See* LINDEN, J. A. VAN DER, *praeses.* Hippocrates de circuitu sanguinis, exercitatio VII. 1660.

ROQUETAILLADE, JEAN DE. *See* JOANNES DE RUPESCISSA [*fl.* 1328-1365]

RORARIO, GIROLAMO [1485-1556] Quod animalia bruta ratione utantur melius homine. Libri duo. Amstelaedami, Apud Joannem Ravesteinium, 1654.
117 p. 14 cm. [9934]
Edited by Gabriel Naudé.
Bound with Cardano, G. De propria vita liber. 1654.

ROSA, ANDREAS [*b.* 1665] *respondent. See* BOESS, D., *praeses.* Dissertatio medica, exhibens aegrum febri quartana intermittente laborantem [1687]; CRAUSE, R. W., *praeses.* Disputatio inauguralis medica de contractura. 1687; WEDEL, G. W. Propempticon inaugurale de naturae ministro medico. 1687.

ROSA, JOÃO FERREIRA DA [*fl.* 1686-1695] Trattado unico da constituiçam pestilencial de Pernambuco of-ferecido a el rey n. s. por servido ordenar por seu governador aos medicos da America, que assistem aonde ha este contagio, que o compusessem para se conferirem pelos coripheos da medicina aos dictames com que he trattada esta pestilencial febre . . . Lisboa, Miguel Manescal, 1694.
[31], 224, [4] p. 21 cm. [9935]

ROSA, JOHANN GEORG [*fl.* 1670-1672] *respondent. See* ISRAEL, J., *praeses.* Dissertatio inauguralis medica de ligatione. 1672.

ROSA, JOHANNES [*fl.* 1601] *respondent.* Themata physiologica de humoribus corporis humani . . . Lipsiae, Michael Lantzenberger [1601]
[23] p. 21 cm. [9936]
Diss. — Leipzig.

ROSACCIO, GIOSEPPE [*ca.* 1530 — *ca.* 1620] Discorsi . . . nelli quali si tratta brevemente dell'eternità, dell'evo, del tempo . . . Con un discorso sopra de'segni che appariscono nel sole, luna, stelli . . . Venetia, Pietro Farri, 1620.
28 p. 14 cm. [9937]
Imperfect: all leaves after B⁶ wanting.
Bound with *his* Il microcosmo. 1620.

— Il medico del dottore in . . . medicina . . . Gioseppe Rosaccio, libre tre. In questo primo si tratta della nobilta [sic] & eccellenza dell'astrologia, et si prova con molte autorità, quanto sia di giovamento al perito medico . . . Aggiuntivi gli Aforismi d'Hippocrate nella volgar lingua . . . Venetia, Pietro Farri, 1621.
[8], 308, [12], [309]-356, [3] 22 cm. [9938]
Libro secondo (p. [57]-308) and Libro terzo (p. [309]-355) have special title pages.
Errata: p. [3] at end.
"Aforismi d'Hippocrate" (p. [32]-56) are partly paraphrased and abridged.

— Il microcosmo . . . Nel quale si tratta brevemente, dell'anima vegetabile, sensibile, & rationale. Dell' huomo sua complessione, & fisionomia. Delle infirmità, che nascono in tutte le parti del corpo, & loro cura. Nuovamente dall'auttore corretto, & ampliato. Venetia, Appresso i Farri, 1607.
40 ll. 16 cm. [9939]

— [The same.] . . . Venetia, Pietro Farri, 1620.
48 ll. 14 cm. [9940]
With this is bound *his* Discorsi. 1620.

—[The same.] . . . Bologna, Per gl'eredi d'Antonio Pisarri, 1688.

80 p.   14 cm.   **[9941]**

ROSAEUS, Clemens [*fl.* 1621-1622] *respondent.* Theses medicae inaugurales de paralysi . . . Lugduni Batavorum, Ex officina Isaaci Elzevirii, 1622.

[12] p.   21 cm.   **[9942]**

Diss. — Leyden.

—*See* Vorstius, A. E., *praeses.* Theses medicae de convulsione. 1621.

ROSARIUM philosophorum.

133-252 p., vol. 2.   illus.   17 cm.   (*In* Artis aurifeare. Basileae, 1610)   **[9943]**

Caption title.

—[German tr.]

185-368 p., part 2.   illus.   19 cm.   (*In* Morgenstern, Philipp, *ed.* and *tr.* Turba philosophorum. Basel, 1613)   **[9944]**

Caption title.

ROSCIUS, Joannes Victorius. *See* Rossi, Gian Vittorio [1577-1647]

ROSE, Ludwig Günther [*fl.* 1668-1670] *respondent.* *See* Meibom, H., *praeses.* Disputatio medica inauguralis de suffusione. 1670.

ROSELL, Juan Francisco. *See* Rossell, Juan Francisco [*fl.* 1593-1632]

ROSENAU, Lorenz Scholtz von. *See* Scholtz, Lorenz [1552-1599]

ROSENBERG, Georg Heinrich [*fl.* 1696-1697] *respondent. See* Crause, R. W., *praeses.* Dissertatio inauguralis medica de signaturis vegetabilium. 1697; Wedel, G. W., *praeses.* Dissertatio medico-chimica de oleis destillatis. 1696.

ROSENBERG, Johann Karl [*fl.* 1622-1628] Rhodologia; seu, Philosophico-medica generosae rosae descriptio: flosculis philosophicis, arcanis politicis, chymicis, &c. adornata. Ed. nov. corr. . . . Francofurti ad Moenum, Sumptibus Wilhelmi Fitzeri, typis haered, Hartmanni Palthenii, 1631.

[40], 403, [1] p.   port.   17 cm.   **[9945]**

—Rosa nobilis iatrica; seu, Animadversiones et exercitationes medicae, Hippocraticae & Hermeticae,

novae ac notatu dignae . . . Argentorati, Sumptibus Eberhardi Zetzneri [1624]

[30], 130 p.   14 cm.   **[9946]**

—*ed. See* Setalla, L. Animadversionum et cautionum medicarum libri septem. 1625.

ROSENCREUTZER, Marcus Friedrich, *pseud. See* Ritter, Franz [*d.* 1641]

ROSENKREUZ, Marcus Friedrich, *pseud. See* Ritter, Franz [*d.* 1641]

ROSENROTH, Christian Knorr von. *See* Knorr von Rosenroth, Christian [1636-1689]

ROSENSCHILD, Jacob Henrik Paulli von. *See* Paulli, Jacob Henrik [1637-*ca.* 1702]

ROSET, Ludovicus [*fl.* 1688] *respondent.* Disputatio medica inauguralis, de pleuritide . . . Trajecti ad Rhenum, Ex officina Francisci Halma, 1688.

11, [1] p.   22 cm.   **[9947]**

Diss. — Utrecht.

ROSETHINOS, Petrus. *See* Rostinio, Pietro [16th cent.]

ROSETINI. *See* Rostinio.

ROSICRUCIANS. *See* Libavius, A. [*d.* 1616] Appendix necessaria Syntagmatis arcanorum chymicorum. 1615; Schalling, J. Ὀφθαλμια; sive, Disquisitio Hermetico-Galenica de natura oculorum. 1615.

ROSICRUTIAN BROTHERHOOD. *See* Rosicrucians.

ROSINUS. Rosinus ad Euthiciam [&] Rosini ad Sarratantam episcopum [&] . . . Liber definitionum . . .

158-204 p., vol. 1.   17 cm.   (*In* Artis auriferae. Basileae, 1610)   **[9948]**

Caption titles.

—[German tr.] Rosinus ad Eutichiam [&] Secundus ad Eutichiam [&] Das erste [-ander] Buch Rosini an den Bischoff Saratantam geschrieben [&] [. . . Beschreibung von den göttlichen Ausslegungen]

199-268 p., part 1.   19 cm.   (*In* Morgenstern, Philipp, *ed.* and *tr.* Turba philosophorum. Basel, 1613)   **[9949]**

Caption titles and title from table of contents.

ROSINUS, Antonius. *See* Deusing, A. Vindiciae foetus. 1644.

ROSITINI. *See* Rostinio.

ROSLER, Jacobus. *See* Röseler, Jakob [*fl.* 1654]

ROSNEL, Joannes Baptista de [*fl.* 1682] *respondent. See* Chirac, P., *praeses.* Dissertatio academica. 1692.

ROSS, Alexander [1590–1654] Arcana microcosmi; or, The hid secrets of mans body disclosed; first, in an anatomical duel between Aristotle & Galen, about the parts thereof. Secondly, by a discovery of the ... diseases, symptomes, and accidents of mans body. With a refutation of Doctor Browns vulgar errors, and the ancient opinions vindicated ... London, Printed by Thomas Newcomb, and sold by George Latham, 1651.

[18], 292 p.   13 cm.   **[9950]**

—[The same.] ... With a refutation of Doctor Brown's vulgar errors, the Lord Bacon's Natural history, and Doctor Harvy's book De generatione, Comenius, and others. Whereto is annexed a letter from Doctor Pr[imrose] to the author, and his answer thereto, touching Doctor Harvey's book De generatione. By A[lexander] R[oss] London, Tho. Newcomb, 1652.

[15], 267, [7] p.   18 cm.   **[9951]**

"An appendix ... wherein are contained divers passages; as of fishes, presages ..." (p. [209]–267) has special title page.

—Medicus medicatus; or, The physicians religion cured, by a lenitive or gentle potion: with some Animadversions upon Sir Kenelme Digbie's Observations on Religio medici ... London, James Young, 1645.

[14], 112 p.   15 cm.   **[9952]**

The Animadversions has special title page.

—The philosophicall touch-stone; or, Observations upon Sir Kenelm Digbie's discourses of the nature of bodies, and of the reasonable soule. In which his erroneous paradoxes are refuted ... And the weak fortifications of a late Amsterdam ingeneer, patronizing the soules mortality briefly slighted ... London, Printed for James Young, and sold by Charles Green, 1645.

[15], 131 p.   19 cm.   **[9953]**

Bound with Digby, *Sir* K. Two treaties. 1645.

ROSSBACH, Nikolaus [*fl.* 1623] *respondent. See* Sennert, D., *praeses.* De scorbuto disputatio. 1623.

ROSSELL, Juan Francisco [*fl.* 1593–1632] Ad sex libros Galeni De differentiis, et causis morborum, & symptomatum commentarii ... Vol. 1. Huic subjunctae sunt ejusdem authoris epistolae, altera ad Andream Laurentium ... altera ad Johannem de Caravajal ... Barcinonae, Apud Sebastianum & Jacobum Matheuat, 1627.

[23] p., 1296 col., 12, [26] p.   31 cm.   **[9954]**

The Galenic text is in the translation of Niccolò Leoniceno.

—El verdadero conocimiento de la peste, sus causas, señales, preservacion, i curacion ... Barcelona, Sebastian i Jaime Matheuad, 1632.

[8], 121 ll.   20 cm.   **[9955]**

ROSSELLO, Timotheo. Della summa de i secreti universali in ogni materia ... Parte prima [-seconda] Si per huomini, & donne di alto ingegno, come ancora per medici, & ogni sorte di artefici industriosi, & a ogni persona virtuosa accommodate. Di nuovo ristampati, et ricorretti. Venetia, Pietro Miloco, 1619.

[8], 152 ll; [8], 52 ll.   illus.   15 cm.   **[9956]**

Part 2 has special title page.

—[The same.] De' secreti universali ... parte prima [-seconda] ... si per huomini, & donne di alto ingegno, come ancora per medici, & ogni sorte di artefici industriosi & ad ogni persona virtuosa accomodati ... Venetia, Il Barezzi, 1644.

[8], 136 ll.; [8], 132 ll.   17 cm.   **[9957]**

Part 2 has special title page.

—[The same.] ... Venetia, Antonio Tivani, 1677.

[16], 238 p.; [16], 239 p.   16 cm.   **[9958]**

Part 2 has special title page.

ROSSELLUS, Johan Francisco. *See* Rossell, Juan Francisco [*fl.* 1593–1632]

ROSSEN, Jan van [*fl.* 1693] *respondent.* Disputatio medica inauguralis de polypo cordis ... Lugduni Batavorum, Apud Abrahamum Elzevier, 1693.

[12] p.   19 cm.   **[9959]**

Diss.—Leyden.

ROSSETINI, Pietro. *See* Rostinio, Pietro [16th cent.]

ROSSETUS, Franciscus. *See* Rousset, François [1535–1590?]

ROSSI, Bastiano de [*fl.* 1585–1605] *See* Crescenzi, P. de. Trattato del'agricoltura. 1605.

ROSSI, Francesco [*b.* 1576] Discorso . . . intorno di curar la peste con brevità di tempo . . . Genova, Giuseppe Pavoni, 6131 [colophon: 1631]

28, [1] p. 15 cm. **[9960]**

Last leaf (blank?) wanting.

—Nocturnae exercitationes in medicas historias, quae plurimum conducunt ad artem praedicendi in morbis acutis. Auctore Francisco Rubeo . . . Joannes Garmers denuo edidit & praefationem notasque & indicem . . . adjunxit. Hamburgi, Typis Pfeifferianis, sumptibus Joh. Naumanni, 1660.

[32], 489, [32] p. 17 cm. **[9961]**

"Joannis Garmeri Annotationes . . .": p. [453]-489. Errata: p. [32] at end.

—Copy 2. 17 cm.

With this is bound Welsch, G. Rationale vulnerum lethalium judicium. 1660.

—*ed. See* Rossi, Girolamo. Annotationes in libros octo Cornelii Celsi De re medica. 1616.

ROSSI, Gian Vittorio [1577-1647] De diuturna aegrotatione toleranda oratio . . . Romae, Apud Carolum Vulliettum, 1605.

[16] p. 25 cm. **[9962]**

ROSSI, Giovanni Battista de [*fl.* 1639] De salubri potu liber . . . In cujus fine continetur De climactericis annis disputatio . . . Velitris, Apud Alphonsum de Insula, 1639.

[16], 96 p. 19 cm. **[9963]**

ROSSI, Giovanni Domenico [*fl.* 1685] *tr. See* [Gaya, L. de] Cerimonie nuzziali di tutte le nationi del mondo. 1685.

ROSSI, Girolamo [1539-1607] Annotationes in libros octo Cornelii Celsi De re medica. Auctore . . . D. Hieronymo Rubeo . . . Nunc primum in lucem editae. Quibus omnia quae ad universam medicinam spectant dilucide, & compendiose explicantur . . . Venetiis, Apud Joannem Guerilium, 1616.

[20], 234 (i.e. 244) ll. 23 cm. **[9964]**

Dedication signed: Franciscus Rubeus.

—De destillatione sive de stillatitiorum liquorum, qui ad medicinam faciunt, methodo, atque virebus . . . 4. ed. . . . multis locis locupletatus . . . Venetiis, Apud Joannem Baptistam Ciottum, 1604.

[16], 181, [1] p. illus. 19 cm. **[9965]**

ROSSI, Lodovico. *See* Rostinio, Lodovico [16th cent.]

ROSSI, Matteo. *See* Rossi, Pietro Matteo [*fl.* 1607]

ROSSI, Perseo, *ed. See* Zecchi, G. In primam D. Hipp. Aphorismorum sectionem . . . lectiones. 1629.

ROSSI, Pietro. *See* Rostinio, Pietro [16th cent.]

ROSSI, Pietro Matteo [*fl.* 1607] Observationes med., chirurgicae & practicae, hoc est: de consultandi; sive, ut vulgo dicitur, collegiandi arte in morbis omnibus . . . ad chirurgiam pertinentibus tractatus; adjectis consultationibus et observationibus selectis pro morbis . . . curandis. Autore . . . Mattaeao Rossio . . . nunc primum a Victoria Rossio, filio . . . editus . . . Francoforti, Typis Wolffgangi Richteri, impensis Jon Theobaldi Schönwetteri, 1608.

[24], 199, [14] p.; [24], 167, [8] p. 18 cm. **[9966]**

Part 2 has special title page: Consultationes et observationes selectae.

—Consultationes & observationes selectae. *In* Borel, P. Historiarum et observationum medicophysicarum centuriae IV. 1676.

ROSSINIO, *See* Rostinio.

ROSSIO, Victorio [*fl.* 1606-1607] *ed. See* Rossi, P. M. Observationes med., chirurgicae & practicae. 1608.

ROSSO, Francesco. *See* Rossi, Francesco [*b.* 1576]

ROSSUM, Johannes van [*fl.* 1688] *respondent.* Disputatio medica inauguralis, de vertigine . . . Trajecti ad Rhenum, Ex officina Francisci Halma, 1688.

11, [1] p. 22 cm. **[9967]**

Diss. — Utrecht.

ROST, Georg [1582-1629] Practica medendi theologico-medica; oder, Guidener Griff, wie man allerley Kranckheiten von Grund aus heylen und vertreiben sol . . . Gosslar, Gedruckt bey Johann Vogt, in Verlegung Johann Hallervorden, 1625.

[96] p. 20 cm. **[9968]**

ROSTAGNY, Jean de [*fl. ca.* 1686] *tr. See* Boyle, Hon. R. Nouveau traité de Monsieur Boyle. 1689; Primrose, J. Traité de Primerose sur les erreurs vulgaires de la medecine. 1689.

ROSTINIO, Lodovico [16th cent.] *See* Rostinio, P. Compendio di tutta la cirugia. 1607, 1677.

ROSTINIO, Pietro [16th cent.] Compendio di tutta la cirugia, per Pietro & Lodovico Rostini ... estrato da tutti coloro, che di essa hanno scritto. Et dall'eccell. ... Leonardo Fioravanti ... ampliato di ... Discorsi: & aggiuntovi un nuovo Trattato a' professori di tal'arte ... utile ... Nuovamente ristampato, & con ogni diligenza corretto. Venetia, Lucio Spineda, 1607.

[24], 175 ll. illus. 15 cm. [**9969**]

Revised and corrected by Borgaruccio Borgarucci.

"Discorso dello ... Leonardo Fioravanti ... sopra la cirugia ..." (p. 129-175) has caption title.

—[The same.] ... Di nuovo ristampato, & con diligenza corretto ... Venetia, Gio: Battista Brigna, 1677.

[48], 368 p. illus. 16 cm. [**9970**]

—Trattato di mal francese; nel quale si discorre di ducento, e trentaquattro sorti di esso male; & à quanti modi si può prendere, & causare, & guarire. Et evidentemente si mostra chi hà il gallico male, & chi nò ... Raccolto, & tradotto da quanti han scritto di mal francese, & massime dal Brassavola; & di più molte cose vi sono di nuovo aggiunte ... Vicenza, Per Il Megietti, 1623.

[16], 174 p. 15 cm. [**9971**]

"Quesiti di Allessandro Fontana, con le risposte del Brasavola": p. 135-151.

A modified translation, with additions, of De morbi Gallici vocati curatione, by Antonio Musa Brasavola, which formed the principal portion of his Examen omnium decoctionum, which, in turn, was published as the final part of his Examen omnium loch, id est linctuum ... ubi de morbo Gallico ... tractatur.

ROT, Jacobus. *See* Roth, Jakob [1637-1703]

ROTA, Julianus Martianus, *tr. See* Tidicaeus, F. De theriaca et ejus multiplici utilitate. 1607.

ROTA, Michelangelo [1589-1662] De peste veneta, anno MDC XXX ... Quaestiones disputatae; sive, apologeticum ad syllogisticam disputationem. Venetiis, Apud Ghirardum de Imbertis, 1634.

[12], 194 p. [**9972**]

Leaf following page 194 (blank?) wanting.

ROTARIO, Sebastiano [*d.* 1742] Ragioni ... contra l'uso del salasso, fondate non solo su le dottrine degli antichi, e moderni scrittori, ma tratte eziandio dalle ragioni medesime colle quali pretende sostenerlo l'autore della medicina ventilata. Verona, Fratelli Merli, 1699.

8, 168, 10 p. 22 cm. [**9973**]

Imperfect: p. 5-8 of the third group of paging wanting.

ROTARIUS, Jan [*fl.* 1682] *respondent.* Disputatio medica inauguralis de cephalalgia calida ... Lugduni Batavorum, Apud Abrahamum Elzevier, 1682.

[12] p. 22 cm. [**9974**]

Diss.—Leyden.

ROTENDORF, Bernard. *See* Rottendorff, Bernhard [*fl.* 1643]

ROTH, Eberhard Rudolph [1646-1715] De velamine capitis virili exercitatio historica ... Jenae, Ex officina Jo. Jacobi Bauhoferi, 1673.

[60] p. 20 cm. [**9975**]

Diss. pro loco—Jena (J. Lorentz, *respondent*)

ROTH, Jakob [1637-1703] *praeses.* Disputationem physico-medicam generalia regni vegetabilis enucleantem ... submittit ... Emanuel König ... Basileae, Typis Emanuelis König & filiorum, 1680.

[8], 84 p. 20 cm. [**9976**]

Diss.—Basel (E. König, *respondent*)

—*respondent.* Theses inaugurales medicae ... Basileae, Typis Joh. Jacobi Deckeri [1665]

[12] p. 22 cm. [**9977**]

Diss.—Basel.

—*See* Bauhin, J. K., *praeses.* Historiam venaesectionis ... in publicum eruditorum examen offert ... J. R. [1662]

—*See* Flores poetici. 1687.

ROTH, Johann Jakob [*fl.* 1665] *respondent. See* Cellarius, T., *praeses.* Disputatio physica de tactu. 1665.

ROTH, Johann Valentin [*fl.* 1671] *respondent. See* Schneider, T. Τριχολογία seu, Dissertatio physica de pilis. 1671.

ROTH, Samuel [*fl.* 1695] *respondent. See* Wedel, G. W., *praeses.* Dissertatio medica de hydrophobia. 1695.

ROTHE, Gottfried [*fl.* 1691] *respondent. See* Berger, J. G. von, *praeses.* Dissertationem inauguralem de leienteria ... p. p. 1691.

ROTHENBURG OB DER TAUBER. Or-
DINANCES, LOCAL LAWS, ETC. Ernstliche, trewhertzige
Ordtnung und Befelch, welcher massen sich alle Einwohner der Statt Rotenburg ob der Tauber . . . bey
der . . . eingerissenen . . . Seuchen der Pestilentz, zu
ihrer selbsten Versicherung zuverhalten. Neben . . .
Bericht, wie sich vor derselben mit bewehrten guten
Artzney Mitteln zuverwahren . . . Aus eines . . .
Raths daselbsten, von dero ordentlichen, provi-
sionirten Medicinae Doctoribus gestellt . . . Rotenburg ob der Tauber, Hieronymo Körnlein [1625]

    [18] p. 20 cm.   **[9978]**

    Signed: Bernhardt Steiber, Joannes Benedictus Berger, Bern-
hardt Suevus.

ROTHLOEBEN, JOHANN MARTIN [1657-1701] *ed.*
See PHARMACOPOEIA HOLMIENSIS. 1686.

ROTHOCHS, JOHANN CHRISTIAN. *See* RODOCHS,
Johann Christian [*fl.* 1684]

ROTMUND, JOHANN CASPAR [*fl.* 1629-1631]
respondent. Positiones medicae, de diaeta sanorum . . .
Basileae, Typis Johan. Jacobi Genathii, 1629.

    [64] p.   **[9979]**
    Diss. — Basel.

ROTTENBERGER, JOHANNES [*fl.* 1674] *respon-*
dent. See WEDEL, G. W., *praeses.* Diaeta literatorum.
1674.

ROTTENDORFF, BERNHARD [*fl.* 1643]
Dreyfaches Consilium oder Gutachten. 1. Von dem
Wesen, Art, Natur, Eigenschafft, und Uhrsprung der
neuen Fiebersucht und epidemischer Haupt-
Kranckheit. 2. Von der einreissenden Rohten-Ruhr.
3. Von der Pest . . . Ossnabrück, J. G. Schwänder,
1679.

    [1], 462 p. 16 cm.   **[9980]**
    The title page is a cancel.
    Leaf following page 462 (blank?) wanting.

    —, *ed. See* LOMMIUS, J. Observationum
medicinalium libri tres. 1643, 1688.

ROUEN. Estat des maisons [des personnes] de la
ville de Rouen, & fauxbourgs d'icelle, qui ont estê
affligées de la maladie contagieuse, [et le nombre des
personnes qui sont morts] depuis le septiéme de
septembre 1668. jusques au [18 janvier 1669] . . .
Rouen, J. Viret, 1668-[1669]

    19 single leaves. 25 cm.   **[9981]**
    Caption titles.
    Published weekly.

—Recit de ce qui s'est passé en l'establissement des
Hospitaux de Saint Louis & de S. Roch de la ville
de Roüen; pour les maladies & convalescents de la
peste. Avec la description particuliere, & la figure
de [sic] tous les bastimens commencés en l'année 1654.
Paris, Charles Savreux, 1654.

    28 p. plate. 26 cm.   **[9982]**

ROUILLARD, SÉBASTIEN. *See* ROULLIARD
SÉBASTIEN [*d.* 1639]

ROULLIARD, SÉBASTIEN [*d.* 1639] Capitulaire
auquel est traicté qu'un homme nay sans testicules
apparens, & qui ha neantmoins toutes les autres marques de virilité: est capable des oeuvres du mariage
. . . Dern. ed. rev. & augm. de quelques autres
opuscules du mesme autheur. Paris, François Jacquin, 1604.

    [1], 140 p. 16 cm.   **[9983]**

—Le grand aulmosnier de France . . . Paris, David
Douceur, 1607.

    372, [60] p. 17 cm.   **[9984]**
    "Catalogue de tous les hostels-Dieu, et maladeries de France,
estans de fondation Royalle. Dressé par Messire Jean d'Aussy . . .":
p. [7-60]

—Les gymnopodes; ou, De la nudité des pieds,
disputée de part & d'autre . . . Paris, L'Olivier, 1624.

    [6], 326 (i.e. 366), [10] p. port. 25 cm.
         [9985]

ROUSE, LEWIS. *See* ROWZEE, Lodwick [*b.* 1586]

ROUSSEAU, ABBÉ. *See* ROUSSEAU, Henri de
Montbazon, *Father* [*ca.* 1643-1694]

ROUSSEAU, HENRI DE MONTBAZON, *Father* [*ca.*
1643-1694] Secrets et remedes éprouvez, dont les
préparations ont été faites au Louvre . . . Avec
plusieurs experiences nouvelles de physique & de
medecine . . . Paris, Jean Jombert, 1697.

    [94], 141 p. 17 cm.   **[9986]**
    Edited by Rousseau de la Grangerouge.

ROUSSEAU, NICOLAS [*fl.* 1614] *respondent. See*
PIETRE, S., *praeses.* Quaestio medica. 1647.

ROUSSEAU DE LA GRANGEROUGE [*fl.* 1697]
ed. See ROUSSEAU, H. de Montbazon, *Father.* Secrets
et remedes éprouvez. 1697.

ROUSSET, FRANÇOIS [1535-1590?] Exsectio foetus
vivi ex matre viva sine alterutrius vitae periculo, &
absque foecunditatis ablatione, à Francisco Rosseto;

Gallice conscripta. Casparo Bauhino . . . reddita, & variis historiis aucta. Adjecta est Joan. Albosii . . . . Foetus per ann. XXIIX. in utero contenti & lapide facti historia. Franc. item Rosseti tractat. hujus indurationis causas explicans. Francofurti, Excudebat Melchoir Hartmannus, Sumptibus Nicolai Bassaei, 1601.

[23], 396 (i.e. 398), [8] p.   16 cm.   **[9987]**

"Matthiae Cornacis . . . Historia gestationis foetus mortui . . ." (p. 228–267) has caption title; "Portentosum lithopaedion; sive, Embryum in utero materno per annos 28. contentum . . . Auctore Joann. Albosio . . . Cui accessit Simonis Provancherii . . . & Francisci Rosseti de eadem re opinio." (p. [287]–396), has half title.

ROUVERIUS, Ludovicus. *See* Rowzee, Lodwick [*b.* 1586]

ROUVEROY, de [*fl.* 1685–*ca.* 1698]Petit traité enseignant la vraye & assurée methode pour boire les eaux chaudes & froides mineralles, qui sortent des rochers qui sont dedans & aux environs du lieu de Plombière . . . Revue de nouv. & augm. par . . . le sieur de Rouveroy, medecin à Plombiere . . . de quelques curiosités & annotations. 2. ed. Épinal, Jean Bouchard & Estienne Le Gros [1698]

136 (i.e. 128) p.   16 cm.   **[9988]**

Date supplied from Eloy, v. 4, p. 122.

ROUVIÈRE, Henry. *See* Rouvière, Henry Louis de [*d.* 1712 *or* 13]

ROUVIÈRE, Henry Louis de [*d.* 1712 *or* 13] *ed.* See Descartes, R. Le monde de Mr. Descartes. 1664.

—, *tr. See* Arberius. La physique d'uzage. 1664.

—*See* Nouveau cours de medecine. 1669, 1683.

ROUVIÈRE, Lud. Henric. *See* Rouvière, Henry Louis de [*d.* 1712 *or* 13]

ROUVROY, N. *See* Rouveroy, de [*fl.* 1685–*ca.* 1698]

ROUW-KLACHTEN over de dood van den eerwaarden godsaligen en wydberoemden . . . Cornelis Ploegh, in sijn leven ledesetter en regeerend burgermeester: tot Jisp . . . Purmerent, Pieter Baars, 1696.

[44] p.   21 cm.   **[9989]**

ROUZAEUS, Ludovicus. *See* Rowzee, Lodwick [*b.* 1586]

ROUZÉ, Louis. *See* Rowzee, Lodwick [*b.* 1586]

ROVAI, Francesco [1605–1647] *See* Castellini, G. De dura cerebri vestiente męninge. 1646; Rondinelli, F. Relazione del contagio stato in Firenze l'anno 1630. e 1633. 1634.

ROWLAND, John, *M. D., ed.* and *tr. See* Pharmacopoeia Belgica. 1659.

—, *ed. See* Topsell, E. The history of four-footed beasts and serpents. 1658.

ROWLAND, William [*fl.* 1652–1655] *tr. See* Feyens, J. A new and needful treatise of spirits and wind offending mans body. 1668, 1676; Rivière, L. The practice of physick. 1655, 1658–61, 1672, 1678; Schröder, J. The compleat chymical dispensatory. 1669.

— *See* Platter, F. [1536–1614] A golden practice of physick. 1662.

ROWLANDS, Richard. *See* Verstegen, Richard [*ca.* 1548–1640]

ROWZEE, Lodwick [*b.* 1586] The queenes welles; that is, A treatise of the nature and vertues of Tunbridge water. Together, with an enumeration of the chiefest diseases, which it is good for, and against which it may be used, and the manner and order of taking it . . . London, John Dawson, 1632.

[8], 79 p.   16 cm.   **[9990]**

STC 21426.

—[The same.] . . . London, Gartrude Dawson, 1656.

[8], 79 p.   15 cm.   **[9991]**

Different setting of type.
View of Tunbridge Wells inserted before the title page.

—[The same.] . . . London, Robert Boulter, 1671.

[8], 79 p.   16 cm.   **[9992]**

Different setting of type.

—*respondent.* Theses medicae inaugurales de epilepsia . . . Lugduni Batavorum, Excudebat Godefridus Basson, 1616.

[8] p.   20 cm.   **[9993]**

Imperfect: upper margins trimmed.
Diss.—Leyden.

ROXAS, Juan Domingo Trigo de. *See* Trigo de Roxas, Juan Domingo.

ROY, Hendrik de. *See* Regius, Henricus [1598–1679]

ROY, JEAN LUCAS DE, *ed. See* BÉGUIN, J. Les elemens de chymie. 1620, 1627, 1658, 1665.

ROYAL ACADEMY OF SCIENCES, Paris. *See* ACADÁMIE ROYALE DES SCIENCES, Paris.

ROYAL COLLEGE OF PHYSICIANS, London. Certain necessary directions, as-well for the cure of the plague, as for preventing the infection; with many easie medicines of small charge, very profitable to His Majesties subjects; set downe by the Colledge of Physicians by the Kings Majesties speciall command. With sundry orders . . . for prevention of the plague. Also certaine select statutes . . . together with His Majesties proclamation for further direction therein and a decree in starre-chamber, concerning buildings and in-mates. London, Robert Barker and John Bill, 1636.

    [72] p.   18 cm.   **[9994]**
    Signatures: A–S⁴.
    Semicolon at end of seventh line; catchword on sig. C1 reads: demenour.
    Imperfect: title page mutilated.
    STC 16769.

    — Another issue.

                               [9995]
    Punctuation of title page differs: period at end of seventh line; catchword on sig. C1 reads: demenour.
    Imperfect: outer and upper margins trimmed.
    STC 16769.5.

    — Another issue.

                               [9996]
    Punctuation of title page differs: comma at end of seventh line; catchword on sig. C1 reads: demenour.
    Imperfect: title page mutilated; outer and upper margins trimmed; first preliminary leaf wanting.
    STC 16769.6.

    — Certain necessary directions, as well for the cure of the plague, as for preventing the infection: with many easie medicines of small charge, very profitable to His Majesties subjects. Set down by the Colledge of Physicians. By the Kings Majesties special command. London, John Bill and Christopher Barker, 1665.

    [8], 35 p.   19 cm.   **[9997]**
    Without catchword on p. 34.

    — Another issue, with catchword on p. 34.
                               [9998]
    Imperfect: first preliminary leaf wanting; upper margins trimmed.

With this is bound London. Ordinances, local laws, etc. Orders. 1665?

    — A short account of the proceedings of the College of Physicians, London, in relation to the sick poor of the said city and suburbs thereof, with the reasons which have induced the College to make medicines for them at the intrinsick value. London, 1697.

    [2], 16 p.   20 cm.   **[9999]**

    — *See* BADGER, J. The case between Doctor John Badger and the College of Physicians London. [1693]; CULPEPER, N. A physicall directory. 1649, 1650, 1651; Pharmacopoeia Londinensis. 1653, 1654, 1659, 1661, 1665, 1669, 1672, 1675, 1679, 1683, 1695; [GARTH, Sir S.] The dispensary; a poem. 1699, 1700; GOODALL, C. The Colledge of Physicians vindicated. 1676 [and] The Royal College of Physicians of London founded and established by law. 1684; GT. BRIT. LAWS, STATUTES, ETC. Certaine statutes especially selected, and commanded by His Majestie. 1630; MERRET, C. A collection of acts of Parliament. 1660; PECHEY, J. The London dispensatory. 1694; PHARMACOPOEIA COLLEGII REGALIS LONDINI. 1677; PHARMACOPOEIA LONDINENSIS. 1639, 1650, 1662, 1678, 1682, 1685, 1691, 1696; [SOCIETY OF APOTHECARIES OF LONDON] The principles of the chymists of London stated. 1676; THE STATUTES OF THE COLLEDGE OF PHYSICIANS LONDON. 1693; [YONGE, J.] Sidrophel vapulans. 1699.

ROYAL COLLEGE OF SURGEONS OF EDINBURGH. The grants and acts of Parliament, in favours of the College and Corporation of Surgeons of Edinburgh. [Edinburgh? 1696]

    [1], 39 p.   26 cm.   **[10000]**
    Half title.
    Latin and English.

ROYAL HOSPITAL OF ST. BARTHOLOMEW, London. *See* ST. BARTHOLOMEW'S HOSPITAL, London.

ROYAL SOCIETY OF LONDON. Museum Regalis Societatis; or A catalogue & description of the natural and artificial rarities belonging to the Royal Society and preserved at Gresham Colledge. Made by Nehemiah Grew. Whereunto is subjoyned The comparative anatomy of stomachs and guts. By the same author. London, Printed by W. Rawlins, for the author, 1681.

[12], 386, [2]p.; [2], 43 p. front. (port.), plates. 34 cm. **[10001]**

Part [2] has special title page.

—[The same.] . . . London, Hugh Newman, 1694.

[12], 386, [2] p.; [2], 43 p. front. (port.), plates. 33 cm. **[10002]**

A reissue of the 1681 edition with new title page and portrait.

—Philosophical transactions. London 1665/66–1886.

177 v. in 176. illus. 22 cm. **[10002.1]**

Publication suspended 1679–82. Replaced during this period by seven numbers of Philosophical collections issued by Robert Hooke.

Original title-pages incorrectly numbered in some editions (some later corrected)

Vols. 1–21 are for the years 1665–1699 printed by various printers between 1665 and 1700.

Imperfect: vol. 16 (1688–1690) wanting.

Issues for Mar. 1665–Dec. 1699 called also no. 1–259.

Indexes: vols. 1–12, 1665–77, with v. 12; vols. 12–17, 1677–93, with v. 17.

—*See* [HOLDER, W.] A supplement to the Philosophical transactions. 1678; SPRAT, T., *Bp. of Rochester.* The history of the Royal-Society of London. 1667; [French tr.] 1669; STUBBS, H. A censure upon certain passages contained in the history of the Royall Society. 1671; WALLIS, J. A defence of the Royal Society. 1678.

ROYLANDUS, ANTONIUS [*fl.* 1631] *respondent. See* BURGERSDIJCK, F. P., *praeses.* Collegium physicum. 1642.

ROZENS, LEWIS. *See* ROWZEE, Lodwick [*b.* 1586]

RUBBENS, AEGIDIUS [*fl.* 1663] *respondent.* Disputatio medica inauguralis de scorbuto . . . Lugduni Batavorum, Apud Gerardum van der Marse, 1663.

[11] p. 23 cm. **[10003]**

Diss.—Leyden.

RUBEAQUENSIS, SEBASTIANUS. *See* AUSTRIUS, Sebastianus [*d.* 1550]

RUBEIS, DOMINICUS DE [*fl.* 1639] Tabulae physiognomicae . . . Venetiis, Apud Gasparem Corradicium, 1639.

[13], 144 p. 16 cm. **[10004]**

—[German tr.] *In* Höchstfürtreflichtes

chiromantisch-und physiognomisches Klee-Blat. 1695.

RUBEIS, JOANNES BAPTISTA. *See* ROSSI, Giovanni Battista de [*fl.* 1639]

RUBER, ANTON. *See* RÜBER, Anton [*fl.* 1620]

RUBEUS. *See* ROSSI.

RUBNERUS, ANDREAS. *See* RÜBNER, Andreas [*fl.* 1669]

RUCKERT, Abraham [*fl.* 1685] *respondent.* Disputatio medica inauguralis, de spasmo . . . Trajecti ad Rhenum, Ex officina Francisci Halma, 1685.

15, [1] p. 22 cm. **[10005]**

Diss.—Utrecht.

RUDBECK, OLOF [1630–1702] Insidiae structae Olai Rudbeckii . . . ductibus hepaticis aquosis, & vasis glandularum serosis. Arosiae editis, a Thoma Bartholino . . . Lugduni Batavorum, Ex officina Adriani Wingaerden, 1654.

[1], 164 p. illus. 16 cm. **[10006]**

An answer to Martin Bogdan's Insidiae structae Thomae Bartholini Vasis lymphaticis ab Olao Rudbekio.

—Nova exercitatio anatomica, exhibens ductus hepaticos aquosos et vasa glandularum serosa. In Hemsterhuis, S. Messis aurea triennalis. 1654, 1659.

—[The same, *as subject.*] *See* BOGDAN, M. Insidiae structae Cl. V. Thomae Bartholini . . . Vasis lymphaticis. 1654.

—Variae anatomicae observationes. In Hemsterhuis, S. Messis aurea triennalis. 1654, 1659.

—*respondent.* Disputatio medica inauguralis, de fundamentali plantarum notitia rite acquirenda . . . Trajecti ad Rhenum, Ex officina Francisci Halma, 1690.

25, [3] p. 21 cm. **[10007]**

Diss.—Utrecht.

—*See* VESLING, J. Syntagma anatomicum. 1666, 1677, 1696.

RUDEL, SIGISMUND [*fl.* 1609–1610] *See* PLATTER, F. [1536–1614] Felix Platerus . . . decreto. 1610.

RUDIO, Eustachio [1551–1611] De affectib. externarum corporis humani partium libri septem: in quorum primis quinque de morbis; in duobus reliquis de symptomatibus . . . disseritur . . . Venetiis,

Apud Joan. Antonium & Jacobum de Franciscis, 1606.

[4], 200, [22] ll; [4], 54, [7] ll.   33 cm.

[10008]

Signatures: pars 1: a⁴, A-20⁶; pars 2: a⁴, A-I⁶, K⁸ (last leaf blank)
Part [1] includes five books.
Part [2] has special title page: De affectibus externarum comporis humani partium pars posterior, in qua de symptomatibus tractatur.

—De morbis occultis, et venenatis, libri quinque ... Venetiis, Apud Thomam Baglionum, 1610.

[12], 227 p.   32 cm.   **[10009]**

—De ulceribus libri tres, non minus physicis, quam chirurgis vocatis medicis utilissimi ... Patavii, Apud Franciscum Bolzettam, ex officina Laurentii Pasquati, 1602 [1601]

[4], 89, [3] ll.   21 cm.   **[10010]**

Errata: ll. [3] at end.

—Liber de anima. In quo probatur Galenum de vegetalis, & sentientis animae substantia reliquis omnibus rectius sensisse, veriora, tum vitae, tum mortis principia, & causae traduntur, nec non rationalis animae immortalitas ... probatur ... Patavii, Apud Petrum Bertellum [Ex typographia Laurentii Pasquati] 1611.

[4], 242, [1] p.   21 cm.   **[10011]**

With this are bound: *his* De virtutibus. Venetiis, 1587; Polo, Antonio. Abbreviatio veritatis animae rationalis. Venetiis, 1578; Mancini, Celso. De cognitione hominis. Ravennae, 1586.

RUDNICIUS, Christian [*fl.* 1661] *respondent.* Disputatio medica inauguralis, peripneumonici historiam & curam proponens ... Lugduni Batavorum, Typis Boxianis, 1661.

[16], p.   19 cm.   **[10012]**

Diss.—Leyden.

RUDOLPH, Johann Gabriel [*fl.* 1690-1708?] Medicus ad aegri palatum varium in materia medica, imprimis universali evacuante adaptatus. Lugduni Batavorum, Apud Jordanum Luchtmans, 1699.

[8], 143 p.   16 cm.   **[10013]**

—, *respondent. See* Bohn, J., *praeses.* Specimen primum medicinae forensis. 1690.

RÜBER, Anton [*fl.* 1620] *respondent. See* Sebisch, M. [1578-1674?] *praeses.* Disputatio de purgatione quarta. 1620 [and] Disputationes de recta ratione purgandi. 1621.

RÜBNER, Andreas [*fl.* 1669] *respondent. See* Saltzmann, J. R. [*fl.* 1637-1670?] *praeses.* Dissertatio solennis de lupo. 1669, 1688.

RÜDIN, Jakob [*fl.* 1649] *respondent. See* Stupanus, E., *praeses.* Signorum medicorum doctrina. 1649.

RÜDIN, Johann Jacob [*fl.* 1686] *respondent.* Dissertationem inauguralem medicam in diabetis naturam inquirentem ... publico ... examini proponit M. Joh. Jacobus Rüdinus ... Basileae, Typis Joh. Rodolphi Genathii [1686]

[20] p.   19 cm.   **[10014]**

Diss.—Basel.

RÜEL, Christopher Friedrich [*fl.* 1681] *respondent.* Disputatio medica inauguralis de scorbuto ... Groningae, Typis Remberti Huysman, 1681.

[28] p.   19 cm.   **[10015]**

Diss.—Groningen.

RÜEL, Heinrich Emanuel [*fl.* 1693] *respondent. See* Franck von Franckenau, G., *praeses.* Dissertationem inauguralem de hydrope ... publice ... examinandam sistit ... H. E. R. 1693.

—*See* Berger, J. G. von. Ordinis medici ... decanus ... lectori ... S. P. D. 1693.

RÜFF, Jakob [1500-1558] [Hebammen Buch. Dutch] 't Boeck vande vroet-wijfs ... Overgheset uyt den Hoogh-duytsche in onse Nederlandtsche spraecke, door Martyn Everaert ... Amstelredam, Broer Jansz, 1633.

74 (i.e. 66), [4] ll. illus.   20 cm.   **[10016]**

Bibl. Belg. R52.

Translation of *his* Hebammen Buch published by Siegmund Feyerabend in Frankfurt am Main in 1580. This is an enlarged edition of the author's Ein schön lustig Trostbüchle von den Empfengknussen und Geburten der Menschen, published in 1554.

—[The same.] ... Amstelredam, Broer Jansz, 1648.

74 (i.e. 70), [5] ll. illus.   19 cm.   **[10017]**

Bibl. Belg. R53.

—[The same.] ... Amsterdam, Jan Jacobsz. Bouman, 1668.

73 (i.e. 69), [3] ll. illus.   21 cm.   **[10018]**

Bibl. Belg. R55.

—[The same.] ... Amsterdam, Michiel de Groot, 1680.

74 (i.e. 70), [2] ll. illus.   20 cm.   **[10019]**

Bibl. Belg. R58.

—[English tr.] The expert midwife; or, An excellent and most necessary treatise of the generation and birth of man ... Also the causes, signes, and various cures, of the most principall maladies and infirmities incident to women. Six bookes ... London, Printed by E. G[riffin] for S. B[urton] and sold by Thomas Alchorn, 1637.

[16], 192, 120 p. illus. 19 cm. [10020]

STC 21442.
Title page mutilated.

RUEFF, JAMES. See RÜFF, Jakob [1500-1558]

RUEL, CHRISTOPHORUS FRIDERICUS. See RÜEL, Christopher Friedrich [fl. 1681]

RUEL, HENRICUS EMANUEL. See RÜEL, Heinrich Emanuel [fl. 1693]

RUEL, JEAN [1474?-1537] tr. See MATTIOLI, P. A. Opera quae extant omnia. 1674.

RUELLE, JEAN DE LA. See RUEL, Jean [1474?-1537]

RUELLIUS, JOANNES. See RUEL, Jean [1474?-1537]

RÜMELIN, JOHANNES. See REMMELIN, Johann [1583-1632]

RUEUS, FRANCISCUS. See LA RUE, François [ca. 1520-1585]

RUFF, JAKOB. See RÜFF, Jakob [1500-1558]

RUFFUS, of Ephesus. See RUFUS, of Ephesus.

RUFINE, JAMES [b. ca. 1649] respondent. Disputatio medica inauguralis de passione coeliaca ... Lugduni Batavorum, Apud viduam & haeredes Joannis Elsevirii, 1671.

[12] p. 23 cm. [10021]

Diss.—Leyden.

RUFUS, of Ephesus. See VESALIUS, A. Anatomia. 1604.

RUICES DE FONTECHA, JUAN ALFONSO. See ALONSO Y DE LOS RUYZES DE FONTECHA, Juan [1560-1620]

RUINI, CARLO [d. 1598] Anatomia del cavallo, infermita, et suoi rimedii. Opera nuova ... Venetia, Fioravante Prati, 1618.

2 v. in 1. illus. 34 cm. [10022]

Previously published also under title: Dell'anotomia, e dell'infermita del cavallo.

—[German tr.] Anatomia & medicina equorum nova; das ist, Neuwes Rossbuch oder von der Pferden Anatomy, Natur, Cur, Pflegung unnd Heylung, zwey ausserlesene Bücher ... Auss dess ... italianischer Edition ... ins Teutsch gebracht, durch Petrum Uffenbach ... Franckfurt am Mayn, Gedruckt bey Matthias Beckern in Verlegung Peter Fischers seligen Erben, 1603.

2 v. in 1. illus. 34 cm. [10023]

—See FRANCINI, H. de. Hippiatrique. 1607.

RUIZ, FRANCISCO [fl. 1625] Discurso sobre la composicion del azucar rosado solutivo, defendiendo las ordinaciones reales, y las del collegio de médicos y cirujanos ... Çaragoça, Pedro Verges, 1628.

[8], 45, [1] p.; 40 p. 20 cm. [10024]

Part [2] has caption title and colophon dated 1625.
With this is bound his Nobilissimae Caesaraugustanae civitatis Aragonum coronae jussu cujusdam apologeticae censurae repulsio. 1629.

—Nobilissimae Caesaraugustanae civitatis Aragonum coronae jussu cujusdam apologeticae censurae repulsio ... Caesaraugustae, Apud Petrum Verges, 1629.

[6], 25 p. 20 cm. [10025]

Bound with his Discurso. 1628.

RULAND, JOHANN DAVID [fl. 1636] respondent. See WEIDNER, G., praeses. De lue sive lepra venerea disputatio. 1636.

RULAND, MARTIN [1532-1602] [Balnearium restauratum. Abridgments. etc. German.] III. Bücher, von Wasserbädern, Aderlassen, und Schrepffen. In welchen, wie alle Kranckheiten durch Wasser, Wild unnd Schweissbäder, Laugen &c. item durch Aderlassen und Schrepffen geheilt werden sollen, angezeigt ... Jetzt ... gebessert, und ubersehen ... Basel [Getruckt durch Sebastian Henricpetri, 1613]

[14], cclxxxvii, [15] p. 16 cm. [10026]

A shortened and rearranged version of the Latin work published in 1597 in Basel under title: Balnearium restauratum.
Bound with Etschenreutter, G. Von den aller heilsamsten ... Bädern, 1616.

—Curationum empiricarum et historicarum, in certis locis & notis personis optime expertarum, &

rite probatarum, centuria prima, emendatius impressa ... Basileae [Per Sebastianum Henricpetri, 1610]

[29], 162, [28] p.   12 cm.   **[10027]**

A page for page reprint of the same publisher's edition of 1581. With this are bound *his*: Curationum ... centuria secunda. Basileae [1580]; Curationum ... centuria III. Basileae [1591]; Curationum ... centuria quarta. Basileae [1593]

—Curationum empyricarum & historicarum, in certis locis & notis personis optime expertarum, & rité probatarum, centuriae decem. Quibus adjuncta de novo ejusdem authoris Medicina practica ... Lugduni, Sumpt. Petri Ravaud, 1628.

[8], 794, [13] p.; 165 (i.e. 175) p.   19 cm.   **[10028]**

"De phlebotomia morbisque per eam curandis" [and] "De scarificatione et ventosatione, morbisque per eam curandis" p. [732]–794.

The Medicina practica and Appendix de dosibus (part [2], p. 105–175) have special title pages.

—[The same.] Thesaurus Rulandinus. Hoc est ... Curationes empiricae; quae antea in decem centurias dissectae prodierunt, nunc vero, in compendiosum ordinem secundum partium corporis seriem redactae, lucem aspiciunt. Accesserunt hisce, ejusdem alii Tractatus tres: I. De phlebotomia. II. De scarificatione & ventosatione. III. Oratio de ortu animae. Omnia studio & opera Joh. Scretae & Georgii Spörlini ... Basileae, Typis Henricpetrinis, 1628.

[48], 408, [11] p.; [16], 119 p.   17 cm.   **[10029]**

Part [2] has special title page with imprint: Basileae, Apud Henricpetrinos, 1627.

—[The same.] ... Curationum ... centuriae decem. ... Rothomagi, Sumptibus Joannis Berthelin, 1650.

[8], 794, 13 p.; 175 p.   18 cm.   **[10030]**

A page for page reprint of the 1628 Lyon edition.

—[The same.] Thesaurus Rulandinus ... Ed. 3. Budissae, Sumptibus Friderici Arnstii, typis Andreae Richteri, 1680.

[26], 118, 434, [12] p.   17 cm.   **[10031]**

Added engraved title page.

The Tractatus tres ([13–26], 118 p., with special title page) is placed ahead of the Curationes.

Identical in contents with the edition published in Basel in 1628, except that the extensive preliminary matter of the earlier edition is here replaced by a new dedication by the present publisher, dated 1679.

—[Dutch tr.] Empirica. Tres centuriae; ofte, Drie honert curatien of genesingen, by ervarentheyt ende geloofwaerdige geschiedenissen in seeckere plaetsen ende welbekenden persoonen versocht nae het behooren, ende goet bevonden ... Nu eerst uyt het Latijn inde Nederlantsche tale overgeset door Jan Pauwelsz Vriese ... Amsterdam, De weduw van Joost Broersz, 1660.

78, [10], [79]–178, [14], [179]–250, [10] p.   16 cm.   **[10032]**

Centuriae 2–3 have special title pages dated 1661.
Centuria 3 is translated by M. Ja. Co. vande Camp.

—[English tr.] Experimental physick; or, Seven hundred famous and rare cures. Being part of the physitian's library. Containing a collection of the most useful parts of the works of M. Ruland. L. Riverius. D. Sennertus. F. Plater ... By Nich. Culpeper ... and Abdiah Cole ... London, Peter Cole, 1662.

[24], 736 (i.e. 726), [15] p.   15 cm.   **[10033]**

Contains "ten centuries" of cures, translated mainly from Martin Ruland's Curationum empyricarum & historicarum ... centuriae decem.

—Lexicon alchemiae; sive, Dictionarium alchemisticum, cum obscuriorum verborum, & rerum hermeticarum, tum Theophrast-Paracelsicarum phrasium, planam explicationem continens ... [Francofurti] Cura ac sumtibus Zachariae Palhenii, 1612.

[7], 471 (i.e. 487) p.   illus.   22 cm.   **[10034]**

Epistola dedicatoria dated 1611 and signed by Martin Ruland, the younger. Attributed to him by BN and Bibl. Waller.

—[The same.] ... Francofurti, Prostat apud Johannem Andream, & Wolfgangi Endteri junioris haeredes, 1661.

[7], 471 (i.e. 487) p.   illus.   23 cm.   **[10035]**

Imperfect: wormholes on p. 363–[487].
A reissue of the 1612 edition with preliminary materials reset.

—Medicina practica recens et nova continens omnes totius humani corporis morbos, per alphabeticum ordinem collectos quibus $\kappa\alpha\theta$ '$\dot{\epsilon}\kappa\alpha\sigma\tau\sigma\nu$ sunt addita medicamenta omnia composita $\tau\alpha$ $\epsilon\nu\pi\sigma\varrho\iota\sigma\tau\alpha$ & quae ubique locorum hodie in pharmacopoeis, seu apothecis semper extant parata: nunc denuo emendatior edita & auctior ... Cum certa compositorum omnium dosi sub finem appensa ... Hanoviae, Apud Guilielmum Antonium, 1610.

169, [7] p.; [2], 104 p.   13 cm.   **[10036]**

Part [2] has special title page: Appendix de dosibus.

—[The same.] . . . Francofurti, Apud Joannum Stôckle, 1625.

169, [7] p.; [2], 104 p. 14 cm.   **[10037]**

Part [2] has special title page: Appendix de dosibus.

—Progymnasmata alchemiae; sive, Problemata chymica, nonaginta & una quaestionibus dilucidata: cum Lapidis philosophici vera conficiendi ratione . . . Francofurti, E Collegio Musarum Paltheniano, 1607.

[16], 254, 136 p.; 165, [1] p. 16 cm. **[10038]**

Dedicatio dated 1606 and signed by Martin Ruland, the younger. Attributed to him by the BNC.

"Elenchus remediorum spagyricorum . . .": p. 227-254.

Part [2] has special title page: Lapidis philosophici vera conficiendi ratio, gemino eruta tractatu, dated 1606.

—See SALMON, W. Iatrica. 1681, 1684, 1694; SPINDLER, P. Observationum medicinalium centuria. 1691.

RULAND, MARTIN [1569-1611] De morbo Ungarico recte cognoscendo et foeliciter curando. Tractatus novus recognitus & auctus, tum curationibus historicis, tum quaestionibus hactenus inter medicos controversis . . . Lipsiae, Sumtibus Jacobi Apelii, 1610.

[19], 743, [35] p. 17 cm.   **[10039]**

Published in Frankfurt in 1600 under title: De perniciosae luis Ungaricae tecmarsi.

—[The same.] Tractatus de morbo Ungarico recte cognoscendo & foeliciter curando. Tum curationibus historicis, tum quaestionibus hactenus inter medicos controversis . . . Ed. 2. recognita & aucta. Stettini, Impensis & sumptibus Jeremiae Mamphrasii, 1651.

[19], 743, [35] p. 16 cm.   **[10040]**

Imperfect: p. [35] wanting.

A reissue of the 1610 Leipzig edition, with title page and preliminary matter reset.

Problematum medico-physicorum liber primus [-pars secunda] . . . Francofurti, E Collegio Musarum Paltheniano, 1608.

189, [18] p.; 2, 152, [14] p. 16 cm. **[10041]**

Part 2 has special title page.

—Lapidis philosophici vera conficienda ratio. *In* Ruland, M. [1532-1602] Progymnasmata alchemiae. 1607.

—, *ed. See* RULAND, M. [1532-1602] Lexicon alchemiae. 1612, 1661 [and] Thesaurus Rulandinus. 1628, 1680.

RUMBAUM, GEORG [*fl.* 1592-1606] *respondent. See* STUPANUS, J. N., *praes.* De febre ephemera. 1606.

RUMELIUS OF NEW MARKET. *See* RUMMEL, Johann Konrad [1597-1661]

RUMLER, JOHANN UDALRICH [*fl.* 17th cent.] Observationes medicae, e bibliotheca Georgii Hieronymi Velschii, cum ejusdem notis.

63, [12] p. 20 cm. (Part [4] *in* Welsch, Georg Hieronymus. Sylloge curationum. Aug. Vindel., 1667)   **[10042]**

RUMMEL, JOHANN KONRAD [1574-1630] Historia morbi, qui ex Castris ad Rastra, a Rastris, ad Rostra, ab his ad aras & focos in Palatinatu superioris Bavariae se penetravit anno MDCXXI. et permansit MDCXXII. MDCXXIII . . . Norimbergae, Typis Simonis Halbmayeri, 1625.

[16], III p. 16 cm.   **[10043]**

—Partus humanus; sive, Dissertatio perbrevis de humani partus natura, temporibus, et causis . . . Noribergae, Cura Simonis Halbmayeri, 1624.

64 p. table. 17 cm.   **[10044]**

—Prophylace medico-practica luis epidemiae εγ κεφαλονοξου, exhibita . . . Una cum apotrope: id est Centuria curationum medicarum . . . factarum in Novo-Foro septemviralis Palatinatus, a Jano-Chunrado Rhumelio . . . conscripta a filio cognomine medicinae studioso. Norimbergae, Sumptibus itemque chalcographicis Simonis Halbmayeri, 1624.

174 p. 16 cm.   **[10045]**

RUMMEL, JOHANN KONRAD [1597-1661] *See* COLSON, L. Philosophia maturata. 1668; RUMMEL, J. K. [1574-1630] Prophylace medico-practica. 1624.

RUMMEL, JOHANN PHARAMUND [*fl.* 1630-1648] Magni libri naturae & artis, tractatus sextus, de phalaia microcosmi; das ist, Gründlicher Bericht, wie man auss der kleinen Welt eine Panaceam oder einige Medicin . . . bereiten soll . . . Das erste Mal gantz new verfertiget, und sonsten vor niemals in den Druck publicirt . . . Nürnberg, In Verlegung Wolff Endters, 1632.

[150] p. 17 cm.   **[10046]**

Erster Theil only.

". . . Phalaia tripartita; das ist, Gründlicher Bericht, wie man die Mumiam microcosmici ohne Gefahr erlangen" (p. [105-150]) has half title.

—Medicamenta militaria dogmatica, hermetica et magica; das ist, Ausserlesene und experimentirte Kriegs Artzney ... Nürnberg, Wolffgang Endter, 1632.

[228] p.   14 cm.   [10047]

—Medicina spagyrica; oder, Spagyrische Artzneykunst. In welcher I. Compendium hermeticum ... II. Antidotarium chymicum ... III. Jatrium chymicum ... gelehret wird ... Erstlich von Johanne Pharamundo Rhumelio, stückweiss an Tag geben, jetzo aber mit hinzuthuung Pharmacopoea chymica und Herbarii hermetici zusammen gelesen, und in gewisse Ordnung gebracht ... Franckfurt, In Verlegung Johann Hüttners, 1648.

[57], 769, [23] p.   15 cm.   [10048]

Added engraved title page.
With this is bound Kunckel, J. Chymische Anmerckungen. 1677.

—[The same.] ... Ed. 2. ... Franckfurt, In Verlegung Christian Hermsdorffs, 1662.

[60], 169 (i.e. 769), [23] p.   15 cm.   [10049]

Added engraved title page.

—Nymphographia; das ist, Kurtze und gründliche Beschreibung, dess heylsamen Wildbads der hochlöblichen Reichs Statt Nürnberg ... [n. p., 1632]

[40] p.   19 cm.   [10050]

—Opuscula chymico-magico-medica ... [n. p.] 1635.

[8], 1-240, [21], 242-456 + p.   13 cm. [10051]

Imperfect: all pages before p. 237, and all pages after p. 456 wanting; p. 237-240 misbound after p. 456.
Title, imprint and collation partially supplied from Ferguson (A).
"Medicamenta militaria dogmatica, hermetica et magica; das ist, Ausserlesene und experimentirte Kriegs Artzney ... 1634" (p. [1-21], 242-338); "De gravidarum, parientium et puerperarum affectibus & morbis ..." (p. [339]-428) have special title pages. "... Phalaia tripartita ... Sampt beygefügtem Bericht, was Phalaia ... seye. Item, wie man ... alle Unfruchtbarkeit und impotentiam curiren solle ..." (p. [429]-456) has half title.

RUMPEL, GEORG FRIEDRICH [*b.* 1662] *respondent.* See WEDEL, G. W., *praeses.* Dissertatio inauguralis medica de purpura puerperarum. 1690.

—*See* WEDEL, G. W. Propempticon inaugurale de morbo et herba solstitiali. 1690.

RUMPEL, JOHANN HEINRICH [*fl.* 1672] *praeses.* Dissertationem meteorologico-physicam de terrae motu ... censurae publice sistent Joh. Heinricus

Rumpelius ... & Nicolaus Daniel Früe-auff ... Lipsiae, Typis Johannis Erici Hahnii [1672]

[12] p.   19 cm.   [10052]

Diss.—Leipzig (N. D. Früeauff, *respondent*).

RUMPEL, JOHANN WILHELM [*b.* 1665] *respondent.* See WEDEL, G. W., *praeses.* Dissertatio inauguralis medica, de arthritide. 1695.

—*See* WEDEL, G. W. Propemticon inaugurale de febri magna. 1695.

RUMPEL, PHILIPP JAKOB [*fl.* 1695] *respondent.* Dissertatio medica inauguralis, de tabe scorbutica ... Trajecti ad Rhenum, Ex officina Francisci Halma, 1695

15 p.   25 cm.   [10053]

Diss.—Utrecht.

RUMPEL, VALENTIN [*fl.* 1600] Einfeltiger Bericht, von der gefehrlich grassenden Seuche der Pestilentz, was diselbe sey, was dero unterschiden Ursachen, Art und Eigenschafft, Vorboten, Kennzeichen, und Prognosticken seyn: mit Unterricht und Verordnung der praeservativ und curativ Mittel ... [Coburgh, Justus Hauck] 1611.

[79] p.   19 cm.   [10054]

RUMPFF, CHRISTIAAN CONSTANTIJN [1633-1706] *ed. See* SCHMITZ, J. A. Medicinae practicae compendium. 1666, 1688, 1691.

RUMSEY, WALTER [1584-1660] Organon salutis. An instrument to cleanse the stomach, as also divers new experiments of the virtue of tobacco and coffee: how much they conduce to preserve humane health. By W[alter] R[umsey] ... London, Printed by R. Hodgkinsonne, for D. Pakeman, 1657.

[24], 56 p.   15 cm.   [10055]

Includes letters from *Sir* Henry Blount and James Howell.

—[The same.] ... The 2d ed., with new additions ... London, D. Pakeman, 1659.

[24], 68 p.   14 cm.   [10056]

—[The same.] ... Instrument to cleanse the stomack ... The 3d ed., with new additions ... London, S. Speed, 1664.

[24], 68 p.   15 cm.   [10057]

Imperfect: upper margins of p. [19-21] trimmed.
A reissue of the 1659 edition with new title page.

RUMSEY, WILLIAM. *See* RUMSEY, Walter [1584-1660]

RUND, Martin [*fl.* 1681] *respondent.* Disputationem inauguralem, de lue jam temporis multas civitates atque regiones de populante, videlicet peste ... publicae ... censurae submittit Martinus Rund ... Erfordiae, Typis Johannis Georgii Hertzii [1681]

[15] p. 19 cm. **[10058]**

Diss.—Erfurt.

RUOFF, Christoph Abraham [*fl.* 1695] *respondent.* See Zeller, J. G., *praeses.* Dissertationem medicam posteriorem de morbis ex strictura glandularum p. n. natis ... exhibit C. A. R. 1695.

RUOFF, Christophor [*fl.* 1623–1626] *respondent.* See Sebisch, M. [1578–1674?] *praeses.* Exercitationes medicae. 1639.

RUOFF, Jakob. See Rüff, Jakob [1500–1558]

RUPERT, Christoph Adam [1612–1647] See Reinesius, T. Ad viros clariss. D. Casp. Hoffmannum. Christ. Ad. Rupertum ... epistolae. 1660.

RUPERTI, Christopher Heinrich [*fl.* 1672–1675] *praeses.* Dissertatio medica de syncope ... Erfurti, Literis Hertzianis [1675]

[16] p. 19 cm. **[10059]**

Diss.—Erfurt (J. P. Eysel, *respondent*)

—*respondent.* See Rolfinck, W., *praeses.* Disputatio medica inauguralis de hydrope ascite. 1672.

RUPERTI, Johann Valentin [*fl.* 1697] *respondent.* Dissertatio inauguralis medica de febre intermittente tertiana convulsiva exanthematica ... Groningae, Typis Joh. Lens, 1697.

[14] p. 20 cm. **[10060]**

Diss.—Groningen.

RUPESCISSA, Joannes de. See Joannes de Rupescissa [*fl.* 1328–1365]

RUPITZ, Heinrich [*fl.* 1628–1629] *respondent.* See Mochinger, G., *praeses.* Sesqui-decas thematum medicorum miscellaneorum ... subjicit. 1629.

RUPITZ, Valentin [*fl.* 1623] *respondent.* De praefocatione hysterica ... Lipsiae, Ex Officina Bavarica [1623]

[28] p. 19 cm. **[10061]**

Diss.—Leipzig.

RUPITZ, Valentin Kaspar [1630–1697] *respondent.* Disputationem medicam inauguralem de asthmate ... examini sistit Valentinus Casparus Rupitz ...

Lugduni Batavorum, Apud viduam & haeredes Joannis Elsevirii, 1670.

[72] p. 23 cm. **[10062]**

"Carmina votiva in honorem ... Valentini Caspari Rupitii" (p. [63–72]) has special title page.

Diss.—Leyden.

RUROCK, Johann Christian [*fl.* 1679] *praeses.* Disputatio medica de haemorrhoidibus ... Regiomonti, Typis Friderici Reusneri haeredum [*ca.* 1680]

[20] p. 20 cm. **[10063]**

Diss.—Königsberg (M. Mönch, *respondent*)

RUSCELLI, Girolamo [*d.* 1566] See Alessio Piemontese, *pseud.*?

RUSCHI, Giovani Battista [*fl.* 17th cent.] De visus organo libri quatuor. Affixa est De oculi dignitate palaestra. Pisis, Francisci Tanaglii, 1631.

[6], 104 p. illus. 23 cm. **[10064]**

RUSSEL, Richard, *chymist.* See Russell, Richard [*fl.* 17th cent.]

RUSSELL, Richard [*fl.* 17th cent.] See Headrich, J. Arcana philosophica; or, Chymical secrets. 1697.

RUSSELL, William [1634–1696] A physical treatise ... consisting of three parts. The first, a manuduction, discovering the true foundation of the art of medicine. The second, an explanation of the general natures of diseases. The third, a proof of the former positions by practice ... London, John Williams, 1684.

[14], 179, [13] p. 17 cm. **[10065]**

—See Headrich, J. Arcana philosophica; or, Chymical secrets. 1697.

RUSTICUS, Christophorus [*fl.* 1650] Excolenda rusticitas per octo gradus philosophicae, ac medicae disciplinae ... Senis, Apud Bonettos, 1650.

[8], 175 p. illus. 23 cm. **[10066]**

RUSTINGH, Salomon van [*fl.* 1693–1705] Chirurgyns leger-kist, voorsten met in-en uytwendige medicamenten ... Amsterdam, Jan ten Hoorn, 1693.

15 p. 16 cm. **[10067]**

Bound with (as issued) *his* Nieuwe veld-medicine en chirurgie. 1693.

—Nieuwe veld-medicine en chirurgie, gegront op reden en ervarentheyt: verhandelende de genesing der ordinare leger-siekten, geschote wonden, beenbreuken, extirpatien, geswellen, en ulceratien ... Amsterdam, Jan ten Hoorn, 1693.

[12], 232. 16 cm.   [**10068**]

Added engraved title page.

With this is bound (as issued) *his* Chirurgyns leger-kist. 1693.

RUTGERSZ. VAN NIEUSTADT, PIETER. *See* NIEUSTADT, Pieter Rutgersz. van.

RUTTÖRFFER, JOHANN JEREMIAS [*fl.* 1665–1666] *respondent. See* FRIDERICI, J. A., *praeses.* Dissertatio medica de incubo. 1665; SCHENCK, J. T., *praeses.* Dissertatio medica inauguralis de phrenitide. 1666.

RUYCH, MARCUS [*fl.* 1650–1651] *See* CLAUDER, G. Ad ... Doxt. Marcum Ruych ... De observatione practico-anatomica mirabili. 1661.

RUYNA, CHARLOT. *See* RUINI, Carlo [*d.* 1598]

RUYSCH, FREDERIK [1638–1731] Dilucidatio valvularum in vasis lymphaticis, et lacteis ... Accesserunt guaedam Observationes anatomicae rariores. Hagae-Com., Ex officina Harmani Gael, 1665.

[18], 94 p. plates. 14 cm.   [**10069**]

Imperfect: plates 4, 5, 8 wanting.

With this is bound Tachenius, O. Tractatus de morborum principe. 1678.

—[The same.] ... Lugd. Batav., Apud Jacobum Moukee, 1687.

[8], 88 p. plates. 14 cm.   [**10070**]

Bound with Schuyl, F. Pro veteri medicina. 1670.

—Observationum anatomico-chirurgicarum centuria. Accedit Catalogus rariorum, quae in Museo Ruyschiano asservantur. Adjectis ubique iconibus aeneis naturalem magnitudinem repraesentantibus. Amstelodami, Apud Henricum & viduam Theodori Boom, 1691.

[16], 138, [2] p; 120 p. illus., plates. 24 cm.
[**10071**]

Imperfect: p. 137–138 and [2] p. wanting.

Part [2] has special title page: Museum anatomicum Ruyschianus; sive, Catalogus rariorum, dated 1689.

Imperfect: fig. 38 (opposite p. 51), fig. 53 (op. p. 82), fig. 75 (op. p. 121) wanting.

—Another issue.

[**10072**]

Title page of part [2] dated 1691 has different setting of type. Dedicatory epistle inserted after title page of part [2]

Imperfect: fig. 1 (opposite p. 45), figs. 2, 3, 4 (op. p. 63), fig. 5 (op. p. 76), figs. 6, 7, 8 (op. p. 94), fig. 9 (op. p. 103) wanting. Bound with Malpighi M. Opera posthuma. 1698.

—Responsio ad Godefridi Bidloi libellum, cui nomen vindicarum inscripsit. Amstelaedami, Apud Joannem Wolters, 1697.

47, [1] p.   22 cm.   [**10073**]

—, *ed. See* COMMELIN, J. Horti medici Amstelodamensis. 1697–1701.

—*See* AANMERKINGEN. 1677; BIDLOO, G. Vidiciae quarundam delineationum anatomicarum. 1697; CAMPDOMERCUS, J. J. Epistola anatomica. 1696; De koeckoecx-zangh. 1677; Dortmont, B. van. Nootwendigh bericht. 1677; *See* ETTMÜLLER, M. E. Epistola anatomica. 1699; FRENTZ, G. Epistola anatomica, problematica quinta. 1696; GAUB, J. Epistola problematica. 1696; GÖLICKE, A. O. Epistola anatomica. 1679 (i.e. 1697); GRAETZ, J. H. Epistola anatomica. 1696, 1697; KEERWOLFF, B. Epistola anatomica. 1697; RAU, J. J. Responsio. 1699, 1700; REGISTER DER BOECKJENS. [1677–1678]; STAETKUNDIGE BEDENCKING, over het verschil tusschen den Heer Bonaventura Dortmond. 1677; VERHEYEN, P. Corporis humani anatomia. 1697, 1699; VESLING, J. Syntagma anatomicum. 1666, 1677, 1696; WEDEL, C. Epistola anatomica. 1700; WOLFF, J. C. Epistola anatomica. 1698.

RUYTER, NICOLAAS [*fl.* 1674] *respondent.* Disputatio medica inauguralis de paralysi ... Lugduni Batavorum, Apud viduam & heredes Johannis Elsevirii, 1674.

[17] p.   22 cm.   [**10074**]

Diss.—Leyden.

RUYZ, FRANCISCO. *See* RUIZ, Francisco [*fl.* 1625].

RUYZES DE FONTECHA, JUAN ALONSO Y DE LOS. *See* ALONSO Y DE LOS RUYZES DE FONTECHA, Juan [1560–1620]

RYCKARTS, N. [*b.* 1641] Eygene kleyne beknopte huys apoteeck, voorsien met seer bequame heyl ende deughtsame medicamenten. Met eet Appendix van de principaelste, krachtigste ende soo hedendaegse gebruyckelijkste chimicae en Galinesche medicamenten. Dordrecht, Niclaes de Vries, 1698.

[16], 94, [20] p.; 150, [24] p. 14 cm. [**10075**]

The Appendix has special title page.

RYCKE, Theodor [1640-1690] *praeses.* Disputatio medica inauguralis de nephritide ... Lugduni Batavorum, Apud Abrahamum Elzevier, 1682.

[20] p.   22 cm.   [**10076**]

Diss.—Leyden (T. Aylwin, *respondent*)

—Disputatio medica inauguralis de sanguificatione ... Lugduni Batavorum, Apud Abrahamum Elzevier, 1682.

[16] p.   22 cm.   [**10077**]

Diss.—Leyden (N. van der Kappen, *respondent*)

RYCKEGEM, Aegidius van [*fl.* 1687] *respondent.* Disputatio medica inauguralis, de epilepsia ... Trajecti ad Rhenum, Ex officina Francisci Halma, 1687.

II, [1] p.   22 cm.   [**10078**]

Diss.—Utrecht.

RYCKEWAERT, Theophil [*fl.* 1683] *respondent.* Disputatio medica inauguralis de diabete ... Lugduni Batavorum, Apud Abrahamum Elzevier, 1683.

[16] p.   22 cm.   [**10079**]

Diss.—Leyden.

RYCKEWAERT, Willem [*fl.* 1677] *respondent.* Disputatio medica inauguralis de surditate & gravitate auditus ... Lugduni Batavorum, Apud viduam & heredes Johannis Elsevirii, 1677.

[16+] p.   19 cm.   [**10080**]

Imperfect: all after p. [16] wanting.
Diss.—Leyden.

RYDER, Henry. *See* Ryder, Hugh [*fl.* 1673-1697]

RYDER, Hugh [*fl.* 1673-1697] New practical observations in surgery, containing divers remarkable cases and cures ... London, James Partridge, 1685.

[13], 96 p.   16 cm.   [**10081**]

RYFF, Jakob. *See* Rüff, Jakob [1500-1558]

RYFF, Peter [1552-1629] Gratiosus ... ordo medic. Basileens. Petro Ryff ... promotore rite electo, decrevit ut ... Gregorio Mättigio ... Petro Vietori ... Danieli Sstyrkolsky ... Martino Webelio ... gradus doctoratus medic. conferretur. Quapropter omnes literarum literarumque amatores ... ut huic agonismo inqugurali, qui ad XII. Aprilis horis locoque consuetis instituetur, adesse ... rogamus ... Basileae, Typis Johannis Schroeteri, 1610.

broadside.   36 x 24 cm.   [**10082**]

Bound with Stupanus, J. Discurus medicus. 1609.

RYFF, Walther Hermenius [*d.* 1548] Ein ausserlesen schön Artzney- und Kräuter Buch, von mancherley bewehrten Experimenten und Artzneyen, dadurch dem menschlichen Cörper, in zutragenden Fällen, da man die Medicos nicht haben kan ... mag Rath schaffen ... In drey Bücher abgetheilet, unter welchen das letzte absonderlich von Pestilentz Kräutern handelt. Erstlich durch ... Q. Apollinarem [pseud.] ... zusammen getragen, jetzundt aber von newen ubersehen, und mit lebendiger Abcontrafactur der fürnemsten Kräuter, neben Beschreibung der Krafft, deren daraus gebrandten Wasser, gebessert und vermehret. Erffurdt, Gedruckt und vorlegt, durch Tobiam Fritzschen, 1629.

Three parts in 1 v.   illus.   20 cm.   [**10083**]

Parts 2 and 3 have special title pages. That of part 3 has title: Warhafftige Beschreibung aller ... Pestilentz Kräuter und Wurtzeln deren an der zahl zwantzig unnd durch ... D. Tarquinium Ocyorum, alias Schnellenberg von Dortmund ... wider die abschewliche Seuche der Pestilentz ... befunden sind. Jetzund auff newe übersehen, und ... verbessert ... Erffurdt, Gedruckt und vorlegt, durch Tobiam Fritzschen, 1629.

—[The same.] Kurtzes Hand-Büchlein, und Experiment, vieler Artzneyen durch den gatzen Cörper dess Menschens ... Sampt lebendiger Abcontrafactur etlicher ... Kräutter, und darauss gebrandten und distillierten Wassern, Krafft und Tugend. Durch ... Q. Apollinarem [pseud.], selbs erfahren und bewehret. Jetzund ... gemehret und gebessert. Sampt dem Experimentbüchlein von zwanzig Pestilentz Wurtzlen, dess ... Tarquinii Ocyori [pseud., i.e. Tarquinius Schnellenberg] ... Strassburg, Bey Johann Philipp. Mülben, und Josia Städeln, 1651.

[2], ccxii, [17] ll.   illus.   16 cm.   [**10084**]

—[The same.] ... Strassburg, Verlegt und gedruckt bey Tobias Grädel, 1677.

[2], 212, [17] ll.   illus.   16 cm.   [**10085**]

—Confectbuch unnd Hauss Apoteck, künstlich zu bereyten, einmachen, unnd gebrauchen, wess in ordenlichen Apotecken unnd Hausshaltungen zur Artzney, täglicher Notturfft, unnd auch zum Lust, dienlich und nutz. trewliche Underrichtung ... in acht Theil ... abgetheilet ... Franckfurt am Mäyn, Getruckt bey Johan Saurn, 1610.

284, [9] ll.   illus.   16 cm.   [**10086**]

—Newe aussgerüste deütsche Apoteck, darinnen aller ... Artzneyen, als Kräutter, Gewürtz, Mineralien, etc. Natur und Vermögen, auch was von denselbigen allen und jeden für apoteckische Stuck, und dergleichen vilfaltige Compositiones, und Vermischungen, bereit werden mögen, als Syrup, Latwergen, Confect . . . und wie solche dem Menschen, zu seiner Gesundheit jeder Zeit zu gebrauchen seyen. Item von nutzlichem Gebrauch, und ordenlicher Zubereitung aller Laxativen, oder purgierenden Artzneyen, einfacher und vermischter, sammt einem . . . Regiment, wie man sich in Sterbensläuffen und pestilentzischen Febern, bewahren soll . . . Auff das new . . . ubersehen, verbessert . . . Beneben einer . . . Beschreibung der vier Hauptstücken der Holtz Churen . . . gemehrt . . . Durch Nicolaum Agerium . . . Strassburg, In Verlegung Lazari Zetzners, 1602.

[12], 721, [25] p.; 302, [8] p.   illus.   36 cm.
[10087]

—Urin und Pulss. *In* Brian, T. Der englische Wahrsager aus dem Urin. 1693.

—, *ed. See* ALBERTUS MAGNUS. Von Weibern und Geburten der Kinder. 1601, 1608, 1613, 1629, 1659.

—*See* BODENSTEIN, A. von. Bericht von der Kranckheit Podagra. 1611; COLUMELLA, L. J. M. Agricultur; oder, Ackerbaw. 1612.

RYQUIUS, THEODORUS. *See* RYCKE, Theodor [1640–1690]

S

S . . . , *docteur en medecine. See* SAULNIER.

S., A. D. A., *pseud. See* LETI, Gregorio [1630–1701]

S., D. B. *See* BUSSOTTI, Dionigi, *Bp. of Borgo San Sepolcro* [*d.* 1654]

S., D. J. *See* SCHREYER, Johann [*fl.* 1655–1694]

S., D. J., *tr. See* BLANKAART, S. Gründliche Beschreibung vom Scharbock. 1690, 1693.

S., H. *See* PEST-BESCHRIJVING. 1664.

S., J. *See* SERGEANT, John [1622–1707]

S., J. *See* SHIPTON, James.

S., J. *See* STARSMARE, J.

S., J. C. *See* STRAUSS, Johann Christoph [1645–1718]

S., J. F. H. *See* HARPRECHT, Johann [*b.* 1610?]

S., M. *See* STANHOPE, Michael [*fl.* 1626–1631]

S., N. *See* SPARK, Nathaniel.

S., S. *See* SORBIÈRE, Samuel [1615–1670]

S., S. [*fl.* 1647] *See* DISCOURS sceptique sur le passage du chyle. 1648.

S., S. I. E. D. V. M. W. A. *See* HIPPOLYTUS redivivus. 1644.

S., T. *See* SHERLEY, Thomas [1638–1678]

S., T. [*fl.* 1633] *tr. See* LESSIUS, L. Hygiasticon. 1634 [and] The temperate man. 1678.

S., T. P. G. L. M., *ed. See* ERBEN VON BRANDAU, M. Warhaffte Beschreibung von der Universal-Medicin. 1689.

S., W. *See* STANES, William [*ca.* 1609–1679]

S., W. C. M. *See* COCKBURN, William [1669–1739]

S. M. *See* M., S.

S. P. D. D. *See* PARKER, Samuel, *Bp. of Oxford* [1640–1688]

S. W. A. *See* SHERARD, William [1659–1728]

SAALMAN, JAKOB [*fl.* 1668] *respondent.* Disputatione inaugurali pleuritin . . . eruditorum disquisitioni . . . exponit Jacobus Saalman . . . Argentorati, Literis Johannis Welperi [1668]
26, [2] p.   20 cm.   **[10088]**
Diss.—Strasbourg.

SAAVEDRA, JUAN DE [*fl.* 1599–1622] Parecer que dieron los dotores consultados en la ciudad de Sevilla, en un accidente de corta vista. [Sevilla? 1622?]
22 ll.   21 cm.   **[10089]**
Caption title.

SABUCO, MIGUEL DE. *See* SABUCO U ÁLVAREZ, Miguel [*fl.* 1563–1590]

SABUCO BARRERA, OLIVA DE NANTES. *See* SABUCO DE NANTES BARRERA, Oliva [1562–1622?]

SABUCO DE NANTES BARRERA, OLIVA [1562–1622?] Nueva filosofia de la naturaleza del hombre, no conocida, ni alcançada de los grandes filosofos antiguos ... con las addiçiones de la segunda impression, y (en esta tercera) expurgada. Braga, Por Fructuoso Loueço de Basto, 1622.

[4], 347, [13] ll.   14 cm.   **[10090]**

Attributed also to Oliva's father, Miguel Sabuco y Álvarez.

SABUCO Y ÁLVAREZ, MIGUEL [*fl.* 1563–1590] *See* SABUCO DE NANTES BARRERA, O. Neuva filosofia de la naturaleza del hombre. 1622.

SACCHETTI, GIULIO, *Cardinal* [1587–1663] *See* ROME (CITY) ORDINANCES, LOCAL LAWS, ETC. Bando per causa di contagio. 1656.

SACCHI, POMPEIUS. *See* SACCO, Giuseppe Pompeo [1634–1718]

SACCO, GIUSEPPE POMPEO [1634–1718] Iris febrilis. Foedus inter antiquorum & recentiorum opiniones de febribus promittens ... Genevae, Sumptibus Leonardi Chouët & Socii, 1685.

[30], 304 p.   18 cm.   **[10091]**

With this is bound (as issued?) *his* Nova methodus febres curandi. 1685.

—[The same.] ... Ed. 2. ... Venetiis, Apud Joseph Mariam Ruinetti, 1695.

[14], 127–384 p.   17 cm.   **[10092]**

Signatures: H–Z⁸, Aa⁸.

With this is bound (as issued?) *his* Nova methodus febres curandi. 1695.

—Medicina theorico-practica ad saniorem saeculi mentem centenis, & ultra consultationibus digesta ... Parmae, Ex typographia Galeatii Rosati, sumptibus Joseph de Rossettis, 1686.

[20], 389, [1] p.   port.   28 cm.   **[10093]**

—Another issue, with date changed to 1687.

          [10094]

Imperfect: title vignette excised.

—Nova methodus febres curandi. Fundamentis alchali & acidi superstructa ... Genevae, Sumptibus Leonardi Chouët & socii, 1684.

[6], 146, [8] p.   18 cm.   **[10095]**

—Another issue, with date changed to 1685.

          [10096]

Bound with (as issued?) *his* Iris febrilis. 1685.

—[The same.] ... Ed. 2. ... Venetiis, Apud Joseph Mariam Ruinetti, 1695.

[8], 124 p.   17 cm.   **[10097]**

Bound with (as issued?) *his* Iris febrilis. 1695.

—Novum systema medicum ex unitate doctrinae recentiorum, & antiquorum ... Parmae, Litteris, ac sumptibus Josephi ab Oleo, per Hippolytum, & fratres de Rosatis, 1693.

[24], 395, [1] p.   23 cm.   **[10098]**

SACCUS, JOSEPHUS POMPEIUS. *See* SACCO, Giuseppe Pompeo [1634–1718]

SACHS, ESAIAS [*fl.* 1602–1605] *respondent.* Theses de dolore colico ... Basileae, Typis Jani Excertier, 1605.

[12] p.   20 cm.   **[10099]**

Diss. — Basel.

SACHS, PHILIPP JAKOB. *See* SACHS VON LEWENHAIMB, Philipp Jakob [1627–1672]

SACHS VON LEWENHAIMB, PHILIPP JAKOB [1627–1672] Αμπελουραφια; sive, Vitis viniferae ejusque partium consideratio physico-philologico-historico-medico-chymica, in qua tam de vite in genere, quam in specie de ejus pampinis, flore, lachryma, sarmentis, fructu, vini multivario usu, de spiritu vini, aceto, vini faece, & tartaro, curiosa notata plurima ... Lipsiae, Impensis Viti Jacobi Trescheri, 1661.

[31], 670 p.; 70, [34] p.   illus.   16 cm.

          [10100]

Added engraved title page.

Part [2] has caption title: Ampelographiae appendix.

Catalogus authorum: [34] p.

—Beschrijvinge achtende dat de melk een troost der podagristen is. *In* Blankaart, S. Verhandelinge van het podagra en vliegende jicht. 1684; [German tr.] 1690, 1692.

—Γαμμαρολογια, sive; Gammarorum vulgo cancrorum consideratio physico-philologico-historico-medico-chymica ... Francofurti & Lipsiae, Sumptibus Esaiae Fellgibelii, 1665.

[49], 962, [2] p.   plates.   17 cm.   **[10101]**

Added engraved title page has title: Gammarologia curiosa.
Imperfect: outer and lower margins of plates trimmed.

—Oceanus macro-microcosmicus; seu, Dissertatio epistolica de analogo motu aquarum ex & ad oceanum, sanguinis ex & ad cor. ... Vratislaviae, Sumtibus Esaiae Fellgiebelii, 1664.

152 p.   16 cm.   **[10102]**

Added engraved title page inserted after title page.

—*respondent.* See Hopp, J., *praeses.* Diatribe medica de phthisi. 1648; Walther, J., *praeses.* Συμπόσιον φιλοσοφικόν nutritionis physicae varios missus exhibens. 1647.

—*See* Major, J. D. Dissertatio epistolica de cancris et serpentibus petrefactis. 1664.

SACHSE DE LEWENHEIMB, Philippus. *See* Sachs von Lewenhaimb, Philipp Jakob [1627–1672]

SACRI ROMANI IMPERII ACADEMIA NATURAE CURIOSORUM. *See* Academia Naturae Curiosorum.

SADER, Georg. *See* Forberger, Georg [16th cent.]

SADLER, John [*ca.* 1615–1664] Praxis medicorum; vel, Formula remediorum, per alphabeticum ordinem digesta ... Londini, Apud Ric [sic] Oulton impensis Phil. Stephens & Christ. Meredith, 1637.
    [19], 250, [1] p. 14 cm.   **[10103]**
Errata: p. [1] at end.
STC 21543.
—[English tr.] Enchiridion medicum: an enchiridion of the art of physick, methodically prescribing remedies ... Written in Latine ... translated, rev., corr. and augm. by R[obert] T[urner]. London, Printed by J. C. for R. Moone and Henry Fletcher, 1657.
    [15], 208 p. 15 cm.   **[10104]**
Imperfect: pages 187–188 wanting; supplied in photocopy from the University of Wisconsin library.
—The sicke womans private looking-glasse wherein methodically are handled all uterine affects, or diseases arising from the wombe ... London, Printed by Anne Griffin, for Philemon Stephens and Christopher Meredith, 1636.
    [23], 164, [2] p. 15 cm.   **[10105]**
Added engraved title page.
STC 21544.

SAFFORD, Jedidja [*fl.* 1689] *respondent.* Disputatio medica inauguralis de dysenteria ... Trajecti ad Rhenum, 1689.
    15, [1] p. 22 cm.   **[10106]**
Diss.—Utrecht.

SAGGI d'anatomia. *See* Beddevole, D.

SAGITTARIUS, Caspar [1643–1694] *praeses.* De nudipedalibus veterum ... Jenae, Typis

Gollnerianis, 1675.
    [48] p. 20 cm.   **[10107]**
Diss.—Jena (J. W. Leidenfrost, *respondent*)
—De sale philologemata ... Jenae, Grammate Kempffiano [1650]
    48 p. 19 cm.   **[10108]**

SAGUGERIUS, Franciscus. *See* Saguyer, François [*fl.* 1547–1604]

SAGUYER, François [*fl.* 1547–1604] *See* Fernel, J. Pharmacia. 1605

SAINCT-YON, Antoine de [*fl.* 1670] *respondent.* See Puylon, C. [*fl.* 1660–1696] *praeses.* Quaestio medica ... An conformatio temperiei nota. 1670.

ST. ALBANS, Francis Bacon, *Viscount. Sir* Bacon, Francis, *viscount St. Albans* [1561–1626]

SAINT-AMAND, Jean de [13th cent.] *See* Mesuë [924 *or* 5–1015] Opera. 1602, 1623.

SAINT ANDRÉ, François de [*fl.* 1677–1725] Entretiens sur l'acide et sur l'alkali, où sont examinées les objections de Mr. Boyle contre ces principes. Avec une replique à la lettre de Mr. S[aulnier] docteur en medecine ... touchant la nature de ces deux sels ... Paris, Lambert Roulland, 1677.
    [12], 3–205 p. 16 cm.   **[10109]**
—[The same.] ... 2. ed. rev., corr. & augm. ... Paris, Lambert Roulland, 1680.
    [12], 189 p. 16 cm.   **[10110]**
—Reflexions nouvelles sur les causes des maladies, et de leurs symptomes ... Paris, Laurent d'Houry, 1687.
    [12], 394, [36] p. 17 cm.   **[10111]**
—Another issue, without title vignette. **[10112]**
—Reflexions sur la nature des remedes, leurs effets, et leur maniere d'agir ... Rouen, Paris, Edme Couterot, 1700.
    [16], 378, [38] p. 17 cm.   **[10113]**
Errata: p. [37–38]
Original imprint covered with slip cancel.

SAINT-AUBIN, Jacques de. *See* Santalbinus, Jacobus [*d.* 1597]

ST. BARTHOLOMEW'S HOSPITAL, London. *See* London. Corporation. Court of Common

Council. The order of the hospitalls of K. Henry the viijth. Not before 1690.

SAINT GERMAIN, Charles de [*fl.* 1650-1655] L'Eschole methodique et parfaite des sages-femmes; ou, L'Art de l'accouchement. Divisé en quartre parties ... Paris, Gervais Clousier, 1650.

[45], 352 p.   17 cm.   **[10114]**

Imperfect: upper margins of p. [29-32] trimmed.

—Le medecin royal; ou, Le parfait medecin charitable. Divisé en trois parties. Enseignant par ordre alphabetique les noms, qualitez ... des medicamens simples, le formulaire ou methode d'ordonner, la maniere de faire & preparer en la maison ... les remedes internes & externes ... Paris, Cardin Besongne, 1655.

[60], 535, [1] p.; 93 p.   18 cm.   **[10115]**

Second group of paging has caption title: Traitté des fausses couches.

—[The same.] ... Nouvelle ed. rev. & corr. ... Paris, Cardin Besongne et Augustin Besongne, 1668.

[55], 535 p.   19 cm.   **[10116]**

Without the traitté des fausses couches.
Different setting of type.

—[English tr.] The royal physician; or, The perfect charitable physician divided in three parts. Teaching by order alphabetical, the names, qualities ... of simple medicaments, the form or method to prescribe, the manner to make and prepare at home ... remedies external and internal ... Edinburgh, John Reid, 1689.

[36], 260 p.   14 cm.   **[10117]**

Translated by Alexander Hay.

—, *tr. See* Fernel, J. La methode generale de guerir les fievres. 1655 [and] Les VII. livres de la physiologie. 1655.

SAINT-GERY, Joseph de [1590-1674] Disquisitio physica de finibus corporis et spiritus. Parisiis, E typographia viduae Edmundi Martini, 1673.

[8], 36 p.   22 cm.   **[10118]**

Bound with *his* Disquisitiones physicae de motu cordis et cerebri. 1673.

—Disquisitiones physicae de motu cordis et cerebri. Parisiis, E typographia viduae Edmundi Martini, 1673.

[12], 88 p.; 87 p.   22 cm.   **[10119]**

Each part has half title.

With this is bound *his* Disquisitio physica de finibus corporis et spiritus. 1673.

[SAINT HILAIRE, *sieur de, fl.* 1665-1698] L'anatomie du corps humain, avec ses maladies, et les remedes pour les guerir, selon les auteurs anciens & modernes ... Paris, Jean Couterot, 1680.

2 v. in 1.   18 cm.   **[10120]**

Vol. 2 has title: Les remedes des maladies du corps humain, selon les auteurs anciens & modernes.

—[The same.] ... Nouv. ed. augm. de plusieurs observations de phisique curieuses & recherchées, & de figures anatomiques & chimiques. Avec les maladies externes sujettes à la chirurgie, & un grand nombre de remedes specifiques, & experimentez. Paris, Jean Couterot, Louis Guerin, 1684-85.

2 v.   illus.   19 cm. (vol. 1); 20 cm. (vol. 2.)
                                         [10121]

Vol. [1] has added engraved title page.
Vol. [2] has title: Les remedes des maladies du corps humain.

—[The same.] ... 3. ed. rev. & augm. ... Paris, Barthelemy Girin, 1698.

2 v.   illus.   20 cm.   **[10122]**

Vol. 1 has added engraved title page.

SAINT MARTIN, Michel de [1614-1687] Moiens faciles et éprouvés, dont Monsieur de l'Orme ... s'est servi pour vivre prés de cent ans ... Caen, Marin Yvon, 1682.

[44], 432 p.; 48, [6] p.   16 cm.   **[10123]**

Part [2] has caption title: Portrait en petit de Monsieur de Lorme.

—[The same.] ... 2. ed. Caen, Marin Yvon, 1683.

[64], 298, [20] p.   15 cm.   **[10124]**

Without the Portrait en petit de Monsieur de Lorme.

SAINT-ROMAIN, G. B. de. La science naturelle, dégagée des chicanes de l'école: ouvrage nouveau, enrichi de plusieurs experiences curieuses tirées de la medecine & de la chymie; & de quelques observations utiles à la santé du corps ... Paris, Antoine Cellier, 1679.

[18], 391 p.   15 cm.   **[10125]**

—[Latin edition.] Physica; sive, Scientia naturalis, scholasticis tricis liberata. Opus novum. Curiosis plurimis, ex medicina & chymia depromtis experimentis, nec non observationibus nonnullis ad corporis sanitatem utilibus adornata. Lugd. Batavor, Apud Petrum vander Aa, 1684.

[16], 367, [24] p.   15 cm.   **[10126]**

Added engraved title page.

—*See* ABERCROMBY, D. Methode asseurée. 1690.

ST. THOMAS'S HOSPITAL, LONDON. *See* LONDON. Corporation. Court of Common Council. The order of the hospitalls of K. Henry the viijth. Not before 1690.

SAINT-VINCENT, GRÉGOIRE DE, *Father* [1584–1667] *See* AYNSCOM, F. X. Expositio. 1656.

SAINTE-MARTHE, ABEL DE [1630–1706] *tr. See* SAINTE-MARTHE, S. de. La maniere de nourrir les enfans a la mammelle. 1698.

SAINTE-MARTHE, GAUCHER II DE. *See* SAINTE-MARTHE, Scévole de [1536–1623]

SAINTE-MARTHE, SCÉVOLE DE [1536–1623] La maniere de nourrir les enfans a la mammelle. Traduction d'un poeme latin . . . Par . . . Abel de Sainte-Marthe . . . Paris, Chez Guillaume de Luyne, Claude Barbin, et Laurent d'Houry, [Imprimerie de Jean Cusson] 1698.

 [24], 135, [1] p. 18 cm. **[10127]**
In Latin and French.

—*See* HIPPOCRATES. [Jusjurandum. Greek and Latin.] 1643.

SAL, lumen, & spiritus mundi philosophici. 1657. *See* [HESTEAU, C., *sieur de Nuisement*]

SALA, ANGELO [1576–1637] Opera medico-chymica quae extant omnia. Frustulatim hactenus, diversisque linguis excusa, nunc in unum collecta Latinoque idiomate edita . . . Francofurti, Sumptibus Joannis Beyeri, 1647.

 [8], 856 (i.e. 860), [15] p. illus. 21 cm.
           [10128]
Added engraved title page.
Contents.—Anatome essentiarum vegetabilium.—Hydraeleologia.—Tartarologia.—Saccharologia.—Septem planetarum terrestrium explicatio.—Aphorismi chymiatrici.—Chrysologia.—Descriptio auri potabilis.—Tractatus de antimonio.—Anatomia vitrioli.—Tractatus de natura, & proprietate vitrioli.—Tractatus de peste.—Antidotus preciosa.—Ternarius triplex hemeticorum, bezoardicorum, & laudanorum.—Exegesis chymiatrica.—Myrothecium spagyricum.—Appendix de pulvere rosae vitae.
Edited by Joannes Beyer.

—[The same.] . . . Ed. postrema auct. & emend. . . . Huic ultima editioni accessit tractatus peculiaris . . . de erroribus pseudochymicorum & Galenistarum, multum desideratus, & nunquam nisi

seorsim editus . . . Rothomagi, Sumptibus Joannis Berthelin, 1650.

 [8], 749, [11] p.; 50 p. illus. 25 cm.
           [10129]
Added engraved title page.
 Imperfect: p. 1–2 of part [1] in duplicate. Duplicate of p. 729–730 bound after p. 2. Index of part [2] misbound after p. 2 of part [1]
 Part [2] has special title page: Tractatus duo: de variis tum chymicorum, tum Galenistarum erroribus, in praeparatione medicinali commissis.
 Contents as in the 1647 edition with the addition of Tractatus duo.

—[The same.] Opera omnia medico-chymica . . . hac editione non solum a mendis quamplurimis correcta, sed etiam juxta originalia . . . D. Johannis Schröderi . . . rev. & emend. . . . Francofurti, Apud Hermannum a Sande, typis Johannis Andreae, 1682.

 [14], 927, [25] p. illus. 21 cm. **[10130]**
Added engraved title page.
Contents as in the 1647 edition with the addition of Tractatus duo and Compositio & formula antidoti pretiosi, aliorumque nonnullorum medicamentorum autoris, the latter translated from the Italian by Ludwig Combach.

—Anatomia vitrioli, in duos tractatus divisa: in quibus vera ratio vitrioli in diversas substantias resolvendi accuratissime traditur. Accedit arcanorum complurium ex substantiis istis deductorum . . . sylva . . . Ex Italica in Latinam linguam translatus, studio & opera J. P. C. R. Ed. 3, ab authore recognita. Lugduni Batavorum, Ex officina Godefridi Basson, 1617.

 [8], 107 p. 15 cm.   **[10131]**
Tractatus alter (p. [27]–107) has special title page.

—Descriptio brevis antidoti pretiosi, qua antiquissimae ejus virtutes, usuque multiplex variis in morbis, & humani corporis affectibus, recensentur, nunc primum luci commissa. Marpurgi, Typis Pauli Egenolphi, 1620.

 63 p. 16 cm.   **[10132]**

—Emetologia; ou, Enarration du naturel et usage des vomitoires. En laquelle est demonstré . . . combien est utile et necessaire l'usage des medicamens vomitifs . . . Delphis, Apud Joannem Andreae, 1613.

 [8], 101, [1] p. 16 cm.   **[10133]**
Imperfect: title page mutilated.

—Essentiarum vegetabilium anatome. Darinnen von den fürtrefflichsten Nutzbarkeiten der vegetabilischen Essentzen in der Artzney . . . und von andern nützlichen, zu dieser Matery gehörigen Stücken gelehret unnd gehandelt wird . . . Rostock,

Gedruckt bey Joh. Richels Erben, in Verlegung Johan Hallervords, 1630.

[24], 255 p.   15 cm.   [**10134**]

—Hydrelaeologia, darinnen, wie man allerley Wasser, Oliteten, und brennende Spiritus der vegetabilischen Dingen, durch gewisse chymische Regeln und Manualia, in ihren besten Kräfften distillieren und rectificiren soll ... Rostock, In Verlegung Johann Hallerfords, 1639.

[320] p.   15 cm.   [**10135**]

—Myrothecium, Ex quo omnis generis, praeparantium sc. emeticorum, catharticorum diureticorum hydroticorum ... aliorumque pretiosorum chymicorum, variis humani corporis morbis inservientium medicaminum dosis & utendi modus candide docetur & ... demonstratur [&] Pulvis rosae vitae, sive excellentissimarum prolixa, virtutum pulveris purgantis, rosa vita dicti, enarratio, modique utendique clara informatio ...

770-918 p.   20 cm.   (*In* Thom, J. D., *ed.* Collectanea chimica curiosa. Francofurti, 1693)
[**10136**]

Caption title.

—Opiologia; ou, Traicté concernant le naturel, proprietés, vraye preparation, & seur usage de l'opium, pour le soulagement de maints malades, qui sont travaillés d'extremes douleurs internes ... La Haye, Hillebrant Jacobssz., 1614.

[22], 69 p.   illus.   16 cm.   [**10137**]

Imperfect: pages 63-69 wanting.

—Processus ... de auro potabili, novo, paucisque adhuc cognito: cui quidam alii ex Basilii Valentini, Josephi Quercetani, Portae, & aliorum scriptis excerpti, cum commentariolis propter affinitatem ut adjungerentur, non in, consultum visum fuit. Argentorati, Sumptibus Johannis-Philippi Sartorii, 1630.

[54] p.   16 cm.   [**10138**]

Bound with Brendel, Z. Chimia in artis formam redacta. 1641.

—Processus de auro potabili [&] Anatomia antimonii [&] Anatomia vitrioli [&] Tractatus de peste [&] Descriptio brevis antidoti pretiosi [&] Ternarius hermeticorum [&] Ternarius bezoardicorum [&] Ternarius laudanorum.

270-626 p.   20 cm.   (*In* Thom, J. D., *ed.* Collectanea chimica curiosa. Francofurti, 1693) [**10139**]

Caption titles.

—Saccharologia, darinnen erstlich von Natur, Qualiteten, nützlichem Gebrauch, und schädlichem Missbrauch des Zuckers: darnach, wie von demselben ein weinmässiger starcker Getranck, Brandwein und Essig, als auch unterschiedliche Art hochnützlicher Medicamenten damit können bereitet werden, beschrieben ... wird ... Rostock, In Verlegung Johann Hallervordts, gedruckt bey Nicolao Keyl, 1637.

[24], 190, [45] p.   16 cm.   [**10140**]

—Spagyrische Schatzkammer, darinnen von unterschiedlichen, alss vorbereitenden ... purgirenden ... und anderer Arth hochbewehrten kräfftigen spagyrischen Medicamenten ... gelehret wird. Hierbey ist auch ein Appendix von Bereitung anderer Gattungen und besonderer gemeiner Artzneyen, die da nebenst den gemeldten Hauptstücken in Vollführung der Curen nothwendig zugebrauchen fürfallen. Rostock, Gedruckt bey Johan Reusnern, in Verlegung Johann Hallervords, 1637.

[16], 223, [21] p.   16 cm.   [**10141**]

—Tartarologia, Das ist: Von der Natur und Eigenschafft des Weinsteins; welcher Gestalt auss demselben underschiedliche hochbewehrte Medicamenten zu bereiten ... Rostock, Gedruckt bey Johan Richels Erben, in Vorlegung Joh. Hallervords, 1632.

[12], 112 (i.e. 114) p.   16 cm.   [**10142**]

Imperfect? Another title page dated 1631 wanting?

—[The same.] ... Rostock, Gedruckt bey Jochim Fuessen s. Wittwen, in Vorlegung Joh. Hallervords, 1636.

[16], 111 p.   16 cm.   [**10143**]

—Ternarius bezoardicorum, & hemetologia; seu, Triumphus vomitoriorum ... e Gallico sermone Latinitate κατα ποδας donati cum Exegesi chymiatrica Andreae Tentzelii ... Erfurti, Impensis Johannis Birckneri, typis haeredum Mechlerianotum, 1618.

[54], 278 p.; [6], 122 p.   illus.   16 cm.   [**10144**]

Part [2] has special title page.

—[The same.] Ternarius ternariorum hemeticorum bezoardicorum laudanorum ... Erfurti, Impensis Johannis Birckneri, 1630.

[16], 684 p.   illus.   16 cm.   [**10145**]

Added engraved title page.

—Traicte de la peste. Concernant en bref les causes & accidents d'icelle, & la description de plusieurs excellents remedes, tant pour se preserver de son infection, que pour guerir les pestiferez . . . Leyden, Godefroy Basson, 1617.

[8], 150, [6] p. 16 cm.   [10146]

—[Latin tr.] Tractatus, de praeservatione et curatione pestis, primum Gallice conscriptus, nunc vero Latine redditus, a Gregorio Horstio . . . Marpurgi, Typis Casparis Chemlini, 1641.

[1], 72 p. 20 cm.   [10147]

—[The same.] *In* Horst, G. [1578-1636] Operum medicorum tomus primus [-tertius] 1660, 1661.

—Tractatus duo; de variis tum chymicorum, tum Galenistarum erroribus, in praeparatione medicinali commissis. Opus Italice primum ab auctore conscriptum, jam vero . . . in Latinam linguam . . . translatum, labore, & conatu, M. A. R. . . . [n. p.] 1608.

[4], 178, [2] p. 16 cm.   [10148]

—[The same.] . . . Francofurti, Apud Joannem Beyerum, 1649.

64, [12] p. 20 cm.   [10149]

"Compositio et formula antidoti pretiosi, aliorumque non nullorum medicamentorum Angeli Salae Vicentini" (p. 5-12) translated from the Italian by Ludwig Combach.

—Von etlichen kräfftigen und hochbewerthen spagyrischen Medicamenten, ein gründliche Erklärung, wie dieselben mit grosser Nutzbarkeit wider vielerley Kranckheiten und Leibs Beschwernissen sollen gebraucht werden. Wandesbeck, Gedruckt durch Hieronymum Rauschern, 1624.

[14], 159, [1] p. 20 cm.   [10150]

—*See* COLSON, L. Philosophia maturata. 1668; LAVATER, H. Defensio medicorum Galenicorum. 1610; TENTZEL, A. Exegesis chymiatrica. 1693.

SALA, GIOVANNI DOMENICO [1579-1644] Ars medica . . . in qua methodus et praecepta omnia medicinae curatricis & conservatricis explicantur . . . Venetiis, Apud Evangelistam Deuchinum, 1620.

[7], 232 p. 20 cm.   [10151]

—[The same.] . . . in hac 2. ed. aucta, correcta . . . Patavii, Apud Franciscum Bolzetta, ex typographia Jo. Baptistae Pasquati, 1641.

[47], 299 p. 24 cm.   [10152]

—[The same.] . . . Patavii, Typis Matthaei Cadorini, M DC LVIX [i.e. 1659?]

[47], 299 p. 24 cm.   [10153]

A reissue of the 1641 edition, title page and preliminary matter reset.

—De alimentis et eorum recta administratione liber . . . in quo primo ex recensu omnium differentiarum alimentorum, tum optima eliguntur tum idonea pro quacumque constitutione, deinde rectae administrationis praecepta traduntur. Patavii, Apud Jo. Bapt. Martinum, 1628.

[8], 152 p.; 48 p. 22 cm.   [10154]

Part [2] has special title page: Sectio altera in qua agitur de recta alimentorum administratione, quae consistit in inventione loci, modi, quantitatis, & temporis tum nutritionis, tum ipsorum alimentorum. Venetiis.

SALADIN, AUGUSTUS [*fl.* 1632-1634] *respondent.* Disputatio inauguralis medica. De passione colica . . . Argentorati, Excudebat Joannes Georgius Simon, 1634.

[16] p. 21 cm.   [10155]

Diss. — Strasbourg.

—*See* SEBISCH, M. [1578-1674?] *praeses.* Exercitationes medicae. 1639 [and] Galeni Ars parva in disputationes triginta resoluta. 1633.

SALADINO FERRO D'ASCOLI. *See* SALADINUS, Asculanus [*fl. ca.* 1430-1448]

SALADINUS, ASCULANUS [*fl. ca.* 1430-1448] *See* MESUË [924 or 5-1015] Opera. 1602, 1623.

SALADO GARCÉS Y RIBERA, FRANCISCO [*fl.* 1644-1654] Varias materias, de diversas facultades, y sciencias: politica contra peste, govierno en lo espiritual, temporal, y medico, essencia, y curacion del contagio del año passado de 1649 . . . Utrera, Juan Malpartida, 1655.

[7], 249, [1] ll. 21 cm.   [10156]

SALAH ED-DIN. *See* SALADINUS, Asculanus [*fl. ca.* 1430-1448]

SALANDI, FERDINANDO [1561-1630] Consilium . . . de melancholia hypocondriaca, de catharro salso, de diminuta purgatione mensium, de vomitu, ac de aliis affectibus praeter naturam, ac de causis, & curationibus eorum in mag. muliere . . . Veronae, Typis Tamianis, 1607.

63 p. 21 cm.   [10157]

—Tractatus de purgatione . . . Veronae, Ex Angeli Tami officina, 1607.

131 p.   21 cm.   **[10158]**

Imperfect: p. [5-6] mutilated.

"Epitome libri primi [-secundi] Galeni de purgantium medicamentorum facultatibus": p. 93-120.

—Trattato . . . sopra la regola del vivere, nelle sei cose chiamate da' medici non naturali . . . Verona, Angelo Tamo, 1607.

[29] p.   20 cm.   **[10159]**

—Copy 2.

With this is bound *his* Trattato . . . sopra li vermi. 1607.

—Trattato . . . sopra li vermi, cause, differenze, pronostico, & curatione . . . Verona, Angelo Tamo, 1607.

31 p.   20 cm.   **[10160]**

Bound with copy 2 of *his* Trattato . . . sopra la regola del vivere. 1607.

SALAT, VICENTE GARCIA. *See* GARCIA SALAT, Vicente [*d.* 1614]

SALAZAR, AMBROSIO DE [*b. ca.* 1575] Thesoro de diversa licion . . . en el qual ay XXII. historias . . . y otras cosas tocantes a la salud del cuerpo humano . . . Tresor de diverses lecons . . . dans laquel il y a XXII. histoires . . . & autres choses touchant la santé du corps humain . . . Paris, Louys Boullanger, 1637.

[14], 270, [8] p.   front. (port.)   17 cm.
                          [10161]

Imperfect: lower margin of title page trimmed.

In Spanish and French.

SALDO, GIOVANNI BATTISTA [*d.* 1652] Pro solemni medicinae artis auspicio . . . Genuae, Apud Petrum Joannem Calenzanum, 1650.

16 p.   19 cm.   **[10162]**

Imperfect: p. 13-16 mutilated.

SALDO, GIOVANNI FRANCESCO [17th cent.] Artis medicae liber primus. In quo ex Hipp. De natura humana, ea quae ad cognitionem subjecti medicinae faciunt accurate tractantur . . . Genuae, Apud Josephum Pavonem, 1628.

[8], 64, [3] p.; [3], 112 p.   24 cm.   **[10163]**

Part [2] has half title: Disputatio philosophica de mistione.

Errata: p. [1] at end of 1st group of paging and p. [3], 2d group of paging.

—De natura aquae vitae libri duo . . . Genuae, Apud Josephum Pavonem, 1620.

[4], 101, [2] p.   20 cm.   **[10164]**

Imperfect: upper corner of p. 67-68 mutilated.

SALER, HIERONYMUS. *See* BRUNSCHWIG, Hieronymus [*ca.* 1450-*ca.* 1512]

SALERNE, LUC ANTOINE DE [*fl.* 1668] *tr. See* GERARDUS, Cremonensis, of Sabbioneta [*fl. ca.* 1255-1259]

SALERNO. SCHOLA MEDICA SALERNITANA. Regimen sanitatis Salernitanum. *See* Regimen sanitatis Salernitanum.

SALIUS DIVERSUS, PETRUS [16th cent.] Commentaria in Hippocratis libros quatuor De morbis luculentissima . . . Quibus non solum difficillima artis medicae capita explicantur, sed Hippocratis quoque obscuriora loca quamplurima ita enarrantur, ut, his delibatis, ad reliqua etiam ejusdem scripta facilis lectori pateat aditus . . . Francoforti, Sumptibus Nicolai Bassaei, typis Melchioris Hartmanni, 1602.

[1], 398, [14] p.   34 cm.   **[10165]**

Includes Latin text of De morbis in the version of Janus Cornarius.

—[The same.] Commentaria luculentissima in Hippocratis . . . De quaesitis universalibus ad medicinam spectantibus, sive, De morbis libros IV. In quibus author quasi manuductionem medicam proponit ad caetera Hippocratis & Galeni scripta tum recte intelligenda, tum rite explicanda . . . Francofordiae, Impensis Joannis Treudelii [Typis Melchioris Hartmanni, sumptibus Nicolai Bassaei] 1612.

[1], 398, [14] p.   33 cm.   **[10166]**

A reissue (with cancel title page and conjugate leaf paged 9-10) of the 1602 edition. The lower part of the final leaf has been cut away to remove the printer's device and date from the original colophon.

Bound with Marziani, P. Magnus Hippocrates. 1626.

—[The same.] Commentaria in Hippocratis libros quatuor De morbis luculentissima . . . Francofurti, Apud Johannem Davidem Zunnerum, 1646.

[2], 398, [14] p.   33 cm.   **[10167]**

A reissue (with cancel title page and conjugate leaf paged 9-10) of the 1602 edition. The verso of the final leaf bears the original colophon: Francofurti, Typis Melchioris Hartmanni, sumptibus Nicolai Bassaei, Anno. M.DCII.

—De febre pestilenti tractatus, et curationes quorundam particularium morborum, quorum tractatio ab ordinariis practicis non habetur. Atque annotationes in artem medicam, De medendis humani corporis malis, a Donato Antonio ab Altomari . . .

conditam ... Ed. 3., praecedentibus multo tersior. Hardevici, Ex officina Societatis Typographicae, 1656.

[8], 523, [29] p. 18 cm.   **[10168]**

—[The same.] Opuscula medica continentia tractatum De febre pestilenti et curationes quorundam particularium morborum, quorum tractatio ab ordinariis practicis non habetur. Necnon annotationes in artem medicam, De medendis humani corporis malis, à Donato Antonio ab Altomari conditam. Editio nova emendatior. Amstelodami, Apud Henricum & viduam Theodori Boom, 1681.

[8], 523, [28] p. 16 cm.   **[10169]**

A reissue of the 1656 edition with new title page and index partly reset.

—In Avicennae librum tertium de morbis particularibus totius corporis, et eorum curatione. Annotationes luculentissimae. Opus posthumum, nunc primum in lucem editum. Patavii, Typis Petri Mariae Frambotti, 1673.

[8], 453, [5] p.   34 cm.   **[10170]**

With this is bound Magati, Caesar. De rara medicatione vulnerum. 1673.

SALLO, Jean Denis de [1626–1669] *ed. See* Le journal des sçavans. 1684.

SALMASIUS DE BURGUNDIA. *See* Saumaise, Claude de [1588–1653]

SALMASIUS, Claudius. *See* Saumaise, Claude de [1588–1653]

SALMON, William [1644–1713] Annotations and observations. *In* A new method of curing the French-pox. 1690.

—Ars chirurgica. A compendium of the theory and practice of chirurgery. In seven books. Containing I. The instruments and operations of the art. II. The removal of defilements. III. The cure of tumors. IV. The cure of wounds. V. The cure of ulcers. VI. The cure of fractures. VII. The cure of dislocations ... To which is added, Pharmacopoeia chirurgica; or, The medical store, Latin and English, which contains an absolute sett of choice preparations or medicaments ... London, Printed for J. Dawks, and sold by S. Sprint and G. Conyers, 1699.

1 v. in 2 ([18], 1352, [18] p.) front. (port.), plates. 18 cm.   **[10171]**

Portrait and title page backed.

Imperfect: upper margins trimmed: p. 939–940 mutilated.

—Doron medicum; or, A supplement to the new London dispensatory. In III. books. Containing a supplement I. to the materia medica. II. to the internal compound medicaments. III. to the external compound medicaments. Compleated with the art of compounding medicines ... London, T. Dawks, T. Bassett, F. Wright, and R. Chiswell, 1683.

[16], 720, [64] p. 18 cm.   **[10172]**

—[The same.] ... The 2d ed. corr. ... London, T. Dawks, T. Bassett, R. Chiswell, M. Wotton, and G. Conyers, 1688.

[14], 776, [56] p. 18 cm.   **[10173]**

—Iatrica; seu, Praxis medendi. The practice of curing, being a medicinal history of above three thousand famous observations in the cure of diseases ... Together with several of the choicest observations of other famous men, taken from Crato, Forestus, Hildanus, Skenkius, Rulandus, Zacutus, Platerus, Riverius, Willis, and several others which are falln into the author's hands in manuscript, all of them digested under their proper heads ... London, Printed for Th. Dawks [and L. Curtis, sold by T. Bassett, J. Wright, and R. Shiswel] 1681.

[8], 64, 37–52, 73–120, 129–762, [14] p. front. (port.) 25 cm.   **[10174]**

Colophon on sig. K2.

—[The same.] ... London, Printed for Th. Dawks, sold by T. Passinger, 1684.

[18], 64, 37–52, 73–120, 129–762, [14] p.   25 cm.
                                            [10175]

A reissue of the 1681 edition with new title page and Index added. Imperfect: title page and p. [3–4] mutilated.

—[The same.] ... To which is newly added, as an appendix, Observations upon the lethargy, carus, frenzy, madness, defects of the internal senses, and hurts of the external senses ... London, Nath. Rolls, 1694.

[18], 64, 37–52, 73–120, 129–762, [14], 763–795, [1] p. 25 cm.   **[10176]**

A reissue of the 1681 edition with new title page, Index, and Appendix added.

—Medicina practica; or, Practical physick. Shewing the method of curing the most usual diseases happening to humane bodies ... To which is added, the philosophick works of Hermes Trismegistus, Kalid Persicus, Geber Arabs, Artefius Longaevus, Nicholas Flammel, Roger Bachon, and George Ripley. All translated out of the best Latin editions, into English ... Together with a singular comment upon the first book of Hermes ... In three books ... London, Printed by W. Bonny, for Tho. Howkins and John Harris, 1692.

[28], 696 p.   plates.   19 cm.   [**10177**]

Books 2 and 3 titled Clavis alchymiae have special title pages. Book 2 has date: 1691.

—Παρατηρήματα; or, Select physical and chyrurgical observations, containing divers remarkable histories of cures, done by several famous physicians. And above seven hundred eminent cures, in the most usual diseases happening to humane bodies, performed by the author hereof ... London, Printed for Thomas Passinger, and John Richardson, and sold by Randal Taylor, and Josias Mitchel, 1687.

[16], 523, [35] p.   front. (port.), plates.   18 cm.   [**10178**]

—Phylaxa medicina: a supplement to the London-dispensatory, and Doron: being, a cabinet of choice medicines collected, and fitted for vulgar use ... The 2d ed. London, Simon Neale, 1688.

[1], 100 p.   18 cm.   [**10179**]

—Seplasium. The compleat English physician; or, The druggist's shop opened. Explicating all the particulars of which medicines at this day are composed and made ... In X. books ... London, Matthew Gilliflower and George Sawbridge, 1693.

[70], 1207 p.   illus.   19 cm.   [**10180**]

—Synopsis medicinae; or, A compendium of astrological, Galenical, & chymical physick. Philosophically deduced from the principles of Hermes and Hippocrates. In three books. The first, laying down signs and rules how the disease may be known. The second, how to judge whether it be curable or not ... The third, shewing the way of curing, according to the precepts of Galen and Paracelsus ... London, Printed by W. Godbid, for Richard Jones, 1671.

[24], 352, [317]-784, [11] p.   illus.   15 cm.   [**10181**]

Books 2 and 3 have special title pages. "Tabulae declinationum, ascensionum rectarum, & logarithmorum logisticorum" (p. [749]-784) has caption title.
Errata: p. [10-11] at end.

—[The same.] ... Synopsis medicinae. A compendium of physick, chirurgery, and anatomy. In

IV. books ... The 2d ed. Enlarged ... London, Printed for Th. Dawks, sold by L. Curtiss, 1681.

[80], 1207, [1] p.   illus., plates.   19 cm.   [**10182**]

Added engraved title page.
Books 2, 3 and 4 have special title pages; book 2 dated 1679; books 3 and 4 dated 1680. Latter has title: Synopsis medicina. Anatomica ... Liber quartus.
Imperfect: plate 1 (book 1) and plate 8 (book 4) mutilated; plates 3 and 7 (book 4) wanting.
Plates bound after books 1 and 4.

—Copy 2.

Imperfect: title page, added engraved title page, plate 13 (book 2) wanting.

—[The same.] ... The 2d ed. Enlarged ... London, Printed for Th. Dawkes, 1685.

[80], 1207, [1] p.   illus., plates.   19 cm.   [**10183**]

Imperfect: leaf [1] at beginning wanting.
A reissue of the 1681 edition, recto and verso of title page reset; plates bound after books 2 and 4.

—Synopsis medicinae; or, A compendium of the theory and practice of physick. In seven books. Containing, I. The elements ... of the art. II. The cure of infants diseases. III. The cure of diseases of the head. IV. The cure of ... brest. V. The cure of ... belly. VI. The cure of diseases universal. VII. The cure of all sorts of fevers ... The 3d ed. ... besides the addition of nearly the whole first book, there are several hundreds of other additions, alterations and amendments, throughout the whole work ... London, J. Dawks, 1695.

[32], 1064 p.   18 cm.   [**10184**]

—[The same.] ... London, Printed by J. D. for S. and J. Sprint and G. Conyers, 1699.

[32], 1064 p.   19 cm.   [**10185**]

Imperfect: p. 347-8, 629-30 and 705-6 mutilated.
A reissue of the 1695 edition with new title page.

—, ed. and tr. See PHARMACOPOEIA LONDINENSIS. 1678, 1682, 1685, 1691, 1696.

—, ed. See BATE, G. Pharmacopoeia Bateana. 1694, 1700; THE LONDON ALMANACK. 1699.

—, tr. See DIEMERBROECK, I. van. The anatomy of human bodies. [1689], 1694; SYDENHAM, T. Practice of physick. 1695.

—See DICTIONAIRE HERMETIQUE. 1695; DOLÄUS, J. Systema medicinale, a compleat system of physick. 1686; [YONGE, J.] Sidrophel vapulans. 1699.

SALMUTH, HEINRICH [1522–1576] *ed. See* PANCIROLI, G. Rerum memorabilium. 1646.

SALMUTH, JOHANN HEINRICH [*fl.* 1699] *respondent. See* WEDEL, E. H., *praeses.* Dissertatio medica de morbis concionatorum. 1699.

SALMUTH, PHILIPP [*d.* 1626] Observationum medicarum centuriae tres posthumae. Cum Hermanni Conringii praefatione de doctrina pathologica. Accedit Rolandi Capelluti libellus De peste a mendis liberatur. Brunsvigae, Sumptibus Gotfridi Mulleri, excudit Andraeas Dunckerus, 1648.
    [16], 160, [8] p.; 16 p.   20 cm.   **[10186]**
    Part [2] has special title page.

SALOM DE AZEVEDO, MOYSES. *See* AZEVEDO, Moyses Salom de [*fl. ca.* 1661]

SALOMO. *See* SOLOMON, *king of Israel.*

SALOMON, NICOLAS. *See* DICTIONAIRE HERMETIQUE. 1695.

SALOMON & Marcolphus Justiniano-Gregoriani. 1678. *See* [REHEBOLD, C.]

SALT-WATER sweetned. 1683. *See* FITZGERALD, R.

SALTZMANN, JOHANN. *See* SALZMANN, Johann [1679–1738]

SALTZMANN, JOHANN PHILIPP [*fl.* 1681] De claudendis aedibus peste infectorum … disputationem solennem eruditorum examini exhibet M. Joh. Philippus Saltzmann … respondente Martino Luthero Fasterling … LL. stud. … Altdorffii, Literis Henrici Meyeri [1681]
    32 p.   19 cm.   **[10187]**
    Diss.—Altdorf (M. L. Fasterling, *respondent*)

SALTZMANN, JOHANN RUDOLPH [1573–1656] Varia observata anatomica hactenus inedita. Edente Theodoro Wynants … Amstelodami, Apud Jacobum Konynenberg, 1669.
    72 p.   14 cm.   **[10188]**
    Added engraved title page.

Dissertations — Strasbourg

—*praeses.* Decas quaestionum physicarum de temperamento … Athenis Alsaticis, Typis Johan. Philip Mülbii, 1647.
    [32] p.   19 cm.   **[10189]**
    G. G. Zillinger, *respondent.*

—Discursus medicus, de peste … Argentorati, Typis Mauritii Caroli, 1637.
    [27] p.   20 cm.   **[10190]**
    J. V. Wille, *respondent.*

—Disputatio medica de calculo renum et vesicae … Argentorati, Typis Johannis Caroli, 1617.
    [24] p.   20 cm.   **[10191]**
    M. Hirschvogel, *respondent.*

—Disputatio medica de dysenteria … Argentorati, Typis Friderici Spoor, 1647.
    [21] p.   18 cm.   **[10192]**
    J. Frey, *respondent.*

—Disputatio medica de fame praeter-naturali et corrupta … Argentorati, Typis Johannis Georgii Simonis, 1632.
    [24] p.   19 cm.   **[10193]**
    Imperfect: title page mutilated.
    L. Eisenheim, *respondent.*

—Disputatio medica de speciali dignotione et curatione morborum totius corporis humani … Argentorati, Typis Johannis Reppii, 1617.
    [43] p.   19 cm.   **[10194]**
    N. P. Scheidt, *respondent.*

—Disputatio medica de urinarum causis in genere, de que earum differentiis … Argentorati, Typis Eberhardi Welperi, 1638.
    [20] p.   19 cm.   **[10195]**
    Imperfect: p. [19–20] mutilated.
    J. W. Hochstatt, *respondent.*

—Dissertatio de mixtione … Argentorati, Typis Johan-Henrici Mittelii, 1654.
    [2], 26 p.   19 cm.   **[10196]**
    Imperfect: title page mutilated; upper margins of p. 1–10 trimmed.
    J. H. Hönig, *respondent.*

—Exercitationum medicinalium ex Fernelio tertia: De abdominis, infimi I. ventris, partibus naturalibus, nutritione et generationi inservientibus organis. Quam ex ejusdem Physiologiae lib. I. cap. VI. & VII. … inclusam … submittit M. Jacobus Bartschius … [Argentorati] Typis Joannis Reppii [1622]
    [32] p.   19 cm.   **[10197]**
    J. Bartsch, *respondent.*

—Exercitationum medicinalium ex Fernelio quinta: De capitis, supremi III. ventris, partibus animalibus, sensui atque motioni inservientibus organis. Quam ex ejusdem Physiologiae lib. I. cap. IX . . . inclusam . . . submittit M. Jacobus Bartschius . . . [Argentorati] Typis Rihelianis [1623]

[16] p. 19 cm.					**[10198]**

J. Bartsch, *respondent.*

— Exercitationum medicinalium ex Fernelio septima: De symptomatis, eorumq. differentiis generalibus et causis. Quam ex ejusdem Pathologiae lib. II. capp. VI. . . . inclusam . . . submittit M. Jacobus Bartschius . . . [Argentorati] Typis Joannis Reppii [1624]

[12] p. 19 cm.					**[10199]**

J. Bartsch, *respondent.*

SALTZMANN, JOHANN RUDOLPH [*fl.* 1637-1670?] *praeses.* Dissertatio solennis de lupo . . . Argentorati, Literis Johannis Welperi, 1669.

35 p. 26 cm.					**[10200]**

Diss. — Strasbourg (A. Rübner, *respondent*)

— [The same.] . . . Argentorati, Literis Welperianis, 1688.

32 p. 26 cm.					**[10201]**

— *respondent. See* SEBISCH, M. [1578-1674?] *praeses.* Examinis vulnerum partium dissimilarium pars I [-IV. & ultima] 1636 [i.e. 1637]

SALTZMANN, LUDWIG [*fl.* 1671] *respondent.* Disputatio inauguralis medica qua abscessum internum insignis magnitudinis (ein innerlich Gewächs) cum hydrope & aliis notatu dignis in muliere Argentorati nuper observatum . . . exhibet Ludovicus Saltzmann . . . Argentorati, Typis Johannis Pastorii [1671]

[28] p. 20 cm.					**[10202]**

Diss. — Strasbourg.

SALTZTHAL, SOLINUS. Discursus . . . de potentissima philosophorum medicina universali. Lapis philosophorum Trismegistus dicta, anno M.DC.LIV. Germanice scriptus, nunc vero in linguam Latinam translatus . . . [&] Brevis descriptio admirandae virtutis et operationis summae medicinae lapis philosophorum dictae . . . [&] Discursus, de philosophico fonte salino . . .

675-714 p., vol. 6. 20 cm. (*In* Zetzner, Lazarus, *ed.* Theatrum chemicum. Argentorati, 1659-61)					**[10203]**

Caption titles.

SALVADOR, HIERONYMUS VINCENTIUS [*fl.* 1624] *ed. See* GALENUS. Αιτιολογικη και παθολογικη; sive, De morborum et symptomatum differentiis, et causis, libri sex. 1624.

SALVADOR BORRÁS, GUILLERMO. *See* INSA, A. J. Officina medicamentorum. 1601 [colophon: 1603], 1698.

SALVATICO, BENEDETTO, *conte di* [1575-1658] Consiliorum et responsorum medicinalium centuriae quatuor. Quibus rari casus proponuntur, pluresque difficultates elucidantur . . . Accessit ejusdem methodus consultandi . . . Patavii, Typis Pauli Frambotti, 1656.

[26], 620, [13] p. 33 cm.					**[10204]**

Errata: p. [13] at end.

— [The same.] . . . Genevae, Sumpt. Joannis Antonii & Samuelis de Tournes., 1662.

[25], 390, [25] p. front. (port.) 36 cm.					**[10205]**

— Copy 2. 33 cm.

With this is bound Major, J. D. Historia anatomes Kiloniensis primae. 1666.

SALVATICO, GIOVANNI BATTISTA. *See* SELVATICO, Giovanni Battista [*d.* 1621]

SALVATOR, HIERONYMUS VINCENTIUS. *See* SALVADOR, Hieronymus Vincentius [*fl.* 1624]

SALVI, TARDUCCIO [*fl.* 1608-1613] Il chirurgo, trattato breve . . . Aggiontovi Il ministro del medico . . . Roma, Stefano Paolini, 1613.

[8], 196 p.; [8], 64 p. illus. 21 cm. **[10206]**

Part [2] has special title page with imprint: Roma, Guglielmo Facciotto, 1608.

— [The same.] . . . Di nuovo ristampato . . . Et un Breve, & utile discorso di chirurgia di Pietro di Piazza . . . Roma, Nella stamperia di Domenico Manelfi, ad istanza di Calisto Ferrante, 1650.

[8], 168 p.; [4], 59 p.; [4], 79 p. illus. 21 cm.					**[10207]**

Imperfect: p. 79 at end mutilated.
Parts [2] and [3] have special title pages.

— [The same.] . . . Roma, Gregorio e Giovanni Andreoli, 1669.

[8], 168 p.; [4], 59 p.; 80 p. illus. 22 cm.					**[10208]**

Different setting of type.
Parts [2] and [3] have special title pages.

—[The same.] ... Bologna, Giuseppe Longhi, 1688.

[10], 168 p.; [4], 16, 21–58 p.; 80 p. illus. 22 cm.   **[10209]**

Added engraved title page.
Parts [2] and [3] have special title pages.
Different setting of type.

SALZBURG, Austria (Diocese) Archbishop. 1668–1686 (Maximilian Gandolf) Instructio practica, de officio parochorum aliorumque curatorum pro tempore pestis expositorum, cum Appendice medica ... Salisburgi, Ex typographeo Jo. Bapt. Mayr, 1680.

[6], 84, 49–92, [5] p. 14 cm.   **[10210]**

Signatures:)(³, A–C¹², D⁶, E¹², F¹⁰, G³.
Imperfect: p. 5–6 mutilated.

SALZMANN, Joannes. See Saltzmann, Johann Rudolph [fl. 1637–1670?]

SALZMANN, Joannes Rudolphus. See Saltzmann, Johann Rudolph [1573–1656]

SALZMANN, Johann [1679–1738] respondent. See Sebisch, M. [1664–1704] praeses. Dissertatio academica de urinatoribus atque arte urinandi. 1700.

SÁMBOKY, János. See Sambucus, Johannes [1531–1584]

SAMBUCUS, Johannes [1531–1584] Veterum aliquot ac recentium medicorum philosophorumque icones; ex bibliotheca Johannis Sambuci; cum ejusdem ad singulas elogiis. Praemisso hac editione, vitae singulorum & scriptorum indiculo; additis sub finem, diversorum de eisdem encomiis. [Leyden] Ex officina Plantiniana Raphelengii, 1603.

[6], 67, [5] ll. front., ports. 35 cm. **[10211]**

Imperfect: four portraits blank.

—[The same.] Veterum aliquot ac recentium medicorum philosophorumque icones; ex bibliotheca Johannis Sambuci; cum ejusdem ad singulas elogiis. Amsterodami, Ex officina Guilielmi Janssonii, 1612.

[1], 67 ll. ports. 32 cm.   **[10212]**

Imperfect: four portraits blank.
Without the biographical sketches.

SAMMARTHANUS, Scaevola. See Sainte-Marthe, Scévole de [1536–1623]

SAMMONICUS, Quintus Serenus. See Serenus Sammonicus, Quintus.

SAN GALLO, Pietro Paolo da [fl. 1679] Experienze intorno alla generazione delle zanzare fatte da Pietro Paolo da Sangallo ... e da lui scritte in una lettera all'illustrissimo sig. Francesco Redi. Firenze, Vincenzo Vangelisti, 1679.

22 p. plate. 25 cm.   **[10213]**

SAN JUAN, Juan Huarte de. See Huarte de San Juan, Juan [1529?–1588]

SAN JUAN Y DOMINGO, Nicolás Francisco [fl. 1663–1686] De morbis endemis Caesar-Augustae ... Caesar-Augustae, Apud haeredes Didaci Dormer, 1686.

[26], 151 p. 21 cm.   **[10214]**

SÁNCHEZ, Dionisio [17th cent.] ed. See Sánchez, F. Opera medica. 1636.

SÁNCHEZ, Francisco [ca. 1550–1623] Opera medica. His juncti sunt Tractatus quidam philosophici non insubtiles. Tolosae Tectosagum, Apud Petrum Bosc., 1636.

[17], 943 p.; 134, [23] p. illus., plates, port. 24 cm.   **[10215]**

Added engraved title page.
"De officio medici; sive, De vita ... Domini Francisci Sanchez, quam ... Raymundus Delassus ... exaravit": p. [10–17]
Part [2] has half title.
Imperfect: title page mutilated.
Edited by Dionisio Sanchez and Guillermo Sanchez.
Based on the works of Aristoteles, Colombo, Galenus, Falloppio, Hippocrates, and Vesalius.

—Tractatus philosophici: Quod nihil scitur. De divinatione per somnum ad Aristotelem. In libr. Aristotelis Physiognomicon commentarius. De longitudine & brevitate vitae. Roterodami, Ex officina Arnoldi Leers, 1149 (i.e. 1649)

[1], 5–420 p. 14 cm.   **[10216]**

SÁNCHEZ, Guillermo [17th cent.] ed. See Sánchez, F. Opera medica. 1636.

SÁNCHEZ, Pedro Jerónimo, de Lazarazo. See Sánchez de Lizarazo, Pedro Jerónimo [d. 1614]

SÁNCHEZ DE LIZARAZO, Pedro Jerónimo [d. 1614] Generalis et admirabilis methodus, ad omnes scientias facilius, et scitius addiscendas, in qua ... Raimundi Lullii Ars brevis, explicatur; & multis exemplis, variisque quaestionibus, circa facultates, quae in scholis docentur, ad praxim (quod nunquam (actum legitur) apertissime reducitur D. D. Petro Hieronymo Sanchez de Liçaraço . . . interprete . . . Turiasonae, Per Carolum à Lavayen, 1619.

[48], 426, [1] p. illus., plates. 20 cm. **[10217]**

Includes the text of Lull's Ars brevis.
Rogent and Duràn 186.

SANCTA CLARA, ABRAHAM. *See* ABRAHAM A SANCTA CLARA, *Father* [1644-1709]

SANCTA CRUZ, ANTONIUS PONZE. *See* PONCE DE SANTA CRUZ, Antonio [*d. ca.* 1650]

SANCTO AMANDO, JOANNES. *See* SAINT-AMAND, Jean de [13th cent.]

SANCTO FINCENTIO, GREGORIUS DE. *See* SAINT-VINCENT, Grégoire de, *Father* [1584-1667]

SANCTORIUS, SANCTORIUS. *See* SANTORIO, Sanorio [1561-1636]

SANCTUS BAROLITANUS, MARIANUS. *See* SANTO, Mariano [*b. ca.* 1490]

SAND, GOTTFRIED [1647-1710] *praeses.* Disputatio academica de areae generibus, alopecia & ophiasi . . . Regiomonti, Praelo Reusneriano [1683]

[16] p. 20 cm. **[10218]**

Diss.—Königsberg (D. Boess, *respondent*)

—Dissertatio academica de incertitudine signorum conceptionis . . . Regiomonti, Typis Friderici Reusneri haeredum [1682]

[44] p. 22 cm. **[10219]**

Diss.—Königsberg (W. von Lenten, *respondent*)

—Fungus cerebri in generoso equitum Prussorum viro anno . . . M DC XCVI inventus & extirpatus . . . Regiomonti, Typis Friderici Reusneri haeredum, 1700.

[4], 36 p. plate. 20 cm. **[10220]**

Diss.—Königsberg (G. A. Stoltz, *respondent*)

SANDAEUS, MAXIMILIANUS. *See* SANDT, Maximilien vander [1578-1656]

SANDEN, HEINRICH VON [1672-1728] *praeses.* Dissertatio medica de molis . . . Regiomonti, Typis Friderici Reusneri haeredum [1697]

[24] p. 23 cm. **[10221]**

Imperfect: sig. C¹⁻⁴ wanting; sig. D¹⁻² repeated; p. [7-10] mutilated.

Diss. - Königsberg (A. F. Lischovini, *respondent*)

—*respondent.* Dissertatio medica inauguralis de ptyalismo . . . Regiomonti, Typis Friderici Reusneri haeredum [1696]

[14] p. 20 cm. **[10222]**

Diss.—Königsberg.

SANDEN, MAXIMILIAN VAN DEN. *See* SANDT, Maximilien vander [1578-1656]

SANDERS, RICHARD. *See* SAUNDERS, Richard [1613-1687?]

SANDERSON, ROBERT, *Bp. of Lincoln* [1587-1663] Physicae scientiae compendium . . . Ed. 2, multo correctior. Oxoniae, Excudebat L. Lichfield, impensis Ri. Davis, 1690.

[4], 124 p. 16 cm. **[10223]**

SANDHOLZER, HIERONYMUS. *See* KALT, A. Discursus medicus de mola ejus causis, signis, generatione et curandi modo. 1611.

SANDIVOGIUS, MICHAEL JAKOB. *See* SENDIVOGIUS, Michael [1566-1636]

SANDT, MAXIMILIEN VANDER [1578-1656] Theologia medica. In qua, principis, tam ecclesiastici, quam politici officia, exemplo medici declarantur, & de morbis a Christo humani generis archiatro sanatis, eorumque remediis disseritur . . . Coloniae Agrippinae, Apud Stephanum Breyelium, 1635.

3 parts in 1 v. 22 cm. **[10224]**

Added engraved title page dated 1637.

SANFFTLEBEN, PETER [*fl.* 1697-1699] *respondent.* *See* HOFFMANN, F. [1660-1742] *praeses.* Dissertatio medico-practica inauguralis sistens historiam febris malignae epidemicae petechizantis hactenus Halae grassantis. 1699.

SANGALLO, PIETRO PAOLO. *See* SAN GALLO, Pietro Paolo da [*fl.* 1679]

SANLORINI, ALESSANDRO [*fl.* 1654] La polvere schernita; overo, Invettiva contr'al tabacco . . . Con l'aggiunta delle postille di Lattanzio Rigogoli dalla Nibbiaia . . . Firenze, Francesco Onofri, 1654.

[72] p. illus. 14 cm. **[10225]**

SANPELLEGRINO, TITO, *tr. See* COLLEGIO DEI MEDICI, Bergamo. La farmacopea o'antidotario dell'eccellentissimo Collegio de' signori medici de Bergomo. 1680.

SANS-MALICE, Martin [1539–1588] *See* Akakia, Martin [1539–1588]

SANSOVINO, Francesco [1521–1586] *tr. See* Bairo, P. Secreti medicinali. 1602, 1629.

SANTA CRUZ, Alfonso de. *See* Ponce de Santa Cruz, Alfonso [*fl. ca.* 1600]

SANTA CRUZ, Antonio Ponce *de. See* Ponce de Santa Cruz, Antonio [*d. ca.* 1650]

SANTALBINUS, Jacobus [*d.* 1597] *tr. See* Hippocrates. [Collected works. Greek and Latin.] Tà εὑρισκόμενα. 1621, 1624, 1657, 1662.

SANTINELLI, Bartolomeo [*b.* 1644] Confusio transfusionis; sive, Confutatio operationis transfundentis sanguinem de individuo ad individuum ... Romae, Apud sucess. Mascardi, sumptibus Josephi Baronii, 1668.

[16], 139, [4] p.   17 cm.   **[10226]**

Errata: p. [4] at end.

—Dissertationum medicarum ... decas ... Romae, Ex typographia Jo. Francisci de Buagnis, 1690.

[8], 123, [7] p.   23 cm.   **[10227]**

Imperfect: p. [3–4] (at beginning), 3–4, 11–12 mutilated.

SANTINI, Giuseppe. Ricettario medicinale ... Nel quale si descrivono i modi di comporre medicine, elettuarii, siroppi ... & altre cose necessarie per l'uso della speciaria. Con un pieno trattato intorno alla cognitione del provedere ... e comporre ogni sorte di medicamento ... Serravalle di Vinetia, Appresso Marco Claseri, Vinetia, Ad instanza di Gio. Battista Ciotti, 1604.

[20], 504 p.   illus.   21 cm.   **[10228]**

Partly based on Ricettario fiorentino.

SANTO, Mariano [*b. ca.* 1490] Compendium in chirurgia. *In* Vigo, G. de. La prattica universale in cirugia. 1605, 1622, 1639, 1647, 1669, 1685.

—*See* Uffenbach, P. Thesaurus chirurgicae. 1610.

SANTORELLI, Antonio [1583–1653] Antepraxis medica. In libros viginti, & unum distributa, in quibus, ea omnia, quae praxim medicinae aggressuris, praenoscere, est necessarium, summa brevitate examinantur ... Neapoli, Apud Lazzarum Scoriggium, 1622.

[24], 533, [3] p.   22 cm.   **[10229]**

—[The same.] ... 2. ed. et duobus libris multisque capitibus ... adaucta. Neapoli, Apud Dominicum Maccaranum, 1633.

[4], 648 (i.e. 656), [24] p.   21 cm.   **[10230]**

—[The same.] ... Prodit, tertia in lucem emendatior. Neapoli, Apud Camillum Cavallum, expensis Caroli de Valle, 1651.

[32], 462, [2] p.   front. (port.)   32 cm.   **[10231]**

—De sanitatis natura lib. XXIV. In quibus explicantur quaecumque ad partem physiologicam vocatam a medicis pertinent, & de sanitate tuenda ... Prodit nunc primum in lucem ... opera Dominici Maccarani. Neapoli [Domenico Maccarani?] 1643.

[4], 556, [14] p.   32 cm.   **[10232]**

—Postpraxis medica; seu, De medicando defuncto, liber unus. In quo, quaecumque prudens, & Christianus medicus debet defuncto praestare, explicantur ... Neapoli, Apud Lazarum Scorigium, 1629.

[14], 159, [1] p.   21 cm.   **[10233]**

SANTORIO, Santorio [1561–1636] Opera omnia ... [Venetiis, Apud Franciscum Brogiollum, 1660]

4 v.   illus., port.   23 cm.   **[10234]**

General half title.

Contents.—v. 1. Commentaria in Artem medicinalem Galeni.—v. 2. Methodi vitandorum errorum omnium, qui in arte medica contingunt libri quindecim.—v. 3. Commentaria in primam fen primi libri Canonis Avicennae.—v. 4. Commentaria in primam sectionem Aphorismorum Hippocratis. De remediorum inventione. De statica medicina. Last item has special title page.

Includes Latin translation by Niccolò Leoniceno of the Galenic and Hippocratic texts and Gerardus Cremonensis' Latin version of Avicenna's Canon.

The Ad Staticomasticem (vol. 4, p. 27–28 at end) is a reply to Ippolito Obizzi's Staticomastix.

—Ars Sanctorii Sanctorii ... de statica medicina, aphorismorum sectionibus septem comprehensa. Accessit Staticomastix, sive ejusdem artis demolitio Hippolyti Obicii ... Lipsiae, Excudebat Gregor. Ritzsch, sumptibus Zachariae Schüreri & Matthiae Götzen [1624]

[407] p.   14 cm.   **[10235]**

Closely trimmed, with some loss of text.

Bound with Grüling, P. Florilegium chymicum. 1631.

—[The same.] . . . Venetiis, Apud Marcum Antonium Bregiollum, 1634.

[II], 71 ll.   14 cm.   [10236]

Without Obizzi's Staticomastix.

—[The same.] . . . Aphorismorum sectionibus octo comprehensa. Lugduni Batavorum, Apud Davidem Lopes de Haro, 1642.

20, 135 p.   illus.   13 cm.   [10237]

—[The same.] De statica medicina . . . Ed. ultima correctior. Hagae-Comitis, Ex typographia Adriani Vlacq., 1657.

20, 135 p.   illus.   13 cm.   [10238]

Different setting of type.

—[The same.] . . . Ed. ult. correctior. Hagae-Comitis, Ex typographia Adriani Vlacq, 1664.

[18], 135 p.   front.   14 cm.   [10239]

Bound with copy 2 of Deusing, A. Fasciculus dissertationum selectarum. 1660.

—[The same.] . . . & Hippolyti Obicii . . . Staticomastix . . . Accessit Tractatus physicus. Ed. ultima correctior. Lipsiae, Apud haered. Schüreri, Götzianorum, & Joh. Fritzschium, 1670.

[406] p.; 424, [4] p.   14 cm.   [10240]

Errata: [4] p. at end.
Part [2] has caption title: Manualis physici prooemium.

—[The same.] . . . Editio postrema prioribus emendatior. Lugduni, Sumptibus Antonii Cellier, 1690.

22, 155, [1] p.   illus.   12 cm.   [10241]

A reprint of the 1642 Leyden edition.
Without Obizzi's Staticomastix and the Tractatus physicus.

—[The same.] . . . Aphorismorum sectionibus septem comprehensa. Bononiae, Typis HH. Antonii Pisarii, 1694.

96 p.   15 cm.   [10242]

—[Dutch tr.] De ontdekte doorwaasseming des menschen lichaams; door een naauwkeurige dertig-jaarige ondervinding ontdekt op de weegschaal . . . De 2. druk. Vermeerdert met Aphorismen; of, Korte spreuken, raakende de genees- en heelkunst, toegepast op ons Nederland . . . Amsterdam, Jacob van Royen en Abraham Vittenbogaart, 1684.

[12], 186, [16] p.   front.   14 cm.   [10243]

Dedication signed by translator: Philippus La Grüe.
The Aphorismen (p. [143]-186) translated by Steven Blankaart has half title.

—[English tr.] Medicina statica: or, Rules of health, in eight sections of aphorisms . . . English'd by J[ohn] D[avies] London, John Starkey, 1676.

[12], 180 p.   front.   15 cm.   [10244]

Includes Santorio's reply (p. 172-180) to the Staticomastix of Ippolito Obizzi.

—[French tr.] Science de la transpiration; ou, Medecine statique, C'est a dire, maniere ingenieuse de se peser pour conserver & rétablir la santé par la connoissance exacte du poids de l'insensible transpiration . . . Traduction de M. Alemand . . . Lyon, Jaques Lyons, 1694.

[22], 156 p.   illus.   16 cm.   [10245]

Includes Santorio's reply (p. 150-156) to the Staticomastix of Ippolito Obizzi.

—Commentaria in Artem medicinalem Galeni . . . Venetiis, Apud Jacobum Antonium Somaschum, 1612.

[8] p., 785 (i.e. 784) columns, [22] p., 418 (i.e. 408) columns.   30 cm.   [10246]

Includes Latin text of the Ars medicinalis, translated by Niccolò Leoniceno.

—[The same.] . . . Lugduni, Ex officina Joannis Pillehotte, sumpt. Joannis Caffin et Francisci Plaignard, 1631.

[8], 878, [24] p.   26 cm.   [10247]

—Commentaria in primam fen primi libri Canonis Avicennae . . . Venetiis, Apud Marcum Antonium Brogiollum, 1646.

[40] p., 1120 (i.e. 1118) columns.   illus.   24 cm.   [10248]

Includes Latin text from the Canon of Avicenna, translated by Gerardus Cremonensis.

—Commentaria in primam sectionem Aphorismorum Hippocratis . . . De remediorum inventione. Venetiis, Apud Marcum Antonium Brogiollum, 1629.

[24] p., 532 columns, [1] p.; 170 columns, [1] p.   23 cm.   [10249]

Includes Latin text of book 1 of the Aphorismi, translated by Niccolò Leoniceno.

—Methodi vitandorum errorum omnium, qui in arte medica cintingunt libri quindecim, quorum principia sunt ab auctoritate medicorum & philosophorum principum desumpta, eaque omnia experimentis, & rationibus analyticis comprobata . . . Venetiis, Apud Franciscum Barilettum, 1603.

[6], 230, [16] ll.   illus.   32 cm.   [10250]

Errata: leaf [16]
Based on the works of Galenus.

—[The same.] . . . Multa in hac nova editione ab ipso auctore addita & emendata . . . Venetiis, Apud Marcum Antonium Brogiollum, 1630.

[64] p.; 972 (i.e. 976) columns. 23 cm.

[10251]

—[The same.] . . . Nunc primum accessit ejusdem authoris De inventione remediorum liber . . . Genevae, Apud Petrum Aubertum, 1630.

[16], 605, [50] p.; 108 p. illus. 23 cm.

[10252]

Imperfect: title page and p. 82-III mutilated.

—Another issue, with date changed to 1631.

[10253]

—*See* BROWN, A. A vindicatory schedule. 1691; GRANDI, J. De laudibus Sanctorii oratio. 1671?; OVERKAMP, H. Alle de medicinale . . . werken. 1694.

SAPORTA, ANTOINE [*d.* 1573] De tumoribus praeter naturam, libri quinque. Ex instructissima bibliotheca Ranchiniana eruti, & publici juris facti, cura, & studio Henrici Gras . . . Accessit Joannis Saportae Tractatus de lue venerea. Lugduni, Sumptibus Petri Ravaud, 1624.

[19], 710 p. 15 cm. [10254]

SAPORTA, JEAN [*d.* 1605] *See* SAPORTA, A. De tumoribus praeter naturam. 1624.

SARACENO, GIOVANNI, *ed.* and *tr. See* GALENUS. Recettario. 1611, 1645, 1666, 1676, 1683, 1686.

SARASIN, JEAN [1610-1676] *respondent. See* SEBISCH, M. [1578-1674?] *praeses.* Disputatio medica de plethora et cacochymia. 1631.

SARNELLI, POMPEO, *Bp. of Bisceglie* [1649-1724] *tr. See* PORTA, G. B. della. Della chirofisonomia. 1677.

SARNICO, CANDIDO DA. *See* BROGNOLI, Candido [1607-1677]

SARRASIN, JANUS. *See* SARASIN, Jean [1610-1676]

SARRATI, ANTONIO [*fl.* 1630] Apologia . . . de gli ordini di medicare nelli lazaretti presentati alla . . . signoria di Venetia dal . . . Sig. Girolamo Thebaldi, stampati per commissione dell'eccellentiss. Collegio . . . Bologna, Clemente Ferroni, 1631.

58, [1] p. 21 cm. [10255]

Concerns controversy with Mondino Mondini.

SARTES, ANTOINE DE [*fl.* 1658] *See* LE GIVRE, P.

Le secret des eaux minerales acides. 1667; [Latin tr. 1682 [and] Traité des eaux minerales de Provins. 1659

SARTORIUS, JOHANN GEORG [*d.* 1696] Admiranda narium haemorrhagia, nuper observata & percurata . . . Altdorffii Noricorum, Typis Henric. Meyeri, 1682.

22 p. 20 cm. [10256]

SARTORIUS, PETRUS [*fl.* 1644] Frantzosen Artzt: das ist, Was die Frantzosen für eine Kranckheit, wo sie herkommen, wie sie fortgeflantzt worden, und endlich sampt ihren mancherley Zufällen auff unterschiedliche Wege zu curiren seye. Auss der bewertesten Authoren und eigener vielfältiger Erfahrung zusammen getragen . . . Erffurth, In Verlegung Christiani von Sahern, druckts Caspar Freyschmied, 1658.

[16], 144, [8] p. 17 cm. [10257]

—[The same.] . . . jetzo auffs neue auffgelegt, mit Fleiss übersehen, und mit nöthigen Anmerckungen erörtert. Leipzig und Franckfurth, In Verlegung Michael Russworms, 1676.

[18], 166, [8] p. 17 cm. [10258]

—[The same.] . . . Leipzig und Franckfurt, In Verlegung Joh. Herbordt Klossen, gedruckt bey Joh. Wilhelm Krügern, 1685.

[18], 166, [8] p. 17 cm. [10259]

Different setting of type.

SASSONIA, ERCOLE [1551-1607] Pantheum medicinae selectum; sive, Medicinae practicae templum, omnibus omnium fere morborum insultibus commune, libris undecim distinctum, omnibusque ad genuinam medicinae praxin necessarii pammechaniis instructum & adornatum . . . Nunc primum in lucem editum ab ejus discipulo Petro Uffenbachio . . . Francofurti, Paltheniana [epistola dedicatoria 1603]

[20], 1063 (i.e. 1051), [30] p. 33 cm. [10260]

Contents. — De affectibus capitis.-De affectibus thoracis.- De affectibus infimi ventris.- De morbis mulieribus.- De pulsibus.- De urinis.- De signis et symptomatibus febrium putridarum.- De febribus.- De lue venerea.- De plica.- De phoenigmis.

—Opera practica. Quibus hac novissima editione praeter alia accesserunt ejusdem auctoris tractatus de morbis mulierum, & de pulsibus, ac urinis. Omnia quam ante cura emendatiore. Patavii, Apud Franciscum Bolzettam, 1639.

5 parts in 1 v. 32 cm. [10261]

Contents. — Praelectionum practicarum pars prima [-tertia]- [2] De febribus.- [3] De lue venerea.- [4] De melancholia.- [5] De sphygmis (De pulsibus) [and] De urinis. Each work has caption title and separate paging except the last two, which are called liber V and liber VI of the Opera.

— Opera practica. Quibus hac octava editione accesserunt quae pagina versa indicantur. Omnia quam ante cura emendatiore. Patavii, Ex typographia Matthaei de Cadorinis, 1658.

     8 parts in 1 v.   34 cm.   [**10262**]

Contents. — [1] Praelectiones practicae in tres partes distinctae.- [2] De febribus.- [3] De melancholia.- [4] De lue venerea.- [5] De pulsibus [and] De urinis.- [6] De plica Polonica.- [7] De putredine.- [8] Disputatio de phoenigmorum. Parts [2], [6], [7] and [8] have special title pages; part [8] dated 1660.

— [The same.] . . . Quibus hac nona editione accesserunt quae pagina versa indicantur . . . Patavii, Ex typographia Jacobi de Cadorinis, 1681.

     [12], 572 p.   34 cm.   [**10263**]

— De febribus tractatus numeris omnibus absolutus . . . Adjectus est capitum index & aquam cordialem componendi ratio, commentario illustrata . . . Venetiis, Apud Alexandrum Polum, & Franciscum Bolzettam, 1620.

     [6], 172 p.   31 cm.   [**10264**]

— De melancholia tractatus perfectissimus & in cap. digestus . . . Cui etiam adjectus est tractatus alius De lue venerea ejusdem authoris . . . Venetiis, Apud Alexandrum Polum, 1620.

     44 p.; 30 p.   31 cm.   [**10265**]

De lue venerea was published in 1597 under title: Luis venereae perfectissimus tractatus.

— De pulsibus libri tres nunc primum in lucem editi . . . Patavii, Apud Franciscum Bolzettam, ex typographia Laurentii Pasquati, 1603.

     [35], 286, [2] ll.   21 cm.   [**10266**]

An unauthorized text was published in the author's Tractatus triplex, edited by Peter Uffenbach, Frankfurt, 1600.
Based on the works of Galenus.

— [The same.] De pulsibus tractatus absolutissimus . . . Priori non solum uberior, sed & tersior, ita ut alius omnino ab ipso videatur. Revisus, emaculatus et indice copioso instructus a Petro Uffenbachio . . . Francofurti, Officina Paltheniana, 1604.

     [8], 164, [6] p.   34 cm.   [**10267**]

With this is bound *his* Prognoseon practicarum libri duo. 1610.

— Prognoseon practicarum libri duo. Novi, reconditi ac a Pantheo ipsius longe alieni, de ratione dignoscendi ac curandi omnes interiores affectus praeter naturam, qui tum singulas corporis humani partes, tum corpus universum divexare consueverunt. A Leandro Vailato . . . singulari attentione & industria cum auctoris authographo collati ac revisi . . . Francofurti, Apud Zachariam Palthenium, 1610.

     [8], 323 p.   34 cm.   [**10268**]

Caption and running titles: Praelectionum pars prima [-secunda] Bound with *his* De pulsibus tractatus. 1604.

— [The same.] . . . Vicentiae, Apud Franciscum Bolzetam, bibliopolam Patavinum, 1620.

     [4], 233, [2] p.   34 cm.   [**10269**]

Colophon: Vicentiae, Ex typographiae [sic] Francisci Grossi, 1619.

SATTLER, CHRISTOPH WILHELM [*b.* 1665] *respondent. See* HOFFMANN, F. [1660-1742] *praeses.* Disputatio inauguralis medica sistens novam febrium intermittentium hypothesin. 1694 [and] Exercitatio physico-medica, de infusi veronicae efficacia praeferenda herbae thee. 1694.

— *See* HOFFMANN, F. [1660-1742] Propempticon inaugurale de febrium novahypothesi. 1694.

SATTLER, WOLFFGANG [*fl.* 1609] *respondent.* Theses de jure et privilegiis medicorum . . . Basileae, Typis Joan. Jacobi Genathii, 1609.

     [20] p.   20 cm.   [**10270**]

Diss. — Basel.

SAUBER, PHILIPP ADAM WOLFFGANG [*fl.* 1693-1695] *respondent. See* WEDEL, G. W., *praeses.* Dissertatio inauguralis medica de fundamentis lethalitatis vulnerum. 1695 [and] Dissertatio medica de nyctalopia. 1693.

SAUERBREI, JOHANN [1644-1721] *praeses.* Diatriben academicam de foeminarum eruditione posteriorem . . . proponit . . . Jacobo Smalcio . . . Lipsiae, Literis Johannis Erici Hahnii [1671]

     [40] p.   19 cm.   [**10271**]

Diss. — Leipzig (J. Schmaltz, *respondent*)

— [The same.] . . . Lipsiae, Revisa & emendatior prodit sumptibus Johannis Erici Hahnii, 1676.

     [48] p.   20 cm.   [**10272**]

—, *respondent. See* THOMASIUS, J. [1622–1684] *praeses.* Diatriben academicam de foeminarum eruditione priorem . . . proponit J. S. 1671, 1676.

SAUERUS, WILHELMUS. *See* SAUR, Wilhelm [*fl.* 1650]

SAULNIER. *See* SAINT ANDRÉ, F. de. Entretiens sur l'acide et sur l'alkali. 1677, 1680.

SAUMAISE, CLAUDE DE [1588–1653] De annis climactericis et antiqua astrologia diatribae. Lugd. Batavor. Ex officina Elzeviriorum, 1648.

[128], 844, [18] p.   illus.   17 cm.   **[10273]**

—De sanguine vetito judicium. *In* Bartholin, T. De sanguine vetito disquisitio medica. 1673.

—Disquisitio de mutuo. Qua probatur non esse alienationem. Auctore S[almasio] D[e] B[urgundia] Lugduni Batavorum, Ex officina Joannis Maire, 1645.

[38], 434, [12] p.   16 cm.   **[10274]**

With this are bound (as issued): Wissenbach, J. J. Confutatio diatribae de mutuo. 1645;- Fabrot, C. A. Epistola . . . de mutuo. 1645.

—Interpretatio Hippocratei aphorismi LXIX. sectione IV. de calculo. Additae sunt epistolae duae Joh. Beverovicii M. D. quibus respondetur. Lugduni Batavorum, Ex officina Joannis Maire, 1640.

[20], 220, [1] p.   16 cm.   **[10275]**

Errata: p. [1] at end.

—[The same, *as subject.*] *See* BEVERWIJCK, J. van. Exercitatio in Hippocratis aphorismum de calculo. 1641.

—Claudii Salmasii Plinianae exercitationes in Caii Julii Solini Polyhistora. Item Caii Julii Solini Polyhistor ex veteribus libris emendatus. Accesserunt huic editioni De homonymis hyles iatricae exercitationes antehac ineditae, nec non De manna & saccharo . . . Trajecti ad Rhenum, Apud Johannem vande Water, Johannem Ribbium, Franciscum Halma, & Guilielmum vande Water, 1689.

2 v.   illus.   41 cm.   **[10276]**

Colophon (vol. 2, part [1]): Ultrajecti, Apud Ernestum Voskuyl, 1688.

Part [2] of vol. 2 has special title page.

"Joannis Baptistae Lantini . . . ad Commentarium de homonymis hyles iatricae prolegomena": vol. 2, part [2], p. [7]–12]

Prefatory epistle by Samuel Pitiscus, the editor.

—*See* FABROT, C. A. Epistola . . . de mutuo. 1645; PLINIUS Secundus, C. Naturalis historiae, tomus primus [-tertius] 1668–1669.

SAUNDERS, RICHARD [1613–1687?] The astrological judgment and practice of physick. Deduced from the position of the heavens at the decumbiture of the sick person: wherein the fundamental grounds thereof are most clearly displayed . . . shewing by an universal method not only the cause, but the cure and end of all manner of diseases . . . London, Printed for L. C. and sold by Thomas Sawbridge, 1677.

[40], 208, 214 p.   illus., plate.   19 cm.   **[10277]**

Imperfect: p. 97–98 mutilated.

—[The same.] . . . The 2d ed., augm. and amend., wherein the receipts which were before in Latine, are rendered into English . . . London, Tho. Sawbridge, 1681.

[40], 208 p.; 214 p.   illus.   20 cm.   **[10278]**

Title page backed.

A reissue of the 1677 edition with new title page.

—Palmistry, the secrets thereof disclosed; or, A . . . new method, whereby to judge of the most general accidents of man's life from the lines of the hand . . . Also many particulars added, discovering the safety and danger of child-bed. With some choice observations of physiognomy; the moles of the body, and other . . . conclusions. The 4th time imprinted; and much inlarged . . . London, Printed by H. Bruges, for G. Sawbridge, 1676.

[34], 299 p.   front., illus.   15 cm.   **[10279]**

The title page is a cancel.

—Physiognomie, and chiromancie, metoposcopie, the symmetrical proportions and signal moles of the body, fully and accurately handled; with their natural-predictive-significations. The subject of dreams; divinative steganographical, and Lullian sciences. Whereunto is added The art of memorie . . . London, Printed by R. White, for Nathaniel Brooke, 1653.

[24], 279 p.; 39, [4] p.   front. (port.), illus.   28 cm.   **[10280]**

"The second part, or second book: wherein is treated of physiognomy, metoposcopy, oneirocracy . . ." (p. [137]–256) has special title page.

"A treatise of the moles" at end is separately paged.

—[The same.] ... The 2d ed. very much enlarged ... London, Printed by H. Brugis, for Nathaniel Brook, 1671.

[27], 160 p.; [1], 155–156, 161–377, [4] p. illus., plate. 27 cm. **[10281]**

Imperfect: p. 287–288 wanting; p. 9–10, 179–180, 213–214, 217–218, 225–226, 275–276 mutilated; lower margins trimmed.

"The second part, or second book, wherein is treated of physiognomy, metoposcopy, oneirocracy ...": p. [155]–281; "A treatise of the moles of the body of man and woman ...": p. [307]–369. Items have special title pages with imprints: London, Printed for Nathaniel Brooks, 1670.

SAUNIER, Jean [*fl.* 1432] *See* Castaigne, G. de, *Father*. Les oeuvres. 1661.

SAUR, Wilhelm [*fl.* 1650] *respondent. See* Sperling, J., *praeses*. Dissertatio physica, de visu. 1650.

SAUTER, Bonifacius. Regiment, Verhütung und Curation, der erschröcklichen Kranckheit der Pestis zu Nutz ... der ... Stett Wasserburg ... verzaichnet ... München, Gedruckt durch Nicolaum Henricum, 1607.

[2], 27 p. 16 cm. **[10282]**

SAUVAGEON, Georges. *See* Sauvageon, Guillaume [*fl.* 1630–1649]

SAUVAGEON, Guillaume [*fl.* 1630–1649] Traicté chymique contenant les preparations, usages, facultez & doses des plus celebres & usitez medicamens chymiques. Rev. & augm. en cette derniere éd. ... Paris, Jean Jost, 1648.

[4], 97, [10] p. 18 cm. **[10283]**

—[The same.] *In* Bauderon, B. Pharmacopee de Bauderon. 1644, 1650, 1655, 1663, 1672, 1681.

—Traité anatomique des valvules. *In* Gelée, T. L'anatomie françoise. 1654, 1668, 1679.

—Traité anatomiques des valvules [&] Des veines lactées. *In* Gelée, T. L'anatomie françoise. 1656, 1658, 1668, 1671.

—, *ed. See* Du Laurens, A. Toutes les oeuvres. 1639, 1646, 1661; Pardoux, B. Bartholomaei Perdulcis ... Ars sanitatis tuendae. 1637 [and] Bartholomaei Perdulcis ... Universa medicina. 1640, 1649.

—, *tr. See* Guibert, P. Medici officiosi opera. 1649.

SAUVALLE [*fl.* 1682] *tr. See* Malpighi, M. Discours anatomiques sur la structure des visceres. 1683, 1687 [and] La structure du ver a soye. 1686.

SAUVALLE, Michael [*fl.* 1687–1706?] *respondent. See* Alliot, F. F. Quaestio medica. 1691.

SAUVIN, François [17th cent.] *tr. See* Riolan, J. [1580–1657] Manuel anatomique et pathologique. 1661, 1672; Wirtz, F. La chirurgie. 1672, 1689.

SAVAGE, John [1673–1747] *ed. See* Connor, B. The history of Poland. 1698.

SAVARIEGO, Juan Ximenez. *See* Jiménez Savariego, Juan [*b.* 1568]

SAVINIEN D'ALQUIÉ, François. *See* Alquié, François Savinien d' [*fl.* 17th cent.]

SAVIOLO, Ottavio [1653–1693] A capite ad cor animo revolvet ... Patavii, Ex typographia Sebastiani Spera, 1690.

[7] p. 23 cm. **[10284]**

—Litterarius hujus saeculi dum se sua per vestigia nonagesimus volvitur annus, Patavini archilycaei ... publica in exedra febrium physiologiam, & pathologiam disserendo, sic priscorum nedum, sed modernorum placita animo revolvam ego ... Patavii, Typis Sebastiani Spera, 1689.

[7] p. 23 cm. **[10285]**

—Lucubrationes physicae, et medicae, duabus comprehensae sectionibus in quarum prima principiorum naturalium genesis meditatur. In secunda ex supposito principiorum systemate cordis eae, quae naturaliter exercentur vires perpenduntur, ac in spetie de vitali fermentatione, generatione, & circulatione sanguinis, nec non de motu cordis disseritur ... Venetiis, Typis Joannis Cagnolini, 1686.

[16], 176 p.; 214, [14] p. 19 cm. **[10286]**

SAVONA, Filippo [*d.* 1636] Decisiones medicinales quo ad diagnosim, et prognosim ... In quinque partes distinctae ... Panormi, Apud Angelum Orlandi, 1624.

[8], 170, [8] p. 29 cm. **[10287]**

SAVOT, Louis [1579–1640] Nova, seu verius nova-antiqua de causis colorum sententia ... Ejusdem, De tetragoni Hippocratici significatione contra chymicos observatio. Parisiis, Ex Officina Plantiniana, apud Hadrianum Perier, 1609.

[4], 23 ll.; 16 p. 18 cm. **[10288]**

Imperfect: [4] ll. (sheet a with title page) misbound at end. 16 p. misbound before 23 ll.

Part [2] has special title page.

SAVOTIUS, Ludovico. *See* Savot, Louis [1579-1640]

SAXONIA, Hercules. *See* Sassonia, Ercole [1551-1607]

SAXONY. Laws, statutes, etc. Des . . . Herrn Johann Ernstens, Hertzogs zu Sachsen . . . Anordnung . . . wegen besorgender ansteckenden Seuchen und Kranckheiten, so wohl auch da Gott dergleichen darüber verhängen solte, in einem und andern zu halten . . . Weimar, Joh. Andreas Müller, 1680.

 48 p. 19 cm.   **[10289]**

"Consilium medicum de peste": p. 25-45.

—Fürstliche sachs. bothaische [sic] medicinische Verordnung wegen hin und wieder sich ereignenden Seuchen . . . Altenburg, Gedruckt bey Gottfried Richtern, 1680.

 16 p. 19 cm.   **[10290]**

Enacted by Friederich, prince of Saxony.

—Nothwendig- und nützlicher Unterricht, wornach sich die in des . . . Herrn Bernhards, Hertzogen zu Sachsen . . . Landen, bestelte Hebammen oder Kind-Frauen, oder deren Stelle vertretende, und sonst männiglich, bey den schwangeren, kreysenden und gebährenden Weibern, vor-in-und nach der Geburth, richten und halten sollen. Nebst einer Anzeige etlicher Sprüche, Psalmen, Seufftzer und Gebethe . . . Meiningen, Gedruckt bey Niclaus Hasserten, 1682.

 72 p. 22 cm.   **[10291]**

SCACCHI, Cesare [16th-17th cent.] *tr. See* Scacchi, D. Sussidio di medicina. 1609.

SCACCHI, Durante [16th cent.] Sussidio di medicina . . . Tradotto dal latino in lingua volgare, dal . . . M. Cesare Scacchi . . . Venetia, Francesco Rampazetto, 1609.

 89, [1] ll. illus. 23 cm. **[10292]**

SCACCHI, Francesco [16th-17th cent.] De salubri potu dissertatio . . . Rome, Apud Alexandrum Zannettum, 1622.

 [10], 235, [12] p. illus. 22 cm. **[10293]**

Engraved title page.

SCACCHO DA TAGLIACOZZO, Filippo [*fl. ca.* 1591] Trattato di mescalzia . . . diviso in quattro libri, ne' quali si cintengono tutte le infermita de' cavalli cosi interiori, come esteriori, & li segni da conoscerle, & le cure con potioni, & untioni & sanguigne per essi cavalli . . . Venetia, Vincenzo Somasco, 1603.

 146, [6] p. illus. 22 cm. **[10294]**

SCACCO, Filippo. *See* Scaccho da Tagliacozzo, Filippo [*fl. ca.* 1591]

SCADIUS, Johannes Valentinus. *See* Schade, Johann Valentin [*fl.* 1673]

SCAFFIGLIONO, Ippolito [17th cent.] *ed. See* Baldi, C. De humanarum propensionum ex temperamento praenotionibus. 1664 [and] De naturali ex unguium inspectione praesagio comment. 1629.

SCALA, Domenico la. *See* La Scala, Domenico [1632-1697]

SCALA philosophorum. *See* [Montanor, G. de]

SCALIGER, Joseph Juste [1540-1609] Loci cujusdam Galeni difficillimi explicatio doctissima, nunc primum in lucem edita, ex museo Joachimi Morsii. Lugduni Batavorum, Excudebat Jacobus Marci, 1619.

 [8] p. 21 cm.   **[10295]**

Editor's presentation copy, signed.

—*See* [Matman, R.] Tres capellae. 1608; Plinius Secundus, C. Naturalis historiae, tomus primus [-tertius] 1668-1669.

SCALIGER, Julius Caesar [1484-1558] Epistola duo lectu dignissima, nunc primum edita, cura ac diligentia Joachimi Morsii. Lugduni Batavorum, Excudebat Jacobus Marci, 1619.

 [16] p. 21 cm.   **[10296]**

—Exotericarum exercitationum liber XV de subtilitate, ad Hieronymum Cardanum . . . Hanoviae, Typis Wechelianis, apud Danielem & Davidem Aubrios, & Clementem Schleichium, 1620.

 [16], 1076, [82] p. illus. 20 cm. **[10297]**

—In librum De insomniis Hippocratis commentarius auctus nunc & recognitus. Amstelaedami, Sumptibus Joannis Ravesteinii, 1659.

 [8], 136 p. 15 cm.   **[10298]**

The imprint date has apparently been altered from 1658.

A reprint of the 1651 Geneva and Lyons edition, edited by Robert Constantin; includes Scaliger's Latin translation of De insomniis.

—Another issue with different title page. Some typographical differences in sheet A. **[10299]**

Bound with Sennert, D. Epitome naturalis scientiae; editio ultima. 1651.

—*See* Aristoteles. Περι ζωων ιστοριας . . . Historia de animalibus. 1619; Theophrastus. De historia plantarum libri decem, Graece & Latine. 1644.

SCANAROLI, Giovanii Battista, *Aph.* [1579-1665] De visitatione carceratorum libri tres. Quibus omnia ad visitationem, patrocinium, & liberationem carceratorum spectantia explanantur . . . Romae, Typis Reverendae Camerae Apostolicae, 1655.

[16], 588, [139] p.; [4], 122, [14] p. illus. 34 cm. **[10300]**

Part [2] has special title page: Appendix ad tres superiores libros; De visitatione carceratorum.

SCARABICIO, Sebastiano [1609-1686] De lapidis concretione in homine . . . Patavii, Apud Petrum Lucianum, 1655.

[12], 90, [17] p. 14 cm. **[10301]**

—De ortu ignis febriferi historia physica medica ad Avicennae ordinem . . . Patavii, Apud Andream Barutium, 1655.

[8], 522, [10] p. 22 cm. **[10302]**

SCARAMUCCI, Giovanni Battista [1650-*ca.* 1710] De motu, et circuitu sanguinis tractatus iatrophisicus . . . adversus disertationem logicoempyricam nuper editam de eodem argumento N[icolo] O[rfeo] P[aoloni] Firmi, Apud Andream de Montibus, 1677.

186 p. 15 cm. **[10303]**

Errata: p. 183-186.

—Theoremata familiaria viros eruditos consulentia de variis physico medicis lucubrationibus juxta leges mecanicas . . . Urbini, Apud Joannem Baptistam Bustum, 1695.

[44], 314, [2] p. illus. 22 cm. **[10304]**

Errata: [2] p.

SCARANO, Lucio [*fl.* 1605] *ed. See* Casaleno, G. A. Disputatio. 1605.

SCARBOROUGH, *Sir* Charles [1615 *or* 16-1694] Syllabus de universis corporis humani musculis. In Browne, J. Myographia nova. 1684, 1687, 1694.

SCARBURGH, *Sir* Charles. *See* Scarborough, *Sir* Charles [1615 *or* 16-1694]

SCARLATTINI, Ottavio [*d.* 1699] L'huomo, e sue parti figurato, e simbolico, anatomico . . .

raccolto, e spiegato con figure, simboli, anatomie . . . opera . . . in due libri distinta . . . Bologna, Giacomo Monti, 1683.

[14], 464 p.; 328 p. front., illus., port. 34 cm. **[10305]**

Liber 2 has half title: Dell' huomo indiviso, e nel suo tutto considerato.

—[Latin tr.] Homo et ejus partes figuratus & symbolicus, anatomicus . . . collectus et explicatus cum figuris, symbolis, anatomiis . . . Tomus primus [-secundus] . . . Nunc primum ex Italico idiomate Latinitati datum a R. D. Matthia Honcamp . . . Augustae Vindelicorum, & Dilingae, Sumptibus Joannis Caspari Bencard, 1695.

2 v. in 1. front., illus. 38 cm. **[10306]**

SCARMIGLIONI, Guido Antonio [*d.* 1620] De coloribus, libri duo, nunc primum in lucem editi. Marpurgi Cattorum, Typis Pauli Egenolphi, 1601.

192, [22] p. 17 cm. **[10307]**

SCARMILIONUS, Vidus Antonius. *See* Scarmiglioni, Guido Antonio [*d.* 1620]

SCARUFFI, Paolo [*fl.* 1611] *See* Reggio Emilia (City) Ordinances, local laws, etc. Bando in occasione di peste. 1611 [and] Bando sopra la peste. 1611.

SCATOLON, Gratian. *See* Croce, Giulio Cesare [1550-1609]

SCATTELONE, Gratiano. *See* Croce, Giulio Cesare [1550-1609]

SCELLIER, Carolus le. *See* Lescellier, Charles.

The **SCEPTICAL** chymist. 1680 [i.e. 1679] *See* Boyle, *Hon.* R.

SCHAACK, Wilhelm van [*fl.* 1686] *respondent.* Disputatio medica inauguralis, de cholorosi . . . Ultrajecti, Ex officina Francisci Halma, 1686.

16, [2] p. 22 cm. **[10308]**

Diss.—Utrecht.

SCHAAP, Michael [*fl.* 1693] *respondent.* Disputatio medica inauguralis de colica . . . Lugduni Batavorum, Apud Abrahamum Elzevier, 1693.

[12] p. 19 cm. **[10309]**

Imperfect: p. [3-6] mutilated.

Diss.—Leyden.

SCHACHER, POLYCARP GOTTLIEB [1674–1737] *praeses.* Hominis loquelam … exponit … Ernst Gottlob Bergmann … Lipsiae, Praelo Goeziano [1696]

[24] p. 19 cm.   **[10310]**

Diss.—Leipzig (E. G. Bergmann, *respondent*)

SCHACHT, HERMANNUS OOSTERDIJK. *See* OOSTERDIJK SCHACHT, Hermannus [1672–1744]

SCHACHT, LUCAS [1634–1689] Oratio funebris … in obitum Francisci de Le Boe Sylvii. *In* Le Boë, F. de. Opera medica. 1679, 1680, 1681, 1693, 1695, 1698.

—, *praeses.* Disputatio medica de chlorosi … Lugduni Batavorum, Apud viduam & haeredes Joannis Elzevirii, 1681.

[24] p. 20 cm.   **[10311]**

Diss.—Leyden (C. Udemans, *respondent*)

—Disputatio medica de rabie hydrophobica … Lugduni Batavorum, Apud viduam & haeredes Joannis Elsevirii, 1676.

[12] p. 22 cm.   **[10312]**

Diss.—Leyden (A. Nuck, *respondent*)

—*respondent.* Disputatio medica inauguralis, mulieris artuum contortione ac rigiditate laborantis historiam & curam describens … Lugduni Batavorum, Apud Petrum Didier, 1661.

[12] p. 19 cm.   **[10313]**

Diss.—Leyden.

—*See* GRAAF, R. de. Tractatus anatomico-medicus de succi pancreatici natura & usu. 1671; MORLEY, C. L. De morbo epidemico. 1680.

SCHACHTLER, ANTON [*fl.* 1682] *respondent. See* FRANCK VON FRANCKENAU, G., *praeses.* Disputatio inauguralis medica, de carbunculo. 1682.

SCHAD, JOHANN DAVID [*fl.* 1696] *respondent.* Disputatio inauguralis medica, tradens historiam et curam pleuritici … Giessae Hassorum, Typis Christophori Hermanni Kargeri [1696]

19 p. 20 cm.   **[10314]**

Diss.—Giessen.

SCHADE, JOHANN VALENTIN [*fl.* 1673] *respondent. See* FRANCK VON FRANCKENAU, G., *praeses.* Disputatio inauguralis medica de sterilitate muliebri. 1673.

SCHÄFFER, AUGUST [*fl.* 17th cent.] Saltz-Proben, dadurch man wissen kan ob ein Saltz gut und wie viel es besser oder geringer, als ein ander Saltz sey … Magdeburg, Zufinden bey Johann Daniel Müllern, 1685.

[18] p. plate. 18 cm.   **[10315]**

SCHÄFFER, CHRISTIAN [*fl.* 1663] *respondent. See* SCHENCK, J. T., *praeses.* Disputatio inauguralis medica de pleuritide. 1663.

SCHAEFFER, JOHANN DANIEL [*fl.* 1700] *See* SCHEFFER, Johann Daniel [*fl.* 1700]

SCHAEVE, HEINRICH [1624–1661] *respondent. See* ROLFINCK, W., *praeses.* Phrenitidem publico … subjicit. 1650.

—*See* WIRTZ, F. Practica der Wundartzney. 1659, 1670, 1675.

SCHAFFER, FRIEDRICH WILHELM [*fl.* 1677] *respondent.* De passione iliaca disputatio medica inauguralis … Altdorffii, Typis Joh. Henrici Schönnerstaed [1677]

20 p. 18 cm.   **[10316]**

Diss.—Altdorf.

SCHAFFER, KARL AUGUST [*fl.* 1698] *respondent.* Disputatio medica inauguralis de dysenteria maligna … Trajecti ad Rhenum, Ex officina Francisci Halma, 1698.

16 p. 22 cm.   **[10317]**

Diss.—Utrecht.

SCHAFFNICHT, JOHANN BENJAMIN [*fl.* 1683] *respondent. See* WALDSCHMIDT, J. J., *praeses.* Exercitatio physica de igne perpetuo. 1683.

SCHAGEN, CORNELIS [*fl.* 1668] *respondent.* Disputatio medica inauguralis de paralysi … Lugduni Batavorum, Apud viduam & haeredes Joannis Elsevirii, 1668.

[10] p. 23 cm.   **[10318]**

Diss.—Leyden.

SCHAGEN, CORNELIS VAN [*fl.* 1687] *respondent.* Exercitatio medica inauguralis de haemoptoe … Trajecti ad Rhenum, Ex officina Francisci Halma, 1687.

16 p. 22 cm.   **[10319]**

Diss.—Utrecht.

SCHAGEN HOOGHLANT, CORNELIS. *See* HOOGHLANT, Cornelis Schagen [*fl.* 1655]

SCHALKEN, CORNELIUS [*fl.* 1631] *respondent. See* BURGERSDIJCK, F. P., *praeses.* Collegium physicum. 1642.

SCHALLER, Hieronymus [*fl.* 1538] *See* Scholtz, L. Epistolarum philosophicarum: medicinalium, ac chymicarum ... volumen. 1610.

SCHALLER, Isaac. *See* Scholtz, L. Consiliorum medicinalium ... liber singularis. 1610.

SCHALLER, Jakob [1604-1676] Dissertatio moralis de sobrietate ... Argentorati, Typis Josiae Staedelii, 1656.

    [12] p.   20 cm.   [**10320**]
Diss.—Strasbourg (J. P. Süess, *respondent*)

SCHALLER, Johannes [*fl.* 1610] *respondent. See* Bauhin, K., *praeses.* Assertiones medicae de catarrho. 1610; Stupanus, J. N. Gratiosi medicorum Basiliens. collegii decreto. 1610.

SCHALLER, Wolfgang [*fl.* 1608-1625] *praeses.* Centuria positionum medicarum de passione colica ... [Wittenbergae] Typis Christiani Tham [1622]

    [28] p.   19 cm.   [**10321**]
Diss.—Wittenberg (M. Friderici and F. Gerstmann, *respondents*)

—Disputatio medica qua hypotyposis universae medendi methodi breviter proponitur ... Wittebergae, Ex officina Christiani Tham, 1625.

    [38] p.   19 cm.   [**10322**]
Diss.—Wittenberg (J. Janus, *respondent*)

—Positionum medicarum semicenturia de syncope ... Wittebergae, Typis Johannis Gormanni, 1618.

    [20] p.   18 cm.   [**10323**]
Diss.—Wittenberg (M. Eccius and M. Crusius, *respondents*)

—Sesquicenturia positionum medicarum de arthritide ... Wittebergae, Excusa typis Johannis Gormanni, 1625.

    [42] p.   19 cm.   [**10324**]
Diss.—Wittenberg (G. Bayer, D. Gesner, J. Janus, M. Mayer, *respondents*)

—*respondent. See* Horst, G. [1578-1636] *praeses.* Problematum medicorum θεραπευτικων decades priores quinque. 1608; Sennert, D., *praeses.* Positiones medicae de vertigine. 1610.

SCHALLING, Jacob [*fl.* 1615] Ὀφθαλμια; sive, Disquisitio Hermetico-Galenica de natura oculorum eorumque visibilibus characteribus morbis & remediis. Censurae ... ordinis ... Rosatae Crucis oblata & repraesentata. Augentrost, darinn von Natur, sichtbaren Bildnissen, Kranckheiten und Artzeneyen der Augen Trewlich und fleissig gehandelt

wird ... Erffurdt, In Verlegung Johann Bischoffs, 1615.

    [10], 169 (i.e. 179) p.   illus.   33 cm.   [**10325**]
In Latin and German.

SCHAMBERG, Johann Christian [1667-1706] Ad orationem professionis chymiae inauguralem ... habendam ... invitat Johannes Christianus Schamberg ... [Lipsiae, Literis Joh. Georg, 1699]

    [8] p.   20 cm.   [**10326**]

—Disputationem medicam de respiratione laesa ... proponit Johannes Christianus Schamberg ... respondente Martino Naboth ... Lipsiae, Literis Johannis Georgii [1693]

    [40] p.   plate.   22 cm.   [**10327**]
Diss. pro loco—Leipzig (M. Naboth, *respondent*)

—*praeses.* Disputatio medica inauguralis de paralysi scorbutica ... Lipsiae, Typis Christoph. Fleischeri [1694]

    [20] p.   21 cm.   [**10328**]
Diss.—Leipzig (K. F. Zimmermann, *respondent*)

—Disputatio physica de gustu ex recentiorum philosophorum hypothesi explicato ... Lipsiae, Typis Wittigavianis [1689]

    [20] p.   19 cm.   [**10329**]
Diss.—Leipzig (G. Boenigk, *respondent*)

—Disputationem inauguralem medicam de peripneumonia ... publico ... examini submittit M. Johannes Christianus Lehmann ... Lipsiae, Typis Christoph. Fleischeri [1698]

    [32] p.   22 cm.   [**10330**]
Diss.—Leipzig (J. C. Lehmann, *respondent*)

—*respondent. See* Ammann, P., *praeses.* Dissertatio inauguralis de remediis stomachicis. 1689.

—*See* Friess, M. F. Facultatis Medicae in Academia Lipsiensi h. t. pro-cancellarius Martinus Fridericus Friess ... L. S. 1689.

SCHAMMEL, Johann Martin [*fl.* 1689] Disputationem physicam de aquae marinae salsugine ... proponunt ... Joh. Martinus Schammelius ... & ... Johann Gabriel Poppo ... Lipsiae, Literis Johannis Georgii [1689]

    [19] p.   19 cm.   [**10331**]
Diss.—Leipzig (J. G. Poppo, *respondent*)

SCHAPER, Johann Ernst [1668-1721]

Programs — Rostock

—Decanus Facultatis Medicae . . . Johannes Ernestus Schaperus . . . ad disputationem inauguralem de valvularum vasorum lacteorum, lymphaticorum ac sanguiferorum dilucidatione a . . . Johanne Jacobo Döbelio . . . habendam . . . invitat. Rostochii, Typis Joh. Wepplingii [1694]

[8] p.   19 cm.   [**10332**]

With vita of J. J. Doebel.

—Facultatis Medicae . . . decanus Johannes Ernestus Schaperus . . . ad disputationem inauguralem de viscido, sanitatis offendiculo . . . candidati Dn. Johannis Christophori Gottwalds . . . habendam . . . invitat. Rostochii, Typis Joh. Wepplingii [1695]

[12] p.   19 cm.   [**10333**]

For J. C. Gottwald.

—Programma quo Facultatis Medicae . . . decanus Johannes Ernestus Schaperus . . . ad disputationem inauguralem de morbo arquato a . . . candidato Dn. Jacobo Barthelmaei . . . habendam . . . invitat. Rostochii, Typis Joh. Wepplingii [1694]

[8] p.   19 cm.   [**10334**]

For J. Barthelmaei.

Dissertations — Rostock

—*praeses.* Disputatione inaugurali valvularum vasorum lacteorum lymphaticorum, sanguiferorum dilucidationem . . . submittit Joh. Jacobus Döbelius . . . Rostochii, Typis Joh. Wepplingii [1694]

[28] p.   19 cm.   [**10335**]

J. J. Doebel, *respondent.*

—Dissertatio de digitis manus dextrae in quadam foemina per conquassationem nodositate, spina ventosa & atheromate monstrosis . . . Rostochii, Typis Joh. Wepplingii [1698]

[14], 42, [2] p.   plates.   19 cm.   [**10336**]

K. F. Below, *respondent.*

—Dissertatio inauguralis de viscido, sanitatis offendiculo . . . Rostochii, Typis Joh. Wepplingii [1695]

[24] p.   19 cm.   [**10337**]

J. C. Gottwald, *respondent.*

—Dissertatio medica inauguralis de morbo arquato . . . Rostochii, Typis Joh. Wepplingii [1714] (i.e. 1694)

[20] p.   19 cm.   [**10338**]

J. Barthelmaei, *respondent.*

—Dissertatio solennis medica, de caduco muliebri . . . Rostochii, Typis Joh. Wepplingii [1699]

[2], 38 p.   19 cm.   [**10339**]

K. F. Below, *respondent.*

—Medicinae curiosae specimen quatuor quaestionum enodatione ostensum . . . exponit . . . Ernestus Heinricus Fecht . . . Rostochii, Typis Jacobi Richelii [1698]

[68] p.   19 cm.   [**10340**]

E. H. Fecht, *respondent*

SCHARANDAEUS, Johann Jakob [1630-1682] De ratione conservandae sanitatis liber . . . Amstelaedami, Apud Joannem Blaeu, 1649.

157, [3] p.   15 cm.   [**10341**]

—Modus & ratio visendi aegros. Solodori, Sumptibus Joannis Jacobi Bernardi, per Petrum Josephum Bernardum, 1670.

[6], 289, [2] p.   14 cm.   [**10342**]

SCHARDINEEL, Adolph [*fl.* 1682] *respondent.* Disputatio medica inauguralis de chylificatione . . . Groningae, Apud Dominicum Lens, 1682.

[11] p.   22 cm.   [**10343**]

Diss. — Groningen.

SCHARFF, Benjamin [1651-1702] Antidotus prophylactica; das ist, Sichere Bewahrungs-Mittel wieder itzt einschleichende Gifft-Mischer . . . Erffurth, Bey Johann Georg Starcken, 1698.

[1], 121 p.   16 cm.   [**10344**]

—’Αρκευθολογια; seu, Juniperi descriptio curiosa ad norman . . . Academiae Naturae Curiosorum elaborata et variis medicamentis ac observationibus referta . . . Francofurti & Lipsiae, Sumptibus Caroli Wollffii, 1679.

[1], 380, [12] p.   illus., plates.   17 cm.   [**10345**]

—Kürtzliche doch gründliche Erinnerung von Erkenn- Bewahr- und Heilung der Pest, benebenst einem Anhang von hitzigen Fiebern und der Ruhr, welche denen sämtlichen gräflichen schwartzburgischen Unterthanen alhier, bey itzo höchstgefährlichen Zeiten und immer näher rückenden Seuchen zur Nachricht wohlmeinend vorstellen, und wie man sich darbey verhalten solle, treulich eröffnen wollen . . . Mühlhausen, Johan Hüters Witwe, 1680.

[2], 25 p.   20 cm.   [**10346**]

—[The same.] Gründliche und unvorgreifliche Erinnerung von Erkenn- Bewahr- und Heilung der Pest, welche bey jetzo höchstgefährlichen Zeiten und immer näher rückenden Seuchen jederman zur Nachricht wohlmeinend vorstellen, und wie man sich dabey verhalten solle, treulich eröfnen wollen ... Jena, Gedruckt und verlegt durch Johann Gollnern, 1681.

[4], 127 p.   14 cm.   [10347]

—Τοξιχολογια; seu, Tractatus physico, medico-chymicus de natura venenorum in genere, in quo venenorum vires ac qualitates considerantur ... Jenae, Typis Gollnerianis, 1678.

189 p.   16 cm.   [10348]

—Unvorgreifliche Gedancken von denen bissher heimlich- und unerforschlich-gehaltenen magnetischen Curen nach gründlicher Anleitnng [sic] der Natur wohlmeinend erwogen und dem curieusen Liebhaber der natürlichen Dinge samt andern so wohl hierbey, als sonst bey der Medicin vorgehenden Fehlern, sonderlich von der Inspection des Urins und Besuchung der Krancken unmassgeblich forgetragen ... Sondershausen, In Verlegung des Autoris, druckts Ludwig Heinrich Schönermarck, 1700.

[16], 9–196, [2] p.   17 cm.   [10349]

"... V. Capita, aus des Hrn. D. Primerosii verdeutschtem andern Buch, De erroribus vulgi in medicina": p. 121–196.

—respondent. See FRIDERICI, J. A., praeses. Disputatio medica de conceptione. 1670.

SCHARFF, JOHANN [1595-1660] praeses. Disputatio physica de auditu et olfactu ... Wittebergae, Excusa typis Johannis Gormanni, 1626.

[15] p.   18 cm.   [10350]

Imperfect: title page mutilated.
Diss. — Wittenberg (D. Sennert, respondent)

SCHARFF, JOHANN FRIEDRICH [fl. 1664-1702] Vindiciae pro assertione physica, elementorum formas actu in misto manere; contra disputationem nuper in vicinia habitam ... Argentorati, Typis Joh. Pastorii, 1664.

[12] p.   20 cm.   [10351]

—praeses. Miraculum naturae magnes ... [Wittenbergae] Literis Matthaei Henckelii [1674]

[12] p.   19 cm.   [10352]

Diss. — Wittenberg (J. C. Viebeg, respondent)

SCHARMANN, ANDREAS [1644-1674] respondent. Disputatio medica inauguralis de lochiis ... [Altdorffii] Typis Johannis Leonhardi Winterbergeri [1669]

24 p.   18 cm.   [10353]

Diss. — Altdorf.

SCHARPE, CLAUDE [fl. 1638] ed. See SCHARPE, G. Institutionum medicarum pars prima. 1638.

SCHARPE, GEORGE [d. 1638] Institutionum medicarum pars prima a Claudio authoris filio ... in lucem edita ... Bononiae, Apud Jacobum Montium, 1638.

[8], 149 (i.e. 249), [2] p.   21 cm.   [10354]

Added engraved title page.
Imperfect: title page mutilated.
Contains Liber primus & secundus.

SCHATTENBERG, CONRAD [fl. 1604-1605] respondent. See SENNERT, D., praeses. De methodo medendi disputatio VI, de purgatione. 1604 [and] De methodo medendi disputatio XI, de repellentibus. 1604.

SCHATZKAMMER rarer und neuer Curiositäten. 1689. See [CHAMBERLAYNE, J.] comp.

SCHEEL-HANS. See GERSDORFF, Hans von [d. 1529]

SCHEEMANN, GEORG ADRIAN [fl. 1679] respondent. Disputatio medica inauguralis de podagra ... Lugduni Batavorum, Apud viduam & heredes Johannis Elsevirii, 1679.

[14] p.   21 cm.   [10355]

Without the dedication on the verso of the title page.
Diss. — Leyden.

SCHEER, JOACHIM. See CURÄUS, Joachim [1532-1573]

SCHEER, JOHANNES [fl. 1668] respondent. Disputatio medica inauguralis, de arthritide ... Trajecti ad Rhenum, Ex officina Antonii Smytegelt, 1668.

[7] p.   20 cm.   [10356]

Diss. — Utrecht.

SCHEFERUS, JOHANNES DANIEL. See SCHEFFER, Johann Daniel [fl. 1700]

SCHEFFEL, MARTIN [*fl.* 1684] *respondent.* Disputatio inauguralis medica virginem chlorosi ... Altdorffii, Literis Schönnerstaedtianis [1684]

16 p.   21 cm.   [**10357**]

Diss. — Altdorf.

SCHEFFER, BARTHOLDUS [*fl.* 1642] *respondent. See* SEBISCH, M. [1578–1674?] *praeses.* Disputatio de variolis et morbillis prima [-sexta & ultima] 1642.

SCHEFFER, JOHANN ANDREAS [*fl.* 1657] *respondent. See* BERG, J., *praeses.* Disputatio psychologica. 1657.

SCHEFFER, JOHANN DANIEL [*fl.* 1700] *respondent.* Disputatio medica inauguralis de chamomilla ... Argentorati, Literis Johannis Friderici Spoor [1700]

[2], 30 p.   21 cm.   [**10358**]

Diss. — Strasbourg.

SCHEFFER, JOHANN WILHELM [*fl.* 1690–1691] *respondent. See* DILLENIUS, J. F., *praeses.* Disputatio medica de pulsu. 1690.

SCHEFFER, JOHANNES [1621–1679] *ed. See* OBSEQUENS, J. De prodigiis liber. 1679.

SCHEFFER, JOHANNES GERHARD. *See* SCHEFFER, Johannes [1621–1679]

SCHEFFER, MARTIN [*fl.* 1605–1610] *respondent.* Disputatio medica de hydrophobia ... Basileae, Typis Joan. Jacobi Genathii, 1610.

[16] p.   20 cm.   [**10359**]

Diss. — Basel.

—*See* SENNERT, D., *praeses.* De febribus disputatio III. De febribus putridis in genere. 1605 [and] Quaestiones medicae controversae quinque, pro disputatione quinta propositae. 1607.

—*See* BAUHIN, K. Hygiae et panaceae parente ... Casparus Bauhinus. 1610.

SCHEFFER, SEBASTIAN [1631–1686] *respondent. See* TAPPE, J., *praeses.* Disputatio medica de melancholica desipientia. 1652.

—, *ed. See* GALENUS. Praxis medica curiosa. 1680; HOFMANN, C. Tractatus tres. 1664? [and] Vita medica, hoc est Galeni ὑγιεινῶν. 1680; MARTINI, H. Anatomia urinae Galeno-spagyrica. 1658; MORONE, M. Directorium medico-practicum. 1663.

—*See* CONRING, H. In universam artem medicam singulasque ejus partes introductio. 1687.

SCHEFFER, WILHELM ERNST [1590?–1664] *respondent. See* HOFFMANN, S., *praeses.* Disputatio medica de lumbricorum in humano corpore generatione. 1620.

SCHEFFERUS, JOANNES. *See* SCHEFFER, Johannes [1621–1679]

SCHEFFRICHIUS, JAKOB [*fl.* 1650] *respondent. See* POMARIUS, S., *praeses.* De modo visionis disputatio secunda. 1650.

SCHEIBNER, CHRISTIAN [*fl.* 1693] *respondent. See* KIRCHMAYER, G. K., *praeses.* Ad Plin. Secund. Hist. nat. 1693.

SCHEID, JOHANNES VALENTIN [1651–1731] *praeses.* De duobus ossiculis in cerebro humano mulieris apoplexia extinctae repertis ... Argentorati, Literis Johannis Friderici Spoor [1687]

[2], 26 p.   table.   21 cm.   [**10360**]

Diss. — Strasbourg (M. Mapp, *respondent*)

—Quaestionum de visu dodecas ... Argentorati, Literis Johannis Pastorii [1684]

24 p.   18 cm.   [**10361**]

Diss. — Strasbourg (J. M. Faust, *respondent*)

—Quaestionum decades duae de magnete ... Argentorati, Literis Staedelianis [1683]

[2], 26, [4] p.   20 cm.   [**10362**]

Diss. — Strasbourg (J. J. Kast, *respondent*)

—*respondent.* Visus vitiatus, ejusque demonstratio mathematico-medica ... Argentorati, Typis Josiae Staedelii [1676]

[8], 70, [1] p.   19 cm.   [**10363**]

Diss. — Strasbourg.

—*respondent. See* Mapp, M. Ζητηματων περι φυσωγ δεκας; h. e., De flatibus quaestiones decem. 1675.

SCHEIDER, BALTHASAR [*fl.* 1556–1562] *See* SCHOLTZ, L. Consiliorum medicinalium ... liber singularis. 1610 [and] Epistolarum philosophicarum: medicinalium, ac chymicarum ... volumen. 1610.

SCHEIDLIN, PHILIPP JAKOB [*fl.* 1667–1668] *respondent. See* SCHENCK, J. T., *praeses.* Dissertatio academica. 1667.

SCHEIDT, JEAN VALENTIN. *See* SCHEID, Johannes Valentin [1651–1731]

SCHEIDT, NIKOLAUS PHILIPP [*fl.* 1617] *respondent. See* SALTZMANN, J. R. [1573–1656] *praeses.* Disputatio medica de speciali dignotione et curatione morborum totius corporis humani. 1617.

SCHEINER, CHRISTOPH, *Father* [1575-1650]
Oculus; hoc est, Fundamentum opticum, in quo . . . radius visualis eruitur; sua visioni in oculo sedes decernitur; anguli visorii ingenium aperitur . . . Oeniponti, Apud Danielem Agricolam, 1619.

[14], 254 p.   illus.   20 cm.   **[10364]**

—[The same.] . . . Londini, Excudebat J. Flesher, & prostant apud Cornelium Bee, 1652.

[12], 254 p.   illus.   21 cm.   **[10365]**
Different setting of type.

SCHEINER, PAUL [*fl.* 1652-1653] *praeses.* Dissertatio physica de ignis elemento . . . Lipsiae, Excudebat Quirinus Bauch [1653]

[16] p.   19 cm.   **[10366]**
Diss. — Leipzig (H. Elmenhorst, *respondent*).

SCHELE, JOACHIM [*fl.* 1626-ca. 1650] *ed. See* DORNCRELIUS, T. Medulla totius praxeos medicae aphoristica. 1656.

SCHELHAMMER, CHRISTOPH [1620-1652]
Dissertationum de humani corporis humoribus biga . . . Jenae, Literis Steinmannianis, excudebat Christianus Laurentius Kempff, 1652.

[8], 64 p.   **[10367]**

—*praeses.* Disputatio medica inauguralis de epilepsia . . . Jenae, E Chalcographeo Lobensteiniano, 1644.

[44] p.   18 cm.   **[10368]**
Imperfect: upper and lower margins trimmed.
Diss. — Jena (J. G. Macasius, *respondent*)

—Disputationem medicam de febre ardente . . . publice exponit Christian Buncke . . . Jenae, Typis Sengwaldi & Freyschmidii, 1646.

[44] p.   19 cm.   **[10369]**
Diss. — Jena (C. Buncken, *respondent*)

—Dissertatio medica inauguralis de colicodolore . . . Jenae, Excudebat Casparus Freyschmid, 1651.

[38] p.   20 cm.   **[10370]**
Diss. — Jena (S. H. Cravelius, *respondent*)

—Hydrops tympanites . . . Jenae, E calcographeo Blasii Lobensteins, 1644.

40 p.   19 cm.   **[10371]**
Diss. — Jena (J. Zencker, *respondent*)

—*respondent. See* SCHLEGEL, P. M., *praeses.* Ophthalmographiam et opsioscopiam thesibus succincte comprehensam . . . subjicit . . . C. S. 1640.

SHELHAMMER, Günther Christoph [1649-1716]
Ad . . . Georgium Wolfgangum Wedelium epistola, qua pulsus ratio omnis diligentius expenditur, & ad mechanicae naturalis aeternas leges exigitur, simul Laurentii Bellini . . . de eodem novae sententiae partim confirmantur, partim ulteriori subjiciuntur examini. Helmestadii, Typis & sumptibus Georgii Wolfgangi Hammii, 1690.

87 p.   18 cm.   **[10372]**

—De auditu liber unus . . . Lugduni-Batavorum, Apud Petrum de Graaf, 1684.

[40], 274, [4] p.   plates.   17 cm.   **[10373]**
Added engraved title page.

—De genuina febres curandi methodo dissertatio in tres partes divisa . . . Jenae, Apud Johannem Bielckium, 1693.

[23], 220, [12] p.   20 cm.   **[10374]**

—De lymphae ortu et lymphaticorum vasorum causis ad . . . Dn. Le Clerc & Manget medicos Genevenses epistolica dissertatio. Helmestadii, Typis Georg-Wolfgangi Hammii, 1683.

[29] p.   20 cm.   **[10375]**

—De spiritibus animalibus disquisitio cum capitis historiam naturalem & morbosam auditoribus suis publice tradere cepisset, in eorum usum conscripta. Helmestadii, Typis Georg-Wolfgangii Hammii, 1682.

[24] p.   20 cm.   **[10376]**

—In physiologiam introductio cum id studium primum aggrederetur publicis praelectionibus praemissa. Helmestadii, Typis & sumtib. haeredum Henrici Davidis Mülleri, 1681.

[35] p.   19 cm.   **[10377]**

—Ογκολογια parva; seu, De humani corporis tumoribus eorumque . . . curatione liber . . . Jenae, Sumtu Jo. Bielkii, litteris Nisianis, 1695.

[36], 179 p.   20 cm.   **[10378]**
With this is bound *his* Programma anatomicum. 1695.

[—] Phocae maris anatome in Academia Kiloniensi suscepta, mense Decembri MDCXCIX.

Ibidem [i.e. Kilonii] Literis Bartholdi Reutheri [1699?]

　　24 p.　20 cm.　　　　　　　　　**[10379]**

　　Author's name from 1707 edition.
　　At head of title: G. C. S.

—Programma anatomicum, quo philiatros suos postremum allocutus est. Jenae, Sumptibus Johannis Bielke, litteris Krebsianis, 1695.

　　12 p.　20 cm.　　　　　　　　　**[10380]**

　　Bound with *his* Ογχολογια parva. 1695.

—Programma rei herbariae professioni in horto medico solenniter auspicandae praemissum, quo medicae artis & naturalium rerum studiosos ad demonstrationes plantarum perhumaniter invitat. Jenae, Literis Krebsianis [1690]

　　[8] p.　18 cm.　　　　　　　　　**[10381]**

Programs — Jena

—Programma conscriptum occasione inauguralis ... Adami Gottlieb Koehleri, disputationis de fulmine tactis. Jenae, Litteris Krebsianis [1694]

　　[8] p.　20 cm.　　　　　　　　　**[10382]**

　　With vita of A. G. Koehler.

—Programma ... inaugurali disputationi D. J. C. Wenzelii praemissum. [Jenae] Literis Nisianis [1694]

　　14 p.　20 cm.　　　　　　　　　**[10383]**

　　With vita of J. C. Wenzel.

Dissertations — Helmstedt

—*praeses.* De peste ... Helmestadii, Typis Georg-Wolfgangi Hammii [1682]

　　100 p.　20 cm.　　　　　　　　　**[10384]**

　　D. C. Meineke, *respondent.*

Jena

—Disputationem inauguralem de suffusione vulgo vom Staar ... examini subjiciet Johannes Georgius Hast. Jenae, Literis Krebsianis [1691]

　　28 p.　20 cm.　　　　　　　　　**[10385]**

　　J. G. Hast, *respondent.*

—Dissertatio inauguralis medica de aqua pericardii ... Jenae, Litteris Joh. Zach. Nisii [1694]

　　57 (i.e. 55) p.　19 cm.　　　　　　　**[10386]**

　　J. C. Wenzel, *respondent.*

—Dissertatio inauguralis medica de dyspepsia ... Jenae, Typis Pauli Ehrichii [1695]

　　32 p.　19 cm.　　　　　　　　　**[10387]**

　　G. C. Wolff, *respondent.*

—Dissertatio inauguralis medica de morbis aetatum ... Jenae, Litteris Joh. Zach. Nisii [1694]

　　56 p.　19 cm.　　　　　　　　　**[10388]**

　　J. E. Waltsgott, *respondent.*

—Dissertatio inauguralis medica de tabe dorsali ... Jenae, Literis Krebsianis [1691]

　　28 p.　19 cm.　　　　　　　　　**[10389]**

　　C. A. Tornesi, *respondent.*

—Dissertationem inauguralem medicam de febrifugorum natura agendi et applicandi modo ... publicae ... disquisitioni sistit Christophorus Hagedorn ... Jenae, Literis Krebsianis [1694]

　　32, [4] p.　20 cm.　　　　　　　　**[10390]**

　　C. Hagedorn, *respondent.*

—Dissertationem medicam inauguralem de lethargo ... submittit Michael Schramm ... Jenae, Typis Krebsianis [1692]

　　36 p.　19 cm.　　　　　　　　　**[10391]**

　　M. Schramm, *respondent.*

—Dissertationem medicam inauguralem de paresi sive paralysi ex colica ... publicae ... disquisitioni sistit Jacobus L'Hommart ... Jenae, Litteris Jo. Zach. Nisii [1693]

　　51 p.　20 cm.　　　　　　　　　**[10392]**

　　J. L'Hommart, *respondent.*

—Dissertationem medicam inauguralem de tremore ... submittit Johannes Philippus Krauss ... Jenae, Typis Krebsianis [1692]

　　24 p.　19 cm.　　　　　　　　　**[10393]**

　　J. P. Krauss, *respondent.*

—Exercitatio medica de capitis dolore ... Jenae, Literis Johannis Jacobi Bauhoferi [1678]

　　[47] p.　20 cm.　　　　　　　　　**[10394]**

　　T. Kemper, *respondent.*

—Exercitationem inauguralem de epulide & parulide cum annexa dentium & gingivarum ἐξερευνησει ... p. p. Georgius Fridericus Francus ... Jenae, Literis Krebsianis [1692]

　　[4], 64 p.　20 cm.　　　　　　　　**[10395]**

　　G. F. Franck von Franckenau, *respondent.*

Kiel

—Dissertatio inauguralis de spina ventosa ... Kiliae, Literis Joachimi Reumanni [1698]

　　44 p.　20 cm.　　　　　　　　　**[10396]**

　　F. Jonsius, *respondent.*

—Exercitationum medicarum quinta continens theses selectas de principio motus animali ... Kilonii, Literis Bartholdi Reutheri, 1700.

[16] p.　19 cm.　　　　　　　　　**[10397]**

C. M. Burchard, *respondent*.

—, *See* WEDEL, G. W., *praeses*. Dissertatio inauguralis medica de voce. 1677.

—, *ed. See* CONRING, H. In universam artem medicam singulasque ejus partes introductio. 1687.

SCHELHASS, ERNST FRIDEMANN [*fl.* 1670–1674] *respondent. See* WEDEL, G. W., *praeses*. Dissertationem inauguralem de paronychia ... subjicit E. F. S. ... anno M DC LXXIV. 1686.

SCHELIGIUS, ALBERTUS., *ed. See* MERCURIALE, G. Tractatus varii de re medica. 1618, 1623.

SCHELIUS, JOACHIMUS. *See* SCHELE, Joachim [*fl.* 1626–*ca.* 1650]

SCHELKENS, DANIEL [*fl.* 1631?] *respondent. See* BURGERSDIJCK, F. P., *praeses*. Collegium physicum. 1642.

SCHEMBERGER, ANDREAS [*fl.* 1677–1678] *respondent. See* FASCH, A. H., *praeses*. Dissertatio medica de latice. 1677; WEDEL, G. W., *praeses*. Disputationem medicam inauguralem, de archeo ... subjicit A. S. 1678.

SCHENCK, EUSEBIUS [1569–1622 or 8] *praeses*. De crisibus, et diebus criticis ... Jenae, Typis Johannis Weidneri, 1620.

[20] p.　19 cm.　　　　　　　　　**[10398]**

Diss. — Jena (J. G. Obele, *respondent*)

—Decas problematum medicorum ... Jenae, Typis Johannis Weidneri, 1621.

[20] p.　19 cm.　　　　　　　　　**[10399]**

Diss. — Jena (J. Eichorn, *respondent*)

—Disputatio medica, de dysenteria ... Jenae, Typis Johannis Beithmanni, 1619.

[16] p.　19 cm.　　　　　　　　　**[10400]**

Diss. — Jena (J.-C. Weber, *respondent*)

—Disputatio medica inauguralis de pleuritide ... Jenae, Typis Johannis Weidneri, 1619.

[16] p.　19 cm.　　　　　　　　　**[10401]**

SCHENCK, JOHANN ANDREAS [*fl.* 1608] *ed.* and *tr. See* COLOMBO, R. Anatomia. 1609; FEDRO VON RODACH, G. Opuscula iatro chemica quatuor. 1611.

SCHENCK, JOHANN FRIEDRICH [*fl.* 1637] *respondent. See* SPERLING, J., *praeses*. De somniis dissertatio physica. 1637.

SCHENCK, JOHANN GEORG [*d.* 1620] Biblia iatrica; sive, Bibliotheca medica macta, continuata, consummata, qua velut favissa, auctorum in sacra medicina scriptis cluentium, reique medicae monumentorum, ac divitiarum thesaurus cluditur ... Francofurti, Typis Joannis Spiessii, sumptibus Antonii Hummii, 1609.

[12], 517 (i.e. 511) p.　17 cm.　　　　**[10402]**

Arranged alphabetically by the given names of the authors.

—Exotericorum experimentorum ad varios morbos. Centuriae VII. In quibus remedia rara, selecta ... exhibentur. Nunc primum e Schenckiana bibliotheca publici juris facta ... Francofurti, Typis Joannis Spiessii, sumptibus Gothofredi Tampachii, 1607.

[44], 454 p.　17 cm.　　　　　　　　**[10403]**

—Lithogenesia; sive, De microcosmi membris petrefactis, et de calculis eidem microcosmo per varias matrices innatis, pathologica historica, per theorian & autopsian demonstrata. Accessit analogicum argumentum ex macrocosmo De calculis brutorum corporib. innatis ... Francofurti, Ex officina typographica Matthiae Beckeri, sumptibus viduae Theodori de Bry, & duorum ejus filiorum, 1608.

[14], 69, [7] p.　illus.　21 cm.　　　**[10404]**

—Pinax auctorum in re medica qui gynaecia scriptis excoluerunt & illustrarunt. *In* Guinterius, J. A. Gynaeciorum commentarius. 1606.

—, *ed.* Monstrorum historia memorabilis, monstrosa humanorum partuum miracula ... vivis exemplis, observationibus, & picturis, referens. Accessit analogicum argumentum De monstris brutis. Supplementi loco ad Observationes medicas Schenckianas edita a Joanne Georgio Schenckio a Grafenberg filio ... Francofurti, Ex officina typographica Matthiae Beckeri, impensis viduae Theodori de Bry, & duorum ejus filiorum, 1609.

[6], 135 p.　illus.　21 cm.　　　　　**[10405]**

—, *ed. See* GUILANDINUS, M. Hortus Patavinus. 1600 [1608]; GUINTERIUS, J. A. Gynaeciorum commentarius. 1606; SCHENCK VON GRAFENBERG, J.

Observationum medicarum rariorum, libri VII. 1643, 1644, 1665 [and] Παρατηρήσεων; sive, Observationum medicarum. 1609.

SCHENCK, JOHANN THEODOR [1619-1671] Anatomen ... artium & scientiarum studiosis commendat, eosque ad demonstrationem fabricae muliebris ... invitat. [Jenae] Typis Johannis Nisii [1656]

[16] p.   19 cm.   **[10406]**

—Anatomen foemineam artium & scientiarum studiosis intimat ... Jenae, Literis Nisianis, 1658.

[8] p.   19 cm.   **[10407]**

—Anatomen localem a calumniis defendit; ejusque utilitatem ... demonstrat ... [Jenae] Literis Nisianis [1657]

[16] p.   19 cm.   **[10408]**

—Catalogus plantarum horti medici Jenensis earumque quae in vicinia proveniunt ... Jenae, Samuel Krebs, 1659.

[95] p.   plates.   13 cm.   **[10409]**

—[Exercitationes anatomicae ad usum medicum accommodatae. Jenae, Apud Johan. Ludovicum Neuenhahn, 166?]

452 + p.   18 cm.   **[10410]**

Imperfect: all pages before p. 1 (including title page), p. 25-33, 341-444, and all pages after p. 452 wanting; p. 452 mutilated. Title and imprint supplied from Linden.

—Humorum corporis humani historia generalis, cognoscendi et curandi principiis illustrata. Jenae, Typis ac sumptibus Johannis Jacobi Bauhoferi, 1663.

[18], 180, [1] p.   21 cm.   **[10411]**

Errata: p. [1] at end.
With this is bound *his* Schola partium humani corporis. 1664.

—Schola partium humani corporis, usum earundem & actionem secundum situm, connexionem, quantitatem ... atque substantiam continens ... Jenae, Sumptibus Johannis Ludovici Neuenhahns, typis Samuelis Krebsii, 1664.

[6], 254 (i.e. 252), [54] p.   21 cm.   **[10412]**

Imperfect: p. 27-28 mutilated.
Bound with *his* Humorum corporis humani historia generalis. 1663.

—Seri sanguinis historia ex veterum & recentiorum scriptis eruta ... una cum disputatione De natura lactis & exercitatione De materia turgente,

aucta & secundum edita. Jenae, Sumtibus Johannis Fritschii, excudebat Joh. Werther, 1671.

[8], 120, [12] p.   20 cm.   **[10413]**

—Structuram corporis humani artium & scientiarum, cumprimis sacrae medicinae cultoribus commendat, eosque ad anatomen publicam in cadavere foemenino ... administrandam ... invitat ... Jenae, Typis Johannis Nisii [1662]

[8] p.   19 cm.   **[10414]**

Dissertations — Jena

—*praeses*. De gravissimo et rarissimo capitis affectu caro disputatio inauguralis medica ... Jenae, Typis Johannis Wertheri, 1665.

[44] p.   19 cm.   **[10415]**

G. A. Dummer, *respondent.*

—De sero sanguinis ... historia ... Jenae, Typis Johannis Nisii, 1655.

63 p.   21 cm.   **[10416]**

S. G. Hausmann, *respondent.*
Bound with Rolfinck, W. Ordo et methodus medicinae specialis consultatoriae ὡς ʼεν ʼατομω. 1669.

—Disputatio dioptrico-anatomica de oculo ... Jenae, Prelo Nisiano, 1654.

[40] p.   20 cm.   **[10417]**

C. Listorp, *respondent.*

—Disputatio inauguralis medica de melancholiae διαγνωει, προγνωσει, και θεραπεια genere ... Jenae, Literis Samuelis Krebsii, 1662.

[4], 43, [5] p.   19 cm.   **[10418]**

K. Eckhard, *respondent.*

—Disputatio inauguralis medica de palpitatione cordis ... [Jenae] Literis Samuelis Krebsii [1662]

[1], 48, [2] p.   18 cm.   **[10419]**

C. Gigas, *respondent.*

—Disputatio inauguralis medica de ... pestilentia ... Jenae, Literis Johannis Wertheri [1668]

[2], 37, [5] p.   19 cm.   **[10420]**

J. A. Harssleben, *respondent.*

—Disputatio inauguralis medica de pleuritide ... Jenae, Literis Samuelis Krebsii [1661]

[40] p.   19 cm.   **[10421]**

J. G. Sommer, *respondent.*

—Disputatio inauguralis medica de pleuritide . . .
Jenae, Literis Samuelis Krebsii, 1663.
    [60] p. 19 cm.   **[10422]**
  C. Schäffer, *respondent.*

—Disputatio inauguralis medica de signultu . . .
Jenae, Ex officina Johannis Wertheri [1667]
    38, [6] p. 19 cm.   **[10423]**
  J. C. Hübner, *respondent.*

—Disputatio inauguralis medica . . . de tartaro
microcosmico, secundum principia Hippocratica,
Galenica, Paracelsica atque Helmontiana considerato
. . . [Jenae] Typis Johannis Nisii [1658]
    [32] p. 19 cm.   **[10424]**
  V. Eckhard, *respondent.*

—Disputatio inauguralis medica de vermibus intestinorum . . . Jenae, Stanno Wertheriano [1670]
    45, [3] p. 20 cm.   **[10425]**
  I. W. Ayrer, *respondent.*

—Disputatio medica de causo . . . Jenae, Typis
Samuelis Krebsii [1664]
    [30] p. 20 cm.   **[10426]**
  M. Jacobi, *respondent.*

—Disputatio medica inauguralis, de dysenteria,
veterum & recentiorum principiis, tum cognoscitivis
tum curativis illustrata . . . Jenae, Literis Krebsianis,
1664.
    [48] p. 18 cm.   **[10427]**
  W. Schultz, *respondent.*

—Disputatio medica inauguralis de ephemera . . .
Jenae, Typis Georgii Sengenwaldianis, 1658.
    [36] p. 19 cm.   **[10428]**
  J. Schreyer, *respondent.*

—Disputatio medica inauguralis de lassitudine . . .
Jenae, Typis Samuelis Krebsii, 1664.
    [64] p. 18 cm.   **[10429]**
  S. Zigemarius, *respondent.*

—Another issue, with laudatory poems.
    [66] p. 19 cm.   **[10430]**

—Disputatio medica inauguralis de vulneribus . . .
Jenae, Literis Krebsianis [*ca.* 1664]
    [1], 36, [2] p. 19 cm.   **[10431]**
  A. Thymius, *respondent.*

—Disputatio medico-chirurgica de fonticulis . . .
Jenae, Joannis Nisii, 1657.
    36 p. 20 cm.   **[10432]**
  J. Crusius, *respondent.*

—Disputationem inauguralem de cholera . . . sub-
jicit Hermannus Fridericus Körber . . . Jenae, E
Calcographeo Nisiano, 1653.
    44 p. 19 cm.   **[10433]**
  H.F. Körber, *respondent.*

—Disputationem inauguralem de macie puerorum
ex fascino . . . submittit Ehrenfridus Hagendornius
. . . Jenae, Literis Krebsianis [1667]
    [2], 33, [5] p. 19 cm.   **[10434]**
  E. Hagendorn, *respondent.*

—Disputationem inauguralem de malo hypochon-
driaco . . . publicae disquisitioni sistit Laurentius
Theill . . . [Jenae] Literis Wertherianis [1668]
    [28] p. 19 cm.   **[10435]**
  L. Theill, *respondent.*

—Disputationem medicam inauguralem de imbecillitate ventriculi . . . publico sistit examini . . .
Franciscus Peters . . . Jenae, Typis Johannis Wertheri, 1669.
    33, [3] p. 19 cm.   **[10436]**
  F. Peters, *respondent.*

—Dissertatio academica, illustrium problematum
circa venaesectionem occurrentium decades duas
continens . . . Jenae, Literis Wertherianis [1667]
    [1], 74 p. 19 cm.   **[10437]**
  P. J. Scheidlin, *respondent.*

—Dissertatio inauguralis medica de bulimo . . .
[Jenae] Typis Johannis Wertheri [1669]
    45, [3] p. 19 cm.   **[10438]**
  L. Schroeck, *respondent.*

—Dissertatio inauguralis medica de catalepsi . . .
Jenae, Typis Johannis Nisii, 1671.
    [51] p. 20 cm.   **[10439]**
  P. C. Möbius, *respondent.*

—Dissertatio inauguralis medica περι της
ανορεξιας; sive, De inappetentia ventriculi . . .
[Jenae] Typis Joh. Nisii, 1660.
    [56] p. 19 cm.   **[10440]**
  J. A. Bossert, *respondent.*

—Dissertatio medica de ambulatione in somno . . .
Jenae, Literis Müllerianis [1671]
    [8], 32 p. 20 cm.   **[10441]**
  Prefatory epistle dated 1671.
  J. J. Theisner, *respondent.*

—Dissertatio medica de cinnamomo . . . Jenae, Literis Wertherianis [1670]

    53, [3] p. 19 cm.   **[10442]**

J. P. Hoechstetter, *respondent.*

—Dissertatio medica de conceptione . . . Jenae, Literis Johannis Wertheri [1664]

    [84] p. 20 cm.   **[10443]**

A. H. Cummius, *respondent.*

—Dissertatio medica de phrenitide, aliquot thematibus comprehensa . . . [Jenae] Literis Wertherianis [1667]

    [32] p. 19 cm.   **[10444]**

S. Ledel, *respondent.*

—Dissertatio medica de poris corporis humani . . . Jenae, Typis Krebsianis [1670]

    56 p. 19 cm.   **[10445]**

M. Frick, *respondent.*

—Dissertatio medica inauguralis de phrenitide . . . [Jenae] Literis Sengenwaldianis [1666]

    [48] p. 19 cm.   **[10446]**

J. J. Ruttörffer, *respondent.*

—Dissertatio methodum cognoscendi & curandi obstructiones continens . . . Jenae, Typis Johannis Nisii [1665]

    [80] p. 20 cm.   **[10447]**

G. Gigas, *respondent.*

—Dissertatio physico medica de tribus coctionibus corporis humani . . . Jenae, Typis Samuelis Krebsii, 1658.

    78, [2] p. 18 cm.   **[10448]**

J. C. Mack, *respondent.*

—Dissertationem inauguralem de paralysi . . . submittit . . . Friedericus Kaltschmied . . . [Jenae] Literis Wertherianis [1668]

    [1], 38 p. 19 cm.   **[10449]**

F. Kaltschmied, *respondent.*

—Dissertationem inauguralem de passione hypochondriaca . . . submittit Samuel Ochlitius . . . Jenae, Charactere Wertheriano, 1666.

    [1], 53 (i.e. 51), [3] p. 19 cm.   **[10450]**

S. Ochliz, *respondent.*

—Dissertationem inauguralem quae sistit aegrum laborantem malo hypochondriaco scorbutico . . . subjicit Godofredus Schultzius . . . Jenae, Typis Johannis Wertheri [1670]

    [28] p. 19 cm.   **[10451]**

G. Schultz, *respondent.*

—Exercitatio anatomica . . . de partibus generationi inservientibus masculis . . . Jenae, Typis Johannis Nisii [1662]

    56, [6] p. 19 cm.   **[10452]**

J. Schröter, *respondent.*

—Exercitatio medica cura vexatorum ad veterum & recentiorum mentem exstructa . . . Jenae, Typis Wertherianis, 1670.

    32 p. 18 cm.   **[10453]**

J. K. Fuchs, *respondent.*

Imperfect: upper margin of last leaf trimmed with possible loss of pagination.

—Exercitationem academicam de moscho . . . submittit Lucas Schroeckius . . . [Jenae] Typis Johannis Wertheri [1667]

    [1], 89, [1] p. plates. 18 cm.   **[10454]**

L. Schroeck, *respondent.*

—Guerneri Rolfincii . . . Epitomes methodi cognoscendi & curandi affectus corporis humani particulares, secundum ordinem Abubetri Rhazae ad regem Mansorem, lib. 9. Hippocratis, Paracelsis & Harveanis principiis illustratae recognitae dissertatio decima tertia, de dolore jecoris, cachexia, ictero et hydrope . . . Jenae, Typis Johannis Nisii, 1655.

    [2], 217–236, [2] p. 19 cm.   **[10455]**

Pages 217–236 of Rolfinck's Epitomes with preliminary and laudatory materials added.

V. Eckhard, *respondent.*

—Historia plantarum generalis, in synopsin redacta, & ad usum medicum concinnata . . . Jenae, Typis Joannis Nisii, 1656.

    [44] p. 20 cm.   **[10456]**

Z. Ennichmann, *respondent.*

—Μαραθρολογια; sive, De foeniculo dissertatio . . . Jenae, Literis Nisianis, 1665.

    [2], 88, [2] p. 19 cm.   **[10457]**

F. Kaltschmied, *respondent.*

—Medico-chirurgicam dissertationem de fistularum vera natura & recta ratione curandarum . . . submittit Jacobus Jodocus Raab . . . Jenae, Typis Johannis Nisii, 1656.

    [44] p. 19 cm.   **[10458]**

J. J. Raabe, *respondent.*

—Thematum theoretico-practicorum de dolore capitis, sesqui-decas . . . Jenae, Typis Johannis Nisii [1665]

    [12] p. 19 cm.   **[10459]**

J. Loss, *respondent.*

—Trigam simplicium medicamentorum illustrem: fermentantium, sedativorum, et praecipitantium ... subjicit ... Johannes Georgius Arens ... Jenae, Literis Johannis Wertheri, 1671.

[4], 24 p. 20 cm. **[10460]**

J. G. Arens, *respondent.*

SCHENCK, JOHANNES. *See* SCHENCK VON GRAFENBERG, Johannes [1530-1598]

SCHENCK VON GRAFENBERG, JOHANNES [1530-1598] Παρατηρήσεων; sive, Observationum medicarum, rararum, novarum, admirabilium, & monstrosarum, volumen, tomis septem de toto homine institutum. In quo, quae medici ... abdita, vulgo incognita, gravia, periculosaque, circa humani corporis anatomen & fabricam, ejusdemque morborum causas, signa, eventus, & curationes accidere compererunt, exemplis ut plurimum & historiis proposita exhibentur ... Retractatius vero a Joanne Georgio Schenckio, ... per tertiationem illustratum ... Francofurti, E typographeo Nicolai Hoffmanni, impensa Jonae Rhodii, 1609.

[36], 1018, [53] p. illus., port. 34 cm.

[10461]

Contents.—De capillis capitis et barbae.—De partibus vitalibus thorace contentis.—De partibus naturalibus nutritioni servientibus, et imo ventre conclusis.—De genitalibus partibus utriusque sexus.—De partibus externis.—De febribus.—De venenis.

—Observationum medicarum rariorum, libri VII. In quibus nova, abdita ... monstrosaque exempla, circa anatomen, aegritudinum causas ... curationes ... proponuntur ... Opus ... a Joan. Georgio Schenckio ... tertium accuratiss. illustratum. Modo vero ab innumeris praecedentium editionum mendis, Car. Sponii ... opera vendicatum. Lugduni, Sumptibus Joannis-Antonii Huguetan, 1643.

[44], 892, [46] p. port. 37 cm. **[10462]**

A revision of the 1609 Frankfurt edition.

—[The same.] ... Opus ... a Joan Georgio Schenckio fil. ... tertium ... illustratum. Modo vero ab innumeris praecedentium editionum mendis, Car. Sponii ... opera vendicatum. Lugduni, Sumptibus Joannis-Antonii Huguetan, 1644.

[44], 892, [46] p. port. 36 cm. **[10463]**

A reissue of the Frankfurt edition with date changed to 1644.

—[The same.] ... Opus ... a Joan. Georgio Schenckio, fil. ... tertium ... illustratum. Ante annos vero XX. ab innumeric praecedentium edi-

tionum mendis ... Car. Sponii ... opera vindicatum, & nunc passim novis recentiorum autorum observationibus auctum, a Laur. Straussio ... Francofurti, Sumptibus Joannis Beyeri, excudebat Hieronymus Polichius, 1665.

[36], 981, [50] p. 36 cm. **[10464]**

Revision of the 1644 Lyons edition.

—*See* ALBINUS, S. Kurtzer Bericht und Handgrieff. 1675.

SCHENCKEL, LAMBRECHT THOMAS [*b.* 1547] *See* PAËPP, J. Vita M. Tullii Ciceronis. 1618.

SCHENFELDER, PHILIPPUS JACOBUS. *See* SCHÖNFELD, Philipp Jakob [*fl.* 1662-1686]

SCHENK, JOHANNES. *See* SCHENCK VON GRAFENBERG, Johannes [1530-1598]

SCHENKEL, LAMBERTUS THOMAS. *See* SCHENCKEL, Lambrecht Thomas [*b.* 1547]

SCHENNIS, HEINRICH VON [*fl.* 1628] *ed. & tr. See* SINICKER, E. Keiser Rudolff des andern ... Spagyrische Hauss und Reiss-Apothec. 1646.

SCHEPLER, TOBIAS [*fl.* 1674] *respondent. See* FRENZEL, S. F., *praeses.* Monstrum humanum ventribus sine proportione et mutilis artubus. 1674.

SCHERB, CHRISTIAN [*fl.* 1660] *respondent. See* SEBISCH, M. [1578-1674?] *praeses.* Disputatio solennis de colica passione. 1660.

SCHERB, JACOB CHRISTOPH [*fl.* 1683] *respondent.* Disputatio medica inauguralis de lienteria ... Basileae, Typis Jacobi Bertschii [1683]

[20] p. 19 cm. **[10465]**

Diss.—Basel.

SCHERB, PHILIP [1555-1605] Theses medicae collectae & editae a Casp. Hofmanno ... Lipsiae, Excudebant haeredes Valentini am Ende, impensis Johannis Börneri & Eliae Rehefeldii, 1614.

[14], 199, [1] p. 17 cm. **[10466]**

Bound with Donati, M. De historia medica. 1613.

—, *ed. See* CESALPINO, A. De metallicis libri tres. 1602.

SCHERER, JAKOB [*fl.* 1626] *respondent. See* SEBISCH, M. [1578-1674?] *praeses.* Exercitationes medicae. 1639.

SCHERER, Johann Jacob [*fl.* 1692–1696] *respondent.* Dissertatio medica inauguralis de actionibus corporis humani viventis plerisque . . . Basileae, Typis Jacobi Bertschii [1696]

[60] p.   20 cm.   **[10467]**

Diss.—Basel.

SCHERPFF, Matthias [*fl.* 1676] *respondent.* Disputatio medica inauguralis exhibens febrem petechialem, quae ante biennium Argentoratum & viciniam infestavit . . . Argentorati, Typis Johannis Welperi [1676]

[8], 28 p.   19 cm.   **[10468]**

Diss.—Strasbourg.

SCHEUBAN, Paul [*fl.* 1664] *respondent. See* Sennert, D., *praeses.* Disputatio anatomica de ossibus in genere. 1664.

SCHEUCHZER, Hans Jakob [1645–1688] *respondent.* Disputatio medica inauguralis de lactatione laesa . . . Lugduni Batavorum, Apud viduam & haeredes Joannis Elsevirii, 1669.

[15] p.   23 cm.   **[10469]**

Diss.—Leyden.

—*See* Applausus gratulatori honoribus . . . Joh. Jacobi Schychzeri. 1669.

SCHEUEBANUS, Paulus. *See* Scheuban, Paul [*fl.* 1664]

SCHEUNEMANN, Henning [*fl.* 1594–1613] Hydromantia Paracelsica; hoc est, Discursus philosophicus de novo fonte in Saxonia Electorali circa oppidum Annebergam reperto, olim S. Annae Fons dicto . . . Francofurti, Prostat in officina Zachariae Palthenii, 1613 [colophon 1615]

[12], 114, [1] p.   illus.   20 cm.   **[10470]**

—Kurtzer Bericht, wie . . . die jetztregierende Pest mit dreyen durch chymische Kunst praeparirte und astralisch gemachte Pulverlein zu curiren und heilen sey . . . Magdeburgk, Joachim Böl, 1611.

[15] p.   18 cm.   **[10471]**

—Medicina reformata; seu, Denarius hermeticus philosophicus medico-chymicus . . . In quo mira brevitate dilucide docetur, decem entibus omnium morborum radices, productiones, transplantationes, astra, signa, indicationes & curationes compleri & absolvi. Francofurti, Typis & impensis Joannis Bringeri, 1617.

122, [2] p.   17 cm.   **[10472]**

Editor's preface, signed I.H.P.M., has initials I.H. only in caption title. P.M. may stand for Protomedicus.

Bound with Duchesne, J. Tetras gravissimorum totius capitis affectuum. 1617.

—Paracelsia . . . de morbo mercuriali contagioso, quem pestem vulgus nominat, ex quintuplici ente, Dei nimirum, astrorum, pagoyi, veneni & naturae prognato: in qua vera curandi ratio recensetur. Babenbergae, Excusa per Antonium Horitzium, 1608.

[6], 66 p.   table.   20 cm.   **[10473]**

—*See* Libavius, A. [*d.* 1616] Appendix necessaria Syntagmatis arcanorum chymicorum. 1615.

SCHEUNERUS, Fabianus [*fl.* 1594] De catharris. Von allerley Flössen und Catharren, so beydes intra Calvam, aus dem Gehirn und seinen Capaciteten etspringen und . . . auch extra Calvam . . . Wie man . . . sich praeserviren, darnach . . . denselben widerumb recht curiren, und letzlichen auch seine dess Catharri Symptomata wider ablehnen sol . . . Leipzig [In Vorlegung Henningi Grossen, gedruckt durch Jacobum Gaubisch, typis haeredum Zachariae Berwaldi, 1601]

[16], 262, [1] p.   17 cm.   **[10474]**

With this is bound Brunschwig, H. Thesaurus pauperum. Franckfort am Mayn, 1598.

—[The same.] . . . Eissleben [In Vorlegung Henningi Grossen, Leipzig; gedruckt durch Jacobum Gaubisch, 1605]

[16], 238, [1] p.   17 cm.   **[10475]**

SCHIAVETTI, Andrea [*fl.* 1583] Breve ragionamento . . . sopra l'acque, & bagni di San Casciano. Con gli ordini da osservarsi nel bevere, & bagnarse in dette acque. Et di nuovo aggiuntovi nel fine alcune antichita ritrovate quest'anno. Orvieto, Per Antonio Colaldi, 1618.

24 p.   illus.   20 cm.   **[10476]**

Imperfect: wormholes on p. 11–24.

SCHICKART, Johann Sebastian [*fl.* 1671] *respondent.* Theses inaugurales de diarrhoea . . . Argentorati, Typis Johannis Pastorii [1671]

[1], 34 p.   20 cm.   **[10477]**

Imperfect: last leaf mutilated.

Diss.—Strasbourg.

SCHIEFORDEGHER, Bernhard [*fl.* 1700] *respondent. See* Vater, C., *praeses.* De ulceribus fistulosis. 1700.

SCHIFFART, HENRICUS VON [*fl.* 1693] *respondent.*
See HERMANN, P., *praeses.* Disputatio medica de
hydrope. 1693.

SCHIFFMAN, JOSEPH [*fl.* 1679] Corpus juris
medicinalis in tres libros divisum, quo medicus
naturae accusantis, et morbi accusati judex propositas lites secundum neuthericorum fundamenta
dirimere sciat . . . Venetiis, Apud Antonium Bosium,
1679.

    [10], 128 p.   front.   23 cm.   **[10478]**
Contains Liber primus.

SCHIFNER, ANDREAS [*fl.* 1610] *respondent.* Περι
του της καρδιας πολμου themata [De palpitatione seu
tremore cordis disputatio] . . . Basileae, Typis Joan.
Jacobi Genathii [1610]

    [12] p.   20 cm.   **[10479]**
Diss. — Basel.

—*See* PLATTER, F. [1536-1614] Felix Platerus . . .
decreto. 1610.

SCHILHANS, HANS. *See* GERSDORFF, Hans von
[*d.* 1529]

SCHILLER, HEINRICH [*fl.* 1600] Von der
Pestilentz. Erster Tractat: Von den pestilentzischen
Funcken, ihrer Art, Underschiedt, Zunder . . . II.
Vom Regiment oder Lebens-Ordnung bey der Pest.
III. Von den bezoartischen Gifftreibern, beyde zur
Versicherung unnd zur Heylung . . . Hanaw,
Gedruckt durch Johannem Halbeyen, 1606.

    87, [1] p.   16 cm.   **[10480]**

SCHILLING, ANDREAS [*fl.* 1651] *respondent.*
Disputatio medica de urinae suppressione . . . Argentorati, Typis Eberhardi Welperi, 1651.

    [40] p.   20 cm.   **[10481]**
Diss. — Strasbourg.

SCHILLING, CHRISTOPH [*d.* 1583] *See* SCHOLTZ,
L. Epistolarum philosophicarum: medicinalium, ac
chymicarum . . . volumen. 1610.

SCHILLING, FLORENTIN [*fl.* 1624] *respondent. See*
SEBISCH, M. [1578-1674?] *praeses.* Exercitationes
medicae. 1639.

SCHILLING, FRIEDRICH [*fl.* 1678] *respondent.*
Disputatio inauguralis medica, qua celebris quaestionis anatomicae de circulatione sanguinis
negativam . . . proponit Fridericus Schilling . . .

Basileae, Typis Jacobi Bertschii [1678]
    [16] p.   21 cm.   **[10482]**
Diss. — Basel.

SCHILLING, HEINRICH SIEGMUND [*fl.* 1629-1668]
Discursus medicus de conservanda sanitate auctius
secunda vice editus . . . Dresdae, Impensis Andreae
Löfleri, typis Melchioris Bergen, 1655.

    [28] p.   19 cm.   **[10483]**
Imperfect: upper margin of p. [25-28] trimmed.

—[The same.] Discursus physiologico-medicus de
vigore sanitatis conservando . . . Dresdae, Typis
Seyffertinis, 1668.

    [23] p.   19 cm.   **[10484]**

—Tractatus osteologicus; sive, Osteologia
microcosmica, de ossium corporis humani admiranda
structura, cui denuo adjicitur Discursus physiologico-
anatomicus, hominem μικροκοσμον, sive cognitionem
sui considerans . . . Dresdae, Impensis haeredum
Melchioris Bergen, 1668.

    [6], 88, 24 p.   19 cm.   **[10485]**

SCHILLING, JAKOB [*fl.* 1666] *respondent. See* KOR-
MART, G., *praeses.* De spiritu animalium corporeo
vero s. vitali. 1666.

SCHILLING, JOANNES [*fl.* 1644] *respondent. See*
SEBISCH, M. [1578-1674?] *praeses.* Disputatio de
naturalibus facultatibus prima [-octava & ultima] 1644
[i.e. 1645]

SCHILLING, JOHANN [*fl.* 1675-1676] *respondent.*
Disputatio inauguralis medica aegrum ex amore
catalepticum factum proponens . . . Giessae, Ex
calcographeo Friderici Kargeri, 1676.

    34, [2] p.   20 cm.   **[10486]**
Diss. — Giessen.

—*See* STRAUSS, L., *praeses.* Dissertatio medica, de
necessaria morbi cognitione ad curandum. 1675.

SCHILLING, LAURENT [*fl.* 1672-1675] Anti-
corollarium Kippingianum; seu, Animadversiones
physico-medicae, in corollarium de sanguinis motu
M. Henrici Kippingi . . . Erffurti, Ex typographeo
Kirschiano, 1673.

    [38] p.   19 cm.   **[10487]**
Previously published as the author's dissertation. Erfurt, 1672.

—*respondent.* Disputatio medica inauguralis de obstructionibus . . . Basileae, Typis Jacobi Bertschii [1675]

[28] p.   20 cm.   **[10488]**

Diss. — Basel.

SCHILLING, SIGISMUND [1575–1622] *praeses.* Themata disputationis ordinariae de gonorrhoea . . . Lipsiae, In officina typographica Tobiae Beyeri [1614]

[32] p.   19 cm.   **[10489]**

Diss. — Leipzig (F. Kest, *respondent*)

SCHINTZNACHER Bad. *See* [ZIEGLER, H. J.] *ed.* Heil-Brunnen. 1663.

SCHIPPEL, JOHANN NIKOLAUS [*b.* 1649] *respondent. See* MAJOR, J. D., *praeses.* Disputatio medica inauguralis quam de usu et abusu mercurii in lue venerea . . . defendam suscipiet Joh. Nicolaus Schippel. 1673.

SCHIRLAEUS, THOMAS. *See* SHERLEY, Thomas [1638–1678]

SCHIURFF, AUGUSTIN. *See* SCHURFF, Augustin [1494–1548]

SCHLAM, GUMB [*fl.* 1684] *respondent.* Disputatio medica inauguralis de dysenteria . . . Lugduni Batavorum, Apud Abrahamum Elzevier, 1684.

[16] p.   22 cm.   **[10490]**

Diss. — Leyden.

SCHLANHOVIUS, JOHANNES JOACHIMUS [*fl.* 1635] *respondent. See* SEBISCH, M. [1578–1674?] *praeses.* Collegii therapeutici disputatio I[–XIV] 1634 [i.e. 1635]

SCHLAPPERITIUS, JOHANN LUDWIG [*fl.* 1671–1673] *respondent. See* BROTBECK, J. K., *praeses.* Scrutinium pepasmi sive disquisitio physico-medica de coctione materiae febrilis. 1671; WEDEL, G. W., *praeses.* Disputatio inauguralis medica de vomitu. 1673 [and] Disputatio medico-consultatoria de mania. 1673.

SCHLAPRIZ, JOHANN LUDWIG. *See* SCHLAPPERITIUS, Johann Ludwig [*fl.* 1671–1673]

SCHLEGEL, GOTTFRIED SIGMUND [*fl.* 1691] *respondent.* Disputatio medica inauguralis de incubo . . . Trajecti ad Rhenum, Ex officina Francisci Halma, 1691.

10 p.   21 cm.   **[10491]**

Diss. — Utrecht.

SCHLEGEL, JOHANN [*fl.* 1667–1668] *respondent. See* ROLFINCK, W., *praeses.* Dissertatio medica de phthisi. 1667.

SCHLEGEL, JOHANN ANDREAS [*fl.* 1657–1681] Dissertatio medico-practica de venenis et morbis venenosis, eorumque curationibus et alexipharmacis . . . Erfordiae, Stanno Kirschiano [1679]

[88] p.   21 cm.   **[10492]**

Imperfect: p. [87–88] mutilated.

—Scriptum apologetico-politicum de podagra; oder, Das so benahmte politische . . . Zipperlein, für alle Podagrams-Gedultige . . . geschrieben, darinnen . . . von . . . Ankunfft, Ursprung . . . des . . . Fräuleins-Podagrae, medico-historicoque jocose discuriret wird . . . Weisenfels, Druckts u. Verlegts Joh. Brühl, 1687.

237, [96] p.   front.   14 cm.   **[10493]**

—Tractatus anti-dysentericus; oder, Eigendliche Abhandlung, Anleit- und Beschreibung . . . wie in grassirender epidemischen Seuche, und Beschwerung der Rothen-Ruhr, Dysenteria, ins gemein der Durchlauff genand, sich so wol Gesunde praeservative, und Krancke curative, mit Artzneyen und andern . . . Stücken, recht verhalten, auch . . . wohl verwahren sollen. Benebst einem Anhange von gifftigen Kranckheiten, Bericht von der Pest, Febribus malignis . . . und wie dieselben . . . curiret werden können, aus vornehmer Medicorum Schrifften und eigener Experienz . . . heraus gegeben . . . Weissenfels, Druckts Joh. Brühl, 1681.

[168] p.   19 cm.   **[10494]**

Imperfect: sig. A¹ (blank?) wanting?

SCHLEGEL, JOHANN JACOB [*fl.* 1690] *respondent. See* VESTI, J., *praeses.* Dissertationem inauguralem medicam de pleuritide . . . proponit J. J. S. 1690.

SCHLEGEL, PAUL [*fl.* 1694] *respondent. See* CRAUSE, R. W., *praeses.* Disputatio inauguralis medica de scirrho lienis. 1694.

SCHLEGEL, PAUL MARQUARD [1605–1653] De sanguinis motu commentatio, in qua praecipue in Joh. Riolani, V. C. sententiam inquiritur . . . Hamburgi, Typis Jacobi Rebenlini, sumptu Zach. Hertelii, 1650.

[16], 133, [2] p.   19 cm.   **[10495]**

Dissertations — Jena

—*praeses.* Disputatio medica de epilepsia . . . Jenae, Typis Lobensteinianis, 1642.

[24] p. 19 cm. **[10496]**

G. Gartz, *respondent.*

—Disputatio medica de erysipelate vulgo rosa dicta . . . Jenae, Typis Ernesti Steinmanni, 1640.

[16] p. 21 cm. **[10497]**

J. W. Hopfner, *respondent.*

—Disputatio medica, de saluberrimo venarum, in corpore humano secandarum, delectu . . . Jenae, Typis Johann. Christoph. Weidneri, 1641.

[16] p. 20 cm. **[10498]**

J. C. Eisenmenger, *respondent.*

—Disputatio medica inauguralis, de ascite . . . Jenae, Typis Steinmannianis, 1640.

[28] p. 20 cm. **[10499]**

J. Dammenhan, *respondent.*

—Disputatio medica inauguralis, de empyemate . . . Jenae, Literis Steinmannianis, 1639.

[19] p. 19 cm. **[10500]**

C. P. Tham, *respondent.*

—Disputatio solemnis et inauguralis medica, de haemorrhagia in genere . . . Jenae, Typis Ernesti Steinmanni, 1640.

[23] p. 18 cm. **[10501]**

Imperfect: upper margins trimmed.
J. W. Hopfner, *respondent.*

—Ophthalmographiam et opsioscopiam thesibus succincte comprehensam . . . subjicit Christophorus Schelhammer . . . Jenae, Prelo Steinmannio, 1640.

[20] p. illus. 19 cm. **[10502]**

C. Schelhammer, *respondent.*

SCHLEHER, JOHANN [*fl.* 1611] Ein nutzlicher Bericht und Regiment, wie zu disen gefährlichen Sterbensläuffen vor der Pestilentz umb uns herumb und andern Ohrten eingerissen, Gesunde zu verwahren, unnd Krancke widerumb zu curieren seyen . . . Costantz am Bodensee, Getruckt bey Jacob Straub, 1611.

[8], 132, [2] p. table. 20 cm. **[10503]**

SCHLEMM, JOHANN [1636-1718] Schirm- und Schutz-Flügel, des allmächtigen Gottes, unter welchen man sich zu jederalso absonderlich zur Pestilentz-Zeit zu verbergen, ausgebreitet und

vorgestellet aus dem XCI. Psalm Davids . . . Nebenst angehengten kurtzen, doch nützlichen Fragen von der Pest, Nicolai Selnecceri, D. Jena, Bey Johann Bielken, 1681.

[8], 128 p. 21 cm. **[10504]**

SCHLET, JOHANN HEINRICH [*fl.* 1689] *praeses.* Disputatio medica inauguralis de cephalalgia particulari . . . Trajecti ad Rhenum, Ex officina Francisci Halma, 1689.

42 p. 22 cm. **[10505]**

Diss. — Utrecht.

SCHMALKALDEN, CHRISTIAN GÜNTHER [*fl.* 1683-1694] *respondent. See* BOHN, J., *praeses.* Dissertationes chymico-physicae. 1685; HOFFMANN, F. [1660-1742] *praeses.* Disputatio inauguralis medico-chymica de nitro. 1694.

—*See* VESTI, J., *praeses.* Disputatio medica de epilepsia. 1687.

SCHMALTZ, JAKOB [*fl.* 1671-1676] *respondent. See* ITTIG, J. F., *respondent.* Dissertatio de fontibus. 1672; SAUERBREI, J., *praeses.* Diatriben academicam de foeminarum eruditione posteriorem . . . proponit. 1671, 1676.

SCHMALTZ, QUIRINUS [*fl.* 1622-1629] *praeses.* Theses medicae, de colica . . . Erfurti, Typis Georgi Hertzi, 1629.

[23] p. 19 cm. **[10506]**

Diss. — Erfurt (S. Ortel, *respondent*)

SCHMALZIUS, QUIRINUS. *See* SCHMALTZ, Quirinus [*fl.* 1622-1629]

SCHMEDES, ARNOLD [*fl.* 1697] *respondent.* Disputatio inauguralis medica de chordapso. Et in specie de subjecto ex hoc malo mortuo ac hicce locorum per anatomiam publicam examinato . . . Duisburgi ad Rhenum, Typis Johannis Sas, 1697.

32 p. 20 cm. **[10507]**

Diss. — Duisburg.

SCHMEER, CHRISTIAN [*fl.* 1683] *respondent. See* ORTLOB, J. F., *praeses.* Analogiam nutritionis plantarum & animalium . . . exponet C. S. 1683.

SCHMELTZ, FERDINAND GOTTLIEB [*fl.* 1688-1690] *respondent. See* CAMERARIUS, E. R., *praeses.* Positiones has medicas publico . . . submittit F. G. S. 1690 [and] Theses medicae de tremore a cessante scabie. 1688.

SCHMELTZER, CHRISTIAN [*fl.* 1695] *respondent.*
See PLANER, J. A., *praeses.* De nive dissertatio secunda.
1695.

SCHMER, CHRISTIAN [*fl.* 1680] *respondent. See*
LANI, G., *praeses.* Διάσκεψις philosophiae naturalis
de unguento armario. 1680.

SCHMID, BERNHARD. *See* SCHMIDT, Bernhard [*ca.*
1634-1697]

SCHMID, CHRISTIAN [1651-1705] . . . Resurectio
rerum artificialis . . . [Lipsiae] Excudebat Samuel
Spörel [1677]
    [16] p.   19 cm.   **[10508]**
    Diss. pro loco — Leipzig.

    —*praeses.* De iride . . . Lipsiae, Literis Johannis
Coleri [1673]
    [28] p.   20 cm.   **[10509]**
    Diss. — Leipzig (F. W. Tüchel, *respondent*)

SCHMID, CHRISTOPH [*fl.* 1684] *praeses.* Dissertatio
physica de prodigiis sanguineis vulgo creditis . . .
Lipsiae, Literis Christophori Fleischeri [1684]
    [20] p.   20 cm.   **[10510]**
    Diss. — Leipzig (J. C. Hesse, *respondent*)

SCHMID, ERASMUS. *See* SCHMIED, Erasmus
[1570-1637]

SCHMID, HEINRICH [*fl.* 1674-1676] *respondent. See*
WEDEL, G. W., *praeses.* Dissertatio medica proponens
aegrum palpitatione cordis laborantem. 1674.

SCHMID, JAKOB [*fl.* 1674-1680] *respondent. See*
WEDEL, G. W., *praeses.* Aegrum tertianarium . . .
publico . . . examini sistet J. S. 1674.

SCHMID, JOACHIM [*fl.* 1667] *respondent. See*
WAGNER, G., *praeses.* Problematum physicorum
senarius de margaritis . . . subjicit J. S. 1667.

SCHMID, JOHANN [*fl.* 1697] *respondent. See* DEK-
KERS, F., *praeses.* Disputatio medica de epilepsia. 1697.

SCHMID, JOHANN ANDREAS [1652-1726] Miscellaneorum physicorum fasciculus, XVI. dissertationes
variorum argumentorum continens una cum totius
scientiae naturalis delineatione loco corollariorum addita . . . publico examini submissus . . . Ed. 2.
[Helmstedt] Sumtibus Joh. Jac. Ehrten [1700?]
    [8], 206 p.   20 cm.   **[10511]**
    Imprint partly supplied from BMC.

Dissertations — Helmstedt

    —*praeses.* Dux foemina facti haereseos vel autor vel
fautor; sive mulier heterodoxa . . . ad locum
Hieronymi in epist. ad Ctesiphontem . . . Helmestadii, Typis Georg-Wolfgangi Hammii [1697]
    [4], 56, [4] p.   19 cm.   **[10512]**
    J. W. Offeney, *respondent.*

    —Mulier orthodoxa . . . Helmstadii, Typis Georg-
Wolfgangi Hammii [1698]
    [4], 36 p.   19 cm.   **[10513]**
    G. E. Büsch, *respondent.*

Jena

    —*praeses.* Auris θεοδείκτος . . . Jenae, Literis Kreb-
sianis [1694]
    24 p.   20 cm.   **[10514]**
    E. H. Wedel, *respondent.*

    —Coecus de colore judicans . . . Jenae, Typis
Johannis Jacobi Bauhoferi [1682]
    [24] p.   22 cm.   **[10515]**
    O. J. M. Neovin, *respondent.*

    —Discursus physicus de cerevisia ut est alimen-
tum . . . Jenae, Literis viduae Wertherianae [1680]
    [12] p.   19 cm.   **[10516]**
    H. Weiss, *respondent.*

    —Discursus physicus de lacrymis . . . Jenae,
Literis Wertherianis [1680]
    [12] p.   19 cm.   **[10517]**
    M. Lüder, *respondent.*

    —Dissertatio academica de sectis physicorum in
genere . . . Jenae, Typis Joannis Wertheri [1676]
    [27] p.   19 cm.   **[10518]**
    M. Gebauer, *respondent.*

    —Dissertationem de thermometris . . . submittit
Jo. Ditericus Winckelmann . . . Jenae, Literis
Bauhoferianis [1684]
    22 p.   plates.   19 cm.   **[10519]**
    Imperfect: p. [15-16] mutilated.
    J. D. Winckelmann, *respondent.*

    —Geomantia, olim pulveri inscripta . . . Jenae,
Litteris Mullerianis [1695]
    [4], 96 p.   illus.   19 cm.   **[10520]**
    G. Büching, *respondent.*

    —Lapsus naturae in genere humano . . . Jenae,
Literis Joh. Dav. Wertheri [1689]
    [30] p.   19 cm.   **[10521]**
    A. D. Schrödter, *respondent.*

—Medicinam affectuum ... proponet ... Samuel Antoni ... Jenae, Litteris Mullerianis [1694]

[2], 36 p.   20 cm.   [**10522**]

S. Antoni, *respondent.*

—Surdus de sono judicans ... Jenae, Ex Officina Krebsiana [1690]

20 (i.e. 32) p.   19 cm.   [**10523**]

J. C. Bartholomaei, *respondent.*

SCHMID, JOHANN GABRIEL. *See* SCHMIEDT, Johann Gabriel [*d.* 1686]

SCHMID, JOHANN TOBIAS [*b.* 1675] *respondent. See* WEDEL, G. W., *praeses.* Dissertatio inauguralis medica de asthmatis mechanica. 1700.

—*See* SLEVOGT, J. A., *praeses.* Facultatis Medicae decani Jo. Hadriani Slevogtii ... prolusio inauguralis de natura morborum effectrice. 1700.

SCHMID, JOHANN ULRICH [*fl.* 1678–1680] *respondent. See* WEDEL, G. W., *praeses.* Disputatio medica, de gialapa. 1678.

SCHMID, JOHANNES [1643–1675] Pulveris sympathetici, examen physicum ... Erffurti, Ex Typogr. Johann-Georg. Hertzen, 1668.

[20] p.   19 cm.   [**10524**]

Diss. pro loco—Erfurt (J. W. Andreae, *respondent*)

SCHMID, JOSEPH [*b.* 1601] Examen chirurgicum; das ist, Wie alle junge angehende Feldscherer, Barbier und Wundärtzt sollen befragt werden, wie sie sich in allen begebenden Verwundungen ... verhalten sollen. Ingleichem wie alle chirurgische Instrumenten zugericht, und gebraucht werden, in Kupffer vor Augen gestellt ... Augspurg, Gedruckt durch Johann Schultes, in Verlegung Johann Weh, 1649.

[20], 497, [15] p.; [24], 208 p.   fronts., plates. 14 cm.   [**10525**]

Part [2] has special title page.

Imperfect: part [1]: front., sig.):(12 wanting; part [2]: plates 9, 76, 80, 81 wanting, plate 12 misbound after plate 14.

—[The same.] ... Franckfurt am Mayn, Gedruckt durch Mattheus Kempffern, in Verlegung Johannes Weh in Augsburg, 1660.

[24], 497, [14] p.; [24], 208 p.   front., plates, port.   14 cm.   [**10526**]

Added engraved title page.

Different setting of type.

Imperfect: the texts of parts 1 and 2 interchanged; part [1]: plate 40 misbound after p. 52; part [2]: plates 51–60 wanting.

—Kriegs-Artzney, wessen sich alle junge Wund-Artzt oder Feldscherer bey jetzigen Feldzug wider den Türcken in allem zu bedienen haben ... Franckfurt, Gedruckt bey Matthäo Kempffer; in Verlag Johannes Weh in Augspurg [1664]

[35], 259 p.   front. (port.)   14 cm.   [**10527**]

Added engraved title page.

Imperfect: p. [19–20] mutilated.

—Kurtzer jedoch eigendlicher Bericht, von denen drey ... Seucht, oder Kranckheiten, als die Pest, Frantzosen, und der Scharbock wie solche mögen curirt und gehailt werden ... Augsburg, Gedruckt bey Johann Schultes, in Verlegung Johann Wehen, 1667.

[30], 441 (i.e. 445), [6] p.   plates.   14 cm.
                                             [**10528**]

Added engraved title page.

Errata: p. [6] at end.

—Speculum chirurgicum; oder, Spiegel der Wund-Artzney; darinnen sich alle junge Wund Aertzt zu ersehen, wie allerhand Verwundugen, sie kommen durch Hawen, Stechen, Schiessen, Werfen oder Schlagen ... auch allerley Arthen der offnen Schäden und Kranckheiten, die dem Menschen wiederfahren, innerlich und äusserlich, in Manglung eines Medici, mögen curirt werden. Neben einer Feld- oder Reiss-Apotheken ... Ulm, In Verlegung Johann Wehe, in Augsburg, 1656.

[10], 904, [23] p.   plates.   21 cm.   [**10529**]

Added engraved title page.

—Spiegel der Anatomiae. Darinnen die sinnreiche, künstliche Auffschneidung ... eines menschlichen Leibs ... durch alle desselbigen ... Glidmassen so mit aigentlicher Beschreibung erklärt, als mit lebendigen Contrafacturen fürgebild. Auss den aller vornembsten Autoribus zusammen getragen, und in das kleine Compendium versetzt ... Franckfurt, Bey Johann Friederich Weitz, in Verlegung Johann Weh, 1654.

[24], 455 p.   plates., port.   14 cm.   [**10530**]

Added engraved title page with imprint: Augspurg, in Verlegung Johann Weh, 1646.

Imperfect: p. 17 mutilated; plates 3–6 and 81–83 wanting.

—Another issue.   [**10531**]

Contains only engraved title page and 83 plates.

SCHMID, JUSTUS ANDREAS [*fl.* 1677–1681] *respondent. See* FASCH, A. H., *praeses.* Disputatio medica inauguralis de suffocatione uterina. 1681; WEDEL, G. W., *praeses.* De medicamentorum facultatibus. 1677.

SCHMID, PAUL [*fl.* 1620] *respondent. See* SEBISCH, M. [1578-1674?] *praeses.* Disputatio de hirudinibus, 1620.

SCHMIDEL, JOHANN [1635-1672] *respondent. See* THOMASIUS, J. [1622-1684] *praeses.* De mandragora disputatio philologica. 1671.

SCHMIDICHEN, CHRISTIAN [*fl.* 1658-1659] *praeses.* Disputatio physica de psittaco . . . [Lipsiae] Literis Christiani Michaelis [1659]

[12] p. 19 cm. **[10532]**

Diss.—Leipzig (L. Thilo, *respondent*)

—, *respondent. See* THOMASIUS, J. [1622-1684] *praeses.* Dissertatio philosophica de hibernaculis hirundinum. 1671.

SCHMIDLIN, JOHANN JAKOB [*fl.* 1679-1680] *respondent. See* CAMERARIUS, E. R., *praeses.* Disputatio inauguralis medica, cur epilepsia hodie inter nos tam frequens sit? 1680; METZGER, J. J., *praeses.* Thesium chiriatricarum sylloge VII & ultima, de vesicatoriis. 1679.

SCHMIDLIN, JOHANN ULRICH [*fl.* 1685] *respondent. See* METZGER, G. B., *praeses.* Scrutinium λυθογενεσιαξ in humano corpore ex occasione singularis casus institutum. 1685.

SCHMIDT, BERNHARD [*ca.* 1634-1697] *praeses.* Exercitatio physiologica de hominis aetatibus . . . [Lipsiae] Ex Officina Wittigiana [1655]

[16] p. 19 cm. **[10533]**

Diss.—Leipzig (A. V. Mavius, *respondent*)

SCHMIDT, ELIAS [*fl.* 1658] *respondent. See* MICHAELIS, J., *praeses.* Anatomiam martis; seu, Dissertationem medico-chymicam de ferro . . . subjicit. 1658.

SCHMIDT, ERASMUS. *See* SCHMIED, Erasmus [1570-1637]

SCHMIDT, FRIEDRICH [*fl.* 1654] *respondent. See* EGENOLF, J. A., *praeses.* Disputatio physica de mistione. 1654.

SCHMIDT, GOTTFRIED [*fl.* 1670-1671] *respondent. See* BOHN, J., *praeses.* Exercitationum physiologicarum prima . . . [-decima tertia] 1674?

SCHMIDT, HEINRICH JOACHIM [*fl.* 1678] *respondent. See* CRAUSE, R. W., *praeses.* Disputatio medica de sphacelo. 1678.

SCHMIDT, JAKOB. *See* SCHMID, Jakob [*fl.* 1674-1680]

SCHMIDT, JOHANN [*fl.* 1693-1697] *respondent. See* HARTMANN, P. J., *praeses.* Exercitationum anatomicarum in publicas lectiones de iis quae contra peritiam veterum anatomicam afferuntur in specie, secunda. 1693.

SCHMIDT, JOHANN ANDREAS. *See* SCHMID, Johann Andreas [1652-1726]

SCHMIDT, JOHANN GABRIEL. *See* SCHMIEDT, Johann Gabriel [*d.* 1686]

SCHMIDT, JOHANN HEINRICH [*fl.* 1684-1691] *respondent.* Dissertationem inauguralem de febre petechiali . . . submittet . . . Joh. Henricus Schmidt . . . Altdorffii, Literis Schönnerstaedtianis [1685]

24 p. 20 cm. **[10534]**

Diss.—Altdorf.

—THOMASIUS, G., *praeses.* Dissertationem academicam de aeris gravitate ad aquam comparati p. p. . . . J. H. S. 1684.

SCHMIDT, JOHANN WILHELM [*fl.* 1673] *respondent. See* MAJOR, J. D., *praeses.* Disputatio medica inauguralis de amaurosi vell gutta serena. 1673.

SCHMIDT, JOSEPH. *See* SCHMID, Joseph [*b.* 1601]

SCHMIDT, PAUL CHRISTOPH [*fl.* 1700] *respondent. See* CRAUSE, R. W., *praeses.* Dissertatio inauguralis medica de phthisi. 1700.

SCHMIDT, WILHELM [*fl.* 1627] *respondent. See* FABRICIUS, J., *praeses.* Theses medicae de ephialte. 1627.

SCHMIDTS, MARGARETA [*ca.* 1661] *defendant,* Acten gemässe relatio facti & juris über den zu Braunschweig wider Margareten Schmieds . . . in puncto verdächtigen Kindermords geführten Inquisitions: wie auch wider dero Advocatum D. Justum Oldekoppen, gegen seine damals ordentliche Obrigkeit begangener Widersetzligkeit und eussersten Ungehorsambs halber vollstreckten Verfestungs-Process, zu steuer der Warheit, uff Urtel und Recht daselbst öffentlich mit Ruthen gestrichener Dirnen jetzt benanten Advocato, und dessen in Druck gegebener Famos-Schrifft entgegen gesetzet . . . Braunschweig, Gedruckt durch Christoff-Friederich Zilligern, 1664.

144 p. 18 cm. **[10535]**

SCHMIED, Erasmus [1570–1637] *tr. See* Sennert, D. Practicae medicinae liber primus [-sextus] 1628–1635, 1629–36, 1632, 1636–54, 1653–62.

SCHMIED, Gottfried [*fl.* 1670–1674] *respondent. See* Petermann, D., *praeses.* Disputationem de glacie . . . exponit G. S. 1670; Vehr, I., *praeses.* Disputatio inauguralis medica de gonorrhoea. 1674.

SCHMIED, Johann [*fl.* 1682] *respondent. See* Meibom, H., *praeses.* Disputatio medica inauguralis de concoctione ventribuli laesa. 1682.

SCHMIED, Margareta. *See* Schmidts, Margareta [*ca.* 1661]

SCHMIEDELING, Konrad [*fl.* 1650] *respondent.* Theses inaugurales de angina . . . Argentorati, Typis Eberhardi Welperi, 1650.

    [12] p. 19 cm.   **[10536]**
Diss. — Strasbourg.

SCHMIEDT, Johann Gabriel [*d.* 1686] *respondent. See* Meibom, H., *praeses.* Disputatio medica inauguralis de febribus malignis. 1679 [and] Exercitatio anatomico-medica de valvulis seu membranulis vasorum earumque structura et usu. 1682.

SCHMILAUER, Peter [*fl. ca* 1608] *respondent. See* Tandler, T., *praeses.* De melancholia ejusque speciebus. 1608.

SCHMIT, Peter [*fl.* 1671] *respondent.* Disputatio medica inauguralis de dysenteria . . . Duisburgi ad Rhenum, Apud Franconem Sas, 1671.

    [36] p. 20 cm.   **[10537]**
Diss. — Duisburg.

SCHMITNER, Ahasver [*d.* 1654] *praeses.* Disputatio medica de paresi ex colica . . . Regiomonti, Typis Johannis Reusneri, 1644.

    [20] p. 20 cm.   **[10538]**
Diss. — Königsberg (J. D. Koch, *respondent*)

SCHMITNER, Asver [*fl.* 1610] *respondent. See* Crüger, B., *praeses.* Disputatio medica prima. 1610.

SCHMITZ, Johann Andreas [*d.* 1652] Medicinae practicae compendium. Hardervici, Ex typographia Joannis Tollii, 1653.

    [14], 243, [1] p. 14 cm.   **[10539]**
Preface by Georg Horn, the editor.

—[The same.] . . . Genevae, Sumptibus Petri Chouët, 1659.

    [12], 250, [11] p. 14 cm.   **[10540]**

—[The same.] Opus posthuman quamplurimis supplementis auctum & recensitum a Ch. Constantino Rompfio . . . Accessit . . . D. Ant. Menjotii . . . Epistola apologetica de variis sectis amplectendis. Lutetiae Parisiorum, Apud Joannem d'Houry, 1666.

    [48], 102 (i.e. 402), [42] p. 16 cm.   **[10541]**
Includes Louis Le Vasseur's letter to the editor.

—Another issue. 17 cm.   **[10542]**
Title page and one line on p. [15] at beginning reset.
Interleaved.
Imperfect: all pages after p. 192 wanting.

—[The same.] . . . 4. ed. longe auct. & corr. Lugd. Batavorum, Apud Johannem de Vivie, 1688.

    [44], 495, [42] p. 15 cm.   **[10543]**

—[The same.] . . . Ed. nov. Pluribus morborum hactenus omissorum descriptionibus locupletata, a Joh. Jac. Mangeto . . . Genevae, Apud Joan. Anton. Chouët, 1691.

    [19], 250 p.; 298, [11] p. 14 cm.   **[10544]**

—*See* Deusing, A. De motu cordis et sanguinis. 1655.

SCHMITZ, Peter Heinrich [*fl.* 1694] *respondent.* Disputatio medica inauguralis de lienteria . . . Duisburgi ad Rhenum, Apud Johannem Sas, 1694.

    16 p. 20 cm.   **[10545]**
Diss. — Duisburg.

—*See* Barbeck, F. G., *praeses.* Disputatio medica de vita. 1694.

SCHMOL, Gottfried [*fl.* 1607] *respondent. See* Möller, S., *praeses.* Themata de dysenteria. 1607.

SCHMOLLER, Johann Daniel [*fl.* 1680] *respondent. See* Ammann, P., *praeses.* Disputatio inauguralis de palpitatione cordis. 1680.

—*See* Friess, M. F. Martinus Fridericus Friess . . . pro-cancellarius, L. S. 1680.

SCHMOLLER, Johann Heinrich [*fl.* 1680] *respondent. See* Wedel, G. W., *praeses.* Disputatio medica, aegrum nephritide laborantem, exhibens. 1680.

SCHMUCK, Martin [*d.* 1640?] De occulta magico-magnetica morborum quorundam curatione naturali, tractatus, das ist, wie man auff verborgene natürliche Weise . . . vielerley Kranckheiten . . .

heilen soll. Ein kurtzes Tractätlein . . . durch L. M[artin] S[chmuck] L. Erstlich gedruckt zu Schleusingen, etc. [1636?]

[2], 78 p. 17 cm. [10546]

The dedication signed: H. T. Autor.

—[The same.] . . . Nürnberg, Gedruckt bey Jeremia Dümlern, 1649.

[2], 76 p. 17 cm. [10547]

The dedication signed: H. T. Autor.

Bound with Kessler, Thomas. Fünffhundert . . . chymische Process. 1645.

—Secretorum naturalium, chymicorum & medicorum, thesauriolus; oder, Schatzkästlein, darinnen 20, natürliche, 20. chymische, und 20. medicinische Secreta . . . zu befinden . . . Nürnberg, Gedruckt bey Jeremia Dümlern, 1649.

79 p.; [8], 103 p. 17 cm. [10548]

Part [2] has special title page: Thesaurioli, secretorum naturalium, chymicorum & medicorum, pars altera.

Bound with Kessler, T. Fünffhundert . . . chymische Process. 1645.

—[Excerpts] In Dolhopff, G. A., comp. Lapis animalis microcosmicus. 1681.

SCHMUCKER, MARTIN. See SCHMUCK, Martin [d. 1640?]

SCHMUTZEN, Doctor. See SCHMUZ, Michael Raphael [fl. 1638–1672]

SCHMUZ, MICHAEL RAPHAEL [fl. 1638–1672] Exorcismus medicus manium, larvarum & maleferiatorum spirituum Zwelferianorum, sub personati Friderici Müller a Lewenstein [pseud., i.e. N. Spaenholz] . . . Qui invito fato, exegesi philosophicae Doctoris Schmuzen . . . exorcizandi & abominandi missi & commissi sunt. [n. p.] 1673.

63, [2] p. 18 cm. [10549]

Errata: 2 p. at end.

With this is bound his Jus retorquendi. 1673.

—Jus retorquendi; seu, Apologiae Schmuzianae pars altera Germanica, hoc est, vera et rationalis veteris dispensatorii Augustani restitutio. Contra Joannem Zwelferum pseudo Hippo-Galenicum medicum . . . [n. p.] 1672.

[20], 5–158 p. 18 cm. [10550]

Bound with his Exorcismus medicus manium, larvarum & maleferiatorum spirituum Zwelferianorum. 1673.

—respondent. See HOEVER, W., praeses. Disputatio medica de angina. 1638.

—See ZWELFER, J. Discursus apologeticus. 1668, 1675.

SCHNEEBERGER, ANTON [1530–1581] Catalogus medicamentorum simplicium & facile parabilium pestilentiae veneno ad versantium, Antonii Sneebergeri . . . recognitus & multorum remediorum accessione adauctus. Opera & studio Henrici a Bra . . . Franekerae, Apud Aegidium Radaeum, 1605.

[19], 186 p. 15 cm. [10551]

—[The same.] . . . Leovardiae, Typis Abrahami Radaei, apud Johannem Starterum, 1616.

[19], 186 p. 16 cm. [10552]

A reissue of the 1605 Franeker edition, with title page and preliminary matter reset.

Bound with copy 2 of Bra, H. van. De curandis venenis. 1616.

SCHNEIDER, CONRAD VICTOR. See SCHNEIDER, Konrad Victor [1614–1680]

SCHNEIDER, JOHANN [fl. 1604–1610] respondent. Inauguralia theoremata de syncope . . . Basileae, Typis Johannis Schroeteri, 1608.

[16] p. [10553]

Diss.—Basel.

SCHNEIDER, KONRAD VICTOR [1614–1680] Liber primus [-quintus et ultimus] de catarrhis . . . Wittebergae, Sumptibus haered. D. Tobiae Mevii & Elerdi Schumacheri, excudebat Michael Wendt, 1660–62.

6 parts in 2 v. plates. vol. 1, 20 cm.; vol. 2, 21 cm. [10554]

Parts 5–6 have special title pages.

Parts 1–2 have date: 1660; pts. 3–4: 1661; pts. 5–6:1662. Pts. 2–5 were printed by Johann Hake and pt. 6 by Matthäus Henckel.

Part 5 has title: Liber quintus [Sectio 1]; pt. 6 has title: Liber quintus et ultimus [Sectio 2]

—Liber de catarrhis specialisimus quo juxta Hippocratem libro De gland. & De locis in homine, septem catarrhi . . . pertractantur, cui alius, ad sextum catarrhum spectans, liber De arthritide, podagra & ischiagra, ac de horum morborum curatione jungitur, item Anacephalaeosis . . . Wittebergae, Impensis haered. D. Tobiae Mevii, & Elerdi Schumacheri, typis Matthaei Henckelii, 1664.

[26], 948 p. 20 cm. [10555]

Does not include Anacephalaeosis.

—Liber de morbis capitis; seu, Cephalicis illis, ut vocant, soporosis, atque horum de curatione conditus, quo quidam loci ex medicina praecipue tractantur ... ut: somni naturalis causa proxima ... facultates animae principes ... vertigo ... cataphora ... lethargus ... carus ... apoplexia ... Wittenbergae, Sumptibus haered. D. Tobiae Mevii, & Elerdi Schumacheri, typis Matthaei Henckelii, 1669.
[76], 443, [16] p.; 535, [12] p.   22 cm. [10556]

—Liber de nova gravissimorum trium morborum curatione, de apoplexia ... lipopsychia ... paralysi ... Anacephalaeoses duae, hic subjectae, quarum altera ad apoplexiam spectat, altera ad paralysin. Francofurti, Apud Erasmum Philippum Bakium, literis Michaelis Meyeri, 1672.
[10], 1141, [62] p.   20 cm.   [10557]
Added general title page.

—Liber de osse cribriformi, & sensu ac organo odoratus, & morbis ad utrumque spectantibus, de coryza, haemorrhagia narium, polypo, sternutatione, amissione odoratus. Wittebergae, Typis Jobi Wilhelmi Fincelii, impensis heraed. D. Tobiae Mevii, & Elardi Schumacheri, 1655.
[18], 531 p.   14 cm.   [10558]

—Liber de spasmorum natura et subjecto, nec non et de causis eorum spasmorum ac earum motionum spasticarum et epilepticarum, quae aliquando in recens defunctis ac in occisis corporibus ... manifestantur ... Wittebergae, Typis Johannis Borckardi, excudebat Simon Lieberhirt, 1678.
1 v.   20 cm.   [10559]
Various pagings.

Dissertations — Wittenberg

—*praeses.* Cachexiam ... publice disputandam sistit ... Joh. Christoph. Strauss ... Wittebergae, Typis Michaelis Wendt [1669]
[36] p.   20 cm.   [10560]
J. C. Strauss, *respondent.*

—De pleuripneumonia dissertatio medica in qua statuitur veram sedem peripneumoniae esse utrumque, pleuritidis vero alterutrum tantum latus pulmonum: quae sententia rationibus, Hippocratisque auctoritate imprimis stabilitur ... proponit Christophorus Schrödter ... die 24 April, Ao. 1662. Wittenbergae, Typis Matthaei Henckelii, 1679.
[48] p.   19 cm.   [10561]
C. Schrödter, *respondent.*

—De pleuritide ... Wittebergae, Excudebat Johannes Röhnerus, 1648.
[24] p.   19 cm.   [10562]
G. Loth, *respondent.*

—Disputatio de vera natura & recta ratione curandae phthiseωs conscripta ... Wittebergae, Typis Michaelis Wendt, 1648.
[20] p.   19 cm.   [10563]
S. Grass, *respondent.*

—Disputatio inauguralis de fracturis cranii ... [Wittenbergae] Literis Matthaei Henckelii [1673]
[36] p.   18 cm.   [10564]
A. Homberg, *respondent.*

—Disputatio inauguralis de partu difficili ... [Wittenbergae] Literis Matthaei Henckelii [1675]
[24] p.   19 cm.   [10565]
Z. Mittlacher, *respondent.*

—Disputatio inauguralis de phthisi ... Wittebergae, Typis Johannis Röhneri [1661]
[4], 50 p.   20 cm.   [10566]
J. Föggler, *respondent.*

—Disputatio inauguralis medica de angina ... Wittebergae, Typis Johannis Haken, 1666.
[3], 27 p.   19 cm.   [10567]
J. Friedel, *respondent.*

—Disputatio medica de arthritide ... Wittebergae Typis Friderici Wilhelmi Fincelii, 1663.
[40] p.   18 cm.   [10568]
J. Brewer, *respondent.*

—Disputatio medica de peste, morborum principe ... Wittenbergae, Typis Christiani Schrödteri [1680]
[74] p.   19 cm.   [10569]
J. Gerdes, *respondent.*

—Disputatio medica de sanguine, ut de parte corporis principe, ac tanquam de causa, & sede morborum; tandemque de via illos curandi, instituta ... Wittenbergae, Literis Johannis Wilckii [1679]
[30] p.   18 cm.   [10570]
M. Pauli, *respondent.*

—Disputatio medica de spasmorum subjecto ... Wittebergae, Typis Johannis Borckartdi [1676]
[42] p.   19 cm.   [10571]
J. J. Muller, *respondent.*

—Disputatio medica inauguralis de hydrope . . .
[Wittenbergae] Literis Matthaei Henckelii [1663]
    [40] p. 20 cm.   [10572]
  M. Tiling, *respondent.*

—Disputatio medica inauguralis, dogmatica juxta
& hermetica, de fluxu alvi colliquativo, qui febri est
consectarius . . . Wittebergae, Typis Johannis
Röhneri, 1641.
    [70] p. 20 cm.   [10573]
  J. Bertram, *respondent.*

—Disputationem inauguralem de epilepsia . . .
submittit Johannes Christianus Nettelbach . . . [Wit-
tenbergae] Literis Matthaei Henckelii [1667]
    [1], 54 p. 18 cm.   [10574]
  J. C. Nettelbach, *respondent.*

—Disputationem inauguralem de ictero flavo . . .
publice habebit Johannes Brewer . . . [Wittebergae]
Literis Matthaei Henckelii [1664]
    [62] p. 18 cm.   [10575]
  J. Brewer, *respondent.*

—Disputationem medicam . . . contra ineptam
opinionem Nicolai Chesneau, de spasmorum subjecto . . . habebit Georgius Himselius . . . Wittebergae, Typis Johannis Borckardi, excudebat
Simon Liberhirt [1676]
    [44] p. 20 cm.   [10576]
  Imperfect? all after p. [44] wanting.
  G. Himselius, *respondent.*

—Dissertatio de morbo comitiali medica . . . Wittebergae, Typis Johannis Haken [1664]
    75 (i.e. 77), [1] p. 18 cm.   [10577]
  J. Köckert, *respondent.*

—Dissertationem inauguralem de melancholia seu
delirio tristi . . . submittit M. Christianus Vater . . .
Wittenbergae, Ex officina Christiani Schrödteri [1680]
    [40] p. 19 cm.   [10578]
  C. Vater, *respondent.*

—Lapidem bezoar . . . submittit . . . Gottlieb
Becker . . . Wittebergae, Typis Johannis Haken
[1673]
    [64] p. 19 cm.   [10579]
  G. Becker, *respondent.*

—Paralysin . . . solenni disputationi submittit . . .
Andreas Christoph. Muller . . . [Wittenbergae]
Literis Meyerianis [1670]
    [33] p. 19 cm.   [10580]
  A. C. Müller, *respondent.*

—*See* VESLING, J. Syntagma anatomicum. 1666,
1677, 1696.

SCHNEIDER, THEODOR [*fl.* 1671] Τριχολογία;
seu, Dissertatio physica de pilis quam . . . publicae
disquisitioni ventilandam subjiciunt M. Thedorus
Schneider . . . et Johannes Valentinus Roth . . .
respondens . . . Jenae, Typis Bauhoferianis [1671]
    [40] p. 20 cm.   [10581]
  Diss.—Jena (J. V. Roth, *respondent*)

SCHNELLENBERG, TARQUINIUS [*fl.* 1546] Von
zwantzig Pestilentz Wurtzeln. Bewisse und bewerte
Experiment durch den . . . Herrn, Tarquinium
Ocyorum, alias Schnellenbergium. Franckfurt an der
Oder, Friderich Hartman, 1613.
    [31] p. 16 cm.   [10582]
  Imperfect: wormholes throughout.

—[The same.] Experimenta von zwantig Pestilentz
Wurtzeln. *In* Ryff, W. H. Ein ausserlesen schön
Artzney- und Kräuter Buch. 1629, 1651, 1677.

SCHNETTER, JOHANN [*fl.* 1608] *respondent. See*
LIBAVIUS, A. [*d.* 1616] *praeses.* De syrophoenissa
haemorrhousa. 1608.

SCHNETTER, JOHANN CHRISTOPH [*fl.* 1686]
respondent. See FASCH, A. H., *praeses.* Disputatio inauguralis medica de praedictione mortis. 1686.

SCHNITZER, SIGISMUND [*fl.* 1586–1620] *See* HOR-
NUNG, J., *ed.* Cista medica. 1626?

SCHNIZERUS, SIGISMUNDUS. *See* SCHNITZER,
Sigismund [*fl.* 1586–1620]

SCHNORF, FRANZ BERNHARD [*d.* 1678] Ostentum
Dolanum. *In.* Collectanea de diuturna graviditate.
1662.

SCHNURR, BALTHASAR [1572–1624] Appendix;
oder, Anhang der Schatzkammer menschlicher
Gesundtheit, von allen und jeden so wol gemeinen
als sonderbaren Kranckheiten, Anligen und
Gebresten dess gantzen menschlichen Leibs, innerlichen und eusserlichen Gliedern desselbigen . . .
wie dieselbige beydes durch gemeine Medicamenten
. . . als, Oel, Balsam, Pulver, etc. . . . mögen curirt
. . . werden. In fünff unterschiedliche Theil verfasset
. . . Franckfurt am Mayn, Bey Wolffgang Richtern,
in Verlegung Antonii Hummen, 1613.
    [8], 240 p. 20 cm.   [10583]
  Part [2] of Kunst und Wunderbuch Schazkammer menschlicher
Gesundheit, published in 1611.

—Kunst- Hauss- und Wunderbuch, darinnen allerhand nutzliche Sachen, Wunder- und Kunststücke begriffen . . . Uffs new jetzo verbessert, vermehrt . . . Franckfurt am Mayn, Wilhelm Serlin, 1657.

[12], 960, [35] p.   plates.   17 cm.   **[10584]**

Added engraved title page.

Imperfect: sig. A1 (blank?) wanting? Plates 2 and 3 wanting.

SCHNURREN VON LENDSIDEL, BALTHASAR. *See* SCHNURR, Balthasar [1572-1624]

SCHOBART, CHRISTOPH [*fl.* 1602] *respondent. See* MÖLLER, S., *praeses.* Theses medicae de vertigine. 1602.

SCHOBINGER, BARTHOLOMAEUS [1610-1675] *respondent. See* SEBISCH, M. [1578-1674?] *praeses.* Galeni Ars parva in disputationes triginta resoluta. 1633.

SCHOBINGER, DAVID [*fl.* 1613] *respondent. See* STUPANUS, J. N., *praeses.* De comatibus somnolento ac vigili. 1613.

SCHOBINGER, HEINRICH, *tr. See* FABRICIUS VON HILDEN, W. Lithotomia vesicae. 1640 [and] Opera. 1646, 1682.

SCHOBINGER, JEREMIAS [*fl.* 1650] *respondent.* Disputatio medica inauguralis de morbo strangulatorio; seu maligno faucium carbunculo . . . Athenis Rauracorum, Typis Georgii Deckeri [1650]

[31] p.   20 cm.   **[10585]**

Diss. — Basel.

SCHOCHIUS, ENGELHARD [*fl.* 1623] *respondent. See* INNICHENHÖFER, H., *praeses.* Γπνολογια; sive, Tractatus jucundus physiologicus. 1624.

SCHOCKWITZ, JOHANN [*fl.* 1692-1699] *respondent. See* HOFFMANN, F. [1660-1742] *praeses.* Dissertatio inauguralis chymico-medica de mirabili sulphuris antimoniati fixati efficacia in medicina. 1699; KIRCHMAYER, G. K., *praeses.* Ferax metallor. 1692.

SCHODER, JOHANN SAMUEL [1660?-1740] *respondent.* Prudentiae medicae decus quaesitum; sive, Dirus hydrops, medicor, scandalum, inauguralis dissertatio . . . [Altdorffii] Excudebat Henricus Meyer [1695]

64 p.   20 cm.   **[10586]**

Diss. — Altdorf.

SCHÖN, GREGOR [*fl.* 1595-1610] *respondent.* Theses hasce chirurgico-medicas de fonticulis . . . proponit . . Gregorius Schön. Basileae, Typis Joan. Jacobi Genathii, 1609.

[15] p.   20 cm.   **[10587]**

Diss. — Basel.

With this is bound Platter, F. Felix Platerus . . . decreto die Jovis. 1610.

—*See* PLATTER, F. [1536-1614] Felix Platerus . . . decreto. 1610.

SCHÖN, MICHAEL [*fl.* 1605] *respondent.* Inaugurale medicinae faciendae specimen in erysipelate . . . Basileae, Typis Jani Excertier, 1605.

[12] p.   21 cm.   **[10588]**

Diss. — Basel.

SCHÖNBORN, SAMUEL [*fl.* 1630] Manuale medicinae practicae Galeno-chymicae. Accessere purgantia secundum humores peccantes disposita. Argentorati, Sumptibus Eberhardi Zetzneri, 1657.

[8], 338, [20] p.   14 cm.   **[10589]**

Engraved title page.

SCHÖNEBERG, SEBASTIAN [*fl.* 1634] *respondent. See* BRUNN, J. J. von, *praeses.* Manuductio ad consultationem medicam recte instituendam. 1634.

SCHÖNFELD, DANIEL [*fl.* 1692] *respondent.* Disputatio medica inauguralis de sterilitate . . . Lugduni Batavorum, Apud Abrahamum Elzevier, 1692.

[20] p.   24 cm.   **[10590]**

Diss. — Leyden.

SCHÖNFELD, PHILIPP JAKOB [*fl.* 1662-1686] Historiarum, enarrationum et curationum. Medicarum in certis locis & notis personis observatarum una cum annotationibus theorico-practicis epistolis ad praxin medicam perquam proficuis liber primus [-secundus] Ratisponae, Sumptibus Pauli Dalnsteineri, 1681-86.

2 v.   ports.   17 cm.   **[10591]**

Vol. 2 has imprint: Ratisponae, Typis Joann. Georgii Hofmann, 1686.

—Kurtze Anmahnungen und Lehrstuck in XI. Regl bestehend, an die Hebammen. Allen gebärenden Matronen und Frawen, zu sondern Trost, gezogen auss . . . Balthasaro Timaeo von Gulden Klee . . . und mit . . . Mittlen in ein rechte Ordnung gebracht . . . [Ingolstatt] Gedruckt bey Johann Ostermayr, 1678.

[1], 29 p.   16 cm.   **[10592]**

Bound with *his* Tractatus brevis de hieronosologia. 1675.

—Synopsis medica super Pharmacopoeiam Augustanam pro praecipuis humani corporis affectibus ... cui accessit magni Hippocratis Coi Jusjurandum ... Ingolstadii, Typis Joannis Philippi Zinck, 1677.

[16], 280, [8] p. 17 cm.   [**10593**]

Interleaved.

Jusjurandum, in the Latin version by Johan van Heurne: p. 278-280.

—Tractatus brevis de hieronosologia; seu, Morbo sacro, aut comitiali infantium, puerorum, juvenum et foeminarum. Kurtzer ... Tractat von der Kinderwehe, Fraiss, unnd Hinfallen der Jünglingen, Knaben, Mägdlein, und Weibspersohnen ... Ingolstatt, Gedruckt bey Johann Ostermayr, 1675.

[18], 154, [1] p. 16 cm.   [**10594**]

Errata: p. [1] at end.

With this are bound: *his* Kurtze Anmahnungen und Lehrstuck. 1678; [Brem, W. S.] Nützliche, bewehrte ... Hauss-Mittel. 1665.

SCHÖNFELD, Victorin [1525-1591] *See* Scholtz, L. Consiliorum medicinalium ... liber singularis. 1610.

SCHOENFELDER, Philipp Jacob. *See* Schönfeld, Philipp Jakob [*fl.* 1662-1686]

SCHÖNFELDT, Melchior [*fl.* 1621-1623] *respondent.* Disputatio inauguralis medica de tussi ... Lipsiae, Ex Officina Bavarica [1623]

[16] p. 19 cm.   [**10595**]

Diss.—Leipzig.

—*See* Sultzberger, J. R. De urinis disputato medica. 1621.

SCHÖNGAST, Christoph Andreas [*fl.* 1668] *respondent. See* Sultzberger, S. R., *praeses.* The rickets Anglorum. 1668.

SCHÖNLIN, Johann Theodor [*fl.* 1600-1620] *tr. See* Du Laurens, A. Discursus de visus nobilitate et conservandi modo. 1618 [and] Discursus philosophicus et medicus de melancholia et catarrho. 1620.

SCHÖNWALDER, Melchior [*fl.* 1607-1611] *respondent. See* Stupanus, J. N., *praeses.* De rebus praeternaturam ὑπομνηματισμος pathologicos. 1607.

—*See* Horst, G. [1578-1636] Dissertatio de natura amoris. 1611.

SCHÖPF, Johannes [*fl.* 1622] Ulmischer Paradiss Garten; das ist: Eine Ferzeichnuss unnd Register, der Simplicien an der Zahl uber die 600. welche inn Gärten unnd nechstem Bezirck umb dess ... Statt Ulm zufinden ... Ulm, Gedruckt durch Johann Medern, 1622.

[8], 62 p. 16 cm.   [**10596**]

Bound with Hornung, J. Notwendiger chirurgischer Unterricht. 1622.

SCHOEPFFER, Johann Joachim [1661-1719] *praeses.* Disputatio juridica de haemorrhagia vulneratorum von Verblutung der Verwundeten ... [Rostochii, 1696]

116 (i.e. 152) p. 19 cm.   [**10597**]

Imperfect: lower margin of title page mutilated.

Diss.—Rostock (L. G. von Stötteroggen, *respondent*)

SCHÖPFFER, Peter [*b.* 1662] *respondent. See* Wedel, G. W., *praeses.* Disputatio inauguralis medica de febribus intermittentibus. 1692 [and] Exercitatio medica de phthisi. 1688.

—*See* Wedel, G. W. Propempticon inaugurale de vini dulcis plenis. 1692.

—**SCHOLA** medica in qua Hippocratis, Galeni, Avicennaeque medicinae facile principum, pro tyronibus habentur fundamenta: quibus ad eorundem intellectus magis dilucidandos nonnulla capita materiarum addita sunt. Venetiis, Apud Turrinum, 1663.

3 parts in 1 v. 11 cm.   [**10598**]

Each part has special title page.

Contents.—Pt. [1] Hipocratis [sic] Aphorismi, cum annotationibus Joannis Manelphi. Hippocratis Jusjurandum. Hippocratis Prognosticorum libri tres. [Alexandri Benedicti] Collectiones medicinae, de medici atque aegroti officio.—pt. [2] Galeni Ars medicinalis.—pt. [3] Avicennae fen I, lib. I Canonis.

—[The same.] ... Patavii, Apud Cadorinum, 1682-84.

3 parts in 1 v. 12 cm.   [**10599**]

Parts [2-3] have special title pages.

Part [1] has caption title: Galeni Ars medicin. Nicolao Leoniceno intetprete [sic] ad Graecorum veterum exemplarium fidem ab Augustino Gadaldino aliquibus in locis emendati [sic]

Leaves paged 5-8 and 25-28 in pt. [1] of this copy are either cancels or supplied from another edition.

Contents.—Pt. [1] Galeni Ars medicinalis.—pt. [2] Avicennae Fen I, lib. I Canonis.—pt. [3] Hippocratis Aphorismorum sectiones septem, quibus adjecta fuit & octava. Hippocratis Prognosticorum libri tres.

SCHOLA ALDORFIANA. *See* ACADEMIA ALDORFIANA.

SCHOLA curiositatis. *See* ANTIDOTUM melancholiae. 1670.

SCHOLA MEDICA PARISIENSIS. *See* UNIVERSITÉ DE PARIS. Faculté de médecine.

SCHOLA SALERNITANA. *See* REGIMEN SANITATIS SALERNITANUM. Schola Salernitana. 1649, 1657, 1667, 1683, 1625, 1672. [Dutch tr.] 1658.

SCHOLIN, JOHANN VOLRAD [*fl.* 1700] *respondent. See* VESTI, J., *praeses.* Disputatio inauguralis medica, de arthritide erratica. 1700.

SCHOLTZ, ADAM SIGISMUND [*fl.* 1671–1672] *respondent. See* CRAUSE, R. W., *praeses.* Mars salutifer omnigenum morborum debellator. 1672; ETTMÜLLER, M., *praeses.* Cerebrum orcae vulgari supposititia spermatis ceti larva develatum. 1678.

SCHOLTZ, HEINRICH [*fl.* 1610–1612] *respondent.* Thema de evacuationibus seqq. thesibus explicatum . . . Basileae, Typis Johannis Schroeteri, 1612.

    [II] p.   20 cm.   **[10600]**
Diss. — Basel.

SCHOLTZ, LORENZ [1552–1599] *comp.* Aphorismorum medicinalium, cum theoricorum, tum practicorum . . . sectiones octo. Quarum priores quinque theoricam medicinae partem, ut ex Arabum distinctione appellatur, posteriores vero tres practicam, sic ab iisdem dictam complectuntur . . . Francofurti ad Moenum, Typis & sumptibus Wechelianorum, apud Danielem & Davidem Aubrios & Clementem Schleichium, 1626.

    [36], 437, [I] p.   13 cm.   **[10601]**

—*ed.* Consiliorum medicinalium, conscriptorum a praestantiss. atque exercitatiss. nostrorum temporum medicis liber singularis . . . Nunc primum studio & opera. Laurentii Scholzii a Rosenaw med. Vratisl. hoc modo in lucem editus. Hanoviae, Typis Wechelianis, apud haeredes Joannis Aubrii, 1610.

    [67] p., 1164 cols., [18] p.   illus.   35 cm.
                               [10602]
    Pages [15–16] in second group of paging, blank.
    A corrected reprint of the 1598 Frankfurt am Main edition.
    "Joannis Cratonis, a Kraftheim . . . Μικροτέχνη, seu parva ars medicinalis": p. [29–37]; "Analogismus, sive artificiosus transitus a generali methodo ad exercitationem particularem [ejusdem]": p. [38–67]; "[Ejusdem] De vera praecavendi, & curandi febrem pestilentem contagiosam ratione, ex idiomate Germanico in Latinam linguam conversa, a Dn. M. Martino Weinrichio, M. C.": cols. 1069–1127; "Assertio [ejusdem] . . . pro tractatu praecedente de peste, in quo pestilentem febrem putridam ab ea, quae a contagione oritur, lateque disseminatur, discernit [dated August 1585]": cols. 1128–1157; "Hieronymi Capivaccii . . . De recta cauteriorum administratione": cols. 1158–1164.

    The Consilia (cols. 1–1068) include contributions by Johann Aichholtz, Martin Akakia the younger, Julius Alexandrinus, G. C. Aranzi, Joachim Baudis, Albertino Bottoni, Girolamo Capivaccio, Diomedes Cornarius, Matteo Corti, Johann Crato von Krafftheim, Joachim Curäus, Rembert Dodoens, Girolamo Donzellini, Jacques Dubois, Thomas Erastus, Antonio Fracanzano, Andrea Gallo, Caspar Hofmann, Thomás Jordán, P. A. Mattioli, G. P. Merenda, Philippus Michaelis, Petrus Monavius, Johann and Kaspar Neeffe (Naevius), Helidaeo Padoano, Bernardino Paterno, Johann Pfeil, Matthäus Ratzenberger, Horatius Reserius, Guillaume Rondelet, Isaac Schaller, Balthasar Scheider, Victorin Schönfeld, Augustin Schurff, Abraham Seyller, Petrus Sibyllenus, Johannes Sigismundus, Henricus Stapedius, Matthias Stoius, Hieronimus Stromair, Jean Tagault, Andreas Vesalius, Stanislaus Weiskopf, and Theodor Zwinger.
    With this is bound *his* Epistolarum philosophicarum: medicinalium, ac chymicarum . . . volumen. 1610.

—Epistolarum philosophicarum: medicinalium, ac chymicarum a summis nostrae aetatis philosophis ac medicis exaratarum, volumen . . . Nunc primum labore, ac industria, Laurentii Scholzii a Rosenaw . . . foras datum. Hanoviae, Typis Wechelianis, apud haeredes Joannis Aubrii, 1610.

    [12] p., 536 (i.e. 538) cols., [15] p.   35 cm.
                               [10603]

    Pages [12–13] in second group of paging, blank.
    A corrected reprint of the 1598 Frankfurt am Main edition.
    Includes letters of G. C. Aranzi, [Guillaume] Arragos, Michael Barth, Girolamo Capivaccio, Bartholomaeus Chrysaeus, Paulus Closius, Valerius Cordus, Johann Crato von Krafftheim, Girolamo Donzellini, András Dudith, Thomas Erastus, Hieronymus Herold, Caspar Hofmann, Caspar Lindner, [Arnold] Manlius "Constantinopolitanus", Girolamo Mercuriale, Thomas Moffet, Petrus Monavius, Adolf Occo, Carolus Oslevius, Justinus Petzold, Christoph Pithopoeius, Hieronymus Schaller, Balthasar Scheider, Christoph Schilling, Johannes von Schröter, Abraham Seyller, Georgius Uberus and Theodor Zwinger.
    Bound with *his* Consiliorum medicinalium . . . liber singularis. 1610.

—*See* CRATO VON KRAFFTHEIM, J. Consiliorum & epistolarum medicinalium . . . liber. 1620, 1671.

SCHOLZ, JOHANN [1621–1687?] Prophylaxis circa praesentem & futurum sanitatis statum oratione proposita . . . Noribergae, Typis Michaëlis Endteri, 1665.

    [10], 62 p.   13 cm.   **[10604]**

—Trichiasis admiranda; sive, Morbus pilaris mirabilis observatus ... Noribergae, Literis Michaelis Enderi, 1658.

[12], 95, [1] p. plates. 14 cm. [10605]

—, *tr.* See FABRICIUS, H., ab Aquapendente. Wund-Artznei. 1672, 1673, 1684.

SCHOLZ, LORENZ [*fl.* 1606-1609] *respondent. See* SENNERT, D., *praeses.* Quaestiones medicae controversae sex. 1607.

SCHOLZIUS À ROSENAU, LAURENTIUS. *See* SCHOLTZ, Lorenz [1552-1599]

SCHOMBART, JAKOB [*fl.* 1669] *respondent.* Disputatio medica inauguralis de phthisi ... Lugduni Batavorum, Apud viduam & haeredes Joannis Elsevirii, 1669.

[16] p. 23 cm. [10606]
Diss. — Leyden.

SCHOMBART, JOHANN THEODOR [*fl.* 1693-1694] *respondent.* Disputatio medica inauguralis de respiratione, ejusque difficultatibus & vitiis ... Duisburgi ad Rhenum, Apud Franconem Sas, 1694.

28 p. 20 cm. [10607]
Diss. — Duisburg.

—See BARBECK, F. G., *praeses.* Disputatio medica de generatione animalium. 1693.

SCHOMBURG, JOHANN [*fl.* 1690-1692] *respondent. See* CRAUSE, R. W., *praeses.* Disputatio inauguralis medica de febre quotidiana intermittente. 1692; WEDEL, G. W., *praeses.* Dissertatio medica de catalepsi. 1690.

SCHONAEUS, ADRIANUS [*fl.* 1660] *respondent. See* LINDEN, J. A. van der, *praeses.* Hippocrates de circuitu sanguinis, exercitatio X. 1660.

SCHONDORFF, JOHANN BALTHASAR [*b.* 1672] *respondent. See* HOFFMANN, F. [1660-1742] *praeses.* Disputatio inauguralis medica de chinae chinae modo operandi. 1694; VATER, C., *praeses.* Historiam & curam sarcomatis monstrosi ... subjiciet J. B. S. 1693.

—See HOFFMANN, F. [1660-1742] Propemticon inaugurale de chinae chinae modo operandi, usu. 1694.

SCHONFELD, MELCHIOR. See SCHÖNFELDT, Melchior [*fl.* 1621-1623]

SCHONHOLTZER, JOHANN BALTHASAR [*fl.* 1605-1609] *respondent. See* STUPANUS, J. N., *praeses.* Theses medicae de arthritide. 1606.

SCHONWELDER, MELCHIOR. *See* SCHÖN-WALDER, Melchior [*fl.* 1607-1611]

SCHOOCK, ISAAC [*ca.* 1650-1681] I. Dissertatio physica de nive, cum rarissimis adhaerentibus quaestionibus, de meteoris aqueis. II. Centuria rariorum problematum historico-medico-physicorum. III. Disputatio philosophica inauturalis de honore. Cum mantissa positionum ex universa philosophia selectarum. IV. Oratio singularis de admiratione cum annexa gratiarum actione. V. Oratiuncula qua ornatissmos juvenes a beanissmo absolvit. [Frankfurt an der Oder] Sumptibus Eichornianis, 1673.

[4], 56 + p. 19 cm. [10608]
Imprint partly supplied from BMC.
Imperfect: includes only part I; all pages after p. 56 wanting.

SCHOOCK, MARTIN [1614-1667] De ecstasi tractatus singularis. Quo plurima huc pertinentia, & ab aliis praeterita non modo tractantur; sed & variae quaestiones, qua theologicae, qua philosophicae, & medicae uberius discutiuntur. Groningae Frisiorum, Jacobus Sipkes, 1661.

[8], 146, [2] p. 20 cm. [10609]

—De fermento et fermentatione liber, complectens multa singularia, speciatim rationem coctionis cibi in ventriculo. Groningae, Typis Johannis Cöllenii, 1663.

670 p. 14 cm. [10610]

—De sternutatione tractatus copiosus, omnia ad illam pertinentia, juxta recentia inventa proponens. Ed. alt. priori & emend. & uberior. Amstelodami, Apud Petrum vanden Berge, 1664.

[24], 164 p. 14 cm. [10611]

—Dissertatio de ovo & pullo. Ed. alt. priori auct. & emend. Ultrajecti, Apud Wilhelmi Strick, 1643.

[6], 183, [1] p. 13 cm. [10612]

—Tractatus de butyro. Accessit ejusdem Diatriba de aversatione casei, hac alt. ed. aucta & vindicata. Groningae, Typis Johannis Cölleni, 1664.

[12], 312 p. 14 cm. [10613]
Bound with copy 2 of Deusing, A. Fasciculus dissertationum selectarum. 1660.

SCHOOLA SALERNITANA. *See* REGIMEN SANITATIS SALERNITANUM. [Dutch] Schoola Salernitana. 1658.

SCHOON, THEODORUS, *ed. See* CRAANEN, T. Tractatus physico-medicus de homine. 1689.

SCHOPFF, ABRAHAM [*fl.* 1588–1623] Katholou omnium praesidiorum medicorum universalium et topicorum disquisitio. *See* MÜNSTER, J. Discussio eorum quae ab Abrahamo Schopffio ... scripta sunt. 1603.

SCHOPPE, KASPAR [1576–1649] Consultationes de scholarum & studiorum ratione deque prudentiae & eloquentiae parandae modis. Patavii, Apud Paulum Frambottum, 1636.

 112 p. 14 cm.   **[10614]**
Bound with Pona, F. Ferdinandi Quarto prudentiam medicam ... d. d. 1650.

 — De paedia humanarum ac divinarum literarum ... Aureliae, 1647.

 [1], 59 p. 14 cm.   **[10615]**
Bound with Pona, F. Ferdinando Quarto prudentiam medicam ... d. d. 1650.

SCHOPPEN is troef, of t'samen-spraak tussen een docter en chyrurgijn. [n. p., 1678]

 28 p. 16 cm.   **[10616]**
Occasioned by the controversy between Andreas Boekelman and Bonaventura van Dortmont.

SCHORBOCKS SPIEGEL. *See* VIEL-VERGRÖSTER UND HELLERPOLIRTER SCHORBOCKS-SPIEGEL. 1659.

SCHORER, CHRISTOPH [1618–1671] Bedenken, wie man sich, nechst göttlicher Hülff, vor dem Schlag, oder Gewalt Gottes, versehen und bewahren solle. Sampt einem kurtzen Bericht, was im Nothfall, und in Abwesenheit eines Medici, bey einer vom Schlag getroffenen Person, zu thun seye ... Jetzunder vermehret, und zum dritten Mal gedruckt. Ulm, Bey Balthasar Kühnen, 1665.

 [8], 166 p. 16 cm.   **[10617]**

 — Bericht vom Nutzen und Gebrauch der Fontanellen, und wie man allerley Zufäll darbey theils verhüten, theils begegnen solle ... Ulm, Gedruckt und verlegt durch Balthasar Kühnen, 1664.

 64 p. 17 cm.   **[10618]**

 — [The same.] ... Augspurg, In Verlegung Gottlieb Göbels, gedruckt durch Jacob Koppmayer, 1671.

 64 p. 16 cm.   **[10619]**
Different setting of type.

 — Medicina peregrinantium; oder, Artzney der Raisenden, worinnen begriffen, wie sich die Rai-sende in Essen und Trincken, etc. verhalten, und zugleich allerley Kranckheiten begegnen sollen ... Ulm, Gedruckt und verlegt durch Balthasar Kühnen, 1663.

 [16], 218 (i.e. 220), [11] p. 17 cm. **[10620]**

 — [The same.] ... Anjetzo zum andern Mal getruckt und vermehrt. Ulm, Bey Balthasar Kühnen, 1666.

 [1], 249, [13] p. 16 cm. **[10621]**

 — Reglen der Gesundheit ... Erster Theil [-Anderer Theil] Ravenspurg, Getruckt bey Johann Jacob Wehrlin, in Verlegung dess Authoris, und zufinden bey Hans Jacob Fridawer, 1668.

 [22], 61 p.; [1], 115, [14] p. 14 cm. **[10622]**
Errata: p. [14] at end.
Part [2] has special title page.
Bound with Gufer, J. Tabulae medicae. 1679.

SCHORKOPFF, JUSTUS THEODOR [*fl.* 1685] *respondent.* Dissertatio medica inauguralis de hydrope ovarii muliebris ... Basileae, Literis Jacobi Bertschii [1685]

 [23] p. 19 cm.   **[10623]**
Diss. — Basel.

SCHOTNOVIUS A ZAVORZIZ, HENRICUS SCRETA. *See* SCRETA, Heinrich [1637–1689]

SCHOTNOVIUS A ZAVORZIZ, JOANNES SCRETA. *See* SCRETA, Johannes [*d.* 1651?]

SCHOTT, CASPAR. *See* SCHOTT, Gaspar, *Father* [1608–1666]

SCHOTT, GASPAR, *Father* [1608–1666] Anatomia physico-hydrostatica fontium ac fluminum, libris VI, explicata ... Accedit in fine Appendix de vera origine Nili ... Herbipoli, Excudit Jobus Hertz, sumptibus viduae Jo. Godefridi Schönwetteri Francofurtensis, 1663.

 [22], 433, [15] p. plates. 18 cm. **[10624]**
Added engraved title page.

 — Magia universalis naturae et artis; sive, Recondita naturalium & artificialium rerum scientia ... Opus quadripartitum. Pars I. continet Optica, II. Acoustica, III. Mathematica, IV. Physica ... Herbipoli, Excudebat Henricus Pigrin, sumptibus haeredum Joannis Godefridi Schönwetteri Francofurtens. 1657–77.

 4 parts in 2 v. illus., plates. 22 cm. **[10625]**

Each part has special title page. Parts 1 and 2 dated 1657; parts 3 and 4 dated 1677.

Each part has added engraved title page: those of parts 1 and 3 are undated, part 4 has date 1659.

Imperfect: plates 19 and 21 of part 2 wanting; added engraved title page of part 2 wanting.

— Physica curiosa; sive, Mirabilia naturae et artis libris XII. comprehensa, quibus pleraque, quae de angelis, daemonibus, hominibus ... rara, arcana, curiosaque circumferuntur, ad veritatis trutinam expenduntur ... Herbipoli, Sumptibus Johannis Andreae Endteri & Wolffgangi Jun. haeredum, excudebat Jobus Hertz, 1662.

[55], 1583, [24] p.   illus., plates.   21 cm.
[10626]

Engraved title page.

— [The same.] ... Ed. alt. auctior. Herbipoli, Sumptibus Johannis Andreae Endteri & Wolfgangi Jun. haeredum, excudebat Jobus Hertz, 1667.

[56], 1389, [23] p.   illus., plates.   21 cm.
[10627]

Added engraved title page.
Errata: p. [22-23] at end.

SCHOTT, Johann Adam [*fl.* 1678] *respondent. See* Crause, R. W., *praeses.* Disputationem inauguralem medicam de febre quartana intermittente ... subjiciet J. A. S. 1678; Wedel, G. W. Dissertatio medica de variolis et morbillis. 1678.

SCHOTT, Reinhard Moritz [*fl.* 1694] *respondent.* Disputatio medica inauguralis de dysenteria ... Giessae Hassorum, Typis Henningi Mülleri, 1694.

24 p.   20 cm.
[10628]
Diss. — Giessen.

SCHOTTELIUS, Elias [*fl. ca.* 1655] *ed. See* Nardi, G. Noctes geniales. 1656.

SCHOTUS, Michaelis. *See* Scott, Michael [1175?-1234?]

SCHOUTEN, Wouter [1638-1704] Het gewonde hooft; of, Korte verhandeling van de opper-hoofts-wonden en bekkeneelsbreuken. Van den wonden des aangesigts en van de wonden des hals ... Door aanmerkelijke voorvallen bevestigt ... Amsterdam, Abraham van Someren, 1694.

[32], 3-296 p.   17 cm.
[10629]

— [German tr.] Walter Schultzens ... Verletzter Kopff; das ist, Kurtze und gründlich untersuchte

Heil-Kunst aller und jeder Kopff-Wunden und Brüche der Hirnschaalen, ingleichen der Wunden des Angesichts, und des Halsses ... Aus den holländischen in die hochteutsche Sprache übersetzet von D. Joh. Christian Rothochs. Leipzig, Joh. Ludwig Gleditsch, und M. G. Weidmanns seel. Erben, 1695.

[28], 279, [9] p.   front. (port.)   17 cm.
[10630]

Imperfect: p. [9-12] wanting.

SCHRADER, Friedrich [1657-1704] De admiranda naturae in operibus suis subtilitate oratio, habita die xxvii. Sept. anno CIC ICC LXXXIII. Helmestadi, Typis Georg-Wolfgangi Hammii, 1684.

[22] p.   20 cm.
[10631]

— Dissertatio epistolica de microscopiorum usu in naturali scientia & anatome ... Gottingae, Typis Johannis Christophori Hampii [sic], sumptibus Bartholdi Fuhrmanns, 1681.

36 p.   16 cm.
[10632]

— Programma cum anatomen publicam in viril cadavere anno M DCC institueret P. P. d. IV. Februarii. Helmestadii, Typis Georg-Wolfgang Hammii, 1700.

[8] p.   20 cm.
[10633]

— Programma quo exercitationes medicas publice habendas significat ad easque ... invitat Fridericus Schraderus ... Helmestadii, Typis Georg Wolfgang Hammii, 1699.

[16] p.   19 cm.
[10634]
Program — Helmstedt (with vita of D. A. Herstelle)

Dissertations — Helmstedt

— *praeses.* De frigoris natura ... Helmestadii Typis Georg-Wolfgangi Hammii [1684]

[28] p.   20 cm.
[10635]
J. B. Slepper, *respondent.*

— De regularum sanitatis prudenti application dissertatio ... Helmestadii, Typis Georgii Wolfgang Hammii [1698]

[58] p.   18 cm.
[10636]
S. C. Rimpau, *respondent.*

— De signis medicis exercitatio prima [-tertia] .. Helmestadii, Typis Georg-Wolfgangi Hammii 1699-1700.

3 vols.   19 cm.
[10637]
D. A. Herstelle, *respondent.*

—Disputatio medica de febre quartana ... Helmstadii, Typis Salomonis Schnorrii [1694]

[24] p. 18 cm.   [**10638**]

G. Loffhagen, *respondent.*

—Disputatio medica de hemicrania ... Helmstadii, Typis Georg-Wolfgangi Hammii [1690]

[30] p. 18 cm.   [**10639**]

J. H. Kreienberg, *respondent.*

—Disputatio medica de vulnerum cura ... Helmstadii, Typis Georg-Wolfgangi Hammii [1695]

[24] p. 20 cm.   [**10640**]

J. H. La Roche, *respondent.*

—Disputatio medica inauguralis de idiosyncrasiis ... Helmestadii, Typis Georg-Wolfgangi Hammii [1696]

[48] p. 20 cm.   [**10641**]

D. V. Kramer, *respondent.*

—Disputatio medica inauguralis de venae sectionis usu et abusu in febribus ... Helmestadii, Typis Georg-Wolfgangi Hammii [1686]

[24] p. 19 cm.   [**10642**]

A. P. Conradi, *respondent.*

—Disputatio medica inauguralis lympham et glandulas pathologice considerans ... Helmstadii, Typis Georg-Wolfgangi Hammii [1686]

[20] p. 20 cm.   [**10643**]

H. Neubaur, *respondent.*

—Dissertatio medica inauguralis de senectutis praesidiis ... Helmestadii, Typis Georg-Wolfgangi Hammii, 1699.

[44] p. 20 cm.   [**10644**]

J. H. Blume, *respondent.*

—Dissertatio physica de habitaculis animantium ... Helmestadii, Literis Henrici Hessii [1685]

[32] p. 20 cm.   [**10645**]

J. G. Lesch, *respondent.*

—Exercitatio academica de aeris in corpus humanum effectibus ... Helmestadii, Apud Henricum Hessium [1685]

[32] p. 20 cm.   [**10646**]

G. C. Wolff, *respondent.*

—Exercitatio academica de insipidorum efficacia ... Helmestadii, Typis Georg-Wolfgangi Hammii [1687]

[40] p. 20 cm.   ⌜**10647**⌝

O. A. Ripenhausen, *respondent.*

—Exercitatio medica de cognoscendis medicamentorum facultatibus ... Helmestadii, Typis Georg-Wolfgangi Hammii [1685]

[34] p. 20 cm.   [**10648**]

G. E. Crauel, *respondent.*

—Exercitatio medica de doloribus ... Helmstadii, Typis Georg-Wolfgangi Hammii [1688]

[35] p. 20 cm.   [**10649**]

R. Hake, *respondent.*

—*respondent.* See CELLARIUS, J., *praeses.* Exercitatio academica de natura panis. 1676.

SCHRADER, JOHANN DANIEL [*fl.* 1678] *respondent.* See WEDEL, G. W., *praeses.* Dissertatio medica de urinis. 1678.

SCHRADER, JUSTUS [*b.* 1646] *ed. See* LE BOË , F. de. Praxeos medicae liber quartus, de morbis infantum. 1674.

—*See* HARVEY, W. Observationes et historiae omnes & singulae e Guilielmi Harvei libello De generatione animalium excerptae. 1674.

SCHRADER, MATTHIAS [*fl.* 1686] *respondent.* See HARDT, J. G., *praeses.* Dubium physicum quoad ignis receptum calorem extricatum. 1686.

SCHRAGE, JOHANN GUALTER [*fl.* 1691] *respondent.* Disputatio medica inauguralis de lue venerea ... Franequerae, Apud Johannem Gyselaar, 1691.

16 p. 19 cm.   [**10650**]

Diss. — Franeker.

SCHRAMM, GOTTLIEB GEORG [1640–1673] *respondent.* Disputatio inauguralis medica de angina ... Lugduni Batavorum, Ex officina Salomonis Wagenear, 1665.

[16] p. 20 cm.   [**10651**]

Diss. — Leyden.

—*See* SENNERT, M., *praeses.* Disputationem anatomicam de cerebro ... subjicit G. G. S. 1662.

SCHRAMM, MICHAEL [*fl.* 1692] *respondent.* See SCHELHAMMER, G. C., *praeses.* Dissertationem medicam inauguralem de lethargo ... submittit M.S. 1692.

SCHRECK, CHRISTIAN HEINRICH [*fl.* 1698] *respondent. See* VESTI, J., *praeses.* Diatribe inauguralis medica, de mictu cruento. 1698.

SCHREIBER, Christoph [*fl.* 1682] Der Engel, der Verderber im Volck; das ist, Die traurige Geschicht von der grossen Pest in Israel, zu Davids Zeiten ... erkläret ... in sechzehn Predigten, als der gerechte Gott mit gleicher Plage dieselbe Anheim gesuchet hatte, im Jahr Christi MDCLXXX ... Budissin, Bey Andreas Richtern, 1682.

[8], 400, [7] p. 21 cm. **[10652]**

SCHREIBER, Johann Christoph [*fl.* 1678] *respondent. See* Thomasius, J. [1622-1684] *praeses.* Dissertatio historica de Pertro Dresdensi. 1678.

SCHREIBER, Johann Christoph [*fl.* 1685] *respondent.* Disputatio medica inauguralis de aerumnis archei in negotio phantasiae ad praxin clinicam accommodata ... Giessae Hassorum, Literis Kargerianis [1685]

28 p. 19 cm. **[10653]**

Diss. — Giessen.

SCHREIBER, Johann Wolffgang [*fl.* 1658] *respondent. See* Frommann, J. C., *praeses.* Exercitationem physico-medicam de consensu partium corporis humani ... publicae eruditiorum censurae sistunt ... J. C. F. ... ac ... J. W. S. 1658.

SCHREINER, George Eberhard [*fl.* 1631-1638] *ed. See* Theodorus, *medicus.* Diaeta. 1632.

SCHREY, Caspar Heinrich [*fl.* 1678-1696] Neugefasster uhralter wolckensteinischer Warmen-Bad- und Wasserschatz, sambt angehengten einigen ... Curen, nebst Herr D. Hauptmanns Admonition an die Herren Badegäste, wie auch solches Warmenbades neue Befestigung wider Herrn D. Melchiors ... Hydrologiam, mit Erörterung der Fragen ob unser wolckenst. Frauenbad wider Unfruchtbarkeit und alzufrühzeitig Gebähren der Weiber, auch wenn solche von Zauberey herkomme, dienlich? ... Leipzig, Zufinden bey Jeremias Schreyen, 1696.

47, [1] p. plate. 16 cm. **[10654]**

Does not include the test of Hauptmann's Admonition.
Bound with Hauptmann, A. Uhralter wolckensteinischer ... Wasser-Schatz. 1657.

—[The same.] Neugefaster uhralter wolckensteinischer Warmer-Bahd- und Wasser-Schatz; das ist, Kurtze ... Beschreibung des so genanten Warmen-Bahdes zu unserer lieben Frauen aufn Sande samt angehängten einigen ... Curen ... nebst Hn. D. Augusti Hauptmanns ... Admonition

an die Herren Bahde-Gäste ... Franckfurt an der Oder, Zufinden bey Jeremias Schrey, druckts Tobias Schwartze, 1696.

[12], 100 p. plate. 17 cm. **[10655]**

Imperfect: plate wanting.

—Ortus sterilitatis et abortus e fascino in ejusdem ultionem. Oder progressum generationis humanae dass ist Erörterung der Frage ob und wie Unfruchtbarkeit und allzu frühzeitig Gebähren, so von Zauberey herkommet, durch unser wolckensteinisches Frauen-Bad, als sonst Sterilitas und Abortus cururet werde? ... Leipzig, Bey Jeremias Schreyer, 1696.

47, [1] p. 17 cm. **[10656]**

—Thermarum contenta rejecta & retenta; das ist, Des uhralten-neugefassten Warmen-Bad- und Wasser-Schatzes, so wohl neue Befestigung wider die von Herrn Doct. Melchiorn ... herausgegebenen Hydrologiam; als auch Erörterung der Frage, ob temperirte Bäder so kräfftig, ja besser, als heisse sind? ... Leipzig, Zufinden bey Jeremias Schreyen, 1696.

72 p. 17 cm. **[10657]**

—*respondent.* Ortus morborum e fermento ventriculi in eorum ultionem ad vitam sanam ... Altdorffii, Typis Johannis Henrici Schönnerstaedt [1678]

27 p. 20 cm. **[10658]**

Dis. — Altdorf.

—*ed. See* Discursus medicus de impotentia virili theoretico-practicus. 1698.

SCHREYER, Johann [*fl.* 1655-1694] Erörterung und Erläuterung der Frage, ob es ein gewiss Zeichen wenn eines todten Kindes Lunge im Wasser intersincket, dass solches in Mutter-Leibe gestorben sey? ...[Zeitz] Gedruckt durch Johann Heinrich Ammersbachen, 1690.

35 p. 19 cm. **[10659]**

With this is bound *his* Erörterung. Halle, 1745.

—, *respondent. See* Schenck, J. T., *praeses.* Disputatio medica inauguralis de ephemera. 1658.

—, *tr. See* Neues Liecht vor die Apothecker. 1690, 1700; Overkamp, H. Neues Gebäude der Chirurgie. 1689, 1692 [and] Oeconomia animalis. 1690.

SCHRIJVER, PIETER [1576–1660] Saturnalia. *In* Regiman sanitatis Salernitanum. Schola Salernitana. 1649, 1657, 1667, 1683.

SCHRIZMEIER, HEINRICH [*fl.* 1662] *respondent.* Disputatio medica inauguralis, de asthmate . . . Lugduni Batavorum, Apud Philippum de Croy, 1662.

   [16] p.   21 cm.   **[10660]**

Diss. — Leyden.

SCHROECK, LUCAS [1646–1730] Historia moschi, ad normam Academiae Naturae Curiosorum conscripta . . . Augustae Vindelicorum, Impensis Theophili Göbelii, excudit Johann. Jacob. Schönigkius [1682]

   [13], 224, [5] p.   front., plates.   21 cm.
                                       [10661]

Errata: p. [5] at end.

— Hygea Augustana; seu, Memoria secularis Collegii Medici Augustani . . . Augustae Vindelicorum, Typis Koppmayerianis excudi curabat Theophilus Göbelius [1682]

   [24] p.   20 cm.   **[10662]**

— Memoria Welschiana; sive, Historia vitae . . . Georgii Hieronymi Welschii . . . Augustae Vindelicorum, Impensis Theophili Göbelii, typis Koppmayerianis, 1678.

   90 p.   21 cm.   **[10663]**

—, *respondent. See* ROLFINCK, W., *praeses.* Ad chimiam in artis formam redactam . . . expositae . . . 1669; SCHENCK, J. T., *praeses.* Dissertatio inauguralis medica de bulimo. 1669 [and] Exercitationem academicam de moscho . . . submittit . . . L. S. 1667.

—, *ed. See* HELLWIG, J. Observationes physico-medicae. 1680; WELSCH, G. H. Curationum propriarum . . . decades X. 1681.

— *See* FELIX, A. *Father.* De ovis cochlearum epistola. 1684; MARSIGLI, A. F. De ovis cochlearum epistola. 1684; MURALT, J. von. Chirurgische Schrifften. 1691; PHARMACOPOEIA AUGUSTANA. 1684, 1694; SPAENHOLZ, N. Eilfertiges Gutachten Philonis Nasturtii Zwelferischen Bundesgenossen. 1673.

SCHRÖDER, AUGUST KONRAD [*fl.* 1695] *respondent. See* MEIBOM, H., *praeses.* Exercitatio medica inauguralis de hydrope ascite. 1695.

SCHROEDER, CASPAR, *pseud. See* HELLWIG, Christoph von [1663–1721]

SCHRÖDER, CHRISTOPH PAUL [*fl.* 1692] *praeses.* Dissertatio inauguralis medica de requisitis veri medici . . . Erfordiae, Typis Kindlebii [1692]

   63 p.   19 cm.   **[10664]**

Diss. — Erfurt (J. M. Kniphof, *respondent*)

SCHRÖDER, HEINRICH [*fl.* 1663] *respondent. See* ROLFINCK, W., *praeses.* Dissertatio medica de chylificatione laesa. 1663.

SCHRÖDER, JOHANN [1600–1664] Pharmacopoeia medico-chymica; sive, Thesaurus pharmacologicus, quo composita quaeque celebriora, hinc mineralia, vegetabilia & animalia chymico-medice describuntur, atque insuper principia physicae Hermetico-Hippocraticae . . . exhibuntur . . . Ulmae, Sumptibus Johannis Gerlini, 1641.

   1 v.   illus.   20 cm.   **[10665]**

Various pagings.
Imperfect: p. 155–158 in Liber IV mutilated.

— [The same.] . . . Ed. 3 . . . auctum ac emend. . . . Ulmae Suevorum, Impensis Johannis Gerlini, 1649.

   [26], 516, 348, [60] p.   illus.   21 cm.   **[10666]**

Added engraved title page dated 1650.

— [The same.] . . . Ed. 4 . . . auctum, ac emend. Lugduni, Sumptibus Petri Regaud, 1656.

   [52], 742, [30] p.   illus.   24 cm.   **[10667]**

Added engraved title page.

— [The same.] . . . Ed. 5. . . . auctum. corr. & emend. . . . Ulmae Suevorum, Impensis Johannis Görlini, typis Joh. Wyrichl Rösslini, 1662.

   [26,] 516, 348, [60] p.   illus.   20 cm.   **[10668]**

Added engraved title page has date: 1655.
A reprint of the 1649 edition.

— [The same.] . . . Ed. ult. . . . auctum, corr. ac emend. Lugduni, Sumpt. Philippi Borde, Laurentii Arnaud, Petri Borde, Guill. Barbier, 1665.

   [52], 742, [30] p.   illus.   24 cm.   **[10669]**

A reprint of the 1656 edition.

— [The same.] . . . Ed. ult. corr., tribus linguis Gallica, Anglica & Belgica, totidemque indicibus aucta . . . Lugduni-Batavorum, Apud Felicem Lopez d'Haro [ex typographia Severini Matthiae] 1672.

   [64], 872, [74] p.; [1], 4-33, [1], [58] p.   illus.   20 cm.   **[10670]**

Added engraved title page.
Part [2] has half title: Appendix pharmacorum in Schröderi Pharmacopoeia omissorum.
Imperfect: p. 23-24 at end mutilated.

—[The same.] ... Opus ... post editionem Horstio-Witzelianam, qua Appendix, & ... linguae Gallicae, Anglicae, & Belgicae, nomina, & indices accessere. Hac septima emendatum, omissis locupletatum, notisque auctum a Joanne Ludovico Witzelio ... Francofurti, Sumptibus viduae Joan. Görlini, typis Joan. Görlini, 1677.

[68], 508, 384, [99] p.; 32, [88] p. illus. 21 cm. **[10671]**

—[The same.] ... Juxta editonem Witzelianam synopsi, Appendice ... locupletatam ... Lugduni, Sumptib. Petri Borde, Joan. & Petri Arnaud, 1681.

[24], 44, 786, [132] p. illus. 24 cm. **[10672]**

— [The same.] Pharmacopoea Schrödero-Hoffmanniana illustrata et aucta, qua composita quaeque celebriora, hinc mineralia, vegetabilia & animalia chimico-medice describuntur, atque insuper principia physicae Hermetico-Hippocraticae ... exhibentur. Opus ... tum pharmacologorum & chimiatrorum, tum celeberrimorum inter recentiores practicorum, tum operum variorum miscellaneorum ... ditatum. Compilavit Johannes Jacobus Mangetus ... Genevae, Sumptibus Samuelis de Tournes, 1687.

[55], 800, [96] p. illus., plates. 38 cm. **[10673]**

"Appendix ... continens tractatus duos: ... Frederici Hoffmanni Thesaurum pharmaceuticum ... et Martini Bernhardi de Bernitz ... Fasciculum medicamentorum singularium ... Andreae Cnöffelii ... & aliorum ... medicorum arcana et experimenta specifica": p. [649]-800.

"D. Andreae Cnöffelii ... Consilium; sive, Prognosis et curatio affectionum ... Vladislao IV. familiarium": p. 705-776.

The Excerpta e pharmacopoea Persica and Excerpta e laboratorio Ceylonico are by François Bernier (p. 780 [i.e. 778]-800)

—[English tr.] The compleat chymical dispensatory, in five books, treating of all sorts of metals, precious stones, and minerals, of all vegetables and animals ... and how they are to be used in physick; with their several doses ... Written in Latin ... and Englished, by William Rowland ... London, Printed by John Darby, for Richard Chiswell, and Robert Clavell, 1669.

[5], 283, 385-545, [12] p. illus. 31 cm. **[10674]**

—[French ed.] La pharmacopée raisonnée ... commentée par Michel Ettmuller. Tome premier [-second] Lyon, Thomas Amaulry, 1698.

2 v. 20 cm. **[10675]**

—[German tr.] Trefflich-versehene medicin-chymische Apotheke; oder, Höchstkostbarer Arzeneÿ-Schatz ... Dabey ferner zu mehrerm Verständnis aller Materien, ein zumahl höchstdienlich-nöthig- und nützlicher Schlüssel in ... Friedrich Hoffmanns ... Anmerkungen bestehend ... auch rarester Arzneymittel der fürtreflichsten Herrn Medicorum, insonderheit des ... D. Johann Michaelis beygefüget ... mit einem pharmaceutischen Schatz der ruhmwürdigsten Arzneymittel dieser Zeit ausgeschmücket, in die hochteitsche Sprache übersetzet und ans Licht gegeben wird von Johann Ulrich Müllern ... Nürnberg, Verlegts Johann Hoffman, gedruckt zu Jena mit Nisiussischen Schrifften, 1685.

[8], 1526, [32] p. illus. 22 cm. **[10676]**

Added engraved title page.

—[The same.] Vollständige und nutzreiche Apotheke; das ist, D. Johannis Schroederi treflich-versehener medicin-chymischer ... Artzney-Schatz nebst D. Friderici Hoffmanni ... Anmerckungen ... aus denen itziger Zeit ... berühmtester Medicorum und anderer gelahrtesten Männer ... Schrifften ... zusammen getragen und vermehret ... Teutscher Nation zu sonderem Nutzen eröffnet von George Daniel Koschwitz ... Nürnberg, In Verlegung Johann Hoffmans, gedruckt bey Andreas Knortzen seel. Wittib., 1693.

[13], 1340, 120, [52] p. front. (port.), plates. 34 cm. **[10677]**

Added engraved title page.

Includes the translation of Pharmacopoea Schrödero Hoffmanniana.

Imperfect: p. 1323-24, and p. 1329-30 wanting.

—as subject. See HOFFMANN, F. [1626-1675] Clavis pharmaceutica Schröderiana. 1675, 1681.

—Ζωολογια; or, The history of animals as they are useful in physick and chirurgery ... London, Printed by E. Cotes for R. Royston, 1650 (i.e. 1659?)

[6], 159, [9] p. 19 cm. **[10678]**

Imperfect: first preliminary leaf wanting.

Translator's address to the reader signed: T. B[ateson]

— ed. See DUCHESNE, J. Quercetanus redivivus. 1648, 1679; HAYNE, J. Drey unterschiedliche neue Tractätlein. 1663; SALA, A. Opera omnia medico-chymica. 1682.

—See ETTMÜLLER, M. Opera medica theoretico-practica. 1696-1697 [and] Opera omnia. 1688 [and]

Opera omnia medico-physica, theoretica et practica. 1700 [and] Operum omnium medico-phisicorum. 1690 [and] Opera pharmaceutico-chymica. 1686; MICHAELIS, J. Opera. 1698.

SCHRÖDTER, ADOLPH DIETRICH [*fl.* 1689] *respondent. See* SCHMID, J. A., *praeses.* Lapsus naturae in genere humano. 1689.

SCHRÖDTER, CHRISTOPH [1641–1706] *respondent. See* SCHNEIDER, K. V., *praeses.* De pleuripneumonia dissertatio medica. 1679.

SCHRÖER, JOHANN CHRISTOPH [*fl.* 1691–1704] *respondent. See* ORTLOB, J. F., *praeses.* Exercitium anatomico-physiologicum . . . exponit J.C.S. 1691.

SCHROEER, SAMUEL [1669–1716] Brevis, sat tamen curiosa in naturam opii inquisitio; h. e., Opii intima & accurata examinatio, in qua variis ratiociniis & experimentis demonstratur . . . Lipsiae, Typis atque impensis Joh. Wilhelmi Krügeri, 1696.
80, [1] p. 17 cm. **[10679]**
Errata: p. [1].

—*respondent.* Disputationem inauguralem de opii natura et usu . . . submittit . . . Samuel Schroeerus . . . Erfurti, Typis Joh. Henrici Kindlebii [1693]
16 p. 19 cm. **[10680]**
Diss.—Erfurt.

SCHRÖN, DÁNIEL CHRISTIAN [*fl.* 1688–1690] *respondent. See* CRAUSE, R. W., *praeses.* Disputatio inauguralis medica de ulceribus uteri. 1690.

SCHRÖTER, CASPAR, *pseud. See* HELLWIG, Christoph von [1663–1721]

SCHRÖTER, ERNST FRIEDRICH [1621–1676] *praeses.* Dissertationem de stylo curiae . . . publicae disquisitioni subjicit Christophorus Reichardus . . . ad d. XXVII Mart. anno M DC LXXII. Jenae, Recusa a Jeremia Neppio, 1688.
[40] p. 21 cm. **[10681]**
Diss.—Jena, 1672 (C. Reichard, *respondent*)

SCHRÖTER, JOHANN [*fl.* 1662] *respondent. See* SCHENCK, J. T., *praeses.* Exercitatio anatomica . . . de partibus generationi inservientibus masculis. 1662.

SCHRÖTER, JOHANN CHRISTIAN [*b.* 1662] *respondent. See* FASCH, A. H., *praeses.* De chylificatione laesa. 1689.

—*See* CRAUSE, R. W. Decanus Collegii Medici

Rudolfus Wilhelmus Crausius . . . Lectori benevolo salutem plurimam. 1689.

SCHRÖTER, JOHANN FRIEDRICH [1559–1625] *praeses.* Αγωνισμα medicum, De sanitate et indicationibus . . . Jenae, Typis Tobiae Steinmanni, 1609.
[22] p. 19 cm. **[10682]**
Diss.—Jena (J. E. Flösserus, *respondent*)

—Dysenteriae αποθεραπεια ιατρικη . . . Genae, Typis Christophori Lippoldi [1602]
[8] p. 20 cm. **[10683]**
Diss.—Jena (P. Krauss, *respondent*)

SCHRÖTER, JOHANNES VON [1513–1593] *See* SCHOLTZ, L. Epistolarum philosophicarum: medicinalium, ac chymicarum . . . volumen. 1610; SENNERT, D. De febribus libri IV. 1628, 1633, 1641, 1653.

SCHRÖTER, MORITZ [*fl.* 16th–17th cent.] *See* JUDICIA e multis quaedam virorum reverendorum . . . de laboribus Dn. Petri Kirstenii. 1611.

SCHRÖTER, PHILIPP JAKOB [1553–1617] *praeses.* De diaeta aegrorum themata medica . . . Jenae, Typis Lippoldianis, 1607.
[22] p. 19 cm. **[10684]**
Diss.—Jena (C. Fulda, *respondent*)

—De incubone disputatio medica . . . Genae, Tobias Steinman, 1602.
[8] p. 20 cm. **[10685]**
Diss.—Jena (J. Fabricius, *respondent*)

SCHROTERUS, JOANNES. *See* SCHRÖTER, Johannes von [1513–1593]

SCHUBART, TOBIAS [*fl.* 1696–1698] *respondent. See* VATER, C., *praeses.* Exercitatio chimica de spiritibus chimicis. 1696.

SCHUBARTH, GEORG [*fl.* 1698] *respondent.* Disputatio medica inauguralis de apoplexia . . . Trajecti ad Rhenum, Ex officina Francisci Halma, 1698.
22 p. 19 cm. **[10686]**
Diss.—Utrecht.

SCHUCHMANN, CHRISTIAN [1652–1719] *respondent. See* PETRI VON HARTENFELS, G. C., *praeses.* Dissertatio inauguralis medica de febre hectica. 1679.

SCHUCHZER, JOHANNES JACOBUS. *See* SCHEUCHZER, Hans Jakob [1645–1688]

SCHUCK, JOHANN GOTTFRIED [*fl.* 1685–1687] *respondent. See* LEICHNER, E., *praeses.* Dissertationem inauguralem de cancro ... sistit ... J. G. 1687.

SCHUCKMANN, CHRISTIAN. *See* SCHUCHMANN, Christian [1652–1719]

SCHÜLER, CONRAD. *See* MEISNER, L. Gemma gemmarum alchimistarum. 1608.

SCHÜTTE, FRIEDRICH [*fl.* 1686] *respondent. See* HELWIG, C., *praeses.* Delineatio medica apoplexiae. 1686.

SCHÜTZ, JOHANN CASPAR [*fl.* 1694–1696] *respondent.* Disputatio inauguralis medica de aphthis ... [Altdorffii] Literis Henrici Meyeri [1696]

20 p.   20 cm.   **[10687]**
Diss. — Altdorf.

SCHÜTZ, MICHAEL. *See* TOXITES, Michael [1515–1581]

SCHÜTZ, WOLFGANG PETER [*fl.* 1667] Thema doctoratus medici de podagra ... [Herbipoli] Typis Eliae Michaelis Zinck [1667]

32, [12] p.   19 cm.   **[10688]**
"Analysis quaestionis inauguralis": [12] p.
Diss. — Würzburg.

SCHÜTZE, GOTTHELFF [*fl.* 1698] *respondent. See* LEHMANN, G., *praeses.* De apotheosi naturae dissertationem priorem ex historia naturali ... defendere constituit G. S. 1698.

SCHÜTZE, TOBIAS [*b.* 1616 *or* 7] Harmonia macrocosmi cum microcosmo; das ist, Eine obereinstimmung der grossen mit der kleinen Welt als dem Menschen, in zwey Theil abgetheilet. Franckfurt am Mäyn, Verlegt von Daniel Reicheln, 1654.

[28], 124 p.; [7], 106, [18] p.   plates, port.   15 cm.   **[10689]**
Part [2] has half title.

SCHUIRMAN, ISAAK [*fl.* 1688] *respondent.* Disputatio medica inauguralis de asthmate ... Trajecti ad Rhenum, Ex officina Francisci Halma, 1688.

24 p.   22 cm.   **[10690]**
Diss. — Utrecht.

SCHUKIUS, JOH. GODOFREDUS. *See* SCHUCK, Johann Gottfried [*fl.* 1685–1687]

SCHULTE, JOACHIM [*fl.* 1605] *respondent. See* LIDDEL, D., *praeses.* Disputatio de apoplexia. 1605.

SCHULTES. *See* SCULTETUS.

SCHULTETUS, JOHANNES. *See* SCHOLZ, Johann [1621–1687?]

SCHULTZ, BALTHASAR [1569–1627] Consilium medicum pro curanda valetudine, aphoristica forma ... aeditum. Cui accedit Epistola prophylactica Dioclis ad Antigonum regem paucis scholiis exornata ... Wittebergae, Excudebat Johan. Schmidt [impensis Clementis Bergeri] 1606.

48 p.; 23 p.   14 cm.   **[10691]**

SCHULTZ, CHRISTOPH [*fl.* 1691] *praeses.* Dissertatio academica, de chiromantiae vanitate ... Regiomonti, Typis Reusnerianis, 1691.

[45] p.   20 cm.   **[10692]**
Diss. — Königsberg (P.C. Engelbrecht, *respondent*)

SCHULTZ, GOTTFRIED [1643–1698] Scrutinium cinnabarinum; seu, Triga cinnabriorum quae sistit naturam cinnabaris, antimonii nativae & factitiae vulgaris. Nec non specifici cephalici ... Johann. Michaelis, cum Appendice de emplastro magnetico hernias scrotales curante, ad enchiresin chemicam & clinicam praxin accommodatum ... Hall. Saxon., Sumptibus Simon Joh. Hübneri [1679?]

[26], 192, [3] p.   front.   17 cm.   **[10693]**
Errata: [3] p. at end.
Includes an excerpt from Friedrich Hoffmann's Opus de methodo medendi quae sistit naturam cinnabaris, and letters addressed to Friedrich Hoffman with his replies.

—*respondent. See* ROLFINCK, W., *praeses.* Dissertatio medica sistens aegrum laborantem febre tertiana intermittente scorbutica. 1669; SCHENCK, J. T., *praeses.* Dissertationem inauguralem quae sistit aegrum laborantem malo hypochondriaco scorbutico ... subjicit ... G. F. 1670.

—, *ed. See* MICHAELIS, J. Dissertatio pharmaceutico-therapeutica. 1678.

SCHULTZ, GOTTFRIED [*fl.* 1693] *respondent. See* PETRI VON HARTENFELS, G. C., *praeses.* Disputatio inauguralis medica, de strangulatione a vaporibus externis. 1693; WOLF, JAKOB, *praeses.* Dissertatio medica de crusta lactea. 1697.

SCHULTZ, JEREMIAS [*fl.* 1650] *respondent. See* POMARIUS, S., *praeses.* De noctambulis disputatio posterior. 1650.

SCHULTZ, JOHANN [*fl.* 1655] *respondent. See* ITTIG, J., *praeses.* Disputatio physica. 1655.

SCHULTZ, Johann [*d.* 1704] *praeses.* Disputatio juridica de contractu medici cum aegroto . . . Gedani, Typis Davidis Friderici Rhetii [1689]

[59, [1] p. 20 cm. [**10694**]

Diss.—Danzig (M. D. Laurens, *respondent*)

SCHULTZ, Johann Georg [*fl.* 1694–1696] *respondent. See* Hoffmann, F. [1660–1742] *praeses.* Disputatio inauguralis medica de apepsia. 1696.

SCHULTZ, Simon [*fl.* 1650] *respondent.* Disputatio medica inauguralis de scorbuto . . . Lugduni Batavorum, E typographeo Francisci Hackii, 1650.

[24] p. 19 cm. [**10695**]

Diss.—Leyden.

SCHULTZ, Wenzel [*fl.* 1664] *respondent. See* Schenck, J. T., *praeses.* Disputatio medica inauguralis, de dysenteria. 1664.

SCHULTZE, Andreas [*fl.* 1657] *respondent.* Disputatio medica inauguralis de pleuritide. Basileae, Typis Georgii Deckeri, 1657.

[16] p. 20 cm. [**10696**]

Diss.—Basel.

SCHULTZE, Balthasar. *See* Schultz, Balthasar [1569–1627]

SCHULTZE, Georg [*fl.* 1678] Dissertatio academica de blanda mulierum rhetorica . . . Lipsiae, Literis Johannis Georgii, prostat apud Johann. Fuhrman [1678]

109, [2] p. 19 cm. [**10697**]

SCHULTZE, Gottfried [*fl.* 1673] *respondent. See* Frenzel, S. F., *praeses.* Causas corporum cruentorum, superioribus non modo annis, sed elapso cum maxime in Misnia, vicinisque oris conspicuorum . . . exponet G. S. 1673.

SCHULTZE, Hans. *See* Praetorius, Johann [1630–1680]

SCHULTZE, Joachim. *See* Schulte, Joachim [*fl.* 1605]

SCHULTZE, Joachim Friedrich [*b.* 1675] *respondent. See* Vesti, J., *praeses.* Dissertatio inauguralis medica, exhibens aegrum phthisi laborantem. 1699.

—*See* Vesti, J. Facultatis Medicae . . . decanus Justus Vesti benevolo lectori S. P. P. [sic] 1699.

SCHULTZE, Johann Christoph [*fl.* 1699] *respondent. See* Vater, C., *praeses.* Dissertationem inauguralem medico-chirurgicam de cerebri commotione . . . exponet J. C. S. 1699.

SCHULTZE, Johannes Georgius. *See* Schultz, Johann Georg [*fl.* 1694–1696]

SCHULTZE, Nikolaus [*b.* 1649] *respondent. See* Helwig, C. Dissertationem inauguralem medicam de sanguine . . . submittit Nicholaus Schultz. 1683.

—*See* Helwig, C. Facultatis Medicae decanus Christophorus Helvigius . . . ad inauguralem de sanguine disputationem quam . . . habebit . . . Nicolaus Schultze . . . invitat. 1683.

SCHULTZE, Simon. *See* Schultz, Simon [*fl.* 1650]

SCHULTZE, Walther. *See* Schouten, Wouter [1638–1704]

SCHULTZEN, Georg. *See* Schultze, Georg [*fl.* 1678]

SCHULZ, Christoph. *See* Schultz, Christoph [*fl.* 1691]

SCHULZ, Godofredus. *See* Schultz, Gottfried [1643–1698]

SCHULZE, Balthasar. *See* Schultz, Balthasar [1569–1627]

SCHUMACHER, Georg [*fl.* 1686–1687] *respondent. See* Waldschmidt, J. J., *praeses.* Exercitatio medica de chylo et sanguine. 1686.

SCHUMACHER, Petrus. *See* Griffenfeld, Peder Schumacher, greve af [1635–1699]

SCHUMANN, Christian Friedrich [*b.* 1659] *respondent. See* Wedel, G. W., *praeses.* Disputatio inauguralis medica de catarrho suffocativo laborante. 1686.

—*See* Wedel, G. W. Propempticon inaugurale de sudore Christi cruento. 1686.

SCHUNCK, Johann Christian [*fl.* 1675–1677] *respondent.* Disputatio medica inauguralis de phthisi . . . Giessae Hassorum, Typis Friderici Kargeri, 1677.

16, [4] p. 20 cm. [**10698**]

Diss.—Giessen.

—*See* WALDSCHMIDT, J. J., *praeses.* Disputatio medica exhibens intricatam hodierno tempore quaestionem de sanguificatione. 1675.

SCHURFF, AUGUSTIN [1494-1548] *See* SCHOLTZ, L. Consiliorum medicinalium . . . liber singularis. 1610.

SCHURMAN, ANNA MARIA VAN [1607-1678] *See* BEVERWIJCK, J. van. Epistolica quaestio de vitae termino, fatali, an mobili? 1636, 1651.

SCHURPF, AUGUSTIN. *See* SCHURFF, Augustin [1494-1548]

SCHURTZFLEISCH, KONRAD SAMUEL [1641-1723] *praeses.* De nive . . . [Wittenbergae] Typis Johannis Borckardi [1665]

    [6] p.   18 cm.   **[10699]**
Diss.—Wittenberg (J. G. Hofmann, *respondent*)

SCHUSLER, CONRADUS [*fl.* 1644] *respondent. See* SEBISCH, M. [1578-1674?] *praeses.* Disputationes de dentibus quatuor. 1645.

SCHUSS frey in dem Krieg Gottes; das ist, Geistlich- und natürliche Mittel wider die Pestilentz, nutzlich zu gebrauchen, sambt etlichen schönen Fragstucken, und der Infections-Ordnung so zu Palermo, und Florenz gehalten worden. Auss dem Lateinischen gezogen durch Ferdinandum Antonium Hauck. Wienn, Gedruckt bey Johann van Ghelen, in Verlegung Johann Friderich Hartung, 1692.

    [2], 192 p.   13 cm.   **[10700]**

SCHUSTER, JOHAN-JAKOB [*fl.* 1657-1658] *respondent.* Disputatio inauguralis medica de pica sive malacia . . . Argentinae, Typis Eberhardi Welperi [1658]

    [16] p.   19 cm.   **[10701]**
Diss.—Strasbourg.

—*See* SEBISCH, M. [1578-1674?] *praeses.* Disputatio solennis de stranguria. 1657.

SCHUSTER, JOHANN CHRISTOPH [*b.* 1664] *respondent. See* CRAUSE, R. W., *praeses.* Dissertatio inauguralis medica de vertigine. 1690.

SCHUSTER, MICHAEL GOTTREICH [*fl.* 1690-1691] *respondent. See* GÖSGEN, D., *praeses.* Dissertatio physica de monstris. 1690; PETERMANN, A., *praeses.* Dissertatio physiologica de visu. 1690; PETRI VON HARTENFELS, G. C., *praeses.* Dissertatio inauguralis medica, de dolore hypochondriaco. 1691.

SCHUT, ASSUERUS [*fl.* 1660] *respondent.* Disputatio medica inauguralis de catarrho . . . Lugduni Batavorum, Apud Johannem Elsevirium, 1660.

    [11] p.   21 cm.   **[10702]**
Diss.—Leyden.

[**SCHUTS,** JACOBUS, *fl.* 1682-1692] De betoverde Bekker; ofte, Een overtuygent bewijs dat het boek vande Heer Bekker, genaemt De betoverde weerelt, doorsaeyt is met de onredelijkste redenering, notoirste onwaaheeden en andere schadelijcke gevogeln . . . 's Gravenhage, Barent Beek, 1661 (i.e. 1691?)

    [6], 88 p.   19 cm.   **[10703]**
Linde 146, dated 1619 (i.e. 1691?)

[—] Missive, aen D. Balthazar Bekker, in 't korte ontdekkende de gronden van sijn mis-grepen, begaen in sijn drie tractaten De betooverde weereld, over den prophete Daniel, en van de Cometen . . . 's Gravenhage, Barent Beek, 1692.

    [20], 69 p.   20 cm.   **[10704]**
Linde 147.

[—] Tweede missive aen d'Heer Balthasar Bekker, over sijn Betooverde weereld, Daniel, en den 2den druk van de Cometen . . . Met den korten inhoud van de eerste Missive . . . 's Gravenhage, Barent Beek en Meinard Uitwerf, 1692.

    [24], 72 p.   20 cm.   **[10705]**
Linde 148.

SCHUYL, FLORENTIUS [1619-1669] Pro veteri medicina. Lugd. Bat. & Amstelod., Apud Gaasbequios, 1670.

    [6], 185, [1] p.   plate.   14 cm.   **[10706]**
Concerns the controversy between Frans de Le Boë and Louis Le Vasseur.

Includes extracts from Hippocrates.

With this is bound Ruysch, F. Dilucidatio valvularum in vasis lymphaticis. 1687.

—*praeses.* Disputatio medica inauguralis, de gonorrhoea . . . Lugduni Batavorum, Ex officina Cornelii Driehuysen, 1666.

    [16] p.   19 cm.   **[10707]**
Imperfect: upper margins trimmed with possible loss of pagination.

Diss.—Leyden (H. Grube, *respondent*)

—Disputatio medica inauguralis de natura et usu lienis . . . Lugduni Batavorum, Ex officina Petri & Cornelii Hackii, 1664.

    [14] p.   21 cm.   **[10708]**
Diss.—Utrecht.

—, *tr. See* DESCARTES, R. De homine figuris. 1662, 1664.

— *See* DESCARTES, R. L'homme . . . et un traitté De la formation du foetus. 1664, 1677, 1680 [and] De verhandeling van den mensch, en de makinge van de vrugt in 's moeders lichaam. 1695.

SCHUYL, HERMAN [*fl.* 1688] *respondent.* Disputatio philosophica inauguralis de vi corporum elastica . . . Lugduni Batavorum, Apud Abrahamum Elzevier, 1688.

    [16] p.   24 cm.   **[10709]**
  Diss.—Leyden.

SCHWALENBERG, ANTON ULRICH [*fl.* 1687–1689] *respondent. See* MEIBOM, H., *praeses.* Exercitatio medica de fluxu humorum ad oculos naturali et praeternaturali hujusque curatione. 1687.

SCHWARTZ, CHRISTOFF. *See* GABELKOVER, O. Kurtzer Bericht: der fürstlichen Württembergischen Hoff Medicorum. 1608, 1626.

SCHWARTZ, WILHELM HEINRICH [*fl.* 1655] *respondent. See* ROLFINCK, W., *praeses.* Dissertatio inauguralis medica, qua . . . catarrhum suffocativum . . . proponit W. H. S. 1655.

SCHWARTZERD, PHILIPP. *See* MELANCHTHON, Philipp [1497–1560]

SCHWARTZWALDT, JOHANN [*fl.* 1682] *respondent. See* ZIEGRA, C. S., *praeses.* Disputatio physica de annis climactericis vitae humanae posterior. 1682.

SCHWARZMANN, JOHANN BALTHASAR [*fl.* 1695] *respondent.* Disputatio medica inauguralis de siti morbosa . . . [Altdorffii] Henricus Meyer [1695]

    20 p.   19 cm.   **[10710]**
  Diss.—Altdorf.

SCHWEDLER, JOHANN CHRISTOPH [1672–1730] *praeses.* Dissertatio praeliminaris de naturali hominis oeconomia, quatenus doctrinae de affectibus & necessario & utiliter praemittenda est . . . [Lipsiae] Literis Immanuelis Titii [1697]

    [32] p.   19 cm.   **[10711]**
  Diss.—Leipzig (J. T. Vopel, *respondent*)

SCHWEICKARD VON CRONENBERG, JOHANN. *See* SCHWEIKARD VON KRONENBERG, Johann, *Abp. of Mainz* [*d.* 1626]

SCHWEIKARD VON KRONENBERG, JOHANN, *Abp. of Mainz* [*d.* 1626] *See* MAINZ. Or-

dinances, local laws, etc. Reformatio, und ernewerte Ordnung deren Apotecken. 1618.

SCHWEITZER, JOHANN FRIEDRICH. *See* HELVETIUS, Johann Friedrich [1629 *or* 30–1709]

SCHWEITZER, JOHANN HEINRICH [1644–1705] Compendium physicae Aristotelico-Cartesianae, in usum tironum methodo erotematica adornatum. Accedit Breve & succinctum theoreticae philosophiae theatrum ed. alt. recognita & emend. Amstelaedami, Apud Henri. Wetstenium, apud Guil. Graves, 1695.

    [8], 236, [10] p.; [34 +] p.   14 cm.   **[10712]**
  Imperfect: all pages after p. [34] wanting.

SCHWENDI, PETRUS [*fl.* 1685] *respondent. See* BARTHOLIN C., *praeses.* Dissertatio medica inauguralis de cruditate ventriculi. 1685.

SCHWERTNER, MARTIN [*fl.* 1661] *respondent. See* KIRCHMAYER, G. K., *praeses.* De vitae humanae unitate. 1661.

SCHWIGER, JOHANN [*fl.* 1668] *respondent. See* MEYER, P. Disputationem physicam de anima . . . exhibet J. S. 1668.

SCHWELING, HEINRICH. Kurtzer und nützlicher Bericht wie sich ein jeder . . . bey dieser . . . gifftigen Seuche so wohl praeservando als auch einiger Massen curando zuverhalten . . . Halberstadt, Gedruckt bey Johann-Erasmo Hynitzsch, 1681.

    [12] p.   19 cm.   **[10713]**

SCHWELING, JOHANN EBERHARD [1645–1714] *praeses.* Bartholdus Baltzers . . . dissertationem hydrographico-physicam de maribus . . . submittet . . . Bremae, Typis Hermanni Braueri, 1676.

    72 p.   19 cm.   **[10714]**
  Diss.—Bremen. Gymnasium (B. Baltzers, *respondent*)

—Disputatio physica de materia mundi subtilissima, ejusque effectibus . . . Bremae, Typ. Hermanni Braueri, 1690.

    36 p.   20 cm.   **[10715]**
  Diss.—Bremen. Gymnasium (J. Tiling, *respondent*)

—Sol obscuratus; quod est, Dissertatio astronomico-philosophica de generatione macularum in sole et fixis . . . Bremae, Typis Hermanni Braueri, 1674.

    20 p.   19 cm.   **[10716]**
  Diss.—Bremen. Gymnasium (J. H. Molanus, *respondent*)

SCHWENCK, JOHANN SIGMUND [*d.* 1670] Disputatio ... secunda ... de echo ... Lipsiae, Typis haeredum Timothei Hönii [1649]

[15] p. 19 cm.   **[10717]**

Diss. pro loco — Leipzig.

— *praes.* Decuria positonum physicarum, exhibens ὑετόλογίαν. Lipsiae, Literis Johann-Erici Hahnii, 1662.

[16] p. 20 cm.   **[10718]**

Diss. — Leipzig (E. Pfautz, *respondent*)

— Disputatio philosophica exhibens metallographian generalem ... Lipsiae, Typis Johannis Erici Hahnii [1659]

[28] p. 20 cm.   **[10719]**

Diss. — Leipzig (S. Vogt, *respondent*)

SCHWENCKFELD, KASPAR [1563-1609] Hirschbergischen warmen Bades in Schlesien ... Neben einem allgemeinen Bericht von mineralischen Wassern und wild Bädern. Und kurtzem Verzeichniss derer Kräuter und Berg Arthen ... Görlitz, J. Rhambaw, 1607.

[24], 236, [4] p. plate. 16 cm.   **[10720]**

Title and imprint supplied from Wellcome.

Imperfect: p. [1-18] including title page wanting; plate mutilated.

— Thermae Teplicenses. Von dess Töplitzen warmen Bades in Böhmen ... gelegen. Ursprung, Gelegenheit, Abetheilung, Natur, Eigenschafft, und rechtem Gebrauch ... Görlitz, Johann Rhambaw, 1607.

[12], 34 p. 15 cm.   **[10721]**

Imperfect: p. 1-2 mutilated.

— [The same.] ... Lignitz, Gedruckt durch Nicloaum [sic] Schneider [In Vorlegung Georg Opitz in Hirschberg] 1619.

[12], 34, [1] p.   **[10722]**

Different setting of type.

SCHWENDENDÖRFFER, GEORG TOBIAS [1597-1681] *praeses.* Pervigilium philologico juridicum medicorum anatomen jure divino-humano licitam ... ad. d. 4. Septembr. ... 1663 ... defendet ... Joachimus Andreas Corvinus ... Lipsiae, Recusa typis Goezianis, 1690.

[24] p. 19 cm.   **[10723]**

Diss. — Leipzig, 1663 (J. A. Corvinus, *respondent*)

SCHWETKIUS, GOTTFRIED [*fl.* 1668] *respondent.* Disputatio medica inauguralis de mola ... Lugduni Batavorum, Apud viduam & haeredes Joannis Elsevirii, 1668.

[16] p. 24 cm.   **[10724]**

Diss. — Leyden.

SCHWIMMER, JOHANN MICHAEL [*d.* 1704] Ex physica secretiori curiositates ... enucleatae ... Jenae, Apud Jo. Bielken [1672]

[8], 256, [8] p. 18 cm.   **[10725]**

Date supplied from BMC.

Imperfect: lower margin of title page trimmed with loss of imprint date.

Based on 14 dissertations concerning sympathy and antipathy.

— [The same.] ... Tractatus physicus in quo nobiliores ex physica secretiori curiositates exhibentur ... Jenae, Apud Jo. Jac. Bauhofern, 1673.

[8], 256, [8] p. 19 cm.   **[10726]**

A reissue of the 1672 edition with new title page and preliminary matter.

— Physicalischer Lust-Garten, worinen ... sehr viele ... Natur-Fragen ... untersuchet, und gründlich erörtert ... verden. Jena, Verlegts Johann Jacob Ehrt, Rudolstatd [sic] Drukts Johann Rudolph Löw, 1690.

[96], 480 p. 14 cm.   **[10727]**

— *praeses..* Disputatio physica de antipathia ... [Jenae] Samuel Adolphus Müller [1669]

[44] p. 19 cm.   **[10728]**

Date changed by hand from MDCLXIV to MDCLXIX.

Diss. — Jena (J. Hellwig, *respondent*)

— Dissertatio physica de generatione ... Salana, Formis Mullerianis [1669]

[32] p. 20 cm.   **[10729]**

Diss. — Jena (P. G. Wanckelmuth, *respondent*)

SCHWINUTZKI, JOHANNA ELISABETH VON, *tr.* See MULTIBIBUS, B. Jus potandi; oder, Zech Recht. 1616.

SCHYCHZER, JOHANNES JACOBUS. *See* SCHEUCHZER, Hans Jakob [1645-1688]

SCHYLHANS, HANS. *See* GERSDORFF, Hans von [*d.* 1529]

SCHYRON, JEAN [*d.* 1556] Methodi medendi; seu, Institutionis medicinae faciendae una cum tractatu de curatione febrium putridarum libri quatuor ... quibus accessit tractatus medicamentorum simplicium et compositorum una cum ipsorum dosibus . . . Monspelii, Apud Franciscum Chouët, 1609.

[31], 542 p. 13 cm.   [**10730**]
Edited by J. Blezinus.

—[The same.] . . . Ed. nova corr. & emend . . . Coloniae Allobrogum, Apud Petrum & Jacobum Chouët, 1623.

[32], 542 p. 12 cm.   [**10731**]
Different setting of type.

SCIALOJA, Donato [17th cent.] Praxis novissima purgandi infirmos . . . utilis, & necessaria, non solum in scholis profitentibus, sed etiam praestantissimis practicantibus, ad sciendum, quando purgatio est indicata . . . Neapoli, Ex typographia Lucae Antonii de Fusco, 1666.

[13], 140, [4], 141-311, [36] p. 31 cm. [**10732**]
Book 2 is preceded by a second title page and dedicatory epistle on two leaves inserted between p. 140 and 141.

SCIELTA di notabili avvertimenti, pertinenti a'cavalli. 1610. *See* Grisone, F.

La SCIENCE curieuse. 1667. *See* [Taisnier, J.]

SCIENTIA, Giuseppe, *ed. See* Zapata, G. B. Li maravigliosi secreti di medicina. 1602, 1611, 1618, 1629, 1641, 1656, 1677, 1700; [Latin tr.] 1696; [German tr.] 1603, 1605.

SCIOPPIUS, Caspar [1576-1649] *See* Schoppe, Kaspar [1576-1649]

SCLANOFIUS, Hector [*fl.* 1601] Quaestiones hasce medicas publice examinandas proponit . . . Hector Sclanofius . . . Marpurgi Cattorum, Excudebat Paulus Egenolphus, 1601.

[16] p. 20 cm.   [**10733**]
Diss. — Marburg.

SCLOPETARIUS, Buldrianus. De peditu; ejusque speciebus crepitu & visio, discursus methodicus, in theses digestus, quas praeside . . . Bombardo Strevarzio . . . defendere conabitur Buldrianus Sclopetarius . . . Disputabuntur autem aedibus Divae Cloacinae, a summo mane, ad noctem usque mediam . . . Clareforti, Apud Stancarum Cepollam, 1671.

[16] p. 19 cm.   [**10734**]

SCOLA SALERNITANA. 1630, 1662, 1666, 1677. *See* Regimen sanitatis Salernitanum.

SCOT, Reginald [1538?-1599] The discovery of witchcraft: proving that the compacts and contracts of witches with devils and all infernal spirits or familiars, are but erroneous novelties and imaginary conceptions . . . Whereunto is added an excellent discourse of . . . devils and spirits, in two books: the first by the aforesaid author: the second now added in this third edition, as succedaneous to the former . . . London, Printed for A. Clark, and sold by Dixy Page, 1665.

[18], 292, [11] p.; [1], 72 p. illus. 28 cm.
                                        [**10735**]
Imperfect: title page mutilated.
Part [2] has special title page: A discourse concerning the nature and substance of devils and spirits.

SCOTUS, Michael. *See* Scott, Michael [1175?-1234?]

SCOTT, Michael [1175?-1234?] Quaestio curiosa de natura solis et lunae . . .

713-722 p., vol. 5. 20 cm. (*In* Zetzner, Lazarus, *ed.* Theatrum chemicum. Argentorati, 1659-61)   [**10736**]
Caption title.

—Tractatus . . . de secretis naturae. Francofurti, Excudebat Johannes Bringerus, opera & impensa Petri Musculi, 1615.

188, [8] p. 14 cm.   [**10737**]
Bound with (as issued?) Albertus Magnus. Tractatus . . . de secretis mulierum. 1615.

—Physionomia. *In* Albertus Magnus. De secretis mulierum. 1601, 1607, 1615, 1637, 1643, 1648, 1655, 1665, 1669; [German tr.] 1678.

—*See* Mensa philosophica. 1602.

SCOTT, Robert [*fl.* 17th cent.] Catalogus librorum ex variis Europae partibus advectorum . . . Londini, Venales prostant apud . . . Robertum Scott, 1674.

[6], [3]-206 p. 23 cm.   [**10738**]

SCOUGALL, J., *tr. See* Beddevole, D. Essayes of anatomy. 1691, 1696.

SCRAMUCCIA, Giovanni Battista. *See* Scaramucci, Giovanni Battista [1650-*ca.* 1710]

SCRETA, Heinrich [1637-1689] Kurzer Bericht fon der allgemainen anstekenden Lagersucht; das ist, Fon dem giftigen und hizigen Haubt-Hals-, Brust-, Magen- und Bauch-Wehe, mit und one Fleken, aus aigner Erfahrung . . . aufgesezet . . . Schafhausen,

In Ferlag Onofrions fon Waldkirch, getrukt bei Alexander Rieding, 1676.

[16], 160 p. 16 cm.   **[10739]**

—[The same.] ... in disem andern Druk um fil fermehrt und ferbessert ... Schafhausen, In Ferlag Joh. Martin Maisters, gedrukt bei Joh. Martin Oschwald, 1685.

[16], 308, [4] p. 16 cm.   **[10740]**

—[Latin tr.] De febri castrensi maligna; seu, Mollium corporis humani partium inflammatione dicta, liber singularis. In Latinum versus, ab auctore recognitus, & auctus. Scafusii, Impensis Joh. Martini Meisteri, typis Joh. Martini Osvaldi, 1686.

[12], 352, [4] p. 16 cm.   **[10741]**

—*respondent.* Dissertatio inauguralis physico-medica de laesa auditione ... Basileae, Apud Jacobum Werenfelsium [1671]

[2], 16 p. 22 cm.   **[10742]**
Diss.—Basel.

—*See* Piens, F. H. Tractatus de febribus in genere. 1689.

SCRETA, Johannes [*d.* 1651?] *ed. See* ruland, M. [1532–1602] Thesaurus Rulandinus. 1628, 1680.

SCRIBANI, Jacobus Antonius [*fl.* 1647] Ovum philosophicum medicinale ... Mediolani, Ex typographia Ludovici Modoetiae, 1647.

76, [1] p. illus. 17 cm.   **[10743]**

SCRIBONIUS, Wilhelm Adolph [16th cent.] Naturall philosophy; or, A description of the world, and of the severall creatures therein contained ... By Daniel Widdowes. 2. ed., corr. and enl. ... London, Printed by Tho. Cotes and sold by Beniamine Allen, 1631.

[14], 65 p. 20 cm.   **[10744]**
Translated and abridged from the Rerum naturalium doctrina methodica of W. A. Scribonius by Daniel Widdowes.
The epistle dedicatory is signed by I. Wyddowes, alias Woodhouse.
STC 22112.5.

SCRIBONIUS LARGUS. Compositiones medicae. Joannes Rhodius recensuit ... Lexicon Scribonianum adjecit. Patavii, Typis Pauli Frambotti, 1655.

[22], 144 p.; 465, [42] p. illus. 23 cm. **[10745]**
Errata: p. [41]

SCRIVERIUS, Petrus. *See* Schrijver, Pieter [1576–1660]

SCRUTINIUM ingeniorum. 1637. *See* Huarte de San Juan, Juan.

SCUDALUPIS, Petrus Arlensis de. *See* Petrus Arlensis de Scudalupis.

SCULTETUS, Johann Martin [*fl.* 1682] *respondent. See* Metzger, G. B., *praeses.* Disputatio medica de fistulis. 1682.

SCULTETUS, Johannes [1595–1645] Χειροπλοθήχη, seu ... Armamentarium chirurgicum ... Opus posthumum ... in quo tot, tam veterum ac recentiorum instrumenta ab authore correcta, quam noviter ab ipso inventa, quot fere hodie ad usitatas operationes manuales feliciter peragendas requiruntur ... depicta reperiuntur ... Nunc primum in lucem editum, studio et opera Joannis Sculteti, authoris ... nepotis ... Ulmae Suevorum, Typis & impensis Balthasari Kühnen, 1655.

[1], 10, 132, [3] p. illus. 37 cm.   **[10746]**

—[The same.] ... Hagae-Comitum, Ex officina Adriani Vlacq, 1656.

[22], 328 (i.e. 330), [14] p. illus. 20 cm. **[10747]**

—[The same.] ... Ed. 3. Hagae-Comitum, Ex officina Adriani Vlacq, 1662.

[24], 328 (i.e. 330), [14] p. illus. 21 cm. **[10748]**
Added engraved title page has date 1657.
Different setting of type.

—[The same.] ... Amstelodami, Ex Officina Janssoniana, 1662.

[16], 343, [21] p. illus. 20 cm.   **[10749]**
Added engraved title page.

—[The same.] ... Ed. 5. Venetiis, Typis Combi, & La Noù, 1665.

[24], 317, [11] p. plates. 19 cm.   **[10750]**
Added engraved title page.
Imperfect: plate 42 wanting.

—[The same.] Armamentarium chirurgicum bipartitum ... reformatum, correctum & auctum ... Francofurti, Sumptibus viduae Joan. Gerlini, bibliop. Ulm, typis Joannis Gerlini, 1666.

[8], 3-156, 144, [27] p. plates. 22 cm.

     [10751]

—[The same.] Armamentarium chirurgicum renovatum & auctum ... Una cum observationum medico-chirurgicarum centuria ... annotata, & collecta opera & studio Joannis Baptistae à Lamzweerde ... Amstelodami, Apud Joannem à Someren, 1672.

3 parts in 1 v.   illus.   19 cm.   [**10752**]

Added engraved title page.

Each part has special title page.

Appendix ad Armamentarium chirurgicum was published in 1672 under title: Chirurgiae veteris ac modernae promptuarium.

Contents.—[pt. 1] Joannis Sculteti Armamentarium chirurgicum. 1672.—[pt. 2] Auctarium ad Armamentarium chirurgicum Johannis Schulteti. Opera defuncti haeredum editum. 1669.—[pt. 3] Appendix ad Armamentarium chirurgicum Joannis Sculteti opera & studio Joannis Baptistae à Lamzweerde. 1671.

—[The same.] ... Nunc vero observationibus ... denuo locupletatum, & ab innumeris mendis expurgatum studio Johannis Tilingii ... Lugdun. Batav., Apud Cornelium Boutesteyn, Jordanum Luchtmans, 1693.

4 parts in 1 v.   illus.   21 cm.   [**10753**]

Imperfect: plate 18 of Appendix wanting.

Added engraved title page.

Parts [2–4] have special title pages.

Part [4] has title: Auctarium II. Continens Petri Hadriani f. Verduin ... Observationes chirurgicas.

—[Dutch tr.] Magazyn, ofte Wapen-huys ... Den 2. druck verb., en met verduytsinge van alle de recepten, tot naerder behulp der ongeleerden, verm. Dordrecht, Jacobus Savry, 1657 [i.e. 1658]

[12], 272 p.; [2], 224, [42] p. illus. 16 cm.   [**10754**]

Added engraved title page dated 1658.

—[English tr.] The chyrurgeons store-house ... faithfully Englished, by E. B. London, John Starkey, 1674.

[16], 389, [11] p.   illus.   19 cm.   [**10755**]

Imperfect: title page mutilated; p. 219–220, 241–242 wanting.

—[French tr.] L'arcenal de chirurgie ... Ouvrage posthume ... Renouvellé, corr., et augm. ... Mis en françois par Mre François Deboze ... Avec la description d'un monstre humain exposé à Lyon le 5. de mars 1671. Lyon, De l'imprimerie d'Antoine Galien; & se vend chez le traducteur, 1672.

[20], 385, [25] p.   illus.   23 cm.   [**10756**]

Added engraved title page.

—[The same.] ... Lyon, Antoine Cellier fils, 1674.

[20], 385, [25] p.   illus.   24 cm.   [**10757**]

Imperfect: added engraved title page wanting, p. [5] mutilated.

Different setting of type.

—Another issue, with date changed to 1675.   [**10758**]

Added engraved title page.

—[German tr.] Wund-artzneyisches Zeug-Hauss ... welches auss dem Lateinischen von dess authoris Brudern Sohn, Herrn Johann Schultes ... reformirtem, verbessert- und an vielen Orten vermehrtem ... in die teutsche Sprach übersetzet hat ... Amadeus Megerlin ... Franckfurt, In Verlegung Daniel Gerlins, Buchhändlers in Ulm, 1679.

[11], 4–263, 238, [56] p.   illus., plates.   22 cm.   [**10759**]

SCULTETUS, JOHANNES [d. 1663] ed. and tr. See VIGO, G. de. Wund-Artznei. 1677.

—, ed. See SCULTETUS, J. [1595–1645] Χειροπλοθήκη. 1655, 1656, 1662, 1666 [and] The chyrurgeons storehouse. 1674 [and] Wund-artzneyisches Zeug-Hauss. 1679.

SCULTETUS, JOHANNES. See also SCHOLZ, Johan [1621–1687?]

SCULTZIUS, GODOFREDUS. See SCHULTZ, Gottfried [fl. 1693]

SCUOLA MEDICA SALERNITANA. REGIMEN SANITATIS SALERNITANA. See REGIMEN SANITATIS SALERNITANUM.

SCURRON, JEAN. See SCHYRON, Jean [d. 1556]

SCUTRON, JEAN. See SCHYRON, Jean [d. 1556]

SEBASTIANUS ALETOPHILUS, pseud. See SORBIÈRE, Samuel [1615–1670]

SEBASTIANUS AQUILANUS. See AQUILANO, Sebastiano [d. 1543]

SEBISCH, JOHANN ALBERT [1614–1685]

Dissertations—Strasbourg

—*praeses.* Disputatio cheirurgica de tumoribus praeter naturam in genere ... Argentorati, Literis Johannis Welperi, 1669.

[2], 40, [2] p.   20 cm.   [**10760**]

J. K. Rasor, *respondent.*

—Disputatio exhibens problemata quaedam anatomica ... Argentorati, Typis Eberhardi Welperi, 1662.

[23] p.   19 cm.   [**10761**]

T. J. Haintzel, *respondent.*

—Disputatio exhibens problemata quaedam anatomica ... Argentorati, Typis Josiae Staedelii, 1665.

[23] p. 19 cm.   [**10762**]

Date has been altered from 1664 to 1665.
J. K. Hammerer, *respondent.*

—Disputatio medica de syncope ... Argentorati, Typis Eberhardi Welperi, 1659.

[24] p. 19 cm.   [**10763**]

J. A. Beza, *respondent.*

—Dissertatio anatomica de jecore ... Argentorati, Typis Eberhardi Welperi, 1655.

[1], 46 p. 19 cm.   [**10764**]

F. Rayger, *respondent.*

—Dissertatio anatomica de ventriculo ... Argentorati, Typis Friderici Spoor, 1660.

[2], 44 (i.e. 34) p. 19 cm.   [**10765**]

M. H. Zollicofer, *respondent.*

—Dissertatio medica de inedia ... Argentorati, Literis Joannis Friderici Spoor, 1664.

69 (i.e. 71), [1] p. 19 cm.   [**10766**]

K. Rayger, *respondent.*

—Dissertatio medica de paralysi ... Argentorati, Typis Eberhardi Welperi, 1657.

[36] p. 18 cm.   [**10767**]

J. M. Welsch, *respondent.*

—Dissertatio philologico-medica de Aesculapio inventore medicinae ... Argentorati, Literis Johannis Welperi, 1669.

[8], 71 p. 19 cm.   [**10768**]

J. L. Engelhardt, *respondent.*

—Dissertatio solennis de instrumento olfactus ... Argentorati, Typis Johannis Pastorii, 1662.

36 p. 19 cm.   [**10769**]

A. Khonn, *respondent.*
Bound with Mapp, M., *praeses.* Tractationis medicae de potu calido. 1673.

—Exercitationum pathologicarum dissertatio undecima ... Argentorati, Literis Johannis Welperi, 1672.

[1], 233–254, [2] p. 20 cm.   [**10770**]

J. C. Sparr, *respondent.*

—Theoremata anatomica miscellanea de variis humani corporis partibus ... Argentorati, Ex typographeo Friderici Spoor, 1653.

[38] p. 20 cm.   [**10771**]

J. K. Knogler, *respondent.*

—Theses anatomicae miscellaneae ... Argentorati, Johannes Pickel, 1663.

[12] p. 19 cm.   [**10772**]

G. Cramer, *respondent.*

—*respondent. See* SEBISCH, M. [1578–1674?] *praeses.* Collegii therapeutici disputatio I[–XIV] 1634 [i.e. 1635]

SEBISCH, JOHANN PAUL [*fl.* 1677] *respondent. See* FAUST, J. *praeses.* Exercitatio academica. 1677.

SEBISCH, MELCHIOR [1578–1674?] Beschreibung und Widerlegung etlicher Missbräuche und Irrthumb, so biss anhero in dem Gebrauch der Saurbrunnen, und andern ... Bädern bey uns fürgangen ... Strassburg, Bey Johan Philipp Mülben, 1647.

[4], 140 p. 16 cm.   [**10773**]

Added engraved title page.

—De alimentorum facultatibus libri quinque, ex optimorum authorum monumentis conscripti & editi ... Argentinae, Ex officina Joh. Philippi Mulbii, & Josiae Stedelii, 1650.

[27], 1552, [48] p. plate. 21 cm.   [**10774**]

Added engraved title page.

—Discursus medico-philosophicus de casu adolescentis cujusdam Argentoratensis mirabili, qui anno M. DC. XVII ... mortuus in quodam paternarum aedium loco, adjacente ipsi serpente ... inventus fuit; publice ... habitus ... Argentorati, Excudebat Antonius Bertramus, impensis Pauli Ledertz, 1617.

[140] p. illus. 21 cm.   [**10775**]

Signatures: (§)⁴, B-R⁴, S².

—Another issue, with date changed to 1618.

[**10776**]

—[The same.] ... Nunc ... denuo recusus, & appendice de quibusdam serpentum generibus, auctus. Argentorati, Typis & sumptibus Friderici Spoor, 1660.

[140] p. illus., plate. 21 cm.   [**10777**]

Signatures: ¶⁴, B-R⁴, S².
Different setting of type.
Bound with copy 2 of Marci von Kronland, J. M. Liturgia mentis. 1678.

—Dissertatio περι θειου, de divino, quod Hippocrates in morbis considerandum in prognosticorum suorum vestibulo praecepit ... Argentorati, Typis Joannis Philippi Mülbii, 1643.

[68] p. 20 cm. **[10778]**

—Dissertationum de acidulis sectiones duae, in quarum priore agitur de acidulis in genere, in posteriore vero de Alsatiae acidulis in specie ... Argentorati, Excudebat Wilhelmus Christianus Glaserus [1627?]

[24], 713, [4] p. 16 cm. **[10779]**
Engraved title page.

—Galeni Methodus medendi in quatuordecim disputationes resoluta, & in inclyta Argentoratensium Academia ad exercenda medicinae studiosorum ingenia proposita ... Argentorati, Apud heredes Lazari Zetzneri, 1639.

[32] p. 20 cm. **[10780]**

—Historia memorabilis de foemina quadam Argentoratensi, quae ventrem supra modum tumidum atque distentum ultra decennium gestavit, & tum hydrope uterino, tum molis carnosis 76, tum ea hydropis specie conflictata fuit, quae ascites dicitur ...Argentinae, Typis Marci ab Heyden, sumptibus Jacobi ab Heyden, 1627.

[62] p. plates. 19 cm. **[10781]**

—Manualis; sive, Speculi medicinae practici ... tomus prior [-posterior] ... Argentorati, Typis & impensis Friderici Spoor, 1661.

[29], 3169 (i.e. 3177), [24] p. 17 cm. **[10782]**
Added engraved title page.
Tomus posterior has special title page.
"Emblematis quod isti manuali praefixum, declaratio": p. [17–29]

Dissertations — Strasbourg

Collections

—*praeses.* Collegii therapeutici disputatio I [–XIV]. continens praeludia in Galeni Methodum medendi ... Argentorati, Typis Eberhardi Welperi, 1634 [i.e. 1635]

[354] p. 21 cm. **[10783]**
Each dissertation has special title page dated 1634 or 1635. (*Respondents*: E. Leichner, no. 1; J. A. Sebisch, no. 2; Adam Gerner, no. 3; A. C. Enckelmann, no. 4; G. Hilling, no. 5; A. Verbezius, no. 6; J. R. Widt, no. 7; J. N. Stupan, no. 8; J. G. Zachmann, no. 9; J. G. Stephanus, no. 10; Adam Gerner, no. 11; J. V. Wille, no. 12; J. J. Schlanhovius, no. 13; P. Fuchs, no. 14)

—Disputatio de naturalibus facultatibus prima [-octava & ultima] continens trium librorum Galeni De naturalibus facultatibus argumentum, divisionem in partes majores ac minores, subjectum, inscriptionem, locum quem in medicina habent ... Argentorati, Typis Johannis Reppii, 1644 [i.e. 1645]

[184] p. 20 cm. **[10784]**
Each dissertation has special title page dated 1644 or 1645. (*Respondents*: C. Harder, no. 1; J. Schilling, no. 2; J. A. Remmelin, no. 3; J. Frey, no. 4; F. Stiber, no. 5; G. Coschwicius, no. 6; J. Peltre, no. 7; J. W. Agricola, no. 8)

—Disputatio de variolis et morbillis prima [-sexta & ultima] Argentorati, Typis Joannis Philippi Mülbii, 1642.

[131] p. 19 cm. **[10785]**
Each dissertation has special title page. (*Respondents*: B. Nagelius, no. 1; J. Becker, no. 2; J. J. Wepfer, no. 3; B. Scheffer, no. 4; M. Ramelov, no. 5; P. Barbette, no. 6)

—Disputationes de dentibus quatuor ... Argentorati, Typis Eberhardi Welperi, prostant apud Casparum Dietzelium, 1645.

[141] p. 21 cm. **[10786]**
Each dissertation has special title page. (*Respondents*: Z. Andreas, S. Closius, C. Schusler, J. Becker)

—Disputationes de recta ratione purgandi, docentes quos, quibus pharmacis, et quo tempore, purgare deceat ... Argentorati, Typis Joannis Reppii, 1621.

[210] p. 19 cm. **[10787]**
Contains 13 dissertations each with special title page dated 1620 or 1621. (*Respondents*: J. Seidel, no. 1; A. Opala, no. 2; E. Geiselbrunner, no. 3; A. Rüber, no. 4; J. L. Gans, no. 5; U. Rietmann, no. 6; J. J. Faber, no. 7; J. Steinicher, no. 8; D. Widholz, no. 9; J. R. Faber, no. 10; J. F. Regulus, no. 11; B. Malleolus, no. 12; J. Langenauer, no. 13)
Bound with copy 2 of Lauremberg, P. Porticus Aesculapii. 1630.

—Disputationes de respiratione tres ... Argentorati, Typis Eberhardi Welperi, Prostant apud Casparum Dietzelium, 1643.

[148] p. 20 cm. **[10788]**
Each dissertation has special title page. (*Respondents:* G. H. Welsch, J. K. Beuttel, J. Becker)

—Examinis vulnerum partium dissimilarium pars I[-IV. & ultima] ... Argentorati, Typis Eberhardi Welperi, 1636 [i.e. 1637]

[199] p. 20 cm. **[10789]**
Each dissertation has special title page dated 1636 or 1637. (*Respondents:* A. C. Enckelmann, J. R. Saltzmann, J. W. Hochstatt, J. Kueffer)

—Exercitationes medicae ... Argentorati, Apud heredes Lazari Zetzneri, 1639.

I v.   20 cm.   **[10790]**

Contains 56 dissertations each with special title page. Dates range from 1622 to 1636. (*Respondents:* J. C. Wesener, no. 1; P. Thomas, no. 2 & 24; B. Haeberlin, no. 3; J. J. Faber, no. 4; N. Ager, no. 5 & 22; J. R. Faber, no. 6; V. Charstadius, no. 7; J. Steinicher, no. 8; J. Bartsch, no. 9; J. M. Zittelin, no. 10; B. Malleolus, no. 11; J. J. Hartig, no. 12; J. J. Seubertus, no. 13 & 32; C. Ruoff, no. 14; C. Hartig, no. 15; J. N. Furich, no. 16; J. N. Baumann, no. 17; J. L. Münster, no. 18; F. Hörscher, no. 19 & 25; J. C. Osiander, no. 20; J. K. Wegelin, no. 21; N. Walther, no. 23; C. Klein, no. 26; J. C. Heppius, no. 27 & 37; F. Schilling, no. 28; J. G. Halbmayer, no. 29; G. F. Widmann, no. 30 & 36; A. Lay, no. 31; H. Platz, no. 33; J. J. Meyer, no. 34; L. von Heyden, no. 35; J. Scherer, no. 38; P. Hiltmann, no. 39; A. Boxbarter, no. 40; J. Rötenbeck, no. 41; M. R. Besler, no. 42; P. Spindler, no. 43; T. Merclin, no. 44; P. Leytinger, no. 45; G. S. Widemann, no. 46 & 47; C. Hartmann, no. 48; E. Habrisch, no. 49; A. Nitzsch, no. 50; G. B. Wolfarth, no. 51; L. Eisenheim, no. 52; A. Saladin, no. 53; M. Wagner, no. 54; G. Kirsten, no. 55; J. C. Creuzauer, no. 56)

—Galeni Ars parva in disputationes triginta resoluta ... Argentorati, Typis Eberhardi Welperi, 1633.

[488] p.   16 cm.   **[10791]**

Each dissertation has special title page dated 1632. (*Respondents:* B. Schobinger, no. 1, 13; M. Wagner, no. 2, 18, 28; J. B. Tagius, no. 3, 14; A. Saladin, no. 4, 15; P. Ansorg, no. 5, 16, 29; J. H. Arcularius, no. 6, 17, 30; J. R. Widt, no. 7, 19; L. Eisenheim, no. 8, 20; J. G. Leyttersperger, no. 9, 21; J. G. Erhardt, no. 10, 22; W. E. Fesel, no. 11, 23; D. Chabrey, no. 12, 24; J. G. Zachmann, no. 25; J. Maclaeus, no. 26; A. Gerner, no. 27)

—Galeni quinque priores libri De simplicium medicamentorum facultatibus in sedecim disputationes resoluti. In quibus primum summa et analysis totius operis, undecim libris comprehensi, continetur. Deinde doctrina quinque priorum librorum problematice & syllogistice traditur. Tertio disputationibus ipsis corolaria numero 183. subjunguntur ... Argentorati, Typis Eberhardi Welperi, 1651.

[672] p.   16 cm.   **[10792]**

Contains 16 dissertations, each with special title page. Dates range from 1646–1651. (*Respondents:* J. Frey, no. 1; J. J. Comezius, no. 2; J. L. Witzel, no. 3; S. Reisel, no. 4; S. Closius, no. 5; M. K. Metzger, no. 6; G. G. Zillinger, no. 7; J. A. Planer, no. 8; J. K. Epplin, no. 9; C. L. Hetzer, no. 10; G. F. Stoffel, no. 11; J. M. Faber, no. 12; V. Riedlin, no. 13; C. Briccius, no. 14; T. Grossmann, no. 15; C. Buckisius, no. 16)

—Libri sex Galeni De morborum differentiis, morborum causis, symptomatum differentiis et causis, in theses partim contracti, partim in epitomas redacti

& ad disputandum in academia Argentoratensi propositi ... Argentorati, Typis Eberhardi Welperi, 1632.

[246] p.   20 cm.   **[10793]**

Each dissertation has special title page dated 1630 or 1631. (*Respondents:* G. Arthusius, A. Hartig, A. Nitzsch, J. G. Jäger, L. Kepler, J. Wolff)

—Prodromi examinis vulnerum singularum humani corporis partium, quatenus vel lethalia sunt & incurabilia, vel ratione eventus salutaria & sanabilia, pars I [–III] vulnerum nomenclaturas definitiones, differentias, subjecta & efficientes causas explicans ... Argentorati, Typis Eberhardi Welperi, 1632.

[132] p.   20 cm.   **[10794]**

Each dissertation has special title page dated 1632 or 1633. (*Respondents:* D. Chabrey, W. E. Fesel, J. G. Zachmann)

Individual dissertations

—*praeses.* Disputatio cheirurgica de ulceribus ... Argentorati, Typis Eberhardi Welperi, 1647.

[28] p.   20 cm.   **[10795]**

D. Espich, *respondent.*

—Disputatio de alimentorum facultatibus prima. Continens generalem de forma, materia, efficiente, & fine alimentorum doctrinam ... Argentorati, Typis Johannis Reppii, 1618.

[28] p.   19 cm.   **[10796]**

L. Mattsperger, *respondent.*

—Disputatio de alimentorum facultatibus secunda. Continens qualitates & vires eorum alimentorum quae a plantis petuntur ... Argentorati, Praelo Reppiano, 1618.

[64] p.   19 cm.   **[10797]**

D. Dinckel, *respondent.*

—Disputatio de alimentorum facultatibus tertia. Continens qualitates & vires eorum ciborum, qui ab animalibus petuntur ... Argentorati, Praelo Reppiano, 1619.

[88] p.   19 cm.   **[10798]**

M. Kohler, *respondent.*

—Disputatio de alimentorum facultatibus quarta et ultima. Continens qualitates & vires potuum ... Argentorati, Typis Johannis Reppi, 1620.

[68] p.   19 cm.   **[10799]**

B. Malleolus, *respondent.*

—Disputatio de arteriotomia ... Argentorati, Typis Joannis Reppii, 1620.

[12] p.   21 cm.   **[10800]**

J. Kisling, *respondent.*

—Disputatio de crisibus posterior: continens doctrinam eorum specialem ... Argentorati, Typis Johannis Andreae, 1627.

[24] p.   20 cm.   **[10801]**

L. von Heyden, *respondent.*

—Disputatio de diebus criticis prior: continens doctrinam eorum generalem ... Argentorati, Typis Johannis Andreae, 1626.

[32] p.   20 cm.   **[10802]**

N. Ager, *respondent.*

—Disputatio de diebus criticis posterior continens doctrinam eorum specialem ... Argentorati, Typis Johannis Andreae, 1626.

[32] p.   20 cm.   **[10803]**

Imperfect: last leaf mutilated.
M. Zschoesy, *respondent.*

—Disputatio de dolore ... Argentorati, Typis Eberhardi Welperi, 1652.

[40] p.   19 cm.   **[10804]**

H. A. Höffer, *respondent.*

—Disputatio de hirudinibus, scarificatione, & cucurbitulis ... Argentorati, Typis Joannis Reppii, 1620.

[16] p.   21 cm.   **[10805]**

P. Schmid, *respondent.*

—Disputatio de morbis contagiosis et contagio ... Argentorati, Typis Eberhardi Welperi, 1650.

[48] p.   19 cm.   **[10806]**

G. H. Cratzmann, *respondent.*

—Disputatio de pilis posterior, continens problemata varia, & curam, qua pili extirpari, reparari, augeri, formari & colorari queunt ... Argentorati, Typis Eberhardi Welperi, 1651.

[40] p.   19 cm.   **[10807]**

D. Stoll, *respondent.*

—Disputatio de purgatione secunda ... Argentorati, Typis Joannis Reppii, 1620.

[16] p.   21 cm.   **[10808]**

A. Opala, *respondent.*
This and succeeding dissertations through Disputatio de purgatione decima tertia also issued in *his* Disputationes de recta ratione purgandi. Argentorati, 1621.

—Disputatio de purgatione quarta ... Argentorati, Typis Johannis Reppii, 1620.

[16] p.   20 cm.   **[10809]**

Signatures: C-D⁴.
A. Rüber, *respondent.*

—Disputatio de purgatione quinta ... Argentorati, Typis Joannis Reppii, 1621.

[16] p.   20 cm.   **[10810]**

J. L. Gans, *respondent.*

—Disputatio de purgatione sexta ... Argentorati, Typis Joannis Reppii, 1621.

[16] p.   20 cm.   **[10811]**

Signatures: G-H⁴.
U. Rietmann, *respondent.*

—Disputatio de purgatione septima ... Argentorati, Typis Joannis Reppii, 1621.

[16] p.   20 cm.   **[10812]**

Signatures: I-K⁴.
J. J. Faber, *respondent.*

—Disputatio de purgatione octava ... Argentorati, Typis Joannis Reppii, 1621.

[16] p.   20 cm.   **[10813]**

Signatures: L-M⁴.
J. Steinicher, *respondent.*

—Disputatio de purgatione undecima ... Argentorati, Typis Joannis Reppii, 1621.

[16] p.   20 cm.   **[10814]**

Signatures: R-S⁴.
J. F. Regulus, *respondent.*

—Disputatio de purgatione duodecima ... Argentorati, Typis Joannis Reppii, 1621.

[16] p.   21 cm.   **[10815]**

Signatures: T-V⁴.
B. Malleolus, *respondent.*

—Disputatio de purgatione decima tertia ... Argentorati, Typis Joannis Reppii, 1621.

[16] p.   20 cm.   **[10816]**

Signatures: X-Y⁴.
J. Langenauer, *respondent.*

—Disputatio de senectutis et senum statu ac conditione ... Argentorati, Typis Eberhardi Welperi, 1645.

[68] p.   20 cm.   **[10817]**

G. H. Welsch, *respondent.*

—Disputatio de spiritibus humani corporis theorica & practica ... Argentorati, Typis Eberhardi Welperi, 1660.

[32] p. 19 cm. [**10818**]

J. D. Widt, *respondent.*

—Disputatio de venae sectione vigesima sexta ... Argentorati, Typis Johannis Reppii, 1620.

[18] p. 21 cm. [**10819**]

A. Opala, *respondent.*

—Disputatio de venae sectione vigesima septima ... Argentorati, Typis Joannis Reppii, 1620.

[8] p. 20 cm. [**10820**]

U. Rietmann, *respondent.*

—Disputatio de venae sectione vigesima octava ... Argentorati, Typis Joannis Reppii, 1620.

[8] p. 20 cm. [**10821**]

J. Steinicher, *respondent.*

—Disputatio de voce hominis ... Argentorati, Typis Johannis Andreae, 1623.

[23] p. 19 cm. [**10822**]

V. Charstadius, *respondent.*

—Disputatio medica de affectione hypochondriaca ... Argentorati, Typis Eberhardi Welperi, 1661.

[32] p. 19 cm. [**10823**]

J. P. Huth, *respondent.*

—Disputatio medica de calculo renum ... Argentorati, Typis Eberhardi Welperi, 1647.

[60] p. 19 cm. [**10824**]

C. Harder, *respondent.*

—Disputatio medica de causis, cur quidam morbi prorsus non, aliqui difficulter, nonnulli cito & facile, alii tarde admodum longoque tempore curentur? ... Argentorati, Typis Eberhardi Welperi, 1662.

32 p. 19 cm. [**10825**]

D. Eckolt, *respondent.*

—Disputatio ... medica de ophthalmia ... Argentorati, Typis Eberhardi Welperi, 1662.

31 p. 19 cm. [**10826**]

S. Geidelin, *respondent.*

—Disputatio medica de plethora et cacochymia ... Argentorati, Typis Eberhardi Welperi, 1631.

[23] p. 20 cm. [**10827**]

J. Sarasin, *respondent.*

—Disputatio medica solennis, de ictero, seu morbo regio ... Argentorati, Typis Eberhardi Welperi, 1663.

32 p. 19 cm. [**10828**]

J. S. Otto, *respondent.*

—Disputatio solennis de asthmate et orthopnoea ... Argentorati, Typis Eberhardi Welperi, 1664.

31 p. 19 cm. [**10829**]

P. J. Waldschmidt, *respondent.*

—Disputatio solennis de colica passione ... Argentorati, Typis Eberhardi Welperi, 1660.

[39] p. 19 cm. [**10830**]

C. Scherb, *respondent.*

—Disputatio solennis de constipatione alvi ... Argentorati, Typis Eberhardi Welperi, 1664.

29 (i.e. 30) p. 19 cm. [**10831**]

F. S. Assmann, *respondent.*

—Disputatio solennis de fame et siti ... Argentorati, Typis Eberhardi Welperi [1655]

[60] p. 19 cm. [**10832**]

J. C. Kisling, *respondent.*

—Disputatio solennis de singultu ... Argentorati, Typis Friderici Spoor, 1659.

[32] p. 20 cm. [**10833**]

M. Mapp, *respondent.*

—Disputatio solennis de stranguria ... Argentorati, Typis Eberhardi Welperi, 1657.

[32] p. 20 cm. [**10834**]

J.-J. Schuster, *respondent.*

—Disputatio solennis de sudore ... Argentorati, Typis Eberhardi Welperi, 1657.

[48] p. 19 cm. [**10835**]

J. Wepfer, *respondent.*

—Disputatio solennis de variis medicae artis curationis problematibus ... Argentorati, Typis Eberhardi Welperi, 1660.

[23] p. 19 cm. [**10836**]

J. A. Beza, *respondent.*

—Examen vulnerum partium similarium ... Argentorati, Typis Eberhardi Welperi, 1635.

[64] p. 19 cm. [**10837**]

J. G. Stephanus, *respondent.*

—Examen vulnerum singularum humani corporis partium, quatenus vel lethalia sunt et incurabilia, vel ratione eventus salutaria, et sanabilia. Cui tractatulus additus de sinovia, seu meliceria C. Celsi, quam vulgus cheirurgorum das Gliedwasser appellare solet ... Argentorati, Apud heredes Lazari Zetzneri, 1639.

[40] p.   20 cm.   **[10838]**

Imperfect: the second tract mentioned on the title page is not present.

Part 1 has special title page with imprint: Argentorati, Typis Eberhardi Welperi, 1632.

Diss., 1632. D. Chabrey, *respondent.*

—Exercitatio medica ... Argentorati, Typis excribebat Joannis Andreae, 1623.

[12] p.   20 cm.   **[10839]**

J. C. Osiander, *respondent.*

—Exercitatio medica prima ... Argentorati, Typis Josiae Rihelii haeredum, 1622.

[8] p.   19 cm.   **[10840]**

A reprint, dated 1623, was published in M. Sebisch's Exercitationes medicae, 1639.

J. C. Wesener, *respondent.*

—Exercitatio medica secunda ... Argentorati, Typis Rihelianis, 1622.

[8] p.   19 cm.   **[10841]**

A reprint, dated 1623, was published in M. Sebisch's Exercitationes medicae, 1639.

P. Thomas, *respondent.*

—Exercitationum medicinalium ex Fernelio prima: De nutritione, concoctionibus & humoribus, cujus ex ejusdem Physiologiae lib. VI. tabulis, aphorismis, & quaestionibus inclusae capita IV. priora ... [Argentorati] Typis Joannis Reppii [1622]

[16] p.   19 cm.   **[10842]**

J. Bartsch, *respondent.*

—Exercitationum medicinalium ex Fernelio secunda: De nutritione, concoctionibus & humoribus, cujus ex ejusdem Physiologiae lib. VI. tabulis, aphorsmis, & quaestionibus inclusae capita V. posteriora ... [Argentorati] Typis Joannis Reppii [1622]

[16] p.   19 cm.   **[10843]**

J. Bartsch, *respondent.*

—Exercitationum medicinalium ex Fernelio sexta: de morbis, eorumque differentiis generalibus: quam ex ejusdem Pathologiae lib. I. capp. X. prioribus tabulis, aphorismis et quaestionibus inclusam ... submittit M. Jacobus Bartschius ... [Argentorati] Typis Joannis Reppii [1623]

[20] p.   20 cm.   **[10844]**

J. Bartsch, *respondent.*

—Liber Galeni de differentiis morborum in theses contractus ... Argentorati, Typis Eberhardi Welperi, 1630.

[31] p.   19 cm.   **[10845]**

G. Arthusius, *respondent.*

—Liber Galeni De tumoribus praeter naturam ... Argentorati, Typis Eberhardi Welperi, 1633.

[28] p.   21 cm.   **[10846]**

J. Maclaeus, *respondent.*

—Problemata medica de infantium et puerorum morbis ... Argentorati, Typis Eberhardi Welperi, 1649.

[44] p.   19 cm.   **[10847]**

G. G. Zillinger, *respondent.*

—Problemata medica miscellanea ... Argentorati, Typis Eberhardi Welperi, 1661.

32 p.   19 cm.   **[10848]**

J. C. Freyburger, *respondent.*

—Problemata medica miscellanea ... Argentorati, Typis Eberhardi Welperi, 1662.

[44] p.   19 cm.   **[10849]**

J. M. Hornung, *respondent.*

—Problemata medica varia ... Argentorati, Typis Eberhardi Welperi, 1662.

36 p.   19 cm.   **[10850]**

U. F. von Gudenus, *respondent.*

—Problemata phlebotomica, ex Galeni libro De curandi ratione per sanguinis missionem deprompta ... Argentorati, Typis Johannis Reppii, 1631.

[23] p.   20 cm.   **[10851]**

A. Kisling, *respondent.*

—*See* PINEAU, S. De integritatis et corruptionis virginum notis. 1640, 1641, 1650, 1663, 1690; STUPANUS, J. N. Gratiosi medicorum Basiliens. collegii decreto, 1610.

SEBISCH, MELCHIOR [1664-1704] *praeses.* Dissertatio academica de urinatoribus atque arte urinandi ... Argentorati, Literis Danielis Maagii [1700]

[2], 38 p.   plate.   20 cm.   **[10852]**

Diss.—Strasbourg (J. Salzmann, *respondent*)

—*respondent.* Dissertatio medica inauguralis de sudore ... Argentorati, Literis Johannis Welperi [1688]

[51] p.   20 cm.   **[10853]**

Diss.—Strasbourg.

SEBITZ. *See* SEBISCH.

SEBIZ. *See* SEBISCH.

SEBIZIUS. *See* SEBISCH.

SECHS Bücher auserlesener Artzney und Kunst-Stück, fast vor alle dess menschlichen Leibes Gebrechen und Kranckheiten, auss vielen beschriebenen Artzney Büchern, so bey fürstlichen und andern hohen Personen verwahret werden, mit sonderm Fleiss zusammen getragen . . . Erstlich auff Fürstlichen Bevhelich gedruckt zu Jhena . . . Zerbst, Bey Zacharias Dörffern, 1613.

[27], 746 p.   21 cm.   **[10854]**

Compiled under the direction of Eleonora, *Landgravine of Hesse-Darmstadt.*

Most bibliographers consider the "Sechs Bücher" an earlier edition of the "Freywillig-aufgesprungener Granat-Apffel" which was compiled by Eleonora Maria Rosalia, Duchess of Troppau and Jägerndorf. The two works, however, are basically different in text.

With this are bound: Hauss Apoteck. 1613.–Herlitz, D. De cura gravidarum. 1613.–Albertus Magnus, Saint, Bp. of Ratisbon. Ein newer Albertus Magnus, von Weybern und Geburten der Kinder. 1608.

—[The same.] Weymarisches Artzney-Buch, das ist: Sechs Bücher auserlesener Artzney und Kunst-Stücke, fast vor alle des menschlichen Leibes Zufälle, Gebrechen und Kranckheiten vom Haupt biss auff die Fuss-Solen. Aus vielen beschriebenen Artzney-büchern, so bey fürstlichen und andern hohen Personen verwahret werden, mit sonderbahren Fleiss zusammen getragen, jetzo aber von neuen von etlichen vornehmen Medicis durchsehen, auch umb ein Grosses vermehret . . . Franckfurt und Leipzig, Lorentz Sigismund Cörner, 1678.

[16], 916, [20] p.   21 cm.   **[10855]**

Added engraved title page.

SECONDE apologie. 1653. *See* [CATTIER, I.]

SECRETI nobilissimi dell'arte profumatoria. 1672. *See* [PELLEGRINI, B.]

Les SECRETS de la medecine des chinois, consistant en la parfaite connoissance du pouls. Envoyez de la Chine par un françois, homme de grand merite . . . Grenoble, Philippes Charuys, 1671.

[12], 135, [6] p.   14 cm.   **[10856]**

Attributed to Louis Augustin Alemand, Micha Piotr Boym and Julien Placide Hervieu. These attributions denied by M. D. Grmek. Les reflets de la sphygmologie chinoise dans la médecine occidentale. Biologie médicale vol. 51, 1962, numéro hors série, p. lix-lxiii.

The SECRETS of physick and chirurgery. *See* [WOOD, O.] Choice and profitable secrets both physicall, and chirurgical. 1658.

SECRETS touchant la medecine. 1668 (i.e. 1678) *See* [AUVERGNE, A.-M.]

SECRETUS, HENRICUS. *See* SCRETA, Heinrich [1637–1689]

SECTIO altera in qua agitur de recta alimentorum administratione. *See* SALA, G. D. De alimentis et eorum recta administratione liber. 1628.

SEELMANN, CHRISTIAN [*fl.* 1649–1650] *praeses.* Mors homini inevitabilis; h. e., Dissertatio physica in qua vitam nullo vel subsidio vel remedio in perpetuum prolongari adeoque mortem vitari posse demonstratur . . . Wittebergae, Typis Johannis Röhneri, 1650.

[16] p.   19 cm.   **[10857]**

Diss. pro loco—Wittenberg (C. Hagius, *respondent*)

SEERUP, GEORG NICOLAUS [*fl.* 1678–1700] *praeses.* Triumphus lithargyriatorum; seu, Dissertatio medico-chemica, qua vindicantur saccharum Saturni & Mercurius lithargyrii ab animadversionibus . . . Joh. Victoris Jaegerschmidii . . . Havniae, Ex typographeo Reg. Majest. & Universitatis [1700]

[2], 50 p.   20 cm.   **[10858]**

Diss.—Copenhagen (E. Møinichen, *respondent*)

—*respondent. See* BARTHOLIN, C. [1655–1738] *praeses.* De cordis structura & motu disquisitio. 1678 [and] De olfactus organo disquisitio anatomica. 1679.

SEGARRA, JAIME [*d.* 1598] *See* GALENUS. Αιτιολογικη και παθολογικη; sive, De morborum et symptomatum differentiis, et causis, libri sex. 1624.

SEGER, GEORG [1629–1678] Dissertatio anatomica de Hippocratis orthodoxia in doctrina de nutritione foetus humani in utero. Cui accessere ejusdem dissertatiunculae binae; quarum altera De democriti heterodoxia in doctrina de nutritione foetus in utero, altera De cotyledonibus uteri . . . Basileae, Typis Georgii Deckeri, 1660.

[4], 50, [2] p.; [2], 9, [1] p.; 8 p.   20 cm.

[10859]

Includes 2 Basel dissertations, each with special title page.

—Dissertatio anatomica, de quidditate & materia lymphae Bartholinianae, cui accessere epistolae doctorum virorum de eadem lympha. Hafniae, Sumptibus Petri Hauboldi, excudebat Petrus Hakius, 1658.

[4], 61 (i.e. 59), [1] p.   21 cm.   **[10860]**

—Dissertatio de Hippocratis libri περι καρδιης ortu legitimo. Basileae, Apud Joannem König, 1661.

32 p.   20 cm.   **[10861]**

—Triumphus . . . cordi, post felicissime tandem ceptam duce . . . Thoma Bartholino ex totali hepatis clade victoriam. Hafniae erectus . . . literis Georgii Lamprechtii, anno 1654. Francofurti, Prostant apud Petrum Hauboldum [1655?]

[80] p.   20 cm.   **[10862]**

Imperfect: first 2 preliminary leaves backed.

—Triumphus et querimonia cordis. Basileae, Apud Joannem König, 1661.

[1], [4], 44, [1] p.; 40, [1] p.   20 cm. **[10863]**

Part [1] has special title page: Triumphus . . . cordi, post felicissime tandem obtentam duce . . . Thoma Bartholino ex totali hepatis clade victoriam. Part [2] has special title page: Querimonia nobilissimi visceris cordis, querimoniae hepatis, autore Joanne Riolano ad medicos Parisienses habitae, opposita, interprete Georgio Segero.

—*respondent.* Dissertatio inauguralis de Hippocratis orthodoxia in doctrina de nutritione foetus humani in utero . . . Basileae, Typis Georgii Deckeri [1660]

[4], 50, [2] p.   20 cm.   **[10864]**

Diss.—Basel.

Published also as part [1] of his Dissertatio anatomica de Hippocratis orthodoxia.

—*respondent. See* BECKHER, D. [1627-1670] *praeses.* Dissertatio medica de opio. 1652.

SEGNI, GIULIANO [*fl.* 17th cent.] Questio de gangraenae et sphaceli diversa curatione ab . . . Ant. Baldesio . . . ex colloquiis, & controversiis a Juliano Signio . . . familiariter cum plurimis doctoribus in S. Marie Novę Xenodochio habitis collecta . . . Per Jo. Castellinum . . . in lucem aedita. In fine addita ejusdem Juliani de ossium capitis occultis noscendis lesionibus secundum Hippocratem tabula . . . Florentiae, In officina Marescotti, 1613.

96 p.   16 cm.   **[10865]**

Imperfect: tables wanting.

SEGNITZ, MICHAEL [*fl.* 1698] *respondent. See* HOFFMANN, F. [1660-1742] *praeses.* Dissertatio inauguralis medica de remediorum evacuantium mechanica operandi ratione. 1698.

SEGUNDO discurso serio-jocoso sobre la neuva invencion de la agua de la vida. 1682. *See* [GONZÁLEZ DE GODOY, P.]

Ein SEHR nöttiger Zettel, auff alle Jar gerichtet, vom Aderlassen, Schröpffen und Artzneyen, auch Haar, und Nägel abschneiden . . . Augspurg, Getruckt bey David Francken, in Verlegung Steffan Michelspachers, 1617.

broadside.   55 x 33 cm.   **[10866]**

Bound with Strobelberger, J. S. Kurtze Instruction und Bad-Regiment. 1630.

SEIDEL, BRUNO [*ca.* 1530-1591] Liber, morborum incurabilium causas . . . explicans . . . Accessit Fabritii de Paduanis tractatus De morbis in quibus praesentaneis uti convenit remediis . . . Lugd. Bat., Apud Petrum Hackium, & veneunt Parisiis, apud Robertum de Ninville, 1662.

[18], 190 (i.e. 198) p.; 34, [14] p.   16 cm.**[10867]**

Part [2] has half title.
The Praefatio is by Zacharias Palthenius.
Edited by Hadrianus Foppens.

—Physica, cum supplemento Rodolphi Goclenii . . . ex ejusdem recognitione edita . . . Francofurti, E Collegio musarum Paltheniano, 1656.

[12], 549, [46] p.   17 cm.   **[10868]**

SEIDEL, CHRISTIAN EPHRAIM [*fl.* 1699] Disputatio medica inauguralis de haemorrhagia narium . . . Lugduni Batavorum, Apud Abrahamum Elzevier, 1699.

[18] p.   21 cm.   **[10869]**

Diss.—Leyden.

SEIDEL, JACOB [1546-1615] *See* LYSER, M. Culter anatomicus. 1665, 1679.

SEIDEL, JAKOB [*fl.* 1657] *respondent. See* EICHSTÄD, L., *praeses.* Disputatio physiologica publica extraordinaria de peste. 1657.

SEIDEL, JOHANN [*fl.* 1620] *respondent. See* SEBISCH, M. [1578-1674?] *praeses.* Disputationes de recta ratione purgandi. 1621.

SEIDEL, MICHAEL [*fl.* 1610] *respondent.* Theses hasce medicas de ictero flavo et nigro . . . publice exponit . . . Michael Seidel . . . Basileae, Typis Joan. Jacobi Genathii, 1610.

[8] p.   20 cm.   **[10870]**

Diss.—Basel.

See BAUHIN, K. Hygiae et panaceae parente . . . Casparus Bauhinus. 1610.

SEIDELL, JOACHIM ERNST [*fl.* 1653] *respondent. See* SUEVUS, G., *praeses.* Disputatio juridica de peste. 1653.

SEIDEMANN, MARTIN [*fl.* 1651] *See* CALISIUS, A. Dissertatio de aere. 1651.

SEIDLER, JOHANN GOTTFRIED [*fl.* 1670] *respondent.* Disputatio medica inauguralis de passione haemoptoica . . . Lugduni Batavorum, Apud viduam & haeredes Joannis Elsevirii, 1670.

[39] p.   23 cm.   **[10871]**
Diss. — Leyden.

SEIFERT, CHRISTOPH [*fl.* 1654-1697] *praeses.* Ανεμολογια; sive, Dissertatio de ventis . . . Lipsiae, Exscribebat Quirinus Bauch [1654]

[23] p.   19 cm.   **[10872]**
Diss. — Leipzig (G. Sternberger, *respondent*)

SEILER, JOHANN DANIEL [*fl.* 1644] *respondent.* De affectu gravissimo ileo seu chordapso . . . Regiomonti, Typis Johannis Reusneri, 1644.

[28] p.   18 cm.   **[10873]**
Diss. — Königsberg.

SEITZ, ALEXANDER [*ca.* 1470-1540?] Manuale medicum; oder, Rüstkamer für die jenigen Personen so Aderlassens und Schrepffens zugebrauchen benötiget . . . In latheinischer Sprach beschrieben. Jetzund aber meniglich zu guttem, neben anderen . . . Experimenten . . . zusamen gebracht und . . . transferiert durch Melchiorn Finold . . . Augspurg, Bey Christoff Mang, 1605.

[126] p.   16 cm.   **[10874]**

SELECTA poemata Italorum. *See* ΑΝΘΟΛΟΓΙΆ; seu, Selecta quaedam poemata Italorum. 1684.

SELIGMANN, GOTTLOB FRIEDRICH [1654-1707] *praeses.* Sciagraphiam virium imaginationis . . . publice exhibebit Johannes Postel. Rostochii, Prelo Jacobi Richelii [1682]

[28] p.   18 cm.   **[10875]**
Diss. — Rostock (J. Postel, *respondent*)

SELNECCER, NICOLAUS [1530-1592] *See* SCHLEMM, J. Schirm-und Schutz-Flügel. 1681; ZWEYER VORTREFF-LICHER THEOLOGEN. 1680.

SELVA di maravigliosi secreti curiosi, e necessarii cosi à gli huomini, come alle donne. Raccolti, &

esperimentati da diversi autori. Palermo, Napoli & Venetia, 1651.

[8] p.   15 cm.   **[10876**

SELVATICO, GIOVANNI BATTISTA [*d.* 1621] Collegii Mediolanensium medicorum origo, antiquitas, necessitas, utilitas, dignitates, honores, privilegia, e viri illustres . . . Mediolani, Apud Hieronymum Bordonum, Petrum Martyrem Locarnum, & Bernardinum Lantonum, 1607.

91 p.   22 cm.   **[10877**
"Clementis Octavi Pontificis Maximi diploma, quo Mediolanensis Collegii medicos, Sacri Palatii, & Aulae Lateranensis comites aurataeque militiae equites creavit" (dated Feb. 23, 1597): p. 86-88

—Controversiae medicae numero centum . . . Francofurti, Typis Wechelianis apud Claudium Marnium, & heredes Joannis Aubrii, 1601.

[8], 470, [26] p.   34 cm.   **[10878**

—[The same.] . . . Mediolani, Typis Societati Hieronymi Bordonii & Petri Martyris Locarni, 1601

[44], 762 (i.e. 764) p.   26 cm.   **[10879**

—De anno climacterico tractatus . . . Ticini, Apud Andream Vianum, 1615.

[6], 94 p.   17 cm.   **[10880**

—Galeni historiae medicinales a Jo. Baptista Silvatico . . . enarratae . . . Hanoviae, Typis Wechelianis, apud Claudium Marnium & haerede Johannis Aubrii, 1605.

[12], 422, [18] p.   34 cm.   **[10881**
Based on case histories selected from Galen's works.
Bound with Valles, F. de. Controversiarum medicarum . . . libri X. 1606.

—Institutio medica de iis, qui morbum simulant deprehendendis. Francofurti ad Moenum, Sumptibus haered. Schürerianor. & Joh. Fritzschi., 1671

[10], 215 p.   14 cm.   **[10882**
Imprint printed on slip cancel.

—Medicus . . . Mediolani, Apud Hieronymum Bordonum, 1611.

[15], 394 (i.e. 344) p.   18 cm.   **[10883**
With this is bound: Settala, L. De naevis liber. 1606.

SEMEDO, JOÃO CURVO. *See* CURVO SEMMEDO João [1635-1719]

SEMINARIUS, JOHANN CHRISTIAN [*fl.* 1664-1666 *respondent.* Dissertationem hanc inauguralem de morbo virgineo . . . submittit Johannes Christianu

Seminarius ... Marpurgi Cattorum, Typis Salomonis Schadewitzii, 1666.

39 p. 19 cm. [10884]

Diss. — Marburg.

—*See* ROLFINCK, W., *praeses.* Casus practicus medicus. 1664.

SEMMEDO, JOÃO CURVO. *See* CURVO SEMMEDO, João [1635-1719]

SEMPRONIUS GRACCHUS MASSILIENSIS, *pseud. See* MANITIUS, Samuel Gotthelf [*d.* 1698]

SENAULT, JEAN FRANÇOIS [1601-1672] De l'usage des passions ... [Leyden?] Suivant la copie imprimée a Paris, 1643.

[36], 559 p. 15 cm. [10885]

Engraved title page.

—[The same.] ... Paris, Laurens Raveneau, 1669.

[70], 492 p. 16 cm. [10886]

Engraved title page.

—[English tr.] The use of passions. Written in French ... and put into English by Henry Earl of Monmouth. London, Printed by W. B. for John Sims, 1671.

[46], 510 p. front. (port.) 17 cm. [10887]

Ein **SEND-SCHREIBEN.** 1700. *See* [LUFNEU, J.]

SENDIVOGIUS, *filius. See* HARPRECHT, Johann [*b.* 1610?]

SENDIVOGIUS, MICHAEL [1566-1636] Les oeuvres du Cosmopolite, divisez en trois parties. [Paris, Jean d'Houry, 1669-1671]

4 parts in 1 v. 16 cm. [10888]

Each part has special title page, part [4] dated 1671.

—Cosmopolite; ou, Nouvelle lumiere chimyque, divisée en douse traitez. Avec un dialogue du mercure, de l'alchymiste, & de la nature. Rev. & ... corr. Paris, Jean d'Houry, 1669.

[13], 118 p. 16 cm. (Part [1] *in* his Les oeuvres. [Paris, 1669]) [10889]

—Duodecim tractatus de lapide philosophorum: authore me, qui Divi Leschi Genus Amo (i.e. Michael Sendivogius) ... [&] ... Aenigma philosophorum [&] Dialogus mercurii, alchemistae, et naturae.

420-456 p., vol. 4. 20 cm. (*In* Zetzner, Lazarus, *ed.* Theatrum chemicum. Argentorati, 1659-61) [10890]

Caption titles.

[—] Lettre philosophique, traduite d'alleman en françois. Par Antoine Du Val. Paris, Jean d'Houry, 1671.

[1], 84 p. 16 cm. (Part [4] *in* his Les oeuvres. [Paris, 1669]) [10891]

[—] Novum lumen chymicum, e naturae fonte & manuali experienta depromptum, in duas partes divisum. Quarum prior XII. tractatibus de mercurio agit, posterior de sulphure, altero naturae principio. Author sum qui Divi Leschi Genus Amo [i.e. Michael Sendivogius] Genevae, Typis & sumpt. Joan. de Tournes, 1628.

202, [1] p. 14 cm. [10892]

—Novum lumen chemicum, e naturae fonte et manuali experientia depromptum. Cui accessit tractatus De sulphure ...

[545]-645 p. 22 cm. (*In* Musaeum Hermeticum. Francofurti, 1678) [10893]

Includes his Aenigma philosophicum (p. 585-590), Dialogus mercurii, alchimistae et naturae (p. 590-600), Novi luminis chemici tractatus alter de sulphure (p. [601]-645).

—[The same.] *In* Aubigné de la Fosse, N. Bibliotheca chemica. 1653; Béguin, J. Novum lumen ad Tyrocinium chymicum. 1625; Müller, Philipp. Miracula & mysteria chymico-medica. 1614, 1616, 1623, 1656.

—*as subject. See* ORTHELIUS. Orthelius commentator in Novum lumen chymicum Michaelis Sendivogii. 1659.

—[English tr.] A new light of alchymie, taken out of the fountaine of nature, and manuall experience. To which is added a treatise of sulphur ... Also nine books Of the nature of things, written by Paracelsus ... Also A chymicall dictionary ... Translated out of the Latin into the English tongue, by J[ohn] F[rench] M. D. London, Printed by Richard Cotes, for Thomas Williams, 1650.

[16], 147, [3] p.; [8], 145 p.; [1], [48] p. 19 cm. [10894]

Parts [2] and [3] have special title pages.

—[The same.] ... London, Printed by A. Clark, for Tho. Williams at the Golden Ball, 1674.

[16], 351 p.   18 cm.   [**10895**]

"Of the nature of things" and "A chymical dictionary" have special title pages.

[—] Traité du sel. Troisiéme principe des choses minerales. De nouveau mis en lumiere. Paris, Jean d'Houry, 1669.

[6], 87 p.   16 cm.   (Part [3] *in* his Les oeuvres. [Paris, 1669])   [**10896**]

[—] Traité du soulphre second principe de la nature ... Rev. & corr. Paris, Jean d'Houry, 1669.

[13], 105 p.   16 cm.   (Part [2] *in* his Les oeuvres. [Paris, 1669])   [**10897**]

SENF, Michael Aloysius. *See* Sinapi, Mihály Alajos [*fl.* 1693-1696]

SENGUERD, Arnold [1610-1667] Discursus de ostento Dolano. *In* Collectanea de diuturna graviditate. 1662.

—Osteologia corporis humani. Amstelodami, Apud Joannem Janssonium, 1662.

[16], 170, [6] p.   13 cm.   [**10898**]

—*praeses.* Disputatio physica de peste ... Amstelodami, Apud Joannem Ravesteinium, 1663.

[12] p.   18 cm.   [**10899**]

Diss. — Amsterdam (C. de Vogel, *respondent*)

SENGUERD, Wilhelm Arnold [*fl.* 1661-1662] *respondent. See* Blasius, G., *praeses.* Exercitationum medicarum de humoribus prima [-secunda, – tertia] 1661, 1662.

SENGUERDIUS, Wolferdus [1646-1724] In- quisitiones experimentales, quibus praeter par- ticularia nonnula phaenomena, atmosphaerici aeris natura explicatius traditur ... Adjectae sunt Ephemerides ... a calendis Februariis, anni 1697 ... ad finem subsequentis a. 1698. exhibentes. Ed. 2, priore plusquam altera parte auctior. Lugduni Batavorum, Apud Cornelium Boutesteyn, 1699.

[8], 3-158, [48] p.   illus., plates.   22 cm.   [**10900**]

The Ephemerides ([48] p.) has half title.
Imperfect: sig. X¹⁻⁴ misbound after Y⁴.

—Philosophia naturalis, quatuor partibus primarias corporum species, affectiones, differentias, productiones, mutationes, & interitus, exhibens. Ed.

2 priore auctior. Lugd. Batav., Apud Danielem à Gaesbeeck, 1685.

[28], 432, 32 p.   illus., plates.   20 cm.   [**10901**]

Added engraved title page.

—Tractatus physicus de tarantula. In quo praeter ejus descriptionem, effectus veneni tarantulae, qui hactenus fuerunt occultis qualitatibus adscripti, ra- tionibus naturalibus deducuntur & illustrantur. Lugduni Bat., Apud Gaasbeeckios, 1668.

87 p.   14 cm.   [**10902**]

"... Oratio inauguralis de usu et dignitate philosophiae ...": p. [71]-87.

Added engraved title page.

—*praeses.* Disputationum physicarum selectarum decima quae est de rabie canum prior ... Lugduni Batavorum, Apud viduam & heredes Johannis Elsevirii, 1674.

[8] p.   17 cm.   [**10903**]

Imperfect: upper margins trimmed.
Diss. — Leyden (G. ab Ophoven, *respondent*)

—Exercitium experimentale duodecimum, de aëris elasticitate secundum ... Lugduni Batavorum, Apud Abrahamum Elzevier, 1696.

[12] p.   19 cm.   [**10904**]

Diss. — Leyden (J. Bovie, *respondent*)

—Exercitium experimentale quartum decimum, quod est de aëris gravitate primum ... Lugduni Batavorum, Apud Abrahamum Elzevier, 1697.

[12] p.   19 cm.   [**10905**]

Diss. — Leyden (J. van Slingerlandt, *respondent*)

—Exercitium experimentale septimum decimum, quod est de aëreae elasticitatis & resistentiae passivae effectis ... Lugduni Batavorum, Apud Abrahamum Elzevier, 1698.

[14] p.   19 cm.   [**10906**]

Diss. — Leyden (S. Voorhoff, *respondent*)

SENNERT, Daniel [1572-1637] Opera omnia in tres tomos distincta. [Parisiis, Apud Societatem, 1641]

3 v.   illus., port.   38 cm.   [**10907**]

Title from general half title.
Edited by Guy Patin.

Contents.—v. 1. De origine et natura animarum in brutis. Epitome naturalis scientiae. Physica hypomnemata. Institutiones medicinae. Tabulae institutionum. De chymicorum cum Aristotelicis et Galenicis consensu et dissensu liber. Appendix de constitutione chymiae.—v. 2. Medicinae practicae, pars 1, 2 [&] De febribus. Fasciculus medicamentorum pestilentia grassante. — v.

3. Medicinae practicae, pars 3–6 [&] De arthritide. Tragopodagra Luciani. De infantium curatione tractatus. Appendix libri VI. Miram veneficii historiam exhibens.

The De origine et natura animarum in brutis concerns his acquittal from the charge of heresy and blasphemy, made by Johann Freitag.

—Opera omnia [Tomus primus-tertius] Venetiis, Apud Franciscum Baba, 1641.

    3 v. illus., port. 33 cm.   [**10908**]

Title from general half title.

The following items have special title pages: Institutionum medicinae, De chymicorum, Epitome naturalis scientiae, De febribus. The Physica hypomnemata has caption title.

Contents as in the 1641 Paris edition with the omission of De origine et natura animarum in brutis and Tabulae institutionum.

Imperfect: Physica hypomnemata wanting.

—Another issue, with different title page.

                                          [**10909**]

Vol. 1 only.

Imperfect: Physica hypomnemata wanting.

—Copy 2.

Vol. 1 only (Includes the Physica hypomnemata) Imperfect: general half title wanting.

—Operum tomus primus [-tertius] Ed. nov. caeteris omnibus auct. & corr. Lugduni, Sumptibus Joannis Antonii Huguetan, & Marci Antonii Ravaud, 1650.

    3 v. illus. 36 cm.   [**10910**]

Imperfect: first preliminary leaf of vol. 1 (general title page?) wanting.

Contents as in the 1641 Paris edition with the omission of Tabulae institutionum, and the addition of Vita Danielis Sennerti, Methodus discendi medicinam, Exoterica, and Judicia virorum clarissimorum. The Tragopodagra Luciani is in Latin and Greek.

—Operum tomus I, quo continentur Methodus discendi medicinam, Exoterica, Institutionum medicinae libri V., Liber chymicorum, Epitome naturalis scientiae, Hypomnemata physica ... Ed. caeteris omnibus auct., & corr., cum ultima impressione Lugdunensi diligentissime collata ... Venetiis, Apud Franciscum Baba, 1651.

    1 v. 34 cm.   [**10911**]

General half title.

Imperfect: title page mutilated.

Includes: Appendix de constitutione chymiae.

—Operum tomus primus [-quartus] ... Ed. nov., caeteris omnibus auct. & corr. ... Lugduni, Sumptibus Joannis Antonii Huguetan, & Marci Antonii Ravaud, 1656.

    4 v. in 2. illus., port. 38 cm.   [**10912**]

General half title.

Contents as in the 1650 Lyons edition.

—Operum in quinque tomos divisorum ... Ed. nov., caeteris omnibus tum corr., tum auct. tomo uno ... Lugduni Sumptibus Joannis Antonii Huguetan Marci Antonii Ravaud, 1666.

    5 v. in 3. illus., port. 37 cm.   [**10913**]

General half title.

Contents as in the 1641 Paris edition with the omission of Tabulae institutionum, and the addition of Vita Danielis Sennerti, Judicia virorum clarissimorum, De arthritide, Tragopodagra Luciani (in Greek and Latin), Exoterica, Epistolarum medicinalium una cum responsorii D. Michaelis Doringei centuriae duae, Epitome institutionum medicinae, Epitome librorum de Febribus, Panegyricus dictus in obitum D. Dan. Sennerti a ... Henningo Grosse. The two Epitomes are reprinted from the Epitome edited by Claude Bonnet.

Imperfect: p. 101–178 of v. 1 wanting.

—Operum in sex tomos divisorum tomus primus [-sextus] ... Ed. nov., caeteris omnibus tum corr., tum auct. tomo uno. ... Lugduni, Sumptibus Joannis Antonii Huguetan, 1676.

    6 v. in 3. illus., port. 37 cm.   [**10914**]

General half title.

Contents as in the 1641 edition with the omission of Tabulae institutionum, and the addition of Vita Danielis Sennerti, Judicia virorum clarissimorum, Methodus discendi medicinam, De curatione infantium, De arthritide, Tragopodagra Luciana (in Greek and Latin), Exoterica, Epitome librorum de febribus, Epistolarum medicinalium una cum responsorii D. Michaelis Doringei centuriae duae. The Epitome is reprinted from the Epitome edited by Claude Bonnet.

—Aphorismi ex institutionibus medicis Sennerti, magna diligentia collecti, opera Joannis Joachimi Becheri ... Francofurti, Sumptibus Johannis Beyeri, typis, Balthasari-Christophori Wustii, 1663.

    [22], 430, [28] p. 14 cm.   [**10915**]

—De arthritide tractatus. *In his* Practicae medicinae liber primus [-sextus]. 1628–1635.

—De chymicorum cum Aristotelicis et Galenicis consensu ac dissensu liber, cui accessit Appendix de constitutione chymiae ... Wittebergae, Sumtibus viduae & haered. Zachariae Schüreri Senioris [typis haeredum Salomonis Auerbach] 1629.

    [19], 434, [11] p. 23 cm.   [**10916**]

Includes a discussion of Paracelsus' therapeutics.

Bound with *his* De febribus.1628.

—[The same.] ... Ed. 3 ab authore adhuc recensita. Francofurti & Wittebergae, Sumptibus haered. D. Tobiae Mevii, & Elerdi Schumacheri, 1655.

[20], 374 + p. 23 cm. [10917]

Imperfect: all pages after p. 374 wanting.
Bound with *his* De febribus. 1653.

—De dysenteria tractatus ... Wittebergae, Apud Zachariam Schürerum, typis Jobi Wilhelmi Fincelii, 1626.

[8], 162, [6] p. 18 cm. [10918]

With this is bound *his* De scorbuto tractatus. 1624.

—De febribus libri IV ... Wittebergae, Apud Zachariam Schurerum [Impressum typis haeredum Johannis Richteri] 1619.

[16], 1090, [35] p. 18 cm. [10919]

—[The same.] ... Accessit ad calcem, ejusdem De dysenteria tractatus. Lugduni, Sumptibus Joannis Lautret, 1627.

[8], 994, [11] p.; [1], 147, [10] p. 18 cm. [10920]

Part [2] has half title.

—De febribus libri IV ... Ed. 2. auct., cui accessit Fasciculus medicamentorum contra pestem. Wittebergae, Sumtibus viduae & haered. Zachariae Schüreri Senioris [Typis haeredum Salomonis Auerbach] 1628.

[12], 704, [7] p. 23 cm. [10921]

The Fasciculus medicamentorum pestilentia grassante (p. [593]-704) includes recipes by Petrus Sibyllenus, Johann Neeffe, Johannes von Schröter, Joannes Guinterius, Andernacus, Johannes Kentmann, Jacobus Theodorus, and Sigismund Kohlreuter.
Errata: p. [7] at end.
With this is bound *his* De chymicorum ... liber. 1629.

—[The same.] ... Ed. 3. auct. ... Parisiis, Apud Societatem, 1633.

[6], 646 [i.e. 648] p. 22 cm. [10922]

—[The same.] ... Ed. nov. ... Venetiis, Apud Franciscum Baba, 1641.

[4], 248, [6] p. 34 cm. [10923]

—[The same.] ... Ed. 3., ab autore adhuc recensita ... Francofurti & Wittebergae, Sumptibus Balthasaris Mevii, 1653.

[8], 700, [14] p. 23 cm. [10924]

With this is bound *his* De chymicorum ... liber. 1655.

—De infantium curatione tractatus. *In his* Practicae medicinae liber primus [-sextus]. 1628-1635.

—De scorbuto tractatus ... Cui accesserunt ejusdem argumenti tractatus & epistolae Balduini Ronssei, Johannis Echthii, Johannis Wieri, Johannis Langii, Salomonis Alberti, Matthaei Martini. Wittebergae, Apud Zachariam Schurerum [Typis Jobi Wilhelmi Fincelii] 1624.

[16], 755 (i.e. 746), [22] p. illus. 18 cm. [10925]

"Balduini Ronssei ... De magnis Hippocratis lienibus, Pliniique stomacace ac sceletyrbe, seu vulgo dicto Scorbuto commentarius. Ejusdem epistolae quinque ejusdem argumenti": p. [233]-353.
"De schorbuto praeside Salomone Alberto ... Respondebit M. Ernestus Hettenbach ...": p. [541]-573.
The two letters of Johannes Lange (p. 343-353) are epist. 13 and 14 in book 2 of his Epistolarum medicinalium miscellanea.
Bound with *his* De dysenteria tractatus. 1626.

—De unguento armario.

585-598 p. 21 cm. (*In* Theatrum sympatheticum auctum. Norimbergae, 1662) [10926]

Caption title.

—Duo tractatus de dignotione & curatione scorbuti & reliquorum ab eo dependentium affectuum hypochondriacorum, quorum prior ... Danielis Sennerti ... posterior ... Matthaei Martini ... Nunc demum ... impressi. Jenae, Typis Johannis Beithmanni, sumptibus Johannis Birckneri, 1624.

[10], 169 p. 16 cm. [10927]

—Epitome institutionum medicarum ... disputationibus XVIII. comprehensa. Witteberge, Sumptibus haered. Zachariae Schüreri Senioris, typis Ambrosii Rothi, 1631.

[928] p. 14 cm. [10928]

Imperfect: upper margins trimmed with possible loss of pagination.

—Epitome institutionum medicinae et Libr. de febribus ... [Wittebergae] Sumptib. haered. Zach. Schüreri [typis haered Georgii Mulleri, 1634]

[32], 936 p.; [1], 249, [2] p. table. 14 cm. [10929]

Engraved title page.
Part [2] has half title: Epitome librorum de febribus.
Imperfect: wormholes in outer margins.

—[The same.] ... Amstelodami, Apud Jodocum Jansonium, 1644.

[24], 710 p.; 188 p. plate. 14 cm. [10930]

Added engraved title page.
Part [2] has special title page: Epitome librorum de febribus.

—[The same.] . . . Patavii, Typis Pauli Frambotti, 1644.

[19], 624, [16] p.; 169, [7] p.   15 cm.   [**10931**]

Part [2] has special title page: Epitome librorum de febribus.

—Epitome institutionum medicinae. Lugduni, Sumptib. Petri Ravaud, 1645.

[24], 932 p.   table.   15 cm.   [**10932**]

—Epitome institutionum medicinae, et Libr. de febribus . . . Amstelodami, Apud Jodocum Janssonium, 1653 [i.e. 1655]

[24], 711 p.; 192 p.   table.   15 cm.   [**10933**]

Part [2] has special title page: Epitome librorum de febribus, with date 1655.
Imperfect: first preliminary leaf wanting.

—[The same.] . . . Ed. 2. ab autore adhuc recensita & aucta. Wittebergae, Sumtibus haered. D. Tobiae Mevii, & Elerdi Schumacheri, typis Matthaei Henckelii, 1664.

[32], 936 p.; [1], 248 p.   table.   14 cm.
[**10934**]

—[English tr.] The institutions or fundamentals . . . of physick and chirurgery, divided into five books . . . The nature of all diseases, their causes . . . and cures. Also The grounds of chymistry, and the way of making all sorts of salves, and preparing of medicines according to art . . . Englished by N. D. B. P. late of Trinity Colledge in Cambridge. London, Published for Ludowick Lloyd, 1656?

[8], 472 (i.e. 474), [5] p.   17 cm.   [**10935**]

Imprint date altered (in manuscript) to 1686.
Imperfect: the first three preliminary leaves mutilated and mounted.

—Epitome naturalis scientiae . . . Witebergae, Impensis Caspari Heiden, 1618.

[16], 643, [20] p.   illus.   17 cm.   [**10936**]

Errata: p. [20]

—[The same.] . . . Ed. ultima . . . Amstelaedami, Ravensteninius, 1651.

[14], 679, [22] p.; [89] p.   15 cm.   [**10937**]

Engraved title page.
Part [2] has special title page: Auctarium epitomes physicae.
With this is bound another issue of Scaliger, J. C. In librum De insomniis Hippocratis commentarius. 1659.

—Epitome universam Dan. Sennerti doctrinam . . . complectens, ex triplici volumine in unum congestam . . . purgata ab illis, quae orthodoxae fidei puritati visa sunt adversari . . . Per Claudium Bonnetium . . . Coloniae Allobrogum, Excudebat Philippus Gamonetus, 1655.

[27], 944, [15] p.   34 cm.   [**10938**]

—[The same.] . . . Per Claudium Bonnetium . . . Avenione, Ex typographia Petri Offray, 1660.

[27], 944, [15] p.   36 cm.   [**10939**]

Different setting of type.

—Institutionum medicinae libri V . . . Witebergae, Apud Zachariam Schurerum, typis Wolfgangi Meisneri, 1611.

[24], 1194, [40] p.   plate, port.   20 cm.
[**10940**]

—[The same.] . . . Ultimum recogniti et auct. ac 3. ed. . . . Witebergae, Apud haeredes Zach. Schüreri Sen. [Typis haeredum Salomonis Auerbach, 1628]

[44], 1518, [62] p.   plate, port.   22 cm.
[**10941**]

Engraved title page.
Errata: p. [61–62]

—[The same.] . . . ult. aucti, recogniti, jamque ter editi in Germania, nunc primum in Gallia. Parisiis, 1631.

[40], 1363, [45] p.   plate.   23 cm.   [**10942**]

—[The same.] . . . Ab autore postremoque omnium recogniti ac quartum jam editi. Witebergae, Sumptibus haered. Tobiae Mevii [Excudebat Michael Wendt] 1644.

[50], 1523, [51] p.   front. (port.), plate.   22 cm.   [**10943**]

Added engraved title page.

—Medicamenta officinalia praecipua, cum Galenica, tum chymica, ex vegetabilibus, animalibus, & mineralibus desumta tabulis . . . legentium oculis subjiciantur . . . quas ad tabulas Institutionum medicinae . . . Danielis Sennerti . . . nuper editas in tyronum medicinae gratiam appendicis loco adjecit Christianus Winckelmannus. Ed. 2. Witebergae, Impensis haered. D. Tobiae Mevii, & Elerdi Schumacheri, literis Matthaei Henckelii, 1670.

[32] ll.   tables.   35 cm.   [**10944**]

Bound with *his* Tabulae institutionum medicinae. 1673.

—Paralipomena, cum praemissa Methodo discendi medicinam. Tractatus posthumus . . . Accesserunt . . . Vita b. autoris . . . Judicia cl. virorum . . . Wittebergae, Sumptibus haered. Zachariae Schüreri, Senioris, Excudebat Michael Wendt, 1642.

[II], 223, [36] p.   22 cm.   **[10945]**

Bound with vol. 6, copy 2 of *his* Practicae medicine. 1628-1635.

—[The same.] . . . Lugduni, Sumptib. Joan. Antonii Huguetan, 1643.

[16], 460, [50] p.   18 cm.   **[10946]**

—Physica hypomnemata. I. De rerum naturalium principiis. II. De occultis qualitatibus. III. De atomis & mistione. IV. De generatione viventium. V. De spontaneo viventium ortu . . . Lugduni, Sumptibus Petri Ravaud, 1637.

[32], 471, [23] p.   19 cm.   **[10947]**

—Podagra tragice producta a Luciano. *In his* Practicae medicinae liber primus [-sextus] 1628-1635.

—Practicae medicinae liber primus [-sextus] . . . [Wittebergae] Sumtibus viduae et haered. Zachariae Schureri senioris [Typis haeredum Salomonis Auerbach, 1628-1635]

6 v. in 5.   port.   21 cm.   **[10948]**

Engraved title pages. Vols. 4 and 5 have added title pages dated 1632 and 1634 respectively. Vols. 6 is dated 1635. Vol. 4-6 were printed by Ambrosius Rothe.

Vol. 4 at end includes "De infantium curatione tractatus" (p. [1-96] with half title).

—Copy 2.   22 cm.

Vols. 2-4 and 6 in 2 volumes.

Vol. 3 (dated 1631) at end includes "De arthritide tractatus" and "Podagra tragice producta a Luciano," both with special title pages. The latter (in Greek and Latin) is translated by Erasmus Schmied.

Imperfect: engraved title page of vol. 6 wanting.

With vol. 6 is bound *his* Paralipomena. 1642.

—[The same.] Medicina practica. Olim in Germania; nunc vero de novo typis excusa, multisque quibus scatebat erroribus repurgata. Lugduni, Sumptibus Petri Ravaud, 1629-36.

3 v.   illus.   18 cm.   **[10949]**

Vol. 3 has title: Practicae medicinae liber tertius . . . 1633.

Vol. 3 at end includes *his* De arthritide tractatus (with half title) and Tragopodagra Luciani (with special title page). The latter (in Greek and Latin) is translated by Erasmus Schmied.

—[The same.] . . . Parisiis, Apud Societatem, 1632.

5 v.   24 cm.   **[10950]**

Vols. 3 & 4 are second edition.

Vol. 3, at end, includes De arthritide tractatus (with special title page) and Podagra tragice producta a Luciano. The latter (in Latin only) is translated by Erasmus Schmied.

Vol. 4, at end, includes De infantium curatione tractatus, with half title.

—[The same.] Practicae medicinae . . . Ed. 2. ab autore secundum recensitus. [Wittebergae, Sumptibus haered. Zachariae Schureii, typis Ambrosii Rothi] 1636-54.

6 v. in 3.   illus., port.   23 cm. (v. 1-2); 22 cm. (v. 3-4 & 5-6)   **[10951]**

Vol. 1, 2, 4 & 5 have added engraved title pages; that of vol. 5 has been changed from Liber quartus to Liber Quintus.

Vol. 2 printed by Johann Röhner; vol. 3 by Tobias Mevius; vol. 4 by the heir of Tobias Mevius and Michaelis Wendt; vol. 5 by the heir of Tobias Mevius.

Imperfect: vol. 6, sig. a² (blank) wanting.

Part [2] of vol. 3 (with special title page) includes the 2d ed. of *his* De arthritide tractatus and Tragopodagra Luciani. The latter (in Greek and Latin) is translated by Erasmus Schmied.

"De infantium curatione tractatus . . .": (vol. 4, p. [1]-96 at end) has half title.

"Appendix libri VI . . . Miram veneficii historiam exhibens", at end, contains Epistolae duae by Balthasar Han and De casu isto judicium & consilium by Joachim Colbe.

Errata: vol. 1 at end.

—[The same.] . . . ab authore tertium recensitus. [Wittebergae, Sumptibus haered. D. Tobiae Mevii & Elerdi Schumacheri, typis Matthaei Henckelii, 1653-62] [v. 1, 1654]

4 v. in 3.   illus., plate, port.   23 cm.   **[10952]**

Imperfect: first preliminary leaf of vol. 2 wanting.

Vol. 1 has added engraved title page.

Vol. 4 includes the 2d ed. of *his* De arthritide tractatus and Tragopodagra Luciani. The latter (in Greek and Latin) is translated by Erasmus Schmied.

"De infantium curatione tractatus . . .": (vol. 4, at end) has half title.

—Practical physick; or, Five distinct treatises of the most predominant diseases of these times . . . scurvey . . . dropsie . . . feavers and agues . . . French pox . . . gout . . . Written in Latine . . . In English, by Nich. Culpeper, and H. Care . . . London, William Whitwood, 1679.

[16], 151, [5], 176, [5], 279 p.   18 cm.   **[10953]**

—Quaestionum medicarum controversarum liber, cui accessit Tractatus de pestilentia . . . Witebergae, Ex officina Martini Henckelii, 1610.

[15] p.; 478, [1] p.   16 cm.   **[10954]**

Imperfect: p. 403-418 wanting.

—Tabulae institutionum medicinae . . . Danielis Sennerti . . . summam breviter & succincte exhibentes in tyronum medicinae gratiam concinnatae & editae a Christiano Winckelmanno . . . Ed. 2. Wittebergae, Impensis haered. D. Tobiae Mevii & Elerdi Schumacheri, typis Matthaei Henckelii, 1673.

[60] p. tables. 35 cm.   [**10955**]

With this is bound *his* Medicamenta officinalia praecipua. 1670.

—Two treatises. The first of the venereal pocks . . . the second treatise of the gout . . . Written in Latin and English. By Daniel Sennert . . . Nicholas Culpeper . . . Abdiah Cole . . . London, Peter Cole, 1660.

[1], 75, [1] p.; 87, [1] p. 27 cm.   [**10956**]

In English.

"Mris. Culpepers information, vindication, and testimony, concerning her husbands books to be published after his death": p. [1] at end of part [1].

Part [1] is a translation of *his* De lue venerea; part [2] is a translation of *his* De arthritide tractatus.

—[The same.] *In* Platter, F. [1536-1614] A golden practice of physick. 1622.

—Verhandelingh der toover-sieckten. Geschil van de schôot-en steeck-vrije. Geschil van de wapen-salve. Paracelsi vrye-konst. Wt verscheyde Latijnsche boecken . . . vertaelt, en by een geschickt door D[aniel] Jonctys. Dordrecht, Hendrick van Esch, 1638.

[31], 343, [8] p. illus. 15 cm.   [**10957**]

Added engraved title page.

"Van de krachten des inbeeldinghs": p. 303-343.

—[The same.] . . . t'Amsterdam, By Gijsbert Jansz van Veen [gedruckt by Pieter Dirckss Boeteman] 1646.

[14], 331, [8] p. 16 cm.   [**10958**]

Added engraved title page.

"Van de krachten des inbeeldinghs": p. 293-331.

Dissertations — Wittenberg

—*praeses*. De caussis morborum disputatio prior . . . Witebergae, Excudebat Johan. Schmidt, 1605.

[12] p. 21 cm.   [**10959**]

J. Wanckel, *respondent*.

—De caussis morborum disputatio altera . . . Witebergae, Excudebat Johan. Schmidt, 1605.

[12] p. 21 cm.   [**10960**]

B. Psichholtz, *respondent*.

—De differentiis morborum, disputatio prima . . . Suscepit . . . ad diem 19. Januarii. Wittebergae, Excudebat Johan. Schmidt, 1605.

[12] p. 21 cm.   [**10961**]

M. Boecher, *respondent*.

—De differentiis morborum disputatio altera . . . Suscepit . . . ad diem 26. Januarii. Witebergae, Excudebat Johan. Schmidt, 1605.

[12] p. 21 cm.   [**10962**]

M. Boecher, *respondent*.

—De differentiis symptomatum disputatio . . . Witebergae, Excudebat Johan. Schmidt, 1605.

[12] p. 21 cm.   [**10963**]

G. Hebenstreit, *respondent*.

—De febribus disputatio III. De febribus putridis in genere, et temporibus febrium . . . Witebergae, Excudebatur a Johanne Schmidt, 1605.

[11] p. 21 cm.   [**10964**]

M. Scheffer, *respondent*.

—De febribus disputatio VIII. & ultima, de febre hectica . . . Witebergae, Excudebat Johan. Schmidt, 1605.

[7] p. 21 cm.   [**10965**]

M. Boecher, *respondent*.

—De febrium malignarum differentiis & signis disputatio . . . Witebergae, Typis Martini Henckelii, 1607.

[23] p. 21 cm.   [**10966**]

M. Döring, *respondent*.

—De febrium malignarum natura & causis disputatio . . . Witebergae, Typis Martini Henckelii, 1607.

[28] p. 21 cm.   [**10967**]

M. Döring, *respondent*.

—De ileo theses disputationis medicae . . . Wittebergae, Ex typographeo Christiani Tham, 1622.

[15] p. 20 cm.   [**10968**]

J. G. Pelshofer, *respondent*.

—De methodo medendi disputatio prima, de methodo et indicationibus . . . Witebergae, Ex Officina Cratoniana, 1603.

[15] p. 21 cm.   [**10969**]

W. Weis, *respondent*.

—De methodo medendi disputatio II. de indicantibus . . . Witebergae, Ex Officina Cratoniana, 1603.
[16] p. 21 cm. **[10970]**
G. Viebing, *respondent.*

—De methodo medendi disputatio III, de indicantium consensu ac dissensu, et de indicatis . . . Witebergae, Ex Officina Cratoniana, 1604.
[16] p. 21 cm. **[10971]**
J. Köppe, *respondent.*

—De methodo medendi disputatio IV, de causus morborum, quatenus toto genere praeter naturam sunt, tollendis, et de sanguinis abundantia hirudinibus, cucurbitulis, scarificatione &c. minuenda . . . Witebergae, Ex Officina Cratoniana, 1604.
[16] p. 21 cm. **[10972]**
B. Psichholtz, *respondent.*

—De methodo medendi disputatio V, de venae sectione . . . Witebergae, Ex Officina Cratoniana, 1604.
[20] p. 21 cm. **[10973]**
T. Ulrich, *respondent.*

—De methodo medendi disputatio VI, de purgatione . . . Witebergae, Ex Officina Cratoniana, 1604.
[16] p. 21 cm. **[10974]**
C. Schattenberg, *respondent.*

—De methodo medendi disputatio VII, de morbi tempore purgationi apto . . . Witebergae, Ex Officina Cratoniana, 1604.
[15] p. 21 cm. **[10975]**
J. Coler, *respondent.*

—De methodo medendi disputatio VIII, de humorum coctione et praeparatione . . . Witebergae, Ex Officina Cratoniana, 1604.
[12] p. 21 cm. **[10976]**
J. Pesserl, *respondent.*

—De methodo medendi disputatio IX, de purgationis quantitate, et loco, per quem fieri debet atque de evacutione per urinam & sudores . . . Witebergae, Ex Officina Cratoniana, 1604.
[16] p. 21 cm. **[10977]**
C. Hartwig, *respondent.*

—De methodo medendi disputatio X, de revulsione et derivatione . . . Witebergae, Excudebat Joan Faber, 1604.
[16] p. 21 cm. **[10978]**
F. Omich, *respondent.*

—De methodo medendi disputatio XI, de repellentibus, intercipientibus, discutientibus, mollientibus, & suppurantibus . . . Witebergae, Excudebat Joan. Faber, 1604.
[12] p. 21 cm. **[10979]**
C. Schattenberg, *respondent.*

—De pestilentia disputatio . . . Witebergae, Typis Martini Henckelii, 1607.
[40] p. 19 cm. **[10980]**
T. Ulrich, *respondent.*

—De pleuritide disputatio . . . Wittebergae, Typis haeredum Salomonis Auerbach, 1627.
[28] p. 19 cm. **[10981]**
J. Girnt, *respondent.*

—De scorbuto disputatio . . . Witebergae, Exscripta typis Johannis Haken [1623]
[50] p. 19 cm. **[10982]**
M. Heider, N. Rossbach, D. Winckler, *respondents.*

—De symptomatum caussis disputatio prima . . . Witebergae, Excudebat Johan. Schmidt, 1605.
[12] p. 21 cm. **[10983]**
A. Gartner, *respondent.*

—De symptomatum caussis disputatio secunda . . . Witebergae, Excudebat Johan. Schmidt, 1605.
[12] p. 21 cm. **[10984]**
J. Degenhard, *respondent.*

—De symptomatum caussis disputatio quarta . . . Witebergae, Excudebat Johan. Schmidt, 1605.
[7] p. 21 cm. **[10985]**
C. Cholius, *respondent.*

—Disputatio anatomica de ossibus in genere . . . Wittebergae, Typis Johannis Haken, 1664.
[24] p. 19 cm. **[10986]**
P. Scheuban, *respondent.*

—Disputatio medica de cardialgia . . . Wittebergae, Excusa typis Johannis Gormanni, 1627.
[16] p. 20 cm. **[10987]**
Z. Polner, *respondent..*

—Disputatio medica de dysenteria . . . Wittebergae, Typis Johannis Gormanni, 1611.
[16] p. 19 cm. **[10988]**
J. Kluge, *respondent..*

—Disputatio medica de hydrope . . . Wittebergae, Ex officina typographica Johannis Richteri, 1616.
[28] p. 19 cm. **[10989]**
M. Syssenbach, *respondent.*

—Disputatio medica, de inflammatione ... Witebergae, Typis Martini Henckelii, 1610.

[14] p. 19 cm. **[10990]**

G. Eberlin, *respondent.*

—Disputatio medica de ophthalmia ... Witebergae, Typis Martini Henckelii, 1608.

[15] p. 20 cm. **[10991]**

P. Hepner, *respondent..*

—Disputatio medica, de pleuritide et ejus in empyema μεταπτωσει ... Wittebergae, Typis M. Georgii Mulleri, 1611.

[12] p. 19 cm. **[10992]**

E. Fischer, *respondent.*

—Dissertatio medica de cephalagia ... Witebergae, Typis haeredum Christiani Tham, 1630.

[24] p. 19 cm. **[10994]**

J. Specht, *respondent.*

—Exercitatio medica de vigiliis nimiis ... Wittebergae, Ex officina Christiani Tham, 1626.

[23] p. 19 cm. **[10995]**

B. Cörner, *respondent.*

—Hasce theses de febre quartana ... Witebergae, Typis Jobi Wilhelmi Fincelii, 1624.

[16] p. 19 cm. **[10996]**

H. Lysius, *respondent.*

—Positiones medicae de colica ... Wittebergae, E typographia Christiani Tham, 1625.

[15] p. 18 cm. **[10997]**

F. Moller, *respondent.*

—Positiones medicae de dysenteria ... Wittebergae, Ex officina Christiani Tham, 1624.

[28] p. 19 cm. **[10998]**

H. Dietrich, *respondent.*

—Positiones medicae de singultu ... Wittebergae, Ex officina typographica Christiani Tham, 1624.

[20] p. 19 cm. **[10999]**

M. Mayer, *respondent.*

—Positiones medicae de vertigine ... Witebergae, Excudebat Johann. Schmidt, 1610.

[12] p. 19 cm. **[11000]**

W. Schaller, *respondent.*

—Quaestiones medicae controversae quinque, pro disputatione prima propositae ... Witebergae, Typis Martini Henkelii, 1607.

19 p. 21 cm. **[11001]**

J. Köppe, *respondent.*

—Quaestiones medicae controversae quinque, pro disputatione tertia propositae ... Witebergae, Typis Martini Henckelii, 1607.

[18] p. 21 cm. **[11002]**

G. Titschard, *respondent.*

—Quaestiones medicae controversae quinque, pro disputatione quinta propositae ... Witebergae, Typis Martini Henckelii, 1607.

[20] p. 21 cm. **[11003]**

M. Scheffer, *respondent.*

—Quaestiones medicae controversae quinque, pro disputatione octava propositae ... Witebergae, Typis Martini Henckelii, 1608.

[20] p. 21 cm. **[11004]**

M. Walther, *respondent.*

—Quaestiones medicae controversae sex ... Witebergae, Typis Martini Henckelii, 1607.

[19] p. 21 cm. **[11005]**

L. Scholz, *respondent.*

—Quaestiones medicae controversae septem ... Witebergae, Typis Martini Henckelii, 1607.

[22] p. 21 cm. **[11006]**

M. Döring, *respondent.*

—Theses de catarrho ... Wittebergae, Typis Johannis Gormanni [1626]

[20] p. 19 cm. **[11007]**

K. Amthor, *respondent.*

—*respondent. See* SCHARFF, J., *praeses.* Disputatio physica de auditu et olfactu. 1626.

—*See* CONRING, H. De sanguinis generatione, et motu naturali. 1646; CRAANEN, T. Observationes. 1687; JONSTONUS, J. The idea of practical physick. 1657, 1661; MAGATI, C. De rara medicatione vulnerum. 1673; MOCHINGER, G. Compendium institutionum medicarum. 1631; SPERLING, J. Tractatus physico-medicus, de calido innato. 1634.

SENNERT, MICHAEL [*fl.* 1639–1681]

Dissertations — Wittenberg

—*praeses.* Disputatio anatomica de intestinis ... Wittebergae, Typis Johannis Haken, 1664.

[34] p. 19 cm. **[11008]**

A. C. Müller, *respondent.*

—Disputatio inauguralis ... casum geminum lactis e vena aperta educti tractans ... Wittebergae, Literis Michaelis Meyeri, 1670.

[24] p.   19 cm.   [11009]

C. Nitzschke, *respondent.*

—Disputatio inauguralis medica de dysenteria ... Wittebergae, Typis Christiani Schrödteri [1677]

[32] p.   19 cm.   [11010]

G. C. Pfeifer, *respondent.*

—Disputatio medica de syncope ... Wittebergae, Typis Joh. Borckardi, excudebat Simon Lieberhirth, 1679.

[20] p.   20 cm.   [11011]

C. E. Creutzmann, *respondent.*

—Disputatio medica inauguralis de suppressione mensium ... Wittebergae, Typis Johannis Haken [1664]

[52] p.   18 cm.   [11012]

M. Cleophas, *respondent.*

—Disputatio physico-anatomica de sanguine ... Wittebergae, Literis Johannis Röhneri [1664]

[60] p.   18 cm.   [11013]

J. L. Loelius, *respondent.*

—Disputationem anatomicam de cerebro ... subjicit Gottlieb Georg Schramm ... Wittebergae, Literis Michaelis Wendt [1662]

[32] p.   18 cm.   [11014]

G. G. Schramm, *respondent.*

—Disputationem inauguralem de imbecileitate ventriculi ... publico ... examini exponit Johannes Voigt ... Wittebergae, Typis Joh. Sigismundi Ziegenbeins [1676]

[24] p.   20 cm.   [11015]

J. Voigt, *respondent.*

—Disputationem inauguralem de lue venerea ... proponit M. Adam Purpius ... [Wittenbergae] Typis Johannis Sigismundi Ziegenbeins [1679]

[48] p.   19 cm.   [11016]

A. Purpius, *respondent.*

—Dissertatio medica de febre petechiali ... Wittenbergae, Typis Matthaei Henckelii [1681]

[44] p.   20 cm.   [11017]

M. G. Ziegra, *respondent.*

—Hemicraniam ... publicae ... disquisitioni submittit Henricus Vollgnad ... Wittebergae, Typis

Johannis Röhneri, 1662.

[48] p.   19 cm.   [11018]

H. Vollgnad, *respondent.*

SENS. Laws, statutes, etc. Reglement politi sur l'ayde et subvention des pauvres malades de pest de la ville & faulx-bourgs de Sens, & sur autres chose en despendans. Sens, George Niverd, 1627.

34 p.   18 cm.   [11019]

SENTIMENTS d'un voyageur sur plusieur libelles de ce temps. [n. p., 1677]

8 p.   16 cm.   [11020]

Concerns controversy between Andreas Boekelman an Bonaventura van Dortmont.

SEPTALIUS, Ludovicus. *See* Settala, Ludovic [1552-1633]

SEPTALIUS, Senator. *See* Settala, Senatore [*d* 1636]

SEQUEIRA, Gaspar Cardoso de. *See* Cardos de Sequeira, Gaspar [16th—17th cent.]

SERAFINI, Herofilo [*fl.* 1617] *See* Vecoli, B Della preparatione della pietra lazzoli. 1617.

SERAPHINUS, Polidorus. Anagyrica medicus aegrotis vero grata, & utilis collectio de manifesti quibusdam erroribus in usu medendi ... Venetiis Apud Evangelistam Deuchinum, 1608.

51 ll.   17 cm.   [11021]

SERDONATI, Francesco [1540-1603] *ed. Se* Marzio, G. Della varia dottrina. 1615.

SERENUS, Quintus. *See* Serenus Sammonicus Quintus.

SERENUS SAMMONICUS, Quintus. De medi cina praecepta saluberrima. Robertus Keuchenius e veteri libro restituit, emendavit, illustravit .. Amstelodami, Apud Petrum van den Berge, 1662

[16], 295, [21] p.   17 cm.   [11022]

Added engraved title page.
"Q. Rhemnii Fannii Palaemonis De ponderibus et mensuri liber": p. 39-44.

—Liber medicinalis. *In* Celsus, A. C. De r medica libri octo. 1608, 1625.

SERGEANT, John [1622-1707] The method t science. By J. S. London, Printed by W. Redmayn for the author, and sold by Thomas Metcalf, 169t

[70], 429 p.   19 cm.   [11023]

A SERIOUS debate. *See* Maynwaring, E.

SERMON, William [1629?–1679] A friend to the sick; or, The honest English mans preservation. Shewing the causes, symptoms, and cures of . . . diseases . . . With a particular discourse of the dropsie, scurvy, and yellow jaundice . . . Whereunto is added, a true relation of some . . . cures effected by the author's . . . cathartique and diuretique pills . . . London, Printed by W. Downing for Edward Thomas, 1673.

[22], 275, [1] p. 18 cm.   [**11024**]
Imperfect: first preliminary leaf (blank?) wanting.

SERNA, Juan Gallego de la. *See* Gallego de la Serna, Juan [*fl.* 1621–1640]

SERRANO, Antonio Pablo, *tr. See* Houllier, J. Tratado de la materia de cirurgia. 1624, 1651.

SERRANUS, Ludovicus. *See* Serres, Louys de [*fl.* 1625]

SERRES, Louys de [*fl.* 1625] Discours de la nature, causes, signes, & curation des empeschemens de la conception, & de la sterilité des femmes . . . Lyon, Antoine Chard, 1625.

[16], 486 p. 18 cm.   [**11025**]

—, *ed. See* Liddel, D. Operum omnium iatro-Galenicorum . . . tomus unicus. 1624; Vega, C. de. Opera omnia. 1626.

—, *tr. See* Renou, J. de. Le grand dispensaire medicinal. 1624, 1626, 1637.

SERRIER, Trophime. Observationes medicae, pluribus praesidiis Galenicis & chymicis ornatae, ampla & pernecessaria theoria, novisque opinionibus illustratae . . . Lugduni, Apud Antonium Jullieron, 1673.

[6], 548 p. 16 cm.   [**11026**]

—Pyretologia. In duos libros divisa, quorum primus gravissimis De febribus quaesitis satisfacit, secundus cujusque febris diagnosin, prognosin & therapiam chymicis praesidiis illustratam complectitur . . . Lugduni, Sumptibus Joan. Antonii Huguetan, & Marci-Antonii Ravaud, 1663.

[16] 322, [14] p. 18 cm.   [**11027**]

SERRURIER, Joseph [*fl.* 1690–1718] *respondent.* Disputatio medica inauguralis de febribus in genere

. . . Lugduni Batavorum, Apud Abrahamum Elzevier, 1690.

[16] p. 23 cm.   [**11028**]
Diss.—Leyden.

SERVI, Pietro [*d.* 1648] Persii Trevi [pseud.] Ad librum de sero lactis Stephani Roderici Castrensis Lusitani declamationes, seu, Privatae quaedam ac domesticae exercitationes . . . Parisiis, Apud Sebastianum Cramoisy, 1634.

[8], 103, [1] p. 18 cm.   [**11029**]

— [The same.] . . . Ed. 2., quam auctor suam agnoscit, auxit, emendavit. Romae, Ex typographia Francisci Corbelletti, 1634.

153, [7] p. 16 cm.   [**11030**]
Bound with Duchesne, J. Jos. Quercetani . . . Ad veritatem hermeticae medicinae . . . adversus cujusdam anonymi phantasmata responsio. 1605.

—Dissertatio de unguento armario; sive, De naturae artisque miraculis. Romae, Typis Dominici Marciani, 1643.

[8], 179, [5] p. 17 cm.   [**11031**]

— [The same.]
532–566 p. 21 cm. (*In* Theatrum sympatheticum auctum. Norimbergae, 1662)   [**11032**]
Caption title.

—Dissertatio philologica de odoribus . . . Romae, Apud Franciscum Caballum, 1641.

[16], 149, [3] p. 16 cm.   [**11033**]

—*See* Digby, *Sir* K. Eröffnung unterschiedlicher Heimlichkeiten der Natur. 1664, 1671.

SESSA, Giovanni Bernardo, *ed. See* Capivaccio, G. Medicina practica. 1601.

SETTALA, Ludovico [1552–1633] . . . Animadversionum, & cautionum medicarum libri septem . . . Mediolani, Apud Jo. Bapt. Bidell, 1614.

[14], 260, [41] p. port. 17 cm.   [**11034**]

—[The same.] . . . Primo Mediolani in lucem editi, nunc vero revisi, emaculati & ab innumeris, quibus prior scatebat ed., mendis perpurgati, nunc primum in tanto exemplarium defectu pariter ac desiderio philiatris communicati, studio & opera Joannis Caroli Rosenberg . . . Argentinae, Sumptibus Eberhardi Zetzneri, 1625.

[36], 330, [41] p. 14 cm.   [**11035**]

—[The same.] . . . Denuo ab auctore recogniti. Adjecimus hac postrema editione ejusdem Librum de naevis. Mediol., Apud Jo. Bapt. Bidell., 1626-29.

2 v.   13 cm.   [11036]

The De naevis liber (at end of vol. 1) has special title page and separate pagination.

Vol. [2] has title: Animadversionum, & cautionum medicarum libri duo. Septem aliis jam editis additi.

—[The same.] . . . Argentinae, Sumptibus Eberhardi Zetzneri, 1629.

[36], 330, [41] p.; [6], 35, [4] p.   14 cm.
                                       [11037]

Part [1] is a reissue of the 1625 edition with new title page. Part [2] has special title page.

—[The same.] . . . hac postrema editione expurgatis quamplurimis mendis, novo nitori restituti. Patavii, Ex typographia Jo. Thuilii, prostant apud Paulum Frambottum, 1628-30.

2 v. in 1.   16 cm.   [11038]

Vol. [2] has title page: Animadversionum, & cautionum medicarum, libri duo. Septem aliis jam editis additi . . . Patavii, Apud Paulum Frambottum, typis Josephi Sardi, & fratrum, 1630.

De naevis liber (1628) is bound with vol. 2.

—[The same.] Animadversionum, & cautionum medicarum libri novem, denuo a J. Perio recogniti, & hac postrema editione, expurgatis quamplurimis mendis, novo nitori restituti . . . Quibus accessit ejusdem auctoris Liber de naevis . . . Dordrechti, Apud Vinçentium Caimax, 1650.

3 parts in 1 v.   15 cm.   [11039]

Imperfect: lower portion of final leaf (index) of part [2] excised; p. [3-4] of pt. [3] wanting.

Each part has special title page.

Contents. — [pt. 1] Animadversionum & cautionum medicarum libri septem. — [pt. 2] Animadversionum & cautionum medicarum libri duo. — [pt. 3] De naevis liber. Ed. postrema emendatior.

—[The same.] Animadversionum et cautionum medicarum libri IX. Postremae huic editioni 4. accedunt Joannis Rhodii Analecta et notae. Patavii, Apud Paulum Frambottum, 1652.

2 parts in 1 v.   16 cm.   [11040]

"De naevis liber. Ed. postrema emend." (p. [575]-608 of pt. [1]) has special title page with date 1651.

—[Italian tr.] In Antidotario romano latino, et volgare. 1635.

—Cura locale de' tumori pestilentiali, che sono il bubone, l'antrace, ò carboncolo, & i furoncoli. Con-

tenente tutto quello, che si hà da fare esteriormente nella cura di questi mali. Tolta dal libro della cura della peste . . . Milano, Giovan Battista Bidelli, 1629.

32 p.   17 cm.   [11041]

Bound with his Preservatione dalla peste. 1630.

—De margaritis nuper ad nos allatis. Judicium . . . [Mediolani, Typis Pandulphi Malatestae, 1618]

21, [1] p.   23 cm.   [11042]

—De morbis ex mucronata cartilagine evenientibus liber unus. Opus novum, et de noviter cognitis morbis editum . . . Mediolani, Ex typographia Georgii Rollae, 1632.

[6], 44 (i.e. 46), [4] p.   16 cm.   [11043]

—De naevis liber . . . Mediolani, Apud Petrum Martyrem Locarnum, 1606.

85, [1] p.   16 cm.   [11044]

—[Another issue.] . . . Mediolani, Apud Hieronymum Bordonum, 1606.

85, [1] p.   18 cm.   [11045]

Bound with Selvatico, G. B. Medicus. 1611.

—[The same.] . . . Ed. postrema emend. & indiculo auct. Patavii, Ex typographia Jo. Thuilii, prostat apud Paulum Frambottum, 1628.

[8], 36, [4] p.   16 cm.   [11046]

Bound with his Animadversionum . . . medicarum libri septem. 1628-30.

—[The same.] In Baillou, G. de. Labyrinthi medici extricati. 1687.

—[Italian tr.] In Porta, G. B. della. Della fisionomia dell'huomo. 1644, 1668.

—De peste, & pestiferis affectibus. Libri quinque . . . Mediolani, Apud Joannem Baptistam Bidellium, 1622.

[16], 343, [16] p.   22 cm.   [11047]

"Erectio magistratus sanitatis cum institutis ei rei consentaneis. Per . . . Mediolani Ducem Franciscum Sfortiam [die 11. Aprilis 1534]": p. 322-343.

—Preservatione dalla peste . . . Milano, Giovan Battista Bidelli, 1630.

60 p.   17 cm.   [11048]

With this is bound his Cura locale de'tumori pestilentiali. 1629.

—See NÚÑEZ, A. Assertio judicii Ludovici Septalii . . . De margaritis nuper ex India allatis. 1620.

SETTALA, SENATORE [d. 1636] ed. See ASELLIO, G. De lactibus. 1627, 1640.

SETTALI, LODOVICO. *See* SETTALA, Ludovico [1552-1633]

SEUBERTUS, JOANNES JACOBUS [*fl.* 1623-1636] *respondent.* Discursum buncce theoretico-practicum inauguralem, de peste ... proponit ... Joannes Jacobus Seubertus ... Argentorati, Typis Eberhardi Welperi [1636]

[20] p. 19 cm. [**11049**]
Diss. — Strasbourg.

—*See* CHARSTADIUS, V., *praeses.* Disputationum medicarum septima de symptomatibus, eorundemque differentiis et causis. 1626; SEBISCH, M. [1578-1674?] *praeses.* Exercitationes medicae. 1639.

SEÜBERT, JOANNES JACOBUS. *See* SEUBERTUS, Joannes Jacobus [*fl.* 1623-1636]

SEUMENICHT, ADRIAN VON. *See* MYNSICHT, Adrian von [1603-1638]

SEURING, KONRAD [*fl.* 1612] *respondent.* Miscellas sequentes ... statuit Chunradus Seuringius ... Basileae, Typis Johan. Jacobi Genathii [1612]

[8] p. 22 cm. [**11050**]
Diss. — Basel.

SEVERINI, MICHAEL [*fl.* 1678] *respondent. See* BARTHOLIN, C. [1655-1738], *praeses.* Exercitatio anatomica de corporis humani oeconomia. 1678.

SEVERINO, MARCO AURELIO [1580-1656] Antiperipatias, hoc est adversus Aristoteleos de respiratione piscium diatriba. De piscibus in sicco viventibus. Commentarius in Theophrasti ... libellum hujus argumenti. Phoca illustratus, scilicet anatome spectatus ... De radio turturis marini, ejusque vi, medicina, veneno ... Accessit vitae authoris synopsis. Neapoli, Apud haeredes Camilli Cavalli, expensis Joannis Alberti Tarini, 1655-59 [v. 1, 1659]

2 v. in 1. 31 cm. [**11051**]
De piscibus in sicco viventibus commentarius in libellum Theophrasti ... autore M. Aurelio Severino (v. [2]) is dated 1655.
Edited by Giovanni Alberto Tarino.

—De efficaci medicina libri III. ... Opus ... nunc primum in lucem datum. Francofurti, Sumptibus Joannis Beyeri, typis vero Antonii Hummii, 1646.

[16], 297, [14] p. illus. 33 cm. [**11052**]
Added engraved title page.
Published also as part [2] of Fabricius von Hilden, Wilhelm. Opera quae extant omnia. 1646, 1682.

—[French tr.] De la medecine efficace; ou, La maniere de guerir les plus ... dangereuses maladies ... par le fer & par le fev. Divisée en III. livres ... Et traduite ... de Latin en François ... Geneve, pour Pierre Chouët [imprimé par Philippe Gamonet] 1668.

[44], 654 p. illus., plates. 22 cm. [**11053**]
"Introduction methodique a la chirurgie. Par Jean van Horn ...": p. [21-44]

—Another issue. 23 cm. [**11054**]
Title page, preliminary matters, and index at end reset.
Signatures of sheet H wrongly imposed.

—[The same.] *In* Bonet, T., ed. Corps de medecine et de chirurgie. 1679.

—De recondita abscessuum natura libri VII. ... Neap., Apud Octavium Beltranum, 1632.

1 v. illus. 20 cm. [**11055**]
Various pagings.
Engraved title page.
Errata at end.

—De recondita abscessuum natura, libri VIII. ... Variis additamentis, eorundemque iconibus ... adaucti ... Accesserunt clarissimorum virorum judicia super hunc ... tractatum. [Ed. 2. ... auct. & corr. ab ipso autore reddita] Francofurti, Impensis Joannis Beyeri, typis Casparis Rotelii, 1643.

[28], 468, [20] p. illus. 23 cm. [**11056**]
Added engraved title page.

—Copy 2. 22 cm.
With this are bound his: Τριβοήτητος ή τρισερειστος. 1653; Seilo-phlebotome castigata. 1654; Volckamer, J. G. Collegium anatomicum. 1654.

—Quaestiones anatomicae quatuor. *In* Jasolino, G. Collegium anatomicum. 1668; Volckamer, J. G. [1616-1693] Collegium anatomicum. 1654.

—Seilo-phlebotome castigata; sive, De venae salvatellae usu & abusu. Censore Marco Aurelio Severino ... Hanoviae, Typis Joannis Aubry, sumptibus Christophori Le Blon, 1654.

[16], 192, [23] p. illus., plates. 23 cm. [**11057**]
Two title pages with identical text but different setting of type.
"Joannis Trullii ... De serie venarum ... epistola": p. 150-154.
"Petri Castelli responsio ad ... Marcum Aurelium Severinum. De venae seilem-phlebotome adversis Spigelium disputatiunculum": p. 155-168.
"Ad ... Petrum Castellum ... Marci Aurelii Severini ... pro sua seilomastyge epistola": p. 169-192.
Bound with copy 2 of his De recondita abscessuum natura. 1643.

—Synopseos chirurgiae libri sex. Amstelodami, Apud Elizeum Weyerstraeten, 1664.

135, [1] p. 14 cm. [11058]

Engraved title page.

—[Italian tr.] *In* Fabricius, H. ab Aquapendente. Le opere chirurgiche. 1684.

—Therapeuta Neapolitanus; seu, Veni mecum consultor curandarum febrium, & internorum omnium morborum. Inclusa Paedanchone affectu pestilente, ac peuros praefocante. Cum Commentario Cl. Thomae Bartholini ... Aedidit Gregorius Villanus ... Neapoli, Typis Roberti Molli, sumptibus Joannis Alberti Tarini, 1653.

[24], 257, [7] p.; 118 (i.e. 128) p. 17 cm. [11059]

Part [2] has half title.

—Τριβοήτητος ἡ τρισέρειοτος. Trimembris chirurgia, in qua diaetetico-chirurgica pharmaco-chirurgica, & chymico-chirurgica traditio est ... Francofurti, Impensis Joannis Godefridi Schönwetteri, 1653.

[8], 268, [10] p. 23 cm. [11060]

Bound with copy 2 of his De recondita abscessuum natura. 1643.

—Vipera Pythia; id est, De viperae natura, veneno, medicina, demonstrationes, & experimenta nova. Patavii, Typis Pauli Frambotti, 1651.

[18], 522, [24] p. front. (port.), illus. 23 cm. [11061]

Added engraved title page.
Errata: p. [23–24]

—Zootomia democritaea; id est, Anatome generalis totius animantium opificii, libris quinque distincta, quorum seriem sequens facies delineabit ... Noribergae, Literis Endterianis, 1645.

[24], 408, [34] p. illus., ports. 20 cm. [11062]

Added engraved title page.
Includes portrait of Giulio Jasolino.
Edited by J. G. Volckamer.

—, *tr. See* COLMENERO DE LEDESMA, A. Chocolata inda. 1644.

—*See* FIERA, B. Coena notis illustrata a Carolo Avantio. 1649.

SEVERINUS, PETRUS. *See* SØRENSEN, Peder [1540 or 42–1602]

SEXTUS EMPIRICUS. Σεξτου Ἐμπειριχου τα σωζομενα ... Opera quae extant ... Pyrrhoniarum Hypotypωσεωn libri III. ... Henrico Stephano interprete, Adversus mathematicos, hoc est, eos qui disciplinas profitentur, libri X, Gentiano Herveto Aurelio interprete, Graece nunc primum editi. Adjungere visum est Pyrrhonis ... Eliensis ... vitam, nec non Claudii Galeni ... De optimo docendi genere librum, quo adversus academicos Pyrrhoniosque disputat ... Genevae, Typis ac sumptibus Petri & Jacobi Chouët, 1621.

[20], 168 p.; 520, [42] p. 36 cm. [11063]

Place of publication "Aurelianae" blocked out.
In Greek and Latin.
"... Pyrrhonis Eliensis ... vita, ex Diogene Laertio": p. 481–495; "... Galeni ... De optimo docendi genere liber ... Erasmo Roterodamo interprete ...": p. 497–503; "In Sexti philosophi Pyrrhon. Hypotyp. libros tres, annotationes Henrici Stephani ...": p. 505–520; "In Pyrronis vitam ex Diog. Laertio ejusdem Henr. Stephani annotationes ...": p. [521]

SEXTUS PLACITUS. *See* PLACITUS, Sextus Papyriensis.

SEXTUS PLATONICUS. *See* PLACITUS, Sextus Papyriensis.

SEYFART, DAVID [*fl.* 1698] *respondent. See* EYSEL, J. P., *praeses.* Disputatio inauguralis medica, de epilepsia. 1698.

SEYFRIED, JOHANN HEINRICH [*fl.* 17th cent] *tr. See* HELMONT, J. B. van. Tumulus pestis; das ist, Gründlicher Ursprung der Pest. 1681.

SEYLER, ABRAHAM. *See* SEYLLER, Abraham [*d.* 1583]

SEYLER, BALTHASAR [*fl.* 1654] *respondent. See* FRIDERICI, V., *praeses.* Disputatio physica de sapore. 1654.

SEYLER, JOHANN ADOLPH [*fl.* 1685] *respondent. See* BOHN, J., *praeses.* Dissertationes chymico-physicae. 1685 [and] Dissertationum chymico-physicarum duodecima de calcinatione. 1685.

SEYLLER, ABRAHAM [*d.* 1583] *See* SCHOLTZ, L. Consiliorum medicinalium ... liber singularis. 1610 [and] Epistolarum philosophicarum: medicinalium, ac chymicarum ... volumen. 1610.

SEYMAR, WILLIAM, *pseud. See* RAMSYE, William.

SFORTIA, Nathanael, *pseud. See* Zwinger, Theodor [1658–1742]

SFORZINO, Francesco Carcano. *See* Carcano, Francesco [*ca.* 1500–1580]

SGAMBATI, Giovanni Andrea [*fl.* 17th cent.] De pestilente faucium affectu Neapoli saeviente opusculum … Neapoli, Excudebat Tarquinius Longus, 1620.

 [8], 71 p. 21 cm.   **[11064]**
 Imperfect: p. 28–29 mutilated.

SGOBBIS DA MONTAGNANA. Antonio de [*b. ca.* 1603] Nuovo, et universale theatro farmaceutico. Fondato sopra le preparationi farmaceutiche scritte da' medici antichi, greci, & arabi; principalmente da Galeno, e Mesue … Ampliato oltre le fabriche … contenute ne gli antidotarii Veneti de Giorgio Melichio, aumentato da Alberto Stecchini … con quelle … compositioni ancora … da gli piu lodati scrittori … Venetia, Stamparia Juliana, a spese dell'authore, si vende Gio. Giacomo Hertz, 1667.

 [12], 62 p.; [6], 880, [32] p. plates, ports., table. 34 cm.   **[11065]**
 Added engraved title page.

 — [The same.] Universale theatro farmaceutico … Venetia, Paolo Baglioni, 1682.

 [10], 820 p. plates (incl. ports.), table. 33 cm.   **[11066]**
 Added engraved title page: Nuovo, et universale theatro farmaceutico.

SHARROCK, Robert [1630–1684] Judicia; (seu, Legum censurae) de variis incontinentiae speciebus … Addita insuper explicatione qui ex communi rationis jure delicta haec inhonesta, & humanae felicitati inimica esse arguantur … Oxoniae, Excudebat H. Hall, impensis Thom. Robinson, 1662.

 [16], 112 p. 17 cm.   **[11067]**

SHEFFLER, Joannes Ernestus. *See* Hippocrates. Aphorismorum sectiones octo. 1633.

SHERARD, William [1659–1728] *ed. See* Tournefort, J. P. de. Schola botanica. 1689.

SHERLEY, Thomas [1638–1678] A philosophical essay, declaring the probable causes, whence stones are produced in the greater world. From which occasion is taken to search into the origin of all bodies, discovering them to proceed from water, and seeds.

Being a prodromus to a medicinal tract concerning the causes, and cure of the stone in the kidneys, and bladders of men … London, William Cademan, 1672.

 [16], 143 p. 18 cm.   **[11068]**

 —[Latin tr.] Dissertatio philosophica, explicans causas probabiles lapidum in macrocosmo, qua occasione in originem corporum omnium inquiritur atque ostenditur eam deberi aquae & seminibus, praemissa tractatui medico de causis et curatione calculi tam renum quam vesicae, Anglice primum edita … nunc … Latine reddita. Hamburgi, Impensis Christiani Guthii, 1675.

 128 p. 17 cm.   **[11069]**
 Imperfect: outer margin of title page trimmed affecting date.

 —, *tr. See* Elsholtz, J. S. The curious distillatory. 1677; Mayerne, Sir T. T. de. Medicinal councels. 1677 [and] A treatise of the gout. *1676;* Moellenbrock, V. A. Cochlearia curiosa. 1676.

SHERLOCK, William [1641?–1707] The nature and measure of charity. A sermon … London, W. Rogers, 1697.

 [1], 30, [2] p. 20 cm.   **[11070]**

SHIPTON, Jacob. *See* Shipton, James.

SHIPTON, James, *ed. See* Bate, G. Pharmacopoeia Bateana. 1688, 1691, 1700; [Dutch tr.] 1698; [English tr.] 1694, 1700.

 —*See* Pharmacopoeiae Collegii Regalis Londini remedia. 1678, 1689, 1699.

[SHIRLEY, John, *fl.* 1680–1702] The accomplished ladies rich closet of rarities; or The ingenious gentlewoman and servant-maids delightful companion. Containing many excellent things for the accomplishment of the female sex, after the exactest manner and method, viz. 1. The art of distilling … 9. Physical and chirurgical receipts. 10. The duty of a wet nurse; and to know and cure diseases in children, &c … To which is added a second part, containing directions for the guidance of a young gentlewoman … 5th ed. with large additions, corr. and amended. London, W. Wilde and J. Blare, 1696.

 192 p. plates. 15 cm.   **[11071]**
 Added engraved title page wanting.
 Imperfect: title page mutilated, affecting imprint date. Date supplied from Wing S 3501.
 Bound with Beauties treasury. London, 1705.

SHIRLEY, Thomas. *See* Sherley, Thomas [1638–1678]

SHORT, Richard [1603?–1668] Περι ψυχροποσιας, of drinking water, against our novelists, that prescribed it in England ... Whereunto is added Περι θερμοποσιας of warm drink, and is an answer to a treatise of warm drink printed in Cambridge. London, John Crook, 1656.

[32], 173 p. 14 cm. **[11072]**

A **SHORT** account of the proceedings of the College of Physicians. *See* Royal College of Physicians, London.

A **SHORT-METHOD** of physick, shewing the cure of fourty-five severall diseases ... Collected out of severall authors ... By the practice of C. B. Gent. ... London, Printed by M. S. for Thomas Jenner, 1659.

[3], 40 p. plate. 20 cm. **[11073]**

SHORTE, R. *See* Short, Richard [1603?–1668]

SIBBALD, *Sir* Robert [1641–1722] Phalainologia nova; sive, Observationes de rarioribus quibusdam balaenis in Scotiae littus nuper ejectis ... Edinburgi, Typis Joannis Redi, vaeneunt apud M. Robertum Edward, 1692.

[4], 44 p. 20 cm. **[11074]**

Imperfect: title page mutilated.

With this is bound Le Boë, Frans de, praeses. Disputatio medica de variis tabis speciebus. 1661.

—Scotia illustrata; sive, Proromus historiae naturalis in quo regionis natura, incolarum ingenia & mores, morbi iisque medendi methodus, & medicina indigena accurate explicantur ... Edinburgi, Ex officina typographica Jacobi Kniblio, Josuae Solingensis & Johannis Colmarii [1684]

3 parts in 1 v. plates. 38 cm. **[11075]**

Each part has separate title page; that of part (1) has imprint: Edinburgi, In officina typographica Davidis Lindesii, Jacobi Kniblio, Josuae Solingensis & Johannis Colmarii, 1683.

Contents.—pt. [1] Nuncius Scoto-Britannus; sive, Admonitio de atlante Scotico.—pt. [2] De plantis Scotiae.—pt. [3] De animalibus Scotiae ... et de mineralibus metallis et marinis Scotiae.

—*respondent. See* Le Boë, F. de, *praeses.* Disputatio medica de variis tabis speciebus. 1661.

SIBENHAR, Martinus. Nothwendig, kurtz, und gründlicher Bericht, wie man sich jetzt in pestilentzischen Sterbensleufften vorhalten soll. Damit die Gesunden vor Gefahr vorwahrnet und worwahret; und die so mit der tödtlichen Seuche angegrieffen ... geheilet werden mögen ... Jetzo wieder auffs newe gedruckt, und neben angehengten nothwendigen Regeln an etlichen Orthen vormehret Neyss, Gedruckt durch Casparum Sigfried, 1601.

[36] p. 20 cm. **[11076]**

Imperfect: wormholes throughout; all pages after sig. E2 wanting.

SIBER, Balthasar [*fl.* 1696–1698] *respondent. See* Planer, J. A., *praeses.* De nive dissertatio quarta. 1696; Sperling, P. G., *praeses.* Dysenteriam ... exponit M. B. S. 1698.

SIBER, Johann Georg [*b.* 1667] *respondent. See* Wedel, G. W., *praeses.* Dissertatio inauguralis medica de terreorum natura. 1697.

—*See* Crause, R. W. Propemticum inaugurale de calendario valetudinariorum perpetuo. 1697.

SIBMACHER, Hans. *See* Sibmacher, Johann [*d.* 1611]

SIBMACHER, Johann [*d.* 1611] *illus. See* Camerarius, J. Symbolorum et emblematum centuriae tres. 1605.

SIBSCOTA, George, The deaf and dumb man's discourse; or: A treatise concerning those that are born deaf and dumb, containing a discovery of their knowledge or understanding; as also the method they use, to manifest the sentiments of their mind. Together with an additional tract of the reason and speech of inanimate creatures ... London, Printed by H. Bruges, for William Crook, 1670.

[1], 89, [5] p. 16 cm. **[11077]**

Signatures: first leaf unsigned, B-F8, G2⁻8.

SIBYLLENUS, Petrus [*fl.* 1548–1564] *See* Scholtz, L. Consiliorum medicinalium ... liber singularis. 1610; Sennert, D. De febribus libri IV. 1628, 1633, 1641, 1653.

SICILY, Protomedico. Constitutiones, capitula, jurisdictiones, ac pandectae Pegii Protomedicatus officii, prius jam a Spect. Joanne Philippo Ingrassia, olim hujus Siciliae Regni . . . Protomedico . . . refor-matae, renovatae, ac elucidatae: nunc a . . . Paulo Pizzuto . . . in ampliorem forman redactae, et quamplurimis adnotationibus . . . juxta temporum indigentiam, refertae. Panormi, Ex typographia Nicolai Bua, 1657.

238, [22] p.   20 cm.   [11078]

Earlier edition by Ingrassia, published in Palermo in 1584 under title: Constitutiones et capitula, nec non et jurisdictiones Regii Protomedicatus officii cum pandectis ejusdem refermatis. Con-tains the ordinances of the protomedici, Antonio d'Alessandri and Giovanni Filippo Ingrassia, with annotations on them by Paolo Pizzuto (p. 1-158) and "Regia, imperatoriaque Protomedicatus of-ficii diplomata, sive privilegia, quae in Regiae Cancellariae Con-servatoris, Protonotariique registris, atque actis invenire huius-que licuit, anno salutis 1564", supplemented by later acts dating through 1653 (p. [159]-230) Some of the later records are in Italian.

SICLER, ADRIAN [*fl.* 1669-1670] La chiromance royale et nouvelle . . . Lyon, Chez Daniel Gayet, et se vendent chez l'autheur, 1666.

[26], 227 p.   illus., plate.   15 cm.   [11079]

—Histoire inoüye, d'un accouchement de dix-neuf moys. Ouvrage grandement utile aux medecins, chyrurgiens . . . Au Puy, Estienne Bleigeac, 1670.

[32], 158 (i.e. 168) p.   illus.   17 cm.   [11080]

Imperfect: title page mutilated.

SICMAN, JOHANNES, *respondent. See* DEUSING, A., *praeses.* Synopsis medicinae universalis. 1649.

SIDOBRE, ANTOINE [*fl.* 1694] Tractatus de variolis et morbillis . . . Lugduni, Apud Anisson, & Posuel, 1699.

[6], 246, [1] p.   16 cm.   [11081]

—*respondent.* Almae medicorum Monspeliensium Academiae hoc primum specimen . . . Monspelii, Apud Joannum Martel, 1694.

131, [1] p.   plate.   15 cm.   [11082]

Errata: p. [1]
Half title reads: Dissertatio academica proposita . . . Petro Chirac . . . sub hac verborum serie An passioni iliacae globuli plumbei hydrargyro praeferendi.
Running title reads: Dissertatio de ileo.
Diss. — Montpellier.

SIEBENB, C. DE. *See* URBIGERUS, Baro.

SIEBMACHER, JOHANN. *See* SIBMACHER, Johann [*d.* 1611]

SIEBOLD, JOHANN. *See* SIEBOLDT, Johannes [*fl.* 1662-1694]

SIEGEMUND, JUSTINE DITTRICH [1648-1705] An Herrn D. Andream Petermann . . . wegen eines corollarii, multae hactenus insolitae laudatae en-chireses in libro, cui titulus est, Die Chur-Brandenburgische Hof-Wehe-Mutter, nituntur vana speculatione, in praxi enim sunt absurdae. Hinc jure miramur, quomodo liber sustinere potuerit censuram totius Collegii Medici. Zu Deutsch also lautend, viele bisshero ungewöhnliche gepriesene Handgriffe in dem Buch, Die Chur-Brandenb. Hof-Wehe-Mutter benennet, bestehen auf eine eitele Ipeculation [sic], dann in der Ubung seyn sie ungereimt . . . So in der Disputation de Gonorrhaea unter seinem Praesidio zu Leipzig gehalten 1690. d. 5. Dec. abgelasenes send-schreiben . . . Cölln an der Spree, Ulrich Liebpert, 1692.

[12] p.   plates.   20 cm.   [11084]

Imperfect: plates 8-12, 14, 20-22 wanting.
Bound with her Die Chur-Brandenburgische Hoff-Wehe-[Mut-ter] Cölln an der Spree, 1690.

—[Die Chur-Brandenburgisch] Hoff-Wehe-[Mut-ter]; das ist, Ein höchst-nöthiger Unterricht, von schweren und unrecht-stehenden Geburten in einem Gespräch vorgestellet . . . Cölln an der Spree, Gebruckt bey Ulrich Liebperten, 1690.

[39], 260, [14] p.   front., plates., port.
                                                          [11085]

Imperfect: front. and port. wanting; title page mutilated.
Title partly supplied from Waller.
With this are bound *her*: Wider Herrn D. Andrea Peterman. 1692; An Herrn D. Andream Petermann. 1692.

—[Dutch tr.] Spiegel der vroed-vrouwen, behelsende een klaer onderrigt van sware verloss-ingen der kramende vrouwen, soo om de selve te helpen, als ook om in veel sware toevallen behulpelijk te zyn . . . Als mede een onderrigt ontrent het Ampt en pligt der vroed-vrouwen. Door Cornelis Solingen . . . Amsterdam, Jan Ten Hoorn, 1691.

[32], 242, [6] p.; [8], 84, [4] p.   plates.   21 cm.
                                                          [11086]

Part [2] has half title.

—Wider Herrn D. Andreae Peterman ... von ihm also-genante gründliche Deduction vieler Handgriffe, die er aus dem Buche Die Chur-Brandenburgische Hoff-Weh-Mutter genant, als speculationes und ungereimt, ja gefährlich zu seyn, vermeinet zu erweisen, nöthiger Bericht, an den geneigten Leser. Cöln an der Spree, Gedruckt bey Ulrich Liebpert, 1692.

36 p.   20 cm.   **[11087]**

Bound with *her* Die Chur-Brandenburgisch Hoff-Wehe-Mutter. 1690.

SIEGFRIED, CASPAR ESAIAS [*fl.* 1655–1681] *praeses.* De mari ejusque salsedine, ut & fluxu & refluxu dissertatio physica ... [Lipsiae] Typis Ritzschianis [1655]

[20] p.   20 cm.   **[11088]**
Diss.—Leipzig (T. Wachsmuth, *respondent*)

—Disputatio physica de terra ... Lipsiae, Literis Christiani Michaelis, 1660.

[16] p.   20 cm.   **[11089]**
Diss.—Leipzig (C. Heider, *respondent*)

SIEGFRIED, CASPAR ESAIAS [*fl.* 1673] *praeses.* Disputatio physica de magnete ... Leucopetrae, Literis viduae Hildebrandianae, excudebat Joh. Brühl [1673]

[28] p.   19 cm.   **[11090]**
Diss.—Weissenfels. Gymnasium (E. Pfundt, *respondent*)

SIEGFRIED, HEINRICH [*fl.* 1683–1685] *respondent. See* BOHN, J., *praeses.* Dissertationes chymicophysicae. 1685 [and] Dissertationum chymico-physicarum septima de comminutione. 1683; LANGE, C. J. Disputationem medicam de haemorrhagia ... subjicit C. J. L. 1685.

SIEGFRIED, JOHANNES [1556–1623] *praeses.* Disputatio de melancholia ... Helmaestadii, Ex officina Jacobi Lucii, 1607.

[24] p.   19 cm.   **[11091]**
Diss.—Helmstedt (D. Finxius, *respondent*)

—Disputationum anatomicarum decima octava. De oculis ... Helmaestadii, Typis impressa Jacobi Lucii, 1600.

[15] p.   21 cm.   **[11092]**
Signatures: A–B⁴.
Diss.—Helmstedt (H. Loss, *respondent*)

—Themata de melancholia ejusque curatione ... Helmaestadii, Typis Jacobi Lucii, 1613.

[16] p.   20 cm.   **[11093]**
Diss.—Helmstedt (J. Cravelius, *respondent*)

SIEMENS, HENNING JOHANN [*b.* 1670] *See* HOFFMANN, F. [1660–1742] Propemticon inaugurale, de vapore carbonum fossilium innoxio. 1695.

SIFILINUS, HUGO, *pseud. See* FABRI, Honoré [1606–1688]

SIGBERT, JAKOB [*fl.* 1652] *respondent. See* TACKE, J., *praeses.* De anima rationali. 1652.

SIGFRID, JOHANN [*fl.* 1631] *praeses.* Positiones physicae de principiis ... [Lipsiae] Typis haeredum Friderici Lanckisch [1631]

[24] p.   18 cm.   **[11094]**
Diss.—Leipzig (V. U. Barger, *respondent*)

SIGFRIDUS, JOANNES. *See* SIEGFRIED, Johannes [1556–1623]

SIGISMUNDUS, JOHANNES. *See* SCHOLTZ, L. Consiliorum medicinalium ... liber singularis. 1610.

SIGNIUS, JULIANUS. *See* SEGNI, Giuliano [*fl.* 17th cent.]

SIGNORETUS, JOANNES. Excerpta aphoristica, cum symbola. *In* HIPPOCRATES. [Aphorismi. Greek and Latin] 1668.

SIKARDUS, GODOFREDUS [*fl.* 1698] *respondent. See* HOFFMANN, F. [1660–1742] *praeses.* Dissertatio inauguralis medica de anthelminthicis. 1698.

SILATAN, FRANÇOIS [*fl.* 1655?] L'interprete de la nature; ou, La science physique tirée d'Aristote, & de Saint Thomas, & de l'experience. Divisée en huit livres, par François Silatan [pseud. of François Noël?] Laval, Jean Ambroise, 1655.

[8], 499, [12] p.   19 cm.   **[11095]**
The first Approbation is dated 1656.

SILENTO, PETRUS DE. *See* PETRUS DE SILENTO.

SILESIA. Laws, statutes, etc. Der hoch-und löblichen Herren Fürsten und Stände im Hertzogthum Ober- und Nieder Schlesien neue Infections-Ordnung, darinnen ausführlich enthalten wie Jedermann ... wegen der ... Pest, zu verhalten, anbey auch der bresslauischen Physicorum medicinisch-entworffenes Pest-Consilium, sambt Anzeigung der ... Zufalle der Pest-Kranckheit, und wie solche zu curiren, nebenst Anhand einer Verzeichnüss derer Medicamenten, so in dem Consilio Medico ge-gemeldet [sic] worden. Bresslau, 1680.

[1], 140, [9] p. 20 cm. [11096]

"Taxa . . . in den bresslauischen Apothecken verhandenen Artzneyen . . .": p. [5-9]

—[The same.] Der hoch- und löblichen Herren Fürsten und Stände, im Hertzogthumb Ober- und Nieder-Schlesien, wie auch bresslauischer Physicorum, neue Infections-Ordnüng, und medicinisches Consilium abgefasset und entworffen. Erffurth, Bey Benjamin Hempeln [1681]

96 + p. 19 cm. [11097]

Imperfect: all pages after p. 96 wanting.

SILLIG, JOHANN BENEDIKT [*fl.* 1690] *respondent.* *See* WELSCH, C. L., *praeses.* De sono. 1690.

SILVATICUS, BENEDICTUS. *See* SALVATICO, Benedetto, conte di [1575-1658]

SILVATICUS, JOANNES BAPTISTA. *See* SELVATICO, Giovanni Battista [*d.* 1621]

SILVESTRE, PETER [*ca.* 1662-1718] *See* [BRUNET, C.] Le progrès de la medecine. 1699.

SILVIUS, DETHLEVUS. *See* SYLVIUS, Dethlevus [*fl.* 1573]

SILVIUS, JACOBUS. *See* DUBOIS, Jacques [1478-1555]

SIMEO Sethus. Σύνταγμα κατὰ στοιχείων περὶ προφῶν δυνάμεων . . . Volumen de alimentorum facultatibus juxta ordinem literarum digestum . . . emend., auct. & Latina versione donatum, cum difficilium locorum explicatione a Martino Bogdano . . . Lutetiae Parisiorum, Ex offic. Dion. Bechet & Lud. Billanii, 1658.

[8], 174 p. 19 cm. [11098]

In Greek and Latin.

SIMMLER, JOSIAS [1530-1576] Vallesiae et Alpium descriptio. Lugduni Batavorum, Ex officina Elzeviriana, 1633.

377, [7] p. 12 cm. [11099]

Engraved title page.

"Appendix descriptionis Vallesianae . . . De thermis & fontibus medicaetis Vallesianorum liber, Gasparo Collino . . . auctore": p. 340-370.

SIMON, BALTHASAR [*fl.* 1618] *respondent.* Τῆς γαγγραίνας και τοῦ σφακέλου διάγνωσις, πρόγνωσις και

δεραπεία . . . Basileae, Typis Johannis Schroeteri [1618]

[32] p. 21 cm. [11100]

Diss. — Basel.

SIMON, BARTHOLD [*fl.* 1668-1670] *respondent.* *See* ROLFINCK, W., *praeses.* Dissertatio practica de curatione hydropis ascitis. 1668.

SIMON, JOHANN [*fl.* 1616] *respondent.* *See* HAWENREUTER, J. L., *praeses.* Disputatio physica de primis corporum naturalium principiis. 1616

SIMON, JOHANN [*fl.* 1659-1694] *praeses.* Diversicolor ovium foetus opera Jacobi patriarchae productus in causis suis naturalibus consideratus . . . Wittebergae, Literis Matthaei Henckelii, 1675.

[16] p. 20 cm. [11101]

Diss. — Wittenberg (J. E. Weber, *respondent*)

—Ex physicis de generatione aequivoca . . . disputabit Johannes Ernestus Hering . . . Wittebergae, Johannes Röhnerus [1659]

[24] p. 19 cm. [11102]

Diss. — Wittenberg (J. E. Hering, *respondent*)

SIMON, JOHANN GEORG [1636-1696] Brevis delineatio impotentiae conjugalis, diu hactenus desiderata, nunc vero denuo revisa et in lucem edita. Jenae, Typis Samuelis Adolphi Mülleri, 1672.

[120] p. 20 cm. [11103]

—[The same.] . . . Nunc vero denuo revisa et opposita spuriis exemplaribus quae vulgo circumferuntur . . . Jenae, Impensis Joh. Theodori Fleischeri, 1675.

[16], [3]-182 p. 20 cm. [11104]

—[The same.] . . . Jenae, Impensis Joh. Theordori Fleischeri, 1682.

209 p. 19 cm. [11105]

Imperfect: title page mutilated and partly backed.

—*praeses.* Faciem humanam ad similitudinem pulchritudinis coelestis figuratam occasione L. 17. si quis. C. de poenis . . . exponit Gothofredus Ebhardt . . . Halae Magdeburgicae, Literis Christiani Henckelii [1696]

[24] p. 20 cm. [11106]

Diss. — Halle (G. Ebhardt, *respondent*)

—Jura obstetricum . . . [Jenae] Typis Nisianis [1671]

[40] p. 20 cm. [11107]

Diss. — Jena (J. H. Lots, *respondent*)

SIMON 11108-11115 SINAPI

SIMON, RICHARD [1638-1712] See VOSSIUS, I. Observationum ad Pomp. Melam appendix. 1686.

SIMON À CORDO. See SIMON GENUENSIS.

SIMON GENUENSIS, tr. See MESUË [924 or 5-1015] Opera. 1602, 1623.

SIMON JANUENSIS. See SIMON GENUENSIS.

SIMONE DA GENOVA. See SIMON GENUENSIS.

SIMONIS, JOHANNES [fl. 1646] respondent. See FRANKENIUS, J., praeses. De occultis medicamentorum. 1646.

SIMOTTA, GEORGE. A theater of the planetary houres for all dayes of the yeare. Wherein may be gathered from the earth, under the coelestiall influences, divers sorts of hearbs, rootes, leaves, barkes ... for the use of physick, whereby both suddenly, and happily infirmities may be cured ... Translated out of Greeke, into French, and now into English ... London, Printed by August Matthewes, and solde by George Baker, 1631.

[4], 31 p. 18 cm. [11108]
STC 22561.

SIMPSON, W. See SIMPSON, William [fl. 1665-1677]

SIMPSON, WILLIAM [fl. 1665-1677] Hydrologia chymica; or, The chymical anatomy of the Scarbrough, and other spaws in York-shire. Wherein are interspersed, some animadversions upon Dr. Wittie's lately published treatise of the Scarbrough-spaw. Also, a short description of the spaws at Malton and Knarsbrough. And a discourse concerning the original of hot springs ... with the causes and cures of ... diseases ... Also, a vindication of chymical physick ... Lastly ... an Appendix of the original of springs; with the author's Ternary of medicines ... London, Printed by W. G. for Richard Chiswel, 1669.

[19], 374 p. plates. 17 cm. [11109]

—[The same, as subject.] See WITTIE, R. Pyrologia mimica, 1669 [and] Scarbroughs spagyrical anatomizer. 1672.

—Hydrological essayes; or, A vindication of hydrologia chymica, being a further discovery of the Scarbrough spaw ... And of the sweet spaw and sulphur-well at Knarsbrough. With a brief account

of the allom works at Whitby. Together with ... some queries, propounded by ... Dr. Dan. Foot, concerning mineral waters. To which is annexed, an answer to Dr. Tunstal's book, concerning the Scarbrough spaw. With an Appendix of ... the German spaw. And ... observations on the dissection of a woman who died of the jaundice ... London, Printed by J. D. for Richard Chiswel, 1670.

[16], 3-159 p. 18 cm. [11110]

—Philosophical dialogues concerning the principles of natural bodies ... London, Printed by T. Hodgkin, for Dorman Newman, 1677.

[16], 173 p. 16 cm. [11111]
Imperfect: title pages [2] and 173 mutilated and backed; title page also supplied in photocopy.

—Zymologia physica; or, A brief philosophical discourse of fermentation, from a new hypothesis of acidum and sulphur ... With an additional discourse of the sulphur-bath at Knarsbrough ... London, Printed by T. R. & N. T. for W. Copper, 1675.

[15], 147, [3] p.; [1], 28 p. 17 cm. [11112]
Part [2] has special title page.
Imperfect: upper and lower margins trimmed; lower outer corner of p. 67-68 wanting.

—respondent. Disputatio medica inauguralis de dolore colico ... Lugduni Batavorum, Apud viduam & haeredes Joannis Elsevirii, 1670.

[12] p. 23 cm. [11113]
Diss.—Leyden.

SINAPI, MIHÁLY ALAJOS [fl. 1693-1696] Absurda vera occasione potissimarum quarundam controversiarum quae neotericis cum Galenicis intercedunt ... In compendio denuo exhibita ... Varsaviae, 1693.

[15], 147 p. 16 cm. [11114]

—Absurda vera; sive, Paradoxa medica quorum pars I. Theoremata & quaestiones controversas varias quae hodie neotericis cum Galenicis intercedunt proponit cum dissertatione ... de spirituum effluviis & animae communis transmigratione juxta modernos Pythagoricos. Pars II. Occasione morborum certorum septentrionalium easdem quaestiones controversas continuat cum dissertatione de falso titulo ... morbi gallici. Pars III. Continet Tractatum de vanitate, falsitate, & incertitudine Aphoris. Hippocratis ... Genevae, Sumptibus Cramer & Perachon, 1697.

3 parts in 1 v. 18 cm. [11115]

Parts 2 and 3 have special title pages.

Dedicatory epistle in pt. 1 dated from Warsaw in 1693. An edition of pt. 1 only appeared in Warsaw in 1693 under title: Absurda vera occasione potissimarum quarundam controversiarum quae neotericis cum Galenicis intercedunt.

Pars tertia includes the Latin text of Hippocrates' Aphorismi, bks. 1–4 in Janus Cornarius' translation.

—Ars diu vivendi, pauca cum medicina . . . n. p. [not before 1689]

[32] p.   17 cm.   [11116]

Text refers to Johann Doläus' Encyclopaedia chirurgica rationis, first published in 1689.

—Tractatus de remedio doloris; sive, Materia anodynorum. Nec non opii, causa criminali in foro medico. Accessit visio Alethophili advocati de secta et religione empyricorum panacaeistarum. Amstelaedami, Apud Janssonio-Waesbergios, 1699.

[1], 172 p.   16 cm.   [11117]

SINCERA, Rege. See Rege Sincera.

SINCERUS, Iatrophilus. See Riedlin, Veit [1656–1724]

SINIBALDI, Giacomo [1630–1704] Apollo bifrons medicas, & amenas dissertationes Latino, & Aetrusco sermone promiscuas exponens. Romae, Typis & expensis Francisci de' Laz. fil. Ignatii, 1690.

[8], 354 p.   front.   21 cm.   [11118]

SINIBALDI, Giovanni Benedetto [1594–1658] Geneanthropeiae; sive, De hominis generatione decateuchon . . . Romae, Ex typographia Francisci Caballi, 1642.

[14] p., 1050 columns, [43] p.   32 cm. [11119]

Added engraved title page.

—[The same.] . . . Adjecta est Historia foetus Mussipontani. Francofurti, Sumptibus Johannis Petri Zubrodt, 1669.

1 v.   21 cm.   [11120]

Various pagings.

Part [2] has special title page: Historia foetus Mussipontani extra uterum in abdomine reperti et lapidescentis cum adjectis variorum . . . commentis. This includes Anton Deusing's Consideratio physico anatomica foetus Mussipontani . . . ad Johan. Daniel. Horstium; Anton Deusing's Foetus Mussipontani . . . secundinae detectae; Honoré Maris Lautier's Prodigium . . . foetum humanum extra loco conceptum . . . Muscipontana exhibet civitas; Anton Deusing's Vindiciae foetus . . . contra . . . Bernhardum a Doma, sub Blottesandaei [pseud. of Oluf Borch] personati vexillo larvato gregarium stratioten; Laurentius Strauss' Judicia varia . . . de foetus Mussipontani explicatione; Johann

Christoph Eisenmenger's De foetu Mussipontano . . . ad Joh. Danielem Horstium. Items have half titles.

Imperfect: title page mutilated.

—Copy 2.

Imperfect: lower margin of title page trimmed, affecting date of imprint.

With this is bound Jasolino, G. Collegium anatomicum. 1668.

—Hippocratis . . . antiphωnωn libri quinque. In quibus celebriores, & a nemine consulto adhuc enadratae, ejusdem contradictiones . . . conciliantur . . . Romae, Typis Ludovici Grignani, 1650.

[16], 338, [31] p.   25 cm.   [11121]

Includes Latin extracts from various Hippocratic works.

SINICKER, Emanuel [fl. 1600] Keiser Rudolff des andern . . . Spagyrische Hauss und Reiss-Apothec, auss . . . lateinischem . . . Exemplar . . . verteutscht, und . . . vermehrt. Darzu ist kommen ein Appendix . . . Durch Weylund H. Heinrich von Schennis . . . Zurich, Getruckt bey Johann Jacob Bodmer, 1646.

[12], 310, [14] p.   plates.   17 cm. [11122]

SINT, Lucas [fl. 1688] respondent. Disputatio medica inauguralis de lienteria . . . Trajecti ad Rhenum, Ex officina Francisci Halma, 1688.

[8] p.   22 cm.   [11123]

Diss.—Utrecht.

SIRENA, Francesco [fl. 1677] L'arte dello spetiale con la quale . . . ogni mediocre ingegno puo senza maestro apprendere la vera maniera di comporre i medicamenti tanto Galenisti, quanto chimici. Opera nova . . . Pavia, Gio. Ghidini, 1679.

[16], 965, [1] p.   plates.   35 cm. [11124]

—[The same.] . . . Venetia, Appresso Nicolo Pezzana, 1680.

[16], 1040, [23] p.   plates.   24 cm. [11125]

—See Friggio, O. Ricette Galenistiche agionte al libro intitolato L'arte del spetiale. 1692.

SIRICIUS, Michael [1628–1685] See Wirdig, S. Victrix veritas in censuris theologico-medicis de nova spirituum medicina. 1684.

SISINIUS, Joannes. See Amabile, Giovanni Sisinio [fl. 1615]

SISMUS, Cornelis [fl. 1695] respondent. Disputatio medica inauguralis de suffocatione stomachica . . .

Lugduni Batavorum, Apud Abrahamum Elzevier, 1695.

[23] p. 23 cm. [11126]
Diss.—Leyden.

SISMUS, Paulus [*fl.* 17th cent.] Tractatus de diaeta ... Hagae-Comitis, Apud Aegidius á Limburg, CIƆ.IƆƆ.IV [1604?]

[12], 68 p. 16 cm. [11127]
Date of imprint may be in error: work dedicated to Johann van der Meer (1589-1652); Prefatio refers to 1619.

SITONI, Giovanni Battista [1605-1681] Iatrosophiae miscellanea ... Opus hac 2. ed. mendis, quibus scatebat expurgatum, et tertia plusquam parte adauctum. Primo ex originalibus secundum duas partes Patavii impressum, nunc vero denuo recusum. [Einsiedeln] Typis Monasterii Einsidlensis, Per Nicolaum Wagenmann, 1649 [i.e. 1669]

[16], 361 p. 22 cm. [11128]
Dedicatory epistle and Privilege dated 1669.

—[The same.] ... Miscellanea medico-curiosa ... Opus hac 2. ed. mendis, quibus scatebat expurgatum, et tertia plusquam parte adauctum. Primo ex originalibus secundum duas partes Patavii impressum, nunc vero denuo recusum. Coloniae Agrippinae, Apud Joannem Wilhelmum Friessem, 1677.

[16], 361, [33] p. 21 cm. [11129]
Added engraved title page has imprint: ... Sumptibus Joannis Wilhelmi Friessem Junioris, 1676.
A reissue of the 1649 (i.e. 1669) edition with new title page and preliminary matters partly reset.

SIX severall orders of the Lords and Commons assembled in Parliament. 1643.

See Gt. Brit. Parliament.

SIX VAN CHANDELIER, Johann [*b.* 1612] Poësy ... Verdeelt in ses boeken en eenige opschriften. Amsterdam, Joost Pluimert, 1657.

[3], 631, [2] p. 17 cm. [11130]

SIXESMITH, Thomas [*fl.* 1628] *ed.* See Brerewood, E. Tractatus quidam logici de praedicabilibus et praedicamentis. 1637.

SIXTUS Papa IV. Ad perpetuam rei memoriam. 1675? See Catholic Church. *Pope,* 1471-1484 (Sixtus IV)

SIZÉ, François [*fl.* 1610] *tr.* See Du Laurens, A. L'histoire anatomique. 1631.

SKINKER, Tannakin. See A certaine relation of the hogfaced gentlewoman. 1640.

SKLERANDER, Philipp Jacob. See Hartmann, Philipp Jakob [1648-1707]

SKOVG, Jan [*fl.* 1692] *respondent.* See Drossander, A., *praeses.* Dissertatio physica de motu musculari. 1692

SKRETA, Heinrich. See Screta, Heinrich [1637-1689]

SLADE, Matthew [1628-1689] Dissertatio de generatione animalium. In Jasolino, G. Collegium anatomicum. 1668.

SLEESWYCK, Sixtus à [*fl.* 1664] *respondent.* Disputatio medica inauguralis, de menstruorum suppressione ... Trajecti ad Rhenum, Ex officina Everhardi ab Eede, 1664.

[16] p. 20 cm. [11131]
Diss.—Utrecht.

SLEGEL, Paulus Marquartus. See Schlegel, Paul Marquard [1605-1653]

SLEGELIUS, Vincentius. See Deusing, A. Resurrectio hepatis asserta. 1662.

SLEPPER, Justus Bernhard [*fl.* 1684] *respondent.* See Schrader, F., *praeses.* De frigoris natura. 1684.

SLESCOVIUS, Sebastianus. See Sleszkowski, Sebastyan [1569-1648]

SLESZKOWSKI, Sebastyan [1569-1648] Incomparabilis thesaurus alexitericus; in quo ... remedia selecta ... contra omnis generis venena mortifera ... proponuntur ... Brunsbergae, In chalcographia Georgii Schönfels, 1621.

[9], 271 ll. 17 cm. [11132]

—Opera medica duo; unum, Praxis phlebotomiae ... Alterum, De febribus liber ... Cracoviae, In chalcographia Antonii Wosinski, 1617.

[13], 114, [12] ll.; [2], 85 ll. 16 cm. [11133]
Imperfect: wormholes on p. [1-6]

SLEVOGT, Johann Adrian [1653-1726] Programma ... de fatis chirurgiae lectionibus publicis privatisque praemissum. [Jenae] Litteris Nisianis, 1695.

[8] p. 20 cm. [11134]

Cariem cranii memorabili exemplo et medica ἐξηγήσει tractatum ... pro loco publicae ... disquisitioni ... sistit Jo. Hadrianus Slevogtius ... Jenae, Literis Jo. Zach. Nisii [1695]

[4], 15, [1] p. plates. 20 cm.   **[11135]**

Imperfect? Fig. 1 wanting?
Diss. pro loco—Jena.

Programs—Jena

—Decani Facultatis Medicae Jo. Hadriani Slevogtii ... invitatio publica ad dissertationem inauguralem de defectu lactis. Jenae, Literis Christoph. Krebsii, 1699.

8 p. 20 cm.   **[11136]**

With vita of C. G. Lehmann.

—Decani Facultatis Medicae Jo. Hadriani Slevogtii ... invitatio publica ad dissertationem inauguralem de ulceribus crurum antiquis. Jenae, Literis Christoph. Krebsii, 1699.

8 p. 20 cm.   **[11137]**

With vita of N. C. Bezold.

—Decani Facultatis Medicae Jo. Hadriani Slevogtii ... praelusio inauguralis de lapide bezoar. Jenae, Litteris Krebsianis [1698]

[8] p. 20 cm.   **[11138]**

With vita of J. D. Ehrhard.

—Decani Facultatis Medicae Jo. Hadriani Slevogtii ... prolusio de polypodio ad dissertationem inauguralem de polypis capitis. Jenae, Litteris Ehrichianis, 1699.

[8] p. 20 cm.   **[11139]**

With vita of J. K. Muller.

—Decani Facultatis Medicae Jo. Hadriani Slevogtii ... prolusio inauguralis de antichetico poterii ... Jenae, Literis Müllerianis [1695]

[8] p. 20 cm.   **[11140]**

With vita of J. A. Eggert.

—Decani Facultatis Medicae Jo. Hadriani Slevogtii ... prolusio inauguralis de fonticulo futurae coronalis, insigni vitiorum memoriae remedio. Jenae, Literis Mullerianis [1694]

[8] p. 19 cm.   **[11141]**

With vita of C. J. Wolff.

—Decani Facultatis Medicae Jo. Hadr. Slevogtii ... prolusio inauguralis de motore cordis. Jenae, Literis Joh. Jacobi Krebsii [1696]

[8] p. 20 cm.   **[11142]**

With vita of K. C. Leisner.

—Decani Facultatis Medicae Jo. Hadriani Slevogtii ... prolusio inauguralis de publicis utriusque Americae sudatoriis. Jenae, Literis Wertherianis [1693]

[8] p. 19 cm.   **[11143]**

With vita of J. G. Pillling.

—Decani Facultatis Medicae Jo. Hadriani Slevogtii ... prolusio inauguralis de scarificatione hydropicorum remedio paracentesis succedaneo. Jenae, Literis Gollnerianis [1697]

[8] p. 20 cm.   **[11144]**

With vita of J. T. Musaeus.

—Decani Facultatis Medicae Jo. Hadriani Slevogtii ... prolusio inauguralis qua argumenta potiora aequivocam generationem assertium proponuntur. Jenae, Literis Wertherianis [1697]

[8] p. 20 cm.   **[11145]**

With vita of R. Genaspe.

—Decani Facultatis Medicae Jo. Hadriani Slevogtii ... prolusio inauguralis quas ostenditur nucem methel Avicennae esse daturam modernorum. Jenae, Literis Wertherianis [1695]

[8] p. 19 cm.   **[11146]**

With vita of M. F. Cunisius.

—Facultatis Medicae decani Jo. Hadriani Slevogtii ... prolusio inauguralis, de exceptionibus medicis, sive permissione prohibitorum, et prohibitione permissorum, Jenae, Literis Ehrichianis [1700]

[11] p. 20 cm.   **[11147]**

With vita of J. J. Baier.

—Facultatis Medicae decani Jo. Hadriani Slevogtii ... prolusio inauguralis de natura morborum effectrice. Jenae, Literis Krebsianis [1700]

[8] p. 19 cm.   **[11148]**

With vita of J. T. Schmid.

—Facultatis Medicae decani Jo. Hadriani Slevogtii ... prolusio inauguralis de natura morborum per morbos curatrice. Jenae, Literis Krebsianis [1700]

[8] p. 20 cm.   **[11149]**

With vita of S. G. Hausdorff.

—Facultatis Medicae decani Jo. Hadriani Slevogtii ... prolusio inauguralis, de partu thamaris difficili et perinaeo inde rupto. [Jenae] Literis Ehrichianis [1700]

[8] p. 19 cm.   **[11150]**

With vita of C. G. Koch.

—Facultatis Medicae Jenensis decani Jo. Hadriani Slevogtii . . . prolusio inauguralis de utero per sarcoma ex corpore protracto, et postmodum resecto. [Jenae] Literis Krebsianis [1700]

[8] p.   20 cm.   [11151]

With vita of F. Winckler.

—Facultatis Medicae decani Jo. Hadriani Slevogtii . . . publica invitatio ad dissertationem inauguralem de puella, variolis malignis laborante. Jenae, Litteris Wertherianis [1699]

[8] p.   20 cm.   [11152]

With vita of J. M. Floribus.

Dissertations—Jena

—*praeses.* Aegram lochiorum fluxu nimio vel potius haemorrhagia uteri laborantem . . . publico . . . examini exponet Wilhelmus Christoph. Paulus Petz . . . [Jenae] Litteris Nisianis [1699]

[6], 28 p.   20 cm.   [11153]

W. C. P. Petz, *respondent.*

—Aegram ex lochiorum retentione graviter decumbentem . . . publico eruditorum examini exhibebit Arnoldus Fridericus Beier. Literis Krebsianis [1697]

23, [1] p.   19 cm.   [11154]

A. F. Beier, *respondent.*

—De crepatura viscerum . . . Jenae, Literis Christophori Krebsii [1699]

35 p.   20 cm.   [11155]

M. H. Dencker, *respondent.*

—De paracentesi thoracis et abdominis . . . Jenae, Typis Gollnerianis [1697]

[24] p.   20 cm.   [11156]

J. T. Musaeus, *respondent.*

—Diatribe physiologica de affectibus animi . . . [Jenae] Litteris Nisianis [1695]

20, [4] p.   20 cm.   [11157]

J. G. Möller, *respondent.*

—Disputatio inauguralis de torminibus infantium . . . Jenae, Literis Wertherianis [1695]

24 p.   20 cm.   [11158]

M. F. Cunisius, *respondent.*

—Disputatio medica inauguralis de epilepsia infantili . . . Jenae, Literis Wertherianis [1696]

24 p.   19 cm.   [11159]

W. D. Lupin, *respondent.*

—Disputatio medica inauguralis de sudoribus . . . Jenae, Literis Wertherianis [1697]

30 p.   20 cm.   [11160]

J. G. Pilling, *respondent.*

—Dissertatio inauguralis medica exhibens foeminam mola laborantem . . . Jenae, Literis Ehrichianis [1700]

24 p.   20 cm.   [11161]

C. G. Koch, *respondent.*

—Dissertatio medica de dura matre . . . Jenae, Literis J. Dav. Wertheri [1690]

[28] p.   20 cm.   [11162]

K. C. Xylander, *respondent.*

—Dissertatio medica inauguralis de cachexia . . . Jenae, Typis Christophori Kresbsii [1697]

23, [1] p.   20 cm.   [11163]

J. W. S. Eck, *respondent.*

—Dissertatio medico-chirurgica inauguralis de ambustione ejusque remediis . . . Jenae, Typis Gollnerianis [1698]

[32] p.   20 cm.   [11164]

C. G. Goldammerus, *respondent.*

—Mulierem gravidam lapsu vagina uteri laborantem . . . examini sistit Fridericus Winckler . . . Jenae, Literis Krebsianis [1700]

[26] p.   20 cm.   [11165]

F. Winckler, *respondent.*

—Polypos capitis . . . exponit Jo. Caspar Muller . . . Jenae, Typis Pauli Echrichii [1699]

28 p.   20 cm.   [11166]

J. K. Muller, *respondent.*

—Puellam variolis malignis laborantem . . . publico eruditorum examini sistit Joh. Mart. Floribus . . . Jenae, Litteris Wertherianis [1699]

24 p.   20 cm.   [11167]

J. M. Floribus, *respondent.*

—Rhonchum infantis, ex ulcerum paroticorum intempestiva curatione variis symptomatibus stipatum . . . Jenae, Literis Gollnerianis [1699]

[30] p.   20 cm.   [11168]

J. S. Büchelmann, *respondent.*

—*respondent. See* FASCH, A. H., *praeses.* Ἄνθραξ pestilens dissertatione inaugurali explicatus. 1681; GRÜBEL, J. G., *praeses.* Dissertatio anatomica de ductu chylifero pecquetiano. 1674.

—*See* Fasch, A. H. Decanus Collegii Medici, Augustinus Henricus Faschius ... S. P. D. benigno lectori. 1681; Frischmuth, J. Epistola gratulatoria ad ... Joh. Hadrianum Slevogtum. 1681; Stahl, G. E. Dissertatio epistolica ad ... Johannem Adrianum Slevogt ... de motu tonico vitali. 1692

SLINGERLANDT, Jan van [*fl.* 1697] *respondent. See* Senguerdius, W., *praeses.* Exercitium experimentale quartum decimum. 1697.

SLINGERLANT, Abraham [*fl.* 1659] *respondent. See* Linden, J. A. van der, *praeses.* Hippocrates de circuitu sanguinis, exercitatio III. 1659.

SLOANE, Sir Hans, *bart.* [1660-1753] Catalogus plantarum quae in insula Jamaica sponte proveniunt ... cum earundem synonymis & locis natalibus; adjustis aliis quibusdam quae in insulis Maderae, Barbados, Nieves ... nascuntur. Seu prodromi Historiae naturalis Jamaicae pars prima ... Londini, Impensis D. Brown, 1696.

[11], 232, [43] p. 18 cm. **[11169]**

SLOANE, Johann. *See* Sloane, Sir Hans, *bart.* [1660-1753]

SLÖTEL, Johann Georg [*fl.* 1689] *respondent. See* Albinus, B. Dissertatio inauguralis de pravitate sanguinis. 1689.

SMALCALD, Valentin Friedrich [*fl.* 1652] *respondent. See* Steger, W. A., *praeses.* Disputationem physicam de nive ... ventilandam exponunt ... V. F. S. 1652.

SMALCIUS, Jacobus. *See* Schmaltz, Jakob [*fl.* 1671-1676]

The **SMALL** herbalist. *See* Pharmacopoea Belgica. 1659.

SMALTZ, Jan [*fl.* 1687] *respondent.* Disputatio medica inauguralis de convulsione ... Lugduni Batavorum, Apud Abrahamum Elzevier, 1687.
[16] p. 21 cm. **[11170]**
Diss.—Leyden.

SMARAGISIUS, Sebaldus, *pseud. See* Bruxius, Adam [*fl.* 1604-1630]

SMARUGIUS, Sebaldus, *pseud. See* Bruxius, Adam [*fl.* 1604-1630]

SMET, Heinrich [1537-1614] Miscellanea ... medica, cum praestantissimis quinque medicis. D.

Thoma Erasto ... Henrico Brucaeo ... Levino Batto ... Joanne Weyero ... Henr. Weyero ... communicata, et in libros XII. digesta ... Francofurti, Impensis Jonae Rhodii, 1611.

[16], 736, [40] p. 20 cm. port., table.**[11171]**

"De occultis medicamentorum proprietatibus: quid, et quotuplices eae sint: quibus in morbis, quomodo, quando, quem usum habeant. Authore Thoma Erasto": p. 61-144. Published as pt. 1 of his De occultis pharmacorum potestatibus in Basel 1574. Includes eight 16th century dissertations.

—Prosodia ... quae syllabarum positione & diphthongis carentium quantitates, sola veterum poetarum auctoritate, adductis exemplis, demonstrat. Ab auctore reformata, locisque innumeris emend., & quarta sui parte adaucta. Ed. 18. ... Cum Appendix aliquot vocum ab ecclesiasticis poetis aliter usurpatarum ... Francofurti, Sumptibus viduae Jonae Rosae, 1660.

[16], 23, 652 p. port. 19 cm. **[11172]**

"Methodus dignoscendarum syllabarum ex Georg. Fabricii ... De re poetica lib. 1. aliquot locus a nobis castigata ...": p. 4-23 of first group of paging.

SMETIUS A LEDA, Henricus. *See* Smet, Heinrich [1537-1641]

SMEUR, Jakob [*fl.* 1687] *respondent.* Disputatio medica inauguralis de gangraena et sphacelo ... Trajecti ad Rhenum, Ex officina Francisci Halma, 1687.

8 p. 22 cm. **[11173]**

Diss.—Utrecht.

SMID, Henrick. *See* Smith, Henrik [*d.* 1563]

SMIDIUS, Justus Andreas. *See* Schmid, Justus Andreas [*fl.* 1677-1681]

SMIDS, Ludolf [1649-1720] Romanorum imperatorum pinacotheca; sive, Duodecim imperatorum simulacra, elogiis, numismatibus, & historia Suetoniana illustrata ... Amstelaedami, Ex officina Henrici Desbordes & Petri Sceperi, 1699.

[60] p. illus. 21 cm. **[11174]**

Added engraved title page.

SMIDT, Henrick. *See* Smith, Henrik [*d.* 1563]

SMIDT, Jan Baptista de [*fl.* 1669] *respondent.* Disputatio medica inauguralis, continens illustres, ex variis medicinae partibus desumptas positiones ...

Lugduni Batavorum, Apud viduam & haeredes Joannis Elsevirii, 1669.

[12] p. 23 cm. [11175]

Diss. — Leyden.

SMILOVIUS, CHRISTIAN [*fl.* 1614-1617] *respondent.* *See* AMPSING, J. A., *praeses.* Disputatio de calculo. 1617.

SMIT, HENRICK. *See* SMITH, Henrik [*d.* 1563]

SMITH, GULIELMUS. *See* SMITH, William [*fl.* 1684]

SMITH, HENRIK [*d.* 1563] En bog om pestilentzis aarsage forvaring oc laegedom der imod, tilsammen dragen aff laerdemaends bøger … Kiøbenhaffn, 1650.

[12], 73, [1] p. 15 cm. [11176]

SMITH, JOHN [1630-1679] Γϱοχομια Βασιλιϰη King Solomons portraiture of old age. Wherein is contained a sacred anatomy both of soul and body. And a perfect account of the infirmities of age, incident to them both. And all those mystical and aenigmatical symptomes, expressed in the six former verses of the 12th chapter of Ecclesiastes, are here paraphrased … London, Printed by J. Hayes for S. Thomson, 1666.

[16], 266, [5] p. table. 17 cm. [11177]

Imperfect: first preliminary leaf (blank?) wanting.

— [The same.] The pourtract of old age … 2d ed. corr. … London, Printed by J. Macock, for Walter Kettilby, 1666.

[15], 266; [6] p. table. 18 cm. [11178]

Running title: King Solomon's portraicture of old age.
Different setting of type.

— Another issue, with new title page: The 2d ed. corr. … London, Printed by J. Macock, for Walter Kettilby, 1676.

[15], 266, [6] p. table. 18 cm. [11179]

SMITH, THOMAS [1638-1710] *See* RAUWOLFF, L. A collection of curious travels & voyages. 1693.

SMITH, WILLIAM [*b.* 1660 *or* 61] *respondent.* Disputatio medica inauguralis de conceptu humano & quibusdam phaenomenis exinde consecquentibus … Lugduni Batavorum, Apud Abrahamum Elzevier, 1684.

[8] p. 22 cm. [11180]

Diss. — Leyden.

SMOLL, GOTTFRIED [*fl.* 1609-1610] Manuale rerum admirabilium et abstrusarum: continens venerandae antiquitatis: Assyriorum, Chaldaeorum, Persarum, Aegyptiorum, Arabum & Graecorum philosophorum & medicorum … philosophica & medica principia … edita per D. Godfrid Smoll … Hamburgi, Ex Bibliopolio Frobeniano, 1610.

[18], 211, [7] p. table. 14 cm. [11181]

Imperfect: p. 175-194 wanting.
With this is bound (as issued?) *his* Trias maritima. 1610.

— Trias maritima, proponens, per introductionem trium aegrotantium; sororum morbosarum domesticarum, hypochondriacae, spleneticae … meseraicae … phantasticae; ortum & interitum. Hamburgi, Ex Bibliopolio Frobeniano. 1610.

67, [1] p. 14 cm. [11182]

Bound with (as issued?) *his* Manuale rerum admirabilium. 1610.

SNAAKENBURG, PETER [*fl.* 1687] *respondent.* Disputatio medica inauguralis de renum & vesicae affectionibus … Lugduni Batavorum, Apud Abrahamum Elzevier, 1687.

[24] p. 22 cm. [11183]

Diss. — Leyden.

SNAPE, ANDREW, Jr. [*b.* 1644] The anatomy of an horse … To which is added an Appendix, containing two discourses, the one, Of the generation of animals; and the other, Of the motion of the chyle, and the circulation of the bloud … London, Printed by M. Flesher for the authour, and by T. Flesher, 1683.

[12], 237 p.; 45, [5] p. front. (port.), plates. 34 cm. [11184]

Part [2] has half title.

SNEEBERGER, ANTON. *See* SCHNEEBERGER, Anton [1530-1581]

SNELL, FRIEDRICH KONRAD [*fl.* 1697] *respondent.* *See* WEDEL, G. W., *praeses.* Dissertatio medica inauguralis de oleosorum natura. 1697.

SNIZER, SIGISMUND. *See* SCHNITZER, Sigismund [*fl.* 1586-1620]

SNYDER, JOHANNES DE MONTE. *See* MONTE-SNYDER, Johannes de [*fl.* 17th cent.]

SOARES FEYO, FRANCISCO. Tratado de scurbuto. *In* Cruz, A. de. Recopilaçam de cirurgia. 669 [i.e. 1669]

SOBREMONTE RAMIREZ, Gaspar Bravo de. *See* Bravo de Sobremonte Ramirez, Gaspar [1603-1683]

SOCIETAS ROSICRUCIANA. *See* Rosicrucians.

[SOCIETY OF APOTHECARIES OF LONDON] The principles of the chymists of London stated, with the reasons of their dissent from the Colledge of Physicians; as they were unanimously agreed on by them, at a meeting in London; and are now published, for the information of the said Colledge, and satisfaction of those that intend the practice of physick; and also for the instructing the people in what is most useful for their preservation. Part I . . . [London?] Printed for the authors, 1676.

[4], 63 p.   16 cm.   **[11185]**

"A supplement to The principles of the chymists of London stated, &c.": p. 33-47.

"An appendix to The supplement to The principles of the chymists of London stated, &c." p. 49-63.

SØRENSEN, Peder [1540 *or* 42-1602] Idea medicinae philosophicae. Continens fundamenta totius doctrinae Paracelsicae, Hippocraticae & Galenicae . . . Hagae-Comitis, Ex typographia Adriani Vlacq, 1660.

[8], 212, [2] p.   21 cm.   **[11186]**

—[The same, *as subject.*] *See* Davison, W. Commentariorum in . . . Petri Severini Dani [i.e. Peder Sørensen] Ideam medicinae philosophicae. 1660; Rhode, A. Disputationes supra Ideam medicinae philosophicae Petri Severini. 1643.

SÖRGEL, Christian [*fl.* 1668] *respondent. See* Rolfinck, W., *praeses.* Specimen inaugurale de dolore capitis, secundum ordinem & methodum medicinae specialis commentatoriae. 1668.

SOERS, Martinus. Stricturae in ceritum quemdam Eburonem inconditum blateronem controversiae de curanda tertiana inter D. D. Petrum Barbam et V. F. Plempium . . . Lovanii, Typis ac sumptibus Jacobi Zegeri, 1642.

14 p.   20 cm.   **[11187]**

Bound with Plemp, V. F. Animadversio. 1642.

SOLÁ, Fernando [*fl.* 1618-1630] Parecer a la muy noble, y muy leal ciudad de Sevilla . . . acerca de los polvos venenosos de Milan. [Sevilla, 1630]

[8] p.   21 cm.   **[11188]**

Caption title.

SOLDAN, Johann Hartmann [*fl.* 1674] *respondent. See* Franck von Franckenau, G., *praeses.* Disputatio inauguralis de soldana. 1674.

SOLDI, Jacopo [*d. ca.* 1440] Antidotario per il tempo di peste, composto in lingua latina Nuovamente tradotto in lingua toscana da D[ionigi] B[ussotti] S. . . . Firenze, Pietro Nesti, 1630.

75 p.   21 cm.   **[11189]**

SOLENANDER, Hermann [*fl.* 1610] *respondent.* De dysenteria & chirurgicis problematis adjunctis disputationem . . . proponit Hermannus Solenander . . . Basileae, Typis Joan. Jacobi Genathii, 1610.

[19] p.   20 cm.   **[11190]**

Diss. —Basel.

—*See* Platter, F. [1536-1614] Felix Platerus . . . decreto. 1610.

SOLENANDER, Reiner [1524-1601] Consiliorum medicinalium . . . sectiones quinque. Quarum prima ante annos trigintaocto, a Joanne Francisco de Gabiano . . . edita, & cum consiliis celeberrimi medici Joannis Montani in 16 excusa. Reliquae quatuor ab auctore jam recens additae. Ed. 2. . . . Hanoviae, Typis Wechelianis, apud Claudium Marnium & heredes Joan. Aubrii, 1609.

[20], 516, [24] p.   33 cm.   **[11191]**

SOLEYSEL, Jacques Labessie de. *See* Solleysel, Jacques de [1617-1680]

SOLINGEN, Cornelis [1641-1687] Alle de medicinale en chirurgicale werken mitsgaders Embryulcia vera, beneffens het ampt en pligt der vroedvrouwen, en Bysondere aanmerkingen de vrouwen en kinderen betreffende, ofte ware oeffeningen der doode vruchten . . . Amsterdam, Jan ten Hoorn, 1698.

[24], 396, [24] p.; 448 (i.e 248), [8] p. plates.   22 cm.   **[11192]**

Part [2] has half title.

—Embryulcia; ofte, Afhalinge eenes dooden vruchts door de handt van den heel-meester . . . s'Graven-Hage, Joh. en Daniel Steucker, 1673.

[14], 340, [4] p.   15 cm.   **[11193]**

— [German tr.] Embryulcia; oder, Herausziehung einer Todten-Frucht durch die Hand des Chirurgi . . . Nunmehro aber auss dem Holländischen ins Hochteutsche übersetzet, von Tob. Peucero . . . Franckfurt und Leipzig, Verlegts

Jeremias Schrey und Heinrich Johann Meyers seel. Erben, 1693.

[6], 175, [2] p.   21 cm.   **[11194]**

Errata: [2] p. at end.

— Manuale operatien der chirurgie, beneffens het ampt en pligt der vroedvrouwen, midsgaders besondere aenmerkingen, de vrouwen en kinderen betreffende ... Amsterdam, Jan Bouman, 1684.

1 v.   plates.   21 cm.   **[11195]**

Various pagings.
Part [2] has half title.
Imperfect: added engraved title page wanting.

—, *tr. See* SIEGEMUND, J. D. Spiegel der vroedvrouwen. 1691.

SOLINUS, CAIUS JULIUS [3d cent.] *See* SAUMAISE, C. de. Claudii Salmasii Plinianae exercitationes in Caii Julii Solini Polyhistora. 1689.

SOLINUS, JOHANNES [*fl.* 1683] Oratio de dignitate & officio veri medici ... Delphis, Apud Jacobum Plantenburg, 1683.

28 p.   21 cm.   **[11196]**

SOLIS DE FONSECA, FERNANDO. *See* FONSECA, Fernando Solis da [*fl.* 1584–1585]

[SOLLEYSEL, JACQUES DE, 1617–1680] Le mareschal methodique, qui traite des moyens de découvrir les défauts des chevaux, & de connoistre leurs maladies. Il donne ensuite les remedes pour les guerir, & enseigne à les dispenser fort exactement, avec leur application au temps le plus propre pour leur entiere guerison ... Par le Sieur de la Bessée [pseud., i.e. Jacques de Solleysel] ... Paris, Gervais Clouzier, 1675.

[16], 341, [2] p.   20 cm.   **[11197]**

— Le parfait mareschal, qui enseigne a connoistre la beauté, la bonté, et les defauts des chevaux, les signes & les causes des maladies, les moyens de les prévenir, leur guerison, & le bon ou mauvais usage, de la purgation & de la saignée ... Ensemble un traité de haras, pour élever de beaux & de bons poulains ... Reveu ... & augm. 9 ed. ... Bruxelles, Lambert Marchant, 1691.

2 v. in 1.   front., illus., plate.   22 cm.   **[11198]**

— [English tr.] The compleat horseman: discovering the surest marks of the beauty, goodness, faults and imperfections of horses: the signs and causes of their diseases, the true method both of their preservation and cure: with reflections on the regular and preposterous use of bleeding and purging ... To which is added, A ... supplement of riding ... With an alphabetical catalogue ... in English, French and Latin. By Sir William Hope ... Made English from the 8th ed. ... London, Printed for M. Gillyflower, R. Bentley, H. Bonwick, J. Tonson, W. Freeman, T. Goodwin, M. Wotton, J. Walthoe, S. Manship and R. Parker, 1696.

2 v. ([36], 261, [17], [4], 86, [1] p.; [16], 300, [4] p.)   fronts., plates.   31 cm.   **[11199]**

"A supplement of horsemanship ... by Sir William Hope ... Printed at Edinburgh" has special title page.
Vol. 2 has frontispiece only.

SOLLEYSEL, *sieur Du Clapier. See* SOLLEYSEL, Jacques de [1617–1680]

SOLMS, JOHANN GEORG [*fl.* 1676] *respondent.* Flumen dysentericum ... Erfurti, Praelo Kirschiano [1676]

[16] p.   19 cm.   **[11200]**

Diss. — Erfurt.

SOLOMON, *king of Israel. See* GLAUBER, J. R. Explicatio; oder, Ausslegung über die Wohrten Salomonis. 1663; [Latin tr.] 1664.

SOLON. *See* MEURS, J. van [1579–1639] Solon, sive, de ejus vita. 1632.

SOLON DE VOGE, *pseud. See* LE BON, Jean [*d.* 1588?]

ΣΩΜΑΤΟΓΡΑΦΙΑ ἀνθρωπινη; or A description of the body of man. 1616, 1634. *See* [CROOKE, H.]

SOME considerations touching the usefulnesse of experimental naturall philosophy. 1663. *See* BOYLE, *Hon.* R.

SOME observations. 1682. *See* [PEACHIE, John, *fl. ca.* 1683–*ca.* 1690]

SOME observations made upon the Cylonian plant. 1695. *See* MULLINS, J., *physician.*

SOMEREN, ADRIAAN VAN [*fl.* 1647] *respondent.* Disputatio medica inauguralis de convulsione ... Lugduni Batavorum, Ex officina Bonaventurae & Abrahami Elsevir, CIↃ CIↃ XLVII [i.e. 1647]

[8] p.   21 cm.   **[11201]**

Diss. — Leyden.

SOMERSET, SAFFORD JEDIDJA. *See* SAFFORD, JEDIDJA [*fl.* 1689]

SOMMAIRE de la medecine chymique. 1632. *See* [GERZAN, F. du *Soucy, sieur de*]

SOMMAIRE des bandes et bandages. *See* MARQUE, J. de. Methodique introduction à la chirurgie. 1639.

SOMMER, FABIAN [*fl.* 1571–1589] De inventione, descriptione, temperie, viribus, et inprimis usu thermarum D. Caroli IIII. imperatoris libellus brevis . . . Nunc tertia vice recusus . . . Lipsiae, Michael Lantzenberger, 1609.

[46], 103, [10] p. 16 cm. [11202]

— [German tr.] Ein kurtzes und sehr nützliches Büchlein von Keyser Carls Warmenbade, desselben Erfindung, Eigenschafften, Krefften, und zuvoraus von seinem heilsamen Gebrauch, in Latein beschrieben . . . Auffs kürtzest . . . verdeutscht durch M. Matthiam Sommer . . . Jetzo auffs new wieder in Druck verfertigt . . . Leipzig [Gedruckt bey Michael Lantzenberger] 1609.

[28], 145, [8] p. 15 cm. [11203]

— [The same.] Thermae Carolinae . . . Anjetzo auffs new übersehen und in Truck verfertiget, mit . . . Instruction und Bad-Regiment D. Joh. Stephani Strobelbergers . . . Nürnberg, Gedruckt durch Jeremian Dümlern, 1647.

[22], 141, [6] p. 16 cm. [11204]

Added engraved title page dated 1648.

SOMMER, HEINRICH GOTTFRIED [*b.* 1666] *respondent. See* WEDEL, G. W., *praeses.* Dissertatio inauguralis medica, de mania. 1693.

— *See* WEDEL, G. W. Propempticon inaugurale de nummis Jani ratitis I. 1693.

SOMMER, JOHANN GEORG [1634–1705] Nohtwendiger Hebammen-Unterricht, wie eine Hebamme gegen schwangere, gebehrende und entbundene Weiber und deren Kinderlein, so wohl bey natürlichen als unnatürlichen Geburten sich zuerweisen; wie auch, wie sie bey solcher Weiber und Kinder Zufällen im Nohtfall einige diensame Mittel anzuwenden habe . . . Welchem noch beygefügt ist ein Weiber und Kinder Pfleg-Büchlein, wie auch eine Anleitung zur christlichen Kinderzucht . . . Arnstadt,

Druckts Heinrich Meurer, zufinden bey Matth. Bircknern in Jehna, 1676.

[33], 192 p.; [8], 252, [4] p.; 72 p. plates. 14 cm. [11205]

Parts [2] and [3] have special title pages.

— [The same.] Hebammen-Schul; oder, Gründlicher Unterricht, wie eine Hebamme gegen schwangere, kreistende und entbundene Weiber, und deren Kinderlein, so wohl bey natürlichen als unnatürlichen Geburten, sich zu verhalten. Nebenst einem nützlichen Weiber- und Kinder-Pfleg-Büchlein, und einer neuen Anführung, wie den meisten Kinder-Kranckheiten zu begegnen, wie auch einer Anleitung zur christlichen Kinder-Zucht. Zum andern Mahl mit Figuren aussgefertiget . . . Arnstadt, Zufinden bey Augusto Boëtio in Gotha, 1693.

[22], 240, [24] p. front., illus. 14 cm. [11206]

Part [1] only.

— Kurtzes und nützliches Weiber- und Kinder-Pflege-Büchlein, wie noch unverheyrathete Weibs-Personen, Eheleute, Schwangere, Sechswöchnerin und Ammen sich zu verhalten, wie auch, wie dieselben nebenst neugebohrnen, entwehnten und ältern Kindern, bey gesunden Zustande zu pflegen, und bey Vorfallen den Zufällen mit guten Mitteln zu versorgen. Neben einer beygefügten Anführung, wie den meisten Kinder-Kranckheiten mit hierinn beschriebenen vornehmen Artzneyen . . . zubegegnen . . . Rudolstadt, In Verlegung des Autoris, 1691.

416, [24] p. 15 cm. [11207]

"Anderer Theil des Weiber- und Kinder-Pflege-Büchleins" (p. [265]-416) has special title page with imprint: Rudolstadt, Druckts Joh. Rudolph Löwe, 1692.

— *respondent. See* ROLFINCK, W., *praeses.* Dissertationes chimicae sex de tartaro. 1660; SCHENCK, J. T., *praeses.* Disputatio inauguralis medica de pleuritide. 1661.

SOMMER, MARTIN, *pseud. See* SCHENCKEL, Lambrecht Thomas [*b.* 1547]

SOMMER, MATTHIAS [*fl.* 1580] *ed.* and *tr. See* SOMMER, F. Ein kurtzes und sehr nützliches Büchlein von Keyser Carls Warmenbade. 1609, 1647.

SON, CORNELIS VAN [*fl.* 1670–1683] *respondent.* Disputatio medica inauguralis de spirituum animalium natura & vitiis ... Lugduni Batavorum, Apud viduam & haeredes Joannis Elsevirii, 1670.

[31] p.   23 cm.   [11208]

Diss. — Leyden.

SONDERBAHRE nutzliche auch nöthige Anmerkungen eine sorgfältige Aufferziehung der jungen Kinder und deren Gebrechen betreffend. Allen sorgfältigen Müttern zur nöthigen Unterricht mitgetheilet von J. H. J. Nürnberg, In Verelegung Johann Ziegers, 1688.

180, [23] p.   14 cm.   [11209]

Imperfect: p. 5-6 mutilated.

SONDERSHAUSEN, Johann Gerlach [b. 1675] *respondent. See* Crause, R. W., *praeses.* Dissertatio medica de carminativis. 1699.

— *See* Crause, R. W. Propempticum inaugurale de meteoris microcosmi. 1699.

SONNET, Thomas, *sieur de Courval* [1577-1627?] Satyre contre les charlatans, et pseudomedecins empyriques. En laquelle sont amplement descouvertes les ruses & tromperies de tous theriacleurs, alchimistes, chimistes, paracelsistes, distillateurs extracteurs de quintescences, fondeurs d'or potable, maistres de l'elixir ... En laquelle d'ailleurs sont refutees les erreurs, abus, & impietez des iatromages, ou medecins magiciens ... Paris, Jean Milot, 1610.

[30], 335 p.   port.   18 cm.   [11210]

SONNEVELT, Daniel à [*fl.* 1631] *respondent. See* Burgersdijck, F. P., *praeses.* Collegium physicum. 1642.

SONTA PAGNALMINO, Gio., *pseud. See* Lampugnani, Agostino [*ca.* 1586-*ca.* 1666]

SORACI, Placide [*fl.* 1698-1703] Reponse a la lettre ecrite par Mr. Chatelain [sic] ... sur la singuliere structure des cheveux qu'il a découverte, & dont il a fait des leçons publiques dans l'Université de Montpellier l'an 1686. [Marseille?] 1699.

110 p.   14 cm.   [11211]

Imperfect: p. 109 mutilated. Leaf following page 110 (blank?) wanting.

SORAND, Francisco [*fl.* 1667-1681] *praeses.* Quaestio medica ... An calculus a caseo? [Parisiis, Apud Franciscum Muguet, 1681]

4 p.   23 cm.   [11212]

Diss. — Paris (J. Poisson, *respondent*)

SORANUS, *of Ephesus. See* Hippocrates. The aphorismes. 1655; Vesalius, A. Anatomia. 1604.

SORAPÁN DE RIEROS, Juan [*fl.* 1615-1638] Medicina española contenida en proverbios vulgares de nuestra lengua. Muy provechosa para todo genero de estados, para philosophos, y medicos, para theologos, y juristas ... [Granada] Por Martin Fernandez Zambrano, 1616.

[41], 517 p.; 75 (i.e. 77), 27 p.   22 cm.

                                                     [11213]

Part 2 has special title page with imprint: Granada, Impresso por Juan Muñoz, 1615.

SORBAIT, Paul de [1624?-1691] Commentaria & controversiae in omnes libros Aphorismorum Hippocratis ... Viennae Austriae, Typis Joannis van Ghelen, 1680.

[14], 1039 (i.e. 1019), [35] p.   front.   21 cm.

                                                     [11214]

Includes Latin text of the Aphorismi.

—Consilium medicum; seu, Dialogus loimicus de peste Viennensi, ejusque origine, causis ... accidentibus, & observationibus. Item de vera praeservatione, & cura per medicamenta saepissime probata, & selecta, cum requisita diaeta, nec non de locis, & numero cryptarum, & mortuorum ... Viennae, Typis Joannis van Ghelen [1679]

[8], 168, [38] p.   14 cm.   [11215]

Sig. H6 dated 1680.

—[German tr.] Freundliches Gespräch, uber den ... Zustand der ... Haupt-Stadt Wienn in Oesterreich, bey dieser ... Contagion ... mit ... Befragund Antwortungen von deren Ursprung, Ursachen ... [Vienna] 1679.

[119] p.   14 cm.   [11216]

Imprint partly supplied from Haller.

—[The same.] Consilium medicum, dialogus; oder, Freundliches Gespräch, über den ... Zustand der ... Haupt- Statt Wienn in Oesterreich, bey dieser gefährlichen ... Contagion; mit ... Befragund Antwortungen, von deren Uhrsprung, Uhrsachen ... von dero praeservation oder Verhüttung ... Wienn, Gedruckt bey Johann von Gehlen [1679?]

[8], 86, [10] p.   17 cm.   [11217]

Imperfect: first preliminary leaf (blank?) wanting.

"Die Tax, in was für einem Werth, und wie theur die vorgeschriebene Medicamenta Alexipharmaca ... zubekommen seynd": p. 77-82.

—[The same.] Freundliches Gespräch . . . [Vienna] 1680.

    [142] p.   14 cm.   [11218]

Imprint partly supplied from Eloy.
Leaf following page [142] (blank?) wanting.

—[The same.] . . . Berlin und Cöllin, Auffgeleget von Ruperto Völckern, 1681.

    [143] p.   15 cm.   [11219]

—Praxios medicae, auctae, et a plurimis typi mendis, ab ipso auctore, castigatae. Tractatus primus. In quo morborum . . . curationes . . . traduntur . . . Secundus. De lue venerea . . . Tertius. De febribus, cum controversiis . . . Quartus. De morbis puerorum . . . Quintus. De chirurgia, cum examine chirurgorum . . . Sextus. De methodo medendi, cum quaestionibus & dosibus medicamentorum . . . Septimus. De modo bene consultandi, & rarioribus observationibus. Ultimo. De modo promovendi doctores Viennae, aliquot discursibus exornato . . . Viennae, Apud Leopoldum Voigt [1680]

    [22], 621, [43] p.   38 cm.   [11220]

Added engraved title page.
The Modus promovendi doctores (text in Latin and German) has special title page dated 1679.

—Universa medicina . . . Tam theorica quam practica, nempe, isagoge institutionum medicarum et anatomicarum, methodus medendi, cum controversiis, annexa sylva medica. Deinde sequuntur curationes omnium morborum . . . et tractatus De febribus, peste et venenis . . . denique Modus Viennae doctores creandi . . . Noribergae, Sumptibus Michael. & Johan. Friderici Endterorum, 1672.

    [35], 782, [37] p.   32 cm.   [11221]

Imperfect: first preliminary leaf and p. [21-22] at end wanting.
Added engraved title page has title: Opera medica theorico-practica.
Errata: p. [37]
There are 2 special title pages beginning with "In nomine SS. Triados": one inserted after sig. A3, the other p. [203] The latter is dated 1671.
The Modus promovendi doctores (p. [763]-782) has special title page.

—, ed. See MANNAGETTA, J. W. Pest-Ordnung. 1679, 1680.

—See PFENDTNER, E. Oesterreicherischer Galenus. 1691?; STEIN, G. Wolgemeintes Consilium Antiloimicum. 1680.

SORBERIUS, SAMUEL. See SORBIÈRE, Samuel [1615-1670]

[**SORBIÈRE**, SAMUEL, 1615-1670] Discours sceptique sur le passage du chyle, & sur le mouvement du coeur. Où sont touchees quelques difficultés sur les opinions des veines lactees, & de la circulation du sang. Leyde, Jean Maire, 1648.

    154 p.   14 cm.   [11222]

Signed at end: S[amuel] S[orbière]

—Discours . . . touchant diverses experiences de la transfusion du sang. Paris, Jean Cusson, 1668.

    12 p.   23 cm.   [11223]

—Extraict d'un discours . . . touchant l'estat des sciençes en Hollande . . . [n. p., 166-?]

    [8] p.   19 cm.   [11224]

Caption title.
Concerns the works of Lodewijk de Bils and his medical contemporaries.

—Lettres et discours . . . sur diverses matieres curieuses. Paris, François Clousier, 1660.

    [28], 731 p.   illus.   24 cm.   [11225]

—Relation d'un voyage en Angleterre, où sont touchées plusieurs choses, qui regardent l'estat des sciences, & de la religion, & autres matieres curieuses. Cologne, Pierre Michel, 1666.

    [8], 180, [3] p.   plate.   14 cm.   [11226]

—Sorberiana; ou, Bons mots, recontres agreables, pensées judicieuses, et observations curieuses . . . Paris, La veuve Mabre-Cramois, 1694.

    [48], 246 p.   15 cm.   [11227]

Memoirs of Samuel Sorbière and Jean Baptiste Cotelier presented in the form of a letter by François Graverol.

—See GASSENDI, P. Opera omnia. 1658.

SORDES, PIERRE [*fl.* 1624] Discours de la goutte et des fluctions qui tombent sur les joinctures . . . Lyon, Claude Chastelard, 1626.

    [12], 126 p.; 24, [4] p.   14 cm.   [11228]

Imperfect: outer margin of title page trimmed.
Part [2] has special title page: Traicté de la peste.

SORDI, GIOVANNI PIETRO [*d.* 1598] Tractatus de alimentis plenissimus . . . in quo universa alimentorum materia, nempe cui & a quibus, quando, quomodo, qualiter, quandiu, ea praestari . . . debeant, vel durante lite, vel eadem cessante, additis cum specialibus eorundem privilegiis, tum praeceptis generalibus, 379 quaestionibus . . . absolvitur . . . Opus nunc excusum, & . . . repurgatum . . . Seorsim excusus Tractatus de sententiis praejudicialibus seu provisionalibus . . . authore D. Petro Rebuffo . . .

Coloniae Allobrogum, Petrus de la Roviere, 1613.

[12], 736, [83] p.   35 cm.   [**11229**]

Rebuffi's treatise has half title (p. [697])

SOREL, CHARLES [*ca.* 1602-1674] De la perfection de l'homme, ou les vrays biens sont considerez, et specialement ceux de l'ame; avec les methodes des sciences ... Paris, Robert de Nain, 1655.

16, 397, [2] p.   tables.   24 cm.   [**11230**]

Errata: p. [2] at end.

—Des talismans; ou, Figures faites sous certaines constellations, pour faire aymer & respecter les hommes ... Avec des observations contre le livre des Curiositez inouyes de M. I. Gaffarel. Et un traicté de l'unguent des armes ... pour sçavoir si l'on en peut guerir une playe ... Le tout tiré de la seconde partie de la Science des choses corporelles. Par le sieur de L'Isle [pseud., i.e. Charles Sorel] Paris, Anthoine de Sommaville, 1636.

[8], 417, [3] p.   18 cm.   [**11231**]

SORI, GIOVANNI BATTISTA [*d. ca.* 1632] Tesoro di chirurgia ... Nel quale si contengono nove libri. 1. De quali dice delle ferite, e contusioni, & commotioni del capo. 2. Delle ferite anco per morso d'animali dal volto a basso. 3. Dell'ulcere in generale. 4. Dell'ulcere nel particolare per i luochi. 5. Delle aposteme callide, e frigide. 6. Delle rotture d'ossa e stocature. 7. De gl'aiuti per tutte le infirmita dal capo alle piante. 8. Della flebotomia. 9. & ultimo de peste. Pavia, Gio. Andrea Magri [Heredi di Gio. Maria Magri] 1632.

582, [15] p.   16 cm.   [**11232**]

SORIANO, GERÓNIMO [*b.* 1575] Libro de experimentos medicos, faciles, y verdaderos. Recopilados de gravissimos autores ... Alcala, Juan Gracian, 1612 [1616]

[8], 108, [4] ll.   15 cm.   [**11233**]

—[The same.] ... Va muy enmendado en esta impression. Valencia, Jayme de Bordazar, 1700.

[8], 192 p.   15 cm.   [**11234**]

—Methodo y orden de curar las enfermedades de los niños ... Corregido en esta ultima impression de los yerros antecedentes, y añadido (por un amigo de la salud) el remedio del bolo armeno, para los carbunculos, con escolios sobre la curacion dèl ... Zaragoça, Por Domingo Gascon, acosta de Antonio Cabeças, 1690.

[4], 192, [3] p.   16 cm.   [**11235**]

SORIANO, MATTEO [16th-17th cent.] Trattato curioso ... Discorso utilissimo del male della podagra, ò chiragra, gotta calda, fredda, e mista, & sue specie ... Palermo, Alfonzo dell'Isola, 1635.

70 p.   21 cm.   [**11236**]

SORIS, GIOVANNI BATTISTA. *See* SORI, Giovanni Battista [*d. ca.* 1632]

SOSPENSIONE della città di Granoble, e di Gap. 1664. *See* MILAN (Duchy) Laws, statutes, etc.

SOSPENSIONE per occasione di peste. 1636. *See* REGGIO EMILIA (City) Ordinances, local laws, etc.

SOSSIUS, GULIELMUS [*fl.* 17th cent.] De vita Henrici Magni libri IV. Parisiis, Apud Petrum Chevalerium, 1522 [i.e. 1622]

[8], 148 ll.   17 cm.   [**11237**]

Bound with copy 2 of Goclenius, R. Mirabilium naturae liber. 1625.

SOTO, JUAN DE [*fl.* 1616] Libro del conocimiento, curacion y preservacion de la enfermedad de garrotillo, donde se trata lo que a de hacer cada uno, para curarse y preservarse desta enfermedad segun su complexion edad y naturaleça ... Granada, Juan Munoz, 1616.

[16], 304 p.   21 cm.   [**11238**]

Engraved title page.

SOTOMAYOR, ANTONIO DE, *Abp.* [1548-1648] *See* QUIÑONES, J. de. Al illustrissimo ... Señor Don Fray Antonio de Sotomayor. 1632?

Le SOUVERAIN a donné la science aux hommes, pour estre honoré en ses merveilles: celuy qui guerit par telles choses, adoucira la douleur ... [Paris? 1696?]

4 p.   33 cm.   [**11239**]

Caption title.

Concerns medicines used by Nicola Cevoli, *marquis del Carretto.*

SOZZI, FRANCESCO JACOPO [*fl.* 1639] *See* TUSCANY. Laws, statutes, etc. Bando contro a chl [sic] fraudolentemente dispenserà l'orvietano di Francesco di Jacopo Sozzi. 1639.

SPAAR, JOHANN CASPAR. *See* SPARR, Johann Caspar [*fl.* 1672-1674]

SPACH, ISRAEL [1560-1610] *ed.* and *tr. See* FRAGOSO, J. Aromatum, fructuum, et simplicium aliquot medicamentorum ex India utraque. 1601.

SPACHER, STEPHAN MICHAEL [*fl.* 1613–1619] *See* [REMMELIN, J. Catoptrum microcosmicum.] 1613, 1614, 1615, 1619, 1645, 1660; [English tr.] 1675 [and] Elucidarius. 1614 [and] Visio prima [-tertia] 1613.

SPADONI, NICOLA [*fl.* 17th cent.] Studio di curiositá nel quale si tratta fisonomia, chiromantia, metoposcopia . . . Venetia, Camillo Bortoli, 1662.

192 p. illus. 15 cm. **[11240]**

Parte seconda has special title page (p. [151]) and was printed by Giacomo Batti.

—[The same.] . . . Venetia, Francesco Busetto, 1675.

191 p. illus. 14 cm. **[11241]**

— [German tr.] In Höchstfürtreflichtes chiromantisch-und physiognomisches Klee-Blat. 1695.

SPÄNHOLTZ, ANDREAS. *See* SPENHOLZ, Andreas [*fl.* 1634]

SPAENHOLZ, N. [*fl.* 1661–1673] Eilfertiges Gutachten Philonis Nasturtii [pseud., i.e. N. Spaenholz] Zwelferischen Bundesgenossen, über die hochbedenckliche Attentata . . . Defensions-Schrifft eines Raphaël Schmuz . . . so er aufgerichtet zu . . . Lob und . . . Siegs-Preiss des Augspurgischen Dispensatorii, wie dann auch zu schändlichem Nachtheil, Hohn und Schimpff des . . . Herrn Joannis Zwelfers . . . erb- und meisterlichen Correctoris des weltbekanten Augustani. Nebenst zu End angehengter Erinnerung an den in Arte Pharmaceutica gantz seichtgelehrten Lucam Schrökium Lucis filium. [Grein?] 1673.

[12], 59 p. 17 cm. **[11242]**

—Lexicon medico-Galeno-chymico-pharmaceuticum; oder, Gründliche Erklärung achtzehen tausend medicinischer Nahmen . . . Zusammen geschrieben . . . und in solch Format erstmhals zum Druck heraussgegeben durch Fridericum Müllern, von Löwenstein [pseud., i.e. N. Spaenholz] . . . Franckfurt am Mayn, In Verlegung Michael Endters, 1661.

[8], 312 p. illus. 35 cm. **[11243]**

—*See* SCHMUZ, M. R. Exorcismus medicus manium, larvarum & maleferiatorum spirituum Zwelferianorum. 1673.

SPAHER, MICHAEL. *See* SPACHER, Stephan Michael [*fl.* 1613–1619]

SPAIN. Sovereign [1621–1665] (Philip IV) *See* GHENT. Ordinances, local laws, etc. Ordonnantien ende statuten, gemaeckt by heer ende weth der stadt Ghendt. 1685?

SPAN VON SPANAU, LAURENTIUS [1539–1575] *See* GALLO, A. Fascis aureus de peste. 1606, 1608.

SPANO, PIETRO. *See* JOHANNES XXI, *Pope* [*d.* 1277]

SPARK, NATHANIEL. A tract concerning the weather, or change of the aire. Wherein an easie and plain method is discovered to the reader, for judging the aires constitution: whether that tend to cold or heat, rain, snow, or the like . . . By N. S. . . . London, Andrew Kemb, 1653.

[249]-303 p. 19 cm. (*In* Dariot, Claude. Dariotus redivivus: or, A briefe introduction conducing to the judgement of the stars. London, 1653)

[11244]

SPARMAN, ANDREA. Sundhetzens speghel uthi hwilken man beskodhar sundhetzens natur, förnämste orsakerne till alla siukdomar, som sundheten förstöra plägha, såsom ock the medels rätta bruk, hwarigenom hon för them befrijat, til thet bestämda målet kan underhållen warda. På wårt tungomål stält och i liuset gifwin . . . Stockholm, Ignatium Meurer, 1642.

[64], 407, [1] p. 17 cm. **[11245]**

Förste deel and andra deel have special title pages.

SPARR, JOHANN CASPAR [*fl.* 1672–1674] Dissertationes duae medicae de lue venerea . . . Argentorati, Apud J. F. Spoor, & R. Waechtler, 1673.

[1], 72 p. 20 cm. **[11246]**

—*respondent.* See MAPP, M., *praeses.* Disputationem medicam solennem de lue venerea . . . submittit J. C. S. 1673; SEBISCH, J. A., *praeses.* Exercitationum pathologicarum dissertatio undecima. 1672.

SPECHT, JOACHIM [*fl.* 1626–1630] *respondent. See* SENNERT, D., *praeses.* Dissertatio medica de cephalagia. 1630.

SPECHT, NIKOLAUS [*fl.* 1688] *respondent.* Disputatio medica inauguralis de nephritide . . . Trajecti ad Rhenum, Ex officina Francisci Halma, 1688.

19, [1] p. 22 cm. **[11247]**

SPECIMEN medicinae Sinicae. 1682. *See* BOYM, M. P.

A **SPECIMEN** of some animadversions upon a book, entituled, Plus ultra. 1670. *See* STUBBS, H.

SPECIMEN unum atque alterum, e quibus constet, quantopere experimenta chymica. *See* BOYLE, *Hon.* R. Tentamina quaedam physiologica diversis temporibus & occasionibus conscripta. 1668.

SPECIOSA VILLA, EDMUNDUS DE, *pseud. See* GAYTON, Edmund [1608-1666]

SPECKER, JOHANN PHILIPP [*fl.* 1683] *respondent.* Disputatio inauguralis medica de phtisi [sic] . . . Basileae, Typis Jacobi Bertschii [1683]
    [16] p. 20 cm.   **[11248]**
  Diss—Basel.

SPECULUM astrologicum; das ist, Nativität-Spiegel, worinnen . . . entworffen, 1. die Principia und das Fundament der Astrologie. 2. Wie eine rechte Nativität zustellen; und 3. wie man sich derselben gebrauchen und zu Nutz machen könne . . . an den Tag gegeben durch J. C. G. Math. Franckfurt und Leipzig, Verlegts August. Boëtius, 1693.
    [16], 144 p. illus. 17 cm.   **[11249]**
  Bound with Höchstfürtreflichstes chiromantisch und- physiognomisches Klee-Blat. 1695.

SPECULUM Salomonis. *See* LYSECK, J. P. Praeservatibum pestilentiale. 1673.

SPEDALE maggiore di Milano. *See* OSPEDALE MAGGIORE DI MILANO.

SPEIRMAN, GEORG THEODOR [*fl.* 1681] *respondent. See* MEIBOM, H., *praeses.* Exercitatio medica de consuetudinis natura. 1681.

SPEISS, JOANNES CAROLUS. *See* SPIES, Johann Karl [1663-1729]

SPELMAN, *Sir* HENRY [1564?-1641] De sepultura . . . London, Printed by Robert Young, and sold by Matthew Walbancke and William Coke, 1641.
    [1], 38 p. 19 cm.   **[11250]**
  Imperfect: first preliminary leaf (blank?) wanting.

SPELMAN, SAMUEL [*fl.* 1664] *respondent.* Disputatio medica inauguralis de haemorrhoidibus . . . Lugduni Batavorum, Apud Abrahamum Verhoeff, 1664.
    [16] p. 19 cm.   **[11251]**
  Diss.—Leyden.

SPENER, CHRISTIAN MAXIMILIAN [1678-1714] Epistola de novo haemorrhoidum coecarum remedio, muribus scl. marinis, his pauca accedunt de akmella pedraporco & hypecacuanha . . . ad . . . Michaelem Bernhardum Valentini . . . Amstelodami, Typis heredum Hermanni Aaltsz, 1700.
    15, [1] p. plate. 20 cm.   **[11252]**

—*respondent.* Disputatio inauguralis medica, sistens aegrum febri maligna phthisi complicata laborantem . . . Gissae-Hassorum, Typis Henningi Mülleri [1699]
    [4], 24 (i.e. 20) p. 20 cm.   **[11253]**
  Diss.—Giessen.

SPENER, JOHANN JAKOB [*fl.* 1687-1688] *praeses.* De magnete errores variorum . . . Lipsiae, Typis Christophori Fleischeri [1688]
    [24] p. 20 cm.   **[11254]**
  Diss.—Leipzig (J. M. Michaelis, *respondent*)

—*respondent. See* RECHENBERG, A., *praeses.* De gemmis errores vulgares. 1687.

SPENHOLZ, ANDREAS [*fl.* 1634] Kurtzer und klarer Bericht von der Natur und Aigenschafft der grawsamen abschewlichen tyranischen Seucht der Pestilentz, wie dieselbige recht erkennet ordentlich und aigentlich curirt werden möge, sambt angehengter Praeservation . . . Lintz, Getruckt durch Gregorium Kürnern, 1639.
    [3], 198 (i.e. 197) p. 12 cm.   **[11255]**

SPERLING, JOHANN [1603-1658] Dissertatio de principiis corporis naturalis . . . Witenbergae, Impensis Johannis Bergeri, typis Johannis Röhneri, 1647.
    [16], 160 p. 16 cm.   **[11256]**

—Institutiones physicae . . . Wittebergae, Apud Johannem Bergerum, typis Wilhelmi Fincelii, 1639.
    [16], 1309, [1] p. 16 cm.   **[11257]**

—[The same.] Institutiones physicae . . . Ed. 5. auct. & corr. . . . Francf. ac Wittebergae, Sumtibus haered. Johannis Bergeri, litteris Johannis Kuchenbecker, 1664.
    [12], 1162, [22] p. 17 cm.   **[11258]**
  Imperfect: first preliminary leaf (blank?) wanting.

—Oratio auspicialis de physica lugente . . . Wittebergae, Excusum typis Johannis Röhneri [1634]
    [28] p. 19 cm.   **[11259]**

—Physica anthropologia . . . Ed. 3. . . . Wittebergae, Impensis hered. Joh. Bergeri, 1668.

[31], 780 p.; [30] p. [11260]

Previously published as Anthropologia physica. Cf. Eloy.

—Physicae studiosis . . . [Wittenbergae, 1652]

[8] p. 19 cm. [11261]

—Synopsis anthropologiae physicae . . . Wittebergae, Impensis Johannis Bergeri, praelo Johannis Röhneri, 1650.

[11], 178 p. 13 cm. [11262]

—[The same.] . . . Ed. 3. Wittebergae, Impensis viduae Johannis Bergeri, praelo Johannis Haken, 1659.

[11], 178 p. 13 cm. [11263]

Different setting of type.

—Tractatus physico-medicus, de calido innato, pro D. Daniele Sennerto . . . contra D. Johannem Freitagium . . . conscriptus. Wittebergae, Impensis Johannis Helwigii, excudebat Ambrosius Rothius, 1634.

[8], 115 p. 17 cm. [11264]

—Tractatus physicus de formatione hominis in utero . . . Wittebergae, Impensis haered. D. Tobiae Mevii, typis Michaelis Wendt, 1641.

[6], 221, [1] p. 16 cm. [11265]

—[The same.] . . . Ed. 2. Wittebergae, Sumptibus haered. D. Tobiae Mevii, & Elerdi Schumacheri, excudebat Michael Wendt, 1655.

[6], 219, [1] p. 16 cm. [11266]

—[The same.] . . . Ed. 3. Wittebergae, Sumptibus haered. D. Tobiae Mevii, & Elerdi Schumacheri, excudebat Matthaeus Henckelius, 1661.

[6], 219, [1] p. 16 cm. [11267]

Different setting of type.

Dissertations — Wittenberg

—*praeses.* An virgula mercurialis agat ex occulta qualitate disquisitio philosophica . . . Ed. 2. Wittenbergae, Typis Johannis Röhneri, 1666.

[24] p. 19 cm. [11268]

Diss., 1658? J. Klein, *respondent.*

—Aphorismi physici de igne . . . Wittebergae, Typis Johannis Röhneri, 1646.

[8] p. 19 cm. [11269]

J. Heinzelmann, *respondent.*

De somniis dissertatio physica . . . Wittenbergae, Typis Johannis Röhneri, 1637.

[16] p. 20 cm. [11270]

J. F. Schenck, *respondent.*

—De vita & morte. Theses cum explicationibus, axiomata cum distinctionibus, & quaestiones cum responsionibus . . . Wittebergae, Typis Johannis Röhneri, 1638.

[20] p. 19 cm. [11271]

D. Faber, *respondent.*

—Disputatio physica de capite humano . . . Wittebergae, Ex officina typograph. Michaelis Wendt, 1648.

[16] p. 19 cm. [11272]

K. Alsleben, *respondent.*

—Disputatio physica de generatione . . . Wittebergae, Ex officina typograph. Michaelis Wendt, 1649.

[28] p. 19 cm. [11273]

P. Weier, *respondent.*

—Disputatio physica de meteoris aqueis . . . Wittebergae, Typis Matthaei Henckelii [1658]

[12] p. 19 cm. [11274]

M. Hentzschel, *respondent.*

—Disputatio physica de monstris . . . Wittebergae, Typis Johannis Borckarti, 1655.

[12] p. 19 cm. [11275]

C. Wallrich, *respondent.*

—Disputatio physica de monstris . . . Wittebergae, Michael Wendt, 1657.

[15] p. 20 cm. [11276]

J. Kalinka, *respondent.*

—Disputatio physica de voluntate . . . Wittebergae, Ex officina typograph. Michaelis Wendt, 1649.

[16] p. 19 cm. [11277]

G. B. Spudaeus, *respondent.*

—Dissertatio physica de sanguine . . . Wittebergae, Typis Michaelis Wendt [1650]

[20] p. 19 cm. [11278]

Imperfect: date of imprint mutilated.
G. Müller, *respondent.*

—Dissertatio physica, de visu . . . Wittebergae, Typis Michaelis Wendt, 1650.

[16] p. 21 cm. [11279]

W. Saur, *respondent.*

—Λιθολογια . . . Wittebergae, E chalcographeo Michaelis Wendt, 1657.

[28] p.   19 cm.   **[11280]**

G. E. Weigand, *respondent.*

—Θανατολογία; sive, Disputatio philosophica de morte . . . Wittebergae, Typis Fincelianis, 1656.

[16] p.   18 cm.   **[11281]**

P. P. Röber, *respondent.*

—*See* MAJOR, J. D. Historia anatomica calculorum. 1662.

SPERLING, PAUL GOTTFRIED]*d.* 1709] Lectori benevolo S. P. D. eundemque ad anatomen publicam cadaveris masculini officiose invitat Paulus Gottfr. Sperling . . . Wittenbergae, Prelo Christiani Kreusigii [1698]

[8] p.   19 cm.   **[11282]**

Dissertations — Wittenberg

—*praeses.* Chymicam formicarum analysin . . . subjiciet Samuel Gotthilff Manitius . . . Wittenbergae, Imprimebat Matthaeus Henckelius [1689]

[64] p.   plate.   20 cm.   **[11283]**

S. G. Manitius, *respondent.*

—Disputatio inauguralis medica de deliriis febrium continuarum . . . Vitembergae, Prelo Christiani Kreusigii [1696]

[30] p.   19 cm.   **[11284]**

H.S. Weitz, *respondent.*

—Disputatio inauguralis medica de haemoptysi . . . Vitembergae, Typis Christiani Kreusigii [1698]

[24] p.   21 cm.   **[11285]**

J. L. G. Lebrun, *respondent.*

—Disputatio medica aegrum suffusione labornatem exhibens . . . Wittenbergae, Typis Matthaei Henckelii [1684]

[2], 30 p.   19 cm.   **[11286]**

J. K. Spies, *respondent.*

—Disputationem solennem medicam de incontinentia urinae . . . submittet M. Christophorus Daniel Distel . . . Wittebergae, Ex officina Johannis Hakii [1697]

[28] p.   21 cm.   **[11287]**

D. C. Distel, *respondent.*

—Dissertatio inauguralis medica de fame canina . . . Wittenbergae, Typis Christiani Kreusigii [1699]

[18] p.   19 cm.   **[11288]**

A. F. Heunisch, *respondent.*

—Dissertatio inauguralis medica exhibens choleram . . . Wittenbergae, Typis Christiani Kreusigii [1699]

[19] p.   20 cm.   **[11289]**

S. A. Heyder, *respondent.*

—Dissertatio medica inauguralis de vomitu simplici . . . Vitenbergae, Literis Goderitschianis [1700]

[32] p.   20 cm.   **[11290]**

G. H. Liebe, *respondent.*

Dissertatio solennis de vermibus in primis viis . . . Vitembergae, Typis Christiani Gerdesii [1700]

[23] p.   20 cm.   **[11291]**

J. C. Bothius, *respondent.*

—Dissertationem chymicam de arsenico . . . submittit . . . Johann Gunther Tiling . . . Wittenbergae, Typis Matthaei Henckelii, 1685.

[40] p.   20 cm.   **[11292]**

J. G. Tiling, *respondent.*

—Dysenteriam . . . exponit M. Balthasar Siberus . . . Vitembergae, Stanno Schulziano [1698]

24 p.   19 cm.   **[11293]**

B. Siber, *respondent.*

—*respondent. See* WEDEL, G. W., *praeses.* Disputationem inauguralem medicam de pervigilio . . . submittit P.G.S. 1680.

SPIEGEL, ADRIAAN VAN DE [1578–1625] Opera quae extant, omnia. Ex recensione Joh. Antonidae vander Linden . . . Amsterdami, Apud Johannem Blaeu, 1645.

2 v. in 1.   illus., plates, port.   53 cm.   **[11294]**

Engraved title page.

Vol. 1 includes: Giulio Casserio's Tabulae anatomicae LXXVIII, cum supplemento XX tabularum Danielis Bucretii. - Gaspare Asellio's De lactibus and Tabulae De venis lacteis. - William Harvey's De motu cordis. - Johannes Walaeus' Epistolae duae: De motu chyli, et sanguinis ad Thomam Bartholinum. Vol. 2 includes J. A. vander Linden's De monstrosis vermibus, observatio rara.

"Index capitum exercitationis anatomicae, De motu cordis & sanguinis . . ." is affixed to verso of sig. Hh6 (below "Finis" of De motu cordis).

—De formato foetu liber singularis, aeneis figuris exornatus. Epistolae duae anatomicae. Tractatus de arthritide. Opera posthuma studio Liberalis Cremae . . . edita. Patavii, Apud Jo. Bap. de Martinis, &

Livium Pasquatum, expensis ejusdem Liberalis Cremae [1626]

[8], 104 p.   illus.   42 cm.   **[11295]**

Bound with his De humani corporis fabrica libri decem. 1627.

— [The same.] . . . Francofurti, Impensis & caelo Matthaei Meriani, typis Casparis Rötelii, 1631.

[8], 105, [6] p.   illus.   20 cm.   **[11296]**

— [German tr.] *In* Casserio, G. Julii Casserii Placentini Anatomische Tafeln. 1656, 1683.

— De humani corporis fabrica libri decem, tabulis XCIIX aeri incisis . . . exornati . . . Opus posthumum. Daniel Bucretius . . . in lucem profert. Venetiis, 1627.

[12] 328 (i.e. 330), [12] p.   42 cm.   **[11297]**

Engraved title page.
With this are bound: Casserio, G. Tabulae anatomicae. 1627; Fabricius, Hieronymus, ab Aquapendente. De formato foetu. 1600 [i.e. 1606?]; Fabricius, Hieronymus, ab Aquapendente. De locutione et ejus instrumentis liber. 1603; Fabricius, Hieronymus, ab Aquapendente. De brutorum loquela. Patavii, 1603; the author's De formato foetu. [1626]

— [The same.] . . . Francofurti, Impensis & Caelo Matthaei Meriani, 1632.

[16], 390, [21] p.   22 cm.   **[11298]**

Engraved title page.

— [Libri V-VII. English tr.] *In* Paré, A. The workes. 1649, 1665, 1678.

— [*as subject*] *See* RIOLAN, J. [1580-1657] Opera anatomica vetera. 1650 [and] Opuscula anatomica nova. 1649.

— De lumbrico lato liber . . . Accessit ejusdem auctoris epistola De incerto tempore partus . . . Patavii, Typis Laurentii Pasquati, 1618.

[8], 88, [12] p.   plate.   20 cm.   **[11299]**

With this are bound: Liceti, F. De animarum coextensione corpori. 1616; Charleton, Walter. Onomasticon zoicon. 1668.

— De semitertiana libri quatuor. Accessit in fine epistola ejusdem argumenti. Francofurti, Apud haeredes Jo. Theodori de Bry, 1624.

[8], 160, [8] p.   21 cm.   **[11300]**

— Epistola de incerto tempore partus. *In* Nymann, G. Dissertatio de vita foetus in utero. 1644; Plazzoni, F. De partibus generationi inservientibus. 1644, 1664.

— Isagoges in rem herbarium libri duo . . . Patavii, Apud Paulum Meiettum, ex typographia Laurentii

Pasquati, 1606.

[16], 138, [14] p.   19 cm.   **[11301]**

— [The same.] . . . Lugduni Batavorum, Ex Officina Elzeviriana, 1633.

271, [16] p.   12 cm.   **[11302]**

Engraved title page.

— [The same.] . . . ed. prioribus correctior . . . Helmestadii, Typis sumtibus Johannis Heitmulleri, 1667.

[12], 127, [13] p.   20 cm.   **[11303]**

— *See* JASOLINO, G. Collegium anatomicum. 1668; Severino, M. A. Seilo-phlebotome castigata. 1654.

SPIEGEL, JEREMIAS [*fl.* 1611] *respondent. See* TILEMANN, T., *praeses.* Disputationum physiologicarum sexta de motu et quiete. 1611.

SPIELENBERGER, DÁVID [*fl.* 1683-1685] *respondent. See* WEDEL, G. W., *praeses.* Dissertatio medica de αντιπραξει viscerum. 1683.

SPIES, JOHANN KARL [1663-1729] *respondent. See* SPERLING, P. G., *praeses.* Disputatio medica aegrum suffusione laborantem exhibens. 1684.

SPIESMACHER, JOHANN [*fl.* 1685-1686] *respondent. See* HEMPEL, C., *praeses.* Ex ungue hominem publicae eruditorum disquisitioni . . . Christianus Hempelius . . . & . . . Johannes Spiesmacher . . . sistunt. 1685.

SPIESS, JOHANN CHRISTOPH [*fl.* 1694] *respondent.* Disputatio inauguralis medica de arthritide, vulgo: von der Glieder-sucht . . . Basileae, Typis Joh. Rudolphi Genathii [1694]

[36] p.   20 cm.   **[11304]**

Diss. — Basel.

SPIESS, JOHANN ELIAS [*fl.* 1681] *respondent.* Theses medico-chirurgicae, p. t. disputationis inauguralis vicem supplentes, de scrophulis seu strumis . . . Erfordiae, Literis Kirschianis [1681]

[7] p.   19 cm.   **[11305]**

Diss. — Erfurt.

SPIESS, JOHANN HEINRICH [*fl.* 1694-1695] *respondent. See* EYSSEL, A., *praeses.* Chylum secundum & praeter naturam spectatum disputatione medica . . . submittit J. H. S. 1694; VESTI, J., *praeses.* Disputatio inauguralis physico-medica de magnetismis macro-et microcosmi. 1695.

SPIEWACZEK, MATTHIAS. Ἐπίσκεψις; seu, Aegroti consideratio. Generice omnes totius corporis humani partes & morbos perpendens. Specifice pectoris aegritudines earundemque subjecta contemplans ... [Prague?] Impressit Joannes Carolus Gerzabek. 1695.

[112] p. 17 cm. **[11306]**

SPIGELIUS, ADRIANUS. *See* SPIEGEL, Adriaan van de [1578-1625]

SPINA, DAVID DE [1662-1710] Manuale sive lexicon pharmaceutico-chymicum ... partim ex corpore pharmaceut. domini physici Jüngken huc translata. Ed. completa ... Francofurti ad Moenum, Sumptibus Friderici Knochii, 1700.

[11], 1054, [50] p. 18 cm. **[11307]**
Added engraved title page.
Imperfect: upper margins trimmed.

—*praeses.* Disputatio medica de venenis ... Heidelbergae, Typis Joh. David. Bergmanni [1692]

[20] p. 21 cm. **[11308]**
Diss.—Heidelberg (J. C. Mezler, *respondent*)

—*respondent.* Disputatio medica inauguralis de philtromania ... Lugduni Batavorum, Apud Abrahamum Elzevier, 1687.

[24] p. 20 cm. **[11309]**
Diss.—Leyden.

SPINA, GIOVANNI FRANCESCO [*fl.* 1612-1622] De hominis procreatione tractatus in duos libros divisus ... Maceratae, Ex officina Juliani Carboni, 1622.

131, [13] p. 21 cm. **[11310]**
Errata: p. [12]

SPINA, PETER DE [1563-1622] *ed. See* MERCURIALE, G. Medicina practica. 1601, 1602, 1617, 1618, 1623.

—*See* VENATOR, B. Vita Petri de Spina. 1625.

SPINA, PETER DE [1661-1741] *respondent.* Disputatio medica inauguralis de elephantiasi ... Lugduni Batavorum, Apud Abrahamum Elzevier, 1685.

[36] p. 22 cm. **[11311]**
Diss.—Leyden.

SPINDLER, PÁL [*fl.* 1629-1664] Observationum medicinalium centuria ... Accessit D. Martini Rulandi Sen. Thesaurus medicus ... Studio & opera Caroli Raygeri ... Francofurti ad Moenum, Typis & Sumpt. Philippi Fieveti, 1691.

[8], 180 p.; 152 p. 21 cm. **[11312]**

The Thesaurus medicus has half title.
Imperfect: p. 13-14 mutilated.

—*respondent. See* SEBISCH, M. [1578-1674?] *praeses* Exercitationes medicae. 1639.

SPINELLI, GIOVANNI PAOLO [*fl.* 1604] Lectione aureae in omni quod pertinet ad artem phar macopaeam lucubrate ... in libros quatuor digesta ... Barii, Apud Julium Caesarem Venturam, 160 ...

2 v. in 1. 20 cm. **[11313**
Vol. 2 (in Italian) has title: Libro secondo delle auree lettion

SPINOWSKI, CHRISTOPH CRELLE [*fl.* 168 ... *respondent.* Disputatio medica inauguralis de calcul renum et vesicae ... Lugduni Batavorum, Apu Abrahamum Elzevier, 1682.

[16] p. 22 cm. **[11314**
Diss.—Leyden

SPLEISS, DAVID [1659-1716] *ed.* and *tr. See* ZAPATA G. B. Mirabilia. 1696.

SPLENDOR salis & solis. Ein Discurs von de wahren Quinta Essentia und Artzney-Krafft de Vegetabilien und Mineralien; sonderlich vom Aur Potabili. Authoris anonymi eremitae ... Neu Hanau, In Verlegung Johann Eichenbergks [1677

29, [1] p. 16 cm. **[11315**
Imperfect: lower margins of pages 6, 12 and 19 trimmed.

SPÖRLIN, GEORGE, *ed. See* RULAND, M [1532-1602] Thesaurus Rulandinus. 1628, 1680.

SPOLE, ANDREAS [1630-1699] *praeses.* Disputati physica de frigore ... Upsalae, Excudit Henricu Curio [1684]

[6], 55, [2] p. 15 cm. **[11316**
Diss.—Uppsala (L. Algaer, *respondent*)

SPOLIUS, ANDREAS. *See* SPOLE, Andrea [1630-1699]

SPON, CHARLES [1609-1684] *ed. See* CARDANO, C Opera omnia. 1663.

—, *tr. See* HIPPOCRATES. [Prognostica. Adapta tions, etc. Latin.] 1661.

—*See* HOFMANN, C. Institutionum medicarum lib sex. 1645; PEYER, J. K. Parerga anatomica et medic septem. 1681; SCHENCK VON GRAFENBERG, J. Obse vationum medicarum rariorum, libri VII. 1643, 164 1665.

SPON, JACOB [1647-1685] Chymica appendix. *In* Pereda, P. P. In Michaelis Joan. Paschalii, Methodum curandi scholia. 1664.

—Observations sur les fievres et les febrifuges, a l'occasion du livre intitulé, La découverte de l'admirable remede anglois. Lyon, Rue Merciere, a la Victoire, 1681.
    95 p. 14 cm. [**11317**]
    Caption title: Lettre a monsieur l'abbé de Sylvecane, contenant des observations sur les fievres & les febrifuges.
    Signed at end: Spon fils D. M. A. Lyon, ce 12, Dec. 1680.
    Bound with Blegny, N. de. Histoire anathomique d'un enfant. 1679.

—Observations sur les fievres et les febrifuges ... 2. ed. rev., corr., & augm. de plus de la moitié. Lyon, Thomas Amaulry, 1684.
    [12], 264, [10] p. 16 cm. [**11318**]

—[The same.] ... 3. ed. ... Lyon, Thomas Amaulry, 1687.
    [12], 264, [10] p. 16 cm. [**11319**]
    Imperfect: sig. M6 (blank) wanting.
    Different setting of type.

—[Latin tr.] *In* [Nigrisoli, F. M.] *ed.* Febris china chinae expugnata. 1687, 1700.

—*ed.* [Selections, etc. Greek and Latin] *See* HIPPOCRATES. Ἀφορισμοι νεώτεροι. 1684.

—*See* [DUFOURS, P. S.] De l'usage du caphé, du thé, et du chocolate. 1671; MALPIGHI, M. Praeclarissimo ... viro D. Jacobo Sponio ... Marcellus Malpighius S. P. 1684; [MONGINOT, F., *the younger*] Traité de la guérison des fiévres par le quinquina. 1679.

SPONTONE, CIRO [*ca.* 1552-*ca.* 1610] La metoposcopia; overo, Commensuratione delle linee della fronte ... Venetia, Evangelista Deuchino, 1626.
    136, [7] p. illus. 16 cm. [**11320**]
    Engraved title page.
    Edited by Giovanni Battista Spontone.

—[The same.] ... 2. imp. [Venetia, Evangelista Deuchino, 1629]
    104, [6] p. illus. 16 cm. [**11321**]

—[The same.] ... Nuovamente ristampata ... Venetia, Gli heredi dell'Imberti, 1645.
    104, [5] p. illus. 15 cm. [**11322**]
    Different setting of type.

—[The same.] *In* Porta, G. B. della. La fisonomia dell'huomo. 1668.

SPONTONE, GIOVANNI BATTISTA [*fl.* 1625] Conechidne-logia; hoc est, Pulveris viperini discursus. In quo variae praeparationes, medicamenta composita, usu ejusdem pulveris methodus ... demonstrantur. Cum selectorum remediorum centuria ... Papiae, Ex typographia Jo. Andreae Magrii, 1648.
    146, [5] p. illus. 18 cm. [**11323**]
    Appendix: p. 117-146.
    Errata: p. [1-5]

—[The same.] ... In hac 2. ed. opus castigatum, & ab auctore locuplectatum. In quo usus foelicissimus pulveris viperini probatur in omnibus morbis curandis; absque ulla carnis perinae [sic] caliditate, ut neoterici decrevere. [Rome, 1648]
    [12], 196 p. illus. 25 cm. [**11324**]
    Added engraved title page.

—, *ed. See* SPONTONE, C. La metoposcopia. 1626, 1629, 1645.

SPORMARKER, CANUT [*fl.* 1696] *respondent. See* WINSLOW, J. B., *praeses.* Exercitii anatomico-pathologici. 1696.

SPRACKLING, ROBERT [*d. ca.* 1670] Medela ignorantiae; or, A just and plain vindication of Hippocrates and Galen from the groundless imputations of M[archamont] N[edham] wherein the whole substance of his illiterate plea, intituled Medela medicinae is occasionally considered ... London, Printed by W. G. for Robert Crofts, 1665.
    [12], 163 p. 15 cm. [**11325**]

SPRAT, THOMAS, *Bp. of Rochester* [1635-1713] The history of the Royal-Society of London, for the improving of natural knowledge ... London, Printed by T. R. for J. Martyn and J. Allestry, 1667.
    [16], 438, [1] p. plates. 21 cm. [**11326**]
    Errata: p. [1] at end.
    Imperfect: p. 183 mutilated.

—[French tr.] L'histoire de la Societé royale de Londres, establie pour l'enrichissement de la science naturelle e scrite en anglois ... et traduite en françois. Geneve, Jean Herman Widerhold, 1669.
    [16], 542 p. plates. 18 cm. [**11327**]

—The plague of Athens, which happened in the second year of the Peloponnesian war. First described in Greek by Thucydides; then in Latine by Lucretius. Now attempted in English by Tho. Sprat. London, Joanna Brome, 1683.

[5], 34 p.   18 cm.   [11328]

Contents.—The epistle dedicatory.—Thucydides, Lib. II. as it is excellently translated by Mr. Hobbs.- The plague of Athens.

—, *ed. See* COWLEY, A. Poemata Latina. 1668, 1678.

SPRENGER, PHILIPP HERMANN [*fl.* 1636] *respondent. See* RECHPERGER, G., *praeses.* Disputatio medica [de scorbuto] 1636.

SPRÖGEL, MICHAEL [*b.* 1653] *respondent. See* FASCH, A. H., *praeses.* Dissertatio inauguralis de asthmate. 1684; WEDEL, G. W., *praeses.* Dissertatio medica sistens aegrum vomitu cruento laborantem. 1680.

—*See* WEDEL, G. W. Decanus Facultatis Medicae Georgius Wolffgangus Wedelius . . . lectori benevolo S. P. D. 1684.

SPUDAEUS, GEORG BALTHASAR [*fl.* 1649] *respondent. See* SPERLING, J., *praeses.* Disputatio physica de voluntate. 1649.

SPUNTONI, BAPTISTAE. *See* SPONTONE, Giovanni Battista [*fl.* 1625]

SPUNTONUS, JOANNES BAPTISTA. *See* SPONTONE, Giovanni Battista [*fl.* 1625]

SPURSTOW, WILLIAM [1605?–1666] The spiritual chymist; or, Six decads of divine meditations on several subjects . . . London, Philip Chetwind, 1666.

[24], 182 p.; [1], 110 p.   18 cm.   [11329]

Part [2] has special title pages: Σatana nohmata; or, The wiles of Satan in a discourse upon 2 Cor. 2.ii.

—[The same.] . . . London, Printed by E. T. for Simon Miller, 1668.

[24], 260, [2] p.   16 cm.   [11330]

Imperfect: first 2 preliminary leaves (blank?) wanting. Without Σatana nohmata.

SSTYRKOLSKY, DANIEL. *See* STYRKOLSZKY, Daniel [*fl.* 1609–1610]

STADLANDER, MATTHIAS [*fl.* 1662] *respondent.* Disputatio medica inauguralis, de scorbuto . . . Lugduni Batavorum, Apud viduam & haeredes Johannes Elsevirii, 1662.

[14] p.   19 cm.   [11331]

Diss.—Leyden.

STADLANDER, THEODOR FRIEDRICH [*fl.* 1683] *respondent.* Disputatio medica inauguralis de pulmonum vulneribus . . . Franequerae, Apud Johannem Gyselaer, 1683.

[16] p.   19 cm.   [11332]

Diss.—Franeker.

—*See* HARTMANN, P. J., *praeses.* Exercitationum anatomicarum . . . de originibus anatomicae prima [-quarta] 1683.

STADT–und LAND-APOTHEKE. *See* CARDILUCIUS, J. H., *ed.* and *tr.* Neuaufgerichtete Stadt- und Land-Apotheke. 1673 — 80.

STAEDEL, JOANNES FRIDERICUS [*fl.* 1694–1695] *respondent.* Paradoxorum anatomicorum circa hominis generationem specimen . . . Argentorati, Literis Staedelianis [1694]

[3], 28 p.   19 cm.   [11333]

Diss.—Strasbourg.

—Theses medicae de gonorrhoea virulenta . . . Argentorati, Literis Staedelianis [1695]

[2], 34 p.   20 cm.   [11334]

Diss.—Strasbourg.

STAEHELIN, JOHANN JAKOB [*fl.* 1665–1680] *respondent. See* BAUHIN, H. *praeses.* Assertiones medicae de catarrho. 1665.

—, *ed. See* GLASER, J. H. Tractatus posthumus de cerebro. 1680.

STAEHELIN, JOHANN SAMUEL [*fl.* 1678] *respondent. See* MÜLLER, Peter, *praeses.* Dissertatio de hierologia. 1694.

STAETKUNDIGE bedencking, over het verschil tusschen den Heer Bonaventura Dortmond, doctor van het gasthuys . . . en . . . Fredericus Ruysch, en Andries Boeckelman . . . of 'er wel een manspersoon tot het manuael der vroet-vrouwen, in eene welgestelde Republijck toegelaten behoorde te worden. Amsterdam, Jacob van Velsen [1677]

40 p.   illus.   16 cm.   [11335]

STAFFARD, THOMAS [*fl.* 1649–1669] *tr. See* BARTHOLIN, T. Anatomia. [Dutch tr.] 1653, 1656, 1658, 1669, 1688; BECKHER, D. Een besondere genesinge van den Prussiaenschen mes-inslicker. 1649.

STAHL, GEORG ERNST [1660–1734] Dissertatio epistolica ad . . . Johannem Adrianum Slevogt . .

de motu tonico vitali, & independente motu sanguinis particulari; qua demonstratur, stante circulatione, sanguinem, & cum eo commeantes humores, ad quamlibet corporis partem specialem, praealiis, copiosius dirigi & propelli posse ... Jenae, Sumtibus Joh. Jacob Ehrten, 1692.

[32] p.   20 cm.   [11336]

—Georgii Ernesti Stahl ... Observationum chymico-physico-medicarum curiosarum, mensibus singulis ... continuandarum, mensis primus ... Julius [-sextus December 1697; mensis primus Januarius-tertius Martius 1698] ... Francofurti & Lipsiae, Imprimebat Georg. Henr. Müller typogr. Erffurt. [Halae Magdeburgicae, Typis Joh. Jacobi Krebsii] 1697 [1698]

480 p.   17 cm.   [11337]
Each month has special title page.

—Positiones, de aestu maris microcosmici; seu; Fluxu et refluxu sanguinis, tum in pluribus aliis ... um praecipue paroxysmo febrili tertianario ... Halae, Typis Christophori Salfeldii [1696?]

[44] p.   20 cm.   [11338]

— Positiones, de mechanismo motus progressivi sanguinis. Quibus motus tonici partium porosarum necessitas ... ad motum sanguinis, lymphae, seri, particulariter dirigendum ... demonstratur, pro futuris usibus pathologiae variorum affectuum, maxime vero febrium, apodictice evolvendae. Halae, Typis Christophori Salfeldii, 1695.

[40] p.   20 cm.   [11339]

—Problemata practica, febrium pathologiae, & herpiae ... quibus, febrium in genere & specie circumstantiae essentiales ... ex ... observatione, & propria experientia, pervestigatae, recensentur, ut ex llis scientifica connexio, & causalis geneologia febrium, efformari possit. Halae, Literis Christophori Salfeldii, 1695.

[8], 20 p.   20 cm.   [11340]

Programs — Halle

—Prolusio inauguralis de certitudine artis medicae. [Halae, 1698]

[8] p.   21 cm.   [11341]
With vita of G. G. Köhler de Mohrenfeld.

—Propempticon inaugurale de abstinentia et nausea carnium in morbis, praecipue acutis. [Halis Magdeburgicis, 1699]

[8] p.   21 cm.   [11342]
With vita of J. J. Ewald.

—Propempticon inaugurale de aestimatione partium & laesionum. [Halae, 1698]

[8] p.   20 cm.   [11343]
With vita of L. F. Gualther.

—Propempticon inaugurale de cephalalgia iliacohaematitica. Vom Über-Kolck, oder Ober-Colic. [Halae, 1698]

[8] p.   19 cm.   [11344]
With vita of J. C. Tieffenbach.

— Propempticon inaugurale de commotionibus sanguinis activis et passivis ... [Halae, 1698]

[8] p.   21 cm.   [11345]
With vita of C. A. Richter.

—Propempticon inaugurale de cornu cervi deciduo. [Halis Magdeburgicis, 1699]

[8] p.   21 cm.   [11346]
With vita of L. A. Labach.

—Another printing.   20 cm.   [11347]

—Propempticon inaugurale de empeiria. [Halae, 1699]

[8] p.   20 cm.   [11348]
With vita of J. Richter.

—Propempticon inaugurale de morbis contumacibus. [Halae, 1698]

[8] p.   21 cm.   [11349]
With vita of H. P. Juch.

—Propempticon inaugurale de pathologia salsa. [Halis Magdeburgicis, 1698]

[8] p.   19 cm.   [11350]
With vita of J. S. Holl.

— Propempticon inaugurale de sterilitate foeminarum per aetatem. [Halis Magdeburg., 1699]

[8] p.   21 cm.   [11351]
With vita of G. D. Coschwitz.

— Propempticon inaugurale de στοχάσμω medico. [Halis Magdeburgicis, 1698]

[8] p.   20 cm.   [11352]
With vita of J. D. Gohl.

—Propempticon inaugurale, de συνεργεια naturae in medendo. [Halae, 1695]

[8] p.   21 cm.   [11353]
With vita of J. J. Reich.

—Another printing.   19 cm.   [11354]

—Propempticon inaugurale quis bonus theoreticus, malus practicus. [Halae, 1698]

[8] p.   20 cm.   [11355]

With vita of A. C. Rhetius.

—Propempticum inaugurale, de commotione sanguinis translatoria, & eluctatoria. Halae, Literis Salfeldianis [1694]

[8] p.   18 cm.   [11356]

With vita of J. G. Brebiss.

Dissertations — Halle

—*praes.* Disputatio inauguralis medica de mensium muliebrium fluxu, S. n. & suppressione, p. n. ... Halae, Literis Salfeldii [1694]

24 p.   20 cm.   [11357]

J. G. Brebiss, *respondent.*

—Another printing.

28 p.   18 cm.   [11358]

—Disputatio inauguralis medica de morbo retrogrado ... [Halae] Typis Christoph. Andreae Zeitleri [1697]

26, [2] p.   20 cm.   [11359]

J. Lindeman, *respondent.*

—Disputatio medica inauguralis de hectica febre ... Halae Magdeburgicae, Literis Chr. Henckelii [1699]

[3], 21 p.   20 cm.   [11360]

J. J. Ewald, *respondent.*

—Disputatio medica inauguralis de inflammationis vera pathologia ... Halae Magdeburgicae, Literis Christiani Henckelii [1698]

23, [1] p.   19 cm.   [11361]

L. F. Gualther, *respondent.*

—Disputatio medica inauguralis de morbis habitualibus ... Halae Magdeburgicae, Typis Chr. Henckelii [1698]

[2], 30 p.   20 cm.   [11362]

A. C. Rhetius, *respondent.*

—Disputatio medica inauguralis de podagrae nova pathologia ... Halae Magdeburgicae, Literis Christiani Henckelii [1698]

[8], 32 p.   20 cm.   [11363]

Date of imprint supplied from Goetze, J.C. Scripta ... Stahlii. Norimbergae, 1729, p. 36.

J. C. Tieffenbach, *respondent.*

With this are bound: Ewaldt, B. Dissertatio medica inauguralis de podagra. [1697]; Gabuccini, Girolamo. Commentarius de podagra. Venetiis, 1569.

—Disputatio medica inauguralis, quae exhibet venaesectionis patrocinium, simul indicans ejus usum et abusum ... Halae, Typis Christoph. Salfeldii [1698]

[1], 38 p.   18 cm.   [11364]

C. A. Richter, *respondent.*

—Disputatio medica medico-pathologica, de infrequentia morborum personali, sive quod singuli homines raris et paucis morbis laborent ... Halae Magdeb., Literis Johannis Jacobi Krebsii [1697]

28 p.   19 cm.   [11365]

H. P. Juch, *respondent.*

—Disputationem inauguralem de passionibus animi corpus humanum varie alterantibus ... submittit Johannes Jacobus Reich ... Halae, Typis Christophori Salfeldii [1695]

[16] p.   20 cm.   [11366]

J. J. Reich, *respondent.*

—Another printing.   20 cm.   [11367]

Recusa Halae Magdeburgicae, Literis Christiani Henckeli [n. d.]

—Dissertatio inauguralis de motu sanguinis haemorrhoidali, et haemorrhoidibus externis ... Halae Magdeb., Typis Chr. Henckelii [1698]

[8], 32 p.   23 cm.   [11368]

H. P. Juch, *respondent.*

—Dissertatio inauguralis medica de ἀδηφαγια sive intemperantia edendi, nocua ... Halae Magdeb. Literis Chr. Henckelii [1700]

24 p.   21 cm.   [11369]

H. Vogel, *respondent.*

—Dissertatio inauguralis medica de haemorrhoidum internarum motu et ileo haematite Hippocratis ... Halae Magdeb., Typis Chr. Henckeli [1698]

[4], 27, [1] p.   20 cm.   [11370]

J. D. Gohl, *respondent.*

—Dissertatio inauguralis medica de lapide manati ... Halae Magdeburgicae, Typis Christiani Henckelii [1699]

[24] p.   20 cm.   [11371]

L. A. Labach, *respondent.*

—Dissertatio inauguralis medica practica sistens aegrum haemoptysi periodica laborantem . . . Halae Magdeburgicae, Typis Christiani Henckelii [1699]

[20] p.   19 cm.   [11372]

G. D. Coschwitz, *respondent.*

—Dissertatio inauguralis medica tradens novam pathologiam calculi renum . . . Halae Magdeb., Typis Chr. Henckelii [1698]

[1], 20, [2] p.   20 cm.   [11373]

G. G. Köhler de Mohrenfeld, *respondent.*

—Dissertatio medica de impotentia virili . . . Halae, Typis Christophori Salfeldii [1697]

[20] p.   20 cm.   [11374]

B. Ewaldt, *respondent.*

—Dissertatio medica de motibus humorum spasmodicis, a motu pulsus ordinarii diversis . . . Halae, Typis Christophori Salfeldii [1697]

[1], 50 p.   20 cm.   [11375]

G. D. Coschwitz, *respondent.*

—Dissertatio medica de sangvisugarum utilitate . . . Halae Magdeb., Literis Chr. Henckelii [1699]

24 p.   20 cm.   [11376]

J. J. Coler, *respondent.*

—Dissertatio medica inauguralis de calculorum generatione, sive lithogenesi . . . [Halae] Typis Christoph. Andreae Zeitleri [1699]

39 (i.e. 40) p.   20 cm.   [11377]

J. Richter, *respondent.*

—Dissertatio medica inauguralis de requisitis bonae nutricis . . . Halae, Typis Christoph. Andreae Zeitleri [1698]

23, [1] p.   19 cm.   [11378]

J. S. Holl, *respondent.*

—Dissertatio medica inauguralis de vena portae porta malorum hypochondriaco-splenetico-suffocativo-hysterico-colico-haemorrhoidariorum . . Halae Magdeb., Literis Chr. Henckelii [1698]

[4], 55, [1] p.   19 cm.   [11379]

Date of imprint supplied from G. E. Stahl. Theoria medica vera. Lipsiae, vol. 1 (1831) p. xxiii; and from the 1719 reprint.

J. P. Gaetke, *respondent.*

—Dissertatio medica-practica, de αὐτοκρατία naturae, sive spontanea morborum excussione, et convalescentia . . . Anno MDCXCVI, publicae eruditorum disquisitioni sistit Johannes Albertus Lasius . . . Recusa Halae Magdeburgicae, Litteris Christiani Henckelii [1697?]

[48] p.   20 cm.   [11380]

J. A. Lasius, *respondent.*

—Dissertatio medica qua temperamenta physiologico-physiognomico-pathologico-mechanice enucleantur . . . Halae Magdeburgicae, Literis Christophori Salfeldii [1698]

[48] p.   19 cm.   [11381]

C. A. Richter, *respondent.*

—Dissertatio medico-semiotica de facie morborum indice, seu morborum aestimatione ex facie . . . Halae Magdeburg., Literis Johannis Jacobi Krebsii [1700]

31, [1] p.   20 cm.   [11382]

E. G. Struve, *respondent.*

— *See* FASCH, A. H. Augustinus Henricus Faschius . . . Collegii Medici decanus S. P. D. lecturis! 1684.

STAHL, GOTTHILFF CHRISTOPHER [*fl.* 1691] *respondent. See* VESTI, J., *praeses.* Disputatio inauguralis medica de singultu. 1691.

STAHL, PAUL [*fl.* 1666] *respondent.* Disputatio medica inauguralis de dolore capitis . . . Lugduni Batavorum, Apud Felicem Lopes de Haro, 1666.

[15] p.   23 cm.   [11383]

Diss.—Leyden.

STAINER, BERNHARD. Gerocomicon; sive, Diaeteticum regimen, de conservanda senum sanitate, et vitae eorundem ad praefixum terminum (per praxin sex rerum non naturalium) productione . . . per Joannem Neydecker . . . contractum atque concinnatum . . . Wirceburgi, Typis Eliae Michaelis Zinck, 1631.

[16], 58 p.   21 cm.   [11384]

STAINES, WILLIAM. *See* STANES, William [*ca.* 1609-1679]

STAIR, DE. *See* DALRYMPLE, *Sir* James, *1st Viscount Stair* [1619-1695]

STAIR, JAMES, *Viscount. See* DALRYMPLE, *Sir* James, *1st Viscount Stair* [1619-1695]

STALPART VAN DER WIEL, CORNELIS [1620-1702] Hondert seldzame aanmerkingen, so in de genees- als heel- en sny-konst, meest by eygen ondervinding, van tijt tot tijt, vergadert, en opgestelt ... Amsterdam, Johan ten Hoorn, 1682–86.

    2 v. plates, port. 17 cm.   **[11385]**

Vol. 1 has added engraved title page.

Vol. 2 has title: Eerste deel, van het tweede hondert-getalder zeldzame aanmerkingen.

—[Latin tr.] Observationum rariorum medic. anatomic. chirurgicarum centuria prior, accedit De unicornu dissertatio. Utraque tertia parte auct. longeque emend. Lugduni Batavorum, Apud Petrum vander Aa, 1687.

    2 v. front. (port.), plates. 17 cm. **[11386]**

Added engraved title pages.

Vol. 2 has title: Observationum rariorum medic. anatomic. chirurgicarum canturiae posterioris pars prior. It contains 50 observations and Pieter Stalpart van der Wiel's Layden thesis: De nutritione foetus exercitatio. Latter has special title page and separate pagination.

STALPART VAN DER WIEL, PIETER [*fl.* 1686] *See* STALPART VAN DER WIEL, C. Observationum rariorum medic. anatomic. chirurgicarum centuria prior. 1687.

STANES, WILLIAM [*ca.* 1609–1679] Medela medicorum; or, An enquiry into the reasons & grounds of the contempt of physicians, and their noble art. With proposals to reduce them to their wonted repute; maintaining the joynt interest of doctors, chyrurgions, and apothecaries, against all intruders. By S[tanes] W[illiam] ... London, Printed by T. M. for Dorman Newman, 1678.

    [24], 113, [7] p. 16 cm.   **[11387]**

STANGE, JOHANN DANIEL [*fl.* 1697] *praeses.* Diatriba de juvenis medici idea errante philosophico-medica, quae ... a Johanne Daniele Stangio ... subjicitur ... respondente Johanne Daniele Dolaeo ... [Halae] Typis Christoph. Andreae Zeitleri [1697]

    50 p. 20 cm.   **[11388]**

Diss.—Halle (J. D. Doläus, *respondent*)

STANGE, JOHANN JAKOB [*fl.* 1700–1702] *respondent. See* HOFFMANN, F. [1660–1742] *praeses.* Exercitatio physico-medica de mentis morbis. 1700.

STANGIUS. *See* STANGE.

STANGIUS, SAMUEL [*fl.* 1607] *See* KNOBLOCH, T., *praeses.* Disputationes anatomicae. 1608, 1612.

STANHOPE, MICHAEL [*fl.* 1626–1631] Cures without care; or, A summons to all such who finde

little or no helpe by the use of ordinary physick to repaire to the northerne spaw. Wherein ... it is evidenced to the world, that infirmities in their owne nature desperate ... have received perfect recovery, by virtue of minerall waters neare Knaresborow ... Collected ... by M[ichael] S[tanhope] ... London, William Jones, 1632.

    [11], 32 p. 20 cm.   **[11389]**

STC 23226.

—Newes out of York-Shire; or, An account of a journey, in the true discovery of a soveraigne minerall, medicinall water ... neere ... Knaresbrough ... London, Printed by J. H[aviland] for George Gibbes, 1627.

    [15], 30 p. 20 cm.   **[11390]**

STC 23228.

— *See* DEANE, E. Spadacrene Anglica. 1649.

STANIA, VIGER NICOLAAS [*fl.* 1652] *respondent.* Disputatio medica inauguralis exhibens casum laborantis chlorosi sive virgineo morbo ... Lugduni Batavorum, E typographeo Francisci Hackii, 1652.

    [12] p. 22 cm.   **[11391]**

Diss.—Leyden.

STANNIUS, FRIEDRICH CHRISTOPH [*fl.* 1687] *respondent. See* LIMMER, C. P., *praeses.* Collegii Physic. disputatio sexta. 1687.

STAPEDIUS, HENRICUS [d. 1587] *See* SCHOLTZ, L. Consiliorum medicinalium ... liber singularis. 1610

STAPEL, REIMAR NIKOLAUS [*fl.* 1665] *respondent. See* MORHOF, D. G., *praeses.* Princeps medicus. 1665

STAPHORST, NICHOLAS [*fl.* 1676–1700] Officina chymica Londinensis; sive, Exacta notitia medicamentorum spagyricorum, quae apud aulam Societatis Pharmaceuticae Londin. praeparantur, & venalia prostant. Consilio pharmacopoeorum & approbatione Collegii Medicorum Londinensium exhibitum ... [Londini] Prostant venales apud Guiliel. Miller, 1685.

    [8], 145 p.; [30] p. 15 cm.   **[11392]**

"Catalogus medicamentorum quae in aula Pharmacopoeorum Londinensium praeparantur et venalia prostant" ([30] p.) has special title page.

—, *tr. See* RAUWOLFF, L. A collection of curious travels & voyages. 1693.

STARCK, Johann Elias [*fl.* 1676-1680] *respondent.* *See* Becmann, J. C., *praeses.* Dissertatio de prodigiis sanguinis. 1676.

STARCK, Nicolaus [*fl.* 1671] *respondent. See* Stryk, S., *praeses.* Disputatio juridica de jure coecorum. 1671.

STARESMORE, J. *See* Starsmare, J.

STARICIUS, Johannes [*fl.* 1618– *ca.* 1641] *ed. See* Paracelsus. Clavis. 1624 [and] Philosophia de limbo. 1618.

STARKEY, George [1627-1665] The admirable efficacy . . . of true oyl. *In* Collectanea chymica. 1684. A brief examination and censure of several medicines, of late years extol'd for universal remedies . . . by which the art of pyrotechny is in danger of being brought into reproach . . . London, Printed for the author, 1664.

[1], 42 p. 15 cm. **[11393]**

With this is bound Mayerne, *Sir* T. T. de. Tractatus de arthritide. 1676.

[−] Liquor alchahest; or, A discourse of that immortal dissolvent of Paracelsus & Helmont. It being one of those two wonders of art and nature, which radically dissolves all animals, vegitables and minerals into their principles, without being in the least alter'd, either in weight or activity, after a thousand dissolutions, etc. Published by J. A. Pyrophilus [pseud., i.e. James Astell] . . . London, Printed by T. R. & N. T. for W. Cademan, 1675.

[30], 55 p. front. 15 cm. **[11394]**

— Natures explication and Helmont's vindication; or, A short and sure way to a long and sound life, being a necessary and full apology for chymical medicaments, and a vindication of their excellency against those unworthy reproaches cast on the art and its professors (such as were Paracelsus and Helmont) by Galenists . . . London, Printed by E. Cotes for Thomas Alsop, 1657.

[63], 336 p. 16 cm. **[11395]**

— Pyrotechny asserted and illustrated, to be the surest and safest means for arts triumph over natures infirmities. Being a full . . . discovery of the medicinal mysteries studiously concealed by all artists, and only discoverable by fire. With an appendix concerning the nature, preparation . . . of several specifick medicaments . . . London, Printed by R. Daniel, for Samual Thomson, 1658.

[18], 172 p. 15 cm. **[11396]**

— [Dutch tr.] Pyrotechnia; ofte, Vuur-stook-kunde, vast-gesteld en opgehelderd, ofte het sekerste en veiligste middel om de konst te doen triumpheren over de natuurlijke gebreken . . . Met een aanhangsel, aangaande de nature . . . en kragten van verscheide specifique medicamenten . . . Uit het Engels vertaalt door J. vande Velde. Amsterdam, Jacob vande Velde, 1687.

[30], 192 p. front. 14 cm. **[11397]**

— *See* Philoctetes, E. Philadelphia; *or,* Brotherly love to the studious in the hermetick art. 1694.

[STARSMARE, J.] Παίδων νοσήματα; or, Childrens diseases, both outward and inward. From the time of their birth to fourteen years of age. With their natures, causes, signs, presages and cures. In three books . . . Also, the resolutions of many profitable questions concerning children, and of nurses, and of nursing children. By J. S[tarsmare], physician. London, Printed by W. G. and sold by J. Playford and Zach. Watkins, 1664.

[14], 176 p. front. 15 cm. **[11398]**

The initials J. S. are identified as those of J. Starsmare by G. F. Still in his History of paediatrics, London, 1931, p. [251]-260. The work was entered in the registers of the Stationers' Company, London, Nov. 13, 1663, as "By J. Starsmare, physician."

De **STATEN** van den lande van Utrecht. 1668. *See* Utrecht. Laws, statutes, etc.

STATLENDER, Theodor Friedrich [*fl.* 1683-1694] *praeses.* Sanguinis motus circularis ex veterum monumentis erutus . . . Oeniponti, Typis Jacobi Christophori Wagner [1694]

[4], 44 p. 19 cm. **[11399]**

Diss. — Innsbruck (F. C. Steiger, *respondent*)

STATUTA Collegii Medici Bruxellensis. *See* Collegie der Medecyne, Brussels.

STATUTA facultatis medicinae Parisiensis. *See* Université de Paris. Faculté de médecine.

STATUTA vetera, et nova . . . Collegii D. D. phylosophorum, et medicorum . . . Taurini. *See* Collegio dei filosofi e medici, Turin.

The **STATUTES** of the Colledge of Physicians London: worthy to be perused by all men, but more especially physicians, lawyers, apothecaries, surgeons, and all such that either do, or shall study, profess, or practise physick. [London] 1693.

[4], 12, 201 p. 16 cm.   [11400]

Latin and English.

Issued by John Badger in an attack on the College. Cf. G. Clark, History of the Royal College of Physicians, v. 2, p. 467.

STATUTI del venerabile Archiospidale di San Giacomo in Augusta. 1659 [1658] *See* OSPEDALE DI SAN GIACOMO in Augusta, Rome.

STAURINI, HERCOLE [*fl.* 1630] Trattato della peste ... Padova, Gasparo Crivellari, 1630.

[71] p. 19 cm.   [11401]

STEARNE, JOHN [1624-1669] Θανατολογια; seu, De morte dissertatio; in qua, mortis natura, causae ... ac variae de cadavere & anima separata controversiae enodantur ...Dublinii, Typis Gulielmi Bladen, & prostat venalis apud Georgium Sawbridg, 1659.

[16], 288, [8] p. 15 cm.   [11402]

STEARNE, JOHN [1660-1745] Tractatus de visitatione infirmorum, seu de eis parochorum officiis, quae infirmos et moribundos respiciunt. Londini, Prostant apud A. Baldwin, 1700.

[10], 120 p. 17 cm.   [11403]

STECCHINI, ALBERTO [*d.* 1631] *See* SGOBBIS DA MONTAGNANA, A. de. Nuovo, et universale theatro farmaceutico. 1667, 1682.

STECHAN, JOHANN [*fl.* 1675] *respondent. See* CRAUSE, R. W., *praeses.* Disputatio inauguralis medica de hernia scroti a prolapsu intestini orta. 1675.

STECHIUS, GODEFRIDUS. *See* STEEGHIUS, Godefridus [*fl.* 1579-ca. 1600]

STEEB, JOHANN CHRISTOPH [*fl.* 1663-1680] Coelum sephiroticum, Hebraeorum, per portas intelligentiae, Moysi revelatas interiores naturalium rerum characteres ... manifestans, ex vetustissima Hebraica veritate medicinae, chymiae, astronomiae, astrologiae, botanicae, zoologiae, anthropologiae, aliarumque scientiarum nova principia ... explicans ... Moguntiae, Sumptibus Ludovicii Bourgeat, typis Christophori Küchleri, 1679.

[4], 140, [16] p. illus. 34 cm.   [11404]

STEEGHIUS, GODEFRIDUS [*fl.* 1579-ca. 1600] Ars medica ... Tota conscripta methodo divisiva a

Galeno diversis locis proposita, commendata & exemplis illustrata, a recentioribus quibusdam clarissimis inchoata, sed a nemine hactenus absoluta ... Francofurti, Apud Claud. Marnium, & heredes Jo. Aubrii, 1606.

[19], 554, [36] p. port. 37 cm.   [11405]

Imperfect: p. [21-22] mutilated.

STEENBERGEN, HENDRIK À [*fl.* 1700] *respondent.* Dissertatio medica inauguralis de ictero ... Lugduni Batavorum, Apud Abrahammu [sic] Elzevier [1700]

21, [3] p. 19 cm.   [11406]

Imperfect: upper margins mutilated.

Diss.—Leyden.

STEENEVELT, CHRISTIAN A [*fl.* 1694] Dissertatio, de ulcere verminoso ad ... Godefridum Bidloo. Lugduni Batavor., Apud Jordanum Lugtmans, 1697.

[1], 24 p. plates. 19 cm.   [11407]

STEENSEN, NIELS. *See* STENO, Nicolaus, *Bp.* [1638-1686]

STEENWINKEL, PAULUS [*fl.* 1685-1693] *See* BEKKER, B. Brief ... aan ... Joannes Aalstius. 1693.

STEENWYCK, JOHANNES [*fl.* 1690] *respondent.* Disputatio medica inauguralis de chlorosi ... Trajecti ad Rhenum, Ex officina Francisci Halma, cIɔ Iɔc cx [i.e. 1690]

14, [2] p. 22 cm.   [11408]

The dissertation was defended on Jan. 16, 1690. Cf. Album Promotorum Academiae Rheno-Trajectinae 1636-1815. Trajecti ad Rhenum, 1936, p. 54.

Frans Halma was active in Utrecht around 1690.

Diss.—Utrecht.

STEER, JOHN, *tr. See* FABRICIUS VON HILDEN, W. Experiments in chyrurgerie: concerning combustions or burnings. 1643.

STEFANI, GIOVANNI [*fl.* 1624-1653] Opera universa, cum medicinae, philosophiae, tum cultioris literaturae studiosis apprime utilia: suprema manu recognita ... Venetiis, Apud Juntas, 1653.

[27], 533 (i.e. 531) p. 34 cm.   [11409]

Half title: Joannis Stephani ... Opera omnia.

—Ad incolumitatem diu servandam diagoge ... Venetiis, Apud haeredes Joannis de Salis, 1639.

[8], 44 p. 23 cm.   [11410]

Bound with *his* In Hippocratis Coi libellum De hominis structura commentarius. 1633.

—Cosmetice. *In* Prevost, J. Tractatus. 1656, 1666.

—Hippocratis Coi theologia, in qua Platonis, Aristotelis, et Galeni placita Christianae religioni consentanea exponuntur ... Venetiis, Apud haeredes Joannis de Salis, 1638.

[8], 62 p.   23 cm.   [11411]

Bound with *his* In Hippocratis Coi libellum De hominis structura commentarius. 1633.

—In Aristotelis libellum De conservatione sanitatis ad Alexandrum Magnum commentarius ... Venetiis, Apud haeredes Joannis de Salis, 1637.

[8], 39, [1] p.   23 cm.   [11412]

Contains excerpts from the pseudo-Aristotelian text in the Latin translation of Philippus Tripolitanus.
Bound with his In Hippocratis Coi libellum De hominis structura commentarius. 1633.

—In Hippocratis Coi Legem commentarius ... Venetiis, Apud haeredes Joannes de Salis, 1637.

[6], 26 p.   23 cm.   [11413]

Includes Janus Cornarius' Latin translation of Hippocrates' Lex. Stefani's commentary was republished in Venice in 1653 with his edition of the Greek text.
Bound with *his* In Hippocratis Coi libellum De hominis structura commentarius. 1633.

—In Hippocratis Coi libellum De hominis structura commentarius, in quo plurimae difficultates diluuntur ... Venetiis, Apud Marcum Antonium Brogiollum, 1633.

[10], 60, [18] p.   23 cm.   [11414]

Includes Nicolas Petreius' Latin translation of the Hippocratic text.
With this are bound six other works by the author: In Hippocratis Coi libellum De virginum morbis commentarius. 1635; In Hippocratis Coi Legem commentarius. 1637; Hippocratis Coi theologia. 1638; Pyrine; sive, De febris natura dialogus. 1639; In Aristotelis libellum De conservatione sanitatis ad Alexandrum Magnum commentarius. 1637; and Ad incolumitatem diu servandam diagoge. 1639.

—In Hippocratis Coi libellum De virginum morbis commentarius ... Accessere medico philosophica epistolia, carmina, sententia de vesicantibus, & medica consilia ... Venetiis, Apud Marcum Antonium Brogiollum, 1635.

[8], 97 (i.e. 87), [1] p.   23 cm.   [11415]

Includes Janus Cornarius' Latin translation of the De virginum morbis.
Bound with *his* In Hippocratis Coi libellum De hominis structura commentarius. 1633.

—Pyrine; sive, De febribus natura dialogus ... Venetiis, Apud haeredes Joannis de Salis, 1639.

[4], 15 p.   23 cm.   [11416]

Caption title: Πυρινε; sive De febris natura dialogus.
Mounted cancel (manuscript?) on title page correcting "febribus" to "febris."
Bound with *his* In Hippocratis Coi libellum De hominis structura commentarius. 1633.

—*See* PREVOST, J. De remediorum cum simplicium, tum compositorum materia. 1640.

STEFFECIUS, STEPHANUS. *See* STEFFEK A KOLODIEG, Stephan [*fl.* 1620]

STEFFECIUS A KOLODIEG, STEPHEN. *See* STEFFEK A KOLODIEG, Stephan [*fl.* 1620]

STEFFEK A KOLODIEG, STEPHAN [*fl.* 1620] *praeses.* Pentas medica miscella ... Basileae, Typis Joannis Schroeteri [1620]

[18] p.   18 cm.   [11417]

Diss.—Basel (J. Bröcking, *respondent*)

STEGER, WOLFGANG ABRAHAM [*d.* 1665] *praeses.* Disputationem physicam de nive ... ventilandam exponunt ... Valentinus Friderici Smalcald [Lipsiae] Typis Johannis Baueri [1652]

[16] p.   18 cm.   [11418]

Diss.—Leipzig (V. F. Smalcald, *respondent*)

STEGMAN, DAVID [*fl.* 1620] Kurtzer Tractat, von der hochgefahrlichen Kranckheit der Pestilentz, derselben Ursachen, Zaichen, wie man sich ... vor derselben bewahren, und da jemand darmit angegriffen, widerumb vertreiben und curiren möge ... Kempten, Bey Christoff Krausen, 1627.

[39] p.   17 cm.   [11419]

STEHELIN, *See* STAEHELIN.

STEIGER, FRANZ CAJETAN [*fl.* 1694] *respondent. See* STATLENDER, T. F., *praeses.* Sanguinis motus circularis ex veterum monumentis erutus. 1694.

STEIGERTHAL, JOHANN GEORG [*b. ca.* 1667] *respondent.* Dissertatio medica inauguralis de medicamentorum noxis ... Trajecti ad Rhenum, Ex officina Francisci Halma, 1690.

16 p.   22 cm.   [11420]

Diss.—Utrecht.

STEIN, GOTTFRIED [*fl.* 1675-1703] Wolgemeintes Consilium Antiloimicum; oder, Rathschlag, welcher gestalt man sich Zeit grassierender Pestilentz, sowohl in Praeservirung, dass gedachtes Ubel nicht so leichtlich einreisse; als auch in Curirung, wo es schon allbereit eingeschlichen, mit natürlichen Mitteln versehen und verhalten sol, auf Hoch-Fürstl. . . . Befehl, dem gemeinen Nutzen, sonderlich dem armen Land- und Bauers-Mann zum Besten, guten Theils aus . . . Paul de Sorbaits . . . 1679 heraus gegebenen Pest-Concilio gezogen und zum Druck verfertiget . . . Bayreuth, Gedruckt bei Johann Gebhard, 1680.

68 p. 19 cm. [11421]

—respondent. Disputatio medica inauguralis de paralysi scorbutica . . . Altdorfii, Typis Johannis Henrici Schönnerstaedt [1675]

28 p. 20 cm. [11422]
Diss.—Altdorf.

STEIN, Johann Joachim [*fl.* 1695] *respondent.* Disputatio medica inauguralis de morbis haereditariis . . . Lugduni Batavorum, Apud Abrahamum Elzevier, 1695.

[24] p. 20 cm. [11423]
Diss.—Leyden.

STEIN, Kaspar [*fl.* 1618] *respondent. See* Varus, A., *praeses.* Disputatio medica de quartana. 1618.

STEINER, Heinrich [1675–1760] *respondent.* Dissertatio chymico-medica inauguralis de antimonio . . . Basileae, Typis Jacobi Bertschii [1699]

[32] p. 20 cm. [11424]
Diss.—Basel.

— *See* Hottinger, S., *praeses.* Αρτολογια. 1696.

STEINICHER, Johann [*fl.* 1620–1623] *respondent. See* Sebisch, M. [1578–1674?] *praeses.* Disputatio de purgatione octava. 1621 [and] Disputatio de venae sectione vigesima octava. 1620 [and] Disputationes de recta ratione purgandi. 1621 [and] Exercitationes medicae. 1639.

STEININGER, Johann Albert [1598–1649] *respondent. See* Blum, M., *praeses.* Centuria positionum medicarum de melancholia hypochondriaca. 1625.

STELLA, Benedetto [17th cent.] Il tabacco opera . . . nella quale si tratta dell'origine, historia, coltura, preparatione, qualita, natura, virtu, & uso in fumo, in polvere, in foglia, in lambitivo, et in medicina della pianta volgarmente detta tobacco . . . Roma, Filippo Maria Mancini, 1669.

[32], 480 p. illus. 17 cm. [11425]

STELLUTI, Francesco [1577–*ca.*1651] *ed.* and *tr. See* Persius Flaccus, A. Persio tradotto in verso sciolto e dichiarato da Francesco Stelluti. 1630.

—, *ed. See* Porta, G. B. della. Della fisonomia di tutto il corpo humano. 1637.

STELTZNER, Johann Wolffgang [*fl.* 1684] *respondent. See* Bechmann, J. V., *praeses.* De coitu damnato. 1684.

STEMPEL, Christian [*fl.* 1668] *respondent. See* Bohn, J., *praeses.* Exercitationum physiologicarum prima . . . [-decima tertia] 1674?

STEMPEL, Christoph Ernst [*fl.* 1665–1666] *respondent. See* Friderici, J. A., *praeses.* Ordo et methodus cognoscendi & curandi gravissimum intestini tenuioris affectum ileum. 1666.

STENGEL, Carl [*fl.* 1607–1664] Αλεξητηιρον; id est, Historia pestis in qua ejus caussae, dirae grassationes, ac remedia . . . divinitus collata fuse enarrantur . . . Augustae Vindelicorum [Typis Chrysostomi Daberii, 1614]

[16], 126 p. illus. 17 cm. [11426]
Engraved title page.

STENGEL, Georg [1585–1651] De monstris et monstrosis, quam mirabilis, bonus, et justus, in mundo administrando, sit Deus, monstrantibus . . . Ingolstadii, Apud Gregorium Haenlin, sumtu Joannis Wagneri, 1647.

[16], 636, [51] p. 16 cm. [11427]

STENO, Nicolaus, *Bp.* [1638–1686] De musculis et glandulis observationum specimen. Cum epistolis duabus anatomicis. Amstelodami, Apud Petrum le Grand, [e typographia Pauli Warnaer] 1664.

[3], 90 p. plate. 14 cm. [11428]
Includes letters addressed to Paul Barbette and Willem Piso.

—[The same.] . . . Hafniae, Literis Matthiae Godicchenii, 1664.

[5], 84 p. 20 cm. [11429]
Added engraved title page.

—[The same.] . . . Lugd. Batav., Apud Jacobum Moukee, 1683.

[6], III p. illus. 14 cm. [11430]
Imperfect: title page mutilated.
Imprint partly supplied from Linden.

—Dissertatio de cerebri anatome . . . e Gallico exemplari Parisiis edito an. 1669. Latinitate donata, opera . . . Guidonis Fanoisii . . . Ludg. Batav., Apud Felicem Lopez, 1671.

[7], 64 p. 14 cm. [**11431**]

—Elementorum myologiae specimen; seu, Musculi descriptio geometrica. Cui accedunt canis carchariae dissectum caput, et dissectus piscis ex canum genere . . . Florentiae, Ex Typographia sub signo Stellae, 1667.

[8], 123 p. illus., plates. 30 cm. [**11432**]

—[The same.] . . . Amstelodami, Apud Johan. Janssonium a Waesberge, & viduam Elizei Weyerstraet, 1669.

148, [3] p. illus., plates. 17 cm. [**11433**]

—Observationes anatomicae, quibus varia oris, oculorum, & narium vasa describuntur novique salivae, lacrymarum & muci fontes deteguntur, et novum nobilissimi Bilsii de lymphae motu & usu commentum examinatur & rejicitur. Lugduni Batavorum, Apud Jacobum Chouët, 1662.

[12], 108 p. plates. 14 cm. [**11434**]

". . . Responsio ad vindicias hepatis redivivi, qua ela, quae in praesidem celeberr. Dn. Johannem van Horne, direxerat Clar. Antonius Deusingius, a Chesium authore excipiuntur, & evenida ostenduntur": p. [55]-78.

—[The same.] . . . Lugd. Batav., Apud Petrum de Graaf, 1680.

[12], 108 p. plates. 14 cm. [**11435**]

Different setting of type.

—*See* VESLING, J. Syntagma anatomicum. 1666, 1677, 1696.

STENONE, NICCOLÓ. *See* STENO, Nicolaus, *Bp.* [1638-1686]

STENONIS, NICOLAUS. *See* STENO, Nicolaus, *Bp.* [1638-1686]

STENSEN, NILS. *See* STENO, Nicolaus, *Bp.* [1638-1686]

STEPHAN, SAMUEL [*fl.* 1619] *praeses.* Disputatio medica de cerebri natura, ejusque affectibus praeter naturam . . . Giessae, Casparus Chemlinus [1619]

[23] p. 19 cm. [**11436**]

Diss.—Giessen (G. H. Botthius, *respondent*)

STEPHANIDES, ARCHIBALDUS [1629 or 30-1710] *respondent. See* HORNE, J. van, *praeses.* Dissertationis anatoicae de ductu chylifero. 1660.

STEPHANUS ALEXANDRINUS. *See* STEPHANUS ATHENIENSIS [7th cent.]

STEPHANUS ATHENIENSIS [7th cent.] *See* [STEPHANUS MAGNETES] Experiment Buch. 1623.

[**STEPHANUS MAGNETES**, 11th cent.] Experiment Buch; dass ist, Probierter unnd in mancherley Kranckheiten versuchter Artzneyen, Offenbahrung und Beschreibung, auss Dioscoride und Stephano Atheniense verteutschet und mit eigener Erfahrung sehr viel vermehret durch Rodolphum Goclenium . . . Franckfurt am Mayn, In Verlag Johan Carl Unckels, 1623.

[15], 408 p. 17 cm. [**11437**]

The present German translation of Stephanus Magnetes' Alphabeticum empiricum, sive Dioscoridis et Stephani Atheniensis . . . De remediis expertis liber, was made from Caspar Wolf's Latin version of a Greek MS presented to Konrad Gesner by Agostino Gadaldini. For the Greek text, cf. Diels. Also L. Thorndike, in *Janus*, v. 51 (1964) p. 20.

STEPHANUS PHILOSOPHUS. *See* STEPHANUS ATHENIENSIS [7th cent.]

STEPHANUS, HENRICUS. *See* ESTIENNE, Henri [1531-1598]

STEPHANUS, JOANNES. *See* STEFANI, Giovanni [*fl.* 1624-1653]

STEPHANUS, JOHANNES GUILHELMUS [*fl.* 1634-1635] *respondent. See* SEBISCH, M. [1578-1674?] *praeses.* Collegii therapeutici disputatio I[-XIV] 1634 [i.e. 1635] [and] Examen vulnerum partium similarium. 1635.

STEPHANUS, NICOLAUS [*fl.* 1661] Castigatio epistolae maledicae quam . . . Ludovicus De Bils scripsit ad Thomam Bartholinum . . . ubi Bilsianae artes deteguntur . . . Juxta exemplar Hafniensi . . . Amstelaedami, Apud Petrum van den Berge, 1661.

45, [1] p. 13 cm. [**11438**]

STEPHEN, *of Athens. See* STEPHANUS ATHENIENSIS [7th cent.]

STEPHENS, JOHN [*fl.* 1669] *respondent.* Disputatio medica inauguralis de sanitate . . . Lugduni Batavorum, Apud viduam & haeredes Joannis Elsevirii, 1669.

[11] p. 23 cm. [**11439**]

Diss. — Leyden.

STERBEECK, FRANCISCUS VAN [1631-1693] Theatrum fungorum; oft, Het tooneel der camper-noelien . . . Antwerpen, Joseph Jacobs, 1675.

[42], 906, [20] p. front., port., plates. 22 cm.

[11440]

STERNBERG, CHRISTOPH [*fl.* 1652] *respondent.* Disputatio medica inauguralis de suffocatione uteri . . . Lugduni Batavorum, Ex officina Jacobi Lauwicii, 1652.

[12] p. 23 cm. **[11441]**

Diss.—Leyden.

STERNBERGER, GOTTFRIED [*fl.* 1654] *respondent.* *See* SEIFERT, C., *praeses.* Ανεμολογια; sive, Dissertatio de ventis. 1654.

STERNE, JOHN. *See* STEARNE, John [1660-1745]

STERRE, D. L. *See* STERRE, Dionysius van der [*d.* 1691]

STERRE, DIONYSIUS VAN DER [*d.* 1691] Tractatus novus de generatione ex ovo, nec non de monstrorum productione; duabus epistolis comprehensus . . . Amstelodami, Apud Cornelium Blancardum [1687]

[3], 149 p. 13 cm. **[11442]**

Epistola de generatione ex ovo is addressed to Theodorus Craanen; Epistola de monstrorum generatione is addressed to Steven Blankaart.

Imperfect: lower margins trimmed.

—Verhandeling der genees-en heel-konstige prac-tyk der medicynen, steunende op d'onder-vinding van verscheyde aanmerkingen . . . Amsterdam, Jan ten Hoorn, 1687.

[16], 354, [6] p. 16 cm. **[11443]**

"Na-reden, geschreven aan . . . Stephanus Blankaart": p. 333-354.

—Voorstelling van de noodsaakelijkheid der keyserlijke snee, daar neven de verhandelinge van de teeling en baaring . . . Leyden, Daniel van Gaesbeek, 1682.

[1], 48 (i.e. 50), 154 p.; 258 (i.e. 286), [2] p. plates. 14 cm. **[11444]**

Imperfect: upper margins of plates preceding pages 101 and 117 of part [2] trimmed.

STERTHEM, JOSSE VAN [16th cent.] *tr. See* GUY DE CHAULIAC. De chirurgije. 1646.

STERTHEMIUS, JODOCUS. *See* STERTHEM, Josse van [16th cent.]

STETTER, JOHANN KONRAD [*fl.* 1662-1665] *respon-dent. See* ISRAEL, J., *praeses.* Disquisitio inauguralis medica de appetitu. 1662.

STEUBER, JOHANN HEINRICH [*fl.* 1679] *respondent. See* KAHLER, J., *praeses.* Dissertatio hydrographica de oceano ejusque proprietatibus & vario motu. 1679.

STEUDNER, THEODOR [*fl.* 1669] *respondent.* Disputatio medica inauguralis de auditus diminu-tione & abolitione . . . Ludguni Batavorum, Apud viduam & haeredes Joannis Elsevirii, 1669.

[20] p. 23 cm. **[11445]**

Diss.—Leyden.

STEVENSON, ARCHIBALD. *See* STEPHANIDES, Ar-chibaldus [1629 *or* 30-1710]

STIBER, FRIDERICUS [*fl.* 1645] *respondent. See* SEBISCH, M. [1578-1674?] *praeses.* Disputatio de naturalibus facultatibus prima [-octava & ultima] 1644 [i.e. 1645]

STIEBER, BERNHARDT [*fl.* 1625] *See* ROTHENBURG OB DER TAUBER. Ordinances, local laws, etc. Ern-stliche, trewhertzige Ordtnung. 1625.

STIEFEL, JOHANN REINHARD [*fl.* 1689] *respondent. See* WEDEL, G. W., *praeses.* Dissertatio medica in-auguralis de ileo. 1689.

STIERS wreetheydt, gepleeght aen meester ende vrou. En wonderlijck bestiert tot verlossingh hunnes kindts, geschiet tot Sardam. Amsterdam, By Fran-cois van Beusecum, 1647.

broadside. illus. 46 x 35 cm. **[11446]**

—[The same.] . . . Amsterdam, By Frans Sadelaar [1647?]

broadside. illus. 46 x 55 cm. **[11447]**

—[The same.] . . . [Amsterdam? 1647?]

broadside. illus. 23 x 28 cm. **[11448]**

STILLE, JOHANN ERNST [*fl.* 1658] *respondent. See* LÖBER, C. H., *praeses.* Disputatio physica de vita et morte. 1658.

STILSOVIUS, JOHANNES [*fl.* 1659] Alter und newer Schreibkalender, mit der Planeten Lauff, Fort-gang, und Adspecten: sambt dem Zustand dess Gewitters . . . Aderlassens, purgirens Artzneyens, und dergleichen . . . Calculirt, auff das M. DC. LX.

... Jahr ... Erffurdt, Gedruckt bey Martha Hertzin [1659?]

[32] p.   20 cm.   [11449]

With this is bound (as issued?) *his* Prognosticon astrologicum. [1659?]

—Prognosticon astrologicum; oder, Practica auff dass Jahr ... M. DC. LX. Darinnen zufinden 1. Vom Chromocratore, oder Regenten dess Jahre ... 5. Von einfallenden Kranckheiten, Pest, Seuchen und Sterben ... Erffurd, Gedruckt bey Martha Hertzin [1659?]

[23] p.   20 cm.   [11450]

Bound (as issued?) with *his* Alter und newer Schreibkalender, [1659?]

La STIMMIMACHIE. 1656. *See* CARNEAU, É.

STIPITE, LEO A. *See* STOCKLEU, Gottfried von [*d.* 1714]

STIRIUS, GEORGIUS FRIDERICUS [*fl.* 1668] *respondent. See* ETTMÜLLER, M., *praeses.* Dissertationem medicam de chirurgia infusoria ... p. p. G.F.S. 1668.

STIRNN, JAKOB [*fl.* 1686] *respondent. See* WALDSCHMIDT, J. J., *praeses.* Physicae curiosae et utilis specimen de sensibus. 1686.

STISSER, HEINRICH KARL [*fl.* 1664-1668] *respondent. See* CONRING, H., *praeses.* Disputatio medica inauguralis de febre maligna vulgo dicta Ungarica. 1668; MEIBOM, H., *praeses.* Theses medicae ex universa arte depromtae. 1668. TAPPE, J., *praeses.* Disputatio physiologica de somno naturali ejusque causis. 1664.

STISSER, JOHANN ANDREAS [1657-1700] Actorum laboratorii chemici ... in Academia Julia editorum specimen primum [-tertium] ... Helmestadii, Typis & sumptibus Georgii Wolfgangi Hammii, 1690-98.

3 parts in 1 v.   19 cm.   [11451]

Part [2] has date: 1693.

—Aquarum Hornhusanarum examen chemicophysicum ... Helmstadii, Typis Georg-Wolfgangi Hammii, 1689.

[21] p.   20 cm.   [11452]

—Commendatio chemiae ... Helmstadii, Apud Georg-Wolfgangum Hammiium, 1689.

[24] p.   20 cm.   [11453]

Imperfect: title page and p. [7-8] mutilated.

—De variis erroribus, chemiae ignorantia in medicina commissis dissertatio epistolaris ad ... Godefr. Guilielmum Leibnitium. Helmestadii, Typis Georg-Wolfgangi Hammii, 1700.

32 p.   19 cm.   [11454]

—Febrium intermittentium consideratio nova. Iatricae hodiernae placitis accommodata. Brunsvigae, Sumptibus Caspari Gruberi, 1687.

104, [1] p.   21 cm.   [11455]

Errata: p. [1]
Bound with Copy 2 of Rolfinck, W. Ordo et methodus cognoscendi & curandi febres generalis. 1658.

—Horti medici Helmstadiensis catalogus plantas omnes enumerans quarum culturam ab anno MDCXCII usque ad annum MDCXCIX in horto suo instituit ... Helmstadi, Typis Georg-Wolfgangi Hammii, 1699.

42 p.   16 cm.   [11456]

Imperfect: lower and outer margins trimmed.
Pritzel 8980*.

—Solamen arthriticorum; hoc est, De podagra nec non selectioribus quibusdam adversus eam remediis tractatus. Helmestadii, Typis Georg-Wolfgangi Hammii, 1690.   [11457]

STISSER, JOHANN CHRISTIAN [*fl.* 1697-1700] *respondent. See* BERGER, J. G. von, *praeses.* Dissertatio solennis de tympanite. 1700; VATER, C., *praeses.* De machinae humanae organis vitalibus. 1697.

STISSER, KONRAD [*fl.* 1686-1688] *respondent.* Disputatio medica inauguralis de lympha ejusque morbis ... Lugduni Batavorum, Apud Abrahamum Elzevier, 1688.

[28] p.   19 cm.   [11458]

Diss. — Leyden.

—*See* BOHN, J., *praeses.* Dissertatio medica de dyspnoea. 1686.

STISSER, STATIUS FRIEDRICH [*fl.* 1673] *respondent. See* TAPPE, J., *praeses.* Disputatio medica pathologica de sensus tactus depravatione. 1673.

STOCKAR, JOHANN. Empirica; sive, Medicamenta varia, experientia diuturna comprobata et stabilita, contra plerosque omnes corporis humani morbos ... in duos libros distributa ... primum inventa ... a D. Joanne Stockero ... in lucem edita, opera & studio Tobiae Dornkreilii ... Francoforti, Typis Melchioris Hartmanni, impensis Nicolai Bassai, 1601.

[16], 228, [1] p. 17 cm. [11459]

Bound with Gatinaria, M. De medendis humani corporis malis practica uberrima. 1604.

—Praxis aurea, ad corporis humani morbos omnes, tum internos, tum externos, quam recensuit, a mendis repurgavit, & commentariis ad obscuriora loca illustravit, opusque novum fecit, Adrianus Toll ... Lugduni Batavorum, Ex officina Joannis Maire, 1634.

[20], 361, [3] p. 13 cm. [11460]

—Praxis morborum particularium ... E posthumis monumentis nunc primum eruta, & luci publicae dedita. Francofurti, Typis Wolffgangi Richteri, sumptibus heredum Nicolaei Bassaei, 1609.

236, [17] p. 17 cm. [11461]

Bound with Gatinaria, M. De medendis humani corporis malis practica uberrima. 1604.

STOCKER, Johann. *See* Stockar, Johann.

STOCKHAMER, Franz [*fl.* 1677] Bibliotheca medico-philosophico-philologica inclytae nationis Germanae artistarum quae Patavii degit sub ... auspiciis ... bibliothecariis Francisco Stokhamer ... Andrea Bridler ... Patavii, Typis Pasquati, 1677.

[4], 150 (i.e. 154) p. 23 cm. [11462]

With this is bound Farnesius, Georg Theodor. Appendix bibliothecae medico philosophico philologicae. Patavii, 1680.

—Microcosmographia; sive, Partium humani corporis omnium earumque actionum & usuum brevis quidem, accurrata tamen & atoma descriptio novis hujus faeculi inventis exornata. Viennae Austriae, Typis Leopoldi Voigt, 1682.

[12], 244, [12] p. 14 cm. [11463]

Added engraved title page.
Imperfect: text of title mended.

STOCKHAUSEN, Julius Albert [*b.* 1659] *respondent. See* Wedel, G. W., *praeses.* Disputatio medica, aegrum haemoptysi laborantem exhibens. 1679 [and] Dissertatio inauguralis medica, de χλωρωσει; seu, Foedis virginum coloribus. 1681.

—*See* Wedel, G. W. Georgius Wolffgangus Wedelius ... Facultatis Medicae decanus, lectori benevolo S. P. D. 1681.

STOCKHAUSEN, Peter Christoph [*fl.* 1670] *respondent. See* Meibom, H., *praeses.* Disputatio medica inauguralis de haemorrhoidibus. 1670.

STOCKHOLM. Collegium medicum. *See* Collegium medicum, Stockholm.

STOCKLEU, Gottfried von [*d.* 1714] Leonis a Stipite ... Religio mentis pars prima [-secunda] editio emendatior ... Vratislaviae, Apud Joh. Georg. Steck, 1694.

2 v. ([8], 382 p.; [10], 840, 342, [2]) p. 20 cm. [11464]

Vol. 2 has imprint: Vratislaviae, In haeredum Baumanianorum, exprimebat Johannes Güntherus Rörerus, apud Joh. Georg. Steck, 1694.

STOCKMANN, Ernst [1634-1712] Hodegeticum pestilentiale sacrum; sive, Quaestiones quinquaginta ... de peste, generales & speciales, theoretico-practicae, animarum pastoribus in casibus istis periculosissimis ... necessariae ... Lipsiae, Sumpt. Georgii Henr. Frommanni, typis Johannis Georgii, 1667.

[48], 309 p. 13 cm. [11465]

Preface by Johannes Olearius.
Imperfect: title page mutilated.

—[The same.] ... Ed. 2. cui praeter Appendicem quaestionum accesserunt nuperrima rescripta & relationes de officio pastorum tempore pestis, ex consistoriis Saxonicis, electorali, Merseburgensi, & Cizensi. Cizae, Sumtu Joh. Bielckii, Jen.; Exscripsit Frideman Hetstedt, 1681.

[46], 310, [68] p. front. 14 cm. [11466]

Preface by Johannes Olearius.
Frontispiece has imprint: Frankf. u. Leipzig beij Joh. Bielcken in Jena, 1681.

STÖER, Johann Adam [*fl.* 1648] *respondent. See* Upilio, W., *praeses.* Viridarium medicum de febre maligna. 1648.

STÖER, Joannes Adamus. *See* Stöer, Johann Adam [*fl.* 1648]

STÖTTEROGGEN, Leonhard Georg von [*fl.* 1696] *respondent. See* Schoepffer, J. J., *praeses.* Disputatio juridica de haemorrhagia vulneratorum von Verblutung der Verwundeten. 1696.

STOFFEL, Georg Friedrich [*fl.* 1649] *respondent. See* Sebisch, M. [1578-1674?] *praeses.* Galeni quinque priores libri. 1651.

STOIUS, MATTHIAS [1526–1583] *See* SCHOLTZ, L. Consiliorum medicinalium ... liber singularis. 1610.

STOK in 't hondert, of toepassingh aen de krakkelende doctoren en chirurgyns van dese tijdt. [Amsterdam, 1677]

14 p.   16 cm.   [**11467**]

STOKHAMER, FRANCISCUS. *See* STOCKHAMER, Franz, *fl.* 1677.

STOLBERGK, JOHANN CHRISTIAN [*fl.* 1650–1655] *respondent. See* BARTHOLIN, T., *praeses.* Spicilegium ex vasis lymphaticis. 1655.

STOLL, DAVID [*fl.* 1649–1651] *respondent. See* DEUSING, A., *praeses.* Synopsis medicinae universalis. 1649; SEBISCH, M. [1578–1674?] *praeses.* Disputatio de pilis posterior. 1651.

STOLL, JOHANN ADOLPH [*b.* 1676] *respondent. See* WEDEL, G. W., *praeses.* Dissertatio inauguralis chimico-medica de mercurio dulci. 1700.

— *See* WEDEL, G. W. Propempticon inaugurale de resina Aegyptia Plauti. 1700.

STOLLIUS, DAVID. *See* STOLL, David [*fl.* 1649–1651]

STOLTERFOHT, JOHANN JACOB [1665–1718] Dissertatio epistolica de sudore sanguineo ... Lubecae, Literis Mauritii Schmalhertzii [1698?]

[24] p.   20 cm.   [**11468**]

— *praeses.* Disputatio medico-physica de idea errante in monstrorum generatione ... Gryphiswaldiae, Literis Danielis Benjaminis Starckii [1695]

[36] p.   20 cm.   [**11469**]

Diss.—Greifswald (D. G. Heisius, *respondent*)

— Physiologia in nuce ... Gryphiswaldiae, Litteris Danielis Benjaminis Starckii [1697]

[42] p.   20 cm.   [**11470**]

Diss.—Greifswald (S. A. Pfeiffer, *respondent*)

— *respondent. See* GERDES, J., *praeses.* Ideam errantem in ecstasi s. enthusiasmo conspicuam ... sistit ... J. J. S. 1692, 1693; PASCH, J., *praeses.* Dissertationem physicam de brutorum sensibus atque cognitione ... publice opponet ... J.J.S. 1686.

STOLTZ, GEORG ALBRECHT [*fl.* 1700–1707] *respondent. See* SAND, G., *praeses.* Fungus cerebri in generoso equitum Prussorum viro anno ... M DC XCVI inventus & extirpatus. 1700.

STORCK, ADOLPH [*fl.* 1655–1664] *ed. See* PREVOST, J. Johannis Prevotii Artem componendi medicamenta genuinae restitutam integritati exhibet Adolphus Storck. 1665.

STORCK, HENRICH ANTHON [*fl.* 1688] *respondent.* Disputatio medica inauguralis de alimentis, medicamentis et venenis ... Trajecti ad Rhenum, Ex officina Francisci Halma, 1688.

[16] p.   21 cm.   [**11471**]

Diss.—Utrecht.

STORCK, JOHANN CHRISTOPH [*fl.* 1685] *respondent.* Disputatio inauguralis medica de malo hypochondriaco ... Altdorffii, Literis Henrici Meyeri [1685]

32 p.   19 cm.   [**11472**]

Diss.—Altdorf.

STORMS, JEAN. *See* STURMIUS, Joannes [1559–1650]

STORTI, GASPARO [*fl.* 1682] *See* BARBETTE, P. Opera chirurgica. 1682, 1692, 1696.

STOTMEISTER, JOACHIM [*fl.* 1607] *See* KNOBLOCH, T., *praeses.* Disputationes anatomicae. 1608, 1612.

STRANGEHOPES, SAMUEL [*fl.* 17th cent.] A book of knowledge in three parts. The first, containing a brief introduction to astrology ... The second, a treatise of physick, the anatomy of mans body, the diseases ... rules and receipts ... The third, the countrey-mans guide to good husbandry, rules for ... planting of orchards, gardens ... also an almanack ... London, Printed by G. P. for Tho. Passinger, 1671.

[16], 128, [16] p.   illus.   15 cm.   [**11473**]

Imperfect: upper margins trimmed.

STRASBURG, JOHANN GEORG [1621–1681] *praeses.* De dolore colico positiones medicas ... Basileae, Typis Georgii Deckeri [1650]

[8] p.   19 cm.   [**11474**]

Diss.—Basel (J. H. Glaser, *respondent*)

STRASBURG, JOHANN THEODOR [*fl.* 1696–1699] *respondent.* Disputatio medica inauguralis de cachexia ... Ludguni Batavorum, Apud Abrahamum Elzevier, 1699.

[20] p.   24 cm.   [**11475**]

Diss.—Leyden.

— *See* HARWECK, A., *praeses.* Dissertatio medica, de affectu hypochondriaco. 1696.

STRASELIUS, Franciscus [*fl.* 1659] *respondent.*
Disputatio medica inauguralis de calculo renum &
vesicae ... Lugduni Batavorum, Apud Petrum Leffen, 1659.
[16] p. 22 cm. **[11476]**
Diss. — Leyden.

STRATEN, Gerard van der [*fl.* 1659] *respondent.*
Disputatio medica inauguralis, de dysenteria ...
Lugduni Batavorum, Ex officina Francisci Hackii,
1659.
[8] p. 21 cm. **[11477]**
Diss. — Leyden.

STRATEN, Willem van der [1593-1681] Disputationes medicae tres de erroribus popularibus, de
fallaci urinarum judicio. *In* Joannes Actuarius. De
urinis libri VII. 1670.

—*See* Eygel, A. Apologema pro urinis humanis.
1672.

STRAUCH, Johann [*fl.* 1655] *respondent. See*
Michaelis, J., *praeses.* Disputatio medica de rosa.
1655.

[STRAUSS, Johann Christoph] 1645-1718. Thermae Carolinae. Lipsiae, Apu Jo. Frider.
Gleditschium, 1695.
124, [1] p. 16 cm. **[11478]**
Errata: p. [125]

—Beschreibung des Carls-Bades ... in lateinischer Sprache heraus gegeben, und nunmehro
... ins Deutsche übersetzt. Leipzig, Verlegts Joh.
Friedrich Gleditsch und im Carls-Bade zu finden bey
Joh. George Bachman, 1695.
166, [2] p. 16 cm. **[11479]**
Imperfect: lower margin of title page trimmed.

—*respondent. See* Schneider, K. V., *praeses.* Cachexiam ... publice disputandam sistit ... J.C.S. 1669.

STRAUSS, Laurentius [1603-1687] Epistola ad
... Dygbaeum.
127-142 p. 21 cm. (*In* Theatrum sympatheticum
auctum. Norimbergae, 1662) **[11480]**
Running title.

—Exercitatio physica de ovo galli. Gissae, Typis
Friderici Kargeri, 1669.
[1], 40 p. 20 cm. **[11481]**

—Judicia varia celeberriorum virorum de foetus
Mussipontani explicatione. *In* Historia foetus
Mussipontani. 1669; Sinibaldi, G. B. Genean-
thropeiae. 1669.

—Palaestra medica, plurimorum humani corporis
affectuum P. N. cognitionem, atque curationem jux-
ta principia non solum antiquorum, Hippocratis,
Galeni etc. sed etiam recentiorum, Helmontii,
Willisii, Sylvii, & aliorum, inter se collata ...
Trutinaque rationis & experientiae examinata, suc-
cincte exhibens. Gissae, Inpensis & typis Henningi
Mülleri, 1686.
[11], 384 p.; 176 p.; 464, [3] p. 17 cm.**[11482]**
Added engraved title page.

—Resolutio casus Mussipontani foetus extra
uterum in abdomine retenti; cum annexis Judiciis
celeberrimorum virorum. Ed. alt. cui accessit Antonii Deusingii Consideratio physico-anatomica
ejusdem foetus cum replica Strausii & Epistola Joh.
Christophori Eisenmengeri cum responso Joh.
Danielis Horstii ... Darmstadii, Typis Christophori
Abelii, 1662.
[1], 249 p. 20 cm. **[11483]**
Imperfect: title page backed and mended.

—Responsum ad examen pulveris sympathetici
... Deusingii. *In* Digby, *Sir* K. Demonstratio immortalitatis animae rationalis. 1664.

Dissertations — Giessen
—*praeses.* Conatus anatomicus, aliquot disputationibus exhibitus. Gissae Hassorum, Typis Josephi
Dieterici Hampelii, 1666.
[8], 144 p. 21 cm. **[11484]**
Includes seven Giessen theses.

—Conatus anatomici specimen quartum; seu,
Disputatio de ventriculo ... Giessae Hassorum,
Typis Josephi Dieterici Hampelii, 1664.
[2], 49 — 72 p. 19 cm. **[11485]**
Pages 49 — 72 are also included in the same setting of type in
L. Strauss' Conatus anatomicus published in Giessen in 1666.
Diss. — Giessen (J. P. Fabricius, *respondent*)

—Disputatio medica, de suffocatione uterina ...
Gissae Hassorum, Typis Friderici Kargeri [1665]
32 p. 20 cm. **[11486]**
J. P. Gieswein, *respondent.*

—Disputatio physico-medica de potu coffi . . . Giessae Hassorum, Typis Friederici Kargeri, 1666. [2], 15 (i.e. 16), [2] p. illus. 19 cm. [**11487**]

F. Peters, *respondent.*

—Dissertatio medica, de necessaria morbi cognitione ad curandum . . . Gissae Hassorum, Typis Friderici Kargeri, 1675. 24 p. 19 cm. [**11488**]

J. Schilling, *respondent.*

—Physicarum quaestionum decas de elementis . . . Gissae, Litteris Friderici Kargeri [1673] [4], 16 p. 20 cm. [**11489**]

Diss.—Giessen (H. Niemand, *respondent*)

—*See* SCHENCK VON GRAFENBERG, J. Observationum medicarum rariorum, libri VII. 1644; THEATRUM SYMPATHETICUM. 1660, 1661, 1662.

STREITLEIN, JOHANN DAVID [*fl.* 1685–1688] *respondent.* Disputationem inauguralem de dentitione . . . exponet . . . Johann David Streitlein . . . Altdorffii, Literis Schönnerstaedtianis [1688] 22, [2] p. 20 cm. [**11490**]

Diss.—Altdorf.

STREITTER, JOHANN HULDERICH [*fl.* 1612–1618] *respondent.* Disputatio inauguralis de gravissimo cerebri affectu epilepsia . . . Giessae, Typis Casparis Chemlini, 1617. [75] p. 19 cm. [**11491**]

Diss.—Giessen.

—*See* HORST, G. [1578–1636] Dissertatio de causis similitudinis . . . in foetu. 1618.

STREVARZIUS, BOMBARDUS. *See* SCLOPETARIUS, B. De peditu. 1671.

STRICER, JOHANN [*fl.* 1665] *respondent. See* ZIEGRA, C., *praeses.* Disputatio physica de monstro. 1665.

STRIJCK op den bruy een sesjen. [n. p., 1677] [2] p. 16 cm. [**11492**]

Poem concerning the controversy between Andreas Boekelman and Bonaventura van Dortmont.

STROBELBERGER, JOHANN STEPHAN [1592 *or* 3–1630] Brevissima manuductio ad curandos pueriles affectus . . . Norimbergae, Typis Abrahami Wagenmanni, 1625. [5], 66 p. 16 cm. [**11493**]

Bound with copy 2 of Hafenreffer, S. Raphael artem medicam explanans. 1629.

—[The same.] . . . Ed. 2. auct. & corr. Lipsiae, Impens. Eliae Rehefeldii & Joann. Grossi, 1629. [6], 58 p. 17 cm. [**11494**]

Bound with copy 2 of Varanda, J. de. Tractatus de affectibus renum et vesicae. 1617.

—De dentium podagra; seu, Potius de 'οδοντάγρα, doloreve dentium, tractatus absolutissimus . . . Cum collectaneorum, dolori, & extractioni dentium ab autoribus dicatorum appendice. Lipsiae, Impensis Johannis Grosii, typis exscribebat Justus Jansonius, 1630. [1], 238 p. 16 cm. [**11495**]

Imperfect: title page mutilated.

—Dissertationes succinctae de peste tyronibus medicinae in studio Parisiensi privatim quondam praelectae, nunc in eorundem gratiam publici juris factae in quibus brevi & facillima doctrina recensetur, quitquid fere de pestis natura passim apud autores controversum est. Norimbergae, Typis Abrahami Wagenmanni [1625] [55] p. 16 cm. [**11496**]

Imprint partly supplied from Linden.

—Epistolaris concertatio super variis . . . quaestionibus, febrim malignam seu petechialem concernentibus . . . inter D. Joan-Stephanum Strobelbergerum . . . et D. Joachimum Burserum . . . Annexa est & disceptatio de venenorum natura . . . habita inter eundem D. Burserum et M. Valentinum Hertelium . . . Lipsiae, Sumtibus Zachariae Schüreri & Matthiae Götzen, excudebat Gregorius Ritzsch, 1625. [264] p. 16 cm. [**11497**]

Imperfect: title page mutilated.

—Kurtze Instruction und Bad-Regiment, wie das Keyser Carls Bad, sampt guter Diaet zu gebrauchen, etc. Nürnberg, Gedruckt bey Wolffgang Endter, 1630. [28] p. 20 cm. [**11498**]

With this is bound Ein sehr nöttiger Zettel. 1617.

—[The same.] . . . Anjetzo auff das newe an das Liecht gebracht . . . Prag, Gedruckt durch Johann Michael Störitz, zufinden bey Andreas Becher in Carls-Bad, 1692. [1], 36, [1] p. 16 cm. [**11499**]

Bound (as issued?) with Hüllinger, W. Hydriatria Carolina. 1692.

—Mastichologia; seu, De universa mastiches natura dissertatio medica ... Declaratis insuper quibusdam dubiis, ac obscuris autorum lectionibus dicteriisque ... Lipsiae, Impensis Eliae Rehefeldt & Joh. Grosii, typis exscribebat Justus Jansonius, 1628.

[2], 109 p. 16 cm. [11500]

—Recens nec antea sic visa Galliae politica-medica descriptio, in qua de qualitatibus ejus, academiis celebrioribus, urbibus praecipuis ... aquis medicatis ... plantis & herbis ... disseritur ... Jenae, Typis & sumptibus Johan. Beithmanni, 1620.

271 p. 13 cm. [11501]

With this is bound Tommasi, Francesco. Dignitates aphoristicae in re medica. Romae, 1589.

—Systematica universae medicinae adumbratio ... Lipsiae, Impensis Eliae Rehefeldii & Joh. Grosii, typis exscribebat Justus Jansonius, 1627.

[118] p. 17 cm. [11502]

Bound with Gellius, A. Noctes atticae. 1603.

—Tractatus novus in quo de cocco baphica, & quae inde paratur confectionis Alchermes recto usu disseritur. Cui insertus est Laurentii Catelani genuinus ejusdem confectionis apparandae modus, nunc primum in Latinum sermonem e Gallico breviter conversus. Cum censura & approbatione Joannes ab Oberndorff ... Jenae, Typis Johannis Beithmanni, 1620.

[107] p. table. 21 cm. [11503]

—, ed. See SOMMER, F. Thermae Carolinae. 1647.

STRÖSSENREUTER, JOHANN [*fl.* 1624] *respondent. See* INNICHENHÖFER, H., *praeses.* Υπνολογια; sive, Tractatus jucundus physiologicus. 1624.

STROMAIR, HIERONIMUS [*fl.* 1577–1582] *See* SCHOLTZ, L. Consiliorum medicinalium ... liber singularis. 1610.

STROMAYERUS, HIERONYMUS. *See* STROMAIR, Hieronimus [*fl.* 1577–1582]

STROMERUS, HIERONIMUS. *See* STROMAIR, Hieronimus [*fl.* 1577–1582]

STROZA, KYRIACUS. *See* STROZZI, Ciriaco [1504–*ca.* 1565]

STROZZI, CIRIACO, [1504–*ca.* 1565] Libri duo politicorum Graeco Latini. *In* Aristoteles. Τὰ σωζόμενα. Operum ... nova editio. 1605 [1606]

STRUŚ, JÓZEF. *See* STRUTHIUS, Josephus [1510–1568]

STRUTHIUS, JOSEPHUS [1510–1568] Ars sphygmica; seu, Pulsuum doctrina supra M. CC. annos perdita, et desiderata ... libris V. conscripta, & iam primum aucta. Accessit Hieronymi Capivaccei De pulsibus elegans tractatus, & Caspari Bauhini Introductio pulsuum synopsin continens. Basileae, Impensis Ludovici Königs, 1602.

[20], 23, [4], 460, [17] p. illus., table. 17 cm. [11504]

Errata: p. [17] at end.
Imperfect: title page mutilated.

—, *tr. See* NAVARRO, J. B. Commentarii ad libros Galeni De differentiis febrium. 1651.

STRUVE, ERNST GOTTHOLD [*b.* 1679] *respondent. See* STAHL, G. E., *praeses.* Dissertatio medico-semiotica de facie morborum indice. 1700.

STRUVE, JOHANN CHRISTOPH [*fl.* 1695] *respondent. See* CRAUSE, R. W., *praeses.* Disputatio inauguralis medica, exhibens aegrum bulimicum. 1695.

STRUVE, JOHANN PHILIPP [*fl.* 1671–1675] *respondent. See* CRAUSE, R. W., *praeses.* Diatribe inauguralis medica ... de fonticulis. 1675.

STRUZIO, GIUSEPPE. *See* STRUTHIUS, Josephus [1510–1568]

STRYGES DE RUSSIE. *See* SUR LES STRYGES DE RUSSIE. 16--?

STRYK, ELIAS AUGUST [*fl.* 1687–1698] *praeses.* Disputatio juridica de matrimonio ex ratione status, von Staats-Heyrathen ... Kiloni, Typis Joachimi Reumanni [1691]

[48] p. 21 cm. [11505]

Diss.—Kiel (J. Wohlmuth, *respondent*)

STRYK, SAMUEL [1640–1710] *praeses.* Disputatio juridica de jure coecorum ... Francofurti ad Viadrum, Literis Johann Ernesti [1671]

[56] p. 20 cm. [11506]

Diss.—Frankfurt an der Oder (N. Starck, *respondent*)

STUBBE, HENRY. *See* STUBBS, Henry [1632–1676]

STUBBS, HENRY [1632–1676] A censure upon certain passages contained in the history of the Royall Society, as being destructive to the established religion and the Church of England. The 2. ed. corr.

and enlarged. Whereunto is added the letter of a virtuoso in opposition to the censure, a reply unto the letter aforesaid, and a reply unto the praefatory answer of Ecebolius Glanvill ... Also an answer to the letter of Dr. Henry More, relating unto Henry Stubbe physician ... Oxford, Richard Davis, 1671.

    47 p.; 79, [1] p.   21 cm.   **[11507]**

Part [2] has special title page: A reply unto the letter written to Mr. Henry Stubbe in defence of the history of the Royal Society. Whereunto is added a preface against Ecebolius Glanvill; and an answer to the letter of Dr. Henry More.

Manuscript notes in the margins of part [2] of NLM's copy by James Arderne identify him as the author of The letter to Mr. Henry Stubs (p. 3-11, part [2]), according to a statement by E. N. da C. Andrade, attached to the work.

With this is bound (between part [1] and [2]) Term catalogues. A catalogue of books continued, printed and published at London. [1676]

—Directions for such as drink the bath-water. *In* Hall, J. Select observations on English bodies. 1679, 1683.

[—] Lex talionis; sive, Vindiciae pharmacoporum; or, A short reply to Dr. Merrett's book; and others, written against the apothecaries, wherein may be discovered the frauds and abuses committed by doctors professing and practising pharmacy ... London, Moses Pitt, 1670.

    [6], 32 p.   21 cm.   **[11508]**

Imperfect: first preliminary leaf (blank?) wanting.

Generally attributed to Stubbs, but the author or authors seem to have been apothecaries. Cf. R. S. Roberts. Jonathan Goddard. Medical History. vol. 8, 1964, p. 191.

—[The same.] *In* Merret, C. The accomplished physician. 1670.

—The Lord Bacons relation of the sweating-sickness examined, in reply to George Thomson ... Together with a defence of phlebotomy in general, and also particularly in the plague, smallpox, scurvey, and pleurisie. In opposition to the same author, and ... Doctor Whitaker, and Doctor Sydenham. Also A relation concerning the strange symptomes happening upon the bite of an adder. And a reply, by way of Preface to the calumnies of ... Glanvile ... London, Phil. Brigs, 1671.

    [10], 27 p.; [7], 259 (i.e. 260) p.; [6], 11 p.; 32 p.   23 cm.   **[11509]**

Part [2] has special title page: An epistolary discourse concerning phlebotomy; part [3] has special title page: A relation of the strange symptomes happening by the bite of an adder. Part [4] has caption title: A preface to the reader.

—Another issue, with title: A Bacon-face no beauty; or, A reply to George Thomson.   **[11510]**

[—] Medice cura teipsum; or, The apothecaries plea in some short and modest animadversions, upon a late tract entituled A short view of the frauds and abuses of the apothecaries, and the onely remedy by physicians making their own medicines, by Christopher Merret ... London, Printed for W. Miller, 1671.

    [1], 50 p.   20 cm.   **[11511]**

—The miraculous conformist; or, An account of severall marvailous cures performed by the stroaking of the hands of Mr Valentine Greatarick; with a physicall discourse thereupon, in a letter to ... Robert Boyle ... Oxford, Printed by H. Hall for Ric. Davis, 1666.

    [7], 44 (i.e. 40) p.   plate.   27 cm.   **[11512]**

Sheets inlaid and pasted on tabs.

—The plus ultra reduced to a non plus; or, A specimen of some animadversions upon the plus ultra of Mr. Glanvill, wherein sundry errors of some virtuosi are discovered, the credit of the Aristotelians in part re-advanced; and enquiries made about ... the use of chymical medicaments ... London, The author, 1670.

    [15], 179 p.   22 cm.   **[11513]**

Special title page (p. [15]) reads: A specimen of some animadversions upon a book, entituled, Plus ultra.

Imperfect: lower margin of title page trimmed.

—*See* A letter to Mr. Henry Stubs. 1670; TRYE, Mrs. M. Medicatrix. 1675.

STUBENDORFF, JOSEF. *See* EUGALENUS, S. De scorbuto morbo liber. 1604, 1623 [i.e. 1624?], 1658.

STUBENRAUCH, JOHANN RUDOLF [*fl.* 1687-1688] *respondent. See* LIMMER, C. P., *praeses.* Collegii Physici disputatorii disputatio quinta. 1687 [and] Disputatio physica extraordinaria de unione mentis humanae. 1688.

STUBNERUS, GEORGIUS ALBERTUS. *See* STÜBNER, Albert Georg [*fl.* 1699-1700]

STUBS, HENRY. *See* STUBBS, Henry [1632-1676]

STUCKEL, GODOFRIED. *See* STUCKLEW, Godefridus [17th cent.]

STUCKLEW, GODEFRIDUS [17th cent.] Indago pestis, qua luis hujus a putredine cadaverosa conceptae genesis, adultae metamorphosis expenditur adjectis nonnullis observationibus argumentum roborantibus; obiter una nodosum dogma de principiis corporum naturalium pro virili enodatur ... Vratislaviae, In Officina Baumanniana, typis exprimebat Joannes Güntherus Roererus, 1699.

[4], 154 (i.e. 254), [3] p.   20 cm.   [11514]
Errata: [3] p. at end.

STUDBROCKIUS, BERNARDUS, *pseud. See* FABRI, Honoré [1606–1688]

STÜBNER, ALBERT GEORG [*fl.* 1699–1700]

Dissertations — Wittenberg

—*praeses.* De lunae viribus in haec inferiora et inprimis oceanum ... [Witenbergae] Prelo Christiani Kreusigii [1700]
[26] p.   20 cm.   [11515]
F. K. Hagen, *respondent.*

—Dissertatio physica de nigritarum affectionibus ... [Wittenbergae] Prelo Christiani Kreusigii [1699]
[16] p.   19 cm.   [11516]
J. K. Wolff, *respondent.*

—Ex historia et scientia naturali de animalibus noctu videntibus ... [Vitembergae] Prelo Christiani Kreusingii [1700]
[16] p.   19 cm.   [11517]
G. T. Beccius, *respondent.*

—Novem ex philosophia naturali paradoxa, de corporibus mundi totalibus ... Vitembergae, Prelo Christiani Kreusigii [1700]
[8] p.   19 cm.   [11518]
G. B. Klett, *respondent.*

—*respondent. See* ROESCHEL, J. B., *praeses.* Paradoxorum physicorum dodecas. 1699.

STULL, JEAN [*fl.* 1606] Medendi practica generalis, in tres fasciculos contracta ... Ursellis, Typis Cornelii Sutorii; prostant Antverpiae, in bibliopolio Gasparis Belleri, 1606.
[23], 191, [1] p.   13 cm.   [11519]
Imperfect: p. 97–120 wanting.
Includes letter addressed to Petrus Rapaertius.

STUMPF, LUDWIG HERMANN [*fl.* 1682] *respondent. See* CROLL, J. L., *praeses.* Dissertatio academica prima, de esu carnium humanarum ejusque moralitate. [1682]

STUMPHIUS, LUDOVICUS HERMANNUS. *See* STUMPF, Ludwig Hermann [*fl.* 1682]

STUPAN, JOHANN NICOLAUS [*fl.* 1634] *respondent. See* SEBISCH, M. [1578–1674?] *praeses.* Collegii therapeutici disputatio I [-XIV] 1634 [i.e. 1635]

STUPANUS, EMMANUEL [1587–1664]

Dissertations — Basel

—*praeses.* Disputatio medica in universam physiologiam ... Basileae, Typis Georgii Deckeri [1660]
[20] p.   22 cm.   [11520]
N. Eglinger, *respondent.*

—Disputatio physico-medica de humanae mentis facultatibus ... Basileae, Typis Georgii Deckeri [1660]   [11521]
D. Gysendörffer, *respondent.*

—Disputationum menstruarum medicarum exercitatio IIX. & ultima de virilium affectibus cognoscendis ... Basileae, Typis Joh. Jacobi Genathii, 1616.
[8] p.   19 cm.   [11522]
J. S. Küffler, *respondent.*

—Signorum medicorum doctrina, annexa sphygmice, uromantia & crisium theoria, ex praecipuis Galen. & Hippocr. monumentis semeioticis excerpta ... Basileae, Typis Georgii Deckeri, 1649.
[28] p.   22 cm.   [11523]
J. K. Bauhin, J. N. Binninger, M. Birr, J. H. Glaser, E. Hurter, J. Rüdin, J. N. Stupanus, B. Verzasca, *respondents.*

—Theses physico-medicae de lacte ... Basileae, Typis Georgii Deckeri [1659]
[12] p.   20 cm.   [11524]
H. J. Ziegler, *respondent.*

—Τοῦ κατὰ την καρδίαν παλμοῦ διαγνώσεώς τε καὶ θεραπείας διάσκεψις. Basileae, Typis Joh. Jacobi Genathii, 1616.
[24] p.   22 cm.   [11525]
H. Pfendler, *respondent.*

—*respondent. See* STUPANUS, J. N., *praeses.* Σημιωτιces particularis cap. I. De affectibus. 1610.

—, *ed. See* CASTELLI, B. Lexicon medicum Graeco-Latinum. 1628; FUCHS, L. Institutionum medicinae. 1618; RIOLAN, J. [1538?–1605?] Artis medicinalis ... systema. 1629.

STUPANUS, JOHANN NIKLAUS [1542–1621] Gratiosi medicorum Basiliens. collegii decreto jussuque, Joan. Nicolaus Stupanus agonothetes rite electus: doctissimis ... viris, simul & juvenibus, ordinem hunc sorte, & bona fide, citra eruditionis praejudicium ullum obtinentibus, nempe D. Melchiori Sebizio ... Joanni Schallero ... Gulielmo Buleto ... Andreae Malacredae ... Henrico de Fehr ... postquam de somni vigilaeque essentia ... quam ad bonam valetudinem conservandam laedendamque, obtinent. Publici speciminis causa disseruerint: Asclepiadaeos honores, docturaeque medicae ornamenta ... collaturus ... ad XXVI. Junii diem indicta ... Basileae, Typis Johannis Schroeteri, 1610.
    broadside.   34 x 23 cm.   **[11526]**
  Bound with Bauhin, K. Assertiones medicae de catarrho. 1610.

—Medicina theorica: ex Hipp. & Galen. physiolog. patholog. semeioticis libris, post diexodicam enarrationem summatim pro disputationibus ordinariis in theses contracta; nunc demum aucta & correcta conjuctim edita. Basileae, Typis Johannis Schroeteri, 1614.
    [16], 822, [12] p.   17 cm.   **[11527]**

Dissertations — Basel

—*praeses.* Casus medicus theoricopracticus de anasarca ... Basileae, Per Joan. Jacob. Genathium, 1608.
    [16] p.   20 cm.   **[11528]**
  J. Franck, *respondent.*

—De comatibus somnolento ac vigili, theses medicae ... Basileae, Typis Johan. Jacobi Genathii, 1613.
    [28] p.   19 cm.   **[11529]**
  D. Schobinger, *respondent.*

—De febre ephemera. Basileae, Typis Joannis Schroeteri, 1606
    [7] p.   19 cm.   **[11530]**
  G. Rumbaum, *respondent.*

—De morbo subitaneo, quem apoplexiam seu totius corporis resolutionem vocant ... Basileae, Typis Joannis Schroeteri, 1606.
    [15] p.   22 cm.   **[11531]**
  J. Küffer, *respondent.*

—De rubus praeternaturam ὑπομνηματισμος pathologicos ... Melchior Schönwälder ... committit ... Basileae, Typis Joan. Schroeteri, 1607.
    [16] p.   23 cm.   **[11532]**
  M. Schönwalder, *respondent.*

—Discursus medicus febrium naturam ac differentias ... explicans ... Basileae, Typis Joannis Schröteri, 1609.
    [16] p.   20 cm.   **[11533]**
  G. Mättig, *respondent.*
  With this is bound Ryff, P. Gratiosus ... ordo medic. Basileens. 1610.

—Exercitatio physico-medica, de concoctionum trium, constitutione naturali ... Basileae, Typis Johannis Schroeteri, 1612.
    [28] p.   20 cm.   **[11534]**
  P. Blandin, *respondent.*

—Positiones iatricae de phrenitide ... Basileae, E typographeio Jani Schroeteri, 1607.
    [19] p.   20 cm.   **[11535]**
  J. W. Krapff, *respondent.*
  With this are bound: Heimbach, J. von. Specimen inaugurale. 1610; Platter, F. Felix Plateus ... decreto. [1610]

—Σημειωτιces particularis cap. I. De affectibus, quibus, cerebrum obnoxium est, & quibus signis cognoscantur ... Basileae, Ex officina Joannis Schroeteri, 1610.
    [36] p.   20 cm.   **[11536]**
  G. Buletus, Z. Dolder, J. J. Friese, A. Hendel, A. Malacreda, A. Pape, J. B. Rivius, E. Stupanus, *respondents.*

—Theses cheirurgicae de ulceribus ... Basileae, Typis Johannis Schroeteri, 1604.
    [14] p.   20 cm.   **[11537]**
  M. Lembka, *respondent.*

—Theses medicae de arthritide ... Basileae, Typis Joannis Schroeteri, 1606.
    [44] p.   20 cm.   **[11538]**
  J. B. Schonholtzer, *respondent.*

STUPANUS, JOHANN NIKLAUS [*fl.* 1649] *respondent. See* STUPANUS, E., *praeses.* Signorum medicorum doctrina. 1649.

STUPPA, JOHANN NIKLAUS. *See* STUPANUS, Johann Niklaus [1542–1621]

STURM, JOANNE. *See* STURMIUS, Joannes [1559–1650]

STURM, JOHANN CHRISTOPH [1635-1703] Collegium experimentale sive, curiosum, in quo primaria hujus seculi inventa & experimenta physicomathematica . . . partim ab aliis jam pridem exhibita, partim noviter istis superaddita per ultimum quadrimestre anni M.DC.LXXII viginti naturae scrutatoribus, ex parte illustri nobilique prosapia oriundis . . . et ad causas suas naturales demonstrativa methodo reduxit, quodque nunc . . . amicorum quorundam suasu & consilio publicum adspicere voluit . . . Norimbergae, Sumtibus Wolfgangi Mauritii Endteri, & Johannis Andreae Endteri haeredum, 1676.

2 parts in 1 v. ([24], 168, 122, [12] p.; [20], 256, 115, [6] p.) illus., plates. 23 cm. **[11539]**

Imperfect: sheets m-q (p. 89-116, [6]) of the Epistola and sheets m-r (p. 89-122, [12]) of the appendix interchanged in binding.

"Tentaminum collegii curiosi quaedam appendices sive auctaria quibus supplentur ea quae partim in ipso collegio per discursum ad superiora phaenomena . . . annotata fuerunt . . ." (122 p.) has half title.

Pars secunda dated 1685 includes: "Ad . . . Henricum Morum . . . epistola qua de . . . principio hylarchico . . . disseritur . . . 1685" (116 p.). Items have special title pages.

—Epistola . . . ad Joh. Georgium Volckamerum . . . de veritate propositionum in Joh. Alphonsi Borelli lib. I. De motu animalium subtilius demonstratarum . . . Norimbergae, Typis & sumptibus Wolffgangi Mauritii Endteri, 1684.

[12] p. plate. 19 cm. **[11540]**

—Philosophia eclectica; h. e., Exercitationes academicae, quibus philosophandi methodus selectior . . . explicatur . . . Altdorfii, Typis Johannis Henrici Schönnerstaedt, 1686.

[12], 674 (i.e. 672), [20] p. 17 cm. **[11541]**

—Physica electiva sive, hypothetica. Tomus primus partem physicae generalem complexus . . . Accessit . . . Theosophiae sive, cognitionis de Deo naturalis specimen mathematica methodo conceptum. Norimbergae, Sumptibus Wolfgangi Mauritii Endteri, 1697.

[80], 947, [1] p. plates. 21 cm. **[11542]**

Vol. 2 was published in 1722.

Dissertations — Altdorf

—*praeses.* De clepsydrarum . . . phaenomenis & effectibus, horumque omnium genuinis causis, exercitatio physica, quae possit esse instar commentarii ad Aristotelis Problema VIII. sectionis XVI . . . Altdorffii, Typis Henrici Meyeri [1674]

[28] p. illus. 20 cm. **[11543]**

H. Müller, *respondent.*

—Destinatum prolixiori tractatui argumentum de respiratione ὡς ἐν συνόψει hic . . . examinatum ventilationi publicae exponunt . . . respondens Joh. Wolfgangus Oswald . . . Altdorfii, Literis Henrici Meyeri [1686]

[28] p. 21 cm. **[11544]**

J. W. Oswald, *respondent.*

—Diducendi alias uberius argumenti de plantarum animaliumque generatione, σχιαγραφιαν quandam . . . exhibent praeses M. Joh. Christophorus Sturmius & . . . respondens Guilielmus Bechmann . . . Altdorffii, Literis Schönnerstaedtianis [1687]

[1], 24 p. 19 cm. **[11545]**

Diss. — Altdorf (W. Bechmann, *respondent*)

—Disquisitio physica de fulmine & cognatis tonitru ac fulgure . . . Altdorfii, Literis Henrici Meyeri [1696]

32 p. 19 cm. **[11546]**

J. A. Dietericus, *respondent.*

—Dissertatio physica de elephante . . . Altdorffii, Typis Henrici Meyeri [1696]

36 p. 20 cm. **[11547]**

J. H. Burckhard, *respondent.*

—Dissertationem inauguralem de ignibus tantumlucentibus . . . sistet Conradus Höger . . . Altdorfii, Literis Henrici Meyeri [1698]

[16] p. 19 cm. **[11548]**

C. Höger, *respondent.*

—Magnorum mundi corporum magnetismus . . . Altdorffii, Typis Henrici Meyeri [1671]

20 p. 19 cm. **[11549]**

J. M. Hoffmann, *respondent.*

—Oculus θεοσκόπος; h. e., De visionis organo et ratione genuina, dissertatio physica . . . Altdorffii, Literis Henrici Meyeri [1678]

32 p. plate. 19 cm. **[11550]**

J. A. Volland, *respondent.*

—Primaria gravium leviumque phaenomena ad principia causasque suas reducens exercitatio . . . Altdorffii, Typis Johannis Henrici Schönnerstaedt [1685]

[4], 16 p. 20 cm. **[11551]**

J. A. Cöler, *respondent.*

—Visionis sensum nobilissimum ex obscurae camerae tenebris luculenter-illustrans dissertatio optico-physica . . . [Altdorffii] Literis Henrici Meyeri [1699]

44 p.   18 cm.   [11552]

J. G. Doppelmayr, *respondent.*

STURM, MORITZ EUCHAR [*fl.* 1695–1699] *respondent.* Aerem anginae causam efficientem . . . examini sisto . . . M. Mauritius Eucharius Sturmius . . . Altdorff. Nor., Literis Henrici Meyeri, 1699.

20 p.   18 cm.   [11553]

Diss. — Altdorf.

STURM, REGINALD. *See* STURMIUS, Reginaldus [*fl. ca.* 1583]

STURM, ROLAND [*fl.* 1636–1658] Febrifugi Peruviani vindiciarum pars prior [-pars altera]. Pulveris historiam complectens ejusque vires & proprietates . . . exhibens . . . Delphis, Apud Petrum Oosterhout, 1659.

[12], 166 p.; [8], 142, [7] p.   14 cm.   [11554]

STURM, SAMUEL [*d.* 1688] Discursus medicus de medicis non-medicis, in salutem periclitantis proximi . . . Accessit D. J[ohann] D[aniel] M[ajor] Epistola ad autorem; De oraculis medicinae ergo quaesitis, et votivis convalescentium tabellis. Wittebergae, Impensis Andreae Hartmanni, imprimebat Michael Wendt, 1663.

[16], 66, [6] p.   20 cm.   [11555]

"Joh. Danielis Majoris . . . De oraculis medicinae ergo quaesitis et votivis convalescentium tabellis, epistola . . ." (p. 43–54) has special title page. "Ex J. Phil. Thomasini libro De donariis caput XXXIV . . .": p. 55–56.

STURMIUS, JOANNES [1559–1650] Physica; seu, Generalia philosophiae naturalis theoremata, e libris Artistotelis desumpta, quae passim in academiis physicae studiosis memoriae mandanda praescribuntur . . . Lovanii, In officina typographica Gerardi Rivii, 1610.

[8], 250, [34] p.   17 cm.   [11556]

STURMIUS, REGINALDUS [*fl. ca.* 1583] *See* HIPPOCRATES. [Adaptations, etc. Greek and Latin.] Aphorismi. 1619.

STURMIUS, SAMUELUS. *See* STURM, Samuel [*d.* 1688]

STUTHENIUS, GERLACUS [*fl.* 1634] Ψυχολογία; hoc est, Disquisitio physica de anima rationali ejusque affectionibus . . . Lipsiae, Excudebat Henningus Köler, 1634.

[28] p.   17 cm.   [11557]

Diss. — Leipzig (S. Loseus, *respondent*)

STUVE, GOTTFRIED [*fl.* 1691] *respondent.* Disputatio medica inauguralis de virium imbecillitate . . . Lugduni Batavorum, Apud Abrahamum Elzevier, 1691.

[36] p.   22 cm.   [11558]

Diss. — Leyden.

STYLLE, PETRUS VON DER. Handbuch der Chirurgiae, darinn gantz eigentlich . . . gelehret wird . . . was Chirurgia sey, mit einer nützlichen anatomischen Beschreibung . . . Coppenhagen, In Verlegung Peter Haubolds, 1651.

[16], 562 + p.   16 cm.   [11559]

Imperfect: all after p. 562 wanting.

—[The same.] Chirurgisches Hand-Buch, in welchen, durch Frag und Antwort . . . gelehret wird, was die Chirurgie seye, sambt einer anatomischen Beschreibung . . . Zum andern Mahl gedruckt. Frankfurt, Peter Haubold, 1682.

[8], 566, [11] p.   table.   17 cm.   [11560]

STYRKOLSZKY, DANIEL [*fl.* 1609–1610] *respondent.* Disputatio medica de menstruorum fluxu nimio . . . Basileae, Typis Johannis Schroeteri, 1610.

[11] p.   20 cm.   [11561]

Diss. — Basel.

—*See* RYFF, P. Gratiosus . . . ordo medic. Basileens. 1610.

SUÁREZ DE FIGUEROA, CRISTÓBAL [*ca.* 1571–1645] Plaza universal de todas ciencias, y artes, parte traduzida de toscano . . . Perpiñan, Luys Roure, 1629.

[8], 379 ll.   20 cm.   [11562]

Partly translated from Tommaso Garzoni's La piazza universale di tutte le professioni del mondo.

"Encomio al arte del ilustrado doctor Raymundo Lull": ll. [6–8]

SUCHTEN, ALEXANDER VON [*fl.* 1535–1576] Chymische Schrifften alle, so viel deren vorhanden, zum ersten Mahl zusammen gedruckt . . . von vielen Druckfehlern gesäubert, vermehret, und in zwey Theile . . . verfasset. Franckfurt am Mayn, In

Verlegung Georg Wolffs, Druckts Johann Görlin, 1680.

[14], 486, [7] p. front. 17 cm.   [11563]

"... Explicatio tincturae physicorum Theophrasti Paracelsi ...": p. 383-457.

—Mysteria gemina antimonii; das ist, Von den grossen Geheimnissen des Antimonii, in zween Tractat abgetheilet, derer einer die Artzeneyen zu anfallenden menschlichen Kranckheiten offenbahret, der ander aber, wie die Metallen erhöhet und in Verbesserung überzetzet werden ... Publiciret ... durch Johann Thölden ... Nürnberg, Johann Hoffmann, 1675.

[8], 380, [27] p. front., plate. 17 cm.
[11564]

With this are bound: Basilius Valentinus. Triumph-Wagen Antimonii. 1676; Meisner, L. Gemma gemmarum alchimistarum. 1608.

— Of the secrets of antimony: in two treatises. Translated out of High-Dutch by Dr. C[able] ... To which is added B. Valentine's salt of antimony, with its use. London, Moses Pitt, 1670.

[10], 122, [2] p. 15 cm.   [11565]

The second treatise (p. [59-122]) has special title page.

SUCINTO fatto per informatione al trono sereniss.mo nella causa dell'arte della speciaria. 1694. *See* GENOA. Laws, statutes, etc.

SUDECIUS, JOHANNES [*fl.* 1689] *respondent. See* BARBECK, F. G., *praeses.* Disputatio medica altera de veneno. 1689.

SUDUM philosophicum. *See* HARPRECHT, J. Sudum philosophicum, pro secretis chymicis perspiciendis. 1660.

SÜESS, JOHANN PHILIPP [*fl.* 1656] *respondent. See* SCHALLER, J. Dissertatio moralis de sobrietate. 1656.

SÜMENICHT, ADRIAN VON. *See* MYNSICHT, Adrian von [1603-1638]

SUEVUS, BERNHARD [*fl.* 1617-1628] Tractatus de inspectione vulnerum lethalium et sanabilium praecipuarum partium corporis humani ... Marpurgi, Sumtibus Casp. Chemlini, 1629.

[24], 136 p. 16 cm.   [11566]

— *See* ROTHENBURG OB DER TAUBER. Ordinances, local laws, etc. Ernstliche, trewhertzige Ordtnung. 1625.

SUEVUS, GOTTFRIED [1615-1658] *praeses.* Disputatio juridica de peste ... Wittebergae, Apud Jobum Wilhelmum Fincelium, 1653.

[28] p. 19 cm.   [11567]

Diss.—Wittenberg (J. E. Seidell, *respondent*)

SUICER, JOHANN HEINRICH. *See* SCHWEITZER, Johann Heinrich [1644-1705]

SULTANINI, BALDASSARE, *pseud. See* LETI, Gregorio [1630-1701]

SULTZBACH, PAULUS. *See* ECK DE SULTZBACH, Paul [*fl.* 1489?]

SULTZBERGER, JOHANN RUPRECHT [*fl.* 1621-*ca.* 1630] De urinis disputatio medica ... Lipsiae, Excudebat Johann Glück [1621]

[28] p. 19 cm.   [11568]

Diss. pro loco — Leipzig (M. Schönfeldt, *respondent*)

—*praeses.* De cancro συζητησις medico-chirurgica ... Lipsiae, Excudebat Gregorius Ritzsch [1625]

[28] p. 19 cm.   [11569]

Diss.—Leipzig (C. Meissner, *respondent*)

SULTZBERGER, SIEGMUND RUPRECHT [*ca.* 1628-1675]

Dissertations - Leipzig

—*praeses.* De pilis ... Lipsiae, Stanno Wittigiano [1654]

[20] p. 19 cm.   [11570]

M. Winckelmann, *respondent.*

— De rore microcosmi ... Lipsiae, Typis viduae Henningi Coleri [1665]

[56] p. 20 cm.   [11571]

G. Fritsch, *respondent.*

—Disputatio medica inauguralis de ictero flavo ... Lipsiae, Typis Joh. Wittigau [1665]

[44] p. 20 cm.   [11572]

A. L. Crüger, *respondent.*

— Dissertatio medica inauguralis de abortu ... Lipsiae, Literis Johannis Erici Hahnii [1669]

[32] p. 20 cm.   [11573]

C. Crusius, *respondent.*

— Dissertationem inauguralem de morsu viperae ... publico examini submittit M. Michael Ettmüller ... [Lipsiae] Literis Christiani Michaelis [1666]

[40] p. 19 cm.   [11574]

M. Ettmüller, *respondent.*

— [The same.] ... Lipsiae, Denuo excud. Nicolaus Scipio, 1679.

[40] p.   20 cm.   [**11575**]

M. Ettmüller, *respondent.*

— [The same.] ... Lipsiae, Denuo excud. Nicolaus Scipio, 1685.

[40] p.   21 cm.   [**11576**]

M. Ettmüller, *respondent.*

— The rickets Anglorum; seu, De rhachitide dissertationem inauguralem ... examini proponit M. Christoph-Andreas Schöngast ... [Lipsiae] Literis Christiani Michaelis [1668]

[32] p.   19 cm.   [**11577**]

C. A. Schöngast, *respondent.*

SULTZE, GEORG DAVID [*fl.* 1676-1677] *respondent.* Disputatio medica inauguralis de angina, strangulationem aemulante affectu ... Altdorffii, Typis Johannis Henrici Schönnerstaedt [1677]

[2], 22 p.   20 cm.   [**11578**]

Diss. — Altdorf.

SULZBERGER, SIGISMUNDUS RUPERTUS. *See* SULTZBERGER, Siegmund Ruprecht [*ca.* 1628-1675]

SUMMA rhytmorum Germanicorum de opere universali ex coelo soloque prodeunte ...

511-513 p., vol. 6.   20 cm. (*In* Zetzner, Lazarus, *ed.* Theatrum chemicum. Argentorati, 1659-61)

[**11579**]

Caption title.
Running title: Rhytmi de lapide philosophorum.

SUMMA rhytmorum parvorum Germanicorum, qui sunt ejusdem tenoris & sensus cum praecedentibus picturis, ad verbum expressa.

521-522 p., vol. 6.   20 CM. (*In* Zetzner, Lazarus, *ed.* Theatrum chemicum. Argentorati, 1659-61)

[**11580**]

Caption title.

SUMMA statutorum, facultatum, privilegiorum, & jurisdictionis aromatariorum a summis pontificibus concess, confirmat. 1693. *See* COLLEGIO DEGLI SPEZIALI, Rome.

SUMMER. *See* SOMMER.

SUPPLEMENT du volume des Journaux de Médecine de l'année M. DC. LXXXVI. 1687. *See* BRUNET, C.

A SUPPLEMENT to the Philosophical transactions. 1678. *See* [HOLDER, W.]

SUR les stryges de Russie. [n. p., 16—?]

107 p.   14 cm.   [**11581**]

Imperfect?: title page wanting?
Caption title.
Bound with Blegny, N. de. Histoire anathomique d'un enfant. 1679.

SURDUS, JOANNES PETRUS. *See* SORDI, Giovanni Pietro [*d.* 1598]

SURGANT, JOHANN MICHAEL [*fl.* 1692] *respondent.* Disputatio inauguralis medica de arthritide vaga ...Basileae, Typis Emanuelis & Joh. Georgii König [1692]

[36] p.   22 cm.   [**11582**]

Diss. — Basel.

SURIANO, MATTEO. *See* SORIANO, Matteo [16th-17th cent.]

SUSCHKY, JOHANN SIGMUND [*fl.* 1694] *respondent.* *See* KETTNER, F. G., *praeses.* Dissertatio historica de mumiis Aegyptiacis. 1694.

SUSIO, GIOVANNI BATTISTA [1519-1583] Liber de sanguinis mittendi ratione. Quo ostendit in quibus hodie medici contra Hippocratis, & Galeni sententiam peccent circa phlebotomiam. Nunc iterum editus à Josepho Trullerio ... Romae, Ex typographia Cam. Apost., sumptibus Octavii Ingrillani, 1628.

[60], 130, [24] p.   15 cm.   [**11583**]

SUTER, HENRICUS [*fl.* 1691] *respondent.* Disputatio medica inauguralis de scorbuto ... Hardervici, Apud Albertum Sas, 1691.

[16] p.   20 cm.   [**11584**]

Diss. — Harderwijk.

SUTHERLAND, JAMES [1639?-1719] Hortus medicus Edinburgensis; or, A catalogue of the plants in the Physical garden at Edinburgh; containing their most proper Latin and English names ... Edinburgh, Printed by the heir of Andrew Anderson and sold by Henry Ferguson and the author, 1683.

[16], 367, [62] p.   16 cm.   [**11585**]

Last leaf (blank) wanting.

al-SUYŪTĪ [1445-1505] De proprietatibus ac virtutibus medicis animalium, plantarum, ac gemmarum, tractatus triplex. Auctore Habdarrahmano

Asiutensi Aegyptio. Nunc primum ex Arabico idiomate Latinitate donatus ab Abrahamo Ecchellensi ... Ex MS. codice bibliothecae ... Cardinalis Mazarini. Parisiis, Apud Sebastianum Cramoisy et Gabrielem Cramoisy, 1647.

[16 +], 179, [17] p.   20 cm.   [11586]

Imperfect: preliminary pages following p. [16] wanting.
Translation of the Dīwān al-ḥayawān.

SVICARDUS, JOANNES. *See* SCHWEIKARD VON KRONENBERG, Johann, *Abp. of Mainz* [*d.* 1626]

SWALMIUS, JAN [*fl.* 1687] *respondent.* Disputatio medica inauguralis de tenesmo ... Lugduni Batavorum, Apud Abrahamum Elzevier, 1687.

[16] p.   22 cm.   [11587]

Diss. — Leyden.

SWALVE, BERNHARD [*ca.* 1625–1680] Alcali et acidum; sive, Naturae et artis instrumenta pugilica, per neochmum & palaephatum hinc inde ventilata, et praxi medicae superstructae praemissa ... Amstelodami, Apud Johannem Janssonium à Waesberge, & haeredes Elizei Weyerstraet, 1670.

[22], 275, [1] p.   14 cm.   [11588]

Added engraved title page.

—[The same.] Naturae et artis instrumenta pugilica, alcali et acidum, per Neochmum et Palaephatum hinc inde ventilata & praxi medicae superstructae praemissa ... Ed. alt. corr. ... Francofurti, 1677.

[15], 320, [24] p.   14 cm.   [11589]

Added engraved title page.

—Disquisitio therapeutica generalis. Amstelodami, Apud Aegidium Janssonium Valkenier, 1657.

[10], 216, [8] p.   13 cm.   [11590]

Engraved title page.
Imperfect: p. 213-214 wanting.

—[The same.] Disquisitio therapeutica generalis; sive, Medendi methodus ad recentiorum dogmata adornata ... Ed. alt. emaculatior ... Jenae, Typis Gollnerianis, 1677.

[11], 208, [20] p.   13 cm.   [11591]

Added engraved title page.

—Pancreas pancrene; sive, Pancreatis et succi ex eo profluentis commentum succinctum ...

Amstelodami, Apud Joannem Janssonium a Waesberge, & viduam Elizei Weyerstraet, 1667.

[14], 271, [8] p.   14 cm.   [11592]

—Another issue, with date changed to 1668.   [11593]

Imperfect: title page mutilated.

—[The same.] ... Ed. postrema, priore correctior. Jenae, Typis Gollnerianis, 1678.

[10], 346 p.   14 cm.   [11594]

Bound with Hofmann, C. Tractatus de usu lienis cerebri. 1682.

—Querelae & opprobria ventriculi; sive προσοποποιια [sic] ejusdem naturalia sua sibi vendicantis, & abusus tam diaeteticos, quam pharmaceuticos perstringentis ... Amstelodami, Ex officina Joannis Janssonii à Waesberge, & Elizei Weyerstraten, 1664.

[16], 321, [11] p.   14 cm.   [11595]

Added engraved title page.

—[The same.] ... Amstelaedami, Apud Joannem Janssonium à Waesberge, 1675.

[12], 286, [10] p.   16 cm.   [11596]

Added engraved title page.

—Copy 2.   14 cm.

Imperfect: first five leaves mutilated.
With this is bound Malpighi, M. Exercitationes de viscerum. 1677.

SWALVE, OTTO [*fl.* 1683] *respondent.* Disputatio medica inauguralis de epilepsia ... Lugduni Batavorum, Apud Abrahamum Elsevier, 1683.

[16] p.   22 cm.   [11597]

Diss. — Leyden.

SWAMMERDAM, JAN [1637–1680] Ephemeri vita; of, Afbeeldingh van 's menschen leven, vertoont in de wonderbaarelijcke en nooyt gehoorde historie van het vliegent ende een-dagh-levent haft of oever-aas ... Hier is achter bygevoeght, een ... verhandeling van den waaren stant des menschen, soo voor als na sijn val ... Amsterdam, Abraham Wolfgang, 1675.

[32], 422, [8] p.   plates.   17 cm.   [11598]

—Historia insectorum generalis; ofte, Algemeene verhandeling de bloedeloose dierkens ... 1. deel ... Utrecht, Merinardus van Dreunen, 1669.

[28], 168 p.; 48 p.   table, plates.   20 cm.   [11599]

Added half title.

Part [2] has half title (p. ɪɪ): Verclaringe, ofte uitlegginge, van de vier orderen der veranderingen, deur middel van afbeeldingen.

Bound with *his* Miraculum naturae. 1672.

—[Latin tr.] Historia insectorum generalis . . . Ex Belgica Latinam fecit Henricus Christianus Henninius . . . Lugd. Batavorum, Apud Jordanum Luchtmans, 1685.

[20], 212 (i.e. 210), [17] p. plates, table. 21 cm.   [**11600**]

—[The same.] . . . Adjicitur Dilucidatio, qua specialia cujusvis ordinis exempla figuris accuratissime, tam naturali magnitudine, quam ope microscopii aucta illustrantur . . . Ed. 2. Ultrajecti, Ex officina Otthonis de Vries, 1693.

[20], 212 (i.e. 210), [17] p. plates, table. 23 cm.   [**11601**]

A reissue of the 1685 edition with new title page and preliminaries reset.

—[French tr.] Histoire generale des insectes . . . Utrecht, Jean Ribbius, 1685.

[8], 215 p. table, plates. 22 cm.   [**11602**]

—Miraculum naturae; sive, Uteri muliebris fabrica, notis in D. Joh. van Horne prodromum illustrata . . . Adjecta est nova methodus, cavitates corporis ita praeparandi, ut suam semper genuinam faciem servent . . . Lugduni Batavorum, Apud Severinum Matthaei, 1672.

[6], 57, [1] p. plates. 20 cm.   [**11603**]

With this is bound *his* Historia insectorum generalis. 1669.

—[The same.] . . . Lugduni Batavorum, Apud Cornelium Boutesteyn, 1679.

[6], 57, [1] p. plates. 22 cm.   [**11604**]

A reissue of the 1672 edition with new title page.

—[The same.] . . . Londini, Typis Johannis Gellibrand & Roberti Sollers, 1680.

[8], 148, [4] p. plates. 18 cm.   [**11605**]

—Tractatus physico-anatomico-medicus de respiratione usuque pulmonum. In quo, praeter primam respirationis in foetu inchoationem, aëris per circulum propulsio statuminatur, attractio exploditur; experimentaque ad explicandum sanguinis in corde tam auctum quam diminutum motum in medium producuntur. Lugduni Batavorum, Apud Danielem, Abraham, & Adrian. à Gaasbeeck, 1667.

[16], 121, [22] p. illus. 17 cm.   [**11606**]

Added engraved title page.

Imperfect: p. [9–16] wanting.

With this is bound copy 2 of Thruston, Malachi. De respirationis usu primario diatriba. Lugd. Batavor., 1708.

—[The same.] . . . Lugduni Batavorum, Apud Joannem vander Linden, 1679.

[16], 121, [23] p. illus. 16 cm.   [**11607**]

Added engraved title page.

A corrected reprint of the 1667 edition.

—*See* HOFFMANN, J. M. Dissertationes anatomico-physiologicae. 1685; LAMSWEERDE, J. B. van. Respirationis Swammerdammianae exspiratio. 1674.

SWAN, JOHN [*ca.* 1600–1671] Speculum mundi; or, A glasse representing the face of the world; shewing both that it did begin, and must also end: the manner how, and time when, being largely examined. Whereunto is joyned an Hexameron, or a serious discourse of the causes . . . of things in nature . . . The 2d ed. enl. . . . Cambridge, Roger Daniel, 1643.

[15], 504, [28] p. illus. 18 cm.   [**11608**]

Added engraved title page has imprint: Cambridge, R. D. for John Williams, 1644.

SWEDEN. Laws, statutes, etc. Kongl. May:tz i nader uthgifne sidste medicinal-ordningar, af trycket utgangne ahr 1699 . . . Constitutiones medicae, publicatae anno M.DC.XCIX . . . Medicinal Ordnungen, durch den Druck herausgegeben Anno 1699. Stockholmiae [1699]

[77] p. 21 cm.   [**11609**]

Contains decrees signed by Carolus XI and Carolus XII.

With this is bound Collegium medicum, Stockholm. Catalogus. [1698?]

SWEERTS, EMANUEL [*b. ca.* 1552] Florilegium . . . tractans de variis floribus et aliis indicis plantis ad vivum delineatum in duabus partibus et quatuor linguis concinnatum . . . Francofurti ad Moenum, Impressum apud Anthonium Kempner, sumptibus autoris, 1612.

[40] p. 67 plates; [1] p., 43 plates., port. 40 cm.   [**11610**]

Engraved title page.

Part 2 has special title page with imprint: Francofurti, Ex officina typographica Erasmi Kempfferi, 1614.

Text in Latin, Dutch, German and French.

SWELING, JOHANN EBERHARD. *See* SCHWELING, Johann Eberhard [1645–1714]

SWETSERTJE, Jan Frederik. *See* Bontekoe, C. Een nieuw bewys van d'onvermijdelijke noodsakelijkheid. 1685.

SWINNAS, Willem [1620-1672] Kinder pocken en maselen. *In* Beverwijck, J. van. Wercken der geneeskonste. 1664, 1672.

SWYCHHUISEN, Hermann [*fl.* 1698] *respondent.* Inaugurale disputatie in de medicine van de rode loop genaemt dysenteria ... Groningen, Johannes Lens, 1698.

    [II] p.   21 cm.   **[11611]**
Diss.—Groningen.

SYBILLENUS, Petrus. *See* Sibyllenus, Petrus [1548-1564]

SYDENHAM, Thomas [1624-1689] Opuscula quotquot hactenus separatim prodiere omnia. Nunc primum junctim edita, a plurimis mendis repurgata ... Amstelaedami, Apud Henricum Wetstenium, 1683.

    [42], 273, [43] p.; 353-489 p.   17 cm.   **[11612]**
Contents.—Observationes medicae.—Epistolae responsoriae duae.—Dissertatio epistolaris.
Each treatise has half title.

    —[The same.] ... Amstelaedami, Apud Henricum Wetstenium, 1683.

    [42], 273, [43] p.; 365-782, [55] p.   port. 17 cm.   **[11613]**
Contents.—Observationes medicae.—Epistolae responsoriae duae.—Dissertatio epistolaris.—Tractatus de podagra et hydrope.—Schedula monitoria de novae febris ingressu.—Processus integri.
The first treatise has half title.

    — [The same.] Opera universa. In quibus non solummodo morborum acutorum historiae & curationes nova & exquisita methodo ...traduntur, verum etiam morborum fere omnium chronicorum curatio brevissima ...exhibetur. Ed. alt., priori multum auct. & emend. reddita ... Londini, Typis R. N., impensis Walteri Kettilby, 1685.

    [41], 321, [41] p.; [1], 277, [56] p. 19 cm.   **[11614]**
Contents.—Observationes medicae.—Epistolae responsoriae duae.—Dissertatio epistolaris.—Tractatus de podagra et hydrope.
Items have special title pages.

    —Additamenta nova ad Thomae Sydenham Opera universa ex nupera Londinensi editione excerpta. [n. p.] 1689.

    68 p.   14 cm.   **[11615]**
Bound with Frick, M. Icon podagrae. 1693.

    — Opera universa. Quibus accedunt additiones novae ex nupera Londinensi ed. excerptae ... Amstelaedami, Apud Henricum Wetstenium, 1687.

    1 v.   port. 17 cm.   **[11616]**
Various pagings.
Contents.—[1] Observationes medicae.—[2] Epistolae responsoriae duae.—[3] Dissertatio epistolaris.—[4] Schedula monitoria de novae febris ingressu.—[5] Tractatus de podagra et hydrope.—[6] Additiones novae. Item [4] has special title page; other items have half titles.

    —[The same.] Praxis medica experimentalis; sive, Opuscula universa, quotquot hactenus ab autore ipso ultimum revisa & aucta in lucem prodierunt, nunc primum in unum collecta volumen ... repurgatum ... Lipsiae, Apud J. Thom. Fritsch, excudebat Christianus Goezius, 1695.

    [62], 782, [55] p.   18 cm.   **[11617]**
Contents as in the 1685 London edition with the addition of Elenchus rerum de hydrope, Schedula monitoria de novae febris ingressu, and Processus integri.

    — [The same.] Opera omnia medica. Ed. nov. omni alia auctior ... Genevae, Apud fratres de Tournes, 1696.

    [72], 733, [51] p. port. 18 cm.   **[11618]**
Contents as in the 1695 Leipzig edition.

    — [The same.] ... Patavii, Typis Seminarii, apud Joannem Manfre, 1700.

    [77], 783 p.   17 cm.   **[11619]**

    —[English tr.] The whole works ... Wherein not only the history and cures of acute diseases are treated of, after a new and accurate method, but also the shortest and safest way of curing most chronical diseases. Translated from the original Latin, by John Pechey ... London, Richard Wellington, 1696.

    [24], 248, 353-592 p.   20 cm.   **[11620]**

    —[The same.] ... The 2d ed. corr. from the original Latin, by John Pechey ... London, Richard Wellington, 1697.

    [16], 232, 323-561, [1] p. 20 cm.   **[11621]**

    —Dissertatio epistolaris ad ... Guilielmum Cole ... de observationibus nuperis circa curationem variolarum confluentium nec non de affectione hysterica ... Londini, Typis M. C. impensis Walteri Kettilby, 1682.

    [1], 193, [1] p. 19 cm.   **[11622]**

    —[The same.] ... Genevae, Apud Samuelem de Tournes, 1684.

    141 p.   15 cm.   **[11623]**
Bound with *his* Epistolae responsoriae duae. 1683.

—Epistolae responsoriae duae . . . Prima de morbis epidemicis ab anno 1675, ad annum 1680. ad
Robertum Brady . . . Secunda de luis venereae
historia & curatione. Ad . . . Henricum Paman . . .
Londini, Typis M. C., impensis Walteri Kettilby,
1680.

[1], 129, [1] p.   19 cm.   [**11624**]

Errata: p. [1] at end.

Includes the letters of Brady and Paman.

—[The same.] . . . Genevae, Apud Samuelem de
Tournes, 1683.

[1], 100 p.   front. (port)   15 cm.   [**11625**]

With this are bound *his:* Dissertatio epistolaris. 1684; Tractatus
de podagra et hydrope. 1686.

—Methodus curandi febres propriis observationibus superstructa. Ed. 2., priori multo auct. ac
emend.; cui etiam accessit Sectio quinta de peste sive
febre pestilentiali . . . Londini, Impensis J. Crook,
1668.

[15], 218, [4] p.   17 cm.   [**11626**]

Imperfect: sig. P8 (blank?) wanting.

—[The same.] Observationes medicae circa morborum acutorum historiam et curationem . . . Londini, Typis A. C. impensis Gualteri Kettilby, 1676.

[54], 425, [53] p.   19 cm.   [**11627**]

The third edition, enlarged.

—[The same.] Observationes medicae circa morborum acutorum historiam et curationem . . . Accesserunt Epistolae ejusdem duae responsoriae,
prima de morbis epidemicis ab anno 1675. ad ann.
1680. secunda de luis venereae historia & curatione.
Genevae, Apud Samuelem de Tournes, 1683.

[53], 458, [61] p.   front. (port.)   15 cm.
[**11628**]

Imperfect: p. 269-270 mutilated.

Lacks the two letters called for on the title page.

— Processus integri in morbis fere omnibus curandis . . . Quibus accessit graphica symptomatum
delineatio. Londini, Impensis Sam. Smith. Benj.
Walford, & Ja. Knapton, 1693.

[11], 108 p.   15 cm.   [**11629**]

—[The same.] Integri processus in morbis fere omnibus curandis . . . Quibus accessit graphica symptomatum delineatio. Amstelodami, Apud Henricum
Wetstenium, 1694.

[16], 96 p.   16 cm.   [**11630**]

—[The same.] Processus integri in morbis fere omnibus curandis . . . Quibus accessit graphica symptomatum delineatio, una cum quamplurimis obser-
vatu dignis. Necnon de phthisi tractatulo nunquam
antehac edito. Londini, Impensis Sam. Smith &
Benj. Walford & J. Knapton, 1695.

[11], 108 p.   15 cm.   [**11631**]

"Tabis descriptio & cura": p. 98-108.

—[The same.] . . . Ed. nov. plurib. articuli aucta
nec non de phthisi tractatulo nunquam ante hac
edito. Genevae, Sumptibus Cramer & Perachon,
1696.

[8], 44 p.   22 cm.   [**11632**]

—[English tr.] Compleat method of curing almost
all diseases, and description of their symptoms. To
which are now added, five discourses of the same
author concerning the pleurisy, gout, hysterical passion, dropsy and rheumatism. Abridg'd and . . .
translated out of . . . Latin. With . . . notes . . . written by a late learned physician, and never before
printed. London, H. Newman and Rich. Parker,
1695.

[8], 202, [6] p.   15 cm.   [**11633**]

Imperfect? sig. A5-12 wanting?

Pages 1-90 are the translation of Processus integri in morbis fere
omnibus curandis.

"Short and useful notes on Dr. Sydenham's Method of curing
diseases. By a late learned physician": p. 91-202.

—Practice of physick. The signs, symptoms,
causes and cures of diseases . . . His discourses of
consumptions gouts, &c. never before publish'd . . .
Translated into English . . . By William Salmon . . .
London, Sam. Smith and Benj. Walford and J.
Knapton, 1695.

[12], 192 p.   17 cm.   [**11634**]

—Schedula monitoria de novae febris ingressu . . .
Londini, Typis R. N. impensis Gualt. Kettilby, 1686.

[8], 115 p.   19 cm.   [**11635**]

—[The same.] . . . Ed. 2. ab authore adhuc vivo
emend. & auct. reddita . . . Londini, Typis R. N.
impensis Gualt. Kettilby, 1688.

[13 +], 127 p.   20 cm.   [**11636**]

Imperfect: first preliminary leaf wanting.

—Processus in morbis ac De phthisi. *In* Morton,
R. Opera medica. 1696, 1697.

—Schedula monitoria de novae febribus ingressu. English. *In* Pechey, J. Collections of acute diseases. 1687.

—Tractatus de podagra et hydrope . . . Londini, Typis R. N. impensis Gualt. Kettilby, 1683.

[9], 201, [1] p.   18 cm.   **[11637]**

—[The same.] . . . Genevae, Apud Samuelem de Tournes, 1686.

147 p.   15 cm.   **[11638]**

Bound with *his* Epistolae responsoriae duae. 1683.

—Verhandelinge van de pokken. *In* Blankaart, S. Venus belegert en ontset. 1684, 1688, 1696; [German tr.] 1689.

—*See* Brown, A. A. vindicatory schedule. 1691; In speculo teipsum contemplare Dr. Black. 1692; Jüngken, J. H. Modernae praxeos medicae vade mecum. 1694; A new method of curing the French-pox. 1690; Pechey, J. A collection of chronical diseases. 1692; Stubbs, H. The Lord Bacons relation of the sweating-sickness examined. 1671.

SYEN, Arnold [1640–1678] *respondent.* Disputatio medica inauguralis, de hydrope ascite . . . Lugduni Batavorum, Apud Isaacum de Waal, 1659.

[8] p.   19 cm.   **[11639]**

Diss. — Leyden.

SYLBURG, Friedrich [1536–1596] *ed. See* Gorris, J. de [1505–1577] Definitionum medicarum libri XXIII. 1601.

SYLVATICUS, Benedictus. *See* Salvatico, Benedetto, *conte di* [1575–1658]

SYLVATICUS, Joannes Baptista. *See* Selvatico, Giovanni Battista [*d.* 1621]

SYLVESTRE, Peter. *See* Silvestre, Peter [*ca.* 1662–1718]

SYLVIUS, Dethlevus [*fl.* 1573] *ed. See* Rantzau, H. De conservanda valetudine liber. 1604, 1617.

SYLVIUS, Franciscus. *See* Le Boë, Frans de [1614–1672]

SYLVIUS, Jacobus [1478–1555] *See* Dubois, Jacques [1478–1555]

SYLVIUS, Jacobus [1648?–1689] Novissima idea de febribus et earundem dogmatica, ac rationalis cura, mechanicis rationibus suffulta. Accessit dissertatio de insensibili transpiratione mechanice probata

. . . Dublinii, Sumptibus Zachariae Conzatti, 1694

[16], 174 p.   13 cm.   **[11640]**

Presumably printed in Lucca instead of Dublin. Cf. T. P. C Kirkpatrick, The Novissima idea de Febribus of Jacobus Sylvius in: The Irish Journal of Medical Science (1933) p. 673.

SYLVIUS, Nathanael [*fl.* 1687] *respondent* Disputatio medica inauguralis de fluore muliebri . . . Lugduni Batavorum, Apud Abrahamum Elzevier, 1687.

[16] p.   21 cm.   **[11641]**

Diss. — Leyden.

SYLVIUS, Zacharias [1608–1664] *ed. See* Heurne, J. van. Praxis medicinae nova ratio. 1650; Regimen sanitatis Salernitanum. Schola Salernitana. 1649 1657, 1667, 1683.

—*See* Harvey, W. Exercitatio anatomica de motu cordis. 1648; [English tr.] 1653; 1673.

SYLVIUS DE LE BOË, Franciscus. *See* Le Boë Frans de [1614–1672]

SYMEON SETH. *See* Simeo Sethus.

SYMNICHT, Adrian von. *See* Mynsicht, Adrian von [1603–1638]

SYMPSON, William. *See* Simpson, William [*fl* 1665–1677]

SYNESIUS, *alchemist. See* Arnauld, P. Troi traitez de la philosophie naturelle. 1612.

SYNESIUS, *Greek abbot.* A true book concerning the philosopher's stone. *In* Basilius Valentinus. Triumphant chariot of antimony. 1678.

SYNONYMA XXIII. *See* Mesuë [924 *or* 5–1015] Opera. 1602, 1623.

SYNOPSIS doctrinae ac medicinae vulnerum . . . Conscripta a J. G. R. M. C. . . . Wittenbergae Literis Johannis Wilckii, 1690.

[46] p.   19 cm.   **[11642]**

SYSSENBACH, Melchior [*fl.* 1611–1616] *re* spondent. *See* Sennert, D., *praeses.* Disputatio medica de hydrope. 1616.

SYTZ, Alexander. *See* Seitz, Alexander [*ca.* 1470–1540?]

SZULECKI, Johann. *See* Schultz, Johann [*d.* 1704]

T

T., A., *practitioner in physicke and chirurgerie. See* A RICH storehouse or treasurie for the diseases. 1616, 1630, 1631, 1650.

T., B. *See* CULPEPER, N. Arts master-piece. 1660

T., E. W. D. *See* TSCHIRNHAUS, Ehrenfried Walther von [1651-1708]

T., G., *tr. See* A BRIEFE discourse of the hypostasis. 1612?

T., H., *autor. See* SCHMUCK, M. De occulta magicomagnetica morborum quorundam curatione naturali, tractatus. 1636?, 1649.

T., H., P. R. M. *See* TENQUE, Jérôme [*d.* 1687]

T., I. G. D., *ed. and tr. See* HÖCHSTFÜRTREFLICHTES chiromantisch-und physiognomisches Klee-Blat. 1695.

T., J. *See* GILPIN, R. The comforts of divine love. 1700.

T., J., *esq. student in physick. See* THOMPSON, James [*fl.* 1657]

T., P., *ed. See* CORDUS, V. Dispensatorium. [Dutch ed.] 1632, 1656.

T., P., *Med. Doct. See* CHEMIA RATIONALIS RATIONIBUS PHILOSOPHICIS. 1687.

T., P. M. [*fl.* 1688] *See* RAMBALDUS, J. Compendiaria tractatio de febris. 1689?

T., R. *See* THORIUS, Raphael [*d.* 1625]

T., V. J. B. *See* BARTHOLIN, Thomas [1616-1680]

T., W. *See* DIGBY, *Sir* K. Medicina experimentalis Digbaeana. 1672-1676, 1687.

T., W., *philo-astro-medicus. See* THRASHER, William.

T. A. *See* A., T.

T. P. M. C. G. L. *See* PEUCER, Tobias [*fl.* 1690-1691]

TAAL, ANTON [*fl.* 1682-1686] *respondent.* Disputatio medica inauguralis de paralysi ... Lugduni Batavorum, Apud Abrahamum Elzevier, 1686.
[16] p.   22 cm.   **[11643]**
Diss. – Leyden.

TABERNAEMONTANUS, JACOBUS THEODORUS. *See* THEODORUS, Jacobus [*d.* 1590]

TABERNARIUS, NICOLAUS. *See* TAVERNIER, Nicolas [*fl.* 1608]

TABLEAU de l'amour consideré dans l'estat du mariage. 1687. *See* [Venette, N.]

TABOR, JOHANN OTTO [1604-1674] *See* WISSENBACH, J. J. Confutatio diatribae de mutuo. 1645.

TABOR, *Sir* ROBERT. *See* TALBOR, *Sir* Robert [1642-1681]

TABULA smaragdina; seu, Verba secretorum Hermetis.
p. 715, vol. 6.   20 cm.   (*In* Zetzner, Lazarus, *ed.* Theatrum chemicum. Argentorati, 1659-61)
    [11644]
Caption title.

TABULAE chiromanticae, lineis montibus et tuberculis manus constitutionem hominum, & fortunae vires ostendentes. Nunc primum luci datae. [Francofurti, Excudebat Wolffgangus Richterus?] 1613.
23 p.   illus., table.   21 cm.   **[11645]**
Bound with (as issued?) Geuss, W. Methodus curandorum morborum mathematica. 1613.

TACHENIUS, OTTO [*fl.* 1644-1699] Antiquissimae Hippocraticae medicinae clavis manuali experientia in naturae fontibus elaborata, qua per ignem & aquam inaudita methodo, occulta naturae, & artis ... manifesta fiunt ... Francofurti, Imp. Jo. Petri Zubrod., 1669.
286, [2] p.   15 cm.   **[11646]**

—[The same.] ... Venetiis, Combi, & La Nou, 1669.
286, [2] p.   16 cm.   **[11647]**
Errata: p. [2]
Different setting of type.

—[The same.] ... Ed. 3. ... emend. ... Lugduni Batavor., Apud Felicem Lopez, Adrianum Severinum, 1671.
[24], 202, [14] p.   14 cm.   **[11648]**

—[The same.] ... Lutetiae Parisiorum, Apud Joannem d'Houry, 1672.
[12], 273, [3] p.   16 cm.   **[11649]**

—Another issue, with new title page dated 1673.
[**11650**]

Bound (as issued?) with *his* Hippocrates chymicus. 1673.

—[The same.] ... Ed. 4. ... emend. ... Neapoli, Typis Josephi Roselli, sumptibus Franc. Ant. Peratii, 1697.

[16], 196, [18] p.   15 cm.   [**11651**]

Imperfect: first preliminary leaf (blank?) wanting.

—Hippocrates chimicus, qui novissimi viperini salis antiquissima fundamenta ostendit ... Venetiis, Combi, & La Noù, 1666.

[36], 239, [1] p.   18 cm.   [**11652**]

—[The same.] ... Brunsvigae, Sumpt. Thomae Henrici Hauensteinii, typis Johann. Henrici Dunckeri, 1668.

[40], 271, [1] p.   14 cm.   [**11653**]

—[The same.] Hippocrates chymicus, omnibus a mendis vindicatus. In quo novissimi viperini salis antiquissima fundamenta simul & acidi alcalique natura fuse ac dilucide explicantur ... Lutetiae Parisiorum, Apud Joannem d'Houry, 1669.

[36], 259, [5] p.   16 cm.   [**11654**]

—[The same.] Hippocrates chimicus, qui novissimi viperini salis antiquissima fundamenta ostendit ... Ed. 3. emend. ... Lugd. Batavor., Apud Felicem Lopez, Adrianum Severinum, 1671.

[48], 190, [2] p.   14 cm.   [**11655**]

Added engraved title page.

—[The same.] ... Lutetiae Parisiorum, Apud Joannem d'Houry, 1673.

[36], 259, [14] p.   16 cm.   [**11656**]

With this is bound (as issued?) *his* Antiquissimae Hippocraticae medicinae clavis manuali experientia in naturae fontibus elaborata. 1673.

—[The same.] Hippocrates chimicus, per ignem & aquam methodo inaudita novissimi salis viperini antiquissima fundamenta ostendens. Ed. 2. auct. & emend. Accessit ejusdem authoris De morborum principe tractatus ... Venetiis, Typis Combi & La Nouii, 1678.

[36], 473, [4] p.   16 cm.   [**11657**]

Added engraved title page.
Imperfect: last leaf (blank?) wanting.

—[English tr.] Otto Tachenius *his* Hippocrates chymicus discovering the ancient foundation of the late viperine salt with his Clavis thereunto annexed

Translated by J. W. London, Nath. Crouch, 1677.

2 v.   20 cm.   [**11658**]

Engraved title page.
Imperfect: first preliminary leaf (blank?) wanting.
Vol. [2] has special title page: ... Otto Tachenius his Clavis to the ancient Hippocratical physick or medicine; made by manual experience in the very fountains of nature. Whereby through fire and water, in a method unheard of before, the occult mysteries of nature and art are unlocked and clearly explained by a compendious way of operation ... London, Printed by Tho. James, and sold by Nath. Crouch, 1677.

—[The same.] ... Translated by J. W. London, W. Marshall, 1690.

[18], 122, [9] p.; [5], 120, [13] p.   20 cm.
[**11659**]

Engraved title page.
A reissue of the 1677 edition with new title pages and preliminary matter. The special title page of part [2] is bound in after the engraved title page: ... His Clavis to the antient Hippocratical physick ...

—Tractatus de morborum principe, in quo plerorumque gravium ac sonticorum praeter naturam affectuum, dilucida enodatio, & hermetica, id est, vera & solida eorundem curatio proponitur ... Osnabrugi, Apud J. G. Schwänderum, 1678.

[16], 187, [1] p.   14 cm.   [**11660**]

Bound with Ruysch, F. Dilucidatio valvularum in vasis lymphaticis. 1665.

—*See* BERTRAND [*fl.* 1683] Reflexions nouvelles sur l'acide et sur l'alcali. 1683; ETTMÜLLER, M. Opera omnia theoretica et practica. 1685; Pharmacopoeia Augustana reformata cum ejus mantissa & appendice. 1672; ZWELFER, J. Discursus apologeticus. 1668, 1675.

TACKE, JOHANN [1617-1675] Coeli anomalon; id est, De cometis, sive stellis crinitis, praeter universi ordinem in coelo multoties visis ἐπίκομμα physicum, in quo de generatione, varia apparitione & praesagiis cometarum, atque inprimis de cometa, quem non sine ingenti terrore mortales praeterito anno 1652 mense Decembri observarunt, ejusque praesagio, fundamentis non tam e coelo quam aliunde petitis, iisque verioribus, solide & pie agitur ... Gissae Hassorum, Ex Officina Typographica Chemliniana, 1653.

[8], 66 (i.e. 64) p.   18 cm.   [**11661**]

—*praeses.* De anima rationali ... Gissae, Typis Josephi Dieterici Hampelii [1652]

[39] p.   19 cm.   [**11662**]

Diss. — Giessen (J. Sigbert, *respondent*)

—, *tr. See* Lotichius, J. P. Gynaicologia. German. 1645

—*See* Horst, J. D. Judicium de chirurgia infusoria Jo. Danielis Majoris. 1655; [Petersen, J. W.] Elegia propemptica. 1675.

TACKE, Ludwig Christian [*fl.* 1675] *respondent.* Disputatio inauguralis de podagra . . . [Gissae-Hassorum] Typis Friderici Kargeri, 1675.

[4], 48, [4] p. 20 cm. **[11663]**
Diss. — Giessen.

—*See* [Petersen, J. W.] Elegia propemptica. 1675.

TACKENIUS. *See* Tachenius, Otto [*fl.* 1644-1699]

TACKIUS, Joannes. *See* Tacke, Johann [1617-1675]

TACKIUS, Ludovicus Christianus. *See* Tacke, Ludwig Christian [*fl.* 1675]

TADDEL, Simon [*fl.* 1659] *respondent. See* Faust, J., *praeses.* Quarta figura quam Galenus medicus et logicus doctissimus invenit. 1659.

TADINI, Alessandro. *See* Tadino, Alessandro [1580?-1661]

TADINO, Alessandro [1580?-1661] Raguaglio dell'origine et giornali successi della gran peste contagiosa . . . seguita nella città di Milano, & suo ducato dall'anno 1629, sino all'anno 1632. Con le loro successive provisioni, & ordini . . . Diviso in due parti . . . Milano, Per Filippo Ghisolfi, ad instanza di Gio. Battista Bidelli, 1648.

[8], 151 p. 22 cm. **[11664]**

—, *ed. See* Asellio, G. De lactibus. 1627; 1640.

—, *tr. See* Antidotario romano latino, et volgare. 1635.

TAGAULT, Jean [*d.* 1546] [De chirurgia institutione libri quinque. French.] La chirurgie . . . Diligemment rev. & corr. en cette derniere ed. Avec plusieurs figures des instrumens necessaires pour l'operation manuelle . . . Paris, Anthoine de Sommaville, 1629.

[47], 738, [14] p. illus. 18 cm. **[11665]**
Imperfect: p. 239-240 wanting.
In 6 books, the last of which is a translation by Siméon de Provanchères of Jacques Houllier's De materia chirurgica.

—[The same.] . . . Rouen, Daniel Loudet, 1645. [49], 845, [15] p. illus. 18 cm. **[11666]**

—[Italian.] Institutione di cirugia . . . distinta in libri cinque. Aggiuntovi il sesto libro Della materia di cirugia, di Giacomo Hollerio. Opera piena di grave dottrina, & degna d'esser letta con sommo studio . . . Venetia, Lucio Spineda, 1607.

[20], 421 (i.e. 413), [1] ll. illus. 15 cm. **[11667]**

—[The same.] *In* Croce, G. A. della. Cirugia universale e perfetta. 1605, 1661.

—*See* Banister, J. A treatise of chirurgerie. 1633; Scholtz, L. Consiliorum medicinalium . . . liber singularis. 1610; Uffenbach, P. Thesaurus chirurgicae. 1610.

TAGEREAU, Vincent [*fl. ca.* 1611] Discours sur l'impuissance de l'homme et de la femme. Auquel est declaré, que c'est qu'impuissance empeschant & separant le mariage . . . Paris, Anthoine de Brueil, 1611.

[8], 191 p. 16 cm. **[11668]**

—[The same.] . . . Rev. & augm. en ceste 2. ed. Paris, La veufue Jean du Brayet, et Nicolas Rousset, 1612.

[8], 226 p. 17 cm. **[11669]**

TAGIUS, Joannes Balthasar [*fl.* 1632-1636] *respondent. See* Rehefeld, J., *praeses.* Exercitatiuncula posterior de lipyriae cura. 1636; Sebisch, M. [1578-1674?] *praeses.* Galeni Ars parva in disputationes triginta resoluta. 1633.

TAGLIACOZZI, Gaspare [1545-1599] *See* Cortesi, G. B. Miscellaneorum medicinalium decades denae. 1625; Read, A. Chirurgorum comes. 1687.

TAILEPIED, Noël [1540-1589] Traicté de l'apparition des esprits. A sçavoir, des ames separees, fantosmes, prodiges, & autres accidens merveilleux, qui precedent quelquefois la mort des grands personnages, ou signifient changement de la chose publique . . . Paris, Jean Corrozet, 1616.

[16], 295, [21] p. 15 cm. **[11670]**
Previously published under title: Psychologie; ou Traité de l'apparition des esprits.

[TAISNIER, Joannes, *b.* 1509] La science curieuse; ou, Traité de la chyromance, récueilly des plus graves

autheurs qui ont traité de cette matiere, & plus exactement recherché qu'il n'a esté cy-devant par aucun
autre ... 2. ed. Paris, François Clousier, 1667.

[8], 212 p.   plates.   23 cm.   [11671]

Attributed to Joannes Taisnier. Cf. Sabattini 589.

TALBOR, *Sir* ROBERT [1642–1681] The English
remedy; or, Talbor's wonderful secret, for cureing
of agues and feavers. Sold by the author Sir Robert
Talbor, to the most Christian king, and since his
death, ordered by his Majesty to be published in
French ... And now translated into English ...
London, Printed by J. Wallis for Jos. Hindmarsh,
1682.

[7], 112 p.   16 cm.   [11672]

Attributed to Nicolas de Blegny by NUC.

—Πυρετολογία; A rational account of the cause &
cure of agues. With ... a successful method ... for
the cure of ... quartans ... Whereunto is added a
short account ... of feavers, and the gripping in the
guts ... London, R. Robinson, 1672.

[11], 77, [3] p.   15 cm.   [11673]

—*See* LES ADMIRABLES QUALITEZ DU KINKINA. 1689,
1694; [Italian tr.] 1694.

TALBOT, EDWARD. *See* KELLY, EDWARD
[1555–1595]

TALBOT, ROBERT. *See* TALBOR, *Sir* Robert
[1642–1681]

TALIACOTIUS, GASPAR. *See* TAGLIACOZZI,
Gaspare [1545–1599]

TAMAYO, ANDRÉS DE [*fl.* 1621–*ca.* 1625] Tratados
breves de algebra, y garrotillo ... Con una Instruccion de los barberos flobotomianos. Por Alonso
Munoz ... Valencia, Por Juan Chrysostomo Garriz, a costa Filipo Pincinali, 1621.

[8], 58, [2] ll.; [1], 17, [2] ll.   15 cm.   [11674]

Part [2] has special title page.

—*See* CALVO, J. Primera y segunda parte de la
cirugia universal. 1647, 1674, 1690.

TAMBURINI, GERONIMO [*fl.* 1613–1621] *ed. See*
ALDROVANDI, U. De piscibus libri V. 1613; BALDI, C.
In Physiognomica Aristotelis commentarii. 1621.

TAMITIUS, ANDREAS [*fl.* 1622] Disputatio
physica de anima ... Lipsiae, Excudebat

Hieronymus Rauscher, 1622.

[12] p.   18 cm.   [11675]

Diss.—Leipzig (E. Fischer, *respondent*)

TANCKE, JOACHIM [1557–1609] Viro nobilissimo
... Dn. Bernhardo G. Penoto ... S. P. Epistola ...

998–999 p., vol. 4.   20 cm.   (*In* Zetzner,
Lazarus, *ed.* Theatrum chemicum. Argentorati,
1659–61)   [11676]

Caption and running title.

—, *ed. See* WARENIUS, H., *praeses.* Νοσολογια. 1605.

—, *tr. See* RESCH, J. U. Osiandrische Experiment
von Sole. 1659.

—*See* REUDEN, M. Bedencken. 1605.

TANCREDI, LATINO [*fl.* 1606] De fame, et siti
lib. III, physicis, ac medicis reconditis controversiis
parsim respersi ... Venetiis, Apud Jac. Antonium
Somaschum, 1607.

[24], 183 ll.   23 cm.   [11677]

TANDLER, TOBIAS [1571–1617] Dissertationes
physicae-medicae: I. De spectris, quae vigilantibus
obveniunt. II. De fascino & incantatione. III. De
melancholia & hujus amolitione. IV. De melancholicorum vaticiniis, aliisque mirandis operibus. V.
De noctisurgio ... Quibus accesserunt ... Hieron.
Nymanni VI. De imaginatione oratio, & D. Martini Biermanni VII. De magicis actionibus ἐξέτα-
σις... Leucoreis Athenis [Witebergae] Impensis
Zacher. Schureri, ex Officina Meisneriana, 1613.

[16], 296 p.   16 cm.   [11678]

—*praeses.* De melancholia ejusque speciebus ...
Witebergae, Typis Cratonianis exscribebat Johan.
Gorman [*ca.* 1608]

[51] p.   18 cm.   [11679]

Diss.—Wittenberg (J. J. Anomoeus and P. Schmilauer
respondents)

TANNER, JOHN [*fl.* 1659–1667] The hidden
treasures of the art of physick; fully discovered: in
four books. Containing a physical description of man
The causes ... of all diseases ... The general cure
of wounds ... A general rule for making all kind of
medicines ... To which is added three necessary
tables ... London, George Sawbridge, 1659.

[16], 543, [36] p.   15 cm.   [11680]

Errata: p. [35–36]

—[The same.] . . . The 3d ed., with additions . . . London, Printed by John Streater and sold by George Sawbridge, 1672.

[14], 324, [22] p.   17 cm.   [11681]

TANSO MAGNALPINA, Gio., *pseud. See* Lampugnani, Agostino [*ca.* 1586-*ca.* 1666]

TANTIUS, Regulus Antonius. *See* Tanzi, Regolo Antonio [1665-1745]

TANZI, Regolo Antonio [1665-1745] Luna in puteo, et sophismatum medico-physicorum apologitica anacrisis; sive, Iatromachia therapeutica de antiphthisico radicis Chinae usu . . . Tractatus chinencomiasticus veterum, & recentiorum placitis accommodatus, methodica ratione, atque multijugo clarissimorum auctorum testimonio decoratus, & comprobatus . . . Venetiis, Typis Aloysii Pavini, 1698.

163, [2] p.   16 cm.   [11682]

TAPARO, Ottavio. Compendio delli casi di chirurgia . . . Di nuovo ristampato . . . Roma, Fabio di Falco, 1663.

47 p.   15 cm.   [11683]

TAPISSIER, Estienne [*fl.* 1646] *defendant. See* Lambert, N., *defendant.* Factum, pour les sieurs conseillers de la chambre de ville de Nancy appellans de deux sentences. 1647.

TAPPE, Jakob [1603-1680] Oratio de tabaco ejusque hodierno abusu . . . Helmestadii, Typis Henningi Mulleri, 1653.

[32] p.   20 cm.   [11684]

—[The same.] . . . 2. ed. auct. Helmestadii, Typis & sumptibus Henningi Mulleri, 1660.

[36] p.   19 cm.   [11685]

Imperfect: sig. E2-3 wanting.
Bound with Pechlin, J. N. Theophilus Bibaculus. 1684.

—[The same.] . . . 3. ed. auct. Helmestadii, Typis & sumtibus Henrici Davidis Mülleri, 1673.

[43] p.   20 cm.   [11686]

—[The same.] . . . 3d ed. auct. & corr. Helmstadii, Typis & sumptibus Georg-Wolfgangi Hammii, 1689.

[40] p.   19 cm.   [11687]

Dissertations — Helmstedt

—*praeses.* Disputatio inauguralis medica de ileo . . . Helmaestadii, Typis Henningi Mulleri, 1664.

[44] p.   19 cm.   [11688]

B. Horne, *respondent.*

—Disputatio medica de amore insano . . . Helmestadii, Typis Henning Mulleri, 1661.

[20] p.   18 cm.   [11689]

J. Wollin, *respondent.*

—Disputatio medica de apoplexia . . . Helmestadi, Typis Henningi Mulleri, 1663.

[32] p.   20 cm.   [11690]

B. Lembken, *respondent.*

—Disputatio medica de febri ephemera . . . Helmestadii, Typis Henningi Mulleri, 1662.

[42] p.   20 cm.   [11691]

F. Heye, *respondent.*

—Disputatio medica de hydrophobia . . . Helmaestadii, Typis Henningi Mulleri, 1659.

[32] p.   18 cm.   [11692]

H. Meibom, *respondent.*

—Disputatio medica de mania . . . Helmestadii, Excudit Henningus Mullerus, 1644.

[28] p.   20 cm.   [11693]

G. Huhn, *respondent.*

—Disputatio medica de melancholica desipientia . . . Helmaestadii, Typis Henningi Mulleri, 1652.

[28] p.   19 cm.   [11694]

S. Scheffer, *respondent.*

—Disputatio medica de phrenitide . . . Helmaestadii, Typis Henningi Mulleri, 1643.

[27] p.   19 cm.   [11695]

J. P. Muller, *respondent.*

—Disputatio medica inauguralis de arthritide . . . Helmestadii, Typis Henningi Mulleri, 1664.

[35] p.   19 cm.   [11696]

J. J. Müller, *respondent.*

—Disputatio medica pathologica de comate et caro . . . Helmestadii, Typis Henningi Mülleri, 1668.

[24] p.   20 cm.   [11697]

E. Barnstorff, *respondent.*

—Disputatio medica pathologica de sensus tactus depravatione . . . Helmestadii, Typis Henningi Mulleri, 1673.

[30] p.   20 cm.   [11698]

S. F. Stisser, *respondent.*

—Disputatio physiologica de somno naturali ejusque causis ... Helmaestadii, Typis Henningi Mulleri, 1664.

[39] p. 18 cm.   [11699]

H. K. Stisser, *respondent.*

TARANTA, Valescus de. *See* Valesco de Taranta [*fl.* 1382–1418]

al-TĀRASŪSĪ, Jābir ibn Haiyān. *See* Jabir ibn Ḥaiyān, al-Ṭarasūsī.

TARDI, Claude. *See* Tardy, Claude [1607–1670]

TARDIGRADO. *See* Stelluti, Francesco [1577–*ca.* 1651]

TARDIN, Jean [*fl.* 1609] Disquisitio physiologica de pilis. Turnoni, Claudius Michael, 1609.

[16], 280, [22] p. 17 cm.   [11700]

Imperfect? Last leaf (blank?) wanting.

TARDY, Claude [1607–1670] An biliosis purgatio ante cibum? [Paris? 1661?]

4 p.   22 cm.   [11701]

Caption title.
Imperfect: p. 3–4 mutilated.
"Quaestio medica. Cardinalitiis disputationibus mane discutienda in scholis medic. die Jovis X. Martii. M. Claudio Tardy ... moderatore."
At end: Probonebat Lutetiae Joannes Baptista Ferrand ... M. DC. LXI.

—An morbi omnes a vitiato circulari motu sanguinis? [Paris? 1660?]

8 p.   23 cm.   [11702]

Caption title.
"Quaestio medica. Quodlibetariis disputationibus mane discutienda, in scholis medicorum, die Jovis 22. Januarii. M. Claudio Tardy ... moderatore."
At end: Proponebat Lutetiae Petrus Pourret ... M. DC. LX.
Bound with *his* Traitté du mouvement circulaire du sang et des esprits. 1654.

—Hippocratica purgandi methodus ... Parisiis, Apud Carolum Chastelain, 1646.

[8], 40 p.   23 cm.   [11703]

Caption title, p. 2: An morbis a pituita, vomitus? a bile, dejectio?
"Quaestio medica, quodlibetariis disputationibus mane discutienda, in scholis medicorum, die Jovis 18. Januarii. M. Claudio Tardy, doctore medico, praeside."
"Proponebat Lutetiae Tussanus Foucault Paris. A. R. S. H. M.DC.XLVI."
Bound with *his* Traitté du mouvement circulaire du sang et des esprits. 1654.

—In libellos Hippocratis De septimestri et octimestri partu. Commentarii, quibus universa partuum doctrina propriis rationibus demonstratur ... Parisiis, Apud Carolum Du Mesnil, 1651.

48 p.   23 cm.   [11704]

—In libellum Hippocratis De virginum morbis commentatio paraphrastica. Ubi de morbis capitis et aliis qui prodeunt ex intercepto, imminuto, depravato & adaucto circulari motu sanguinis. Ac eorum curatione. Idque expositione continua difficillimorum contextuum ex variis Hippocratis libris ... Parisiis, Apud Jacobum de Senlecque, et apud Carolum du Mesnil, 1648.

40 p.   23 cm.   [11705]

Bound with *his* Traitté du mouvement circulaire du sang et des esprits. 1654.

—Observationes anatomicae ... [165–?]

7 p.   23 cm.   [11706]

Caption title.
Bound with *his* Traitté du mouvement circulaire du sang et des esprits. 1654.

—Tempus infusionis animae ... [Paris? 165–?]

8 p.   22 cm.   [11707]

—Traitté de la monarchie du coeur en l'homme, des quatre humeurs & de leurs sources, des usages du foye, et des vaisseaux qui contiennent le chyle ... Paris, La vefve Du Puys et Jean Guignard, 1656.

[2], 12 p.   23 cm.   [11708]

Bound with *his* Traitté du mouvement circulaire du sang et des esprits. 1654.

—Traitté des moyens de conserver en santé les hommes bilieux ... [Paris? 165–?]

8 p.   22 cm.   [11709]

Caption title.

—Traitté du mouvement circulaire du sang et des esprits. Qui est le principal des trois moyens dont la nature se fert à perfectionner l'homme ... Paris, Charles Du Mesnil et Jean Guignard, 1654.

[16], 119, 32, [2] p.   23 cm.   [11710]

"Seconde partie du traitté du mouvement circulaire du sang et des esprits" (32, [2] p. at end) includes, Commentaire avec paraphrase du troisiéme livre de la diette du grand Hippocrate and Commentaire avec paraphrase du livre des songes du grand Hippocrate.
With this are bound *his*: Traitté de la monarchie du coeur en l'homme. 1656; Hippocratica purgandi methodus. 1646; In libellum Hippocratis De virginum morbis commentatio paraphrastica. 1648;

An morbi omnes a vitiato circulari motu sanguinis? [1660?]; Observationes anatomicae. [165-?]

—, *ed.* and *tr. See* HIPPOCRATES. [Collected works. French] Les oeuvres du grand Hippocrate. 1667.

—*See* BARTHOLIN, T. Opuscula nova anatomica. 1670.

TARENTA, VALESCO DE. *See* VALESCO DE TARANTA [*fl.* 1382-1418]

TARGIER, JOACHIM [*fl.* 1687] *respondent.* Exercitationis medicae specimen inaugurale de abortu . . . Trajecti ad Rhenum, Ex officina Francisci Halma, 1687.

    22, [2] p.   22 cm.   **[11711]**
Diss—Utrecht.

TARGIRUS, JOACHIMUS [*fl.* 1697] Medicina compendiaria, in qua, propositis veterum sententiis, nova & verissima artis medicae forma ac ratio breviter & dilucide explicatur. Lugduni in Batavis, Apud Fredericum Haringium, 1698.

                                                 [11712]

—*See* REVERHORST, M. van. Dissertatio anatomico-medica de motu bilis. 1696.

TARIFFA et prezzi da vendere, & apprezzare le robbe. 1619. *See* PERUGIA. Magnifica arte delli spetiali.

TARINO, GIOVANNI ALBERTO [*fl.* 1655-1659] *tr. See* SEVERINO, M. A. Antiperipatias. 1655-1659.

TARNOV, JOHANN [*fl.* 1649-1652] *respondent. See* GRASS, S., *praeses.* Exercitatio medica de pleuritide. 1649.

TASGRESTI, GIOVANNI BATTISTA. *See* GRASSETTI, Giovanni Battista [1609-1684]

TASSA delle robbe medicinali. 1677. *See* MODENA. Ordinances, local laws, etc.

TASSIN, LÉONARD [*d.* 1687] Les administrations anatomiques . . . Sedan, François Chayer, 1676.

    [5], 226 p.   17 cm.   **[11713]**
"Myologie": p. 137-226.

—[The same.] Les administrations anatomiques, et la myologie . . . 3. ed. Paris, Michel Vaugon, 1688.

    [8], 314 (i.e. 304) p.   16 cm.   **[11714]**
With this is bound *his* La chirurgie militaire. 1688.

—[The same.] . . . Derniere ed. Lyon, La veuve de Jean-Bapt. Guillimin, 1696.

    [8], 304 p.   16 cm.   **[11715]**
With this is bound (as issued) *his* La chirurgie militaire. 1696.

—La chirurgie militaire; ou, L'art de guarir les playes d'arquebusades . . . Paris, Michel Vaugon, 1688.

    57 p.   16 cm.   **[11716]**
Bound with *his* Les administrations anatomiques. 1688.

—[The same.] . . . Lyon, La veuve de Jean-Bapt. Guillimin, 1696.

    57, [1] p.   16 cm.   **[11717]**
Different setting of type.
Bound with (as issued) *his* Les administrations anatomiques. 1696.

—[German tr.] *In* Botallo, L. Zwey chirurgische Bücher. 1676.

TASSONI, ALESSANDRO [1565-1635] Dieci libri di pensieri diversi . . . ne' quali per via di quisiti con nuovi fondamenti, e ragioni si trattano le più curiose materie naturali, morali, civili, poetiche, istoriche, e d'altre facolta . . . corretti . . . e arricchiti in questa 8. impr. . . . Venezia, Marc'Antonio Brogiolo, 1636.

    [104], 551 (i.e. 547) p.   21 cm.   **[11718]**

TATAI KOVÁTS, GYÖRGY. *See* KOVÁCS GYÖRGY, *tatai* [*b.* 1645]

TATE, NAHUM [1652-1715] Panacea: a poem upon tea: in two canto's . . . London, J. Roberts, 1700.

    [16], 34, [5] p.   19 cm.   **[11719]**
Imperfect: title page mutilated affecting imprint.

—, *ed. See* A MEMORIAL FOR THE LEARNED. 1686.

—, *tr. See* FRACASTORO, G. Syphilis. 1686, 1693.

TATINGHOFF, MICHAËL FREDERIK [*d.* 1673] *respondent.* Disputatio medica inauguralis, de pleuritide & peripneumonia . . . Lugduni Batavorum, Ex officina Severini Matthaei, 1659.

    [8] p.   19 cm.   **[11720]**
Diss. — Leyden.

—, *tr. See* HIPPOCRATES. [Aphorismi. Dutch.] 1658.

TATTER, GEORG MARTIN [*fl.* 1673-1678] *respondent. See* MAJOR, J. D., *praeses.* Disputationem anatomicam de sanguine peridromo . . . intimant . . . Joh. Daniel Major . . . & . . . Georgius Martinus

Tatter. 1673; Pechlin, J. N., *praeses.* Disputatio medica inauguralis de epilepsia 1678.

TATTI, Francesco, *pseud. See* Sansovino, Francesco, [1521–1586]

TATTI, Giovanni, *pseud. See* Sansovino, Francesco [1521–1586]

TAUBE, Christoph Ernst [*fl.* 1694] *respondent.* Dissertatio medica inauguralis de recens natorum sanitate tuenda . . . Trajecti ad Rhenum, Ex officina Francisci Halma, 1694.

    16 p. 21 cm.   **[11721]**
Diss. — Utrecht.

— *See* Rolfinck, W., *praeses.* Disputatio inauguralis medica de plica Polonica. 1658.

TAUBENHEIM, Johann Casimir [*fl.* 1682–1685] *respondent. See* Bohn, J., *praeses.* Dissertationes chymico-physicae. 1685.

TAUCHER, Pierre [*fl.* 1680] *See* Alsace, Conseil Souverain. Arrest. 1680.

TAURELLUS, Andreas [*fl.* 1630–1641] De peste Italica, libri duo. Quibus discutiuntur ortus, progressus causae . . . remedia, cum in genere pestilentiae, tum in specie epidemiae, quae anno MDCXXX. contagiose grassari coepit per aliquot Italiae provincias. Additae narratione praesidiorum politicorum, quibus . . . Bononia languentem populum sustinuit . . . Bononiae, Typis Nicolai Tebaldini, 1641.

    [16], 170 (i.e. 160), [16] p. plate. 24 cm.
                            [11722]
Added engraved title page.

TAUVONIUS, Abraham Georg. *See* Thauvonius, Abraham Georg [*ca.* 1622–1679]

TAUVRY, Daniel [1669–1701] Nouvelle anatomie raisonnée; ou, Les usages de la structure du corps de l'homme, et de quelques autres animaux, suivant les loix des mechaniques . . . Paris, Estienne Michallet, 1690.

    [25], 379, [5] p. plates. 17 cm.   **[11723]**
Errata: p. [25]

— [The same.] . . . 2. ed., rev., corr., & augm. par l'auteur. Paris, Estienne Michallet, 1693.

    [12], 417, [14] p. front., plates. 17 cm.**[11724]**

— [The same.] . . . 3. ed., rev., corr. & augm. par l'auteur . . . Paris, Barthelemy Girin, 1698.

    [12], 422, [15] p. front., plates. 17 cm.**[11725]**

— [Latin tr.] Nova anatomia ratiociniis illustrata, quibus usus structurae partium corporis humani, & quorundam aliorum animalium, secundum leges mechanicae explicantur . . . Latinitate donata, a Melchiore Friderico Geudero . . . juxta exemplar Parisiense. Ulmae, Sumptibus Georgii Wilhelmi Kühnii, typis haered. Christ. Balth. Kühnens, 1693.

    [31], 472, [23] p. front., plates. 16 cm.**[11726]**

— Another issue, with new title page dated 1694
                             [11727]
Imperfect? front wanting?

— Nouvelle pratique des maladies aigues, et de toutes celles qui dependent de la fermentation des liqueurs . . . Paris, Laurent d'Houry, 1698.

    2 v. 17 cm.   **[11728]**

— Traité de la generation et de la nourriture du foetus . . . Paris, Barthelemy Girin, 1700.

    [20], 215 p.; [6], 75, [7] p. 17 cm.   **[11729]**
Part [2] has caption title: Replique aux réponses de Mr Mery

— Traité des medicamens, et la maniere de s'en servir pour la guerison des maladies, suivant les experiences des medecins modernes. Avec les formules pour la composition des medicamens . . . Paris, Estienne Michallet, 1691.

    [16], 385 (i.e. 389), [2] p. plate. 17 cm.**[11730]**

— [The same.] . . . 2. ed., rev. corr. & augm. . . . Paris, Estienne Michallet, 1695.

    [24], 596, [21] p. 17 cm.   **[11731]**

— [The same.] . . . Nouv. ed., rev., corr. & augm. . . . Paris, Barthelemy Girin, 1699.

    2 v. 18 cm.   **[11732]**

— [English tr.] A treatise of medicines, containing an account of their chymical principles, the experiments made upon 'em, their various preparations, their vertues, and the modern way of using them . . . Written originally in French . . . Translated from the last ed. London, Richard Wellington, Arthur Bettesworth, and Bernard Lintott, 1700.

    [15], 287, 291, [4] p. 20 cm.   **[11733]**

—, *respondent. See* Poirier, L., *praeses.* Quaestio medica . . . An dysenteriae, mochlica purgatio? 1695

TAVARES, Manuel dos Reys. *See* Reys Tavares, Manuel dos [*fl.* 1667]

TAVERNIER, Nicolas [*fl.* 1608] *respondent.* Theses iatricae de lapide calculo ... Basileae, Typis Johannis Schroeteri, 1608.

    [12] p.   20 cm.   **[11734]**
Diss.—Basel

TAVOLA de prezzi delle robbe di spetiaria per tutto lo Stato Ecclesiastico. 1648. *See* Vatican. Protomedico generale.

TAXA pharmaceutica officinar. *See* Leipzig. Ordinances, local laws, etc. Raths der Stadt Leipzig ... Ordnung und Taxa. 1689.

TAXA; seu, Pretium omnium officinis marchiae usualium medicamentorum. *See* Dispensatorium Brandenburgicum. 1698.

TAXATIO; seu, Valor medicamentorum omnium, tam simplicium, quam compositorum, quae in officina pharmaceutica Isnacensi prostant. Tax; oder, Werth aller Artzeneyen ... welche in der Apotheken zu Eisenach zu finden. Jena, Gedruckt bey Joh. Nisien, 1681.

    87, [1] p.   19 cm.   **[11735]**
In Latin and German.

TAXIL, Jean [*fl.* 1602–1608] Traicté de l'epilepsie, maladie vulgairement appellée au pays de Provence, la gouttete aux petits enfans. Avec plusieurs belles, & curieuses questions, touchant les causes prognostiques, & cure d'icelles ... Lyon, Robert Renaud, 1602.

    24, 296, [32] p.   18 cm.   **[11736]**
  Imperfect: last 2 leaves of index and errata leaf at end wanting. Supplied in photocopy from the copy of the 1603 issue in the New York Academy of Medicine Library.
  Author's portrait wanting from last prelim. page, although space was left for it, and the title and poem to accompany it are printed there.

TAYLOR, Jeremy, *Bp. of Down and Connor* [1613–1667] Ductor dubitantium. *See* [Dugard, S.] The marriages of cousin Germans. 1673.

TAYLOR, John, *apothecary, York. See* Deane, E. Spadacrene Anglica. 1649.

TAYLOR, Thomas [1670?–1735] *tr. See* Malebranche, N. Treatise concerning the search after truth. 1694.

TECENENSIS, Guilhelmus [*fl.* 16th-17th cent.] Liber ... qui lilium tanquam de spinis evulsum appellatur.

    887–912 p., vol. 4.   20 cm. (*In* Zetzner, Lazarus, *ed.* Theatrum chemicum. Argentorati, 1659–61)   **[11737]**

TECKOP, Peter [*fl.* 1661] *respondent.* Disputatio medica inauguralis de motus difficultate affectioni hypochondriacae juncta ... Lugduni Batavorum, Ex officina Isaaci de Waal, 1661.

    [12] p.   21 cm.   **[11738]**
Diss.—Leyden.

TECTORIIS, Franciscus Maria de [*fl.* 16th cent.] *See* Melich, G. Dispensatorium medicum. 1601.

TEICHER, Christoph [*fl.* 1671–1676] *respondent.* Disputatio medica inauguralis de epilepsia ... Lugduni Batavorum, Apud viduam & haeredes Joannis Elsevirii, 1671.

    [16] p.   22 cm.   **[11739]**
Diss.—Leyden.

TEICHMEYER, Hermann Theodor [*fl.* 1674] *praeses.* Dissertatio inauguralis medica de hydrope ascite ... Erffurti, Charactere Kirschiano [1674]

    [36] p.   19 cm.   **[11740]**
Diss.—Erfurt (J.A. Beck, *respondent*)

TEIL, Bernard du. *See* Du Teil, Bernard [*fl.* 1636–*ca.* 1659]

TELESIO, Antonio [1482–1533?] De coloribus. *In* Joannes Actuarius. De urinis libri VII. 1670; Willich, J. Exercitationes et probationes de urinis libri IV. 1688.

TEIXEIRA, António [1602–1687] Epitome das noticias astrologicas para a medicina ... Lisboa, Ioam da Costa, 1670.

    [11], 407, [12] p.   20 cm.   **[11741]**
  Imperfect: sheet E bound after sheet F; sig. ****2 bound between sig. 3Fl and 2.

TELL-TROTH, Tim. The knavery of astrology discover'd, in observations upon every month, of the year 1680. Together with the nature of the seven planets, &c. By Tim. Tell-Troth, star-gazer to the great mogul ... London, Printed for T. B. and R. E., 1680.

    20 p.   22 cm.   **[11742]**

[**TEMPLE**, *Sir* WILLIAM, *bart.,* 1628-1699] Miscellanea. I. A survey of the constitutions and interests of the empire, Sueden, Denmark, Spain, Holland, France, and Flanders; with their relation to England, in the year 1671. II. An essay upon the original and nature of government. III. An essay upon the advancement of trade in Ireland. IV. Upon the conjuncture of affairs in Octob. 1673. V. Upon the excesses of grief. VI. An essay upon the cure of the gout by moxa. By a person of honour. London, Printed by A. M. and R. R. for Edw. Gellibrand, 1680.

    [8], 238 p. 19 cm.   **[11743]**

    —Miscellanea. The first part [-third part]. London, 1690—1701.

    3 v. in 2. 19 cm., 20 cm.   **[11744]**

    Imprint varies: Vol. 1. 3d ed. Jacob Tonson and John Churchill, 1691; vol. 2. 2d ed. Printed by J. R. for Ri. and Ra. Simpson, 1690; vol.3. Benjamin Cooke, published by Jonathan Swift, 1701.

TEN RHIJNE, WILLEM. *See* RHIJNE, Willem ten [1647-1700]

TENCKE, HENRICUS. *See* TENQUE, Jérôme [*d.* 1687]

TENCKE, JÉRÔME. *See* TENQUE, Jérôme [*d.* 1687]

TENISON, THOMAS, *Abp. of Canterbury* [1636-1715] *ed. See* BACON, F., *viscount St. Albans.* Baconiana. 1679; BROWNE, *Sir* T. Certain miscellany tracts. 1683, 1684.

TENORIO DE LEÓN, ALVARO [*fl.* 17th cent.] Atomos que nuevamente se han descubierto con las luzes de Apolo, en la controversia cèlebre del uso de las sangrias, assi en los afectos superiores, como en las calenturas. Respondese a los argumentos con que . . . Juan Moyano pretende impugnar la comun sentientia de los autores, que venera el arte por principes, cuya doctrina se explica . . . [Sevilla? ca. 1650]

    [4], 71, [1] p. 20 cm.   **[11745]**

    Errata: p. [72]
    Imperfect: outer margins trimmed.
    Concerns controversy with Juan Moyano de Medina and Luis Pérez Ramírez.

TENQUE, JÉRÔME [*d.* 1687] Instrumenta curationis morborum deprompta ex pharmacia, chyrurgia & diaeta. Pars prima. De instrumentis pharmaceuticis, Galenicis & chymicis . . . Authore

Hieronymo Tenque . . . Monspelii, Apud Danielem Pech, venaeunt apud Stephanum Marret, 1679.

    452, [1] p. 15 cm.   **[11746]**

    Errata alia: p. [453]
    Imperfect: title page mutilated, with loss of imprint; p. 49-132 wanting.
    Apparently complete. Later editions omit "Pars prima" from title.

    —Another issue, with undated title page: Authore H[ieronymo] T[enque] P[rofessore] R[egio] M[onspeliensi] Monspelii, Apud Danielem Pech, venaeunt apud Stephanum Marret [1679?]

    452, [1] p. 16 cm.   **[11747]**

    Imperfect: Errata alia (p. [453]) wanting.

    —[The same.] . . . Lugduni, Apud Caesarem Chappuis, 1684.

    [6], 363, [15] p. 16 cm.   **[11748]**

    —[The same.] . . . Venetiis, Typis Joseph Mariae de Ruinettis, 1686.

    [24], 343, [15] p. 16 cm.   **[11749]**

    —[The same.] . . . Ed. 2. . . . Authore H[ieronymo] T[enque] P[rofessore] R[egio] M[onspeliensi] Biterris, et venaeunt Monspelii, Apud Petrum Peronnet, 1486 (i.e. 1686).

    560 (i.e. 561) p. 16 cm.   **[11750]**

    Errata: p. 554-560.

    —[The same.] . . . Ed. 2., plurimis tum remediis, tum cautionibus aucta . . . Authore H[ieronymo] T[enque] P[rofessore] R[egio] M[onspeliensi]. Lugduni, Apud Joannem Certe, 1687.

    [20], 413, [33] p. 15 cm.   **[11751]**

    Special title page (p. [15]) reads: Formules de medecine tirées de la pharmacie, galenique et chymie . . . Par H. Tencke . . . Et nouvellement traduites en françois. Lyon, Jean Certe, 1686.
    Text in Latin.

    —[French tr.] Formules de medecine tirées de la pharmacie galenique et chymique: où il est traité de la méthode d'ordonner toute sorte de remedes pharmaceutiques, & de les adapter à chaque maladie . . . Traduites en françois. 3. ed. rev. & corr. Lyon, Jean Certe, 1690.

    [18 +], 498, [45] p. 16 cm.   **[11752]**

    Imperfect: first preliminary leaf (blank?) wanting.

TENTAMEN medicum, de natura, causis, temporibus, differentiis, signis diacriticis, prognosticis, medelaque variolarum ... Lugduni Batavorum, Apud Felicem Lopez, & Arnoldum Doude, 1675.

84 p. 14 cm.   [**11753**]

TENTZEL, ANDREAS [*fl.* 1614-1625] Exegesis chymiatrica ... qua in ... Angeli Salae libris tacta quidem, attamen plane detecta non sunt, multaque alia διεξοδικως interpolata ...

627-769 p. illus. 20 cm. (*In* Thom, J. D. ed. Collectanea chimica curiosa. Francofurti, 1693)

[**11754**]

Caption title.

—[The same.] *In* Sala, A. Ternarius bezoardicorum & hemetologia. 1618, 1630.

—Medicina diastatica; hoc est, Singularis illa et admirabilis ad distans, & beneficio mumialis transplantationis operationem & efficaciam habens, quae ipsa loco commentarii in tractatum tertium De tempore seu philosop. D. Theoph. Paracelsi, multa, eaque selectissima abstrusioris philosophiae & medicinae arcana continet Jehnae, Sumtibus Johannis Birckneri, 1629.

[16], 188 p. 14 cm.   [**11755**]

Added engraved title page.
Sudhoff 331.

—[The same.] ... Erfurti, Sumtibus Johanni Birckneri, excud. Johann Georg. Hertz, 1666.

[16], 188 p. 14 cm.   [**11756**]

Different setting of type.
Sudhoff 396.

—, *ed. See* THEATRUM SYMPATHETICUM AUCTUM. 1662.

—*See* PARACELSUS. Of the chymical transmutation. 1657.

TENZEL, ANDREAS. *See* TENTZEL, Andreas [*fl.* 1614-1625]

TEOFILO PAMIO, *pseud. See* MONIGLIA, Giovanni Andrea [1624-1700]

TERENTIUS, JOANNES [1576-1630] *See* HERNÁNDEZ, F. Rerum medicarum Novae Hispaniae thesaurus. 1628, 1651.

TERILLI, DOMENICO [*fl.* 1607-1615] De causis mortis repentinae distinctiss. tractatio, in qua etiam disputatur quid sit mors, & vita in genere, & quae

mortis causae communes ... Venetiis, Apud haeredem Damiani Zenarii, 1615.

[16], 118 p. 23 cm.   [**11757**]

Imperfect: wormholes on p. [1]-38.

—De vesicantibus dilucida, ac familiaris antilogia. In qua de vesicantium recto usu, de utilitatibus, mirificisque in praxi eorum fructibus fuse pertractatur ... Venetiis, Apud Joan. Baptistam Bertonum, 1607.

96, [4] p. 23 cm.   [**11758**]

Bound with Casserio, G. Tabulae anatomicae LXXIIX. 1632.

TERM catalogues. A catalogue of books continued, printed, and published at London in Michaelmas-term, 1676. Numb. 9. [London, 1676]

[10] p. 32 cm.   [**11759**]

Signatures: O-P², Q¹.
Edited by Robert Clavell.
Bound with (between part [1] and [2]) Stubbs, H. A censure upon certain passages. 1671.

TERRANOVA, FRANCESCO DI, *Father* [*fl.* 1658] Brevis ampla methodus pro morbis humani corporis in particulari curandis secundum recentiorum usum. Ad medicorum majus commodum disposita elaborato studio Fr. Francisci Cangemii de Terranova ... Romae, Typis Angeli Bernabò á Verme, 1658.

[12], 318 p. 17 cm.   [**11760**]

TERRANUOVA, TOMMASO, *tr. See* VITTORI, B. Prattica d'esperienza. 1624.

TERRENTIUS, JOANNES. *See* TERENTIUS, Joannes [1576-1630]

TERTIIS, JOSEPHUS DE [*fl.* 1685] De curiositatibus physicis tractatus. In quo natura stramentorum foenateorum, & qualitates odoris, & effluviorum, elementorumque mutatio, & praecipue aëris examinantur ... Medioburgi, Apud Aegidium Horthemels juniorem, 1686.

[8], 114, [6] p. front. 17 cm.   [**11761**]

Another issue, with imprint: Lugd. Batavorum, Apud Jacobum Mocque, 1686.   [**11762**]

Without frontispiece.

TERTRE DE LA MARCHE, MARGUERITE DU. *See* LA MARCHE, Marguerite Du Tertre de [1638-1706]

TERUD, JEAN. *See* LAGNEAU, D. Traicté pour la conservation de la santé. 1650.

TESORO delle gioie. *See* ARNOBIO, C.

TESSERAR, JEREMIAS [*fl.* 1626-1627] *respondent. See* CHARSTADIUS, V., *praeses.* Disputationum medicarum tertia de animae facultatibus et earum functionibus. 1626 [and] Disputationum medicarum octava de signis diagnosticis et prognosticis. 1626 [and] Disputationum medicarum duodecima de chirurgia. 1626.

TESTI, LODOVICO [1640-1707] Disinganni, overo ragioni fisiche fondate sù l'autorità, ed esperienza, che provano l'aria di Venezia intieramente salubre . . . Colonia [Venice], Per Giovanni Wilelmo Schell, 1694.

[16], 160 p.   25 cm.   **[11763]**

TESTORI, GIUSEPPE. *See* TESTORI DE CAPITANI, Giuseppe.

TESTORI DE CAPITANI, GIUSEPPE, *ed.* and *tr. See* CRISTINI, B. Pratica medicinale. 1680-1681.

TETTERODE, JAN À [*fl.* 1646-1647] *respondent. See* WALAEUS, J., *praeses.* Disputatio medica de phthisi. 1646.

TETZEN, JOHANN VON. *See* JOHANN VON TETZEN.

TEUBERUS, JOANNES. *See* TEÜBER, Johann [*fl.* 1653]

TEÜBER, JOHANN [*fl.* 1653] Arthritis; sive, De natura, ortu, causis, signis, incrementis, & practica curatione podagrae, tractatus physicus singularis . . . Pragae, Typis Caesareo-Academicis, 1653.

[15], 119 p.   20 cm.   **[11764]**

TEVETIO CRUFENAS, CARIOLLINUS. *See* CRUFENAS, Cariollinus Tevetio, *pseud.*

TEXEIRA, ANTONIO. *See* TEIXEIRA, António [1602-1687]

Le TEXTE d'alchymie. 1695. *See* [BERNARDUS TREVIRENSIS]

TEYLINGEN, JAN VAN [*fl.* 1676] *respondent.* Disputatio medica inauguralis de angina . . . Lugduni Batavorum, Apud viduam & haeredes Johannis Elsevirii, 1676.

[10] p.   22 cm.   **[11765]**

THAM, CHRISTOPH PAUL [*fl.* 1639] *respondent. See* SCHLEGEL, P. M., *praeses.* Disputatio medica inauguralis de empyemate. 1639.

THAMM, JOHANN GEORG [*fl.* 1696] *respondent. See* LANGE, C. J., *praeses.* Valetudinarium gravidarum. 1696.

—*See* RIVINUS, A. Q. L. S. D. Facultatis Medicae . . . procancellarius, Augustus Quirinus Rivinus. 1696.

THARANTA, VALESCUS DE. *See* VALESCO DE TARANTA [*fl.* 1382-1418]

THAUVONIUS, ABRAHAM. *See* THAUVONIUS, Abraham Georg [*ca.* 1622-1679]

THAUVONIUS, ABRAHAM GEORG [*ca.* 1622-1679] *praeses.* Disputatio physica de sensibus . . . Aboae, Impressa a Petro Hanson [1655]

[24] p.   20 cm.   **[11766]**

Diss. — Åbo (P. J. Eck, *respondent*)

THAYER, THOMAS. THAYRE, Thomas [*fl.* 1603-1625]

THAYRE, THOMAS [*fl.* 1603-1625] An excellent and best approved treatise of the plague. Containing, the nature, signes, and accidents of the same . . . London, Thomas Archer, 1625.

[8], 54, [2] p.   19 cm.   **[11767]**

STC 23930.

THEATINES. Congregazione di Palermo. Regole osservate da PP. Theatini di Palermo in S. Gioseffo nel tempo del contagio. [n. p., 1624?]

9 p.   20 cm.   **[11768]**

Caption title.

THEATRUM botanicum. *See* MATTIOLI, P. A.

THEATRUM chemicum. *See* ZETZNER, L., *ed.*

THEATRUM sympatheticum, in quo sympathiae actiones variae . . . exhibentur, & . . . occasione pulveris sympathetici, ita quidem elucidantur, ut illarum agendi vis & modus, sine qualitatum occultarum, animaeve mundi, aut spiritus astralis magnive magnalis, vel aliorum commentariorum subsidio ad oculum pateat. Opusculum . . . Digbaei, Papinii, Helmontii, aliorumque recentiorum scriptorum prolata exhibens & trutinans, atque ipsius pulveris sympathetici . . . descriptionem simul exponens. Norimbergae, Impensis Joh. And. & Wolffg. Jun. Endterorum haered., 1660.

[20], 377, [4] p.   double front.   14 cm.
[11769]

Dedication signed: Joh. Andreas Endter.

'Explicatio tituli aenei" (p. [3–7], in verse) signed: L. S. M. D. [. Laurentius Strauss?]

Contains Oratio de vulnerum per pulverum sympatheticum [c]atione, by Sir Kenelm Digby (a translation by Laurentius [Str]auss of his Discours touchant la guérison des plaies par la poudre [de] sympathie); a letter by Laurentius Strauss to Digby, dated 1659 [(p.] 193–252); De pulvere sympathico, by Nicolas Papin; and Pulvis [sym]patheticus, by Henri Mohy. No work by Helmont is included.

—[The same.] ... Ed. alt. priori emendatior. [A]mstelaedami, Impensis Thomae Fontani, 1661.

[12], 259 p. 15 cm.   [11770]

Apparently the pirated edition referred to in the note "Ad in[i]quos & Christianos bibliopolas" in the enlarged edition published [by] the original Nuremberg publishers in 1662.

With this is bound: Maxwell, W. De medicina magnetica libri [III]. 1679.

—[The same.] THEATRUM sympatheticum auctum, [ex]hibens varios authores, de pulvere sympathetico, [qu]idem: Digbaeum, Straussium, Papinium, et [M]ohyum. De unguento vero armario: Goclenium, [R]obertum, Helmontium ... Praemittitur his [Sy]lvestri Rattray, Aditus ad sympathiam et an[tip]athium. Ed. nov. corr. auct. multisque parasangis [m]elior. Norimbergae, Apud Johan. Andream End[te]rum, & Wolfgangi Junioris haeredes, 1662.

[8], 722, [42] p. illus. 21 cm.   [11771]

The four works by Sir Kenelm Digby, Laurentius Strauss, [Ni]colas Papin and Henri Mohy, which were contained in the [or]iginal edition of the collection published by the same press in [16]60, are here reprinted on p. [72]–176.

Sylvester Rattray's "Aditus novus ad occultas sympathiae et [an]tipathiae causas inveniendas" (p. [1]–71) was first printed [se]parately in Glasgow in 1658.

The editorship of this enlarged edition has been ascribed to [An]dreas Tentzel.

—[Dutch ed.] Theatrum sympateticum; ofte, [W]onder-toneel des natuurs verborgentheden. [Be]helsende een uitstekende oratie, over het gebruik [de]s poeders de sympathie ... door Kenelmus Digby [..]. Benevens twee waardige vervolgen, van vele [ze]ldzame antipathien en sympathien ... Door N. [P]apinius, en A. Kircherus. Amsterdam, Jacob van [R]oyen en Timotheus ten Hoorn, 1681.

[8], 439 (i.e. 437), [25] p. 15 cm.   [11772]

Added engraved title page.

Tweede deel (p. [147]) and Derde deel (p. [219]) have special title [pa]ges.

—[The same.] ... Den 2. druk, verm. en verb. [L]eeuwarden, Hendrik Rintjes, Amsterdam, Jan ten

Hoorn, 1697.

[8], 320 p.; 169 (i.e. 196), [20] p. 16 cm.   [11773]

Imperfect: first preliminary leaf wanting.

Part 2 has special title page: Nieuwe beproefde en wel ondersochte genees-middelen ... Getrokken uyt de gedenk-schriften van den ... Kenelmus Digby.

—[The same, as subject.] See DEUSING, A. Sympathetici pulveris examen. 1662.

THEBALDI, GIROLAMO [*fl.* 1630] See SARRATI, A. Apologia. 1631.

THEILL, LORENZ [*fl.* 1668] *respondent.* See SCHENCK, J. T., *praeses.* Disputationem inauguralem de malo hypochondriaco ... publicae disquisitioni sistit ... 1668.

THEISNER, JOHANN JAKOB [*fl.* 1671–1673] See SCHENCK, J. T., *praeses.* Dissertatio medica de ambulatione in somno. 1671.

THEOCRITUS, A GANDA, *pseud.* See HEINSIUS, Daniel [1580–1655]

THEODIDACTUS, EUGENIUS [*pseud.*] See HEYDON, John [*b.* 1629]

THEODORICUS, ALBERT [*fl.* 1608] *respondent.* See LIBAVIUS, A. [*d.* 1616] *praeses.* De mundi corporumque mixtorum elementis. 1608.

THEODORUS, *medicus.* Diaeta; sive, De salutaribus rebus liber, Georg-Eberhardus Schreinerus recensuit ... Halis Saxonum, Apud Melchiorem Oelschlegelium, 1632.

[7], 81, [6] p. 16 cm.   [11774]

Attributed also to Theodorus Priscianus. Cf. Thomas Reinesius. Variarum lectionum libri III. Altenburgi, 1640. p. 510.

THEODORUS, JACOBUS [*d.* 1590] Neuw vollkommentlich Kreuterbuch, mit schönen ... Figuren, aller Gewächs der Bäumen, Stauden und Kräutern ... eygentlich beschrieben ... darinn viel ... Artzney vor allerley innerlichen unnd eusserlichen Kranckheiten, beyde der Menschen, und dess Viehes ... beschrieben werden ... Jetzt widerumb ... gemehret, durch Casparum Bauhinum ... Franckfurt am Mayn, Durch Nicolaum Hoffman [Matthias Beckers seligen Wittib] in Verlegung Johannis Bassaei und Johann Dreutels, 1613.

2 v. in 1. illus. 39 cm.   [11775]

Title page of vol. 2 lists Nicolas Braun as joint author.

—[The same.] ... Franckfurt am Mayn, Gedruckt durch Paulum Jacobi, in Verlegung Johann Dreutels, 1625.

    3 v. in 1. illus. 39 cm.   **[11776]**

    Imperfect: sig.):(i,):(ij,):(v wanting; supplied in photocopy from College of Physicians of Philadelphia library.

    Title page of vol. 2 lists Nicolas Braun as joint author.

—[The same.] ... Vohrmals ... verbessert, durch Casparum Bauhinum ... Jetz widerumb ... vermehret, durch Hieronymum Bauhinum ... Basel, Gedruckt durch Jacob Werenfels, in Verlegung Johann Königs, 1664.

    2 v. in 1. illus. 38 cm.   **[11777]**

    Added illustrated title page.

    Imperfect: added engraved title page mutilated.

    Title page of vol. 2 lists Nicolas Braun as joint author.

—*See* SENNERT, D. De febribus libri IV. 1628, 1633, 1641, 1653.

THEODORUS VERAX, *pseud. See* WALKER, Clement [1595-1651]

THEODOSIUS, OF TRIPOLIS. *See* CHALES, C. F. M. de, *Father.* Cursus seu mundus mathematicus. 1690.

THEOPHILUS. *See* FAUST, Johann Michael [1663-1707]

THEOPHILUS A GANDA, *pseud. See* HEINSIUS, Daniel [1580-1655]

THEOPHILUS PROTOSPATHARIUS [7th cent.] Ἰατροσοφιστου περι οὐρων. Iatrosophistae de urinis lib. singularis. Fed. Morellus ... nunc primum prodeuntem Latine vertit. Lutetiae, Apud Fredericum Morellum, 1608.

    70, [1] p. 14 cm.   **[11778]**

    Errata: p. [71]

    In Greek and Latin.

—[The same.] *In* Hippocrates. [De medicamentis purgatoriis. Greek and Latin.] 1617.

THEOPHILUS, CHRISTIANUS, *pseud. See* BARTHOLIN, Thomas [1616-1680]

THEOPHRASTUS. Θεοφράστον ... ἅπαντα. Theophrasti ... Graece & Latine opera omnia. Daniel Heinsius textum Graecum ... emendavit ... interpretationem passim interpolavit ... Lugduni Batavorum, Ex typographio Henrici ab Haestens,

impensis Johannis Orlers, And. Gloucq, & Joh. Maire, 1613.

    [16], 508 p. 33 cm.   **[11779]**

    Translated by Theodorus Gaza.

    "Theophrasti ... opuscula Graece & Latine, emendatoria ..." (p. [389]-494) has special title page and contains short treatises translated by Daniel Furlanus, Adrien Turnebe and Isaac Casaubon.

—De historia plantarum libri decem. Graece & Latine. In quibus textum Graecum variis lectionibus ... Latinam Gazae versionem nova interpretatione ad margines: totum opus ... commentariis ... illustravit Joannes Bodaeus à Stapel ... Accesserunt Julii Caesaris Scaligeri ... animadversiones et Roberti Constantini annotationes ... Amstelodami, Apud Henricum Laurentium, 1644.

    [20], 1187, [88] p. illus. 37 cm.   **[11780]**

    Imperfect? First preliminary leaf wanting?

    Edited by Egbertus Bodaeus, with a preface by Johannes Arnoldi Corvinus.

—De piscibus. *In* Severino, M. A. Antiperipatias. 1655-1659.

—De vertigine [Greek and Latin.] *In* Baillou, G. de. Commentarius in libellum Theophrasti de vertigine. 1640.

THERMAE CAROLINAE. 1695. *See* [STRAUSS, J. C.]

THESAURUS HIPPOCRATICUS. 1639. *See* HIPPOCRATES. Aphorismi. Latin. 1639.

THESORO DE POBRES. *See* JOHANNES XXI, *Pope.* Libro de medicina llamado Thesoro de pobres. 1611.

THÉVART, JACQUES [1600-1674?] Defense [-Deuxiéme defense] de la Faculté de medecine de Paris, contre Me François Blondel. Dans laquelle il est prouvé ... que l'emetique composé d'antimoine est un souverain remede pour la guerison de plusieurs maladies, & que ceux qui s'en servent ne sont point empiriques, heretiques, ny empoisonneurs ... Paris, Emmanuel Langlois, 1668.

    [2], 20 p.; [2], 31, [1] p.; 24, 4, 2, 3 p. 22 cm.

    [11781]

—, *ed. See* BAILLOU, G. de. Commentarius in libellum Theophrasti De vertigine. 1640 [and] Consiliorum medicinalium libri II. 1635-1636; 1635-1649 [and] De convulsionibus libellus. 1640 [and] De virginum et mulierum morbis liber. 1643 [and] Definitionum medicarum liber. 1639 [and] Epidemiorum . . . libri duo. 1640 [and] Opuscula medica. 1643.

—*See* [BLONDEL, F.] Alethophanis archiatri ad Jacobum Thevartum. 1655.

THÉVENIN, FRANÇOIS [*d.* 1656] Les oeuvres . . . Contenant un Traité des operations de chirurgie, un Traité des tumeurs, & un Dictionnaire etymologique de mots grecs servans à la medecine. Recüeillies par . . . Guillaume Parthon . . . Paris, P. Rocolet, 1658.

[24], 335, [23] p.; 206, [14] p.   37 cm.   **[11782]**

"Dictionnaire etymologique de mots grecs servans à la medecine, avec leur transcription . . . leur explication en françois, & quelques definitions tirées & traduites de celles de monsieur Desgorris": 206 p.

—[The same.] . . . Nouv. ed. rev. & corr. Paris, En la boutique de P. Rocolet, chez Damien Foucault, 1669.

[16], 560 p.   25 cm.   **[11783]**

"Dictionnaire etymologique . . .": p. 341–533.

—[The same.] . . . Nouv. ed. rev. & corr. Lyon, Jean Certe, 1691.

[16], 469, [3] p.   24 cm.   **[11784]**

"Dictionnaire etimologique . . .": 289–442.

THIBAUT, PIERRE [*fl.* 17th cent.] Cours de chymie . . . Paris, Thomas Jolly, 1667.

[16], 285 (i.e. 287), [15] p.   20 cm.   **[11785]**

—Cours de chymie . . . Augmenté de la composition du baume vert vulneraire, avec son emplastre stiptique; du febrifuge de F. Delboe Sylvius; d'un excellent emetique: d'une eau ophthalmique, & du merveilleux onguent Manus Dei . . . Paris, Jean d'Houry, 1674.

[16], 285 (i.e. 287) p.; [7], [1], 16, [15] p.   plates.   19 cm.   **[11786]**

Part [1] is of the same setting as the 1667 edition.

—[English tr.] The art of chymistry: as it is now practised. Written in French . . . and now translated into English by a fellow of the Royal Society. London, John Starkey, 1675.

[31], 279 p.   16 cm.   **[11787]**

THIELEN, JOHANNES [*fl.* 1662] *respondent.* Disputatio medica inauguralis, de passione hysterica

. . . Lugduni Batavorum, Ex officina Jacobi à Mylendonck, 1662.

[12] p.   19 cm.   **[11788]**

Diss. — Leyden.

THIEME, JOHANN PHILLIPP [*fl.* 1692] *respondent.* See VESTI, J., *praeses.* Disputatio inauguralis medica de phrentide. 1692.

THIEMEN, WILLEM VAN. *See* ATHENIUS, Gulielmus.

THIENEN, WILLEM VAN. *See* ATHENIUS, GULIELMUS.

THIERMAIR, FRANZ IGNAZ [1626–1680] Scholia medica ad totidem & ante nunquam vulgatas consultationes et responsiones, quas partim author, partim alii . . . archiatri . . . exararunt, noviter concinnata . . . Monachii, Typis & impensis Joannis Jaecklini, 1673.

[26], 196, [8], 200, [15] p.   illus.   28 cm.   **[11789]**

Added half title.

—, *ed. See* MERMANN VON SCHÖNBURG, T. Consultationes. 1675.

THILAU, GOTTFRIED. *See* THILO, Gottfried [1646–1724]

THILE, Johann [*ca.* 1646–1688]

Dissertations — Wittenberg

—*praeses.* Disputatio medica de purgatorio actu . . . Wittenbergae, Typis Matthaei Henckelii, 1683.

[18] p.   19 cm.   **[11790]**

C. W. Dam, *respondent.*

—Disputatio medico-chymica, qua sal tartari volatile coagulatum . . . Wittenbergae, Literis Johannis Wilckii [1683]

[24] p.   20 cm.   **[11791]**

J. G. Rebentrost, *respondent.*

—Dissertatio medica inauguralis de purpura epidemia scorbutica . . . Wittenbergae, Typis Matthaei Henckelii [1685]

[32] p.   19 cm.   **[11792]**

J. E. Egerland, *respondent.*

—Dissertatio medico-chymica de minera martissolari; seu, Acidularum artificialium materia . . . Wittebergae, Literis Brüningianis [1682]

[24] p.   20 cm.   **[11793]**

J. E. Egerland, *respondent.*

—Theelogia medica; i.e., De usu & abusu potus calidi cum herba thee, exercitatio ... publico expositurus est ... D. XXXI Decembr. A. M.DC.LXXXVII ... Wittenbergae, Typis Christiani Schrödteri, 1690.

[1], 18, [4] p. 20 cm. [11794]

K. C. Kirchmajer, *respondent.*

—Theses inaugurales de tussi ... Wittebergae, Literis Bruningianis [1685]

[24] p. 20 cm. [11795]

J. D. Gütner, *respondent.*

THILEN, GERHARD [*fl.* 1656] *respondent.* Disputatio medica inauguralis, de ictero ... Gissae Hassorum, Typis Ghemlinianis, 1656.

20 p. 19 cm. [11796]

Diss. — Giessen.

THILEN, JOHANN GERHARD [*b.* 1664] *respondent.* See WEDEL, G. W., *praeses.* Dissertatio medica inauguralis de cucurbitula sicca. 1691.

—See WEDEL, G. W. Propempticon inaugurale de balsamatione corporis Christi. 1691.

THILESIUS, ANTONIUS. *See* TELESIO, Antonio [1482-1533?]

THILL, GYÖRGY ERIK [*b.* 1655] *respondent. See* WEDEL, G. W., *praeses.* Dissertatio medica inauguralis de fluore albo. 1682.

—See CRAUSE, R. W. Rudolffus Wilhelmus Krauss ... Collegii Medici decanus lectori benevolo S. P. D. 1683.

THILO, GOTTFRIED [1646-1724] *praeses.* Exercitatio e philosophia naturali de succino ... Wittebergae, Typis Matthaei Henckelii, 1668.

[16] p. 19 cm. [11797]

Diss. — Wittenberg (K. Gräber, *respondent*)

THILO, ISAAC [*fl.* 1659-1677] Dissertatio physico-historica de succino Borussorum prima nomina, descriptionem & materiam ejus exhibens ... Lipsiae, Literis Christiani Michaelis [1663]

[36] p. 20 cm. [11798]

Diss. pro loco — Leipzig.

—See KLIPPER, J. P., *respondent.* Respirationem ... disputabunt M. Johannes Petrus Klipperus ... et Isaacus Thilo. 1659; SCHMIDICHEN, C., *praeses.* Disputatio physica de psittaco. 1659.

THILO, JOHANN MELCHIOR [*fl.* 1685-1688] *respondent. See* GERBER, G. S., *praeses.* Driff Helmontii ... disputatione inaugurali ... publice examinandum proponit ... J. M. T. 1685.

THÖLDE, JOHANN [*fl.* 1599-1624?] *ed. See* BASILIUS VALENTINUS. Von den natürlichen unnd übernatürlichen Dingen. 1603.

—*See* BASILIUS VALENTINUS. Triumph-Wagen Antimonii ... 1676; SUCHTEN, A. von. Mysteria gemina antimonii. 1675.

THOFALL, PETER [*fl. ca.* 1672] *respondent.* Disputatio medica inauguralis de apoplexia ... Regiomonti, Typis Friderici Reusneri [*ca.* 1672]

[20] p. 20 cm. [11799]

Friedrich Reusner was active between 1666 and 1678. Cf. Benzing(A), p. 246.

Diss. — Königsberg.

—*See* ALBERTUS UNIVERSITÄT. Medizinische Fakultät. Decanus senior [*ca.* 1672]

THOLDIUS, JOHANNES. *See* THÖLDE, Johann [*fl.* 1599-1624?]

THOM, J. D., *ed.* Collectanea chimica curiosa quae veram continent rerum naturalium anatomiam sive analisin e triplici regno tam vegetabili animali quam & minerali unde generosa hactenus a neotericis hinc inde tradita resultant & traduntur medicamina, adversus omnes corporis morbos ... Opera & studio J. D. Thom. A. Francofurti, Apud viduam Hermanni a Sande, 1693.

[8], 927, [25] p. illus. 20 cm. [11800]

THOMAE Hobbes Angli Malmesburiensis philosophi vita. Carolopoli, Apud Eleutherium Anglicum sub signo Veritatis, 1682.

[12], 67, [1] p. port. (front.) 22 cm. [11801]

Fictitious imprint. Published in London by William Crook or Crooke. Cf. Wing. H2268-9.

Contains three lives: the first by an unidentified author, the second, entitled Vitae Hobbianae auctarium, by Richard Blackburne, and the third, in verse, by Hobbes himself.

THOMAI, THOMASO. *See* TOMAI, Tommaso [*d.* 1593]

THOMAIUS, CAMILLUS. *See* TOMAI, Camillo [*d.* 1549]

THOMAS AQUINAS, *Saint* [1225?-1274] In libros Aristotelis De generatione et corruptione expositio

In Díaz de los Llanos, F. De generatione, et corruptione tractatus. 1699.

—Liber lilii benedicti . . .

960-974 p. vol. 4. 20 cm. (*In* Zetzner, Lazarus, *ed.* Theatrum chemicum. Argentorati, 1659-61) cm. [11802]

Caption title.

— [. . . Secreta alchemiae magnalia: de corporibus supercoelestibus, quod in rebus inferioribus inveniantur, quoque modo extrahantur]

267-283 p., vol. 3. 20 cm. (*In* Zetzner, Lazarus, *ed.* Theatrum chemicum. Argentorati, 1659-61) [11803]

Title from table of contents.

—[The same.] *In* Broekhuizen, D. van. Secreta alchimiae magnalia D. Thomae Aquinatis. 1602.

—Tractatus sextus, de esse et essentia mineralium . . .

806-814 p., vol. 5. 20 cm. (*In* Zetzner, Lazarus, *ed.* Theatrum chemicum. Argentorati, 1659-61) [11804]

Caption title.

—*See* Campanella, T. Astrologicorum libri VII. 1630; Silatan, F. L'interprete de la nature. 1655.

THOMAS DE BONONIA. *See* Thomas, *of Bologna* [*ca.*1320-*ca.* 1384]

THOMAS DE PISAN. *See* Thomas, *of Bologna* [*ca.* 1320-*ca.* 1384]

THOMAS, *of Bologna* [*ca.* 1320-*ca.* 1384] *See* Bernardus Trevirensis. Ein Antwort Bernhardi Trevirensis, an Thomam von Bononia. 1613 [and] Bernardi Trevirensis [responsio] S ad Thomam de Bononia. 1610.

THOMAS, *of Pisa. See* Thomas, *of* Bologna [*ca.* 1320-*ca.* 1384]

THOMAS, Christian. *See* Thomasius, Christian [1655-1728]

THOMAS, Paul [*fl.* 1622-1624] *respondent. See* Sebisch, M. [1578-1674?] *praeses.* Exercitatio medica secunda. 1622 [and] Exercitationes medicae. 1639.

THOMASAY, Thomas. *See* Tomai, Tommaso [*d.* 1593]

THOMASINI, Jacobus Philippus. *See* Tomasini, Jacopo Filippo [1597-1654]

THOMASIUS, Christian [1655-1728] *praeses.* Dissertatio inauguralis de jure circa pharmacopolia civitatum . . . [Halae] Typis Christoph. Andreae Zeitleri [1697]

68 p. 20 cm. [11805]

Diss. — Halle (C. L. Fritsch, *respondent*)

THOMASIUS, Gottfried [1660-1746] *praeses.* Dissertationem academicam de aeris gravitate ad aquam comparati p. p. . . . Jo. Henricus Schmidt . . . Lipsiae, Literis Johannis Georgii [1684]

[16] p. 20 cm. [11806]

Diss. — Leipzig (J. H. Schmidt, *respondent*)

—*respondent. See* Berger, J. G. von, *praeses.* Exercitationem inauguralem de animi deliquiis . . . p. p. G. T. 1689; Bohn, J., *praeses.* Dissertationes chymico-physicae. 1685 [and] Dissertationum chymico-physicarum quarta de aëre. 1683.

— *See* Franck von Franckenau, G. De medicis philologis epistola. 1691.

THOMASIUS, Jakob [1622-1684] Contemplatio luminis . . . Lipsiae, Typis Timothei Ritzschii, 1645.

[16] p. 19 cm. [11807]

Diss. pro loco — Leipzig.

Dissertations — Leipzig

—*praeses.* De barba . . . Lipsiae, Typis Ritzschianis [1671]

[26] p. 20 cm. [11808]

G. Barth, *respondent.*

—[The same.] De barba disputatio, quam sub moderamine . . . Dn. M. Jacobi Thomasii . . . die VI. Decembr. anno M.DC.LXXI proposuit ac defendit Gothofredus Barthius . . . Jenae, Sumptibus Christoph. Enoch. Buchta, recusa emendatius anno 1672.

[31] p. 20 cm. [11809]

G. Barth, *respondent.*

—De mandragora disputatio philologica . . . A. O. R. MDCLV examini eruditorum commissa a Johanne Schmidelio . . . nunc recusa & aucta . . . Lipsiae, Typis & sumptibus Johann-Erici Hahnii [1671]

[23] p. 20 cm. [11810]

J. Schmidel, *respondent.*

—De transformation hominum in bruta dissertationem philosophicam ... publicae ... ventilationi subjicit ... Anno C. 1667, Fridericus Tobias Moebius ... Lipsiae, Typis & sumptibus Joh. Erici Hahnii, recusa 1673.

[40] p. 19 cm. [**11811**]

F. T. Möbius, *respondent.*

—De visu talparum discursus physicus, quem ... publicae eruditorum ventilationi ... A. 1659 ... subjecit Joachimus Corthum ... Altenburgi, Literis Richterianis curabat Christoph. Enoch. Buchta, 1671.

[**11812**]

J. Corthum, *respondent.*

—Diatriben academicam de foeminarum eruditione priorem ... proponit Johannes Sauerbrei ... Lipsiae, Literis Johannis Erici Hahnii [1671]

[28] p. 19 cm. [**11813**]

J. Sauerbrei, *respondent.*

—[The same.] Diatriben academicam de foeminarum eruditione priorem ... A. O. R. cIc Icc LXXI ... proponit Johannes Sauerbrei ... Lipsiae, Revisa & emendatior prodit sumptibus Johannis Erici Hahnii, 1676.

[36] p. 20 cm. [**11814**]

J. Sauerbrei, *respondent.*

—Disputatio physica de origine animae humanae, quam ... anno M DC LXIX respondendo tuebitur Johannes Vake ... Ed. 2, priori auct. & corr. Lipsiae, Typis Johannis Georgii [1669?]

72 p. 19 cm. [**11815**]

J. Vake, *respondent.*

—Disputatio physica de putredine ... Lipsiae, Literis Ritzchianis [1660]

[19] p. 20 cm. [**11816**]

J. Bohn, *respondent.*

—Dissertatio historica de Petro Dresdensi ... Lipsiae, Literis Christiani Michaelis [1678]

[40] p. 20 cm. [**11817**]

J. C. Schreiber, *respondent.*

—Dissertatio philosophica de hibernaculis hirundinum ... subjecit ... anno ... M.DC.LVIII. [Lipsiae] Literis Richteri curabat, Christoph Enoch Buchta, 1671.

[30] p. 19 cm. [**11818**]

C. Schmidichen, *respondent.*

—Exercitatio philosophica de morte in undis, contra servium & synesium ... Lipsiae, Literis Christiani Michaelis [1667]

[24] p. 19 cm. [**11819**]

S. Corfinius, *respondent.*

THOMASIUS, Johannes [*fl.* 1664] *respondent.* Disputatio medica inauguralis de lue venerea ... Altdorffii, Typis viduae Johannis Göbelii [1664]

20 p. 18 cm. [**11820**]

Diss.—Altdorf.

THOMASSEAU, Joseph [1648?–1710] *praeses.* Quaestio medica ... Ad ab exlege inspirati aëris motu, febres? [Parisiis, Apud Franciscum Muguet, 1695]

4 p. 25 cm. [**11821**]

Caption title.

Diss.—Paris (H. Michelet, *respondent*)

—Quaestio medica ... An vivat miserè, qui vivit medicè? [Lutetiae, Apud Franciscum Muguet, 1693]

[4] p. 25 cm. [**11822**]

Caption title.

Diss.—Paris (A. N. Chemineau, *respondent*)

—Quaestio medica ... Est-ne uterus pars ad vitam necessaria? [Parisiis, 1677]

[4] p. 25 cm. [**11823**]

Caption title.

Diss.—Paris (J. Des Prez, *respondent*)

—*respondent. See* Hellot, M. A., *praeses.* Quaestio medica ... An demorsis a cane rabido colocynthis? 1676; Jouvanci, N. de, *praeses.* Quaestio medica. 1675; Rainssant, N., *praeses.* Quaestio medica ... Est-ne optima vivendi lex sua unicuique consuetudo? 1676.

THOMASSIN, Louis [1619–1695] Traitez historiques et dogmatiques sur divers points de la discipline de l'Eglise, & de la morale chrétienne. Tome premier ... Divisé en deux parties. 2. ed., rev., corr., & augm. ... Paris, François Muguet, 1685.

[16], 565 p. 20 cm. [**11824**]

THOMPSON, George. *See* Thomson, George [1619–1677]

THOMPSON, James [*fl.* 1657] Helmont disguised; or, The vulgar errours of impericall and unskilfull practisers of physick confuted. More especially, as they concern the cures of the feavers, stone, plague, and other diseases. In a dialogue between Philiatrus, and Pyrosophilus ... By J[ames]

T[hompson] esq. student in physick. London, Printed by E. Alsop, for N. Brook, 1657.

[8], 134, [10] p.   15 cm.   [11825]

Imperfect: wormholes on p. [2]-16.

THOMSCHLÄGER, Caspar [*fl.* 1689] *respondent.* *See* Wartenberg, E. C., *praeses.* De anima humanum corpus informante. 1689.

THOMSON, George [1619–1677] Αἱματιασις; or, The true way of preserving the bloud in its integrity, and rectifying it . . . wherein Dr. Willis his errour of bleeding is reprehended, and offered to be confuted by practice and frequent experiments; and certain opinions of Dr. Betts in physick rejected and proved dangerously false . . . Whereunto are added a stomachical spirit . . . The nature . . . of the griping of the guts . . . [London] Nath. Crouch, 1670.

[16], 180, [3] p.   front. (port.)   17 cm.[11826]

—Chymiatrorum acus magnetica; sive, Recta chymice curandi methodus . . . nunc Latino sermone commonstrata a Gottf. Hennicken . . . Francofurti ad Moenum, Sumpt. Georgii Erhardi Martii, Marburgi Cattorum, Typis Joh. Henrici Stockenii, 1686.

[12], 261 p.   14 cm.   [11827]

—Epilogismi chymici observationes nec non remedia Hermetica longa in arte hiatrica exercitatione constabilita. Item essentiae nostrae stomachicae vires insignes medicae explicantur, ejusque materia, modus ac methodus praeparationis ad Galeno-chymicorum elenchum . . . describuntur . . . Lugduni Batav., Apud A. Doude & A. Severinus, 1673.

[8], 87, [1] p.   13 cm.   [11828]

—Galeno-pale; or, A chymical trial of the Galenists, that their dross in physick may be discovered. With the grand abuses and disrepute they have brought upon the whole art of physick and chirurgery, in their method touching phlebotomy and purgation . . . To which is added An appendix de litho-colo; or, An history of three large stones excluded the colon by chemical remedies . . . London, Printed by R. Wood, for Edward Thomas, 1665.

[15], 120 p.   18 cm.   [11829]

—Λοιμοτομια; or, The pest anatomized . . . Together with the author's apology against the calumnies of the Galenists, and a word to Mr. Nath.

Hodges, concerning his late Vindiciae medicinae . . . London, Nath. Crouch, 1666.

[16], 189, [3] p.   front.   15 cm.   [11830]

—'Ορθομεθοδος ιατροχυμικη; or, The direct method of curing chymically. Wherein is conteined the original matter, and principal agent of all natural bodies. Also the efficient and material cause of diseases in general, their therapeutick way and means. I. Diaetetical by rectifying eating, drinking, &c. II. Pharmaceutick . . . To which is added, the art of midwifery chymically asserted. The character of an ortho-chymist, and pseudo chymist. A description of the sanative virtues of our stomach-essence. Also, Γαληνο-μεμψις; or, A just complaint of the method of the Galenists . . . London, B. Billingley, and S. Crouch 1675.

[14], 40 (i.e. 200) p.   front.   17 cm. [11831]

—*See* Cocke, T. Kitchin-physick. 1675, 1676; Stubbs, H. The Lord Bacons relation of the sweating-sickness examined. 1671.

THONER, Augustin [1567–1655] Appendix epistolarum medicinalium quae pro mantissa, cum observationes illius ante annum secunda vice praelo subjectae caeteris . . . incorporari non potuerunt, jam seorsim sunt excusae cum adjuncta querimonia . . . adversus quendam antagonistam. Tubingae, Typis Johann Alexandri Cellii, impensis Johann Heinrici Reisii, 1653.

64 p.   19 cm.   [11832]

—Observationum medicinalium, haud trivialium, libri quatuor . . . Hisce adjuncti sunt consultationum, cum diversarum regionum medicis habitarum & epistolarum de variis rebus medico-philosophicis, disserentium, libri duo . . . Ulmae, Sumptibus Johannis Gerlini, 1649.

[16], 368, [23] p.   21 cm.   [11833]

—[The same.] . . . Ulmae, Sumptibus Johannis Gerlini, 1651.

[16], 368, [23] p.   22 cm.   [11834]

Text partly reset.

With this are bound Alessi, A.: Consilia medica. 1660; Preservatione dalla peste. 1660.

THOR, George, *astromagus.* Cheiragogia heliana. A manuduction to the philosopher's magical gold . . . To wich is added: 'Αντρον Μιτρας; Zoroaster's cave . . . Together with the famous catholic epistle of John Pontanus upon the minerall fire ... London, Humphrey Moseley, 1659.

[II], 96 p.   15 cm.   [**11835**]

THOREAU, ANDREA. *See* TAURELLUS, Andreas [*fl.* 1630–1641]

THORER, LAURENTIUS [*fl.* 1631] *respondent. See* BURGERSDIJCK, F. P., *praeses.* Collegium physicum. 1642.

THORIUS, RAPHAEL [*d.* 1625] Hymnus tabaci ... Lugd. Bat., Typis Isaaci Elsevirii, 1625.

[8], 55 p.   22 cm.   [**11836**]
Engraved title page.

—[The same.] *In* Everard, G. De herba panacea. 1644.

—[English tr.] Hymnus tabaci; a poem in honour of tabaco ... Made English by Peter Hausted ... London, Printed by T. N. for Humphrey Moseley, 1651.

73 p.; [6], 8 p.   15 cm.   [**11837**]
Part [2] has special title page: Cheimonopegnion; or, A winter song, by Raphael Thorius; newly translated.

[—] Medici Londinensis eximii, epistola de ... Isaaci Casauboni morbi mortisque causa. Edita ex museo Joachimi Morsii. Lugduni Batavorum, Excudebat Jacobus Marci, 1619.

[4] p.   21 cm.   [**11838**]
The London physician is identified as R. T., i.e. Raphael Thorius. Cf. printer's note on p. [2]

THORMANN, MICHAEL FRIEDRICH [*fl.* 1683] *respondent. See* HARTMANN, P. J., *praeses.* Disquisitio de phoca sive vitulo marino. 1683.

A THOUSAND notable things of sundrie sorts. 1631. *See* [LUPTON, T.]

THRASHER, WILLIAM. The marrow of chymical physick; or, The practice of making chymical medicines. Divided in three books: viz. shewing the true ... order to distil ... from vegetables, minerals, and metals ... Whereunto is added at the end of every such preparation, its ... medicinal use ... By W[illiam] T[hrasher] philo-astro-medicus, and student in chymistry. London, Printed by T. J. for Peter Parker, 1669.

[4], 188 p.   illus.   15 cm.   [**11839**]

THRASTER, WILLIAM. *See* THRASHER, William.

THRIVERUS, HIEREMIAS. *See* DRYVERE, Jérémie de [1504–1554]

THRUSTON, MALACHI [*fl.* 1665–1681] De respirationis usu primario, diatriba ... Accedunt Animadversiones a cl. viro [Georgio Entio] in eandem conscriptae, una cum responsionibus auctoris. Londini, Apud Johannem Martyn, 1670.

[30], 206, [1] p.   17 cm.   [**11840**]
Errata: p. [207]
Imperfect: first preliminary leaf (blank?) wanting.
The Animadversiones has half title (p. [121]).

—[The same.] ... Lugd. Batav., Apud Felicem Lopez de Haro, Cornelium Driehuysen, 1671.

[10], 165, [8] p.   16 cm.   [**11841**]
The Animadversiones has half title (p. [99]).

—*See* ENT, *Sir* G. 'Αντιδιατριβη. 1679, 1685 [and] Opera omnia medico-physica. 1687.

THUCYDIDES. *See* MARCHINI, F. Belli divini; sive, Pestilentis temporis accurata. 1633; PAULINUS, F. Praelectiones Marciae. 1603; SPRAT, T., *Bp. of* Rochester. The plague of Athens. 1683.

THUILLE, JOHANN [1590–1630] Funus ... Hieronymi Fabricii ab Aquapendente ... die 23 Maii ... M.DCXIX ... celebratum a Joanne Thuilio ... Patavii, Typis Petri Pauli Tozzii, 1619.

[24] p.   21 cm.   [**11842**]

—, *ed. See* GALENUS. [Ars medico. Latin.] 1622, 1642.

THUILLIER, CHARLES [*fl.* 1684–1703] Lettre ... a ... Demetrius Ammirally ... sur les maladies veneriennes & les antiveneriens. [Paris] 1693.

[2], 94 p.   17 cm.   [**11843**]
Bound with *his* Observations pour bien connoistre ... le maladies veneriennes. 1693.

—Observations sur les maladies veneriennes et sur un remede qui les guerit seurement et facilement ... Imprimées à Roüen, & se trouvent a Paris, Chez l'Auteur, 1684.

[2], 108, [2] p.   19 cm.   [**11844**]

—Observations pour bien connoistre, et bien traiter les maladies veneriennes, avec des experiences d'un remede qui les guerit seurement, & facilement ... 2. ed., rev., & corr. Paris, L'auteur, 1693.

[40], 112 (i.e. 114), [2] p.   17 cm.   [**11845**]
With this is bound *his* Lettre ... a ... Demetrius Ammirally 1693.

THUMM, Theodor [1586-1630] Tractatus theologicus, de sagarum impietate, nocendi imbecilitate et poenae gravitate . . . Nunc secunda cura . . . auctus. Tubingae, Apud Johann-Georgium Cottam, typis Johann Henrici Reisii, 1667.

[12], 107 p. 21 cm. [**11846**]

Bound with Frommann, J. C. Tractatus de fascinatione. 1675.

THURINGUS, H. Aquila. *See* Aquila, H., Thuringus.

THURN, Leonhard Thurneisser zum. *See* Thurneisser zum Thurn, Leonhard [1531-1596]

THURNEISSER ZUM THURN, Leonhard [1531-1596] Methodus brevis et dilucida, von rechter und warhaffter Extraction der seelischen . . . Kräfften, aus allerley Kräutern, Baumfrüchten . . . Mineren und Edelgesteinen, etc. . . . Wittenberg, In Verlegung Clement Bergers, 1619.

[1], 70 p. plates. 21 cm. [**11847**]

Imperfect: p. 1-2 mutilated.

—Reise und Kriegs-Apotecken, darinnen nicht allein die . . . Kranckheiten an des Menschen Leibe . . . vermeldet, sondern auch die . . . Medicamenta Chimica, an Tincturen, Essentien, Oelen . . . und dergleichen . . . beschrieben werden . . . Durch Agapetum Kozerum Austropedium . . . in Druck verfertiget. Leipzigk, In Vorlegung Jacob Apels [Zerbst, Gedruckt durch Johann Schleern] 1602.

[4], 124 (i.e. 134), [5] p. 16 cm. [**11848**]

With this is bound: Duchesne, J. Spagirica. 1608.

—Zehen Bücher von kalten, warmen, minerischen und mettalischen Wassern . . . Auffs new durchsehen . . . und verbessert. Dem ein Kurtze Beschreibung des Selbacher Brunnens . . . hinzugethan . . . Strassburg, In Verlegung Lazari Zetzners, 1612.

[18], 324, [47] p.; [5], 13 p. 29 cm. [**11849**]

Part [2] has special title page: Kurtze Beschreibung des heylsamen Bronnens der Sahlbronnen.
Edited by Johann Ludwig Hawenreuter.

—*See* Martini, H. Anatomia urinae Galenospagyrica. 1658; Panckow, T. Herbarium. 1673.

THURRIANUS, Bartholomaeus. *See* Torre, Bartolomeo della [*fl.* 1599-1602]

THYLESIUS, Antonius. *See* Telesio, Antonio [1482-1533?]

THYMIUS, Andreas [*fl. ca.* 1664-1665] *praeses.* Magni Hippocratis Coi Aphorismi XLV. sectionis VI. ulcerum antiquorum statum et prognosin continentis, resolutio . . . [Jenae] Typis Johannis Nisii [1665]

[2], 22 p. 20 cm. [**11850**]

Diss.—Jena (J. C. Neuberger, *respondent*)

—, *respondent. See* Schenck, J. T., *praeses.* Disputatio medica inauguralis de vulneribus. 1664.

THYRAEUS, Petrus [1546-1601] Daemoniaci cum locis infestis et terriculamentis nocturnis. Id est, libri tres, quibus spirituum homines obsidentium atque infestantium genera, conditiones, &, quas adferunt, molestiae, molestiarumque causae atque modi explicantur . . . Coloniae Agrippinae, Ex officina Materni Cholini sumptibus Gosuini Cholini, 1604.

[40], 210, [1] p.; 356 p. 22 cm. [**11851**]

Part [2] has caption title.

—[The same.] Daemoniaci; hoc est, De obsessis a spiritibus daemoniorum hominibus, liber unus. In quo daemonum obsidentium conditio: obsessorum hominum status, rationes & modi, quibus ab obsessis daemones exiguntur . . . discutiuntur & explicantur, denuo omnia repurgata & aucta . . . Lugduni, Apud Joannem Pillehotte, 1626.

324, [4] p. 18 cm. [**11852**]

Date has been altered to 1626. Printer's preface dated 1603.

—De apparitionibus spirituum tractatus duo: quorum prior agit de apparitionibus omnis generis spirituum, Dei, angelorum, daemonum, et animarum humanarum libri uno . . . Posterior continet Divinarum; seu, Dei in Veteri Testamento apparitionum & locutionum tam externarum, quam internarum libros quatuor, nunc primum editos. Coloniae Agrippinae, Ex officina Mater. Cholini, sumptibus Gosuini Cholini, 1605.

[15], 486 p. 21 cm. [**11853**]

TICINENSIS, Johannes. *See* Johann von Tetzen.

TIDICAEUS, Franciscus [1485-1565] De theriaca et ejus multiplici utilitate, ac recta conficiendi ratione, in Andromachi senioris . . . Carmen Graecum de theriaca ex viperis inscriptum, commentarius . . . Thorunii, Ex officina typographica Andreae Cotenii, 1607.

[4], 320, [15] p. 20 cm. [**11854**]

"Andromachi . . . theriaca ex viperis facta, quae vocatur quies sive tranquillitas" (p. 3-13) includes Greek text.

"Andromachi ... theriaca Latino Carmine ex carmine ipsius Graeco descripta; interprete Julio Martiano Rota ...": p. 14–21.

TIEFFENBACH, JOHANN CONRAD [*b.* 1673] *respondent. See* STAHL, G. E., *praes.* Disputatio medica inauguralis de podagrae nova pathologia. 1698.

—*See* STAHL, G. E. Propempticon inaugurale de cephalalgia iliaco-haematitica. 1698.

TIELEMAN, JOHANN WENNEMAR [*fl.* 1699] Disputatio inauguralis medica de morborum transmutatione ... Duisburgi ad Rhenum, Typis Johannis Sas, 1699.

     36 p.   20 cm.   **[11855]**

Diss.—Duisburg.

TIELENS, PAUL [*fl.* 1691] *respondent.* Disputatio medica inauguralis de urinis ... Lugduni Batavorum, Apud Abrahamum Elzevier, 1691.

     [12] p.   22 cm.   **[11856]**

Diss.—Leyden.

TIERBYENS, OLAUS ANDREAS. *See* ANDREAS, Olaus [*fl.* 1656]

TIETZE, GEORG [*fl.* 1683] *respondent.* Disputatio medica inauguralis de pleuritide vera ... Ultrajecti, Ex officina Rudolphi a Zyll, 1683.

     [16] p.   20 cm.   **[11857]**

Diss.—Utrecht.

TIGURINUS, ABRAHAMUS [*fl.* 1671] *respondent.* Disputatio medica inauguralis, de febribus intermittentibus in genere ... Trajecti ad Rhenum, Ex officina Antonii Smytegelt, 1671.

     [12] p.   20 cm.   **[11858]**

Diss.—Utrecht.

TILEMANN, JOHANNES [*fl.* 1635–1664] Aphorismi Hippocratis facili methodo digesti cum ipso textu, aliisque insuper therapeuticis pro curatione morborum omium totius humani corporis. Denuo eduntur auctiores & correctiores, ut & Appendix de materia medica. Ab Johanne Tilemanno ... Marpurgi, Typis Chemlinianis, 1650.

     2 v. in 1.   front. (port.)   11 cm.   **[11859]**

Imperfect: leaf paged 289–290 in v. [1] mutilated; text restored in manuscript.

Appendix de materia medica (v. [2]) has special title page.

The main work was published by the same press in 1643 under title: Synopsis Aphorismorum Hippocratis, facili methodo digestorum. Cf. Linden, p. 694.

"Aphorismi Hippocratis ... ex recognitione A. Vorstii": [2]–60, [1] p. at end of v. [1]. Last page contains Aphorismi skipped on p. 29 of text.

—[The same.] ... Giessae, Sumptibus Caspari Vulpii, typis Friderici Kargeri, 1660.

     2 v. in 1.   front. (port.)   12 cm.   **[11860]**

Appendix de materia medica (v. [2]) has special title page dated 1666.

A page-for-page reprint of the 1650 Marburg edition.

"Aphorismi Hippocratis ... ex recognitione A. Vorstii": [2]–60, [1] p. at end of v. [1]. Last page, containing Aphorismi skipped on p. 29 of text, bound facing p. 29 in this copy.

—Cantilenae cygneae diu compressae, nunc ante mortem ebuccinatae ... Oeniponti, Jacobus Christofforus Wagner, 1680.

     [12], 287 (i.e. 286) p.   13 cm.   **[11861]**

—Experimenta circa veras, & irreducibiles auri solutiones, addenda suo Lapidi ignis Basilii, antehac typis jam divulgato. Amstelodami, Apud Joannem Jansonium, 1669.

     [3], 3–46 p.   14 cm.   **[11862]**

Bound with Prevost, J. Hortulus medicus selectioribus remediis. 1681.

[—] Guldiner Apffel. Von dem Goldbaum dess irrdischen Lebens decerpiret, durch welches Anatomi die geheime und verborgne Universal-Medicin, sampt anderen hierzu nöttigen Wissenschafften geoffenbahret ... an Tag gegeben. Durch Johannem Henricum Menni ... Tübingen, Bey Johann Cunrad Geysslern, 1635.

     [119] p.   14 cm.   **[11863]**

Bound with Jonstonus, J. Idea hygieines recensita. 1661.

—[The same.] Lapis ignis Basilii; das ist, Guldiner Apffel ... Anjetzo auf das neu recidiret, corrigieret ... und vermehret worden. Augspurg, Johann Schultes, 1666.

     [40] p.   20 cm.   **[11864]**

—Oratio de medicinae restauratione, memoriter habita Moguntiae, die 1. Maji, anno ... 1656 ... Herbipoli, Ex officina typographica Jobi Hertzii, 1657.

     [52] p.   19 cm.   **[11865]**

—*praeses.* Harmoniae physico-medicae de numero elementorum disputatio II ... Marpurgi Cattorum, Typis haeredum Casparis Chemlini, 1645.

     [3], 24 p.   19 cm.   **[11866]**

Diss.—Marburg (J. L. Witzel, *respondent*)

TILEMANN, TOBIAS [1586?–1614] *praeses.* Disputationum physiologicarum sexta de motu et quiete ...

Witebergae, Ex officina typographica Martini Henckelii, 1611.

[12] p.   19 cm.   **[11867]**

Diss.—Wittenberg (J. Spiegel, *respondent*)

TILESIO, ANTONIO. *See* TELESIO, Antonio [1482-1533?]

TILGER, KONRAD [*fl.* 1625] *respondent. See* AGER, N. Disputatio physica de monstris. 1625.

TILING, JOHANN [1668-1715] *respondent. See* SCHWELING, J. E., *praeses.* Disputatio physica de materia mundi subtilissima. 1690

—, *ed. See* NUCK, A. Operationes & experimenta chirurgica. 1692, 1696, 1698; SCULTETUS, J. [1595-1645] Armamentarium chirurgicum. 1693.

TILING, JOHANN GÜNTHER [*fl.* 1685-1686] *respondent. See* SPERLING, P. G., *praeses.* Dissertationem chymicam de arsenico . . . submittit . . . J. G. T. 1685.

TILING, MATHIAS [1634-1685] Anatomia lienis, ad circulationem sanguinis, aliaque recentiorum inventa, accommodata. Rinthelii, Impensis Thomae Henrici Hauensteinii, typis G. C. Wächter, 1673.

[23], 511, [9] p.   14 cm.   **[11868]**

—Anchora salutis sacra; seu, De laudano opiato, medicamine isto divino . . . liber singularis. In quo ineffabiles . . . medicamenti hujus . . . virtutes . . . partim secundum rationis normam considerantur, partim observationibus permultis . . . adornantur ac confirmantur . . . Francofurti, Impensis Wilhelmi Richardi Stockii, 1671.

[14], 554, [5] p.   18 cm.   **[11869]**

Imperfect: wormholes on p. 45-58.

—[The same.] Opiologia nova modernis artis medicae principiis superstructa ineffabiles opii sane divini vires et effectus ad omnes corporis cruciatus juxta rationis leges accommodans. Autore T[ilingio] M[edicinae] P[rofessore] Cum praefatione Joh. Helff. Jungken . . . Francofurti ad Moenum, Sumptibus Joh. Adolphi & Phil. Wilh. Stockii, 1697.

[8], 554, [5] p.   18 cm.   **[11870]**

A reissue of Anchora salutis sacra, with new title and new dedicatory epistle.

—Cinnabaris mineralis; seu, Minii naturalis scrutinium physico-medico-chymicum . . . Francofurti ad Moenum, Sumptib. Jacobi Gothofredi

Seyleri, typis Balth. Christ. Wustii, 1681.

[8], 250 p.   17 cm.   **[11871]**

—De febribus petechialibus tractatus curiosus, duabus sectionibus comprehensus, universam . . . hujus morbi historiam . . . breviter exhibens. Francofurti, Impensis Jacobi Gothofredi Seyleri, 1676.

[42], 362, [5] p.   18 cm.   **[11872]**

Added engraved title page.

—De placenta uteri disquisitio anatomica, novis in medicina hypothesibus illustrata. Rinthelii, Impensis Thomae Henrici Hauensteinii, typis G. C. Wächter, 1672.

[16], 458 (i.e. 438), [1] p.   14 cm.   **[11873]**

Errata: p. [439]

—De recidivis tractatus aureus, uterum & neotericorum medicorum fundamentis superstructus, & ad usum practicorum insignem accommodatus. Mindae, Impensis Thomae Henrici Havensteinii, typis Johannis Pileri, 1679.

[24], 489, [2] p.   13 cm.   **[11874]**

—De tuba uteri deque foetu nuper in Gallia extra uteri cavitatem in tuba concepto, exercitatio anatomica, cui duorum monstrorum . . . nuper editorum, relatio est innexa. Rinthelii, Impensis Thomae Henrici Hauensteinii, Typis G. C. Wächter, 1670.

108 p.   14 cm.   **[11875]**

Imperfect: p. 98 and 107 mutilated.

—Disquisitio physico-medica de fermentatione; sive, De motu intestino particularum in quovis corpore, ex fundamentis Willisianis & Moebianis in philiatrorum gratiam adornata, principiis quinque Paracelsicis accommodata, variis observationibus illustrata . . . Bremae, Sumptibus Antonii Güntheri Schwertfegers, 1674.

[12], 276 p.   14 cm.   **[11876]**

—Lilium curiosum; seu, Accurata lilii albi descriptio, in qua ejus natura & essentia mirabilis . . . secundum leges & methodum S. R. I. Academiae Naturae Curiosorum explicantur . . . Francofurti ad Moenum, Sumptibus Jacobi Gothofredi Seyleri, typis Balthas. Christoph. Wustii, sen., 1683.

[32], 576 p.   17 cm.   **[11877]**

—Παρέχβασις; seu, Digressio physico-anatomica curiosa de vase brevi lienis ejusque usu nobili . . .

in corporis humani oeconomia. Mindae, Impensis Thomae Henrici Havensteinii, typis Johannis Pileri, 1676.

[16], 740, [4] p.   14 cm.   **[11878]**

—Prodromus praxeos chimiatricae; seu, Liber singularis, in quo praescribitur variorum mysteriorum chimicorum & medicamentorum . . . conficiendorum certa ratio . . . Rintelii, Sumptibus Thomae Henrici Hauensteinii, typis G. C. Wächter, 1674.

[30], 1004, [52] p.   plates.   17 cm.   **[11879]**

—*praeses.* Disputatio inauguralis de apoplexia . . . Rinthelii, Literis Godofr. Casp. Wächters, 1682.

24 p.   19 cm.   **[11880]**

Diss.—Rinteln (B. H. Wallman, *respondent*)

—Dissertatio medica de dysenteria principiis Hippocraticis, Galenicis, Paracelsicis, Helmontianis, Harveanis, Sylvianis, Tackenianis & Willisianis illustrata . . . Rinthelii, Literis G. C. Wächters, 1677.

48, [3] p.   illus.   21 cm.   **[11881]**

Diss.—Rinteln (J. M. Trost, *respondent*)
Bound with Cortnumm, J. De morbo attonito. 1677.

—*respondent. See* SCHNEIDER, K. V., *praeses.* Disputatio medica inauguralis de hydrope. 1663.

TILKOWSKI, ADALBERTUS. *See* TYLKOWSKI, Adalbert [1625-1695]

TIL-LANDZ, ELIAS [1640-1693] *respondent.* Disputatio medica inauguralis de atrophia . . . Lugduni Batavorum, Apud viduam & haeredes Joannis Elsevirii, 1670.

[15] p.   23 cm.   **[11882]**

Diss.—Leyden.

TIMAEUS, CHRISTIAN. *See* TIMAEUS VON GÜLDENKLEE, Christian [*fl. ca.* 1653]

TIMAEUS, GOTTLOB [*fl.* 1699] *praeses.* Disputatio prior de metallurgia rerum gerendarum nervo . . . Vitembergae, Prelo Christiani Kreusigii [1699]

[16] p.   20 cm.   **[11883]**

Diss.—Wittenberg (J. C. Viertel, *respondent*)

—Disputatio posterior, de metallurgia rerum gerendarum nervo . . . Wittenbergae, Prelo Christiani Kreusigii [1699]

[16] p.   20 cm.   **[11884]**

Diss.—Wittenberg (J. G. Meiner, *respondent*)

TIMAEUS, JOANNES EDWARDUS. *See* TIMAEUS VON GÜLDENKLEE, Johann Edward [*fl.* 1653-1668]

TIMAEUS VON GÜLDENKLEE, BALTHASAR [1600-1667] Opera medico-practica. I. Casus & observationes practicae triginta sex annorum. II. Descriptiones medicamentorum singularium. III. Epistolae & consilia. IV. Consilium de peste. V. Responsa. VI. Consilium diaeticon. Quibus accessit Egidii van der Myle Hortolini Timaeani topographia & inscriptiones. Lipsiae, Impensis Johannis Herebordi Klosii, 1691.

[30], 1157 (i.e. 1218) p.   22 cm.   **[11885]**

Items I-II and V-VI have special title pages, both bound after the title page. The special title page of item III. is dated 1677. Item IV has half title: Superpondium alexicacon; seu, Consilium de peste, lingua Germanica editum Dantisci anno M.DC.XXX . . . et denuo excusum Sedini anno M.DC.LIII. Latinitate donatum a Christiano Timaeo von Güldenklee.

The Responsus was edited by Johann Edward Timaeus von Güldenklee.

—Casus medicinales praxi triginta sex annorum observati. Accessere et Medicamentorum singularium quae in casibus proponuntur descriptiones. Lipsiae, Impensis Christiani Kirchneri, typis Johann-Erici Hahnii, 1662.

[24], 433 (i.e. 483), [9] p.   20 cm.   **[11886]**

Each Casus has half title.

—[The same.] . . . Lipsiae, Impensis Christiani Kirchneri, literis Christiani Michaelis, 1667

[24], 433 (i.e. 483), [9] p.   20 cm.   **[11887]**

Different setting of type.
Bound with *his* Baldassaris Timaei von Guldenklee . . . epistolae et consilia, 1665.

—[The same.] . . . Lipsiae, Impensis Johannis Herebordi Klosii, 1691.

[24], 433 (i.e. 483), [9] p.   20 cm.   **[11888]**

Different setting of type.

—Baldassaris Timaei von Guldenklee medici electoralis et celebrium quorundam Germaniae, Galliae et Italiae medicorum epistolae et consilia. Accessit & Hortolini Timaeani topographia metrica & inscriptiones. Lipsiae, Impensis Christiani Kirchneri, typis Johann Erici Hahnii, 1665.

[16], 464 (i.e. 496), [8] p.   20 cm.   **[11889]**

The second work is by Aegidius van der Myle.
With this is bound *his* Casus medicinales. 1667.

—Responsa medica, et diaeteticon opus posthumum. Lipsiae, Impensis Christiani Kirchneri, literis Christiani Michaelis, 1668.

[8], 188 p.   20 cm.   **[11890]**

—See BONET, T., ed. Corps de medecine et de chirurgie. 1679; SCHÖNFELD, P. J. Kurtze Anmahnungen . . . an die Hebammen. 1678. WALDSCHMIDT, J. J. Praxis medicinae rationalis succincta. 1690, 1691.

TIMAEUS VON GÜLDENKLEE, CHRISTIAN [*fl. ca.* 1653] *tr.* See TIMAEUS VON GÜLDENKLEE, B. Opera medico-practica. 1691.

TIMAEUS VON GÜLDENKLEE, JOHANN EDWARD [*fl.* 1653-1668] *respondent.* Analysis thematis philosophici et medici. Accedit ad casum medicum de febre putrida maligna in juvene responsio . . . Patavii, Typis Pauli Frambotti, 1655.

26 p.   18 cm.   **[11891]**
Diss. — Padua, 1653.

—, *ed.* See TIMAEUS VON GÜLDENKLEE, B. Opera medico-practica. 1691.

TIMARETES, PHILELEUTHERUS. See ALMELOVEEN, Theodoor Jansson van [1657-1712]

TIMME, THOMAS. See TYMME, Thomas [*d.* 1620]

TIMPLER, CLEMENS [*fl.* 1604-1617] Opticae systema methodicum per theoremata et problemata selecta concinnatum & duobus libris comprehensum. Cui subjecta est Physiognomia humana, itidem duobus libris breviter & perspicue pertractata . . . Hanoviae, Apud Petrum Antonium, 1617.

[22], 240 (i.e. 248) p.   18 cm.   **[11892]**
Special title page (Physiognomiae humanae, libri duo) and index (4 leaves) inserted between p. 128 and 129.

TINCTORIUS, CHRISTOPH [1604-1662] *praeses.* Generationem hominis ut & reliquorum animantium ex semine . . . subjiciet . . . Christophoro Tinctorio . . . Johannes Masius . . . Regiomonti, Typis Laurentii Segebadii [1637]

[20] p.   20 cm.   **[11893]**
Diss. — Königsberg (J. Masius, *respondent*)

TINELLI, ZOROASTRO. Medicarum consultationum juxta magni Hyppocratis doctrinam. Tomus primus . . . Senis, Apud Sylvestrum Marchettum, 1605.

[16], 397, [21] p.   22 cm.   **[11894]**
No more appears to have been published.

TINTA, LORENZO. *See* Tinti, Lorenzo [1626 *or* 34-1672]

TINTI, LORENZO [1626 *or* 34-1672] *See* BORBONI, M. Teatro anatomico di Bologna. 1668?

TIRELLI, MAURIZIO [*fl.* 1630] De historia vini, et febrium, libri duo . . . Venetiis, Apud Jacobum Scaleam, 1630.

[8], 395 p.   20 cm.   **[11895]**

TIRION, KRISTOFFEL [*fl.* 1695] *respondent.* Disputatio medica inauguralis de cordis palpitatione . . . Trajecti ad Rhenum, Ex officina Francisci Halma, 1695.

15 p.   22 cm.   **[11896]**
Diss. — Utrecht.

TISENIUS, GEORGIUS [*fl.* 1610] *respondent.* See CRÜGER, B., *praeses.* Disputatio medica secunda. 1610.

TITI, PLACIDO [*d.* 1668] De diebus decretoriis et aegrorum decubitu . . . Epitome astrosophica physicis maxime rationibus, deinde Galeni, Aristot. & Ptolemaei praeceptis contexta . . . Tomus primus [-secundus] Ticini, Ex officina Joannis Andreae Magrii, 1660-65.

2 v. in 1.   fronts., illus.   22 cm. **[11897]**
Vol. 2 has imprint: Ticini, Ex officina Joannis Ghidini, 1665.

TITIANO. See TIZIANO VECELLI [1477-1576]

TITIS, PLACIDUS DE. See TITI, Placido [*d.* 1668]

TITSCHARD, GEORG [*fl.* 1606-1610] *respondent.* Assertiones medicae de renum et vesicae urinariae calculo . . . Basileae, Typis Joan. Jacobi Genathii, 1610.

[12] p.   20 cm.   **[11898]**
Diss. — Basel.

—See SENNERT, D., *praeses.* Quaestiones medicae controversae quinque, pro disputatione tertia propositae. 1607.

—[*as subject*] See BAUHIN, K. Hygiae et panaceae parente . . . Casparus Bauhinus. 1610.

TIXEDAS, CHRISTOVAL [*fl.* 1688] Verdad defendida, y respuesta de Fileatro, a la Carta medico chymica, que contra los medicos de la Junta, de la Corte, y contra todos los Galenicos, le escrivo el Doctor . . . D. Juan de Cabriada . . . Barcelona, Antonio y Balthasar Ferrer, 1688.

[22], 460, [8] p.   20 cm.   **[11899]**

TIZIANO VECELLI [1477-1576] *See* [VESALIUS, A.] Notomie di Titiano. *ca.* 1670.

TOBAR, SIMÓN DE. *See* TOVAR, Simón [*fl.* 1565–*ca.* 1590]

TOELASTH, HEINRICH [*fl.* 1677] *respondent.* Disputatio medica inauguralis, de peste ... Ultrajecti, Apud Guilielmum Clerck, 1677.

[20] p.   20 cm.   **[11900]**
Diss. — Utrecht.

TOEPFER, BENEDICT [*fl.* 1607] *ed.* and *tr. See* PARACELSUS. Zween underschiedene Tractat. 1608.

—, *ed. See* KHUNRATH, H. De igne magorum philosophorumque secreto externo. 1608.

TÖPFFER, JOHANN [*fl.* 1652-1653] *respondent. See* FRIDERICH, A. G., *respondent.* Disputatio physica de nutritiva facultate. 1652.

TOGNI, MICHIEL [*fl.* 1675] Raccolta delle singolari qualità del caffè ... Venetia, Gio. Francesco Valvasense, 1675.

[3]—48 p.   illus.   14 cm.   **[11901]**
Includes excerpts from Prosper Alpini's De plantis Aegypti liber.

TOLEDO, GONDISALVUS [*fl.* 1496-1508] *See* GANIVET, J. Amicus medicorum. 1614.

TOLEDO, GONZALO DE. *See* TOLEDO, Gondisalvus [*fl.* 1496-1508]

TOLET, FRANÇOIS [1647-1724] Traité de la lithotomie, ou de l'extraction de la pierre hors la vessie ... Paris, L'autheur, 1682.

249, [7] p.   plates.   15 cm.   **[11902]**

— [The same.] ... 3. ed. Paris. L' autheur, 1686.

249, [7] p.   illus., plates.   16 cm.   **[11903]**
A reissue of the 1682 edition with new title page.
Imperfect: plates facing p. 88, 104, 105, 119, 120, 137, 140, 144-146 and 159 wanting.

— [The same.] ... avec les appareils, les remedes preservatifs du calcul, & les medicamens pour les taillez ... Dern. ed. Suivant la copie à Paris. La Haye, Barent Beek, 1686.

172, [6] p.   plates.   17 cm.   **[11904]**
Added engraved title page.

—[The same.] ... 4. ed. Paris, L'autheur, 1689.

249, [7] p.   plates.   16 cm.   **[11905]**
A reissue of the 1682 edition with new title page.

—[The same.] ... Avec les appareils, les remedes preservatifs du calcul, & les medicamens pour les taillez ... 4. ed. Suivant la copie à Paris. Utrecht, Antoine Schouten, 1693.

172, [6] p.   illus.   16 cm.   **[11906]**
Added engraved title page.
A reissue of the 1686 La Haye edition with new title page and preliminary matter reset.

— [Dutch tr.] Tractaat van de lithotomia, of de uythalinge van de steen uyt de blaas ... Beneffens de toesteltsels, de preservative remedien tegen de steen, en de medicamenten voor de geene die gesneden sijn ... Uyt het Frans vertaalt. 's Gravenhage, Barent Beeck, 1686.

155 (i. e. 261), [7] p.   illus., plates.   16 cm.
                    [11907]
Added engraved title page reads: Tractat vant steensnyden.

—[The same.] ... Utrecht, Anthoni Schouten, 1693.

[14], 19-155 (i.e. 261), [7] p.   illus., plates.   17 cm.   **[11908]**
Imperfect: engraved title page, p. 53-54 and 59-62 wanting.
A reissue of the 1686 edition with "Waerschouwinge" reset.

— [English tr.] A treatise of lithotomy; or, Of the extraction of the stone out of the bladder. Written in French ... Translated into English by A. Lovell. London, Printed by H. H. for William Cademan, 1683.

[8], 185, [6] p.   plates.   17 cm.   **[11909]**
Imperfect: plate illustrating text on p. 61-62 wanting.

— [German tr.] Tractätlein von der besten Art und Weise den Blasen-Stein zu schneiden ... Hannover und Wolffenbüttel, Bey Gottlieb Heinrich Grentzens seel. Wittwe und Erben, 1694.

[1], 200 (i.e. 198), [5] p.   front., plates.   17 cm.   **[11910]**
Frontispiece reads: Tractat von Stein-schneiden.
With this are bound: Momber, Anton. Tractat vom Nier- und Blasen-Stein. Helmstädt [dedication 1735] - Hellwig, Christoph von. Der curieuse und vernünfftige Zauber-Artzt. Franckfurt und Leipzig, 1725.

— [Another German tr.] Verhandlung von der Lithotomie; oder, Einer zahrten und sichern Weise von Ausziehung des Steins auss der Blase ... Im Francoistschen beschrieben ... in Teutsch übersetzet durch D. B. Medecinae Doctor. Wesell, Johann Cattepoel und Jacobus von Wesell, 1700.

[1], 7, 160 p. plates., illus. 16 cm. **[11911]**

Added engraved title page.
Plate 6 bound after plate 17.

TOLET, Pierre [1502–1586] tr. See Galenus. Les six principaux livres de la methode therapeutique. 1605.

TOLL, Adrianus [d. 1675] ed. See Boodt, A. B. de. Gemmarum et lapidum historia. 1636 [and] Le parfaict joaillier. 1644; Galenus. [In Hippocratis Aphorismos. Greek and Latin] 1633; Stockar, J. Praxis aurea. 1634.

TOLLIUS, Jacobus [1633–1696] Manuductio ad caelum chemicum. Amstelaedami, Apud Janssonio-Waesbergios, 1688.

16 p. 16 cm. **[11912]**

With this is bound *his* Sapientia insaniens. 1669.

— Sapientia insaniens; sive, Promissa chemica . . . Amstelaedami, Apud Janssonio-Waesbergios, 1689.

64 p. plate. 16 cm. **[11913]**

Bound with *his* Manuductio ad caelum chemicum. 1688.

TOLON, Maurice de. See Maurice de Toulon, *Father* [d. 1668]

TOMAI, Camillo [d. 1549] Compendiosa methodus, tum pathologica, tum therapeutica. In Dispensatorium chymicum. 1626; Vittori, B. De curandis morbis ad tyrones practica magna. 1628.

TOMAI, Tommaso [d. 1593] Discorso del vero modo di preservare gli huomini dalla peste . . . Bologna, Presso Clemente Ferroni, ad instanza di Sebastiano Balestra, 1630.

16 p. 20 cm. **[11914]**

— Idea del giardino del mondo . . . ove oltre molti secreti maravagliosi di natura, sono posti varii, & soavissimi frutti curiosissimi secondo la diversità del gusto degli huomini . . . Novamente ristampata, & . . . corretta. Aggiuntovi di nuovo una tavola di tutti li nomi de gli auttori . . . Venetia, Nella stamperia del Miloco, a spese del Turrini, 1648.

[24], 179 p. 14 cm. **[11915]**

— [French tr.] Abregé curieux, des plus beaux secrets de la nature, par Thomas Thomasay . . .

Traduict d'italien en françois, par M. Nicolas Le Moulinet . . . Paris, Eustache Daubin, 1648.

[2], 228 p. 16 cm. **[11916]**

Title page is a cancel; cancelandum title page is also present, with title: Idée du jardin du monde.

TOMASINI, Jacopo Filippo [1597–1654] De donariis ac tabellis votivis liber singularis . . . Utini, Ex typographia Nicolai Schiratti, 1639.

[8], 266, [22] p. illus., plates. 22 cm. **[11917]**

— Gymnasivm Patavinvm . . . libris V. comprehensum . . . Utini, Ex typographia Schirati, 1654.

[16], 497, [45] p. illus., plate. 23 cm. **[11918]**

— Illvstrivm virorvm elogia; iconibus exornata. Patavii, Apud Pasquardum, 1630.

[16], 373, [48] p. illus., ports. 21 cm. **[11919]**

Added engraved title page.

— See Fabricius, H., *ab Aquapendente*. Opera chirurgica. 1647, 1666; Sturm, S. Discursus medicus de medicis non-medicis. 1663.

The TOMB of Semiramis. See Collectanea chymica. 1684.

TOMLINSON, Richard [b. ca. 1633] tr. See Renou, J. de. A medicinal dispensatory. 1657. See A physical dictionary. 1657.

TONDI, Bonaventura [fl. 17th cent.] Aforismi di morte in ricette di medico; overo, I languori della natura accresciuti dall'arte. Opera protofisica . . . Trevigi, Il Righettini, 1689.

[6], 171 p. 15 cm. **[11920]**

Imperfect: first preliminary leaf (blank?) wanting.

TONJOLA, Nikolaus [1668–1707] *respondent.* Dissertatio medica de ictero flavo . . . Basileae, Typis Joh. Rudol. Genathii, 1692.

[20] p. 20 cm. **[11921]**

Diss. — Basel.

TONSTALL, *Doctor.* See Tonstall, George [b. 1616]

TONSTALL, George [b. 1616] A new-years-gift for Doctor Witty; or, The dissector anatomized, which is a reply to the discourse intituled, An answer to all that Doctor Tonstall has writ, or shall hereafter write, against Scarbrough spaw ... London, Printed by J. M. for the author, 1672.

[29], 162 p.   14 cm.   [11922]

—Scarbrough spaw spagyrically anatomized ... London, Printed by J. M. for the author, 1670.

63, [6] p.   14 cm.   [11923]

— *See* SIMPSON, W. Hydrological essayes. 1670; WITTIE, R. Scarbroughs spagyrical anatomizer dissected. 1672.

TOORNBURG, KLAAS [*b. ca.* 1657] Kort vertoog van de anatomia. Bestaande in een korte verhandeling van de melk-making, en omloop des bloeds, en af-scheyding der sappen. Dienende tot een grond-slag om een grondige kennis van de genees- en heel-konst te bekomen ... Amsterdam, Timotheus ten Hoorn, 1691.

[12], 59, [1] p.   16 cm.   [11924]

Bound with Goodschalk, D. Prodromus de ossium tum generatione, tum corruptione interna. 1691.

TOPPI, NICOLÒ [1603?-1681] Biblioteca napoletana, et apparato a gli huomini illustri in lettere di Napoli, e del regno, delle famiglie, terre, citta, e religioni, che sono nello stesso regno. Dalle loro origini, per tutto l'anno 1678. ... Divisa in due parti. Nelle quali vengono molte famiglie forastiere lodate, e varii autori illustrati, & emendati. Napoli, Appresso A. Bulifon, 1678.

[16], 400, [56] p.   31 cm.   [11925]

Part 2 has special title page (p. [261]).
With this is bound *his* Addizioni. 1683.

— Addizioni copiose di Lionardo Nicodemo alla Biblioteca napoletana del dottor Niccolo Toppi. Napoli, Per S. Castaldo, 1683.

[8], 250, [5] p.   31 cm.   [11926]

Compiled with the assistance of Francesco Nicodemo.
Bound with N. Toppi's Biblioteca napoletana. 1678.

TOPSELL, EDWARD [1572-1625?] The history of four-footed beasts and serpents ... Collected out of the writings of Conradus Gesner and other authors, by Edward Topsel. Whereunto is now added, The theater of insects; or, lesser living creatures ... by T. Muffet ... Rev., corr., and inl. ... by J[ohn] R[owland] M. D. London, Printed by E. Cotes for G. Sawbridge, T. Williams and T. Johnson, 1658.

[16], 818, [6] p.; [12], 889-1130, [6] p.   illus.   35 cm.   [11927]

Added half title.
Part [1] is mainly a translation of books 1 and 5 of Gesner's Historia animalium, with additions by Topsell. "The history of serpents" (p. [587]-818) has special title page.
Part [2] has special title page: "The theater of insects; or, lesser living creatures ... by Tho. Mouffet ..."

TORELLI, ANDRÉ. *See* TAURELLUS, Andreas [*fl.* 1630-1641]

TORIBIO ALFONSO MOGROVEJO, *Saint. See* MOGROVEJO, Toribio Alfonso de, *Saint* [1538-1606]

TORNESI, CAROLUS AMATON [*fl.* 1690-1691] *See* SCHELHAMMER, G. C. Dissertatio inauguralis medica de tabe dorsali. 1691; WEDEL, G. W. Dissertatio chimica de antimonio diaphoretico. 1690.

TORRAEUS, GEORGIUS [*fl.* 1625] Epileptica consideratio; hoc est, Morbi comitialis (quem vocant) qua theoretica, qua practica medicina ... Francofurti ad Moenum, Typis Egenolphi Emmelii, 1625.

39 p.   20 cm.   [11928]

TORRE, BARTOLOMEO DELLA [*fl.* 1599-1602] Iatrobulia, sive Βουλιατρεία; hoc est, De medica consultatione libri quatuor ... Francofurti, E Collegio Paltheniano, 1606.

[8], 330, [19] p.   17 cm.   [11929]

— *See* LICETI, F. De ortu animae humanae libri tres. 1602.

TORRE, GEORGIUS VAN. *See* TORRAEUS, Georgius [*fl.* 1625]

TORRE, GIORGIO DALLA [1607-1688] Junonis, et nestis vires in humanae salutis obsequium traductae. Dissertatio qua aeris, et aquae natura summatim consideratur, atque expenditur ... Patavii, Typis ac impensis heredum Pauli Frambotti, 1668.

[14], 105 p.   22 cm.   [11930]

Imperfect: signatures b4 (blank?) and N6 (blank?) wanting.

TORRE Y BALCARCEL, JUAN DE LA. *See* TORRE Y VALCARCEL, Juan [*fl.* 1666]

TORRE Y VALCARCEL, JUAN [*fl.* 1666] Espejo de la philosophia y compendio de toda la medicina theorica, y practica ... Amberes, Imprenta Plantiniana de Baltasar Moreto, 1668.

[6], 190, [14] ll.   29 cm.   [11931]

TORREBLANCA Y VILLALPANDO, FRANCISCO DE [*d.* 1645] Daemonologia; sive, De magia naturali, daemonica, licita, & illicita, deque aperta & occulata, interventione & invocatione daemonis libri quatuor ... Moguntiae, Impensis Joh. Theowaldi Schönwetteri, 1623.

[24], 636, [42] p.   19 cm.   **[11932]**

TORRESANI, GIOVANNI BENEDETTO [*fl.* 1623] Discorso sopra il male delle petecchie, peste, e ghiandussa, con il modo, che si deve tenere à curare le febri pestilentiali, & altri simili mali ... Raccolta da varii auttori ... Bologna, Theodoro Macheroni, & Clemente Ferroni, 1623.

53, [3] p.   21 cm.   **[11933]**

Imperfect: upper margins of title page and p. 51-[56] mutilated.

TORTEBAT, FRANÇOIS, *pseud. See* PILES, Roger de [1635-1709]

TORTONI, CARLO ANTONIO [*fl.* 1686] Nuovo composto apopletico chiamato balsamo Tortoniano ... Roma, Mascardi, 1689.

[3]-33 p.   16 cm.   **[11934]**

TORTUOSENSIS, ABRAHAM JUDAEUS. *See* ABRAHAM BEN SHEM-TOB [13th cent.]

TORZOLO, RUTILIO [*fl.* 1627] Manipolo universale di chirurgia ... Dell'anatomia del capo ferite, e curatione di esse ... Bracciano, Andrea Fei, 1627.

[16], 110 p.   16 cm.   **[11935]**

Last leaf (blank?) wanting.

TOSSOFFACAN, ASDRYASDUST, *pseud. See* GAYTON, Edmund [1608-1666]

A TOUCH-STONE for physick. 1667. *See* WALWYN, W.

TOULLIEU, PAUL DE [*fl.* 1691-1692] *respondent. See* DES PREZ, J., *praeses.* Quaestio medica. 1691.

TOULON, MAURICE DE. *See* MAURICE DE TOULON, *Father* [*d.* 1668]

TOULOUSE (City). Capitoul. *See* RIVEYRON, L., *Father.* Secrets. 1641.

TOULOUSE. UNIVERSITÉ, FACULTÉ DE MÉDECINE. *See* UNIVERSITÉ DE TOULOUSE. Faculté de médecine.

TOURNEFORT, JOSEPH PITTON DE [1656-1708] Elemens de botanique; ou, Methode pour connoître les plantes ... Paris, Imprimerie royale, 1694.

3 v.   front., plates.   22 cm.   **[11936]**

Vols. 2-3 have engraved title pages only.

— [Latin tr.] Institutiones rei herbariae. Ed. alt. Gallica longe auctior ... Tomus primus [-tomus III] Parisiis, E Typographia regia [Curante Joanne Anisson] 1700-1703.

3 v.   illus.   23 cm.   **[11937]**

Vols. 2-3 have engraved title pages only.

— Histoire des plantes qui naissent aux environs de Paris, avec leur usage dans la medecine ... Paris, Imprimerie royale [Par les soins de Jean Anisson] 1698.

[56], 543, [19] p.   20 cm.   **[11938]**

Imperfect: p. 241-244 and 249-250 mutilated.

— Schola botanica; sive, Catalogus plantarum, quas ab aliquot annis in Horto regio Parisiensi studiosis indigitavit ... Joseph Pitton Tournefort ... ut et Pauli Hermanni ... Paradisi Batavi prodromus ... Edente in lucem S. W. A. [i.e. Simon Warton Anglus? pseud. of William Sherard?] Amstelaedami, Apud Henricum Wetstenium, 1689.

[12], 386, [26] p.   15 cm.   **[11939]**

Special title page bound before title page reads: Schola botanica ut et Paradisi Batavi prodromus ... Edente in lucem Simone Wartono, Anglo.

— *See* RAY, J. De variis plantarum methodis. 1696 [and] Synopsis methodica stirpium Britannicarum. 1696.

TOURNERIUS. *See* TOURNIER, JEAN [*fl.* 1609-1613]

TOURNIER, JEAN [*fl.* 1609-1613] *See* CANTEREL, R. L'Aesculape francois hymne. 1614.

TOUSTALL, GEORGE. *See* TONSTALL, George [*b.* 1616]

TOVAR, SIMÓN [*fl.* 1565-*ca.* 1590] Hispalensium pharmacopoliorum recognitio. *In* Du Boys, J. Methodus miscendi & conficiendi medicamenta. 1640.

TOXITES, MICHAEL [1515-1581] *ed. See* CARRICHTER, B. Horn dess Heyls menschlicher Blödigkeit. 1673 [and] Kräuter und Artzeneybuchs erster [-dritter] Theil. 1652-1631; LULL, R. Testamentum. 1663?; PARACELSUS. Liber de occulta philosophia. 1686.

TOZZI, LUCA [1638-1717] In Hippocratis Aphorismos commentaria; ubi universae medicanae, tum theoreticae, tum practicae celebriores quaestiones perpenduntur, atque nedum recentiorum inventis, sed & genuinae ejusdem Hippocratis menti congruentes, quam dilucide explicantur ... Neap., Ex nova officina sociorum Dom. Ant. Parrino & Michaëlis Aloysii Mutii, sumptibus haeredum Cosimi Fioravanti, 1693.

   2 v. front. 23 cm.   [11940]
   Contains commentaries on books 1-4 of the Aphorismi, with the Latin text in Niccolò Leoniceno's version.

— Medicinae pars prior Θεωρητική, curiosa quaequae tum ex physiologicis, tum pathologicis deprompta; veterum, recentiorumque medendi methodum complectens. Nunc primum in lucem prodit. Lugduni, Apud Anissonios, & Joan. Posuel, 1681.

   [24], 267, [2] p. 18 cm.   [11941]

— Medicinae pars altera πρακτική, quae hactenus adversus morbos adinventa sunt ... brevissime explicans. Nunc primum in lucem prodit. Avenione, Apud Jacobum Duperier, 1687.

   2 v. 19 cm.   [11942]
   Vol. 2 has half title: Tractatus de natura, et curatione singulorum morborum, pars secunda.

— [The same.] ... Nunc primum in lucem prodit. Avenione, Apud Jacobum Duperier, 1688.

   [16], 360 p.; [1], 387 p. 18 cm.   [11943]
   Part 2 has half title: Tractatus de natura, et curatione singulorum morborum, pars secunda.

— [The same.] ... Nunc primum in lucem prodit. Bononiae, Typis Longi, 1697.

   [16], 596 p. 16 cm.   [11944]
   "... Tractatus de natura, et curatione singulorum morborum. Pars secunda" has half title (p. [277]).

TRABER, ZACHARIAS [1611-1679] Nervus opticus; sive, Tractatus theoricus, in tres libros opticam catoptricam dioptricam distributus. In quibus radiorum a lumine, vel objecto per medium diaphanum processus, natura ... figuris, demonstrationibusque exhibentur ... Viennae Austriae, Typis Joannis Christophori Cosmerovii, 1675.

   [24], 225, [1] p. plates. 30 cm.   [11945]
   Added engraved title page.

—[The same.] ... Viennae Austriae, Sumptibus Philippi Fieveti, 1690.

   [24], 225, [1] p. plates. 31 cm.   [11946]
   Added engraved title page.
   A reissue of the 1675 edition with new title page and dedicatory epistle.

TRACTÄTLEIN und kurtzer Bericht. *See* MAINZ. Ordinances, local laws, etc.

TRACTATUS aliquot chemici singulares summum philosophorum arcanum continentes. 1647. *See* [COMBACH, L.] *ed.* and *tr.*

TRACTATUS aureus de lapide philosophico. *See* [GRASSHOFF, J.] Aureus tractatus de philosophorum lapide. 1677.

TRACTATUS de barometris. *See* ALENCÉ, J. d'. Neu-erfundene mathematische Curiositäten. 1695.

TRACTATUS novi de potu caphe, de Chinensium the, et de chocolata. 1685. *See* [DUFOUR, P. S.]

TRACTATUS quid pro quo. *See* MESUË [924 *or* 5-1015] Opera. 1602, 1623.

TRACTATUS varii de morbis, ad recentiorem mentem concinnati nunc primum in unum collecti, notulis aucti, & publici juris facti ... Ferrariae, Bernardini Pomatelli, 1690.

   [14], 315 p. 17 cm.   [11947]

TRAICTÉ de la dissolution du mariage par l'impuissance ... de l'homme. 1610. *See* [HOFMAN, A.]

TRAICTÉ de la peste. 1606. *See* COLLÈGE DES MAÎTRES CHIRURGIENS JURÉS DE PARIS.

TRAICTÉ des abus qui se commettent sur les procedures de l'impuissance des hommes & des femmes. 1620. *See* [GUILLEMEAU, C.]

TRAICTÉ du divorce par l'adultere. Sçavoir, s'il est permis a l'homme ou à la femme en ce cas de se remarier. Paris, Nicolas Rousset, 1629.

   79, [1] p. 17 cm.   [11948]
   With this is bound: Tagereau, V. Discours sur l'impuissance. 1612.

TRAITÉ de la circulation des esprits animaux. 1682. *See* JAMET, N. P.

TRAITÉ de la connoissance des causes magnetiques. *See* VALLEMONT, P. Le Lorrain, *abbé de.* La physique occulte. 1696.

TRAITÉ de la guérison des fiévres par le quinquina. 1679. *See* [MONGINOT, F., *the younger*]

TRAITÉ de la longue vie, dans lequel, par des principes nouveaux de médecine, on donne des moyens certains pour conserver long-tems la vie . . . Rouen, Jacques Besogne, 1698.

[32], 366 p.   18 cm.   **[11949]**

Dedication signed: A. D.

TRAITÉ des blesseures et playes faites par armes a feu. 1668. *See* [PLAZZONI, F.]

TRAITÉ des eaux minerales d'Attancourt. 1696. *See* BAUGIER, E.

TRAITÉ des maladies veneriennes. *See* RIOLAN, J. [1538?–1605?] Chirurgie. 1669.

TRAITÉ des qualitez du kinkina. P. M. M. Amsterdam, Theodore Labbé, 1685.

[6], 28 p.   16 cm.   **[11950]**

TRAITÉ du scorbut. 1671. *See* [VENETTE, N.]

TRAITÉ du sel. 1669. *See* [SENDIVOGIUS, M.]

TRAITÉ du soulphre second principe de la nature. 1669. *See* [SENDIVOGIUS, M.]

TRAITÉE des fiévres. 1682. *See* BONTEKOE, C.

TRAITÉS nouveaux de medecine. 1684, 1688. *See* BARBEYRAC, C. de.

TRAITTÉ de l'aiman. 1687. *See* ALENCÉ, J. d'.

TRAITTEZ des barometres. 1688. *See* ALENCÉ, J. d'.

TRALLES, Alexandre de. *See* ALEXANDER TRALLIANUS [6th cent.]

TRALLES, JOHANN CHRISTIAN [d. 1698] *respondent. See* MAJOR, J. D., *praeses.* Disputatio medica inauguralis de malacia. 1677.

TRALLES, *Phlegon of. See* PHLEGON OF TRALLES [*fl.* 2d cent.]

TRALLIANUS, ALEXANDER. *See* ALEXANDER TRALLIANUS [6th cent.]

TRALLIANUS, PHLEGON. *See* PHLEGON OF TRALLES [*fl.* 2d cent.]

TRANAEUS, JOHANNES GOTZCHALCHUS [*fl.* 1685] *respondent.* Dissertatio chymico-medica inauguralis de calce viva . . . Lutetiae Parisiorum [1685]

[64] p.   20 cm.   **[11951]**

Diss. — Paris.

TRAPHAM, THOMAS [d. 1692?] A discourse of the state of health in the island of Jamaica . . . London, R. Boulter, 1679.

[16], 149, [3] p.   17 cm.   **[11952]**

TRASGRESTI, GIOVANNI BATTISTA. *See* GRASSETTI, Giovanni Battista [1609–1684]

TRAVAGINUS, FRANCISCUS [*fl.* 1669] Super observationibus a se factis tempore ultimorum taerremotuum, ac potissimum Ragusiani physica disquisitio; seu, Gyri terrae diurni indicium. Juxta exemplar Venetiis impressum. [Francofurti?] 1673.

[5], 17+ p.   illus.   19 cm.   **[11953]**

Imperfect: all after p. 17 wanting; lower margins trimmed; p. 16-17 mutilated.

—*See* PETREUS, P. P. Musaeum Travaginianum. 1679.

TRAVO, SEBASTIANO [*fl.* 1618] Scholia in theoremata medica, physica, metaphysica, & moralia paradoxi naturam referentia; his Animadversiones cum antithesibus, in propositiones physicas, & medicas, ex cujusdam authoris manuscriptis decerptas, adjecit . . . Taurini, Apud HH. Jo. Dominici Tarini, 1618.

[32], 785, [38] p.; 256, [36] p.   19 cm.   **[11954]**

TRAVUS, SEBASTIANUS. *See* TRAVO, Sebastiano [*fl.* 1618]

The **TREASURE** of health. *See* [DURANTE, C.] A family-herbal; or, The treasure of health. 1689.

A **TREATISE** concerning the plague and the pox. *See* A RICH CLOSET OF PHYSICAL SECRETS. 1652.

A **TREATISE** of mathematicall physick. Or a briefe introduction to physick, by judiciall astrologie . . . Written by G. C. London, Andrew Kemb, 1653.

[135]-184 p.   19 cm.   (*In* Dariot, C. Dariotus redivivus; or, A briefe introduction conducing to the judgement of the stars. London, 1653)   **[11955]**

A **TREATISE,** wherein is declared the sufficiencie of English medicines. 1615. *See* [BRIGHT, T.]

TREEK, JOHANNES VAN DEN [*fl.* 1689] *respondent.* Disputatio medica inauguralis de phthisi . . . Trajecti ad Rhenum, Ex officina Francisci Halma, 1689.

[8] p.   22 cm.   **[11956]**

Diss. — Utrecht.

TREFEL, Jean Malbec de. *See* Malbec de Tresfel Jean [*fl.* 1668]

TRÉGUIER, France (*Diocese*) *Bishop* [1646–*ca.* 1679] (Baltazar Grangier) Remedes pour les pauvres gens ... Mandement de feu Monseigneur l'Evesque de Treguyer ...Baltazar Grangier ... [n. p.] 1678.
    4 p.   24 cm.   **[11957]**
Caption title.

TREMOSINUS, Salomon. *See* Trismosin, Salomon, *pseud?*

Le **TRÈS-ANCIEN** duel des chevaliers. *See* [Uralter Ritter-Krieg. French] 1699.

TRES tractatus de metallorum transmutatione. 1668. *See* [Philalethes, E.]

TRESEL, Petrus. *See* Trezel, Peter [*fl.* 1694]

TRESEL, Galenus. *See* Trezel, Galenus [*fl.* 1661–1695]

TRESFEL, Jean Malbec de. *See* Malbec de Tresfel, Jean [*fl.* 1668]

TRESSINA, Aloysius. *See* Trissino, Alvise [1519–1544]

TREU, Abdias. *See* Trew, Abdias [1597–1669]

TREUCHSES, Philipp Heinrich [*fl. ca.* 1665] *tr. See* May, P. La chiromancie medicinale. 1665.

TREVICO, Ferrante Loffredo, *marchese di. See* Loffredo, Ferrante, *marchese di Trivico* [16th cent.]

TREVISAN. *See* Bernardus Trevirensis [14th cent.]

TREVUS, Persius, *pseud. See* Servi, Pietro [*d.* 1648]

TREW, Abdias [1597–1667] Nucleus astrologiae correctae; das ist, Kurtzer Bericht vom Nativitätstellen, wie darmit umbzugehen, und was es nutze ... Nürnberg, Jeremia Dümler, 1651.
    [12], 95, [2] p. illus. 21 cm.   **[11958]**
Errata: p. [97]
Added engraved title page reads: Gründlicher Bericht von dem Nativitaetstellen.

TREWMUNDT, Christian. Dess Christiani Trewmundts [pseud.] Gewissen-loser Juden-Doctor, in welchem erstlich das wahre Conterfeit eines christlichen Medici, und dessen nothwendige Wissenschafften, wie auch gewissenhaffte Praxis, zweytens die hingegen abscheuliche Gestalt dess Juden-Doctors ... vorgestellet wird. Frayburg, 1698.
    [19], 140 p. 18 cm.   **[11959]**
Imperfect: p. 123-126 mutilated.

TREZEL, Galenus [*fl.* 1661] *respondent.* Disputatio medica inauguralis de epilepsia ...Lugduni Batavorum, Ex officina Francisci Moyaert, 1661.
    [12] p. 21 cm.   **[11960]**
Diss.—Leyden.

TREZEL, Galenus [*fl.* 1695] *respondent.* Disputatio medica inauguralis de arthritide ... Trajecti ad Rhenum, Ex officina Francisci Halma, 1695.
    15, [1] p. 23 cm.   **[11961]**
Diss.—Utrecht.

TREZEL, Peter [*fl.* 1694] *respondent.* Disputatio medica inauguralis de fluido nervorum ... Lugduni Batavorum, Apud Abrahamum Elzevier, 1694.
    [16] p. 24 cm.   **[11962]**
Diss.—Leyden.

The **TRIALL** of tabacco. 1610. *See* Gardiner, E.

TRIBBECHOV, Johann [1678–1712] *praeses.* De lectione fontium ut vulgo appellatur cursoria ... Jenae, Typis Mullerianis [1699]
    24 p. 20 cm.   **[11963]**
Diss.—Jena (F. H. Jacobs, *respondent*)

TRIBUDENIUS, *pseud. See* Mynsicht, Adrian von [1603–1638]

TRIBUNALE DELLA SANITÀ DI MILANO. Instruttione generale per purgare ogni sorte di robba, tanto per la città di Milano, quanto per ogni altro luogo. [Milano, Gio. Battista Malatesta, e ristampato in Bologna per l'herede del Benacci, 1630]
    12 p. 20 cm.   **[11964]**
Caption title.

TRICHARD, Claude [*fl.* 1699–1700] *respondent. See* Denyau, A. M., *praeses.* Quaestio medica ... An oculi sint pathematum idola? 1700.

TRIER. Ordinances, local laws, etc. *See* Kurtze medicinalische Nachricht. 1666.

TRIGG, Dr. *See* Philanthropos, E., *ed.* Dr. Trigg's secrets. 1665.

TRIGGE, Stephen. *See* Paracelsus. Of the chymical transmutation. 1657.

TRIGO DE ROXAS, JUAN DOMINGO. Memorial christiano, y politico sobre la permanencia del dotor Juan Joseph Lopez en la ciudad de Valencia, a fin de averiguarse practicamente su metodo de curar las calenturas ardientes, por el medio del agua fria, proponida con varias circunstancias . . . Valencia, Francisco Mestre, 1684.

[4], 19 p.   32 cm.   **[11965]**

TRILLA, ANTONIO DE. *See* TRILLA Y MUÑOZ, Antonio [*fl.* 1677]

TRILLA Y MUÑOZ, ANTONIO [*fl.* 1677] Perfecto practicante medico y nueva luz de facil enseñança. Toledo, Agustin de Salas Zaço, 1677.

8, [12], 9-108 ll.   16 cm.   **[11966]**

TRILLER, JOHANN MORITZ [*fl.* 1686-1701] *respondent.* Dissertatio inauguralis de officio medici praesentibus contraindicationibus . . . Altdorffii, Literis Henrici Meyeri [1689]

32 p.   21 cm.   **[11967]**
Diss. — Altdorf.

— *See* WEDEL, G. W., *praes.* Dissertatio medica de consensu partium. 1686.

TRIMARCHI, ANDREA [*ca.* 1580-1660] Discorso anatomico capriccio . . . Messina, Gl' heredi di Pietro Brea, 1644.

[24], 447, [8] p.   port.   22 cm.   **[11968]**
Imperfect: title page mutilated.

TRINCAVELLI, VITTORE [1496-1568] Controversiarum medicinalium practicarum libri quinque. Quibus quaestiones maxime controversae & abstrusae, doctrinam inprimis de sanguinis missione innoxia, concernentes, dexterrime explicantur . . . Opus posthumum . . . Nunc primum publici juris factum . . . Francofurti, Apud Nicolaum Rothium, 1617.

[12], 291, [25] p.   20 cm.   **[11969]**
Edited by Johann Münster.

TRINCKHUS, GEORG [1643-1673] Dissertatiuncula de caecis sapientia ac eruditione claris, mirisque caecorum quorundam actionibus . . . Gerae, Literis Georgii Henrici Mülleri, 1672.

[31] p.   20 cm.   **[11970]**

TRINKHUSIUS, GEORGIUS. *See* TRINCKHUS, Georg [1643-1673]

TRINUM magicum; sive, Secretorum magicorum opus. 1673. *See* LONGINUS, C., *ed.*

Le TRIOMPHE hermetique; ou, La pierre philosophale victorieuse. *See* URALTER RITTER-KRIEG. French. 1699.

TRISMEGISTUS, HERMES. *See* HERMES TRISMEGISTUS.

TRISMOSIN, SALOMON, *pseud?* Aurem vellus. *In* Dariot, C. Die gulden Arch. 1614.

TRISSINO, ALVISE [1519-1544] Problematum medicinalium ex sententia Galeni libri sex posthumi . . . Patavii, Apud Franciscum Bolzettam, 1629.

[20], 212, [24] p.   17 cm.   **[11971]**
Imperfect: sig. + [8] wanting.

TRISSMOSIN, SALOMON. *See* TRISMOSIN, Salomon, *pseud?*

TRITEMIUS, JOANNES. *See* TRITHEMIUS, Johannes [1462-1516]

TRITHEMIUS, JOHANNES [1462-1516] Tractatus . . . chemicus nobilis . . .

585-586 p., vol. 4.   20 cm.   (*In* Zetzner, Lazarus, *ed.* Theatrum chemicum. Argentorati, 1659-61)   **[11972]**
Caption title.

— *See* DORN, G. [Clavis totius philosophiae chemisticae. 1659.]

TRIVICO, FERRANTE LOFFREDO, *marchese di. See* LOFFREDO, Ferrante, *marchese di Trivico* [16th cent.]

TROJEL, JOHANN THOMAS [*fl.* 1695] *respondent. See* WINSLOW, J. B., *praeses.* Exercitii anatomicopathologici. 1695.

TROMBETTA, FILIPPO. *See* TROMBETTI, Filippo [*fl.* 1674-1681]

TROMBETTA, PIETRO MARIA [*fl.* 1688] In consultationem pro illustrissima Genuensi matrona, hypochondriaco-hysterica affectione laborante, a semetipso scriptis mandatam paraphrasis una cum aliorum consulentium responsis. Accessere dissertationes De chalybis natura, & viribus; De macie, ejusque causis in morbis hypochondriacis; De sanguinis missione in emaciatis an in macie hypochondriaca, etiam cum febre, & hecticae suspicione, conveniat chalybs . . . Genuae, Typis Antonii Casamarae, 1689.

251 p.   21 cm.   [11973]

TROMBETTI, FILIPPO [*fl.* 1674-1681] Apologia . . . contro una lettera del sig. Stanislao Omati . . . sopra la cognitione, e cura di passione ipocondriaca. Genova, Ant. Giorgio Franchelli, 1674.

196 p.   15 cm.   [11974]

—La bilancia nella quale si librano autorità, e ragioni, contenute nell'antilogia apologetica, data alle stampe dal sig. Stanislao Omati, appartenenti alla vera cognizione, e buona cura del morbo ipocondriaco . . . Genova, Antonio Casamara, 1682.

314, [1] p.   21 cm.   [11975]

—*See* OMATI, S. Antilogia apologetica. 1677.

TROMBSDORFF, JOHANN NIKOLAUS [*fl.* 1678] *respondent. See* RODIGAST, S., *praeses.* Disquisitio physica, de calore nivis. 1678.

TROPPANNIGER, JOHANNES CHRISTOPHORUS [*ca.* 1651-1729] *respondent. See* ETTMÜLLER, M., *praeses.* Dissertatio medica de malo hypochondriaco. 1684.

TROPPAU UND JÄGERNDORF, ELEONORA MARIA ROSALIA, *Herzogin zu* [1647-1704] Freywillig-auffgesprungener Granat-Apffel dess christlichen Samaritans. Oder, Auss christlicher Lieb dess Nächsten eröffnete Gehaimbnus viler vortrefflichen, sonders bewährten Mitteln und wunder-haylsamen Artzneyen . . . auss viler Artzney-Erfahrner und berühmbter Leib-Artzten oder Medicin-Doctorn lang gepflogener Erfahrenheit . . . zusammen getragen . . . Wienn in Oesterreich, Leopold Voigt, 1695.

[3], 516, [11] p.   31 cm.   [11976]

Imperfect: p. 283-286 wanting.

—[The same.] . . . Auffs neue vermehrt (sambt einer kleinen Diaeta, wie sich bey jeder Kranckheit in Essen und Trincken zu verhalten, wie auch beygefügten neuen Koch-Buch. . .) nun zum dritten-mahl in offentlich Druck verfertiget . . . Wienn in Oesterreich, Leopold Voigt, 1697.

[4], 499 p.   21 cm.   [11977]

Imperfect: Koch-Buch wanting.

—*See* SECHS BÜCHER AUSERLESENER ARTZNEY UND KUNST-STÜCK. 1613, 1678.

TROST, JOHANN MARTIN [*fl.* 1677] *respondent. See* TILING, M., *praes.* Dissertatio medica de dysenteria. 1677.

TROTT, JOHANN GEORG [*fl.* 1662-1663] *respondent. See* ROLFINCK, W., *praeses.* Dissertationem inauguralem de tertiana intermittente . . . proponit J. G. T. 1662.

A TRUE account of the royal bagnio, with a discourse of its vertues. By a person of quality. London, Joseph Hindmarsh, 1680.

8 p.   32 cm.   [11978]

A TRUE gentlewomans delight. *See* KENT, E. (Talbot) G., *countess of.* A choice manuall. 1653, 1654.

A TRUE relation of the wonderful cure of Mary Maillard, (lame almost ever since she was born) . . . With the affidavits and certificates of the girl, and several other . . . persons . . . To which is added, a letter from Dr. Welwood to . . . the Lady Mayoress, upon that subject. London, Richard Baldwin, 1694.

48 p.   16 cm.   [11979]

Imperfect: upper margins trimmed.

—[French tr.] Relation veritable de la guerison miraculeuse de Marie Maillard, qui avoit eté boiteuse presque dés sa naissance . . . Avec les despositions & certificats de la fille, & plusieurs autres personnes . . . où l'on ajoûte une lettre du Docteur Welwood sur ce sujet d [sic] l'epouse du Maire de Londres. Traduit de l'anglois. Amsterdam, Paul Marret, 1694.

68, [2] p.   12 cm.   [11980]

TRÜBE, GOTTFRIED THEODOR [*fl.* 1700] Dissertatio historico-physica de mortus ex affectibus . . . Lipsiae, Literis Gözianis [1700]

[23] p.   20 cm.   [11981]

Diss. — Leipzig (J. W. Loges, *respondent*)

TRULLERI, GIUSEPPE [16th-17th *cent.*] *ed. See* SUSIO, G. B. Liber de sanguinis mittendi ratione. 1628.

TRULLIER, JOSEPH. *See* TRULLERI, Giuseppe [16th-17th cent.]

TRULLIO, GIOVANNI [1597 *or* 8-1661] *See* JASOLINO, G. Collegium anatomicum. 1668; SEVERINO, M. A. Seilo-phlebotome castigata. 1654.

TRUMPH, JOHANN GEORG [*fl.* 1667–1668] *praeses.* Dissertatio medica de salivatione mercuriali … Jenae, Literis Samuelis Krebsii [1668]

   36, [4] p. 18 cm.   **[11982]**
  Diss. – Jena (B. C. Capelle, *respondent*)

—*respondent. See* ROLFINCK, W., *praeses.* Hoc cardialgiae scrutinium … exponit … J. G. T. 1667.

TRUMPH, JOHANN HEINRICH [*b.* 1669] *respondent. See* WEDEL, G. W., *praeses.* Dissertatio inauguralis medica, de aromaticorum natura. 1695.

—*See* WEDEL, G. W. Propemticum inaugurale de medicamine faciei. 1695.

TRUYCK, MARTIN [*fl.* 1652] *respondent. See* DEUSING, A., *praeses.* Disputationum anatomicarum tertia. 1652 [and] Disputationum anatomicarum quarta. 1652 [and] Idea doctrinae de febribus. 1655.

The **TRYAL** of Spencer Cowper. 1699. *See* COWPER, S., *defendant.*

TRYE, *Mrs.* MARY [*fl.* 1674] Medicatrix; or, The woman-physician, vindicating Thomas O'Dowde, a chymical physician … against the calumnies and abusive reflections of Henry Stubbe … A revival of Mr. O'Dowd's medicines … London, Printed by T. R. and N. T. and sold by Henry Broome and John Leete, 1675.

   [8], 126, [10] p. 16 cm.   **[11983]**

[**TRYON**, THOMAS, 1634–1703] A dialogue between an East-Indian brackmanny or heathen-philosopher, and a French gentleman concerning the present affairs of Europe. London, Andrew Sowle, 1683.

   [2], 20 + p. 19 cm.   **[11984]**
  Imperfect: all after p. 20 wanting.
  Bound with copy 2 of *his* The way to health. 1683.

—[The same.] … London, Printed for D. Newman, and R. Baldwin, 1691.

   [1], 18 p. 19 cm.   **[11985]**
  Bound (as issued) with *his* The way to health. 1691.

—The good house-wife made a doctor; or, Health's choice and sure friend being a plain way of nature's own prescribing, to prevent and cure most diseases … by diet and kitchin-physick only … The 2d ed. To which is added some observations on the tedious methods of unskilful chyrurgions … London,

Printed for H. N. and T. S. and sold by Randal Taylor, 1692.

   [12], 285 p. 14 cm.   **[11986]**
  Imperfect? Sig. A⁷⁻¹² wanting?

—Healths grand preservative; or, The womens best doctor. A treatise shewing the nature and operation of brandy, rumm, rack, and other distilled spirits, and the ill consequences of mens, but especially of womens drinking such pernicious liquors and smoaking tobacco. As likewise, of the immoderate eating of flesh … Together, with a … discourse of the excellency of herbs … London, Printed for the author, and sold by Langley Curtis, 1682.

   [1], 22 p. 22 cm.   **[11987]**

—Letters, domestick and foreign … occasionally distributed in subjects, viz. philosophical, theological, and moral … London, Geo. Conyers and Eliz. Harris, 1700.

   [11], 240 p. 19 cm.   **[11988]**
  Imperfect: p. [3–6] wanting, supplied in photocopy from Harvard University library.
  Added title page (p. [11]): … Letters, upon several occasions.

—A new art of brewing beer, ale, and other sorts of liquors … The 2d ed. To which is added, the art of making mault … with several other … profitable things relating to country affairs … London, Tho. Salusbury, 1691.

   [4], 137 p. 16 cm.   **[11989]**
  Imperfect: sig. [A4] "The contents of this book," misbound at end; first preliminary leaf (blank?) wanting?

—A treatise of cleannes in meats and drinks, of the preparation of food, the excellency of good airs … Also of the generation of bugs, and their cure. To which is added a short discourse of the pain of the teeth … London, Printed for the author, and sold by L. Curtis, 1682.

   [1], 21 p. 19 cm.   **[11990]**

—A treatise of dreams & visions, wherein the causes natures and uses of nocturnal representations, and the communications both of good and evil angels, as also departed souls, to mankinde, are theosophically unfolded … To which is added, a discourse of the causes, natures and cure of phrensie, madness or distraction. By Philotheos Physiologus [pseud., i.e. Thomas Tryon] [London, Andrew Sowles, 1689]

   [14], 299, [3] p. 15 cm.   **[11991]**
  Imperfect: last leaf wanting, supplied in photocopy.

—[The same.] . . . By Thom Tryon . . . The 2d ed. London, T. Sowle, 1695.

[14], 299, [3] p. 15 cm.   [11992]

A reissue of the first edition with new title page.

—The way to health, long life and happiness; or, A discourse of temperance and the particular nature of all things requisit for the life of man, as all sorts of meats, drinks, air, exercise, &c. . . . To which is added a treatise of most sorts of English herbs . . . The like never before published . . . By Philotheos Physiologus [pseud., i.e. Thomas Tryon] London, Andrew Sowle, 1683.

[15], 699, [3] p. 19 cm.   [11993]

—Copy 2.

Imperfect: first preliminary leaf and p. 627–630 wanting. With this is bound *his* A dialogue between an East-Indian . . . and a French gentleman. 1683.

—[The same.] . . . The 2d. ed., with amendments. London, Printed by H. C. for R. Baldwin, 1691.

[14], 500 p. 19 cm.   [11994]

With this is bound (as issued) *his* A dialogue between an East-Indian . . . and a French gentleman. 1691.

—Another issue, with imprint: London, Printed by H. C. for D. Newmann, 1691.   [11995]

First preliminary leaf (blank) wanting.

—[The same.] . . . The 3d ed. To which is added A discourse of the philosopher's stone, or universal medicine, discovering the cheats and abuses of those chymical pretenders. London, 1697.

[16], 456 (i.e. 464) p.; 24 p. 19 cm.   [11996]

"A dialogue between an East-Indian brackmanny, or heathen philosopher, and a French gentleman, &c": 1–17 p. at end. Imperfect: p. 183–188 mutilated.

—Wisdom's dictates; or, Aphorisms & rules, physical, moral, and divine, for preserving the health of the body, and the peace of the mind . . . To which is added a bill of fare of seventy five noble dishes of excellent food, far exceeding those made of fish or flesh . . . London, Tho. Salusbury, 1691.

[6], 153, [3] p. 15 cm.   [11997]

—[The same.] . . . London, John Salusbury, 1696.

[6], 144 p. 15 cm.   [11998]

Imperfect: first preliminary leaf (blank?) wanting; p. 143–144 mutilated.

TSCHIENTSCHI, FELIX [*fl.* 1663–1664] *respondent.* Disputatio medica de asthmate . . . Basileae,

Typis Joh. Jacobi Deckeri [1664]

[8] p. 19 cm.   [11999]

Diss. — Basel.

TSCHIRNAUSEN, EHRENFRIED WALTER VON. *See* TSCHIRNHAUS, Ehrenfried Walther von [1651–1708]

[**TSCHIRNHAUS,** EHRENFRIED WALTHER VON, 1651–1708] [Medicina corporis. German] Die curiöse Medicin, darinnen die Gesundheit des Leibes in sehr wahrscheinlichen Gedancken in XII. Reguln vorgestellet, und wie solche durch gar leichte Mittel zu unterhalten, gezeiget wird. Franckfurt und Leipzig, Bey Johann Georg Lippern, 1688.

191 p. 14 cm.   [12000]

—Medicina mentis; sive, Tentamen genuinae logicae, in qua disseritur de methodo detegendi incognitas veritates. Amstelaedami, Apud Albertum Magnum, & Joannem Rieuwerts juniorem, 1687.

[16], 224 p.; [4], 59, [1] p. illus. 21 cm. [12001]

Part [2] has special title page dated 1686: Medicina corporis; seu, Cogitationes admodum probabiles de conservanda sanitate.

—[The same.] Medicina mentis; sive, Artis inveniendi praecepta generalia. Ed. nova, auctior & correctior, cum praefatione autoris. Lipsiae, Apud J. Thomam Fritsch, 1695.

[28], 296 p.; [4], 64 p. illus. 22 cm. [12002]

Part [2] has special title page: Medicina corporis; seu, Cogitationes admodum probabiles de conservanda sanitate.

—Another printing. 23 cm.   [12003]

Identical in contents, but of a different setting of type throughout

TUCCARO, ARCANGELO [*b. ca.* 1535] Trois dialogues . . . Le premier dialogue traicte des exercices gymnastiques, dont les anciens usoient . . . Le second contient plusieurs beaus discours du faut appellé par les anciens cubistique . . . Au troisiesme est fort amplement dicouru des exercices que l'homme peut faire, selon sa nature & complexion, & comme il en doit user pour rendre le corps agile, vigoureux & sain . . . Tours, Georges Griveau, 1616.

[2], 197 ll. illus. 22 cm.   [12004]

TUDECIUS, SIMON ALOYSIUS [*fl.* 1679–1695] Amussis antiloimica ad mentem quorundam clarissimorum archiatrorum tum veterum tum recentiorum . . . concinnata, & practice adhibita . . . Norimbergae, Expensis Johannis Ziegeri, 1695.

[12], 227 p. 13 cm.   [12005]

TÜBINGEN, UNIVERSITÄT. *See* EBERHARD-KARLS-UNIVERSITÄT TÜBINGEN.

TÜCHEL, FRIEDRICH WILHELM [*fl.* 1673] *respondent. See* SCHMID, Christian, *praeses.* De iride. 1673.

TULLEKEN, OSUALD [*fl.* 1694] *respondent.* Disputatio medica inauguralis de catarrho suffocativo ... Lugduni Batavorum, Apud Abrahamum Elzevier, 1694.

    [13] p.   22 cm.   **[12006]**
Diss.—Leyden.

TULP, NICOLAAS [1593-1674] Observationum medicarum, libri tres ... Amstelredami, Apud Ludovicum Elzevirium, 1641.

    [14], 279 p.   illus.   16 cm.   **[12007]**

—Copy 2.
Sig. *⁸ (blank) wanting.
With this is bound Willich, Jodocus. Juditia urinarum. Witebergae, 1560.

—[The same.] Observationes medicae. Ed. nova, libro quarto auctior, et sparsim ... emendatior. Amstelredami, Apud Ludovicum Elzevirium, 1652.

    [16], 403 p.   illus.   17 cm.   **[12008]**
Engraved title page.

—[The same.] ... Amstelredami, Apud Danielem Elzevirium, 1672.

    [16], 392 p.   illus.   17 cm.   **[12009]**
Added engraved title page.
Imperfect: sig. *⁸ (p. [15-16]) wanting.

—[The same.] ... Amstelaedami, Apud Henricum Wetstenium, 1685.

    [14], 382 p.   illus.   17 cm.   **[12010]**
Engraved title page.

—[Dutch tr.] De drie boecken der medicijnsche aenmerkingen, in 't Latijn beschreven ... Amstelredam, Jacob Benjamyn [gedrukt by Jan Jacobsz. Bouman] 1650.

    [16], 279 p.   illus., port.   16 cm.   **[12011]**

— Copy 2.
Imperfect: port. wanting.
Bound with Harvey, W. Vande beweging van 't hert. 1650.

TUNSTAL, GEORGE. *See* TONSTALL, George [*b.* 1616]

TURBA philosophorum [&] Turbae philosophorum alterum exemplar [&] Allegoriae super librum Turbae [&] Aenigma ex visione Arislei

[&] In Turbam philosophorum exercitationes ...

    1-118 p., vol. 1.   17 cm.   (*In* Artis auriferae. Basileae, 1610)   **[12012]**
Caption titles.
Ascribed to Arisleus or Arislaeus by Schmieder (p. 124) and Ferguson (v. 2, p. 477), to Arislaus, pseud. of Guglielmo Grataroli, by BMC and NUC. According to Plessner, it was written around 900; according to Schmieder in the 12th century.

—Turba philosophorum, ex antiquo manuscripto codice excerpta, qualis nulla hactenus visa est editio. Arislei epistola, quam de intentione libri, futuris, ad eorum instructionem, sapientum dictis praemisit ...

    1-52 p., vol. 5.   20 cm.   (*In* Zetzner, Lazarus, *ed.* Theatrum chemicum. Argentorati, 1659-61)
Caption title.   **[12013]**

—[German ed.] Turba philosophorum [&] Das ander Exemplar der Turbae philosophorum [&] Etliche Retzel, oder Aenigmata auss dem Gesicht des Philosophi Arislei unnd auss den Allegoriis der Weissen [&] Ubungen in die Turbam ...

    1-141 p.   19 cm.   (Part 1 *in* Morgenstern, Philipp, *ed.* and *tr.* Turba philosophorum. Basel, 1613)
Caption titles.   **[12014]**

TURIBIUS, *Saint, Archbishop of Lima. See* MOGROVEJO, Toribio Alfonso de, *Saint* [1538-1606]

TURIBIUS ALFONSUS MOGROVEJUS. *See* MOGROVEJO, Toribio Alfonso de, *Saint* [1538-1606]

TURIN. Collegio dei filosofi e medici. *See* COLLEGIO DEI FILOSOFI E MEDICI, Turin.

TURNÈBE, ADRIEN [1512-1565] De vino. *In* Meibom, J. H. De cervisiis. 1668.

—, *tr. See* THEOPHRASTUS. Θεοφράστον ... ἄπαντα. Theophrasti ... Graece & Latine opera omnia. 1613.

TURNER, DANIEL [1667-1741] Apologia chyrurgica. A vindication of the noble art of chyrurgery, from the gross abuses offer'd thereunto by mountebanks, quacks, barbers ... London, J. Whitlock, 1695.

    [16], 140 p.   17 cm.   **[12015]**

TURNER, JOHN, *vicar of Greenwich.* A discourse on fornication: shewing the greatness of that sin, and examining the excuses pleaded for it, from the examples of antient times. To which is added An appendix concerning concubinage; as also a remark on

Mr. Butler's explication of Hebr. xiii. 4. in his late book on that subject ... London, John Wyat, 1698.

[4], 62 p.   21 cm.   [12016]

TURNER, Robert [*fl.* 1654-1665] Βοτανολογια. The Brittish physician; or, The nature and vertues of English plants. Exactly describing such plants as grow naturally in our land, with their ... applications and vertues, physical and astrological uses, treated of, each plant appropriated to the several diseases they cure ... London, Printed by R. Wood for Nath. Brook, 1664.

[14], 363, [20] p.   front.   18 cm.   [12017]

—[The same.] ... London, Obadiah Blagrave, 1687.

[8], 363, [26] p.   front.   18 cm.   [12018]
Imperfect: p. 39-40 mutilated.

—De morbis foemineis, the womans counsellour; or, The feminine physician enlarged ... Whereunto is added The mans counsellonr [sic], healing of ruptures, and particular diseases belonging to men. The 4th ed. London, J. Streater, 1686.

[8], 207 p.   17 cm.   [12019]

—Μιϰϱοϰοσμος. A description of the little-world. Being a discovery of the body of man, exactly delineating all the members, bones, veins, sinews, arteries, and parts thereof, from the head to the foot. Heerunto is added ... the cure of wounds ... London, John Harrison, 1654.

[13], 172 p.   15 cm.   [12020]
Imperfect: p. 5-6 and 27-30 mutilated.

—, *ed.* and *tr. See* MOULTON, T. The compleat bone-setter. 1656, 1666; PARACELSUS. Of the chymical transmutation. 1657; SADLER, J. Enchiridion medicum: an enchiridion of the art of physick. 1657.

—, *tr. See* [HESTEAU, C., *sieur de Nuisement*] Sal, lumen, & spiritus mundi philosophici. 1657.

TURNER, WILLIAM [*d.* 1568] *See* VICARY, T. The English mans treasure. 1613,1633, 1641 [and] The surgions directorie. 1651.

TURNER, WILLIAM [1653-1701] A compleat history of the most remarkable providences, both of judgment and mercy, which have hapned in this present age ... To which is added, whatever is curious in the works of nature and art ... London, John Dunton, 1697.

3 parts in 1 v.   35 cm.   [12021]

Parts II and III have special title pages: The wonders of nature
The curiosities of art.

TURNISER, LEONHARD. *See* THURNEISSER ZUM THURN, Leonhard [1531-1596]

TURQUET DE MAYERNE, THÉODORE. *See* MAYERNE, *Sir* Théodore Turquet de [1573-1655]

TURRE, GAMALIEL DE [*fl.* 1615] Theses medicae cardinalitiae, pro ... doctoratus laurea consequenda propositae, sub hac quaestionis forma; an in peste, cardiaca sint tum medicamentorum, tum praesidiorum omnium praestantissima? Quibus accessere positiones ac assertiones ... ex ... medicinae ... fontibus desumptae ... Monspelii, Joan. Gileti, 1615.

46 p.   16 cm.   [12022]
Imperfect: margins trimmed, affecting text.
Diss. — Montpellier.

TURRE, GIORGIO A. *See* TORRE, Giorgio dalla [1607-1688]

TURRIANUS, BARTHOLOMAEUS. *See* TORRE, Bartolomeo della [*fl.* 1599-1602]

TUSCANY. Laws, statutes, etc. Bando contro a chl [sic] fraudolentemente dispenserà l'orvietano di Francesco di Jacopo Sozzi viperaio di S. A. S. habitante in Pistoia ... [Roma, Firenze, & Pistoia, 1639]

[2] p.   21 cm.   [12023]
Caption title.
Page [2] has caption title: Modo d'adoperare l'orvietano contra veleni vivi, e morti, dispensato da Francesco di Jacopo

TUTHILL, FRANCIS [*fl.* 1698] *See* COLBATCH, *Sir* J. The doctrine of acids. 1689 [i.e. 1698] [and] A relation of a very sudden ... cure. 1698.

TUTIUS, MÁRTON [*d.* 1702] *respondent. See* LOSS, J., *praeses.* Dissertationem medicam de arthritide ... publico ... examini exponit M. T. 1683.

TWEEDE missive aen d'Heer Balthasar Bekker. 1692. *See* [SCHUTS, J.]

De TWEEDE onschult. Zynde een nadere coutenantie tusschen de geesten van imant en niemant. [Amsterdam] Gedruckt te Scheyteldoecks-haven voor de Liefhebbers, 1678.

46 p.   16 cm.   [12024]
Occasioned by the controversy between Andreas Boekelman and Bonaventura van Dortmont.

TWISCK, Pieter Janszoon [1566–1636] Van de peste. Gestelt in ses deelen. Met korte, bondige leeringen, vermaninghen, vertroostingen, en waerschouwingen, tot beteringe des levens, gerustheyt der conscientie, ende een saligh eynde . . . Hoorn, Door Zacharias Cornelissz. [Druckt by Issac Willemsz] 1635.

88 p. 15 cm. [**12025**]

TWYSDEN, John [1607–1688] Medicina veterum vindicata; or, An answer to a book, entituled Medela medicinae; in which the ancient method and rules are defended . . . that there is no such change in the diseases of this age, or their nature in general, that we should be obliged to an alteration of them. Against the calumnies . . . of . . . Mar. Nedham . . . London, Printed by J. G. for John Crook, 1666.

[24], 214, [1] p. 16 cm. [**12026**]

Errata: p. [215]

TYLKOWSKI, Adalbert [1625–1695] Disquisitio physica, ostenti duorum puerorum quorum unus cum dente aureo alter cum capite gyganteo Vilnae in Lithuania regni Poloniae provincia spectabatur. Anno Domini 1673. Olivae, Typis Monasterii Olivensis, 1674.

[84] p. 14 cm. [**12027**]

Imperfect: upper margins trimmed.

TYLKOWSKI, Woyciech. See Tylkowski, Adalbert [1625–1695]

TYMME, Thomas [d. 1620] tr. See Duchesne, J. The practise of chymicall and hermeticall physicke. 1605.

TYROANDRUS, Johannes. See Kesmann, Johann [fl. 1613]

TYSON, Edward [1650–1708] Orang-outang, sive homo sylvestris; or, The anatomy of a pygmie compared with that of a monkey, an ape, and a man. To which is added, A philological essay concerning the pygmies, the cynocephali, the satyrs, and sphinges of the ancients . . . London, Thomas Bennet and Daniel Brown, 1699.

[10], 108 p.; [1], 58 p. plates. 29 cm. [**12028**]

Part [2] has special title page.
Imperfect? First preliminary leaf (blank?) wanting?

—Phocaena; or, The anatomy of a porpess, dissected at Gresham Colledge: with a praeliminary discourse concerning anatomy, and a natural history of animals . . . London, Benj. Tooke, 1680.

[4], 48, [4] p. plates. 24 cm. [**12029**]

U

UBBENIUS, Nicolaas [fl. 1676] respondent. Disputatio medica inauguralis de haemorrhagia narium . . . Lugduni Batavorum, Apud viduam & haeredes Johannis Elsevirii, 1676.

[24] p. 22 cm. [**12030**]

Diss. — Leyden.

UBERTE DE LA CERDA, Marcelino [fl. 1622–1639] Tractatus de inopinata causa variolarum, & morbillorum, febris principio intrinseco, remedioque prophilactico pestis. Quibus accessit De pinguedine cum paradoxa urinae sedimenti. Oscae, Apud Petrum Bluson, 1635.

[8], 171, [1] p. 15 cm. [**12031**]

Imperfect: the second treatise wanting.

UBERTE Y BALAGUER, Anastasio Marcelino [fl. 1678–1681] Noticia dela justa, santa, y zelosa prohibicion del libro de Catanea por la Sacra Congregacion del indice contra el padre fray Juan de Olmo a 31. de marzo 1681. y publicado de 1. de abril 1681. en Roma. Y de consiguiente prohibido tambien el de Valencia. Y respuesta segunda contra su segundo aumentado en Valencia a 31. de diciembre 1679. y su manifesto, ò prologo Praefatium ad opus, que sacò a luz año 1680 . . . [Parma? 1681]

[27] p. 22 cm. [**12032**]

Bound with his La obligacion prevenida. 1678.

—La obligacion prevenida con su primera, y segunda respuesta a un papel manuscrito de 3. de junio 1677. En que un moderno da absolutamente por licito el permisso de las rameras en los castillos de Napoles, y contra otro del mismo autor, impreso a los primeros de noviembre 1677. con titulo de Catania, en que confirma lo mismo . . . Puzol, Geronimo Fasulo, 1678.

[40], 146, [5] p. 22 cm. [**12033**]

With this are bound his: Noticia. [1681]; Respuesta. [1679]

—Respuesta ... al manifiesto intitulado Praefatium ad opus, que le embiarion de Cartagena ... contra su segundo libro, cuio titulo es La obligacion prevenida ... [Napoles? 1680]

[12] p. 22 cm. [12034]

Imperfect: p. [5] wrongly printed, part of text supplied in manuscript.

Bound with *his* La obligacion prevenida. 1678.

UBERTO, Marcelino *See* UBERTE DE LA CERDA, Marcelino [*fl.* 1622-1639]

UBERUS, Georgius [*fl.* 1544-1566] *See* Scholtz, L. Epistolarum philosophicarum ... volumen. 1610.

UCAY, Gervais [*fl.* 1668-1695] Apologie du nouveau traité de la maladie venerienne, contenant des eclaircissemens tres utiles sur le remede de l'autheur ... Avec quelques nouveaux problemes sur cette maladie ... Toulouse, Dominique Desclassan, 1689.

84 p. 14 cm. [12035]

Bound with his Nouveau traité. 1688.

—Nouveau traité de la maladie venerienne. Ou aprés avoir demontré que la methode ordinaire de la guerir est tres-dangereuse ... on en propose une autre fort facile & asseruée ... Toulouse, Dominique Desclassan, 1688.

[24], 180 p. 14 cm. [12036]

Special title page (p. [119]) reads: Problemes curieux dans lesquels on resout les plus belles questions qu'on peut proposer sur la maladie venerienne ...

With this is bound *his* Apologie. 1689.

—[The same.] ... Amsterdam, Daniel Pain, 1699.

[16], 259, [2] p. front. 14 cm. [12037]

UDEMANS, Cornelis [*fl.* 1681] *respondent.* Disputatio medica inauguralis de motus impotentia & in specie de paralysi ... Lugduni Batavorum, Apud viduam & heredes Johannis Elsevirii, 1681.

[28] p. 22 cm. [12038]

Diss.—Leyden.

—*See* Schacht, L., *praeses.* Disputatio medica de chlorosi. 1681.

UDENIUS, Utes, *pseud. See* Wedel, Georg Wolffgang [1645-1721]

ÜBELIUS, Samuel. *See* Uebelin, Samuel [1541-1609]

UEBELIN, Samuel [1541-1609] Positiones physicae ωξὶ τῆς σηψεος; sive, De putredine: quas, D. A. G. consensu & auctoritate amplissimi ... in inclyta Basileens. Academia collegii philosophici, praeside clarissimo ... viro Dn. Joh. Georgio Leone, medico experientissimo ... discutiendas & examinandas publice ... proponit Samuel Übelius ... Basileae, Typis Exertierianis, 1608.

[14] p. 20 cm. [12039]

A mock thesis.

UFFENBACH, Peter [1566-1635] Thesaurus chirurgicae, continens praestantissimorum autorum, utpote Ambrossi Parei ... Joannis Tagaultii ... Jacobi Hollerii ... Mariani Sancti ... Angeli Bolognini, Michaelis Angeli Blondi, Alphonsi Ferrii ... Jacobi Dondi et Guilelmi Fabritii Hildani. Opera chirurgica ... Ante hac ... disjunctim edita, nunc vero in unum collecta ... repurgata ... Francofurti, Typis Nicolai Hoffmanni, impensa Jacobi Fischeri, 1610.

[12], 1164, [31] p. illus., port. 35 cm. [12040]

—*ed.* and *tr.* Ein newes Artzney Buch darinn fast alle eusserliche und innerliche unnatürliche Geschwülste, alle dess gantzen menschlichen Leibs und dessen Gliedmassen Wunden, alle Geschwär und Fisteln aller und jeder Glieder: endlich auch die Beinbrüche selbst, beschrieben, und wie dieselbe ... curiert werden mögen angezeigt wird. Darneben auch drey newer Tractat darvon ... Christoff Wirsung nicht geschrieben: I. Von den Schwachheiten und Gebrechen der jungen Kinder und ihrer Cur. II. Von der Kunst die todten Cörper zu balsamiren. III. Von dem Schorbock und seiner Cur. Alles ... verteutscht und an Tag geben, durch ... Petrum Uffenbach ... Franckfort am Mayn, Gedruckt durch Zachariam Palthenium, 1605.

[12], 222, 261, [3] p. ports. 36 cm. [12041]

Ein newes Artzney Buch is a translation of Hieronymus Fabricius ab Aquapendente's Pentateuchos cheirurgicum; Von den Schwachheiten und Gebrechen der jungen Kinder und ihrer Cur, of Girolamo Mercuriale's De morbis puerorum; Von der Kunst die todten Cörper zu balsamiren, of Pieter van Foreest's Observationum et curationum medicinalium liber XXIX. Observatio XXIX; Von dem Schorbock und seiner Cur, of Hieronymus Reusner's Diexodicarum exercitationum liber de scorbuto.

Bound with Wirsung, C. Ein newes Artzney Buch. 1619.

—, *ed.* and *tr. See* Ferrara, C. Sylva chirurgiae. 1625.

—, *ed. See* Argenterio, C. Opera. 1610; Bernard de Gordon. Lilium medicinae. 1617; Cardoso, F. R.

Tractatus absolutissimus. 1620; DIOSCORIDES, Pedanius, of Anazarbos. Kräuterbuch. 1610; GALLO, A. Fascis aureus de peste. 1606, 1608; GATINARIA, M. De medendis humani corporis malis practica. 1604; GÓMEZ MEIDES, B. Αλογραφια. 1605; MANARDI, G. Ἰατρολογια επιστολιχή; sive, Curia medica. 1611; MONTAGNANA, B. Selectiorum operum ... Montagnanae. 1604; SASSONIA, E. De pulsibus tractatus. 1604 [and] Pantheum medicinae selectum. 1603; VITTORI, B. De curandis morbis ad tyrones practica magna. 1628; WIRSUNG, C. Ein new Artzney Buch. 1605, 1619.

—, tr. See CROCE, G. A. della. Officina aurea. 1607; DURANTE, C. Hortulus sanitatis. 1609; PARÉ, A. Wundt Artzney. 1601, 1635; PORTA, G. B. della. Ars destillatoria. 1611; RUINI, C. Anatomia & medicina equorum nova. 1603;

—See BRUYERIN, J. B. Dipnosophia seu sitologia. 1606.

UGO DE SIENA. See BENZI, Ugo [1376–1439]

ULMANN, DAVID [fl. 1667–1671] praeses. Dissertatio physica de dracone volante ... Lipsiae, Stanno Johannis Georgii [1671]

[16] p.   19 cm.   [12042]

Diss. — Leipzig (D. Lindner, *respondent*)

ULMUS, MARCUS ANTONIUS. See OLMO, Marc' Antonio.

ULOT, BALTHASAR [fl. 1632] respondent. Disputatio inauguralis medica de volvulo sive iliaca passione ... Argentorati, Typis Eberhardi Welperi, 1632.

[16] p.   21 cm.   [12043]

Diss. — Strasbourg.

ULRICH, DANIEL HEINRICH [fl. 1681] respondent. See WEDEL, G. W., praeses. Dissertatio medica exhibens aegrum laborantem peste. 1681.

ULRICH, TIMOTHEUS [fl. 1604–1607] respondent. See SENNERT, D., praeses. De methodo medendi disputatio V, de venae sectione. 1604 [and] De pestilentia disputatio. 1607.

ULRICUS, TIMOTHEUS. See ULRICH, Timotheus [fl. 1604–1607]

ULSTÄTT, JOHANN DAVID [fl. 1662–1665] respondent. See HOFFMANN, M., praeses. Ασκημα ἱατριχόν. 1662.

al-**UMAWĪ,** KHĀLID IBN YAZĪD. See KHĀLID IBN YAZĪD, al-Umawī.

UNIVERSIDADE DE COIMBRA. COLLEGIUM CONIMBRICENSE SOCIETATIS JESU. Commentarii Collegii Conimbricensis Societatis Jesu, in tres libros De anima Aristotelis ... Hac nuper editione summa diligentia, mendis quampluribus expurgati, atque in studiosorum gratiam editi ... Venetiis, Apud Jacobum Vincentium & Ricciardum Amadinum, 1606.

[24] p., 826 col.   23 cm.   [12044]

—Commentarii Collegii Conimbricensis, e Societate Jesu, in duos libros De generatione & corruptione, Aristotelis ... Quibus, praemissa gemina Graeci textus in Latinum translatione, illiusque diligenti explanatione de arduis, & obscuris quaestionibus, causas ortus & interitus rerum naturalium demonstrantibus, admodum erudite in utramque partem disseritur. Superiori tempore in Germania praelo suppositi, hoc vero instanti denuo tertia vice in Italia impressi, summo studio emendati, & ab omnibus erroribus liberati ... Venetiis, Apud Andream Baba, 1616.

[40] p., 760 columns.   24 cm.   [12045]

With this is bound *its* In libros Ethicorum Aristotelis ad Nicomachum ... cursus disputationes. 1616.

—In libros Ethicorum Aristotelis ad Nicomachum, aliquot Conimbricensis cursus disputationes: in quibus praecipua quaedam ethicae disciplinae capita continentur. Hac novissima editione ab omnibus erroribus expurgatae, & summo studio correctae ... Venetiis, Apud Andream Baba, 1616.

71, [8] p.   24 cm.   [12046]

Bound with *its* Commentarii ... De generatione & corruptione, Aristotelis. 1616.

—, FACULDADE DE MEDICINA. See PORTUGAL. Sovereigns, etc. [1598–1621] (Philip II). Regimento dos medicos e boticarios. 1604.

UNIVERSITÀ DI BOLOGNA. See ALIDOSI, G. N. P. I dottori bolognesi. 1623 [and] Li dottori forestieri. 1623.

—, COLLEGIO DE MEDICINA. Antidotarium Bononien[se] a Medicinae Collegio nuperrime auctum et emendatum, et amplissimo ejusdem civitatis Senatui dicatum ... Bononiae, Apud haeredem Victorii Benacii, 1641.

[36], 506, [10] p.   23 cm.   [12047]

Engraved title page.

Compiled by Ulisse Aldrovandi. Published in 1574 under title: Antidotarii Bononiensis ... epitome.

With this is bound *its* Gl'indirizzi dell'arte dello spetiale medicinalista. [1658?]

—[The same.] Antidotarium Bononiense novissimum. Sapientissimis ac illustrissimis DD. Felsineae patriae patribus a jatrophysico ejusdem Collegio dicatum. Bononiae, Ex Typographie Manolessia, 1674.

    [8], 408, [16] p. 24 cm.   **[12048]**

—Conventioni fra l'eccelentiss. Collegio de'medici, et l'honorabile Compagnia delli speciali medicinalisti di Bologna. Bologna, Vittorio Benacci, 1606.

    16 p. 21 cm.   **[12049]**

—Gl'indirizzi dell'arte dello spetiale medicinalista, cioè un dispensatorio copiosissimo, ed alfabetico delle materie di quella in varie classi distinto, colla enumeratione de i termini, e ministeri più principali della medema, ed alcuni di loro esemplificati, acommodo dell' honoranda Compagnia de gli maestri spetiali medicinalisti di Bologna, per instruire più metodicamente i discepoli, e gargioni loro. Ordinati dagli eccellentiss. signori protomedici del Collegio di Bologna ... 1658. Bologna, Herede di Vittorio Benacci [1658?]

    32 p. 23 cm.   **[12050]**

Bound with *its* Antidotarium Bononien[se], 1641, to which it forms an appendix. Cf. p. 32.

—Liber pro recta administratione protomedicatus, in quo plura notanda subjiciuntur, & offeruntur excellentissimis DD. prioribus Colllegii [sic] Medicinae, et ejus protomedicis pro tempore futuris, ut statuta praecipue. A multis summis pontificibus confirmata observentur, & secundum justitiam clare jus reddatur. Bononiae, Ex Typographia Ferroniana, 1666.

    87, [7] p. 20 cm.   **[12051]**

"Die 3. Novembris 1665, in pleno Collegio legitime congregato, &c. fuerunt declarati assumpti pro nova impressione Constitutionum protomedicatus ...": p. [89]

"Catalogo de'ss. filosofi medici viventi, tanto bolognesi, quanto forastieri ... 1666, secondo l'ordine de i loro dottorati": p. [91]-[94]

—*See* Grandi, P. Illustriss. Gabellae syndicorum nomenclatura pro parte ... Collegii Medicae Facultatis ab anno Domini 1508. usque ad annum 1641 inclusive. 1641.

UNIVERSITÀ DI PADOVA. *See* Tomasini, J F. Gymnasivm Patavinvm ... libris V. comprehensum. 1654.

UNIVERSITÄT KÖNIGSBERG. *See* Albertus-Universität.

UNIVERSITÄT LEIPZIG. Decanus com munitatis studii bonarum artium et philosophiae i Academia Lipsiensi ad auscultandam orationem, qua gratiosi medici adversus obtrectatores defenduntur lectorem benevolum officiose invitat. [Lipsiae, Literis Wittigavianis, 1661]

    [4] p. 32 cm.   **[12052**

Invitation to an oration by Jakob Holtzapfel.

With this is bound Holtzapfel, J. Medicina ab opprobriis vin dicata. 1661.

—, Medizinische Fakultät. *See* Vieussens, R. Epistola de sanguinis humani cum sale fixo. 1698.

UNIVERSITÄT TÜBINGEN. *See* Eberhard-Karls-Universität Tübingen.

UNIVERSITÄT WITTENBERG. Medizinische Fakultät. Kurtzer Bericht und Ordnung: wie männiglich in Pestilentz Zeiten sich verhalten solle und mit was Mitteln und Artzneyen ... ein jeder sich ... möge verwahren ... Gestellet durch das Collegium Medicum zu Wittenberg. Anno 1626. [Wittenberg] Gedruckt bey Christian Tham [1626]

    [46] p. 19 cm.   **[12053**

Imperfect: all after p. [46] wanting.

—[The same.] ... Jtzo zum andern Mahl in Druck gegeben und ... corrigirt. Wittenberg, In Verlegung Paul Helwigs, 1626.

    [1], 46 p. 20 cm.   **[12054**

—Kurtzer Bericht, wie die Artzneyen, welche in vorstehender Sterbens Gefahr, alhier zu Wittenberg, in der Apotheken angeordnet ... Gestellet von dem Collegio Medico doselbst. Wittenberg, In Verlegung Paul Helwigs [gedruckt by Martin Henckel] 1607.

    [23] p. 20 cm.   **[12055**

UNIVERSITAS HAVNIENSIS. *See* Universitas Regia Hafniensis. Facultas medica.

UNIVERSITAS LUGDUNO BATAVA. *See* Rijksuniversiteit te Leiden.

UNIVERSITAS REGIA HAFNIENSIS.

FACULTAS MEDICA. Kurtzer Unterricht vom Blut- oder Hoffgang, welcher gestalt demselben, vermitelst göttlicher Hülffe kan vorgekommen, und durch gute Cur abgeholffen werden. Auff Ihr: Kön. M. Friderici III . . . Befehl dem gemeinen Mann zum Besten gestellet und verordnet von der Facultate Medica zu Kopenhagen anno 1652. Kopenhagen, Gedruckt bey Georg Lamprecht, auff Jochim Moltkens Bekostung, 1652.

[16] p.   16 cm.   **[12056]**

Bound with Charleton, W. Spiritus gorgonicus. 1650.

UNIVERSITATIS MEDICORUM VILLE MONTISPESSULANI. *See* UNIVERSITÉ DE MONT- PELLIER. Faculté de médecine.

UNIVERSITÉ DE MÉDECINE DE MONT- PELLIER. *See* UNIVERSITÉ DE MONTPELLIER. Faculté de médecine.

UNIVERSITÉ DE MONTPELLIER. FACULTÉ DE MÉDECINE. *See* CHASTELAIN, J. Quaestiones medicae duodecim. 1668 [and] Quaestiones medico- chymico-practicae duodecim. 1697; DEIDIER, A. Quaestiones medico-chymico-practicae duodecim. 1697; FABRE, J. Quaestiones medico-chymico- practicae duodecim. 1697; GAUTERON, A. Quaestiones medico-chymico-practicae duodecim. 1697; PICHON, P. Quaestiones medicae duodecim. 1673; RICOME, L. Quaestiones medico-chymico-practicae. 1696; RIDEUX, P. Quaestiones medico-chymico-practicae duodecim. 1697; [RIOLAN, J. [1580-1657] Curieuses recherches sur les escholes en medecine de Paris. 1651; RIVIÈRE, G. Quaestiones medico-chymico-practicae duodecim. 1696.

UNIVERSITÉ DE PARIS. Decretum almae Universitatis Parisiensis, anno salutis M DC XXVI, die XII. kal. Majas, in maturinensi, scribendo ad- fuerunt rector . . . universitas studiorum. Parisiis, Apud Petrum Durand, 1626.

8 p.   16 cm.   **[12057]**

Bound with copy 2 of Goclenius, R. Mirabilium naturae liber. 1625.

—, — FACULTÉ DE MÉDECINE. Codex medicamen- tarius; seu, Pharmacopoea Parisiensis . . . in lucem edita Philippo Harduino de S. Jacques, Decano.

Lutetiae Parisiorum, Sumptibus Olivarii de Varen- nes, 1638.

[16], 128, [8] p.   22 cm.   **[12058]**

"Catalogus doctorum . . . 1638": p. [12-16]

—Another issue, with date changed to 1639.   **[12059]**

—[The same.] . . . Lutetiae Parisiorum, Sump- tibus Olivarii de Varennes, 1645.

[16], 128, [8] p.   21 cm.   **[12060]**

Different setting of type.

—Statuta facultatis medicinae Parisiensis . . . Parisiis, Apud Franciscum Muguet, 1660.

[1], 90, [14] p.   15 cm.   **[12061]**

Engraved title page.
Edited by François Blondel.

—Statuta facultatis medicinae Parisiensis. Parisiis, Franciscum Muguet, 1696.

[1], 190, [24] p.   15 cm.   **[12062]**

Added engraved title page.
With this are bound: France. Parlement (Paris). Arrest de la cour de Parlement. [Paris 1718]—Université de Paris. Faculté de médecine. Ritus et insigniora. Parisiis, 1716.

—Statuts de la Faculté de medecine en l'Univer- sité de Paris, avec les pieces justificatives de ses privileges & ses droits & soumissions à elle deubs par les apothicaires & chirurgiens. Ensemble les jugemens rendus contre les empiriques & les medecins non approuvez par ladite Faculté de medecine, & les reglemens pour la visite des bouti- ques & drogues & compositions de medicamens . . . fait & mis en ordre par maistre Denis Puylon . . . Paris, François Muguet, 1672.

Various pagings.   25 cm.   **[12063]**

Each part has special half title or caption title.

—*See* COLLÈGE DES MÉDECINS, Dijon. Dissertation sur les fievres pourprées. 1685; DU VAL, G. Historia monogramma. 1643; FRANCE. Sovereigns, etc. [1643-1715] (Louis XIV) Declaration du roy. 1695, 1696; RIOLAN, J. [1580-1657] Curieuses recherches sur les escholes en medecine de Paris. 1651; THÉVART, J. Defense [-Deuxiéme defense] de la Faculté de medecine de Paris. 1668.

UNIVERSITÉ DE TOULOUSE. FACULTÉ DE MÉDECINE. *See* CODEX MEDICAMENTARIUS. 1648.

UNIVERSITY OF OXFORD. *See* WOOD, A. à. [Historia et antiquitates Universitatis Oxoniensis. 1674]

UNON, OLOF [*d.* 1666] *praeses.* Generalis physiologiae ratio leviter libita . . . Ubsaliae, Typis Eschilli Matthiae, 1647.

[48] p. 18 cm. [**12064**]

Imperfect: upper margins trimmed.

Date has been altered to 1647.

Diss. — Uppsala (O. Magnel, *respondent*)

UNSEN, JOHANNES [*fl.* 1671] *respondent. See* LEICHNER, E., *praeses.* Dissertationem inauguralem de υστερομανια . . . offert . . . Johannes Unsenius. 1671.

UNTERSCHIEDLICHE heylsame Mittel, so zur Zeit der Infection und Pest, nutzlich mögen angewendet, und gebraucht werden. Zusamen gezogen auss unterschiedlicher . . . Medicorum Gutachten . . . Erstlich herauss gegeben zu Wienn . . . Saltzburg, Durch Johann Baptist Mayr, 1679.

[2], 88, [3] p. 14 cm. [**12065**]

UNTZELMANN, ADAM [*fl.* 1690–1692] *respondent.* Dissertatio medica inauguralis de anasarca . . . [Altdorffi] Literis Henrici Meyeri [1692]

24 p. 20 cm. [**12066**]

Diss. — Altdorf.

— *See* HOFFMANN, J. M., *praeses.* Exercitatio medica de salivatione mercuriali. 1692.

UNTZER, MATTHIAS [1581–1624] Opus chymico-medicum, in quo anatomia spagirica trium principiorum, nec non corporis humani affectus, cum succinctis curis & remediis specificis . . . explicantur. Continet septem tractatus, quorum tres priores inscribuntur De sale, sulphure & mercurio, reliqui De nephritide, seu calculo renum, De peste & epilepsia. Hactenus singuli seorsim sunt excusi, jam vero in unum volumen redacti, & . . . ab ipso autore correcti & aucti . . . Halae Saxonum, Sumtibus et typis Melchioris Oelschlegelii, 1634.

[16] p., 756 col., 757–761 p., 762–2511 col., [48] p. 20 cm. [**12067**]

— Anatomia mercurii spagirica; seu, De hydrargyri natura, proprietate, viribus atque usu, libri duo . . . Hallae-Saxonum, Impensis Michaelis Oelschlegelii, typis excudit Petrus Faber, 1620.

[38], 264 p. plate. 20 cm. [**12068**]

— Antidotarium pestilentiale in duos libros tributum. Hallae-Saxonum, Impensis Michaelis Oelschlegelii, 1621.

[28], 277, [1] p. port. 21 cm. [**12069**]

— De nephritide seu renum calculo. Florilegium medico-chymicum in duos libros tributum . . . Halae Sax., Prostat apud Joach. Krusiken [Excudebat Christophorus Bismarc] 1614.

[16], 239 p. 19 cm. [**12070**]

— De renum calculo florilegium medico-chymicum denuo recognitum & auctum. Magdeburgi, Typis Andreae Bezelii, impensis Michaelis Oelschlegelii, 1623.

[23], 300 p. port. 20 cm. [**12071**]

Engraved title page.

Running title: De nephritide liber.

With this is bound *his* De sulphure tractatus. 1620.

— De sulphure tractatus medico-chymicus nunc noviter in lucem emissus. Hallae-Saxonum, Prostat apud Michaelem Oelschlegelium, typis exscribebat Petrus Faber, 1620.

[20], 101, [1] p. 20 cm. [**12072**]

Bound with *his* De renum calculo. 1623

Ἱερονοσολόγια chymiatrica. Hoc est epilepsiae seu morbi sacri, accuratissima, juxta Hippocratico-Galenica atque Hermetica principia, descriptio, ejusdemque per remedia . . . cum dogmaticorum, tum chymicorum, methodica curatio. Duobus libris comprehensa . . . Halae-Saxonum, Christophorus Bismarcus, 1616.

[20], 255, [1] p. port. 21 cm. [**12073**]

— Κάτοπτρον λοιμῶσες; hoc est, De lue pestifera libri tres . . . Hallae Saxonum [Christoph, Bismarcus] 1615.

[19], 271, [1], p. port. 20 cm. [**12074**]

Engraved title page.

— Physiologia salis; seu, De salis natura, ejusque prima origine, differentiis, proprietate atque usu . . . Opus posthumum. [Halae Saxonum] Impensis Michaelis Oelschlegelii, 1624.

[20], 166 p. 19 cm. [**12075**]

— *respondent.* Disputatio medica de mola matricis . . . Basileae, Imprimebat Johannes Schroeter [1605]

[18] p. 32 cm. [**12076**]

Diss. — Basel.

UNZER, GOTTHELFF ANDREAS [*fl.* 1676–1680] *respondent. See* CRAMER, C., *praeses.* Specimen inaugurale de spiritu mundi Nitneriano . . . subjicit Gotthelff Andreas Unzerus. 1680.

UPILIO, Wolfgang [*fl.* 1648] *praeses.* Viridarium medicum de febre maligna ... Herbipoli, Ex officina typographica H. Pigrini [1648]

    [4], 33 (i.e. 34), [1] p.   19 cm.   **[12077]**
    Diss.—Würzburg (J. A. Stöer, *respondent*)

[URALTER Ritter-Krieg. French] Le triomphe hermetique; ou, La pierre philosophale victorieuse ... Amsterdam, Henry Wetstein, 1699.

    [13], 153 p.   17 cm.   **[12078]**
    Added half title (p. [13]) reads: L'ancienne guerre des chevaliers; ou, Entretien de la pierre des philosophes avec l'or & le mercure ... Composé originairement en alleman ... & traduit nouvellement du latin en françois. At end: Le nom de l'autheur est en latin dans cette anagramme: Dives Sicut Ardens S***.
    Published also under title: Le très-ancien duel des chevaliers; ou, Dialogue chymique de la pierre physique.
    Translation of the Uralter Ritter-Krieg first published at Leipzig, in 1604, appended to Basilius Valentinus' Triumphwagen Antimonii. CF. Ferguson (A). Vol. 2, p. 466, and p. 486–487.

URBIGERUS, Baro. Aphorismi Urbigerani; or, Certain rules, clearly demonstrating the three infallible ways of preparing the grand elixir or circulum majus of the philosophers, discovering the secret of secrets, and detecting the errors of vulgar chymists in their operations: contain'd in one hundred and one aphorisms, to which are added, the three ways of preparing the vegetable elixir or circulatum minus ... London, Henry Faithorne, 1690.

    [10], 86 p. front. 16 cm.   **[12079]**
    "Circulatum minus Urbigeranum; or, The philosophical elixir of vegetables ... 1690" (p. [55]–86) has special title page.

URBINO (Duchy) **Ordinances, local laws,** etc. Bando sopra le guardie delle marine per causa di peste. Il Cardinale Cantelmo legato ... Pesaro, Nella Stamperia dell reverenda Camera Apostolica, 1690.

    broadside.   57 × 43 cm.   **[12080]**

— Bando sopra quelli, che essercitano la medicina, la chirurgia, cavano, sangue, fanno spetiaria, e drogheria, cavano pietre, saltano in banco, fanno stufe, confetterie, e simili. Il Cardinale Carlo Barberini Legato ... Pesaro, Nella Stamparia della reverenda Camera Apostolica, 1680.

    broadside.   56 × 41 cm.   **[12081]**

URIN Büchlein. *See* Brian, T. Der englische Wahrsager aus dem Urin. 1693.

URIN- und Hauss-Artzney-Büchlein. *See* Mueller, S. Vade-Mecum botanicum. 1687.

URSIN, Georg Heinrich [*d.* 1707] *respondent. See* Kirchmajer, T., *praeses.* De locustis ex zoologia physica. 1669?

URSIN, Joachim [*fl.* 1606–1615] Kurtzer, gründlicher und vollkommener Bericht, von Erkentnuss und Unterscheidung aller Fieber ins gemein, welche fast alle Jahr ... den Menschen anfechten. Nebenst einem kurtzen Anhang, von dem ... gifftigen ... pestilentzischen Fieber ... Rostock, Joh. Hallerf[ordius] 1616. [Gedruckt durch Hans Witten, 1613]

    [20], 176 (i.e. 191), [3] p.   16 cm.   **[12082]**

URSIN, Johann Christian [*b.* 1659] *respondent. See* Crause, R. W., *praeses.* Disputatio inauguralis medica de vulneribus per se lethalibus. 1684; Wedel, G. W., *praeses.* Dissertatio medica de venenis & bezoardicis. 1682.

— *See* Wedel, G. W. Propempticon inaugurale de vulnere ‎שׁרֹת חֹ - לאֹ‎ seu in quinta costa. 1684.

URSIN. Leonhard [1618–1664] De corporis humani proportione ... Lipsiae, Typis haered. Friderici Lanckisch [1643]

    [14] p.   19 cm.   **[12083]**
    Diss. pro loco—Leipzig.

— *respondent. See* Michaelis, J., *praeses.* Disputatio medica inauguralis, de morbis metallariorum. 1652.

URSIN, Paul Christoph [*fl.* 1679] *respondent. See* Vehr, I., *praeses.* Disputatio inauguralis medica, de anima foetida. 1679.

URSIN, Simon Christoph [1644–1702] *praeses.* Quaestum meretricium, Germ. Hüren-Lohn ... Francofurti ad Viadrum, Typis Johannis Coepselii [1682]

    [4], 48, [4] p.   20 cm.   **[12084]**
    Diss.—Frankfurt an der Oder (J. W. Lüder, *respondent*)

— Another printing.

    [8], 48 p.   20 cm.   **[12085]**

URSINUS, Fulvius. *See* Orsini, Fulvio [1529–1600]

URSINUS, Joannes [16th cent] *ed. See* Fabricius, H., *ab Aquapendente.* De locutione et ejus instrumentis liber. 1603.

URSINUS, Johann Conrad [*fl. 1676*] *respondent.* Inauguralis de ephemera disputatio ... Basileae, Typis Jacobi Bertschii [1676].

    [24] p.   19 cm.   **[12086]**

Diss. — Basel.

USLEBERUS, Johannes. *See* Ussleber, Johann [*fl. 1669–1672*]

USSLEBER, Johann [*fl. 1669–1672*] *respondent.* Disputationem medicam ... de sterilitate utriusque sexus ... p. p. Johannes Usleberus ... Altdorffii, Ex officina Johannis Henrici Schönnerstaedt [1672]

    30, [2] p.   20 cm.   **[12087]**

Diss. — Altdorf.

— *See* Friderici, J. A. Anatomia lienis. 1669.

UTENHOVE, Carolus [1536–1600] *See* Fabricius von Hilden, W. De combustionibus. 1607.

UTERVERIUS, Joannes Cornelius, *ed. See* Aldrovandi, U. De piscibus libri V. 1613, 1638 [and] De quadrupedibus solidipedibus volumen integrum. 1639 [and] Quadrupedum omnium bisulcorum historia. 1642.

UTRECHT. (City) **Ordinances, local laws, etc.** Cort bericht, tot voor-cominge ende genesinge vande peste, beraemt ter begeerte van de E. heeren regeerders der stadt Utrecht, door haer E, ordinaris medecijns. Utrecht, Amelis Janssz, 1636.

    [16] p.   21 cm.   **[12088]**

— Ordonnantie van de vroedschap der stadt Utrecht, op't apothekers-gildt binnen deselve stadt, als oock op de medicamenten, die sy-luyden in hare winckels moeten hebben; midsgaders het praepareren, vermengen, ende uyt-leveren van dien. Gepubliceert den xxxiij^en Julij 1655. Utrecht, Williem van Paddenburgh, 1679.

    [8] p.   21 cm.   **[12089]**

— Ordonnantie van de vroedschap der stadt Utrecht, op't stuck van de peste, ende begravinge der dooden. Gepubliceert den xxvj^en Julij 1655. Utrecht, Willem van Paddenburgh, 1679.

    [16] p.   21 cm.   **[12090]**

— Ordonnantie vande vroedschap der stadt Utrecht, waer naer de doctoren in de medicijne binnen de selve stadt practiserende, haer sullen hebben te reguleren. Gepubliceert den xxiij^en Julij 1665. Utrecht, Amelis van Paddenburgh, 1655.

    [6] p.   21 cm.   **[12091]**

— Ordonnantie, waer nae de doctoren in de medicijne binnen de stadt Utrecht practiferende, haer sullen hebben te reguleren. [Utrecht, 1655]

    [4] p.   21 cm.   **[12092]**

Caption title.

— Waerschouwinge wegens het verkopen van arsenicum ofte rotte-kruyt ... Actum den 12 Februar, 1669. [&] Placaet jegens het in brengen ende uyt geven van quade of uyt-heemsche duyten. [Utrecht 1670]

    [2] p.   21 cm.   **[12093]**

Caption titles.

UTRECHT. (Province) **Laws, statutes, etc.** De staten van den lande van Utrecht, in ervaringe komende, dat ten platten lande door persoonen de chirurgie aldaer exercerende, als die sig onderstaen medicamenten aen andere voor te schrijven ende in te geven, groote abuysen tot nadeel van het leven ende de gesondheyd van de opgesetenen werd gepleegt ... [Utrecht, 1668]

    [2] p.   21 cm.   **[12094]**

Issued without title page; title from beginning of text.

— Another printing.

                          [12095]

V

V., A. V. V. *See* Rochas, H. de. Notabilia excerpta. 1663.

V., E. *See* Venette, Nicolas [*ca. 1631–1698*]

V., I. *See* Veyras, Jacques [*fl. ca. 1625*]

V., P. A. *tr. See* Lessius, L. Kunst lang zu leben. 1697.

V., R. *See* Verstegen, Richard [*ca. 1548–1640*]

V. J. B. T. *See* Bartholin, Thomas [1616–1680]

VACA DE ALFARO, Enrique [*fl. 1618*] Proposicion chirurgica, i censura judiciosa entre las dos vias curativas de heridas de cabeça comun, i particular, i elecion desta. Con dos epistolas al fin, una de la naturaleza del tumor preternatural, i otra de la patria i origen de Avicena . . . Sevilla, Gabriel Ramos Vejarano, 1618.

[8], 126, [13] ll. 21 cm. **[12096]**

VACCA, Girolamo Capo di. *See* Capivaccio, Girolamo [1523–1589]

VACCHERIUS, Horatius. *See* Vachiero, Orazio [*b.* 1606]

VACCHIERI, Orazio. *See* Vachiero, Orazio [*b.* 1606]

VACHIERO, Orazio [*b.* 1606] De sanguinis missione in vulneribus, disceptatio apologetica . . . Taurini, Ex typographia Joannis Baptistae Zavattae, 1650.

62 p. plate. 22 cm. **[12097]**

VADE-MECUM curiosum medicum et chirurgicum. *See* Mueller, S. Vade-Mecum botanicum. 1687.

VADILLO, Pedro Gago de. *See* Gago de Vadillo, Pedro [*fl.* 1630]

VAENIUS, Ernestus. Tractatus physiologicus de pulchritudine. Juxta ea quae de sponsa in Canticis canticorum mystice pronunciantur . . . Bruxellis, Typis Francisci Foppens, 1662.

[8], 60, [1] p. illus. 15 cm. **[12098]**

VAILATUS, Leander, *ed. See* Sassonia, E. Prognoseon practicarum libri duo. 1610, 1620

VAILLANT, Jean-Foi [1632–1706] Numismata imperatorum Romanorum praestantiora a Julio Caesare ad postumum et tyrannos . . . Tomus primus [-secundus] . . . Lutetiae Parisiorum, Sumptibus Joannis Jombert, 1692.

2 v. in 1. illus. 25 cm. **[12099]**

VAIX, monsieur du. *See* Du Vair, Guillaume [1556–1621]

VAKE, Johann [*d.* 1709] *respondent. See* Thomasius, J. [1622–1684] *praeses.* Disputatio physica de origine animae humanae. 1669?

VAKO, Jean. *See* Falcon, Jean [*fl.* 1491–1541?]

VALAGUER, Anastasio Marcelino Uberte. *See* Uberte y Balaguer, Anastasio Marcelino [*fl.* 1678–1681]

VALANSI, David. *See* Valenza, David [*fl.* 1656–1680]

VALASCO DE TARENTA. *See* Valesco de Taranta [*fl.* 1382–1418]

VALCKENIER [*fl.* 1682] Remedie voor de brandende kreeft: geëxtraheert uyt de missive van de Heer resident Valckenier uyt Franckfort. Van dato den 26 July, des jaers 1682 . . . Amsterdam, Johannes van Lamsvelt, 1683.

broadside. 42 x 34 cm. **[12100]**

VALCKENISSE, André Eugène de [1630–1701] *See* Antwerp. Ordinances, local laws, etc. Gheboden ende uyt-gheroepen by mijne heeren den schouteth . . . ende raedt der stadt van Antwerpen. 1668?

VALCKENISSE, Philippe de [1596–1665] *See* Antwerp. Ordinances, local laws, etc. Gheboden ende uyt-gheroepen by mijne heeren, den onderschouteth . . . ende raedt der stadt van Antwerpen. 1646?

VALDECEBRO, Andres. *See* Ferrer de Valdecebro, Andrés [1620–1680]

VALDER, David [*fl.* 1674] *respondent. See* Beier, G., *praeses.* Erotematum medicorum de peste, decades quatuor. 1674.

VALDÉS, Benito Daza de. *See* Daza de Valdés, Benito [*fl.* 17th cent.]

VALENCIA. Laws, statutes, etc. Real crida y edicte, manat publicar per . . . Don Luys Faxardo de Requesens y Zuñiga, Marques de los Velez . . . lloctinent y capita general en la present ciutat y regne de Valencia. Sobre la guarda de la peste, y poluos pestilencials della . . . Valencia, Juan Batiste Marçal, 1630.

[8] p. 30 cm. **[12101]**

Palau 86320, 251016.

VALENTINI, Innocenzio [*fl.* 17th cent.] *See* Moniglia, G. A. Risposte. 1663.

VALENTINI, Johann Matthäus [*fl.* 1667–1668] *respondent.* Disputatio inauguralis medica de passione colica . . . Giessae Hassorum, Typis Friderici Kargeri, 1668.

30, [2] p. 20 cm. **[12102]**

Diss. — Giessen.

VALENTINI, MICHAEL BERNHARD [1657-1729] De monstrorum Hassiacorum ortu atque causis, epistola ad . . . Joh. Danielem Dorstenium . . . Marburgi Cattorum, Typis Johannis Henrici Stockenii [1684?]

[49]-68 p.   21 cm.   [12103]
Includes J. D. Dorsten's response.

—Epistola de nova matricis et morbonae muliebris anatome aliisque observationibus curiosae . . . Giessae Hassorum, Typis Academicis Kargerianis, 1683.

24 p.   16 cm.   [12104]

—Polychresta exotica in curandis affectibus contumacissimis probatissima . . . ut et Nova hernarium cura. Accedunt seorsim olim editae, nunc autem . . . conjunctim denuo prodeuntes Dissertationes epistolicae varii argumenti . . . Francofurti ad Moenum, Sumptibus Johannis Davidis Zunneri, 1700.

[8], 293, [1] p.   plates.   21 cm.   [12105]
Errata: p. [294]

—Historia physices experimentalis . . . Gissae Hassorum, Typis & impensis Henningi Mülleri, 1688.

44 p.   20 cm.   [12106]
Imperfect: error in printing: pages 34-39 wrongly imposed.
Diss. pro loco — Giessen.

—*praeses*. Discursus academicus de china chinae . . . Gissae Hassorum, Ex officina Henningi Mülleri, 1695.

[4], 10 (i.e. 20) p.   18 cm.   [12107]
Diss. — Giessen (P. Wolfart, *respondent*)

—Disputatio medica, de ipecuanha, novo Gallorum antidysenterico . . . Gissae-Hassorum, Typis Henningi Mülleri, 1698.

24 p.   20 cm.   [12108]
Diss. — Giessen (C. F. Kneussel, *respondent*)

—Disputatio medico-chirurgica de herniis arcano regis Galliarum absque sectione curandis . . . Gissae Hassorum, Typis Henningi Mülleri, 1697.

[4], 24 p.   20 cm.   [12109]
Imperfect: title page mutilated.
Diss. — Giessen (A. Raumburger, *respondent*)

—Disputatio physico-mechanica, de vacuo in vacuo . . . Gissae-Hassorum, Typis Henningi Mülleri, 1698.

24 p.   20 cm.   [12110]
Diss. — Giessen (J. M. Verdries, *respondent*)

—*See* Spener, C. M. Epistola de novo haemorrhoidum coecarum remedio. 1700.

VALENTINUS, *magister*. Opus praeclarum . . . quod pro testamento dedit filio suo adoptivo, qui etiam ostum tractatulum propria manu scripsit Joanni Apot.

941-954 p., vol. 4.   20 cm. (*In* Zetzner, Lazarus, *ed.* Theatrum chemicum. Argentorati, 1659-61)   [12111]
Caption title.

VALENTINUS, BASILIUS. *See* BASILIUS VALENTINUS.

VALENTINUS, BENEDICTUS PERERIUS. *See* PEREIRA, Benito [*ca.* 1535-1610]

VALENTINUS, JOHANNES [*fl. ca.* 1672] Curriculum analyticum; h. e. Syllabus lucubrationum, quas inde usque ab A. M.DC.XLIV in Academia . . . Erfurtina ejusd. non ita pridem rector . . . Eccardus Leichnerus . . . in gratiam studiosae juventutis, exercite pariter ac signate, ad studium apodicticum manuducendae, publico commisit . . . Erfurti, Typis Kirschianis [*ca.* 1673]

[32] p.   16 cm.   [12112]

[**VALENTINUS**, PETRUS POMARIUS] Enchiridion medicum, containing an epitome of the whole course of physicke, with the examination of a chyrurgian . . . by way of dialogue betweene the doctor and the student . . . And an antidotary of many excellent and approved remedies for all diseases . . . The 2d impr., enlarged with a second part, containing . . . the flowers of Celsus . . . London, Printed by N. O. for John Royston, and William Bladon, 1612.

[4], 172, 169, [5] p.   19 cm.   [12113]

"The examination of a chyrurgion . . . By S. H." has special title page (p. [73])
STC 24578.

VALENZA, DAVID [*fl.* 1656-1680] Ligulogio aforistico; overo, Promptuario methodico di preservatione, & curatione contra la peste. In cui brevemente, ma à pieno si propone l'essenza . . . e pronostici di esso male, ma sopra ogn'altra cosa si dà la vera regola di medicarlo, fondata sopra ragionevole esperienza, pratticata nel contaggio di

Venetia, che principio di luglio 1630. & fini di novembre 1631 ... Venetia, Per i Giunti, 1656.

76, [4] p. 24 cm. [12114]

VALENZO, DAVID. *See* VALENZA, DAVID [*fl.* 1656-1680]

VALERIANO, PIERIO. *See* VALERIANO BOLZANI, Giovanni Pierio [1477-1560]

VALERIANO BOLZANI, GIOVANNI PIERIO [1477-1560] Hieroglyphica; sive, De sacris Aegyptiorum aliorumque gentium litteris, commentariorum libri LVIII, cum duobus aliis ab eruditissimo viro [C. A. Curione] annexis. Ed. nov., variis ... hieroglyphicis adornata; pluribus item ejusdem Pierii opusculis ... locupletata ... Coloniae Agrippinae, Ex officina Hieratorum ff., 1631.

1 v. (various pagings) illus. 25 cm. [12115]

Contents. — [1] Hieroglyphica. — [2] Hieroglyphicorum collectanea. — [3] Hieroglyphica Horapollinis a Davide Hoeschelio. — [4] Pro sacerdotum barbis declamatio. — [5] Poemata varia. — [6] De litteratorum infelicitate libri duo. — [7] Antiquitatum Bellunensium, sermones quattuor.

Items 2 and 4 have special title pages.

—[The same.] ... Accesserunt loco auctarii, Hieroglyphicorum collectanea ... item Horapollinis hieroglyphicorum libri duo ex postrema Davidis Hoeschelii correctione. Praeterea ejusdem Pierii Declamatiuncula pro barbis sacerdotum; De infelicitate literatorum libri duo; denique Antiquitatum Bellunensium sermones quatuor. Ed. ad novissimas Germaniae composita ... Francofurti ad Moenum, Sumptibus Christiani Kirchneri, typis Wendelini Moewaldi, 1678.

1 v. (various pagings) front. (port.), illus. 26 cm. [12116]

The Hieroglyphicorum collectanea has special title page.

VALERIANUS, JOANNES PIERIUS. *See* VALERIANO BOLZANI, Giovanni Pierio [1477-1560]

VALERIIS, VALERIUS DE [*fl.* 1589] Opus aureum in quo explicantur quae R. Lullus tam in Scientiarum arbore quam in Arte generali tradit. *In* Lull, R. Opera. 1617, 1651.

VALERIOLLE, NICOLAS DE [*fl.* 1629] L'ordre politique teneu en la ville d'Arles, en temps de la peste, année 1629 ... Avignon, Jean Bramerau, 1632.

23, 322 p. 15 cm. [12117]

VALESCO DE TARANTA [*fl.* 1382-1418] Philonium pharmaceuticum et chirurgicum, de medendis omnibus ... humani corporis affectibus, a Valesco de Taranta ... deinde post Guidonis Desiderii editionem ... emendatum ... opera et studio Joannis Hartmanni Beyeri ... cum praefatione Georgii Wolfg. Wedelii ... editum ... Francofurti & Lipsiae, Sumtibus Joannis Adami Kästneri, Typis Joannis Nisii, 1680.

[14], 871, [27] p. 20 cm. [12118]

VALESCO DE TARANTA [*fl.* 1382-1418] Practica, quae alias Philonium dicitur. *In* Dodoens, R. Medicinalium observationum exempla rara. 1621.

VALESIUS DUBOURGDIEU, CAROLUS. *See* DUBOURGDIEU, Carolus Valesius.

VALET, ANTOINE [*d.* 1607] *ed. See* HOULLIER, J. Ad libros Galeni De compositione medicamentorum. 1603 [and] De morbis internis libri II. 1603 [and] Omnia opera practica. 1623, 1635, 1664.

VALLE, BARTOLOMÉ DEL [*fl. ca.* 1619] Avisos, y remedios preservativos de peste ... [Granada, 1690]

[12] p. 21 cm. [12119]

Caption title.
Imperfect: pages [9-12] mutilated.
Palau 349875.

VALLEGIO, GIOVANNI BATTISTA [*d.* 1678] Discorso a favore dell'aqua fredda ... Palermo, Per Diego Bua, impr. Martinez Rubio, 1664.

71 p. 19 cm. [12120]

VALLEMOND, *l'Abbé de. See* VALLEMONT, Pierre Le Lorrain, *abbé de* [1649-1721]

VALLEMONT, PIERRE LE LORRAIN, *abbé de* [1649-1721] La physique occulte; ou, Traité de la baguette divinatoire, et de son utilité pour la découverte des sources d'eau, des miniéres, des tresors cachez, des voleurs & des meurtriers fugitifs ... Augmenté en cette edition, d'un Traité de la connoissance des causes magnetiques des cures sympathiques, des transplantations & comment agissent les philtres. Par un curieux de la nature ... Paris, Jean Boudot, 1696.

[14], 422, 34, [7] p. front., plates. 14 cm. [12121]

VALLENSIS, ROBERTUS [*d.* 1567?] De veritate et antiquitate artis chemicae [& Pulveris sive medicinae philosophorum vel auri potabilis, testimonia & theoremata ex variis auctoribus]

7-27 p., vol. I 20 cm. (*In* Zetzner, Lazarus, *ed.* Theatrum chemicum, Argentorati, 1659-61)

[**12122**]

Caption title, partly supplied from table of contents.

—*See* BERNARDUS TREVIRENSIS. Ein Antwort Bernhardi Trevirensis, an Thomam von Bononia. 1613.

VALLERIOLA, FRANÇOIS [1504-1580] Artis medicae fundamina secundum Galenum. Lugduni, Apud Ambrosium Traversarium, 1626.

[16], 566 (i.e. 562), [25] p. port., diagr. 18 cm. [**12123**]

A reissue (with newly printed preliminaries) of the 1577 Geneva edition under title: Commentarii in librum Galeni De constitutione artis medicae. Includes Latin text of Galen, in the version of Joannes Guinterius, Andernacus.

—Loci medicinae communes, tribus libris digesti. Quibus accessit Appendix, universa complectens ea, quae ad totius operis integritatem deesse videbantur … [Genevae] Sumptibus Francisci Fabri Lugdun. & Samuelis Crispini, 1604.

[24], 830 (i.e. 848), 137, [78] p. 18 cm. [**12124**]

Franciscus Faber was located in Geneva after 1590. Cf. H. L. Baudrier, Bibl. lyonnaise, v. 5, p. 351.
Includes extracts in Latin from Hippocrates and Galen.

—Observationum medicinalium lib. vi. Denuo editi, & emendatiores quam antea in lucem emissi: in quibus multorum gravissimorum morborum historiae, eorundem causae, symptomata atque eventus, tum etiam curationes miro, utili & compendioso ordine describuntur … [Genevae], Apud Franciscum Fabrum, Lugdun., 1605.

[16], 399, [29] p. 16 cm. [**12125**]

Imperfect: p. 55-58 and 169-172 wanting.

—Another issue. 18 cm. [**12126**]

"Genevae" hand-stamped at foot of title page.

VALLERIOLE, NICOLAS. *See* VALERIOLLE, Nicolas de [*fl.* 1629]

VALLERIUS, Nicolaus [*fl.* 1699] Tentamina physico-chymica circa aquas thermales Aquisgranenses quibus adjecta ex Anglico ab eo versa R[oberti] B[oylei] Specimina historiae naturalis & experimentalis aquarum mineralium. Atque Joh. Floyeri Inquisitio in usum & abusum calidorum,

frigidorum & temperatorum balneorum. Lugduni Batavorum, Apud Cornelium Boutesteyn, 1699.

[16], 282, [22] p. 17 cm. [**12127**]

—*respondent.* Disputatio medica inauguralis de mammis … Trajecti ad Rhenum, Ex officina Guilielmi vande Water, 1699.

[4], 30, [4] p. 21 cm. [**12128**]

Imperfect: upper margin of last page trimmed.
Diss.—Utrecht.

VALLES, FRANCISCO DE [1524-1592] Commentaria in Prognosticum Hippocratis, nunc primum in Galliis excusa; multoque quam antea emendatiora, textu Hippocratis ad Graecum exemplar recognito, & innumeris erroribus repurgato. Opera & studio S. Gaudei … Aureliae, Apud Stephanum Potet, patrem & filium, 1655.

[4] p., 134 columns, [4] p. 33 cm. [**12129**]

Includes Latin text of the Prognostica.
With this is bound *his* Commentaria in quatuor Hippocratis libros De ratione victus in morbis acutis. 1655.

—Commentaria in quatuor Hippocratis libros De ratione victus in morbis acutis. Nunc primum in Galliis excusa, multoque quam antea emendatiora, textu Hippocratis ad Graecum exemplar recognito, & innumeris erroribus repurgato. Opera & studio S. Gaudei … Aureliae, Apud Stephanum Potet, patrem & filium, 1655.

[8] p., 239 (i.e. 236) columns, [6] p. 33 cm. [**12130**]

Includes Latin text of De victus ratione in morbis acutis.
Bound with *his* Commentaria in Prognosticum Hippocratis. 1655.

—In Hippocratis libros De morbis popularibus commentaria magnam utriusque medicinae, theoricae inquam, et practicae partem continentia. Ed. 3. … Neapoli, Ex typographia Lazari Scorigii, sumptibus Petri Antonii Reae, 1621.

[6], 449, [28] p. 30 cm. [**12131**]

Engraved title page.
Includes Latin text of De morbis popularibus, i.e. Epidemiorum libri VII.

—[The same.] Commentaria in septem Hippocratis libros Epidemiorum; seu, De morbis popularibus; magnam utriusque medicinae theoricae inquam, & practicae partem continentia. Ed. 4. … Neapoli, Typis Camilli Cavalli, Lazari Scorigii, sumptibus Caroli de Valle, 1652 [i.e. 1653]

[8], 449, [28] p. 32 cm. [**12132**]

Different setting of type.
Bound with Marziani, P. Magnus Hippocrates. 1652.

—[The same.] Commentaria, in septem libros Hippocrat. De morbis popularibus, nunc primum in Galliis excusa, multoque quam antea emendatiora, textu Hippocratis ad Grecum exemplar recognito, & innumeris erroribus repurgato, nonnullisque additis scholiis, opera & studio S. Gaudei ... Aureliae, Apud Claudium et Jacobum Borde, 1654 [i.e. 1655]

[6] p., 914 (i.e. 912) columns, [28] p.   34 cm.

[12133]

On last page: Achevé d'imprimer ce 12. Janvier 1655.

—Imber aureus; sive, Chilias aphorismorum, ex libris Epidemiων Hippocratis, eorumque Francisci Vallesii commentariis extracta. In gratiam praxeos studiosae juventutis colligebat ... Petrus a Castro, D. Med. Ulmae, Typis & impensis Balthasar Kühnen, 1661.

370 p.   14 cm.   [12134]

Contains two thousand aphorisms extracted and paraphrased from Valles' commentaries.

—Controversiarum medicarum et philosophicarum ... libri X. Accessit libellus De locis manifeste pugnantibus apud Galenum, eodem Vallesio autore. Ed. 4. ... Hanoviae, Typis Wechelianis, apud Claud. Marnium & haeredes Joannis Aubrii, 1606.

[8], 452, [9] p.   34 cm.   [12135]

With this is bound Selvatico, G. B. Galeni historiae medicinales. 1605.

—[The same.] ... Venetiis, Apud Joannem Guerilium, 1609.

[20], 452 p.   33 cm.   [12136]

Different setting of type.

—[The same.] ... Ed. postrema, praecedentibus multo correctior ... Lugduni, Sumptib. Antonii Chard, 1625.

[16], 640, [16] p.   25 cm.   [12137]

—Methodus medendi ... [Alcala de Henares, Impresso por Francisco Sanchez] Ex typographia Ludovici Martinez Grande, 1614.

[15], 416, [32] p.   15 cm.   [12138]

Imperfect: last leaf mutilated.

—[The same.] ... In quatuor libros divisa. Quorum I. continet victum aegrotantium. II. Rationem curandi per indicationes simplices. III. Per compositas, & cum aliquid eorum, quae indicare possunt nos latet. IV. Occasiones curandi, & abstinen-

di a curationibus. Lovanii, Typis Hieronymi Nempaei, 1647.

[6], 296 p.   17 cm.   [12139]

—[The same.] ... Parisiis, Apud Hieremiam Boüillerot, 1651.

[11], 320, [36] p.   15 cm.   [12140]

Edited by I. S. A. D. M.

—[The same.] ... Val[entiae] Typ. haered. Benedicti Macè, a costa de Claudio Macè, 1696.

[8], 298, [28] p.   16 cm.   [12141]

—, ed. and tr. See GALENUS. Francisci Vallesii ... Commentaria illustria, in Cl. Galeni Pergameni libros. 1645.

VALLISNIERI, ANTONIO [1661-1730] Dialoghi ... sopra la curiosa origine di molti insetti ... Venezia, Girolamo Albrizzi, 1700.

[8], 268, [7] p.   17 cm.   [12142]

VALNASI, DAVID. See VALENZA, David [fl. 1656-1680]

VALOIS, HENRI DE [1603-1676] See HARPOCRATION, V. Λεξικὸν τῶν δέκ α ῥητόρων ...Lexicon decem oratorum. 1683.

VALOIS DU BOURGDIEU, CHARLES. See DUBOURGDIEU, Carolus Valesius.

VALTHER, DAVID [fl. 1678] respondent. See FASCH, A. H., praeses. Dysenteriam ... disquisitioni proponit ... D. V. 1678.

VALVERDE, JUAN DE. Anotomia del corpo humano ... co' discorsi del medesimo, novamente ristampata e con l'aggiunta d'alcune tavole ampliata. Vinetia, Giunti, 1606.

[18], 154 ll.   port., illus.   31 cm.   [12143]

Engraved title page.

First published under title: Historia de la composicion del cuerpo humano.

Cushing VI.D.-39.

— Another issue with date changed to 1608.

[12144]

Cushing VI.D.-40.

— [The same.] ... Venetia, Nicolo Pezzana, 1682.

[14], 152 ll.   port., illus.   32 cm.   [12145]

Engraved title page.

Cushing VI.D.-42.

— [Latin tr.] Anatome corporis humani . . . Nunc primum a Michaele Columbo Latine reddita, et additis novis aliquot tabulis exornata. Venetiis, Studio, et industria Juntarum, 1589 [colophon 1607]

[36], 340 (i.e. 339) p.   port., illus.   33 cm.

[12146]

Engraved title page.

— Another issue, with date on title page changed to 1607.   **[12147]**

Cushing VI.D.-41.

— A. Vesalii en Valverda Anatomie; ofte, Afbeeldinghe van de deelen des menschelijcken lichaems, en derselver verklaringhe. Met een aenwijsinghe om het selve te ontleden volgens de leeringe Galleni, Vesalii, Fallopii en Arantii. Amstelredam, Cornelis Danckertz, 1647.

[4], 196 (i.e. 198), [1] p.   plates.   30 cm.

[12148]

Added engraved title page.

The text accompanying the plates is translated from Valverde's Vivae imagines partium corporis humani.

"Het epitome, oft kort verhael van de boecken van Andries Vesalius . . . van de fabrijcke van d'menschelijcke lichaemen": p. 141-196.

"De differentien van alle de partien oft deelen des lighaems deur Jacob Grevin": p. [199]

Cushing VI.D.-46.

With this is bound: Mauden, D. van. Bedieninghe der anatomien. 1646.

[VALVERDE DE HOROZCO, Diego de, 17th cent.] Controversia medica, en que se disputa, si conforme al arte y methodo de medicina, se ha de variar la parte, do se ha de sangrar, segun las diferencias de las enfermedades, y partes afectas: o si siempre en qualquiera enfermedad, se aya de començar sangrando del touillo. [n. p., 1652?]

[38] p.   20 cm.   **[12149]**

Caption title.

— Proteccion de la doctrina de Hippocrates y Galeno, acerca del methodo de curar por sangrias, segun las diferencias de las enfermedades, y partes afectas, y aniquilacion de la nueva opinion de sangrar de los tovillos . . . Sevilla, Juan Lorenço Machado, 1653.

[6], 64 p.   20 cm.   **[12150]**

VÁM, xó hó. *See* Wang, Shu-ho [*fl.* 280]

VANCIO, Angelo [*fl.* 1625] *ed. See* colonna, E. De humani corporis formatione. 1626.

VANDE CAMPE, M. Ja. Co. *See* Camp, M. Ja. Co. vande.

VANDER WIEL, Cornelis Stalpart. *See* Stalpart van der Wiel, Cornelis [1620–1702]

VAN FOREEST, Pieter. *See* Foreest, Pieter van [1522–1597]

VAN GUTSCHOVEN, Gérard. *See* Gutschoven, Gérard van [1615–1668]

VAN HELMONT, Jean Baptiste. *See* Helmont, Jean Baptiste van [1577–1644]

VANINI, Giulio Cesare [1585–1619] De admirandis naturae reginae deaque mortalium arcanis. Liber quatuor. Lutetiae, Apud Adrianum Perier, 1616.

[16], 495, [1] p.   illus.   18 cm.   **[12151]**

VANINI, Lucillo. *See* Vanini, Giulio Cesare [1585–1619]

VAN LOM, Josse. *See* Lommius, Jodocus [*ca.* 1500–*ca.*1564]

VAN LOMMEN, Josse. *See* Lommius, Jodocus [*ca.* 1500–*ca.* 1564]

VAN LOOM, Jodocus. *See* Lommius, Jodocus [*ca.* 1500–*ca.* 1564]

VANSELOW, Michael [*fl.* 1696] *respondent. See* Eysel, J. P., *praeses.* Disputatio medica inauguralis exhibens historiam de ruptura lienis. 1696.

VANTIUS, Angelus. *See* Vancio, Angelo [*fl.* 1625]

VÁRADI, Mátyás [*fl.* 1667–1669] *respondent. See* Matthaeus, P., *praeses.* Disputatio medica de variolis et morbillis. 1667.

VARANDA, Jean de [1563 or 4–1617] Opera omnia theorica et practica . . . 2. ed. corr. & emend. Genevae, Apud Petrum & Jacobum Chouët, 1620.

[6], 56 p.; [16], 475 p.; 164, [2] p.; 159 p.   18 cm.   **[12152]**

Imperfect: wormholes on the first seven leaves.

Part [1] has running title: Tractatus de diagnosi. Part [2] has special title page: Physiologia et Pathologia. Quibus accesserunt ejusdem Tractatus prognosticus: item Tractatus de indicationibus curativis.

— Copy 2.   17 cm.

Incomplete: contains part [1] only (Tractatus de diagnosi).

With this are bound *his*: Tractatus de elphantiasi. Genevae, 1620; Tractatus de affectibus renum & vesicae. Genevae, 1620.

— Opera omnia. Ad fidem codicum ipsius authoris manuscriptorum recognita & emendata, postrema hac editione multis tractatibus nunquam antea editis auctiora. Cura & studio Henrici Gras ... Lugduni, Sumptibus Christophori Fourmy, 1658.

[12], ccxxviii, 834 (i.e. 842), [17] p.   37 cm.

[12153]

"Editio prima perfecta est die 1. Octobris, 1657": p. [12] (1st group). Includes Greek and Latin texts of Hippocrates' De natura hominis (incomplete) Aphorismi (book 5, sect. 1–6) and Epidemiorum libri (book 3, case histories 1–12).

— Posthumus ... in lucem editus De morbis & affectibus mulierum. Opera Petri Mylaei ... Huic accessit ... epilepsiae, podagrae, hydrop. & leprae curatio. Lugduni, Sumptibus Bartholomaei Vincentii, 1619.

[8], 228, 176, 86, [1] p.; [4], 34, [2] p.   18 cm.

[12154]

Imperfect: printing not clear on several pages; photocopy supplied from copy 2.

— Copy 2.   17 cm.

Last part wanting.

— [The same.] De morbis mulierum lib. III ... Nunc primum in lucem editi opera Romani a Costa ... Genevae, Apud Petrum & Jacobum Chouët, 1620.

[20], 511, [4] p.   17 cm.   [12155]

With this is bound *his* Tractatus therapeuticus. Genevae, 1620.

— Another issue, with imprint: Monspessuli, In officina Francisci Chouët, 1620.   [12156]

Imperfect: p. 369–380 mutilated.
Bound with copy 2 of *his* Tractatus therapeuticus. 1620.

— [French tr.] Traité des maladies des femmes ... Rev., augm. ... & traduit ... par I. B[onamour] ... Paris, Robert de Ninville, 1666.

[16], 620, [12] p.   18 cm.   [12157]

— Formulae remediorum internorum et externorum ... ante annos aliquot medicinae studiosis traditae ... nunc vero publicae factae, per Petrum Janichium ... Hanoviae, Typis Petri Antonii, 1617.

[32], 129 p.   17 cm.   [12158]

— [The same.] ... 2. ed., genuina & ab innumeris ... erroribus emendata. Genevae, Apud Petrum & Jacobum Chouët, 1620.

[8], 134, [2] p.   17 cm.   [12159]

Imperfect: wormholes on p. [1]–20.
With this is bound Morel, P. Systema parascevasticum. 1628.

— Physiologia et Pathologia ... Quibus accesserunt ejusdem I. Tractatus prognosticus. II. Tractatus de indicationibus. Opera Petri Janichii ... in lucem edit ... Hanoviae, Apud Petrum Antonium, 1619.

[20], 296, 171, [1] p.; 164 p.; 159 p.   18 cm.

[12160]

Parts [2] and [3] have special title pages.

— [The same.] ... 2. ed. corr. & emend. Genevae, In officina Francisci Chouët, 1620.

[16], 475 p.; 164, [2] p.; 159 p.; 56 p.   17 cm.

[12161]

Original place of imprint blocked out.

— Tractatus de affectibus renum et vesicae, ad mentem inprimis Hippocratis & Galeni accuratissime conformatus; publicique juris factus a Petro Janichio ... Hanoviae, Apud Petrum Antonium, 1617.

205, [2] p.   16 cm.   [12162]

— Copy 2.   17 cm.

With this is bound Strobelberger, J. S. Brevissima manuductio. 1629.

— [The same.] ... 2. ed. corr. & emend. Monspessuli, In officina Francisci Chouët, 1620.

[8], 167 p.   17 cm.   [12163]

Bound with copy 2 of *his* Tractatus therapeuticus. Monspessuli, 1620.

— Another issue, with imprint: Genevae, Apud Petrum & Jacobum Chouët, 1620.   [12164]

Bound with copy 2 *of his* Opera omnia. 1620.

— Tractatus de elephantiasi seu lepra, item De lue venerea, et hepatitide, seu hepatis ἀτονία. Nunc primum in lucem editi. Monspessuli, In officina Francisci Chouët, 1620.

174, [2] p.   17 cm.   [12165]

With this is bound *his* Tractatus de morbis ventriculi. 1620.

— Another issue, with place of imprint (Monspessuli) blocked out and new place name (Genevae) added.   [12166]

Bound with copy 2 of *his* Opera omnia. 1620.

— Tractatus de morbis ventriculi ... nunc primum in lucem editus, opera Claudii Dubost ... Lugduni, Sumptibus Bartholomaei Vincentii, 1620.

[8], 152 p.   17 cm.   [12167]

Imperfect: p. 81-96 wanting; wormholes on p. 135-152. Bound with *his* Tractatus de elephantiasi. 1620.

—Tractatus therapeuticus primus de morbis ventriculi. Nunc primum in lucem editus, Romani a Costa ... Monspessuli, In officina Francisci Chouët, 1620.

[8], 168 p.   17 cm.   **[12168]**

—Copy 2.
With this are bound *his*: Tractatus de affectibus renum & vesicae. Monspessuli, 1620; De morbis mulierum. Monspessuli, 1620.

—Another issue, with imprint: Genevae, Apud Petrum & Jacobum Chouët, 1620.   **[12169]**
Bound with *his* De morbis mulierum. Genevae, 1620.

VARANDAEUS, JOANNES. *See* VARANDA, Jean de [1563 or 4-1617]

VARANDAL, JEAN. *See* VARANDA, Jean de [1563 or 4-1617]

VARANDÉ, JEAN DE. *See* VARANDA, Jean de [1563 or 4-1617]

VARCIN, AIMÉ [1630-1702] *ed. See* CHALES, C. F. M. de, *Father*. Cursus seu mundus mathematicus. 1690.

VARDADERA medicina, cirugia, y astrologia. 1607. *See* BARRIOS, J. de.

VARENBÜLER, ULRICH. *See* VARNBÜLER, ULRICH [*fl.* 1618]

VARIORUM tractatus theologici de peste. Lugd. Batav., Apud Johannem Elsevirium, 1655.

[2], 380 p.   14 cm.   **[12170]**

Contains treatises by Théodore de Bèze, André Rivet, Gijsbert Voet and Johannes Hoornbeek.

VARNBÜLER, ULRICH [*fl.* 1618] *respondent.* Theses de peste ... Basileae, Excudebat Joh. Jacobus Genathius [1618]

[12] p.   22 cm.   **[12171]**
Diss.—Basel.

VARUS, ANTON [1557-1637]

Dissertations — Jena

—*praeses.* Disputatio inauguralis medica de dysenteria ... Jenae, Typis Weidnerianis, 1635.
[15] p.   19 cm.   **[12172]**
H. Plancus, *respondent.*

—Disputatio medica de quartana ... Jenae, Typis Tobiae Steinmanni, 1618.
[32] p.   19 cm.   **[12173]**
K. Stein, *respondent.*

—Disputatio medica de venae sectione ... Jenae, Typis Tobiae Steinmanni, 1607.
[16] p.   21 cm.   **[12174]**
P. Macasius, *respondent.*

—Disputatio medica inauguralis de peripneumonia ... Jenae, Typis Johannis Beithmanni [1619]
[11] p.   19 cm.   **[12175]**
L. Maenius, *respondent.*

—Themata medica περι της φρενιτιδος ... Jenae, Tobias Steinman [1607]
[16] p.   20 cm.   **[12176]**
P. Gallus, *respondent.*

—Theses medicae de febri maligna ... Jenae, Ex officina Tobiae Steinmanni, 1605.
[11] p.   20 cm.   **[12177]**
J. P. Brendel, *respondent.*

VASCO CASTELLO, PEDRO. *See* CASTELLO, Pedro Vasco [*fl.* 1616]

VASMAR, DANIEL PHILIPP [*fl.* 1698-1701] *respondent. See* CUNRAD, C., *praeses.* Dissertatio medica de colica flatulenta. 1698; PANTELIUS, M., *praeses.* Disputatio medico-chymica de mercurio. 1698.

VASSEUR, LOUIS LE. *See* LE VASSEUR, Louis [*fl.* 1658-1674]

VASSEUR DU VAUGOSSE, AEGIDIO LE. *See* LE VASSEUR DU VAUGOSSE, Gilles [*fl.* 1612]

VASTENOU, BERNHARD [*fl.* 1652] *respondent.* Disputatio medica inauguralis, de paralysi ... Trajecti ad Rhenum, Typis Gisberti à Zijll & Theodori ab Ackersdijck, 1652.
[8] p.   20 cm.   **[12178]**
Diss.—Utrecht.

VASTRICK, THOMAS [*fl.* 1686] *respondent.* Disputatio medica inauguralis de morbis in genere ... Lugduni Batavorum, Apud Abrahamum Elzevier, 1686.
[14] p.   22 cm.   **[12179]**
Diss.—Leyden.

VATER, CHRISTIAN [1651–1732] Cadaveris virilis anatomen et condituram publicam lustraturis intimat ... Wittenbergae, Stanno Kreusigiano [1693]

   [8] p. 19 cm.   **[12180]**

—Collegii Medici decanus Christianus Vater ... benevolo lectori S. P. D. [Wittenbergae, 1693]

   [12] p. 19 cm.   **[12181]**

  Program—Wittenberg (with vita of G. P. Juch)

—Collegii Medici ... decanus Christianus Vater ... L. B. S. P. D. [Wittenbergae, 1696]

   [11] p. 19 cm.   **[12182]**

  Program—Wittenberg (with vita of H. S. Weitz)

Dissertations — Wittenberg

—*praeses.* De chymicorum principio, quod sal vocant ... Wittebergae, Typis Johannis Borckardi, excudebat Simon Liberhirt [1676]

   [16] p. 20 cm.   **[12183]**

  J. M. Helmich, *respondent.*

—De dyspnoea ... Wittebergae, Literis virduae Brüningianae [1684]

   [20] p. 20 cm.   **[12184]**

  A. C. Georgi, *respondent.*

—De machinae humanae organis vitalibus, secundum αὐτοψιαν delineatis ... Wittenbergae, Typis Martini Schultzii [1697]

   [4], 68 p. 20 cm.   **[12185]**

  J. C. Stisser, *respondent.*

—De mercurialibus medicamentis ... Vitembergae, Stanno Christiani Kreusigii [1695]

   [1], 27, [3] p. 20 cm.   **[12186]**

  J. C. Pezold, *respondent.*

—De transpiratione insensibili corporis humani ... Vitembergae, Typis Christiani Kreusigii [1695]

   [28] p. 20 cm.   **[12187]**

  C. Berndt, *respondent.*

—De ulceribus fistulosis ... Vitembergae, Literis Goderitschianis [1700]

   [32] p. 20 cm.   **[12188]**

  B. Schiefordegher, *respondent.*

—Disputatio inauguralis medica, de affectibus soporosis ... Vitembergae, Prelo Christiani Kreusigii [1699]

   28 p. 20 cm.   **[12189]**

  J. G. Hugo, *respondent.*

—Disquisitionem physico-medicam de vermibus intestinorum ... instituet Henricus Ernestus Muscovius ... [Wittenbergae] Aere Martini Schultzii [1687]

   [32] p. 20 cm.   **[12190]**

  H. E. Muscov, *respondent.*

—Dissertatio inauguralis medica de venenis eorundemque antidotis ... Wittenbergae, Litteris Fincelianis [1700]

   27 p. 20 cm.   **[12191]**

  J. F. Helwich, *respondent.*

—Dissertatio physico-medica de febrium natura, causis, differentiis & symptomatibus ... Wittebergae, Literis Schultzianis [1685]

   [24] p. 19 cm.   **[12192]**

  A. Jacobaeer, *respondent.*

—Dissertatio solennis de pulmonum vomica ... [Wittembergae] Literis Fincelianis [1700]

   [23] p. 20 cm.   **[12193]**

  J. C. Minner, *respondent.*

—Dissertationem inauguralem de morbo laterali acuto, pleuritis dicto ... publico ... examini subjicit Johannes Andreas Gormann ... Wittenbergae, Typis Christiani Kreusigii [1695]

   [34] p. 19 cm.   **[12194]**

  J. A. Gormann, *respondent.*

—Dissertationem inauguralem de vertigine ... publico ... examini exponet Martinus Francisci ... Witenbergae, Typis C. Fincelii [1698]

   [32] p. 20 cm.   **[12195]**

  M. Francisci, *respondent.*

—Dissertationem inauguralem medico-chirurgicam de cerebri commotione ... exponet Joh. Christoph Schultze ... Vitembergae, Prelo Christiani Kreusigii [1699]

   24 p. 21 cm.   **[12196]**

  J. C. Schultze, *respondent.*

—Dissertationem physiologicarum quinta qua motus animalis e fundamentis genuinis erutus ... publico eruditorum examini sistitur a Joh. Adolpho Mühlpfort ... Wittenbergae, Typis Martini Schultzii [1694]

   [32] p. 19 cm.   **[12197]**

  J. A. Mühlpfort, *respondent.*

—Examen sulphuris vitriolo anodyni . . . Wittebergae, Typis viduae Augusti Brüningii [1683]

[24] p.   19 cm.   **[12198]**

J. E. Böchm, *respondent.*

—Exercitatio chimica de spiritibus chimicis . . . Wittenbergae, Typis Christiani Kreusigii [1696]

[24] p.   19 cm.   **[12199]**

T. Schubart, *respondent.*

—Exercitationem medicam de hemiplegia . . . exhibebit A. R. Balth. Meno Hannekenius . . . Vitembergae, Ex officina Christiani Schrödteri [1700]

[4], 39 p.   19 cm.   **[12200]**

B. M. Hanneken, *respondent.*
Imperfect: p. 34–39 wanting.

—Existentiam & motum spirituum animalium in nervis . . . defendet Johannes Glosemeyer . . . Wittenbergae, Literis Martini Schultzii, 1687.

[24] p.   20 cm.   **[12201]**

J. Glosemeyer, *respondent.*

—Historiam et curam bubonis inguinalis cum perforatione intestini & eruptione lumbricorum . . . submittit Gustavus Prosper Juch . . . Witenbergae, Literis Christiani Kreusigii [1693]

[24] p.   20 cm.   **[12202]**

Imperfect: lower margin of title page trimmed.
G. P. Juch, *respondent.*

—Historiam & curam sarcomatis, monstrosi & cancrosi . . . subjiciet Jo. Balthasar Schondorff . . . Wittenbergae, Typis Christiani Schrödteri [1693]

[20] p.   20 cm.   **[12203]**

J. B. Schondorff, *respondent.*

—Inauguralis dissertatio medica de contracturis . . . Vitembergae, Typis Christiani Kreusigii [1696]

[24] p.   20 cm.   **[12204]**

C. Berndt, *respondent.*

—Judicium e sanguine per venae sectionem emisso . . . Vittebergae, Prelo Goderitschiano [1693]

[20] p.   19 cm.   **[12205]**

J. A. Jormann, *respondent.*

—Machinae humanae organa animalia in specie dicta . . . Wittenbergae, Typis Martini Schulzii [1700]

[1], 71–112 p.   20 cm.   **[12206]**

J. F. Helwich, *respondent.*

—Motum sanguinis per venam portae . . . exponet Joan. Friedrich Beyer . . . [Wittenbergae] Literis Brüningianis [1685]

[24] p.   20 cm.   **[12207]**

J. F. Beyer, *respondent.*

—Naturam et curam memoriae . . . exhibet . . . Gottlieb Budaeus . . . Wittenbergae, Excudebat Martinus Schultze [1686]

[32] p.   20 cm.   **[12208]**

G. Budaeus, *respondent.*

—Rationes et curationes dolorum . . . Wittenbergae, Literis Goderitschianis [1696]

[23] p.   20 cm.   **[12209]**

J. C. Pezold, *respondent.*

—*respondent. See* FRENZEL, S. F., *praeses.* Disquisitionem naturalem de unicornu . . . publicae ventilatione sistit . . . C. V. 1679; SCHNEIDER, K. V., *praeses.* Dissertationem inauguralem de melancholia seu delirio tristi . . . submittit . . . M.C.V. 1680.

VATICAN. Protomedico generale. Tavola de prezzi delle robbe di spetiaria per tutto lo Stato Ecclesiastico . . . Fatta dall'eccellentiss. sig. Protomedico Generale [i.e. Dominicus Guidarellus] . . . Roma, Stamparia della Rev. Cam. Apost., 1648.

[8] p.   22 cm.   **[12210]**

VATTIER, PIERRE [1623–1667] Le coeur dethroné. Discours de l'usage du foye, où il est monstré que le coeur ne fait pas le sang, & qu'il n'est pas mesme une des principales parties de l'animal. Prononcé dans une assemblée de physiciens . . . Paris, François Clousier, 1660.

[8], 56 p.   17 cm.   **[12211]**

—Nouvelles pensees sur la nature des passions, ou leurs vrayes differences, & les dependances qu'elles ont les unes des autres, sont methodiquement descourvertes, & leur nombre infiny mis en ordre . . . Paris, L'autheur, 1659.

[12], 188 p.   23 cm.   **[12212]**

—, *tr. See* AVICENNA. Abugalii filii Sinae . . . de morbis mentis tractatus. 1659.

VAUDOULEURS, MATTHAEUS MAHEULT DE. *See* MAHEULT, Mathieu [1630–1700]

VAUGHAN, THOMAS [1622–1666] The man-mouse taken in a trap, and tortur'd to death for gnawing the margins of Eugenius Philalethes [pseud., i.e. Thomas Vaughan] . . . London, [H. Blunden] 1650.

[3], 116 p.   15 cm.   **[12213]**

A satire on Henry More.

— *See* A HERMETICALL BANQUET. 1652; *See* PHILALETHES, E.

VAUGHAN, WILLIAM [1577-1641] Directions for health, both naturall and artificiall: approved and derived from the best physitians, as well moderne as auncient . . . Divided into 6 sections. 1. Ayre, fire, and water. 2. Meate, drinke with nourishment. 3. Avoydance of excrements . . . 4. Remedies for common sickness. 5. The soules qualities and affections. 6. Quarterly, monethly, and daily diet. Newly enriched with large additions by the author. The 5th ed. London, Printed by T. S. for Roger Jackson, 1617.

[8], 300, [3] p. 15 cm. [12214]

STC 24616.

The 1600 London edition was published under title: Naturale and artificial directions for health.

—[The same.] . . . The 6th ed. reviewed by the author. Whereunto is annexed Two treatises of approved medicines for all diseases of the eyes; and preservation of the eye-sight. The first written by Doctor Baily . . . the other collected out of those two famous phisitians, Fernelius and Riolanus. London, Printed by John Beale, for Francis Williams, 1626.

[6], 169 (i.e. 171) p.; [4], 38 p. 19 cm. [12215]

Part [2] has special title page.
STC 24617.

—[The same.] . . . The 7th ed. reviewed by the author . . . London, Printed by Thomas Harper, for John Harison, 1633.

[6], 169 (i.e. 171) p.; [4], 38 p. 18 cm. [12216]

Imperfect: last leaf (blank?) wanting.
Part [2] has special title page.
STC 24618.
A partly corrected reprint of the 6th edition.

VAUGOSSE, AEGIDIO. *See* LE VASSEUR DU VAUGOSSE, Gilles [*fl.* 1612]

VAUGUION, DE LA. *See* LA VAUGUION, de.

VAULX, BARTHOLOMÉ ALEXANDRE [*fl.* 17th cent.] La verité descouverte; ou, Esclaircissement pour cognoistre la vraye methode de guerrir. Contenant quelques-unes des principales differences, qu'il y a entre la vielle & nouvelle idée de la medecine, touchant le traitement des malades . . . Bruxelles, Pierre de Dobbeleer, 1676.

[30], 187, [13] p. 12 cm. [12217]

VAUROÜY, HENRY DE BOYVIN DU. *See* BOYVIN DU VAUROÜY, Henry de [*b.* 1623]

VAUSSARD, G. L'operateur des pauvres; ou, La fleur d'operation necessaire aux pauvres . . . Ou se monstre un discours des operateurs, avec les remedes de purgation, le prix que couste les drogues, & les moyens de les appliquer. Ensemble le secret du baulme policreston, sa vertu, & autres secrets admirables . . . Rev. & corr. par l'autheur . . . Troyes, Nicolas Oudot, 1642.

42 p. 17 cm. [12218]

Imperfect: all pages after p. 42 wanting.
With this are bound: Guibert, P. L'apothiquaire charitable. [*ca.* 1640]; another issue of Guibert, P. Toutes les oeuvres charitables. 1640.

—[The same.] *In* Guibert, P. L'apotiquaire charitable. 1646.

VAUTIER, FRANÇOIS [1589-1652] *See* REFLEXIONS. 1652.

VAUX, JEAN DE. *See* DEVAUX, Jean [1649-1729]

VAUX, LOUIS DE [*fl.* 1690] *respondent. See* MARAIS, P., *praeses.* Quaestio medica. 1690.

VECELLI, TIZIANO. *See* TIZIANO VECELLI [1477-1576]

VECOLI, BERNARDINO [*fl.* 1617] Della preparatione della pietra lazzoli per la confettione Alchermes . . . Lucca, Ottaviano Guidoboni, e Baldassari del Giudice, 1617.

[4], 36 p. 22 cm. [12219]

—[The same.] . . . Con alcune considerationi di Nicolo Mazza, & di Herofilo Serafini . . . Lucca, Ottaviano Guidoboni, & Baldassar del Giudice, 1617.

48 p. 21 cm. [12220]

—*See* MACCIONI, G. Risposta. 1631.

VECOLI, PAOLO ANTONIO [*fl.* 1647] Innoxiae medicinae defensio in qua probatur praegnantiam ex signis tuto cognosci non posse, & pharmaca solventia, & saphenae sectionem etiam in ultimis mensibus pregnantiae convenire . . . Lucae, Apud Peregrinum Bidellium, 1647.

[8], 20 p. 20 cm. [12221]

VEELER wonderens wonderbaarelijck lof. Behelsende het lof van het hatelick podagra. Het lijfbergende zwemmen. Dat gruwelick groot beest den

oliphant. Dat verachtelicke slijck. Die mensch-
lievende luys. Dat moeyelicke zwijgen. Dat hert-
kittelende lacchen. Die plaeghlicke derden-daeghse-
koorts. De stantreckelicke bruyloft. De nyverige
mier. Dien alder-treffelicksten uyl. Dien alder-
zedestichtelicksten ezel. Amsterdam, Samuel Im-
brechts, en Adam Snewater, 1664.

[15], 221 p. illus., plates. 15 cm.   **[12222]**

Added engraved title page.

Includes treatises by Ulisse Aldrovandi, Celio Calcagnini,
Girolamo Cardano, Justus Lipsius and Wilibald Pirckheimer.

VEEZAERDT, PAULUS [*d. ca.* 1670] *ed.* and *tr.*
See GOEDAERT, J. Metamorphosis et historia naturalis
insectorum. 1667–70.

VEEZAERDT, PETRUS. *See* VEEZAERDT, Paulus
[*d. ca.* 1670]

VEGA, CRISTÓBAL DE [1510?–1573?] Christophori
a Vega . . . Opera omnia: nunc denuo publici juris
facta, recens recensita, ab erroribus typographicis . . .
repurgata, & annotationibus . . . illustrata; opera &
labore Ludovici Serrani . . . Lugduni, Sumptibus
Antonii Chard, 1626.

[10], 894 (i.e. 892), [28] p.   38 cm.   **[12223]**

"Pars altera" (p. [441]–894) has half title.

Includes Latin text of Hippocrates' Aphorismi and Prognostica
(both translated by Vega), and of Galen's De differentiis febrium
and In Hippocratis Prognostica (both translated by Lorenz
Laurenziani).

VEGA, PETRUS DE. *See* VEGE, Petrus de [*fl. ca.*
1619]

VEGA, THOMAS RODRIGUEZ DE. *See* RODRIGUES DA
VEIGA, Tomás [1513–1579]

VEGE, PETRUS DE [*fl. ca.* 1619] Pax fidissima, et
probatissima methodicorum, seu Galenicorum cum
spagyricis. De medicinae pura veritate . . . Huic accessit gemmula de epilepsiae, podagrae, hydrop. &
& [sic] leprae curatione, cum medicamentorum
descriptione . . . Lugduni, Sumptibus Bartholomaei
Vincentii, 1619.

[4], 34, [2] p.   18 cm.   **[12224]**

(*In* Varanda, Jean de. Posthumus in lucem editus De morbis
& affectibus mulierum. Lugduni, 1619)

—Pax methodicorum, cum spagyricis . . . Cum
epilepsiae, podagrae, hydrop. & leprae curatione. Accessit Conr. Gesneri Thesaurus Euonymi [pseud.]
de remediis secretis nunc in lucem editus, diligentia

Casp. Wolffii . . . Lugduni, Apud Bartholomaeum
Vincentium, 1620.

59, [1] p.; 531, [27] p. illus. 13 cm. **[12225]**

Part [2] has special title page.

—Tractatus duo. I. Pestis praecavendae & curandae methodus certissima. II. Pax dogmaticorum cum
spagyricis. Genevae, Typis Joan. de Tournes, 1628.

72 p.   14 cm.   **[12226]**

—, *ed. See* VARANDA, J. de. Posthumus . . . in
lucem editus De morbis & affectibus mulierum. 1619.

VEHR, IRENAEUS [1646–1710]

Dissertations—Frankfurt an der Oder

—*praeses.* Delirium ex ventriculo . . . disputatione
inaugurali . . . sistitur ab Adolpho Fried. Ger-
resheimio . . . Francofurti ad Oderam, Ex officina
typographica Joh. Coepselii [1682]

24 p.   20 cm.   **[12227]**

A. F. Gerresheim, *respondent.*

—Diatriben inauguralem de minis medicis . . . offert Lucas Kühn . . . Francofurti ad Viadrum, Ex
chalcographeo Academico-Coepseliano [1693]

[2], 82, [2] p.   20 cm.   **[12228]**

L. Kühn, *respondent.*

—Disputatio inauguralis, de hydrope sicco . . .
Francofurt. [sic] ad Viadrum, Typis Joh. Coepselii
[1686]

24 p.   19 cm.   **[12229]**

C. Peichel, *respondent.*

—Disputatio inauguralis de suspirio et suspirioso
. . . Francofurti ad Viadr., Typis Joh. Coepselii
[1689]

[58] p.   19 cm.   **[12230]**

J. C. Kletwich, *respondent.*

—Disputatio inauguralis medica de affectione marmorea . . . Francofurti ad Viadrum, Typis Johannis Coepselii [1698]

64 p.   21 cm.   **[12231]**

W. H. Nehmitz, *respondent.*

—Disputatio inauguralis medica, de anima foetida
. . . [Francofurti ad Viadrum] Literis excudit Johannes Coepselius [1679]

[64] p.   20 cm.   **[12232]**

P. C. Ursin, *respondent.*

—Disput. inauguralis medica, de febre virginum amatoria . . . Francofurti ad Viadrum, Typis Joh. Coepselii [1688]

[4], 30, [1] p.   20 cm.   [**12233**]

J. H. Hübner, *respondent.*

—Disputatio inauguralis medica de gonorrhoea . . . [Francofurti ad Viadrum] Typis Friderici Eichhornii [1674]

[28] p.   20 cm.   [**12234**]

G. Schmied, *respondent.*

—Disputationem inauguralem, de laeta ac laesa spiritus mundi parvi in cerebro generatione . . . publicae . . . disquisitioni subjiciet Caspar Friderich Vehr . . . Francofurti ad Viadrum, Imprimebat Johannes Coepselius [1698]

23 p.   18 cm.   [**12235**]

Imperfect: Upper margins trimmed.

K. F. Vehr, *respondent.*

—Disputationem inauguralem medicam, qua casus aegri sanguinam vomentis, resolutus sistitur . . . submittit Johannes Augustus Leddin . . . Francofurti ad Viadrum, Literis Christophori Zeitleri [1696]

[1], 42 p.   20 cm.   [**12236**]

J. A. Leddin, *respondent.*

—Dissertatio inauguralis medica de leucorrhoea . . . Francofurti ad Oderam, Typis Joh. Coepselii [1686]

34, [2] p.   20 cm.   [**12237**]

F. Maschow, *respondent.*

—Dissertatio inauguralis medico-chirurgica, de gangraena et sphacelo . . . Francofurti ad Viadrum, Imprimebat Joh. Coepelius [1698]

27 p.   20 cm.   [**12238**]

G. Wiedemann, *respondent.*

—Dissertatio medica inauguralis de astrobolismo . . . Francofurti ad Viadrum, Literis excudebat Joh. Coepselius [1690]

[6], 5-73, [1] p.   18 cm.   [**12239**]

A. Müller, *respondent.*

—Dissertationem medicam inauguralem de soffocatione hysterica . . . exhibet Johannes Joachimus Lincke . . . Francofurti ad Viadrum, Typis haered. J. Ernesti [1678]

[28] p.   20 cm.   [**12240**]

J. J. Lincke, *respondent.*

—Dissertationem physico medicam de oxyregmia . . . exponit . . . Johann. Christoph. Kletwich . . . Francofurt. ad Oderam, Typis Joh. Coepselii [1689]

19, [1] p.   18 cm.   [**12241**]

J. C. Kletwich, *respondent.*

—*respondent.* De erysipelate . . . Altdorphii, Typis Schönnerstaedtianis [1667]

[2], 59 (i.e. 60), [2] p.   20 cm.   [**12242**]

Diss.—Altdorf.

VEHR, Kaspar Friedrich [*fl.* 1698] *respondent. See* Vehr, I., *praeses.* Disputationem inauguralem, de laeta ac laesa spiritus mundi parvi in cerebro generatione . . . subjiciet C. F. V. 1698.

VEIEL, Elias [1635-1706] Dissertatio epistolica de summa dignitate et praestantia studii medici juxta mentem ductumque SS. Graecorum et Latinorum patrum . . . Ulmae, Literis Gassenmejerianis, 1692.

56 p.   21 cm.   [**12243**]

VEIEL, Samuel [*fl.* 1692-1694] *respondent. See* Bohn, J. Facultatis Medicae in Academia Lipsiensi p. t. pro-cancellarius, D. Johannes Bohn . . . L. S. D. 1694; Lange, C. J., *praeses.* Disputatio inauguralis medica de morbis endemiis. 1694; Rivinus, A. Q., *praeses.* Dissertatio therapeutica de medicamentorum proprietatibus. 1692.

VEIGA, Thomas a. *See* Rodrigues da Veiga, Tomás [1513-1579]

VEIGA, Tomás Rodrigues da. *See* Rodrigues da Veiga, Tomás [1513-1579]

VELDE, Jacob van de [*fl.* 1686] *respondent.* Disputatio medica inauguralis de angina . . . Lugduni Batavorum, Apud Abrahamum Elzevier, 1686.

[14] p.   22 cm.   [**12244**]

Diss.—Leyden.

—*See* Maets, C. L. de., *praeses.* Disputatio chemico-medica de calculo renum & vesicae. 1686.

VELDE, Jacob van de, *bookseller* [*fl.* 1687-1709] *tr. See* Starkey, G. Pyrotechnia; ofte, Vuur-stookkunde. 1687.

VELDE, Jacobus van den [*fl.* 1700-1717] *respondent. See* Hoffmann, F. [1660-1742] *praeses.* Specimen medicum solenne de mercurio et medicamentis mercurialibus selectis. 1700.

VELDE, Jason van de. *See* Pratensis, Jason [1486-1558]

VÉLEZ DE ARCINIEGA, Francisco [*fl.* 1593-1613] Historia de los animales mas recebidos en el uso de medicina: donde se trata para lo que cada uno entero, ò parte del aprovecha, y de la manera de su preparacion ... Madrid, Imprenta real, 1613.

[16], 454, [1] p. 21 cm. [12245]

—Theoria pharmaceutica. *In* Insa, A. J. Officina medicamentorum. 1698.

VELIUS, petrus [*fl.* 1664] *See* Baldi, C. De humanarum propensionum ex temperamento praenotionibus. 1664.

VELSCHIUS, Georgius Hieronymus. *See* Welsch, Georg Hieronymus [1624-1677]

VELSEN, Henricus à [*fl.* 1659-1660] *respondent.* Disputatio medica inauguralis, de angina ... Hardervici, Ex typographia viduae Gualtheri Rampen, 1660.

[11] p. 21 cm. [12246]
Diss.—Harderwijk.

VELSERUS, antonius. *See* Welser, Anton [*d.* 1618]

VELTHUIS, tobias [*fl.* 1631] *respondent. See* Burgersdijck, F. P., *praeses.* Collegium physicum. 1642.

VELTHUSIUS, Lambertus. *See* Velthuysen, Lambert van [1622-1685]

VELTHUYSEN, Lambert van [1622-1685] Tractatus duo medico-physici, unus de liene, alter de generatione ... Trajecti ad Rhenum, Typis Theodori ab Ackersdijck, & Gisberti à Zyll, 1657.

[56], 162 p.; 286, [1] p. 14 cm. [12247]
Errata: p. [287]

—Tractatus moralis de naturali pudore & dignitate hominis in quo agitur, de incestu, scortatione voto caelibatus, conjugio, adulterio, polygamia & divortiis ... Trajecti ad Rhenum, Ex officina typographica Rudolphi à Zyll, 1676.

[8], 146 (i.e. 148) p. 22 cm. [12248]

VELUMIUS, Sebastianus [*fl.* 1618] Medicorum tetras operum; ex doctissimorum medicorum assiduis vigiliis, & accurata theoriae & praxis observatione,

elucubrata ... Cracoviae, In chalcographia Matthiae Andreou, 1618.

[13], 167, [1] ll. 15 cm. [12249]

VENATOR, Adolph [*fl.* 1618] *respondent.* Theses medicae inaugurales de triplici melancholia ... Lugduni Batavorum, Excudit Jacobus Patius, 1618.

[19] p. 20 cm. [12250]
Imperfect: upper margins trimmed.

VENATOR, Balthasar [*fl.* 1620-1674] Vita Petri de Spina ... [Argentorati?] 1625.

[42] p. 20 cm. [12251]

VENDELINUS, Gottifredus. *See* Wendelin, Godefroid [1580-1667]

VEN. Collegii physicorum Mediolanensium antiquitas. [1645?] *See* Collegio dei fisici, Milan.

VENERIUS, Joannes Antonius [*fl.* 1617-*ca.* 1628] Opusculum de homine humanae speciei dicatum. In quo de humana felicitate ... disseritur, & quae tandem sit humana infelicitas secundum etnicorum sententiam concluditur. Venetiis, Ex typographia Ambrosii Dei, 1617.

30 p. 20 cm. [12252]

VENEROSIUS, Hieronymus. *See* Veneroso Lomellino, Girolamo [1545-1625]

VENEROSO, Hieronimo. *See* Veneroso Lomellino, Girolamo [1545-1625]

VENEROSO LOMELLINO, Girolamo [1545-1625] Consultatio responsiva. *In* A Puteo, Z. Clavis medica rationalis spagyrica. 1612.

VENETIANO, Jacomo. Specchio universale ... Opera à chi brama la sanità utilissima, & necessaria nelli corpi humani. Dove si tratta della generatione dell'huomo, & proportione sua. Con il modo di conservarsa in sanità, & rimedii di tutte l'infirmità dal capo fir'à'piedi. Ristampato in Firenze. Stampato in Padoua & in Brescia [*ca.* 1601]

[8] p. 22 cm. [12253]

[VENETTE, Nicolas, *ca.* 1631-1698] Tableau de l'amour consideré dans l'estat du mariage. Divisé en quatre parties ... Amsterdam, Jean & Gilles Jansson, 1687.

[24], 552, [23] p. 16 cm. [12254]

— [The same.] De la generation de l'homme; ou, Tableau de l'amour conjugal. Divisé en quatre parties ... 7. ed., rev., corr., augm. & enrichie de figures par l'auteur. Cologne, Claude Joly, 1696.

[28], 642, [28] p.   illus., plates., port.   16 cm.

[**12255**]

— [Dutch tr.] Venus minsieke gasthuis, waer in beschreven worden de bedryven der liefde in den staet des houwelijks, met de natuurlijke eygenschappen der mannen en vrouwen, hare siekten, oirsaken en genesingen. Door J. V. E. ... Den 3. druk. Amsterdam, Timotheus ten Hoorn, 1688.

[22], 654, [28] p.   front.   17 cm.   [**12256**]

— [German tr.] Von Erzeugung der Menschen ... Leipzig, Thomas Fritsch, 1698.

[62], 608 p.   front. (port.), plates.   18 cm.

[**12257**]

[—] Traité du scorbut, ou l'on peut connoistre fort exactement la plus-part des maladies, qui arrivent sur la mer, leurs causes, leurs signes, et les remedes, dont on se doit servir, pour les combatre. La Rochelle, Toussains de Goüy, 1671.

[17], 219, [3] p.   16 cm.   [**12258**]

Dedicatory letter signed N[icolas] V[enette]

— Another issue, with new title page and imprint: La Rochelle, Jacob Mancel & Louys Chuppin, 1671.   [**12259**]

Imperfect: p. [3] at end (Privilege) wanting.

Bound with Harvey, G. Ars curandi morbos expectatione. 1695.

VENICE (Republic, to 1797) **Laws, statutes, etc.** *See* CAMERARIUS, J. Unterricht von der Pest. 1626?

—, Magistrato della sanità. Raccolta di avvertimenti & raccordi per conoscer la peste: per curarsi, & preservarsi; & per purgar robbe, & case infette. Presentata al magistrato ill.^{mo} della sanità di Venetia, & di ordine di quello mandata alla stampa ... Venetia, Appresso i Ciera, 1630.

63 p.   22 cm.   [**12260**]

— [The same.] ... mandata alla stampa l'anno 1630. Venetia, Presso Combi, & La Noù, 1682.

125 p.   18 cm.   [**12261**]

VENNER, THOMAS. *See* VENNER, Tobias [1577?-1660]

VENNER, TOBIAS [1577?-1660] A briefe and accurate treatise, concerning the taking of the fume of tobacco, which very many, in these dayes, doe too licentiously use. In which, the immoderate, irregular, and unseasonable use thereof is reprehended, and the true nature and best manner of using it, perspicuously demonstrated ... London, Printed by W[illiam] J[ones] for Richard Moore, 1621.

[25] p.   19 cm.   [**12262**]

Signatures: 2 leaves unsigned, B-D⁴ (last leaf (blank) wanting)

STC 24642.

— Via recta ad vitam longam; or, A plaine philosophical discourse of the nature, faculties, and effects, of all such things, as by way of nourishments, and dieteticall observations, make for the preservation of health ... Wherein also ... the true use of our famous bathes of Bathe is ... demonstrated ... London, Edward Griffin for Richard Moore, 1620.

[4], 195, [8] p.   19 cm.   [**12263**]

STC 24643.

— [The same.] ... The 2d ed., corr. and enl. ... London, Printed by T. S[nodham] for Richard Moore, 1622-23.

2 v. in 1.   20 cm.   [**12264**]

Signatures: [v. 1] A², B-2C⁴, 2D² (last leaf blank); v. 2, A-E⁴, F².

Vol. 2 has imprint: London, Printed by George Eld for George Winder, 1623.

STC 24644.

— [The same.] ... London, Imprinted by Felix Kyngston, for Richard Moore, 1628.

[11], 226 (i.e. 224) p.; [4], 24 p.   19 cm.

[**12265**]

Signatures: A⁴, (a)², B-2F, A-C⁴, D².

Part [2] has special title page.

STC 24645.

— [The same.] ... Whereunto is annexed ... a ... treatise of the famous baths of Bathe, with a censure of the medicinable faculties of the water of Saint Vincent's Rocks neere the city of Bristoll. As also an accurate treatise concerning tobacco. London, Printed by R. Bishop, for Henry Hood, 1637.

[13], 364 p.   19 cm.   [**12266**]

Signatures: A³, a⁴, B-2Z⁴, 2A².

"The baths of Bathe" and "A briefe and accurate treatise concerning the taking of the fume of tobacco" have special title pages.

STC 24646.

— [The same.] ... London, Printed by R. Bishop, for Henry Hood, 1638.

[13], 364 p.   19 cm.   [**12267**]

Signatures: A³, a⁴, B-2Z⁴, 2A².

A reissue of the 1637 edition with date changed to 1638.

STC 24647.

—[The same.] . . . All which are likewise amplified since the former impressions. London, Printed by James Flesher for Henry Hood, 1650.

[12], 417 (i.e. 387) p.   19 cm.   [12268]

—[The same.] . . . The 4th impr. . . . with many . . . additions . . . London, Printed [by T. R.] for Abel Roper, 1660.

[6], 404, [8] p.   front. (port.).   20 cm.

[12269]

VENOSTA, Antonio Maria. *See* Venusti, Antonio Maria [16th cent.]

VENTURA, Laurentius. De ratione conficiendi lapidis philosophici, liber . . .

215–312 p., vol. 2.   20 cm. (*In* Zetzner, Lazarus, *ed.* Theatrum chemicum. Argentorati, 1659–61)

[12270]

Caption title.

VENTURINI, Alessandro. Zomista; overo, Secretario degli animali . . . Roma, Per gli Mascardi, ad instanza di Pompilio Totti, 1636.

[12], 178, [1] p.   15 cm.   [12271]

Imperfect: p. 21–22 mutilated.

—[The same.] Secretario de gl'animali; cioe, Secreti medicinali, che dalle parti d'ogn'uno d'essi si cavano, incominciando dall' huomo . . . Milano, Per Filippo Ghisolfi, ad instanza di Gio. Battista Bidelli [1649?]

142 p.   15 cm.   [12272]

Imperfect: p. 15–16 wanting.

—[The same.] Le medicine che da tutti gl'animali si può cavar à beneficio dell' huomo; altre volte intitolato il Zomista, e secretario de gl'animali . . . Hora accresciuto d'importanti secreti da Francesco Pignoccati . . . 4. imp. Venetia, Il Turrini, 1654.

[28], 126 p.   14 cm.   [12273]

—[The same.] Secreti medicinali . . . ne' quali si contengono i più scelti rimedi, che si cavano da gli animali per salute dell' huomo. Nuovamente accresciuti d'importanti secreti dal sig. Francesco Pignocatti . . . Bologna, Gio. Recaldini, 1672.

[8], 136 p.   15 cm.   [12274]

—[The same.] Le medicine che da tutti gl'animali si può cavar à beneficio dell' huomo; altre volte intitolato il Zomista, e secretario de gl'animali . . . Hora accresciuto d'importanti secreti da Francesco

Pignocatti . . . 6. impr. Venetia, Il Curti, 1674.

[24], 154 p.   14 cm.   [12275]

VENUS minsieke gasthuis. 1688. *See* [Venette, N.]

VENUSTI, Antonio Maria [16th cent.] Consilio medica. *In* Lautenbach, J., *ed.* Consilia medicinalia. 1605, 1660.

—Discorso generale . . . intorno alla generatione, al nascimento de gli huomini, al breve corso della vita humana, & al tempo . . . Milano, Gio. Battista Bidelli, 1614.

[32], 312 p.   15 cm.   [12276]

VERA relazione, e ritratto di portento maraviglioso operato da dio in una bambina mostruosa nata . . . anno 1687 nella città del Campo in Spagna con due corpi in uno, due teste, delle quali una sola hadenti, quattro braccia, etrè gambe, figlia di Francesco Garzia, e di Maria Martinez . . . Tradotta del spagnuolo in italiano. [Madrid, Torino, Venetia, Milano, & Bologna, Giacomo Monti, 1687]

[4] p.   illus.   20 cm.   [12277]

VERADIANUS. *See* Jābir ibn Ḥaiyān, al-Ṭarasūsī. Gebri . . . Summa perfectionis magisterii in sua natura. 1682.

VERAX, Theodorus, *pseud. See* Walker, Clement [1595–1651]

VERBEECK, Damasus [*fl.* 1687] *respondent.* Disputatio medica inauguralis de concoctione ventriculi integra & laesa . . . Lugduni Batavorum, Apud Abrahamum Elzevier, 1687.

[12] p.   21 cm.   [12278]

Diss. — Leyden.

VERBEZIUS, Alexander [*fl.* 1634] *respondent. See* Sebisch, M. [1578–1674?] *praeses.* Collegii therapeutici disputatio I [–XIV] 1634 [i.e. 1635]

VERBEZIUS, David [1577–1644] Exercitationum medicarum, super disputatione quadam de peste. Liber unus . . . [Kempten] Typis Christophori Kraus, 1618.

[16], 179, [1] p.   port.   19 cm.   [12279]

Engraved title page.

—Pro Raymundi Mindereri . . . disquisitione iatrochymica de chalcantho, ad Dodecaporii Chalcanthini Petri Castelli . . . partem priorem responsio. Qua simul Aetii Cleti … disputatio de chalcantho, in R. Mindererum … examinatur. Augustae Vindelicorum, Apud Sebastianum Mylium [Typis Johannis Praetorii] 1626.

[16], 198, [1] p. 19 cm.   **[12280]**

VERBRIGGE, Johannes. *See* Verbrugge, Johannes.

VERBRUGGE, Johannes. Chirurgijn of heel-meesters reys-boek, bestaande in II. deelen; I. van sijn sheeps-medicament of reys-kist; en van sijn sheeps-kost of alimenten. II. Van de algemeene gebreeken … Item: Van de crisie, urine, en hare teykenen … Den alderlaetsten druk. Middelburg, Anthony de Winter [167–?]

[16], 126 p.; [6], 56 p.; [2], 18 p. 15 cm.
                                              [12281]

Parts 2 and [3] have special title pages.

—Chirurgyns scheeps-kist. *In* Bondt, J. de. Oost-Indische warande. 1673; Voorde, C. van de. Lichtende fakkel der cheirurgia. 1668.

—De nieuwe verbeterde chirurgyns scheeps-kist. *In* Bondt, J. de. Oost-en West-Indische warande. 1694.

—Examen van land- en zee-chirurgie, handelende van alle de voornaemste hooft-stucken die de … chirurgie aengaen … Als oock de land en scheeps-kist, met de kraghten der medicamenten van dien … Amsterdam, Jan ten Hoorn, 1687.

[12], 373 (i.e. 430), [5] p. 17 cm.   **[12282]**

—[The same.] … Den 4. druk vermeerdert. Amsterdam, Jan ten Hoorn, 1686 (i.e. 1696).

[14], 426, [6] p. 16 cm.   **[12283]**

Printer's preface dated 1696.
Imperfect: first preliminary leaf (blank?) wanting.

—Zee-chirurgie, waer in de gronden der heel-konst ende voornaemste gebreecken, soo te welde, als by der zee door-vallende, verhandelt werden, in verscheyden deeltjens begrepen … Amsterdam, Johannis ten Hoorn, 1680.

[16], 533, [7] p. 17 cm.   **[12284]**

—, *ed.* and *tr.* See Guillemeau, J. Hondert en der-tien gebreken en genesinge der oogen. 1678.

VERDEMANUS, Ludolphus. *See* Ludolphus, Verdemanus.

VERDRIES, Johann Melchior [1679–1735] *respondent. See* Valentini, M. B., *praeses.* Disputatio physico-mechanica. 1698.

VERDUC, Jean Baptiste. Discours sur l'utilité du microscope. *In* Brunet, C. Le progrès de la medecine. 1695.

[—]Nouvelle osteologie, où l'on explique méca-niquement la formation & la nourriture des os. Avec Le squelete du foetus, et une Dissertation sur le mar-cher de l'homme & des animaux, sur le vol des oyseaux, & sur le nager des poissons. Paris, Laurent d'Houry, 1689.

[16], 414, [2] p. plates. 17 cm.   **[12285]**

Le squelete du foetus is based on Theodor Kerckring's Osteogenia foetuum which was published as part of his Spicilegium anatomicum; Dissertation sur le marcher de l'homme & des animaux is based chiefly on Giovanni Alfonso Borelli's De motu animalium.

[—] Les operations de chirurgie, par une methode courte & facile. Avec deux traitez, l'un des maladies de l'estomach, & l'autre des maux veneriens. Paris, Laurent d'Houry, 1691.

[20], 356 (i.e. 354) p. 16 cm.   **[12286]**

—[The same.] Nouvelle methode d'operations de chirurgie, avec deux traitez, l'un de la nouvelle maniere de guerir la verole, et l'autre les maladies de l'estomach. Paris, Laurent d'Houry, 1693.

324, [12] p. front. 15 cm.   **[12287]**

Ascribed by BMC. to Joseph de La Charrière.

[—] Les operations de la chirurgie. Avec une pathologie, dans laquelle on explique toutes les maladies externes du corps humain, & leurs remedes, selon les principes de la physique moderne … Divisé en deux parties. Tome premier [-second] Paris, Laurent d'Houry, 1694.

[88], 622, [60] p.; [621]–1142, [4] p. front. (port.) 20 cm.   **[12288]**

Tome second has title page: Suite de la pathologie de chirurgie.

—Suite de la nouvelle osteologie, contenant un traité de myologie raisonnée; où, aprés avoir parlé du mouvement des muscles selon les modernes, on fait une exacte description de tous les muscles du corps … Paris, Laurent d'Houry, 1698.

[8], 235, [4] p. 17 cm.   **[12289]**

VERDUC, Jean Philippe. *See* Verduc, Jean Baptiste.

VERDUC, Laurent [*d.* 1695] La maniere de guerir toutes les fractures et les luxations qui arrivent au corps humain, par le moyen des bandages ... Paris, L'autheur, 1685.

 [24], 370 p. 17 cm.   [**12290**]

—[The same.] ... 2. ed. Rev., corr. & augm. d'un nouveau Traité des playes d'arquebusades. Paris, Laurent d'Houry, 1689.

 [16], 436, [6] p. 16 cm. [**12291**]

—[Dutch tr.] Het Parische verband-huis, waar in getoont werd, de wyse om alle fracturen en luxatien, van alle de deelen des linghaams door maniere van swagtelen te genesen ... Als mede Hippocrates over de fracturen en luxatien. Amsterdam, Jan ten Hoorn, 1691.

 [8], 306, [4] p. plates. 17 cm. [**12292**]
Added engraved title page.
Imperfect: p. 147-148 mutilated.

—*ed. See* Guy de Chauliac. Le maistre en chirurgie. 1691, 1697; [Italian tr.] 1697.

VERDUC, Laurent [*d.* 1703] *See* Guy de Chauliac. Le maistre en chirurgie. 1691, 1697; [Italian tr.] 1697; Malpighi, M. Discours anatomiques sur la structure des visceres. 1687.

VERDUYN, Pieter Adriaanszoon [1625?-*ca.* 1700] Dissertatio epistolaris de nova artuum decurtandorum ratione ... Amstelaedami, Apud Joannem Wolters, 1696.

 32 p. plates. 18 cm. [**12293**]

—*See* Scultetus, J. [1595-1645] Armamentarium chirurgicum. 1693.

La **VERGE** de Jacob; ou, L'art de trouver les tresor, les sources, les limites, les metaux, les mines, les mineraux, & autres choses cachées, par l'usage du bâton fourché. Par I. N. Lyon, Hilaire Baritel, 1693.

 [28], 137, [5] p. front. 15 cm. [**12294**]
Errata: p. [4-5] at end.

[**VERGILIUS**, Polydorus, *d.* 1555] A pleasant and compendious history of the first inventers and instituters of the most famous arts, misteries, laws, customs and manners in the whole world ... To which is added, several curious inventions, peculierly attributed to England & English-men ... London, John Harris, 1686.

 [15], 159, [4] p. 15 cm. [**12295**]

Preface signed: J[ohn] H[arris]
"This is Langley's translation arranged alphabetically, with some alterations, omissions, and additions." Cf. J. Ferguson. Bibliographical notes on the English translation of Polydore Vergil's work, "De inventoribus rerum." Westminster, 1888, p. 32.

VERHEYEN, Philipp [1648-1710] Corporis humani anatomia, in qua omnia tam veterum, quam recentiorum anatomicarum inventa methodo nova & intellectu facillima describuntur ... Lovanii, Apud Aegidium Denique, 1693.

 [12], 300, [11] p. plates. 21 cm. [**12296**]

—[The same.] ... Accessit ejusdem appendix cum Animadversionibus in anatomiam Blancardianam, & obiter in quasdam alias: item Epistola anatomica ad ... Fredericum Ruyschium ... Lovanii, Apud Aegidium Denique, 1697.

 [12], 152, 8, 153-300, [11], 24 p. plates, port. 21 cm.   [**12297**]

—[The same.] ... Lipsiae, Apud Thomam Fritsch, 1699.

 [17], 622, [18] p. front. (port.), plates. 16 cm.
            [**12298**]

"Philippi Verheyen Animadversiones in anatomiam Blancardianam: et obiter in quasdam alias. Accessit ejusdem Epistola ad ... D. Friedericum Ruyschium ..." (p. [577]-622) has half title.

VERHEYEN, Philipp [1648-1710] *See* [Brunet, C.] Le progrès de la medecine. 1699.

VERHOOFD, Lucas, *ed.* and *tr.* See Hippocrates. Ἀφορισμοί [Aphorismi. Greek and Latin.] 1675?, 1685.

VERHOOFT, Pieter [*fl.* 1694] *respondent.* Disputatio medica inauguralis de vomitu ... Lugduni Batavorum, Apud Abrahamum Elzevier, 1694.

 [8] p. 22 cm.   [**12299**]
Diss. — Leyden.

VERLA, Jean. *See* Verle, Giovanni Battista [17th cent.]

VERLE, Giovanni Battista [17th cent.] Anatomia artifiziale dell'occhio umano, inventata, e fabbricata nuovamente ... Firenze, Per il Vangelisti Stamp. Arcivescóvale, 1679.

 45, [2] p. front., plate. 13 cm. [**12300**]
Imperfect: lower part of plate wanting.

—[Latin tr.] Anatomia artificialis oculi humani inventa & recens fabricata ... Ex Italico in Latinum

sermonem conversa. Amstelaedami, Apud Henricum
Wetstenium, 1680.

[6], 63 p.   illus.   14 cm.   **[12301]**

—[The same.] *In* Cellier, A., *ed.* Opuscula nova
anatomica. 1680.

't VERMAKELIJCK landt-leven. I [-twaelfde]
deel. Den Nederlandtsen hovenier, door J. van der
Groen ... Amsterdam, Gysbert de Groot, 1686.

[30], 103, [3] p.; [8], 84, [4] p.; 88 p.   illus.
21 cm.   **[12302]**

Engraved title page.

Deel I includes: Twee hondert modellen, voor de liefhebbers
van hoven en thuynen, with special title page (p. [41])

Deel II has engraved title page and special title page: Den
verstandigen hovenier ... door P. Nyland.

Deel III has special title page: De medicyn-winckel, of ervaren
huys-hounder ... door P. Nyland, followed by Nyland's Den
naerstigen byen-houder, and the anonymous De verstandige kock,
each with special title page (p. [39] and p. [57]).

With this is bound Nylandt, P. De Nederlandtse herbarius of
kruydt-boeck. 1682.

VERMEER, CORNELIS [*fl.* 1689] *respondent.*
Disputatio medica inauguralis de angina ... Tra-
ecti ad Rhenum, Ex officina Francisci Halma, 1689.

12, [2] p.   22 cm.   **[12303]**
Diss.—Utrecht.

VERMEIREN, NICOLAUS [*fl.* 1662] Oratio in
laudem medicinae. Amstelodami, Ex officina Henrici
Stam, 1662.

[8] p.   18 cm.   **[12304]**

VERMEY, JOHANNES [*fl.* 1667] *respondent.*
Disputatio medica inauguralis de paralysi ... Ultra-
ecti, Ex officina Johannis à Sambix, 1667.

[8] p.   20 cm.   **[12305]**
Diss.—Utrecht.

VERMOST, DANIEL. *See* PLEMP, V. F. Fundamenta medicinae ad scholae acribologiam aptata.
1644, 1654.

VERNEUERTE GESETZ, Ordnung und Tax ...
less ... Reichs Statt Nürmberg. 1624, 1700. *See*
NUREMBERG. Ordinances, local laws, etc.

VERNEUERTE Leich Ordnung der Statt Nürmberg. 1625, 1662. *See* NUREMBERG. Ordinances, local
laws, etc.

VERNEY, PIERRE [16th cent.] L'antidote
apologetic de la peste ... Avec les remedes

esprouvez, preservatifs, & curatifs manifestes, occultes ou specifics, faciles en leur usage & preparation. Et la composition & usage aggreable du syrop
catholique de cassia. Dole, Antoine Binart, 1629.

[16], 174 p.   16 cm.   **[12306]**
The second treatise has special title page: De recto syrupi de
cassia usu epilogismus.

—*See* HIPPOCRATES. [Prognostica. English.] 1611
[1612], 1634, 1655.

VERNON, FRANCIS [1637?–1677] *See* RAUWOLFF, L.
A collection of curious travels & voyages. 1693.

VERNY, FRANÇOIS, *ed. See* BAUDERON, B. La pharmacopée de Bauderon. 1663, 1672.

—*See* PHARMACOPOEIA AUGUSTANA REFORMATA CUM
EJUS MANTISSA & APPENDICE. 1672; ZWELFER, J. Discursus apologeticus. 1668, 1675.

Il VERO et pretioso thesoro di sanità. [1630?] *See*
CROCE, G. C.

Il VERO ritrato di un giovine con due teste. *See*
MOBILISSIMI SIGNIORI. 1695.

VERONA (City) **Ordinances, local laws, etc.**
Regolatione de pretii delle cose medicinali semplici,
e composte, che vendono nelle speciarie della magn.
città di Verona, e suo distretto riformata nuovamente
da gli eletti giusto parti del magn. conseglio di XII.
3, aprile 1669. & 28 giugno 1692 ... Verona, Fratelli
Merli [1696]

16 p.   31 cm.   **[12307]**

VERONICI, ANDREA [*fl.* 1695] In defensionem
Anconae typis editam a quodam in arte chirurgica
viro, gratis asserente, rotulam transversim fractam
sine restitante claudicationis incommodo nequaquam
posse curari, responsio ... Maceratae, Typis Michaelis Archangeli Silvestri, 1695.

99, [4] p.   16 cm.   **[12308]**

VERPOORTEN, GODFRIED [*fl.* 1693] *respondent.*
Disputatio medica inauguralis de hydrope ascite ...
Lugduni Batavorum, Apud Abrahamum Elzevier,
1693.

[42] p.   22 cm.   **[12309]**
Diss.—Leyden.

VERRI, GIOVANNI BATTISTA [*fl.* 1662] Sanitatis
prodomus vitae nuncius rurales lucubrationes pestilentiae tempore ... Neapoli, Apud Novellum de
Bonis, 1662.

[12], 328, [19] p.   port.   31 cm.   **[12310]**

VERRYN, GISBERT [*fl.* 1687] *respondent.* Dissertatio medica inauguralis de haemorrhagia ... Lugduni Batavorum, Apud Abrahamum Elzevier, 1687.

[15] p.   21 cm.   **[12311]**

Diss.—Leyden.

De **VERSTANDIGE** kock. *See* 't VERMAKELIJCK LANDT-LEVEN. 1686.

VERSTEEG, GODEFROID. *See* STEEGHIUS, Godefridus [*fl.* 1579–*ca.* 1600]

VERSTEGEN, RICHARD [*ca.* 1548–1640] A restitution of decayed intelligence: in antiquities. Concerning the most noble and renowned English nation. By the studie and travell of R[ichard] V[erstegen] ... London, John Bill, 1628.

[22], 338, 12 p.   illus.   19 cm.   **[12312]**

Preface signed: Richard Verstegan.
Title page backed, text partly mutilated and mended.
STC 21362.

VERTUA, GIOVANNI BATTISTA [*d.* 1630] De morte retardanda tractatio ... Mediolani, Apud Jo. Jacobum Cumum, 1616.

[16], 260, [1] p.   17 cm.   **[12313]**

Errata: p. [261]

VERULAM, FRANCIS BACON, baron. *See* BACON, Francis, *viscount St. Albans* [1561–1626]

VERVECEIDOS libri duo. 1636. *See* [LICETI, F.]

VERVOLG van de Aardige duyvelary, voorvallende in dese dagen. Begrepen in een twede brief van een heer t'Amsterdam, geschreven aan een van sijn vrienden te Leeuwaarden, in Vriesland. Rotterdam, Pieter van Veen, 1691.

[1], 45 p.   19 cm.   **[12314]**

Not in Linde.
Concerns controversy with Balthasar Bekker.
Bound with Aardige duyvelary. [1691?]

VERWEY, REINER [*fl.* 1687] *respondent. See* ESCHENBACH, A. C., *praeses.* De unctionibus gentilium. 1687.

VERWOUT, JAN [*fl.* 1669] *respondent.* Disputatio medica inauguralis de mensium suppressione ... Lugduni Batavorum, Apud viduam & haeredes Joannis Elsevirii, 1669.

[11] p.   23 cm.   **[12315]**

Diss.—Leyden.

VERZASCA, BERNHARD [1628–1680] Exercitatio de apoplexia et paralysi. Basileae, Typis Joh. Jacobi Deckeri [1662?]

[7], 68, [3] p.   18 cm.   **[12316]**

—Observationum medicarum centuria. Cui accesserunt celeberrimorum virorum consilia & epistolae ... Basileae, Typis Johannis Jacobi Deckeri, 1677.

[16], 311, [17] p.   16 cm.   **[12317]**

Includes correspondence with Johann Jakob Wepfer.

—*respondent. See* STUPANUS, E., *praeses.* Signorum medicorum doctrina. 1649.

—, *ed. See* MATTIOLI, P. A. Neu vollkommenes Kräuter-Buch. 1678, 1696; MEYSSONNIER, L. Breviarum medicum. 1664; RIVIÈRE, L. Medicina practica in succinctum compendium redacta studio & sumptibus Bernhardi Verzaschae. 1663.

VESALIUS, ANDREAS [1514–1564] Anatomia. Venetiis, Apud Joan. Anton. et Jacobum de Franciscis [1604]

[8], 510, [65] p.; [19] p.   plates.   33 cm.

                                                    [12318]

Engraved title page.
Cushing VI.A.–5.
"Universa antiquorum anatome tam ossium, quam partium & externarum, & internarum: ex Rufo Ephesio ... tribus tabellis explicata per Fabium Paulinum. Quibus accessit quarta ex Sorani ... fragmento Graeco non antehac Latino facto. De matrice": [19] p.
First published in 1543 under title: De humani corporis fabrica.

—De humani corporis fabrica librorum epitome: cum iconibus elegantissimis juxta Germanam authoris delineationem artifitiose jampride ex aere expressis ... Opus perinsigne, nunc primum in Germania renatum, hacque forma quam emendatissime editum. Colonie Ubiorum, Formis et expensis Joan. Buxmacheri et Georgii Meutingi, 1600 [i.e. 1601]

[98] p.   port., plates.   39 cm.   **[12319]**

Engraved title page.
Colophon: Coloniae Agrippinae, Typis Stephani Hemmerdeu, 1601.
Cushing VI.D.–10.
Edited by Hendrik Botter.

—[The same.] Epitome anatomica. Opus redivivum cui accessere, notae ac commentaria F. Paaw ... Lugduni Batavorum, Ex officina Justi à Colster, 1616.

[8], 226, [1] p.   illus.   20 cm.   **[12320]**

Cushing VI.D.–19.

—[The same.] Anatomia ... in qua tota humani corporis fabrica, iconibus elegantissimis, juxta genuinam auctoris delineationem aeri incisis, lectori ob oculos ponitur ... Opus perinsigne et utilissimum, nunc primum quam emendatissime editum. Amstelodami, Excudebat Joannes Jansonius, 1617.

[98] p. port., plates. 38 cm. [12321]

Imperfect: 4th prelim. leaf (poem and port.) wanting.
Cushing VI.D.–12.
A reissue, with new title page, of the Cologne 1600 [i.e. 1601] edition.

—[The same.] Librorum ... de humani corporis fabrica epitome: cum annotationibus Nicolai Fontani ... Amstelodami, Apud Joannem Janssonium, 1642.

[14], 112 (i.e. 110) p. port., plates. 41 cm. [12322]

Cushing VI.D.–13.

[—] Notomie di Titiano ... [Bologna? *ca.* 1670]

[1] p. 17 plates. 45 cm. [12323]

Engraved title page.
Edited and engraved by Domenico Bonaveri. Includes the 3 skeletal plates and the 14 muscle plates from Vesalius' Fabrica, formerly attributed to Tiziano Vecelli, but now generally conceded to have been drawn by Jan Stephan van Calcar.
Cushing VI.D.–9.

—[Dutch excerpts.] *In* Valverde, J. de. A. Vesalii en Valverda Anatomie. 1647.

—[The same; illustrations based on Vesalian plates.] *In* COLOMBO, R. Anatomia. 1609; *In* MORO, G. Anatomia ridotta all'uso de' pittori. 1679.

—*See* GALENUS. De ossibus ad tirones. Greek and Latin. 1665; PILES, R. de Abregé d'anatomie. 1667; PLATTER, F. [1536–1614] De corporis humani structura et usu libri III. 1603; SÁNCHEZ, F. Opera medica. 1636; SCHOLTZ, L. Consiliorum medicinalium ... liber singularis. 1610.

VESLING, JOHANN [1598–1649] De plantis Aegyptiis observationes et notae ad Prosperum Alpinum, cum additamento aliarum ejusdem regionis. Patavii, Apud Paulum Frambottum, 1638.

[12], 80 p. illus. 23 cm. (Vol. 3 in Alpini, P. De plantis Aegypti. Patavii, 1638–40) [12324]

Nissen 20.
Includes the illustrations of Alpini's work, but from different woodcuts presumably based on Vesling's drawings. Cf. Haller's comparison of Alpini's and Vesling's illustrations in his Bibl. bot., v. I, p. 456.
Also published separately in the same year. Cf. Hunt 231; Nissen 2057; Pritzel 9745.

Contains brief commentary (p. 63, 67, 71, and 75) on Alpini's De plantis exoticis, published posthumously by the author's son in Venice in 1627.

—Observationes anatomicae & epistolae medicae ex schedis posthumis selectae & editae a Th. Bartholino. Hafniae, Apud Petrum Hauboldum, 1664.

[8], 248 p. 15 cm. (Part [2] in Bartholin, Thomas. De insolitis partus humani viis ... Hafniae, 1664) [12325]

—Opobalsami veteribus cogniti vindiciae. Patavii, Typis Pauli Frambotti, 1644.

[24], 108 p. 22 cm. [12326]

"... Paraeneses ad rem herbariam publicis plantarum ostensionibus praemissae" (p. [61]-108) has special title page.

—Syntagma anatomicum publicis dissectionibus, in auditorum usum, diligenter aptatum. Patavii, Typis Pauli Frambotti, 1641.

[12], 194, [1] p. 16 cm. [12327]

Errata: p. [195]

—Syntagma anatomicum, locis plurimis auctum, emendatum ... Patavii, Typis Pauli Frambotti, 1647.

[15], 274, [14] p. illus. 26 cm. [12328]

Added engraved title page.

—[The same.] ... 2. ed. ab extrema auctoris manu. Patavii, Typis Pauli Frambotii, 1651.

[16], 274, [12] p. port., illus. 24 cm. [12329]

Added engraved title page dated 1647.

—Syntagma anatomicum, commentariis illustratum a Gerardo Leonardi Blasio ... Amstelodami, Apud Joannem Janssonium, 1659.

[23], 274, [14] p.; 228, [19] p. illus. 26 cm. [12330]

Added engraved title page.
Part [2] has special title page: Gerardi Leon. Blasii Commentaria, in Syntagma anatomicum.

—Syntagma anatomicum, commentario atque appendice ex veterum, recentiorum, propriisque, observationibus, illustratum & auctum a Gerardo Leon. Blasio ... Ed. 2. priori emend. ... Amstelodami, Apud Joannem Janssonium a Waesberge, & Elizeum Weyerstraet, 1666.

[25], 558, [16] p. front. (port.), illus. 24 cm. [12331]

Added engraved title page.
Includes contributions by Gaspare Asellio, Thomas Bartholin, Lorenzo Bellini, Reinier de Graaf, Nathaniel Highmore, Marcello Malpighi, Jacob Henrik Paulli, Olof Rudbeck, Frederik Ruysch, Konrad Victor Schneider, Nicolaus Steno and Thomas Willis.

—Copy 2.

Imperfect: portrait wanting.

Date on engraved title page altered by hand to 1669, on title page to 1673.

—[The same.] ... Cui addita noviter fuit erudita epistola Georgii Hieronymi Velschii ... Patavii, Apud Petrum Mariam Frambottum, 1677.

[8], 248 (i.e. 482), [16] p.   plates.   24 cm.
                                                    [**12332**]
Added engraved title page.

—[The same.] ... Ed. nov. priori emend. ... Trajecti ad Rhenum, Apud Antonium Schouten, 1696.

[12], 560, [16] p.   front. (port.), illus.   23 cm.
                                                    [**12333**]
Added engraved title page.

—Another issue.   25 cm.   [**12334**]

Frontispiece not present; added engraved title page dated 1695.

—[Dutch tr.] Konstige ontleding des menschelijcken lichaems; in 't Latijn beschreven ... vertaelt door Gerardus Blasius ... Amsterdam Gerret Sweerman, 1661.

[20], 259, [21] p.   17 cm.   [**12335**]

Imperfect: first preliminary leaf (blank?) wanting.

—[English tr.] The anatomy of the body of man: wherein is exactly described every part thereof ... Published in Latin ... and Englished by Nich. Culpeper ... London, Peter Cole, 1653.

[16], 192 (i.e. 92) p.   tables, plates.   28 cm.
                                                    [**12336**]

Imperfect: table 1, and plates 1, 2, 7 and 21 wanting; p. [4] mutilated.

—[The same.] ... London, George Sawbridge, 1677.

[8], 192 (i.e. 92) p.   tables, plates.   30 cm.
                                                    [**12337**]
Different setting of type.

—[German tr.] Künstliche Zerlegung des gantzen menschlichen Leibes. Anfangs in lateinischer Sprache beschrieben ... jetzo aber ... ins Teutsche übersetzt durch Gerhardum Blasium ... Nürnberg, In Verlegung Johann Hoffmanns, 1676.

[14], 333, [32] p.   plates.   17 cm.   [**12338**]

Added engraved title page reads: Neuherausgegebene Anatomia.

—[The same, as subject] See MARCHETTI, D. de. Anatomia. 1652, 1654, 1656, 1688; RIOLAN, J.

[1580–1657] Opera anatomica vetera. 1650 [and] Opuscula anatomica nova. 1649.

—See JASOLINO, G. Collegium anatomicum. 1668; LICETI, F. De motu sanguinis. 1647; PANUZZI, F., *ed.* Francesco Panuzzi ... a i lettori. 1640.

VESTI, JUSTUS [1651–1715] Compendium institutionum medicarum IV. disputationibus comprehensum & in perantiqua Electorali ad Hieram Academia propositum ... Erfurti, Typis Joh. Henr. Groschii, 1686.

188 p.   12 cm.   [**12339**]

Contents. —Praeliminaria et physiologia, respondente, J. S. Brehm. —De pathologia, respondente Christoph. Helbigio. —De semiologia atque therapeutica, respondente J. T. Ehrlich. —De diaetetica, pharmaceutica atque chirurgica, respondente J. M. Thilo.

—[The same.] ... Ed. 2. Erfurti, Chalcographeo Joh. Henr. Groschii, Sumptibus Joh. Caspar. Birckneri, 1688.

188 p.   13 cm.   [**12340**]
Different setting of type.

—Institutiones medicae reformatae, hoc est, fundamenta medica olim luci publicae exposita, jam vero revisa, aucta, in variis immutata & ... denuo edita ... Francofurti & Lipsiae, Sumtibus Joh. Caspar. Bircknieri; Erfurti, Typis Joh. Heinrici Kindlebii, 1697.

192, [24] p.   15 cm.   [**12341**]

A 3d ed., rewritten in part, of *his* Compendium institutionum medicarum.

—De purgatione doctrina theoretico-practica, brevis & succincta, secundum neotericorum mentem adornata & medicinae studiosis, practicisque junioribus apprime utilis & summe necessaria. Erfurti, Typis Johann. Henr. Groschii, 1686.

[10], 50 p.   13 cm.   [**12342**]

—Oeconomia corporis humani, in qua octo dissertationibus functiones ... proponuntur ... Accesserunt duo tractatus, alter De purgatione, alter De medicamentorum ... Jenae, Sumptibus Joh. Jacobi Ehrt. Efordiae, Typis Joh. Henrici Groschii [1688]

[8], 112 p.; 58 (i.e. 60) p.; 76 p.   16 cm.   [**12343**]

Imprint partly supplied from Eloy.

Bound with Eysel, J. P. Compendium physiologicum [1698]

—Facultatis Medicae . . . decanus, Justus Vesti . . . benevolo lectori S. P. D. . . . Erfordiae, Typis Groscianis [1689]

[8] p.   19 cm.   [**12344**]

Program—Erfurt (with vita of C. M. Horlacher)

—Facultatis Medicae . . . decanus Justus Vesti . . . benevolo lectori S. P. D. . . . Erfordiae, Typis Joh. Henrici Kindlebii [1694]

[12] p.   21 cm.   [**12345**]

Program — Erfurt (with vita of J. M. Kniphof)

—Facultatis Medicae . . . decanus Justus Vesti benevolo lectori S. P. P. [sic] . . . Erfurti, Stanno Kindlebiano [1699]

[6] p.   21 cm.   [**12346**]

Program — Erfurt (with the vita of J. F. Schultze)

Dissertations — Erfurt

—*praeses*. Diatribe inauguralis medica, de mictu cruento . . . Erfordiae, Praelo Groschiano [1698]

16 p.   19 cm.   [**12347**]

C. H. Schreck, *respondent*.

—Disputatio inauguralis medica de abortu . . . Erfordiae, Typis Johann-Henrici Groschii [1690]

[22] p.   18 cm.   [**12348**]

G. C. Habermass, *respondent*.

—Disputatio inauguralis medica de anorexia . . . Erfurti, Literis Kindlebii [1691]

24 p.   19 cm.   [**12349**]

C. Richter, *respondent*.

—Disputatio inauguralis medica, de arthritide erratica . . . Erfordiae, Stanno Groschiano [1700]

24 p.   20 cm.   [**12350**]

J. V. Scholin, *respondent*.

—Disputatio inauguralis medica de atrophia . . . Erfurti, Typis Kindlebianis [1694]

16 p.   19 cm.   [**12351**]

C. Fischer, *respondent*.

—Disputatio inauguralis medica de motu sanguinis circulari naturali & praet. naturali . . . Erfurti, Literis Kindlebianis [1700]

28 p.   19 cm.   [**12352**]

V. J. Burchard, *respondent*.

—Disputatio inauguralis medica de phrenitide . . .

Erfurti, Typis Kindlebianis [1692]

20 p.   20 cm.   [**12353**]

J. P. Thieme, *respondent*.

—Disputatio inauguralis medica de singultu . . . Erfurti, Typis Kindlebii [1691]

[1], 30 p.   19 cm.   [**12354**]

G. C. Stahl, *respondent*.

—Disputatio inauguralis medica de suffocatione hysterica . . . Erfurti, Literis Groschianis [1685]

[35] p.   20 cm.   [**12355**]

J. J. Braun, *respondent*.

—Disputatio inauguralis medica de ventriculi inflatione . . . Erfurti, Typis Joh. Georg. Hertzi [1686]

[24] p.   19 cm.   [**12356**]

A. Buxbaum, *respondent*.

—Another issue.

[26] p.   19 cm.   [**12357**]

More laudatory poems added.

—Disputatio inauguralis medica qua aegrum artuum tremore correptum . . . Erfurti, Literis Kindlebianis [1694]

16 p.   21 cm.   [**12358**]

J. M. Kniphof, *respondent*.

—Disputatio inauguralis medica, qua hectica cardiaca . . . examini submittitur a Johanne Gottlob Reymmanno . . . Erfurti, Literis Kindlebianis [1697]

24 p.   19 cm.   [**12359**]

J. G. Reymann, *respondent*.

—Disputatio inauguralis physico-medica de magnetismis macro- et microcosmi . . . Erfordiae, Stanno Kindlebiano [1695]

32 p.   20 cm.   [**12360**]

J. H. Spiess, *respondent*.

—Disputatio medica, de diarrhoea . . . Erfurti, Literis Hertzianis, 1682.

[20] p.   20 cm.   [**12361**]

G. Bergmann, *respondent*.

—Disputatio medica de epilepsia . . . Erfurti, Typis Johann-Henrici Groschii [1687]

24 p.   20 cm.   [**12362**]

C. G. Schmalkalden, *respondent*.

—Disputatio medica inauguralis de medico felici et infelici . . . Erfordiae, Typis Groschianis [1689]

19, [1] p.   20 cm.   [**12363**]

J. G. Haberland, *respondent*.

—Disputatio physico-medica de pulvere sympathetico ... Erfurti, Typis Johann-Henrici Groschii [1687]

19 p. 18 cm.   [12364]

J. C. Müller, *respondent.*

—Disputationem inauguralem medicam de pollinctura ... submittit Joh. Fridericus Brebisius ... Erfurti, Typis Georgii Henrici Mülleri [1695]

[24] p. 20 cm.   [12365]

J. F. Brebis, *respondent.*

—Disquisitio inauguralis medica de febre Hungarica, quam vulgus cephalalgiam epidemiam vocitat ... Erfurti, Literis Groschianis, 1687.

28 p. 20 cm.   [12366]

A. C. Georgi, *respondent.*

—Dissertatio inauguralis medica, exhibens aegrum phthisi laborantem ... Erfurti, Literis Joh. Heinrici Kindlebii [1699]

28 p. 20 cm.   [12367]

J. F. Schultze, *respondent.*

—Dissertatio inauguralis medica, exhibens casum de doloribus vehementissimis partum praegredientibus ... Erfurti, Stanno Kindlebiano [1696]

20 p. 21 cm.   [12368]

G. S. Cronpusch, *respondent.*

—Dissertatio inauguralis physico-medica, de anime habitudine ad corpus, speciatim quoad mixtionis corporeae conservationem, subnexis genuinae praxeos fundamentis ... Erfordiae, Typis Groschianis [1699]

60 (i.e. 80) p. 20 cm.   [12369]

C. Isermann, *respondent.*

—Dissertatio medica de colica ... Erfordiae, Typis Johann-Henrici Groschii [1690]

24 p. 20 cm.   [12370]

F. C. Florus, *respondent.*

—Dissertatio medica de febri ardente maligna ... Erfurti, Typis Joh. Henr. Groschii [1686]

28 p. 19 cm.   [12371]

J. T. Ehrlich, *respondent.*

—Dissertatio medica de mictione cruenta ... Erfordiae, Charactere Groschiano [1686]

[16] p. 19 cm.   [12372]

J. C. Müller, *respondent.*

—Dissertatio medica inauguralis, de apoplexia ... Erfordiae, Excudebat Joh. Henr. Grosch [1698]

24 p. 19 cm.   [12373]

J. G. Wagner, *respondent.*

—Dissertatio medica inauguralis de dyspepsia ... Erfordiae, Typis Groschianis [1689]

16 p. 18 cm.   [12374]

J. J. Zimmermann, *respondent.*

—Dissertatio medica inauguralis de lue venerea ... Erfordiae, Typis Johann Henrici Groschii [1689]

16 p. 20 cm.   [12375]

J. E. Jacobi, *respondent.*

—Dissertatio medica inauguralis, proponens casum aegri ascitici ... Erfordiae, Praelo Groschiano [1697]

32 p. 19 cm.   [12376]

D. S. Bockshammer, *respondent.*

—Dissertationem inauguralem de variolis ... subjicit ... Johann Wilhelm Gottfried ... Erfordiae, Charactere Kindlebiano [1698]

20 p. 20 cm.   [12377]

J. W. Gottfried, *respondent.*

—Dissertationem inauguralem medicam de pleuritide ... proponit Johannes Jacobus Schlegel ... Erfurti, Typis Kindlebii [1690]

24 p. 19 cm.   [12378]

J. J. Schlegel, *respondent.*

—Exercitium medicum inaugurale, proponens chlorosin, vulgo die Jungfer-Kranckheit ... exponet Ericus Hesterberg ... Erfurti, Typis Kindlebii [1691]

16 p. 19 cm.   [12379]

E. Hesterberg, *respondent.*

—Inaugurales de hydrocephalo theses ... Erfordiae, Typis Groschianis [1688]

39 p. 18 cm.   [12380]

J. S. Brehm, *respondent.*

VETTORI. *See* VITTORI.

VEYRAS, JACQUES [*fl. ca.* 1625] *tr. See* NEANDER, J. Traicté du tabac. 1626.

VEZELIUS, THEODORUS BEZA. *See* BÈZE, Thédore de [1519–1605]

VIANA, ANTONIO DE. Espejo de cirugia en tres exercitacions de theorica, y practica, que tratan de los tiempos del apostema sanguineo; como se han de

observar, para el uso recto de los remedios ...
Sevilla, Juan Perez Berlanga [1696]

[12], 216, [7] p.   21 cm.   **[12381]**

First published in Lisbon in 1631. Cf. Hernández Morejón, vol.
5, p. 158.

VIANA, JUAN DE. *See* VIANA MENTESANO, Juan de
[*fl.* 1636–1649]

VIANA MENTESANO, JUAN DE [*fl.* 1636–1649]
Tratado de peste, sus causas y curacion, y el modo
que se ha tenido de curar las secas y carbuncos
pestilentes, que han oprimido a esta ciudad de
Malaga este año de 1637 ... Malaga, Juan Serrano
de Vargas, 1637.

[4], 98, [8] ll.   21 cm.   **[12382]**

VIARDEL, COSME [*fl.* 1671–1647] Observations sur
la practique des accouchemens naturels, contre
nature & monstreux, avec une methode tres-facile
pour secourir secourir les femmes en toute sorte d'accouchemens, sans se servir de crochets, ny d'aucun
instrument, que de la seule main ... Avec un traitté
des principalles maladies qui arrivent ordinairement
aux femmes & aux filles, & des maladies des mam-
melles ... Paris, Edme Couterot, Nicolas Bessin,
François Mauger, 1671.

[44], 371 p.   18 cm.   **[12383]**

—[The same.] ... Rev., corr., enrichy & augm.
de quantité de figures en taille douce ... 2. ed. Paris,
L'autheur et Jean d'Houry, 1673.

[44], 371 p.   front. (port.), plates.   18 cm.
                                          [12384]

A reissue of the 1671 edition with new title page and plates added;
the errata are uncorrected.

—Another issue, with date changed to 1674.
                                          [12385]

—[German tr.] Anmerckungen von der weiblichen
Geburt, so wohl der natürlichen, als unnatürlichen,
wie auch Missgeburt; benefenst einem kurtzen und
leichten Unterricht denen Weibern in allerley
Geburten zu helffen, also dass man weder die
Hacken, oder einig ander Instrument, sondern allein
die blosse Hand gebrauche ... Nebenst einem
kleinen Anhang von den vornehmsten Krancheiten,
welche so wohl bey den Frauen als Jungfrauen zu
entstehen pflegen ... Im Jahr 1671. in frantzösischer
Sprache beschrieben, und auss derselben in die
Teutsche übersetzet. Franckfurt, In Verlegung

Johann Peter Zubrodt, gedruckt bey Johann Andrea,
1676.

[24], 212 p.   illus.   17 cm.   **[12386]**

VICARIUS, JOHANN JACOB FRANZ [1664–1716]
Basis universae medicinae in quinque libros institutionum pro veteri more divisa, ac juxta neotericos
in principiis mathematicis, mechanicis & anatomicis
fundata ... Constantiae, Typis Francisci Xav.
Straub, 1698.

[16], 333, [11] p.   17 cm.   **[12387]**

—Hydrophilacium novum; seu, Discursus de
aquis salubribus mineralibus ... Ulmae Suevorum,
Impensis Laurentii Kronigeri & haeredum Theophili
Goebelii, 1699.

[16], 272 p.   17 cm.   **[12388]**

—*praeses.* Disceptatio medica ... de malo
hypochondriaco ... Friburgi Brisgoiae, Typis Joannis Jacobi Handler [1699]

[4], 24 p.   19 cm.   **[12389]**

Diss.—Freiburg im Breisgau (J.J. König, *respondent*)

VICARY, THOMAS [*d.* 1561] The English mans
treasure. With the true anatomie of mans bodie: compiled by ... Thomas Vicary ... Whereunto are annexed many secrets appertaining to chirurgerie, with
divers excellent approved remedies for all captaines
and souldiers ... and for all diseases ... with
emplaisters of speciall cure: with other potions and
drinks approved in physicke. Also the rare treasure
of the English bathes. Written by William Turner
... Gathered ... by William Bremer ... Now sixtly
augmented and enlarged, with almost a thousand ...
medicines ... by G. E. practitioner in physicke and
chyrurgerie ... London, Thomas Creede, 1613.

[8], 224, [8] p.   illus.   18 cm.   **[12390]**
STC 24710.

Vicary's anatomical treatise (p. 1–54) was first published in an
edition of 1548 no longer extant. It appears to be based largely on
a medieval English compilation dating from 1392, now Wellcome
MS. 564. This anonymous text was itself an abridged version of
passages in Henri de Mondeville and Lanfranco of Milan. The
"annexed secrets" (p. 55–110) include extracts taken without
acknowledgement from John Hester's translation of Leonardo
Fioravanti, A short discours ... uppon chirurgerie (London, 1580
and William Ward's translation of The secretes of ... Alexis of
Piemont [pseud.? i.e. Girolamo Ruscelli?] (London, 1562)

—[The same.] ... Now eightly augmented and
enlarged, with almost a thousand ... medicines ...
by W[illiam] B[oraston] practitioner in physicke and

chyrurgerie ... London, Bar. Alsop and Tho. Fawcet, 1633.

[8], 264, [8] p. illus. 19 cm.   [12391]

Imperfect: p. 231–232 wanting.

Vicary's anatomical treatise (p. 1–57) is a word by word reprint of the 1613 edition.

STC 24712.

—[The same.] ... Now ninthly much augmented, corrected and enlarged, with almost a thousand ... medicines ... by W[illiam] B[oraston] practitioner in physicke and chyrurgerie ... London, B. Alsop and Tho. Fawcet, 1641.

[11], 292, [15] p. illus. 18 cm.   [12392]

Vicary's anatomical treatise (p. 1–57) is word by word reprint of the 1613 edition.

—The surgions directorie, for young practitioners, in anatomie, wounds, and cures, &c. shewing, the excellencie of divers secrets belonging to the noble art ... Divided into X. parts ... London, Printed by T. Fawcet and sold by J. Nuthall, 1651.

[16], 332 p. 14 cm.   [12393]

Imperfect: lower margins trimmed including part of imprint.

Basically a reprint of The English mans treasure, published in 1613.

VICENTE DE ALHAMBRA, BALTASAR. *See* MERCATI, M. Instruccion sobre la peste. 1648.

VICO, GIOVANNI DI. *See* VIGO, Giovanni de [1460?–1525?]

VICTORIUS, ANGELUS. *See* VITTORI, Angelo [*d.* 1640?]

VICTORIUS FAVENTINUS, BENEDICTUS. *See* VITTORI, Benedetto [*d.* 1561]

VIDIUS, VIDUS. *See* GUIDI, Guido [*ca.* 1500–1569]

VIDMAYER, WOLFFGANG ANDREAS. Hygiene; seu, Dissertationes philosophico-medicae de aere, cibo, & potu ... Labaci, Typis Josephi Thaddaei Mayr, 1692.

[28], 280, [19] p. 13 cm.   [12394]

Errata: p. [19] at end.

VIDÓS Y MIRÓ, JUAN DE [*fl.* 1674–1699?] Memorial y manifiesto a la augusta, y imperial ciudad de Zaragoça, cerca la oposicion, que el Colegio de medicos, y cirujanos de dicha ciudad haze a los remedios, que aplica, y usa el licenciado Juan de Vidós ... declaracion de la firma, que la ilustrissima corte del señor justicia de Aragon declarò

à su favor; y firma que le concediò en prueva de los constitos; en processo contradictorio, y resolucion que el iluste capitulo, y consejo de dicha ciudad tomó para usar de dichos remedios. Çaragoça, Tomas Gaspar Martinez 1683.

[8], 46 p. 21 cm.   [12395]

—Primera parte de medicina, y cirugia racional, y espagirica, sin obra manual de hierro, ni fuego, purificada con el de la caridad, en el crisol de la razon, y experiencia, para alivio de los enfermos, Con su antidotario de rayzes, yervas, flores semilla. frutos ... Zaragoça, 1699.

[12], 391, [7] p. illus. 21 cm.   [12396]

Imperfect: sig. Bb8 at end (blank?) wanting.

La VIE de Mr Des-Cartes. 1692. *See* [BAILLET, A.]

VIEBEG, JOHANN CHRISTOPH [*fl.* 1674] *respondent.* *See* SCHARFF, J. F., *praeses.* Miraculum naturae magnes. 1674.

VIEBEG, Theodor [*fl.* 1670] *respondent. See* EBBLE, J. L., *praeses.* Principia entis naturalis intrinseca in fieri et facto esse ... dissertatione physica ... exponunt ... T. V. 1670.

VIEBING, GOTTFRIED [*fl.* 1603] *respondent. See* SENNERT, D., *praeses.* De methodo medendi disputatio II. de indicantibus. 1603.

VIEL-VERGRÖSTER und hellerpolirter Schorbocks-Spiegel, oder eigentliche und ausführliche Beschreibung dess nunmehr weitreissenden Schorbocks, in vier auffs neue unterschiedlichen Tractätlein verfasset ... Nürnberg, In Verlegung Johann Andreas, und Wolffgang Endters, des Jüngern, seligen Erben, 1659.

[22], 701, [19] p. front., plates. 14 cm.   [12397]

Frontispiece has title: Schorbocks Spiegel.

Imperfect: p. 119–120 (blank?) wanting.

With this is bound Cellarius, Kurtzer Bericht. 1675.

VIELHEUER, CHRISTOPH. Gründliche Beschreibung fremder Materialien und Specereyen Ursprung, Wachsthum, Herkommen und deroselben Natur und Eigenschafften ... in drey Theil unterschieden. Der Erste handelt von Metallen und Mineralien, etc. Der ander Theil, von Kräutern, Wurtzeln und Blumen, etc. Der dritte Theil, von

Thieren und was davon kommt . . . Leipzig, Johann Fritzsche, 1676.

[4], 12, [16], 240 p.   20 cm.   [12398]

Added engraved title page.

VIERTEL, JOHANN CHRISTIAN [*fl.* 1699] *respondent. See* TIMAEUS, G., *praeses.* Disputatio prior de metallurgia rerum gerendarum nervo. 1699.

VIERZIGMANN, JOHANN [*fl.* 1695] *respondent.* Disputatio inauguralis medica de phimosi . . . [Altdorffii] Typis Henrici Meyeri [1695]

23 p.   20 cm.   [12399]

Diss. — Altdorf.

See HOFFMANN, J. M., *praeses.* Disputatio medica publica de omento. 1695.

VIETOR, PETRUS [*fl.* 1607-1610] *respondent.* Theses medicae de praefocatione uteri . . . Basileae, Typis Joan. Jacobi Genathii, 1610.

[8] p.   20 cm.   [12400]

Diss. — Basel

VIETOR, PETRUS [*fl.* 1607-1610] *See* RYFF, P. Gratiosus . . . ordo medic. Basileens. 1610.

VIEUSSENS, RAYMOND [1641-1715?] Deux dissertations . . . La premiere touchant l'extraction du sel acide du sang. La seconde sur la proportion de quantité de ses principes sensibles. Montpelier, Honoré Pech, 1698.

[28], 162 p.   17 cm.   [12401]

With this is bound his Réponse. 1698.

— Epistola de sanguinis humani cum sale fixo, spiritum acidum suggerente, tum volatili, in certa proportione sanguinis phlegma, spiritum subrufum ac oleum foetidum ingrediente, nec non de bilis usu ad Facultatem Medicam Lipsiensem perscripta, una cum hujus responso. Lipsiae, Apud Joh. Ludovicam Gleditschium, 1698.

[22] p.   22 cm.   [12402]

— Neurographia universalis; hoc est, Omnium corporis humani nervorum simul & cerebri, medullaeque spinalis descriptio anatomica . . . Ed. nova. Lugduni, Apud Joannem Certe, 1685.

[20], 252, [2] p.   illus., plates.   port.   35 cm.   [12403]

Errata: [2] p.

— [The same.] . . . Editio in Germania prima . . . Francofurti, Prostat apud Georgium Wilhelmum Kühnium, 1690.

[38], 492, [12] p.   plates, port.   18 cm.   [12404]

Errata: p. [11-12] at end.

— Réponse . . . a trois lettres . . . du sieur Chirac . . . Montpelier, Honoré Pech, 1698.

163, [8] p.   17 cm.   [12405]

Includes letters from Guy Crescent Fagon, Richard Lower, William Briggs and others.

Bound with his Deux dissertations. 1698.

— Tractatus duo. Primus de remotis et proximis mixti principiis in ordine ad corpus humanum spectatis. Secundus de natura, differentiis, subjectis . . . & causis fermentationis . . . Lugduni, Apud Joannem Certe, 1688.

[12], 348 p.   plates.   26 cm.   [12406]

Date altered from M.DC.LXXXVII to M.DC.LXXXVIII. Privilege du roy dated: Le 6. Janvier 1688.

— *See* CHIRAC, P. De motu cordis adversaria analytica. 1698.

VIGENÈRE, BLAISE DE [1523-1596?] Tractatus de igne et sale . . . in Latinam linguam translatus . . .

1-139 p., vol. 6.   20 cm.   (*In* Zetzner, Lazarus, *ed.* Theatrum chemicum. Argentorati, 1659-61)   [12407]

Caption title.

Translated by Johann Jacob Heilmann.

VIGIER, JEAN [*fl.* 1608?] Opera medico-chirurgica quae continent Chirurgiam magnam, Thesaurum & armamentarium medico-chirurgicum, Enchiridion anatomicum, Historiam foetus . . . Ex variis authoribus Graecis, Latinis, Arabibus & neotericis compilata, Gallico idiomate primum edita, nunc vero Latina facta, recognita, & multum aucta, cum variis observationibus & operationibus, a Joanne Vigierio filio . . . Hagae-Comitum, Ex typographia Adriani Vlacq, 1659.

3 parts in 1 v.   table.   21 cm.   [12408]

Parts [2-3] have special title pages.

— Enchiridion anatomic, auquel est . . . descripte l'histoire anatomique du corps humain . . . Corr. & augm. en ceste derniere ed., de plusieurs annotations . . . avec un nouveau Traicté des valvules du corps humain . . . Paris, Jean Jost, 1628.

[24], 335 p.   15 cm.   [12409]

Edited by François de Long-Pré.

—La grande chirurgie des tumeurs, en laquelle, selon les anciens Grecs, Latins, Arabes, & modernes approuvez, est contenue la theorie & practique tres parfaicte de toutes les maladies externes, qui surviennent au corps humain. Le tout composé de nouveau, & curieusement recerché ... Lyon, Jean Anth. Huguetan, 1611.

[20], 613 (i.e. 603), [33] p. 15 cm. **[12410]**

Errata: p. [31–33]

—[The same.] ... Le tout curieusement rev. & corr. de nouveau en cette dernier ed. ... Lyon, Jean Champion & Christophle Fourmy [1657?]

[16], 528, [38] p. 18 cm. **[12411]**

—[The same.] ... Lyon, Pierre Compagnon & Robert Taillandier, 1670.

[16], 528, [38] p. 17 cm. **[12412]**

Different setting of type.

—La grande chirurgie des ulceres. En laquelle, selon les anciens Grecs, Latins, Arabes & modernes approuvez, est contenuë la theorie & practique des ulceres de tout le corps humain ... 2. ed. rev. & corr. Lyon, Jean Champion & Christophle Fourmy, 1656.

[40], 571, [29] p. 18 cm. **[12413]**

—[The same.] ... Lyon, Pierre Compagnon & Robert Taillandier, 1674.

[40], 571, [29] p. 18 cm. **[12414]**

A reissue of the 1656 edition with new title page.

—Tractatus absolutissimus et accuratissimus de catarrho, rheumatismo, vitiis dentium, linguae, vocis, de immodica & indecora salivatione, & aliis a cerebro destillationibus, de variis authoribus compilatus. Item Andreae Laurentii ... Tractatus ... de catarrho e Gallico sermone in Latinum conversus ... Genevae, Apud Joannem Bouchereau, 1620.

120 (i.e. 220) p. 18 cm. **[12415]**

—, tr. See CHAUMETTE, A. Le parfaict chirurgien. 1628.

VIGIER, JEAN [fl. 1658] ed. and tr. See HIPPOCRATES. [Aphorismi. French.] 1620, 1666; VIGIER, J. [fl. 1608?] Opera medico-chirurgica quae continent Chirurgiam magnam. 1659.

VIGILANTIUS DE MONTE CUBITI, ed. and tr. Dreyfaches hermetisches Kleeblat, in welchem begriffen dreyer vornehmen Philosophorum herrliche Tractätlein. Das erste von dem geheimen waaren Salz der Philosophorum, und allgemeinen Geist der Welt, H. Nuysement ... Das andere Mercurius redivivus, Unterricht von dem philosophischen Stein so wol den weisen als rohten aus dem Mercurio zu machen, Samuelis Nortoni sonsten Rinville. Und das dritte von dem Stein der Weisen Marsilii Ficini ... In unser teutsche Mutterschprach übersetzet, und ... zum Druck verfertiget. Durch Vigilantium de Monte Cubiti [pseud.] Nürnberg, In Verlegung Michael und Johann Friderich Endtern, 1667.

[24], 448, [32] p. plates. 17 cm. **[12416]**

Added engraved title page, illustrated.

Includes Samuel Norton's Catholicon physicorum (p. [231]–246); Venus vitriolata (p. [247]–262); Elixir; seu, Medicina vitae (p. [263]–282); Saturnus saturatus disolutus & Coelo restitutus (p. [283]–312); Metamorphosis lapidum ignobilium in gemmas quasdam pretiosas (p. [313]–328); Alchymiae complementum, et perfectio (p. [329]–354); Ein Tractätlein, welches von den philosophischen Schrifften handlet (p. [355]–372). All have half titles.

VIGNERIUS, BLASIUS. See VIGENÈRE, Blaise de [1523–1596?]

VIGNOLA, GIACOMO BAROZZIO, called [1507–1573] Le due regole della prospettiva pratica di M. Jacomo Barozzi da Vignola con i comentarii del R. P. M. Egnatio Danti ... Roma, Nella stamparia del Mascardi, ad instanza di Filippo de Rossi, 1644 [1642]

[12], 145, [5] p. illus. 34 cm. **[12417]**

Engraved title page.

Half title: Prospettiva del Vignola.

VIGO, GIOVANNI DE [1460?–1525?] [Practica in arte chirurgica copiosa & Practica in arte chirurgica compendiosa. Dutch] Medecyn boec, ende chyrurgie ... Welck een principael fondament van alle chyrurgijen is, beyde in de theorijcke ende practijcke ... Noch is hier achter by-gevoeght een grondigh ende ervaren medecijn-boeck inhoudende veel schoone ende versochte remedien. Eertijts ghestelt ende ghepractiseert door M. Joannis Hagius ... ende nu uyt des autheurs eyghen schriften met aller neersticheydt af-ghevaerdight. Dordrecht, Peeter Verhaghen, 1614.

[4], 202 (i.e. 203), [2], 28, [1] ll. 30 cm. **[12418]**

—[French tr.] La practique et chirurgie ... divisee en deux parties ... Traduict de latin en françois, par M. Nicolas Godin ... Le tout de nouveau rev., & exactement corr. Lyon, Pierre Rigaud, 1610.

[12], 960, [12] p.; 106 p. 15 cm. **[12419]**

Part 2 has special title page.

—[German tr.] Wund-Artznei, in zwey Theile merckwürdig eingetheilet: allwo der erste, Die grosse Practica in neun Büchern abgehandelt wird; der andere, oder Die kleine Practica, helt in sich fünff Bücher, von gleicher, jedoch weit kurtzer gefaster Materi, mit beygefügten von dem Authore selbsten jedes Orths experimentirten Artzneien. Aus gestimmelten zweyen Exemplarien, einem nehmlich An. 1540 zu Vincentz, den andern zu Leiden ... An. 1561, auf sehr eiveriges und lang gesuchtes Begehren in bessere und heut zu Tag weit deutlichere Red-Arth übersetzet, und eines Theils mit Anmerckungen versehen ... Zum öffentlichen Druck gebracht durch Johannem Scultetum ... Nürnberg, In Verlegung Johann Hoffmanns, gedruckt bey Christoph Gerhard, 1677.

[29], 1292, [144] p.; [1], 227, [18] p. 22 cm. **[12420]**

Added engraved title page.

Part 2 has special title page.

—[Italian tr.] La prattica universale in cirugia ... Di nuovo riformata, & dal latino ridotta à la sua vera lettura con le figure in disegno de semplici nel settimo libro. Appresso vi è un bellissimo Compendio, che tratta dell'istessa materia, composto per m. Mariano Santo ... Con due trattati de m. Giovanni Andrea dalla Croce, l'uno in materia delle ferite, l'altro del cavar l'armi e le saette fuori della carne ... Et di nuovo aggiuntivi molti capitoli estratti dalle opere dell'eccellentissimo dottor ... Leonardo Fioravanti ... i quali sono multo necessarii alla medicina, & cirugia per bene operare ... Venetia, Domenico Imberti, 1605.

[8], 566 p. illus. 21 cm. **[12421]**

La prattica universale in cirugia is a translation by Lorenzo Chrisaorio of Practica in arte chirurgia copiosa and Practica in arte chirurgia compendiosa.

The "Due trattati" by G. A. della Croce, first published with the 1560 edition of Vigo's Prattica universale, were revised to form books 5-7 in the 1573 edition of Croce's Chirurgiae libri septem.

—[The same.] ... Venetia, Ghirardo, & Iseppo Imberti, 1622.

[8], 566 p. illus. 21 cm. **[12422]**

Different setting of type.

—[The same.] ... Venetia, I Bertani, 1639.

[8], 504 p. illus. 24 cm. **[12423]**

—[The same.] ... Venetia, Marco Ginammi, 1647.

[8], 485, [3] p. illus. 23 cm. **[12424]**

—[The same.] ... Venetia, Nicolò Pezzana, 1669.

[8], 478 (i.e. 484) p. illus. 25 cm. **[12425]**

Imperfect: p. 481-484 mutilated.

—[The same.] ... Venetia, Nicolò Pezzana, 1685.

[8], 484 p. illus. 24 cm. **[12426]**

Different setting of type.

—[Spanish tr.] Teorica y pratica en cirugia ... Hecha de latina castellana, por el ... Miguel Juan Pascual ... Y agora nuevamente impressa, y de las faltas ... corregida ... Perpiñan, Luys Roure, 1627.

[8], 222 ll. illus. 29 cm. **[12427]**

Imperfect: ll. 222 mutilated.

VILANOVA, ARNALDUS DE. *See* ARNALDUS DE VILLANOVA [*d.* 1313?]

VILLA, FRAY ESTEBAN DE [*d.* 1660] Examen de boticarios. *In* Insa, A. J. Officina medicamentorum. 1698.

—Libro de simples incognitos en la medicina ... Burgos, Pedro Gomez de Valdivielso, 1643-54.

2 v. ([16], 114, [5] p.; [8], 42, [2] ll.) 21, 20 cm. **[12428]**

—Ramillete de plantas ... Burgos, P[edro] Gomez de Baldivielsso, 1637.

[5], 148, [4] ll. 20 cm. **[12429]**

Engraved title page.

VILLALPANDO, FRANCISCO DE TORREBLANCA. *See* TORREBLANCA Y VILLALPANDO, Francisco de [*d.* 1645]

VILLAMEDIANA, ANDRÉS DE [*fl.* 1662] Consulta de los carbuncos que corren en la villa de Alaexos ... Valladolid, Imprenta de Valdivielso, 1663.

[21], 72 ll. 20 cm. **[12430]**

Imperfect: first preliminary leaf wanting.

VILLANOVA, ARNALDO DE. *See* ARNALDUS DE VILLANOVA [*d.* 1313?]

VILLANUEVA, ANDRES. *See* VILLAMEDIANA, Andrés de [*fl.* 1662]

VILLANUS, GREGORIUS [17th cent.] *ed. See* SEVERINO, M. A. Therapeuta Neapolitanus. 1653.

VILLARS, *abbé de. See* VILLARS, Nicolas Pierre Henri de Montfaucon [*ca.* 1635-1673]

VILLARS, Nicolas Pierre Henri de Montfaucon [*ca.* 1635-1673] Le Comte de Gabalis; ou, Entretiens sur les sciences secrets. Renouvellé & augmenté d'une lettre sur ce sujet . . . Cologne, Pierre Marteau [1675?]

[1], 161 p. 16 cm. **[12431]**

VILLAS, Fr. Estevaõ de. *See* Villa, Fray Esteban de [*d.* 1660]

VILLE. *See* Deville.

VINCENT, Thomas [1634-1678] Gods terrible voice in the city. Wherein you have I. the sound of the voice, in the history of the two late dreadful judgments of plague and fire in London. II. The interpretation of the voice . . . The 5th ed. corr., with the addition of a sermon preached at the funeral of Mrs. [sic] A. F. [i.e. Mr. Abraham Faneway, minister of the Gospel] . . . London, George Calvert, 1667.

[6], 242 (i.e. 226) p. front. 18 cm. **[12432]**

The Sermon has special title page (p. [217]).

—[The same.] . . . The 6th ed. corr. . . . London, George Calvert, 1668.

[5], 225 p.; 77 p. 17 cm. **[12433]**

The Sermon has special title page (p. [199]). Part [2] has half title: Annus mirabilis: the year of wonders, MDCLXVI.

VINCENTIUS, Athanasius. *See* Lyser, Johann [1631-1684]

VINCENTIUS, Nicolaus, *pseud. See* Scaliger, Joseph Juste [1540-1609]

VINCENTIUS, Theophilus. *See* Lyser, Johann [1631-1684]

VINDICIANUS. *See* Celsus, A. C. De re medica libri octo. 1608, 1625.

VINTHER, Philipp Jakob [*fl.* 1670-1678] *respondent.* Dissertatio medica inauguralis περὶ τῶν ἀπράκτων μορίων . . . Argentorati, Typis Johannis Welperi [1678]

[8], 56 p. 18 cm. **[12434]**

Diss.—Strasbourg.

VIOLET, Fabien, *sieur de Coqueray* [*fl.* 1635] La parfaicte et entiere cognoissance de toutes les maladies du corps humain, causées par obstruction . . . Paris, Pierre Billaine, 1635.

[16], 350, [2] p. 17 cm. **[12435]**

VIOLETTE, Joseph Duchesne, *seigneur de la. See* Duchesne, Joseph [*ca.* 1544-1609]

VION D'ALIBRAI, Charles. *See* Dalibray, Charles Vion, *sieur de* [*ca.* 1600–*ca.* 1655]

VIRDUNG, Paul [*fl.* 1608] *respondent.* Discursus medicus de ventis in microcosmo seu spiritu flatulento & affectuum hinc in humano corpore nascentium διαγνωσει ac θεραπεια . . . Basileae, Per Joan. Jacob. Genathium [1608]

[40] p. 20 cm. **[12436]**

Diss. — Basel.

VIRDUNG VON HARTUNG, Hieronymus Konrad [*fl.* 1679] *praeses.* Congressus inauguralis Herculeus quem cum Herculeo morbo id est epilepsia . . . Herbipoli, Typis Eliae Michaelis Zinck [1679]

[5], 19 p. 20 cm. **[12437]**

Diss. — Würzburg (J. P. Ernst, *respondent*)

VIRDUNG VON HARTUNG, Philipp Wilhelm [1664-1708] *praeses.* Disputatio inauguralis medica de colica . . . Herbipoli, Typ. haer. Zinck. topogr. per Martinum Richter [1694]

[2], 17 p. 20 cm. **[12438]**

Diss. — Würzburg (P. L. Kirchenn, *respondent*)

—Disputatio medica de ictero flavo . . . Herbipoli, Typis haeredum Zinck, per Martinum Richter [1692]

[2], 12 p. 20 cm. **[12439]**

Imperfect: ink stains throughout.
Diss. — Würzburg (J. G. Jaeger, *respondent*)

—*respondent. See* Lucas, J. M., *praeses.* Disputatio medica inauguralis de palpitatione cordis. 1686.

VIRIDET, Jean [1655-1736] Tractatus novus medico-physicus de prima coctione praecipueque de ventriculi fermento . . . Genevae, Sumptibus Leonardi Chouët & socii, 1691.

[16], 336, [28] p. 18 cm. **[12440]**

—Another issue, with date changed to 1692. **[12441]**

VIRNA, Samuel [*fl.* 1659] *respondent. See* Kirchmayer, G. K., *praeses.* Τετρας quaestionum illustrium anthropologico-physicarum. 1659.

VIRUES, Gerónimo [*fl.* 16th cent.] *tr. See* Montemayor, C. Medicina y cirugia de vulneribus capitis. 1664.

VISCARDI, JACOPO. Explanationes aromatum, quae supersunt in primo Dioscoridis lib. De medica materia ... [Patavii, Apud Cadorinum, 1687]

[8] p.   23 cm.   **[12442]**

Caption title.

Half title reads: Explanationes in pr. lib. Dioscoridis.

VISCERUS, JOANNES. *See* VISCHER, Johann [1524-1587]

VISCHER, HIERONYMUS [*fl.* 1619] *respondent.* Positiones medicae de peripneumonia ... Basileae, Typis Joannis Schroeteri [1619]

[12] p.   19 cm.   **[12443]**

Diss. — Basel.

VISCHER, JOHANN [1524-1587] *See* HIPPOCRATES. [Aphorismi. Latin.] 1681.

VISSEMBACHIUS, JOHANNES JACOBUS. *See* WISSENBACH, Johann Jacob [1607-1665]

VISSENDIEP, QUIRYN VAN [*fl.* 17th cent.] *tr. See* HORNE, J. van. Kort-begrijp der ontleed- en heel-konst. 1669.

VISVLIET, MEINERD EGBERT VAN [*fl.* 1658] *respondent.* Disputatio medica inauguralis, de empyemate ... Lugduni Batavorum, Ex officina Francisci Moyardi, 1658.

[12] p.   21 cm.   **[12444]**

Diss. — Leyden.

VITALE, GIOVANNI ANTONIO [*b.* 1633] Quaestiones prooemiales chyrurgiae, quaestionesve de capitis vulneribus secundum Hippocratis mentem, etiam cum parte ipsiusmet capitis anatomica ... Neapoli, Ex typographica Joannis Francisci Paci, 1676.

[26], 245, [17] p.   port.   22 cm.   **[12445]**

VITO, GIOVANNI DE [*fl.* 1602] De causis nostrarum calamitatum: et de morbis epidemicis qui vulgabantur per totum regnum Neapolitanum anno Domini 1600. Cum pronosticis usque ad annum 1608. Neapoli, Apud Jo. Jacobum Carlinum, 1602.

[20], 167, [9] p.   23 cm.   **[12446]**

VITRIOLI, ALESSANDRO [17th cent.] *tr. See* COLMENERO DE LEDESMA, A. Della cioccolata ... Tradotto ... con aggiunta d'alcune Annotationi da Alessandro Vitriolo. 1667.

VITTORI, ANGELO [*d.* 1640?] Medica disputatio. De palpitatione cordis, fractura costarum aliisque affectionibus B. Philippi Nerii ... Qua ostenditur praedictas affectiones fuisse supra naturam ... Romae, Ex typographia Camerae Apostolicae, 1613.

[8], 43, [3] p.   22 cm.   **[12447]**

With this are bound: copy 3 of Rudio, E. De virtutibus, et viciis cordis, libri tres. Venetiis, 1587; Rudio, E. De usu totius corporis humani liber. Venetiis, 1588.

— Medicae consultationes post obitum auctoris in lucem editae a Vincentio Mannuccio ... Romae, Ex officina typographica Caballina, 1640.

[16], 449, [25] p.   33 cm.   **[12448]**

"Palpitationem cordis et fracturam costarum, quas per annos quinquaginta substinuit S. Philippus Nerius supra ordinem naturae fuisse demonstratur": p. 415-443.

VITTORI, BENEDETTO [*d.* 1561] De curandis morbis ad tyrones practica magna, in duos tomos divisa, opus ... in Germania nusquam visum ... nunc demum Petrum Uffenbachium ... a primae & antiquae editionis mendis emaculatum ... Francofurti, Impensis Joannis Theobaldi Schönwetteri, typis Erasmi Kempfferi, 1628.

[16], 1006 (i.e. 1106), [14] p.; [4], 477, [43] p.   19 cm.   **[12449]**

Published in Venice in 1562 under title: Practicae magnae ... de morbis curandis, ad tyrones, tomi duo.

Part [2] contains Benedetto Vittori's Medicationis empiricae, Camillo Tomai's Compendiosa methodus, tum pathologica, tum therapeutica, and Nicolaus Epiphanius' Empyrica. This section was originally published as part 3 of the 1626 Frankfurt edition of Dispensatorium chymicum.

— De morbi gallici curandi ratione. *In* his Prattica d'esperienza. 1624.

— [Exhortatio ad medicum recte sancteque medicari cupientem. Italian] Prattica d'esperienza ... nella quale si contengono maravigliosi remedii, da lui istesso, & da molto altri ... medici esperimentati in tutte l'infermità, che occorrer possono nel corpo humano. Tradotta in lingua volgare dall'eccellente medico m. Tomaso Terranuova. Vicenza, Antonio Megietti, 1624.

[6], 264 ll.   15 cm.   **[12450]**

Apparently reprinted from the 1570 Venice edition.

— Medicationis empeiricae. In *his* De curandis morbis ad tyrones practica magna. 1628; *In* Dispensatorium chymicum. 1626.

VIVA, JACOBUS [1622-1650] *ed. See* KIRCHER, A. Musurgia universalis. 1650.

VIVIANI, VIVIANO [*fl.* 1626-1644] Opere . . .
Venetia, Heredi di Gio. Salis, 1644.

[6], 56 (i.e. 64) p.   23 cm.   **[12451]**

Contains his Oratione, Consiglio sopra le febri pestilentiali, and Modo di purificar le robbe infette.

—De peste; sive, Viviani Viviani . . . Apologia.
Syllogisticae disputationis editae anno MDCXXX
. . . Venetiis, Apud Jacobus Sarzinam, 1633.

[8], 71 p.   22 cm.   **[12452]**

Bound with *his* Opusculum de peste. 1634.

—Opusculum de peste . . . Venetiis, Apud Rubertum Meiettum, 1634.

[8], 76 p.   22 cm.   **[12453]**

With this is bound *his* De peste. 1633.

—Trattato del custodire la sanità . . . Venezia,
Girolamo Piuti, 1626.

205, [7] p.   16 cm.   **[12454]**

VIVIER, DANIEL DU. *See* DU VIVIER, Daniel.

VIVO MORTO, ACCADEMICO DELLA CRUSCA, *tr.*
See REGIMEN SANITATIS SALERNITANUM. Scola Salernitana. 1630, 1662, 1666, 1677.

VLACQ, THEODOR [*fl.* 1616] *respondent. See*
VORSTIUS, A. E., *praeses.* These medicae de ictero.
1616.

VOCHETIUS, ANASTASIUS. *See* HILARIUS A
SANCTO ANASTASIO [*fl.* 1637]

VOCKERODT, BENJAMIN [*fl.* 1694] *respondent.*
Disputatio medica inauguralis, de diarrhoea . . .
Harderovici, Apud Albertum Sas, 1694.

[8] p.   19 cm.   **[12455]**

Diss. — Harderwijk.

VÖLCKER, DANIEL CHRISTOPH [*fl.* 1688] *respondent. See* PETRI VON HARTENFELS, G. C., *praeses.*
Disputatio inauguralis medica, de morbo comitiali.
1688.

VÖLTER, CHRISTOPH [1616 *or* 17–*ca.* 1682] Neu
eröffnete Heb-Ammen-Schuhl; oder, Nutzliche
Unterweisung christlicher Hebammen und Wehe-Müttern, wie solche sich vor- in- und nach der
Geburt bey Schwangern und Gebährenden, auch
sonst gebrächlichen Frauen zu verhalten haben.
Sambt beygesetztem Unterricht, wie todte Kinder,
die in Mutterleib abgestanden, ohne Gefahr
ausszuziehen . . . Stuttgart, In Verlegung Johann

Gottfriedt Zubrodt, gedruckt bey Paulus Trew, 1679.

[29], 328, [35] p.; 172, [3] p.   front., plates.   18
cm.   **[12456]**

Errata: p. [35]

Part [2] has half title: Christlicher Bericht . . . von den Heb-Ammen, deren Ahnnahm, Ampt, Ayd, Freyheiten, Besoldungen, und dergleichen.

—[The same.] . . . Anjetzo aber von neuem mit
Fleiss übersehen . . . verbessert, besonders mit einem
sehr nutzlichen Anhang, von der Hebammen Beruff
und Stand, vermehret . . . Stutgart, In Verlegung
Johann Gottfried Zubrods, gedruckt durch Melchior
Gerhard Lorbern, 1687.

[24], 448, 79, [29] p.   front., illus., plates.   17
cm.   **[12457]**

Imperfect: on p. 127, explanatory text of plate facing that page wanting; plate facing p. 291 wanting.

VOET, GIJSBERT [1589-1676] *See* DESCARTES, R.
Meditationes de prima philosophia. 1650; Variorum
tractatus theologici de peste. 1655.

VOGEL, CHRISTIAN ANDREAS [*fl.* 1671] *respondent.*
See DONAT, C., *praeses.* Dissertatio physica de somniis. 1671.

VOGEL, CHRISTOPH [*fl.* 1660] *respondent. See*
CALVISIUS, S. Theses physicae de sermone . . .
publicae proponit M. Sethus Calvisius, Jun. . . .
respondente Christophoro Vogelio. 1660.

VOGEL, CHRISTOPH [*d.* 1678] *praeses.* Theorema
geographicum de physica telluris rotunditate . . .
Jenae, Typis Johannis Nisii, 1658.

[20] p.   19 cm.   **[12458]**

Diss.—Jena (G. C. Eimmart, *respondent.*)

VOGEL, CORNELIUS DE [*fl.* 1662-1672] *respondent.*
See BLASIUS, G., *praeses.* Disputatio medica de peste,
prior [-posterior] 1663 [and] Exercitium anatomicum
de pulmone. 1662; SENGUERD, A., *praeses.* Disputatio
physica de peste. 1663.

VOGEL, DAVID [*fl.* 1695] *respondent. See* HELWICH,
C. Exercitatio academica. 1695.

VOGEL, EWALD. Liber de lapidis physici conditionibus [quo abditissimorum auctorum Gebri &
Raymundi Lullii methodica continetur explicatio]

527-648 p., vol. 3.   20 cm. (*In* Zetzner,
Lazarus, *ed.* Theatrum chemicum. Argentorati,
1659-61)   **[12459]**

Caption title, partly supplied from table of contents.

VOGEL, Hermann [*fl.* 1700] *respondent. See* Stahl, G. E., *praeses.* Dissertatio inauguralis medica de αδη-φαγια. 1700.

VOGEL, Johann Valentin [*fl.* 1700] *respondent. See* Hoffmann, F. [1660-1742] *praeses.* Dissertatio inauguralis medico-practica de podagra retrocedente. 1700.

VOGLER, Carl de. *See* Gogler, Carl von [17th cent.]

VOGLER, Johann Ehrenfried [*fl.* 1700] *respondent. See* Eysel, J. P., *praeses.* Disputatio inauguralis medica, sistens aegrum haemoptyseos malignae. 1700.

VOGLER, Valentin Heinrich [1622-1677] De rebus naturalibus ac medicis quarum in scripturis sacris fit mentio commentarius. Accessit ejusdem Physiologia historiae passionis Jesu Christi. Helmaestadii, Typis & sumptibus Georg-Wolfgangii Hammii, 1682.

 [24], 472, [6] p. 20 cm. **[12460]**
 Imperfect: part [2], the Physiologia, wanting.

—De valetudine hominis cognoscenda liber ... Helmestadii, Apud Henricum Davidem Mullerum, 1674.

 [1], 118, [24] p. 19 cm. **[12461]**

—Diaeteticorum commentariorum liber unus. Addita est ejusdem De vi imaginationis in pestilentia producenda perbrevis dissertatio. Helmestadii, Typis & sumtibus Henningi Mulleri, 1667.

 [12], 307, [35] p. 20 cm. **[12462]**

—Institutionum physiologicarum liber primus. Quo natura elementorum, mistionis, ac temperamenti dilucidatur. Helmestadii, Typis Henningi Mulleri, 1661.

 [4], 148 p. 20 cm. **[12463]**

—*praeses.* Disputatio medica de tussi ... Helmestadii, Typis Henningi Mülleri, 1667.

 [80] p. 20 cm. **[12464]**
 Diss.—Helmstedt (K. C. Mylius, *respondent*)

—Disputatio medica de venenis ... Helmestadii, Typis Henningi Mulleri, 1661.

 [88] p. 20 cm. **[12465]**
 Diss.—Helmstedt (J. H. Brechtfeld, *respondent*)

—Disputatio medica inauguralis de haemorrhagia narium ... Helmstadii, Typis Henrici Davidis

Mulleri, 1673.

 [48] p. 20 cm. **[12466]**
 Diss.—Helmstedt (J. T. Willerding, *respondent*)

—Dissertatio medica de pleuritide ... Helmestadii, Literis Jacobi Mülleri, 1669.

 [32] p. 20 cm. **[12467]**
 Diss.—Helmstedt (J. K. Axt, *respondent*)

—*respondent. See* Conring, H., *praeses.* De vertigine disputatio medica. 1650 [and] Delacte exercitatio physiologica. 1678.

VOGT, Gottfried. *See* Voigt, Gottfried [1644-1682]

VOGT, Johannes Casparus Ignatius. *See* Voigt, Johann Kaspar Ignaz [*fl.* 1678]

VOGT, Samuel [*fl.* 1659] *respondent. See* Schwenck, J. S., *praeses.* Disputatio philosophica exhibens metallographian generalem. 1659.

VOIGT, Gottfried [1644-1682] Curiositates physicae, de resuscitatione brutorum ex mortuis, resurrectione plantarum, cantione cycnea, congressu et partu viperarum, chamaeleontis victu, aliisque rebus jucundis raris novis, accurata methodo conscriptae ... Gustrovii, Prostat ap. Joach. Wilden, exscribebat Sceippelius, 1668.

 [8], 184, [8] p. 17 cm. **[12468]**

—*praeses.* Disputatio physica de amore ovis et lupi, quem sympathiam vocant ... Wittebergae, Typis Johannis Borckardi [1667]

 [16] p. 21 cm. **[12469]**
 Diss.—Wittenberg (P. H. Möhring, *respondent*)

—Disputatio physica prima de stillicidio sanguinis ex interemti hominis cadavere, praesente occisore ... Wittebergae, Typis Johannis Borckardi, 1667.

 [16] p. 19 cm. **[12470]**
 Diss.—Wittenberg (C. R. Cnuppius, *respondent*)

—*respondent. See* Faselt, C., *praeses.* Exercitatio physica. 1665.

VOIGT, Hartuicus [*fl.* 1700] *respondent. See* Dollmann, J. C., *praeses.* Acquae supra-caelestes quas ex principio domestico demonstratas. [1700]

VOIGT, Johann [*fl.* 1676-1681] *respondent. See* Sennert, M., *praeses.* Disputationem inauguralem de imbecileitate ventriculi ... exponit. J. V. 1676.

—*See* KUNCKEL, J. Chymischer Probier-Stein. 1686.

VOIGT, JOHANN KASPAR IGNAZ [*fl.* 1678] Tractatus medicus Galeno-chymicus, de passione seu affectione hypochondriaca, authoritatibus Galeni et Hippocratis suffulsus ... Pragae, Sumptibus authoris, typis Georgii Czernoch, 1678.
[104] p.   20 cm.   **[12471]**

VOITA, JOANNES IGNATIUS FRANCISCUS [*fl.* 1684] *respondent. See* DOBRZENSKY, J. J. W., *praeses.* Hippocrates redivivus. 1684.

VOLCAMERUS, JOANNES GEORGIUS. *See* VOLCKAMER, Johann Georg [1616–1693]

VOLCK, JOHANN [*fl.* 1642] *respondent. See* ROLFINCK, W., *praeses.* Disputatio medica de febre maligna. 1642.

VOLCKAMER, JOHANN GEORG [1616–1693] Opobalsami orientalis in theriaces confectionem Romae revocati examen, doctiorumque calculis approbati sinceritas ... Norimbergae, Typis Wolfgangi Enderi, 1644.
[6], 224, [8] p.   front.   13 cm.   **[12472]**
Bound with (as issued?) Colmenero de Ledesma, A. Chocolata inda. 1644.

—Oratio. *In* Galenus. [Selected works. Latin.] 1680.

—ed. Collegium anatomicum. Clarissimorum trium virorum Julii Jasolini ... Marci Aurelii Severini ... Bartholomaei Cabrolii ... per quos singulos collatae operae posteriore paginae facie patescent collect. & promot. Joanne Georgio Volcamero ... Hanoviae, Sumptibus Christophori Le-Blon, typis Joannis Aubry, 1654.
[6], 20 (i.e.68) p.; 54, [2] p.   plates.   23 cm.   **[12473]**
Cover title.
Part [2] has special title page: Marci Aurelii Severini Quaestiones anatomicae quatuor prima, De aqua pericardia. Secunda, De cordis adipe. Terria [sic], De poricsholidochis. Quarta, Osteologia pro Galeno adversus argutatores epidochae in totidem alias Julii Jasolini.
Bound with copy 2 of Severino, M. A. De recondita abscessum natura. 1643.

—, *ed. See* COLMENERO DE LEDESMA A. Chocolata inda. 1644; SEVERINO, M. A. Zootomia democritaea. 1645.

—*See* HOFMANN, C. Vita medica, hoc est Galeni ὑγιεινῶν. 1680; *See* STURM, J. C. Epistola ... ad Joh. Georgium Volckamerum. 1684.

VOLCKAMER, JOHANN GEORG [1662–1744] *respondent.* Dissertatio medica inauguralis de lethargo ... Altdorffii, Typis Henrici Meyeri [1684]
24 p.   20 cm.   **[12474]**
Diss.—Altdorf.

VOLDER, BURCHARDUS DE [1643–1709] *respondent.* Disputatio medica inauguralis de natura ... Lugduni Batavorum, Apud Severinum Matthiae, 1664.
[24] p.   18 cm.   **[12475]**
Diss.—Leyden.

VOLDER, BURCHER DE. *See* VOLDER, Burchardus de [1643–1709]

VOLKAMER. *See* VOLCKAMER.

VOLLAND, JOHANN ANDREAS [*fl.* 1678] *respondent. See* STURM, J. C., *praeses.* Oculus Θεοσκόπος; h. e. De visionis organo et ratione genuina, dissertatio physica. 1678.

VOLLAND, JOHANN JONAS [*b.* 1665] *respondent. See* CRAUSE, R. W., *praeses.* Disputatio inauguralis medica de tinnitu aurium. 1694.

VOLLANDT, JOHANN JONAS. *See* VOLLAND, Johann Jonas [*b.* 1665]

VOLLGNAD, HEINRICH [1634–1682] *respondent. See* SENNERT, M., *praeses.* Hemicraniam ... publicae ... disquisitioni submittit H. V. 1662.

VOLLHARDT, JOHANN JEREMIAS [*fl.* 1654] *respondent.* Disputatio medica inauguralis de melancholia ... Argentorati, Typis Eberhardi Welperi, 1654.
23 p.   19 cm.   **[12476]**
Diss.—Strasbourg.

Der VOLLKOMMENE und wolerfahrne Wundarzt; oder, Gründliche Erörterung aller und jeder chyrurgischen Fragen ... des gantzen menschlichen Leibes ... Aus der holländischen Sprach in Teutsch übergesetzet. Minden, Verlegts Johann Heudorn, 1687.
[12], 212, [13] p.   17 cm.   **[12477]**
Bound with copy 2 of Purmann, M. G. Kurtze, doch gründliche Anweisung. 1686.

VOLPINO, Giovanni Battista [1644–*ca.* 1722] Haemophobiae triumphus; sive, Erasistratus vindicatus. Ubi veterum phlebotomiae scopi ad trutinam revocantur ... Lugduni, Typis Benedicti Vignieu, 1697.

[37], 155 p. front. (port.) 16 cm. **[12478]**

VON DER PESTILENTZ, zwei kurtze Tracätlin, deren das eine begreifft einen Bericht, was für Artzneyen man zur Zeit der Pestilentz nutzlich gebrauchen könne. Das ander: Zwo Predigen ... Sampt einer nutzlichen Vorred. Zürych, Joh. Jacob Bodmer, 1629.

[24], 143 p. 16 cm. **[12479]**

"Kurtzer Bericht von der Pestilentz": p. 1–42. "Medicamenta contra pestem": p. 43–55.
The "Vorred" is by Johann Jacob Breitinger.

VON gemeiner Hauss-Artzney. *See* Hauss Apoteck. 1613; Ein nutzliches Hand-Büchlein. 1684.

VON KEIL, Andreas. *See* Keil, Andreas von [*fl.* 1665–1688]

VOORD VAN DUVERDEN, Johan van. *See* Duverden van Voord, Johan van.

VOORDE, Cornelis van de [*ca.* 1630–1678] Lichtende fakkel der cheirurgia, onsteken ten profijte van alle die gene welke genegen zijn de heel-konst ... in haar volkomen perfectie te leeren, gestelt by vrage, en antwoorde. Verdeeld in drie deelen ... Hier achter is by-gevoeght, de Chirurgijns scheepskist, zijnde een catalogus ofte lijste der medicamenten, die yder chirurgijn naer Oost of West-Indien gemeenlijk mede voert ... door J. V. B. [i.e. Johannes Verbruge] ... Amsterdam, By Jacob Vinckel [Gedruckt by Jacob van Velsen] 1668.

[24], 603, [5], 31 p. port. 22 cm. **[12480]**

The Chirurgyns scheeps-kist (31 p.) has special title page.

—[The same.] Nieuw lichtende fakkel der chirurgie of hedendaagze heel-konst ... Nu in dezen laatsten druk ... verbeterd en vermeerderd ... door Antonius de Heyde ... Verrijkt met een Chirurgijns of heel-meesters zee-compas ... Middelburg, Wilhelmus Goeree, 1680.

[12], 797, [19] p. 25 cm. **[12481]**

Imperfect: p. 581–582 (blank?) wanting.
"Chirurgijns zee-compas verdeeld in XVI streken ... door Cornelis vande Voorde ... Middelburg ... 1679" (p. [583]–797) has special title page.

VOORHOFF, Seger [*fl.* 1698] *respondent. See* Senguerdius, W., *praeses.* Exercitium experimentale septimum decimum. 1698.

[**VOORN,** Jacob] Catalogus antiquarum et novarum rerum ex longe dissitis terrarum oris quarum visendarum copia Lugduni in Batavis in anatomia publica ... Lugduni Batavorum, Apud Jacobum Voorn [1690?]

14, [2] p. 19 cm. **[12482]**

In his prefatory epistle Voorn takes credit for the authorship.
The text is generally similar to, and some pages agree word for word with, Gerardus Blancken's work of the same title published in 1700.

VOPEL, Johann Tobias [*fl.* 1697] *respondent. See* Schwedler, J. C., *praeses.* Dissertatio praeliminaris de naturali hominis oeconomia. 1697.

VORST, Johannes [1623–1676] De generatione animantium conjectura, observationi cuidam Harveanae, ne vetus pervulgataque omnium gentium opinio per hanc concidat, submissa a Jano Orchamo [pseud.] Coloniae Brandenburgicae, Typis Georgii Schultzii, 1667.

58, [1] p. 14 cm. **[12483]**
Errata: p. [1]

VORSTELICK geschenck; dat is, Een medecynboeck, inhoudende vele ... medecijnstucken, om veelerhande sieckten ende gebreken des lichaems, te genesen ... Amstelredam, Johannes van Ravesteyn, 1662.

206, [8] p. 16 cm. **[12484]**
Previously published in 1621 and 1628.

VORSTER, Franz Sebastian [1666–1738] *respondent.* Experimenta de pleuro peri pneumonia epidemica cum polypo cordis ... Basileae, Typis Jacobi Bertschii [1689]

[24] p. 19 cm. **[12485]**
Diss. — Basel.
With this is bound Harder, J. J. Alexander Pfisterus. [1689]

—*respondent. See* Brunner, J. C., *praeses.* Exercitatio anatomica de glandula pituitaria. 1688.

—*See* Harder, J. J. Alexander Pfisterus. 1689.

VORSTIUS, Adolph [1597–1663] *praeses.* Aphorismorum Hippocrateorum decades duae ... Lugduni Batavorum, Apud Johannem Elsevirium, 1659.

[7] p. 19 cm. **[12486]**
Diss. — Leyden (Z. Ennichman, *respondent*)

—, *ed.* and *tr.* *See* HIPPOCRATES. [Aphorismi. Greek and Latin.] 1628.

—, *ed.* *See* BÈZE, T. de. De pestis contagio & fuga dissertatio. 1636; HIPPOCRATES. [Aphorismi. Greek and Latin.] 1661.

—, *tr.* *See* LORENZ, G. F. Georgii-Friderici Laurentii Exercitationum in non nullos minus absolute veros Hippocratis Aphorismos. 1647.

—, *See* HIPPOCRATES. [Aphorismi. Latin.] 1639, 1681; TILEMANN, J. Aphorismi Hippocratis. 1650, 1660.

VORSTIUS, AELIUS EVERHARDUS [1565–1624] Oratio funebris in obitum ... Caroli Clusii ..: Accesserunt variorum epicedia. [Lugduni Batavorum] In Officina Plantiniana Raphelengii, 1611.

   39 p. 23 cm.   [**12487**]

   Published also as part [2] of L'Écluse, Charles. Curae posteriores. 1611.

Dissertations — Leyden

—*praeses.* Disputatio medica de apoplexia ... Lugduni Batavorum, Ex officina Zachariae Smetii, 1621.

   [8] p. 21 cm.   [**12488**]

   Benedicto de Castro, *respondent.*

—Disputatio medica de crisibus et diebus decretoriis ... Lugduni Batavorum, Ex officina Jacobi Patii, 1616.

   [8] p. 20 cm.   [**12489**]

   G. Bruno, *respondent.*

—Disputatio medica de regio morbo ... Lugduni Batavorum, Ex officina Zachariae Smetii, 1621.

   [8] p. 20 cm.   [**12490**]

   A. Andla, *respondent.*

—Theses medicae de convulsione ... Lugduni Batavorum, Ex officina Zachariae Smetii, 1621.

   [8] p. 21 cm.   [**12491**]

   C. Rosaeus, *respondent.*

—Theses medicae de convulsione quarum patrocinium volente ... Lugduni Batavorum, Ex officina Jacobi Patii, 1616.

   [8] p. 21 cm.   [**12492**]

   Philippus a Gennip, *respondent.*

—Theses medicae de ictero ... Lugduni Batavorum, Excudebat Godefridus Basson, 1616.

   [12] p. 20 cm.   [**12493**]

   T. Vlacq, *respondent.*

—Theses medicae de melancholia ... Lugduni Batavorum, Ex officina Zachariae Smetii, 1621.

   [8] p. 20 cm.   [**12494**]

   J. Le Piper, *respondent.*

—Theses medicae de natura morbi ... Lugduni Batavorum, Godefridus Basson, 1616.

   [12] p. 20 cm.   [**12495**]

   D. Danius, *respondent.*

VORSTIUS, EVERHARDUS. *See* VORSTIUS, Aelius Everhardus [1565–1624]

Der VORTREFFLICHE Tractat und Hauptschlüssel aller Hermetischen Schrifften genannt. 1676. *See* [PHILALETHES, E.]

VOS, ABRAHAM LENERTSZ. *See* VROLINGH, Abraham Lenertsz [*fl.* 1621–1646]

VOSSIUS, ISAAC [1618–1689] De lucis natura et proprietate ... Amstelodami, Apud Ludovicum & Danielem Elzevirios, 1662.

   [8], 85, [2] p. illus. 20 cm.   [**12496**]

—De motu marium et ventorum liber. Hagae-Comitis, Ex typographia Adriani Vlacq, 1663.

   [12], 123 p. 22 cm.   [**12497**]

   With this is bound *his* Observationum ad Pomp. Melam appendix. 1686.

—Observationum ad Pomp. Melam appendix. Accedit ejusdem ad tertias P. Simonii objectiones responsio. Subjungitur Pauli Colomesii ad Henricum Justellum epistola. Londini, Prostant apud Robertum Scott, 1686.

   [1], 136, [1] p. 22 cm.   [**12498**]

   Errata: p. [137]
   Bound with *his* De motu marium. 1663.

—Variarum observationum liber. Londini, Prostant apud Robertum Scott, 1685.

   [6], 397, [1] p. illus. 23 cm.   [**12499**]

   Errata misbound at end.

—*See* BRUYN, J. de. Epistola ad ... Isaacum Vossium. 1663; PLINIUS SECUNDUS, C. Naturalis historiae, tomus primus [-tertius] 1668–1669.

VOTA amicorum, ad ... Joh. Kisnerum, cum post habitam de suffocatione hypochondriaca disputationem eruditissimam summo cum auditorum applausu gradum doctoratus consequeretur, decantata ... Lugduni Batavorum, Apud viduam & haeredes Joannis Elsevirii, 1670.

[8] p. 23 cm. **[12500]**

VOTIVI applausus amicorum in honorem eximii ... Dn. Pauli Edingh, cum in inclyta Gelro-Zutphanica, quae est Hardervici, Academia, publice declararetur medicinae doctor ... Harderovici, Apud Albertum Sas, 1683.

[8] p. 18 cm. **[12501]**

VRANCKHEIM, MARCELL [*fl.* 1612] Ἐπίκρισις σοχαστικη. *In* Burggrav, J. E. Achilles πανοπλος redivivus. 1612.

VRAYE et parfaicte chyromancie et phisionomis. 1620. *See* [INDAGINE, J. ab]

VREESWYK, GOOSSEN VAN [1626–*ca.* 1689] Het cabinet der mineralen, metalen, en berg-eerts; hare gangen, en natuur; ook wat instrumenten daer toe behooren, om in vremde gewesten te gebruiken. Hier is noch by-gevoegt een uitlegging over de onderste deelen van de tafel Hermetis ... Amsterdam, Joannes Janssonius van Waesberge, 1670.

[8], 56 p. illus. 16 cm. **[12502]**

With this is bound *his* Vervolg van 't cabinet der mineralen. 1675.

—Silvere rivier; ofte, Konings fontein. Waar-in ontdekt worden veele notable medicijnen der oude philosophen; ook van't sout en ♃ der metalen, ende wat voor krachten der medicijnen daar-in verborgen zijn; als mede het leven en de dood vande metalen en mineralen, haar verwen en tinctuur ... 's Gravenhage, Pieter Haagen, 1684.

[24], 132, [12] p. 16 cm. **[12503]**

—Vervolg van 't cabinet der mineralen, of de goude son der philsophen; waer in alle bewerckingen der metalen en mineralen, met de gereedschappen daer toe dienende, hare openingen, verwen, en tincturen, nevens verscheide heerlijke medicijnen ... aen 't licht gegeven ... Amsterdam, Gedruckt voor den autheur, zijn mede te bekomen by Johannes Janssonius van Waesberge, 1675.

[16], 325 (i.e. 225), [14] p. illus. 16 cm. **[12504]**

Added illustrated title page.
Imperfect: p. 325 wanting; supplied in photocopy.
Bound with *his* Het cabinet der mineralen. 1670.

VRIES, BAUKE CLAASES DE. Nuttelyke consideratien of sedige aanmerkingen over het heedendaags tabak-suigen ... als ook eenige aanmerkingen tegen verscheide stellingen, vervat in het tractaat ... door J. J. W. Beintema van Peyma M. D. [pseud., i.e. Johan Ignaz Worb] tot lof van den tabak, voerende den tijtul Tabacologia ... Hier aan volgen dan noch ook verscheide maat-gedichten over aanmerkelijke saken. Alles door B. C. de Vries ... Amsterdam, Gedrukt by Cornelis van Hoogenhuisen en zijn te bokomen by Jacobus van Nieuwenveen, 1692.

[32], 280, [16] p. 19 cm. **[12505]**

VRIES, WILLEM VAN [*fl.* 1666] *respondent.* Disputatio medica inauguralis, de dysenteria ... Ultrajecti, Ex officina Johannis à Sambix, 1666.

[8] p. 20 cm. **[12506]**

Diss.—Utrecht.

VRIESE, JAN PAUWELSZOON. *See* PAUWELSZOON, Jan.

VROLINGH, ABRAHAM LENERTSZ [*fl.* 1621–1646] Der matroosen ghestontheydt; ofte, De goede dispositie der zee-varende luyden. Waer in ghehandelt wordt nevens andere siechten, den matroosen ghemeen: vande aerdt, nature en eyghenschap des scheurbuycks: anders schimmelsieckte ghenaemt ... Zaerdam, By Heyndrick Jacobsz [Ghedruckt by Symon Cornelisz tot Alckmaer, 1646]

[4], 211, [16] p. 15 cm. **[12507]**

Imperfect: title page mutilated; sig. A3–? (of the unnumbered leaves) wanting.

—[The same.] Matroosen gesontheyt; of, Goede dispositie der zee-varende lieden, handelende van veelderley siechten en gebreken der menschen in 't gemeen: maer bysonderlijck van de scheurbuyck of schimmel-siechte, den zee-lieden meest onderworpen ... Vermeerdert met Putmans manuael ... Amsterdam, Michiel de Groot, 1680.

[8], 230, [2] p.; 76, [2 +] p. 15 cm. **[12508]**

Imperfect: all after p. [78] at end wanting.
The Putmans manuael has special title page.

—, *ed. See* PUTMAN, E. Puthmans manuael. 1646?

VROMANS, PIETER [*fl.* 1695] *respondent.* Disputatio philologico-medica inauguralis de balneis ... Lugduni Batavorum, Apud Abrahamum Elzevier, 1695.

[15] p. 22 cm. **[12509]**

Diss.—Leyden.

VROOM, Joachim [*fl.* 1669] *respondent*. Disputatio medica inauguralis de fluore albo … Lugduni Batavorum, Apud viduam & haeredes Joannis Elsevirii, 1669.

[12] p. 23 cm. **[12510]**
Diss.—Leyden.

VRY, Sebastian Egbertszoon de [1563-1621] *ed. See* Dodoens, R. *In* D. Remberti Dodonaei Praxin artis medicae scholia. 1640 [and] Praxis medica. 1616.

VUECKERUS, Joannes Jacobus. *See* Wecker, Johann Jakob [1528-1586]

VULPINUS, Joannes Baptista. *See* Volpino, Giovanni Battista [1644-*ca.* 1722]

VULPIUS, Johannes Christophorus [*fl.* 1686] *respondent. See* Posner, C., *praeses.* Disputatio physica de ignibus lambentibus. 1686.

VULSON, Marc, *sieur de La Colombière. See* Vulson de la Colombière, Marc [*d.* 1658]

VULSON DE LA COLOMBIÈRE, Marc [*d.* 1658] Le palais des curieux, ou, l'algebre et le sort donnent la decision des questions les plus douteuses: et ou les songes et les visions nocturnes sont expliquez selon la doctrine des anciens. 2. ed., rev., corr., & augm. d'un Traité de la physiognomie. Imprimé à Orleans, & se vend a Paris, Pierre Lamy, 1660.

[15], 52, [2] p.; 120 (i.e. 210), [4] p.; 168 p. 18 cm. **[12511]**
Parts [2] and [3] have special title pages.

VULTEJUS, Justus Hermann [1654-1701] *respondent. See* Posner, C., *praeses.* Diatribe academica de longaevitate hominum. 1673.

VUOLPHIUS, Casparus. *See* Wolf, Caspar [1532-1601]

VUSON, Marc, *sieur de la Colombière. See* Vulson de la Colombière, Marc [*d.* 1658]

W

W., B. *See* Wells, Benjamin [1616?-1678]

W., D. *See* Waldschmidt, Johann Jakob [1644-1689]

W., G. H., *med. doct., tr. See* Blankaart, S. Neuscheinende Praxis der Medicinae. 1700.

W., I., *tr. See* Guibert, P. The charitable physitian with The charitable apothecary. 1639.

W., J. [17th cent.] *tr. See* Basilius Valentinus. The last will and testament. 1671; Muys, J. A rational practice of chyrurgery. 1686; Tachenius, O. Otto Tachenius *his* Hippocrates chymicus. 1677, 1690.

W., O., *professour in physick and chirurgery. See* Wood, Owen.

W., T. *See* Wright, Thomas, D. D.

W., T., *master of arts. See* Walkington, Thomas [*d.* 1621]

W., V. W. *See* Waldschmidt, Wilhelm Ulrich [1669-1731]

W., W. *See* Walwyn, William [*fl.* 1667-1696]

W., W., *philosophus, student in the coelestial sciences. See* Williams, William, *astrologer.*

W., W., *surgeon. See* Novum lumen chirurgicum extinctum. 1695.

Wr., Th. *See* Wright, Thomas, D. D.

W. I. *See* I., W.

W. M. *See* M., W.

W. R. *See* Rand, William [*fl.* 1656]

WAAS, Hendrik Hieronymus [*fl.* 1684] *respondent.* Disputatio medica inauguralis de hydrope ascite … Franequerae, Apud Johannem Gyselaar, 1684.

8 p. 21 cm. **[12512]**
Diss. — Franeker.

WACHENDORF, *tr. See* Blankaart, S. Die belägert-und entsetzte Venus. 1689.

WACHSMUTH, Tobias [*fl.* 1655] *respondent. See* Siegfried, C. E. [*fl.* 1655-1681], *praeses.* De mari ejusque salsedine. 1655.

WACHTEL, Joachim Friedrich [*fl.* 1698-1710] *respondent. See* Werckmeister, F. H., *praeses.* Dissertatio medica filum Ariadneum in studio medico. 1698.

WACHTEL, Johann Christoph [*fl.* 1697-1702] *respondent. See* Eysel, J. P., *praeses.* Exercitatio medica de pleuritide. 1697; FASCH, A. H., *praeses*. Disputatio inauguralis medica exhibens mulierem melancholia hypochondriaca loborantem. 1674.

WACHTEL, JUSTIN [*fl.* 1700] *respondent. See* ADOLPHI, C. M. Specimen physicum. [1700]

WACHTER, GEORG [*fl.* 1672] *respondent. See* MÖGLING, J. L. [*fl.* 1662-1685] *praeses*. Vigilia. 1672.

WACHTER, JACOB [*fl.* 1671] *respondent. See* METZGER, G. B., *praeses*. Disputatio inauguralis medica. 1671.

WADSWORTH, THOMAS [*d.* 1733] *respondent*. Theses medicae inaugurales de secretionibus in genere ... Lugduni Batavorum, Apud Abrahamum Elzevier, 1699.

　[12] p. 24 cm. **[12513]**
Diss. — Leyden.

WÄCHTLER, CHRISTOPH JAKOB [*fl.* 1691] *respondent*. Verisimilia de stellis novis ... ostendunt ac defendunt M. Christophorus Jacobus Wächtler ... & Godofredus Günzius ... Vitembergae, Literis viduae Matthaei Henckelii [1691]

　[16] p. 19 cm. **[12514]**
Diss. — Wittenberg (G. Günz, *respondent*)

—*See* RÖHRENSEE, C., *praeses*. Propositas theses physicas defendendas suscipit M. Christoph. Jacobus Wächtler, 1691.

WAECHTLER, JOHANN CONRAD. *See* WECHTLER, Johann Conrad [*fl.* 1656-1659]

WAEIJEN, JOHAN. *See* WAEYEN, Johannes van der [1639-1701]

WAERSCHOUWINGE wegens het verkopen van arsenicum ofte rotte-kruyt. 1670. *See* UTRECHT. Ordinances, local laws, etc.

WAERT, ADRIAAN VAN [*fl.* 1669] *respondent*. Disputatio medica inauguralis de phthisi ... Lugduni Batavorum, Apud viduam & haeredes Joannis Elsevirii, 1669.

　[8] p. 23 cm. **[12515]**
Diss. — Leyden.

WAEYEN, JOHANNES VAN DER [1639-1701] *See* [ANDALA, R.] Uiterste verleegentheid van Doctor Balt. Bekker. 1696; BEKKER, B. Brief ... aan den ... prinsse Hendrik Kasimyr. 1693 [and] En insonderheyd syner voedsterlingen onkunde. 1696.

WAEYEN, OTTO VAN DER [*fl.* 1674] *respondent*. Disputatio medica inauguralis de pleuritide ... Ultrajecti, Ex officina Meinardi a Dreunen, 1674.

　[14] p. 24 cm. **[12516]**
Diss. — Utrecht.

WAFER, LIONEL [1660?-1705] A new voyage and description of the Isthmus of America, giving an account of the author's abode there ... The Indian inhabitants, their features ... customs ... With remarkable occurrences in the South Sea ... London, James Knapton, 1699.

　[8], 224, [16] p. plates. 18 cm. **[12517]**

WAGENISIUS, MELCHIOR ERNST. *See* WAGNITZ, Melchior Ernst [*fl.* 1693-1702]

WAGENSEIL, JOHANN CHRISTOPH [1633-1705] Belehrung der jüdisch-teutschen Red- und Schreibart ... Unter andern jüdischen Büchern, wird dargestellet ... Das talmudische Buch von dem Aussatz ... Zur Zugabe ... ein Bedencken ... ob die Heil. Schrifft einem Mann erlaube zwey Schwestern nacheinander zu heyrathen ... Königsberg, Paul Friedrich Rhode, 1699.

　[82], 334, 56, [3] p. plates., port. 21 cm.
　[12518]
Das talmudische Buch von dem Aussatz (Mishna: Tohoroth Nega'im) is in Hebrew and German in parallel columns, p. 1-80.

—Exercitationes sex varii argumenti ... Ed. alt. Altdorfii Noricorum, Jodocus Wilhelmus Kolesius excudit, 1697.

　[8], 244 p. illus. 21 cm. **[12519]**
Exercitationes 2-4 and 6 are in Hebrew and Latin in parallel columns.

WAGNER, CHRISTIAN HEINRICH [*fl.* 1649] *respondent. See* LEICHNER, E., *praeses*. De calibo innato exercitatio II. 1649.

WAGNER, GEORG [1630-1683] *praeses*. Problematum physicorum senarius de margaritis ... subjicit Joachimus Schmid ... Wittebergae, Typis Johannis Borckardi, 1667.

　[16] p. 20 cm. **[12520]**
Diss. — Wittenberg (J. Schmid, *respondent*)

WAGNER, JOHANN [*fl.* 1697] *respondent*. Exegesis medico-inauguralis casus synochi putridae ... Basileae, Literis Jacobi Bertschii [1697]

　[14 + ?] p. 19 cm. **[12521]**
Imperfect: last leaf (blank?) wanting.
Diss. — Basel.

WAGNER, Johann Erhard [*fl.* 1690] *respondent.* See Camerarius, R. J., *praeses.* Continuatio tentaminum circa lignum nephriticum. 1690.

WAGNER, Johann Georg [*fl.* 1698] *respondent. See* Vesti, J., *praeses.* Dissertatio medica inauguralis, de apoplexia. 1698.

WAGNER, Matthaeus [*fl.* 1632-1634] *respondent. See* Sebisch, M., [1578-1674?] *praeses.* Exercitationes medicae. 1639 [and] Galeni Ars parva in disputationes triginta resoluta. 1633.

WAGNER, Michael [*fl.* 1663-1667] *praeses.* Disputatio medica de colica ... Herbipoli, Ex officina typographica Jobi Hertzii, 1663.

    [22] p.   20 cm.   **[12522]**
    Diss. — Würzburg (J. P. Zinck, *respondent*)

WAGNER, Paul [*fl.* 1615] *respondent.* Disputatio inauguralis medica de haemorrhoidibus ... Basileae, Typis Joh. Jacobi Genathii, 1615.

    [36] p.   22 cm.   **[12523]**
    Diss. — Basel.

—*See* Burser, J., *praeses.* Assertiones medicae de phlegmone renum & vesicae. 1615.

WAGNER, Reinhold [*fl.* 1694-1695] *respondent. See* Bartholin, C. [1655-1738], *praeses.* Dissertatio inauguralis chirurgico-medica de meliceria Celsi sive synovia. 1695; Gottsched, J., *praeses.* Dissertatio physiologica de motu musculorum. 1694.

WAGNER, Wolffgang Ernest [*fl.* 1698] *respondent.* Specimen inaugurale medicum de oculo ... [Altdorffii] Literis Henrici Meyeri [1698]

    28 p.   plate.   20 cm.   **[12524]**
    Diss. — Altdorf.

WAGNITZ, Melchior Ernst [*fl.* 1693-1702] *respondent.* Dissertatio inauguralis medica de hemicrania ... [Altdorffii] Literis Henrici Meyeri [1697]

    20 p.   20 cm.   **[12525]**
    Diss. — Altdorf.

WAHRMUND, Ursinus. *See* Gohl, Johann Daniel [1674-1731]

WALAEUS, Johannes [1604-1649] Medica omnia, (quae hactenus inveniri potuere,) ad chyli & sanguinis circulationem eleganter concinnata ... In lucem nunc primum proferre voluit C. Irvinus ...

Londini, Excudebat J. C. & prostant venales apud T. Davies & T. Sadler, 1660.

    [16], 288 p.   19 cm.   **[12526]**
    Imperfect: title page mutilated.

—Epistolae duae de motu chyli et sanguinis. In Bartholin, C. [1585-1629] Institutiones anatomicae. 1641, 1645; [French tr.] 1647; Bartholin, T. Anatomia. 1651, 1655, 1660, 1663, 1666, 1669,1674, 1677, 1684, 1686; — [Dutch tr.]: 1653, 1656, 1658, 1669, 1688; [English tr.] 1665, 1668; [German tr.] 1677; Harvey, W. De motu cordis. 1643, 1660; Recentiorum disceptationes de motu cordis. 1647; Riolan, J. [1580-1657] Opera anatomica vetera. 1650 [and] Opuscula anatomica nova. 1649; Spiegel, A. van de. Opera quae extant, omnia. 1645.

—[Dutch tr.] Twee brieven van de beweginge des chyls ende des bloeds ... Nu eerst uit het Latijn vertaalt, door N. van Assendelft. Amstelredam, van Cornelis Last [Gedrukt by Adriaan Roest] 1650.

    62, 24 p.   16 cm.   **[12528]**
    "Beschrijvinge der melk-aderen, van Asellius": p. 21-24 at end. Bound with Harvey, W. Vande beweging van 't hert. 1650.

—Methodus medendi brevissima, ad circulationem saguinis adornata, ac ante annos XII. in academia, quae Lugduni Batavorum est, studiosae juventuti privatim praelecta ... Ulmae, Typis & impensis Balthas. Kühnen, 1660.

    172, [8] p.   14 cm.   **[12529]**

—[The same.] ... Georg. Hieronymi Welschii ... animadversionibus illustrata. Augustae Vindelicorum, Impensis Theophili Goebelii, typis Koppmayerianis, 1679.

    [10 + ?], 348, [25] p.   14 cm.   **[12530]**
    Imperfect: first preliminary leaf (blank?) wanting; last leaf misbound before p. 1.

—*praeses.* Disputatio medica de circulatione naturali seu cordis & sanguinis motu circulari. Pro Cl. Harveio ... Lugduni Batavorum, Ex officina Wilhelmi Christiani, 1640.

    [18] p.   19 cm.   **[12531]**
    Diss. — Leyden (R. Drake, *respondent*)

—[The same.] Theses de circulatione naturali, seu cordis & sanguinis motu circulari. Pro Cl. Harveio ...

    14 p.   20 cm.   (Part [2] in Recentiorum disceptationes de motu cordis. Lugduni Batavorum, 1647)
                                     [12532]

Caption title.

Diss. — Leyden, 1640 (R. Drake, *respondent*)

—Disputatio medica de phthisi ... Lugduni Batavorum, Apud Franciscum Moiardum, 1646.

[8] p.   20 cm.   [12533]

Diss. — Leyden (J. à Tetterode, *respondent*)

WALCH, HIERONYMUS [*fl.* 17th cent.] Kurtze Beschreibung der Bergsäffte und Tugenden dess heilsamen und berühmten Sawer-Brunnens, bey der Stadt Göppingen ... sampt einem ... Begriff etlicher gelehrten Leute hiervon, zu unterschiedlichen Zeiten, in Druck aussgegangener Meinungen, verfertigt ... Nürnberg, Michael Endter, 1644.

[31] p.   16 cm.   [12534]

Imperfect: upper margins of p. [7] and [25] trimmed.

WALCH, JOHANN. *See* Grasshoff, Johann [*d.* 1623]

WALD, GEORG AM [*fl.* 1580-1596] Gemehrter Bericht, wie und was Gestalt die new erfundne ... Terra Sigillata ... wider die Pestilentz ... und viel andere schwere Kranckheiten ... zu gebrauchen sey ... Zu Stutgarten, Getruckt durch Marx Fürstern, 1601.

[4], 72, [3] p.   20 cm.   [12535]

Imperfect: p. 65-66 mutilated.

WALDBURGER, DIETRICH GEBHARD [*fl.* 1670-1674] *respondent. See* ROLFINCK, W., *praeses.* Non ens chimicum. 1670.

WALDMANN, DANIEL. *See* GEIGER, Daniel [1595-1664]

WALDSCHMIDT, Johann Jakob [1644-1689] Opera medico-practica, quibus continentur I. Institutiones medicinae rationalis ... II. Praxis medicinae rationalis succincta, per casus tradita. III. Monita medico-practica necessaria ... IV. Notae ad praxin chirurgicam Barbettae. V. Notae ad casus Baldas. Timaei a Guldenklee. VI. Disputationes medicae varii argumenit [sic]. VII. Decas epistolarum de rebus medicis & philosophicis. Omnia ad mentem Cartesii. Francofurti ad Moenum, Sumptibus Friederici Knochii, 1695.

[7], 652, [16] p.; 354, [6] p.; 268 p.   22 cm.
                                                  [12536]

Added engraved title page.

Part [2] has caption title: Disputationes medicae varii argumenti.

Part [3] has special title page: Joh. Jacobi Waldschmidt ... et

Johannis Dolaei ... Ἐπιστολαι αμοιβαιαι, sive; Dissertationes epistolicae de rubus medicis & philosophicis ... 1689. This part includes: Thee domi militiaeque valetudinis custos ... Vorgestellet von D. W. (with half title, p. 181) and Decas epistolarum de rubus medicis et philosophicis ... 1689 (with special title page, p. [245]).

—Anchora salutis pro variolosis. Offenbarung ... eines gewissen ... Medicaments, nicht allein die Kinder vor denen also genannten Kinds-Pocken oder Blattern damit zu praeserviren, sondern auch selbige gantz sicher zu curiren. Worbey zugleich der rechte Grund der Artzney-Kunst aus der also gennannten Cartesianischen Philosophie gezeiget, und der Thée-Tranck von denen falschen ... Imputationibus freygeschprochen wird ... Geschrieben von D[octor] W[aldschmidt] Franckfurt am Mayn, Zufinden bey Friedrich Knochen, 1689.

24 p.   20 cm.   [12537]

—Commercium literarium virorum ... Joh. Jacobi Waldschmidii ... et ... Joh. Dolaei ... Lugd. Batav., Apud Petrum vander Aa, 1688.

[3], 159 p.   13 cm.   [12538]

Each Epistola has special title page.

—Dissertationes epistolicae de rubus medicis et philosophicis. *In* Doläus, J. Encyclopaedia chirurgica rationalis. 1695.

—Fundamenta medicinae, ad mentem neotericorum delineata. Lugd. Batavorum, Apud Adrianum Marston, 1685.

[16], 199 p.   16 cm.   [12539]

—Institutiones medicinae rationalis, recentiorum theoriae & praxi accommodatae. Marburgi, Sumpt. Friderici Knochii, typis Joh . Henrici Stockii, 1688.

[36], 245 (i.e. 345) p.   15 cm.   [12540]

—[The same.] ... Lugduni Batavorum, Apud Fredericum Haaring, 1689.

[16], 252, [2] p.   17 cm.   [12541]

—[The same.] ... Ed. 4 ... corr. Lugduni Batavorum, Apud Fredericum Haaring, M.DC.LXCI [1691?]

[16], 237, [3] p.   17 cm.   [12542]

[—Monita medica de morbis chronicis. English] Advice to a physician: containing particular directions relating to the cure of most diseases. With reflections on the nature and uses of the most celebrated remedies . . . Done from the Latin. London, H. Newman, 1695.

[5], 116 p. 15 cm. [12543]

Imperfect: front. (port.) wanting; supplied in photocopy; title page mutilated.

Edited by Wilhelm Ulrich Waldschmidt.

—Praxis medicinae rationalis succincta, per casus tradita, et in appendice Monitis medico-practicis necessariis illustrata per plurimos morbos. Quibus accesserunt notae ejusdem ad praxin chirurgicam Barbette; nec non ad casus Baldas. Timaei a Güldenklee. Omnia ad mentem Cartesii. Cum praefatione Johannis Dolaei . . . Francofurti, Sumpt. Friderici Knochii, 1690.

[16], 1140, [29] p. illus. 19 cm. [11544]

Edited by Wilhelm Ulrich Waldschmidt.

—[The same.] . . . Parisiis, Sumptibus Societatis, 1691.

[12], 874, [19] p. 16 cm. [12545]

Added engraved title page.

Edited by Wilhelm Ulrich Waldschmidt.

—Vade mecum Waldschmidianum; hoc est, Institutiones medicinae rationalis . . . per quaestiones ac responsiones sub forma tabellarum ita distincta . . . conscriptae ab H. H. S. I. C. Francofurti ad Moenum, Sumptibus Friderici Knochii, 1696.

[8], 370, [19] p. 17 cm. [12546]

Dissertations — Marburg

—praeses. Astrologus medicus, catarrhorum theoriae et praxi astrorum vim et influxum in microcosmum . . . exhibens . . . Marpurgi Cattorum, Typis Johannis Jodoci Kürsneri, 1681.

[2], 22 p. 18 cm. [12547]

Imperfect: lower margin trimmed with loss of date; date supplied from B. M. C.

J. P. Fabricius, respondent.

—Chirurgus Cartesianus, detegens aliquot in chirurgia errores, hactenus ex ignorantia philosophiae commissos . . . Marburgi Cattorum, Typis Joh. Henrici Stockenii, 1687.

24 p. 19 cm. [12548]

W. U. Waldschmidt, respondent.

—Disputatio decima tertia de phthisi et empyemate . . . Marpurgi Cattorum, Typis Johannis Jodoci Kürsneri [1683]

[8] p. 20 cm. [12549]

C. Kürsner, respondent.

—Disputatio inauguralis physico-hydroscopica, de vera origine fontium dulcium et salinorum . . . Marburgi Cattorum, Typis Johannis Henrici Stockenii, 1686.

20 p. 20 cm. [12550]

J. N. Cnyrim, respondent.

—Disputatio medica de chylificatione, sive, cibi in chylum mutatione . . . Marburgi Cattorum, Typis Salomonis Schadewitzii, 1674.

[2], 28 p. 19 cm. [12551]

B. W. Geilfus, respondent.

—Disputatio medica de epilepsia, von der schweren Noht . . . Marburgi Cattorum, Typis Salomonis Schadewitzii, 1676.

28 p. 20 cm. [12552]

J. Dinckgreue, respondent.

—Disputatio medica de glandulae pinealis statu naturali & praeternaturali . . . Marpurgi Cattorum, Typis Salomonis Schadewitzii, 1680.

[2], 20 p. 19 cm. [12553]

J. W. Beutler, respondent.

—Disputatio medica, de mania vulgo die Tobsucht oder Wahnwitzigkeit . . . Marburgi Cattorum, Typis Salomonis Schadewitzii, 1680.

20 p. 18 cm. [12554]

L. G. Buelius, respondent.

—Disputatio medica de morbis aulicis . . . Marburgi Cattorum, Typis Johannis Jodoci Kürsneri [1686]

24 p. 19 cm. [12555]

W. U. Waldschmidt, respondent.

—Disputatio medica de phthisi, Schwind-oder Lungensucht . . . Marburgi Cattorum, Typis Salomonis Schadewitzii, 1675.

30 p. 20 cm. [12556]

A. Erni, respondent.

—Disputatio medica de veneni pestilentialis, ut et alexipharmacorum natura et in corpus humanum agendi modo, ex verae philosophiae principiis perspicue demonstrato, multisque experimentis suffulto . . . Marburgi Cattorum, Typis Salomonis Schadewitzii, 1675.

[1], 16 p. 20 cm. [12557]

H. Horch, respondent.

—Disputato medica de ventriculi et intestinorum morbis ... Marpurgi Cattorum, Typis Joh. Jodoci Kürsneri [1684]

40 p. 20 cm. [12558]

M. Harmes, *respondent.*

—Disputatio medica exhibens intricatam hodierno tempore quaestionem de sanguificatione ... Marpurgi Cattorum, Typis Salomonis Schadewitzii, 1675.

24 p. 20 cm. [12559]

J. C. Schunck, *respondent.*

—Disputatio physica de causa partus monstrosi nuperrime nati, hujusque occasione de monstrorum humanorum causis in genere ... Marburgi Cattorum, Joh. Jodoci Kursneri [1684]

32 p. 18 cm. [12560]

C. Kürsner, *respondent.*

—Disputatio physica de colore Aethiopium, qui vulgo nigritae ... Marburgi Cattorum, Typis Joh. Jodoci Kürsneri, 1683.

[1], 18 p. 20 cm. [12561]

M. E. Lucan, *respondent.*

—Disquisitio medica de haemorrhagia narium ... Marb. Cattorum, Typis Johannis Henrici Stockenii, 1686.

12 p. 19 cm. [12562]

K. P. Lombard, *respondent.*

—Dissertatio medica de potu theae ... Marburgi Cattorum, Typis Johannis Jodoci Kürsneri [1685]

24 p. 20 cm. [12563]

C. Kürsner, *respondent.*

—Dissertatio physica de primaevo et ho dierno telluris statu ... Marburgi Cattorum, Typis Johannis Jodoci Kürsneri [1684]

24 p. 19 cm. [12564]

C. Kürsner, *respondent.*

—Exercitatio medica de chylo et sanguine ... Marburgi Cattorum, Typis Johannis Jodoci Kürsneri [1686]

28 p. 19 cm. [12565]

G. Schumacher, *respondent.*

—Exercitatio medica de cura lactis podagricorum solatio et certo podagrae remedio ... Marburgi Cattorum, Typis Salomonis Schadewitzii, 1675.

32 p. 20 cm. [12566]

L. K. Jacobi, *respondent.*

—Exercitatio physica de igne perpetuo ... Marburgi Cattorum, Typis Joh. Jodoc. Kürsneri, 1683.

20 p. 20 cm. [12567]

J. B. Schaffnicht, *respondent.*

—Exercitationem medicam de acidulis, vulgo den Sauerbrunnen, examini publico exponit ... Ludovicus Gothofredus Buelius ... Marpurgi Cattorum, Ex chalcographeo Joh. Jodoci Kürsneri, 1682.

12, [2] p. 19 cm. [12568]

L. G. Buelius, *respondent.*

—Medicus Cartesianus, detegens aliquot in medicina errores, hactenus ex ignorantia philosophiae commissos ... Marburgi Cattorum, Typis Joh. Jodoci Kürsneri, 1687.

16 p. 20 cm. [12569]

J. J. Baier, *respondent.*

—Monita medic circa opii et opiatorum usum vulgo Schlaff-Tränck ... Marpurgi Cattorum, Typis Salomonis Schadewitzii, 1679.

24 p. 19 cm. [12570]

P. H. Chuno, *respondent.*

—Physicae curiosae et utilis specimen de sensibus ... Marburgi Cattorum, Typis Johannis Henrici Stockenii, 1686.

16 p. 19 cm. [12571]

J. Stirnn, *respondent.*

—*respondent.* Disputatio inauguralis medica de affectione hypochondriaca ... Giessae, Typis Friederici Kargeri, 1666.

19 p. 20 cm. [12572]

Diss. — Giessen.

—*See* DOLÄUE, J. Opera omnia. 1695.

WALDSCHMIDT, PHILIPP JACOB [*fl.* 1664–1665] *respondent. See* SEBISCH, M. [1578–1674?] *praeses.* Disputatio solennis de asthmate et orthopnoea. 1664.

WALDSCHMIDT, WILHELM ULRICH [1669–1731] Facultatis Medicae ... decanus Wilhelmus Huldericus Waldschmiedt ... ad audiendam dissertationem inauguralem de usu & abusu potus thee in genere praecipue vero in hydrope quam ... examini submittet ... Jeremias Muller ... invitat. Kiliae, Joachimus Reuman [1692]

[8] p. 18 cm. [12573]

Program - Jena (with vita of J. Müller)

—*praeses*. Dissertatio chymico-medica de salis volatilis cornu cervi crystallisatione volatili essentiali ... Kiliae, Typis Joachimi Rheumanni, 1697.

20 p.   20 cm.   **[12574]**

Diss.—Kiel (J. Hartmann, *respondent*)

—Dissertatio inauguralis exhibens pathologiae animatae specimen ... Kilonii, Literis Joach. Reumanni, 1697.

48 p.   20 cm.   **[12575]**

Letter on last page misdated 1699.

Diss.—Kiel (T. T. M. J. D. Hanneman, *respondent*)

—Dissertatio inauguralis medica de usu & abusu potus thee in genere praecipue vero in hydrope ... Kiliae, Joachimus Reumann [1692]

24 p.   19 cm.   **[12576]**

Diss.—Kiel (J. Müller, *respondent*)

—Dissertatio medica, de ignorantia et nequitia empiricorum ... Kiliae, Typis Joachimi Reumanni, 1692.

[12] p.   20 cm.   **[12577]**

Diss.—Kiel (J. Müller, *respondent*)

—*respondent*. See WALDSCHMIDT, J. J., *praeses*. Chirurgus Cartesianus. 1687 [and] Disputatio medica de morbis aulicis. 1686.

—, *ed. See* [WALDSCHMIDT, J. J.] Advice to a physician. 1695 [and] Praxis medicinae rationalis. 1690, 1691.

WALDSCHMIEDT. *See* WALDSCHMIDT.

WALDUNG, WOLFGANG [1555-1621] Lagographia. Natura leporum, qua prisci autores et recentiores prodidere quidve utilitatis in re medica ab isto quadrupede percipiatur. Liber singularis ... Ambergae, Typis & sumptibus Joh. Schönfeldii, 1619.

82 (i.e. 91), [4] p. illus. 19 cm.   **[12578]**

WALE, JAN de. *See* WALAEUS, Johannes [1604-1649]

WALKER, CLEMENT [1595-1651] *See* MAIER, M. Themis aurea. 1656.

[WALKER, OBADIAH, 1616-1699] Propositions concerning optic-glasses, with their natural reasons, drawn from experiments. Oxford, At the Theater, 1679.

[4], 46 p. illus. 19 cm.   **[12579]**

Attributed also to Robert Cooper. Cf. Madan, vol. 3, p. 370-371.

WALKER, THOMAS [*b. ca.* 1665] *respondent.* Disputatio medica inauguralis de hydrope intercute, seu anasarca ... Lugduni Batavorum, Apud Abrahamum Elzevier, 1688.

[24] p.   21 cm.   **[12580]**

Diss.—Leyden.

WALKINGTON, THOMAS [*d.* 1621] The optick glasse of humors; or, The touchstone of a golden temperature, or the philosophers stone to make a golden temper. Wherein the foure complections sanguine, cholericke, phligmaticke, melancholicke are succinctly painted forth and their externall intimates laid open ... by T[homas] W[alkington] master of artes ... London, Printed for [and by] J. D[awson] and are to be sould [sic] by L[awrence] B[laiklock] 1639.

[25], 168 p. plates. 15 cm.   **[12581]**

Engraved title page.

Imperfect: lower margin of title page trimmed including date of imprint.

STC 24969.

—[The same.] ... London, Printed for G. Dawson and sold by Edward Man, 1664.

[26], 168 p. plate. 15 cm.   **[12582]**

Added engraved title page has imprint: London, Printed for I. D. and sould by E. M., 1663.

WALL, W. A new system of the French disease. With an easy and familiar method of curing it, unknown to the ancients or moderns ... Together, with an epistle dedicatory to the president and censors, &c. of the learned College of Physicians ... Together, with ... commendatory verses ... London, John Baker [1696?]

[24], 30 p. 18 cm.   **[12583]**

The imprint date is that proposed by Watt, vol. 2, 944m, and Wing, no. W490.

With this are bound The tomb of Venus. London, 1710; copy 2 of Boerhaave, Herman. A treatise on the venereal disease. London, 1729.

WALLE, PIETER VAN DE [*fl.* 1694-1697] *respondent.* Disputatio medica inauguralis de hydrocephalo ... Lugduni Batavorum, Apud Abrahamum Elzevier, 1697.

[17] p.   21 cm.   **[12584]**

Diss.—Leyden.

WALLENBERGER, VALENTIN [*fl.* 1620] Trias quaestionum controversarum. I. De animae mortalitate. II. De fidei naturalis in morborum curatione tempore Christi & apostolorum operatione. III. De tribus substantialibus sive essentialibus hominis partibus. Ἀνασκευαστικῶς opposita Dyadi mysticae Christiani Theophili [pseud., i.e. Valentin Weigel] ... Erffordiae, Typis Joannis Röhbock, impensis Joannis Bischoffs, 1621.

25 ll.   20 cm.   [**12585**]

WALLER, RICHARD [*d.* 1714 *or* 15] *tr. See* ACADÉMIE ROYALE DES SCIENCES, Paris. Memoires for a natural history of animals. 1687, 1688; ACCADEMIA DEL CIMENTO, Florence. Essayes of natural experiments. 1684.

WALLERIUS, NICOLAUS. *See* VALLERIUS, Nicolaus [*fl.* 1699]

WALLETIUS, GUALTERUS. *See* WELLESIUS, Walter [*b. ca.* 1582]

WALLICH, GEORG TOBIAS [*fl.* 1667-1670] *respondent. See* FRIDERICI, J. A., *praeses.* Disputatio inauguralis medica de lienteria. 1670 [and] Disputationem medicam de mania ex philtro ... publicae censurae submittit G. T. W. 1670.

—*See* WEDEL, G. W. Diatriben medicam de diebus criticis ... subjiciunt G. W. W. ... & G. T. W. 1667, 1678.

WALLIS, JOHN [1616-1703] A defence of the Royal Society, and the Philosophical transactions, particularly those of July, 1670. In answer to the cavils of Dr. William Holder ... In a letter to the right honourable William Lord Viscount Brouncker. London, T. S. for Thomas Moore, 1678.

33 p.   20 cm.   [**12586**]

—Grammatica linguae Anglicanae. Cui praefigitur de loquela sive sonorum formatione, tractatus grammatico-physicus. Et (nunc primum) subjungitur, praxis grammatica. Ed. 4. prioribus auctior. Oxoniae, Typis L. Lichfield, et prostant venales apud Joh. Crosley, 1674.

[23], 190 (i.e. 191) p.   18 cm.   [**12587**]

—*See* [HOLDER, W.] A supplement to the Philosophical transactions. 1678.

WALLMAN, BALTHASAR HEIDENREICH [*fl.* 1682] *respondent. See* TILING, M., *praeses.* Disputatio inauguralis de apoplexia. 1682.

WALLNER, ELIAS, *tr. See* BARTHOLIN, T. Neu-ver-besserte künstliche Zerlegung dess menschlichen Leibes. 1677.

WALLRICH, CHRISTOPH [*fl.* 1655] *respondent. See* SPERLING, J., *praeses.* Disputatio physica de monstris. 1655.

WALTEN, ERICUS [1663-1697] *See* P[OST] S[CRIPTUM] of, na-courier, van de Tweede missive aen Dr. Balthasar Bekker. 1692.

WALTER, GOTTFRIED [*fl.* 1688] *respondent. See* DRELINCOURT, C., *praeses.* Disputatio medica inauguralis de suffocatione hypochondriaca in viro. 1688; ROLFINCK, W., *praeses.* De inundatione microcosmi. 1652.

—De melancholia. *In* Rolfinck, W., *praeses.* Methodus cognoscendi & curandi adfectus capitis particulares. 1653.

WALTHER, GEORG DAVID [*b.* 1664] *respondent. See* CRAUSE, R. W., *praeses.* Disputationem inauguralem, de morbis spirituum in genere ... proponit G. D. W. 1688.

—*See* WEDEL, G. W. Propempticon inaugurale de quadragesima medica. 1688.

WALTHER, GOTTFRIED. *See* WALTER, Gottfried [*fl.* 1652]

WALTHER, JOHANN [1618-1679] *praeses.* Disputatio physica de lapidibus in genere ... Lipsiae, Literis heredum Timothei Hönii [1648]

[16] p.   19 cm.   [**12588**]
Diss.—Leipzig (J. H. Müller, *respondent*)

—Disquisitio physica de pluvia ... Lipsiae, Typis Hönianis [1648]

[16] p.   19 cm.   [**12589**]
Diss.—Leipzig (K. Exner, *respondent*)

—Συμπόσιον φιλοσοφικόν nutritionis physicae varios missus exhibens ... Lipsiae, Typis haeredum Timothei Hönii [1647]

[28] p.   19 cm.   [**12590**]
Diss.—Leipzig (P. J. Sachs von Lewenhaimb, *respondent*)

WALTHER, JOHANN GEORG [*fl.* 1639-1679] Sylva medica opulentissima ... in qua ... ex aliquot centenis autoribus medicis ... quotquot hactenus inveniri potuerunt, omnia morborum nomina & synonyma ... litera sua initiali ordine alphabetico ita sunt collecta, ut extemplo . . . videri possit, quid, quinam & quot autores de unoquoque morbo scripserint . . . Budissae, Sumptibus Friderici Arnsti, typis Andreae Richteri, 1679.

[15], 1438, [35] p. front. (port.) 21 cm.

[12591]

WALTHER, KONRAD [1609-1658] *respondent. See* FREITAG, J., *praeses.* Disputatio medica calidi innati essentiam juxta veteris medicinę & philosophiae decreta explicans. 1632; HORST, G. [1578-1636] *praeses.* Problematum medicorum θεραπευτικων decades priores quinque. 1608; SENNERT, D., *praeses.* Quaestiones medicae controversae quinque, pro disputatione octava propositae. 1608.

WALTHER, NOAH [*fl.* 1624] *respondent. See* SEBISCH, M. [1578-1674?] *praeses.* Exercitationes medicae. 1639.

WALTHER, WOLFGANG DIETRICH [*fl.* 1671] *respondent. See* PURPIUS, A., *praeses.* De sede vitae in calido innato dissertatio. 1671.

WALTON, ERICUS. *See* WALTEN, Ericus [1663-1697]

WALTSGOTT, JOHANN ERNST [*b.* 1671] *respondent. See* SCHELHAMMER, G. C., *praeses.* Dissertatio inauguralis medica de morbis aetatum. 1694.

WALTZ, JOHANN CASPAR [*fl.* 1672-1688] *See* HOELTICH, F. H. Quaest. foemina non est homo. 1672? 1688?

WALTZIUS, JOHANN CASPAR. *See* WALZ, Johann Caspar [*fl.* 1668]

WALWIJK, PAUL VAN [*fl.* 1687-1707] *respondent.* Disputatio medica inauguralis de cacochymiae sanguinis pituitosae symptomatis . . . Lugduni Batavorum, Apud Abrahamum Elzevier, 1687.

[24] p. 21 cm.   **[12592]**
Diss. — Leyden.

WALWYK, PAUL. *See* WALWIJK, Paul van [*fl.* 1687-1707]

WALWYN, WILLIAM [*fl.* 1667-1696] Physick for families, discovering a safe way, and ready means, whereby every one at sea or land, may . . . be in capacity of curing themselves . . . London, Printed by J. Winter, and sold by Robert Horn, 1669.

[6], 118, [1] p. 17 cm.   **[12593]**

—[The same.] . . . London, Printed by J. R. and sold by John Starky, 1681.

[14], 144 p. 15 cm.   **[12594]**
Imperfect: front. (port.) wanting.

—[The same.] . . . London, Printed by J. R. and sold by the author, 1696.

[13], 144 p. front. (port.) 15 cm.   **[12595]**
Different setting of type.
Imperfect: front. (port.) wanting.

—A touch-stone for physick, directing by evident marks and characters to such medicines, as without purgers, vomiters . . . or any other disturbers of nature, may be securely trusted for cure in all extremities . . . London, Printed by J. W. for Benjamin Billingsley, 1667.

[11], 110 (i.e. 100) p. 15 cm.   **[12596]**

WALZ, JOHANN CASPAR [*fl.* 1668] *respondent. See* FROMMANN, J. C., *praeses.* Problemata miscellanea tria. 1668.

WANCKEL, AUGUST [*fl.* 1651-1654] *respondent. See* BANZER, M., *praeses.* Disputatio medica de incubo. 1651.

WANCKEL, JOHANN [*fl.* 1605-1608] *respondent. See* SENNERT, D., *praeses.* De caussis morborum disputatio prior. 1605.

WANCKELMUTH, PAUL GABRIEL [*fl.* 1669] *respondent. See* SCHWIMMER, J. M., *praeses.* Dissertatio physica de generatione. 1669.

WANDAL, HANS [1656-1710] Vindiciae libertatis Christianae circa sanguinem escarium, recentiorum quorundam superstitiosis novitatibus praecipue vero Christiani cujusdam Theophili disquisitioni uberiori pro Thomae Bartholino, oppositae . . . Wittebergae, Sumtibus autoris, typis vero Matthaei Henckelii, 1678.

[1], α-ν, 286, [18] p. 17 cm.   **[12597]**
Bound with Fedele, F. Schola jure-consultorum medica. 1679.

WANDALIN, JANUS JOHANN [*fl.* 1649] *See* BARTHOLIN, T. Ad secundum N. T. paralyticum omnium ordinum auditores opposituros pro disputatione ordinaria. 1649.

WANDALINUS, JOHANNES. *See* WANDAL, Hans [1656-1710]

WANG, SHU-HO [*fl.* 280] *See* [BOYM, M. P.] Specimen medicinae Sinicae. 1682.

WANGNERECK, HEINRICH [1595-1664] Conclusiones selectae ex Parvis naturalibus Aristotelis ... Dilingae, Apud Casparum Sutorem, 1628.

    [4], 16 p.   19 cm.   **[12598]**

—*praeses.* Conclusiones philosophicae ex libris De generatione [Aristotelis] ... Dilingae, Impensis Caspari Sutoris, 1628.

    [2], 13, [1] p.   19 cm.   **[12599]**

    Diss.—Dillingen (F. Nusser and H. Riedmiller, *respondent*)

WANSLEBEN, ANSELMUS [*fl.* 1653] *respondent.* De catarrho. *In* Rolfinck, W., *praeses.* Methodus cognoscendi & curandi adfectus capitis particulares. 1653.

WANTSCHER, CHRISTOPH [*fl.* 1666] *respondent. See* WOLFF, Christian, *praeses.* Disputatio zoologica de lupo et lycanthropia. 1666.

WARD, WILLIAM [1534-1609] *tr. See* ALESSIO PIEMONTESE, *pseud.?* The secrets. 1615; VICARY, T. The English mans treasure. 1613, 1633, 1641 [and] The surgions directorie. 1651.

WARDE, WILLIAM. *See* WARD, William [1534-1609]

WARENBURGIUS, SINCERUS. *See* LYSER, Johann [1631-1684]

WARENIUS, HENRICUS [*d. ca.* 1604] *praeses.* Νοσολογια; seu, Adfectuum humanorum curatio Hermetica et Galenica thesibus comprehensa, ac consentiente senatu medico in Academia Rostochiense disceptata ... Post obitum autoris ... collecta & publicata studio & opera Joachimi Tanckii ... Lipsiae, Excudebat Michaël Lantzenberger, sumtibus Johannis Rosae, 1605.

    [22], 240 p.   16 cm.   **[12600]**

    Contains 22 Rostock theses by 8 respondents.

WARLITZ, CHRISTIAN [1648-1717] Exercitatio medico-sacra, de senio Salomonaeo ad Ecclesiastae Cap. XII. Lipsiae, Apud Johann Herebord Klosium, 1700.

    [53] p.   20 cm.   **[12601]**

WARNATIUS, HENRICUS [*fl.* 1668-*ca.* 1670] *respondent. See* BOHN, J., *praeses.* Exercitationum physiologicarum prima ... [-decima tertia] 1674?; ETTMÜLLER, M., *praeses.* Medicina Hippocratis chymica. 1678, 1684; WIESSNER, G. Dissertationem

medicam theoretico-practicam de malo pestifero ... p.p. G. W. 1668.

WARTENBERG, ERNST CHRISTIAN [1665-*ca.* 1720] *praeses.* De anima humanum corpus informante ... Lipsiae, Christian Scholvin [1689]

    [16] p.   21 cm.   **[12602]**

    Diss.—Leipzig (C. Thomschläger, *respondent*)

WARTENBERG, FRIEDRICH JAKOB ILLMER VON UND ZU. *See* ILLMER, Friedrich Ferdinand [*fl.* 1698]

WARTON, SIMON. *See* SHERARD, William [1659-1728]

WASMUHT, JOHANN HEINRICH [*fl.* 1691] *respondent.* Disputatio medica inauguralis de laeso ... Duisburgi ad Rhenum, Apud Franconem Sas, 1691.

    18 p.   20 cm.   **[12603]**

    Diss.—Duisburg.

WASMUTH, MATTHIAS [*d.* 1693] *respondent.* Disputatio medica inauguralis de febribus ardentibus ... Lugduni Batavorum, Apud Abrahamum Elzevier, 1691.

    [16] p.   20 cm.   **[12604]**

    Diss.—Leyden.

WASSENAAR, JAN VAN [*fl.* 1660] *respondent.* Disputatio medica inauguralis de convulsione ... Lugduni Batavorum, Apud Joannem Elsevirium, 1660.

    [12] p.   23 cm.   **[12605]**

    Diss.—Leyden.

WASSILEWITZ, JOANNES NICOLAUS [*fl.* 1671] *respondent.* Disputatio medica inauguralis de variolis ... Lugduni Batavorum, Apud viduam & haeredes Joannis Elsevirii, 1671.

    [32] p.   23 cm.   **[12606]**

    Diss.—Leyden.

WATESON, GEORGE [*fl.* 1598-1607] *See* A RICH STOREHOUSE OR TREASURIE FOR THE DISEASED. 1616, 1630, 1631, 1650.

WATS, GILBERT [*d.* 1657] *See* BACON, F., *viscount* St. Albans. Of the advancement and proficience of learning. 1640.

WATSON, GEORGE [*fl.* 1598-1607] *See* WATESON, George [*fl.* 1598-1607]

WATTS, GILBERT. *See* WATS, Gilbert [*d.* 1657]

WAXMANN, ZSIGMOND [*fl.* 1687–1688] *respondent.* See FASCH, A. H., *praeses.* Disputatio inauguralis medica de suffocatione hysterica. 1687.

WAXMUTH, JOHANN GEORG [*fl.* 1670] *respondent.* Disputatio medica inauguralis de abortu ... Lugduni Batavorum, Apud viduam & haeredes Joannis Elsevirii, 1670.

[28] p. 23 cm. **[12607]**
Diss. — Leyden.

WEBEL, MARTIN [*fl.* 1610] *See* RYFF, P. Gratiosus ... ordo medic. Basileens. 1610.

WEBER, ANTON [*fl.* 1646] *respondent.* Disputatio medica inauguralis de scorbuto ... Lugduni Batavorum, Ex officina Joannis Maire, 1646.

[16] p. 19 cm. **[12608]**
Diss. — Leyden.

WEBER, CHRISTIAN HEINRICH [*fl.* 1678] *respondent.* See PETRI VON HARTENFELS, G. C., *praeses.* Dissertationem inauguralem de abortu ... submittit. 1678.

WEBER, JAN-CHRISTIAN [*fl.* 1619] *respondent.* See SCHENCK, E., *praeses.* Disputatio medica de dysenteria, 1619.

WEBER, JOHANN CONRAD, *pseud.* See NIGRISOLI, Francesco Maria [1648–1727 or 8]

WEBER, JOHANN CORNELIUS [*d.* 1684] Anchora sauciatorum; hoc est, Liquor stypticus, sanguinem confestim et miraculose sistens ... Wratislaviae, Apud Joh. Kaestnerum, 1680.

[7], 126 p. plate. 17 cm. **[12609]**

WEBER, JOHANN ERNST [*fl.* 1675] *respondent.* See SIMON, J., *praeses.* Diversicolor ovium foetus opera Jacobi patriarchae productus. 1675.

WEBER, PHILIPP [*fl.* 1609–1617] Thermarum Wisbadensium descriptio. Complectens antiquitatem et utilitatem harum thermarum, victus commoditatem, regimen utentium, modum adhibendi cum et sine acidulis Langenschwalbacensibus, accidentia thermarum, eorundemque remedia ... Oppenheimio, Ex officina typographica Hieronymi Galleri, sumptibus Johannis Theodori de Bry, 1617.

[8], 146 p. table. 20 cm. **[12610]**

— *respondent.* Problematum medicorum triades tres cum corollariis tribus ... Basileae, Typis Joan. Jacobi Genathii, 1610.

[12] p. 20 cm. **[12611]**

Diss. — Basel.
With this is bound Bauhin, K. Hygiae et panaceae parente ... Casparus Bauhinus. 1610.

— *respondent.* See HORST, G. [1578–1636] *praeses.* Tractatus de scorbuto. 1609.

— See BAUHIN, K. Hygiae et panaceae parente ... Casparus Bauhinus. 1610.

WEBSTER, JOHN [1610–1682] The displaying of supposed witchcraft. Wherein is affirmed that there are many sorts of deceivers and impostors, and divers persons under a passive delusion of melancholy and fancy ... Wherein also is handled, the existence of angels and spirits ... London, J. M., 1677.

[15], 346, [4] p. 31 cm. **[12612]**
Imperfect: p. 117–118 mutilated.

— Copy 2. 30 cm.
Imperfect: first preliminary leaf wanting.

— Metallographia; or, An history of metals. Wherein is declared the signs of ores and minerals ... As also, the handling and shewing of their vegetability, and the discussion of ... questions belonging to mystical chymistry, as of the philosophers gold ... Gathered forth of the most approved authors ... London, Printed by A. C. for Walter Kettilby, 1671.

[16], 388, [2] p. 21 cm. **[12613]**

WECHTLER, Johann Conrad [*fl.* 1656–1659] De unguenti armarii difficultatibus.

598–604 p. 21 cm. (*In* Theatrum sympatheticum auctum. Norimbergae, 1662) **[12614]**
Caption title.

— Homo oriens et occidens, duobus actibus et libris in scenam publicam ita datus et productus ... Omnia ex optimis quibusque partim medicis partim philosophis desumpta ... accedit ... appendix ... de statu animae separatae ex lumine naturae deducta ... Francofurti ad Moenum, Impensis Caspari Wechtleri, ut & sumptibus typisque Balthasaris Christophori Wustii, 1659.

[4], 524, [20] p.; 475, [20] p. 32 cm. **[12615]**
Errata: p. [20] at end.
Added engraved title page dated 1660.

WECKER, ANNA [*fl.* 1588–1596] New, köstlich und nutzliches Kochbuch. In welchem kurtzlichen begriffen, wie allerhand künstliche Speisen ... für Gesunde und Krancke ... für schwangere Weiber,

Kindbettherinnen ... mit geringem Kosten zubereiten und zuzurichten ... Jetzo ... mit vielen, newen ... Trachten vermehrt und gebessert. Basel, In Verlegung Ludwig Königs Erben, 1652.

[16], 459, [5] p.   17 cm.   **[12616]**

WECKER, HANS JACOB. *See* WECKER, Johann Jakob [1528–1586]

WECKER, JOHANN JACOB [1528–1586] Antidotarium generale et speciale: ex opt. authorum ... scriptis ... congestum & dispositum. Nunc vero supra priores editiones omnes multis novis & optimis formulis, maxime vero extractis auctum ... Basileae, Per Conr. Waldkirch, sumptibus Episcopianorum, 1601.

[15] p., 222 col., [4] p.; [12] p., 1210 col., [29] p. illus. 26 cm.   **[12617]**
Part [2] has special title page.

—[The same.] ... Venetiis, Apud Georgium Variscum, 1608.

[16] p., 222 col., [5] p.; [12] p., 1210 col., [42] p. illus. 26 cm.   **[12618]**
Part [2] has special title page.
Different setting of type.

—[The same.] ... Basileae, Per Joan. Jacobum Genathium, sumptibus Ludovici König, 1617.

[15] p., 222 col., [4] p., [12] p., 1210 col., [29] p. illus. 25 cm.   **[12619]**
Part [2] has special title page.
Different setting of type.

—[The same.] ... Basilae, Typis Joan. Jacobi Genathii, sumptibus haeredum Ludovici König, 1642.

[15] p., 222 col., [4] p., [12] p., 1210 col., [29] p. illus. 24 cm.   **[12620]**
Part [2] has special title page.
Different setting of type.
Imperfect: error in binding: title pages and preliminary leaves of Antidotarium generale and Antidotarium speciale are interchanged.

—[French tr.] Le grand dispensaire; ou, Thresor general et particulier des preservatifs ... enrichi d'annotations en suitte du texte, de nottes en marge ... Plus d'une methode ... d'extraire les facultez des medicaments purgatifs ... Le tout par Jan du Val ... Geneve, Estienne Gamonet, 1609.

[16] p., 286 col., [8] p., 1336 col. illus. 24 cm.   **[12621]**
Part [2] has special title page.

—[The same.] ... Geneve, De l'imprimerie d'Estienne Gamonet [S'en vend a Lyon de Paul Frellon & Jan. Ant. Huguetan] 1610.

[24] p., 286 col.; [17] p., 1336 col. illus. 24 cm.   **[12622]**
A reissue of the 1609 edition with new title page and other preliminary matter. Both title pages have been retained from the 1609 edition. Part [2] has also a special title page dated 1610.

—[The same.] ... Cologny, Estienne Gamonet, 1616.

[16] p., 286 col., [14] p.; [1] p., 1336 col. illus. 24 cm.   **[12623]**
Original place of publication blocked out and "A Geneve" printed below.
Part [2] has special title page.

—De secretis libri XVII. Ex variis authoribus collecti, methodiceque digesti, & aucti ... Basileae, Typis Conradi Waldkirchii, sumptibus Episcopianorum, 1604.

[15], 667, [27] p. illus. 18 cm.   **[12624]**
A reprint, for the most part page for page, of the same publisher's edition of 1598.

—[The same.] ... Basileae, Sumptibus Ludovici Regis, 1629.

[15], 667, [27] p. illus. 17 cm.   **[12625]**
Different setting of type.

—[The same.] ... Basileae, Sumptibus Ludovici Regis, 1642.

[15], 667, [27] p. illus. 19 cm.   **[12626]**
Different setting of type.

—[The same.] ... Basileae, Sumptibus Johannis Regis, excudebat Joh. Rodolphus Genath, 1662.

[15], 667, [27] p. illus. 17 cm.   **[12627]**
Imperfect: p. 93–94 wanting.
Different setting of type.

—[English tr.] Eighteen books of the secrets of art & nature, being the summe and substance of naturall philosophy ... now much augm. and inlarged by Dr. R. Read ... London, Simon Miller, 1661.

[8], 346, [11] p. front. (ports.), illus. 28 cm.   **[12628]**

—[French tr.] Les secrets et merveilles de nature. Recueillies de divers autheurs, & divisez en XVII. livres ... Rev., corr. & augm. ... Rouen, Claude Le Villain, 1620.

[15], 858, [45] p. illus. 17 cm.   **[12629]**
Imperfect: p. 803–4 mutilated.
Edited by Pierre Meyssonier.

—[The same.] ... Rouen, Claude Le Villain, 1627.

[15], 1012 (i.e. 1014), [41] p.   illus.   17 cm.[**12630**]

[The same.] ... Rouen, Richard Lallemant, 1699.
[15], 1012 (i.e. 1014), [41] p.   illus.   17 cm.[**12631**]
Different setting of type.

—De secretis liber octavus de artificiosis vinis liber. *In* Alessio Piemontese, pseud.? De secretis libri septem. 1603.

—Medicinae utriusque syntaxes, ex Graecorum, Latinorum, Arabumque thesauris ... singulari fide, methodo ac industria collectae & concinnatae. Ed. ult., prioribus correctior ... Basileae, Per Sebastianum Henricpetri [1601]

[7], 752, [26] p.   34 cm.   [**12632**]
Signatures: α⁴, a-z, A–2P⁶, 2Q⁴, 2R–2S⁶, 2T⁸ (last leaf blank). Imperfect: sig 2T7–8 wanting. Sig. 2T7, containing end of index, colophon, and printer's mark, is supplied in photocopy from the New York Academy of Medicine Library.

—[English tr.] A compendious chyrurgerie. *In* Banister, J. The workes. 1633.

—Ein nutzliches Büchlein von mancherleyen künstlichen Wassern, Ölen und Weinen, jetzt newlich inn Teutsch gebracht ... Basel, Conrad Waldkirch, 1605.

[6], 86, [3] p.   17 cm.   [**12633**]

—[The same.] *In* Alessio Piemontese, pseud. Mirabilia magna naturae. 1622.

—Practica medicinae generalis ... septimis libris explicata ... Tarvisii, Apud Fabritium Zanettum, 1602.

[80], 542 p.   11 cm.   [**12634**]

—[The same.] ... Lugduni, Apud haeredes Guilliel. Rouillii, 1606.

[32], 593, [22] p.   13 cm.   [**12635**]

—[The same.] ... Venetiis, Apud Franciscum Bolzettam, 1608.

[32], 337 (i.e. 437), [27] p.   11 cm.   [**12636**]

—[The same.] ... Venetiis, Apud Donatum Pasquardum, & socium, 1630.

[80], 542 p.   11 cm.   [**12637**]

—[The same.] Practica Wekerii. Venetiis, Combi, 1644.

482, [22] p.   11 cm.   [**12638**]

Engraved title page.

The dedication and the commendatory verses have been omitted from this edition of the Practica medicinae generalis.

—, *tr. See* ALESSIO PIEMONTESE. De secretis libri septem. 1603.

—*See* COLUMELLA, L. J. M. Agricultur; oder, Ackerbaw. 1612; CULPEPER, N. Arts master-piece. 1660.

WECKERLIN, KASPAR [*fl.* 1615] *respondent.* Quaestiones medicae variae ... Basileae, Per Joan. Jacobum Genathium, 1615.

[28] p.   23 cm.   [**12639**]
Diss.—Basel.

WEDEKIND, JOHANN KASPAR [*fl.* 1685] Dissertatio inauguralis medica de alkahest ... Erfordiae, Typis Groschianis [1685]

20 p.   20 cm.   [**12640**]
Diss.—Erfurt (C. Helbigk, *respondent*)

WEDEL, CHRISTIAN [1678-1714] Epistola anatomica, problematica, tertia & decima ... Ad ... Fredericum Ruyschium ... De oculorum tunicis. Amstelaedami, Apud Joannem Wolters, 1700.

40 p.   plate.   22 cm.   [**12641**]
"Frederici Ruyschii responsio ...": p. [9]-34.

—*praeses.* Centuria thesium de theriaca ... Jenae, Literis Ehrichianis [1700]

16 p.   20 cm.   [**12642**]
Diss.—Jena (H. E. Hartmann, *respondent*)

—*respondent. See* HAMBERGER, G. A., *praeses.* Dissertatio physica de elatere. 1699; WEDEL, G. W., *praeses.* Dissertatio medica de aneurismate. 1699 [and] Dissertatio medica inauguralis de terebinthina. 1700; WEDEL, J. A., *praeses.* Dissertatio medico-physiologica de temperamento mixti. 1698.

—*See* CRAUSE, R. W. Propempticum inaugurale de temerario quorundam simplicium remediorum, apriscis commendatorum, contemtu. 1700.

WEDEL, ERNST HEINRICH [1671-1709] *praeses.* Dissertatio anatomico-medica de peritonaeo ... Jenae, Litteris Nisianis [1696]

26, [2] p.   20 cm.   [**12643**]
Diss.—Jena (J. K. Muller, *respondent*)

—Dissertatio chimico-medica de tinctura martis helleborata ... Jenae, Litteris Krebsianis [1695]

20 p.   20 cm.   [**12644**]
Diss.—Jena (J. A. Wedee, *respondent*)

—Dissertatio medica de ephemera ... Jenae, Typis Christophori Krebsii [1698]

20 p.   20 cm.   [12645]

Diss.—Jena (S. G. Paulsen, *respondent*)

—Dissertatio medica de morbis concionatorum ... Jenae, Literis Christophori Krebsii [1699]

32 p.   19 cm.   [12646]

Diss.—Jena (J. H. Salmuth, *respondent*)

—*respondent. See* HOFFMANN, M., *praeses.* Theses summariae medicae de procidentia uteri. 1695; SCHMID, J. A., *praeses.* Auris Θεοδείκτος. 1694. WEDEL, G. W., *praeses.* Dissertatio inauguralis chimico-medica de sale ammoniaco. 1695. [and] Dissertatio medica de spectris. 1693, 1698.

—*See* WEDEL, G. W. Propemticum inaugurale de corchoro Theophrasti in specie. 1695.

WEDEL, GEORG WOLFFGANG [1645-1721] Amoenitates materiae medicae. Jenae, Sumptibus Johannis Bielkii, typis viduae Samuelis Krebsii, 1684.

[13], 512, [14] p.   front.   (port.)   20 cm.
                                            [12647]

Imperfect: last leaf (blank?) wanting.

—Aphorismi aphorismorum; id est, Aphorismi Hippocratis in porismata resoluti, ut & mens textus, & usus facile patere queat. Jenae, Sumptibus Johannis Bielkii, 1695.

[46], 362 (i.e. 360) p.   14 cm.   [12648]

With this are bound: *his* Diaeta literatorum. 1695; Franck von Franckenau, Georg. De studiorum noxa. 1695.

—De medicamentorum compositione extemporanea, ad praxin clinicam & usum hodiernum accommodata, liber, tribus sectionibus distinctus. Jenae, Sumptibus Johannis Bielkii, typis Samuelis Krebsii, 1678.

[8], 212, [11] p.   20 cm.   [12649]

—Another issue, with date changed to 1679.
                                            [12650]

—[The same.] ... Ed. 2. Jenae, Sumptibus Johannis Bielkii, typis viduae Samuelis Krebsii, 1693.

[8], 212, [11] p.   21 cm.   [12651]

Different setting of type.

With this is bound *his* Syllabus materiae medicae selectioris. Jenae, 1701.

—De medicamentorum facultatibus cognoscendis & applicandis, libri duo. Jenae, Sumptibus Johannis Bielckii, excudebat Samuel Krebsius, 1678.

[14], 238, [10] p.   20 cm.   [12652]

Imperfect? Sig a4 wanting?

—[The same.] ... Ed. 2. Jenae, Sumtu Joannis Bielckii literis Nisianis, 1696.

[24], 238, [10] p.   20 cm.   [12653]

Imperfect: first leaf (blank?) wanting.

"Catalogus librorum et scriptorum editorum a Georgio Wolffgango Wedelio." (p. [3-6] inserted after title page) has special title page.

—[English tr.] An introduction to the whole practice of physick, shewing the natures and faculties of medicines ... directing the more unskilful in the true method of physick; according to the most successful practice of several modern physicians in general, and of ... Dr. Willis in particular; being chiefly a translation of ... Wedelius ... London, William Thackery and Thomas Yeate, 1685.

[7], 322, [6] p.   19 cm.   [12654]

—Duae orationes, quarum prior de causis diritatis pestilentiae ... altera de diritatis pestilentiae antidoto ... Norimbergae, 1683.

[20] p.   21 cm.   [12655]

—Exercitationes pathologico-therapeuticae. Jenae, Sumptibus Johannis Bielckii, 1697.

[16], 162, [6] p.   21 cm.   [12656]

Bound with *his* Physiologia reformata. 1688.

—Exercitationes semiotico-pathologicae. Jenae, Sumptibus Johannis Bielckii, literis Christophori Krebsii, 1700.

[16], 214, [6] p.   21 cm.   [12657]

—Exercitationum medico-philologicarum decades duae. Jenae, Sumptibus Johannis Bielckii, literis viduae Samuelis Krebsii, 1686.

[8], 80 p.   21 cm.   [12658]

Bound with Bellini, L. De urinis. 1685.

—Exercitationum medico-philologicarum sacrarum et profanum decas quarta ... Jenae, Sumptibus Johannis Bielckii, literis viduae Samuelis Krebsii, 1689.

[4], 52 p.   20 cm.   [12659]

—Exercitationum medico-philologicarum sacrarum et profanarum decas quinta. Jenae, Sumptibus Johannis Bielckii, literis viduae Samuelis Krebsii, 1691.

[16], 56 p.   21 cm.   [12660]

—Exercitationum medico-philologicarum sacrarum et profanarum decas septima. Jenae, Sumtibus Joh. Bielckii, literis Jo. Zach. Nisii, 1694.

[8], 72 p. illus. 21 cm.   [**12661**]

—Experimentum chimicum novum de sale volatili plantarum, quo latius exponuntur, specimine ipso exhibita. Jenae, Sumptibus Johannis Fritschii, literis Samuelis Krebsii, 1675.

[24], 96 p. 14 cm.   [**12662**]

—Opiologia ad mentem Academiae Naturae Curiosorum. Jenae, Sumptibus Johannis Fritschii, typis Samuelis Krebsii, 1674.

[8], 170, [2] p. 19 cm.   [**12663**]

—[The same.] ... Jenae, Sumptibus Johannis Bielkii, typis viduae Samuelis Krebsii, 1682.

[16], 170, [20] p. 20 cm.   [**12664**]

The main text is a reissue of the 1674 edition.

—Pathologia medica dogmatica. Jenae, Sumptibus Johannis Bielkii, typis Krebsianis, 1692.

[16], 694, [10] p. 21 cm.   [**12665**]

Imperfect: all p. after index wanting.
Bound with *his* Physiologia reformata. 1688.

—Pharmacia acroamatica. Jenae, Sumptibus Johannis Bielckii, literis viduae Samuelis Krebsii, 1686.

[16], 520, [14] p. 21 cm.   [**12666**]

—Pharmacia in artis formam redacta, experimentis, observationibus et discursu perpetuo illustrata. Jenae, Sumptibus Joh. Bielckii, typis Samuelis Krebsii, 1677.

[14], 245, [9] p. 18 cm.   [**12667**]

—[The same.] ... Ed. 2. Jenae. Sumptibus Johannis Bielkii, typis viduae Samuelis Krebsii, 1693.

[16], 245, [9] p. 19 cm.   [**12668**]

Different setting of type.

—Physiologia medica, quatuor sectionibus distincta. Jenae, Sumptibus Johannis Bielkii, typis Samuelis Krebsii, 1680.

[15], 328, [8] p. front. (ports.) 20 cm.   [**12669**]

With this is bound *his* Physiologia medica. Jenae, 1704.

—Physiologia reformata. Jenae, Sumptibus Johannis Bielkii, typis Krebsianis, 1688.

[16], 616, [16] p. 21 cm.   [**12670**]

With this are bound *his*: Pathologia medica dogmatica. 1692; Exercitationes pathologico-therapeuticae. 1697.

—Propempticon anatomicum, de epispasmo Judaeorum. Jenae, Literis Krebsianis, 1690.

8 p. 19 cm.   [**12671**]

—Specimen experimenti chimici novi, de sale volatili plantarum, quo demonstratur, posse ex plantis modo peculiari parari sal volatile verum & genuinum. Francofurti, Sumpt. haered. Shurerianorum & Joh. Fritzschii, 1672.

[24], 96 p. 14 cm.   [**12672**]

Bound with copy 2 of Rhijne, Willem ten. Meditationes in magni Hippocratis textum xxiv De veteri medicina. 1672.

—Tabulae pathologico-therapeuticae, omnium morborum synopsin, quo ad effectus, phaenomena, causas & curationem uno intuitu facillimaque methodo exhibentes. Jenae, Sumptibus Johannis Bielkii, literis Krebsianis, 1687.

[4] p. 10 tables. 33 cm.   [**12673**]

—Theoremata medica; seu, Introductio ad medicinam, certis theorematibus, juxta ductum institutionum medicarum, absoluta, ad legendum & disputandum proposita. Jenae, Sumptibus Johannis Bielkii, typis Samuelis Krebsii, 1677.

[23], 240 p. tables. 14 cm.   [**12674**]

Imperfect: added engraved title page wanting.
With this are bound: Horne, J. van. Μικροκοσμος. 1675; Molitor, J. H. Tractatus de thermis artificialibus. 1676.

—[The same.] ... Ed. 2. auct. & corr. Jenae, Sumptibus Johannis Bielckii, typis viduae Samuelis Krebsii, 1692.

[23], 240 p. tables. 14 cm.   [**12675**]

Added engraved title page.
Different setting of type.

Dissertation — Pro loco — Jena

—Exercitationem medico-chirurgicam de setaceis ... submittit Georgius Wolffgangus Wedelius ... Jenae, Literis Samuelis Krebsii [1673]

24 p. 20 cm.   [**12676**]

—Another printing, without pagination and running title.   [**12677**]

Programs — Jena

—Decanus Facultatis Medicae Georgius Wolffgangus Wedelius ... lectori benevolo S. P. D. [Jenae, 1683]

[8] p. 18 cm.   [**12678**]

With vita of B. Kruger.

—Decanus Facultatis Medicae Georgius Wolff-gangus Wedelius ... lectori benevolo S. P. D. [Jenae, 1684]

[8] p. 20 cm. [12679]

With vita of M. Sprögel.

—Georgius Wolffgangus Wedelius ... Facultatis Medicae decanus, lectori benevolo S. P. D. [Jenae, 1681]

[8] p. 19 cm. [12680]

With vita of J. L. Dresler.

—Georgius Wolffgangus Wedelius ... Facultatis Medicae decanus, lectori benevolo S. P. D. [Jenae, 1681]

[8] p. 19 cm. [12681]

With vita of J. A. Stockhausen.

—Georgius Wolffgangus Wedelius ... Facultatis Medicae decanus, lectori benevolo S. P. D. [Jenae, 1683]

[8] p. 19 cm. [12682]

With vita of G. Grundel.

—Propempticon inaugurale de amello Virgilii. Jenae, Literis Krebsianis, 1686.

8 p. 20 cm. [12683]

With vita of H. A. Kestner.

—Propempticon inaugurale de anil, indico, glasto. Jenae, Litteris Krebsianis [1689]

8 p. 20 cm. [12684]

With vita of J. J. Fick.

—Propempticon inaugurale de animalitate hominis. Jenae, Literis Krebsianis, 1690.

8 p. 20 cm. [12685]

With vita of J. L. Hechtel.

—Propempticon inaugurale de balsamatione corporis Christi. Jenae, Litteris Krebsianis, 1691.

8 p. 20 cm. [12686]

With vita of J. G. Thilen.

—Propempticon inaugurale de balsamatione corporum in genere. Jenae, Litteris Krebsianis, 1691.

8 p. 19 cm. [12687]

With vita of E. G. Bremer.

—Propempticon inaugurale de bile, fermento intestinorum. Jenae, Literis Krebsianis, 1684.

8 p. 20 cm. [12688]

With vita of J. J. Hoffmann.

—Propempticon inaugurale de cirsio Dioscoridis. Jenae, Typis Krebsianis [1700]

8 p. 20 cm. [12689]

With vita of J. Heimreich.

—Propempticon inaugurale de contractura daemoniaca. Jenae, Litteris Krebsianis, 1691.

8 p. 20 cm. [12690]

With vita of J. J. Baier.

—Propemticun inaugurale de corchoro Theophrasti in specie. Jenae, Litteris Krebsianis [1695]

8 p. 19 cm. [12691]

With vita of E. H. Wedel.

—Propempticun inaugurale de decimatione operum. Jenae, Litteris Krebsianis [1695]

8 p. 19 cm. [12692]

With vita of G. C. Wolff.

—Propempticon inaugurale de demonstratione Hippocratica. Jenae, Litteris Krebsianis [1689]

8 p. 20 cm. [12693]

J. Eichel, *respondent.*

—Propempticum inaugurale de expectatione medica. Jenae, Literis Wertherianis [1696]

8 p. 19 cm. [12694]

With vita of W. D. Lupin.

—Propempticon inaugurale de faecula coa ... [Jenae] Litteris Nisianis [1693]

[8] p. 19 cm. [12695]

With vita of J. L'Hommart.

—Propemticum inaugurale de febri magna. Jenae, Litteris Krebsianis [1695]

8 p. 20 cm. [12696]

With vita of J. W. Rumpel.

—Propempticon inaugurale de fortuna medici. Jenae, Literis Krebsianis, 1686.

8 p. 20 cm. [12697]

With vita of A. S. Backhauss.

—Propempticon inaugurale de fundamentis empiricorum. Jenae, Literis Krebsianis, 1686.

8 p. 20 cm. [12698]

With vita of J. M. Ehrlich.

—Propempticon inaugurale de fundamentis methodicorum. Jenae, Literis Krebsianis, 1684.

[8] p. 20 cm. [12699]

With vita of C. W. Förster.

—Propempticon inaugurale de hyperico mystico. Jenae, Literis Krebsianis, 1686.

8 p.   20 cm.   **[12700]**

With vita of J. C. Cummius.

—Propemticum inaugurale de medicamine faciei. Jenae, Litteris Krebsianis [1695]

8 p.   19 cm.   **[12701]**

With vita of J. H. Trumph.

—Propemticum inaugurale de minio lunari. Jenae, Litteris Krebsianis [1695]

8 p.   19 cm.   **[12702]**

With vita of G. Held.

—Propempticon inaugurale de morbis senum Salomonaeis ... Jenae, Literis Krebsianis, 1686.

[8] p.   20 cm.   **[12703]**

With vita of J. E. Kisner.

—Propempticon inaugurale de morbo crasso Hippocratis. Jenae, Literis Krebsianis, 1688.

8 p.   19 cm.   **[12704]**

With vita of K. F. Nester.

—Propempticon inaugurale de morbo et herba solstitiali. Jenae, Litteris Krebsianis, 1690.

8 p.   20 cm.   **[12705]**

With vita of G. F. Rumpel.

—Propempticon inaugurale de morbo hiobi. Jenae, Literis Krebsianis [1689]

8 p.   19 cm.   **[12706]**

With vita of C. Pezold.

—Propempticon inaugurale de morbo nabalis. Jenae, Litteris Nisianis [1696]

[8] p.   19 cm.   **[12707]**

With vita of F. W. von Rhoda.

—Propempticon inaugurale de Mose chimico. Jenae, Typis Christophori Krebsii [1698]

8 p.   19 cm.   **[12708]**

With vita of C. G. Goldammerus.

—Propempticon inaugurale de naturae ministro medico. Jenae, Literis Krebsianis, 1687.

8 p.   21 cm.   **[12709]**

With vita of Andreas Rosa.
Bound (as issued) with Crause, R. W. Disputatio inauguralis medica de contractura. 1687.

—Propempticon inaugurale de nummis Gothicis. Jenae, Typis Christophori Krebsii [1698]

8 p.   21 cm.   **[12710]**

With vita of T. Dehne.

—Propempticon inaugurale de nummis Jani ratitis I. Jenae, Literis Krebsianis, 1693.

8 p.   20 cm.   **[12711]**

With vita of H. G. Sommer.

—Propempticum inaugurale de nummis pileatis. Jenae, Litteris Krebsianis [1695]

8 p.   20 cm.   **[12712]**

With vita of J. L. Müller.

—Propempticon inaugurale de pane quotidiano. Jenae, Litteris Krebsianis [1689]

8 p.   20 cm.   **[12713]**

With vita of G. S. Cotta.

—Propemticon inaugurale de physiologia exidii sodomorum et statuae salis. Jenae, Litteris Krebsianis, 1692.

8 p.   20 cm.   **[12714]**

With vita of J. P. Biester.

—Propempticon inaugurale de quadragesima medica. Jenae, Literis Krebsianis, 1688.

[8] p.   20 cm.   **[12715]**

With vita of G. D. Walther.

—Propempticon inaugurale de radice amara Homeri. Jenae, Litteris Krebsianis, 1692.

8 p.   19 cm.   **[12716]**

With vita of E. K. Judel.

—Propempticum inaugurale de ramo aureo Virgilii. Jenae, Typis Gollnerianis [1699]

[8] p.   19 cm.   **[12717]**

With vita of J. S. Büchelmann.

—Propemticum inaugurale de ramo aureo Virgilii II. Jenae, Literis Christophori Krebsii [1700]

8 p.   20 cm.   **[12718]**

With vita of W. C. P. Pez.

—Propempticon inaugurale de resina Aegyptia Plauti. Jenae, Typis Krebsianis [1700]

[8] p.   20 cm.   **[12719]**

With vita of J. A. Stoll.

—Propempticon inaugurale de sudero Christi cruento ... Jenae, Literis Krebsianis, 1686.

8 p.   20 cm.   **[12720]**

With vita of C. F. Schumann.

—Propempticon inaugurale de suspendio virginum milesiarum. Jenae, Litteris Krebsianis, 1692.

8 p.   20 cm.   **[12721]**

With vita of J. Müller.

—Propempticon inaugurale de tetragono Hippocratis. Jenae, Literis Krebsianis, 1688.

8 p. 19 cm. [**12722**]

With vita of C. F. Hojer.

—Propemticum inaugurale de valvulis conniventibus. Jenae, Litteris Krebsianis [1695]

8 p. 19 cm. [**12723**]

With vita of J. L. Kamper.

—Propempticon inaugurale de vini dulcis plenis. Jenae, Litteris Krebsianis, 1692.

8 p. 19 cm. [**12724**]

With vita of P. Schöpffer.

—Propempticon inaugurale de vulnere אל-תחזמש seu, in quinta costa. Jenae, Literis Krebsianis, 1684.

8 p. 20 cm. [**12725**]

With vita of J. C. Ursin.

Dissertations — Jena

—*praeses.* Aegram pleuriticam ... publico ... examini subjiciet ... Wolfgangus Christophorus Wesenerus ... Jenae, Literis Krebsianis, 1674.

[16] p. 19 cm. [**12726**]

W. C. Wesener, *respondent.*

—Aegram suppressione mensium laborantem ... publicae ... ventilationi exponit Clemens Weigelius ... Jenae, Typis Samuelis Krebsii [1676]

[16] p. 19 cm. [**12727**]

C. Weigel, *respondent.*

—Aegrum hypochondriacum ... publice examinandum proponit ... Johannes Philippus Grauel ... Jenae, Typis Samuelis Krebsii [1675]

[28] p. 19 cm. [**12728**]

J. P. Grauel, *respondent.*

—Aegrum pollutione nocturna laborantem ... examini exponent ... Johannes Justus Bückingius ... Jenae, Typis Samuelis Krebsii [1675]

[20] p. 20 cm. [**12729**]

J. J. Bücking, *respondent.*

—Aegrum singultu ex febri maligna laborantem ... publice examinandum proponit ... Simon Andreas Beckerus. Jenae, Typis Krebsianis [1676]

[20] p. 20 cm. [**12730**]

S. A. Becker, *respondent.*

—Aegrum tertianarium ... publico ... examini sistet Jacobus Schmid ... Jenae, Typis Samuelis Krebsii [1674]

[20] p. 19 cm. [**12731**]

J. Schmid, *respondent.*

—Casum laborantis corysa ... publice ... proponit Augustus Michael Dörmer ... Jenae, Typis Samuelis Krebsii [1673]

[16] p. 19 cm. [**12732**]

A. M. Dörmer, *respondent.*

—De medicamentorum facultatibus, disputatio II. de adstringentibus, aperientibus, incrassantibus, repellentibus, et causticis ... Jenae, Typis Samuelis Krebsii [1677]

[2], 33-66, [2] p. 19 cm. [**12733**]

J. A. Schmid, *respondent.*

—Diaeta literatorum ... Ed. 3., cum additamentis paradoxis. Jenae, Charactere ac impensis Nisianis [1674]

[1], 38 p. 19 cm. [**12734**]

Originally published as a dissertation "exercitii gratia" in Jena in 1674.

J. Rottenberger, *respondent.*

—[The same.] ... Ed. 4., cum additamentis paradoxis. Jenae, Apud Johann. Bielckium, 1695.

112 p. 14 cm. [**12735**]

Bound with *his* Aphorismi aphorismorum. 1695.

—[The same.] ... Ed. 4., cum additamentis paradoxis. Jenae, Charactere ac impensis Nisianis, 1699.

[1], 38 p. 20 cm. [**12736**]

—Diatribe medica exhibens aegrum memoriae debilitate laborantem ... Jenae, Typis Johannis Jacobi Krebsii [1696]

[18], 2 p. 20 cm. [**12737**]

J. G. Maley, *respondent.*

—Diatriben medicam de diebus criticis ... subjiciunt Georgius Wolffgangus Wedelius ... & Georgius Tobias Wallich ... Jenae, Typis Samuelis Krebsii [1667]

[20] p. 19 cm. [**12738**]

Diss. — Jena (G. T. Wallich, *respondent*)

—[The same.] ... Jenae, Typis Samuelis Krebsii, recusa 1678.

[20] p. 20 cm. [**12739**]

—Diatriben medicam diureticis ... subjiciunt Georgius Wolffgangus Wedelius ... & Conradus Theodorus Witte ... Jenae, Typis Samuelis Krebsii [1667]

[24] p. 19 cm. [12740]

—Disputatio inauguralis de arthritide vaga scorbutica ... Jenae, Excudebat Samuel Krebs [1674]

[32] p. 19 cm. [12741]

C. E. Clauder, *respondent.*

—Disputatio inauguralis medica de bulimo ... Jenae, Literis Krebsianis [1691]

18 (i.e. 28) p. 20 cm. [12742]

K. G. Carsten, *respondent.*

—Disputatio inauguralis medica de cardialgia ... Jenae, Literis Krebsianis [1688]

16 p. 20 cm. [12743]

C. F. Hojer, *respondent.*

—Disputatio inauguralis medica, de catarrho suffocativo ... Jenae, Typis viduae Samuelis Krebsii, 1680.

48 p. 20 cm. [12744]

G. F. Aeplinius, *respondent.*

—Another issue, with date changed to 1681.

[12745]

—Disputatio inauguralis medica de catarrho suffocativo laborante ...Jenae, Literis Krebsianis [1686]

16 p. 19 cm. [12746]

C. F. Schumann, *respondent.*

—Disputatio inauguralis medica de empyemate ... Jenae, Literis Krebsianis [1686]

24 p. 20 cm. [12747]

J. E. Kisner, *respondent.*

—Disputatio inauguralis medica de epilepsia hysterica ... Jenae, Typis Nisianis [1676]

[24] p. 19 cm. [12748]

N. L. Heden, *respondent.*

—Disputatio inauguralis medica de febribus intermittentibus ... Jenae, Typis Krebsianis [1692]

32 p. 20 cm. [12749]

P. Schöpffer, *respondent.*

—Disputatio inauguralis medica de hydrope ... Jenae, Literis Krebsianis [1685]

32 p. 19 cm. [12750]

C. L. Göckel, *respondent.*

—Disputatio inauguralis medica de mensium fluxu immodico ... Jenae, Literis Krebsianis [1688]

32 p. 20 cm. [12751]

F. J. Erich, *respondent.*

—Disputatio inauguralis medica de ophthalmia ... Jenae, Literis Krebsianis [1684]

26, [2] p. 20 cm. [12752]

A. Rehme, *respondent.*

—Disputatio inauguralis medica de peripneumonia ... Jenae, Literis Krebsianis [1687]

24 p. 20 cm. [12753]

A. Bechmann, *respondent.*

—Disputatio inauguralis medica, de punctura nervorum ... Jenae, Litteris Krebsianis [1689]

24 p. 20 cm. [12754]

J. Eichel, *respondent.*

—Disputatio inauguralis medica de vomitu ... Jenae, Typis Johannis Nisii, 1673.

[16] p. 18 cm. [12755]

J. L. Schlapperitius, *respondent.*

—Disputatio medica, aegram dysentericam sistens ... Jenae, Prodibat e chalcographeo Samuelis Krebsii [1675]

[20] p. 18 cm. [12756]

J. Röder, *respondent.*

—Disputatio medica aegrum erysipelate laborantem exhibens ... Jenae, Literis Krebsianis [1682]

20 p. 19 cm. [12757]

G. F. Kinner, *respondent.*

—Disputatio medica, aegrum haemoptysi laborantem exhibens ... Jenae, Literis Samuelis Krebsii [1679]

19, [5] p. 18 cm. [12758]

J. A. Stockhausen, *respondent.*

—Disputatio medica aegrum haemorrhoidibus dolentibus et immodicis laborantem exhibens ... Jenae, Literis Samuelis Krebsii [1679]

18, [2] p. 19 cm. [12759]

J. F. Eckhard, *respondent.*

—Disputatio medica, aegrum nephritide laborantem, exhibens ... Jenae, Typis viduae Samuelis Krebsii [1680]

23, [1] p. 20 cm. [12760]

J. H. Schmoller, *respondent.*

—Disputatio medica, casum aegri hernia laborantis exhibens ... Jenae, Literis Krebsianis [1684]
    20 p.   19 cm.   [12761]
J. M. Ehrlich, *respondent.*

—Disputatio medica de aegra dysenteria laborante
... Jenae, Literis Krebsianis [1687]
    16 p.   19 cm.   [12762]
H. M. Bartholomaei, *respondent.*

—Disputatio medica de contagio et morbis contagiosis ... Jenae, Literis Krebsianis [1689]
    40 p.   20 cm.   [12763]
J. F. Breitert, *respondent.*

—Disputatio medica, de gialapa ... Jenae, Typis
Samuelis Krebsii [1678]
    40 p.   19 cm.   [12764]
J. U. Schmid, *respondent.*

—Disputatio medica de purgantibus rite adhibendis ... Jenae, Typis Samuelis Krebsii [1675]
    [40] p.   20 cm.   [12765]
D. de Four, *respondent.*

—Disputatio medica de tussi ... Jenae, Literis
Krebsianis [1688]
    31, [1] p.   20 cm.   [12766]
J. A. Cramer, *respondent.*

—Disputatio medica de venae sectione rite
adhibenda ... Jenae, Literis Samuelis Krebsii [1675]
    [32] p.   20 cm.   [12767]
T. E. Beerwinckel, *respondent.*

—Disputatio medica, exhibens aegrum epilepticum ... Jenae, Typis Samuelis Krebsii [1673]
    [20] p.   19 cm.   [12768]
S. Zeideler, *respondent.*

—Disputatio medica, exhibens aegrum laborantem colica ... Jenae, Literis Krebsianis [1674]
    [20] p.   18 cm.   [12769]
E. Franz, *respondent.*

—Disputatio medica inauguralis de bile ejusque
morbis ... Jenae, Litteris Krebsianis [1689]
    24 p.   20 cm.   [12770]
K. J. Leicker, *respondent.*

—Disputatio medica inauguralis de morbis a
fascino ... Jenae, Literis Krebsianis [1682]
    40 p.   20 cm.   [12771]
F. Käseberg, *respondent.*

—Disputatio medica inauguralis de palpitatione
cordis ... Jenae, Litteris Krebsianis [1690]
    26, [2] p.   20 cm.   [12772]
G. Budaeus, *respondent.*

—Disputatio medica inauguralis de paralysi ...
Jenae, Typis Samuelis Krebsii [1677]
    [1], 37 p.   20 cm.   [12773]
S. Grass, *respondent.*

—Disputatio medica inauguralis, de partu difficili
... Jenae, Literis Samuelis Krebsii [1675]
    [40] p.   20 cm.   [12774]
B. Lohner, *respondent.*

—Disputatio medica inauguralis de raucedine ...
Jenae, Literis Krebsianis [1683]
    41, [3] p.   20 cm.   [12775]
G. F. Kinner, *respondent.*

—Disputatio medica inauguralis de somno
praeternaturali ... Jenae, Literis Krebsianis [1686]
    24 p.   20 cm.   [12776]
K. G. Hartmann, *respondent.*

—Disputatio medica juvenem ictero flavo
laborantem exhibens ... Jenae, Charactere Samuelis
Krebsii, 1675.
    [16] p.   19 cm.   [12777]
J. G. Weller, *respondent.*

—Disputatio medica sistens aegrum laborantem
vertigine ... Jenae, Typis viduae Samuelis Krebsii
[1682]
    22, [2] p.   20 cm.   [12778]
C. F. Gerber, *respondent.*

—Disputatio medica, sistens aegrum quartana
laborantem ... Jenae, Literis Krebsianis [1688]
    19, [1] p.   19 cm.   [12779]
J. F. Herwig, *respondent.*

—Disputatio medico-consultatoria de mania ...
Jenae, Typis Johannis Nisii [1673]
    [16] p.   18 cm.   [12780]
J. L. Schlapperitius, *respondent.*

—Disputationem inauguralem de bubone pesti-
lenti ... subjicit Fridericus Wilhelmus Clauderus ...
Jenae, Typis viduae Samuelis Krebsii [1681]
    [1], 30, [8] p.   19 cm.   [12781]
Includes program with vita of F. W. Clauder by R. W. Crause
[8 p.].
F. W. Clauder, *respondent.*

—Disputationem inauguralem de diarrhoea ... exponit Augustus Michael Dörmer ... Jenae, Typis Samuelis Krebsii [1673]

[36] p. 18 cm. [12782]

A. M. Dörmer, *respondent*.

—Disputationem inauguralem de febri petechiali ... subjiciet Johannes Guilielmus Eichhorn ... Jenae, Typis Samuelis Krebsii [1674]

[32] p. 18 cm. [12783]

J. W. Eichhorn, *respondent*.

—Disputationem inauguralem de scorbuto ... proponit Conradus Rudolphus Hertz ... [Jenae] Literis Georg. Heinr. Mülleri [1687]

38, [2] p. 20 cm. [12784]

C. R. Hertz, *respondent*.

—Disputationem inauguralem medicam de colica scorbutica ... submittit Carolus Fridericus Nesterus ... Jenae, Literis Krebsianis [1688]

32 p. 19 cm. [12785]

K. F. Nester, *respondent*.

—Disputationem inauguralem medicam de pervigilio ... submittit Paulus Gottfried Sperling ... Jenae, Typis Wertherianis [1680]

48 p. 20 cm. [12786]

P. G. Sperling, *respondent*.

—Disputationem medicam inauguralem, de archeo ... subjicit Andreas Schemberger ... [Jenae] Typis Samuelis Krebsii [1678]

36 p. 20 cm. [12787]

A. Schemberger, *respondent*.

—Disputationem medicam inauguralem de dentitione infantum ... subjicit Johannes Ernestus Krausold ... Jenae, Literis Nisianis [1678]

31, [1] p. 19 cm. [12788]

J. E. Krausoldt, *respondent*.

—Dissertatio chimica de antimonio diaphoretico ... Jenae, Literis Krebsianis [1690]

20 p. 20 cm. [12789]

C. A. Tornesi, *respondent*.

—Dissertatio inauguralis chimico-medica de mercurio dulci ... Jenae, Literis Christophori Krebsii [1700]

38 (i.e. 36) p. 20 cm. [12790]

J. A. Stoll, *respondent*.

—Dissertatio inauguralis chimico-medica, de sale ammoniaco ... Jenae, Litteris Krebsianis [1695]

32 p. 19 cm. [12791]

E. H. Wedel, *respondent*.

—Dissertatio inauguralis de morbis tartareis ... Jenae, Litteris Krebsianis [1695]

32 p. 20 cm. [12792]

J. L. Müller, *respondent*.

—Dissertatio inauguralis medica de aegilope ... Jenae, Litteris Krebsianis [1695]

28 p. 20 cm. [12793]

J. F. Hünerwolff, *respondent*.

—Dissertatio inauguralis medica de aegro cachectico ... Jenae, Literis Christophori Krebsii [1700]

20 p. 19 cm. [12794]

S. G. Hausdorff, *respondent*.

—Dissertatio inauguralis medica, de amarorum natura & usu ... Jenae, Typis Krebsianis [1692]

28 p. 20 cm. [12795]

T. R. Rommel, *respondent*.

—Dissertatio inauguralis medica, de apoplexia ... Jenae, Typis viduae Samuelis Krebsii [1680]

32, [8] p. 19 cm. [12796]

With vita of Georg Heinrich Bachov by Augustin Heinrich Fasch ([8] p.).

G. H. Bachov, *respondent*.

—Dissertatio inauguralis medica, de aromaticorum natura, usu et abusu ... Jenae, Litteris Krebsianis [1695]

23, [1] p. 20 cm. [12797]

J. H. Trumph, *respondent*.

—Dissertatio inauguralis medica, de arthritide ... Jenae, Litteris Krebsianis [1695]

38 (i.e. 36) p. 20 cm. [12798]

J. W. Rumpel, *respondent*.

—Dissertatio inauguralis medica de asthmatis mechanica ... Jenae, Literis Christophori Krebsii [1700]

34, [2] p. 20 cm. [12799]

J. T. Schmid, *respondent*.

—Dissertatio inauguralis medica, de Χλωρωσει; seu, Foedis virginum coloribus ... Jenae, Literis Krebsianis, 1681.

28 p. 20 cm. [12800]

J. A. Stockhausen, *respondent*.

—Dissertatio inauguralis medica de defectu lactis .. Jenae, Typis Christophori Krebsii [1699]
28 p.   20 cm.   [**12801**]
C. G. Lehmann, *respondent*.

—Dissertatio inauguralis medica de febri phemera ... Jenae Litteris Nisianis [1696]
35, [1] p.   19 cm.   [**12802**]
F. Liefmann, *respondent*.

—Dissertatio inauguralis medica de febri maligna .. Jenae, Litteris Nisianis [1696]
28 p.   20 cm.   [**12803**]
J. G. Ludwig, *respondent*.

—Dissertatio inauguralis medica de fundamentis lethalitatis vulnerum ... Jenae, Litteris Krebsianis [1695]
24 p.   18 cm.   [**12804**]
P. A. W. Sauber, *respondent*.

—Dissertatio inauguralis medica, de mania ... Jenae, Literis Krebsianis [1693]
24 p.   20 cm.   [**12805**]
H. G. Sommer, *respondent*.

—Dissertatio inauguralis medica de purpura puerperarum ... Jenae, Litteris Krebsianis [1690]
24 p.   20 cm.   [**12806**]
G. F. Rumpel, *respondent*.

—Dissertatio inaguralis medica de terreorum natura, usu et abusu ... Jenae, Literis Krebsianis [1697]
32 p.   21 cm.   [**12807**]
J. G. Siber, *respondent*.

—Dissertatio inauguralis medica de thermis ... Jenae, Litteris Krebsianis [1695]
44 p.   19 cm.   [**12808**]
G. Held von Hagelsheim, *respondent*.

—Dissertatio inauguralis medica de tinctura bezoardica essentificata ... Jenae, Typis Christophori Krebsii [1698]
30, [2] p.   19 cm.   [**12809**]
J. D. Eberhard, *respondent*.

—Dissertatio inauguralis medica de vitiis humorum morbificis ... Jenae, Literis Krebsianis [1684]
32 p.   20 cm.   [**12810**]
M. Lüder, *respondent*.

—Dissertatio inauguralis medica de voce, ejusque affectibus ... Jenae, Typis Samuelis Krebsii [1677]
56 p.   20 cm.   [**12811**]
G. C. Schelhammer, *respondent*.

—Dissertatio medica, aegrum haemorrhagia narium laborantem sistens ... Jenae, Aere Krebsiano, 1679.
16 p.   19 cm.   [**12812**]
J. Block, *respondent*.

—Dissertatio medica, aegrum incubo laborantem sistens ... Jenae, Aere Krebsiano, 1678.
23, [1] p.   19 cm.   [**12813**]
G. F. Aeplinius, *respondent*.

—Dissertatio medica, aegrum ischuria laborantem exhibens ... Jenae, Literis Krebsianis [1699]
19, [1] p.   21 cm.   [**12814**]
J. Á. Gensel, *respondent*.

—Dissertatio medica de acidulis ... Jenae, Literis Krebsianis [1695]
36 p.   20 cm.   [**12815**]
F. W. von Rhoda, *respondent*.

—Dissertatio medica de ambra ... Jenae, Typis Christophori Krebsii [1698]
44 p.   19 cm.   [**12816**]
J. J. Baier, *respondent*

—Dissertatio medica de aneurismate ... Jenae, Literis Christophori Krebsii [1699]
32 p.   19 cm.   [**12817**]
C. Wedel, *respondent*.

—Dissertatio medica de ἀντιπραξει viscerum ... Jenae, Typis viduae Samuelis Krebsii [1683]
32 p.   18 cm.   [**12818**]
D. Spielenberger, *respondent*.

—Dissertatio medica de austerorum et acerborum natura, usu et abusu ... Jenae, Typis Christophori Krebsii [1698]
31, [1] p.   20 cm.   [**12819**]
J. G. Hugo, *respondent*.

—Dissertatio medica, de casu ab alto ... Jenae, Literis Krebsianis [1684]
30, [2] p.   20 cm.   [**12820**]
J. P. Fischer, *respondent*.

Dissertatio medica de catalepsi . . . Jenae, Ex officina Jo. Zach. Nisii [1690]
28 p. 19 cm. [12821]
J. Schomburg, *respondent.*

—Dissertatio medica de clavo pedis . . . Jenae, Literis Krebsianis [1686]
24 p. 20 cm. [12822]
J. R. Fuchs, *respondent.*

—Dissertatio medica de consensu partium . . . Jenae, Literis Krebsianis [1686]
28 p. 20 cm. [12823]
J. M. Triller, *respondent.*

—Dissertatio medica de convulsione, ad praxin clinicam accommodata . . . Jenae, Typis viduae Samuelis Krebsii [1683]
16 p. 20 cm. [12824]
C. L. Göckel, *respondent.*

—Dissertatio medica de epilepsia . . . Jenae, Stanno Wertheriano, 1673.
[42] p. 19 cm. [12825]
J. Röser, *respondent.*

—Dissertatio medica de foetore praeternaturali . . . Jenae, Litteris Nisianis, 1696.
24 p. 19 cm. [12826]
R. Genaspe, *respondent.*

—Dissertatio medica de gibbere . . . Jenae, Typis viduae Samuelis Krebsii [1681]
36 p. 20 cm. [12827]
F. Käseberg, *respondent.*

—Dissertatio medica de hydrophobia . . . Jenae, Litteris Krebsianis [1695]
40 p. 21 cm. [12828]
S. Roth, *respondent.*

—Dissertatio medica de insomniis . . . Jenae, Litteris Krebsianis [1690]
[32] p. 18 cm. [12829]
T. R. Rommel, *respondent.*

—Dissertatio medica de lue venerea . . . Jenae, Stanno Bauhoferiano [1682]
42, [2] p. 20 cm. [12830]
A. Löw, *respondent.*

—Dissertatio medica de morbis praecordialibus . . . Jenae, Litteris Krebsianis [1689]
60 p. 20 cm. [12831]
P. G. Lautitz, *respondent.*

—Dissertatio medica de naevis maternis . . . Jenae, Literis Krebsianis [1688]
32 p. 19 cm. [12832]
J. L. Hechtel, *respondent.*

- Dissertatio medica de notis gravidarum . . . Jenae Literis Krebsianis [1690]
32 p. 20 cm. [12833]
J. P. Biester, *respondent.*

—Dissertatio medica de nutritione et atrophia . . . Jenae, Literis Krebsianis [1682]
31, [1] p. 20 cm. [12834]
P. Ebeling, *respondent.*

—Dissertatio medica de nyctalopia . . . Jenae, Literis Krebsianis [1693]
27 (i.e. 28) p. 20 cm. [12835]
P. A. W. Sauber, *respondent.*

—Dissertatio medica de oblivione . . . Jenae, Litteris Krebsianis [1690]
32 p. 20 cm. [12836]
M. Kauliz, *respondent.*

—Dissertatio medica de pernionibus . . . Jenae, Literis Samuelis Adolphi Mülleri [1680]
28 p. 19 cm. [12837]
W. Müller, *respondent.*

—Dissertatio medica de pleuritide . . . Jenae, Typis Samuelis Krebsii [1673]
28 p. 19 cm. [12838]
J. A. Lentz, *respondent.*

—Dissertatio medica de procidentia ani . . . Jenae, Litteris Nisianis [1696]
32 p. 19 cm. [12839]
W. D. Lupin, *respondent.*

—Dissertatio medica de ructu . . . Jenae, Typis Christophori Krebsii [1698]
31, [1] p. 20 cm. [12840]
J. D. Eberhard, *respondent.*

—Dissertatio medica de scabie . . . Jenae, Typis Samuelis Krebsii [1674]
[32] p. 20 cm. [12841]
J. L. Neuenhahn, *respondent.*

—Dissertatio medica de similitudine morborum . . . Jenae, Litteris Krebsianis [1689]
34, [2] p. 19 cm. [12842]
J. C. Neubich, *respondent.*

—Dissertatio medica de spectris . . . Jenae, Literis Krebsianis [1693]

31, [1] p. 20 cm. [**12843**]

E. H. Wedel, *respondent.*

—[The same.] . . . Proposita . . . ad . . . Maji M DC XCIII. Ed. 2. Jenae, Litteris Krebsianis, 1698.

39, [1] p. 19 cm. [**12844**]

—Dissertatio medica de terrore . . . Jenae, Typis Christophori Krebsii [1697]

36, p. 20 cm. [**12845**]

H. Eckardi, *respondent.*

—Dissertatio medica de urinis, earumque significationibus . . . Jenae, Typis Samuelis Krebsii [1678]

38, [2] p. 20 cm. [**12846**]

J. D. Schrader, *respondent.*

—Dissertatio medica de varice . . . Jenae, Literis Krebsianis [1699]

[44] p. 20 cm. [**12847**]

D. Praetorius, *respondent.*

—Dissertatio medica de variolis et morbillis . . . Jenae, Typis Samuelis Krebsii [1678]

39, [1] p. 19 cm. [**12848**]

J. A. Schott, *respondent.*

—Dissertatio medica de venenis & bezoardicis . . . Jenae, Literis Krebsianis [1682]

31, [1] p. 19 cm. [**12849**]

J. C. Ursin, *respondent.*

—Dissertatio medica de verrucis . . . Jenae, Litteris Nisianis [1696]

32 p. 20 cm. [**12850**]

J. Ziegler, *respondent.*

—Dissertatio medica de vomitoriis rite adhibendis . . . Jenae, Typis Samuelis Krebsii [1676]

[20] p. 19 cm. [**12851**]

J. C. Zopff, *respondent.*

—Dissertatio medica exhibens aegrum laborantem peste . . . Jenae, Typis viduae Samuelis Krebsii [1681]

36, [4] p. 20 cm. [**12852**]

D. H. Ulrich, *respondent.*

—Dissertatio medica inauguralis de camphora . . . Jenae, Typis Christophori Krebsii [1697]

36 p. 20 cm. [**12853**]

J. A. Wedel, *respondent.*

—Dissertatio medica inauguralis de cholera . . . Jenae, Typis Christophori Krebsii [1697]

38, [2] p. 19 cm. [**12854**]

J. H. Ameldung, *respondent.*

—Dissertatio medica inauguralis de chorea S. Viti . . . Jenae, Literis Krebsianis [1682]

[32] p. 19 cm. [**12855**]

G. Profius, *respondent.*

—Dissertatio medica inauguralis de circulatione sanguinis . . . Jenae, Typis Johannis Jacobi Krebsii [1696]

31, [1] p. 20 cm. [**12856**]

K. C. Leisner, *respondent.*

—Dissertatio medica inauguralis de convulsione . . . Jenae, Typis viduae Samuelis Krebsii, 1684.

20 p. 19 cm. [**12857**]

W. Müller, *respondent.*

—Dissertatio medica inauguralis de cucurbitula sicca . . . Jenae, Literis Krebsianis [1691]

24 p. 20 cm. [**12858**]

J. G. Thilen, *respondent*

—Dissertatio medica inauguralis de dulcium natura, usu et abusu . . . Jenae, Literis Krebsianis [1694]

28 p. 20 cm. [**12859**]

J. C. Clauder, *respondent.*

—Dissertatio medica inauguralis de febre intermittente . . . Jenae, Litteris Krebsianis [1690]

32 p. 20 cm. [**12860**]

J. G. Mosdorff, *respondent.*

—Dissertatio medica inauguralis de fluore albo . . . Jenae, Literis Joh. Jac. Bauhoferi [1682]

53, [3] p. 20 cm. [**12861**]

G. E. Thill, *respondent.*

—Dissertatio medica inauguralis de ileo . . .Jenae, Literis Krebsianis [1689]

28 p. 20 cm. [**12862**]

J. R. Stiefel, *respondent.*

—Dissertatio medica inauguralis de inflammatione renum . . . Jenae, Typis Christophori Krebsii [1697]

36 p. 19 cm. [**12863**]

J. Brasche, *respondent.*

—Dissertatio medica inauguralis de natura et usu acidorum . . . Jenae, Typis Krebsianis [1692]

16 + p. 20 cm. [**12864**]

Imperfect: all after p. 16 wanting.

J. P. Biester, *respondent.*

—Dissertatio medica inauguralis de oleosorum natura, usu et abusu . . . Jenae, Typis Christophori Krebsii [1697]

27, [1] p. 18 cm. [**12865**]

F. K. Snell, *respondent.*

—Dissertatio medica inauguralis de procidentia uteri . . . Jenae, Literis Krebsianis [1684]

27, [1] p. 20 cm. [**12866**]

C. W. Förster, ... *respondent.*

—Dissertatio medica inauguralis de spiritu vini . . . Jenae, Literis Christophori Krebsii [1697]

32 p. 19 cm. [**12867**]

S. Closius, *respondent.*

—Dissertatio medica inauguralis de sudore Anglico . . . Jenae, Literis Krebsianis [1697]

31, [1] p. 20 cm. [**12868**]

E. Leupold, *respondent.*

—Dissertatio medica inauguralis de syncope . . . Jeane, Typis Wertherianis [1680]

44 p. 17 cm. [**12869**]

T. Kemper, *respondent.*

—Dissertatio medica inauguralis de terebinthina . . . Jenae, Literis Krebsianis [1700]

52 p. 20 cm. [**12870**]

C. Wedel, *respondent.*

—Dissertatio medica, physiologiam pulsus exhibens . . . Jenae, Literis Krebsianis [1689]

36 p. 20 cm. [**12871**]

J. C. Clauder, *respondent.*

—Dissertatio medica proponens aegrum palpitatione cordis laborantem . . . Jenae, Typis Samuelis Krebsii [1674]

[20] p. 19 cm. [**12872**]

H. Schmid, *respondent.*

—Dissertatio medica propnens juvenem melancholia laborantem . . . Jenae, Ex Typographia Krebsiana [1675]

[28] p. 19 cm. [**12873**]

J. R. Heydenreich, *respondent.*

—Dissertatio medica, sistens aegrum hydropicum . . . Jenae, Stanno Krebsiano [1674]

[28] p. 18 cm. [**12874**]

S. Chemnitz, *respondent.*

—Dissertatio medica, sistens aegrum laborantem dolore ischiadico . . . Jenae, Literis Krebsianis [1681]

24 p. 19 cm. [**12875**]

M. Hohberg, *respondent.*

—Dissertatio medica sistens aegrum laborantem syncope . . . Jenae, Literis Krebsianis [1682]

19, [1] p. 20 cm. [**12876**]

G. Grundel, *respondent.*

—Dissertatio medica sistens aegrum vomitu cruento laborantem . . . Jenae, Literis viduae Samuelis Krebsii [1680]

[1], 19, [1] p. 19 cm. [**12877**]

M. Sprögel, *respondent.*

—Dissertatio medico-chimica de oleis destillatis . . . Jenae, Litteris Nisianis [1696]

23,]1] p. 19 cm. [**12878**]

G. H. Rosenberg, *respondent.*

—Dissertationem inauguralem de malo hypochondriaco . . . ensurae expono Johannes Christophorus Zopff . . . [Jenae] Typis Krebsianis [1676]

[52] p. 19 cm. [**12879**]

J. C. Zopff, *respondent.*

—Dissertationem inauguralem de paronychia . . . subjicit Ernestus Fridemann Schelhass . . . anno M DC LXXIV. Ed. 2. Jenae, Literis Bauoferianis, 1686.

[6], 28, [2] p. 20 cm. [**12880**]

E. F. Schelhass, *respondent.*

—Dissertationem medicam de suffimentis . . . submittet . . . Johannes Hardovicus Hampe . . . Jenae, Stanno Nisiano [1676]

[40] p. 19 cm. [**12881**]

J. H. Hampe, *respondent.*

—Dissertationem medicam inauguralem de melancholia . . . subjicit Johannes Georgius Neuse . . . Jenae, Literis Krebsianis [1685]

40 p. 20 cm. [**12882**]

J. G. Neuse, *respondent.*

—Dissertationem medicam inauguralem de transplantatione morborum . . . submittit M.

Heinricus Andreas Kestner . . . Jenae, Literis Krebsianis [1686]

    28 p. 20 cm.   **[12883]**

  H. A. Kestner, *respondent.*

—Exercitatio chimica de menstruis . . . Jenae,
Literis Krebsianis, 1674.

    [32] p. 20 cm.   **[12884]**

  H. F. Körber, *respondent.*

—Exercitatio medica aegrum paralysi laborantem
sistens . . . Jenae. Literis Krebsianis [1682]

    24 p. 21 cm.   **[12885]**

  J. M. Hoffmann, *respondent.*

—Exercitatio medica, de cephalalgia in genere,
vulgo von Kopff-Wehtagen . . . Jenae, Literis Krebsianis [1686]

    44 p. 19 cm.   **[12886]**

  A. P. Kopff, *respondent.*

—Exercitatio medica de phthisi . . . Jenae, Literis
Samuelis Adolphi Mülleri [1688]

    28 p. 20 cm.   **[12887]**

  P. Schöpffer, *respondent*

—Exercitatio medica, sistens aegrum mictu
cruento laborantem . . . Jenae, Stanno Krebsiano
[1683]

    16 p. 20 cm.   **[12888]**

  J. M. Bertuch, *respondent.*

—Exercitatio medica, sistens aegrum vulnere
capitis laborantem . . . Jenae, Literis Krebsianis
[1684]

    24 p. 19 cm.   **[12889]**

  C. Bekker, *respondent.*

—Exercitationem pathologic-therapeuticarum
disputatio II. de inflammationibus . . . Jenae, Litteris Nisianis [1696]

    [1], 23–34 p. 19 cm.   **[12890]**

  W. D. Lupin, *respondent.*

—Exercitationum pathologico-therapeuticarum
disputatio X de laesionibus motus . . . Jenae, Litteris Nisianis [1697]

    [2], 149–162 p. 20 cm.   **[12891]**

  Signatures [A]¹, T³⁻⁴, V⁴, X¹.

  J. T. Deutgen, *respondent.*

—Lemmata medica . . . Jenae, Litteris Krebsianis
[1699]

    16 p. 20 cm.   **[12892]**

  N. C. Bezold, *respondent.*

—Spicilegium medicum de peste . . . Jenae, Literis
Krebsianis [1685]

    28 p. 19 cm.   **[12893]**

  J. B. Winterbach, *respondent.*

—Venus medica et morbifera . . . Jenae, Literis
Krebsianis [1688]

    40 p. 20 cm.   **[12894]**

  G. W. Blumberg, *respondent.*

—Visum . . . physiologice examinandum . . . disquisitioni sistet . . . Johannes Burg . . . Jenae, Literis
Krebsianis [1674]

    [32] p. 20 cm.   **[12895]**

  J. Burg, *respondent.*

—, *respondent. See* ROLFINCK, W., *praeses.* Dissertatio inauguralis medica de pollutione nocturna. 1667
[and] Dissertatio medica de tussi. 1663.

—, *ed. See* LOMMIUS, J. Observationum
medicinalium libri tres. 1688; LUDWIG, D. De pharmacia moderno seculo applicanda. 1688; MÖBIUS, G.
Fundamenta medicinae physiologica. 1678; ZOBEL, F.
Tartarologia spagirica. 1676.

—*See* ELSHOLTZ, J. S. Destillatoria curiosa. 1674;
ETTMÜLLER, M. Operum omnium medico-
phisicorum. 1690; FRANCK VON FRANCKENAU, G. F.
'Ονυχολογια curiosa. 1695; HOFFMANN, F. [1660–1742]
De affectu cataleptico rarissimo dissertatio. 1692;
KÖNIG, E. Regnum vegetabile . . . enucleatum. 1688;
SCHELHAMMER, G. C. Ad . . . Georgium
Wolfgangum Wedelium epistola. 1690; VALESCO DE
TARANTA. Philonium pharmaceuticum et chirurgic-
um, de medendis omnibus . . . humani corporis af-
fectibus a Valesco de Taranta. 1680.

WEDEL, JOHANN ADOLPH [1675–1747] *praeses.*
Dissertatio medico-physiologica de temperamento
mixti . . . Jenae, Typis Christophori Krebsii [1698]

    24 p. 20 cm.   **[12896]**

  Diss. — Jena (C. Wedel, *respondent*)

—*respondent. See* BOHN, J., *praeses.* Disputatio
therapeutica. 1697; POSNER, C., *praeses.* Dissertatio
physica de igne. 1696; WEDEL, E. H., *praeses.* Dissertatio chimico-medica de tinctura martis helleborata.
1695; WEDEL, G. W., *praeses.* Dissertatio medica inauguralis de camphora. 1697.

WEDMANN, MELCHIOR [*fl.* 1591] *respondent.*
Capita de morbis incurabilibus. *In* Lipsius, D. Tractatus de hydropisis. 1624, 1678.

WEEKLY memorials for the ingenious: or, An account of books lately set forth in several languages. With other accounts relating to arts and sciences. London, Henry Faithorne and John Kersey, 1683.

[8], 390, [8] p. illus., plates. 23 cm. **[12897]**

Numbers 1-50 (January 16, 1682 — January 15, 1683)

—[Another publication] . . . London, Printed for the author, and are to be sold by R. Chiswel, Tho. Basset, W. Crook, and Sam. Crouch, 1683.

[8], 224 p. 23 cm. **[12898]**

Numbers 1-29 (March 20, 1682 — Sept. 25, 1682)

WEERDER, EWALD VAN [*fl.* 1664] *respondent.* Disputatio medica inauguralis de dysenteria . . . Trajecti ad Rhenum, Ex officina Hermanni Rinckenraet, 1664.

[12] p. 20 cm. **[12899]**

Diss.—Utrecht.

WEERDT, G. DE [*fl.* 1647] *See* ANTWERP. Ordinances, local laws, etc. Gheboden ende uytgheroepen by mijne heeren, den schouteth . . . ende raedt der stadt van Antwerpen. 1647?

WEGELIN, JOHANN KASPAR [*fl.* 1624] *respondent. See* SEBISCH, M. [1578-1674?] *praeses.* Exercitationes medicae. 1639.

Den WEGH naar het spaa: maniere van leven aldaar, 't gebruik ende kracht van die wateren. Haarlem, Pieter Castelein, 1655.

11 p. 19 cm. **[12900]**

WEGHORST, HEINRICH [*fl.* 1662] *respondent. See* LINEMANN, A., *praeses.* Disputatio psychologica. 1662.

WEGWEISER, UTOPIANUS. *See* WEIGEL, Valentin [1533-1588]

WEIDEMÜLLER, DANIEL HEINRICH [*fl.* 1699] *respondent. See* LANGE, C. R., *praeses.* Dissertatio medica inauguralis de palpitatione cordis. 1699; *See* RIVINUS, A. Q. L. S. D. Facultatis Medicae . . . procancellarius Augustus Quirinus Rivinus. 1699.

WEIDENFELD, JOHANN SEGER VON. De secretis adeptorum; sive, De usu spiritus vini Lulliani libri IV. Opus practicum per concordantias philosophorum inter se discrepantium, tam ex antiquis, quam modernis philosophiae adeptae . . . Hamburgi, Apud Gothofredum Schultzen, Typis Nicolai

Spieringii, 1685.

[48], 602, [8] p. 14 cm. **[12901]**

—[English tr.] Four books . . . concerning the secrets of the adepts; or, Of the use of Lully's spirit of wine . . . Collected out of the ancient as well as modern fathers of adept philosophy . . . London, Printed by Will. Bonny, for Tho. Howkins, 1685.

[51], 380 p. 23 cm. **[12902]**

Translator's preface signed: G. C.

WEIDLER, FRANZ EHRENFRIED [*fl.* 1684] *respondent. See* WOLF, Jakob, *praeses.* Exercitatio medica de literatorum potu ejusque usu et abusu. 1684.

WEIDNER, GOTTFRIED [*d.* 1639] *praeses.* De lue sive lepra venerea disputatio . . . [Francofurti ad Viadrum] Literis Michaelis Kochii [1636]

[16] p. 19 cm. **[12903]**

Diss.—Frankfurt an der Oder (J. D. Ruland, *respondent*)

WEIER, HEINRICH. *See* WIER, Heinrich [*fl.* 1567-1588]

WEIER, JOHANN [1515-1588] *See* WIER, Johann [1515-1588]

WEIER, JOHANN [*fl.* 1603-1607] *respondent.* Theses . . . inaugurales de difficultate respirandi . . . Basileae, Per Joannem Schroeterum, 1607.

[20] p. 20 cm. **[12904]**

Diss.—Basel.

WEIER, PAUL [*fl.* 1649] *respondent. See* SPERLING, J., *praeses.* Disputatio physica de generatione. 1649.

WEIGAND, GEORG ERNST [*fl.* 1657] *respondent. See* SPERLING, J., *praeses.* Λιθολογια. 1657.

WEIGANMAIER, JOHANN BAPTISTA [*fl.* 1620] *praeses.* Disputatio physica de nutritione . . . Tubingae, Excudebat Eberhardus Wildius, 1620.

[2], 16 p. 19 cm. **[12905]**

Diss.—Tübingen (A. Planer, *respondent*)

WEIGEL, CLEMENS [*fl.* 1676-1677] *respondent. See* WEDEL, G. W., *praeses.* Aegram suppressione mensium laborantem . . . publicae . . . ventilationi exponit C. W. 1676.

WEIGEL, ERHARD [1625-1699] Philosophia mathematica, theologia naturalis solida, per singulas scientias continuata, universae artis inveniendi prima stamina complectens. Jenae, Sumptibus Matth. Birckneri, typis Pauli Ehrichii, 1693.

[40], 156, 262 p.; 512 p.   illus., plates.   18 cm. **[12906]**

Added engraved title page.
Pars altera has half title.

WEIGEL, VALENTIN [1533–1588] *See* WALLEN-BERGER, V. Trias quaestionum controversarum. 1621.

WEINDRICH, MARTIN. *See* WEINRICH, Martin [1548–1609]

WEINHART, FERDINAND KARL [17th–18th cent.] *praeses*. Summa fundamentorum universae medicinae ad mentem tam veterum, quam neotericorum delineata . . . Oeniponti, Typis Benedicti Caroli Reisacher [1688]

[12], 438, [4] p.   16 cm.   **[12907]**
Diss.—Innsbruck (P. Linsing, *respondent*)

—Thesaurus sanitatis inaestimabilis quomodo facili methodo ad plurimos vitae dies integer & incolumis conservari possit . . . Oeniponti, Typis Bened. Carol. Reisacher, 1691.

[10], 287, [8] p.   plate.   16 cm.   **[12908]**
Diss.—Innsbruck (G. Blas, *respondent*)

WEINLIG, GODOFREDUS [*fl.* 1676] *respondent. See* ETTMÜLLER, M., *praeses*. Disputationem medicam de epilepsia . . . submittit G. W. 1676, 1683.

WEINLIN, GEORG NIKOLAUS [*fl.* 1683–1684] *respondent. See* CAMERARIUS, E. R., *praeses*. Disquisitio inauguralis medica de phrenitide. 1684 [and] Historia anatomica renum et vesicae. 1683.

WEINRICH, MARTIN [1548–1609] *tr. See* CRATO VON KRAFFTHEIM, J. Consiliorum & epistolarum medicinalium . . . liber. 1620, 1671; SCHOLTZ, L. Consiliorum medicinalium . . . liber singularis. 1610.

WEINRICH, MARTIN [*fl.* 1603] *respondent. See* MÖLLER, S., *praeses*. Disputatio medica de phthisi. 1603.

WEIS, GEORG FRANZ [*fl.* 1698] Alexiterium; sive, Opusculum continens remedia adversus venena et maleficia . . . Coloniae Agrippinae, Typis Petri Theodori Hilden [1698]

[14], 172, [1] p.   16 cm.   **[12909]**

WEIS, JUCUNDUS. *See* WEIS-ET ROTHWEIN DE REBENSAFFT, Jucundus.

WEIS, WOLFGANG [*fl.* 1603] *respondent. See* SENNERT, D., *praeses*. De methodo medendi disputatio prima. 1603.

WEIS- ET ROTHWEIN DE REBENSAFFT, JUCUNDUS. Novae regulae sanitatis medico-physicae; sive, Disputationes inaugurales de esculentis et poculentis, ad usum mundi moderni: quas praeside . . . Hilario Fresbauch [pseud.] . . . pro consequenda in omni Scibili laurea contra melancolicos & hypocondriacos, suffumabit per tabacum. Jucundus Weis: et Rothwein de Rebensafft, Toubacensis [pseud.] . . . Quibus mixtae sunt admirabiles conclusiones de casei stupendis laudibus, nec non de jure et natura scribarum seu pennalium hujus temporis . . . Gratianopoli, 1657.

[24] p.   18 CM.   **[12910]**

WEISBERGER, JOHANN LORENZ [*fl.* 1671] *respondent*. Disputatio medica inauguralis de sterilitate . . . Lugduni Batavorum, Apud viduam & haeredes Joannis Elsevirii, 1671.

[12] p.   17 cm.   **[12911]**
Imperfect: upper margins trimmed.
Diss.—Leyden.

WEISKOPF, STANISLAUS. *See* SCHOLTZ, L. Consiliorum medicinalium . . . liber singularis. 1610.

WEISS, FRANCISCUS GEORGIUS. *See* WEIS, Georg Franz [*fl.* 1698]

WEISS, GOTTFRIED [*fl.* 1682] *respondent. See* ANTON, P. Exercitationem historicam de circumcisione gentilium [1682]

WEISS, HEINRICH [*fl.* 1680] *respondent. See* SCHMID, J. A., *praeses*. Discursus physicus de cerevisia ut est alimentum. 1680.

WEISS, JOHANN JACOB [*fl.* 1694] *respondent. See* HARDER, J. J., *praeses*. Exercitatio medica de sanguinis motu vitali. 1694.

WEISS, SIMON [*fl.* 1694] Dissertatio physica de excrescentiis plantarum animatis . . . Lipsiae, Literis Christophori Fleischeri [1694]

[24] p.   19 cm.   **[12912]**
Diss.—Leipzig (P. F. Balduin, *respondent*)

WEISS, WOLFGANGUS. *See* WEIS, Wolfgang [*fl.* 1603]

WEISSBERGER, JOHANN LORENZ [*fl. 1658*] *respondent. See* AMMANN, P., *praeses.* Theses physicae de auctione. 1658.

WEISSE, JOHANN SEVERIN [1640-1686] *praeses.* Disputatio physico-philologica de sale . . . [Lipsiae] Literis Christiani Michaelis [1665]

 [28] p. 19 cm.   **[12913]**
Diss.—Leipzig (A. G. Johnius, *respondent*)

WEISSENLÖW, BERNHARD FRIEDRICH VON. *See* ALBINUS, Bernhard [1653-1721]

WEISSENSEHE, PETER [*fl. 1622*] *respondent. See* HOFMANN, C., *praeses.* Theses de pulmone. 1622.

WEISSIUS, GODOFREDUS. *See* WEISS, Gottfried [*fl. 1682*]

WEITZ, HEINRICH SIGMUND [*b. 1671*] *respondent. See* SPERLING, P. G., *praeses.* Disputatio inauguralis medica de deliriis febrium continuarum. 1696.

 —*See* VATER, C. Collegii Medici . . . decanus Christianus Vater . . . L. B. S. P. D. 1696.

WEITZ, JAKOB [*fl. 1665*] *respondent.* Disputatio medica inauguralis de passione hysterica . . . Ultrajecti, Ex officina Meinardi a Dreunen, 1665.

 [10] p. 20 cm.   **[12914]**
Diss.—Utrecht.

WEIZ, JACOB [*fl. 1682*] Meditatio de peste et febribus malignis . . . Norimbergae, 1683.

 [16] p. 21 cm.   **[12915]**

WELBY, HENRY [*d. 1636*] *See* THE PHOENIX OF THESE LATE TIMES. 1637.

WELDON, WILLIAM. A short catalogue of some choice chymical preparations faithfully prepared . . . [London? not before 1675]

 4 p. 35 cm.   **[12916]**

WELLECHIUS, GUALTERUS. *See* WELLESIUS, Walter [*b. ca.1582*]

WELLER, JOHANN GOTTLIEB [*fl. 1675*] *respondent. See* WEDEL, G. W., *praeses.* Disputatio medica juvenem ictero flavo laborantem exhibens. 1675.

WELLES, BENJAMIN. *See* WELLS, Benjamin [1616?-1678]

WELLESIUS, WALTER [*b. ca. 1582*] *respondent.* Disputatio inauguralis de obstructione hepatis . . .

Lugduni Batavorum, Excudebat Godefridus Basson, 1616.

 [7] p. 20 cm.   **[12917]**
Diss.—Leyden.

WELLS, BENJAMIN [1616?-1678] A treatise of the gout, or joint-evil . . . London, Printed by J. M. for Henry Herringman, 1669.

 [7], 148 p. 15 cm.   **[12918]**

 —, *tr. See* BAUDERON, B. The expert phisician. 1657.

WELLWOOD, JAMES [1652-1727] *See* A TRUE RELATION OF THE WONDERFUL CURE OF MARY MAILLARD. 1694. —[French tr.]: 1694.

WELMAN, HEINRICH [1611-1643] *respondent. See* FREITAG, J., *praeses.* Disputatio medico philosophica de formarum origine. 1633.

WELPER, EBERHARD [*fl. 1609-ca. 1630*] Descriptio fabricae et usus instrumenti critici, in usum medicinae studiosorum facta . . . Nunc vero in lucem producta ab Eberhardo Welpero . . . auctoris filio. Argentorati, Sumptibus Johannis Friderici Spoor, 1666.

 [2], 13, [1] p. plates. 19 cm. **[12919]**

WELPER, EBERHARD [*fl. 1664*] *ed. See* WELPER, E. [*fl. 1609-ca. 1630*] Descriptio fabricae et usus instrumenti critici. 1666.

WELPHIUS, GASPARUS. *See* WOLF, Caspar [1532-1601]

WELSCH, CHRISTIAN LUDWIG [1669-1719] Tabulae anatomicae, universam humani corporis fabricam perspicue atque succincte exhibentes . . . Lipsiae, Sumptibus autoris, prostant apud Henricum Christoph. Crökerum, 1697.

 [116] p. 33 cm.   **[12920]**
Interleaved.
Original printer's name [Prostant apud Fridericum Groschii] covered with slip cancel.

 —*praeses.* Compendiosam naturalis hominis status historiam . . . publico eruditorum examini sujiciunt . . . Christianus Ludovicus Welsch . . . et . . . Johannes Conradus de Muralto . . . Basileae, Typis Emanuelis & Joh. Georgii König [1692]

 [24] p. 20 cm.   **[12921]**
Diss.—Basel (J. C. von Muralt, *respondent*)

—De sono . . . Lipsiae, Literis Joh. Georg [1690] [28] p. 19 cm. **[12922]**

Diss.—Leipzig (J. B. Sillig, *respondent*)

—*respondent.* See BERGER, J. G. von, *praeses.* Inauguralem disputationem de angina . . . submittit. 1691.

WELSCH, GEORG HIERONYMUS [1624–1677] Curationum exotericarum chiliades II, et Consiliorum medicinalium centuriae IV, cum adnotationibus . . . nunc primum ex MSS. editae. Ulmae, Ex typographeo Christiani Balthas. Kuenii, 1676. [18], 496, [56] p.; [4], 484, [60] p.   21 cm. **[12923]**

Engraved title page.
Part [1] has special title page: Consiliorum medicinalium centuriae quatuor. Part [2] has special title page: Exotericarum curationum et observationum medicinalium chiliades duae.

—Curationum propriarum, & consiliorum medicorum decades X, cum commentario, sive necessaria exegesi, opus posthumum, astronomiae & medicorum veterum placitis, nec non modernis pharmacorum legibus admensum & accuratum. Augustae Vindelicorum, Apud Theophilum Göbelium, typis Koppmayerianis, 1681. [8], 676, [31] p.   plates.   21 cm.   **[12924]**

Each decas has half title not included in the pagination.
Edited by Lucas Schroeck.

—Dissertatio medico-philosophica de aegagropilis. Augustae Vindelicorum, Typis Joannis Praetorii, impensis Joannis Weh, 1660. [4], 71, [9] p.   plates.   20 cm.   **[12925]**

—[The same.] . . . Cui secunda hac editione emendatiori, auctarii vice altera accedit. Augustae Vindelicorum, Impensis J. Wehe, typis Jacobi Kopmajeri et heredum Jo. Praetorii, 1668. [7], 71, [9] p.; [6], 101, [23] p.   plates.   21 cm. **[12926]**

Engraved title page.
Part [2] has special title page: Dissertatio medico-philosophica II. de aegagropilis. Quae nunc primum priori auctarii vice accedit. [Augustae Vindelicorum] Typis Jacobi Kopmair haered Joannis Praetorii, 1668.
Imperfect: part [2] bound before [1].

—Epistolae mutuae Argonautae [pseud., i.e. J. M. Fehr] ad Nestorem [pseud., i.e. G. H. Welsch] et Nestoris ad Argonautam, de Thesauro experientiae medicae, cujus accedit specimen de abortu. Augustae

Vindelicorum, Typis Joannis Schrönickii, 1677. 32 (i.e. 23), [1] p.   19 cm.   **[12927]**

Prepared for publication by Welsch. Welsch's proposed Thesaurus experientiae medicae, of which the specimen is given on p. 12-19, was never completed.

—Exercitatio de vena medinensi, ad mentem Ebnsinae; sive, De dracunculis veterum. Specimen exhibens novae versionis ex Arabico, cum commentario uberiori. Cui accedit altera, De vermiculis capillaribus infantium. Augustae Vindelicorum, Impensis Theophili Goebelii, 1674. [54], 456, [119] p.   front., port., plates.   21 cm. **[12928]**

"De dracunculis, disputatio medica . . . a M. Georgio Cunelio . . . Basileae, Typis Leonh. Ostenii, 1589" (p. [395]-400) has special title page.
Includes the Arabic text, the Latin translation by Gerardus Cremonensis and Andrea Alpago, and Welsch's new translation of Avicenna's Canon, lib. IV, fen. III, cap. XXI-XXII.

—Hecatosteae II. observationum physicomedicarum . . . Augustae Vindelicorum, Impensis Theophili Goebelii, typis Joannis Schönigkii, 1675. [11], 130, [5] p.; 69, [26] p.   plates.   21 cm. **[12929]**

Added engraved title page.
Each part has half title.

—Observationum medicinalium episagmata centum. 70, [10] p.   plates.   20 cm.   **[12930]**

(Part [6] *in* Welsch, Georg Hieronymus. Sylloge curationum. Aug. Vindel., 1667)

—Another issue, with date changed to 1668. **[12931]**

Somnium vindiciani; sive, Desiderata medicinae, Augustae Vindelicorum, Impensis Theophili Göbelii, typis Joannis Schönigkii, 1676. 44, [4] p.   21 cm.   **[12932]**

—Sylloge curationum et observationum medicanalium centurias VI. complectens, c. notis ejusdem et episagmatum centuria I. Aug. Vindel., Impensis Gottlieb Goebelii, typis Christiani Balthasaris Kuhnii, 1667. 6 parts in 1 v.   plates.   20 cm.   **[12933]**

Engraved title page.

—Another issue, with date altered to 1668.**[12934]**

Imperfect: lower margin or title page.

—, *respondent. See* SEBISCH, M.[1578-1674?] *praeses.* Disputatio de senectutis et senum statu ac conditione. 1645 [and] Disputationes de respirationes tres. 1643.

—, *ed. See* WALAEUS, J. Methodus medendi brevissima. 1679.

See ALMELOVEEN, T. J. van. Bibliotheca promissa et latens. 1688; MEIBOM, H. De medicorum historia scribenda epistola. 1669; SCHROECK, L. Memoria Welschiana. 1678.

WELSCH, GOTTFRIED [1618-1690] Rationale vulnerum lethalium judicium, in quo de vulnerum lethalium natura, & causis ... agitur ... Lipsiae, Sumptibus ac literis Ritzschianis, 1660.

    [199] p. illus. 17 cm. **[12935]**
Signatures:)(⁶, A-L⁸, M⁴, N².
Errata: p. [197]
Bound with copy 2 of Rossi, F. Nocturnae exercitationes in medicas historias. 1660.

—[The same.] ... Ed. 2. Cui accesserunt signa lethalitatis in iis, qui veneno extincti sunt ... Lipsiae, Sumptibus ac literis Ritzschianis, 1662.

    [12], 204 p. 16 cm. **[12936]**
Added engraved title page.

—Copy 2. 15 cm.
With this is bound: Brevis ad materiam medicam ... manuductio. Lipsiae, 1675?

—[The same.] ... Ed. 3. ... Lipsiae, Sumptibus ac literis Ritzschianis, 1674.

    [11], 216 p. 17 cm. **[12937]**
Added engraved title page dated 1662.

Dissertations — Leipzig

—*praeses.* Anatome cerebri humani ... [Lipsiae] Imprimebat Gregorius Ritzsch [1639]

    [12] p. 19 cm. **[12938]**
H. Meyer, *respondent.*

—Discursus physico-medicus de gemellis et partu numerosiore ... Lipsiae, Typis viduae Henningi Coleri [1667]

    [36] p. 20 cm. **[12939]**
C. F. Garmann, *respondent.*

—Disputationem inauguralem de morbis haereditariis in genere ... subjicit Martinus Heer ... Lipsiae, Typis Bauerianis [1665]

    [20] p. 18 cm. **[12940]**
M. Heer, *respondent.*

—Dissertatio medica de singularibus ... Lipsiae, Impensis Nicolai Scipionis [1663]

    32 p. 21 cm. **[12941]**
M. Ettmüller, *respondent.*

—[The same.] ... Lipsiae, Praelo Ritzschiano [1663]

    [35] p. 20 cm. **[12942]**
M. Ettmüller, *respondent.*

WELSCH, GOTTFRIED [1618-1690] *tr. See* MERCURIO, G. La commare dell Scipione Mercurio. Kindermutter oder, Hebammen Buch. 1652, 1653, 1671.

WELSCH, JOHANN MELCHIOR [*fl.* 1695] *respondent. See* ALBINUS, B. Dissertatio inauguralis medicochirurgica, de polypis. 1695; Dissertatio medica de paralysi. 1657.

WELSER, ANTON [*d.* 1618] *See* PIGNORIA, L. De servis, et eorum apud veteres ministeriis, commentarius. 1613.

WELWOOD, JAMES. *See* WELLWOOD, James [1652-1727]

WENCK, GASPAR [1589-1634] Notae unguenti magnetici et ejusdem actionis ... Dilingae, Apud Jacobum Sermodi [1626]

    [2], 89, [4] p. 16 cm. **[12943]**
Errata: p. [4]

—*praeses.* Disputatio philosophica de praecipua passione mobilis ... Dilingae, Apud Udalricum Rem [1622]

    [2], 13 p. 19 cm. **[12944]**
Diss.—Dillingen (K. Albertus, *respondent)*

WENCKER, DANIEL [*fl.* 1693-1695] *respondent.* Dissertatio medica inauguralis de paralysi ... Argentorati, Literis Joh. Friderici Spoor [1695]

    [2], 30 p. 20 cm. **[12945]**
Diss.—Strasbourg.

—*See* MAPP, M., *praeses.* Dissertatio medica de potu cafe. 1693.

WENCKH, GASPAR. *See* WENCK, Gaspar [1589-1634]

WEND, GEORG [*d.* 1705] Silesiam instans pestilentiae malum in gymnasio Wratislav. Magdalenaeo a. d. 28. Novembr. A. Ch. 1680 ante solennem praemiorum distributionem serio deprecantem H. L.

Q. S. introductum iri intimat ... Wratislaviae, In haeredum Braumannianorum typographia exprimebat Godofredus Gründer [1680]

[4] p. 29 cm.   **[12946]**

WENDE, GEORGIUS. *See* WEND, Georg [*d.* 1705]

WENDELAND, KASPAR [*fl.* 1692] *respondent. See* RIVINUS, A. Q., *praeses.* Dissertationem therapeuticam de remediis antepilepticis ... submittit. 1692.

WENDELEN, GODEFROID. *See* WENDELIN, Godefroid [1580-1667]

WENDELER, MICHAEL. *See* WENDLER, Michael [1610-1671]

WENDELIN, GODEFROID [1580-1667] Pluvia purpurea Bruxellensis. Parisiis, Apud Ludovicum de Heuqueville, 1647.

26, [2] p. 17 cm.   **[12947]**
With this is bound La Courvée, J. C. de. Ostentum. 1648.

WENDLER, MICHAEL [1610-1671] Disputationum physico-mathematicarum prima de maris nominibus, definitione, causis, loco, situ, & salsedine quam ... proponunt M. Michael Wendlerus ... & Johannes Durrius ... Witebergae, Ex officina typographica Johannis Haken [1636]

[19] p. 19 cm.   **[12948]**
Diss.—Wittenberg (J. Durrius, *respondent*)

WENTZEL, CHRISTOPH HEINRICH [*fl.* 1698] *respondent. See* CORYLI, S., *praeses.* Disputationem physicam de corylo Jacobi ... defendendam proponent ... C. H. W. 1698; KRAFFT, J. A., *praeses.* Dissertatio physica de objecto visus. 1698.

WENTZEL, JOCHANN CHRISTOPH. *See* WENZEL, Johann Christoph [*b.* 1659]

WENZEL, JOHANN CHRISTOPH [*b.* 1659] *respondent. See* SCHELHAMMER, G. C., *praeses.* Dissertatio inauguralis medica de aqua pericardii. 1694.

— *See* SCHELHAMMER, G. C. Programma ... inaugurali disputationi D. J. C. Wenzelii praemissum. 1694.

WENZLOVIUS, CAROLUS GOTTLIEB [*fl.* 1687-1691] *respondent. See* ALBINUS, B. Dissertatio inauguralis medica de incubo. 1691; LIMMER, C. P. Disputatio chirurgico-medica de fonticulis. 1687.

WEPFER, JOHANN [*fl.* 1657] *respondent. See* SEBISCH, M. [1578-1674?] *praeses.* Disputatio solennis de sudore. 1657.

WEPFER, JOHANN JAKOB [1620-1695] Cicutae aquaticae historia et noxae ... Basileae, Apud Joh. Rodolphum König, imprimebat Joh. Rodolphus Genathius, 1679.

[16], 336 p. plates. 22 cm.   **[12949]**

—Observationes anatomicae, ex cadaveribus eorum, quos sustulit apoplexia, cum exercitatione de ejus loco affecto. Schaffhusii, Typis Joh. Caspari Suteri, 1658.

[16], 304 p. illus. 17 cm.   **[12950]**
Bound with Castro, E. R. de. Variae exercitationes medicae. 1656

—[The same.] ... Novae ed. accessit auctuarium Historiarum & observationum similium, cum scholiis. Schaffhusii, Impensis Onophrii a Waldkirch, typis Alexandri Riedingii, 1675.

[16], 464 p. illus. 17 cm.   **[12951]**
"Historiarum et observationum apoplecticarum & similium, potissimum anatomae subjectarum auctarium cum scholiis ... Cui addita est Epistola ... Johannis Ott ... de scriptis D. G. Holderi De elementis sermonis, D. Morlandi De stentorophonia ..." has special title page (p. [305]).

—[The same.] ... Amstelaedmi, Apud Henricum Wetstenium, 1681.

[16], 464 p. illus. 17 cm.   **[12952]**
Pages [319-320] (blank) wanting.
A reissue of the 1675 Schaffhausen edition with new title page.

—Oratio de thermarum potu in ... inclytae academiae Basiliensis cum solemnitates doctorales subierit publice dicta ... Basileae, Typis Georgii Deckeri [1647]

[23] p. 19 cm.   **[12953]**

—*respondent. See* SEBISCH, M. [1578-1674?] *praeses.* Disputatio de variolis et morbillis prima [-sexta & ultima] 1642.

—*See* PAULLI, J. H. Anatomiae Bilsianae anatome. 1665; VERZASCA, B. Observationum medicarum centuria. 1677.

WERCKMEISTER, FRANZ HEINRICH [*fl.* 1689-1698] *praeses.* Disputatio medica de absoluta lethalitate vulneris arteriae magnae ... Halae, Literis Salfeldianis, 1694.

12 p. 20 cm.   **[12954]**
Diss.—Halle (J. G. Reichhelm, *respondent*)

—Dissertatio medica, de genio, curatione et praeservatione arthritidis; sive, Von dem Reissen in den Gliedern . . . Halae Magdeb., Literis Chr. Henckelii [1697]

[1], 30 + p.   19 cm.   **[12955]**

Imperfect: all after p. 30 wanting.

Diss. — Halle (H. P. Juch, *respondent*)

—Dissertatio medica de imaginatione, morborum causa . . . Halae, Literis Salfeldianis [1694]

[4], 28 p.   20 cm.   **[12956]**

Diss. — Halle (J. N. Röper, *respondent*)

—Dissertatio medica filum Ariadneum in studio medico . . . pertexere & philiatris benevole probandum offerre sustinebit Joachimus Fridericus Wachtel . . . Halae Magdeburgicae, Typis Christiani Henckelii [1698]

31, [1] p.   20 cm.   **[12957]**

Diss. — Halle (J. F. Wachtel, *respondent.*)

WERNER, August [*fl.* 1673] *respondent. See* Beier, G., *praeses.* Dissertatio academica. 1673.

WERNER, Philipp [*fl.* 1614] *respondent. See* Opsopäus, S., *praeses.* Medicam de phrenitide συςτησιν proponit M. Philippus Werner. 1614.

WERNHER, Johann Balthasar, *Freiherr von* [1675–1742] *praeses.* Disputationem physicam de saporibus eorumque differentiis . . . publico . . . examini exponit . . . Joh. Andreas Plohr . . . Lipsiae, Literis Brandenburgerianis [1698]

[44] p.   19 cm.   **[12958]**

Diss. — Leipzig (J. A. Plohr, *respondent*)

WERNHÖFER, Heinrich [*fl.* 1665] *respondent. See* Frommann, J. C. Quaestionis hujus physicae, an sanguis, quem Christus passionis suae initio sudavit, naturaliter promanarit. 1665.

WERNIC, Philipp [*fl.* 1667] *respondent. See* Friderici, J. A., *praeses.* Dissertatio medica inauguralis de stranguria. 1667.

WESEL, Adrianus a [*fl.* 1669–1676] *respondent.* Disputationum selectarum . . . prima de semine mulieris . . . Lugduni Batavorum, Apud viduam & haeredes Joannis Elsevirii, 1676.

[8] p.   21 cm.   **[12959]**

Diss. — Leyden.

WESENER, Johannes Carolus [*fl.* 1622] *respondent. See* Sebisch, M. [1578–1674?] *praeses.* Exercitatio

medica prima. 1622 [and] Exercitationes medicae. 1639.

WESENER, Wolffgang Christoph [*fl.* 1674–1692] Der hällische Messer-Schlucker, sammt dessen Kur, und den 2. Augusti 1692. erfolgte Erledigung von dem am 3. Januarii 1691. eingeschluckten Messer, denen curiösen Liebhabern kürtzlich vorgestellet . . . Bresslau, Zu finden bey George Seydeln [1692?]

[8] p.   illus.   21 cm.   **[12960]**

—*respondent. See* Wedel, G. W., *praeses.* Aegram pleuriticam . . . publico . . . examini subjiciet . . . W. C. W. 1674.

WESENFELD, Arnold [*d.* 1720] Georgica animi et vitae; seu, Pathologia practica, moralis nempe & civilis, ex physicis ubique fontibus, libera neque ad ullam sectam astricta methodo, cohaerentibus tamen ubique principiis deducta . . . Francofurti ad Viadrum, Impensis Johannis Volckeri, 1696.

[8], 688 p.   19 cm.   **[12961]**

WESLINGH, Jan [*fl.* 1694] *respondent.* Dissertatio medica inauguralis de passione hysterica . . . Lugduni Batavorum, Apud Abrahamum Elzevier, 1694.

[40] p.   18 cm.   **[12962]**

Diss. — Leyden.

WESLINGIUS, Johannes. *See* Vesling, Johann [1598–1649]

WESTENBERG, Johann Ortwin [*fl.* 1654] *respondent.* Assertio medica inauguralis de vertigine . . . Lugduni Batavorum, Ex officina Johannis Meyer, 1654.

[8] p.   22 cm.   **[12963]**

Diss. — Leyden.

WESTENBERGH, Ernst Wilhelm [*fl.* 1693] *respondent.* Disputatio medica inauguralis de hydrope . . . Lugduni Batavorum, Apud Abrahamum Elzevier, 1693.

[17] p.   24 cm.   **[12964]**

Diss. — Leyden.

WESTERVELT, Paulus [*fl.* 1661] *respondent.* Disputatio medica inauguralis, de apoplexia . . . Lugduni Batavorum, Ex officina Nicolai Herculis, 1661.

[12] p.   19 cm.   **[12965]**

Diss. — Leyden.

WESTHOFF, RUDGER [*fl.* 1668] *respondent.*
Disputationem inauguralem medicam de affectu hypochondriaco ... examini ... sistet Rudgerus Westhoff ... [Argentorati] Literis Johannis Wilhelmi Tidemann [1668]

    [4], 28 p.   19 cm.   **[12966]**
    Diss.—Strasbourg.

WESTMACOTT, WILLIAM [*b.* 1650]
Θεολοβοτονολογια sive, Historia vegetabilium sacra; or, A scripture herbal; wherein all the trees, shrubs, herbs, plants, flowers, fruits, &c. both foreign and native, that are mentioned in the Holy Bible, (being near eighty in number) are in an alphabetical order, rationally discoursed of, shewing, their names, kinds, descriptions, places ... various uses ... Together with their medicinal preparations ... Galenically and chymically handled ... London, T. Salusbury, 1694.

    [24], 232, [8] p.   15 cm.   **[12967]**

  —[The same.] ... London, John Salusbury, 1695.
    [22], 232, [8] p.   16 cm.   **[12968]**
    First leaf (blank?) wanting.
    A reissue of the 1694 edition with new title page.

WESTPHAL, JOACHIM CHRISTIAN [*fl.* 1684-1687]
Natura peccans septenario problematum numero proposita, de qua ... disputabit M. Joach. Christianus Westphal ... Lipsiae, Typis Christiani Gözii [1687]

    [24] p.   20 cm.   **[12969]**
    Diss. pro loco—Leipzig.

  —*praeses.* De ventis, incendii tempore orientibus ... Lipsiae, Excudebat Christianus Goezius, MLXXXVII [i.e. 1687]

    [20] p.   18 cm.   **[12970]**
    Diss.—Leipzig (H. A. Merk, *respondent*)

WESTPHAL, JOHANN KASPER [*d.* 1722] *respondent.*
See LEICHNER, E., *praeses.* Disputatio medica inauguralis de dysenteria. 1678.

  —, *ed. See* ETTMÜLLER, M. Opera medica theoretico-practica. 1696-1697.

WETENHALL, EDWARD [*fl.* 1684] *respondent.*
Dissertatio medica inauguralis de cordis palpitatione ... Lugduni Batavorum, Apud Abrahamum Elzevier, 1684.

    [12] p.   22 cm.   **[12971]**
    Diss.—Leyden.

WETTSTEIN, JOHANN RUDOLF [1647-1711] *praeses.*
Disputatio theologica de circumcisione ... Basileae, Typis Jacobi Bertschii [1700]

    [16] p.   20 cm.   **[12972]**
    Diss.—Basel (C. Burckard, *respondent*)

WETZEL, JOHANN CASPAR. *See* WITZEL, Johann Kaspar [*fl.* 1675-1676]

WETZEL, JOHANN LUDWIG [*fl.* 1693] *respondent.*
See BODE, H. von, *praeses.* Disputatio inauguralis juridica de juribus infirmorum seu aegrotorum singularibus, 1693.

WEUELICHOVEN, JOHANN [*fl.* 1631] *respondent.*
See BURGERSDIJCK, F. P., *praeses.* Collegium physicum. 1642.

WEYER, HEINRICH. *See* WIER, Heinrich [*fl.* 1567-1588]

WEYER, JOHANN. *See* WIER, Johann [1515-1588]

WEYMARISCHES ARTZNEY-BUCH. *See* SECHS BÜCHER AUSERLESENER ARTZNEY UND KUNSTSTÜCK. 1613, 1678.

WEZ, MICHAEL [*fl.* 17th cent.] *See* KOLLEGIUM DER AERZTE, Regensburg. Kurtzer, sehr nothwendig-und treuhertziger Bericht. 1680.

WHARTON, SIMON. *See* SHERARD, William [1659-1728]

WHARTON, THOMAS [1614-1673] Adenographia; sive, Glandularum totius corporis descriptio ... Londini, Typis J. G., impensis authoris, 1656.

    [16], 287 p.   plates.   18 cm.   **[12973]**

  —[The same.] ... Amstelaedami, Sumptibus Joannis Ravesteinii, 1659.

    [24], 261 p.   plates.   13 cm.   **[12974]**
    Imperfect: title page mutilated.

  —[The same.] ... Noviomagi, Apud Andream ab Hoogenhuyse, 1664.

    [24], 261 p.   plates.   14 cm.   **[12975]**
    Different setting of type.

WHARTON, THOMAS [1614-1673] *See* BARTHOLIN, T. Opuscula nova anatomica. 1670.

WHITAKER, TOBIAS [*fl.* 1666] The tree of humane life; or, The bloud of the grape. Proving the possibilitie of maintaining humane life from infancy to extreame old age without any sicknesse by the use of wine ... London, Printed by I. D. for H. O., 1638.

[15], 73, [3] p.   15 cm.   [**12976**]

—[Latin tr.] Tractatus de sanguine uvae, ejusque natura et usu, diaetetice & pharmaceutice ... Francofurti, Ex officina typographica Wolfgangi Hoffmanni, 1655.

118 p.   17 cm.   [**12977**]

Bound with copy 2 of Hoffmann, M. Synopsis institt. medicinae. 1663.

—*See* Stubbs, H. The Lord Bacons relation of the sweating-sickness examined. 1671.

WHITE, R., *gent.* [*fl. ca.* 1658] *tr. See* Digby, *Sir* K. A late discourse. 1658, 1660.

WHITE, Thomas [1593–1676] *See* Digby, *Sir* K. Demonstratio immortalitatis animae rationalis. 1664; Glanvill, J. Scepsis scientifica. 1665.

WHITELOCKE, Bullstrode [*fl.* 1671] *respondent.* Disputatio medica de dolore nephritico ... Lugduni Batavorum, Apud viduam & haeredes Johannis Elsevirii, 1671.

[8] p.   23 cm.   [**12978**]

Diss.—Leyden.

WHITLOCK, Richard [*b.* 1616?] Ζωοτομία; or, Observations on the present manners of the English: briefly anatomizing the living and the dead. With a useful detection of the mountebanks of both sexes ... London, Printed by Tho. Roycroft, and sold by Humphrey Moseley, 1654.

[33], 568, [14] p.   15 cm.   [**12979**]

Added engraved title page.
Last leaf (blank?) wanting.

WICHGREVE, Albert [*fl.* 1592–1607] Oratio pro ... μιχραμθρωποιϛ, sive homullis ... Francofurti, Apud Casparum Rotelium, 1628.

44 p.   19 cm.   [**12980**]

WICHMANS, Augustin [*fl.* 1625] Diarium ecclesiasticum de sanctis contra pestem tutelaribus, in quo quam plurimae antiquitates ecclesiasticae grata varietate explicantur ... [Antverpiae, 1625?]

[4], 110, [2] p.   20 cm.   [**12981**]

WICHTLER, Johann Conrad. *See* Wechtler, Johann Conrad [*fl.* 1656–1659]

WICKEN, Georg [*fl.* 1674] *respondent. See* Franck von Franckenau, G., *praeses.* Disputatio medica de alapis. 1674 [and] Disputatio medica qua lupanaria

s. v. Huren-Häuser, ex principiis medicis qq. improbantur. 1674.

WIDDOWES, Daniel. *See* Scribonius, W. A. Naturall philosophy. 1631.

WIDDOWES, J. [*fl.* 1606–1640] *See* Scribonius, W. A. Naturall philosophy. 1631.

WIDEBRAM, Friedrich [1532–1585] *See* Goclenius, R. [1547–1628] Physiologia crepitus ventris. 1607.

WIDEBRANDUS, Fridericus. *See* Widebram, Friedrich [1532–1585]

WIDEMANN, Georg Melchior [*fl.* 1681] *respondent. See* Ettmüller, M., *praeses.* Disputatio medica de corpulentia nimia. 1681.

WIDEMANN, Georg Sebastian [*fl.* 1629–1630] *respondent. See* Sebisch, M. [1578–1674?] *praeses.* Exercitationes medicae. 1639.

WIDER, Jakob Samuel [*fl.* 1673] *respondent. See* Friess, M. F., *praeses.* Inauguralis de podagra disputatio. 1673.

—*See* Bohn, J. D. Johannes Bohn ... p. t. procancellarius L. S. 1673.

WIDER, Johannes Karl [*fl.* 1663] *respondent. See* Bruno, J. P., *praeses.* Αίματοξυμωσιλογία. 1663.

WIDHOLTZ, Jeremias [*fl.* 1607] *See* Knobloch, T., *praeses.* Disputationes anatomicae. 1608, 1612.

WIDHOLZ, Daniel [*fl.* 1621] *respondent. See* Sebisch, M. [1578–1674?] *praeses.* Disputationes de recta ratione purgandi. 1621.

WIDMANN, Georg Friedrich [*fl.* 1624] *respondent. See* Sebisch, M. [1578–1674?] *praeses.* Exercitationes medicae. 1639.

WIDMARCKTER, Kaspar [*fl.* 1682] *praeses.* Dissertatio inauguralis medica de inflammatione ... Erfordiae, Typis Joh. Georg. Hertzii [1682]

[20] p.   21 cm.   [**12982**]

Diss.—Erfurt (H. C. Alberti, *respondent*)

WIDT, Johann Daniel [*fl.* 1660–1663] *respondent.* Λιθολογια ... Argentorati, Typis Eberhardi Welperi, 1663.

32 p.   19 cm.   [**12983**]

Diss.—Strasbourg.

—*See* SEBISCH, M. [1578-1674?] *praeses*. Disputatio de spiritibus humani corporis theorica & practica. 1660.

WIDT, JOHANN REINHARD [*fl.* 1632-1634] *respondent. See* SEBISCH, M. [1578-1674?] *praeses*. Collegii therapeutici disputatio I[-XIV] 1634 [i.e. 1635] [and] Galeni Ars parva in disputationed triginta resoluta. 1633.

WIEDEMANN, GOTTFRIED [*fl.* 1698] *respondent. See* VEHR, I., *praeses*. Dissertatio inauguralis medico-chirurgica. 1698.

WIEL, CORNELIUS STALPART VAN DER. *See* STALPART VAN DER WIEL, Cornelis [1620-1702]

WIEL, PETRUS STALPART VAN DER. *See* STALPART VAN DER WIEL, Pieter [*fl.* 1686]

WIELAND, MELCHIOR. *See* GUILANDINUS, Melchior [1519 *or* 20-1589]

WIER, HEINRICH [*fl.* 1567-1588] *See* SMET, H. Miscellanea . . . medica. 1661.

WIER, JOHANN [1515-1588] Opera omnia . . . Ed. nova . . . Amstelodami, Apud Petrum vanden Berge, 1660.

　　[44], 1002, [60] p. illus., port. 21 cm.
　　　　　　　　　　　　　　　　　　　　[12984]
"Vita Joannis Wieri": p. [9-12]
De lamiis liber (p. [667]), De irae morbo (p. [771]), Wieri Medicarum observationum . . . libri II (p. [877]), have special title pages.

—Artzney Buch: von etlichen unbekannteu [sic] und unbeschriebenen Kranckheiten . . .

　　[447]-701 p. plates. 14 cm. (*In* Viel-vergröster und hellerpolirter Schorbocks-Spiegel. Nürnberg, 1659)　　　　　　　　　　　　　**[12985]**
Half title.

—Medicarum observationum rararum liber I. De scorbuto. De quartana. De pestilentiali angina, pleuritide, & peripneumonia. De hydropis curatione. De curatione meatuum naturalium clausorum, & quibusdam aliis. Ult. ed. auctior, & mendatior . . . Amstelodami, Apud Petrum Montanum, 1657.

　　[1], vi, 124, [11] p. illus. 14 cm.　**[12986]**
Bound with Follinus, J. Synopsis tuendae et conservandae bonae valetudinus. 1648.

—Verhandelinge van de pokken. *In* Blankaart, S. Venus belegert en ontset. 1684, 1688, 1696. [German tr.] 1689.

—Von dem Schurbauch. *In* Horst, G. [1578-1636] Büchlein von dem Schorbock. 1615.

—*See* BODIN, J. De magorum daemonomania. 1603; SMET, H. Miscellanea . . . medica. 1661.

WIESSNER, GOTTFRIED [*fl.* 1668] Dissertationem medicam theoretico-practicam, de malo pestifero . . . p. p. Gottfried Wiessner . . . respondente Henrico Warnatio . . . Lipsiae, Literis Joh. Erici Hahnii [1668]

　　[32] p. 19 cm.　　　　　　　　　　　**[12987]**
Diss. pro loco—Leipzig (H. Warnatius, *respondent*)

WIETZEL, JOHANN CASPAR. *See* WITZEL, Johann Kaspar [*fl.* 1675-1676]

WIGANDUS, JOACHIMUS VITUS, *pseud. See* WILLE, Johann Valentin [1651-1677]

WILCKE, JODOCUS. *See* WILLICH, Jodocus [1501-1552]

WILD, JODOCUS. *See* WILLICH, Jodocus [1501-1552]

WILDVOGEL, CHRISTIAN [1644-1728] *praeses*. Disputatio inauguralis de jure manus dextrae vom Rechte der Rechten Hand . . . Jenae, Litteris Mullerianis [1700]

　　[4], 56 p. 20 cm.　　　　　　　　　　**[12988]**
Diss.—Jena (J. A. Gutzmer, *respondent*)

—Dissertatio inauguralis juridica de jure embryonum von ungebohrner Kinder Rechte . . . Jenae, Typis viduae Mullerianae [1693]

　　[124] p. 21 cm.　　　　　　　　　　　**[12989]**
Diss.—Jena (J. E. von der Lange, *respondent*)

WILHELM TECCENENSIS. *See* TECENENSIS, Guilhelmus [*fl.* 16th-17th cent.]

WILHELM, PETER [*fl.* 1619] *respondent. See* CUTENIUS, M. Themata physica de vita & morte. 1619.

WILHELMI, JOHANN [*fl.* 1699] *respondent. See* HOFFMANN, F. [1660-1742] *praeses*. Disputatio inauguralis medica, de terebinthina. 1699.

WILKE, JODOCUS. *See* WILLICH, Jodocus [1501-1552]

WILKOFER, JOHANN [*fl.* 1607] *See* KNOBLOCH, T., *praeses*. Disputationes anatomicae. 1608, 1612.

WILLE, JOHANN VALENTIN [*fl.* 1635-1640] *respondent*. Disputatio medica inauguralis de dysenteria . . .

Argentorati, Typis Johannis Georgii Simonis, 1640.

[16] p.   21 cm.   **[12990]**

Diss. — Strasbourg.

— *respondent. See* Saltzmann, J. R. [1573–1656] *praeses.* Discursus medicus. 1637; Sebisch, M. [1578–1674?] *praeses.* Collegii therapeutici disputatio I[-XIV] 1634 [i.e. 1635]

WILLE, Johann Valentin [1651–1677] Tractatus medicus de morbis castrensibus internis ... Hafniae, Typis Matthiae Godicchenii, 1676.

[16], 94, [2] p.   19 cm.   **[12991]**

Imperfect: p. [9–16] wanting.

— Another issue, with portrait on verso of title page.   **[12992]**

Bound with copy 2 of Marci von Kronland, J. M. Liturgia mentis. 1678.

— *praes.* Synopsis tractatus de morbis castrensibus internis ... Hafniae, Typis Matthiae Godicchenii [1676]

[2], 8, [2] p.   20 cm.   **[12993]**

Diss. — Copenhagen (P. Brand, *respondent*)

— *See* Paulli, S. Epistola votiva ad Johannem Valentinum Willium. 1676.

WILLE, Matthes [*fl.* 1671] De salis origine, ejusque incremento, accremento et decremento tractatus philosophicus; das ist, Von des Saltzes und seiner Qvellen Uhrsprunge, fort- aus und endlichen Untergange. Wobey mit angefügt ... Vera virgulae mercurialis relatio; das ist, Wahrhafftiger ... Bericht von der Wünschel-Ruther. Anitzo ... vermehret und ... zum andern Mahle heraus gegeben ... Jena, Druckts Johann Gollner, verlegts Gottfriedt Schmiedt, 1684.

[85] p.   20 cm.   **[12994]**

Text in German.

The "Vera virgulae mercurialis relatio" has special title page (p. [47]).

WILLERDING, Joachim Theodor [*fl.* 1673] *respondent. See* Vogler, V. H., *praeses.* Disputatio medica inauguralis de haemorrhagia narium. 1673.

WILLIAMS, Ralph. Physical rarities, containing the most choice receipts of physick, and chyrurgerie, for the cure of all diseases ... London, Printed for J. M. and sold by George Calvert, 1651.

[16], 208 p.   15 cm.   **[12995]**

WILLIAMS, William, *astrologer.* Occult physick; or, The three principles in nature anatomized by a philosophical opperation, taken from experience, in three books. The first of beasts, trees, herbs ... The second book containeth most excellent and rare medicines for all diseases ... The third ... is ... shewing how to cure all diseases ... Whereunto is added ... how to judge of a disease by the affliction of the moon ... By W[illiam] W[illiams] philosophus; student in the coelestial sciences. London, Printed by Tho. Leach, for H. Marsh and W. Palmer, 1660.

[8], 160, [4] p.   illus.   18 cm.   **[12996]**

WILLIAMS, William, *student in the cabalistical sciences. See* Williams, William, *astrologer.*

WILLICH, Jodocus [1501–1552] Exercitationes et probationes de urinis libri IV ... His accessere remedia plurima ex urinae desumpta. Amstelodami, Apud Joannem Wolters, 1688.

[1], 460, 308 p.   16 cm.   **[12997]**

"Aristotelis ... De coloribus liber, Coelio Calcagnino interprete, quem ut plurimum ad urinarum differentias intelligendas, studiosis profuturum, huic operi adjungendum putavimus. Cui subjicitur Antonii Thylesii ... De coloribus libellus" (p. [409]–460) has half title.

— Urinarum probationes. *In* Joannes Actuarius. De urinis libri VII. 1670.

WILLIS, Guillaume [*fl.* 1688] *tr. See* Blankaart, S. Traité de la verole. 1688.

WILLIS, Thomas [1621–1675] Opera omnia ... Genevae, Apud Samuelem de Tournes, 1676.

5 parts in 1 v.   plates, port.   22 cm.   **[12998]**

Imperfect: portrait wanting.

Each part has special title page.

Contents. — Diatribae duae medico-philosophicae quarum prior agit de fermentatione, altera de febribus; quibus accessit Dissertatio de urinis. — Cerebri anatome, nervorumque descriptio & usus; quibus accessit viri cujusdam clarissimi [i.e. William Croone] De ratione motus musculorum tractatus singularis. — Pathologiae cerebri & nervosi generis specimen, in quo agitur de morbis convulsivis & de scorbuto. — De anima brutorum. — Pharmaceutice rationalis, sive Diatriba de medicamentorum operationibus in humano corpore [pars prima]

— Opera medica & physica, in varios tractatus distributa ... Lugduni, Sumptibus Joannis Antonii Huguetan, 1676.

2 v.   plates., port.   23 cm.   **[12999]**

Contents. — [v. 1.] De fermentatione. De febribus. De urinis. Cerebri anatome. Nervorum descriptio, & usus. De ratione motus musculorum studio Gulielmi Croone. De morbis convulsivis. De scorbuto. De affectionibus hystericis & hypochondriacis. De sanguinis incalescentia. De motu musculari. — [v. 2.] De anima brutorum exercitationes duae. Pharmaceutice rationalis & de medicamentorum operationibus in humano corpore.

Both parts of Pharmaceutice rationalis have special title pages and separate pagination.

—Opera omnia ... Genevae, Apud Samuelem de Tournes, 1680.

 7 parts in 2 v. plates., port. 23 cm. **[13000]**

Each part has special title page.

Contents as in the 1676 Geneva edition with the addition of Affectionum quae dicuntur hystericae de hypochondriacae pathologia spasmodica cui accesserunt exercitationes medico physicae duae. I. De sanguinis accensione. II. De motu musculari, and Pharmaceutice rationalis, sive Diatriba de medicamentorum operationibus in humano corpore, pars secunda.

—Opera omnia ... Lugduni, Sumptibus Joannis Antonii Huguetan, 1681.

 2 v. plates, port. 24 cm. **[13001]**

Imperfect: plate 3 of Cerebri anatome (v. 1, p. 265) wanting.

A reprint of the 1676 Lyon edition. The Pharmaceutice rationalis has half titles.

—Opera omnia, nitidius, quam unquam hactenus edita, plurimum emendata, indicibus rerum copiosissimis, ac distinctione characterum exornata. Studio & opera Gerardi Blasii ... Amstelaedami, Apud Henricum Wetstenium, 1682.

 6 parts in 2 v. plates, front. (port.) 25 cm. **[13002]**

Vol. 2 has engraved title page.

Contents as in the 1680 Geneva edition without William Croon's De ratione motus musculorum.

—[The same.] ... Hac tandem novissima editione accuratissime recognita ... Coloniae, Sumptibus Gasparis Storti, 1694.

 [16], 586, [17] p. illus., plates., port. 34 cm. **[13003]**

"De ratione motus musculorum, studio Gulielmi Croone": p. 181–188.

—[The same.] Opera omnia. Ed. nova emendatior & tractatu De peste auctior ... Genevae, Apud Samuelem de Tournes, 1695.

 8 parts in 2 v. bound in 1. plates., front. (port.) 24 cm. **[13004]**

Imperfect: title page for second part of Pharmaceutice rationalis and title page for De anima brutorum misbound.

Each part has special title page dated 1694–96.

"Viri cujusdam clarissimi [i.e. William Croone] De ratione motus musculorum tractatus singularis": at end of part [2].

"Perspicua facilisque methodus sanos, benedicente Deo, tuendi a peste vel quolibet morbo contagioso, ut et ea lue infectos ubicunque curandi" (19 p. at end) has special title page.

—[English tr.] Practice of physick, being the whole works of that renowned and famous physician ... The Pharmaceutice new translated, and the whole carefully corr. and amended. London, T. Dring, C. Harper and J. Leigh, 1684.

 6 parts in 1 v. plates. 31 cm. **[13005]**

Imperfect: several leaves mutilated or wanting.

Each part has special title page.

Consists of The remaining medical works ... 1681 [in 3 pts.] Pharmaceutice rationalis ... 1684 [in 2 pts.] Two discourses concerning the soul of brutes ... 1683.

Translated by Samuel Pordage.

—Another issue.

The first and last special title pages of "The remaining medical works" are dated 1684.

 6 parts in 1 v. plates. 34 cm. **[13006]**

—The remaining medical works ... Viz. I. Of fermentation. II. Of feavours. III. Of urines. IV. Of the accension of the bloud. V. Of muscular motion. VI. Of the anatomy of the brain. VII. Of the description and use of the nerves. VIII. Of vonvulsive diseases ... Englished by S[amuel] P[ordage] ... London, Printed for T. Dring, C. Harper, J. Leigh, and S. Martyn, and sold by Robert Clavell, 1681.

 3 parts in 1 v. 34 cm. **[13007]**

Imperfect: last leaf mutilated.

Each part has special title page: [1] A medical-philosophical discourse of fermentation. [2] Five treatises. [3] An essay of the pathology of the brain and nervous stock.

Bound with another issue of *his* Pharmaceutice rationalis. 1679.

—Affectionum quae dicuntur hystericae et hypochondriacae pathologia spasmodica vindicata, contra responsionem epistolarem Nathanael. Highmori, M.D. Cui accesserunt exercitationes medico-physicae duae 1. De sanguinis accensione. 2. De motu musculari ... Lugd. Batav., Apud Cornel. Driehuysen, apud Felicem Lopez, 1671.

 [6], 172 p. plates. 14 cm. **[13008]**

—Cerebri anatome: cui accessit nervorum descriptio et usus ... Londini, Typis Ja. Flesher, impensis Jo. Martyn & Ja. Allestry, 1664.

 [39], 456 p. plates. 21 cm. **[13009]**

Feindel 1.

—Another printing, with imprint: Londini, Typis Tho. Roycroft, impensis Jo. Martyn & Ja. Allestry, 1664.

[28], 240 p. plates. 16 cm. [13010]

Imperfect: plate 10 wanting.

Feindel 2.

The plates are duplicates of those in the Flesher edition, with engraved page numbers altered by hand.

—[The same.] . . . Accessit viri cujusdam clarissimi [i.e. William Croone] De ratione motus musculorum tractatus singularis. Amstelodami, Apud Casparum Commelinum, 1664.

[24], 273 p.; 32 p. illus., plates. 14 cm. [13011]

Imperfect: plate 1 wanting; sign. M6 (blank?) wanting?

Part [2] has special title page.

—[The same.] . . . Amstelodami, Apud Gerbrandum Schagen, 1666.

[15], 342 p.; [4], 37 p. plates. 16 cm. [13012]

Added engraved title page dated 1665.

Imperfect: added engraved title page, 8th prelim. leaf and plates opposite p. 47 and 81 wanting; supplied in photocopy from the New York Academy of Medicine Library.

Part [2] has special title page dated 1665.

—[The same.] . . . Ed. ult. priori emendatior. Amstelodami, Apud Casparum Commelinum, 1667.

[22], 272 p. plates. 14 cm. [13013]

Imperfect: first prelim. leaf (blank?) wanting.

With this is bound (as issued?) Croone, W. De ratione motus musculorum. 1667.

—De anima brutorum quae hominis vitalis ac sensitiva est, exercitationes duae. Prior physiologica ejusdem naturam, partes, potentias & affectiones tradit. Altera pathologica morbos qui ipsam, & sedem ejus primariam, nempe cerebrum & nervosum genus afficiunt, explicat, eorumque therapeias instituit . . . Oxonii, E Theatro Sheldoniano, impensis Ric. Davis, 1672.

[56], 565 (i.e. 547), [11] p. plates. 21 cm. [13014]

Errata: p. [56]

Pars prima physiologica and Pars secunda pathologica have half titles.

—Another issue. Londini, Prostant apud Gulielm. Wells & Robertum Scott, 1672.

[49], 565 (i.e. 547), [18] p. plates. 21 cm. [13015]

A variant issue of the 1672 Oxford edition with different title page, without the Imprimatur, the half title for pars prima physiologica

and the title label; A catalogue of some books . . . sold by Richard Davis, p. 565 is in duplicate.

Errata: p. [18] at end.

—[The same.] . . . Londini, Typis E. F., impensis Ric. Davis, 1672.

[46], 400, [16] p. plates. 16 cm. [13016]

—Another issue, with imprint: Londini, Prostant apud Gulielm. Wells, & Rob. Scot, 1672. [13017]

—Another issue, with imprint: Amstelodami, Apud Joannem Blaeu, 1672. [13018]

Imperfect: plate II. wanting.

—[The same.] . . . Amstelodami, Apud Joannem à Someren, 1674.

[47], 552, [20] p. plates. 14 cm. [13019]

—Diatriba de febribus. See MEARA E. DE. Examen Diatribae Thomae Willisii de febribus. 1665, 1667.

—Distribae duae medico-philosophicae, quarum prior agit de fermentatione, sive de motu intestino particularum in quovis corpore. Altera de febribus sive de motu earundem in sanguine animalium. His accessit Dissertatio epistolica de urinis . . . Londoni, Typis Tho. Roycroft, impensis Jo. Martin, Ja. Allestry & Tho. Dicas, 1659.

[14], 97 p.; [16], 239 p.; [8], 52, [3] p. 17 cm. [13020]

—[The same.] . . . Ed. 2., ab authore recognita atque ab eodem multiplici auctario locupletata. Londini, Typis Tho. Roycrofts, impensis Jo. Martin, Ja. Allestry & Tho. Dicas, 1660.

[36], 376, [3] p. 16 cm. [13021]

—[The same.] . . . Ed. 3., ab authore recognita, atque ab eodem multiplici auctario locupletata. Londini, Typis Tho. Roycroft, impensis Jo. Martin, Ja. Allestry & Tho. Dicas, 1662.

[46], 376 p. illus. 15 cm. [13022]

Different setting of type.

—Another printing. 16 cm. [13023]

Without the first and second prelim. leaves; identical in contents, but of a different setting of type throughout.

—[The same.] . . . Ed. 3., ab authore recognita, atque ab eodem multiplici auctario locupletata. Hagae-Comitis, Ex typographia Adriani Vlacq, 1662.

[32], 376 p. front. 16 cm. [13024]

The text is of the same setting of type.

—[The same.] ... Ed. postrema, prioribus longe emendatior atque auctior. Amstelodami, Gerbrandus Schaghen, 1663.

[30], 376 p. front. 14 cm. [13025]

Different setting of type.

— Copy 2. 15 cm.

Imperfect: front. wanting; supplied in photocopy from other copy in NLM.

With this is bound: Lower, R. Diatribae Thomae Willisii ... De febribus vindicatio. 1666.

—[The same.] ... Amstelodami, Apud Gerbrandus Schagen, 1669.

[34], 408 p. front 13 cm. [13026]

Imperfect: p. 1 and 41-42 mutilated; p. 47 blank, lacks text; p. 48 erroneously printed.

—[The same.] ... Ed. 4., ab authore recognita, atque ab eodem multiplici auctario locupletata. Londini, Typis T. R., impensis J. Martyn, prostant apud Samuelem Carr, 1677.

[48], 146 + p. 15 cm. [13027]

Imperfect: 2 prelim. leaves and all after p. 146 wanting.

—[Dutch tr.] Nieuwe en geneeskundige verhandeling vande fermentatie ofte rysing, hoedanig ons die inde beschouwing aller mineralen, planten, dieren, en andere lichamen, ten aansien harer voort-teeling, aangroejing, verwisseling, sterven en ontdoeninge, als in der selver chymische behandeling voorkomt ... Beneffens een tractaat van Des scheurbuiks oorsprong, soorten, toevallen en konstige genesing, volgens de nieuwe chymische gronden van den selven autheur ... Middelburgh, Wilhelmus Goeree; en sijn mede te bekomen, tot Amsterdam, by Joh. Jansonius van Waasberge, 1676.

[12], 344, [23] p. 17 cm. [13028]

Des scheur-buiks oorsprong has special title page.

—Dissertatio de urinis. *In* Joannes Actuarius. De urinis libri VII. 1670.

—[French tr.] Dissertation sur les urines ... Nouvellement mise en françois par ***. Paris, Laurent d'Houry, 1683.

[14], 162 p. 16 cm. [13029]

—[The same.] ... Nouvellement mis en François, par ***. 2. ed. Paris, Laurent d'Houry, 1687.

[14], 162 p. 16 cm. [13030]

A reissue of the 1683 edition with new title page.

—Pathologiae cerebri et nervosi generis specimen. In quo agitur de morbis convulsivis, et de scorbuto

... Oxonii, Excudebat Guil. Hall, impensis Ja. Allestry, 1667.

[32], 202, [1], 203-316 (i.e. 306) p. port. 21 cm.

Imperfect: portrait wanting (cf. Madan, no. 2793); p. 313-314 in duplicate. [13031]

—[The same.] ... Amstelodami, Apud Danielem Elzevirium, 1668.

[12], 338, [19] p. port. 14 cm. [13032]

— ... Amstelodami, Apud Danielem Elzevirium, 1670.

[11], 338, [19] p. port. 14 cm. [13033]

Different setting of type.

—[The same.] ... Genevae, Apud Samuelem de Tournes, 1676.

[16], 214 p. 22 cm. [13034]

Issued also as part [3] of his Opera omnia.

—Pharmaceutice rationalis; sive, Diatriba de medicamentorum operationibus in humano corpore ... [Oxoniae], E Theatro Sheldoniano, 1674.

2 parts in 1 v. plates. 21 cm. [13035]

Imperfect: plate VIII in part 2 mutilated.

Part 2 has special title page dated 1675.

—[The same.] ... Hagae-Comitis, Ex officina Arnoldi Leers, 1674.

[40], 330, [9] p. illus. 15 cm. [13036]

Added engraved title page.

Imperfect: plates 3-6 wanting.

Part [1] only.

—[The same.] ... Ed. postrema, prioribus emendatior. Hagae-Comitis, Ex officina Arnoldi Leers, 1675.

2 parts in 2 v. plates. 14 cm. [13037]

Added engraved title page dated 1674.

Part 2 has title page dated 1677.

—[The same.] ... Ed. 3. Oxoniae, E Theatro Sheldoniano, 1679.

2 parts in 1 v. plates. 19 cm. [13038]

Imperfect: plate II of part 1 wanting.

Part 2 has special title page dated 1678.

—[English tr.] Pharmaceutice rationalis; or, An exercitation of the operations of medicines in humane bodies. Shewing the signs, causes and cures of most distempers incident thereunto ... As also a treatis of the scurvy, and the several sorts thereof, with their symptoms, causes and cure ... London, Printed for

T. Dring, C. Harper, and J. Leigh, and sold by R. Clavell, 1679.

 2 parts in 1 v. plates, port. 32 cm.
[13039]

Part 2 has special title page.
Imperfect: portrait wanting.

—Another issue, with imprint: London, Printed for Thomas Dring, Charles Harper, and John Leigh, 1679.   [13040]

Imperfect: The table to the Tract of the scurvy wanting.
With this is bound *his* The remaining medical works. 1681.

—A plain and easie method for preserving (by God's blessing) those that are well from the infection of the plague, or any contagious distemper in city, camp, fleet, &c. and for curing such as are infected with it. Written in the year 1666. By Tho. Willis ... With a poem on the virtue of a laurel leaf for curing of a rheumatism, by W[illiam] B[olton]. Never before printed. London, W. Crook, 1691.

 [2], 7, [8], 74 p. 18 cm.   [13041]

Imperfect: sig. F6 (blank?) wanting.
Edited by J. Hemming.
A poem upon a laurel-leaf (7 p. inserted after 2d. prelim. leaf) has half title and colophon dated 1690. Text in Latin and English, the latter "paraphrastically translated by T. F. Gent."

—The London practice of physick: or the whole practical part of physick contained in the works of Dr. Willis. Faithfully made English, and printed together for the publick good. London, Thomas Basset and William Crooke, 1685.

 [10], 672 (i.e. 680), [16] p. 18 cm. [13042]

Preface signed by the editor: Eugenius φιλιατρός.
Synopsis of five treatises contained in the author's Practice of physick: Pharmaceutice rationalis, Of convulsive diseases, Of the scurvy, Of the diseases of the brain and genus nervosum, and Of fevers.

—*See* DOLÄUS, J. Encyclopaedia chirurgica rationalis. 1689, 1690, 1695 [and] Encyclopaedia, medicinae theoretico-practicae. 1684, 1686, 1688, 1690, 1691 [and] Opera omnia. 1695 [and] Systema medicinale, a compleat system of physick. 1686; ETTMÜLLER, M. Opera omnia theoretica et practica. 1685; GRUBE, H. De arcanis medicorum non arcanis commentatio. 1673; HERFELT, H. G. Philosophicum hominis, de corporis humani machina. 1687; HIGHMORE, N. De hysterica & hypochondriaca passione. 1670; LA FONT, C. de. Dissertationes duae medicae de veneno pestilenti. 1670, 1671; LA SCALA, D. Phlebotomia damnata. 1696; LOWER, R. Diatribae

Thomae Willisii. 1665, 1666; MAYNWARING, E. Morbus polyrhizos & polymorphaeus. 1669, 1672, 1679; NOUVEAU COURS DE MEDECINE. 1669, 1683; PESTBESCHRIJVING. 1664; PORZIO, L. A. Erasistratus; sive, De sanguinis missione. 1683; SALMON, W. Iatrica. 1681, 1684, 1694; THOMSON, G. Αἱματιασις; or, The true way of preserving the bloud in its integrity. 1670; VESLING, J. Syntagma anatomicum. 1666, 1677, 1696; WEDEL, G. W. An introduction to the whole practice of physick. 1685.

WILLIUS, JOANNES VALENTINUS. *See* WILLE, Johann Valentin [1651–1677]

WILLIUS, JOHANNES. *See* WILLE, Johann Valentin [*fl.* 1635–1640]

WILLOUGHBY, FRANCIS *See* WILLUGHBY, Francis [1635–1672]

WILLUGHBY, FRANCIS [1635–1672] *See* RAY, J. Observations topographical, moral, & physiological. 1673.

WILMERDING, JOHANN [*fl.* 1682] *respondent.* Disputatio medica inauguralis de cardialgia ... Lugduni Batavorum, Apud Abrahamum Elzevier, 1687.

 [20] p. 22 cm.   [13043]

Diss.—Leyden.

WILRICH, THOMAS [*fl.* 1679] *respondent. See* MEIBOM, H., *praeses.* Disputatio medica inauguralis de cardialgia. 1679.

WILSON, EDWARD. Spadacrene Dunelmensis; or, A short treatise of an ancient medicinal fountain or vitrioline spaw near ... Durham ... By E[dward] W[ilson] ... London, W. Godbid, 1675.

 [29], 88 p. 15 cm.   [13044]

Imperfect: first preliminary leaf (blank?) wanting.

WILTENS, Ambrosius [*fl.* 1631] *respondent. See* BURGERSDICJCK, F. P., *praeses.* Collegium physicum. 1642.

WINCKELMANN, CHRISTIAN [*fl.* 1635] *See* SENNERT, D. Medicamenta officinalia praecipua. 1670 [and] Tabulae institutionum medicinae. 1673.

WINCKELMANN, JOHANN DIETRICH [*fl.* 1684] *respondent. See* SCHMID, J. A., *praeses.* Dissertationem de thermometris ... submittit ... J. D. W. 1684.

WINCKELMANN, MATTHIAS [*fl.* 1654] *respondent. See* SULTZBERGER, S. R., *praeses.* De pilis. 1654.

WINCKLER, DANIEL [*fl.* 1623-1629] Animadversiones in tractatum, qui inscribitur: Dissertatio de vita foetus in utero ... Jenae, Typis Tobiae Steinmanni, sumtibus Blasii Lobensteins, 1630.

88 p. 20 cm. [**13045**]

The Dissertatio de vita foetus in utero is by Gregor Nymann.

—De opio tractatus, in quo simul liber De opio D. Joh. Freitagii examinatur ... Lipsiae, Impensis Henningi Grosii [Excudebat Justus Jansonius] 1635.

[1], 268, [10] p. 16 cm. [**13046**]

WINCKLER, DANIEL [*fl.* 1623-1629] *respondent. See* SENNERT, D., *praeses.* De scorbuto disputatio. 1623.

WINCKLER, FRIEDRICH [*b.* 1677] *respondent. See* SLEVOGT, J. A., *praeses.* Mulierem gravidam lapsu vagina uteri laborantem ... examini sistit F. W. 1700.

—Facultatis Medicae Jenensis decani Jo. Hadriani Slevogtii ... prolusio inauguralis de utero per sarcoma ex corpore protracto. 1700.

WINCKLER, FRIEDRICH CHRISTIAN [*fl.*1665-1684]

Dissertations — Heidelberg

—*praeses.* Casus curati phrenetici ... Heidelbergae, Literis Samuelis Ammonii, 1678.

20 p. 19 cm. [**13047**]

J. P. Elwerth, *respondent.*

—Disputatio inauguralis medica de dysenteria ... Heidelbergae, Litteris Samuelis Ammonii [1681]

12 p. 18 cm. [**13048**]

J. K. Rapp. *respondent.*

—Disputatio inauguralis medica de siriasi ... Heidelbergae, Litteris Samuelis Ammonii [1684]

16 p. 20 cm. [**13049**]

J. K. Kissel, *respondent.*

—Disputatio medica, de ea melancholiae specie ... Heidelbergae, Liter. Abrahami [sic] Ludovici Walteri [1681]

34 p. 19 cm. [**13050**]

W. Ohm, *respondent.*

—Dissertatio inauguralis medica de plica, German: Wichtel-Zopff ... Heidelbergae, Litteris Samuelis Ammonii [1682]

24 p. 19 cm. [**13051**]

S. Kress, *respondent.*

WINCLERUS. See WINCKLER.

WINSLOW, JACQUES BÉNIGNE [1669-1760] *praeses.* Exercitii anatomico-pathologici, circa historiam de solennni alvi solutione ex ira et moerore, particula I. anatomica ... Hafniae, Typis Conradi Hartwigi Neuhofii [1695]

[10] p. 19 cm. [**13052**]

Diss.—Copenhagen (J. T. Trojel, *respondent*)

—Exercitii anatomico-pathologici, circa historiam de solenni alvi solutione ex ira et moerore, particula II. pathologica ... Hafniae, Literis Johannis Philippi Bockenhoffer [1696]

[15] p. 20 cm. [**13053**]

Diss.—Copenhagen (C. Spormarker, *respondent*)

WINSLOW, JACQUES BÉNIGNE [1669-1760] *respondent. See* JACOBAEUS, H., *praeses.* Dissertatio de vermibus et insectis. 1696.

WINSTON, THOMAS [1575-1655] Anatomy lectures at Gresham Colledge ... London, Printed by R. Daniel, for Thomas Eglesfield, 1659.

[8], 256 p. 18 cm. [**13054**]

Imperfect: p. 1-2 and 225-240 wanting.
Preface signed by F. P., the editor.

WINTER, GEORG SIMON [17th cent.] Wolerfahrner Ross-Arzt; oder, Vollständige Ross-Artzney-Kunst, in dreyen Büchern verabfasset ... Nürnberg, Wolffgang Moritz Endter, und Johann Andreae Endters sel. Erben, 1678.

[16], 490, [9] p. illus., plates, port. 34 cm. [**13055**]

Added engraved title page in German; added Latin title page reads: "...Hippiater expertus; seu, Medicina equorum absolutissima, tribus liber comprehensa ..."

WINTER, JAN FEIJO [*fl.* 1691] *respondent.* Disputatio medica inauguralis de phthisi ... Lugduni Batavorum, Apud Abrahamum Elzevier, 1691.

[12] p. 22 cm. [**13056**]

Diss.—Leyden.

WINTER, JOHANN GERHARD. *See* WINTHER, Johann Gerhard [*d.* 1722]

WINTER, JOHANNES, of Andernach. *See* GUINTERIUS, Joannes, Andernacus [1505-1574]

WINTER, Matthias Heinrich [*fl.* 1680] *respondent.* Disputatio inauguralis medico-chirurgica de fonticulis . . . Altdorffii, Literis Henrici Meyeri [1680]

27 p. 20 cm. [**13057**]

Diss.—Altdorf.

—*respondent. See* Hoffmann, J. M., *praeses.* Dissertationem medicam de aepothpia . . . submittit M. H. W. 1680.

WINTERBACH, Johann Bernhard [*fl.* 1685] *respondent. See* Wedel, G. W., *praeses.* Spicilegium medicum de peste. 1685.

WINTERTON, Ralph [1600–1636] *See* Hippocrates. [Aphorismi. Greek and Latin.] Aphorismorum . . . liber primus. 1631 [and] [Aphorismi. Greek and Latin.] Οἱ Ἀφορισμοὶ πεξικοὶ τε καὶ ἔμμετροι. 1633.

WINTHER, Johann, von Andernach. *See* Guinterius, Johannes, Andernacus [1505–1574]

WINTHER, Johann Gerhard [*d.* 1722] *praeses.* De admirando illo affectu catalepsi, dissertationem inauguralem medicam . . . subjicit . . . Johannes Röser . . . Rinthelii, Typis Godofredi Caspari Wächters [1692]

23 (i.e. 24) p. 19 cm. [**13058**]

Diss.—Rinteln (J. Röser, *respondent*)

—Diatribam hanc medicam hydropem ascitem examinantem . . . censurae sistit Johann. Andreas Riesnerus . . . Rinthelii, Typis Hermanni Augustini Enax, 1699.

16 p. 20 cm. [**13059**]

Diss.—Rinteln (J. A. Riesner, *respondent*)

—Dissertat. inauguralem medicam de rabie . . . subjicit . . . Petrus Carita . . . Rinthelii, Typis Hermanni Augustini Enax [1698]

28 p. 19 cm. [**13060**]

Diss.—Rinteln (P. Carita, *respondent*)

—Sermo physicus de sermone seu loquela . . . Rinthelii, Typis Godofredi Caspari Wächter [1688]

20 p. 20 cm. [**13061**]

Diss.—Rinteln (J. Röser, *respondent*)

—*respondent. See* May, H., *praeses.* Disputatio medico-physiologica de calido innato et humido radicali. 1674.

WINTHROP, John. [1606–1676] *See* Philalethes, E.

WINZER, Christian Ehrenfried [*fl.* 1669] *respondent. See* Purpius, A., *praeses.* Reserata geocosmi majestas, per XII exercitationes physicas, quarum primam . . . submittet. 1669.

WIRDIG, Sebastian [1613–1687] Nova medicina spirituum . . . in qua primo spirituum naturalis constitutio, vita, sanitas, temperamenta . . . dehinc spirituum praeternaturalis seu morbosa dispositio, causae, curationes per naturam, per diaetam, per arcana majora . . . magnetissimum seu sympatheismum, transplantationes, amuleta . . . demonstrantur . . . Hamburgi, Ex officina Gothofredi Schulzen, prostant & Amsterodami apud Johannem Jannssonium a Waesberge, 1673.

[42], 238, 3–284, [12 +] p. front. 14 cm. [**13062**]

Imperfect: sig.)(:)(12 and all after p. [12] at end, wanting.

—[The same.] . . . Accedit ob affinitatem argumenti anonymi Philalethae tractatus nunquam editus De liquore alcahest. [Hamburgi] Sumtib. viduae Gothofr. Schultzen, 1688.

[40], 198, [14], 3–236, [14] p. front. 15 cm. [**13063**]

Imperfect: frontispiece wanting.

"Arcanum liquoris immortalis ignis-aquae, seu alkahest; ab anonymo Philaletha . . . per interregationes & responsiones communicatum" ([14] p., between part [1] and [2]) has half title.

— Victrix veritas in censuris theologico-medicis de nova spirituum medicina . . . cum praeloquio Michaelis Siricii . . . Gustrovii, Typis Johannis Spierlingii, 1684.

96 p. 17 cm. [**13064**]

WIRSUNG, Christoph [1500 or 1505–1571] Ein new Artzney Buch darinn fast alle eusserliche unnd innerliche Glieder dess menschlichen Leibs, sampt ihren Kranckheiten und Gebrechen, von dem Haupt an biss zu der Fusssolen, und wie man dieselben . . . curieren soll . . . Erstlich durch . . . Christophorum Wirsung mit sonderm Fleiss auss den berühmptesten Aertzten, so wol der newen, als der alten geschriebenen Büchern, und sonderbarer auff vielen Reichs und Fürsten-Tägen Erfahrung zusammen getragen. An jetzo . . . verbessert. Durch . . . Petrum Urfenbachen . . . Ursel, Gedruckt durch Cornelium Sutorium, 1605.

[42], 316 ll.; 172, [142] p. 35 cm. [**13065**]

Previously published in Heidelberg in 1568 under title: Artzney Buch.

—[The same.] ... Franckfurt am Mayn, Getruckt bey Hartmanno Palthenio, in Verlegung Zachariae Palthenii s. Erben, 1619.

[112], 236 (i. e. 237) ll.; 134 p.   36 cm.   [13066]

With this is bound: Uffenbach, P., ed. and tr. Ein newes Artzney Buch. 1605.

— [Dutch tr.] Medecyn boec. ? ?er inne alle wtwendighe, ende inwendige parthyen aes menschen lichaems, met alle hare sieckten ende ghebreken, van den hoofde af, tot de voeten toe, begrepen zijn, ende daerinne ooc geleert wort, hoe datmen alle deselbe ... door menichderleye remedien, helpen, ende cureren sal ... Door ... Christophorum Wirtsung, wt der beroemster, outster, ende nieuwer doctoren schriften, ende wt zijne langhe experientie (onlancx door den druck) inde Hoochduytache sprake wtghegeven, ende nu wt de vierde editie, in onse ghemeyne Nederlantsche tale, overgheset, door D. Carolum Battum ... Hier achter is by gevoecht, eenen excellenten, nieuwen, geapprobeerden cocboeck. De 3. verbeterde druck. Dordrecht, Isaac Janissz. Canin, 1601.

[19], 676, [82] p.   28 cm.   [13067]

—[The same.] ... De 4. verbeterde druck. Dordrecht, Peeter Verhagen, ende Abraham Canin, 1605.

[19], 676, [72] p.   30 cm.   [13068]

Different setting of type.

—[The same.] ... De 5. verbeterde druck ... Dordrecht, Isaac Abrahamsz. Canin, 1616.

[19], 676, [120] p.   33 cm.   [13069]

A reprint of the 1605 Dordrecht edition, with addition of the third "Register."

—[The same.] ... Dese 7. ed., is van nieus oversien ende van ontallijcke menichfuldige fauten gesuyvert ... oock is hier bij gevoecht, een treffelijcke Observatie end cure van een sware geschoten wonde, mitsgaders een tractaet van de verbrantheyt. In 't Latijn beschreven door Wilhelm Hildanum. Ende nu uyt 't Latijn vertaelt door Johann. Burgundum ... Amsterdam, Jan Eversten Cloppenburg, 1627.

[16], 676, [96] p.; [26] p.; [2], 24 (i.e. 23), [1] ll. illus.   32 cm.   [13070]

De fransoysche chirurgie of Guillemeau bound between Wirsung's Medicyn-boeck and the works with which it was issued.

The appended works of Wilhelm Fabricius von Hilden, paged separately from the main work, but continuously with each other,

have special title pages: Een singuliere end voortreffelijcke observatie ende cure eens sware periculeuse geschoten wondes ... Amsterdam, Jan Evertsz. Cloppenburch, 1627; Cort ende claer tractaet vande verbrantheydt ... (with the same imprint). The first is a translation of De vulnere quodam gravissimo et periculoso, ictu sclopeti inflicto (Oppenhemio, 1614) and the second of De combustionibus (Basiliae, 1607)

"Pulvis catagmaticus ... Observatie venden Euphorbium aen D. D. Caspar Bauhin": [1] leaf at end.

With this is bound: Guillemeau, Jacques. De Fransoysche chirurgie. Dordrecht, 1598.

— [English tr.] The general practise of physicke. Conteyning all inward and outward parts of the body, with all the accidents and infirmities that are incident unto them, even from the crowne of the head to the sole of the foote. Also by what meanes ... they may be remedied ... Written ... in the German tongue, and now translated into English ... corr. and ... augm., by Jacob Mosan ... Londini, Georg. Bishop, 1605.

[20], 790, [121] p.   28 cm.   [13071]

STC 25864.

—[The same.] ... London, Thomas Adams, 1617.

[20], 790, [121] p.   28 cm.   [13072]

Imperfect: p. 471–474 wanting; supplied in photocopy from Yale Medical Library, Historical Library; title page and last two leaves mutilated.

Different setting of type.

STC 25865.

—Another issue, with misnumbered pagination partly corrected.   [13073]

—[The same.] ... In this 4th and last ed. are very many additions added by some of our English physitians ... London, Printed for J. L., Henry Hood, Abel Roper, and Richard Tomlins, 1654.

[21], 818, [123] p.   30 cm.   [13074]

Imperfect: Longitudinal label preceding title page wanting.

—Another issue, with misnumbered pagination partly corrected.   [13075]

WIRTH, Gottfried Erhard [*fl.* 1691] *respondent.* *See* Petri von Hartenfels, G. C., *praeses.* Disputatio inauguralis medica de febre petechiali. 1691.

WIRTZ, Felix [*ca.* 1510–*ca.* 1590] Wund Artzney ... Jetzo auffs newe ... nach dess Authoris eigenen Schrifften ubersehen und mit einem zuvor nie also in Truck gesehenem Hebammenbüchlein vermehret, durch Rudolff Würtz ... Basel, Bey den Petrinischen, 1638.

[55], 872 p. 17 cm. [13076]

First published in 1563 under title: Practica der Wundartzney. Cf. Gurlt. Vol. 3, p. 238–261.

—[The same.] Practica der Wundartzney ... darinnen allerley schädliche Missbrauche ... aussführlichen angedeutet, und umb vieler erheblichen Ursachen, willen abgeschaft werden. Jetzunder alles ... von neuen übersehen, und ... vermehret durch Rudolph Würtzen ... und Hn. D. Heinrich Schaevii anatomischer Abriss hinangethan ... Stettin, In Verlägung Jeremiae Mamphrasen [gedruckt bey Georg Götzken] 1659.

[54], 813 p. 16 cm. [13077]

Added engraved title page.

—[The same.] Wund-Artzney, darinnen allerhand schädliche Missbräuche ... aussführlich angedeutet, und umb vieler erheblichen Ursachen willen abgeschafft werden. Jetzund alles ... von neuem übersehen, mit ... einem ... Hebammen-und Kinder-Büchlein vermehret durch Rudolph Würtzen ... Sampt angehencktem anatomischen Abriss Herrn D. Henrici Schaevii. Basel, In Verlag Emanuel Königs und Söhnen, 1670.

[54], 730, 85 p. 17 cm. [13078]

Added engraved title page.

—[The same.] ... Basel, In Verlag Emanuel Königs und Söhnen, 1675.

[54], 730, 85 p. 17 cm. [13079]

Added engraved title page.

A reissue of the 1670 edition with new title page.

—[English tr.] An experimental treatise of surgerie, in four parts ... Exactly perused after the authors own manuscrip [sic], by Rodolph Wurtz ... Englished and much corrected by Abraham Lenertzon Fox ... Whereunto is added ... the Childrens book ... London, Gartrude Dawson, 1656.

[20], 366 p. 19 cm. [13080]

—[French tr.] La chirurgie ... Nouvellement reveuë & corrigée, selon les propres manuscrits de l'autheur, par Rudolfe Wurtzius ... Traduite d'allemand ... par ... François Sauvin ... Paris, Gaspar Meturas, 1672.

[24], 524, [3] p. 15 cm. [13081]

—[The same.] ... Paris, Laurent d'Houry, 1689.

[24], 524 p. 15 cm. [13082]

A reissue of the 1672 edition with new title page and without Metura's advertisement.

WIRTZ, Rudolf [*fl.* 1612–1620] *ed. See* Wirtz, F. Wund Artzney. 1638, 1659, 1670, 1675; [English tr.] 1656; [French tr.] 1672, 1689.

WIRZ. *See* Wirtz.

WISEMAN, Richard [1622?–1676] Severall chirurgicall treatises ... London, Printed by E. Flesher and J. Macock, for R. Royston, and B. Took, 1676.

[15], 498, 79, [13] p. 37 cm. [13083]

—[The same.] ... The 2d ed. London, Printed by R. Norton and J. Macock, for R. Royston, and B. Took, 1686.

[15], 577, [13] p. 33 cm. [13084]

—[The same.] Several chirurgical treatises on these following heads, viz. I. Of tumours. II. Of ulcers. III. Of diseases of the anus. IV. Of the kings evil. V. Of wounds. VI. Of gun-shot wounds. VII. Of fractures & luxations. VIII. Of the lues venerea ... The 2d ed. London, Samuel Clement, 1692.

[13], 577, [13] p. 33 cm. [13085]

Imperfect: first preliminary leaf wanting. A reissue of the 1686 edition with new title page.

—[The same.] Eight chirurgical treatises, on these following heads, viz. I. Of tumours. II Of ulcers. III. Of diseases of the anus. IV. Of the kings-evil. V. Of wounds. VI. Of gun-shot wounds. VII. Of fractures and luxations. VIII. Of the lues venerea ... The 3d ed. London, Benj. Tooke, and Luke Meredith, 1696.

[12], 563, [13] p. 32 cm. [13086]

Imperfect: first preliminary leaf wanting.

—[The same.] ... The 3d ed. London, Printed for B. T. and L. M. and are sold by W. Keblewhite and J. Jones, 1697.

[14], 563, [13] p. 32 cm. [13087]

A reissue of the 1696 edition with new title page.

WISSENBACH, Johann Jacob [1607–1665] Confutatio diatribae de mutuo, tribus disputationibus ventilatae auctore & praeside Jo. Jacobo Vissembachio ... Lugduni Batavorum, Ex officina Joannis Maire, 1645.

[16], 3–358, [9] p. 16 cm. [13088]

"Elenchus ἐχθέσεως de mutuo, ex jurisprudentiae methodicae partitionibus elementariis Johan. Ottonis Tabor" (p. [305]–358) has special title page.

Fabrot's Epistola, another work bound with Saumaise, is misbound after p. 302.

Bound with (as issued) Saumaise, C. de. Disquisitio de mutuo. 1645.

WITHER, GEORGE [1588-1667] Britain's remembrancer. Containing a narration of the plague lately past; a declaration of the mischiefs present; and a prediction of judgments to come . . . [London] Sold by John Grismond, 1628.

[2], 287 (i.e. 289) p.   15 cm.   **[13089]**

Added engraved half title, preceded by "The meaning of the title page".

Imperfect: outer margin of first leaf trimmed.

In verse.

STC 25899.

—, *tr. See* NEMESIUS, Bp. of Emesa. The nature of man. 1636.

WITICHIUS, JOHANNES. *See* WITTICH, Johann [1537-1596]

WITTE, CONRAD THEODOR [*fl.* 1667] *respondent. See* WEDEL, G. W. Diatriben medicam de ciureticis . . . subjiciunt G. W. W. . . . & C. T. W. 1667.

WITTE, H. T. *See* WITTE, Heinrich Theodor [*fl.* 1697-1699]

WITTE, HEINRICH THEODOR [*fl.* 1697-1699] *respondent. See* FICK, J. K., *praeses.* Dissertationem hanc de abortu epidemico . . . publice ventilandam sistit . . . H. T. Witte. 1697.

WITTE, HENNING [1634-1696] Memoriae medicorum nostri seculi clarissimorum renovatae decas prima [-secunda] . . . Francofurti, Apud Martinum Hallervord, typis Joannis Andreae, 1676.

[1], 175 (i.e. 275) p.   18 cm.   **[13090]**

Added engraved title page.

—Another issue.

[1], 185 (i.e. 285) p.   **[13091]**

Memoria Horstiana is omitted with the addition of Memoria Beckheriana and Memoria Schenckiana.

WITTE, JAN DE [*fl.* 1666-1669] *respondent.* Disputatio medica inauguralis de catarrho . . . Lugduni Batavorum, Apud viduam & haeredes Joannis Elsevirii, 1669.

[12] p.   23 cm.   **[13092]**

Diss. — Leyden.

WITTEN, ALBERT [*fl.* 1688] *respondent.* Disputatio medica inauguralis de pleuritide . . . Duisburgi ad Rhenum, Apud Franconem Sas, 1688.

20 p.   20 cm.   **[13093]**

Diss. — Duisburg.

WITTEN, HENNING. *See* WITTE, Henning [1634-1696]

WITTENBERG. Universität. Medizinische Fakultät. *See* UNIVERSITÄT WITTENBERG. Medizinische Fakultät.

WITTENBERGIUS, BURCHARDUS. Declaratio . . . toti ut propalet universo, novam absque effusione sanguinis dissectionem atque embamma . . . Ludovici de Bils . . . Brugis Flandrorum, Lucas Kerchovius, 1658.

10 p.   19 cm.   **[13094]**

WITTENDEL, PETRUS DE [*fl.* 1589] *ed. See* MERCURIALE, G. Commentarii eruditissimi, in Hippocratis Coï Prognostica. 1602 [and] Tractatus: De compositione medicamentorum. 1601.

WITTICH, CHRISTOPH [1625-1687] *See* DESMARETS, S. Indiculus. 1671.

WITTICH, JOHANN [1537-1596] Bericht von den wunderbaren bezoardischen Steinen, so wieder allerley Gifft krefftiglich dienen, und aus den Leiben der frembden Thier genommen werden: so wol auch von andern Steinen, so aus verborgener eingepflantzter Natur und Kraft, unerhörte und ungleubliche Wirckung verrichten. Dessgleichen von den fürnembsten edlen Gesteinen, unbekandten hartzigen Dingen, und des newen armenischen Balsams, frembden Wunderkreutern, Holtz und Wurtzeln . . . und wie solche inner und ausserhalb des Leibes zugebrauchen. Endlichen auch von der newen schlesischen Terra Sigillata, Axungia Solis genandt. Welche alle . . . aus India Orientali und Occidentali, durch Gartiam ab Horto, und Nicolaum Monardum kündig gemacht worden seind, darbey auch anderer gelehrter Medicorum Meinung mit eingesprengt, zuvor nie Deutsch ausgangen, jtzo aber . . . zusammen gebracht, durch M. Johannem Wittichium . . . [Heidelberg] Gotthard Vögelin [1612]

[6], 120, [7] p.   20 cm.   **[13095]**

Imperfect: title page mutilated; first preliminary leaf (blank?) wanting.

With this is bound *his* Von dem Ligno guayaco. 1603.

—Consilia, observationes atque epistolae medicae . . . Addita est methodus componendi theriacam & praeparandi ambram factitiam D. Johannis Pontani D. . . . Lipsiae, Impensis Henningi Grosii [Excudebant haeredes Francisci Schnelbolzii] 1604.

[16], 645, [2] p.   port.   20 cm.   **[13096]**

—Consilium apoplecticum; seu, De subitanea morte: das ist: ein nützlicher Rathschlag . . . von der . . . schrecklichen Kranckheit . . . den gehenden Todt, Schlag, und Hand Gottes pflegt zu nennen. Vom Ursprung des Namens: was solche Kranckheit sey: wovon sie verursacht; was vor Zeichen vorher gehen; und wie man sich . . . mit gantz heilsamen und krefftigen Mitteln darfür praeserviren möge. Item, was sich ein Christ bey der erschrecklichen Kranckheit des Schlags . . . erinnern, und wie er nach Anweisung göttliches Worts, sich darzu shicken und bereiten soll. Zuvor niemals an Tag kommen . . . Leipzig, In Verlegung Bartholomaei Voigts [Gedruckt durch Frantz Schnellboltzens Erben; typis haeredum Beyeri] 1602.

191, 73, [14] p.   16 cm.   [13097]

A word for word reprint of the 1593 edition.

—Praeservator sanitatis. Ein nützlicher Bericht von den sechss unvormeidlichen Dingen, zur Gesundheit gantz erspriesslichen, wie man sich in denselben beydes zu Hause, und auch uber Land verhalten soll . . . Item, Arcula itineraria; oder, Reyse-Kästlein, für allerhand Kranckheiten. Auch Von der schrecklichen Heuptkranckheit . . . Mit einer Zugabe, Von Meth, Weinmeth, Claret, Lautertranck, Hippocras und Nectar . . . Alles von newem ubersehen, corrigirt und verbessert . . . [n. p.] 1607.

175, [10] p.; [2], 107, [8] p.   16 cm.   [13098]

Lacks the two last items called for on the title page.

—Vade mecum. Das ist; ein künstlich new Artzneybuch, so man stets bey sich haben und führen kan, in fürfallender Noth sich Hülff daraus zuerholen, wider allerhand Kranckheit dess menschlichen Leibes, vom Haupt an bis auff die Fusssohlen . . . Leipzig, In Vorlegung Bartholomaei Voigts, 1601–1607.

2 v. in 1.   20 cm.   [13099]

Vol. 2 has title page dated 1607: Vade mecum. Der ander Theil des künstlichen newen Artzneybuchs, so man stets bey sich haben und führen kan, in allerhand Kranckheiten der Jungfrawen, besonders der ehelichen Weiber, sich vor, in und nach der Geburt, gutes Raths daraus zu erholen, Item: Von allerhandt Kranckheiten der jungen Kinder . . .

The last work, on pediatrics, has special title page (also dated 1607) and separate pagination: Libellus de infantilium aegritudinum medicatione, das ist: Artzneybüchlein, wie man den armen Kinderlein für allerhand Leibs Gebrechen, vom Haupt an, biss auff die Fusssole, helffen und rathen soll . . . Running title: New Artzneybuch Wititchii, von Kleinen Kindern.

Colophon at end of vol. 2: Leipzig, Typis haeredum Beyeri, gedruckt durch Valentin am Ende, 1607.

—[The same.] . . . Leipzig, In Verlegung Bartholomaei Voigts, 1616–1619.

2 v. in 1.   20 cm.   [13100]

Vol. 2 has title page dated 1619: Vade mecum.

The last work, on pediatrics, has special title page (also dated 1619) and separate pagination.

Colophon at end of vol. 2: Leipzig, Typis Lambergianis, gedruckt durch Johann Glück, 1619.

—Von dem Ligno guayaco Wunderbawm, Res Nova genandt, von der China ex Occidentali India, von der Sarsa Parilla, von dem Fenchelholtz Sassafras, und von dem Griessholtz, so man Lignum nephriticum nennet. Welche alle zum Theil wieder die flechtende indianische Seuche, zum Theil für die Flüsse, Zipperle, Wassersucht und reissenden Stein, sampt andren eingewurtzelten Kranckheiten, gantz dienstlichen, und wie dieselben, an denen Orten, da sie wachsen, zubereitet und gebraucht werden, biss daher in Druck also noch nicht kommen . . . [Heidelberg] Typis Voegelinianis, 1603.

[36] p.   20 cm.   [13101]

Bound with his Bericht von den . . . bezoardischen Steinen. 1612.

—, ed. See PADOANO, H. Processus. 1607.

—, ed. and tr. See RANTZAU, H. De conservanda valetudine. 1601.

See AALBORG, N. M. Medicin eller laege-boog. 1640.

WITTICH, NIKOLAUS [fl. 1673] respondent. See JOHRENIUS, J. M., praeses. Disputatio philosophica de sede animae rationalis. 1673.

WITTIE, ROBERT [1613?–1684] Gout raptures. Ἀστρομαχία; or, An historical fiction of a war among the stars: wherein are mentioned the 7 planets, the 12 signs of the zodiack, and the 50 constellations of heaven mentioned by the ancients . . . Cambridge, Printed by John Hayes and sold by John Creed, 1677.

[14], 44, [3] p.   18 cm.   [13102]

Errata: p. [47]

Imperfect: first preliminary leaf (blank?) wanting.

In English, Latin and Greek verse.

—Fons Scarburgensis; sive, Tractatus de omnis aquarum generis origine ac usu. Particulariter de fonte minerali apud Scarbrough . . . Item dissertationes variae tam philosophicae quam medicinales . . . Londini, Typis R. Everingham, ac impensis N. Simmons & J. Edwin, 1678.

[7], 235, [3] p.   17 cm.   [13103]

—Οὐρανοσκοπία; or, A survey of the heavens . . . To which is added The gout-raptures, augmented and improved. In English, Latine, and Greek lyrick verse . . . London, Printed by J. M. for the author, and sold by R. Clavell, J. Robinson, and R. Boulter, 1681.

    [4], 158 p.   16 cm.   **[13104]**
The gout-raptures has special title page (p. [71]).

—Pyrologia mimica; or, An answer to Hydrologia chymica of William Sympson . . . in defence of Scarbrough-spaw. Wherein the five mineral principles of the said spaw are defended . . . Also a vindication of the rational method . . . called Galenical, and a reconciliation betwixt that and the chymical . . . London, Printed by T. N. for J. Martyn, 1669.

    [40], 312 p.   16 cm.   **[13105]**

—Scarbrough spaw; or, A description of the nature and vertues of the spaw at Scarbrough . . . Also a treatise of the nature and use of water . . . London, Charles Tyus and Richard Lambert, 1660.

    [13], 254, [1] p.   15 cm.   **[13106]**
Errata: p. [255]

—Scarbroughs spagyrical anatomizer dissected; or, An answer to all that Dr. Tonstal hath objected in his book against Scarbrough spaw . . . As also reflections upon a late piece, called a vindication of Hydrologia chymica . . . London, Printed by B. G. for Nath. Brooke and R. Lambert, 1672.

    [31], 127 p.   15 cm.   **[13107]**

—, *tr. See* PRIMROSE, J. The antimoniall cup twice cast. 1640 [and] Popular errours. 1651.

—*See* [PEACHIE, John] Some observations made upon the root called nean. 1680?; SIMPSON, W. Hydrologia chymica. 1669; TONSTALL, G. A new-years-gift for Doctor Witty. 1672.

WITTIG, JOHANN JAKOB [*fl.* 1660] *respondent. See* LINDEN, J. A. van der, *praeses.* Hippocrates de circuitu sanguinis, exercitatio VI. 1660.

WITTWER, JOHANN JAKOB [*fl.* 1672] *respondent. See* CRAUSE, R. W., *praeses.* Dissertatio medica inauguralis de cordis palpitatione. 1672.

WITTY, ROBERT. *See* WITTIE, Robert [1613?–1684]

WITZEL, JOHANN KASPAR [*fl.* 1675–1676] *respondent.* Disputatio inauguralis medica de morsibus et

puncturis animalium . . . Argentorati, Literis Joh. Friderici Spoor, 1676.

    40 p.   19 cm.   **[13108]**
Diss.—Strasbourg.

—*See* MAPP, M., *praeses.* Disputatio de fistula genae terminata ad dentem cariosum. 1675.

WITZEL, JOHANN LUDWIG [*fl.* 1645–1668] *respondent.* Λεπτυνσεως s. extenutiationis σκιαγραφίαν . . . exponit Johannes Ludovicus Witzel . . . Argentorati, Typis Eberhardi Welperi, 1651.

    [32] p.   19 cm.   **[13109]**
Diss.—Strasbourg.

— *See* SEBISCH, M. [1578–1674?] *praeses.* Galeni quinque priores libri. 1651; TILEMANN, J., *praeses.* Harmoniae physico-medicae de numero elementorum disputatio II. 1645.

— *ed. See* SCHRÖDER, J. Pharmacopoeia medico-chymica. 1677, 1681.

WÖLFFEL, Gabriel [*fl.* 1688–1692] *respondent.* Dissertatio inauguralis juridica de obligatione medicorum . . . Erfordiae, Stanno Groschiano [1692]

    [16] p.   19 cm.   **[13110]**
Diss.—Erfurt.

WÖRGER, FRANZ [1647–1708] Triga dissertationum sacrarum. I. De signo Filii hominis in coelo. II. De haedis separandis ab ovibus in judicio. III. De mense nascentis Domini contra Bochartum . . . Kilonii, Literis Joachimi Reumanni, 1679.

    31, [1] p.   20 cm.   **[13111]**

WOESTHAUS, HENRICUS JACOBUS. *See* WUYSTHAUS, Henricus Jacobus.

WOESTHOVEN, ABRAHAM [*fl.* 1693–1699] *respondent.* Disputatio medica inauguralis, continens varias miscellaneas theses . . . Lugduni Batavorum, Apud Abrahamum Elzevier, 1699.

    [16] p.   22 cm.   **[13112]**
Diss.—Leyden.

—*See* DEKKERS, F., *praeses.* Disputatio medica de morbis soporosis. 1699.

WOHLMUTH, JOHANN [*fl.* 1691] *respondent. See* STRYK, E. A., *praeses.* Disputatio juridica de matrimonio ex ratione status. 1691.

WOHLRAB, Johann. Von der wunderbarlichen Tugend, Krafft und Würckung der köstlichen Wurtzel Saxifraga, auff Teutsch Steinbrech genandt . . . [Luzern? 16--?]

[2] p.   21 cm.   **[13113]**

At end: Diese Wurtzel findet man bey mir Johann Wohlrab von Lucern . . .

Andreas Matthioli and Joachim Camerarius are mentioned in the text.

WOLF, Caspar [1532–1601] *ed.* and *tr. See* [Stephanus Magnetes] Experiment Buch. 1623.

—, *ed. See* Gesner, K. Historiae animalium liber primus [-liber V] 1617–1621 [v. 1 1620]; Vege, P. de. Pax methodicorum. 1620.

WOLF, Heinrich, *physician of Goslar.* Tractatus und kurtzer Bericht, wie man sich . . . vor der jetzo anfahenden, regierenden Seuche der gifftigen Pestilentz praeserviren, verhalten, dienlichen Mitteln verwahren, und was teglich, so wol ad praeservationem, als dann auch curationem, nötig gebraucht werden könne . . . Gosslar, Johann Vogt, 1625.

[39] p.   20 cm.   **[13114]**

WOLF, Heinrich, *physician of Halberstadt.* Febris malignae anatomia; das ist, Des gifftigen Fleck-Fiebers Zerlegung, worinn beschrieben werden, des Fiebers Natur, Nahme, Unterscheid, Ursachen, Erkennezeichen, Praeservation und Curation . . . Halberstadt, Gedruckt durch Johann-Erasmum Hynitzsch, 1670.

64 p.   21 cm.   **[13115]**

WOLF, Jakob [1642–1694]

Dissertations — Jena

—*praeses.* Disputatio seu judicium medicum de cerevisia Numburgensi. Jenae, Stanno Joh. Dav. Wertheri [1684]

60 p.   20 cm.   **[13116]**

J. R. Pretten, *respondent.*

— Dissertatio medica de crusta lactea, vulgo vom Ansprunge . . . publico examini subjicit . . . Godofredus Scultzius . . . 1697 [sic] Jenae, Ex officina Johannis Gollneri [1697]

27, [1] p.   19 cm.   **[13117]**

Reprint of a dissertation originally published in 1693.
G. Schultz, *respondent.*

— Dissertatio medica de obesitate exsuperante . . .

Jenae, Typis Gollnerianis, 1683.

102 p.   20 cm.   **[13118]**

K. C. Leisner, *respondent.*

— Dissertatio medica de urinae incontinentia . . . Jenae, Literis Georgii Heinrici Mülleri [1688]

48 p.   19 cm.   **[13119]**

J. E. Güth, *respondent.*

— Exercitatio medica de literatorum potu ejusque usu et abusu . . . Jenae, Typis Joh. Dav. Wertheri [1684]

[1], 98 p.   19 cm.   **[13120]**

F. E. Weidler, *respondent.*

—*respondent. See* Ammann, P., *praeses.* Dissertatio medica inauguralis de mictione cruenta. 1673, 1686?; Bohn, J., *praeses.* Exercitationum physiologicarum prima . . . [-decima tertia] 1674?

—*See* Bierling, C. G. Thesaurus theoretico-practicus. 1695.

WOLF, Johann [1537–1616] *ed.* and *tr. See* Gelli, G. B. De naturae humanae fabrica. 1609.

WOLF, Johann [*fl.* 1673–1680] *praeses.* Disputationem physicam evolventem qu. num daemon cum sagis generare possit . . . submittit Johann. Paulus Reineccius . . . Wittenbergae, Typis Christiani Schrödteri [1676]

[16] p.   20 cm.   **[13121]**

Diss.—Wittenberg (J. P. Reineccius, *respondent*)

—*respondent. See* Jahn, P., *praeses.* De lupo disputatio physica. 1673.

WOLF, Johann Christian. *See* Wolff, Johann Christian [1673–1723]

WOLF, Michael [1584–1623] *praeses.* Disputationum acroamaticarum quinta de natura et discrimine physici ac mathematici . . . Jenae, Imprimebat Johannes Weidner, 1618.

[16] p.   19 cm.   **[13122]**

Diss.—Jena (C. Brunner, *respondent*)

— Ἑπτάς problematum physicorum . . . proponit: Balthasar Han . . . Jenae, Typis Henrici Rauchmaule [1613]

[16] p.   19 cm.   **[13123]**

Diss.—Jena (B. Han, *respondent*)

WOLFART, Erasmus [*fl.* 1609] *ed. See* Khunrath, H. Amphitheatrum sapientiae. 1609.

WOLFART, PETER [1675-1726] *respondent. See* VALENTINI, M. B., *praeses.* Discursus academicus de china chinae. 1695.

WOLFARTH, GEORG BALTHASAR [*fl.* 1631] *respondent. See* SEBISCH, M. [1578-1674?] *praeses.* Exercitationes medicae. 1639.

WOLFERSTAN, STANFORD. An enquiry into the causes of diseases in general, and the disturbances of the humors in man's body ... Together with some observations, shewing wherein the venom of vipers, particularly that of the English adder, does consist ... London, Thomas Basset, 1692.

[12], 86, [4] p.   16 cm.   **[13124]**

WOLFF, AUGUST [*fl.* 1651] *praeses.* De quatour anni temporibus dissertationem philosophicam ... P. P. ... Christianus Colerus ... [Lipsiae] Typis haeredum Timothei Hönii, 1651.

[20] p.   19 cm.   **[13125]**

Diss. — Leipzig (C. Coler, *respondent*)

WOLFF, BENEDICT [*fl.* 1619] *respondent. See* COSCANUS, O., *praeses.* Disputationis physicae de substantia corporea mobili. 1619.

WOLFF, CHRISTIAN [*fl.* 1665-1670] *praeses.* Disputatio zoologica de lupo et lycanthropia ... Wittebergae, Typis Michaelis Wendt, 1666.

[16] p.   19 cm.   **[13126]**

Diss. — Wittenberg (C. Wantscher, *respondent*)

WOLFF, CHRISTIAN [*fl.* 1671] *respondent. See* BOHN, J., *praeses.* Exercitationum physiologicarum prima ... [-decima tertia] 1674?

WOLFF, CHRISTIAN [*fl.* 1693] *See* BEYER, G. Bey hochansehnlicher Beerdigung der ... Frauen Annen Sabinen ... 1693.

WOLFF, CHRISTIAN JUSTIN [*b.* 1672] *respondent. See* CRAUSE, R. W., *praeses.* Dissertatio medica inauguralis de memoria ejusque remediorum natura, usu, et abusu. 1696.

— *See* SLEVOGT, J. A. Decani Facultatis Medicae Jo. Hadriani Slevogtii ... prolusio inauguralis de fonticulo futurae coronalis, insigni vitiorum memoriae remedio. 1694.

WOLFF, CHRISTOPH [*fl.* 1661] *respondent.* Inauguralem hanc de septi transversi inflammatione disputationem medicam ... exponit Christophorus

Wolffius ... Argentorati, Typis Johannis Pastorii, 1661.

24 p.   19 cm.   **[13127]**

Diss. — Strasbourg.

WOLFF, ERNST CHRISTOPH [*fl.* 1697] *respondent. See* CRAUSE, R. W., *praeses.* Disputatio medica inauguralis de potu frigido. 1697.

WOLFF, GEORG [*fl.* 1624] *respondent. See* BLUM, M., *praeses.* Decas problematum medicorum. 1624.

WOLFF, GEORG CHRISTIAN [*b.* 1669] *respondent. See* SCHELHAMMER, G. C., *praeses.* Dissertatio inauguralis medica de dyspepsia. 1695.

— *See* WEDEL, G. W. Propempticum inaugurale de decimatione operum. 1695.

WOLFF, GEORG CHRISTOPH [*fl.* 1641] *respondent. See* MÖBIUS, G., *praeses.* Disputatio medica de tertiana intermittente. 1641.

WOLFF, GEORG CONRAD [*fl.* 1685-1687] *respondent. See* ALBINUS, B. Disputatione medica inauguralis de melancholia. 1687; ALBINUS, B. Dissertatio de cervo corde glande plumbea trajecto. 1689; SCHRADER, F., *praeses.* Exercitatio academica de aeris in corpus humanum effectibus. 1685.

WOLFF, HERMANN [*d.* 1620] Beschreibung des mineralischen Brunnen, so newlicher Zeit bey Cassel in Hessen widerumb in Brauch gebracht worden ... Cassel, Wilhelm Wessel, 1609.

[8], 46 p.   20 cm.   **[13128]**

Vorrede signed by Hermann Wolff and Jacob Mosan, the authors.

WOLFF, JAKOB. *See* Wolf, Jakob [1642-1694]

WOLFF, JOHANN [*fl.* 1632] *respondent. See* SEBISCH, M. [1578-1674?] *praeses.* Libri sex Galeni De morborum differentiis. 1632.

WOLFF, JOHANN CHRISTIAN [1673-1723] Epistola anatomica, problematica, undecima ... ad ... Fredericum Ruyschium ... de intestinorum tunicis, glandulis, &c. Amstelaedami, Apud Joannem Wolters, 1698.

13, [2] p.   plate.   22 cm.   **[13129]**

"Frederici Ruyschii responsio ...": p. 7-13.

— *respondent. See* BERGER, J. G. von, *praeses.* Dissertatio solennis de febribus malignis. 1696.

WOLFF, Johann Kaspar [*fl.* 1669] *respondent. See* Crocius, C. F., *praeses.* Exercitatio medica. 1669.

WOLFF, Johann Konrad [*fl.* 1699] *respondent. See* Stübner, A. G., *praeses.* Dissertatio physica de nigritarum affectionibus. 1699.

WOLFF, Pancraz [*fl.* 1674-1726] Cogitationes medico-legales de cogitatione, non excogitatae saltem, sed ex ipsius veritatis floribus, ab Hippocrate maxime, hinc Helmontio, Cartesio, Willisio, Malpighio, aliisque … medicis … congestis, in circulum philosophicum contextae … Cizae, Excudebat Melchior Hucho [1697?]

    [16], 112, [1] p.   17 cm.   **[13130]**
    Errata: p. [113]

— *respondent. See* Bohn, J., *praeses.* Dissertationem medicam de haemorrhagia … submittet P. W. 1674.

WOLFFGANG, György [*fl.* 1642] *respondent. See* Poláni, J., *praeses.* Discursus de origine animae rationalis. 1642.

WOLFFGANG, Johann [*fl.* 1633] *respondent. See* Plachet, J., *praeses.* Disputatio medica de lue. 1633.

WOLFFHART, Ludwig [*fl.* 1631-1632] Experimentum cremoris tartari. *In* Eisenmenger, J. C. Nothwendiger Bericht. 1632?

WOLFFIUS, Michael. *See* Wolf, Michael [1584-1623]

WOLFIUS, Christianus Justinus. *See* Wolff, Christian Justin [*b.* 1672]

WOLFIUS, Johannes. *See* Wolf, Johann [*fl.* 1673-1680]

WOLFROM, Johann [*fl.* 1623] *respondent. See* Innichenhöfer, H., *praeses.* Υπνολογια; sive, Tractatus jucundus physiologicus. 1624.

WOLLEB, Johann [1640-1675] *respondent.* Theses … de cancro mammarum … Basileae, Typis Joh. Jacobi Deckeri [1667]

    [16] p.   20 cm.   **[13131]**
    Diss. — Basel.

WOLLEB, Lukas [*fl.* 1698-1721] *respondent.* Dissertatio medica inauguralis de tympanite … [Basileae] Literis Regiis [1698]

    32 p.   19 cm.   **[13132]**
    Diss. — Basel.

WOLLIN, Johann [*fl.* 1661] *respondent. See* Tappe, J., *praeses.* Disputatio medica de amore insano. 1661.

WOLLITZ, Johann [*fl.* 1662] *respondent. See* Beckher, D. [1627-1670] *praeses.* Disputatio medica de medicamentis purgantibus. 1662.

WOLPHIUS, Casparus. *See* Wolf, Caspar [1532-1601]

WOLPHIUS, Johann Caspar. *See* Wolff, Johann Kaspar [*fl.* 1669]

WOLSELEY, Sir Charles, *bart.* [1630?-1714] The case of divorce and re-marriage thereupon discussed. By a reverend prelate of the Church of England and a private gentleman … London, Nevill Simmons, 1673.

    [6], 155 p.   14 cm.   **[13133]**
    First and last leaf (blank?) wanting.
    Longitudinal label preceding title page: S^r. Charles Wolseley on divorce.

WOLTER, Ambrosius. *See* Wolter a Liebenfeldt, Gualter Ambrosius [*fl.* 1666]

WOLTER A LIEBENFELDT, Gualter Ambrosius [*fl.* 1666] Pyrotechnicum opusculum de cauteriorum; sive, Fonticulorum ad privatos partium affectus medendos usu, & utilitate … Wratislaviae, In haeredum Baumanniorum typographia, exprimebat Joh. Christoph. Jacobi [1672]

    [24] p.   17 cm.   **[13134]**

— Tractatlein für die Krancken. In zwey Theyl getheilet: welcher Theyle, das Erste, ein Unterricht ist, und etliche Artickel fürschreibet, wie, und nach welchen sich die Krancken alle und jegliche in gemein verhalten sollen … Das Andere aber ist eine Ableittung von den falschen Wahnen, Irrthumben, und Miessbräuchen, so gemelten Artickeln zu wieder seyn … Neyss, Ignatius Schubarth, 1666.

    [86] p.   16 cm.   **[13135]**

WOLVERIDGE, James [*fl.* 1670] Speculum matricis Hybernicum. *See* The English midwife enlarged. 1682.

De WONDERLIJCKE en wel geoeffende geneesen heelmeester, leerende alderley siecktens, gebreken, accidenten, wonden … handelende mede van pestilentie en swangere vrouwen. Als oock 't rechte gebruyck van allerley kruyden, wortelen, zaden, oilen, wateren tot gesonheyt. Mitsgaders een nieuw uytgevonden disteleer-konst . . . Door d'overleden Heer J. C. [i.e. Johannes Casteleyn?] Amsterdam, Cornelis Jansz, 1663.

[8], 164 p.   21 cm.   [**13136**]

WONDERS no miracles. 1666. *See* [LLOYD, D.]

WOOD, ANTHONY À [1632-1695] [Historia et antiquitates Universitatis Oxoniensis, duobus voluminibus comprehensae. Oxonii, E Th. Sheld., 1674]

2 v. in 1.   illus.   42 cm.   [**13137**]

Imperfect: t. p. and all other leaves preceding p. 1 wanting; title supplied from Madan. 2996.

Originally written in English and translated into Latin under the direction of Dr. John Fell, by Richard Peers and Richard Reeve.

WOOD, OWEN. An alphabetical book of physicall secrets, for all those diseases that are most predominant and dangerous (curable by art) in the body of man . . . Whereunto is annexed a small treatise of the judgement of urines . . . London, Printed by John Norton for Walter Edmonds, 1639.

[8], 238, [1] p.   14 cm.   [**13138**]

To the reader, signed by Alexander Read.
STC 25955.

—[The same.] An epitomie of most experienced, excellent and profitable secrets appertaining to physick and chirurgery, alphabetically, for all those diseases that are most predominant . . . Also, the judgement of urines . . . By O[wen] W[ood] professour in phisick and chirurgery. The 4th ed. corr. and amend. London, Printed by E. C. for Michael Spark, 1653.

[32], 238, [1] p.   15 cm.   [**13139**]

Imperfect: p. [27-30] and 223-228 wanting.
The text is of the same setting of type.

[—] Choice and profitable secrets both physicall, and chirurgical: formerly concealed, by the deceased Dutchess of Lenox, and now published for the use and benefit of such as live far from physicians and chirurgions: being approved of by eminent doctors, and published by their charitable advice for the publique good. Whereunto is annexed, A discovery of the natures and properties of all such herbs which are most commonly known, and grow in countrey gardens. London, Printed for the use and benefit of William Masters, 1658.

[8], 317 (i.e. 308) p.; 94, [23] p.; 2 + p.   front. (port.)   14 cm.   [**13140**]

Imperfect: p. 197-200, 209-212 and 215-218 of part [1]; all pages of part [3] after p. 2 wanting.

Part [1] has running title: The secrets of physick and chirurgery. Part [2] has caption title: The phisitians help to the chirurgeons salvatory for suddain accidents. Part [3] has caption title: A discourse of the natures and applications of those herbes which are most usually known by countrey-people.

Preface: 5th edition.

WOOD, ZACHARIAH. *See* SYLVIUS, Zacharias [1608-1664]

WOODALL, JOHN [1556?-1643] The surgeons mate; or, Military & domestique surgery. Discovering . . . ye method and order of ye surgeons chest, ye uses of the instruments, the vertues and operations of ye medicines with ye exact cures of wounds made by gun-shott, and otherwise . . . with a treatise of ye cure of ye plague . . . London, Printed by Rob. Young, for Nicholas Bourne, 1639.

[36], 275, [12], 301-412, [11] p.   front., illus., plates.   31 cm.   [**13141**]

Engraved title page.

Imperfect: frontispiece and engraved title page wanting; supplied in photocopy from the copy in the Osler Library, McGill University.

"An epistle congratulatory to . . . Sir Christoper Clitherow" inserted between sig. A2 and A3.

The "Viaticum," "Of the plague," and "A treatise of gangrena" have special title pages with imprint: London, Printed by E. P. for Nicolas Bourne, 1639.

STC 25963.

—[The same.] . . . London, Printed by John Legate for Nicolas Bourne, 1655.

[34], 26, [8], 27-275, [12], 303 (i.e. 301)-412, [11] p.   front., illus., plates.   29 cm.   [**13142**]

Engraved title page.

Imperfect: frontispiece wanting; lower margin of title page trimmed including imprint date; last page of the index wanting.

The "Viaticum," "Of the plague," and "A treatise of gangrena" have special title pages with imprint: London, Printed by J. L. for Nicholas Bourne, 1653.

A reprint of the 1639 edition. "An epistle congratulatory to . . . Sir Christopher Clitherow" omitted.

Imperfect: frontispiece, engraved title page and special title page of "A treatise of gangrena" wanting; third leaf of index mutilated.

WOODHOUSE. *See* WIDDOWES, J. [*fl.* 1606-1640]

WOOLLEY, HANNAH [*fl.* 1670] *See* THE ACCOMPLISH'D LADY'S DELIGHT. 1675; The compleat servant-maid. 1683.

Een **WOORTJE** in transitu, aan den scheuren breuck-meester Andries Boeckelman. [n. p.] 1678.

22 p.   16 cm.   [**13143**]

WORB, Johann Ignaz [*b.* 1666] Tabacologia; ofte, Korte verhandelenge over de tabak, desselvs deugd, gebruyk, ende kennissee: waar door aangeweesen wordt een wegh om lang, vroolijk, ende gesond te leeven. Door J. I. W. Beintema van Peima [pseud.] . . . 's Gravenhage, Levyn van Dyck, 1690.

[14], 175 p.   17 cm.   [**13144**]
Added engraved title page.

WORB, Johan Ignaz [*b.* 1666] *See* Vries, B. C. de. Nuttelyke consideratien of sedige aanmerkingen over het heedendaags tabak-suigen. 1692.

WORK for chimny-sweepers. *See* [Marbecke, R.] 1602.

WORM, Ole [1588-1654] Controversia, quis sit renum usus? *In* Meibom, J. H. De usu flagrorum. 1670.

—De aureo cornu Danico. *In* Bartholin, T. De armillis veterum schedion. 1676.

—Museum Wormianum; seu, Historia rerum rariorum, tam naturalium, quam artificialium, tam domesticarum, quam exoticarum, quae Hafniae Danorum in aedibus authoris servantur . . . Amstelodami, Apud Ludovicum & Danielem Elzevirios, 1655.

[15], 389, [3] p.   illus.   37 cm.   [**13145**]
Added engraved title page.

—*praeses.* Disputatio medica de melancholia hypochondriaca . . . Hafniae, Typis Martzanianis [1623?]

[31] p.   18 cm.   [**13146**]
Diss. — Copenhagen (F. Arnisaeus, *respondent*)

—*respondent.* Selecta controversiarum medicarum centuria . . . Basileae, Typis Johan. Jacobi Genathii, 1611.

[20] p.   20 cm.   [**13147**]
Diss. — Basel.

WORM, Ole [*fl.* 1686] *praeses.* De harmonia sensuum . . . [Hafniae] Literis J. P. Bockenhoffer [1686]

28 p.   19 cm.   [**13148**]
Diss. — Copenhagen (B. Brandt, *respondent*)

WORM, Wilhelm [1633-1704] Oratio in excessum . . . Thomae Bartholini . . . Hafniae, Sumptibus Petri Hauboldi, 1681.

[8], 120 p.   19 cm.   [**13149**]
"Programma in obit. Th. Bartholini" by Hans Bagger on p. 86-109.

—Copy 2.   23 cm.
With this is bound Jacobaeus, H. Oratio in obitum . . . Thomae Bartholini. 1681.

—*respondent. See* Bartholin, T., *praeses.* Tertium N. T. paralyticum. 1653.

WORMBSER, Johannes [*fl.* 1668-1676] *respondent.* Ἀσχημα medicum de suppressione mensium . . . Gissae Hassorum, Typis Josephi Dieterici Hampelii, 1668.

8 p.   20 cm.   [**13150**]
Diss. — Giessen.

—Dissertatio medica inauguralis, de pleuritide . . . Giessae, Typis Frider. Kargeri, 1676.

16 p.   18 cm.   [**13151**]
Diss. — Giessen.

WORMS, Jehosua [*fl.* 1687] *respondent.* Disputatio medica inauguralis de asthmate . . . Lugduni Batavorum, Apud Abrahamum Elzevier, 1687.

[16] p.   21 cm.   [**13152**]
Diss. — Leyden.

WORTH, W. Y. *See* Y-Worth, William [*fl.* 1690-1691]

A WORTHY treatise of the eyes. *See* Guillemeau, J. A treatise of one hundred and thirteene diseases of the eyes. 1622.

WOSCHKI, Christoph [*fl.* 1683] *respondent. See* Hartmann, P. J., *praeses.* Exercitationum anatomicarum . . . de originibus anatomicae prima [-quarta] 1683.

WOTTON, Edward [1492-1555] *See* Moffett, T. Insectorum, sive minimorum animalium theatrum. 1634.

WOTTON, William [1666-1762] Reflections upon ancient and modern learning . . . London, Printed by J. Leake for Peter Buck, 1694.

[32], 359 p.   20 cm.   [**13153**]

—[The same.] . . . The 2d ed. with large additions. With A dissertation upon the epistles of Phalaris, Themistocles, Socrates, Euripides, &c. and Aesop's Fables. By Dr. Bentley. London, Printed by J. Leake for Peter Buck, 1697.

[8], xxxvii, [3], 421, [1] p.; 152 p.   [**13154**]
Part [2] has special title page.

WOUW, HENDRIK VAN [*fl.* 1669] *respondent.* Disputatio medica inauguralis de scorbuto … Trajecti ad Rhenum, Ex officina Joannis van de Water, 1569 (i.e. 1669).

    [32] p. 23 cm.   **[13155]**
Diss. — Utrecht.

WOYNA, JOANNES. *See* MATTHIAE, D. M. Experimentorum medico-chymicorum decades tres. 1683.

WOYSKY, MICHAEL. *See* SENDIVOGIUS, Michael [1566–1636]

WOYSSELL, SYGMUTT. Bericht zweyer bewehrter Artzneyen in bevorstehender Infectionsgefahr, so wol zur praeservation als curation zugebrauchen … Bresslaw, Georg Bawman, 1625.

    [7] p. 19 cm.   **[13156]**

WRIGHT, THOMAS, *D. D.* A succinct philosophicall declaration of the nature of clymactericall yeeres, occasioned by the death of Queene Elizabeth. Written by T[homas] W[right] London, Thomas Thorpe, 1604.

    [1], 17 p. 18 cm.   **[13157]**
Issued also as part [2] of his The passions of the minde, 1601. STC 26043.3.

WÜRTTEMBERG, ELEONORA, *Herzogin von. See* ELEONORA, *consort of* George I, *landgrave of Hesse-Darmstadt* [1551 or 2–1618]

WÜRTZ, FELIX. *See* WIRTZ, Felix [*ca.* 1510 – *ca.* 1590]

WÜRTZ, RUDOLFF. *See* WIRTZ, Rudolf [*fl.* 1612–1620]

WÜESTHUBE, JOHANN [*fl.* 1611] *respondent.* Themata … physica-medica miscellanea … Basileae, Typis Johan. Jacobi Genathii [1611]

    [12] p. 22 cm.   **[13158]**
Diss. — Basel.

WUIST-HAUSZ, HENRICUS JACOBUS. *See* WUYSTHAUS, Henricus Jacobus.

WULSON, MARC, *sieur de La Colombière. See* VULSON DE LA COLOMBIÈRE, Marc [*d.* 1658]

Das WUND-ARTZNEY-BUCH. *See* GÄBELE, J. Dass Ihro käyserl. Majestät Leopoldus die Freyheit mitgetheilt, auch durch die Herren Doctores untersucht und abprobiert worden. 1658.

WUNDER-CUR, an einem von Schlage gerührten Mägden, den 12. May Anno 1697, zu Magdeburg erlebt, und zu nöthigen Nachdencken sonder Vorurtheil warhafftig berichtet. Magdeburg, Zufinden bey Johann Daniel Müllern [1697?]

    [10] p. 20 cm.   **[13159]**

WURFBAIN, JOHANN PAUL [1655–1711] Epistola. Ad amicum anonymum Med. Doct. qua nonnulla in Dn. Joh. Hiskiae Cardilucii … Germanico idiomate, nuper demum edito Tractatus de peste, contenta ad examen revocantur, scripta a J[ohann] P[aul] W[urfbain] D[octor] Norimbergae, Typis Christophori Gerhardi [1679?]

    57, [2] p. 14 cm.   **[13160]**

—Salamandrologia; h. e. Descriptio … salamandrae quae vulgo in igne vivere creditur, S. R. J. Academiae Naturae Curiosis exhibita … Norimbergae, Sumtibus Georgii Scheureri, typis Johannis Michaelis Spörlin, 1683.

    [7], 133 (i.e. 131), [14] p. illus., plates. 21 cm.   **[13161]**
Imperfect: table 4 wanting.
Added engraved title page.

—*respondent. See* BRUNO, J. P., *praeses.* Disputationem medicam de mendicamentis ex homine qua vivo qua mortuo desumtis ductu Schroederiano tractatis … submittit … J. P. W. 1677.

WURFBAIN, JOHANN PAUL [1655–1711] *See* CARDILUCIUS, J. H. Anhang über das … Tractätlein, von der Pestilentz. 1681 [and] Appendix … uber das … Tractätlein, von der Pestilentz. 1679.

WURGER, JOHANN [*fl.* 1687] *respondent.* Disputatio medica inauguralis de mola … Trajecti ad Rhenum, Ex officina Francisci Halma, 1687.

    23 p. 22 cm.   **[13162]**
Diss. — Utrecht.

WURSTSCHMIDT, JOHANN OTTO [*fl.* 1670] *respondent. See* FRIDERICI, J. A., *praeses.* Haemorrhagiae uteri menstruae praeternaturalis, θεωριαν και θεραπειαν ut specimen. 1670.

WURTZIUS, FELIX. *See* WIRTZ, Felix [*ca.* 1510 – *ca.* 1590]

WURTZIUS, RUDOLFE. *See* WIRTZ, RUDOLF [*fl.* 1612–1620]

WUYSTHAUS, HENRICUS JACOBUS, *respondent. See* DEUSING, A., *praes.* Synopsis medicinae universalis. 1649.

WYBERD, JOHN [*b. ca.* 1618] *respondent.* Disputatio medica inauguralis de pica praegnantium ... Franekerae, Uldericus Balck, 1644.

    [8] p.   20 cm.   **[13163]**
    Diss. — Franeker.

WYBURG, GERARD [*fl.* 1686] *respondent.* Disputatio medica inauguralis de febribus ... Lugduni Batavorum, Apud Abrahamum Elzevier, 1686.

    [16] p.   22 cm.   **[13164]**
    Diss. — Leyden.

WYDDOWES, I. *See* WIDDOWES, J. [*fl.* 1606-1640]

WYER, HEINRICH. *See* WIER, HEINRICH [*fl.* 1567-1588]

WYER, JOHANN. *See* WIER, Johann [1515-1588]

WYKHUISE, ANGELUS DANIELIDES VAN [*fl.* 1678] *respondent.* Disputatio medica inauguralis de variolis morbillis ... Lugd. Batav., Apud Petri à Meersche, 1678.

    [12] p.   22 cm.   **[13165]**
    Diss. — Leyden.

WYMIS, AARNOUT VAN, *tr. See* RANCHIN, F. Heelkonstige geschillen. 1662.

WYNANTS, THEODORUS [17th cent.] *ed. See* SALTZMANN, J. R. [1573-1656] Varia observata anatomica hactenus inedita. 1669.

WYNELL, JOHN [*fl.* 1660-1670] Lues venerea. Wherein the names, nature, subject, causes, signes and cure, are handled. Mistakes ... rectified, doubts and questions succinctly resolved ... The 2. ed. ... London, Printed by W. W. for the author, and sold by John Amery, 1670.

    [16], 76, [3] p.   16 cm.   **[13166]**

X

XENIUM a multis saeculis raro exemplo inauditum; seu, Miranda synopsis, omnium humani generis symptomatum, potentiarum & facultatum ... sensuum, ossium, a capite morali et physico usque ad plantam pedis ad adversam declinantium sanitatem ... Adjunctis extraordinariis Hypocratis cepitulationibus & jurejurando cum diis ... Redacta per V. H. Z. ... Francofurti, Sumptibus Georgii Fickwirt, 1660.

    [22] p.   14 cm.   **[13167]**
    Imperfect: last leaf (blank?) wanting.

XYLANDER, GULIELMUS [1532-1576] *tr. See* PHLEGON OF TRALLES. Quae exstant, opuscula. 1620.

XYLANDER, KARL CHRISTIAN [*fl.* 1690-1691] *respondent.* Disputatio medica inauguralis de chlorosi, von de Jüngfern Kranckheit ... Lugduni Batavorum, Apud Abrahamum Elzevier, 1691.

    [19] p.   18 cm.   **[13168]**
    Imperfect: upper margins trimmed.
    Diss. — Leyden.

XYLANDER, KARL CHRISTIAN [*fl.* 1690-1691] *respondent. See* SLEVOGT, J. A., *praeses.* Dissertatio medica de dura matre. 1690.

XIMÉNEZ SAVARIEGO, JUAN. *See* JIMÉNEZ SAVARIEGO, Juan [*b.* 1568]

Y

Y., W. *See* Y-WORTH, William [*fl.* 1690-1691]

Y-WORTH, WILLIAM [*fl.* 1690-1691] Chymicus rationalis; or, The fundamental grounds of the chymical art ... by various examples in distillation, rectification ... tinctures ... and oleosums ... In all which the chymical doctrines are illustrated ... composed agreeable to practical philosophy, and ...

for mysteries treated of by Cartes, Starkey, Sylvius, Glauber, Helmont, Paracelsus, and others ... In which is contained, a philosophical description of the astrum lunare microcosmicum, or phospheros ... London, Thomas Salusbury, 1692.

    [16], 154, [6] p.   plate.   18 cm.   **[13169]**

    Imperfect: plate wanting.

—Introitus apertus ad artem distillationis; or, The whole art of distillation practically stated, and adorned with all the new modes of working now in use. In which is contained, the way of making spirtis, aquavitae, artificial brandy ... To which is added, the true ... way of preparing powers ... London, Joh. Taylor, 1692.

[17], 189, [3] p. plates. 18 cm.   **[13170]**

—A new art of making wines, brandy, and other spirits ... Wherein is laid down full and effectual directions for the making of wholsome and medicinal wines ... Lastly is subjoyn'd, a general treatise concerning the original and nature of diseases, together with their cure by spagirick medicines ... by W[illiam] Y[-Worth] ... London, T. Salusbury, 1691.

[48], 153, [27] p. 15 cm.   **[13171]**

Published also under title: The Britannian magazine; or, A new art of making above twenty sorts of English wines.

YĀ'KŪB IBN ISḤĀK IBN ṢUBBĀḤ, Abū Yūsuf, al-Kindī [*d. ca.* 873] *See* Mesuë [924 *or* 5-1015] Opera. 1602, 1623.

YARWOOD, John [*fl.* 1682] Physick refin'd; or, A little stream of medicinal marrow, flowing from the bones of nature, wherein several signs ... and ... symptoms; whereby the most ordinary diseases may be ... known ... are ... delineated; and the ... cure ... demonstrated ... London, Tho. Passinger [1682?]

120 p. 13 cm.   **[13172]**

Imperfect: first and last three leaves mutilated.

YDELEY, Etienne [*b.* 1540?] Les secrets souverains et vrais remedes contre la peste ... Extraicts nouvellement ... de plusieurs ... autheurs anciens ... Lyon, Vincent de Coeursilly, 1628.

[7], 170, [6] p. 17 cm.   **[13173]**

YDELEZ, Estienne. *See* Ydeley, Etienne [*b.* 1540?]

YONGE, James [1647-1721] Currus triumphalis, e terebintho; or, An account of the many admirable vertues of oleum terebinthinae. More particularly, of the good effects produced by its application to recent wounds ... And lastly, a new way of amputation ... in two letters: the one to ... James Pearse ... chirurgeon to ... the Duke of York ... The

other, to Mr. Thomas Hobbs, chirurgeon in London. London, J. Martyn, 1679.

[24], 120 p. 20 cm.   **[13174]**

[—] Sidrophel vapulans; or, The quack-astrologer toss'd in a blanket. By the author of Medicaster medicatus [i.e. James Yonge]. In an epistle to W[illia]m S[almo]n. With a postscript, reflecting briefly on his late scurrilous libel against the Royal College of Physicians, entituled, A rebuke to the authors of a blue book ... [London, John Nutt, 1699]

[8], 59 p. 19 cm.   **[13175]**

Imperfect: lower margin of title page trimmed affecting imprint; upper margins trimmed with loss of pagination and text.
Wing 42a.

—Wounds of the brain proved curable ... London, Printed by J. M. for Henry Faithorn and John Kersey, 1682.

[20], 132 p. illus. 16 cm.   **[13176]**

"The epilogue to my learned and civil antagonist, Dr. W. Durston of Plimouth": p. 101-132.

YOUNG, James, *Surgeon, of Plymouth, See* Yonge, James [1647-1721]

YOUNGE, James [1647-1721] *See* Hooke, R. Lectures and collections. 1678.

YPELAER, Gabriel [*fl.* 1661] *respondent.* Disputatio medica inauguralis affectionis hypochondriacae historiam & curandi modum continens ... Lugduni Batavorum, Apud Davidem Lopez de Haro, 1661.

[12] p. 19 cm.   **[13177]**

Diss. — Leyden.

YPELAER, Nicolaas [*fl.* 1690] *respondent.* Disputatio medica inauguralis de scorbuto ... Lugduni Batavorum, Apud Abrahamum Elzevier, 1690.

[24] p. 22 cm.   **[13178]**

Diss. — Leyden.

YPEREN, Theodor van. *See* Halling, P. Bekentmakinge aen Doctor van Yperen. 1678.

YSAACUS. *See* Israeli, Isaac [*ca.* 832-*ca.* 932]

YŪḤANNĀ IBN MĀSAWAIH. *See* Mesuë [*d.* 857]

Z

Z., C. H. D. *See* HUYGENS, Christiaan [1629–1695]

Z., V. H. *See* XENIUM A MULTIS SAECULIS RARO EX-EMPLO INAUDITUM. 1660.

ZACAIRE, DENIS [1510–1556] Opusculum philosophiae naturalis metallorum ... [&] Annotata quaedam ex Nicolao Flammello ... [&] Quae ex Democrito collegimus apponere visum est, quo res dilucidiur fiat, ex multorum opinionibus auctorum.

710–794 p., vol. I. 20 cm. (In Zetzner, Lazarus, ed. Theatrum chemicum. Argentorati, 1659–61) **[13179]**
Caption titles.

ZACCAGNI, LELIO [1595–1678] Notabilium medicinae libri duo primus agit de vitae humanae longitudine, ac brevitate ... Secundus inscribitur adversus eos, qui praeter duos in homine testes tertium quoque dari posse opinantur ... Romae, Bernardini Tani, 1644.

[16], 158, [13] p.   22 cm.   **[13180]**

ZACCHAIRE, DENIS. *See* ZACAIRE, Denis [1510–1556]

ZACCHIA, Paolo [1584–1659] De' mali hipochondriaci libri due ... Nel primo s'insegna quanto appartiene alla cognitione, & alla cura di questi mali. Nel secondo si discorre degli accidenti di essi, & de' loro rimedii. Roma, Appresso Pietro Antonio Facciotti, ad instanza di Francesco Corbo, 1639.

[8], 413, [14] p.   22 cm.   **[13181]**
Bound with Argoli, A. De diebus criticis et de aegrorum decubitu libri duo. 1639.

—[The same.] De' mali hipochondriaci libri tre ... 2. impr. corr. ... Roma, Vitale Mascardi, ad instanza di Egidio Ghezzi, 1644.

[12], 527, [12] p.   21 cm.   **[13182]**

—[The same.] ... 3. impr. ricorr. ... Roma, Vitale Mascardi, ad instanza di Egidio Ghezzi, 1651.

[12], 543, [11] p.   23 cm.   **[13183]**

—[The same.] ... Nuova impr. corr. ... Venetia, Paolo Baglioni, 1665.

[10], 374, [8] p.   23 cm.   **[13184]**

—[Latin tr.] De affectionibus hypochondriacis libri tres. Italico idiomate primum ... conscripti nunc in Latinum sermonem translati ab Alphonso Khonn ... Augustae Vindelicorum, Sumptibus viduae Joh. Görlini, typis Jacobi Koppmairii, 1671.

[20], 705, [21] p.   21 cm.   **[13185]**

— Quaestiones medico-legales, liber secundus continens titulos tres. Quorum primus est de dementia, secundus de venenis, tertius in ll. aliquot ff. de aedil. edict. Lipsiae, Impensis Eliae Rehefeldii, 1630.

[16], 428, [52] p.   16 cm.   **[13186]**

— Quaestiones medico-legales. In quibus eae materiae medicae, quae ad legales facultates videntur pertinere, proponuntur, pertractantur, resolvuntur ... Ed. 3., corr., auct. ... subjunctis ... partibus octava & nona. Amstelaedami, Ex typographejo Joannis Blaeu, 1651.

[28], 127, 731, [56] p.   35 cm.   **[13187]**

—[The same.] ... Ed. 4. ... Ab ... mendis repurgata, plerisque additionibus ... locupletior. Avenione, Ex typographia Joannis Piot, 1665.

[36], 127, 788, [84] p.   port.   36 cm.   **[13188]**

—[The same.] ... Ed. 5. ... repurgata, plerisque additionibus ... multisque consultationibus ad rem facientibus locupletior. Avenione, Ex typographia Joannis Piot, 1657.

[32], 127, 324, [12], 325–788, [84] p.   front. (port.)   36 cm.   **[13189]**

—[The same.] Quaestionum medico-legalium tomus prior [-posterior], in hac editione Lugdunensi ab auctore novis additionibus locupletatus ... Lugduni, Sumptibus Joannis-Antonii Huguetan, & Marci-Antonii Ravaud. 1661.

2 v. in 1.   37 cm.   **[13190]**
Added half title.

—[The same.] Quaestionum medico-legalium tomi tres. Ed. nova, a variis mendis purgata, passimque interpolata, et novis recentiorum authorum inventis ac observationibus aucta, cura Joan. Danielis Horstii ... Francofurti, Sumptibus Joannis Baptistae Schönwetteri, 1666.

2 v. in 1.   35 cm.   **[13191]**
Added half title.
The pagination of tomus I and 2 is continuous. Tomus secundus has special title page facing p. 442.

—[The same.] . . . Lugduni, Ex typographia Germani Nanty [Apud Claudium Langloys, & soc.] 1673-74 [v. 1, 1674]

2 v. in 1.   37 cm.   [13192]

Added half title.

The pagination of tomus 1 and 2 is continuous. Tomus secundus has special title page facing p. 442.

Different setting of type.

—[The same.] . . . Olim aucti et emendati a . . . Joh. Daniel. Horstio, nunc . . . emendati atque adaucti a Georgio Franco . . . Francofurti ad Moenum, Sumtibus Johannis Melchioris Bencard, 1688.

3 v.   39 cm.   [13193]

Added half title.

— Il vitto quaresimale . . . Ove insegnasi, come senza offender la sanità si possa viver nella quaresima. Si discorre de'cibi in essa usati, de gli errori, che si commettono nell'usargli, dell'indisposizioni, ch'il lor'uso impediscono, de gli accidenti, che soglion cagionare, e del modo di rimediarui. Roma, Per Pietro Antonio Facciotti, ad istanza Gio. Dini, 1637.

[8], 264, [16] p.   16 cm.   [13194]

ZACCHIA, PAOLO [1584-1659] *See* PANUZZI, F., *ed.* Francesco Panuzzi . . . a i lettori. 1640.

ZACCHIAS, PAUL. *See* ZACCHIA, Paolo [1584-1659]

ZACCHUS, HIERONYMUS [*fl.* 1577] *ed. See* MERCURIALE, G. De pestilentia. 1601.

ZACHARIAS, DIONYSIUS. *See* ZACAIRE, Denis [1510-1556]

ZACHMANN, JOHANN GUILHELMUS [*fl.* 1632-1634] *respondent. See* SEBISCH, M. [1578-1674?] *praeses.* Collegii therapeutici disputatio I[-XIV] 1634 [i.e. 1635] [and] Galeni Ars parva in disputationes triginta resoluta. 1633 [and] Prodromi examinis vulnerum singularum humani corporis partium. 1632 [i.e. 1633]

ZACUTO LUSITANO. *See* ZACUTUS, Abraham, Lusitanus [1575-1642]

ZACUTUS, ABRAHAM, LUSITANUS [1575-1642] Opera omnia, in duos tomos divisa . . . [Lugduni, Sumptibus Joannis-Antonii Huguetan, 1642-43]

2 v.   front. (port.)   37 cm.   [13195]

Title from general half title. Each volume has special title page. Vol. 2 is in two parts; part [2] has half title.

Vol. [2] has general half title: Praxis historiarum, Introitus medici ad praxin, Pharmacopoea, Praxis medica admiranda.

—[The same.] Operum tomus primus [-secundus] . . . Ed. postrema, a mendis purgatissima. Lugduni, Sumptibus Joannis Antonii Huguetan filii & Marci Antonii Ravaud, 1649.

2 v.   38 cm.   [13196]

Imperfect: first preliminary leaf of both volumes, and sig. ã4 of vol. 2 wanting.

Vol. 2 is in two parts.

—[The same.] . . . Lugduni, Sumptibus Joannis-Antonii Huguetan & Marci-Antonii Ravaud, 1657.

2 v.   front. (port.)   37 cm.   [13197]

Vol. 1 has added general title page. Vol. 2 is in two parts.

—[The same.] . . . Lugduni, Sumptibus Joannis-Anthonii Huguetan & Guillielmi Barbier, 1667.

2 v.   38 cm.   [13198]

Vol. 2 is in two parts.

—De medicorum principum historia. Libri sex . . . Quorum primus liber nunc primum in lucem exit . . . Coloniae Agrippinae, Ex officina Johannis Frederici Stam, 1629.

[72], 624, [51] p.   18 cm.   [13199]

—Historiarum medicarum libri quatuor. In quibus medicinales omnes medicorum principum historiae . . . proponuntur . . . & . . . observationibus illustrantur . . . Ed. 2. . . . Amstelodami, Sumtibus Henrici Laurentii, 1642.

[75], 703, [1] p.   18 cm.   [13200]

Imperfect: sheet (d) wrongly imposed.

Constitutes De medicorum principum historia. Liber I.

With this is bound *his* Liber sextus. Amstelodami, 1638.

—Liber sextus. In quo medicinales omnes medicorum principium historiae proponuntur . . . Amstelodami, Sumptibus Henrici Laurentii, 1642.

[16], 348, [4] p.   [13201]

De medicorum principum historia. Liber VI.

Bound with *his* Historiarum medicarum libri quatuor. Amstelodami, 1642.

—De praxi medica admiranda. Libri tres. In quibus, exempla monstrosa, rara . . . circa abditas morborum causas, signa, eventus, atque curationes exhibita, diligentissime proponuntur . . .

Amstelodami, Typis Corneli Breugeli, sumptibus Henrici Laurentii, 1634.

[47], 492, [26] p.   18 cm.   [**13202**]

"Zacuti Lusitani ad philiatros candidissimos exhortatio": p. [23-26] at end.

—[The same.] . . . Praxis medica admiranda . . . Lugduni, Apud Joannem Antonium Huguetan, 1637.

[48], 634, [28] p.   18 cm.   [**13203**]

—Liber octavus. In quo describitur curatio morborum, qui partes vitales, & naturale infestant . . . Amstelodami, Sumptibus Henrici Laurentii, 1641.

[60], 781, [3] p.   18 cm.   [**13204**]

Constitutes Praxis historiarum. Liber VIII.

—*See* SALMON, W. Iatrica. 1681, 1684, 1694.

ZADITH BEN HAMUEL [*fl.* 13th cent.] Tabula chimica . . .

191-239 p., vol. 5.   20 cm.   (*In* Zetzner, Lazarus, *ed.* Theatrum chemicum. Argentorati, 1659-61)   [**13205**]

Caption title.

ZADITH, senior. *See* ZADITH BEN HAMUEL [fl.13th cent.]

ZAESLIN, EMANUEL [1663-1727] *respondent.* Dissertatio inauguralis medica de olfactu ejusque laesione . . . Basileae, Literis Jacobi Bertischii [1687]

[16] p.   19 cm.   [**13206**]

Diss. — Basel.

ZAHALON, JACOB BEN ISAAC [1630-1693] יזר סלאכח הרפואח הרא ספר ארצר החיים . . . חלקנ. Venetia, Stamparia Vendramina, 1683.

[193] p.   30 cm.   [**13207**]

Imperfect: p. 42-43 mutilated.

ZAHN, JOHANN [1641-1707] Oculus artificialis teledioptricus; sive, Telescopium, ex abditis rerum naturalium & artificialium principiis protractum nova methodo, eaque solida explicatum ac comprimis e triplici fundamento physico seu naturali, mathematico dioptrico et mechanico, seu practico stabilitum . . . Herbipoli, Sumptibus Quirini Heyl, 1685-87.

3 v. in 1.   illus., plates.   33 cm.   [**13208**]

Added engraved title age dated 1687.

al-ZAHRĀWĪ, ABŪ AL-QĀSIM KHALAF IBN 'ABBĀS. *See* ABULCASIS [936?-1013?]

ZALDUENDO, JUAN MARTÍNEZ DE. *See* MARTÍNEZ DE ZALDUENDO Y AGUIRRE, Juan [*fl.* 1696]

ZALUŽANSKÝ, ADAM [1555-1613] Methodi herbariae libri tres. Quale suae terrae plantae decus, ordinis usu arti plantarum ponitur ima manus. Francofurti, E Collegio Paltheniano, 1604.

[239] p.   table.   19 cm.   [**13209**]

ZAMBECCARI, GIUSEPPE [1653-1728] Esperienze . . . intorno a diverse viscere tagliate a diversi animali viventi . . . Firenze, Francesco Onofri, 1680.

30, [2] p.   24 cm.   [**13210**]

ZAMORA Y CLAVERÍA, JOSÉ [*b.* 1622] Pathologicae elucubrationes, in quibus explanatur sex Galeni libri de morborum, & symptomatum differentiis, eorumque causis, noviter excultae, variisque quaestionum, dubiorum, & observationum flosculis, lepade, & studiose exornatae . . . Caesaraugustae, Typ. Michaelis de Luna et Joannis de Ybar, 1659.

[24], 256, 212, [8] p.   port.   30 cm.   [**13211**]

ZANETINIS, HIERONYMUS DE. [Conclusio & comprobatio alchymiae, qua dispositioni & argumentis angeli respondetur]

247-248 p., vol. 4.   20 cm.   (*In* Zetzner, Lazarus, *ed.* Theatrum chemicum. Argentorati, 1659-61)   [**13212**]

Title from table of contents.

ZANETTINUS, HIERONYMUS. *See* ZANETINIS, Hieronymus de.

ZANFORTIUS. *See* FORTIS, Raimondo Giovanni [1603-1678]

ZANONI, GIACOMO [1615-1682] Istoria botanica . . . Nella quale si descrivono alcune piante de gl'antichi, da moderni con altri nomi proposte . . . Bologna, Gioseffo Longhi, 1675.

[14], 211, [2] p.   plates.   36 cm.   [**13213**]

Added engraved title page.

ZANTEN, JACOB VAN [*fl.* 1680] *respondent.* Disputatio medica inauguralis de lethargo . . . Lugduni Batavorum, Apud viduam & haeredes Joannis Elzevirii, 1680.

[24] p.   22 cm.   [**13214**]

Diss. — Leyden.

ZAPATA, DIEGO MATHEO [*fl.* 1691] Verdadera apologia en defensa de la medicina racional philosophica, y devida respuesta a los entusiasmos medicos, que publicò en esta corte D. Joseph Gazola ... Madrid, Antonio de Zafra [1691]

[20], 92 p.   21 cm.   [13215]

ZAPATA, GIOVANNI BATTISTA [*b. ca.* 1520] Li maravigliosi secreti di medicina, e chirurgia. Nuovamente ritrovati, per guarire ogni sorte d'infermità. Raccolti ... da Gioseppe Scientia ... Venetia, Nicolò Tebaldini, 1602.

[46], 190 p.   16 cm.   [13216]

—[The same.] ... Venetia, Lucio Spineda, 1611.

[46], 190 p.   16 cm.   [13217]
Different setting of type.

—[The same.] ... Venetia, Gio. Battista Benfadino, 1618.

[46], 190 p.   15 cm.   [13218]
Different setting of type.

—[The same.] ... Venetia, Santo Lanza, 1629.
[46], 190 p.   15 cm.   [13219]

—[The same.] ... Venetia, Giovanni, & Domenico Imberti, 1641.

[48], 190 p.   16 cm.   [13220]
Different setting of type.

—[The same.] ... Venetia, Carlo Conzatti, 1656.
[48], 301 (i.e. 300) p.   17 cm.   [13221]
Dedicetory/epistle dated 1665.

—[The same.] ... Secreti varii di medicina, e chirurgia ... Venetia, Antonio Tivanni, 1677.
[48], 174 p.   15 cm.   [13222]
Imperfect: p. 173-174 mutilated.

—[The same.] ... Bologna, Il Longhi, 1700.
[8], 197, [1] p.   16 cm.   [13223]

—[Latin tr.] Mirabilia; sive, Secreta medico-chirurgica, denuo inventa, ad sanandos omnes humani corporis affectus. Ex Italico idomate, nunc primum in Latinum versa, & annotationibus foecundissimis, ad genium seculi ita adcommodatis illustrata ... per Davidem Spleissium ... Ulmae, Apud Georgium Wilhelmum Kühnen, 1696.

[27], 453, [161] p.   front.   18 cm.   [13224]
Originally edited by Giuseppe Scientia.

—[German tr.] Schlüssel der Artzeney; das ist: Wunderbahre ... Secreta und Künste der Artzeney und Chirurgy. Erstlich von ... Joanne Zepata ... erfunden unnd gebraucht, auch nachmals durch Josephum Scientia ... in italiänischer Sprach in Truck verfertiget. Jetzundt aber durch einen ... geübten Medicum ... in unsere teutsche Sprach transsferiert: dessgleichen in Truck zuvor nicht aussgangen ... Franckfurt am Mayn, Gedruckt durch Joach. Brathering, in Verlegung Johan Spiessen und Johann Ludwig Bitschen, 1603.

[16], 250 p.   17 cm.   [13225]

—[The same.] ... Zum andern Mal in Truck aussgangen. Franckfurt am Mayn, Gedruckt bey Matthias Beckern, Verlegung Johann Ludwig Bitschen, 1605.

[16], 250 p.   16 cm.   [13226]
A reissue of the 1603 edition.

ZAPFF, JOHANN ADAM [*fl.* 1666] *respondent. See* FRIDERICI, J. A., *praeses.* Disputatio medica inauguralis de morbo castrensi seu Hungarico. 1666.

ZAPF, JOHANN GEORG [*fl.* 1689] *respondent.* Dissertatio medica inauguralis de gonorrhoea virulenta ... Erffurti, Chalcographo Johanne Henrico Groschio [1689]

31 (i.e. 32), [4] p.   20 cm.   [13227]

Diss. — Erfurt.

[ZAQUIIAS, *doctor*] El medico caritativo. Que enseña azer los remedios en casa para todas enfermetades mas suaves y seguros y con muy pocogasto. [Rome? 1660?]

[8], 285 p.   14 cm.   [13228]

Dedicatory epistle signed by Doctor Oylime.

ZARA, ANTONIO [1574-1621] Anatomia ingeniorum et scientiarum sectionibus quatuor comprehensa ... Venetiis, Ex typographia Ambrosii Dei, & fratrum, 1615.

[8], 592, [72] p.   port.   23 cm.   [13229]
Each section has half title.

ZAROTTI, CESARE [1610-1670] M. Valerii Martialis epigrammatum, medicae, aut philosophicae considerationis enarratio; sive, De medica Martialis tractatione commentarius ... Venetiis, Apud Baba, 1657.

[12], 413, [22] p.   22 cm.   [13230]

ZAS, NICOLAAS [1610-1663] Brief, aen den grooten Th. Bartholinus ... Rakende de mishandelinge van

... Lowys de Bils ... Rotterdam, Joannes Naeranus, 1661.

22 p.   16 cm.   [13231]

Bound with *his* Den dauw der dieren. 1660.

—Den dauw der dieren, ende de welle des waters ... Tot bevestiginge der ongemeene ontledinge van ... Lowys de Bils ... Rotterdam, Joannes Naeranus, 1660.

[14], 112 p.   plate.   16 cm.   [13232]

With this is bound *his* Brief, aen den grooten Th. Bartholinus. 1661.

—Epistola apologetica ad magnum Th. Bartholinum ... Roterodami, Ex officina Arnoldi Leers, 1661.

26 p.   illus.   20 cm.   [13233]

"Exemplar fusioris codicilli, authore ... Ludovico de Bils ... in quo agitur de vera humani corporis anatomia": p. 11–[19]. "Ludovici de Bils ... epistolica dissertatio: qua verus hepatis circa chylum, & pariter ductus chiliferi hactenus dicti usus, docetur": p. 20–23. "Ludovicus de Bils ... omnibus verae anatomes studiosis": p. 24–26.

Bound with (as issued?) Bils, L. de. Specimina anatomica. 1661.

ZAS, NICOLAAS [1610–1663] *tr. See* BONDT, J. de. Oost-en West-Indische warande. 1694.

ZAS, NICOLAAS [1610–1663] *tr. See* BONDT, J. de. Oost-Indische warande. 1673.

ZAVATTA, GIOVANNI FRANCESCO [*fl.* 1629] *ed. See* MOCCA, C. Discorsi preservativi e curativi della peste. 1630.

ZAVONA, MASSIMIANO [1579–1652] Abuso del tabacco de' nostri tempi, trattato ... Nel quale si dimostra, che con quello si possono curare un'infinito numero di mali, che molestano l'huomo. Bologna, Gio. Battista Ferroni [1650?]

[8], 55, [9] p.   19 cm.   [13234]

—De Ravennatis aeris admirandis auscultationibus opusculum ... Ravennae, Apud impressores Camerales, 1649.

8, 108 p.   21 cm.   [13235]

ZAVORZIZ. *See* SCRETA.

ZEBRIACHER, JOHANN JAKOB [*fl.* 1698] *respondent. See* ILLMER, F. F., *praeses*. Disputatio medica de pulsu et respiratione. 1698.

ZECAIRE, DENIS. *See* ZACAIRE, Denis [1510–1556]

ZECCA, ANDROMACO. *See* ZECCHI, Andromaco [*fl.* 1599]

ZECCHI, ANDROMACO [*fl.* 1599] *ed. See* ZECCHI, G. Liber primus Consultationum medicinalium. 1601, 1617, 1650.

ZECCHI, ERCOLE [*d.* 1622] *ed. See* ZECCHI, G. De urinis brevis. 1613.

ZECCHI, GIOVANNI [1533–1601] Liber primus Consultationum medicinalium ... Andromachi Zecchii ejus filii opera & studio in lucem editus ... Romae, Apud Gulielmum Facciottum, ad instantiam Joannis Martinelli, 1601.

[52], 499 p.   21 cm.   [13236]

No more published.

"De pulsibus brevis methodus": p. 476–499.

—[The same.] Consultationes medicanales, in quibus universa praxis medica exacte pertractatur: Andromachi Zecchii ejus filii opera & studio in lucem editae ... Venetiis, Apud Joannem & Variscum Variscos, & fratres, 1617.

[44], 432 p.   23 cm.   [13237]

—[The same.] ... Accessit tractatus ejusdem De pulsibus ... Francofurti, Sumptibus Johannis Beyeri, 1650.

[7], 955, [77] p.   17 cm.   [13238]

—De urinis brevis, et pulcherrima methodus. Cui de laterali dolore cum febre putrida, necnon mali moris tractatus & consultatio accedunt ... Herculis Zecchii ejus nepotis ... opera, & studio in lucem edita ... Bononiae [Apud heredes] Joan. Rossii, 1613.

[8], 85, [9] p.   21 cm.   [13239]

Title page mutilated, with loss of part of imprint.

— In primam D. Hipp. Aphorismorum sectionem, dilucidissimae lectiones. Quibus accedunt tractatus quatuor insignes, admirabili quadam methodo digesti, De purgatione videlicet, De sanguinis missione, De criticis diebus, ac De morbo Galico. A Scipione ex Mercuriis ... summa diligentia ab ore auctoris excepti. Ejusdem Scip. Merc. ... scholia in singulas lectiones. Nunc denuo ... a Perseo Rossio in lucem editae ... Bononiae, Apud haeredes Joannis Rossii, 1629.

[8], 300, [11], 94, [10] p.   21 cm.   [13240]

The treatises De purgatione, De sanguinis missione, and De criticis diebus are interspersed in the commentary on the Aphorismi.

Includes Latin test of the 1st book of the Aphorismi.

ZEHNER, JOHANNES [*fl.* 1609] *respondent. See* PLATTER, F. [1536–1614] *praeses*. Theses medicae de ἀπεψία. 1609.

ZEIDELER, SIMON [*fl.* 1673-1674] *respondent. See* FASCH, A. H., *praeses.* Dissertatio inauguralis medica purpuram puerperarum exponens. 1674; WEDEL, G. W., *praeses.* Disputatio medica, exhibens aegrum epilepticum. 1673.

ZEIDLER, BERNARDUS NORBERTUS À. *See* ZEIDLERN, Bernhard Norbert von [*fl.* 1686]

ZEIDLER, JOHANN [1596-1645] Kurtzer Bericht, was man in diesen gefährlichen Sterbensäufften, beydes an innerlichen, und denn an eusserlichen Mitteln, so wol zur Praeservation als zur Curation gehörig, in der eylenburgischen Apothecken bekommen kan, neben angehencktem leydlichem Taxt. Auff Anordnung und Begehren eines ehrenvesten und wolweisen Raths der Stadt Eylenbergk gemeiner Bürgerschafft zu besonderm Nutz und Frommen verfertiget . . . Leiptzig, Georgio Liger, 1625.

[8] p.   19 cm.   **[13241]**

—*praeses.* De mania themata medica . . . Lipsiae, Typis exscripta per Gregorium Ritzsch [1630]
[27] p.   19 cm.   **[13242]**
Diss. — Leipzig (C. König, *respondent*)

ZEIDLER, JOHANNES [*fl.* 1690] *respondent. See* LEICHNER, E., *praeses.* Dissertatio inauguralis medica de apoplexia. 1690.

ZEIDLER, SEBASTIANUS CHRISTIANUS À. *See* ZEIDLERN, Sebastian Christian von [*ca.* 1616-*ca.* 1686]

ZEIDLERN, BERNHARD NORBERT VON [*fl.* 1686] *ed. See* ZEIDLERN, S. C. von. Somatotomia anthropologica. 1686, 1692.

ZEIDLERN, SEBASTIAN CHRISTIAN VON [*ca.* 1616-*ca.* 1686] Institutiones medicae libris V . . . in auditorio medico Universitatis Carolo-Ferdinandae Pragensis dictatae, nunc revisae & typis mandatae. Pragae, Apud Joannem Carolum Gerzabek, 1687.

[14], 291, [3] p.   port.   21 cm.   **[13243]**

—Somatotomia anthropologica; seu, Corporis humani fabrica methodice divisa, & controversarum quaestionum discussionibus illustrata, publice . . . celebrata . . . praeparante . . . Bernardo Norberto à Zeidlern . . . Pragae, Typis Johannis Caroli Gerzabek, 1686.

[10], 118, [2] p.   port., plates.   32 cm.   **[13244]**
Imperfect: added engraved title page wanting.

—[The same.] . . . Viennae Austriae, Sumptibus Philippi Fieveti, 1692.

[8], 118, [2] p.   port., plates.   33 cm.   **[13245]**
Added engraved title page bound in at end before plates.
A reissue of the 1686 Prague edition with new title page and preliminaries partly reset.

ZEIDLERN, SEBASTIANUS DE. *See* ZEIDLERN, Sebastian Christian von [*ca.* 1616-*ca.* 1686]

ZEISLER, CHRISTOPH. *See* ZEISSELER, Christoph [*fl.* 1668]

ZEISOLD, JOHANN [1599-1667] *praeses.* Disputatio physica de humoribus corporis humani . . . Jenae, Casparus Freyschmidt, 1652.

[16] p.   18 cm.   **[13246]**
Diss. — Jena (J. C. Kisling, *respondent*)

ZEISSELER, CHRISTOPH [*fl.* 1668] *respondent. See* ZENTGRAF, J. J., *praeses.* Disputatio publica physica de notis genitivis. 1668.

ZELLER, JOHANN. *See* ZELLER, Johann Gottfried [1656-1734]

ZELLER, JOHANN GOTTFRIED [1656-1734] *praeses.* Dissertatio anatomica de vasorum lymphaticorum administratione, observatis ac observandis in hac illorum phoenomenis . . . eorumque causis . . . Tubingae, Typis viduae Johann-Henrici Reisii [1687]
[1], 18 p.   20 cm.   **[13247]**
Diss. pro loco - Tübingen (J. S. Knisel, *respondent*)

Dissertations — Tübingen

—Disputatio inauguralis medica de gonorrhoea virulenta utroque in sexu, vulgo Drûpper, et la chaudepisse . . . Tubingae, Johann. Conradi Reisii [1700]
20 p.   20 cm.   **[13248]**
G. F. Gmelin, *respondent.*

—Dissertationem medicam posteriorem de morbis ex strictura glandularum p. n. natis . . . exhibet Christoph. Abrahamus Ruoff . . . Tubingae, Typis Joh. Conradi Eitelii & viduae Martini Rommeii [1695]
[1], 19-40 p.   21 cm.   **[13249]**
Signatures: A-C⁴.
C. A. Ruoff, *respondent.*

—Infanticidas non absolvit nec a tortura liberat nec respirationem foetus in utero tollit: pulmonum infantis in aqua subsidentia . . . Tubingae, Typis Martini Rommeii [1691]

28 p.   20 cm.   **[13250]**

J. D. Mauchart, *respondent.*

— Vita humana ex fune pendens; h. e., Disquisitio anatomico-physiologica de funiculo umbilicali human. eumque ligandi necessitate, cum famosae istius objectionis, cur in brutis, funiculo non ligato, nulla tamen superveniat haemorrhagia? tentata resolutione . . . Tubingae, Typis Johann-Conradi Reisii, 1692.

18 p.   plate.   20 cm.   **[13251]**

J. W. Müller, *respondent.*

— *respondent. See* METZGER, G. B., *praeses.* Affectuum p. n. haereditariorum theoria. *ca.* 1683.

ZELST, THEODOOR VAN [*fl.* 1700–1738] *respondent.* Dissertatio medica inauguralis de tartaro . . . Lugduni Batavorum, Apud Abrahamum Elzevier [1700]

26, [2] p.   21 cm.   **[13252]**

Diss. — Leyden.

ZENCKER, JOHANN [*fl.* 1643–1644] *respondent. See* SCHELHAMMER, C., *praeses.* Hydrops tympanites. 1644.

ZENDER, JOHANN RUDOLPH [*fl.* 1671] *respondent.* Dissertatio inauguralis medica de haemoptysi seu sputo sanguinis . . . Basileae, Typis Johan. Rodolphi Genathii [1671]

[19] p.   20 cm.   **[13253]**

Diss. — Basel.

ZENIUS, NICOLAUS [*fl.* 1646] *respondent. See* GESTRIN, M. E., *praeses.* Disputatio physica de intellectu humano. 1646.

ZENTGRAF, JOHANN JOACHIM [1643–1707] *praeses.* Disputatio prior de tactu regis Franciae, quo strumis laborantes restituuntur . . . disputabunt . . . D. XXIV Julii, 1667 . . . Wittebergae, Literis Matthaei Henckelii, 1675.

[16] p.   19 cm.   **[13254]**

Articulus primus, historica tractans.
Diss. — Wittenberg, 1667 (G. H. Petri, *respondent*)

— Disputatio posterior de tactu regis Franciae, quo strumis laborantes restituuntur . . . defendet . . . ad d. 23. Octob. 1667 . . . Wittebergae, Literis Matthaei Henckelii, 1675.

[16] p.   19 cm.   **[13255]**

Articulus secundus, physicus.
Diss. — Wittenberg, 1667 (J. A. Metz, *respondent*)

— Disputatio publica physica de notis genitivis . . . Wittebergae, Typis Johannis Borckardi [1668]

[20] p.   19 cm.   **[13256]**

Diss. — Wittenberg (C. Zeisseler, *respondent*)

ZENTGRAVIUS, JOHANNES JOACHIMUS. *See* ZENTGRAF, JOHANN JOACHIM [1643–1707]

ZEPHYRINUS, JOHANNES [*fl.* 1686] *respondent. See* DROSSANDER, A., *praeses.* Tenuis & succincta contemplatio pororum. 1686.

ZERENGHI, FEDERICO [*fl.* 1603–1631] Il vero tesoro da preservarsi dalla peste, di tutte le spetie, & da tutti li veleni naturali, & artefitiali . . . Macerata, Gio. Battista Bonomo, 1631.

[8], 46 p.   21 cm.   **[13257]**

ZESCH, WILHELM [1629–1682] *praeses.* Disputationum physicarum de maximo et minimo rerum naturalium tertia et ultima, de accidentium termino versus maximum et minimum . . . subjiciet Antonius Krecke . . . Jenae, Typis Nisianis, 1656.

[28] p.   20 cm.   **[13258]**

Diss. — Jena (A. Krecke, *respondent*)

ZESEN, PHILIPP VON [1619–1689] *respondent. See* GUEINZ, C., *praeses.* Disputatio de sale. 1639.

—, *tr. See* BEVERWIJK, J. van. Schatz der Gesundheit. 1671.

ZETZNER, LAZARUS [*d.* 1616] *ed.* De magni lapidis; sive, Benedicti compositione & operatione aliquot capita. Secunda hac editione . . . emaculata, atque a mendis liberata . . . Argentorati, Sumptibus Lazari Zetzneri, 1613.

28 p.   18 cm.   **[13259]**

Bound (as issued) with vol. 3 of *his* Theatrum chemicum. 1613–1622.

— Theatrum chemicum, praecipuos selectorum auctorum tractatus de chemiae et lapidis philosophici antiquitate, veritate . . . & operationibus, continens: in gratiam verae chemicae, et medicinae chemicae studiosorum . . . congestum, & in quatuor partes seu volumina digestum . . . Volumen primum [-quintum] Argentorati, Sumptibus Lazari Zetzneri, 1613–1622.

5 v.   illus., plates.   18 cm.   **[13260]**

Imperfect: p. 663–666 and plate at p. 662 of vol. 4 wanting.

Vol. 5 edited by Isaac Habrecht.

Contents as in vols. 1-5 of the 1659-1661 edition, with the exception of "De magni lapidis".

With vol. 3 of this is bound (as issued) *his* De magni lapidis. 1613.

—[The same.] ... In sex ... volumina digestum ... Volumen primum [-sextum] Argentorati, Sumptibus heredum Eberh. Zetzneri, 1659-61.

6 v. illus. 20 cm. [13261]

Imperfect: title page of vol. 5 wanting.

Vol. 5 edited by Isaac Habrecht and vol. 6 edited and translated by Johann Jacob Heilmann.

Analyzed in part. For full contents *see* Ferguson (A). Vol. 2, p. 436-440.

ZEUMER, CASPAR [*fl.* 1656] *respondent. See* MOELLENBROCK, V. A., *praeses*. Disputationum medicarum de ventriculo secunda. 1656.

ZIEGLER, ADRIAN [1584-1654] Pharmacopoea spagyrica, continens selectissima remedia chymica, desumpta ex Basilica chymica Oswaldi Crollii; Pharmacopoea dogmatica restituta Josephi Quercetani ... [Tiguri] Typis Bodmerianis, 1628.

[19], 141, [11] p. 20 cm. [13262]

Imperfect: lower margin of title page trimmed.

With this is bound Gehrig, Christoph. Aegrotans ipse medicus. Schneeberg, 1712.

ZIEGLER, HANS JAKOB, 1640-1683, *ed.* Heil-Brunnen; das ist, Beschreibung dess ... Gesund-Bads bey Schintznacht ... in der mächtigen H. von Bern Landschafft gelegen. Deme beygefügt seynd die mineralischen Proben dieses Wassers ... Zusammen verfasset von Jacob Ziegler ... [Zürich] Hans-Caspar Hardtmeyer, 1663.

[2], 20 p. front. 20 cm. [13263]

Frontispiece has title: Schintznacher Bad.

—*respondent. See* BAUHIN, J. K., *praeses*. Theses medicae de veneni natura. 1659; STUPANUS, E., *praeses*. Theses physico-medicae de lacte. 1659.

ZIEGLER, JAKOB [1591-1670] Beschreibung des Geirenbads, in der Pfarz Hinweil, drey meilen von Zürich, in dero Herrschaft Grüningen ... [Zürich? 1662?]

broadside. 43 × 32 cm. [13264]

Imperfect: mutilated.

—Von dem kostlichen Bad Urdorff, bey Zürich gelegen. Dises Bad führt in dreyen underschiedenlichen Ursprüngen: 1. Schwäbel. 2. Vitriol, oder

Kupfferwasser. 3. Allet, oder Alaun. [Zürich? 1662?]

broadside. 36 × 28 cm. [13265]

—*See* [ZIEGLER, H. J.] *ed.* Heil-Brunnen. 1663.

ZIEGLER, JAKOB *fil. See* ZIEGLER, Hans Jakob [1640-1683]

ZIEGLER, JOHANN [1673-1749] *respondent*. Dissertatio inauguralis, casum viri hypochondriaci exhibens ... Basileae, Typis Jacobi Bertschii [1697]

[12] p. 18 cm. [13266]

Diss. — Basel.

—*respondent. See* WEDEL, G. W., *praeses*. Dissertatio medica de verrucis. 1696.

ZIEGLER, JOHANN BERNHARD [*fl.* 1678] *respondent. See* FASCH, A. H., *praeses*. Disputatio medica inauguralis de dysenteria epidemica. 1678.

ZIEGRA, CHRISTIAN SAMUEL [*fl.* 1678-1687] *praeses*. Disputatio physica de annis climactericis vitae humanae posterior ... Wittenbergae, Matthaeus Henckelius, 1682.

[20] p. 20 cm. [13267]

Diss. — Wittenberg (J. Schwartzwaldt, *respondent*)

—Disputatio physica de morte plantarum ... [Wittenbergae] Aere publico Matthaei Henckelii [1680]

[16] p. 18 cm. [13268]

Diss. — Wittenberg (J. B. Reising, *respondent*)

ZIEGRA, CONSTANTIN [1617-1691] *praeses*. De sympathia atque antipathia rerum naturalium ... Wittebergae, Literis Matthaei Henckelii, 1663.

[26 +] p. 20 cm. [13269]

Imperfect: all after p. [26] wanting.

Diss. — Wittenberg (J. C. Meelführer, *respondent*)

—Disputatio physica de magia ... Wittebergae, Excudebat Joh. Röhnerus, 1665.

[16] p. 19 cm. [13270]

Diss. — Wittenberg (G. F. Magnus, *respondent*)

—Disputatio physica de monstro ... Wittebergae, Excudebat Joh. Röhnerus, 1665.

[20] p. 20 cm. [13271]

Diss. — Wittenberg (J. Stricer, *respondent*)

ZIEGRA, MICHAEL GOTTFRIED [*fl.* 1676-1683] *respondent. See* LOSS, J., *praeses*. Dissertatio inauguralis medica de inflammatione. 1683; SENNERT, M., *praeses*. Dissertatio medica de febre petechiali. 1681.

ZIERVOGEL, JOANNES MARTINUS. *See* ROTHLOEBEN, Johann Martin [1657-1701]

ZIGEMARIUS, STEPHAN [*fl.* 1664] *respondent. See* SCHENCK, J. T., *praeses*. Disputatio medica in-auguralis de lassitudine. 1664.

ZIHN, JOHANN HEINRICH [*fl.* 1681] *respondent. See* CRAMER, C., *praeses*. Dissertatio medica inauguralis de vertigine. 1681.

ZILLINGER, GEORG GOTTFRIED [*fl.* 1647-1649] *respondent. See* SALTZMANN, J. R. [1573-1656] *praeses*. Decas quaestionum physicarum de temperamento. 1647; SEBISCH, M. [1578-1674?] *praeses*. Galeni quin-que priores libri. 1651 [and] Problemata medica de infantium et puerorum morbis. 1649.

ZIMARA, MARCO ANTONIO [1460-1532] Antrum magico-medicum; in quo arcanorum magico-physicorum, sigillorum, signaturarum & imaginum magicarum ... ut & curationum magneticarum ... thesaurus ... reconditus ... Accessit motus perpetui mechanici absque illo aquae, vel ponderis adminiculo conficiendi documentum ... Francofurti, Typis Joannis Friderici Weisii, 1625.

[13], 525 p.; [15], 749, p. 18 cm. **[13272]**

Part 2 has special title page: Pars secunda, in qua arcana naturae, sympathiae & antipathiae rerum in plantis, animalibus ... om-niumque corporis humani morborum ... cura hermetica ... con-tinentur ... Accesserunt Portae intelligentiarum; sive, Canones Hebraeorum, Chaldaeorum, Arabum, Aegypitorum, Orphicorum, Pythagoraeorum, Graecorum et Latinorum priscorum ... Fran-cofurti, Typis & sumptibus Wechelianorum, apud Danielem & Davidem Aubrios, & Clementem Schleichium, 1526 (i.e. 1626).

—Problemata. *In* Aristoteles. Aristotelis, aliorum-que philosophorum, ac medicorum problemata. 1631.

—[English tr.] *In* Aristoteles. The problems of Aristotle. 1670; 1684.

—[French tr.] *In* Aristoteles. Les problemes d'Aristote. 1618; 1683.

—[German tr.] *In* Aristoteles. Problemata. 1604; 1679.

—Tractatus magicus. *In* Longinus, C., ed. Trinum magicum; sive, Secretorum magicorum opus. 1616, 1673.

ZIMERA, MARCO ANTONIO. *See* ZIMARA, Marco Antonio [1460-1532]

ZIMMER, JOHANN PAUL [*fl.* 1700] *respondent. See* HERTEL, J. M., *praeses*. Medicinae theoricae, generalis. 1700.

ZIMMERMAN, MATHAEUS. *See* ZIMMERMANN, Mathäus [*fl.* 17th cent.]

ZIMMERMANN, JOHANN JOACHIM [*fl.* 1689] *respondent. See* VESTI, J., *praeses*. Dissertatio medica inauguralis de dyspepsia. 1689.

ZIMMERMANN, KARL FRIEDRICH [*fl.* 1694] *respondent. See* SCHAMBERG, J. C., *praeses*. Disputatio medica inauguralis de paralysi scorbutica. 1694.

—*See* RIVINUS, A. Q. Facultatis Medicae in Academia Lipsiensi p. t. procancellarius ... L. S. D. 1694.

ZIMMERMANN, MATHÄUS [*fl.* 17th cent.] Unda Jordanis Fabariana. Pfäffesserischer Jordan, oder Piscinaprobatica Fabariana. Eigentlicher Entwurff dess heylreichenden weltberühmbten Pfaeffers Bads, in der oberen Schweitz ... Einsidlen, Joseph Reymann, 1682.

[18], 150 p. 14 cm. **[13273]**

ZINCK, AEGIDIUS [*fl.* 1698] *respondent. See* LUNGERSHAUSEN, J. J., *praeses*. Disputatio physica de imitamentis naturae circa figuras. 1698.

ZINCK, GEORG CHRISTOPH [*fl.* 1671] *respondent*. Disputatio medica inauguralis de dysenteria ... Argentorati, Literis Johannis Wilhelmi Tidemanni, 1671.

24 p. 18 cm. **[13274]**

Diss. — Strasbourg.

ZINCK, JOHANN PETER [*fl.* 1663] *respondent. See* WAGNER, M., *praeses*. Disputatio medica de colica. 1663.

ZINCKE, JOHANNES [*ca.* 1506-1545] De crisibus commentarius. In quo de natura ... utilitate atque necessitate criseǫn, & dierum criticorum; eorumque artificioso judicio ... atque prognostico, ex motu lunae coelique aspectibus cognoscendo agitur. Nunc primum in lucem prolatus ... Francofurti, Impen-sis haeredum Nicolai Bassaei, 1609.

[7], 151 p. illus. 13 cm. **[13275]**

ZIPFFELL, JONAS [*fl.* 1659] Podagrischer Triumph; das ist, Kurtzer doch gründlicher Bericht, vom Griess, Sand, Stein, und Podagra, was sie seyn ... und mit was solche ... zu-curiren? Nebenst zwey dieser Kranckheit halber geschehenen Schreiben von Hr. Christoph Fahrnern ... Altenburgk, In Verlegung des Authoris, 1659.

149 (i.e. 141) p. 16 cm. [13276]

ZITTELIN, JOHANN MICHAEL [*fl.* 1623] respondent. *See* SEBISCH, M. [1578-1674?] *praeses.* Exercitatio medicae. 1639.

ZOAR. *See* AVENZOAR [*d. ca.* 1162]

ZOBEL, FRIEDRICH [*d.* 1647] Tartarologia spagirica; seu, Medicamentorum ex tartaro in laboratorio Gottorpiensi paratorum fidelis descriptio. E bibliotheca Georgii Wolffgangi Wedelii. Jenae, Typis Gollnerianis, 1676.

[II], 96, [6] p. 14 cm. [13277]

ZOLLICOFER, MAXIMILIAN HONORIUS [*fl.* 1660] respondent. *See* SEBISCH, J. A., *praeses.* Dissertatio anatomica de ventriculo. 1660.

ZOLLICOFFERUS, DAVID. *See* ZOLLIKOFER, David [*fl.* 1682-1685]

ZOLLIKOFER, DAVID [*fl.* 1682-1685] respondent. Dissertatio medica inauguralis de polypo cordis ... [Basileae] Typis Emanuelis König & Ludovici König haeredum [1685]

[20] p. 22 cm. [13278]
Diss. — Basel.

—*See* HOFFMANN, J. M., *praeses.* Disputatio medica publica de dolore in genere. 1682.

ZOPFF, JOHANN CHRISTOPH [*fl.* 1676] respondent. *See* WEDEL, G. W., *praeses.* Dissertatio medica de vomitoriis rite adhibendis. 1676 [and] Dissertationem inauguralem de malo hypochondriaco ... censurae expono. J. C. Z. 1676.

ZORN, BARTHOLOMAEUS [1639-1717] respondent. Disputationem de abortu ... submittit Bartholomaeus Zornn ... Altdorffii, Ex officina typographica Johannis Goebelii [1663]

44 p. 20 cm. [13279]
Diss. — Altdorf.

—*See* Hoffmann, M., *praeses.* Theses medicae de venaesectionis necessitate. 1661.

—, *ed. See* PANCKOW, T. Herbarium. 1673.

ZSÁMBOK, JÁNOS. *See* SAMBUCUS, Johannes [1531-1584]

ZSCHOESY, MELCHIOR [*fl.* 1626] respondent. *See* SEBISCH, M. [1578-1674?] *praeses.* Disputatio de diebus criticis posterior. 1626.

ZSCHÜRNER, CHRISTIAN [*fl.* 1683] respondent. *See* CRAUSE, R. W., *praeses.* Disputatio inauguralis medica de atrophia. 1683.

ZUCCARO, MARIO [*d.* 1634] De venenis consilium ... Neapoli, Apud Tarquinium Longum, 1605.

[6], 81, [1] p. 20 cm. [13280]

—De vera ac methodica nutriendi ratione, Neapoli usurpata pro curandis morbis disputatio unica ... Neapoli, Apud Jo. Baptistam Subtilem, 1000 [i.e. 1602]

[8], 71, [1] p. 21 cm. [13281]
Date of imprint supplied from Toppi, p. 207.

—Tractatus de morbis puerorum ... Neapoli, Apud Jo. Baptistam Subtilem, 1604.

[16], 359, [1] p. 21 cm. [13282]

ZUCCHINETTI, DOMENICO [*d. ca.* 1626] *ed. See* CATHOLIC CHURCH. Province of Milan. Constitutiones, et decreta sex provincialium synodorum Mediolanensium. 1603.

ZUCCHINETTI, GIOVANNI DOMENICO. *See* ZUCCHINETTI, Domenico [*d. ca.* 1626]

ZUCHARUS, MARIUS. *See* ZUCCARO, Mario [*d.* 1634]

ZUCKMANTEL, JOHANN CASPAR [*fl.* 1669] respondent. *See* AMMANN, P., *praeses.* Disputatio medica de cancromammarum. 1669.

ZUINGGER, THEODORUS. *See* ZWINGER, Theodor [1533-1588]

ZUNTHUS, HIERONYMUS [*fl.* 1615] De balneo thermali, Lixignano vocato, necnon de luto barboliorum medicato, in ducatu Parmensi ... Venetiis, Apud haeredem Damiani Zenarii, 1615.

[15], 102 p. 23 cm. [13283]
"...Responsio de obstructionibus ingentibus circa mesenterium ... Gabrielis Falloppii, nunc primum edita a Hieronymo Zunthio": p. [99]-102.

ZURNER, NIKOLAUS [*fl.* 1697] *respondent. See* POSNER, C., *praeses.* Dissertatio physica de viventibus mobilibus a seipsis secundum sententiam Aristotelis. 1697.

ZVINGER, JOHANN FRIEDRICH. *See* ZWINGER, Johann Friedrich [*fl.* 1638]

ZVINGER, THEODOR. *See* ZWINGER, Theodor [1658-1724]

ZWELFER, JOHANN [1618-1668] Discursus apologeticus ... adversus ... Ottonis Tackenii, ejusque adulterini salis viperini novissimi fundamenta, ut ait, antiquissima. Cui & accessere ejusdem justissimae Vindiciae contra Franciscum Verny ... Annexo etiam Apologemate epistolico anonymi ... Norimbergae, Sumtibus Michaelis & Johann. Friderici Endterorum, 1668.

[12], 267, [1] p. 34 cm. [**13284**]

"Coronidis loco accessit haec epistola apologetica, contra quendam, Schmuzium a Poystorff ... ab anonymo quodam edita: pro integerrima Zwelferi fama vindicanda": p. 257-267.

Bound with (as issued?) Pharmacopoeia augustana. Animadversiones in Pharmacopoeiam augustanam [1667-68]

—[The same.] ... Norimbergae, Sumtibus Michaelis & Johann. Friderici Endterorum, 1675.

[12], 267, [1] p. 33 cm. [**13285**]

Different setting of type.

Bound with (as issued?) vol. 2 of Pharmacopoeia augustana. Animadversiones in Pharmacopoeiam augustanam. [1675]

—Pharmacopoeia regia. *In* Pharmacopoeia augustana. 1652, 1653, 1667-68, 1675; Pharmacopoeia augustana reformata cum ejus mantissa & appendice. 1672.

—[German tr.] Königliche Apotheck, oder Dispensatorium. Das ist: Neu-bereicherter ganz-angefüllter Schatz-Kasten der ausserlesensten Artzneyen; zusamt einer diesem bewerthesten Artzney-Buch beygefügten spagyrischen oder chymischen Zugabe ... In lateinischer Sprach geschrieben; nun aber ... in unsere teutsche Mutter-Sprach ... übersetzet ... Nürnberg, In Verlegung Martin Endters, 1692.

[6], 780, [26] p. front. (port.), illus. 20 cm. [**13286**]

—Appendix ad Animadversiones in Pharmacopoeiam augustanam, ejusque annexam mantissam. Item ad Pharmacopoeiam regiam seu dispensatorium novum; in qua obscura explicantur ...

Goudae, Sumptibus Gulielmi vander Hoeve, 1658.

[16], 198, [10] p. 18 cm. [**13287**]

Bound with Pharmacopoeia augustana reformata. 1653.

—Vindiciae adversus Franciscum Verny. *In* Bauderon, B. La pharmacopée. 1672.

—*See* SCHMUZ, M. R. Exorcismus medicus manium, larvarum & maleferiatorum spirituum Zwelferianorum. 1673 [and] Jus retorquendi. 1672; SPAENHOLZ, N. Eilfertiges Gutachten Philonis Nasturtii Zwelferischen Bundesgenossen. 1673.

ZWEYER vortrefflicher Theologen, Herrn d. Lutheri, und Herrn D. Selnecceri seel. kurtze Erörterung zweyer Bewissens-Fragen, I. Ob ein Christ vor der grassirenden Seuche der Pestilentz fliehen könne? II. Wie man in solchem Falle gegen die inficirte Oerter und Personen sich christlich bezeigen solle? Bey ietziger betrübten Pest-Zeit ... vorgestellet von einem Leidens-Mitgenossen. Franckfurt, 1680.

[48] p. 14 cm. [**13288**]

ZWINGER, JOHANN FRIEDRICH [*fl.* 1638] *respondent. See* BENTZON, N., *praeses.* Theoria iatrica. 1638.

ZWINGER, JOHANNES [1634-1696] *praeses.* Disputatio theologica de circumcisione ... Basileae, Typis Johan. Jacobi Deckeri [1667]

[12] p. 19 cm. [**13289**]

Diss.—Basel (P. Dodel, *respondent*)

ZWINGER, THEODOR [1533-1588] *ed. See* BAIRO, P. De medendis humani corporis malis enchiridion. 1612.

— *See* SCHOLTZ, L. Consiliorum medicinalium ... liber singularis. 1610 [and] Epistolarum philosophicarum: medicinalium, ac chymicarum ... volumen. 1610.

ZWINGER, THEODOR [1658-1724] Der sichere und geschwinde Artzt; oder, Neues Artzney-Buch, worinnen eine jede Kranckheit des menschlichen Leibs ... beschrieben, und wie sie am geschwindesten und sichersten zu heilen ... Anfänglich zwar under dem verdeckten Nahmen Nathanäelis Sforcia [pseud., i.e. Theodor Zwinger] herauss gegeben, anjetzo aber ... vermehret und verbessert von Theodor Zwingern ... Basel, In Verlag Johann-Philip Richters, Druckts Jacob Bertsche, 1686.

[8], 642, [21] p. 18 cm. [**13290**]

—Oratio panegyrica in obitum ... Jo. Caspari Bauhini ... Basileae, Typis Jacobi Bertschii, 1687.
   91 p. 19 cm.   **[13291]**

—*praeses*. Dissertatio academica de vita hominis sani ... Basileae, Typis Jacobi Bertschii [1699]
   [12] p. 19 cm.   **[13292]**
   Diss.—Basel (D. Brandmüller, *respondent*)

—Dissertationem hanc philosophicam quae est de natura mentis humanae ... tuebitur ... Joh. Ludovicus Frey ... Basileae, Typis Jacobi Bertschii [1699]
   [12] p. 22 cm.   **[13293]**
   Diss.—Basel (J. L. Frey, *respondent*)

—, *ed. See* MATTIOLI, P. A. Theatrum botanicum. 1696.

ZWÖLFER, JOANNES. *See* ZWELFER, Johann [1618-1668]

ZYL, DOMINICUS VAN [*fl.* 1694] *respondent*. Disputatio philosophico-medica inauguralis de memoria, ejusque vitiis ... Lugduni Batavorum, Apud Abrahamum Elzevier, 1694.
   [20] p. 22 cm.   **[13294]**
   Diss.—Leyden.

XYLANDER, GULIELMUS [1532-1576] *tr. See* ANTIGONUS OF CARYSTUS. Historiarum mirabilium collectanea. 1619.

ZYLL, CORNELIUS VAN [*fl.* 1658] *respondent*. Disputatio medica inauguralis, de febre ardente seu causo ... Ultrajecti, Ex officina Adriani van Dam, 1658.
   [8] p. 20 cm.   **[13295]**
   Diss.—Utrecht.

ZYNTHUS, HIERONYMUS. *See* ZUNTHUS, Hieronymus [*fl.* 1615]

ZYPAEUS, FRANCISCUS. *See* ZYPE, Franz van den [*fl.* 1683-1692]

ZYPE, FRANZ VAN DEN [*fl.* 1683-1692] Fundamenta medicinae physico-anatomica. Bruxellis, Apud Aegidium t'Serstevens, 1683.
   [20], 398 p. 16 cm.   **[13296]**
   Added engraved title page.

—[The same.] ... Ed. 2., ex M. S. authoris aucta, corr., & emend. Bruxellis, Apud Aegidius t'Serstevens, 1687.
   [14], 524 p. 16 cm.   **[13297]**
   Added engraved title page.
   Imperfect. Sig. a8 (blank?) wanting.

—[The same.] ... Nunc primum prodeunt in Galliis. Lugduni, Anisson & Posuel, 1692.
   [16], 398 p. 19 cm.   **[13298]**

— Fundamenta medicinae reformata physico-anatomica. Ed. 3. multo auct. & corr. Bruxellis, Apud Aegidium t'Serstevens, 1693.
   [6], 343 (i.e. 334), [7] p. 18 cm.   **[13299]**